BERRY & KOHN'S
OPERATING ROOM TECHNIQUE

FIFTEENTH EDITION

ANITA HORNACKY, BS, RN, CST, CNOR

Perioperative Educator
Surgical Pharmacology and Orthopedics
Lakeland Community College (formally)
Kirtland, Ohio

NANCYMARIE PHILLIPS, RN, BSN, BA, MEd, RNFA, CNOR(E), PhD

Professor Emeritus
Director, Department of Perioperative Education
Perioperative Nursing, Registered Nurse First Assistants, Surgical Technology
Lakeland Community College
Kirtland, Ohio

ELSEVIER

Elsevier
3251 Riverport Lane
St. Louis, Missouri 63043

Notice

Practitioners and researchers must always rely on their own experience and knowledge in evaluating and using any information, methods, compounds or experiments described herein. Because of rapid advances in the medical sciences, in particular, independent verification of diagnoses and drug dosages should be made. To the fullest extent of the law, no responsibility is assumed by Elsevier, authors, editors or contributors for any injury and/or damage to persons or property as a matter of products liability, negligence or otherwise, or from any use or operation of any methods, products, instructions, or ideas contained in the material herein.

Previous editions copyrighted 2021, 2017, 2013, 2007, 2003, 2000, 1996, 1991, 1986, 1978, 1972, 1966, 1960, and 1955.

Senior Content Strategist: Sandra Clark
Content Development Specialist: Susan Callahan
Publishing Services Manager: Deepthi Unni
Project Manager: Thoufiq Mohammed
Design Direction: Patrick Ferguson

Printed in India

Last digit is the print number: 9   8   7   6   5   4   3   2   1

Mary Lou Beatrice Gaeher Kohn (1920–2019)

*An inspiration to all perioperative nurses and caregivers
of the past, present, and future.*

Preface to the Fifteenth Edition

This time-honored text has its roots in the operating room (OR) orientation manual created by Mary Louise Kohn in the late 1940s while working as an OR educator at University Hospitals of Cleveland, Ohio. Her impeccable notes were a source of interest to many OR supervisors and educators who wanted to standardize their teaching techniques in accordance with Mary Louise's orientation tool. Many observers requested copies of her writings, and eventually the cost of providing copies became prohibitive.

In 1951, at the request of her publisher and with the encouragement of her superiors, Mary Louise assembled her orientation material into a manuscript suitable for publication. She spent countless hours writing and revising material until the birth of her daughter. Her dedication to her family led her to seek assistance for this project from Edna Cornelia Berry, who became her willing partner and coauthor through the first four editions.

The first edition of *Introduction to Operating Room Technique* by Edna Cornelia Berry and Mary Louise Kohn was published in 1955. We are fortunate to have obtained first edition copies and have them signed by Mary Louise Kohn before she died. The first edition was dedicated to "those nurses who accept the tension and challenge of coordinated teamwork as they minister to the patient in the operating room." The main emphasis was on intraoperative care of the patient.

Berry and Kohn's Operating Room Technique has been the perioperative text of choice for almost 70 years because it emphasizes the importance of the patient and presents the material in concise, understandable language. The name remains "Operating Room Technique" because that is how it has been commonly known and identified, although the text has a comprehensive perioperative focus. It would be a disservice to our patients to merely describe the intraoperative phase and not include preoperative and postoperative care.

Every new edition of this classic perioperative text has addressed changing roles, needs, and evolving technologies while maintaining the fundamental focus that still remains valid—the care of the perioperative patient. This edition of the text identifies the knowledge and skill needs of the caregiver and strives to incorporate components of patient care from preoperative, intraoperative, and postoperative practice areas. A systems approach is used to help organize patient care to minimize the risk for human error.

Berry and Kohn's Operating Room Technique is designed to meet the needs of educators, learners, caregivers in diverse disciplines, and managerial personnel who care for surgical or interventional patients in many types of environments. Knowing the "why" of patient care is as important as knowing the "how." Additionally, it is important to stress that outcomes must be evaluated to support evidence-based practice. This text is the book of choice for certification preparation in diverse disciplines and incorporates all elements of the core curricula specified by several accrediting and certifying bodies.

Features of the Fifteenth Edition

- A user-friendly 12-section arrangement.
- A logical and sequential order of the subject matter.
- Incorporation of the *AORN Guidelines for Perioperative Practice* (2024) and *AST's Core Curriculum for Surgical Technology*, 6th edition, to reflect modern perioperative practice.
- A focus on the physiologic and psychologic considerations of perioperative patients to provide guidelines and standards for planning and implementing safe individualized care.
- Use of the systems approach as a foundation to support solid evidence-based practice to establish patient care procedures in such a way that all team members can identify their roles in a cooperative spirit of safety and efficiency.
- In-depth discussion of patients with special needs related to age or health status considerations.
- Discussion of perioperative patient care in inpatient, ambulatory, and alternative sites/locations to highlight considerations based on the setting, as well as the surgical procedure.
- Encouragement of the patient care team to identify and examine personal and professional development issues that influence the manner in which care is rendered.
- Detailed information about the fundamentals of perioperative nursing and surgical technology roles.
- Building of knowledge in a logical sequence—from fundamental concepts to implementation during surgical intervention—to enable readers to apply theory to practice.
- Comprehensive coverage of a broad range of essential topics to provide a thorough understanding of fundamental principles and techniques and an understanding of their applications in various surgical procedures.
- Descriptions of specific surgical procedures in each specialty chapter to assist the learner and caregiver in planning and delivering patient care in the perioperative environment.
- An Evolve website that has learning and teaching aids to enhance the classroom experience and support assimilation of knowledge. For the student, this includes tips for the scrub person and circulating nurse, historical perspectives, body spectrum software, student interactive questions, and an audio glossary. For the instructor, this includes a TEACH manual with a lesson plan, lecture outline, case studies, and PowerPoint slides for each chapter; test bank; and collection of all the images in the book.

New to the Fifteenth Edition

- Insightful Pros & Cons boxes throughout the text examine the two sides of a patient care topic and provide references for further reading.
- Updated references highlight the evidence-based practice approach used in the book.
- Terminology and key words have been updated to reflect modern practice.
- Each chapter has been revised to emulate current practice and knowledge.

Organization

Section 1 describes education, learning, and professional issues. The correlation of theory and practice is integral to the success of patient care in the perioperative environment. Fundamental professional and personal attributes of the caregiver are examined, with an emphasis on objectivity in the development of the plan of care. Legal and ethical issues are discussed.

Section 2 delineates the roles of the members of the health care team as both direct and indirect caregivers. Nonphysician first assistant roles and credentials are discussed in a separate chapter. Management of the perioperative patient care areas is described, including Magnet Status.

Section 3 provides in-depth information on patient assessment and the development of an individualized plan of care, with the patient viewed as a unique individual. Special needs are identified by health condition and age. Geriatric and pediatric chapters are included.

Section 4 examines the physical plant of the perioperative environment—both hospital-based, freestanding ambulatory facilities and alternative locations. Diagrams of conventional and nonconventional perioperative suite designs are included with airflow designs. Care of the perioperative environment, occupational hazards, and safety issues are examined in depth.

Section 5 explains microbiology and the importance of microbiologic control in the perioperative environment, with an emphasis on standard precautions. It delineates aseptic and sterile techniques as fundamental to intermediate aspects, such as attire, scrubbing, gowning, and gloving. Separate chapters are provided regarding the sterilization and disinfection of surgical instrumentation and patient care supplies.

Section 6 details the primary surgical instrumentation and equipment used during surgical procedures. The safe use of specialized surgical equipment is presented. Electricity is explained.

Section 7 discusses preoperative patient care and includes the family and significant others in the plan of care. Diagnostic procedures and specimen handling are described.

Section 8 covers methods of anesthetic administration and the role of caregivers during this process. Physiologic patient responses and related potential perioperative complications are discussed in detail. Surgical pharmacology is included.

Section 9 describes intraoperative patient care, including positioning, prepping, and draping. The interactive roles of the circulator and the scrub person are specified in Chapter 25. Economy of motion and the properties of physics are applied. Physiologic monitoring of the perioperative patient is described.

Section 10 focuses on the surgical site. Incisions, hemostasis, and wound closure are discussed in detail. Wound assessment, dressing, and healing throughout the perioperative care period are described.

Section 11 presents an expanded view of postoperative patient care. The postanesthesia care unit is explained. Prevention of patient complications is described. The death of a patient is discussed, and the importance of legal evidence is stressed.

Section 12 covers the surgical specialties. Salient surgical anatomy and procedures are described and illustrated in line drawings for clarity.

Acknowledgments

We want to thank so many people who have made this fifteenth edition possible. First, we want to thank all the reviewers of the previous editions for their time in review and for their input. The identified needs of this group provide the baselines for the growth and effectiveness of this work. The reviews were very detailed and appropriately critical.

We are so grateful to the many nurses, surgical technologists, and readers of previous editions who wrote or called requesting specialty topic coverage in this edition. We welcome feedback at all times.

We want to thank our ongoing students in all disciplines (perioperative nursing, registered nurse first assistant, and surgical technology) for asking hard questions and forcing us to step beyond the classroom to satisfy their learning needs. We see them as the future of patient care and the representatives of the high standards described in this text.

We want to thank our perioperative nursing and surgical technologist colleagues for their professionalism and for making the task of revision exciting and fresh. A special thank you to Joe Fortunato, Jr., who created much of the art for previous editions and other authorship projects.

We want to thank Sandra Clark, Executive Content Strategist; Susan Callahan, Senior Content Development Specialist; and Thoufiq Mohammed, Project Manager, for their support and patience during the production of this edition. Their support made this project possible.

We want to thank Mary Louise Kohn, RN, who trusted us with her wonderful creation. She is the epitome of the perioperative nurse we should strive to be. We put her foremost in mind before we commit any word to paper. We ask ourselves, "How would Mary Lou describe this?" Or, "What would Mary Lou think about adding this?" We do this not only out of reverence for her trust but also because she still exemplifies the highest standards of patient care despite being long retired. Mary Lou was a delightful human being and forever a perioperative nurse.

Anita Hornacky
Nancymarie Howard Phillips

Contents

Section 1: Fundamentals of Theory and Practice

1 Perioperative Education, 1
The Art and Science of Surgery, 2
Perioperative Learner, 3
Perioperative Educator, 5
Application of Theory to Practice, 10
Expected Behaviors of Perioperative Caregivers, 11
Realities of Clinical Practice, 13

2 Foundations of Perioperative Patient Care Standards, 16
Surgical Conscience, 17
Patient Rights, 17
Accountability, 17
Standardization of Patient Care, 18
Recommended Practices, 21
Professionalism, 26
Professional Perioperative Nursing, 27
Evidence-Based Practice, 27
Nursing Process, 28
Standards of Perioperative Nursing Practice, 30
Clinical Competency of the Perioperative Nurse, 33
Scope of Perioperative Nursing Practice, 34
Surgical Technology, 34
Clinical Competency of the Surgical Technologist, 35
Continual Performance Evaluation and Improvement, 35

3 Legal, Regulatory, and Ethical Issues, 37
Legal Issues, 38
Liability, 38
The Joint Commission and Sentinel Events, 42
Consent, 44
Documentation of Perioperative Patient Care, 46
Legal Aspects of Drugs and Medical Devices, 50
Ethical Issues, 51

Section 2: The Perioperative Patient Care Team

4 The Perioperative Patient Care Team and Professional Credentialing, 55
Dependence of the Patient on the Qualified Team, 56

Credentialing of Qualified Caregivers, 56
Perioperative Patient Care Team, 56

5 The Surgical First Assistant, 64
First Assistant's Knowledge and Skill Level, 65
What Does the First Assistant Do?, 66
Disciplines Associated With First Assisting in Surgery, 71

6 Administration of Perioperative Patient Care Services, 79
Establishing Administrative Roles, 79
Interdepartmental Relationships, 84
Patient Care Departments, 85
Patient Services Departments, 85
Departmental Service Divisions, 86
Coordination Through Committees, 88
Surgical Services Management, 91
Budgeting and Financial Responsibility, 95
New Product and Equipment Evaluation, 97

Section 3: The Patient as a Unique Individual

7 The Patient: The Reason for Your Existence, 99
The Patient as an Individual, 99
The Patient With Individualized Needs, 102
The Patient With Cancer, 110
The Patient With Chronic Comorbid Disease, 117
The Patient Who Is a Victim of Crime, 119
End-of-Life Care, 123
Death of a Patient in the Operating Room, 123

8 Perioperative Pediatrics, 125
Indications for Surgery, 125
Considerations in Perioperative Pediatrics, 126
Perioperative Assessment of the Pediatric Patient, 127
Preoperative Psychologic Preparation of Pediatric Patients, 134
Pediatric Anesthesia, 135
Intraoperative Pediatric Patient Care Considerations, 140
Common Surgical Procedures, 142
Postoperative Pediatric Patient Care, 160

9 Perioperative Geriatrics, 161
Perspectives on Aging, 161
Perioperative Assessment of the Geriatric Patient, 164
Intraoperative Considerations, 174
Postoperative Considerations, 175

Section 4: The Perioperative Environment

10 Physical Facilities, 177
Physical Layout of the Surgical Suite, 178
Transition Zones, 179
Peripheral Support Areas, 180
Operating Room, 183
Special Procedure Rooms, 193
Construction or Renovation of the Surgical Suite, 194

11 Ambulatory Surgery Centers and Alternative Surgical Locations, 197
Ambulatory Surgical Setting, 197
Alternative Sites Where Surgery Is Performed, 206

12 Care of the Perioperative Environment, 211
Guidelines for Cleanliness in the Surgical Environment, 211
Establishing the Surgical Environment, 211
Room Turnover Between Patients, 212
Daily Terminal Cleaning, 216

13 Potential Sources of Injury to the Caregiver and the Patient, 218
Environmental Hazards, 218
Physical Hazards and Safeguards, 219
Chemical Hazards and Safeguards, 231
Biologic Hazards and Safeguards, 233
Risk Management, 236

Section 5: Surgical Asepsis and Sterile Technique

14 Surgical Microbiology and Antimicrobial Therapy, 238
Microorganisms: Nonpathogens Versus Pathogens, 239
Types of Pathogenic Microorganisms, 244
Antimicrobial Therapy, 255

15 Principles of Aseptic and Sterile Techniques, 260
What Is the Difference Between Aseptic and Sterile Techniques?, 261
Transmission of Microorganisms, 262
Human-Borne Sources of Contamination, 262
Nonhuman Factors in Contamination, 263
Sources of Infection, 264

Environmental Controls, 264
Standard Precautions, 267
Principles of Sterile Technique, 269
No Compromise of Sterility, 274

16 Appropriate Attire, Surgical Hand Hygiene, and Gowning and Gloving, 275
Appropriate Operating Room Attire, 276
Surgical Hand Hygiene, 285
Gowning and Gloving, 288

17 Decontamination and Disinfection, 295
Central Processing Department, 296
Central Service Personnel, 296
Instrument Cleaning and Decontamination, 297
Disinfection of Items Used in Patient Care, 301
Methods of Disinfection, 302
Disposable Products, 309

18 Sterilization, 312
Sterilization Versus Disinfection, 313
Sterilization, 313
Assembly of Instrument Sets, 315
Packaging Instruments and Other Items for Sterilization, 316
Thermal Sterilization, 320
Chemical Sterilization, 326
Radiation Sterilization, 333
Control Measures, 333
Custom Packs, 335

Section 6: Surgical Instrumentation and Equipment

19 Surgical Instrumentation, 338
Fabrication of Metal Instruments, 338
Classification of Instruments, 339
Handling Instruments, 356

20 Specialized Surgical Equipment, 360
Using Specialized Equipment in Surgery, 361
Electrosurgery, 361
Laser Surgery, 365
Microsurgery, 372
Ultrasonosurgery, 377
Integrated Technologies, 377

Section 7: Preoperative Patient Care

21 Preoperative Preparation of the Patient, 379
Hospitalized Patient, 379
Preoperative Preparation of All Patients, 379
Transportation to the Operating Room Suite, 390
Admission to the Operating Room Suite, 390

22 Diagnostics, Specimens, and Oncologic Considerations, 395
Diagnosing Pathology, 396
Specimens and Pathologic Examination, 396
Radiologic Examination, 399
Magnetic Resonance Imaging, 404
Nuclear Medicine Studies, 405
Ultrasonography, 406
Doppler Studies, 406
Sensory Evoked Potential, 407
Plethysmography, 408
Endoscopy, 408
The Patient With Cancer, 408

Section 8: Pharmacology and Anesthesia

23 Surgical Pharmacology, 420
Pharmacology Baselines, 421
Considerations in Surgical Pharmacology, 424
Surgical Drug and Pharmaceutical Sources, 426
Pharmacologic Forms Used in Surgery, 428
Potential Complications Caused by Pharmaceuticals and Herbal Medicine, 430

24 Anesthesia: Techniques and Agents, 432
The Art and Science of Anesthesia, 433
Choice of Anesthesia, 433
Anesthesia State, 433
Knowledge of Anesthetics, 434
Types of Anesthesia, 434
Alternatives to Conventional Anesthesia, 464

Section 9: Intraoperative Patient Care

25 Coordinated Roles of the Scrub Person and the Circulating Nurse, 466
Division of Duties, 466
Efficiency of the Operating Room Team, 495

26 Positioning, Prepping, and Draping the Patient, 499
Preliminary Considerations, 499
Anatomic and Physiologic Considerations, 504
Equipment for Positioning, 506
Surgical Positions, 512
Physical Preparation and Draping of the Surgical Site, 519

27 Physiologic Maintenance and Monitoring of the Perioperative Patient, 535
Monitoring Physiologic Functions, 535

Section 10: Surgical Site Management

28 Surgical Incisions, Implants, and Wound Closure, 551
The Surgical Incision, 551
Surgical Landmarks, 556
Wound Closure, 559

29 Wound Healing and Hemostasis, 583
Mechanism of Wound Healing, 584
Types of Wounds, 585
Factors Influencing Wound Healing, 586
Hemostasis, 589
Wound Management, 598
Complications of Wound Healing, 604
Postoperative Wound Infections, 606
Wound Assessment, 607
Basic Wound Care, 607

Section 11: Perianesthesia and Postprocedural Patient Care

30 Postoperative Patient Care, 610
Postanesthesia Care, 610
Admission to the Postanesthesia Care Unit, 612
Discharge From the Postanesthesia Care Unit, 614

31 Potential Perioperative Complications, 616
Potential for Complications During and After Surgery, 616
Respiratory Complications, 617
Cardiovascular Complications, 620
Fluid and Electrolyte Imbalances, 632
Blood Volume Complications, 634
Shock, 641
Metabolic Crises, 642
Iatrogenic Injury, 646

Section 12: Surgical Specialties

32 Endoscopy and Robotic-Assisted Surgery, 647
Eight Essential Elements of Endoscopy, 647
Knowledge and Skill for a Safe Endoscopic Environment, 655
Types of Endoscopic Procedures, 655
Care of Endoscopes, 658
Considerations for Patient Safety, 659
Duties of the Assistant for Flexible Endoscopy, 660
Robotic-Assisted Endoscopy, 660

33 General Surgery, 664
Special Considerations for General Surgery, 664

Breast Procedures, 666
Abdominal Procedures, 670
Liver Procedures, 674
Splenic Procedures, 675
Pancreatic Procedures, 675
Esophageal Procedures, 676
Gastrointestinal Surgery, 677
Intestinal Procedures, 682
Colorectal Procedures, 686
Abdominal Trauma, 688
Anorectal Procedures, 691
Hernia Procedures, 692
Amputation of Extremities, 694

34   Gynecologic and Obstetric Surgery, 696
Anatomy and Physiology of the Female Reproductive System, 697
Gynecology: General Considerations, 700
Diagnostic Techniques, 701
Robotic Procedures, 706
Vulvar Procedures, 706
Vaginal Procedures, 707
Abdominal Procedures, 710
Perioperative Obstetrics, 714
Complicated Birth, 718
Assisted Reproduction, 722
Nonobstetric Surgical Procedures and the Pregnant Patient, 725

35   Urologic Surgery, 730
Anatomy and Physiology of the Urinary System, 730
Special Features of Urologic Surgery, 733
Surgical Procedures of the Genitourinary System, 738
Bladder Flap Urethroplasty, 748
Male Reproductive Organs, 749
Endocrine Glands, 758
Transsexual Surgery (Sex Reassignment), 758
Postoperative Complications of Urologic Surgery, 759

36   Orthopedic Surgery, 761
The Art and Science of Orthopedic Surgery, 761
Anatomy and Physiology of the Musculoskeletal System, 762
Special Features of Orthopedic Surgery, 765
Extremity Procedures, 770
Fractures, 771
Joint Procedures, 775
Repair of Tendons and Ligaments, 784
Cast Application, 785
Complications After Orthopedic Surgery, 788

37   Neurosurgery of the Brain and Peripheral Nerves, 790
Anatomy and Physiology of the Brain, 790
Special Considerations in Neurosurgery, 792

Patient Care Considerations for Craniotomy, 795
Surgical Procedures of the Cranium, 799
Peripheral Nerve Surgery, 806

38   Spinal Surgery, 808
Anatomy and Physiology of the Spinal Cord and Vertebral Column, 808
Special Considerations for Spinal Surgery, 811
Pathology of the Vertebrae and Spinal Cord, 816
Surgical Procedures of the Spine, 820

39   Ophthalmic Surgery, 826
Anatomy and Physiology of the Eye, 826
Ophthalmic Surgical Patient Care, 827
Special Features of Ophthalmic Surgery, 829
Ocular Surgical Procedures, 832
Eye Injuries, 844
Ophthalmic Lasers, 845

40   Plastic and Reconstructive Surgery, 847
Special Features of Plastic and Reconstructive Surgery, 847
Skin and Tissue Grafting, 850
Head and Neck Plastic and Reconstructive Procedures, 858
Plastic and Reconstructive Procedures of Other Body Areas, 861
Burns, 867

41   Otorhinolaryngologic and Head and Neck Surgery, 873
General Considerations in Ear, Nose, and Throat Procedures, 873
Ear, 876
Nose, 881
Oral Cavity and Throat, 885
Neck, 889
Face and Skull, 897

42   Thoracic Surgery, 905
Anatomy and Physiology of the Thorax, 905
Physiology, 908
Special Features of Thoracic Surgery, 908
Thoracic Surgical Procedures, 916
Chest Trauma, 919
Intrathoracic Esophageal Procedures, 920
Complications of Thoracic Surgery, 920

43   Cardiac Surgery, 923
Anatomy of the Heart and Great Vessels, 923
Physiology of the Heart, 925
Cardiac Cycle, 925
Special Features of Cardiac Surgery, 926
Cardiac Surgical Procedures, 933
Mechanical Assist Devices, 940
Complications of Cardiac Surgery, 945

44 Vascular Surgery, 947

Anatomy and Physiology of the Vascular System, 947
Vascular Pathology, 949
Diagnostic Procedures, 951
Special Features of Vascular Surgery, 952
Composite Vein Grafts, 955
Conservative Interventional Techniques, 955
Laser Angioplasty, 956
Vascular Surgical Procedures, 958

45 Organ Procurement and Transplantation, 969

Types of Transplants, 969
Tissue Transplantation, 969
Organ Transplantation, 972

Index, 988

1

Perioperative Education

CHAPTER OUTLINE

The Art and Science of Surgery, 2

Perioperative Learner, 3

Perioperative Educator, 5

Application of Theory to Practice, 10

Expected Behaviors of Perioperative Caregivers, 11

Realities of Clinical Practice, 13

CHAPTER OBJECTIVES

After studying this chapter the learner will be able to:

- Compare and contrast the art and science of surgery.
- Identify three characteristics of adult learners.
- Name five educational resources available for the learner.
- Define the difference between andragogy and pedagogy.

- Describe how adult learning principles apply to patient teaching.
- Discuss the problems associated with disruptive behavior in the perioperative environment.

KEY TERMS AND DEFINITIONS

Andragogy Teaching and learning processes for mature adult populations.

Behavior Actions or conduct indicative of a mental state or predisposition influenced by emotions, feelings, beliefs, values, morals, and ethics.

Disruptive behavior (bullying) Power imbalance that involves intimidation, oppression, or aggression and results in a counterproductive atmosphere.

Cognition Process of knowing or perceiving, such as learning scientific principles and observing their application.

Competency Creative application of knowledge, skills, and interpersonal abilities in fulfilling functions to provide safe, individualized patient care.

Critical thinking The mental process by which an individual solves problems.

Disease Failure of the body to counteract stimuli or stresses adequately, resulting in a disturbance in function or structure of any part, organ, or system of the body.

Environmental factors Water, air, soil, and food. Contamination and exposure of any of these factors can lead to disease.

Evaluation A process by which the educator measures performance by standardized indicators established by a school, employer, or professional organization.

Knowledge Organized body of factual information.

Learning style Individualized methods used by the learner to understand and retain new information. These may be visual, auditory, tactile, sensory, kinesthetic, or performance-oriented behaviors.

Mentoring A nurturing, flexible relationship between a more experienced person and a less experienced person that involves trust, coaching, advice, guidance, and support. A sharing relationship guided by the needs of the less experienced person.

Objectives Written in behavioral terms, statements that determine the expected outcomes of a behavior or process.

Occupational hazard A workplace hazard that can cause physical, biologic, or chemical injury, leading to disease or death.

Orientation Period during which a student or new employee becomes acquainted with the environment, policies, and procedures of a professional environment.

Pedagogy Teaching and learning processes for immature and/or pediatric populations. A very directed style is used.

Perioperative Total surgical experience that encompasses preoperative, intraoperative, and postoperative phases of patient care.

Preceptor A person who observes, teaches, and evaluates a learner according to a prescribed format of training or orientation.

Psychomotor Pertaining to physical demonstration of mental processes (i.e., applying cognitive learning).

Role model A person who is admired and emulated for good practices in the clinical environment. The relationship between a role model and a learner can be strictly professional without personalized mentoring.

Skill Application of knowledge into observable, measurable, and quantifiable performance.

Surgery Branch of medicine that encompasses preoperative, intraoperative, and postoperative care of patients. The discipline of surgery is both an art and a science.
Surgical conscience Awareness that develops from a knowledge base of the importance of strict adherence to principles of aseptic and sterile techniques.

Surgical procedure Invasive incision into body tissues or a minimally invasive entrance into a body cavity for either therapeutic or diagnostic purposes; protective reflexes or self-care abilities are potentially compromised during such a procedure.

The main focus of this chapter is to establish the baseline or framework for an in-depth study of perioperative patient care and support the educational process of the learner. Consideration is given to the perioperative educator, who may not have had a formal education in the teaching of adult learners. Both learners and educators should understand that the same learning and teaching principles apply to patient education. The key terms are commonly used terms that the learner should understand as the basis for learning about and participating in the art and science of surgery.

The Art and Science of Surgery

Health is both a personal and an economic asset. Optimal health is the best physiologic and psychologic condition an individual can experience. Disease is the inability to adequately counteract physiologic and psychologic stressors that cause disruption of the body's homeostasis. Additional influences, such as congenital anomalies, infection, trauma, mental disorders, occupational hazard, or environmental factors, interfere with optimal human health and quality of life. As both a science and an art, surgery is the branch of medicine that comprises perioperative patient care, encompassing such activities as preoperative preparation, intraoperative judgment, intervention, management, and postoperative care of patients. As a discipline, surgery combines physiologic management with an interventional aspect of treatment. The common indications for surgical intervention include correction of defects, alteration of form, restoration of function, diagnosis and/or treatment of diseases, and palliation. Table 1.1 describes some of the most common indications for surgery.

In the 1930s, the English physician Lord Berkeley George Moynihan (1865–1936) said, "Surgery has been made safe for the patient; we must now make the patient safe for surgery." Surgical intervention is becoming a safer method of treating physiologic conditions. Most of the former contraindications to surgery that were related to patient age or condition have been reduced because of better diagnostic methodologies, minimally invasive procedures, and drug therapies. More individuals are now considered for surgery; however, each patient and each procedure are unique. Perioperative caregivers should not become complacent with routines but should always be prepared for the unexpected. Surgery cannot be considered completely safe all the time, and patient outcomes are not always predictable.

A surgical procedure may be invasive, minimally invasive, minimal access, or noninvasive. An invasive or minimal access procedure enters the body either through an opening in the tissues or by a natural body orifice. Noninvasive procedures are frequently diagnostic and do not enter the body. Technology has elevated the practice of surgery to a more precise science that minimizes the "invasiveness" and enhances the functional aspects of the procedure. Recovery or postprocedure time decreases, with

TABLE 1.1 Common Indications for Surgical Procedures	
Indication for Surgical Procedure	**Example**
Augmentation	Breast implants
Debulking	Decreasing the size of a mass
Incision	Open tissue or structure by sharp dissection
Excision	Remove tissue or structure by sharp dissection
Diagnostics	Biopsy tissue sample
Repair	Closing of a hernia
Removal	Foreign body
Reconstruction	Creation of a new breast
Palliation	Relief of obstruction
Aesthetics	Facelift
Harvest	Autologous skin graft
Procurement	Donor organ
Transplant	Placement of a donor organ or tissue
Bypass/shunt	Vascular rerouting
Drainage/evacuation	Incision into abscess
Stabilization	Repair of a fracture
Parturition	Cesarean section
Termination	Abortion of a pregnancy
Staging	Checking of cancer progression
Extraction	Removal of a tooth
Exploration	Invasive examination
Diversion	Creation of a stoma for urine
Implantation	Inserting a subsurface device
Replantation	Reattaching a body part
Amputation	Removing a large structure
Stenting	Using an implant as a supporting device
Neoconstruction	Face transplant

less pain, and the patient is restored to functional capacity faster. Improvements in perioperative patient care technology are attributed to the following:
- Surgical specialization of surgeons and teams
- Sophisticated diagnostic and intraoperative imaging techniques
- Minimally invasive equipment and technology

- Ongoing research and technologic advancements

Surgical procedures are performed in hospitals, in surgeons' offices, or in freestanding surgical facilities. Many patients can safely have a surgical procedure as an outpatient and do not require an overnight stay at the facility. The types of surgical procedures performed on an outpatient basis are determined by the complexity of the procedure and the general health of the individual. Procedures performed on patients who remain overnight in the hospital vary according to the expertise of the surgeons, the health of the patient, and the availability of the equipment.

The purpose of this text is to provide a baseline for learning the professional and technical patient care knowledge and skill required to provide safe and efficient care for patients in the perioperative environment.

Perioperative Learner

The learner in the perioperative environment may be a medical, nursing, or surgical technology student enrolled in a formal educational program, or the learner may be a newly hired orientee. Medical students have a surgical rotation that includes participation in surgical procedures. They learn some of the basic principles of surgical technology and sterile technique to ensure the safety and welfare of patients and staff.

Some nursing schools offer basic exposure to perioperative nursing as a short observation period, part of the core curriculum, or an elective. After graduating from nursing school, the nurse needs further education before functioning as a perioperative professional.[1] Education may take place in a postbasic/postgraduate perioperative nursing course offered by a college or a hospital orientation program. Entry-level education for perioperative practice prepares nurses to be generalists. Basic perioperative nursing elective programs focus on the role of the perioperative nurse as both generalist circulator and scrub person. Specialization can follow a period in professional practice in a specific service. The perioperative nurse's role encompasses supervision of unlicensed personnel who scrub in surgery, such as surgical technologists, and requires knowledge of practices and procedures performed under this title.

Surgical technology programs focus primarily on scrubbing in to prepare and maintain the sterile surgical field and handle instruments. Some surgical technology programs offer circulating experiences under the supervision of a registered nurse; however, the role of the circulator requires knowledge and skill not commonly covered in significant depth in shorter training programs. Most surgical technology programs provide scrub experiences in many specialties. After satisfactory completion of the program, many technologists are capable of functioning in the scrub role as a generalist or, in some circumstances, a specialist. Advancing technology indicates the need for specialized competencies for all disciplines of perioperative patient care. Surgeons, perioperative nurses, and surgical technologists should continually strive to learn new procedures and technologies in a team-oriented environment.

Perioperative caregivers new to a particular practice setting should learn the specific performance standards and expectations of that institution. All personnel go through an orientation process to familiarize themselves with the philosophy, goals, policies, procedures, role expectations, equipment, and physical facilities specific to their institution. Departmental orientation is specific to the area in which the caregiver is employed.

Many graduates seek employment in the institutions where they performed clinical rotations. This is usually beneficial to the facility and the employee. Some students are hired into apprenticeships before graduation, enabling them to work in the operating room (OR) in a limited capacity in anticipation of a permanent position. Schools that permit students to work while still in the education process should have a policy in place to delineate the student role from the employee role. The policy should be made known in writing to all clinical facilities hosting students and students performing clinical rotations where apprenticeships are offered. The following are considerations in developing a policy for working students:

- Students may not work for compensation during official clinical hours.
- Students may not wear facility name or identification badges while performing clinical rotations as an agent of the school.
- Students may not wear school name or identification badges while performing work for compensation as an agent of the facility.
- Students may not take time off from classroom or clinical rotations to work for compensation.
- Students are not part of the clinical staff during clinical rotation hours.
- Students are to maintain patient confidentiality at all times.
- Students may be screened by the school or facility by routine background checks and drug testing.
- Students should be subject to health screening and vaccinations followed by titers for proof of immunity (i.e., varicella; rubeola; diphtheria, tetanus, pertussis [DTaP]; and hepatitis B). Some facilities require flu and COVID-19 vaccinations. Tuberculosis testing should be performed before clinical rotation.

All learners in the perioperative environment are adults and perform better if given due respect. This concept applies whether the caregiver is experienced or a novice. Treating an adult learner in a pedagogic manner (pedagogy), as a child is treated, is counterproductive and becomes a barrier to learning. The learner can become resentful and unable to separate feelings of inexperience from feelings of inadequacy. Regardless of the level of learning required, the general characteristics of the adult learner (andragogy) as compared with the child learner (pedagogy) apply (Table 1.2). These concepts also should be applied to patient education programs.

Not everyone learns at the same speed or assimilates information in the same manner. Theoretic knowledge or a skill learned quickly by one individual may be difficult for another. Cognition is premised on the ability to process and retain information. Learning styles vary among individuals and are influenced by internal and external factors. Examples of learning-style influences are listed in Box 1.1. Learning styles were described in the early 1990s by Howard Gardner at Harvard University. Understanding the differences in individual learners is the first step to imparting knowledge and skill.[2] Eight learning skills identified by Gardner are summarized as follows with application of teaching methods for perioperative learners:

1. *Visual-spatial:* Very environmentally aware. Learns well by observation, puzzles, graphics, and modeling.
   - The educator can create poster boards with images of instrument pictures and setups. Posters can have backgrounds of blank sterile fields constructed of felt and cardboard cutouts of instruments with hook and loop backing for students to place on the surface.

TABLE 1.2	Characteristics of the Adult Learner Compared With the Child Learner	
Adult (Andragogy)	**Child (Pedagogy)**	
Is self-directed	Is task oriented	
Uses activities that follow transitions of maturity	Uses activities that follow stages of development	
Uses intrinsic thought processes	Uses extrinsic thought processes	
Uses problem-solving approach	Uses trial-and-error approach	
Values self-esteem	Values self-esteem	

• BOX 1.1 Learning-Style Influences

- Intelligence
- Attentiveness
- Cultural and ethnic background
- Educational preparation
- Motivation to learn
- Concentration and distractibility
- Personality characteristics
- Psychologic strengths or deficiencies
- Social skills, including communication skills
- Manual dexterity
- Physical senses
- Physical health
- Perceptual preferences and sensory partiality (e.g., visual vs. auditory)
- Environment

2. *Bodily kinesthetic:* Keen sense of motion and hands-on sense. Communicates well by physical practice.
   - The educator can provide sterile drapes and instrument trays for students' use in preparing sterile fields and setups. The task can be made more challenging by timing the process and creating competition for the best time with the highest degree of accuracy. Teams competing against each other in table setups and draping make the activity fun and exciting.
3. *Musical:* Learns well by listening and the auditory use of multimedia. Frequently learns better with music in the background.
   - The educator (with the help of the students) can enumerate specific steps to a procedure, such as donning the sterile gown and gloves. The steps are recited to a musical beat provided by rhythmic clapping or to an instrumental background tune. Most students recognize simple childhood tunes and can sing or say the steps to the music. Also, modern musical instrumentals are easy to use for this purpose.
4. *Interpersonal:* Group dynamics and study sessions work well for this learner.
   - The educator can assign topics to groups for exploration and development. The students present their findings to the class in a forum setting. Some students may want to simulate procedures for the class.
5. *Intrapersonal:* Learns well through self-study and independence. Highly self-motivated and disciplined.

   - The educator can guide individual students in the creation of personal flashcards or organization of class notes. Students who learn best by self-study generally seek assistance only when further explanation or clarification is needed.
6. *Linguistic:* Very good with language and auditory skill. Learns effectively through lectures and explanation.
   - The educator presents lectures on specific topics and uses multimedia to reinforce the discussion. PowerPoint presentations enhance the lecture and can be printed for the students to use in following along. Embedded video is useful, and links to webinars and websites provide variety, such as www.youtube.com.
7. *Logical-mathematical:* Prefers to investigate and solve problems. Conceptual thinking precedes detailing with these learners.
   - The educator can use several testing formats to challenge the learners. Tables set up with instruments for identification by category or classification give students the opportunity to determine how each item is used in a particular specialty. An interesting twist to this method involves intentionally omitting a particularly necessary item from the field; the students have to reconstruct the steps of the procedure to figure out which item is missing.
8. *Naturalist:* The naturalist was added to learning styles in 2006. The naturalist is in tune with their surroundings (sounds, smells, temperature, and activity). They respect all living things.[2] Likes balance and is detail orientated. Has the ability to see patterns.
   - The educator can demonstrate a table setup and the student can re-create the setup with the ability to identify and classify instruments in an organized manner.

Each facility should clearly define the role of the perioperative learner of each discipline. Activities of new perioperative nurses and surgical technology students are not the same. The perioperative nurse is involved with more direct patient care and decision-making through physical assessment. The student surgical technologist is concerned primarily with preparing and maintaining the sterile field. Both disciplines of learners help prepare for and assist a qualified preceptor during surgical procedures and cleanup afterward, but they are not considered members of the staff complement.

Instructional staff should observe for and guard against laziness in the preceptor group. Some preceptors may want to sit back in the pretense of "letting the student take over." In essence this is not an improper approach to precepting, but it can be abused if the preceptor continually leaves the student to flounder or delay the progress of the procedure.

Some preceptors and surgeons may "bully" the students and become impatient because of the students' inexperience. Disruptive behavior (bullying) is counterproductive. Students should be taught to speak up when necessary, respect the preceptors and surgeons, but not be afraid to ask questions. Most facilities have developed a "zero-tolerance" policy concerning interprofessional relationships wherein one person causes another person to feel intimidated or fearful. All forms of bullying or violence (psychologic or physical) are unacceptable in the workplace. All incidents should be reported immediately with documentation. Employers are required to follow up to promote a safe work environment.[3]

Some facilities now require a preceptor class to address appropriate behavior, understand student learning styles, and learn what is expected of them and how to help students become successful.

Students should know basic standards and protocol before entering the OR for a clinical rotation. Preceptors may have developed shortcuts with questionable technique not understood by students who are new to the OR environment. Students should not blindly perform tasks directed by preceptors that cause question as to technique or safety without fully understanding what resultant outcome is expected. Students should speak up in a respectable way for clarification.[4]

Educators should discuss the potential for these questionable events and give the student a vehicle for professionally or assertively deferring or opting out of doing something that is nonstandard by the level of education they have experienced in the classroom. This process can be particularly uncomfortable if the student does not feel supported by the educator, who is a mentor in the environment, in doing what has been ingrained as the standard of care. Some examples of this activity include but are not limited to the following (these examples actually happened at a clinical site):

1. *Event:* Preceptor insists on gowning and gloving from the primary sterile field and instructs the student to do so as well. Student deferral vehicle: "My clinical instructor will give me a deficiency grade if I gown and glove from the sterile back table. I am required to gown and glove from a separate sterile surface other than the main field."

2. *Event:* Preceptor is impatient and goes to sit on a stool in the corner because part of the procedure is taking a long time. Student deferral vehicle: "My clinical instructor will give me a deficiency grade if I sit and change the level of sterility of the front of my gown."

3. *Event:* Preceptor instructs the student to offer a towel from the open and biologically contaminated back table to a person who plans to enter the working sterile field. Student deferral vehicle: "My clinical instructor will give me a deficiency grade if I offer a towel from my working sterile back table."

Learners are not expected to assume responsibilities for which they are not fully prepared, but they should be taught to politely speak up when something is not right for the benefit of the team and the patient.[4] Only through continued study and experience can individuals qualify as team members in the perioperative environment.

The new perioperative nurse in a hospital orientation program, who will be functioning in interchangeable scrub and circulating roles, may learn the scrub role first in the learning sequence so as to learn the art of anticipation of surgeon and patient needs during a surgical procedure. This is the closest vantage point by which participation enables the perioperative nurse to be familiarized with the surgical process. An educator, preceptor, or other qualified staff member scrubs in as support and gradually allows the new perioperative nurse to take over more of the work in the sterile field. One of the primary behavioral objectives is to gain knowledge and skill in sterile technique. Performing the scrub role allows repetition of tasks performed within the sterile field and better prepares the perioperative nurse to supervise surgical technologists.

The second component of the perioperative nurse's learning sequence is the circulating role. A registered nurse preceptor is assigned to teach the new nurse the coordination of the scrub and circulating roles. Standard routines are taught under the supervision of an experienced perioperative nurse with comparable knowledge, skill, and educational preparation. Guidance and help from the clinical educator and other experienced staff members help the new perioperative nurse pull it all together. Surgeons and other staff members contribute to the learning process.

Personality traits, such as emotional maturity, social skills, and psychologic characteristics, are continually assessed by the educator. A moody, easily angered, and negative person can be very difficult to deal with as a future team member. The learner who does not possess assertive skills for dealing with stressful events cannot function effectively in a team environment. Subjective responses to all activities should remain on a professional level if the team is to function efficiently. The perioperative nurse in training should be evaluated on a periodic basis to assess for increased competency levels.

Perioperative Educator

Experience in the perioperative clinical setting should be planned and supervised by an experienced perioperative nurse educator. The term *educator* is used throughout this text to refer to the person responsible for planning, implementing, and evaluating the learner's experiences in the classroom and clinical perioperative setting. Other teaching personnel at the clinical site include perioperative nurse preceptors.

The educator should consider the effect on the learner who is seeing the perioperative environment for the first time. The OR can appear cold, large, and overwhelming. A tour of the facility before beginning the program can help decrease the learner's anxiety.

A structured curriculum uses behavioral objectives, written guidelines, and relevant assignments for feedback to ensure that learning has occurred. Learner conferences are held at regular intervals to discuss procedures and progress.

AORN (The Association of periOperative Registered Nurses) offers perioperative nursing education in several courses: AORN Periop 101 offers three courses (OR curriculum, ambulatory surgery center [ASC] curriculum, and cesarean section curriculum). Periop 202 focuses on knowledge and skills needed for specialty services such as cardiac, spine, and orthopedics. A Periop Mastery 2.0 course is available for the experienced nurse or those looking to become travel nurses. These programs are purchased by hospitals for training of new perioperative nurses. Some facilities offer nurse residency or nurse internships programs that can last up to 2 years. More information about perioperative nursing courses can be found at www.aorn.org.

Didactic presentations should be incorporated into the teaching program to provide information concerning the theory and detail of all performed actions in the perioperative environment. Presentations should be offered by knowledgeable presenters who are well prepared to deliver information to the group.

If PowerPoint multimedia are used, the educator should be sure to use accurate and concise terminology when creating the slides.

Handouts can be printed in several formats for distribution to the participants to use when following along with the talk or taking notes. Overloading each slide with wordiness and silly images causes confusion and wastes time. The key elements should be simply worded and should not exceed six lines of text per slide.

The educator should not read exactly from the slides but explain while incorporating the concept the slide imparts. Font style should be simple, and font size should be readable even at the back of the classroom. Avoid typing words in all caps. The slide color scheme and design can be selected from predesigned templates or customized per presentation. Colors such as blue and green are easier on the eyes than reds, oranges, and bright yellows. Time between slide changes should permit questions or examples.

Positive reinforcement helps the learner build confidence and competence. The educator should not punish a learner for making honest errors during supervised learning. Degradation and damage to self-esteem are barriers to learning. The learner should not be required to perform any function for which the learner has not had adequate training or guided practice. The educator should maintain a list of procedures in which the learner has participated and has demonstrated increasing levels of competence.

Whether the learner is in a school-sponsored OR education program or a departmental orientation program, the duration of the program should be sufficient to afford opportunities for adequate experience to facilitate success. The AORN position statement on basic orientation recommends a period of 40 hours in each specialty as part of the orientation process.[1] Novice perioperative nurses can be in orientation from 6 to 12 months. Novice surgical technologists (ST) may have an orientation period of up to 6 months. Orientation time is based on an individual's knowledge and skill level.

Check-off sheets can help track experiential progress during the education process. Fig. 1.1 shows an example of a basic check-off sheet for the evaluation of knowledge and skill in the scrub role. Fig. 1.2 shows an example of a basic check-off sheet for evaluation of knowledge and skill in the circulating nurse's role. This sheet can be modified to apply to specialties as needed. The Association of Surgical Technologists (AST) and AORN have developed skills checklists available through the organizations.

Behavioral Objectives

The learner takes an active role in the teaching/learning process by helping identify behavioral objectives. Effective and organized educational experiences are identified and based on these objectives. The identified behavioral objectives are attained through critical-thinking exercises. Skill in questioning and encouragement in making discoveries allow the learner to use critical thinking as a learning tool.

Evaluation of the learner's progress is measured by how successfully the learner has met the behavioral objectives. Behavioral objectives are identified and written in behavioral terms and based on standards of expected performance and accepted standards of patient care. In 1956, Benjamin Bloom described the measurement of cognitive learning. He detailed six levels of learning, ranging from simple recall to advanced abstract thinking.

Bloom's taxonomy provides a framework for structuring cognitive and affective learning. Therefore the concepts to be learned and the behavioral objectives to be met should form the foundation on which all perioperative caregivers build their practice. Each behavioral objective in Box 1.2 is measurable and is evaluated by performance standards.

Elements of Effective Instruction

The organization of the instructional material and the learning experience are further enhanced by the way the program is presented. The elements of effective instruction are summarized as follows:

- Set clear and concise behavioral objectives measurable in cognitive terminology that describes knowledge, comprehension, application, analysis, understanding, and evaluation.
- Establish a learning environment that is controlled by the educator.
- Provide variation in presenting material. Computer modules, webinars, animated computer programs, podcasts, video, and photographs can be alternated with lectures and hands-on practice. Handling instruments and supplies in a classroom is less intimidating than handling them in the perioperative environment for the first time.
- Encourage the exchange of questions and answers as an assessment tool. Learners often ask exactly what they need to know. The educator can determine areas of deficient knowledge.
- Reinforce learning. After a skill has been taught in a didactic manner, provide guided practice in the clinical laboratory before the task is performed in the perioperative environment. Provide positive support for desired behaviors. Self-assessment tools and performance evaluations provide feedback about the learner's progress. One method may include videoing the learner performing a task like a setup and playing it back for self-assessment.
- Computerized modules with testing may be used to evaluate comprehension.
- Summarize the learner's accomplishments at regular intervals. Reviewing daily activities helps reinforce the learning process by allowing the learner to associate the events of their experience with newly acquired knowledge.

The educator should work closely with the perioperative nurse manager. Classroom hours and clinical experience assignments are coordinated to provide the best experience for the learner. The nurse manager offers suggestions and coordination input for the benefit of the learner and staff members. The educator identifies areas of needed experience for the learner. An effort is made to confer and coordinate any changes in the program with all personnel in the department. The educator and the manager collaborate with the assigned preceptors as needed. These strategies foster a friendly and cooperative relationship among learners, educators, management, and preceptor staff.

All perioperative staff members indirectly assist in teaching the learners within the guidelines of the structured learning experience. The learners gain knowledge by observing and working with members of the entire team. Everyone should be familiar with the knowledge level of the learners, the behavioral objectives, and the teaching roles that staff members are expected to assume. Learners also should be responsible for updating the staff about needed experience and their current level of achievement.

Hospitals or facilities offering the clinical perioperative setting for educational programs have policies and procedures that are adaptations of national standards. All personnel, including faculty members and learners, are expected to adhere to their content.

Evaluation	Meets Standard	Needs Improvement	Improving Yes or No	Does Not Meet Standard	Comments
Reports for duty in a punctual manner					
Wears OR attire properly: Dons personal protective gear Dons radiation badge as needed					
Performs housekeeping duties: Before first procedure of day Between procedures After last procedure of day					
Sterile supplies: Plans and gathers supplies Checks integrity of packages Checks sterility integrator Checks dates on perishables					
Places items on sterile surface: Opening wrapper(s) Peel packages Solution dispensing					
Scrubs for setup and procedure: Hand and arm scrubbing Hand hygiene with hand antiseptic					
Gowning: Gowns self correctly Gowns others					
Gloves: Closed method Open method Changes contaminated glove Gloves others					
Sterile setup: Drapes table and Mayo stand Positions items in the field					
Accountability: Participates in timeout before incision Labels solutions and drugs Reports amount of use Practices safety Maintains the sterile field Responds appropriately to emergent situations					
Anticipates needs of surgeon: Coordinates with circulator Facilitates the first assistant Passes instrumentation Prepares and applies dressing materials					
Counts: Sponges Sharps Instruments					
Assembles instruments: Attaches knife blades on handles Loads or prepares suture Tests drills and devices Other					
Disassembles the table: Follows proper disposal of items Follows decontamination procedures					
Removes gown and gloves: Gown off first Glove-to-glove/skin-to-skin					

• **Fig. 1.1** Performance appraisal of the scrub role.

Evaluation	Meets Standard	Needs Improvement	Improving Yes or No	Does Not Meet Standard	Comments
Reports for the duty in a punctual manner					
Wears OR attire properly: Dons personal protective gear Dons radiation badge as needed					
Performs housekeeping duties: Before first procedure of day Between procedures After last procedure of day					
Sterile supplies: Plans and gathers supplies Checks integrity of packages Checks sterility integrator Checks dates on perishables					
Dispenses or transfers items to sterile surface as appropriate: Opens wrapper(s) and peel packs Opens closed container Solution dispensing Medication dispensing					
Validates implant parameters and documents in the lot log					
Practices aseptic technique: Dons and removes sterile or nonsterile gloves as appropriate for task Hand hygiene with hand antiseptic					
Gowning and gloving of others: Ties gowns for sterile team members Assists with contaminated glove removal Provides additional gowns and gloves as needed					
Accountability: Gathers and checks solutions and drugs for use on the field Documents amount of usage of drugs and solutions on the field Practices safety for the patient and team Monitors the sterile field and the members of the sterile team					
Anticipates needs of patient, anesthesia provider, surgeon, and other team members: Coordinates with the scrub person Obtains additional supplies and instrumentation as needed					
Provides safe and competent direct patient care: Patient advocate Patient identification Assists the anesthesia provider as needed during induction Validates correct site protocol and time out procedures Patient assessment Responds appropriately to emergent situations Supports psychosocial aspects of care Positioning and prepping as appropriate Monitoring physiologic and psychologic responses as appropriate Cares for specimens Patient teaching					
Counts: Sponges Sharps Instruments Documents any other item added to the field intraoperatively					
Attaches and activates surgical machinery and devices for the sterile field: Electrosurgery (ESU) cables, suction, power cords, and other peripheral equipment Activates, sets, and monitors peripheral equipment					
Supervises and manages the room: Plans and implements direct patient care using the nursing process Directs the activities of learners Communicates procedural progress to the control desk Communicates with family members Manages messages for the surgeon and first assistant Prevents inappropriate traffic through the room Documents procedural activities in patient record Computer literacy Uses patient electronic medical record responsibly Maintains patient confidentiality Manages patient charge items responsibly					

• **Fig. 1.2** Performance appraisal of the circulating nurse's role.

- To identify the role and responsibility of each team member
- To define current standard terminology associated with perioperative patient care through use of the perioperative nursing data set (PNDS)
- To compare and contrast knowledge of normal anatomy, physiology, and pathophysiology
- To discuss the interrelationships among physiologic, ethnocultural, and psychosocial factors that affect a patient and family's adaptation to the perioperative experience
- To identify the procedures necessary to prepare each patient as an individual for the intended surgical procedure
- To demonstrate the ability to select appropriate instrumentation, equipment, and supplies according to the individualized plan of care
- To apply the principles of sterilization, disinfection, and aseptic and sterile techniques in the preparation and use of all materials in the perioperative environment to prevent transmission of biologic contamination
- To identify the potential environmental hazards to the patient and team
- To demonstrate knowledge of the basic actions and uses of anesthetic agents, medications, fluid therapies, and electrolytes
- To demonstrate the ability to identify implants, correct size, and proper handling
- To demonstrate knowledge and skill during the surgical procedure by anticipating the needs of the patient and the team
- To discuss the principles of wound management
- To function as a team member by showing consideration for and cooperation with other perioperative caregivers
- To communicate effectively with personnel on other patient care divisions within the facility
- To develop the ability to perform safely and effectively during stressful situations

Media and Print Learning Resources

Books, journals, videos, DVDs, slides, photographs, computers, and audiovisual materials may supplement the lecture approach to perioperative education. Larger teaching institutions may have live closed-circuit television and interactive telecommunication systems that permit educators and learners to communicate from remote locations. Many audiovisual materials, such as videos, webinars, audiotapes, and computer-assisted instruction, are self-contained units for individual study. A bibliography in a text such as this or at the conclusion of a journal article provides references to broaden the learner's database. Accessibility to current medical and scientific literature is without limit. Other sources include websites on the Internet and educational services that provide contact hours online.

The following are useful resources for acquiring and reinforcing knowledge:
1. Library and literature file. Books and current periodicals are available for the learner's reference in the medical library, online, and in learning centers at local colleges and libraries.
2. Educational literature, DVDs, and portable storage devices such as a USB flash drive or jump drive are available from surgical supply and instrument manufacturers. Most manufacturers have their product literature and educational material online. All personnel who will be working with the item should review the new equipment literature. In-services are commonly provided by clinical staff associated with the industry. The purchasing agent is a good resource for these types of references.

PROS/CONS

Perioperative Educator: Engaging the Learner

Pros
- Health care facilities perform better when employees are engaged with what they are doing. Commitment is linked to job satisfaction and better organizational performances.
- Educators and managers must recognize the current culture of their department and find ways for improvement.
- Health care facilities require education on certain topics as part of employee annual training. These competencies may be required yearly and are documented in the employee record.
- As part of continuing education, a facility may have a perioperative educator or manager who follows a structured curriculum according to the facility guidelines and policies.
- Continuing education credit may be given for completion of a test after an educational presentation.
- Scheduled regular in-services are planned when most employees can be present; this usually occurs during the workday. Employees who are not in attendance may need to reschedule with the educator to cover the missed material.
- Staff involvement during in-services increases when they are recognized, part of decision-making, on a unit council, involved in teamwork, involved in training, and recruited to assist.
- A structured presentation keeps the group interested. When knowledge is linked with previous knowledge and preexisting cognitive structure, effective learning occurs.
- People retain information in different ways. Some positive ways to engage staff during an in-service include vary the tone of voice, include positive body language, practice presentation skills, offer refreshments, tell a story, ask questions, role play, use fewer words, and use technology.
- Understanding information is easier through the use of images, color, audiovisual, demonstration, and active participation.
- Set a goal and use critical thinking and decision-making during participation.

- Employees may have preclass preparation such as an article or computer module to read, small group discussions, and simulation. Each employee may be required to demonstrate the simulation during the in-service. This helps build confidence and competence through positive reinforcement.
- Use surveys and committees to engage staff; this encourages participation and a chance to be heard.

Cons
- Low morale and poor job satisfaction lead to low participation in educational activities. Workplace culture is hard to change and often ingrained into the culture of the facility.
- Disruptive behavior (bullying) creates bad employee attitudes and needs to be redirected. Redirection may increase in-service participation, positivity, and a better learning environment.
- Learners forget what was taught and done during boring in-services. They get distracted easily. Use emotion because it is a strong memory stimulus and can be more effective than reading data.
- Large groups tend to be less engaging. Break a large group into smaller groups if possible because they are more productive.
- Some facilities have gone to online remote learning, which creates a challenge to keep the learner from being distracted in their surroundings.

References
1. Tuma F, Malgor R, Nassar A: Actions to enhance interactive learning in surgery, Ann Med Surg 64:102256, 2021.
2. Crowley-Barnett J, Pagano T, Kent M: Engaging perioperative learners using online game-based education, AORN J 112(5):447–456, 2020.
3. Venton J, Pompano R: Strategies for enhancing remote student engagement through active learning, Anal Bioanal Chem 413(6):1507–1512, 2021.

3. Computer database information systems are available in most facilities or through personal Internet access providers for researching topics of interest for self-study or for supplementing classroom presentations. Many web browsers are available, such as Internet Explorer, Microsoft Edge, Mozilla Firefox, Safari, Opera, and Google Chrome, for searching the Internet. Most search engines have an image-finding capability that allows students to associate the image when searching for a surgical procedure. Many prerecorded surgical procedures can be watched on various websites such as YouTube. Search engines such as Google are valuable tools for finding special-interest groups and professional medical associations. Most health-related organizations have a website full of information for professionals and patients. AORN Online can be accessed at www.aorn.org. AST has a website at www.ast.org that provides information about surgical technology. Terms associated with the Internet and computer can be found at http://evolve. elsevier.com/Hornacky/BerryKohn/.

4. Internet broadcasting in podcast format can be uploaded onto a smart device such as MP3 player, phone, watch, or speaker in audio or video format for remote viewing.

5. Netcasts and webinars are online broadcasts for use on smartphones, tablets, PCs, or Macs.

6. Many topics are available via computer programs or downloaded applications (apps). Apps can be downloaded to a device and an account can be set up with a credit card or other online pay service. Both Apple and Android offer apps for research.

7. *Really Simple Syndication* (RSS) feeds are subscription services that provide information via computer and cell phone in the form of email. RSS feeds use minimal data, so they work well with smartphones. A software RSS reader program is needed to receive and open RSS feeds. The readers are free on the Internet and are part of browser packages such as Firefox.

8. Specialty online news groups can be subscribed to through computerized email systems. Referred to as *Listserv*, these groups are communication tools for day-to-day discussions with others who have comparable interests. They are available as daily email entries or as a weekly digest. The specialty assemblies at aorn.org have membership blogs where members share ideas. The surgical technology website has educator and student blog sites to discuss topics of interest for surgical technologists.

9. Literature databases are found on select websites and in most libraries. Examples of online literature databases include but are not limited to the following:
   a. Cumulative Index to Nursing and Allied Health Literature (CINAHL) is a widely used index for nursing and allied health. The database includes indexing by subject headings from virtually all English-language nursing journals and allied health literature from January 1983 to current periodicals.
   b. Medical Literature Analysis and Retrieval System Online (MEDLINE) is a computer-based reference system available at most libraries in the United States and Canada. Many websites on the Internet offer free MEDLINE access. Biomedical journals, including nursing journals, are referenced. References dating from 1966 at the National Library of Medicine are found at www.nlm.nih.gov. PubMed is a government site that shares articles from MEDLINE and publisher websites; access can be found at www.pubmed.ncbi.nlm.nih.gov.
   c. Medscape (www.medscape.com) is a free article subscription service online. This site requires registration. The user selects an identification name and password. Many different educational topics, news, references, and specialty services are represented in print with continuing education credits.

The array of health-related educational materials is endless. The Internet, which is accessible 24 hours a day, has opened many channels of information throughout the world. Many websites can be accessed in a multilingual mode providing translation in most languages. Some websites offer full-text articles that can be downloaded or printed. Some of the articles are in .zip or .pdf format that requires WinZip or Adobe Acrobat Reader to open the file into a readable and/or printable document. WinZip and Acrobat Reader are free programs that can be downloaded and used repeatedly to open zipped or pdf files. These programs are frequently preloaded onto the hard drive of new computer models.

The advancement of computer technology has made computer equipment as small as a wristwatch and devices that easily fit in a pocket or backpack. The average household can now own multiple devices because of their affordability. Tablets and similar devices are good for reading. Multiple articles and documents can be stored on one device.

When researching scientific data on the Internet, it is advisable to review more than one website to support the accuracy of the information. Caution is advised regarding providing personal information such as credit card numbers over the Internet; security may be an issue.

Application of Theory to Practice

Learning is a process of discovery and mastery of skills. Performance-based learning to function competently in an area such as the perioperative environment should take place on three levels: cognitive, psychomotor, and affective. The learner should understand the scientific principles (cognitive learning) underlying the technical skills (psychomotor learning) and should appreciate the necessity of adhering to these principles (affective learning). In simpler terms, the learner should know why to do what (cognitive); how (psychomotor); and when, where, and by whom (affective). The learner should always have a rationale for each action. Learners and practicing perioperative caregivers should always know exactly why they are doing what they are doing—not just blindly perform tasks. This approach enables an intelligent modification of the plan of care in the event of an emergency or other untoward situation. In actual practice this knowledge may be critical for patient safety and attainment of favorable outcomes.

Practice will give learners an opportunity to apply their knowledge of the basic sciences. Theory becomes meaningful and valuable only when put to practical use. Some knowledge is gained through observation, but skills are learned through actual hands-on experience in applying the theory learned in the classroom, laboratory, or self-study.

In the perioperative environment the learner observes living anatomy; its alteration by congenital deformities, disease, or injury; and its restoration or reconstruction. Perioperative experience enables the learner to be a more understanding, observant, and efficient person. In close teamwork with surgeons and anesthesia providers, the nurse and the surgical technologist participate in vital resuscitative measures and learn to care for anesthetized, unconscious, and/or critically ill patients. Learning to function in life-threatening situations is critical to the patient's welfare. In addition, the learner discovers that emergencies such as cardiac arrest are easier to prevent than treat. By learning how theory applies to clinical practice, the student gains valuable experience that is applicable to any patient care situation. The learner should strive to attain the following objectives:

- Appreciate what surgical intervention means to each patient.
- Recognize the importance of optimal physical and psychologic preoperative patient preparation.
- Validate the need for constant patient observation intraoperatively.
- Determine the cause of postoperative pain and/or complications.
- Differentiate between seemingly innocuous occurrences and situations that, if left unrecognized and allowed to progress, lead to injury of the patient or a team member or damage to departmental equipment.
- Demonstrate proficiency in lifesaving techniques and equipment.
- Cope with all situations in a calm, efficient manner, and think clearly and act quickly in an emergency.
- Attend to every detail, observe keenly, and anticipate the needs of the patient and team members.
- Determine the importance of aseptic and sterile techniques, and comprehensively and conscientiously apply knowledge to practice.
- Expect the unexpected. Situations or conditions can change at a moment's notice. The student should use the "what if" philosophy for planning patient care. Thinking ahead and anticipating what to do "if" the patient becomes critical benefit the patient and the team by minimizing the element of surprise when unexpected events occur.

Above all, perioperative experience teaches that no surgical procedure is a minor event to the surgical patient! The only predictable element in the perioperative environment is the potential for an unpredictable occurrence. For practical use, hospitals may classify surgical procedures as major or minor; however, in reality no such distinction exists. Every procedure has a deep personal meaning for each patient and their family, and the possibility of an unfavorable outcome can never be completely excluded. All perioperative procedures carry an element of inherent risk. A relatively safe procedure can rapidly become catastrophic, even fatal, if the patient:

- Is unknowingly allergic or sensitive to a chemical, substance, medication, or anesthetic drug
- Develops uncontrollable bleeding
- Has seizures or blackouts
- Experiences cardiac arrest on the OR bed
- Goes into irreversible shock (cardiogenic, hematologic, hypovolemic, neurogenic, toxic, or vasogenic)
- Develops a metabolic event such as malignant hyperthermia, thyroid storm, hyperglycemia, or hypoglycemia

Although every precaution is taken to foresee and prevent adverse reactions, such reactions do occur on occasion. No matter how simple the procedure, an experienced, conscientious team member is always acutely aware of potential problems and always gives undivided attention to the patient and procedure.

During the learning experience the learner will participate in or observe the preparation of supplies and equipment and learn their intended use. With practical experience the learner will gain an appreciation for the precision of surgical instrumentation and equipment. The learner should understand which piece of equipment on the field gets plugged into a specific power source. Familiarity with the unit and settings is important for patient safety. The facility should provide in-service education for each type of machinery or equipment used in patient care.

In helping carry out a daily schedule of surgical procedures, the learner will become aware of the interdependence of the various departments within the facility and how they work together for the well-being of the patient. One of the most valuable learning experiences in the perioperative environment is the opportunity to see and become a part of real teamwork in action. Chapter 25 explores and explains the coordinated roles of the circulating nurse and the scrub person.

Expected Behaviors of Perioperative Caregivers

Regardless of their respective roles, all perioperative caregivers are expected to be competent and humane. A patient's sense of security is grounded in how the learner perceives the behavior of the team as a whole. This leaves a lasting impression that patients associate with their experiences in the perioperative environment. The behavior of the team reveals self-confidence (or diffidence), interest (or indifference), proficiency (or ineptitude), and authority (or indecision). In addition to possessing technical knowledge and skill, personnel should display appropriate personal attributes and communication skills that inspire confidence and trust in patients and other team members.

Personal Attributes

Personal attributes are manifest in the attitudes displayed by an individual while performing their duties. These inherent characteristics contribute to interrelatedness of the team and the outcome for the patient. Although these concepts are intrinsic to the individual and are certainly open to interpretation, the main premise remains focused on providing safe and efficient patient care through a team effort. Desirable personal attributes are listed in Table 1.3.

Communication

Communication is essential for exchanging information with another person. It is necessary for successful interpersonal relationships and serves to clarify actions. Communication is proactive when an idea or intent is relayed to another person and reactive when a response is received. Communication has taken place when the receiver interprets the message in the manner intended by the sender. Communication is effective only when the patient and caregivers understand one another. A key element is to demonstrate appropriate body language to match the spoken word.

Teamwork

A team is a group of two or more people who recognize common goals and coordinate their efforts to achieve them. Broadly defined, the health care team includes all personnel relating to the patient—those in direct patient contact and those in other departments whose services are essential and contribute indirectly to patient care. Interdependence characterizes a team—without the other members, the goals cannot be met.

TABLE 1.3 Attributes Expected in a Perioperative Caregiver

Desirable Attribute	Measurable Behaviors
Empathy	Develop a sense of what the patient is feeling
Conscientiousness	No compromise in quality of care
Efficiency	Organized and properly prepared; time is not wasted duplicating steps
Sensitivity	Genuine caring and perceptiveness for the patient and the team
Open-mindedness	Accepting of the ideas of others
Flexible and adaptable	Able to cope with changes in routine
Supportive	Nonjudgmental and sincere approach to relationships
Communicative	Exchanges information in a professional manner
Listening	Accepts and receives information in a professional manner
Even-temperedness	Hostility and anger have no place in the perioperative environment
Versatility	Knowledgeable and can troubleshoot
Analytic	Knowing how and why for each task
Creativity	Able to innovate solutions
Sense of humor	Eases tension at appropriate times
Manual dexterity	Good hand-eye coordination
Stamina	Capable of standing for prolonged periods
Good hygiene	Body odors cause discomfort for the team
Ethics	Strong sense of truth, honor, and goodness
Curiosity	Desire to know and learn new things
Observant	Listens, watches, and reacts quickly to changes

The team approach to patient care should be a coordinated effort that is performed with the cooperation of all caregivers. Team members should communicate and should have a shared division of duties to perform specified tasks as a unified body. The failure of any one member to perform their role can have a serious effect on the success of the entire team. Performing as a team requires that each member exert an effort to attain the common goals competently and safely. The actions of each team member are important. No one individual can accomplish the goal without the cooperation of the rest of the team.

Pride in professional work, and in the team as a whole, leads to personal satisfaction. High morale is facilitated by adequate staff orientation, hands-on training, and staff participation in departmental decision-making and problem-solving. The receipt of deserved praise, opportunity for continuing education, and motivation creates an environment to practice at the highest potential.

The common goal of the perioperative team is the effective delivery of care in a safe, efficient, and timely manner. To function efficiently, team members must communicate effectively. Problems such as a break in aseptic or sterile technique must be identified and corrective actions taken. To fulfill expectations, team members must be aware of each other's needs for information. Efforts of other support services, such as radiology,

pathology, intensive care unit (ICU), or postanesthesia unit (PACU), are coordinated with the needs of the patient and the surgeon.

Mutual respect is the foundation of teamwork. It is also a right. Respect is shown through collaboration, cooperation, and truthful communication. Verbal abuse, bullying, violence, disruptive behavior, and harassment are out of place in the professional environment. Behavior that inhibits the performance of team members or threatens patient safety should be factually documented and reported to superiors in the chain of command. The Joint Commission (TJC) requires accredited facilities to establish leadership standards that address disruptive and inappropriate behaviors as follows:

1. Defines a code of conduct to distinguish between acceptable and inappropriate behaviors in interpersonal relationships in the perioperative environment
2. Creates and implements a process for managing behaviors that undermine a culture of safety in the perioperative environment

Teamwork requires the commitment and effort of team members to increase productivity, ensure quality performance, and participate in problem-solving by communicating and cooperating with one another. A team approach is necessary for patient-centered care. Surgeons, assistants, anesthesia providers, patient care staff, and staff of supporting services should coordinate their efforts. Each discipline contributes to successful outcomes of surgical intervention by working together as a team. The following factors contribute to these successful outcomes:

1. Interdepartmental communication is important for cooperation, consideration, and efficient collaboration.
    a. Personnel on patient care divisions and physicians share pertinent information concerning patients. Accurate and complete collected data are documented, thereby protecting the patient, the patient care personnel, and the facility.
    b. Personnel work together in a congenial atmosphere with respect and appreciation for each other's unique skills and contributions. Team members benefit from the expertise of each other. Teamwork is at its finest in the perioperative environment.
    c. Personnel are considerate of each other and the patient.
    • The surgeon should inform the team of any anticipated potential deviation from their regular routine for the scheduled procedure. An advance notice of changes can help avoid delays in obtaining needed equipment.
    • Staff must check all equipment and implants for correct sizes and availability before a surgical procedure. Missing items should be reported to the surgeon and manager.
    • The perioperative team promotes a quiet atmosphere to ensure the surgeon's uninterrupted concentration. Interruptions during the procedure can cause the team to lose concentration and jeopardize the safety of the patient or team members.
    • The anesthesia provider and circulating nurse assist each other with certain procedures such as medication administration and intubation.
2. Adequate preparation and familiarity with the surgeon's preferences and the surgical procedure to be performed are fundamental to teamwork. If the perioperative staff members are unfamiliar with the routine and equipment, the patient or a team member may be at risk for injury. An adequately experienced and skilled team is essential for the effective performance of a safe, efficient procedure.

3. The patient has an unconditional right to the team's complete concentration and attention at all times. The patient is a unique individual who is completely dependent on the perioperative caregivers to work as a team.

Although the ideologic differences of personnel may at times be a source of conflict, the care of the patient should be a priority over personality differences. Complex procedures, busy surgery schedules, or shortages of personnel should not interfere with the delivery of efficient, individualized patient care.

Clinical Competence

Based on experience and performance, patient care personnel can be categorized as novice, competent, proficient, or expert. The novice lacks experience but is expected to perform to the best of their ability with assistance. Most employers provide a formal orientation program for new patient care personnel. During this orientation period, the necessary knowledge, skills, and abilities should be developed to perform at a level of basic competency. As experience is gained, proficiency expands from a minimal competency to an advanced level of expertise. Competent practice requires critical thinking skills and decision-making ability. Statements of clinical competency are established by professional organizations such as AORN and AST. Guidelines are published by each professional organization and made available to practitioners of all disciplines. Competencies are discussed in more detail in Chapter 2.

Realities of Clinical Practice

When a formal educational experience is completed, a learner or orientee is eager to apply their skills and knowledge in an employment setting. A transition from dependent learner to independent practitioner evolves over time. The realities of the work environment and the emotional and ethical dilemmas of some situations are experienced as basic competencies are developed. The development of surgical conscience evolves as experience is gained. Surgical conscience applies the standards of care to ethical situations and makes decision-making more concrete.

It can take 6 months to 1 year to feel confident as a functioning perioperative team member. Many facilities require personnel to take calls for emergencies after business hours; therefore the staff must be competent to fulfill this requirement independent of a preceptor.

Reality Shock

Reality is a sense of actuality, a feeling that this is what the real world is all about. Reality shock sets in as the transition takes place from being a beginning learner to becoming an employed graduate professional nurse or surgical technologist. The familiar educator and peer learners are not always present to give counsel, advice, and moral support. As professional caregivers attempt to adapt to new demands, they need to remember the following:
- Learning does not end with basic education. It is an ongoing process throughout an entire professional career.
- Teaching at various levels is the responsibility of the entire team. New information is developed and shared by the group for the improvement of patient care practices.

- All caregivers were once novices (although some may have forgotten those novice days). They have experienced the feelings and frustrations of being the newest staff member. The experienced caregiver should try to remember these feelings and offer encouragement and guidance to new personnel.
- Patience is an asset while developing work habits and establishing working relationships. Expectations of self and of others should be realistic. Feelings of excitement and anticipation and the fear of failure or making mistakes are normal but should be expressed appropriately. Disruptive behavior distracts the attention of the team from the patient.
- Applying the principles and techniques already learned will enable the caregiver to make sound judgments and appropriate decisions in the perioperative environment.
- It is important to ask questions and acknowledge not knowing how to do something. Seeking help promotes professional growth and reinforces patient safety.

Everyone wants and needs to become an accepted member of both social and work groups. The entire perioperative team, including the surgeon and anesthesia provider, is both a social group and a work group. Ambivalent feelings may arise on entering these groups. The pleasures of functioning as a team member may be offset by uncertainty about the ability to perform well. Initial goals will be task- and skill-oriented as learning focuses on policies, procedures, and routines. Eventually insecurity will be replaced with self-confidence. The display of confidence will increase trust, respect, and recognition from others, as well as the personal satisfaction of accomplishment.

Dynamics of the Psychologic Climate: Preceptors, Mentors, and Role Models

Learning to adapt to the variety of tasks and ever-changing demands in the perioperative environment is difficult. Some anxiety is normal, especially in situations in which feelings of insecurity are generated or a sense of intimidation pervades the environment. At times the demands of the job may seem to outweigh the personal resources of the caregiver. Confidence develops as skills are learned.

An understanding of expected performance is perhaps the most important element in the transition from novice to independent practitioner. Personnel in the perioperative environment play vital roles in the beginner's development. There is a distinction among the roles of preceptor, mentor, and role model. A preceptor works with orientees and learners according to a prescribed task-oriented lesson plan. The process offers minimal flexibility and little personalization for individual needs. Some facilities offer a preceptor program such as the AORN Preceptor Certificate Program. The program defines the preceptor role and the role of the student and objectives.[5]

A mentor has more experience with the personnel and the climate of the OR and can provide insight into the social atmosphere of the department. A mentor develops a relatively personalized relationship with less experienced orientees or learners and fosters a sense of nurturance for their growth and assimilation into the department. A beginner should look for a mentor to help bridge the gap between novice and proficient levels.

Beginners should also look for role models—those experienced staff members who are emulated and respected for their clinical competence—and pattern their emerging professional self after the behaviors of the role model. A personal relationship may not evolve with a role model in the same way as with a mentor.

The beginner should stick with those staff members who are reaping personal rewards and self-satisfaction from their work ethic. Their enthusiasm will be contagious and start the growth of an exciting career. Staff members who have negative attitudes, complain, and do not try to solve problems but instead create them should be avoided.

Eustress Versus Distress

Physical and emotional stresses are part of daily life. Stress is the nonspecific reaction of the body, physiologically and/or psychologically, to any demand. The demand may be pleasant or unpleasant, conscious or unconscious. The intensity of the stressor will dictate adaptation. An individual's perception of a situation will influence the reaction to it.

Stress is not only an essential part of life but also a useful stimulant. Positive stress, referred to as *eustress,* motivates an individual to be productive and efficient. It forces adaptation to the ever-present changes in the perioperative environment. The response should be quick (e.g., when a trauma victim arrives or a patient has a cardiac arrest). To expect the unexpected is part of perioperative patient care. Eustress fosters a sense of achievement, satisfaction, and self-confidence.

Stress that becomes overwhelming and uncomfortable is referred to as *distress.* In the perioperative environment the behavior of others may be perceived as cause for distress. Policies, or a lack of them, can also be a source of distress if they conflict with the caregiver's expectations. Through adaptive mechanisms, the caregiver can cope with the tensions, conflicts, and demands of the perioperative environment in either a collaborative or a nonproductive manner. Even though perceived as distress, some conflict is necessary to stimulate a change in work methods and solve organizational problems. Sometimes it takes dissatisfaction with a situation to spark positive change and prevent stagnation.

Patient care personnel become distressed by the conduct of other team members. For example, it is uncomfortable to be harshly criticized by a surgeon in front of peers or patients. However, much that is said is not personally directed. Often the surgeon is reacting to distress regarding unanticipated circumstances presented by the patient, team member, or equipment during the surgical procedure. The reactions of personnel will be influenced by their attitudes, mood, cultural and religious background, values and ethics, experiences, and concerns of the moment. Outbursts of anger are never appropriate in the OR. However, constant frustration and inner conflict create the distresses that can lead to job dissatisfaction. Behaviors that place patients or personnel at risk, such as throwing objects, should be reported to the nurse manager and documented. Many facilities have developed a zero-tolerance policy for abusive behavior in the OR.

Stress Reduction

Assertive behavior is a useful tool for conflict resolution. Shared professional communication can keep the tension in the environment at a minimum. The caregiver should keep their composure at all times and maintain a professional and assertive (not aggressive) attitude. Personal conflicts between team members should be dealt with privately.

Humor can be an effective method of reducing anxiety. It should be used appropriately to defuse tension. Laughing at oneself helps preserve self-esteem while learning from the experience.

At the end of the work shift the caregiver should evaluate the events of the day, the emotions evoked, and how they were handled. What was done effectively? What coping skills may be needed to improve or enhance positive attitudes and interpersonal relationships in the work environment? Teamwork is essential in the perioperative environment, with every team member obligated to make a positive contribution.

Stress is a reality that need not create a sense of self-defeat. Regardless of the source of stress, the body responds, and the physiologic and psychologic effects can be subtle or intense. The determination of whether a stressor is good or bad depends on an individual's perception of the circumstances. Any event that creates a feeling of impending danger also creates the perception of loss of control. A major factor in stress management is maintaining control, which can be accomplished by learning to tune in to the balance between the body and the mind. The caregiver can learn to be prepared for life's difficulties by understanding how the perception of stress can affect decision-making, self-expression, and subsistence in the world.

Listening to the Body

The caregiver should develop a sense for how the body signals exhaustion, hunger, illness, and/or physical pain. The body is a sensory barometer of the environmental effects on the caregiver, and ignoring physical signals decreases the ability of the body to manage stress. Going without sleep or skipping meals creates physical stress that can be avoided. Sleep deprivation caused by long hours on call can be as dangerous as overuse of alcohol or using illegal drugs. The biologic need for sleep cannot be denied and is important for the health and safety of the individual and the others in the environment. Decision-making, reaction times, memory, and generalized health are impaired by not getting enough rest. Regular sleep of at least 6 hours per day and rest periods, exercise, adequate dietary practices, and routine health checkups provide a sound basis for care of the body. Managers should schedule regular employee breaks when possible to maintain healthy staff.

Maintaining the Mind

Mental relaxation can help the caregiver manage stress. Using meditation and mental imagery on a regular basis provides a break from stressful routines and allows the mind to fortify itself against the negative perceptions of a situation. Creating time to clear confusing thoughts and align productive thinking enables the body and the mind to support an emotional balance and a sense of well-being. This positive interaction can become an influence in a stressful situation and serve as an example to coworkers. Many facilities offer counseling for emotional stress related to trauma or death of patients.

Ⓔ EVOLVE WEBSITE

http://evolve.elsevier.com/Hornacky/BerryKohn/

- Historical Perspective
- Glossary

References

1. Wiggy Z: Educational opportunities, *AORN J* 116(4):374–378, 2022.
2. Sadiku M, Ashaolu T, Musa S: Naturalistic intelligence, *Int J Sci Adv* 1(1), 2020.
3. Croke L: Prevention and management of workplace violence, *AORN J* 116(2):P5–P7, 2022.
4. Carmack A, Valleru J: Empowering perioperative team members to speak up, *AORN J* 116(4):351–355, 2022.
5. Zekveld K: Perioperative nurse recruitment: an OR placement program for fourth-year nursing students in Ontario, *AORN J* 116(2):133–142, 2022.

2

Foundations of Perioperative Patient Care Standards

CHAPTER OUTLINE

Surgical Conscience, 17

Patient Rights, 17

Accountability, 17

Standardization of Patient Care, 18

Recommended Practices, 21

Professionalism, 26

Professional Perioperative Nursing, 27

Evidence-Based Practice, 27

Nursing Process, 28

Standards of Perioperative Nursing Practice, 30

Clinical Competency of the Perioperative Nurse, 33

Scope of Perioperative Nursing Practice, 34

Surgical Technology, 34

Clinical Competency of the Surgical Technologist, 35

Continual Performance Evaluation and Improvement, 35

CHAPTER OBJECTIVES

After studying this chapter the learner will be able to:

- Discuss how standardization influences patient care.
- Describe two professional sources of patient care standards.
- List three main aspects of accountability.
- Identify the components of the nursing process.

KEY TERMS AND DEFINITIONS

Accountability Answering for performance of a service or task.

Accreditation Method of professional evaluation and recognition of an institution for meeting educational, practice, and national standard parameters.

Advocacy Active support of another person.

Benchmark Point of reference that sets the evaluation point of activities.

Competency statement Document based on empirical data that define expected and measurable clinical activities.

Domain Set of knowledge that is specific and clearly identified.

Element Smallest unit of data that is known and can be described and measured.

Guidance statement Document based on empirical data that suggests processes for performance of clinical activities.

Guideline Document or concept based on empirical data that guides clinical activities.

Licensure Approval for practice granted by a governmental agency for a predetermined period, after which the approval process is repeated.

Nomenclature Specialized set of terms.

Nursing diagnosis Identification of patient problem, need, or health consideration, which may be actual or at risk; based on human response patterns according to NANDA International.

Nursing process Organizational framework for planning patient care; this involves assessment, nursing diagnosis, planning, implementation, and evaluation of the plan.

Obligation Duty or promise.

Outcome Effect of an intervention.

PNDS Perioperative nursing data set. Standardized perioperative nursing language.

Position statement Document that describes a particular belief.

Profession Vocation in a specialty requiring specialized education and knowledge.

Recommended practice Activities believed to be the optimal level of professional practice that are achievable.

Responsibility Social, moral, or legal duty.

Rights Power or possession of privilege.

Standard Authoritative statement that describes accountability, values, and priorities.

Taxonomy Orderly classification based on interrelationships.

This chapter establishes the basis for perioperative patient care. The opening section gives a glimpse of historic patient care and progresses to modern perioperative practice.

Surgical Conscience

The essential elements of perioperative practice are caring, conscience, discipline, and technique. Optimal patient care requires an inherent surgical conscience, selflessness, self-discipline, and the application of principles of asepsis and sterile technique. All are inseparably related.

Florence Nightingale is credited with developing the environmental theory of patient care on which all perioperative patient care is based (Box 2.1). According to her theory, the caregiver is accountable for creating and maintaining the best possible environmental conditions to assist natural healing. She emphasized the need for prevention through education and teamwork. In her eyes the team consisted of not only the caregivers but also the patient and family. She often approached her legislators with suggestions for bills and laws designed to protect patients and caregivers. Her numerous letters and writings chronicle her work.

The concept of a surgical conscience is simply a surgical Golden Rule: *Do unto the patient as you would have others do unto you* (Box 2.2). The caregiver should consider each patient as the self or as a loved one. Once an individual develops a surgical conscience, it remains inherent thereafter. Nightingale summarized what is, in essence, its meaning, when she said, "The nurse should keep a high sense of duty in her own mind, must aim at perfection in her care, and must be consistent always in herself."

Patient Rights

As a consumer, the patient may purchase insurance or services to fulfill health care needs and is entitled to certain rights. Access to

---

•BOX 2.1 Nightingale's Environmental Theory

Physical Environment
- Sanitation
- Ventilation
- Lighting
- Noise
- Odors
- Temperature

Psychologic Environment
- Communication
- Advice
- Variety

- Scientific knowledge base
- Creativity
- Spirituality

Social Environment
- Mortality data
- Prevention of disease
- Education of caregiver
- Nursing as distinct from medicine
- Accountability
- Responsibility

•BOX 2.2 Elements of Surgical Conscience

- A sense of moral obligation and responsibility
- Self-regulation and control
- Honesty and integrity in professional practice
- Personal commitment
- Ethical value system
- Admit and remedy errors
- Sincere desire to do the right thing

---

health care is recognized as a right, not a privilege, of every human. Individuals who do not have the means to purchase insurance have the right to all necessary treatments in emergency situations.

Patient Advocacy

In advocacy, a patient advocate recognizes the patient's, the family's, and significant others' need for information and assistance in coping with the surgical experience, regardless of the setting. As an advocate, the perioperative nurse can provide information discovered during patient assessment that identifies specific needs or health concerns requiring action. Advance preparation can help the patient, family, or significant others anticipate events. Assistance in coping acknowledges the anxieties and fears, regardless of how minimally invasive the procedure may seem. No procedure is minor to the patient! Each patient reacts differently. The patient senses some relief in knowing that the caregiver has taken the time to identify specific needs and provide individualized care. The patient advocate is a caregiver who acts in the following ways:

1. Establishes rapport with the patient, family, or significant others in a manner that conveys genuine concern and sincere caring
2. Encourages the patient, family, and significant others to express feelings and ask questions
3. Helps relieve anxiety and apprehension by providing appropriate information regarding what to expect
4. Helps the patient make informed decisions throughout the perioperative experience
5. Acts as a patient representative by communicating pertinent information to other team members
6. Oversees all activities throughout the perioperative experience to ensure the safety and welfare of the patient
7. Keeps the family or significant others informed of events throughout the perioperative experience
8. Protects the patient's rights by compliance with advance directives for care (living will, durable power of attorney, or both). Additional information about advance directives and durable power of attorney can be found in Chapter 3.

Accountability

Accountability means answering to someone for an obligatory action. As both learners and caregivers, perioperative nurses and surgical technologists are accountable to the following people and entities:
- Patients receiving services
- Employer
- Educational institution providing learning experiences
- Profession or vocation to uphold established standards of practice
- Self and other team members

A lack of accountability for behavior in the perioperative environment may result in patient injury or dissatisfaction with care. Health care providers have a legal and moral obligation to identify and correct situations that threaten a patient's safety and well-being. Most incidents that endanger the patient are preventable and could lead to unnecessary legal action. Prevention focuses on the responsible performance of duty and continual performance improvement. The provision of safe care of the patient also protects caregivers and the health care facility from liability. In addition, it upholds the reputation of the professions by maintaining the confidence of the individual consumer and public. Failure of a caregiver to maintain accountability constitutes negligence. If negligence is established, any caregiver can be held liable for acts of omission or commission. Each person is responsible for individual actions leading to neglect.

Standardization of Patient Care

Importance of Standardization

Perioperative patient care personnel should be able to cope with all situations and give patients the best of their skills and knowledge. Although the use of different techniques may achieve the same results, each hospital establishes policies and procedures for all personnel to follow based on standards, recommended practices, and guidelines developed by professional organizations and predicated on scientific research and evidence-based practice. These written policies, procedures, and guidelines help prevent confusion and foster coordination of activities. Deviations from standardization can cause confusion and result in patient or caregiver harm. The guidelines, or guidance statements, are intended to demonstrate a way to incorporate recommended practices in everyday patient care. Uniformity and standardization of procedures help personnel develop skill and efficiency for the following reasons:

- The main purpose is to ensure the safety and welfare of the patient and personnel.
- It is easier for the perioperative educator and preceptors to teach learners consistent methods of patient care.
- Learning is easier if everyone performs procedures in the same way.
- Deviations show a need for evaluation of the procedures or the staff. Do the procedures need revision?
- Consistent procedures provide an efficient check during preparation for any surgical procedure.
- One person can take over for another at any time during the surgical procedure, if necessary, and know exactly where to find instruments and supplies.
- Routine procedures establish habits that increase speed in thought and action. Doing work in a certain way promotes a high level of proficiency.
- Knowing the standards allows intelligent decision-making when a patient's condition requires modification of a routine.

Professional Sources of Standards

Standards of care are defined as those acts that a reasonably prudent person with comparable training and experience would perform under the same or similar circumstances. Professional standards delineate activities related to performance, performance improvement, continuing education, ethical behavior, responsibility, and accountability.

Standards established by regulatory agencies are governed by laws. Standards established by professional associations are voluntary. Standards of practice for perioperative patient care include professional and regulated standards. Several sources of perioperative patient care standards are identified in the following list:

1. Standards of Perioperative Nursing. These standards, which originated as American Nurses Association (ANA) standards of OR practice in 1975, were approved by ANA and AORN (Association of periOperative Registered Nurses) and originally published in 1981. Reviews and revisions are done annually as needed.

   Sets of standards for an optimal level of perioperative nursing practice are published annually in the *AORN Guidelines for Perioperative Practice*. The scaffold of the standards is premised in patient care quality and is primarily trifold—Structure, Process, and Outcome. These three components provide a means for the perioperative nurse to analyze and interpret care. Reviews and revisions are done yearly as needed.

   a. *Standards of Perioperative Administrative Nursing Practice.* These structural standards provide a framework for establishing administrative and organizational practices in a variety of settings.

   b. *Standards of Perioperative Clinical Practice.* These process standards are based on problem-solving techniques using principles and theories of biophysical and behavioral sciences. They describe how the nursing process is used in the perioperative setting. The Perioperative Nursing Data Set (PNDS) provides a means to measure and collect performance improvement data using standardized language.

   c. *Standards of Perioperative Professional Practice.* These process standards describe a competent level of behavior for the professional role of the perioperative nurse. The activities relate to quality practice evaluation, continuing education, collegial relations, collaboration, ethical conduct, and use of resources, evidence-based research, and leadership.

   d. *Quality and Performance Improvement Standards for Perioperative Nursing.* These process standards to assist in the development of methods to measure, assess, and improve patient care.

   e. *Perioperative Patient Outcomes: Standards of Perioperative Care.* These outcome standards reflect desired observable patient outcomes during preoperative, intraoperative, and postoperative phases of patient care. They focus on the patient's, the family's, and significant others' responses to intervention during surgical, diagnostic, or therapeutic intervention. Each outcome has a unique identifier in the PNDS.

2. The Operating Room Nurses Association of Canada (ORNAC, www.ornac.ca) has published the ORNAC Standards, Guidelines, and Position Statements for Perioperative Registered Nurses.

3. Association of Surgical Technologists (AST) Standards of Practice (www.ast.org). These process standards provide guidelines for safe and effective patient care in appropriate preoperative, intraoperative, and postoperative practice settings. They include knowledge, interpersonal skills, environmental safety, and application of principles of surgical technology.

4. The Joint Commission (TJC) standards (www.jointcommission.org). These standards, published in the Accreditation Manual for Hospitals, are functional, performance-based standards that focus on actual clinical care provided directly to patients and on management of the health care organization providing services. They relate to efficiency, effectiveness, safety, and timeliness; appropriateness, trust, lifelong learning, continuity, and availability of care; and patient satisfaction.

a. TJC evaluates compliance with these standards and reviews clinical outcomes of care provided as fundamental criteria for accreditation. Selective clinical indicators serve as outcome measurements for the processes of patient care.

TJC has expanded its accreditation for many health care settings such as surgery centers, doctor's offices, nursing homes, assisted living, behavioral health, and other facilities that care for patients. Information for specific facilities can be found at Joint Commission Resources (www.jcrinc.com). Additional information about error reporting and monitoring of patient care standards is found in Chapter 3.

- TJC established National Patient Safety Goals: The goals are updated as needed. Some of the 2024 goals include:
  - Improve the accuracy of patient identification by using at least two forms of patient identification. Be aware of patient-preferred gendered pronouns (he, she, them, they) to minimize confusion when identifying the patient. Biologic sex may differ from preferred gender identity.
  - Improve the effectiveness between caregivers by using standardized patient "handover" or "handoff" reporting (change from one caregiver to another), verbal reflection, avoiding abbreviations and symbols, and ensuring timely communications.
  - Improve the safety of using medications by identifying potential "sound-alike" or "look-alike" drugs in the facility, labeling all drug containers and delivery devices on and off the field, and decreasing the risk of anticoagulation error.
  - Improve patient specimen identification handling and processing.
  - Reduce the risk for health care–associated infections by meticulous hand hygiene and by recording and reporting as a sentinel event any unanticipated death or loss of function associated with sepsis or health care–acquired infection.
  - Accurately and completely reconcile medications across the continuum of care by comparing patient current medication regimen with medication orders during care in the facility. Patient and subsequent caregivers in and out of the facility are provided a complete list of current medications on discharge.
  - Reduce the patient's risk for harm from falls by implementing a program of safe patient positioning and transport in the OR. Fall prevention programs should have an evaluation process.
  - Encourage the patient's participation in the safe delivery of care by defining and communicating the steps of care and encouraging the patient, family, and significant others to ask questions and voice concerns for safe care.
  - Identification of potential safety risks in the patient population relevant to patients with emotional or behavioral disorders by prevention of self-harm or suicide.
  - Improve recognition and response to changes in the patient's condition by ongoing assessment and immediate access to specially trained individuals when a patient's condition has changed.
5. National Fire Protection Association (NFPA) standards (www.nfpa.org). NFPA 99 includes the codes and standards for health care facilities. These standards apply to environmental safety to reduce, to the extent possible, hazards to patients, personnel, and visitors.

6. Association for the Advancement of Medical Instrumentation (AAMI) device standards (www.aami.org). These standards provide the industry with reference documents on accepted levels of device safety and performance and test methods to determine conformance. AAMI standards also have been established for processing, sterilization, electrical safety, and patient monitoring for health care providers in relation to evaluation, maintenance, and use of medical devices and instrumentation.

7. Clinically based risk-control standards. These standards are written by medical specialty groups and professional liability underwriters. They establish appropriate benchmarks of acceptable practices and outcomes specifically for controlling liability losses. Benchmarking is used for quality improvement leading to better patient outcomes. Benchmarks may be incorporated into the health care facility's risk management program.

Standards From Regulatory Bodies

The standards set by these organizations are enforceable by law, as follows:

1. Federal Medicare Act and all subsequent amendments to this Social Security Act (www.cms.gov). This legislation incorporates the provision that institutions participating in Medicare must maintain the level of patient care recognized as the norm. Specific requirements are included.

a. Health Insurance Portability and Accountability Act (HIPAA) (www.cms.gov). The Department of Health and Human Services (HHS) set national standards for electronic health care transactions and national identifiers for providers, health plans, and employers. It also addresses the security and privacy of health data. Many facilities require their employees to sign a confidentiality agreement upon hire. Schools of nursing and surgical technology, clinical sites, and patient care training sites require students to sign confidentiality agreements. Some schools prohibit tape recording in class because of patient and facility confidentiality issues.

b. Medicare's "No Pay List." Accuracy of documentation of conditions present on admission as differentiated from conditions acquired during hospitalization determines facility reimbursement for patient care. Claims for payment that have no documentation about conditions "present on admission" are immediately rejected without reimbursement. More information can be found at (www.cms.gov). As of October 2008, the Centers for Medicare & Medicaid Services (CMS) decided not to reimburse facilities for acquired conditions. As of 2024, CMS will not reimburse the facility for the following conditions:
   1) Pressure ulcers (stages III and IV)
   2) Falls or trauma
   3) Vascular catheter–associated infection
   4) Retained foreign objects from surgery
   5) Certain surgical site infections (mediastinitis after cardiac surgery, bariatric gastrointestinal procedure, and orthopedic procedures of spine, neck, shoulder, or elbow)
   6) Air embolus
   7) Blood incompatibility
   8) Uncontrolled blood sugar

9) Deep vein thrombosis (DVT) and pulmonary embolus (PE) after knee or hip joint arthroplasty
10) Urinary catheter—associated infection
11) Wrong site surgery
12) Wrong patient surgery
13) Wrong surgery performed on a patient
14) Iatrogenic pneumothorax, venous catheterization

  c. National Quality Forum (NQF) is an organization that measures health care quality through public reporting and measures health care evidence-based practices to promote quality health care. Serious reportable events mirror the CMS "No Pay List," and the updated serious reportable events document can be viewed online at www.qualityforum.org.

The NFQ document details include, but are not limited to, the following events:

a) Surgical events such as wrong site or wrong patient surgery
b) Deaths associated with devices, radiation emittance, or biologic materials (equipment and medication contamination)
c) Patient protection event such as patient suicide
d) Care management event such as wrong drug or blood administration
e) Environmental event such as electrocution or falls
f) Criminal event such as assault or abduction

2. American National Standards Institute (ANSI) standards (www.ansi.org). These standards concern exposures to toxic materials and safe use of equipment such as lasers. ANSI works with both private and public companies to set technology standards to promote uniform safe practices.

3. U.S. Food and Drug Administration (FDA) performance standards (www.fda.gov). Federal Medical Device Amendments regulate the manufacture, labeling, sale, and use of implantable medical devices and many products used in or on patients. The FDA also controls treatment protocols for use of drugs and regulates the reprocessing of medical instrumentation. The manufacturer's lot number and product description of implanted devices are required documentation in the patient's chart.

4. Agency for Healthcare Research and Quality (AHRQ) clinical practice guidelines (www.ahrq.gov). These standards include indicators for performance measurement. They are based on research and professional judgment regarding effectiveness and appropriateness of medical care, including fairness, affordability, safety, efficacy, and effectiveness of technology. This agency was created in provisions of the Consolidated Omnibus Budget Reconciliation Act of 1989.

5. Occupational Safety and Health Administration (OSHA) standards (www.osha.gov). These legally enforceable standards cover public and private industry and include permissible levels of toxic substances in the environment. Although explicitly developed to protect employees by providing safe and healthy working conditions, patients receive secondary benefits from control of hazards in the environment.

Sources of Standardization Data Within the Health Care Facility

Each patient care facility uses multiple sources from which to derive standardization data. Efficient use of time and resources is the end result. Establishing protocols and performance expectations that are specific to the needs of the facility benefits the patient, the caregiver, and the facility. Many of the following documents may be found on the facility's intranet for employee use.

1. *Facility-specific patient care standards.* The patient care services department establishes standards for appropriate patient care based on the standards developed by the ANA. Optimal standards of nursing practice guide the provision of patient care throughout the institution. Written policies and procedures reflect these standards. Institutional standards are based on standards established at national levels by TJC, AORN, ANA, and other nursing organizations and governmental agencies.

  a. Nurses should work within the limitations of the nurse practice act of the state in which they are licensed and practice. The enhanced Nursing Licensure Compact (eNLC) issues multistate nursing licenses for states that pass legislation. As of 2023, more than 42 states are part of eNLC. Licensure is a legal requirement to practice nursing. Copies of facility-specific documents are available for review from the nursing or hospital administration.

2. *Hospital policy and procedure manual.* This manual contains basic and general administrative and patient care policies that apply to all hospital personnel. A copy is retained on each patient care unit and in all departments of the hospital.

3. *Safety plan manual.* The potential hazards and identifiable situations that may cause injury to a caregiver or patient are described in the manual provided by the hospital safety committee. Plans for fire or disaster drills and evacuation routes are outlined.

4. *Safety data sheets (SDS).* Formerly known as material safety data sheets (MSDS). These detailed sheets describe chemicals used in the workplace and actions to take if they are spilled into the environment. Specific cleanup and disposal methods are outlined. Most facilities require a yearly review of the SDS process and where to locate the information quickly. Individual SDS for specific chemicals are online at www.msds.com.

5. *Disaster plan manual.* This manual outlines the plans for both internal and external disasters. Both internal and external disasters require rapid activation of all services within the hospital. Personnel who are off duty will be called to the facility and assigned as needed. Command centers and communications will be critical stations for the entire facility to follow and respond. Triage protocol will be followed carefully as defined by the facility.

  a. An internal disaster is an event that happens within the facility (e.g., an explosion, a fire) and requires employee assistance for control of the situation and evacuation of personnel and patients. An evacuation plan should be part of this planning structure because in-process surgeries cannot be abruptly halted and simply carried out of the building.

  b. An external disaster is an event that happens outside the confines of the facility (e.g., the World Trade Center terrorist actions of September 11, 2001, or an active shooter at a public venue). An external disaster could also be a natural phenomenon such as an earthquake or an accident (e.g., a train derailment).

c. A combined internal-external disaster such as Hurricane Katrina is complex and may have multiple stages of resolution. Extremes of patient casualties may be brought in only to find the facility is to capacity in census. In some circumstances the facility may be out of communication with surrounding communities because of power failure or flooding and cannot easily reroute patients to a safe receiving hospital.

6. *Infection control manual.* This manual contains the policies and procedures designed to minimize the risk for infection and control the spread of disease within the health care facility. It includes state, local, federal, and professional standards for the protection of the patient and the caregiver.

7. *Perioperative policy and procedure manual.* This manual contains the policies pertaining solely to the administration and operation of the perioperative environment or online in the hospital's intranet. A copy is accessible for reference in the manager's office, at the control desk, or in both places. The primary purpose of the perioperative policy and procedure manual is to detail why and how procedures should be specifically performed within the perioperative environment. It includes both supportive activities and practices that involve direct perioperative patient care.

8. *Orientation manual.* This manual is designed to acquaint personnel with the environment, policies, and procedures specific to performance and the position descriptions of all personnel in the department.

9. *Instrument book.* The individual instruments and trays required for each surgical procedure are listed in a central processing computer or in a separate book kept in the instrument processing area. Photographs or catalog illustrations help instrumentation personnel identify the vast number of instruments and how they are compiled into sets. Flashcards and educational instrument textbooks are commercially available. A search engine with an image finder (e.g., Google, Bing, or Yahoo) may be used to find specific instruments. Most instrument companies have online catalogs.

10. *Surgeon's preference cards/case cart sheet.* A preference card is maintained in a computerized database or written note card for each surgical procedure that each surgeon performs. The surgeon's specific preferences and any variance from the procedures are listed on these cards or sheet. Revisions are made as procedures and personal preferences or new technology change. A set of these cards is kept readily available in a central file or in a computer under the surgeon's name, and they are pulled for each day's surgical procedures. In preparing for each surgical procedure, nurses and surgical technologists consult both these cards and the procedure book. A surgical central supply department may use these cards to pack a case cart for each individual procedure. Box 2.3 shows sample case cart sheet components incorporating the surgeon's preference card.

11. *Directories.* Alphabetic listings of the location of supplies and equipment are maintained for the instrument room, general workroom, sterile supply room, and general perioperative storage areas. Regardless of where the storage areas are located, personnel should know the location of supplies and equipment. Directories save time in trying to locate items.

• BOX 2.3   Sample Case Cart Sheet Components With Surgeon's Preferences[a]

Surgeon:
  Dr. Jared
Gloves:
  Size 8
Positioning:
  Supine
Instruments:
  Soft tissue set
Procedure:
  Excision lipoma right anterior thigh
Prep:
  One-step iodophor
Medications:
  1% lidocaine plain
  Sterile saline 1000 mL
Suture:
  3-0 Vicryl PS1
Disposable supplies:
  Extra 4 × 4 sponges available
Patient:
  Martin Alexander
Patient data (e.g., age, sex, allergies):
  26 years old, male, no allergies
Drapes:
  General custom pack
  2 gowns
Sponges:
  2 packs Raytec
Notes or special requests:
  Call family when procedure completed

[a]*Components of computer-generated case cart procedure supply sheet. These sheets are generated at the time the procedure is scheduled using standardized surgeon's preference cards and patient-specific needs. Items listed under each heading are examples only.*

Recommended Practices

Recommended practices are optimum behavioral objectives for caregivers. They may not always be achievable, as standards are, because of limitations in a particular practice setting. Recommended practices state what ideally can be done.

AORN guidelines for perioperative nursing concern sterile and aseptic techniques, and other technical aspects of professional practice are directed toward providing safety in the perioperative environment. They are premised in principles of microbiology, scientific literature, validated research, evidence-based practice, and experts' opinions. Although compliance is voluntary, individual commitment, professional conscience, and the practice setting should guide perioperative caregivers in using these recommended practices. They represent an optimal level of practice and are achievable.

Guidelines and recommended practices of other agencies, including AAMI, the Centers for Disease Control and Prevention (CDC), the National Institute for Occupational Safety and Health (NIOSH), OSHA, and the Environmental Protection Agency (EPA), also are used for environmental, patient, and personnel safety.

Policies and Procedures

Policies and procedures reflect variations in institutional environments and clinical situations. They are established to protect employees, learners, and patients. They establish the facility's standard of care. Policies should be consistent with regulatory and professional standards of practice. Procedures define scope of practice, purposes, and instructions to be carried out and by whom. They should be clearly written, current, dated, and reviewed periodically. Although policies and procedures vary from one institution to another, they provide guidelines for patient care and safety in that specific physical facility. Learning and following policies and procedures are protective measures against potentially litigious actions.

Many facilities document in the employee's personnel file that policies and procedures were reviewed during orientation to the employment setting. Employees are often asked to sign a notation verifying knowledge of a new or revised policy or procedure after its introduction. Some policies and procedures apply to all employees; others refer to a specific department. Because of the potential legal implications, adherence to all policies and procedures is mandatory. Personnel are evaluated on their ability to follow policy and perform procedures correctly. The following examples should be included in the perioperative department manual. These procedures are incorporated into discussions in subsequent chapters.

Universal Protocol

Universal Protocol is a standardized means for keeping a patient safe in surgery. The World Health Organization (WHO) created a basic surgical safety checklist under the guidance of Dr. Atul Gawande and a select team of anesthesiologists, surgeons, and registered nurses. The purpose of the checklist is to globally reduce surgical harms to patients in a manner that can be applied universally in high- and low-income countries. Initial multinational studies of the checklist have demonstrated a one-third reduction in surgical mortality and morbidity.

The initial items require oral confirmation at four critical points during perioperative patient care: (1) the "check-in" in the preoperative area; the patient is identified by the nurse, (2) the "sign in" before induction of anesthesia, (3) "time out" before skin incision, and (4) "sign out" before the patient leaves the OR. The universal checklist provides a means for documentation of each step of care for patients undergoing invasive and noninvasive surgical procedures. AORN incorporated TJC's 2010 Patient Safety Goals and Universal Protocol into the WHO Surgical Safety Checklist to create a Comprehensive Surgical Checklist. Updates to the checklist are made as necessary and can be found on the Comprehensive Surgical Checklist at www.aorn.org. Many facilities use this basic checklist and customize it according to individual needs (Fig. 2.1).

Identifying the Patient

When a patient enters the facility a plastic identification wristband is put on the patient in the admitting area. Care is taken to place the wristband in a location that does not interfere with the surgical site. To verify accuracy the patient should be asked identifying questions: date of birth, full name, spelling, and pronunciation. The circulating nurse and anesthesia provider check the wristband with the patient's and surgeon's names, the patient's chart, and the surgical schedule. The surgeon should visit with the patient before an anesthetic is administered. A parent, legal guardian, or individual with power of attorney can complete this identification process. TJC indicates that at least two methods should be used to identify a patient as part of the patient safety goals.

Identifying the Surgical Site

The surgical site indicated by the consent form should be verified between the circulating nurse and the patient. Universal methods of surgical site verification include asking the patient to describe the planned procedure and acknowledge that the information was presented in an understandable manner. If the procedure is on a particular side of the body, the patient should be asked to point to and clarify the site. The surgeon should mark the site with legible initials and indelible ink that does not wash off during intraoperative skin preparation. Marking with an X is inappropriate and may be misunderstood.

Before an incision is made, the entire team pauses for a "time out" as the patient is identified and the surgical site listed on the consent form is read aloud. The entire team confirms that the information is correct for the patient and that any scans or radiographs reflecting the same body part are displayed in the correct orientation. Allergies, sensitivities, and administered medications are confirmed at this time. During the "time out" process, the availability of the correct implants or special equipment is confirmed (Box 2.4).

The surgical site marking and identification process should be standardized within the facility and written into policy to avoid wrong site procedures. The time out process should be documented in the patient's record by the circulating nurse. More information can be found at www.aorn.org in the official statements section and on the TJC website at www.jointcommission.org. TJC has described factors that contribute to wrong site, wrong patient, and wrong procedure surgery. They are as follows:

- Emergencies
- Morbid obesity
- Physical deformity
- Unusual equipment or setup of the OR
- Multiple surgeons
- Multiple procedures
- Unmarked patients
- Unverified patients
- No checklist
- No assessment
- Staffing issues
- Distractions and disharmony among staff members
- Lack of information about the patient
- Organizational culture of the facility
- Hurrying to complete procedures

Protecting Personal Property

Personnel in preoperative areas are responsible for removing valuables and prostheses before patients go to the OR. The circulating nurse is responsible for double-checking each patient and removing unnecessary items brought to the OR. Personal items such as religious medals, hearing aid(s), eyeglasses, dentures, and eye prostheses are commonly permitted to remain with the patient who is having local or regional anesthesia. The circulating nurse should inform the anesthesia provider and the surgeon of

COMPREHENSIVE SURGICAL CHECKLIST

Blue = World Health Organization (WHO)   Green = The Joint Commission - Universal Protocol 2016 National Patient Safety Goals   Teal = Joint Commission and WHO

PREPROCEDURE CHECK-IN	SIGN-IN	TIME-OUT	SIGN-OUT
In Preoperative Ready Area	**Before Induction of Anesthesia**	**Before Skin Incision**	**Before the Patient Leaves the Operating Room**
Patient or patient representative actively confirms with registered nurse (RN):	**RN and anesthesia professional confirm:**	**Initiated by designated team member:** All other activities to be suspended (except in case of life-threatening emergency)	**RN confirms:**
Identity ❑ Yes Procedure and procedure site ❑ Yes Consent(s) ❑ Yes Site marked ❑ Yes ❑ N/A by the person performing the procedure RN confirms presence of: History and physical ❑ Yes Preanesthesia assessment ❑ Yes Nursing assessment ❑ Yes Diagnostic and radiologic test results ❑ Yes ❑ N/A Blood products ❑ Yes ❑ N/A Any special equipment, devices, implants ❑ Yes ❑ N/A	Confirmation of the following: identity, procedure, procedure site, and consent(s) ❑ Yes Site marked ❑ Yes ❑ N/A by person performing the procedure Patient allergies ❑ Yes ❑ N/A Pulse oximeter on patient ❑ Yes Difficult airway or aspiration risk ❑ No ❑ Yes (preparation confirmed) Risk of blood loss (> 500 mL) ❑ Yes ❑ N/A # of units available _____ Anesthesia safety check completed ❑ Yes Briefing: All members of the team have discussed care plan and addressed concerns ❑ Yes	Introduction of team members ❑ Yes All: Confirmation of the following: identity, procedure, incision site, consent(s) ❑ Yes Site is marked and visible ❑ Yes ❑ N/A **Fire Risk Assessment and Discussion** ❑ Yes (prevention methods implemented) ❑ N/A Relevant images properly labeled and displayed ❑ Yes ❑ N/A Any equipment concerns ❑ Yes ❑ N/A **Anticipated Critical Events** Surgeon: States the following: ❑ Critical or nonroutine steps ❑ Case duration ❑ Anticipated blood loss Anesthesia professional: Antibiotic prophylaxis within 1 hour before incision ❑ Yes ❑ N/A Additional concerns ❑ Yes ❑ N/A Scrub person and RN circulator: Sterilization indicators confirmed ❑ Yes Additional concerns ❑ Yes ❑ N/A RN: Documented completion of time out ❑ Yes	Name of operative procedure: _____ Completion of sponge, sharp, and instrument counts ❑ Yes ❑ N/A Specimens identified and labeled ❑ Yes ❑ N/A Equipment problems to be addressed ❑ Yes ❑ N/A **Discussion of Wound Classification** ❑ Yes To all team members: What are the key concerns for recovery and management of this patient? _____ _____ _____ Debriefing with all team members: Opportunity for discussion of - team performance - key events - any permanent changes in the preference card
Include in Preprocedure check-in as per institutional custom: Beta blocker medication given ❑ Yes ❑ N/A Venous thromboembolism prophylaxis ordered ❑ Yes ❑ N/A Normothermia measures ❑ Yes ❑ N/A			January 2019

The Joint Commission does not stipulate which team member initiates any section of the checklist except for site marking. The Joint Commission also does not stipulate where these activities occur. See the Universal Protocol for details on the Joint Commission requirements.

 AORN
SAFE SURGERY TOGETHER

• **Fig. 2.1** AORN comprehensive surgical checklist. (Reprinted with permission from AORN.org. Copyright © 2019, AORN, Inc, 2170 S. Parker Road, Suite 400, Denver, CO 80231. All rights reserved.)

•BOX 2.4   "Time out" for Prevention of Wrong Site Surgery

- Correct patient?
- Correct position?
- Correct site?
- Correct procedure?
- Correct equipment?
- Correct images? (scans or radiographs in proper orientation)
- Correct implants? (as appropriate)

---

the presence of such items and document them on the patient's chart. Artificial extremities, contact lenses, piercings, undergarments, wigs, hairpins, wristwatches, and rings should be removed. Jewelry could get lost or interfere with the surgical site, or a ring might become stuck on the patient's finger because of postoperative swelling. In addition to the danger of losing or damaging these items, some could cause pressure areas on the anesthetized patient's body.

Any item that is removed should be placed in a rigid container and labeled with the patient's name and identification number. The patient's personal property should not be wrapped in a paper or linen towel that could inadvertently be discarded in a trash receptacle or laundry hamper. The container may be retained by the circulating nurse during the surgical procedure and sent with the patient to the postoperative area. Alternatively, the circulating nurse may immediately ask a nursing assistant to return the container to the patient care unit. This person should obtain a receipt for the patient's personal property from the person receiving it. The receipt is given to the circulating nurse to put in the patient's chart along with a notation of the transaction in the nurse's notes. Patients value their property. A caregiver can be held liable for lost or damaged personal property.

Observing the Patient

Unattended patients may fall from a stretcher or the OR bed. Falls are one of the most frequent causes of avoidable injuries. Side rails, restraints, and safety straps should be used to protect all patients, children as well as adults. A small child could reach and insert a tiny finger into an electrical socket. Patients should be observed at all times in the perioperative environment.

Positioning the Patient

Care is taken when moving all patients to and from the OR bed. The patient should be positioned to ensure adequate exposure of the surgical site for the surgeon but not compromise any body system. The anesthesia provider should determine the physiologic safety of the patient's body systems. Cardiopulmonary functioning should not be impaired. Adequate support of joints and limbs should be provided during movement into the desired position. Pressure areas should be adequately protected and padded with recommended devices to prevent neurovascular damage.

The plan of care should include appropriate numbers of personnel for safe patient movement. Patients who are incapable of assisting with physical motion require a minimum of four people to ensure a safe move from one surface to another. There should be at least one person on either side of the patient, one at the foot, and one at the head to monitor the patient's airway and physiologic response. The person guiding the patient's head, usually the anesthesia provider, should be the one who counts "one—two—three" to pace the synchronized movement from one surface to another.

The surgeon determines the appropriate surgical position in consultation with the anesthesia provider. The circulating nurse and first assistant help position the patient. A stretcher is always kept nearby if a patient is placed in a prone position or any position other than supine. In the event of an emergency the patient will need to be placed in a supine position for treatment such as cardiopulmonary resuscitation (CPR).

Many patients receive a general anesthetic or heavy sedation and are therefore unconscious or not in control of their protective reflexes. Constant vigilance is essential to safeguard patients who are vulnerable and unable to protect themselves. Liability on the part of the team would be difficult to dispute. Everyone in the perioperative environment has a duty to always monitor and protect the patient without exception.

Aseptic and Sterile Techniques

Infection is a serious postoperative complication that may become life-threatening for the patient. Perioperative patient care team members must know and always apply the principles of aseptic and sterile techniques. Established procedures for aseptic technique, sterilization, and disinfection should be followed meticulously. An emergency in which asepsis becomes a secondary concern is a rare occurrence. Asepsis should not be compromised for the sake of convenience of the caregiver. Each team member should consider how personal preferences for care of self or a loved one should be applied to the care of patients.

Postoperative wound infection can originate in the OR from a break in technique by any team member. Inappropriate reuse of disposable items may be indefensible, as can use of an unsterile endoscope introduced into a sterile body cavity. An unsterile scope can disrupt the mucous membrane and come into contact with the patient's vascular system. No area of the body is considered "dirty." Any area of the body is at risk when the vascular system is entered and should be worthy of sterile instrumentation. Microorganisms can be transferred via any access portal to the vascular system, including, but not limited to, the mouth, urethra, penis, vagina, rectum, and ear. Strict asepsis and sterile technique prevent many postoperative complications. The following principle applies: When in doubt about something's sterility, consider it unsterile; hence the phrase, "When in doubt, throw it out."

Accountability of Accurate Counts

The primary responsibility for accounting for all sponges, sharps, and instruments before, during, and after every surgical procedure rests with the circulating nurse and scrub person. Laziness and a cavalier attitude surround the statement, "The incision is too small to lose anything." Do not be fooled by this cavalier statement. It can happen when least expected. There are several reasons to count and be accountable for items used in a surgical procedure. Examples include the following reasons for accountability:

1. Patients have retained items from a surgical procedure regardless of the size or location of the surgical site. This is a serious safety breach that is inexcusable.
2. Instruments are costly and should not "vanish into thin air." It is a shame that some hospitals x-ray all the trash and have metal detectors on the doors of the OR. Instruments stuck in washing machines cause damage to the mechanisms. Accountability significantly decreases this loss.
3. Many instruments and devices have sharp tips or cutting surfaces. If an instrument is in the trash or laundry, it can become a source of injury to unsuspecting housekeepers or laundry workers. Gloves worn for cleaning do not protect from sharp objects. This can result in prolonged illness and inability to work.

Any item put into the patient should be documented as part of the count and reconciled at the end of the procedure. The counts should proceed in an established manner each time. The surgeon and first assistant facilitate the count of the items on the surgical field before closure; however, it is not their job to perform the actual counts. Because accountability for sponges, sharps, and instruments is recognized as essential to safe practice and the standard of care, omission of appropriate counts or a facility's lack of established procedures for counting and accountability could result in a serious injury to a patient and threat of liability for the facility. There is no excuse for any retained foreign object if the entire team follows the systems for accountability.

The circulating nurse should document in writing the outcome of the final counts as correct or incorrect and any unusual incidents concerning them, including the need for an x-ray to look for a lost item. If an x-ray is taken, the name of the radiologist and the findings also should be documented. An incident report should be filed on all counts that remain unresolved. It is not necessary to indicate the actual number of sponges or needles used on the OR record. The documentation of correct or incorrect counts is sufficient. Any questionable count should be documented as resolved or unresolved and to whom the event was reported.

CHAPTER 2 Foundations of Perioperative Patient Care Standards 25

Counting and Accountability

- Every health care organization should define a standardized count procedure that fits their facility. Count sheets may be used as part of the standardized count procedure, but it is up to each facility to determine the appropriate practices to implement.
- The circulating nurse and scrub person should do a count before any procedure in which any item from the sterile field could be retained.
- Some facilities have policies in which the only counted items are those that are small enough to be lost in a wound. Instruments may not be counted for tiny incisions.
- Specific cases such as trauma may be exempt from the counting process because the priority is to save the patient's life.
- Documentation must state the reason for aborting the count in cases in which the count was void. An x-ray may be done after the procedure to determine whether any item was retained.
- Facility standardization and counting protocols are put in place to protect the patient and surgical staff.

- Some organizations do not specify that everything needs to be counted for every procedure. Every facility is responsible for their own policies and procedures determining what items need to be counted in every case.
- Counting is a time-consuming part of the surgical process because it is done before the procedure, during the procedure, before closing the wound, and after the procedure (final count).
- Some cases, such as orthopedic surgeries, have many trays with small parts that are designed to size custom implants. Because there are so many pieces, they are not counted based on the rationale that they will not be removed from their tray.
- Accountability is the responsibility of the surgical team. Lack of accountability can result in patient injury or poor surgical outcome.
- Long procedures with changing staff members can result in inaccurate counts. Some cases may need additional counts and should be done if a staff member believes it is necessary.
- Deviations in the standard counting policies can result in a "never event," which is a retained surgical item. Risk factors that contribute to retained items may include error in the count, unexpected change in procedure, high body mass index, distractions, and change of staff.

1. Cochran K: Guidelines in practice: prevention of unintentionally retained surgical items, *AORN J* 116(5):428–437, 2022.
2. Weprin S, Crocerossa F, Meyer D, et al.: Risk factors and preventive strategies for unintentionally retained surgical sharps: a systemic review, *Patient Saf Surg* 15:24, 2021.
3. AORN: *Guidelines for perioperative practice*, Denver, CO, 2024, The Association.

Facility policy and procedure should determine the disposition of any tally sheets used in the counting process. The tally sheets are merely worksheets and have no value to the permanent record. Some facilities use a wipe-off board to tally sponge, needle, and instrument counts. Additional information about the processes and rationale for counting and being accountable is described in Chapter 25.

All instruments, equipment, and appliances should be used and tested according to the recommendations and instructions of the manufacturer. Safety devices such as personal protective attire or smoke evacuation apparatus should be used as necessary. Electrical and laser equipment also should pass inspection by the biomedical engineering department and be tagged with a dated preventive maintenance sticker. Electrical equipment should be properly grounded to prevent electrical shock and burns. Equipment or devices that are known or suspected to be faulty are not used. Faulty equipment should be removed from circulation immediately and tagged according to policy.

The facility should conduct appropriate training and competency reviews for all equipment used in patient care. Personnel who set up and operate facility-owned equipment may be found negligent if a patient is injured. Great care is critical to prevent injury when using all equipment in the perioperative environment. It is inappropriate to operate equipment or machinery for which the employee has had no training. All personnel should have adequate training on all equipment they are expected to operate during patient care in the OR. Records of such training should be on file within the department.

Preventing Skin Injury

Skin injury may be caused by an electrical or thermal device, chemical agent, sharp objects, or mechanical pressure. Pressure necrosis is possible after any procedure and especially after procedures lasting more than 2 hours. Patients who have been in holding areas or emergency departments may have pressure injury in process before arriving at the OR. The circulating nurse should assess the patient's body for skin injury.

A burn may occur from the use of a hot instrument taken directly out of the autoclave, such as a mouth gag or a large retractor. The best practice is to avoid immediate-use sterilization (IUSS) and obtain a wrapped, processed instrument if available. If immediate sterilization must be used, the scrub person should immerse the hot instrument in a basin of cool, sterile water before handing it to the surgeon. The hot item should not be placed in a damp towel and placed on the patient's skin; the heat from the item will transfer through the towel and cause a burn. Prolonged contact of even moderate temperatures can cause tissue damage. The patient under anesthesia has no protective reflexes to warn of an impending injury. Thermal injury can happen when any device or solution heated beyond 110° F (44° C) comes into contact with a patient's tissues.

A patient may be burned during use of the electrosurgical unit (ESU). Inadequate skin contact or improper placement of the patient return electrode can cause a deep tissue burn that will not manifest immediately in the OR by a superficial reaction. Redness of the skin on removal of the patient return electrode may be caused by the adhesive rather than a burn. In a thermal injury the deep tissue necroses and sloughs from the bottom up, leaving a full-thickness wound that may be insensate because of nerve damage. The tip of the ESU pencil, endoscopic instrument, or suction cautery probe remains hot after it is applied to tissues for hemostasis. Unintended burns may occur if the hot tip touches other body parts or it is activated against a metal retractor or instrument. Use of a dry sponge or towel against an activated tip causes ignition and fire.

Alcohol and other flammable solutions such as some one-step alcohol-based prep chemicals can ignite, causing flash fires if the solutions are pooled under the patient or allowed to saturate drapes, especially in the presence of oxygen. Vapors, fumes, or oxygen can accumulate under drapes and ignite if exposed to an ESU device. A thermal burn also can occur from other types of electrical and laser equipment that are improperly used or maintained. The caregiver should be aware that the effects of some types of lasers on tissue are not readily visible until tissue necrosis takes place several days postoperatively.

Administering Drugs

Any drug or solution used in the surgical site, such as an antibiotic or local anesthetic, is recorded in the perioperative note by the circulating nurse and surgeon. The drug is checked by a registered nurse and the scrub person before it is transferred to the sterile field. The sterile medication cup and syringes (if used) are clearly labeled by the scrub person on the field immediately after the drug is dispensed (Fig. 2.2). The scrub person frequently has more than one drug on the instrument table, and confusion could result if the drugs are not properly marked. The scrub person repeats the name of the drug to the surgeon when passing it. Medications and medication handling are described in more detail in Chapters 23 and 25.

The scrub person should not "spear" a vial held by the circulating nurse because that action places the circulating nurse's hand at risk for a needlestick injury. The drug should be drawn into a syringe by the circulating nurse and dispensed into the sterile medicine cup after removing the needle used to penetrate the vial. Dispensing with the needle in place can cause aerosolization of the drug, potentially causing airborne exposure of a sensitive person.

Before dispensing any medication, consider the "seven rights" of medication administration:
- Right patient
- Right drug
- Right dose
- Right reason
- Right time
- Right route
- Right documentation

Monitoring the Patient

The standard of care indicates that a registered nurse is responsible for monitoring the cardiac and respiratory status of a patient receiving local anesthetic, with or without intravenous (IV) moderate sedation, if an anesthesia provider is not present. The

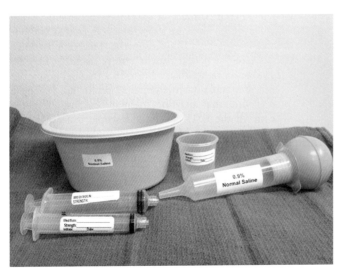

• **Fig. 2.2** Labeled basin with solution and labeled delivery device.

nurse is expected to interpret the monitoring equipment, assess the patient, and initiate interventions promptly if the patient has an untoward reaction. Policies and procedures are delineated by each facility for care of the patient receiving local anesthetic. The nurse who is monitoring the patient should not be assigned circulating duties that would distract attention from the patient. Nurses who monitor patients under moderate sedation should be advanced cardiac life support (ACLS) certified. Patient monitoring is described in more detail in Chapter 27.

Preparing Specimens

With very few exceptions, tissue and objects removed from a patient are sent to the pathology department. The loss of a tissue biopsy specimen could necessitate a second surgical procedure to obtain another one. Incorrectly labeled specimens such as wrong patient or wrong site could result in a mistaken diagnosis, with possible critical implications for two patients. The loss of a specimen could prevent determination of a diagnosis and subsequent initiation of definitive therapy. The pathology report becomes part of the patient's permanent record as added documentation of the diagnosis. Specimens from opposite sides of the body should be sent in separate marked containers. Do not label the lid. Only mark the specimen container to minimize the risk of placing the wrong lid on the wrong container.

Care for foreign bodies according to the policy of the facility. They may have legal significance and frequently are claimed by police, especially if the foreign body is a bullet or something implicated in a crime. A receipt from the person taking them protects personnel and the facility. Chain of custody is a serious subject, and these items are accounted for at all times.

Specimen handling can be hazardous for personnel. Best practices indicate that a sterile container and lid of the appropriate size on the sterile field is the safest way to prevent biologic exposure of other team members. The scrub person should contain the specimen completely before handing off the container to the circulating nurse, who is wearing protective gloves. Dropping a specimen into a cup being held by another is placing that person at risk for exposure. This is avoidable. Specific information about specimen preparation is found in Chapter 22.

Patient Teaching

The patient, family, and significant others need to be informed about treatment options and their roles in the process. The patient has the right to make decisions and contribute to the development of the plan of care. The perioperative nurse can assist with preoperative teaching of deep-breathing exercises for postoperative recovery. Information should be provided verbally and in writing. The patient, family, and significant others should respond appropriately in such a way as to signify understanding of the information. This is particularly important for ambulatory surgery patients who will go home under the care of others. Patient teaching and demonstration of understanding is documented in the chart. More information about patient teaching is in Chapter 21.

Professionalism

Professionals act responsibly in accord with their commitment to public trust and service. Simply stated, the word profession implies a combination and coordination of knowledge, skills, and ideals that are communicated through activities based in higher education. The characteristics of a profession include the following:

- It defines its own purposes and code of ethics.
- It sets its own standards and conducts its own affairs; it is self-regulated and has autonomy.
- Through research, it identifies and develops its own body of knowledge unique to its role.
- It requires critical thinking skills in clinical judgment, as well as problem-solving and decision-making skills in the application of knowledge.
- It engages in self-evaluation and peer review to control and alter its practices and accountabilities.

Professional Perioperative Nursing

Professional nursing is dedicated to the promotion of optimal health for all humans in their various environments. AORN is the leading organization for perioperative nursing and sets the standard for professionalism. In the support of professional perioperative nursing in a wide variety of specialties, AORN has formed specialty assemblies for specialized practice areas and professional interests. The specialty assemblies do not have regular meetings but offer online and newsletter participation. Several times a year the specialty assemblies offer workshops. Assembly meetings are held at the annual AORN Conference. An abbreviated internal specialty assembly governance structure provides a chairperson and other elected officials. A perioperative nurse may belong to as many assemblies as desired.

Local AORN chapters are also available that connect the local perioperative nursing community. Local chapters may have meetings, educational activities, and speakers. They also serve as a discussion platform for current topics, networking, and patient advocacy in the local community.

Nursing in general is both a humanistic art and an applied science. The art of professional nursing practice involves nursing diagnoses and the treatment of human responses to health and illness in all patient care settings. The science behind the paradigm of nursing is based on theories about the nature of humankind, health, and disease. Nursing education prepares nurses to translate the art and science of nursing into relevant knowledge and skill. Professional nursing education is built on a solid base of general education in liberal arts, humanities, and natural and behavioral sciences. AORN Position Statements reflect that the minimal entry level into perioperative nursing should be the baccalaureate degree.

A wise physician once said that the physician's role is to cure sometimes, to relieve often, and to comfort always. The same can be said for the perioperative nurse, who is a registered nurse who embodies all that "nurse" has traditionally meant to a patient—provider of safety and comfort, supporter, and confidante. The patient's safety and welfare are entrusted to the perioperative OR nurse from the moment of arrival in the perioperative environment until departure and the transfer of responsibility for care to another professional health care team member. The perioperative nurse is legally accountable for the delivery of care to patients in the perioperative environment, including interventions that assist the patient in a conscious or unconscious state. The primary emphasis of the nurse's responsibility is to the patient. The perioperative nurse identifies the physiologic, psychologic, and sociologic needs of the patient; develops and implements an individualized plan of care that coordinates interventions; and

evaluates outcomes of the patient's perioperative experience. The nurse is accountable and responsible for delegated patient care.

Patient-Nurse Relationship

To practice in a technologically complex environment, perioperative nurses must be flexible, and their skills must be diverse. Their roles incorporate both the technical and the behavioral components of professional nursing. Competent fulfillment of the perioperative nursing role is based on the knowledge and application of the principles of biologic, physiologic, behavioral, and social sciences and technology. Perioperative nurses develop nursing diagnoses based on patients' problems, needs, and health status. This is essential information in the identification of expected outcomes and in the formulation of a perioperative plan of care.

The perioperative nurse shares a special humanized experience with the patient at a time of great stress and need. This relationship encompasses feelings, attitudes, and behaviors, with mutual trust and understanding as vital components. Effective interaction encompasses concern for the unique personhood of both the patient and the nurse. The length of time spent with the patient is not as important as the quality of the interaction. The level of the interaction may directly affect the patient's perception of the delivery of care in the perioperative environment.

To achieve and maintain a viable cooperative relationship, the patient should be able to sense a feeling of well-being and that the nurse unconditionally cares. The nurse should remain aware that personal interaction is often predicated on culture, lifestyle, attitudes, beliefs, and experiences. Knowledge of the effect of care on the patient's outcome enhances the attainment of the desired result.

Perioperative nursing care is a specialized combination of individualized and standardized care. Individualized care, the art of nursing, demonstrates genuine concern for the patient as a person and is not purely technical. Standardized care, the science of nursing, is derived from a body of scientific knowledge that has been developed through research and clinical practice.

Evidence-Based Practice

The medical model has used tradition or habit to determine the foundations of practice. In the 1980s, medicine adopted an evidence-based framework premised in research as a foundation for patient care practices. Nursing has questioned the best methods for performing patient care and has sought confirmation of the rationale that supports nursing actions. The development of a systematic process involves research that yields evidence of best practices. The essential elements involve obtaining and evaluating evidence and considerations for implementing newly established evidence in practice. AORN has an Evidence Rating Model and Research Appraisal Tool to assist with evaluating recommended practices.

Caregivers should always question why they are doing a particular action and if it is truly effective. Behaviors should continually be evaluated for usefulness as opposed to ritualism. Many practices may no longer be necessary and are not supported by evidence. The following questions should be systematically reviewed when researching for evidence-based practice:

- Which practice area requires evidence?
- What comprises evidence?
- How can evidence be found?
- What is the value of individual increments of evidence?

- Can the increments of evidence be combined into a unit of practice?
- Can the unit of practice be implemented in patient care?

To set up a research project or a systematic review, the following should be well established:

- Who will make up the population to be studied?
- Which intervention will be studied?
- How does one intervention compare with another?
- Which outcomes are preferred?
- Has an investigational review board approved the research project?

Nursing Process

Perioperative patient care requires developing a plan of care and identifying expected outcomes through the nursing process (Box 2.5). The nursing process is a systematic approach to nursing practice using problem-solving techniques. This five-part process provides a systematic foundation for assessing the patient, establishing a nursing diagnosis, planning interventions for desired outcomes, implementing care, and evaluating the success of the plan. Human response patterns to health and illness are vital elements in establishing a nursing diagnosis (Box 2.6).

Integration of the Nursing Process Into Perioperative Patient Care

The five components of the nursing process are integrated into the three phases of the patient's perioperative experience: the preoperative phase, the intraoperative phase, and the postoperative phase. Throughout the entire perioperative period the patient is continually assessed, the plan of care is modified, implementation is effected, and the cycle is evaluated for the attainment of outcomes. The perioperative nurse is responsible for continually assessing the patient by observing and acknowledging parameters identified in Box 2.7. The system and the structure had been traditionally complex until specific data elements of perioperative patient care were clearly stated in a standardized manner.

In 2000, AORN established a Perioperative Patient Focused Model that includes a framework for perioperative care. The primary focus of the model is the patient and the nursing care delivered by the perioperative nurses to ensure optimal patient

---

• BOX 2.6   Human Response Patterns According to NANDA International

- Exchanging
- Communicating
- Relating
- Valuing
- Choosing
- Moving
- Perceiving
- Knowing
- Feeling

• BOX 2.7   Assessment Parameters Monitored Throughout Perioperative Care by the Circulating Nurse

- Physiologic
- Medical diagnosis
- Surgical site and procedure
- Results of diagnostic studies
- Laboratory tests
- Review of systems
- Mobility, range of motion
- Prosthetics (internal or external)
- Sensory impairments
- Allergies
- Skin condition
- Nutritional and metabolic status
- Height and weight
- Vital signs
- Elimination pattern (e.g., continence)
- Sleep, rest, exercise patterns
- Medications
- Substance abuse
- Psychosocial
- Cognition (e.g., mental status)
- Cultural, religious beliefs, and lifestyle
- Perception of procedure
- Expectations of care
- Knowledge base (e.g., informed consent)
- Readiness to learn
- Ability to understand and retain teaching
- Stress level (e.g., anxiety, fears)
- Coping mechanisms
- Support from family or significant others
- Attitude and motivation (e.g., health management)
- Affective responses (e.g., ability to express feelings)
- Speech characteristics (e.g., language)
- Nonverbal behavior

• BOX 2.5   The Nursing Process

Assessment

- Identify the actual or potential problems, needs, and health status considerations through appraisal of the physiologic, psychosocial, objective, subjective, cultural, and ethnic data related to the patient as an individual. Assessment is based on functional health patterns.
- Document assessment data.

Nursing Diagnosis

- Formulate prioritized actual or potential nursing diagnoses unique to the patient. Human response patterns guide the development of nursing diagnoses.

Planning/Identification of Outcomes

- Establish and prioritize a working set of interventions for the actual problems, needs, and health status considerations.
- Establish a contingency plan for the potential problems, needs, and health status considerations that may become actual during the perioperative experience.
- Include the patient's input for the construction of the individualized plan.

- Develop measurable and attainable expected outcomes and mutual goals in collaboration with the patient, family, significant others, and other health care providers.
- Identify realistic time frames in which fulfillment may be accomplished.
- Document the plan of care in a retrievable manner.

Implementation

- Share the plan with the perioperative team for continuity of care.
- Activate the interventions in a systematic order of priority.
- Discontinue any intervention that is ineffective.
- Document the implementation of the interventions and their effectiveness.

Evaluation

- Determine the effectiveness of the plan as the expected outcomes and mutual goals are met.
- Reformulate the plan and implement new interventions as necessary.
- Document the effectiveness of the plan of care in an ongoing, systematic manner.

outcomes. Focused areas reflected in the model describe the perioperative patient's interaction with the health care system, particularly surgery. The four primary domains concerning perioperative nurses and patients are patient safety, physiologic responses, behavioral responses, and the health care system.

Perioperative Nursing Data Set (PNDS)

AORN developed the perioperative-specific nursing vocabulary (known as PNDS) that defines and describes the perioperative patient's experiences from preadmission to discharge from care. The standardized language of data elements (nursing diagnoses, nursing interventions, and patient outcomes), identifies specific common components that are distinctly part of perioperative patient care, and incorporates the Patient Focused Model. Electronic health records (EHRs) represent perioperative nursing care in a unified language that provides feedback in an evidence-based format. The AORN SYNTEGRITY framework was developed to provide a consistent integration of perioperative documentation incorporating PNDS into the perioperative record for minimization of discrepancies and evidence of standards compliance (Fig. 2.3). The PNDS is set into tables used by perioperative information systems. Tables of PNDS values connect assessment and nursing diagnoses, intervention, and outcome data directly to the individual patient via standardized documentation by EHR or paper documentation.

A data element is the smallest unit of descriptive information available that retains its meaning. It allows the reader to conceptualize without added descriptors. The Perioperative Nursing Data Set (PNDS) published by AORN includes perioperative nursing diagnoses, perioperative nursing interventions, and patient outcomes. The PNDS is described in four domains specific to the perioperative nursing process. These are as follows:
- Domain 1: Safety
- Domain 2: Physiologic responses
- Domain 3: Behavioral responses of patient, family, and significant others
- Domain 4: Health system

The PNDS is important for capturing data in a systematic way that can be retrieved, measured, and evaluated for quality of care. Nursing diagnoses have been connected with planning, implementation, and evaluation of nursing interventions and with specific outcomes to further validate the use of a standardized perioperative language. The standardized language has a letter and a number specific to the nursing activity it describes within the particular domain. For example:
- A: Assessment
- Im: Implementation
- E: Evaluation
- O: Outcome

The PNDS was officially recognized by the ANA's Committee on Nursing Practice Information in 1999. The clinical relevance of the PNDS is specific to perioperative patient care and provides a standardized language to validate the value of the role of the professional perioperative nurse. The PNDS is a clinically validated nursing language that is useful for clinical practice, education, and research. According to AORN, the advantages of PNDS use include, but are not limited to, the following:

The AORN Syntegrity® solution is standardized content for perioperative nursing documentation and surgical scheduling that is built into the current electronic health record.

• **Fig. 2.3** AORN SYNTEGRITY Standardized Perioperative Framework. Nurses enter their documentation, and AORN SYNTEGRITY framework provides a guide through a standardized language, PNDS, with your current information system. (Reprinted with permission from AORN. Copyright © 2016, AORN, Inc, 2170 S. Parker Road, Suite 400, Denver, CO 80231. All rights reserved.)

- Identifying essential content for educational and orientation programs
- Providing reliable and valid perioperative nurse-sensitive data
- Providing a universal language for perioperative nursing practice
- Assisting in the measurement and evaluation of patient care outcomes
- Providing a foundation for perioperative nursing research to examine the quality and effectiveness of care
- Informing decisions about the relationship of staffing to patient outcomes
- Providing data about the contributions of nurses to patient outcomes in the perioperative arena

AORN's SYNTEGRITY Perioperative Documentation Solution is compatible with most EHRs and can be found at www.aorn.org/syntegrity. Consult AORN online at www.aorn.org for additional information about the PNDS or SYNTEGRITY Perioperative Documentation Solution system. Other nursing organizations with recognized forms of standardized language are listed online at www.nursingworld.org.

Preoperative Phase

The preoperative phase of the patient's surgical experience begins when the decision is made to undergo surgical intervention, and it ends when the patient is transferred to the OR bed in the OR. During this phase the perioperative nurse performs the assessment, determines the nursing diagnoses, identifies potential outcomes, and develops a plan of care. The nurse assesses the patient to identify any actual or potential physiologic, psychosocial, and spiritual needs, problems, or other health status considerations. In collaboration with the patient, family, and significant others, the nurse then determines the nursing diagnoses and identifies the expected outcomes of the perioperative experience. The perioperative nurse plans, prioritizes, and initiates the patient care necessary for the attainment of the desired outcomes.

Intraoperative Phase

The intraoperative phase begins with placement of the patient on the OR bed and continues until the patient is admitted to a postprocedure or postoperative area, such as the postanesthesia care unit (PACU). Implementation of the plan and evaluation of care continue during this phase. The perioperative nurse either personally carries out the plan of care or supervises others in carrying out the plan with skill, safety, efficiency, and effectiveness. Modification of the plan may be necessary during the procedure.

Postoperative Phase

The postoperative phase begins with admission of the patient to a postprocedure or postanesthesia area (PACU) or an intensive care unit (ICU). Patients admitted to the facility on an ambulatory 1-day-stay basis may return to the ambulatory unit. As indicated by their condition, the patient will transfer from the immediate postoperative patient care division for progressive stages of self-care on a surgical unit before being discharged from the hospital. The postoperative phase ends when the surgeon discontinues follow-up care. Evaluation, the sixth component of the nursing process, is completed during this phase.

Standards of Perioperative Nursing Practice

A standard is an authoritative statement established and published by a profession and by which the performance of practice can be measured. The standards of nursing practice establish parameters and competency levels against which the practice of the profession is compared.

The ANA Standards of Clinical Nursing Practice reflect the nursing process and state the interventions to be performed. These standards are a description of a competent level of practice common to all nurses and form the foundation of all decision-making in the provision of care to all patients. The interpretive statements that accompany each standard provide definitions of terms along with the interventions and guidelines necessary to achieve these standards. Criteria for the achievement of each standard are also stated and remain consistent with current nursing practice.

Nursing practice is based on theory and evidence-based practice. Nursing is constantly evolving with the development of new technology and research. The standards are written in behavioral terms so nurses can measure to what degree each standard has been met.

The *Standards of Perioperative Clinical Practice*, originally published in 1981, are revised by the AORN Board of Directors. The standards are updated annually as necessary to keep pace with changes to validate current practices. The nursing activities inherent in each standard are incorporated in the nursing process during the three phases of surgical care.

Standard I: Assessment

The perioperative nurse collects patient health data from which the nursing diagnoses are derived. Data collection is continual and ongoing. It may be gathered in the preoperative holding area, on the patient care unit, in the clinic, or by a telephone call to the patient at home. Information can be obtained from the patient's chart, by consultation with other members of the health care team (e.g., unit nurses, surgeon, anesthesia provider), through interviews with the patient, family, or significant others, and by observation and physical assessment. Data collection is a progressive and orderly process of gathering meaningful information pertinent to the planned surgical intervention. It includes, but is not limited to, the following parameters:
- Current medical diagnosis and therapy
- Diagnostic studies and laboratory test results
- Physical status and physiologic responses, including allergies and sensory or physical deficits
- Psychosocial status, including education level
- Spiritual needs, ethnic and cultural background, and lifestyle
- Previous responses to illness, hospitalization, and surgery
- Patient's understanding, perceptions, and expectations of the procedure

Pertinent data collected through physiologic and psychosocial assessment are documented. Box 2.7 lists the perioperative assessment parameters. The basic elements of a nursing assessment are described in the sections that follow.
- *Subjective data*: Include the patient's perceptions and expectations of the procedure and may be recorded in the form of a direct quote.
- *Objective data*: Include the nurse's observations of the patient and the interpretation of baseline data.

Physiologic Assessment

The perioperative nurse performs a physical assessment of the patient. Techniques include inspection/observation, auscultation, percussion, palpation, and olfaction. The assessment of major body systems establishes the baseline health status of the patient. It provides a basis for planning appropriate patient care and provides a database for postoperative evaluation.

The perioperative nurse should be familiar with laboratory test norms so that critical deviations can be identified in all phases of perioperative care. Other important parameters for planning perioperative care include knowledge of allergies, skin integrity, sensory or physical limitations, prosthetic devices, nutritional/metabolic status, and chronic illness. The routine use of medications can affect or interact with anesthetic medications and postoperative recovery. A patient who smokes and who will have general anesthesia needs to be taught coughing and deep-breathing exercises. The patient who is dependent on alcohol or other drugs can suffer postoperative physiologic and psychologic manifestations of withdrawal. A chemically dependent person who is recovering from an addiction may refuse preoperative sedation and postoperative narcotics for pain.

Psychosocial Assessment

The perioperative nurse performs a psychosocial assessment. Illness makes a person vulnerable, and individuals vary in their ability to cope with stressful situations. Culture, religion, lifestyle, and socioeconomic factors influence a patient's interpretation of illness and response to the interaction with the perioperative environment. Anticipatory apprehension, although normal to some degree, may diminish critical-thinking and decision-making abilities. Stress may initiate an exaggerated response of normal coping mechanisms for self-protection. Establishing a preoperative psychosocial baseline facilitates prompt recognition of maladaptation to a perioperative event.

Documentation

Pertinent information should be recorded in the patient's chart or EHR for use by the perioperative team. Data collection sets the baseline for ongoing care in the perioperative environment and into the remote postoperative care period.

Computer information systems can be used to establish a computerized patient database. Many facilities have incorporated the Internet to permit the patient access to their own medical record with a personalized log-on and password. Use of the PNDS allows the nurse to use standardized terminology that in turn permits data collection about patient care. This is the foundation of evidence-based practice. A copy of the patient care plan can be viewed in the patient's record. The nurse should review the patient care plan and date and sign it for the permanent record.

Standard II: Diagnosis

The perioperative nurse analyzes the assessment data in determining the nursing diagnoses. Nursing diagnoses are conclusions based on analysis and interpretation of the human response patterns revealed by the assessment data. These are concise written statements about a patient's actual or potential problems, needs, or health status considerations amenable to nursing intervention.

A medical diagnosis defines problems based on a patient's pathologic condition(s). NANDA International (NANDA-I) has developed a long list of nursing diagnoses available at www.nanda.org. This list, known as a taxonomy, classifies human response patterns and standardizes the nomenclature for describing them. It includes definitions and defining characteristics for each diagnosis and leads the nurse to generate assessment data that link to outcomes. The PNDS has more than 93 nursing diagnoses specific to perioperative patients. A NANDA-I nursing diagnosis has three components:

1. *Defining characteristics.* Human responses to altered body processes and other contributing factors describe the acuity of an actual or potential health status deviation. The nurse identifies the characteristics for which nursing interventions can legally be used to maintain current health status or to reduce, eliminate, or prevent its alteration. These interventions are based on human response patterns:
   a. *Problem.* Any health care condition that requires diagnostic, therapeutic, or educational action. Problems can be active (requiring immediate action) or inactive (having been solved). Problem-oriented medical records are built on this premise. An ongoing list is maintained in a database and is used throughout the managed care environment.
   b. *Need.* A lack of something essential for the maintenance of health that may be met through the plan of care. Needs may be actual (in existence at the time of assessment) or potential (anticipated to become actual during the length of stay [e.g., deficient knowledge]). Many of these needs are met through the intervention component of the plan of care.
   c. *Health status considerations.* A personal habit, lifestyle, or influencing agent that if uncontrolled can lead to a decline in physiologic or psychologic well-being (e.g., occupational hazards, exposure to chemical agent or smoke, substance abuse).
2. *Signs (objective) and symptoms (subjective).* Data obtained during the assessment identify the defining characteristics of the patient's actual or potential health problems. The patient's functional health patterns are assessed (Box 2.8). Gordon has suggested that there are 11 functional health patterns that should be assessed. The domains include physiologic, psychologic, and sociologic aspects of observed behavior.
3. *Etiology/related factors.* The causes of problems may be related to physiologic, psychosocial, spiritual, environmental, or other factors contributing to the patient's health status. These causes define relevant risk factors to be considered in planning patient care.

•BOX 2.8   Gordon's Functional Health Patterns of Observable Behaviors

- Health perception/health management
- Nutritional/metabolic
- Elimination
- Activity/exercise
- Sleep/rest
- Cognitive/perceptual
- Self-perception/self-concept
- Role/relationship
- Sexuality/reproductive
- Coping/stress tolerance
- Value/belief

Modified from Gordon M: Manual of nursing diagnosis, 1997-1998, St. Louis, 1997, Mosby.

Documentation

Use of the PNDS terminology helps perioperative nurses establish standard communication when documenting nursing diagnoses. A common language facilitates continuity of patient care.

Standard III: Outcome Identification

The perioperative nurse identifies expected outcomes unique to the patient. Each outcome can be affected by nursing care (also referred to as "nurse sensitive") and is specific to the individual, the family, significant others, and the community. The Nursing Outcomes Classification (NOC) taxonomy is built on five levels: domains, classes, outcomes, indicators, and measures. The standardized terminology gives quantifiable language to the statement of outcomes and has numeric codes that can be used in nursing informatics systems. Each outcome is evidence based and researched using qualitative and quantitative methods.

The nurse measures the patient's responses and uses a five-point Likert scale to tally the score. A numeric baseline range is documented, and the numeric target outcome is identified. This method permits the use of the data in an information system and empiric research. More than 612 outcomes are closely linked and integral with NANDA-I nursing diagnoses and can be used across the care continuum in all branches of nursing, including the perioperative care areas.

Expected perioperative outcomes are the desired and obtainable patient objectives after a surgical intervention. These outcomes occur within specified time frames and have specific criteria for evaluation, as demonstrated in the identified PNDS patient outcomes. They direct patient care to modify or maintain the patient's baseline functional physical capabilities and behavioral patterns. The patient's rights and preferences are the cornerstones for expected outcomes. They should be realistic, attainable, and consistent with medical regimen and patient outcome standards for perioperative nursing.

Documentation

The results of care should be documented in standardized language. Select examples of PNDS documentation include the following:
- The patient's neurologic status is consistent with or improved from baseline levels established preoperatively.
- The patient's respiratory status is consistent with or improved from baseline levels established preoperatively.
- The patient's fluid and electrolyte balance is consistent with or improved from baseline levels established preoperatively.

Standard IV: Planning

The perioperative nurse develops a plan of care that prescribes interventions to attain the expected outcomes. Based on the assessment data, nursing diagnoses, and identified expected outcomes, the perioperative nurse devises a plan of care. The plan should include a provision for all phases of patient care in the perioperative environment. Strategic concepts to consider in planning perioperative patient care include but are not limited to the following:
- Participation of the patient and/or the family and significant others in formulation of the plan
- Medical diagnosis and effect of surgical intervention on the patient's physiology
- Psychosocial and spiritual needs of the patient and their family and significant others
- Environmental safety, comfort, and well-being

- Provision of supplies, equipment, and technical expertise
- Current best nursing practices

The plan of care should reflect current standards, facilitate the prescribed medical care, and work toward the attainment of desired outcomes. The scope of the plan is determined by assessment data. Any unusual data are considered for individualized patient care. Alternative options or interventions, not just routine procedures, are a necessary part of the plan. Regardless of format, the plan of care specifies the following parameters:
- Patient care necessary to achieve expected outcomes
- Interventional priorities and sequence of care
- Availability of resources needed to implement the plan
- How, where, and by whom the care will be delivered
- Specific modifications for individualized aspects of care
- Methods for evaluating the effectiveness of the plan

Documentation

Standardized patient care plans may be developed for patient populations undergoing like procedures, with space provided to note any unique or unusual patient assessment data. These care plans can be organized on preprinted forms to include the usual nursing diagnoses and expected outcomes and may include, but are not limited to, the following:
- The patient will demonstrate understanding of the procedure.
- The patient will be injury free.
- The patient will remain normothermic.
- The patient will be infection free.
- The patient's skin will remain intact.
- The patient will remain physiologically stable.
- The patient will demonstrate psychologic comfort.
- The patient will return to normal activities of daily living.

The format of the record may include checklists and spaces for specific patient data. This record accompanies the patient throughout the perioperative environment and serves as a guide for the perioperative team. Use of a standardized language, such as the PNDS, is beneficial for precise communication. Dissemination of the plan to all personnel involved in providing care to the patient is essential for continuity of care. The plan is modified as indicated by ongoing evaluation data.

Standard V: Implementation

The perioperative nurse implements the direct and indirect interventions identified in the plan of care. A taxonomy of nursing interventions known as the Nursing Intervention Classification (NIC) is the basis for the standardization of terminology. The NIC is linked to NANDA-I and describes more than 566 evidence-based interventions that are grouped into classes. The seven domains of the NIC are Physiologic: Basic, Physiologic: Complex, Behavioral, Safety, Family, Health System, and Community. The standardized terminology of the NIC gives quantifiable language to the nursing interventions and has numeric codes that can be used in nursing informatics systems.

The plan of care is implemented throughout the perioperative care period by the entire team. Scientific principles provide the basis for patient care interventions that are consistent with the plan for continuity of patient care in the perioperative environment. They are performed with safety, skill, efficiency, and effectiveness.

The patient's welfare and individual needs are paramount in every facet of activity and must not be compromised. Seemingly routine details are significant. For example, taking a defective instrument out of circulation may prevent injury to the patient or team member. All preoperative preparations within the perioperative environment provide for the physical safety of the patient and team in an aseptic, controlled manner. The circulating nurse also provides emotional support to the patient before transfer to the OR bed and during induction of anesthesia.

This text focuses primarily on direct and indirect interventions that perioperative and perianesthesia nurses and surgical technologists perform to ensure achievement of expected patient outcomes. Implementation of safe and efficient patient care requires the application of technical and professional knowledge, sound clinical judgment, and a surgical conscience on the part of all team members. Nurses have a responsibility to monitor constantly the physiologic and psychologic responses of patients to care. They control environmental factors that affect outcomes of surgical intervention.

Documentation

All patient care interventions (both routine and individualized), observations of patient responses, and the resultant outcomes delineated in the patient care plan are documented as evidence of the care given. This written documentation becomes part of the patient's permanent record. The circulating nurse accountable for the patient's care is responsible for the documentation either in writing or through the EHR. The person completing the documentation should sign with a complete name and title. Interventions contributing to patient comfort and safety are identified. Activities other than direct patient care that are not recorded elsewhere and may affect patient outcomes are included (e.g., how tissue specimens were handled).

Writing nurse's notes or progress notes on the patient's chart or completing an accurate intraoperative observation checklist provides a profile of what has happened to the patient. The notes should contain what happened and why. Intraoperative records not only have legal value but also are valuable to the postoperative care team. The PNDS provides standardized language to describe nursing interventions. Select PNDS intervention examples include the following:

- Administers care to wound site
- Administers electrolyte therapy as prescribed
- Administers care to invasive device sites
- Evaluates for signs and symptoms of electrical injury
- Manages specimen handling and disposition

Standard VI: Evaluation

The perioperative nurse evaluates the patient's progress toward the attainment of outcomes with an actual outcome statement, as described in the PNDS. Evaluation is a continual process of reassessing the patient and their responses to implementation of the plan of care. Perioperative caregivers accommodate a variety of intense situations within a short time. The perioperative team is always on the alert for, and prepared to respond to, the unexpected. The flexibility of the team is manifest in the quick modifications to the plan of care during emergency situations.

All components of the nursing process are performed concurrently during the intraoperative phase as changes occur in the patient's internal and external environments. The patient is observed during the surgical procedure and evaluated for responses to all interventions.

Determination of patient responses and the realization of expected outcomes can be verified by direct observation of and/or conversation with the patient. The perioperative nurse observes the patient's responses to interventions during the immediate preoperative and intraoperative phases of care in the perioperative environment. The perioperative nurse may accompany the patient to the PACU or postprocedure area to determine the level of attainment of expected outcomes. The "handover" or "handoff" report should be standardized between the perioperative nurse and the postanesthesia nurse. For the purposes of this text, the term *handover* is used to describe the exchange of patient information between professional caregivers. Ideally the perioperative nurse visits the patient postoperatively on the patient care division or phones an ambulatory patient at home within 24 to 48 hours after discharge to complete the assessment of outcomes.

Documentation

The patient's permanent record should reflect the ongoing evaluation of perioperative nursing care and its outcomes. This includes a comparison of expected outcomes to the degree of outcome attainment as determined by the patient's responses to nursing interventions. Documentation using a standardized language provides legal evidence of results of the plan of care and revisions to the plan after reassessment of the patient. Examples of PNDS nursing diagnoses and outcome statements:

- Patient demonstrates knowledge of the expected responses to the procedure.
- Patient has wound/tissue perfusion consistent with or improved from baseline levels established preoperatively.
- Patient is at or returning to normothermia at the conclusion of the immediate postoperative period.
- Patient is free from injury from extraneous objects.

Clinical Competency of the Perioperative Nurse

Using the framework of the nursing process, AORN published Competency Statements in Perioperative Nursing in 1986 and revises them periodically. These broadly written statements of expected competencies can be used to develop position descriptions, generate performance appraisals, and organize orientation and staff development activities. They serve as guidelines for the skills a nurse should reasonably expect to achieve to function as a competent perioperative nurse in the perioperative environment. These statements incorporate the many principles, procedures, and practices elaborated throughout this text for competent care of the surgical patient, as follows:

- Assess the physiologic health status of the patient.
- Assess the psychosocial health status of the patient.
- Formulate nursing diagnoses based on health status data.
- Establish the patient's expected outcomes based on nursing diagnoses.
- Develop a plan of care that identifies patient care interventions to achieve expected outcomes.
- Implement patient care interventions according to the plan of care.
- Evaluate the attainment of expected outcomes and effectiveness of patient care.
- Participation in teaching of the patient, family, or significant others.
- Create and maintain a sterile field.

- Provide equipment and supplies based on patient needs.
- Perform sponge, sharps, and instrument counts.
- Administer drugs and solutions as prescribed.
- Monitor the patient physiologically during the surgical procedure and throughout the perioperative experience.
- Monitor and control the environment.
- Respect the patient's rights.
- Demonstrate accountability.

Scope of Perioperative Nursing Practice

Perioperative nurses care for patients throughout the continuum of the perioperative intervention. The patient's needs are unique during this phase of care and require specific activities particular to the realm of perioperative nursing. Professional nurses render direct care or oversee the implementation of the plan of care through specialized activities that include, but are not limited to, the following:

- Educate staff and peers
- Emotionally support and reassure the patient, family, and significant others
- Serve as patient advocate
- Control a safe and effective environment
- Provide resources
- Maintain asepsis
- Monitor physiologic and psychologic status
- Manage aggregate patient needs
- Supervise ancillary personnel
- Validate and explore current and prospective practices
- Integrate and coordinate care across all disciplines
- Collaborate and consult

These activities are incorporated into the scope of perioperative practice by managers, educators, practitioners, and researchers. These practices take place in hospitals, clinics, educational facilities, physicians' offices, provider organizations, and industry.

Surgical Technology

The activities of registered professional nurses are supplemented and complemented by the services of allied technical health care personnel. The term *allied health care personnel* refers to individuals who have been trained in a health care–related science and have responsibility for the delivery of health care–related services but who are not graduates of schools of medicine, osteopathy, dentistry, podiatry, or nursing. Approximately two-thirds of the health care workforce are designated as allied health professionals. Educational preparation may be offered in colleges, vocational-technical schools, hospital-based programs, or military service schools. Technologists, technicians, and therapists in more than 130 occupational categories work collaboratively with and under the direction of physicians and registered nurses.

The surgical technologist, or ST, is a member of the direct patient care team and works intraoperatively with the surgeon and anesthesia provider under the direction of the circulating nurse. This team is referred to as the *perioperative team*. The surgical technologist prepares instruments, supplies, and equipment to maintain a safe and therapeutic surgical environment for the patient. The surgical technologist performs specific techniques and functions designed to exclude pathogenic microorganisms from the surgical wound.

An accredited surgical technology program includes courses in anatomy and physiology, pathology, and microbiology as prerequisites to courses that involve the theory and application of technology during surgical procedures and for care of the perioperative environment. Other courses in the curriculum, such as pharmacology, help explain the underlying basis for the technical tasks to be performed. Courses in psychology, ethics, and interpersonal communication are fundamental to an appreciation of the humanities.

Association of Surgical Technologists (AST), National Board of Surgical Technology and Surgical Assisting (NBSTSA), Accreditation Review Council on Education in Surgical Technology and Surgical Assisting (ARC-STSA), and the Commission on Accreditation of Allied Health Education Programs (CAAHEP) play a role in program core curriculum, standards for accreditation, certification, and education.

NBSTSA offers a national certification examination for individuals who meet the graduation requirements from an accredited program. After graduation from an accredited program, an application for testing may be submitted for approval. Upon passing the examination, individuals may use the credential Certified Surgical Technologist (CST). As of 2020, the certification cycle is 2 years and the credential renewed by continuing education hours or retaking the examination. Continuing education credits must be specific to surgical technology and may be obtained from AST.

The NBSTSA 2-year recertification cycle by continuing education requires:

- 30 continuing education credits for a CST
- 38 continuing education credits for a Certified Surgical First Assistant (CSFA)
- The renewal fee is reduced to reflect the 2-year cycle

Guidelines for Surgical Technologists

AST has developed evidence-based position statements and guidelines that provide a description of professional topics and guidelines that demonstrate best practices. The quality of the surgical technologist's practice is judged by these guidelines. The authoritative position and practice statements include those in the following section.

Teamwork

Teamwork is essential for perioperative patient care and is contingent on interpersonal skills. Communication is critical to the positive attainment of expected outcomes of care. All team members should work together for the common good of the patient. For the benefit of the patient and the delivery of quality care, interpersonal skills are demonstrated in all interactions with the health care team, the patient and family, superiors, and peers. Personal integrity and surgical conscience are integrated into every aspect of professional behavior.

Preparation

Preoperative planning and preparation for surgical intervention are individualized to meet the needs of each patient and their surgeon. The surgical technologist collaborates with the professional registered nurse in the collection of data for use in the preparation of equipment and supplies needed for the surgical procedure. The implementation of patient care identified in the plan of care is performed under the supervision of a professional registered nurse.

The preparation of the perioperative environment and all supplies and equipment will ensure environmental safety for patients and personnel. The application of the plan of care includes wearing appropriate attire, anticipating the needs of the patient and perioperative team, maintaining a safe work area, observing aseptic technique, and following all policies and procedures of the institution.

Surgical Expertise

Application of basic and current knowledge is necessary for a proficient performance of assigned functions. The surgical technologist should maintain a current knowledge base of procedures, equipment and supplies, emergency protocol for various situations, and changes in scientific technology pertinent to their performance description objectives. It is the responsibility of the surgical technologist to augment their knowledge base by studying recent literature, attending in-service and continuing education programs, and pursuing new learning experiences.

Ethics

Each patient's rights to privacy, dignity, safety, and comfort are respected and protected. Each member of the OR team has a moral and ethical duty to uphold strict observance of the patient's rights. The surgical technologist, like all members of the health care team, is expected to perform as a patient advocate in all situations. This is an accountability subject and should be part of each aspect of patient care.

Aseptic Technique

Every patient is entitled to the same application of aseptic technique within the physical facilities. Implementation of the individualized plan of care for every patient includes the application of aseptic or sterile technique at all times by all members of the health care team. All patients are given the same dedication in their care.

Clinical Competency of the Surgical Technologist

The performance description developed by AST identifies performance objectives against which the surgical technologist may measure clinical competency. According to AST, the surgical technologist can aspire to three levels based on education, experience, and time in service. Each level requires the surgical technologist to be certified and employed in the OR. The employment setting can be a clinic, private practice, or facility, such as a hospital. These levels could be used to structure seniority, promotions, and salaries.

Continual Performance Evaluation and Improvement

Nursing research and experience have shown that quality cannot be ensured, only monitored, and performance can be improved. TJC has adopted a definition of quality as "continual improvement" in patient care services to increase the probability of expected patient outcomes and reduce the probability of undesired outcomes. Outcomes can be defined, monitored, and measured. Patient satisfaction is one outcome measurement that is critical in evaluating quality of performance. Satisfied patients are more cooperative and receptive to therapy and teaching.

Each patient deserves the best possible care. Without the structure provided by the nursing process, health care services would be fragmented and accountability for the quality of services rendered would be made difficult. Society demands the accountability of those who provide patient care services. Patients are protected by laws, standards, and recommended practices. Performance of care should comply with established policies and procedures of the hospital or ambulatory care facility and with professional standards of practice.

Performance Improvement Studies

Most studies are designed to measure compliance with current policies and procedures and identify the need for change in practice guidelines or education of staff. Both strengths and weaknesses in performance are identified. Ultimately the purpose is to correct deficiencies and deviations from expected standards. Important aspects that influence the quality of patient care are identified, and a measurable indicator is established for each aspect. Data sources and methods of data collection should be appropriate for each indicator. Sample size and the frequency of data collection should be sufficient to identify trends or patterns in the delivery of care.

Data are collected either concurrently or retrospectively and are organized for evaluation. A concurrent study begins with a current manifestation and links this effect to occurrences at the same time (i.e., is related to care in progress). This type of study focuses on a systematic series of actions that brings about an outcome. Through concurrent observation, the implementation component of the nursing process can be monitored during perioperative patient care to determine whether interventions are consistent with established standards for care and recommended practices. The interventions performed should protect the welfare and safety of the patient and should meet the identified physiologic and psychologic needs. The environment, including equipment or supplies used in the room, can be evaluated at this time.

A retrospective study focuses on the end result of patient care or on a measurable change in the actual state of the patient's health because of care received. This evaluation of outcomes usually occurs through review of patient records. The study begins with a current manifestation and links this effect to some occurrence in the past (i.e., care previously given). Complications attributable to care in the perioperative environment may be identified (e.g., nerve palsy from poor positioning, infiltration of an IV infusion, postoperative wound infection). The source of these complications may be difficult to identify unless every detail of actual care given and any unusual occurrences are recorded in the patient's record. Accurate and complete documentation is therefore essential for meaningful retrospective studies.

Any method that systematically monitors and evaluates the quality of patient care can enable perioperative nurses and surgical technologists to take corrective action for improvement of performance. Quality improvement studies also assist in the coordination of plans for patient care with surgeons; improve communications with other departments; identify needs for revision of policies and procedures; and reassess equipment, personnel, and other aspects of patient care.

Benchmarking

Benchmarking is a term that is used to continually monitor progress of a competitor to discover methods for performance improvement and how to implement them. According to TJC, when processes within the same facility are measured against each other, this is referred to as *internal benchmarking*. Measuring performance against an outside competitor is referred to as *competitive benchmarking*. If another industry's activities are used as the comparison, the reference is then made to *functional benchmarking*.

When practices are benchmarked, the current level of attainment is clearly identifiable and higher performance attributes can be viewed as the next step in professionalism.

Peer Review

Peer review differs from other quality improvement programs in that it looks at the strengths and weaknesses of an individual practitioner's performance rather than appraises the quality of care rendered by a group of professionals to a group of patients. An associate with the same role expectations and performance description examines and evaluates the clinical practice of a peer. The individual is evaluated by written standards of performance, and the review should offer constructive criticism of the performance observed. Through this framework, caregivers gain feedback for personal improvement or confirmation of personal achievement related to their effectiveness of professional, technical, and interpersonal skills in providing patient care.

EVOLVE WEBSITE

http://evolve.elsevier.com/Hornacky/BerryKohn/

- Historical Perspective
- Glossary

Bibliography

AORN: *Guidelines for perioperative practice*, Denver, CO, 2024, The Association.

Association of Surgical Technologists: www.ast.org. Accessed January 7, 2022.

Benze C, Spruce L, Groah L: *Perioperative nursing scope and standards of practice*, Denver, CO, 2021, AORN.

Makic M, Martinez-Kratz M: *Ackley and Ladwig's nursing diagnosis handbook*, ed 13, St. Louis, 2023, Elsevier.

Moorhead S, Swanson E, Johnson M: *Nursing outcomes classification (NOC)*, ed 7, St. Louis, 2022, Elsevier.

Nightingale F: *Notes on nursing: what it is, and what it is not*, New York, 1969, Dover Publications.

Petersen C: Evolution and revision of the perioperative nursing data set, *AORN J* 93(1):127–132, 2011.

Phillips NM, Hornacky A: *Pass CNOR*, St. Louis, 2019, Elsevier.

3

Legal, Regulatory, and Ethical Issues

CHAPTER OUTLINE

Legal Issues, 38

Liability, 38

The Joint Commission and Sentinel Events, 42

Consent, 44

Documentation of Perioperative Patient Care, 46

Legal Aspects of Drugs and Medical Devices, 50

Ethical Issues, 51

CHAPTER OBJECTIVES

After studying this chapter, the learner will be able to:

- Define negligence as it applies to caregivers.
- Discuss informed consent.
- Describe the importance of patient care documentation.
- List several methods of documentation of patient care.
- Identify three potential events that could lead to litigation.
- Describe the role of The Joint Commission in the promotion of patient safety.

KEY TERMS AND DEFINITIONS

Advance directive Document that indicates wishes concerning health care and usually designates someone to make decisions if the patient is unable to do so for self.

Autonomy Self-government or independence.

Causation Action directly or indirectly causing an injury.

Consent Voluntary, autonomous permission to proceed with an agreed-on course of action.

Damages Compensation awarded to make restitution for an injury or a wrong.

Defendant Person named as the object of a lawsuit.

Deposition Statement given under oath that is a documentation of fact used in a court of law.

Iatrogenic Injury or illness caused by professional intervention of a health care provider.

Indicator A measured increment of performance, process, system, or outcome.

Liability Legally responsible for personal actions.

Malpractice Substandard delivery of care that results in harm.

Near miss An event or situation that just by chance did not cause patient injury. A very close call.

Negligence Careless performance of duty.

Plaintiff Person who initiates a lawsuit.

Proximate cause An act of commission or omission by one or more persons that caused a consequence to another.

Root cause analysis The baseline reason for the occurrence of failure in a process or system.

Sentinel event An unexpected occurrence that involves physiologic or psychologic injury or death. This occurrence signals the need for appropriate reporting and documentation, immediate investigation, and response.

Systems approach A global attitude of improvement and safety that encompasses involvement of individuals and the organization at all levels. Adverse events are attributed not only to individuals but also failure of the interaction of the individual and the organization.

Tort Wrong committed by one person against another; civil action.

Competent patient care is the best way to avoid a malpractice or negligence claim. Unfortunately, even under the best of circumstances, a patient may be injured and recover monetary damages as compensation. Understanding how a liability action starts and how it proceeds is important in the effort to avoid the many pitfalls that can lead to being named and successfully sued in a lawsuit.

Caregivers should consider that liability is not the only rationale behind competent care. The focus should be the desired outcome for the patient and the exemplary delivery of care.

Performing in a particular manner merely to avoid being sued is not an ethical practice.

Legal Issues

Inherent in professional practice is the duty to safeguard the safety and rights of patients. The patient is at risk for harm during any surgical procedure. These factors also may present health care providers with ethical dilemmas complicated by legal issues. Respect for the patient's autonomy and the patient's right to make informed decisions about health care should be considered and balanced by the professional obligations of beneficence (the duty to benefit) and nonmaleficence (not to harm).

Any caregiver can be named in a lawsuit. Being named in a suit does not mean that you have been successfully sued and does not always mean you are liable for anything. Attorneys frequently name everyone involved with the patient in the suit as part of the fact-finding process for building the lawsuit. When in doubt about personal competency for a new or unfamiliar procedure or piece of equipment, seek guidance from the clinical educator, mentor, or immediate supervisor to prevent patient harm.

Regardless of who oversees the team, each team member is responsible for individual actions. When performing duties within the scope of practice and according to facility policy and procedure, the risk for being successfully sued in a malpractice or negligence suit is very limited. Honest mistakes can result in patient injury. If a suit is brought to court, a jury can evaluate a reasonable set of circumstances, facts, and testimony to render a verdict in favor of the caregiver. The plaintiff does not always win. If the verdict is found in favor of the plaintiff, the damages awarded may be a compensatory award. Many states have set limits on the amount of money that can be awarded by the court.

The quality of health care is assessed through the outcome of services rendered. If the outcome is unacceptable, patients tend to take grievances to court. The severity of an injury usually determines whether a claim of merit will arise, but other contributing factors include a breakdown of rapport between the patient and the health care team members and unrealistic expectations about the outcome of care.

Causes for litigation lie with the patient's, family's, or significant others' belief that physicians and/or health care organizations have not provided appropriate diagnosis, treatment, or results. Although the physician is professionally responsible for patient care, other patient care personnel act as part of the health care team, carrying responsibility for their own actions. Medical and surgical vendors and suppliers of equipment and drugs also are indirectly involved in treatment and may be held responsible for product liability.

Liability

To be liable is to be legally bound and responsible for personal actions that adversely affect another person. Every patient care provider should always perform duties in accordance with standards and practice guidelines established by federal statutes, state practice acts, professional organizations, and regulatory agencies and those that are common practice throughout the facility and community. Deviation from these standards and practices that cause injury to a patient can result in liability for negligence or malpractice. For this type of civil suit to be successful, the plaintiff must prove that negligent care or malpractice caused the injury.

Negligence is the failure to use the care or skills that any caregiver in the same or a similar situation would be expected to use. These acts of omission or commission that cause damage to a patient may give rise to tort action, which is a civil lawsuit.

Malpractice is any professional misconduct, unreasonable lack of skill or judgment, or illegal or immoral conduct. Malpractice and negligence claims usually are settled in a civil court; however, depending on the severity of the injury and the extent of the misconduct, they may be taken to criminal court. From the legal point of view of damages or fault, professional negligence is often synonymous with malpractice in a tort action. The following factors contributing to a successful lawsuit on behalf of the plaintiff have been called the "four Ds of malpractice":

1. Duty to deliver a standard of care directly proportional to the degree of specialty training received
2. Deviation (dereliction) from duty by omission or commission
3. Direct causation of a personal injury or damage because of deviation of duty
4. Damages to a patient or personal property caused by the deviation from the standard of care

Statutory laws (laws by legislation) and common laws (laws based on court decisions) differ from state to state. Courts differ at times in their interpretation of laws. Any caregiver who is in some way thought to be responsible for injury to a patient may be sued. The nurse manager or clinical educator responsible for assigning duties to this individual may be included in the suit if delegation and supervision are in question.

Caregivers, such as nurses, surgical assistants, technologists, and technicians, are considered employees of the health care facility. The facility is almost always named in the suit as ultimately responsible for hiring, monitoring credentials, educating, evaluating, and disciplining their employees.

The court may rule that a learner or an experienced practitioner is liable for their own actions. A learner may be held responsible for independent actions in proportion to the amount and type of instruction received and judged by the standard of other learners in training. An instructor can be named with the learner as partially liable.

Medical care and professional liability have become institutional problems. The primary cause of professional liability claims is iatrogenic medical injury—an injury or other adverse outcome sustained by a patient as a result of treatment. Many incidents in the perioperative environment have been causes for a lawsuit.

Liability Prevention for the Facility and the Team

Many factors present challenges in managing risks for liability, such as complex technologies, acuity of hospitalized patients' conditions, short-stay procedures, diverse roles of providers, inadequacy of staffing numbers, misdiagnosis, or delayed care. Many surgeons restrict their practices to avoid patients who have complex diseases or who are at high risk for uncertain outcomes. Others practice defensive medicine, ordering tests principally to protect themselves against possible litigation. Because lawyers have become increasingly sophisticated in representing injured patients, all health care providers need to take measures to protect themselves from litigation. A preventive strategy includes the following:

- Become active within the professional organizations associated with setting the standards for practice. Most organizations provide up-to-date education and resources for improvement of practice. Have a voice in shaping the future of the profession.

- Remain current with continuing education. Become certified, and maintain credentials.
- Establish positive rapport with patients. Patients are less likely to sue if they perceive that they were treated with respect, dignity, and sincere concern. Patients have the right to accurate information and good communication.
- Comply with the legal statutes of the state and standards of accrediting agencies, professional associations, and the health care facility policies.
- Adhere to the policies and procedures of the facility. Seek a position on the policy and procedure committee to have a say in the formation and revision of facility practices.
- Document assessments, interventions, and evaluations of patient care outcomes. Each patient care activity is an indicator of competent care and should be documented. Leave a paper trail that is easy to follow for the reconstruction of the event in question.
- Prevent injuries by adhering to policies and procedures. Shortcuts can be hazardous to the patient and team members.
- Speak up if something does not seem right. Ask for clarification from a supervisor if unsure of an order or procedure.
- If an injury occurs, control further injury or damage by reporting problems and taking corrective action immediately.
- Maintain good communications with other team members.
- In addition to these strategies, the facility as the employer and the caregiver as the employee should take steps to avoid liability. The facility protects the patient, its personnel, and itself by maintaining safe and well-defined policies and procedures based on national standards and recommended practices.

Liability Insurance

Formerly it was thought that patients did not sue nurses and other patient care providers because they had no large assets. Unfortunately, this is no longer true. Increased autonomy increases the risk for liability. Perioperative nurses make independent nursing decisions based on assessments, and they perform and/or delegate certain patient care interventions without a physician's order. No matter how careful the caregiver is, mistakes can happen. An unintentional wrong may cause injury to a patient.

Most facilities carry insurance that covers incidents that result in harm to a patient when policies and procedures are followed; however, they may not cover the employee who fails to follow the established protocol of policies and procedures. In some instances the facility's insurance may not adequately cover all of the expenses associated with a lawsuit, such as a private attorney, time in deposition, and lost wages during suspensions and trial.

The caregiver who accidentally caused the injury may be named in the suit as an individual or as a codefendant. Carrying personal liability insurance protects against a possible discrepancy with the facility's insurance coverage and provides the employee with the opportunity for representation by a personal attorney.

A professional liability policy can be individualized to meet the practice of the insured. The cost of a policy can vary depending on the amount of coverage, but the protection of personal assets and wages may well be worth the price of the coverage. Professional associations recommend individual professional liability insurance and frequently offer discounts to members.

Borrowed Servant Rule

In the past the surgeon was considered the captain of the ship in the perioperative environment and was liable for the negligent acts of servants. In the early 1940s and 1950s, courts held that this doctrine, based on the master–borrowed servant relationship, was applicable by the mere presence of the surgeon. Once having entered the operating room (OR), the surgeon was considered to have complete control over other team members. But courts now recognize that the surgeon does not have complete control over the acts of the perioperative patient care team at all times.

Each member of the team has significant performance autonomy. The surgeon usually is not held responsible when a perioperative caregiver fails to carry out a routine procedure as expected. Courts have decided that certain procedures do not need to be personally performed by the surgeon, such as counts or mixing medications on the sterile field.

According to the borrowed servant rule, the surgeon is liable for acts of team members only when supervising and controlling the way in which a perioperative caregiver performs specific tasks. A good example of this is counting sponges, sharps, and instruments. The facility, not the surgeon, establishes the mechanism and policies by which the employee team accounts for items used during a procedure. The surgeon does share some liability for prohibiting or preventing the team from accomplishing this task. If this is the case, the circulating nurse should clearly document the surgeon's refusal to permit counting in the medical record and report to the immediate supervisor.

Contracted Services

Health care facilities use many different contracted individuals and organizations to help keep a facility running smoothly. A contracted organization may be nonpatient care, such as laundry, groundskeepers, or maintenance. Direct patient care staff may be licensed practitioners, such as nurses, surgical or physician assistants, physicians, or other support staff. The employer may be held responsible for employees under the master-servant rule. However, the current trend is to hold an individual responsible for actions under the principles of the agreed contract. For example, a private scrub person, biomedical technologist, or first assistant may contract with several surgeons to provide services on a fee-for-service basis. These individuals are not directly employed by the facility but are usually credentialed and given permission to work with the surgeon by the medical staff department. A detailed contract explaining all responsibilities and duties should be written and signed by all contracting personnel. Questions may arise concerning the level of responsibility of the facility for credentialing someone who is accused of substandard practice. The facility may take legal action to remove an individual for not practicing under the agreed contract. Contracted personnel are held responsible for following the policies and procedures of the facility.

The Joint Commission (TJC) dictates that a facility that permits contractors, such as private first assistants, interns, residents, or other privately engaged personnel, is responsible for specific standards associated with accountability. All contractors who hold licensing credentials are referred to as "licensed practitioners." TJC's updated standards and definitions are available at www.jointcommission.org. Current standards for contracted licensed practitioners are as follows:

- Have appropriate current credentials for the role
- Must be competent
- Provide care under direct supervision if necessary
- Perform duties only within the scope of the intended role
- Adhere to the policies and procedures of the facility and state
- Complete orientation to the facility's emergency evacuation procedures
- Keep current in immunizations and health screenings
- Always display appropriate identification
- Comply with all background checks, including fingerprinting and drug testing
- Agree to proof of continuing education, practice evaluation, physical ability, and professional performance

Doctrine of the Reasonable Man

A patient has the right to expect that all patient care personnel will use education, knowledge, skill, and unbiased judgment in performing duties that meet standards exercised by other reasonably prudent professionals involved in similar circumstances.

Whenever a mishap occurs in patient care, the cause of the event is compared with local and national standards of care. Experts are consulted by attorneys, and the mishap is studied. The results should show whether the same event performed by someone else of the same or similar education and role would have had the same result under the same or similar circumstances. This is how the courts determine the reasonableness of a caregiver's actions. An example of this might be how drugs are administered. The average nurse in average circumstances would check and recheck to be sure the right patient gets the right drug. A careless nurse might omit checking the patient's identification and administer the wrong drug. This would be considered unreasonable and would be a source of liability.

Doctrine of *Res Ipsa Loquitur*

Translated from Latin, *res ipsa loquitur* means "the thing speaks for itself." Under this doctrine, the courts allow the patient's injury to stand as inference of negligence. The defendant has to prove that the act was not negligent. Before this doctrine can be applied, three conditions must exist:

1. The type of injury would not ordinarily occur without a negligent act.
2. The injury was caused by the conduct or instrumentality within the exclusive control of the person or persons being sued.
3. The injured person could not have contributed to negligence or voluntarily assumed risk.

This doctrine applies to injuries sustained by the patient while in the perioperative environment, such as a retained foreign object (e.g., sponge, towel, needle, or other instrument/item), a fall, or a burn. The defendant must prove that a breach did not occur and the act was not negligent.

Doctrine of *Respondeat Superior*

An employer may be liable for an employee's negligent conduct under the *respondeat superior* master-servant employment relationship. This implies that the master will answer for the acts of a servant. If a patient is injured as a result of an employee's negligent act within the scope of that employment, the employer is responsible to the injured patient. The patient may name both the facility and the employee in a civil suit. The employee could be dropped from the suit if the facility policy, procedure, and actions within the appropriate scope of practice were followed.

A facility may have outdated practices or unsafe procedures. One example might be the labeling of drugs on the sterile field. Instead of requiring the name and dose of the drug to be written on the sterile container and the syringe, the facility may permit the scrub person to place the cap of the syringe into the medicine cup containing local anesthetic to signify the contents of both the syringe and cup. This is a practice that was in effect in some facilities. It is clearly an unsafe practice to require a scrub person to manage drugs on the sterile field in this manner. The facility would be found liable for this action if it required the employee to perform at this unacceptable level.

Doctrine of Corporate Negligence

Under the corporate negligence doctrine, the facility may be liable not for the negligence of employees but for its own negligence in failing to ensure that an acceptable level of care is provided. The facility has a duty to provide services and is responsible for the following:

- Screening and verifying qualifications of all staff members, including medical staff, according to standards established by TJC
- Monitoring and reviewing performance and competency of staff members through established educational activities, personnel appraisal, and peer review procedures
- Maintaining a competent staff of physicians
- Revoking practice privileges of a physician or staff member when the administrators know or should have known that the individual is incompetent or impaired

Corporate negligence includes the use of personnel who are inadequately trained for the position they hold. The Alabama Supreme Court found HealthTrust, Inc. liable for permitting a surgical technologist to perform in the role of first assistant at Crestwood Hospital in 1997 (*Cantrell v. Crestwood*). The surgical technologist was holding a retractor during an open hip procedure on a pediatric patient and permanently injured the sciatic nerve. Her leg was disfigured, and she had to undergo multiple failed surgeries to restore function. The surgeon was not found liable for the acts of the facility's employee.

Extension Doctrine

If the surgeon goes beyond the limits to which the patient consented, liability for assault and battery may be charged. This doctrine implies that the patient's explicit consent for a surgical procedure serves as an implicit consent for any or all procedures deemed necessary to cope with unpredictable situations that jeopardize the patient's health. By medical necessity and sound judgment, the surgeon may perform a different or an additional surgical procedure when unexpected conditions are encountered during an authorized surgical procedure (e.g., finding an abscess near the target organ or finding a tumor extended into adjacent structures).

The surgeon may extend the surgical procedure to correct or remove any abnormal or pathologic condition under the extension doctrine. The court will determine whether the patient consented to a specific procedure or generally to surgical treatment of a health problem. The surgeon may not routinely remove the appendix or gallbladder during a tubal ligation.

Assault and Battery

In legal terms, assault is an unlawful threat to harm another physically. Battery is the carrying out of bodily harm, as by touching without authorization or consent. Lack of informed consent to perform a procedure is an important aspect of an assault-and-battery charge. Informed consent must be obtained by the physician and consent to perform a procedure must be given voluntarily with full understanding of implications by the patient. The purposes of a written, signed, and witnessed consent are to protect the surgeon, anesthesia provider, perioperative team members, and facility from claims of unauthorized procedures and to protect the patient from unsanctioned procedures. Consents are discussed in detail later in this chapter.

Invasion of Privacy

The patient's right to privacy exists by statutory or common law. The patient's chart, medical record, DVD, videotapes, radiographs, and photographs are considered confidential information for use by physicians and other health care personnel directly concerned with that patient's care. The patient should give written consent for videotaping or photographing the surgical procedure for medical education or research. The patient has the right to refuse photographic consent.

The patient has the right to expect that all communications and records pertaining to individualized care will be treated as confidential and will not be misused. This includes the right to privacy during interview, examination, and treatment. The surgery schedule bearing the names of the patients should not be posted in a location where the public or other patients can read it.

Some patients, such as celebrities, may request to be admitted with an alias. Care is taken when identifying these patients so they will not be confused with other patients and receive the wrong procedure. Community hospitals may be admitting people from the surrounding neighborhood. The caregiver may be able to learn private information about a neighbor. Maintaining the confidentiality of patient information is imperative.

Every health care worker has a moral obligation to hold in confidence any personal or family affairs learned from patients. Only personnel with direct patient care have the right to access the patient's records. Many facilities have implemented confidentiality agreements with all health care personnel on the premises. Health care personnel must sign and date the agreement and understand that it is a legal binding document. Violations can lead to punishment or termination of employment. Schools for surgical personnel require students to sign confidentiality agreements before going to a clinical site.

Health Insurance Portability and Accountability Act

The Health Insurance Portability and Accountability Act (HIPAA) was originally published in the *Federal Register* in 2003. The act provides confidentiality of health data (past, present, or future records) involved in research or transmitted and stored by electronic devices or any other means. The release or disclosure of this protected health information (PHI) or electronic PHI (ePHI) requires patient authorization. HIPAA covers far more than PHI—it covers fingerprints, voice prints, and photographic images.

In 2009, HIPAA added the Health Information Technology for Economic and Clinical Health (HITECH) Act because of the increased electronic health record (EHR) sharing of medical information between health care providers and facilities. The HITECH Act enforces the security and privacy of health information. With additional strengthening needed, updates were added in 2021. The Omnibus Act of 2013 added additional rules to HIPAA that strengthened privacy laws to protect health information from unauthorized use or sale.

Since HIPAA has become very complex, the Department of Health and Human Services (HHS) Office of Civil Rights (OCR) enforces, investigates, and sets nationals standards for protecting health information. They operate under several rules: The Privacy Rule, Security Rule, Breach Notification Rule, and Enforcement Rule. Details of each rule can be found at www. hhs.gov/hipaa.[1]

As the world of technology evolves, use of social media and how information is stored, sent, requested, and used requires updated rules for privacy and are in process for 2024.[2] The use of social media, such as X (formerly known as Twitter), Facebook, and Instagram, to discuss patient information is a violation of patient confidentiality. Accessing patient records without authorization is grounds for dismissal from employment. Both of these activities are violations of HIPAA and are punishable by law.

When a victim of crime or a perpetrator is in a health care facility, both have the right to privacy. Caregivers may not speak to news media or any other person concerning either individual. If a crime is discovered by a caregiver, the information must be reported to an appropriate supervisor. At no time is a caregiver to make a promise of secrecy to a suspected perpetrator.

Some circumstances permit the use of health information without authorization, such as reporting suspected cases of child or elder abuse or neglect; sexual assault; abuse of a patient, caregiver, or visitor in a facility; information related to a crime; or cases concerning public health. Specific information can be found in the HIPAA Privacy Rule, No Authorization Required standards at www.hipaasurvivalguide.com.

Abandonment

Abandonment consists of leaving the patient for any reason when the patient's condition is contingent on the presence of the caregiver. If the caregiver leaves the room knowing there is a potential need for care during any absence, even under the order of a physician, the caregiver is liable for that action.

In *Czubinsky v. Doctor's Hospital*, the surgeon ordered the circulating nurse to leave the room to help him start another procedure. During the circulating nurse's absence, the patient had a cardiac arrest. The only team members on hand were the anesthesia provider and the surgical technologist. At the trial, the circulating nurse admitted to knowing that it was wrong to leave the patient but left because of the surgeon's insistence. The expert witness testified that the circulating nurse should not have been ordered away from the patient to work in another room. The court decided that if adequate help for resuscitation had been available in the OR during the crisis, the patient would not have suffered permanent brain damage, which occurred because of this breach of duty. According to the court, the circulating nurse had a duty to remain with the patient.

If an event necessitates leaving a patient, it is important to transfer care to another caregiver of equal status and function. In uncontrollable circumstances, the perioperative manager should be consulted immediately. The patient must not be left unattended. No one, not even a physician, may release a caregiver from a responsibility to a patient. A child or disoriented patient left alone or unguarded in a holding area, for example, may sustain injury by pulling out an IV (intravenous line) or an electric shock from a nearby outlet or by some other hazard. The circulating nurse may be considered negligent by reason of abandonment for failure to monitor a patient in the OR. The circulating nurse should be in attendance during induction of and emergence from anesthesia and throughout the surgical procedure to assist as needed.

The Joint Commission and Sentinel Events

Professional accountability requires professionals to monitor performance as it applies to patient outcomes. The identification of an undesired outcome may be the result of direct or indirect actions of the caregiver. Such an outcome is referred to as a sentinel event—an unexpected event that involves a risk for or the occurrence of death or serious physical or psychologic injury. Serious injury specifically includes loss of limb or function. The term *sentinel* was selected to represent the concept because the seriousness of the event requires immediate investigation and response. These events have a significant effect on patient outcomes; they should be evaluated for root cause, and a plan to prevent its occurrence should be prepared.

Root Cause Analysis

TJC developed and approved a list of sentinel events that should be voluntarily reported and other events that need not be reported (Box 3.1). The TJC publication *Framework for Root Cause Analysis and Action Plan* has been made available to institutions as a guideline for investigating the causes of sentinel events. The objective is to improve the system that has permitted the error to occur. The guidelines include a fill-in-the-blank questionnaire to help track the cause of the event.

The guidelines suggested by TJC allow each facility flexibility in determining the root causes for events specific to the environment. Using flowcharts, the facility can identify one or more of these root causes in identification of the problem or proximate cause of the error. Each facility is encouraged, but not required, to report sentinel events to TJC. Other sources, such as the patient, a family member, significant others, or the media, may generate a report and can find the forms online on TJC's website. If TJC becomes aware of an event, the facility is required to perform a root cause analysis and action plan or other approved protocol within 45 days of the occurrence. A TJC glossary of sentinel event terminology is available at www.jointcommission.org.[3]

Institutional Reporting of Sentinel Events

The Patient Safety and Quality Improvement Act of 2005 encourages a culture of safety in the health care system. TJC indicates that mistakes are minimized by designing a systems approach that anticipates and possibly prevents human error. Each procedure has inherent safety risks that are not always apparent. These tend to surface when procedural guidelines are not established, not effective, or not followed.

The 2005 act references data that show the incidence of reporting to be more accurate when done on a voluntary basis

> **• BOX 3.1 Reportable and Nonreportable Sentinel Events Identified by The Joint Commission**
>
> **Reportable**
> - Any event that results in the loss of life or limb (e.g., death, paralysis, coma) associated with a medication error
> - Suicide of a patient within 72 hours of being in an around-the-clock care setting
> - Elopement or unauthorized departure of an individual from an around-the-clock care facility that results in suicide or homicide or permanent loss of function
> - Abduction from a care facility
> - Rape, sexual assault, or abuse
> - Discharge of an infant to the wrong family
> - Hemolytic transfusion reaction involving the administration of blood or blood products having major blood group incompatibilities
> - Surgery on the wrong patient or the wrong body part
> - Intrapartum maternal death related to the birth process
> - A perinatal death unrelated to a congenital condition in an infant weighing more than 2500 g
> - Assault, homicide, or other crime resulting in patient or staff member death or a major permanent loss of function
> - A fall that results in death or major permanent loss of function as a direct result of the injuries sustained
> - A retained foreign object from surgery
>
> **Nonreportable**
> - Any near miss
> - Full return of limb or bodily function by discharge or within 2 weeks of the initial loss of function
> - Medication errors that do not result in death or the permanent loss of function
> - Any sentinel event that has not affected the recipient of care
> - A death or injury that follows discharge against medical advice (AMA)
> - Unsuccessful suicide attempts
> - Unintentionally retained foreign body without permanent loss of function
> - Minor hemolysis with no clinical sequelae
>
> Adapted from The Joint Commission: Accreditation Committee examples of voluntary reportable sentinel events, 2022.

rather than when reporting is mandatory. Health care facilities have requested protection for reporting information because to rework the system the faults need to be known. This is the main way of studying problems and finding solutions for improved performance. Many states have adopted the National Quality Forum's (NQF) list of adverse events as the foundation for mandatory adverse event reporting.

In 2004, Minnesota was the first state to adopt the adverse events list as mandatory to report. In the first year of mandatory reporting, surgical adverse events were the highest reported of all the categories by early 2006. Other states have followed by implementing reporting systems and including additional categories of adverse events that are mandatory to report. For additional information about the NQF adverse event list, go to www.qualityforum.org.

National Patient Safety Goals

Universal Protocol is incorporated into the National Patient Safety Goals (NPSGs) implemented in July 2010 by TJC (Fig. 3.1). The updated TJC accreditation statements incorporate NPSGs' language to prevent wrong patient, wrong site, and wrong surgery

Speak UP™

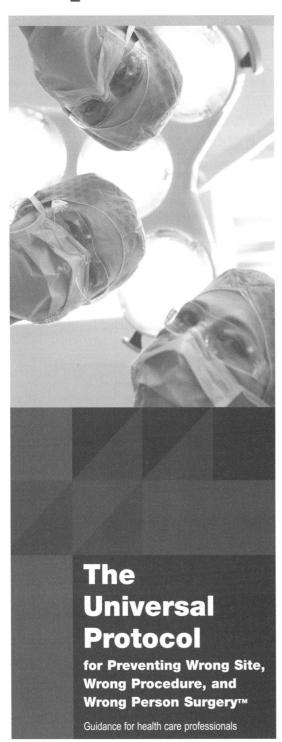

The Universal Protocol

for Preventing Wrong Site, Wrong Procedure, and Wrong Person Surgery™

Guidance for health care professionals

Conduct a pre-procedure verification process

Address missing information or discrepancies before starting the procedure.

* Verify the correct procedure, for the correct patient, at the correct site.
* When possible, involve the patient in the verification process.
* Identify the items that must be available for the procedure.
* Use a standardized list to verify the availability of items for the procedure. (It is not necessary to document that the list was used for each patient.) At a minimum, these items include:
  ☐ relevant documentation
    Examples: history and physical, signed consent form, preanesthesia assessment
  ☐ labeled diagnostic and radiology test results that are properly displayed
    Examples: radiology images and scans, pathology reports, biopsy reports
  ☐ any required blood products, implants, devices, special equipment
* Match the items that are to be available in the procedure area to the patient.

Mark the procedure site

At a minimum, mark the site when there is more than one possible location for the procedure and when performing the procedure in a different location could harm the patient.

* The site does not need to be marked for bilateral structures.
  Examples: tonsils, ovaries
* For spinal procedures: Mark the general spinal region on the skin. Special intraoperative imaging techniques may be used to locate and mark the exact vertebral level.
* Mark the site before the procedure is performed.
* If possible, involve the patient in the site marking process.
* The site is marked by a licensed independent practitioner who is ultimately accountable for the procedure and will be present when the procedure is performed.*
* Ultimately, the licensed independent practitioner is accountable for the procedure – even when delegating site marking.

  * In limited circumstances, site marking may be delegated to son e medical residents, physician assistants (P.A.), or advanced practice registered nurses (A.P.R.N.).

* The mark is unambiguous and is used consistently throughout the organization.
* The mark is made at or near the procedure site.
* The mark is sufficiently permanent to be visible after skin preparation and draping.
* Adhesive markers are not the sole means of marking the site.
* For patients who refuse site marking or when it is technically or anatomically impossible or impractical to mark the site (see examples below): Use your organization's written, alternative process to ensure that the correct site is operated on. Examples of situations that involve alternative processes:
  ☐ mucosal surfaces or perineum
  ☐ minimal access procedures treating a lateralized internal organ, whether percutaneous or through a natural orifice
  ☐ interventional procedure cases for which the catheter or instrument insertion site is not predetermined
    Examples: cardiac catheterization, pacemaker insertion
  ☐ teeth
  ☐ premature infants, for whom the mark may cause a permanent tattoo

Perform a time-out

The procedure is not started until all questions or concerns are resolved.

* Conduct a time-out immediately before starting the invasive procedure or making the incision.
* A designated member of the team starts the time-out.
* The time-out is standardized.
* The time-out involves the immediate members of the procedure team: the individual performing the procedure, anesthesia providers, circulating nurse, operating room technician, and other active participants who will be participating in the procedure from the beginning.
* All relevant members of the procedure team actively communicate during the time-out.
* During the time-out, the team members agree, at a minimum, on the following:
  ☐ correct patient identity
  ☐ correct site
  ☐ procedure to be done
* When the same patient has two or more procedures: If the person performing the procedure changes, another time-out needs to be performed before starting each procedure.
* Document the completion of the time-out. The organization determines the amount and type of documentation.

 The Joint Commission

This document has been adapted from the full Universal Protocol. For specific requirements of the Universal Protocol, see The Joint Commission standards.

• **Fig. 3.1** The Joint Commission poster for the Universal Protocol. (From The Joint Commission: Speak up initiatives, available at www.jointcommission.org.)

events as part of Universal Protocol. The complete list of NPSGs can be viewed at www.jointcommission.org.

Universal Protocol adherence is expected wherever patient care is provided. Examples of accredited facilities accountable for meeting the NPSGs include the following:

- Ambulatory health care facilities
- Critical access hospitals
- Hospital systems
- Office-based surgeries
- Assisted living, nursing care centers, home care
- Behavior health care services
- Laboratory services

Patient safety is a serious concern when the patient's protective reflexes and cognition are impaired by preoperative medications and/or anesthetics. The focus of the applicable patient safety goals includes, but is not limited to, the following points:

- Adequate patient identification
- Accurate marking for surgical procedures
- Eliminating medication errors
- Improving communication between caregivers
- Preventing health care–associated infections
- Preventing injury from falls and pressure points
- Safe and appropriate use of machinery alarms (e.g., electrosurgery, cardiac monitors)
- Identification of patient safety risks

"Never Events" and Reimbursement for Hospitals and Health Care Facilities

The Centers for Medicare & Medicaid Services (CMS) took action in 2009 to improve patient care and decrease errors and injury by denying payment for medical errors that result in serious harm or death for patients. The CMS no longer reimburses for care rendered to patients to remedy the consequences of errors. The CMS generated a list of nonreimbursable conditions, or a "No Pay List," for the following injuries acquired during care:

- Air embolism
- Blood incompatibility
- Catheter-associated urinary tract infection
- Poor control of blood sugar
- Deep vein thrombosis or pulmonary emboli after total knee or total hip surgery
- Falls or trauma while in care
- Removal of a retained object from surgery
- Pressure injury (stages III and IV)
- Surgical site infection after certain orthopedic or bariatric surgery
- Surgical site infection after coronary artery bypass surgery
- Catheter-associated vascular (blood-borne) infection
- Iatrogenic pneumothorax with venous catheterization

Details concerning statistics and trends in CMS programs and rulings can be found at www.cms.gov.

Consent

General Consent

Most facilities require the patient or their legal guardian to sign a general consent form on admission. This form authorizes the attending physician and the staff to render standard day-to-day treatment or to perform generalized treatments and care as the

---

• BOX 3.2 **Examples and Comparison of Consent Form Contents**

General Consent to Treat

Admission to facility
Time and date admitted
Admissions clerk name
Mode of admission
Treating/admitting physician
Person responsible for payment
Contact persons for emergency
Basic care assumptions (such as dietary orders, activity orders, testing, examination by physician)

Informed Consent

Name of patient and legal guardian as appropriate
Name of facility
Specific procedures and who explained them
Specific practitioners and their roles
Risks of the procedure
Alternatives to treatment
Patient's decision and preference
Signatures: patient or legal guardian, surgeon(s), and the witness to the signatures
Date and time the process took place

Data from Centers for Medicare & Medicaid Services, 2024, available at www.cms.gov.

---

physician deems advisable. This general consent is relied on only for activities performed in routine care. Physicians and nurses should be knowledgeable about the statements on the form used in their facility.

Each facility should have policies and procedures in place about the authorization of general consent. Many facilities require the patient or appropriate guardian to sign the general consent document in the admission department before admission to the facility. This is usually facilitated by an admitting clerk, who is a nonmedical person. This in no way equals informed consent. Box 3.2 compares content examples of general consent to treat versus informed consent.

Informed Consent

State statutes differ in their interpretation of the doctrine of informed consent, but all recognize the physician's duty to inform the patient of the risks, benefits, and alternatives of a procedure and to obtain consent before treatment. Failure to do so may be considered a breach of duty. *Informed consent is a process—not a paper document that is signed.* Explanations of the procedure, risks, benefits, and alternative therapy are made verbally to the patient's level of understanding. Some facilities have a special form that is used during this process.

A surgeon or anesthesia provider may be held liable for negligence if the patient can prove failure to disclose significant information that would have influenced a reasonable person's decision to consent. Informed consent is a protective act for the patient and the treating physician and should be documented appropriately. The circulating nurse, as patient advocate, should ensure that an accurate and complete informed consent process has taken place before permitting the patient to be transferred to the OR.

The anesthesia provider also has a responsibility to inform the patient of any potential for unfavorable reactions to any medication or anesthetic agent that may be given during the surgical procedure. The risks of anesthesia should be explained without causing the patient undue stress. If the surgeon intends or wants to perform a procedure not specified on the consent form, the circulating nurse has the responsibility to inform the surgeon and/or proper administrative authority of the discrepancy.

The surgeon may be approved by the U.S. Food and Drug Administration (FDA) as a clinical investigator or by the HHS as a researcher for the controlled experimental use of new drugs, chemical agents, or medical devices. Written consent based on an informed decision to participate in the research should be obtained from the patient before any investigational item, drug, or procedure begins. The surgeon completes an investigator's report that is returned to the supplier of the drug or device and eventually filed with the FDA (www.fda.gov). The patient is free to refuse or withdraw at any time from research performed under the auspices of the HHS. All parties involved with the procedure are bound by HIPAA and the confidentiality implied therein. More information can be found on the HHS website (www.hhs.gov).

Informed Consent for a Surgical Procedure

According to the American College of Surgeons, a reasonable approach to informed consent should involve answering the following patient questions:
- What do you plan to do to me?
- Why do you want to do this procedure?
- Are there any alternatives to this plan?
- What things should I worry about?
- What are the greatest risks or the worst thing that could happen?

The patient has the right to waive an explanation of the nature and consequences of the procedure and has the right to refuse treatment. When a patient signs a consent agreement, consent is given only for the specific procedure indicated on the form. Additional procedures should be listed and signed separately—not added after the patient has already signed the form. Contents documented about informed consent should include, but are not limited to, the following:
- Who will be performing the procedure, including any residents, interns, or first assistants
- Each surgical procedure to be performed, including secondary procedures
- Any procedure for which an anesthetic is administered
- Procedures involving entrance into the body via an incision, puncture, or natural orifice
- Any hazardous therapy, such as irradiation or chemotherapy
- Other persons attending the performance of the procedure, such as students, vendors, or other observers
- Video recording or photography and the disposition of the recorded/photographed images

Responsibility for Informed Consent Before a Surgical Procedure

The surgeon is responsible for obtaining informed consent from the patient, which should include the risks, benefits, and possible complications of all proposed surgical procedures. The explanation should include a discussion of the removal and disposition of body parts, the potential for disfigurement or disability, and what the patient may expect in the postoperative period. The preoperative discussion also should include advice to the patient regarding medications, diet, bathing, smoking, activities of daily living, and other factors that might affect outcome and rehabilitation.

The surgeon has the ultimate responsibility for obtaining informed consent for the procedure and should document this activity in the patient's permanent record according to facility policy and procedure. The patient or appropriate guardian may be required to sign this record in the presence of a witness. All consent documents become a permanent part of the medical record and accompany the patient throughout the perioperative environment. When checking the patient's identity and chart on arrival in the OR, it is the duty of the circulating nurse and the anesthesia provider to be certain of the following:
- The appropriate consents are on the chart and are properly completed, dated, and signed.
- The information on the form is correct concerning the patient, procedure, and personnel performing the procedure.

Validation of Consent

The patient should personally sign the consent if all information is understood. If the patient is a minor, unconscious, mentally incompetent, or is in a life-threatening situation, the next of kin, legal guardian, or other authorized person should sign the consent. The physician gives explanations to the parent of a minor or to the legal guardian of an incompetent adult.

A consent document should contain the patient's name in full, the surgeon's name, the specific procedure to be performed, the signatures of the patient and authorized witness(es), and the date of signatures. A signed consent is regarded as legally valid for as long as the patient still consents to the same procedure. Institutional policy may vary.

The patient giving consent for treatment should be of legal age and mentally competent. Except in life-threatening emergency situations, the patient should sign the consent form before premedication is given and before going to the OR or other procedural/interventional area. This may be done in the surgeon's office, in the facility's admitting office, or on the patient care unit; it is done freely without coercion. If the patient is the following:
- A minor, a parent or legal guardian should sign.
- An emancipated minor, married or independently earning a living, may sign.
- A minor who is the parent of an infant or child who is having a procedure may sign for the child.
- Illiterate, may sign with an X, after which the witness writes, "Patient's mark." Because illiteracy implies the inability to read and write, the patient should indicate an understanding of a verbal explanation.
- Unconscious, a responsible relative or guardian should sign.
- Mentally incompetent, the legal guardian—who may be either an individual or an agency—should sign. A court order may be necessary to legalize the procedure in the absence of the legal guardian.
- An adult or an emancipated minor who is mentally incapacitated by alcohol or other chemical substance, the spouse or responsible person of legal age may sign when the urgency of the procedure does not allow time for the patient to regain mental competence.

Consent documents vary. Policies related to informed consent are developed by the medical staff and governing body in accordance with legal requirements. All personnel involved in the care of patients should be familiar with these policies.

Witnessing a Consent

A witness verifies that the consent was signed without coercion after the surgeon explained the details of the procedure. The patient's or guardian's signature should be witnessed by one or more authorized people. The witnesses may be physicians, nurses, other facility employees, family members, or significant others as established by policy. Checking or witnessing the signature of the patient or other authorized person does not constitute validation of informed consent. The witness assumes no liability or responsibility for the patient's understanding of the procedure. The witness signing a consent document attests only to the following:

- Identification of the patient or legal substitute
- Voluntary signature, without coercion
- Mental state of signatory (i.e., not coerced, sedated, or confused) at the time of signing

Consent in Emergency Situations

In a life-threatening emergency, the consent to treat and stabilize is not essential. Although every effort should be made to obtain consent, the patient's physical condition takes precedence over a procedure permit. The patient's state of consciousness may prevent verbalization or signing a permit for treatment. Permission for a lifesaving procedure, especially for a minor, may be accepted from a legal guardian or responsible relative by telephone, fax, or other written communication. If it is obtained by telephone, two nurses should monitor the call and sign the form, which is signed later by the parent or legal guardian on arrival at the facility.

Right to Refuse a Surgical Procedure

The patient should reconcile the advantages and disadvantages of the surgical intervention. Each patient is entitled to receive sufficient information from which to intelligently base a decision regarding whether to proceed. The patient has the right to decide which procedure will or will not be done. Only after making this decision is the patient asked to sign a written consent for a surgical procedure.

The patient has a right to withdraw written consent at any time before the surgical procedure. The surgeon is notified, and the patient is not taken into the OR. The circulating nurse documents the situation in the patient's record. The surgeon should explain the medical consequences of refusing the surgical procedure. If therapeutically valid, alternative methods of medical management should be offered. The surgical procedure is postponed until the patient makes a final decision. The procedure may be canceled.

The surgeon should document the patient's refusal for surgical treatment. For legal protection, the surgeon should also obtain from the patient, parent, or legal guardian a written refusal for the procedure or other treatment. The physician is required to inform the patient of the consequences of refusing diagnostic tests or therapeutic procedures.

Second Opinion

If the surgeon or patient has doubts about the necessity of a procedure, another opinion should be sought from a qualified specialist in the appropriate field of surgery. Consultation is a common and desirable part of good surgical practice. A second opinion may be required by third-party payers (i.e., insurance carriers) or managed care services. This is particularly indicated if the surgical procedure involves extended disability. Policy may require special consultation or consent for procedures resulting in reproductive sterilization or a pregnancy termination.

Advance Directives

The Patient Self-Determination Act (PSDA) enacted by the U.S. Congress in December 1991 ensures the patient the opportunity to participate in decision-making before a procedure. The law requires that patients be informed of their rights to make their own decisions regarding health care. This act applies to hospitals, nursing homes, home health care agencies, hospice programs, and health maintenance organizations. It does not apply to freestanding ambulatory or office settings. If a patient has advanced directives in place, a conversation with the surgeon and staff should take place to clarify actions in the event of an emergency. In 2016, CMS issued a final rule allowing advanced care planning conversations and counseling to be reimbursed under the physician fee schedule.

Each patient has the right to determine the care received and participate in the selection of delivery methods. The caregiver has the obligation to respect the patient's wishes regarding that care. This right extends to the issue of refusing treatment. Policies should be in place to provide for making patients aware of their right of self-determination.

The term advance directive encompasses durable power of attorney and living wills. The living will concept allows the patient to refuse treatment or nonessential measures to prolong life in a hopeless situation. A *durable power of attorney* document designates the person authorized to make decisions in the event that the patient is incapacitated. It allows the wishes of patients concerning their care needs to be met if they become impaired and cannot make decisions. The durable power of attorney does not apply to pediatric patients or to incompetent adults who are already under legal guardianship. These patients already have decision-makers available to decide treatment options.

On admission to the facility, the patient is asked whether an advance directive or durable power of attorney form has been completed. A federal regulation requires that the institution be aware of whether such a document exists and enact it in the event of impaired cognitive function of the patient. The perioperative team should be made aware of its existence. A copy, not the original, is placed in the patient's record. Advance directives may also indicate the patient's preferences concerning organ donation. The family is still asked for consent before any procurement occurs after the patient's death. In some states, the family has the right to refuse procurement regardless of the patient's last wishes.

Documentation of Perioperative Patient Care

Verbal communication between patients and health care providers does not constitute legal documentation of care. Entries in the record by nurses and physicians provide a history of the patient's clinical course and responses to treatment. The record serves to identify what was done. The broad assumption is that if something is not documented, it was not done. The record serves as a means of communication among providers for continuity of care. Policies and procedures should be in place for documentation. Each patient care facility is responsible for the following:

- Establishing, evaluating, and enforcing policies and procedures for patient care documentation
- Interpreting and outlining standards for care documentation in accordance with accreditation guidelines
- Protecting the privacy of patients by preventing unauthorized access and use of documented patient care data and reports
- Creating forms and charting formats for personnel to use in hard copy, and computer documentation
- Selecting protocol for computerized archives of patient care records and reports
- Providing a timely mechanism for retrieval of archived patient care records and reports for reference in a timely manner for routine or emergency care

All interactions with patients should be documented in the patient's medical record in the appropriate format. Regardless of the format or the media used for the patient's record, all entries should be:

- Documented on the appropriate form (e.g., code sheet, perioperative record, medication sheet, progress note).
- Written legibly in ink without erasures. The charting procedure may be specific (e.g., all entries are to be made in black ink if paper charting is used).
- Stated factually. Documentation of objective data and services rendered should be very specific. Observations and actions should be stated definitively, objectively, and concisely. Record what is seen, heard, felt, or smelled (i.e., the facts without judgment or opinion). Write quotes of the patient's subjective expression.
- Stated in understandable terminology. Abbreviations may be permissible only for very commonly accepted medical terms (e.g., T&A, D&C, TUR). Most institutions provide a standard list of their accepted medical abbreviations for charting purposes.
- Dated (month, day, year), including the time (AM/PM) the note is written and the time an action was performed as appropriate for significant events or changes in the patient's condition. Late entries are documented as per facility policy. Computerized entries are date stamped.
- Signed with the full legal signature, title, and status of the writer, either in permanent ink or electronically.
- Corrected if an error is made. The date, time, and initials of the person making a correction should be noted next to the correction. A single line should be drawn through incorrect information on a paper document without obliterating it (the mistake should not be scribbled out or erased), and the correct information should then be entered. Correction fluid is not acceptable. If an entire page must be recopied, the original is attached to the new copy and not destroyed.

Additional documentation in the patient's record should include the following:

- Execution of the physician's orders and the patient's responses
- Any teaching of the patient, family, or significant others, including documentation of understanding
- Any unusual event, such as a fall, spontaneous change in condition, or injury
- All visitors, especially physicians
- Any notification of physicians or supervisors

The perioperative nurse should be alert to signs that a patient does not clearly understand what is going to happen as a result of surgical intervention. This should be documented and brought to the attention of the surgeon. Significant observations should be recorded in the chart. For example, if a patient verbally withdraws consent for a surgical procedure or expresses a fear of death in the OR, the perioperative nurse is responsible for communicating this information to the surgeon and anesthesia provider and for recording the patient's statement.

Benefits of Documentation to the Facility

There are many reasons for accurate documentation other than those for legal application. Some facilities use the data for strategic planning and growth of the organization. Benefits of accurate documentation to the facility include, but are not limited to, the following:

- Legal permanent record
- Billing and reimbursement
- Performance improvement
- Measurement of clinical pathways
- Budget and financial planning
- Staffing ratios
- Research protocol
- Utilization review
- Risk management
- Patient acuity and census

Standards and Methods for Documentation of Patient Care

The standards for patient care documentation are established by the American Nurses Association (ANA) and TJC. The standard of care requires that patient care documentation reflect the application of the nursing process (assessment, nursing diagnosis, planning/outcome identification, intervention, and evaluation) during the entire length of stay, according to the ANA and TJC. The use of the perioperative nursing data set (PNDS) is the method of choice for perioperative patient care documentation. The PNDS provides a standardized universal language for patient care documentation and is used by many surgical computer information system manufacturers.

Charting Modalities

Many ways of recording patient care information have been used over the years. Changes in technology have created more methods of recording patient care. Examples of documentation methods include the following:

- *Narrative charting.* Expository writing about significant events using third-person commentary, quotes, and standard abbreviations. Entries are sequential, timed, dated, and signed.
- *Block charting.* Short commentary on activity that resembles narrative charting covering a longer period of several hours or days. Entries are sequential, timed, dated, and signed. Some facilities use a checklist format.
- *Focus charting.* Specific documentation directed at a designated aspect of the patient's needs, status, or health considerations. Example: FDAR—focused, data, action, response.
- *Subjective-objective charting (subjective-objective assessment plan [SOAP] or SOAP(IE) [SOAP + intervention and evaluation]).* Multidisciplinary approach to documenting care according to

cues given by a patient with a specific set of signs and symptoms. This approach uses direct quotes and assessment data.

- *Problem-oriented charting (problem-oriented medical record [POMR]).* Approach using a problem list as the working element from which care is planned. Working from the list, patient priorities are investigated, diagnosed, treated, minimized, solved, or remain ongoing. As problems are solved, they are removed from the list.
- *Computer-generated charting.* Use of standardized care plans formulated in the computer and modified for the individual patient. The computer time and date stamps the plan as it is printed for the hard copy record. This form of charting requires the caregiver's signature.
- *Computer information systems, check-off forms, and flow sheets.* Commonly used as shortcuts for recordkeeping. Unfortunately, it is easy to rely on the standardized data on these preprinted records and inadvertently omit potentially important individualized information. Most computerized patient records have secondary documentation fields to complete for individualized data capture.

Computerized Documentation

Many facilities have been using computers for patient admitting, billing, scheduling, and human resource information for several decades. Within the past decade, patient data have been recorded and stored electronically at the patient care unit level. Referred to as *electronic health records* (EHRs) or *electronic medical records* (EMRs), the documentation is transmitted electronically to multiple sites, including the OR, surgeon's offices, patient care areas, and other health care facilities around the world. Only select personnel are permitted to access this information and must log on using employee identification and passwords to enter the computer system. Documenting under another individual's name and password is against facility policy. Passwords are changed at routine intervals as determined by the patient care facility.

Retrievable data recorded and accumulated in these electronic files include patient care information, laboratory results, surgical reports, admission and discharge summaries, and many highly sensitive details about a patient's financial status. Many larger multihospital systems use the internet to permit multiple record access points for office-based physicians, surgeons, and the patient. All authorized users have access to reports and health data as soon as they are entered into the system.

Nurses charged with the responsibility of accessing and contributing to computerized patient data should be aware that security and confidentiality must be protected. Failing to maintain the secrecy of passwords and failing to log off after use are common problems identified with unauthorized access. Some systems have a built-in log-off feature if the workstation is left idle for a prolonged period. If this happens, the user has to reenter the system by logging back on.

Perioperative Documentation

Specific care given in the perioperative environment should be documented on the patient's chart. Most facilities use a preprinted form with a standardized plan of care. Space is provided to add individualized patient needs and to document additional interventions. Data included in the record come from several patient care areas.

PROS/CONS

Computerized Documentation

Pros

- Terminology is standardized.
- Abbreviations are standardized.
- Useful for accumulation of data from many sources.
- Data retrieval is easier and efficient.
- Information is legible and in standard terminology.
- Uses standardized formats, flowcharts, and graphs.
- All entries and printing are time and date stamped.
- Can minimize errors if orders are entered online instead of handwritten.
- Data can be transferred electronically between physician's office and care facility.
- Record updating is more timely and ongoing.
- Can save time, space, and resources.
- Easier to retrieve archived charts from previous admissions.
- Health care organizations with multiple remote sites can transfer patient data online.

Cons

- Can be confusing for inexperienced users.
- Failure to log off can leave the system available to unauthorized use.
- Can be out of service for undetermined periods.
- Needs periodic maintenance and software updates.
- Backups of files are needed in case of failure.
- Paper records must be kept when the system is down.
- Impersonal interaction between patient and caregivers.
- Preoutlined care plans are less individualized.
- Hardware and software can be costly to install.
- Potential for breach of security if files are transferred online.
- Charting can be easily recorded under the wrong patient.
- Detailed information may be left out because the user only clicks on items from a checklist that applies to the patient.

A comprehensive checklist is included with the chart to assist the circulating nurse to determine whether all of the data initiating Universal Protocol are included on the chart (see Fig. 3.1). Expected outcomes should be specified (e.g., the patient is free from injury). The circulating nurse should document specific activities performed to achieve the expected outcomes. The permanent perioperative record should include, but not be limited to, the following:

- Preoperative history and physical (H&P) examination, laboratory reports, consent form(s), and other documents in the chart per policy. Any area on the patient's body with redness or injury before hands-on care begins must be documented as "present on admission."
- Patient identification and surgical site verification, intended surgical procedure, allergies, nothing-by-mouth (NPO) status, and pregnancy status (test if appropriate).
- Significant intraoperative times, such as arrival in and departure from the OR, anesthesia start and finish, and incision and closure.
- Patient's condition on transfer to and from the OR, as well as the method of transport to and from the OR, and by whom. Any change in the patient's skin integrity, such as redness or injury, should be documented as "not present on admission."
- Level of consciousness or anxiety manifested by objective observation.

- Patient position, and types of restraints and supports used for maintaining the patient's position on the OR bed and for protecting pressure areas, and by whom.
- Personal property disposition, such as prosthetics, wigs, jewelry, false eyelashes, religious articles, hearing aid, eyeglasses, contact lenses, and dentures.
- Skin condition and antimicrobials used for skin preparation, and by whom.
- Intravenous (IV) site, time started, type of needle or cannula, solutions administered IV (including blood products and antibiotics), and by whom.
- Medication types and amounts (including local anesthetic agents), irrigating solutions used and amounts, and given by whom.
- Tourniquet cuff location, pressure, inflation duration, identification of unit, and applied by whom.
- Estimated blood loss and urinary output, as appropriate.

- Sponge, sharps, and instrument counts as correct or incorrect. If inconclusive, state steps taken in remedy of the situation and notification steps taken.
- Surgical procedure performed and location of the incision.
- Specific equipment used (e.g., laser), electrosurgical unit, dispersive and monitoring electrode(s), and prosthetic devices implanted, if applicable, including the manufacturer and lot/serial number.
- Specimens and cultures sent to the laboratory.
- Site and types of drains, catheters, and packing as applicable.
- Wound classification is documented at the end of the procedure when all risks for infection have been identified.
- Type of dressing(s) applied and location.
- Any unusual event or complication, and action performed.
- All personnel in the room and their roles, including physicians, visitors, vendors, students, and others as applicable.

PROS/CONS

Patient Handover

Pros
- A handover is defined as a linear transmission of information and responsibility from one qualified caregiver to another.
- TJC recommends a standardized handover in their National Patient Safety Goals. It is called the Targeted Solutions Tool (TST) for Hand-off Communications.
- AORN also has recommendations for transferring patient care information.
- Standardized protocols are recommended because the handover of patients to another health care provider is reported as a high-risk time associated with sentinel events.
- Every facility should establish a format for standardized handoff/handover protocols and policies. Standardized protocols provide critical patient information necessary for safe patient transfer and reduction in communication breakdown.
- Many standardized communication and documentation models exist. Examples of standardized documentation formats include the following:
  1. SBAR (Situation, Background, Assessment, and Recommendation)
  2. I PASS THE BATON (Introduction, Patient, Assessment, Situation, Safety)
  3. Concerns, Background, Actions, Timing, Ownership, Next
  4. SHARED (Situation, History, Assessment, Request, Evaluate, and Document)
  5. SURPASS (SURgical Patient Safety System)
- Handover reporting improved when health care facilities established a format of standardized tools, checklists, and protocols. These protocols can be written, verbal, and or electronic methods of accurate documentation and communication.
- Handover communication improved when personnel were educated about the standardized protocols and policies. Positive education methods include role playing, competency training, case studies, anticipated patient needs, and simulation.

- Professional attributes that improve receiving handover reports include completing all necessary physiologic tasks before report begins (attaching monitors, securing the patient), reducing noise and distractions, improving listening skills, using standard vocabulary, asking questions, taking notes, and reading back information to verify. The person taking the report signs the document and records the names of the personnel giving the report.

Cons
- Communication breakdown has been documented as the root cause of many sentinel events.
- Problems and errors related to poor handover include room noise, rushing, errors on record, distractions, multitasking, change of staff, lack of information, personnel physiologic problems, relationship barriers, lack of experience, reporting before the procedure is finished, and number of personnel involved in the handover process.
- More research is needed to identify an error-free transfer of information to improve patient outcomes. The current standardization protocols still have breakdowns in communication, putting patients at risk for injury.

References
1. Webster K, Keebler J, Chaparro, et al.: Handoffs and teamwork: a framework for care transition communication, *Jt Comm J Qual Patient Saf* 48(6–7):343–353, 2022.
2. Burns S, Parikh R, Schuller K: Utilization of a checklist to standardize the operating room to post-anesthesia care unit patient handoff process, *Periop Care OR Manage* 13:1–5, 2018, 2018.
3. AORN: *Transfer of patient care information: guidelines for perioperative practice*, Denver, CO, 2024, AORN, Inc.
4. Fitzgerald K, Banerji T, Starmer A, et al.: Effect of a multispeciality faculty handoff initiative on safety culture and handoff quality, *Pediatr Qual Saf* 7(2):e539, 2022.

- Falls or unexpectedly finding a patient, visitor, or other personnel lying on the floor
- Injury to patient, visitor, or other personnel
- Needlesticks
- Any fire or smoke event
- Possible theft or loss of an item
- Malfunctioning equipment
- Intruder or unauthorized personnel
- Medication error
- Medication reaction
- Lost sponge or instrument during a procedure (incorrect and unresolved count)
- Object retained within patient

Incident Report

When an accident or unusual incident occurs involving a patient, employee, or property in the facility, the factual details should be reported to the nurse manager and documented according to institutional policy. Details should be objective, complete, and accurate. They should be written as statements of facts without interpretation or opinion. For example, it should be stated that the area of the patient's skin under the inactive dispersive electrode of the electrosurgical unit was mottled and red when the electrode was removed, rather than that the patient's skin appeared burned by the dispersive electrode. The details of equipment used, including the serial number or asset tag identification of the generator and the lot number of the electrode, should be included.

The action performed as a result of any adverse event should be described in detail. Any equipment in question should be removed from service and tagged as "out of order" for repair by the biomedical personnel of the facility. Any suspect device should be inspected and reapproved for use according to institutional policy before it is returned to service. All devices suspected of being defective and their identifying wrappers should be secured for inspection by the facility's risk management personnel.

Incident reports are completed per policy and retained by the risk management department. They should be reviewed as part of the overall institution and departmental quality improvement and risk management programs. Incident reports are considered work products and constitute privileged information. They may serve to refresh an individual's memory of events, however, for preparation of defense in a lawsuit. The fact that an incident report was completed should not be documented in the patient's permanent record. Examples of situations that require incident reporting are included in Box 3.3.

Legal Aspects of Drugs and Medical Devices

In 1906, the U.S. government enacted the Pure Food and Drug Act, with the U.S. Department of Agriculture as the enforcing agency, to ensure the introduction of safe and sanitary foods and drugs to the public. The Food, Drug, and Cosmetic Act of 1938 extended the regulation to include cosmetics, drugs, and medical devices. The FDA, within the Department of Agriculture, became the enforcing agency with authority to implement a preclearance mechanism requiring drug manufacturers to provide evidence of safety before a new drug could be sold. Sutures were classified as drugs.

The Kefauver-Harris Drug Amendments of 1962 added strength to the new drug clearance procedures. Drug manufacturers must prove to the FDA the effectiveness, as well as the safety, of drugs before making them commercially available. These amendments established a mechanism for clinical investigation to evaluate the efficacy of drugs. Depending on the nature of a drug, clinical studies often require several years before the FDA approves commercial sale of a product.

The Medical Device Amendments of 1976 gave the FDA regulatory control over medical devices. A medical device is defined as any instrument, apparatus, or other similar or related article, including any component, part, or accessory, promoted for a medical purpose that does not rely on chemical action to achieve its intended purpose. Under this definition, sutures were reclassified as devices. All the wound closure materials discussed in this chapter are classified as devices.

In 1988, the FDA reclassified the regulation of many devices (single use and reusable), including surgical attire, masks, gloves, and drapes. Medical devices were classified and received FDA approval for safety and effectiveness before they were marketed. Today, a device is given a classification and listed as exempt or nonexempt. Some exempt devices that are similar to already produced devices can be manufactured without FDA approval. The medical devices are categorized into one of three classifications:

- Class I devices are subject to general regulatory controls that ensure they are as safe and effective as similar devices already being sold.
- Class II devices must establish safety and effectiveness performance standards for a new type of product.
- Class III devices are usually life-sustaining or life-supporting implants or external devices. The manufacturer must file for premarket approval before the device is tested clinically to substantiate effectiveness.

A mandatory device-reporting regulation was put into effect in 1984. This regulation requires manufacturers and importers to report to the FDA any death or serious injury to a patient as a result of the malfunction of a medical device. Through the Safe Medical Devices Act of 1990, health care facilities are required to report directly to the FDA and to the manufacturer the probability that a device caused or contributed to a patient's death, serious injury, or serious illness. Additional requirements for tracking certain permanently implantable devices became effective in 1993. Manufacturers are responsible for tracking devices from the manufacturing facility through the chain of distribution (purchasers) to the end users (patients). Health care facilities that implant and explant (remove) these devices must submit reports to manufacturers promptly after devices are received, implanted, and/or explanted. The manufacturer must be able to provide to the FDA the following specific information:

1. Device
   a. Lot, batch, model, and serial numbers or other identification used by the manufacturer
   b. Date(s) of receipt or acquisition within the chain of distribution
   c. Name(s) of person(s) or supplier from whom the device was received
2. Patient
   a. Date of implantation
   b. Name, address, and telephone number of the recipient patient

c. Social Security number, if the patient's permission is obtained to release the Social Security number to the manufacturer

3. Physician(s) who prescribed, implanted, and/or explanted the device

4. End-of-life information about the device, as applicable
   a. Date of explantation
   b. Date of patient's death
   c. Date the device was returned to the distributor or manufacturer
   d. Date the device was permanently retired from use or disposed of

The FDA monitors the voluntary MedWatch program to encourage physicians, nurses, pharmacists, and other health care professionals to report adverse events and defects or problems with regulated drugs and devices. The purpose of MedWatch is to provide a nationwide standardized system for reporting to the FDA any medical device or drug suspected of causing a patient's death, life-threatening injury or illness, disability, prolonged hospitalization, congenital anomaly, and/or experience that required intervention to prevent permanent health impairment. Adverse events can be reported online at www.fda.gov/Safety/MedWatch/. Examples of reportable problems include latex sensitivity, malfunction of drug infusion pumps, failure of an alarm during malfunction of a ventilator, and drug and vaccine reactions.

Surgeons who implant or use medical devices, and nurses, surgical technologists, and others who handle them, must be adequately instructed in the proper care and handling of all devices to ensure patient safety. Most adverse events occur when devices are misused, are defective, or malfunction. However, an adverse patient reaction can occur when the device functions properly and is used appropriately. The FDA is responsible for investigating a report of an adverse event or product problem and for taking corrective action.

Ethical Issues

Professions have codes of conduct and documents that include value statements derived from moral concepts. The Code of Ethics of the Association of Surgical Technologists (AST) provides guidance for surgical technologists. Nursing is regarded as one of the most noble professions according to patient polls. Patients expect nurses to be honest, ethical, and caring. Nurses refer to codes of ethics established by their own professional associations for guidance, such as the International Code of Ethics for Nurses (INC), ANA Code for Nurses, or the Code of Ethics for Nursing of the Canadian Nurses Association. Nurses are required to complete classes in ethics as part of a curriculum or as a requirement for license renewal.

In the statement of the nature and scope of nursing practice titled Nursing, a Social Policy Statement, developed by the ANA Congress of Practice in 1980, nurses committed to respect for human beings "unaltered by social, educational, economic, cultural, racial, religious or other specific attributes of human beings receiving care, including nature and duration of disease and illness." The ethics of a profession establish the role and scope of professional behavior and the nature of relationships with patients and colleagues.

> ### • BOX 3.4 Moral Principles in Decision-Making
>
> **Autonomy:** Self-determination implies freedom of choice and ability to make decisions to determine one's own course of action. Decisions may be made in collaboration with others, based on reasonable and prudent information. Decisions should be acknowledged and respected by others.
> **Beneficence:** Duty to help others seek balance between what is good to do and what might produce harm to another or self.
> **Nonmaleficence:** Duty to do no harm.
> **Justice:** Allocation of human, material, and technologic resources a person has a right to receive or claim (i.e., equality of care).
> **Veracity:** Devotion to truthfulness (i.e., to give accurate information).
> **Fidelity:** Quality of faithfulness, based on trust and honesty, which protects rights of individuals (e.g., dignity, privacy).
> **Confidentiality:** Respect for privileged information received from another person with disclosure only to appropriate others.

Universal moral principles guide ethical decision-making and activities in clinical practice (Box 3.4). These include the following:

- Values are operational beliefs an individual chooses as the basis for behavior. They may change over time. They may create conflicts when value systems are not compatible with the expectations of others. Values reflect ethics. Ethics refers to standards or principles of moral judgment and action. Ethics as a philosophy defines a systematic method of differentiating right from wrong within a specific belief system.
- Professional and societal codes and standards offer guidelines in this determination. Ethics and law are closely related. Legal doctrines often interpret ethical concepts.
- The Bill of Rights of the Constitution of the United States establishes individual rights based on moral principles that respect human worth and dignity. Some states have upheld the right to individual autonomy in making health care decisions, as evidenced by rulings about such issues as abortion, the right to die with dignity, and living wills.

Bioethical Situations

An ethical dilemma arises in the work situation when the choice between two or more alternatives creates a conflict between an individual's value system and moral obligation to the patient, to the family or significant others, to the physician, or to the employer and coworkers. Conflicts can be between rights, duties, and responsibilities.

Students and other caregivers should take the time to review the remaining pages in this chapter and make a personal determination about facing some of these situational ethics in practice. Personal moral-ethical conflicts can be avoided by having a predetermined sense of action when faced with situations involving procedures such as abortion, reproductive sterilization, experimentation, organ procurement, and end-of-life decisions. Actions may be governed by religious or philosophic beliefs. Each caregiver should have the opportunity to abstain or participate according to personal choice.

Both legal and ethical considerations can cause conflicts. Legally, a patient has the right to choose among treatment alternatives or the right to refuse treatment. Philosophically, the patient's preference may be different from that of the health care provider.

The primary responsibility to the patient is to ensure delivery of safe care. This includes use of appropriate and available technology, but only if this is the patient's choice, with informed consent freely given, or is known to be the patient's wish. Conversely, the patient and the caregiver may be forced to face court-ordered procedures or treatments. This may impose the need to assist in a surgical intervention such as a cesarean section on a woman who has moral or religious objections to this form of treatment but who has been ordered by the court to have the procedure performed for the benefit of the unborn fetus. Another example is when a patient refuses a blood transfusion for themselves or their child. The surgeon has to honor the adult patient's decision, even if it results in death. In the case of a minor, some states have laws or can obtain a court order against the parent's/guardian's wishes and provide lifesaving treatment.

These examples are extreme, but the courts are constantly working to define the rights of the unborn and children. In the issue of viability versus possible death, the court usually supports measures necessary to sustain life. The caregiver who participates in a court-ordered procedure is protected by law, provided that the performance of their duties meets the standards of care.

Caregivers should decide for themselves the appropriate course of action when dealing with an ethical dilemma. By developing a personal philosophy and by understanding both professional and institutional philosophies, the caregiver may better answer many personal ethical questions such as the following:

- When does life begin?
- When does it end?
- What is my perception of quality of life between conception and death?
- What is my role in health care?
- What is my role as patient advocate?
- What are my moral rights in relation to my personal beliefs and values and those of others?
- Where are the dividing lines between a patient's personal rights to privacy and confidentiality and a legal or ethical duty of disclosure?

A few of the ethical dilemmas facing physicians and perioperative personnel are mentioned for personal consideration. It also should be noted that some of these issues are regulated by state statutes or federal court decisions. All caregivers should be familiar with statutes in the state in which they practice, particularly those regarding participation and the right to refrain on the basis of personal beliefs. The right to refuse to participate may be covered by a law but not at the expense of a patient's safety and welfare. The patient cannot be harmed by acts of commission or omission.

Reproductive Sterilization

Voluntary reproductive sterilization as a contraceptive method may be contrary to the moral, ethical, or religious beliefs of a caregiver. Consent is required to perform reproductive sterilization. Some facilities require consent from a patient's spouse.

Abortion

Legalized abortion allows for induced termination of pregnancy. In the 1973 decision of *Roe v. Wade*, the U.S. Supreme Court ruled that any licensed physician can terminate pregnancy during the first trimester with the woman's consent. During the second trimester, the Court requires a state statute that regulates abortion on the basis of preservation and protection of maternal health. During the third trimester, legal abortion should consider meaningful life for the fetus outside the womb and endangerment to the mother's life and health. By selective abortion, one or more fertilized ova may be aborted so that others may mature properly in a multiple pregnancy, which is perhaps a result of fertility drugs.

In 2022, the U.S. Supreme Court overturned the *Roe v. Wade* legislation. The change in legislation is now in the hands of each state to make the decision concerning abortion. Many states have fully banned abortion or have restrictions on reproductive care. The change in legislation has caused turmoil for patients who rely on these services and health care providers. Many patients and health care providers must now travel to states where abortion is still legal. The impact of these changes can put patients at risk for finding safe efficient care. In states where abortion is illegal, health care providers can no longer provide services.

In facilities where abortions and other reproductive procedures are performed, employees have the right to refrain from participation because of their moral, ethical, or religious beliefs except in an emergency that threatens the life of the mother. These beliefs should be made known to the employer in writing. Some states have a protective statute for employees and employers regulating good-faith efforts to accommodate employees' beliefs. In other states, laws protect an employee from being forced by an employer to assist in abortions.

Human Experimentation

Procedures still in developmental stages are performed in clinical research—oriented facilities with the patient's informed consent. Human experimentation currently includes cases such as face transplants, uterine transplants, genetic alteration of fetuses, and transplanted organs from other species (xenotransplantation). Those willing to be pioneers in human experimentation have given or will give hope to many patients with poor prognoses. A caregiver should make a personal decision to participate in experimental surgery.

Fetal Tissue and Stem Cell Research

Experimentation with human tissues may be of moral concern to some individuals. The acquisition of the tissues may take place in the OR in the form of embryonic tissue, and the implantation may take place in the OR. Fetal tissue lacks lymphocytes that can cause graft-versus-host response. Advantages of fetal tissue include rapid proliferation of cells, quick reversal of the host's condition, and differentiation in response to cues of the host tissue. Studies have shown promise in the treatment of diabetes mellitus, Parkinson disease, and certain blood disorders and that the fetal tissue used in the treatment of Parkinson disease continues to proliferate and function for many years after transplant. Tissue from spontaneous abortion and ectopic pregnancy has generally undergone pathologic degradation and is not suitable for this use. The use of fetal tissue and organs is subject to state law.

Scientists and researchers are trying to grow cells from animals such as sheep, rats, mice, pigs, and primates to grow organs for transplantation into humans. Stem cells from primates have shown promise because of the similarity to human cells.

Ethical issues may arise for some health care providers in cases of xenotransplantation. Organs from pigs have been transplanted in humans as heart valves, kidneys, and a heart. In 2022, a modified pig heart was transplanted into a human patient who was brain dead and on ventilator. The transplant was successful, but the patient lived for only 61 days. Information about other cases and research on xenotransplantation can be found at www.fda.gov/xenotransplantation.

HIV and Other Infections

The prevalence of human immunodeficiency virus (HIV) infection, with or without acquired immunodeficiency syndrome (AIDS), created devastating health problems with many inherent emotional issues. Unlike other communicable diseases, HIV infection is an illness with no known cure at this time, although current drug therapies may slow its progression and leave the patient with an undetectable viral load. Its mode of transmission and methods of prevention are known. Therefore personal biases and prejudices should not discriminate against the infected patient. However, underlying attitudes about homosexuality and IV drug abuse may subconsciously influence the care of such patients. Are HIV-positive patients any different from patients with hemophilia or those who became infected through a contaminated blood transfusion? Should the infant with HIV be treated any differently from an infant with a congenital anomaly? Does the diagnosis make a difference to the health care provider and to the quality of care that the patient receives?

Knowing that HIV infection is transmitted by blood and body secretions, conscientious application of standard precautions for infection control should provide protection against occupational exposure to HIV, hepatitis, tuberculosis, and other communicable or resistant infections. The ANA Code for Nurses emphasizes that care is given regardless of the nature of health problems.

Other ethical questions concern screening and the reporting of test results versus confidentiality. Do the same considerations apply to team members as to patients? What constitutes valid reasons for restricting or terminating employment based on health status? This question has broader implications than just the issue of being seropositive for HIV. No state mandates by law that a health care worker can refuse to provide care for a patient with HIV infection. Risks versus benefits to self, patients, and team members, plus potential litigation as a result of actions, should be evaluated in making ethical decisions. Confidentiality, privacy, and informed consent are human rights that should be protected, but the right to health care should be protected also.

Both AORN and AST have published statements encouraging health care facilities to provide policies and procedures to ensure the safety of patients and personnel. These organizations believe that providers have a right to know the HIV or other infectious status of patients but that caregivers do not have the right to discriminate against HIV-positive patients. They should follow the Centers for Disease Control and Prevention guidelines in caring for all patients to prevent transmission of infection.

Quality of Life

Surgeons often must make critical decisions before or during surgical interventions regarding the quality of patients' lives after surgical procedures. Palliative procedures may prolong life and relieve pain.[4] Therapeutic procedures may be disfiguring. Life-support systems may sustain vital functions. Life-sustaining therapy may prolong the dying process. Many questions arise regarding care of terminally ill, severely debilitated or injured, and comatose patients. What will be the outcome in terms of mental or physical competence? When should cardiopulmonary resuscitation be initiated or discontinued? Physicians decide, but all team members are affected by the decisions.

Patients with advance directives have made many of these difficult decisions while in a lucid mental state. This saves the family, significant others, or legal guardians the anguish of making the decision during times of duress. This helps provide some closure and a small sense of satisfaction that the loved one's wishes were known and followed.

Euthanasia

How is euthanasia defined? Is mercy killing ethical, legal, or justified? Does the patient, family or guardian, physicians, or courts have the right to decide to abandon heroic measures to sustain life? The patient who is aware of the options and whose decision-making capacity is intact has the right of self-determination. OR personnel develop the plan of care guided by an advance directive.

Euthanasia is derived from the Greek words meaning "good or merciful death." Both active euthanasia and passive euthanasia are intentional acts that cause death, but the methods are different. An act of direct intervention that causes death is active euthanasia. Withholding or withdrawing life-prolonging or life-sustaining measures is passive euthanasia. Death is caused by the underlying disease process, trauma, or physiologic dysfunction. This concept differs from physician-assisted suicide. Suicide involves the person voluntarily causing self-demise.

The idea of euthanasia seems to violate traditional principles of medicine to preserve life, but our modern technologies can prolong life without preserving quality. Quality of life can be interpreted as life that has a meaningful value. Most humans value having cognitive abilities, physical capabilities, or both, and living free of undue pain and suffering. This raises the ethical question of whether physicians should do what they technologically can do.

Right to Die

Courts have determined that patients have a constitutional right to privacy in choosing to die with dignity or a common law right to withhold consent and refuse treatment. A mentally competent adult older than the age of 18 years can execute a living will, an advance directive, directing physicians and other health care providers not to use extraordinary measures to prolong life. Most physicians designate "extraordinary" measures as those that are optional, such as mechanical respiration, hydration, nutrition, medication, or a combination of these and that sustain life. If it is the expressed wish of the patient, the physician writes do-not-resuscitate (DNR) or allow-natural-death (AND) orders.[5]

A living will relieves family members of decision-making when the patient becomes terminally ill, incompetent, or comatose. No laws or court precedents deal specifically with the issue of DNR orders in the perioperative environment. Institutional policy should address this matter. Theoretically, a patient can attempt to sue for compensation for expenses under a negligence or battery charge. In general, courts are reluctant to hold health care workers liable for acts performed to maintain life. In *Anderson v. St. Francis*, defibrillation was performed despite a DNR order. The court found that sustaining life was not considered an injury and rejected the compensatory claim.

A patient who has a standing DNR or AND order may require a procedure to decrease pain or palliate uncomfortable symptoms. Before going to the OR, the DNR or AND order should be reaffirmed with the patient, family, significant others, guardian, or person who has durable power of attorney. The status of the DNR or AND order must be clarified before the patient goes to the OR. In an emergency, if there is doubt about the validity of the DNR order or a question concerning reconsideration of the order, the caregiver should participate in resuscitation. If there is any question about the patient changing their mind, a second chance may not be an option during an emergency. If the patient, family, significant others, or legal guardian is specifically clear about upholding the DNR order in the OR, the team has the responsibility to follow the patient's wishes. A caregiver who has a moral objection to upholding a DNR order may request reassignment through the nurse manager of the department.

The issue of discontinuation of life-sustaining measures becomes more difficult in a comatose, mentally incompetent patient who has not executed an advance directive. Family members or significant others, in consultation with physicians, may request DNR orders. Caregivers are obligated to understand and follow DNR orders.[5]

Organ Donation and Transplantation

As a result of the Uniform Anatomical Gift Act of 1968, many adults carry cards stating that at death they wish to donate their body organs or parts for transplantation, therapy, medical research, or education. Most states include this information on a driver's license. If this legal authority is not available, some states have a required request law. In the event of legally defined brain death, the caregivers are required by this law to ask the family or significant others if they wish to allow organ retrieval for transplantation.

Transplant surgeons rely on the perioperative patient care teams who procure donor organs, eyes, bone, and skin. Organ transplantation has complicated the issue of time of death. Perfusion of oxygenated blood through tissues must be sustained by artificial means during procurement of vital organs with functional viability. Brain death must be clearly established before procurement can proceed.

Legally, death has occurred when an individual has sustained either irreversible cessation of circulation and respiratory functions or irreversible cessation of all functions of the entire brain, including the brainstem. Therefore the accepted definition of irreversible coma for potential donors includes unresponsiveness, no spontaneous movements of respiration, no reflexes, and a flat electroencephalogram.

When brain death is determined by two physicians who are not part of the transplant team, the donor will be taken to the OR with artificial support systems functioning to perfuse organs. Some caregivers have moral questions about assisting with removal of viable organs from seemingly living bodies. When the heart is removed, cardiopulmonary support is discontinued and the anesthesia personnel leave the room. This is a difficult time for the remaining team who may still have the assignment of procuring nonperfused tissues, such as skin, bone, or eyes.

Perioperative caregivers who believe that donation of organs and body parts is a gift of love find it easier and ethically acceptable to participate in procurement procedures. Family members of donors have been encouraged by surgical team members not to focus on their grief, but rather to focus on the gifts of life they are giving unselfishly to the recipients. This does not mean that the donor's family will not go through the grieving process. They will need support. Caregivers learn to cope with feelings associated with the procurement of donor organs in a manner similar to dealing with the sudden death of any patient in the perioperative environment.

Death and Dying

Intellectually we know that death is inevitable. Death can be a difficult burden for caregivers to bear because our education, experience, and philosophy are dedicated to survival. Regardless of religious or cultural beliefs, death is a mystery, a passage from the known to the unknown. Perhaps partially for this reason, the death of a patient in the OR is an unsettling experience, especially if it is unexpected.

One of the most difficult aspects of a death in the OR for the team members is the period after the actual event. The surgeon goes to inform the family. The assistants and anesthesia provider leave the room. Often the perioperative team is left alone with the patient's body. The patient should be prepared so that the family or significant others can view the body in an area adjoining the perioperative environment, where they can have privacy in expressing their feelings. The perioperative nurse may be expected to accompany them and to lend support during the viewing. A chaplain or other clergy should be called if desired by the family. Specific departmental policies should be developed to assist the caregiver with this difficult aspect of patient care. Coping strategies that can help team members may include the following:

- Realize that everyone involved is part of a team effort.
- Believe in a power greater than the skills of the team.
- Share feelings with others. It is helpful for perioperative patient care team members to talk with each other about what happened. Encourage each other to share feelings associated with the loss. Crying is acceptable behavior.
- Deal with the patient's death by identifying personally with the loss. Empathy is a positive emotion. Working through the grieving process brings a sense of closure to the relationship.
- Some facilities provide support groups to help staff members and the bereaved deal with death.
Arrange a visit with the hospital chaplain, clergy, or rabbi.

ⓔ EVOLVE WEBSITE

http://evolve.elsevier.com/Hornacky/BerryKohn/

- Historical Perspective
- Glossary

References

1. Department of Health and Human Services: HIPAA basics for providers: privacy, security, breach notification rules. www.hhs.gov/HIPAA. Accessed January 13, 2023.
2. New HIPAA regulations in 2023. www.hipaajournal.com. Accessed January 14, 2023.
3. Guidance for performing root cause analysis (RCA) with performance improvement projects (PIPs). www.cms.gov. Accessed January 15, 2023.
4. House S: Palliative and end-of-life care. *Conn's current therapy*, St. Louis, 2023, Elsevier, pp. 42–48, Elsevier.
5. Iserson K, Heine C: Bioethics. *Rosen's emergency medicine: concepts and clinical practice*, ed 10, St. Louis, 2023, Elsevier, pp. e51–e63.

Bibliography

AORN: *Guidelines for perioperative practice*, Denver, CO, 2024, AORN, Inc.
Rothrock J. In *Alexander's care of the patient in surgery*, ed 17, St. Louis, 2023, Elsevier.

4

The Perioperative Patient Care Team and Professional Credentialing

CHAPTER OUTLINE

Dependence of the Patient on the Qualified Team, 56
Credentialing of Qualified Caregivers, 56

Perioperative Patient Care Team, 56

CHAPTER OBJECTIVES

After studying this chapter, the learner will be able to:

- Define the concept of the sterile team.
- Define the concept of the nonsterile team.
- Describe the role of the circulating nurse.

- Describe the role of the scrub person.
- Describe the credentialing process for perioperative nurses.
- Describe the credentialing process for surgical technologists.

KEY TERMS AND DEFINITIONS

Anesthesia provider Member of the nonsterile team who administers anesthetics during the surgical procedure; may be a physician (MD, DO), anesthesia assistant (AA), or a specially trained and certified registered nurse anesthetist (CRNA).

Certification A method of professional evaluation and recognition of an individual for meeting educational, practice, and national standard parameters that extend above minimal competency.

Circulating nurse Perioperative registered nurse (RN) member of the nonsterile team who directs and coordinates the activities of the intraoperative environment during the surgical procedure. Role involves patient assessment, planning, and critical thinking skills.

Credentials Validation of professional recognition, such as licensure or certification.

Delegation A registered nurse or physician can assign and supervise tasks performed by a licensed practical nurse/licensed vocational nurse (LPN/LVN), surgical technologist (ST), or other unlicensed assistive personnel (UAP), provided the tasks are not intended for a licensed individual's scope of practice and are within the capabilities of the person being assigned the tasks.

Licensure Governmental regulation of approval to practice in a specific profession to provide specific services. Practicing without a license is illegal and punishable by law. Some license renewals include attainment of continued education in the profession. Licensure is designed to ensure minimal competency of the licensee for the benefit of protecting the safety and welfare of the public. The laws that define the scope of

practice governing a registered professional are called practice acts.

Nonsterile team Intraoperative caregivers who provide direct care from the periphery of the sterile field and environment; do not wear sterile attire (e.g., radiology technician, anesthesia technologist).

Perianesthesia nurse RN who renders care in the preoperative and postoperative environment. Member of the nonsterile team.

Registration Establishing a record of name, address, and qualifications of a professional with a state authority. This does not establish standards of practice, does not require a certain entry level, and does not provide for continued competency verification or continued education. Proof of continued education is required for relicensure and renewal of registration.

Scrub person Member of the sterile team who passes instruments and facilitates the surgical procedure. Is an ST, RN, or LPN/LVN.

Sterile team Intraoperative caregivers who provide direct care within the sterile field; wear sterile attire (e.g., surgeon, first assistant, scrub person).

Surgeon Physician (e.g., MD, DO, DDS, DPM) who performs the surgical procedure.

Surgical assistant Member of the sterile team who provides exposure and hemostasis during a surgical procedure. Is a physician, registered nurse first assistant (RNFA), surgical assistant (SA), physician assistant (PA), or certified surgical technologist specially trained and certified as a first assistant (CST/CFA).

Dependence of the Patient on the Qualified Team

The perioperative team works to always promote the best interests of the patient. For the welfare and safety of the patient, the entire team must work efficiently as a functioning single unit. The members should be thoroughly familiar with procedures, setups, equipment, and policies and should be able to cope with the unpredictable. Individual qualifications must be beyond reproach. Team members should have a high morale, mutual understanding, trust, cooperation, and consideration. Anyone who cannot function wholeheartedly as a qualified team member has no place in the operating room (OR).

All OR personnel should have the proven knowledge, skill, competency, and ability to perform at an optimal level at all times. The validation of clinical competence is an important aspect of providing safe patient care. Once each member of the team has passed the novice stage, other criteria demonstrate and document the knowledge and skills gained through experience and continuing education. Aligning professionally with local, state, and nationally recognized organizations that establish guidelines and standards of practice provides an opportunity for growth. Credentialing and certification may include completing a course of instruction or meeting certain criteria and passing an examination. Other measurements of competence include performance evaluations in a clinical setting.

Credentialing of Qualified Caregivers

Credentialing refers to the processes of accreditation, licensure, and certification of institutions, agencies, and individuals. These processes establish quality, identity, protection, and control for the competency-based education and performance of professional and allied technical health care personnel. Credentialing also protects the public from fraudulent practitioners.

Accreditation of Schools and Facilities

An accrediting body of a voluntary organization evaluates and sanctions an educational program or an institution as meeting predetermined standards and/or essential criteria. Several organizations are involved in the accreditation of nursing schools, such as the National League for Nursing (NLN), the Commission for Nursing Education Accreditation (CNEA), the Commission on Collegiate Nursing Education (CCNE), and the Accreditation Commission for Education in Nursing (ACEN). Surgical technology programs are accredited by the Commission on Accreditation of Allied Health Education Programs (CAAHEP) after a satisfactory review and recommendation by the Accreditation Review Council on Education in Surgical Technology and Surgical Assisting (ARC-STSA).

The National Board of Surgical Technology and Surgical Assisting (NBSTSA) offers certification eligibility to individuals graduating from an accredited surgical technology program. The Accrediting Bureau of Health Education Schools (ABHES) accredits many colleges and vocational settings in the United States. Certifying and licensing bodies require graduation from an accredited program before eligibility criteria are met to take professional certification or licensing examinations.

The Joint Commission (TJC) accredits hospitals and ambulatory care centers. Other professional organizations offer accreditation for special-interest groups.

Licensure and Registration

A license to practice is granted to professionals by a governmental agency, such as the state board of nursing or medicine. Licensure implies a certain amount of appropriate independence in actions. On completion of a formal academic education, nurses and physicians who successfully pass a state examination receive a license to practice in that state. To maintain this license, they must register with the state as required by law; hence the term *registered nurse* (RN). Licensed practical nurses/licensed vocational nurses (LPN/LVNs) also are licensed.

Most states grant a license by reciprocity or endorsement to applicants who wish to practice in their state but who took the examination in another state. Many states allow for multistate nursing licensure with renewal and required continued education. Some states require licensure for some categories of allied health occupations, such as physical therapists, occupational therapists, and radiographers.

Licensure is not offered on an indefinite basis. Applicants apply for renewal at specific time intervals determined by each state. Many states require proof of continuing education for nurses and physicians as a prerequisite for eligibility of relicensure.

Registration is a method of state regulation of practice parameters and designation for disciplinary action. Perioperative nurses are *registered* as well as *licensed*. The goal of registration is to establish a means for protecting the safety parameters for patients and the public.

Certification

A nongovernmental private organization can award a credential that attests to level of knowledge above minimal competency of an individual who meets predetermined qualifications. Certification may be defined as documented validation of an individual's professional achievement of knowledge and skill in identified standards. To be certified is to demonstrate the attainment of more than minimal competency; it is a statement of certification-level knowledge. Certification is an additional or specialized form of a credential.[1]

Certification is granted for a limited time. To retain this credential, an individual must complete the recertification process established by the certifying body. For recertification, some certifying organizations require a specified number of clinical hours, continuing education contact hours, a written or computer-generated examination, or a combination of these in a portfolio format. Maintaining certification by going through this process demonstrates a high level of motivation and commitment to the profession.

Physicians, nurses, and allied health care personnel may be certified by their professional specialty association as competent in knowledge and skills to practice. Applicants take an examination that tests knowledge in the area of specialization. This is often referred to as *board certification*. For example, a surgeon can be board certified in a particular branch of surgery.

Perioperative Patient Care Team

The perioperative patient care team is like a symphony orchestra, with each person an integral entity in unison and harmony with professional colleagues to accomplish the expected outcomes. Communication using a comprehensive surgical checklist and briefing can provide a seamless interface between patient care areas and minimize the risk for error (see Fig. 2.1).

Preoperatively, the perianesthesia nurse or anesthesia provider initiates the use of the comprehensive surgical checklist and performs the preoperative assessment. The surgeon should mark the surgical site with an indelible ink marker. The patient is transferred to the care of the surgical team, and information concerning the patient's condition is communicated verbally and in writing.

In the OR, the patient is surrounded by the surgeon, the surgical assistant, the scrub person, the anesthesia provider, and the circulating nurse. Before the procedure begins, the OR team stops all activities for the "time out" and reaffirms the correct patient is having the correct surgery on the correct body part. Patient participation is recommended before administration of drugs if possible. The circulating nurse documents this collaboration.

Postoperatively, the perianesthesia nurse receives information from the circulating nurse and the anesthesia provider concerning the surgical procedure and the patient's condition in the form of a handover report. The handover report is verbal and a continuation of the comprehensive checklist. A comparison is made of all baseline values with the current condition of the patient. The patient remains in the postanesthesia care unit (PACU) until their physiologic status is deemed stable by the anesthesia provider.

The group of individuals, each with specific functions to perform, creates the perioperative patient care team. The role of the perianesthesia nurse is described in more detail in Chapter 30. More information about perianesthesia nursing is available at www.aspan.org.

U.S. Medicare and Medicaid regulations Title 42, Public Health, describe conditions for participation of individuals in surgical services departments. In Chapter IV, Part 482, Section 482.51, the regulation states that the OR must be supervised by an experienced RN and that the circulator must be an RN. It further states that an LPN/LVN and surgical technologists (STs) may serve as scrub persons or assist with circulating duties under the supervision of the qualified RN. A copy of the updated Center for Medicare & Medicaid Services (CMS) regulation is available at www.ecfr.gov.[2]

Nonsterile and Sterile Team Members

The perioperative team is subdivided according to the functions of its members:

1. The nonsterile team
   a. Anesthesia provider
   b. Circulating nurse
   c. Perianesthesia nurse
   d. Others (e.g., students, vendors, laboratory or radiography personnel)
2. The sterile team
   a. Surgeon
   b. First assistant (second assistant if needed)
   c. Scrub person

The perioperative team also may include biomedical technicians, specialty technicians, and others who may be needed to set up and operate specialized equipment or monitoring devices during the surgical procedure. Specialty technicians are usually considered separately from the main nonsterile and sterile team members. They may not enter the sterile field.

Nonsterile team members do not enter the sterile field; they function outside and around it. They assume responsibility for maintaining sterile and aseptic techniques during the surgical procedure. They handle supplies and equipment that are not considered sterile. Following the principles of aseptic technique, they keep the sterile team supplied, provide direct patient care, and handle situations that may arise during the perioperative care period.

Sterile team members perform a surgical scrub on their hands and arms, don a sterile gown and gloves, and enter the sterile field. The sterile field is the area of the OR that immediately surrounds and is specially prepared for each patient. To establish and maintain a sterile field, all items needed for the surgical procedure are sterile and handled in a sterile manner. Only sterile items and personnel dressed in sterile attire may enter the sterile field.

Nonsterile Team Members

Perianesthesia Team

The perianesthesia team consists of RNs and specially trained patient care assistants who care for the patient in the presurgical and postsurgical areas. In some facilities this incorporates an ambulatory or interventional surgery suite.

Preoperatively, the perianesthesia nurse assesses the patient and documents the findings on the comprehensive surgical checklist that will accompany the patient throughout the surgical experience. Some perianesthesia RNs specialize in the care of the patient before the surgical procedure, and others specialize in the care of the patient postoperatively.

Anesthesia Provider

Anesthesia and surgery are two distinct but inseparable disciplines; they are two parts of one medical entity. Adequate communication between the surgeon and the anesthesia provider is the patient's greatest safeguard. The anesthesia provider is an indispensable member of the perioperative team. Functioning as a guardian of the patient's physiology throughout the entire care period, the anesthesia provider manages the patient's medication, vital signs, and general well-being. Throughout this text the term *anesthesia provider* is used to refer to the person responsible for inducing and maintaining anesthesia at the required levels and managing untoward physiologic reactions throughout the surgical procedure. Functions of medical delegation in the area of anesthesia are performed under the overall supervision of a responsible physician or in accordance with state regulations and individual written guidelines approved within the health care facility.

An anesthesiologist is an MD or a DO, preferably certified by the American Board of Anesthesiology, who specializes in administering anesthetics to produce various states of anesthesia. To become eligible for certification, physicians complete a 4-year anesthesia residency program after successful completion of medical school. The term *anesthetist* refers to a qualified RN, anesthesiologist assistant (AA), dentist, or physician who administers anesthetics.

Anesthesia has become so specialized that as of 2022, the requirements have changed to become a nurse anesthetist, requiring all certified programs to transition to doctorate programs by 2025. An RN is required to have a minimum of a bachelor's degree in nursing or science with intensive care experience for entrance into a school of nurse anesthesia. To become a certified registered nurse anesthetist (CRNA), a graduate of an accredited nurse anesthesia program (a minimum of 3 years) is now required to obtain a doctor of nursing practice (DNP) or doctor of nurse anesthesia practice (DNAP) degree. On completion of an accredited program, the individual must pass the national certification examination. Nurse anesthetists with doctoral degrees must complete 60 continuing education (CE) credits every 4 years and will be recertified every 8 years by examination. More information is available at www.aana.com.[3]

An AA or a certified anesthesiologist assistant (CAA) is a master's degree—prepared nonphysician, nonnurse anesthetist who administers anesthesia under the direction of an anesthesiologist. The AA's education consists of a baccalaureate in biologic science and 2 additional years of specialty training in biophysical science. On completion of a certified program, the individual may sit for the Certifying Examination for Anesthesiologist Assistants to become a CAA. More information on the AA or CAA degree is available at www.anesthetist.org.[4]

Some anesthesia providers prefer to specialize in one area, such as cardiothoracic or obstetric anesthesia. The latter involves the simultaneous care of two patients—the mother and the neonate. In some settings, anesthesia providers participate in teaching and research as well as in clinical practice.

Anesthesia providers are not confined to the perioperative environment, but this is their primary arena. In addition to providing anesthesia during surgical procedures, anesthesia providers oversee the PACU until each patient has regained control of their vital reflexes. They also participate in the hospital's program of cardiopulmonary resuscitation as teachers and team members. They are consultants or managers for problems of acute and chronic respiratory insufficiency that require respiratory therapy, as well as for a variety of other fluid, electrolyte, and metabolic disturbances that require intravenous therapy through a central venous catheter. In the intensive care unit (ICU) or emergency department, their advice may be sought regarding the total care of unconscious, critically ill, or injured patients with acute circulatory disorders or neurologic deficits. Anesthesia providers also are integral staff members of pain therapy clinics.

Circulating Nurse

The circulating nurse is a qualified RN. The circulating nurse is vital to the smooth flow of events before, during, and after the surgical procedure. Physical and psychologic demands of the circulating nurse's role are described in Box 4.1.

The patient's medical record is required to identify who provided circulating duties. The circulating nurse's role as the patient's advocate and protector is critical and extends throughout the entire perioperative environment. A qualified ST or LPN/LVN may assist with circulating duties under the supervision of the RN. The surgeon is in charge at the operating bed but relies on the circulating nurse to monitor and coordinate all activities within the room and to manage the care required for each patient. The RN should be continuously knowledgeable about the status of the patient. To some extent, the circulating nurse controls the physical and emotional atmosphere in the room, which allows other team members to concentrate on tasks without distraction.

The laws in many states and the current AORN position statement specify that one RN circulates in each room (hospital and ambulatory centers combined). A qualified perioperative nurse should be always available to respond to emergencies in the perioperative environment according to the CMS regulations.

"Immediately available" has been interpreted to imply that one RN can supervise an unspecified number of contiguous rooms and be immediately available to assist in each of these rooms at any given moment. The RN who is called to a room to manage a crisis is not immediately available to any other patient who may be in need. The circulating nurse would be abandoning one patient to tend to another. This is highly unsafe and places the nurse and the facility at risk for liability.

The circulating nurse is vital to the provision of care that includes, but is not limited to, the following:

1. Applying the nursing process to directing and coordinating all activities related to the care and support of the patient in the OR. Nursing diagnosis and decision-making skills are essential in assessing, planning, implementing, and evaluating the plan of care before, during, and after a surgical intervention. This is the professional perioperative role of the RN circulating nurse.
2. Creating and maintaining a safe and comfortable environment for the patient by implementing the principles of asepsis. The circulating nurse demonstrates a strong sense of surgical conscience. Any break in technique by anyone in the room should be recognized and corrected instantly. Although sterile technique is the responsibility of everyone in the room, the circulating nurse is on the alert to correct any breaks that others may not have seen. By standing farther away from the sterile field than others, the circulating nurse is better able to observe the entire field and the sterile team members.
3. Aiding any member of the OR team in any manner for which the circulating nurse is qualified. This role requires current knowledge of the legal implications of surgical intervention. The circulating nurse knows the organization of the work and the relative importance of the factors involved in accomplishing it. An effective circulating nurse ensures that the sterile team is supplied with every item necessary to perform the surgical procedure efficiently. The circulating nurse must know all supplies, instruments, and equipment; be able to obtain them quickly; and guard against inadvertent hazards in their use and care. A competent circulator must be able to direct the scrub person.
4. Identifying any potential environmental danger or stressful situation involving the patient, other team members, or both. This role requires constant flexibility to meet the unexpected and to always act in an efficient, rational manner.
5. Maintaining the communication link between events and team members in the sterile field and people who are not in the OR but are concerned with the outcome of the surgical procedure. The latter includes the patient's family or significant others plus other personnel in the perioperative environment and in other departments of the hospital. The ability to recognize and effectively communicate situations involving the patient and/or other team members is a vital link in the continuity of patient care.
6. Directing the activities of all learners. The circulating nurse must have the supervisory capability and teaching skills necessary to ensure maintenance of a safe and therapeutic environment for the patient. Kindly given assistance builds up the learner's confidence. In this capacity the circulating nurse acts as a supervisor, adviser, teacher, or mentor.

CNOR: The Certified Perioperative Nurse

A perioperative nurse who has been in clinical perioperative practice for 24 months and who has successfully passed a national

1. Visual acuity with or without correction is critical to precise observation of the environment, patient, and team and for reading small print. Protective eyewear is always required when in proximity to the surgical field or when at risk for a splash/aerosol exposure. Bright lights or dim lights are commonly used throughout the surgical procedure, and people with photosensitivity or susceptibility to light-mediated eye irritation will find the OR environment problematic. Visual accuracy is imperative.
2. Manual dexterity and accuracy of motion are required for fast action during emergencies. Inability to coordinate body motions could cause injury to the patient, team, or self. Physical ability to maneuver around the periphery of the sterile field without causing contamination or disruption of the surgical procedure is critical.
3. Eye-hand coordination is essential for safe and efficient aseptic delivery of sterile items to the field. Eye-hand coordination is imperative for the safety and preservation of the sterile field.
4. Ability to concentrate and remain alert during long procedures. Thinking on one's feet is a hallmark of the circulating nurse. Multitasking is essential because the coordination of the room, patient care, team, documentation, and anticipation demands clear thinking.
5. Ability to lift instrument trays of at least 20 lb and assist with moving large equipment or incapacitated patients using proper body mechanics.
6. Auditory acuity in both ears with or without amplification is critical for hearing and understanding commands while machinery is running. Voices are kept low during surgery, especially when the patient is awake. Hearing correctly is imperative.
7. Ability to quickly anticipate and discern commands and needs of the team. Must be able to differentiate and prioritize the needs of the surgical team and the anesthesia provider efficiently and to be able to offer appropriate alternatives in extraordinary circumstances.
8. The ability to speak, understand, and document clearly using the English language is critical to safe patient care. Appropriate terminology and use of approved standard accepted abbreviations are essential to communication in the OR.
9. Communication is essential between the team, anesthesia provider, control desk, family waiting room, laboratories, and perianesthesia care areas. The circulating nurse coordinates pertinent information among all areas concerning the care of the perioperative patient.
10. The ability to remain calm and function quickly, safely, and precisely during an emergency. Must be able to make decisions and problem-solve effectively without loss of emotional control.
11. Mental clarity. Use of medications or substances that alter alertness and attentiveness is not acceptable in the OR. Lack of sleep can affect thought processes.
12. Accountability. Takes responsibility for independent actions. Admits error and remedies the situation when breaches in technique or contamination occurs.

examination is certified by the Competency & Credentialing Institute (CCI; www.cc-institute.org) as a certified perioperative nurse, which is credentialed as CNOR. Box 4.2 describes the required eligibility for CNOR certification, and Table 4.1 describes the criteria for recurrent CNOR recertification up to 2028. Changes for recertification are moving toward a more comprehensive performance-based format. CNORs seeking recertification will be required to recertify using points or CE credits. Examination will no longer be used as a recertification measure.

Retired CNOR nurses can accept an emeritus status to retain the credential. They are signified by (E) after the main credential of CNOR [i.e., CNOR(E)]. Certification and recertification information can be found at www.cc-institute.org.

Several nursing specialty organizations, such as the National Association of Orthopaedic Nurses (www.orthonurse.org) and the International Society of Plastic and Aesthetic Nurses (www.ispan.org), offer certification examinations through their certifying bodies as an additional credentialing tool. CNOR certification is valued for its representation of advanced knowledge and upholding high standards of patient care.

Sterile Team Members

Surgeon

The surgeon must have the knowledge, skill, and judgment required to successfully perform the intended surgical procedure and any deviations necessitated by unforeseen difficulties. The American College of Surgeons has stated the principles of patient care that dictate ethical surgical practice. Protection of the patient and quality care are preeminent in these principles. The surgeon's responsibilities include preoperative diagnosis and care, selection and performance of the surgical procedure, and postoperative management of care.

The care of many surgical patients is so complex that considerably more than technical skill is required of a surgeon. The surgeon cannot predict that a surgical procedure will be simple and uncomplicated. The surgeon must be prepared for the unexpected by having knowledge of the fundamentals of the basic sciences and by having the ability to apply this knowledge to the diagnosis and management of the patient before, during, and after surgical intervention. The surgeon assumes full responsibility for all medical acts of judgment and for the management of the surgical patient.

A surgeon is a licensed MD, DO, oral surgeon (doctor of dental surgery [DDS] or doctor of dental medicine [DMD]), or doctor of podiatric medicine (DPM; a podiatrist) who is specially trained and qualified by knowledge and experience to perform surgical procedures. After earning a bachelor's degree, all physicians complete the equivalent of 4 years of medical school. To become a surgeon, a physician completes at least 2 years of general surgical residency training before completing additional years of postgraduate education in a surgical specialty. The surgical residency provides the physician with education and experience in the preoperative evaluation, intraoperative treatment, and postoperative care of patients. Consultation and supervision are available from faculty and attending surgeons.

By virtue of their postgraduate surgical education, most surgeons practice within a specific surgical specialty. Highly trained and qualified surgeons limit themselves to their specialty, except perhaps in emergency situations.

Qualification for surgical practice involves certification by a surgical specialty board approved by the American Board of Medical Specialties. American specialty boards grant certification for surgical practice. All boards governing the surgical specialties require at least 3 years of approved formal residency training, and most set the minimum at 4 or 5 years. Any physician who aspires to become a board-certified surgeon must meet these requirements. The complete list of specialty boards can be found at www.abms.org.

Surgical procedures may be performed by physicians who do not meet the previously discussed criteria. These physicians include those who have had surgical privileges for more than 5 years in a hospital approved by TJC, where most of their surgical practice is conducted; those who render surgical care in an emergency or in an area of limited population where a surgical

BOX 4.2 CNOR Eligibility Criteria

- Licensed RN in state of practice and currently employed full or part time in administrative, teaching, research, or general staff capacity in perioperative nursing.
- Bachelor of science in nursing (BSN) or related degree (BA or BS) is not required for CNOR.
- Two years of perioperative nursing experience (2400 hours).

Roles Eligible for CNOR Certification

- OR staff nurse
- Surgical services administrative nurse manager
- Surgical services nursing coordinator
- Assistant surgical services supervisor
- Surgical services director
- Surgical services information technology specialist
- Surgical services budget and finance manager
- Surgical services central processing manager
- Surgical services materials manager
- Surgical services quality assurance coordinator/auditor
- Surgical services head nurse
- Surgical services assistant head nurse
- Surgical services team leader
- Surgical services charge nurse
- Perioperative educator or staff development director (whether teaching RNs, student nurses, or surgical technologists)
- Private RN scrub nurse
- RN first assistant
- Perioperative administrative supervisor
- Medical-surgical instructor in perioperative nursing
- Perioperative clinical nurse specialist or nurse clinician
- Full-time student who meets applicant status requirements

- Perioperative nurse consultant
- Individual who handles the perioperative role in a noninvasive/invasive procedure setting, such as a radiology suite, a cardiac catheter laboratory, an office surgery setting, or an endoscopy suite
- Clinical education consultant (who provides in-service programs to OR staff)
- Case manager

Roles Ineligible for CNOR Certification

- Nurse anesthetist (eligible only if functioning as a perioperative nurse)
- PACU nurse or manager (eligible only if relieving in the OR as needed or has responsibility for OR/surgical services)
- Emergency department nurse
- OR labor and delivery nurse (eligible only if surgical procedures such as cesarean sections are done in delivery room)
- RN sales representative (eligible only if performing the role of perioperative nurse part time or the role of perioperative educator, e.g., providing in-service programs)
- Director or assistant director of nursing service (eligible only if directly responsible for the OR)
- RN hospital administrator/assistant administrator (eligible only if directly responsible for OR/surgical services)
- Nurse in surgical care or surgical rehabilitation units
- ICU or coronary care unit nurse
- Infection control nurse/nurse epidemiologist (eligible only if directly responsible for OR/surgical services)
- Veterinary OR nurse
- Cardiopulmonary perfusionist (eligible only if performing the role of perioperative nurse)
- Nurse with inactive licensure and/or graduate nurse status

TABLE 4.1 CNOR Recertification

Contact Hour Method	Professional Point Activities
125 approved contact hours in 5 years; one year is January 1 to December 31 of same year 75 contact hours continuing education; must be specific to perioperative nursing 62.5 contact hours may be earned via continuing medical education (CME) (1 CME = 1 contact hour) Must be part of academic credit toward a baccalaureate degree or higher; grade of C or better (1 semester hour = 20 contact hours) (1 quarter hour = 10 contact hours)	Documentation of applied learning to professional activities within the previous 5-year certification period Professional résumé for previous 5 years Select from the following activities to earn points: Educational presentations Academic courses completed or taught Certifications Continued education (50 contact hours) Professional writing Standards application Patient-centered care Precepting, mentoring, coaching Risk mitigation/management Evidence-based practice/research Contributions to: • Professional organization • Volunteering • Institution (committees) (1 contact hour = 2 points) (semester hour/credit hour = 20 points)

Consult www.cc-institute.org for more information and recertification applications.

specialist is not available; and those who by reason of education, training, and experience are eligible for but have not yet obtained certification.

A surgeon must become a member of the medical staff and be granted surgical privileges in each facility to practice. Standards for admission to staff membership and the retention of that membership are clearly delineated in the bylaws formulated by the medical staff and are approved by the governing body of the hospital. The credentials committee has the primary responsibility for thoroughly investigating not only the training of an applicant but also integrity, technical competence, and professional judgment. In making its recommendations, this committee can limit a surgeon's privileges as appropriate, which ensures that each surgeon performs only those services according to credentials and competency.

Patients are entitled to protection and the assurance that a surgeon's surgical privileges are limited to those for which training and competence have been demonstrated. The patient's choice of and confidence in a surgeon, as well as adherence to instructions and advice, are factors in the outcome of surgical intervention. A discerning patient will check the surgeon's qualifications before surgery.

A competent surgeon is a physician who realistically appreciates their own cognitive skills and personal characteristics and can intervene effectively in a patient's illness or injury. Appropriate clinical skills (e.g., data-gathering, decision-making, problem-solving) and appropriate personal characteristics (e.g., humanistic concern, accountability, compassionate interpersonal behavior) are important attributes of a surgeon.

First Assistant

Under the direction of the surgeon, a qualified first assistant helps maintain visibility of the surgical site, controls bleeding, closes wounds, and applies dressings. The first assistant handles and manipulates tissues and uses instruments to provide hemostasis. The role of and need for a first assistant will vary with the type of procedure or surgical specialty, the condition of the patient, and the type of surgical facility. In determining this need, the characteristics of the surgical procedure should be evaluated for anticipated blood loss, anesthesia time for the patient, fatigue factors affecting the OR team, and the potential for complications. This role is critical to the well-being of the patient. All first assistants must be granted privileges to practice by the medical staff department in the facility of employment or practice. Detailed information about the role and duties of the first assistant can be found in Chapter 5.

For many simple procedures, it is unreasonable to insist that a second surgeon assist a competent surgeon. Reimbursement is generally not provided for simple cases. The surgeon should evaluate all factors to determine the need for assistance during the surgical procedure and consider that some insurance providers do not reimburse for a physician first assistant. However, the assistance of another qualified surgeon is usually necessary for procedures requiring considerable judgment or technical skill and those requiring more than one sterile team. The hazards of a surgical procedure may depend more on the condition of the patient than on the complexity of the procedure itself. The surgeon should be able to provide rationale for all decisions if challenged or if not in compliance with medical staff bylaws. More information can be found at the American College of Surgeons website, www.facs.org. Lists of specific surgeries requiring MD/DO or other assistants are located on this website.

Scrub Person

The scrub person is a patient care staff member of the sterile team. The scrub role may be filled by an RN, LPN/LVN, or ST. The term *scrub person* is used throughout this text to designate this role and to elaborate on the specific technical and behavioral functions of the individual performing on the sterile team in this capacity.

The scrub person should not simultaneously function in the role of first or second assistant. Performing additional tasks takes the scrub person's attention away from the primary responsibilities of maintaining the sterile field and facilitating the surgical procedure. Holding retractors, for example, can cause permanent injury to a patient if inappropriately positioned, maintained in alignment exerting pressure, or placed in contact with electrocautery inadvertently.

The scrub person is responsible for establishing and maintaining the integrity, safety, and efficiency of the sterile field throughout the surgical procedure. Knowledge of and experience with aseptic and sterile techniques qualify the scrub person to prepare and arrange instruments and supplies and to facilitate the surgical procedure by providing the required sterile instruments and supplies.

The scrub person must anticipate, plan for, and respond to the needs of the surgeon and other team members by constantly watching the sterile field. Manual dexterity and physical stamina are required. Other important assets include a stable temperament, an ability to work under pressure, a keen sense of responsibility, and a concern for accuracy in performing all duties. Box 4.3 describes the physical and psychologic attributes required of the scrub person in the sterile scrub role.

Two scrub persons may join the team in teaching situations or during extremely complicated or hazardous surgical procedures. One scrub person may pass instruments and supplies to the surgeon while the other prepares the supplies. Two scrub persons should be assigned if two complete teams are working simultaneously.

An experienced preceptor may join the team to teach, guide, and assist the learner functioning as a scrub person. When unexpected, unusual, or emergency situations arise, specific instructions and guidance are received from the surgeon or RN. The ST provides services and assists with patient care always under the supervision of an RN.

Some facilities permit RNs or STs privately employed by surgeons to come into the OR to perform the scrub role for their employers. These private scrub persons should adhere to all hospital policies and procedures and to approved, written guidelines for the functions they may fulfill. They are not covered under the facility's liability insurance and should carry their own policy as independent contractors. There is no such thing as working under someone else's license such as a physician or an RN. Each person is responsible for personal liability. Further discussion of independent practitioners can be found in Chapter 3.

Private scrub persons can create liability for the facility because the facility will be held liable by virtue of permitting them to work within the facility. They should not perform first-assisting tasks or be considered first assistants unless they are appropriately educated and credentialed in the role. Several states have addressed who may and may not first assist in surgery.

CST: The Certified Surgical Technologist

STs who have completed an accredited surgical technology program and successfully passed an examination attesting to their

• BOX 4.3 Physical and Psychologic Attributes of the Scrub Person's Role

1. Visual acuity with or without correction is critical to threading small needles and reading small print. Protective eyewear is always required when at the surgical field. Bright lights or dim lights are commonly used throughout the surgical procedure, and people with photosensitivity or susceptibility to light-mediated eye irritation will find the OR environment problematic. Visual accuracy is imperative.
2. Manual dexterity and accuracy of motion are required for fast action during emergencies. Inability to coordinate body motions could cause injury to the patient, team, or self. Manual dexterity is imperative.
3. Eye-hand coordination and alertness are essential for safe handling of instruments during surgery. Eye-hand coordination is imperative for the efficiency of the procedure.
4. Ability to delay nutritional intake or bathroom breaks for prolonged periods during long procedures.
5. Ability to stand in a confined space for prolonged periods.
6. Ability to lift instrument trays of at least 20 lbs and assist with moving large equipment or incapacitated patients using proper body mechanics.
7. Auditory acuity in both ears with or without amplification is critical for hearing and understanding commands while machinery is running. Voices are kept low during surgery, especially when the patient is awake. Hearing correctly is imperative.
8. Ability to quickly anticipate and discern commands and needs of the team. Must be able to differentiate between instruments and supplies efficiently and to offer appropriate alternatives in extraordinary circumstances.
9. The ability to speak, understand, and document clearly using the English language is critical to safe patient care. Appropriate terminology and use of approved standard accepted abbreviations are essential to communication in the OR.
10. The ability to remain calm and function quickly, safely, and precisely during an emergency. Must be able to make decisions and problem-solve effectively without loss of emotional control.
11. Mental clarity. Use of medications or substances that alter alertness and attentiveness is not acceptable in the OR. Lack of sleep can affect thought processes.
12. Accountability. Takes responsibility for independent actions. Admits error and remedies the situation when breaches in technique or contamination occurs.

• BOX 4.4 Eligibility for Certification by Examination for Surgical Technologists

- STs may recertify by examination every 2 years or 30 CE credits
- Graduate of a CAAHEP-accredited surgical technology program
- Graduate of an ABHES program from the U.S. Department of Health and Human Services. For additional information, visit www.abhes.org
- Graduate of an accredited Alternative Accelerated Delivery program attached to an accredited school of surgical technology
- No minimum practice hour requirement (accredited programs have minimum case number ratings for new graduates)
- Eligibility: limited to graduates of CAAHEP or ABHES accredited surgical technology program
- Renewal: CSTs must renew certification every two years
  - CSTs may renew by earning a total of 30 CE credits (4 being live credits)
  - CSTs may also renew by taking and passing the CST examination.

Consult www.nbstsa.org for additional information.

• BOX 4.5 Calculating Approved Continuing Education (CE) Credits for CST

Lecture
1 CE = 50–60 minutes of lecture
0.5 CE = 30 minutes of lecture
Add 0.25 CE for every 15 minutes over the first 30 minutes of lecture

Independent Study Article
2000 typed words = 1 CE

Go to www.ast.org for information on approved CE credits.

theoretic knowledge are certified by the NBSTSA, the main certifying body for STs. These individuals are entitled to use the designator CST after their names as a credential. Box 4.4 describes eligibility for taking the CST examination.

Graduates of accredited surgical technology programs are required to take the NBSTSA certification examination as a graduation requirement. Application for the certification examination may be made as soon as 30 days before graduation for the graduating class to apply as a group. Certification fees are discounted for Association of Surgical Technologists (AST) members. Special packages are available from AST that include membership and registration for the examination. The results of the examination provide data for measuring an accredited program's effectiveness.

As of 2022, 17 states require the CST credential for employment or specific practice laws. These states are New York, New Jersey, South Carolina, Tennessee, Indiana, Massachusetts, Texas, Nevada, Idaho, Pennsylvania, Virginia, Colorado, North Dakota, Washington, Arkansas, Illinois, and Oregon. Other states are in the process of working to pass legislation to require certification. The map of current required certification states can be found at www.ast.org. STs who were employed before the date of the CST

requirement are permitted to remain in the role of scrub person. Military and federal government employees are exempt. The CSTs are permitted to function under the direction of the RN circulator and may not administer medication or place retractors according to the laws governing CST role activities. Refer to the laws governing CST practice in the individual state of employment.

As of 2023, certification for the CST is valid for 2 years. The CST must be renewed to remain active. It can be renewed by retaking the CST examination or attainment of 30 approved CE credits. Recertification fees are discounted for AST members. Calculations for accruing CE credits can be found in Box 4.5. Providers of CE credits must apply to AST for approval of the offering. Continuing education forms are available for download from www.ast.org.

ⓔ EVOLVE WEBSITE

http://evolve.elsevier.com/Hornacky/BerryKohn/
- Historical Perspective
- Glossary

References

1. ANCC Pathway to Excellence program. www.nursingworld.org. Accessed February 7, 2023.
2. Code of Federal Regulations. www.ecfr.gov. Accessed February 7, 2023.
3. Feeney A: How to become a nurse anesthetist. www.nursejournal.org. Accessed February 8, 2023.
4. Anesthesia as a career. www.asahq.org. Accessed February 8, 2023.

Bibliography

AORN: *Guidelines for perioperative practice*, Denver, CO, 2024, The Association.

AST: *Surgical technology for the surgical technologist*, ed 5, Boston, MA, 2018, The Association.

Hornacky A, Phillips NM: *Pass CNOR*, St. Louis, 2019, Elsevier.

5

The Surgical First Assistant

CHAPTER OUTLINE

First Assistant's Knowledge and Skill Level, 65

What Does the First Assistant Do?, 66

Disciplines Associated With First Assisting in Surgery, 71

CHAPTER OBJECTIVES

After studying this chapter, the learner will be able to:

- Identify key components of the first assistant's knowledge and skill levels.
- List pertinent perioperative activities of the first assistant.
- Describe the patient care disciplines that with appropriate education function in the role of the first assistant.
- Discuss the legal implications of the first assistant role.

KEY TERMS AND DEFINITIONS

Anastomosis Creating a patent connection between two tubular structures by use of suture or specialized staples.

Approximation Bringing the edges of an incision or wound together with closure medium.

Buzzing a forceps A method of applying the active electrode of a monopolar cautery against an instrument clamped to the patient's tissue for the purpose of spot hemostasis. The flat side of a metal cautery blade is placed in contact with a clamped instrument below the level of the operator's hand before activation of the current. The edge of a Teflon-coated cautery blade is placed against an instrument clamped to the patient's tissue below the level of the operator's hand before activation of the current.

Cleavage lines Tissue planes where the natural line of tissue growth permits dissection between areas that maintain anatomic structure.

Debridement Trimming the wound edges of devitalized tissue before packing or closure.

Dissection Separation of tissue planes by sharp or blunt means.

Dynamic tension The stress on skin caused by underlying musculature, joints, and body motion.

"Golden period" An estimated time in which the wound can be closed by primary intention with minimal risk to wound integrity and healing. Influences include anatomic location, mechanism of injury, and amount of contamination in the wound. The golden period is approximately 6 to 8 hours after initial injury for optimal healing.

Hemostasis Preventing the loss of blood. Stopping the flow of blood. The best method is direct pressure. Random clamping of vessels can lead to damage of underlying structures such as nerves, tendons, or other structures.

Incise cut Scalpel is used in a perpendicular position to slice tissue in a linear direction.

Langer lines Natural lines along skin caused by tension inherent in the structure of the dermal-epidermal layers. Healing in the natural lines produces a smaller scar. Transection across the Langer lines does not follow the natural musculofascial tension and will produce a wider scar.

Ligation The act of tying or occluding an anatomic structure.

Palmed Method of holding an instrument in which the working end is nested in the palm of the hand of the assistant and the fingers remain free to grasp other items in the field. The working end can be presented and made functional by a rotation of the wrist. This method can be used for counter-traction with some manual retractors.

Perpendicular The intersection of surfaces at right angles. The scalpel is held perpendicular to the tissue during incision. The belly of the blade is used to incise tissue for best control over the depth of the cut.

Press cut Scalpel is pushed into the tissue rather than slid to incise. Press cutting can be a form of intentional puncture. A precise cut results when the scalpel is held like a pen.

Raising a flap Perpendicular countertraction is placed on superficial tissues as large areas are undermined by dissection. Care is taken not to disrupt vascularization of the elevated tissue.

Retraction Displacement of structures by use of the hand or an instrument to expose the surgical site.

Scrape cut Scalpel is dragged laterally across tissues to separate cell layers rather than full tissue layers.

Skin tension The turgor of the skin that is either static or dynamic. Tension factors largely in the final healing of the incision and the appearance of the scar.

Splitting Separation of muscle tissue along the fascial layers. A form of blunt dissection.

Sponging A method of providing exposure by removal of blood and fluid from the surgical site. The preferred way to sponge is to blot or pat the area so as not to remove biologic clots.

Static tension The constant state of skin position over the framework of the body. Also known as Langer lines.

Suction Negative pressure used to clear the visual field of blood and body substances. Various styles of tips and tip protectors are used. On occasion, a rigid suction tip can be used to remove fluids and retract tissues simultaneously.

Surgical assistant Member of the sterile team who provides exposure and hemostasis during a surgical procedure. A physician, registered nurse first assistant (RNFA), surgical assistant (SA), physician assistant (PA), or certified surgical technologist (CST) specially trained and certified as a certified first assistant (CFA).

Suture (verb) The act of sewing tissues with the goal of approximation, not strangulation. (noun) A thread used for sewing tissue in surgery. Suture knowledge is critical. Types include barbed, absorbable or nonabsorbable, multifilament or monofilament, and natural or synthetic.

Thenar grip Method of holding an instrument in which the ring handle is secured in the palm at the base of the thumb instead of placing the thumb through the ring. A small portion of the ring finger may be situated within the opposing ring of the handle.

Traction-countertraction Displacement of a structure by pulling the tissue in an opposite direction to facilitate sharp or blunt dissection of tissue planes.

Transection Cutting across natural anatomic lines. Can be done by sharp dissection or electrocoagulation.

Triangulation Suturing three opposing points of a tubular structure so that the distance between two points can be approximated in a straight line.

Tripod grip Holding an instrument or scissors in a steady position with the index finger on the box lock hinge and the thumb and ring finger partly in the ring handles for ease of release.

Undermining Dissection of subsurface tissue planes. Care is taken not to devascularize upper layers of tissue or cut nerves. Undermining decreases tension of the overlying tissues. Areas of higher skin tension benefit from this technique.

First Assistant's Knowledge and Skill Level

Surgical Anatomy and Physiology

The patient's body is a complex biosystem. Every surgical procedure interrupts multiple facets of a patient's anatomic structure and physiologic function. Lack of knowledge about each structure and its function could cause untoward disruption and injury. A single injury will affect many aspects of the patient's outcome and could progress to permanent disability or death. Anatomy and physiology are closely intertwined and should be considered as inseparable components of the whole person.

Knowledge of anatomic structures is critical to the first assistant. Tissue manipulation with instruments requires expert working knowledge of what is grossly seen and what is occluded from view. Improper retraction of tissue that has nervous and vascular structures contained within could cause complications, such as neurologic dysfunction or vascular obstruction, resulting in thrombosis or embolization. Lack of this knowledge can lead to permanent nerve damage. For example, a lawsuit was filed against a surgical technologist (ST) who was performing in the role of surgical first assistant and was unable to identify the location of the sciatic nerve and caused serious injury with a retractor. The ST held the retractors where the surgeon placed them. This is an unacceptable and unsafe practice. The ST must work within the designated scope of practice.

The surgical first assistant must absolutely know all the ramifications of every action performed in the role and its effect on the patient's outcome. The actions of the surgical first assistant should reflect the ability to identify all the normal and abnormal structures in the surgical site and make intelligent, informed decisions about patient safety. *Each first assistant is responsible for personal liability.* There is no such thing as "working under someone else's license" as commonly misinterpreted by some surgical staff members.

Pharmacology

Medications taken by the patient can cause complications in the perioperative environment. The first assistant should have a clear understanding of each drug the patient takes and its effect on the surgical procedure. Anticoagulants, for example, could cause intraoperative bleeding or postoperative hematoma. Other drugs such as birth control pills can predispose the patient to deep vein thrombosis, which in turn could lead to pulmonary embolism. Vasoconstrictors in the local anesthetic can delay the normal inflammatory process necessary for incisional healing. Patients who take hypoglycemic medication may be predisposed to metabolic problems during the procedure and poor healing or infections postoperatively. Knowledge of each drug's pharmacologic use and action can help prevent complications throughout the perioperative care period. The first assistant and the circulating nurse should collaborate concerning patient sensitivities and allergies. This should also be part of the surgical "time out."

Psychomotor Dexterity

Precise, purposeful movement at the sterile field is important for the maintenance of the sterile field and the protection of the patient and team. Many instruments used could cause a puncture injury if mishandled, and the resultant contamination could cause transmission of a serious illness such as human immunodeficiency virus (HIV) or hepatitis B or C. Clumsiness can cause instruments to fall into the surgical site or from the field to the floor, resulting in injury or damaged equipment. Use of an item for a purpose other than its intended function can create liability for the facility if someone is harmed.

Efficiency is important to facilitate the procedure. The surgeon relies on the first assistant to help manipulate tissues with instrumentation in both open and endoscopic procedures. For open procedures, the surgical site is visually larger and requires the first assistant to be a "second set of eyes." The surgeon's attention may be focused on a particular organ system, and the first assistant helps by providing exposure and observing for problems in the periphery.

For endoscopic and robotic procedures, the visual field is limited to the image on the video monitor. The first assistant needs a steady hand when using endoscopic or robotic instruments because even the slightest motion can cause the entire surgical field to shift, placing the patient at risk for injury and causing nausea in team members who are viewing the video monitor. Extreme caution is exercised to prevent injury to tissue not in the direct visual field.

Specialized training or certification may be required by some facilities to assist in endoscopic and robotic procedures. Robotic surgery requires the first assistant to be at the surgical field while the surgeon is at a console away from the surgical field. The Association of Surgical Assistants (ASA) provides guidelines and educational requirements approved by the organization's professional standards committee. More information can be found at www.surgicalassistant.org.

Procedure Knowledge and Techniques

The first assistant needs to know each step that will be encountered during the surgical procedure. It is important to anticipate and think in advance about each step to help the procedure move smoothly. The first assistant should have clear knowledge about not only the functional steps but also the indications for the procedure. Refer to Table 1.1 for the most common indications for a surgical procedure.

When the surgeon incises tissue, the first assistant usually provides a clear field by retraction (traction or countertraction), sponging, or suction. Some circumstances require the use of hemostatic actions, such as clamping, suturing, cauterizing, or application of some other pharmacologic preparation to stop bleeding.

The surgeon may request the first assistant to "buzz the forceps," which means placing the active electrode against a forceps that is holding patient tissue and delivering electrical current after the tip is in complete contact with the instrument (Fig. 5.1). The gloved hand holding the forceps should have as much contact with the instrument as possible before the current is delivered. This decreases the amount of current passing over the holder's hand and prevents concentration of electricity at a focal point on the hand. The current is delivered below the holder's hand and as close to the actual patient tissue as possible to minimize the risk for an alternative current pathway. The forceps is not permitted to touch any other part of the patient's tissue or other instrumentation during this process, or the patient will suffer burns to nontarget tissue.

Knowing how and when to perform each action is part of the knowledge base of the first assistant. Random clamping or cautery application can cause serious tissue damage.

Surgical Site Management

Management of the surgical site is a crucial part of the successful outcome of the procedure for both physiologic and aesthetic reasons. Physiologically, a surgical site infection could be devastating to the health of the patient and be an incredible cost factor during the recovery period. Aesthetically, the closure is what the patient sees at the end of the procedure and how the quality of care is judged.

The first assistant commonly assists in closing the skin and applying dressings or supportive materials, such as casts. Improper technique of closure can lead to poor wound healing and unsightly scarring. Securing drains appropriately facilitates surgical site healing and minimizes the risk for dead space where a hematoma or seroma can form (Fig. 5.2).

What Does the First Assistant Do?

Position, Prep, and Drape the Patient

The first assistant is frequently responsible for positioning the patient on the table after the anesthesia provider indicates it is safe to do so. In the absence of the first assistant, other members of the team may perform this function. Provision for safe exposure of the surgical site without compromising the physiology of the patient is the key to a successful procedure.

The dispersive electrode (i.e., patient return electrode; Bovie pad) is placed after the patient is in the final resting position for the procedure. Positioning the patient after the pad (Bovie pad) is in place can cause the pad to slip or gape, preventing full contact with the skin. It should not be removed and reapplied for any reason. The Bovie pad should never be cut to size. The prep solution should not be permitted to pool or drip under the pad. Alcohol-based preps are flammable, so care is taken that the prep is completely dry before drapes are applied. Be sure that the safety straps are correctly positioned. The straps should be over the patient's blanket where they are visible before the drapes are applied.

Keep in mind that the height of the OR bed should be adjusted to suit the reach of the tallest person at the sterile field. Shorter individuals should stand on steps or platforms for ergonomic comfort and adequate visualization of the surgical site. Sitting is appropriate only when the entire team is seated so as not to change the level of the sterile field. Chapter 26 describes the processes for positioning, prepping, and draping the patient.

Handle Instrumentation

The role of the first assistant involves knowledge, skill, and dexterity in handling and using surgical instrumentation. A skilled

• **Fig. 5.1** Buzzing the forceps. The active electrode tip is placed against the forceps to deliver current to a specific spot of bleeding.

• **Fig. 5.2** The surgical drain should be secured with a suture.

first assistant can make the role look easy, but in fact skill is reflected by precise action. Fumbling or struggling indicates lack of knowledge and skill in the role. The standard of care for the use of equipment or instrumentation in the role of first assistant includes the following:

- Knowledge of the equipment and instrumentation
- Knowledge of how and when to use the equipment and instrumentation
- Dexterity of holding and using basic instrumentation (Figs. 5.3 to 5.6)
- Skill in the use or operation of the equipment and machinery
- Knowledge of potential for injury to underlying and surrounding tissues

Provide Exposure

Methods of providing exposure include use of rigid and flexible retractors, grasping instruments (e.g., clamps, forceps), Silastic bands (e.g., vessel loops), rubber drains (e.g., Penrose), umbilical tapes, Raytec sponges, laparotomy tapes, suture traction, plastic isolation bags (bowel bags), and suction, as well as by direct hand positioning.

The method used to provide exposure is carefully selected. Physical attributes of the patient are considered, such as body size, tissue type, adjacent structures, depth, and type of exposure needed. The presence of blood, body fluid, or plume can require the use of suction as part of the exposure process. Prolonged need for surgical exposure may require the use of a self-retaining retractor. Whenever tissues are exposed to air for extended periods, the first assistant should be sure to irrigate the site lightly with an appropriate irrigant.

Use of manual retractors can be physically demanding, and prolonged use can contribute to repetitive stress injuries of the assistant's wrist and arm, causing carpal tunnel syndrome. Most retractors are designed to be held in an ergonomic fashion and do not require the forces associated with a tense, struggling grasp (Fig. 5.7). If the retractor in use causes the assistant to struggle, another style may be indicated for use.

Suction should be used with caution. Evacuation of fluids to clear the field of vision should be done in a manner that is not injurious to adjacent structures. The direct force of the vacuum against tissues can cause suction lesions that can become inflamed and necrose. Blind suctioning should be avoided because organs such as the spleen could be perforated and cause hemorrhage.

Provide Hemostasis

Prevention of active bleeding and blood loss is a major part of every surgical procedure. The surgeon takes great care to avoid vessels and organs during dissection because blood and body fluids obscure vision in the surgical field and the loss of blood is a detriment to the patient. Unfortunately, some maneuvers during the procedure can cause bleeding, and this bleeding must be cleared and controlled. The clearing of the field is part of the exposure process, but the control of bleeding and blood loss is referred to as hemostasis. Prevention of retained pools of blood or serum that could create a nidus for infection in tissues is

• **Fig. 5.3 A,** Holding a needle holder correctly in dorsal view. **B,** Holding a needle holder correctly in palmar view. **C,** Incorrect way to hold a needle holder, with finger in.

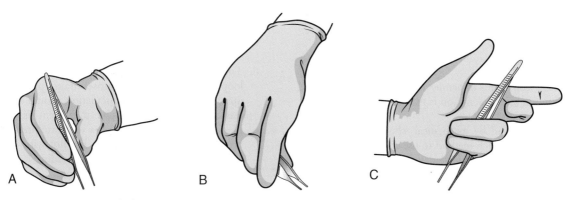

• **Fig. 5.4 A,** Correct way to hold forceps. **B,** Incorrect way to hold forceps. **C,** Palming a forceps.

• **Fig. 5.5 A,** Correct way to hold scissors, using the tripod grip showing dorsal hand view. **B,** Correct way to hold scissors with tripod grip showing the palmar hand view.

• **Fig. 5.6** Using a free tie to occlude a blood vessel.

• **Fig. 5.7** Retractors are ergonomically designed to provide exposure with minimal assistant fatigue.

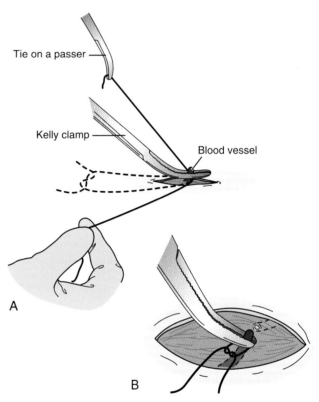

• **Fig. 5.8 A,** Using a clamp to occlude a vessel. **B,** Using a free tie around a clamped vessel.

accomplished by the elimination of dead space when tissues are closely approximated.

Methods and mechanisms of hemostasis are described in detail in Chapter 29, but a brief description is provided here for the first assistant role description.

Hemostasis is provided by mechanical, chemical, or thermal means. The decision of which method to use at a given point in a procedure requires significant knowledge and skill. Examples of each method include, but are not limited to, the following:

1. *Manual hemostasis.* Direct pressure over a part; indirect pressure adjacent to a part.

   a. Clip (metallic, plastic, temporary, permanent, absorbable)
   b. Suture (suture ligature, free tie; see Fig. 5.6)
   c. Clamp and tie (hemostat: crushing or noncrushing; Fig. 5.8)
   d. Tourniquet (Rummel vascular sliding occlusion, vessel loop, umbilical tape, Penrose drain, pneumatic tourniquet). Occlusion of the circulation should be held to the least amount of time possible to prevent tissue damage.
   e. Hand and/or fingers over area to create pressure. Directly hold or blot sponge over site. Do not wipe off the newly formed clot; doing so will cause bleeding to resume.
2. *Chemical hemostasis.* Agent is placed over a localized bleeding surface to control active bleeding. Care is taken not to allow the material to be introduced into the systemic circulation.

Hemostatic materials should not be permitted to contaminate blood salvage systems. The returned blood could potentially cause an embolus. Chemical hemostatic agents are topical (liquid, gelatin sponge, collagen fibers or sponge, cellulose, fibrin glue, or albumin). Epinephrine is commonly added to local anesthetics for its vasoconstrictive properties. (This is contraindicated in small distal vessels of the digits, penis, ears, and nose.)

3. *Thermal hemostasis.* Electrosurgical units (ESU) or lasers are the most common means of thermal hemostasis. Safety is a critical factor in the use of such equipment. Do not use thermal methods in the presence of oxygen exposure (e.g., airway or thoracotomy) to minimize the risk for fire. Care is taken not to allow a dry sponge to contact the active ESU tip. This could also result in a fire. Personnel using thermal hemostatic devices should have appropriate training and credentials. Chapter 20 describes the most used devices for hemostasis in more detail.

    a. *Electrosurgery unit (ESU).* Monopolar ESU requires the use of a return electrode on the patient. An active electrode can be touched directly to tissue or to a forceps holding a segment of tissue. Enhanced monopolar units may have argon beam (argon gas) coagulation properties that are useful for large bleeding surfaces. The tip of the argon beam coagulator is not touched directly to the bleeding surface because it can clog.

    The argon gas is nonflammable and is used to clear blood away as the current flows across the bleeding surface. Bipolar ESU requires no return electrode. The active and inactive electrodes in the tips of the instrument prevent the current from passing through the patient's body.

    b. *Laser.* Extreme caution is always exercised during laser use. Eyewear of the appropriate optical density is worn by everyone, including the patient. The environment should not support inadvertent injury by any stray laser light. Signs should be placed on the outside of OR doors when lasers are in use for the safety of incoming staff.

Handle Tissue With Instrumentation

The first assistant should always be aware of each tissue type and the appropriate way to handle it. All tissue should be handled with care, using the fewest instruments possible. Knowledge of the instrumentation and its intended use is critical. Some instruments are considered crushing and should not be used to handle delicate lumens. Skin edges can be crushed by inappropriate grasping with forceps (Fig. 5.9).

Forceps should be used on tissue with care. Tight grasping can cause perforations, also known as "buttonholes," in tissue that will scar or leave tissue defects that may not heal correctly. Clamps should never be placed randomly because of the potential for structural destruction. The fingers are placed lightly into the ring handles, and the clamp is steadied by an extended index finger used to "tripod" the shanks of the instrument.

The first assistant should always be able to apply a clamp and quickly retract the fingers without entanglement in the rings. A delicate grasp should remain on the instrument as it holds the tissue securely. Traction on the attached instrument is appropriate when the structure is to be removed or excised. No traction should be placed on soft tissue in process of repair.

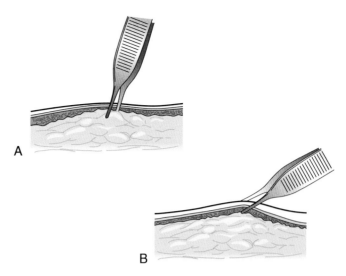

• **Fig. 5.9 A,** Correct way to grasp subcutaneous tissue with forceps. **B,** Incorrect way to grasp tissue by crushing the dermis and epidermis in the jaws of the forceps.

Dissection

The first assistant should be familiar with and skilled in methods of tissue dissection. Procurement of vascular conduit or preparing kidneys for transplant requires the first assistant to know sharp and blunt methods of separating tissue. ESU can be used for dissection.

Sharp methods require the use of a scalpel or scissors. Some tissue is slippery or highly mobile. Use of traction-countertraction maintains enough tightness to prevent excess jagged edges as the primary incision is made using a scalpel. A dry sponge can be used in countertraction to stabilize the skin for a straight incision (Figs. 5.10 and 5.11).

Scalpels are used to sharply open the skin, separate tissues, and create precise incisions. The scalpel blade is held perpendicular to the surface as it cuts. Allowing the blade to lie at an angle causes the incision to bevel the surface, which in turn can undermine the skin, harming the circulation. The grip of the individual fingers provides varying degrees of pivot, balance, and pressure. The size of the blade is determined by the area to be incised. The scalpel is held differently according to the type of tissue and the incision being created. The scalpel can be held like a

1. Pencil with the index finger alongside the superior edge (the dull ridge) of the blade for fine shallow lines made in a "slide" motion; the wrist rests on the surface of the area to be incised and the cutting edge does not have full contact with the skin's surface.
2. Pencil with the index finger over the superior ridge of the blade for a press cut; the finger acts as a stop as the blade enters the tissue.
3. Violin bow for a deeper straight cut with maximum contact with the cutting edge; the hand is positioned over the scalpel, but the wrist is not in contact with the patient's body. When a sawing motion is used, the risk for fat necrosis from devitalized tissue in the incision increases.
4. Pencil with the point of the scalpel directed at the tissue and the entire handle at a right angle to the body for a puncture cut.

• **Fig. 5.10** Using a scalpel to create incision with right hand and exerting traction with the left.

A

B   C

• **Fig. 5.11** Techniques for undermining the skin with scissors. **A,** Skin is peeled back over the left middle finger. Edge is held by delicate skin hook retractor. Scissors are used to nip at subcutaneous tissue. **B,** Closed scissors are placed under the skin at the incision line. **C,** Scissors are opened and spread to first bluntly dissect and separate tissues with the outer edge of blades. Sharp dissection can be used secondarily from within the pocket of dissection.

• **Fig. 5.12** Blunt dissection using a gauze sponge over the first finger.

Pickup

• **Fig. 5.13** Correct way to introduce the suture needle into the skin.

5. Straight razor to use in a sideways scraping motion to debulk or debride tissue.

Scissors use a cross-action to transect tissue. The same physical instrument handling is used in debridement. Care is taken not to completely insert the fingers into the ring handles of the scissors. A delicate balance between the fingertips and the first phalangeal joint of the thumb, index, middle, and ring fingers prevents the fingers from being ensnared in the handles during dissection. The index finger should extend along the back of the blades like a tripod for stability.

The dexterity of opening and closing the scissors permits the user to insert the closed tips between layers and slowly spread the blades to separate tissue planes bluntly followed by precise sharp cutting of the individual layers. The curve of the scissors usually matches the curve of the hand with the tips pointing upward for most cuts. A few backward cuts require the scissors to be held with the curve opposite the curve of the hand. The straight scissors are not often used for cutting tissue.

Blunt methods commonly use dull edges of instruments or a sponge-covered finger (Fig. 5.12). Instruments designed as planar dissectors are used to peel away tissue in blunt dissection fashion.

For small areas, the blunt end of the scalpel can be used to peel back tissue bluntly.

Chapters 19 and 20 describe common instruments and equipment used by the first assistant in surgery.

Suture

The first assistant may be required to suture (Fig. 5.13) and cut suture (Fig. 5.14) during and at the end of the procedure. Suturing is considered a form of closure and can entail the use of conventional suture material and needles, metallic or absorbable clips, staplers, wound tape strips, wound glue, wire, and other materials for joining tissue. Intraoperative suturing is performed for hemostasis, stabilization of a part, traction, or other tissue manipulation. At the end of the procedure, the incision is closed by a closure method using one of the aforementioned devices.

Traumatic wounds have a specific set of criteria for closure. The decision for closure timing and mechanism is determined by degree of contamination, location on the patient's body, the mechanism of injury, and, in some patients, the duration of time between injury and closure, referred to as the "golden period."

• **Fig. 5.14** Correct way to cut suture.

• **Fig. 5.15** Types of knots used in surgical procedures.

This period is based on the previously mentioned factors. Additional discussion of suture and techniques is found in Chapter 28.

Knot tying requires extensive practice and skill (Fig. 5.15). An insecure knot can lead to an obstructed view during the procedure if bleeding is not controlled and to postoperative hemorrhage leading to hematoma. Knot tying for conventional surgery is performed by one of the following methods:

• Two-handed tie (Fig. 5.16)
• Instrument tie (Fig. 5.17)
• One-handed tie (Fig. 5.18)

Recognize Surgical Hazards

Surgical hazards are described in Chapter 13. The first assistant works with the surgeon and the rest of the team to provide a safe environment. Every step of the procedure requires diligence and care. The first assistant should be able to identify potential hazards and prevent them. Should an untoward event occur, the first assistant should know the steps to take to resume a safe environment. Primary hazards are biologic, physical, and chemical. Each hazard has a multitude of manifestations. Examples of hazards include, but are not limited to, the following:

• *Biologic hazards.* Exposure to contamination by both the patient and the team. This can be blood, plume, excreta, transudate, exudate, tissue, semen, or any other physiologic substance.
• *Physical hazards.* Risk for sharps puncture, infection, fire, tissue damage, pressure injury, burns, physical mechanical stress, electrocution, or other physiologic damage to the patient or team.
• *Chemical hazards.* Medications, prep solution, sterilants, anesthetics, cement, cytotoxic material, or any substance not derived from biologic sources.

Respond Appropriately to Emergency Situations

The first assistant should be credentialed in cardiopulmonary resuscitation (CPR), preferably at the advanced cardiac life support (ACLS) level. The first assistant is a key member of the team during lifesaving procedures. Emergencies can be environmental fires or other events that place human life at risk.

Patient Assessment

The assessment of the patient is an ongoing activity practiced by all the professionals rendering direct care. The advanced practice first assistant is master's degree prepared and has extensive education in physiology. Some states have granted prescriptive privileges to disciplines that participate in perioperative patient care.

Orders written by first assistant personnel are cosigned by the surgeon or anesthesiologist; an exception is the physician associate/assistant and nurse practitioner writing a prescription permitted under the authority of each individual state. Physician associates/assistants, nurse practitioners, and advanced practice nurses have a number assigned by the U.S. Drug Enforcement Agency that is included with a written prescription.

Disciplines Associated With First Assisting in Surgery

Registered Nurse First Assistant

A certified perioperative nurse (CNOR) who successfully completed an accepted program based on the Standards for the Education of the Registered Nurse First Assistant by AORN (the Association of periOperative Registered Nurses) may seek a position as a registered nurse first assistant (RNFA) with a private surgeon, hospital, or clinic. An advanced practice registered nurse (APRN) is not required to be a CNOR because certification is part of advanced practice.

A baccalaureate degree (BA or BS) or higher is required to enter an accepted RNFA program as of January 2020. RNFA is a recognized job description that can be credentialed by certification after completing 2000 hours in RNFA practice and taking an examination. A baccalaureate degree is required to sit for the examination. The credential is certified registered nurse first assistant (CRNFA).

Nurses who completed an accepted RNFA program that includes a minimum of 120 hours of internship are eligible to take a separate examination sponsored by the National Assistant at Surgery Certification (NASC) organization. This examination is a form of certification that provides a credential for 3 years while completing the 2000 practice hour requirement for the CRNFA. It can be renewed and does not require a baccalaureate degree. The credential is registered nurse assistant at surgery (RNAS-C). The 3-year certification interval is useful for nurses working toward a baccalaureate degree in compliance with the CRNFA requirement.

The RNFA functions under the direct supervision of a surgeon and is permitted to first assist by the medical service department at the facilities of practice. The RNFA functions solely as the first assistant and should not simultaneously

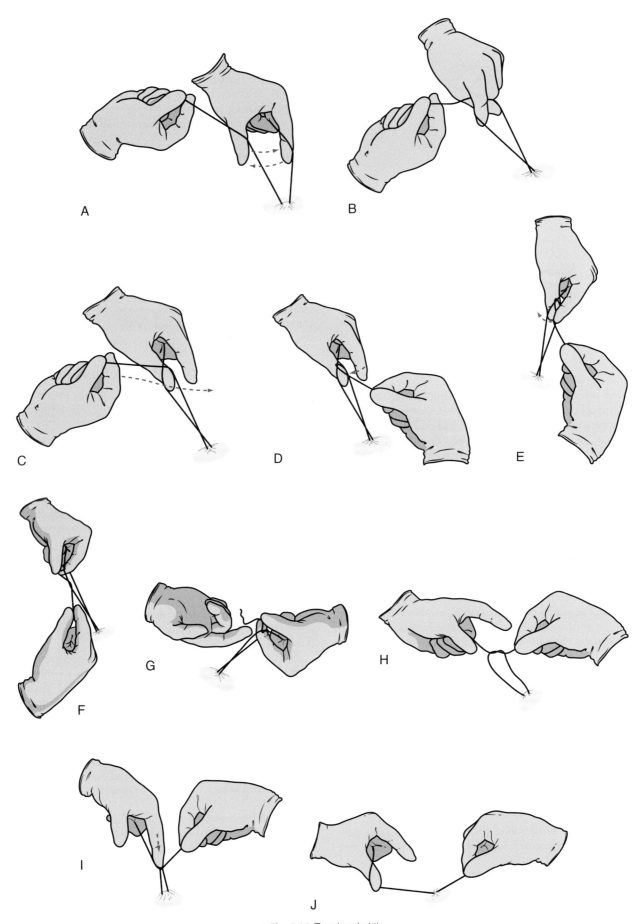

A

B

C

D

E

F

G

H

I

J

• **Fig. 5.16** Two-handed tie.

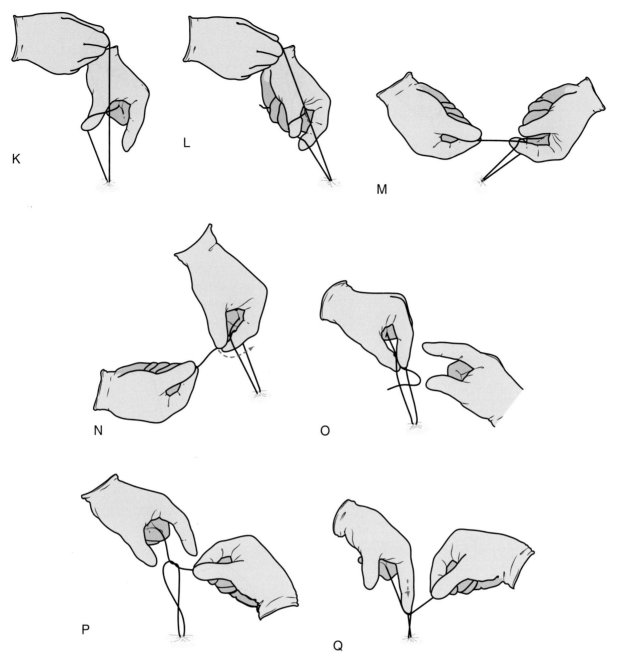

• **Fig. 5.16 cont'd**

perform the functions of a scrub nurse or circulator. Performing both roles diverts attention away from the primary focus of the sterile field and subsequently away from the patient. A sample performance description is shown in Figure 5.19. The qualifications to function as a first assistant should include, but are not limited to, the following:

- Demonstrated competency in both scrub and circulating nurse roles for a minimum of 2 years
- Knowledge and skill in applying the principles of aseptic and sterile techniques to ensure infection control
- Knowledge of surgical anatomy, physiology, fluid and electrolyte balance, acid-base regulation, clinical pathology, and wound healing because these factors relate to surgical procedures

- Comprehension of risk factors and potential intraoperative complications and knowledge of actions to minimize them
- Technical skill and manual dexterity in handling tissue, providing exposure, using instruments and devices, providing hemostasis, tying sutures and knots, and applying dressings
- Ability to recognize safety hazards and initiate appropriate preventive and corrective actions
- Ability to perform cooperatively and effectively with other team members
- Ability to perform effectively in stressful and emergency situations
- CNOR is maintained. Advanced practice nurses are exempt from the CNOR requirement because they have advanced certification.

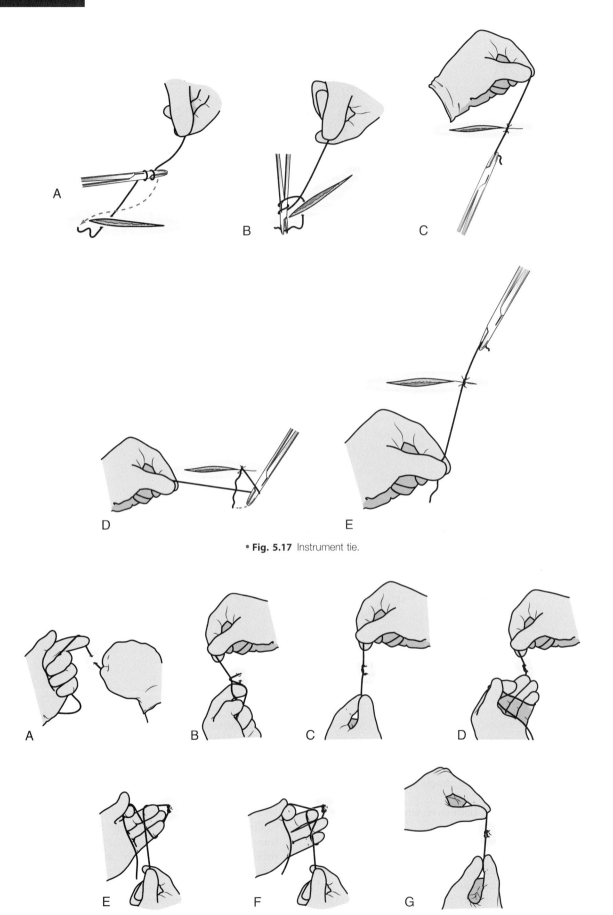

• **Fig. 5.17** Instrument tie.

• **Fig. 5.18** One-handed tie.

- Certification in CPR (basic cardiac life support [BCLS] or ACLS preferred)
- Completion of formal RNFA program based on the AORN RNFA Core Curriculum and the AORN standards for RNFA education

Curriculum for the RNFA

Since 1995, the role of the RNFA is recognized in all 50 states as within the scope of nursing practice as an expanded role of the perioperative nurse. Recognition as an RNFA is controlled by individual state boards of nursing.

Registered Nurse First Assistant Sample Performance Description

Job Title: Registered Nurse First Assistant (RNFA)

Purpose of Position:
Assist under the direction of the primary operating surgeon in the perioperative care of the patient undergoing a surgical experience. The RNFA uses the nursing process in the formulation of the plan of care. The RNFA functions within the policies and guidelines established by the facility and reports directly to the Surgical Unit Manager. The RNFA is an expanded role of the registered nurse and is accountable for exemplifying leadership and professionalism in the implementation of the role.

Qualifications:
1. Graduate of accredited school of nursing
2. Licensed to practice in the state of application.
3. Minimum of 24 months perioperative experience, both scrubbing and circulating
4. Satisfactory completion of CCI approved RNFA program
5. Certification in perioperative nursing (CNOR)
6. Certified in cardiopulmonary resuscitation, basic life-saver BCLS (CPR-ACLS preferred)
7. Accumulation of 125 contact hours of continuing education every 5 years to maintain CNOR status.
8. BSN and 2000 practice hours in role of RNFA if planning certification (CRNFA) credential with CCI.

Functions:	Satisfactory Performance:
1. Preoperative assessment and teaching of the patient and family (significant other)	1. RNFA reviews objective and subjective data. Is aware of lab results and pending tests. The assessment includes the patient as a member of a family unit and a member of society. RNFA is aware of cultural and personal influences in the interpretation of assessment data. RNFA communicates findings to the primary surgeon.
2. Formulation of nursing diagnoses	2. RNFA interprets the assessment data and plans care appropriate to the pending surgical procedure. RNFA collaborates with the primary surgeon and others to facilitate the pending surgical procedure and the attainment of favorable patient outcomes.
3. Recognizes potential hazards and initiates corrective action	3. RNFA is aware of the environment observing for potential sources of injury to self, team, and the patient. RNFA practices universal precautions at all times and is in observance of OSHA regulations.
4. Practices within the guidelines established by the state of licensure	4. RNFA:
	a. Handles tissue
	b. Provides exposure
	c. Uses instrumentation
	d. Sutures
	e. Provides hemostasis
	f. Closes tissue and skin
	Prohibitions:
	a. May not perform the intended procedure
	b. May not perform the task of the surgeon
	c. Does not simultaneously function as scrub nurse

• **Fig. 5.19** Sample performance description for registered nurse first assistant.

5. Demonstrates intraoperative competency as an RNFA	5. Knowledge:
	a. Principles of asepsis and infection control
	b. Surgical anatomy and physiology
	c. Surgical procedures
	d. Recognizes hazards and effects safety measures
	Skill:
	a. Manual dexterity
	b. Suturing and ligating
	c. Providing hemostasis
	d. Exposing the surgical site
	e. Positioning, prepping, and draping
6. Continuous assessment of the patient during the intraoperative phase of the surgical experience	6. RNFA observes condition of patient and initiates emergency measures as needed.
7. Postoperative assessment, evaluation and teaching	7. RNFA accompanies the patient to the postoperative unit as needed and communicates with the patient and family (significant other) as designated by the primary surgeon. RNFA, in collaboration with the primary surgeon and others, evaluates the attainment of expected outcomes.
8. Communicates postoperative information as directed by primary surgeon	8. Writes orders as per policy for verbal orders with the co-signature of the primary surgeon.
9. Adheres to institutional policies and procedures reflecting attendance, registered nurse professional responsibility, standards of care, and communication through chain of command	9. Observes institutional policy and practices the art and science of registered nursing in the expanded role of the RNFA

• **Fig. 5.19 cont'd**

Voluntary certification is attained by successfully passing the national CRNFA examination. CCI has developed a national certification examination for the eligible RNFA that includes the following requirements:
- Licensed as an RN in the state (country or province) of practice
- Baccalaureate degree or higher (copy of diploma must be included in application packet)
- CNOR or certification in advanced practice nursing (APRN)
- Completion of an RNFA program based on the AORN RNFA Core Curriculum and the AORN standards for RNFA education
- Documentation of 2000 hours of first-assisting experience during a period of 5 years
- 1400 hours must be in the intraoperative role; 600 hours may be in preoperative or postoperative settings
- Documentation of clinical competency

After meeting all requirements and successfully passing the certification examination, a certified RNFA may use the title certified registered nurse first assistant (CRNFA) as an official credential. The CRNFA may recertify every 5 years by contact hours, portfolio, or by examination. Eligibility for recertification includes maintenance of CNOR status and documentation of

•BOX 5.1 CRNFA Recertification Requires That the CNOR Credential Is Maintained

Recertification by Contact Hours
- 1000 clinical practice hours (200 contact hours), 150 RNFA/perioperative related
- 500–1000 clinical practice hours (at least 300 contact hours), 225 RNFA/perioperative related

Recertification by Points
- 1000 clinical practice hours (400 points)
- 500–1000 clinical practice hours (500 points)

active clinical practice as an RNFA with continued clinical competency for the 2-year period preceding the recertification date. Recertification can be done through clinical practice hours or points. Box 5.1 describes recertification methods.

For ease of processing, the certifications for CNOR and CRNFA were merged in January 1998 to allow recertification at the same intervals.

Certified Nurse Midwife

Certified nurse midwives (CNMs) are credentialed as advanced practice nurses to provide perinatal care. The CNM is a master's degree—prepared RN who has been licensed and credentialed by the state board of nursing in their practice locale. The scope of practice includes antenatal care, gynecologic care, parturition care, and postnatal care. The CNM works with female patients in wellness centers, preventive settings, and childbirth. Occasionally a pregnant patient will present with complications requiring cesarean delivery. Usually the CNM has been with the patient throughout labor and is present when the determination is made by the physician to perform a surgical delivery. The surgically trained CNM can shorten the interval wait for additional surgical staff to arrive by first assisting in the cesarean birth.

The CNM works collaboratively with an obstetrician who performs the surgical procedure. Most states permit the CNM who has had appropriate additional training to function in the role of first assistant in the cesarean procedure. Training includes surgical anatomy, procedure steps, suturing, and the safe use of surgical instruments. This does not necessarily qualify the CNM as a fully credentialed RNFA for all procedures, but rather only those procedures associated with the female reproductive system during childbirth. Some CNMs first assist during gynecologic procedures on nonpregnant patients with additional training and medical staff credentialing. The CNM does not meet the requirements for certification as an RNFA unless a formal RNFA course has been completed. The CNM in the first assistant role in the cesarean section provides continuity of care within the specialized patient population.

This role is supported by the American College of Nurse-Midwives, the American College of Obstetricians and Gynecologists, and the American College of Surgeons. Some state boards of nursing prohibit the CNM from first assisting. They state that the CNM must also meet the same educational requirements as an RNFA to be permitted to first assist. (More information is available at www.midwife.org/.)

Physician Associate/Assistant

In May 2021, the American Academy of Physician Assistants (AAPA) officially changed the title of the physician assistant to physician associate. The title change was implemented to encompass the multiple roles and functions of the physician associate. The medical staff may approve privileges for an allied health care professional referred to as a physician associate/assistant (PA) who is qualified by academic and clinical training to first assist in the OR and function in other areas of perioperative patient care. The extent of a PA's practice is defined by state law, facility policy, and preference of the employing physician. Prescription authority has been granted at various levels in all 50 states.

Most students entering PA school have at least 4 years of health care experience and a minimum of a bachelor's degree. Many PA programs are housed within medical schools, and graduates are referred to as physician extenders. The first 2 years of the program are accomplished in the same classes with the medical students. The clinical component of their education includes 2000 clinical hours, and practice requirements include registration or licensure by the state in which they practice. The role of the PA evolved in the late 1960s and now incorporates about 300 accredited programs throughout the United States that incorporate 27 months of PA education.

Physician associate/assistant is a generic term with two subcategories: the assistant to the primary care physician in the clinical area and the first assistant to the surgeon. The PA who functions as a first assistant in surgery is required to have surgical training in addition to the baseline PA education. The surgical education process usually encompasses six semesters of clinical surgical experience. Eligibility for acceptance by the medical staff either as a PA or a surgical assistant (SA) is determined by the following criteria:

- Exercising critical thinking within areas of competence, with the physician member of the medical staff having the ultimate responsibility for patient care
- Participating directly in the management of patients under the supervision or direction of a member of the medical staff
- Documenting progress notes on patients' medical records and writing orders to the extent established by the medical staff
- Writing limited prescriptions in 50 states and the District of Columbia (not permitted in Puerto Rico). The educational requirement is a minimum of 75 credit hours in pharmacology, 12 credit hours every 2 years to maintain credentials
- Performing direct patient care in conformity with applicable provisions of medical staff bylaws, which may include obtaining medical histories and performing physical examinations

The SA performs duties under the direct supervision of a surgeon, who maintains the direct responsibility for the patient. The assistant may perform tasks delegated by the surgeon for the care of patients in any setting for which the surgeon assumes responsibility. The SA education program has an intense intraoperative focus.

After completion of a formal Commission on Accreditation of Allied Health Education Programs/Accreditation Review Committee on Education for the Physician Assistant (CAAHEP/ARC-PA)—accredited academic program, the PA or SA should attain national certification by taking the Physician Assistant National Certifying (PANC) exam. The recertification period is 10 years by exam and includes a 100-hour continuing education (CE) requirement every 2 years. The medical staff bylaws delineate the practice privileges of the assistant within the hospital.

Reimbursement for services is determined by role, employer, and case involvement. The PA's reimbursement can now be paid directly to the PA under the 2022 Physician Fee Schedule, whether it is a private physician practice or a hospital surgical department. More information is available at www.aapa.org. (Specific questions can be addressed by email at customercare@aapa.org.)

Surgical Technologist

A certified surgical technologist (CST) may also be trained to first assist in a program of study approved by the Association of Surgical Technologists (AST) and the National Board of Surgical Technology and Surgical Assisting (NBSTSA). An associate degree should be the minimal entry-level requirement for CSTs who enter a postgraduate first-assisting program as described by NBSTSA and the Accreditation Review Council on Education in Surgical Technology and Surgical Assisting (ARC/STSA), the certifying and accrediting bodies for surgical technology. For CSTs with at least 2 years of first-assisting experience during the previous 4 years, a national first-assisting certification examination is available from the NBSTSA. After successfully passing this examination, the CST first assistant may use the initials CST/CFA.

At the time of original certification as a CFA, the CST period of the certification is adjusted to be of the same duration as the CFA portion of the certification. Both aspects of the certification will be adjusted for the same period of 2 years. Recertification as a CST/CFA is accomplished by providing documentation of practicing as a CST/CFA for 2 years during the certification period and by obtaining 38 CE credits approved by the NBSTSA. This includes eight credits in a live setting and advanced credits. Another option is to document 2 years of practice as a first assistant and take the certification examination again.

Several states have indicated that first assisting is not within the role of the ST. The ST should not first assist unless a formal first assistant training program accepted by the ARC/STSA or NBSTSA has been completed. Basic ST programs following the core curriculum for surgical technology do not prepare an ST for first-assisting duties. Random clamping, mishandling of tissue, or holding retractors inappropriately can cause serious injury and should not be taken lightly. (More information is available at www.ast.org.)

ⓔ EVOLVE WEBSITE

http://evolve.elsevier.com/Hornacky/BerryKohn/

- Historical Perspective
- Student Interactive Questions
- Glossary

Bibliography

American College of Nurse-Midwives: *The midwife as first assistant handbook*, Washington, DC, 2001, The Association.

AORN (Association of periOperative Registered Nurses): *Core curriculum for the RN first assistant*, ed 5, Denver, CO, 2014, The Association.

AORN (Association of periOperative Registered Nurses): *Guidelines for perioperative practice*, Denver, CO, 2024, The Association.

Novitsky Y: *Atlas of robotic surgery*, St. Louis, 2022, Elsevier.

Phillips N, Hornacky A: *Surgical instrumentation*, ed 3, Clifton Park, NY, 2019, Cengage.

Trott AT: *Wounds and lacerations: emergency care and closure*, ed 4, St. Louis, 2012, Elsevier.

www.aapa.org. History of the PA profession. Accessed February 12, 2023.

www.aorn.org. AORN standards for the RN first assistant education program. Accessed February 15, 2023.

www.nccpa.net. NCCPA board certification and title change. Accessed February 13, 2023.

6

Administration of Perioperative Patient Care Services

CHAPTER OUTLINE

Establishing Administrative Roles, 79

Interdepartmental Relationships, 84

Patient Care Departments, 85

Patient Services Departments, 85

Departmental Service Divisions, 86

Coordination Through Committees, 88

Surgical Services Management, 91

Budgeting and Financial Responsibility, 95

New Product and Equipment Evaluation, 97

CHAPTER OBJECTIVES

After studying this chapter the learner will be able to:

- Define the role of the perioperative management team.
- Describe the relationship between the perioperative environment and other patient care departments.
- Define the role of intradepartmental surgical services committees.
- Facilitate mediation in conflict resolution.

KEY TERMS AND DEFINITIONS

Administrator Person who directs or manages departmental affairs; may be a nurse or physician.

Capital budget Monies for larger purchases that have lasting-use implications for a time-defined period. Some items depreciate over time and need replacement as technologies change.

Committee Group within the organization that is assembled to perform a specific task.

Evidence-based practice Procedure or activity that is validated with scientific proof in a clinical setting.

In-service education Departmental programs designed to introduce or demonstrate equipment, techniques, or procedures used in perioperative patient care.

Learning organization Functional group that includes all personnel involved with the facility. The organization needs to learn from experience and the environment if it is to survive

and grow. Stagnation and inflexibility are costly and a main cause of failure and financial loss.

Manager Person who plans and executes directives passed down from administration.

Materials Supplies, such as reusable or disposable goods, ordered and maintained in stock for departmental use in patient care.

Operational budget Monies appropriated for the costs of day-to-day business.

"Sacred cow" Practice that continues despite lack of scientific evidence or validation with evidence-based practice.

Systems thinking Process by which the learning organization collectively examines practices and processes during analysis of root causes. This mechanism examines long-term activity, not just one single change. It is a circular process of business and people skills.

Establishing Administrative Roles

The perioperative patient care team surrounds the patient throughout the perioperative experience. This direct team functions within the physical confines of the operating room (OR), which is one part of the physical facilities that comprise the total perioperative environment. Other areas in the perioperative environment include preadmission testing (PAT), the ambulatory

services unit (ASU), and the postanesthesia care unit (PACU). Likewise, the perioperative patient care team makes up only one part of the human activity directed toward the care of the surgical patient.

Many other people function in an indirect relationship with the patient and contribute vital supporting services toward the common goal of ensuring a safe, comfortable, and effective perioperative environment. The relationship and duties of perioperative staff members vary according to the size and extent of the physical facilities and the number of personnel employed. No person's job is insignificant. Each staff member has important functions to perform, and each is responsible for assuming a part of the total workload.

The purpose of this chapter is to acquaint the perioperative staff with the role of the management team and the nature of the job they must perform. This is not a "how-to" chapter on management but rather a descriptive collection of structural and elemental components of the underpinnings of a surgical services department.

Current online leadership-based information keeps managers informed of new developments in the perioperative arena.

Magnet Recognition
Leading the Way to Magnet Status

The Magnet Recognition Program was founded in the early 1990s by the American Nurses Credentialing Center (ANCC) as a way to improve health care management, staffing, and outcomes. Magnet recognition is the highest acknowledgment on a national and international level of ongoing nursing care excellence through education and development.[1] Detailed information and a visual diagram are available at www.nursingworld.org.

Activities in a Magnet hospital are highly visible to the public and point to 14 forces that form the core values of this distinguished title (Box 6.1). The five primary hallmarks of Magnet status fall under the Global Issues in Nursing & Health Care model. Individual manuals are available and include the following:
1. *Transformational leadership:* Demonstrated vision, influence, clinical knowledge, and expertise in professional nursing practice.
2. *Structural empowerment:* Mission, policies, practices, values, and vision are manifest in outcomes through professional partnerships and collaborations with the staff.
3. *Exemplary professional practice:* Application of the nursing process and the emergence of new knowledge are reflected with the response from patients, families and significant others, the team, and the community at large. This is a circular process.

•BOX 6.1 Fourteen Dimensions of Magnet Recognition Status (Known as "Forces of Magnetism")

1. Quality nursing leadership
2. Organizational structure
3. Management style
4. Personnel policies and programs
5. Professional models of care
6. Quality of care
7. Quality improvement
8. Consultation and resources
9. Autonomy
10. Community and the hospital
11. Nurses as teachers
12. Image of nursing
13. Interdisciplinary relationships
14. Professional development

4. *New knowledge, innovation, and improvements:* Continual implementation of improved methods and new information helps refine the system through evidence-based practice. Individualized care uses a blend of new technology and old techniques.
5. *Empirical quality results:* The end result of care is compared with benchmarks established along the way. Making a difference is emphasized through a solid structure, better outcomes, innovation, and creativity. Standards remain, but flexibility is the strategy to gain new learning directed at improved outcomes.

Eligibility for Magnet Status

A formal application is preceded by an analysis of current workplace status. The nursing division must be part of a larger health care organization. A manual is available from the ANCC website (www.nursingworld.org) to assist in determination of eligibility. The process includes a documentation phase and a site visit by the Magnet recognition appraisal committee. The site visit is funded totally by the applicant organization. The Commission on Magnet Recognition renders a decision concerning status within 3 to 4 months of the site visit and a review of all application documentation. Magnet recognition is effective for 4 years, during which time spot inspections may be made to assess for variances.

Some prerequisites to application include, but are not limited to, the following requirements:
1. Data collection concerning quality and outcomes must become part of a national database for benchmarking nurse-sensitive quality indicators at the patient care division level.
2. Commitment to educational preparation of nursing administration:
   a. The Chief Nursing Officer (CNO) is required to be master's degree prepared at minimum when the application is submitted. A doctorate degree is preferred. The baccalaureate, master's degree, or doctorate degree must be in nursing. The CNO must participate in the highest structural governance and be ultimately responsible for all nursing divisions.
   b. Since January 2015, a baccalaureate degree or graduate degree in nursing is required for 100% of nurse managers or nurses in an educational role at the time of application.
3. ANCC's *Nursing Administration: Scope and Standards of Practice* must be in effect for adequate measuring and surveying by Magnet site visitors.
4. The organization must be in full compliance with all local, state, and federal laws and regulations.
5. Compliance with National Safety Patient Goals from The Joint Commission (TJC) is required.
6. Policies and procedures must be in place to permit nurses to voice concerns about the practice environment without retribution.

Maintaining Magnet Status

Ongoing quality improvement and evaluation of performance are documented in writing during the first 2 years of Magnet status. Staff and physician demonstrations of collaborative teamwork are highly valued aspects of the Magnet credential. Changes in management personnel and differences in attainment of expected outcomes may trigger the need for additional reporting or an additional site visit.

During the third year of Magnet recognition a renewed application for the credential is made, complete with arrangement for a site visit. All measurable indicators outlined in the Magnet Application Manual must remain at 100% of Magnet criteria to maintain or request redesignation of the credential of Magnet status.

Benefits of Magnet Status

Nursing care is more clearly defined, which offers the opportunity for professional growth and enrichment and thereby supports recruitment and retention of staff. Nursing turnover is minimized. Cost-saving benefits for retention lead to better outcomes, lower mortality rates, appropriate service reimbursement, and timely discharge planning. Nursing administrators use programs such as the Effective Performance Management Strategies for Nurse Leaders to provide guidance, skills, and strategies for a stable managerial environment. Magnet status can be highly publicized and prized by the marketing department of the facility. Reimbursement sources recognize the credential and use the facility as a referred recommendation to insured groups. The public views the credential as a reassuring atmosphere of safe, efficient care.

Management of Surgical Services
Perioperative Administrative Personnel

Personnel should know the direction of the entire organizational effort as a prerequisite for successful functioning. Administrative personnel are responsible for interpretation and education of hospital and departmental philosophy, objectives, policies, and procedures to the perioperative staff. These terms are generally found in the orientation manual and can be defined as follows:

1. *Philosophy:* Statement of beliefs regarding patient care and the nature of perioperative nursing that clarifies the overall responsibilities to be fulfilled.
2. *Objectives:* Statements of specific goals and purposes to be accomplished during the course of action and definitions of criteria for acceptable performance.
3. *Policies:* Specific authoritative statements of governing principles or actions, within the context of the philosophy and objectives, that assist in decision-making by providing guidelines for action to be taken or, in some situations, for what is not to be done.
   a. *Basic policies:* Statements of the principles of the administration and its approach to functioning. Examples include disallowing smoking by anyone on facility premises.
   b. *General policies:* Guidelines of the principles dealing with everyday situations that affect all personnel within the hospital. Examples include requiring all personnel, regardless of role, to be certified in cardiopulmonary resuscitation (CPR).
   c. *Departmental policies:* Guidelines structured to meet the needs of a specific work unit (e.g., OR policies). Examples include dress codes for specific areas.
4. *Procedures:* Statements of task-oriented and skill-oriented actions to be taken in the implementation of policies.

Perioperative Nurse Manager

In most accredited facilities a registered nurse (RN) is responsible for administration and supervision of all perioperative patient care services. The perioperative environment is a business unit and high-cost center of the hospital. It is usually run by an administrator, director, or vice president and managed as a business to control costs and maintain effectiveness. The title and functions of the perioperative nurse manager is reflected by the size of the facility and complexity of the administrative responsibilities.

In larger hospitals the perioperative nurse manager may hold some variation of the title of director of perioperative services or assistant vice president. Because of the magnitude of the administrative duties, actual supervision of personnel may be delegated to a line manager or charge nurse. In smaller hospitals in which administrative responsibilities focus mostly on one department, the perioperative nurse manager directly supervises personnel. In other situations, one nurse may manage more than one clinical service, such as the OR, PACU, ASU, special procedures room, or central processing department. The term *manager* is used throughout this text to designate the perioperative nurse responsible for coordinating patient care and related support services of the department.

The perioperative nurse manager should have strong knowledge of nursing theory and practice, specialized knowledge of OR technique and management, and knowledge of business and financial management. The manager should possess leadership and people management skills to supervise and direct patient care within the perioperative environment according to established principles and professional standards.[2] The main function of the manager is to provide leadership that promotes a cooperative team effort. Leaders need additional business skills and knowledge, which concern functions of management that include planning, organizing, staffing, directing, and controlling, problem-solving, decision-making, coordinating, and communicating.

Personal Skills and Communications

The perioperative manager works to build a successful surgical department with a cooperative team approach. Communications are fostered through the philosophy extended by those in leadership. Perioperative personnel use many tools to communicate information. Some of the standardized mechanisms for relaying information and enhancing team performance are expressed in the following list:

1. *TeamSTEPPS* (Team Strategies and Tools to Enhance Performance and Patient Safety) was developed for the Department of Defense Patient Safety Program in collaboration with the Agency for Healthcare Research and Quality. It includes core values of teamwork such as leadership, situation monitoring, mutual support, and communication. The outcomes affect performance, knowledge, and attitudes. I PASS THE BATON I is the mnemonic that describes the communication activities as part of TeamSTEPPS. Detailed tools and training programs can be found at www.ahrq.gov/TeamSTEPPS.
2. *Leadership* organizes and articulates clear goals. Decisions are made with input from team members, who feel empowered enough to speak when information needs to be imparted to the group. Team relations are supported, and conflicts are resolved. Events are planned, problems are solved, and performance is improved by evaluating processes.
3. *Situation monitoring* (*STEP: S*tatus of patient, *T*eam members, *E*nvironment, and *P*rogress toward goal) is an ongoing process of constant vigilance for progress or regress of goal attainment. Each team member is responsible for personal safety.
4. *Mutual support* is actively given and received by all team members. Feedback is timely, considerate, and respectful. Information exchanged is specific and directed toward improvement of team performance. Concerns should be voiced and elicit a

response to be certain of successful communication. If a situation is an essential safety breach, any team member may "stop the line," meaning that the activity or procedure immediately halts without fear of repercussions. The goal is still met without compromising relationships.

5. *Communication* ranges from basic information to critical dialogue. One structured communication technique uses *SBAR* (*S*ituation: What is going on with the patient? *B*ackground: What is the clinical context or history related to the patient? *A*ssessment: What is the presumed problem? *R*ecommendation and request: What can the team or I do immediately to correct the situation?). Other communication tools, such as HUDDLE (Healthcare Utilizing Deliberate Discussion Linking Events), SWITCH, or SURPASS, can be used. The method of communication should be standardized, include all team members, and may include a checklist. A briefing should take place before each procedure and a debriefing before the patient is transferred from the OR to the postanesthesia area.[3]

The "call out" and "check back" feedback methods are used to validate the correctness of the received message (e.g., the surgeon asks for 10 mL of lidocaine plain, and the scrub person repeats "10 mL lidocaine plain" as the syringe is passed to the surgeon's hand).[4] The surgeon should acknowledge the correctness of the exchange. "Handover," or patient transfer of care, report is included in this activity. Transitions of care include shift change, breaks, addition of team members to the field, and change of surgeons or anesthesia providers.

Barriers to Effective Communication

Human factors can interfere with communication and team effectiveness. Communication errors and barriers are a leading cause of adverse events.[5] Some problems include rapid turnover in team members, lack of knowledge, personnel who are rushed for time, withholding of information, pecking order, defensive behaviors and insecurity, laziness, complacency, poor follow-through, fatigue, excess workload, distractions, conflicts between team members, lack of role clarity, cultural indifference, and misunderstandings.

Managers must work toward a just culture in the OR to minimize the human factors that affect safe performance of patient care. A continual appraisal of actions and outcomes should focus on accountability for patient and team safety, even if it means losing some productivity.

Managerial Responsibilities

The manager is responsible for the allocation and completion of work but does not do it all or make all the decisions. Qualified personnel are employed, and they are delegated increasing responsibility as they develop competence in their work. An organizational attitude develops that can function well in the manager's absence.

The manager implements and enforces hospital and departmental policies and procedures. Through participation in research, patient care services rendered are constantly analyzed and evaluated to improve the quality of care given. The manager retains accountability for all related activities in the perioperative environment. The scope of this accountability includes the following tasks:

- Provision of competent staff and supportive services that are adequately prepared to achieve quality patient care objectives.
- Delegation of responsibilities to professional nurses and assignment of duties to other patient care personnel.
- Responsibility for evaluation of the performance of all departmental personnel and for assessment and continuous improvement of the quality of care and services.
- Provision of educational opportunities to increase knowledge and skills of all personnel.
- Coordination of administrative duties to ensure proper functioning of staff.
- Provision and fiscal control of materials, supplies, and equipment.
- Coordination of activities between the perioperative environment and other departments.
- Creation of an atmosphere that fosters teamwork and provides job satisfaction for all staff members.
- Identification and resolution of problems in a decisive, timely manner.
- Initiation of data collection and analyses to develop effective systems and to monitor efficiency and productivity.

Clinical Coordinator

An assistant nurse manager aids in administration and supervision of nursing service in the OR and is directly responsible to the perioperative nurse manager. This nurse acts as administrative head in the absence of the manager. The position usually does not exist in small hospitals. In large hospitals one or more clinical coordinators provide leadership to specific services and assist with the management of personnel and material resources.

Head Nurse or Charge Nurse

The head nurse or charge nurse functions in a line management position as a liaison between staff members and administrative personnel. In some hospitals the title of head nurse is given to the person whose position is comparable with that of a coordinator. In other, typically smaller, hospitals the perioperative nurse manager functions more or less in the capacity of a head nurse; for simplicity, the term *head nurse* is used to refer to this role.

In large hospitals with many surgical specialty services a head nurse may be responsible for the administration and direct supervision of patient care in a particular specialty service, such as ophthalmology, neurosurgery, cardiovascular surgery, or urology. With this structure, several head nurses are in the department. These head nurses should have the technical proficiency necessary for the specialty service for which they are responsible and should have sufficient managerial ability to plan for and administer effectively the patient care activities.

The duties of the head nurse include, but are not limited to, the following tasks:

- Planning and supervising patient care activities within the OR suite or assigned rooms.
- Coordinating patient care activities with the surgeons and anesthesia providers.
- Maintaining adequate supplies and equipment and providing for their economic use.
- Observing the performance of all staff members and providing feedback.
- Interpreting the policies and procedures adopted by the department and hospital administration.
- Informing the perioperative manager of needs and problems that arise in the department and assisting with problem-solving.
- Assisting with orientation of new staff members.

Functions vary in different hospitals, but the position of head nurse, with its direct and continuous responsibility for both patients and staff, is an important one.

Perioperative Business Manager

Some hospitals employ a perioperative business manager, who sometimes has the title of unit manager. This person may report to the perioperative manager or directly to the hospital administrator. Lines of authority and responsibility between the business manager and the perioperative nurse manager should be clearly defined regardless of the organizational structure. The business manager directs the management of daily operational and indirect patient care functions in the perioperative environment.

Nonnursing administrative duties should include maintenance of a clean, orderly, safe environment within the department for patients and personnel. This entails more than removing visible dust and dirt.

A safe environment is defined as free of contamination, electrical and fire hazards, and negligence. Formulation of procedures is necessary. Personnel should be trained. However, inspection and follow-up are equally important. The business manager coordinates these efforts with the supporting service departments: housekeeping, maintenance, laundry, and materials management.

A business manager may prepare and administer the department budget. This duty may include maintaining inventories and evaluating supplies and equipment. If the hospital does not employ a business manager, the nurse manager or coordinator assumes responsibility for these duties.

Advanced Practice Registered Nurse or Clinical Nurse Specialist

Within any organization a formal structure of authority and responsibility exists. However, the evolution of technology and the acute illnesses of patients have changed the focus of functions for many nurses within the hospital organization. With experience, the advanced practice registered nurse (APRN) can manage patient care and direct the activities of others. This practitioner may hold the title of perioperative nurse clinician, clinical nurse specialist (CNS), or APRN. Although the term *practitioner* is used to describe any of or all these advanced roles, differentiation is made within the profession on the basis of formal academic education that includes master's degree preparation, doctor of nursing practice (DNP) degree, or specialty certification.

The CNS is comparable with other perioperative APRNs in an advanced role and is a graduate of a master's degree program in nursing (master of science in nursing [MSN]), with a clinical specialty. APRNs and CNSs serve as role models for and consultants to the professional nursing staff and as teachers of patients and other personnel. The CNS conducts research to validate nursing interventions. These skills can be used effectively for advanced practice in the perioperative environment. A nurse with a DNP degree may hold positions in research, education, administration, or private practice.

Some APRNs are registered nurse first assistants (RNFAs), and those who have attained certification in this role are credentialed as certified registered nurse first assistants (CRNFAs). APRNs in this role are not required to concurrently maintain a certified perioperative nurse (CNOR) status because of other advanced certifications. The AORN position statement concerning APRNs as RNFAs requires completion of an RNFA program that meets the AORN standards set for RNFA education.

The APRN is capable of exercising a high degree of discriminative judgment in planning, executing, and evaluating nursing care based on the assessed needs of patients with one or more common clinical manifestations. A practitioner may develop the plan of care for a group of orthopedic patients, for example. This plan is coordinated for each patient with the surgeon, other professional nurses, and allied health care personnel who assist in the performance of functions related to the plan.

Clinical nursing interventions are not necessarily performed by the practitioner. The APRN decides which nursing interventions can be performed by others. These decisions are based on personal interaction with each patient and knowledge of the clinical condition. The practitioner exercises a degree of autonomy and independence within the clinical setting. Some state boards of nursing have permitted select APRNs to have minimal prescriptive powers.

Because a practitioner has advanced academic preparation in theoretic knowledge and clinical experience in a particular clinical patient care setting and is an expert in nursing situations in that setting, qualified clinical coordinators may function as practitioners. In this role they assist in planning the total care for each surgical patient, in coordinating nursing and supportive services, and in participating in the orientation, development, and evaluation of caregivers assigned to direct patient care functions in the perioperative environment.

The APRNs who assess individual patient needs through personal patient interviews and physical examinations and who plan for individualized care in the perioperative environment truly function as perioperative nurse practitioners. Using specialized judgment and skills, they make decisions relative to direct and indirect patient care in the perioperative environment. Solving problems and making decisions are the heart of professional management and professional leadership.

The practitioner may work solely or primarily with the surgeons in a specific surgical specialty. Some APRNs work as independent contractors with a surgical group as a qualifier for APN certification. This concept of nursing specialization coincides with the specialization of surgeons. With practice and formal or informal study, nurses develop expertise in planning and implementing care for patients with comparable surgical problems. Skills and knowledge become highly specialized. Surgeons in that particular specialty rely on these nurses to supervise the care of their patients and to direct less experienced personnel on the perioperative team.

Perioperative Education Coordinator

Planned educational experiences are provided in the job setting to help staff members perform competently and knowledgeably. Most hospitals have a staff development department committee to plan, coordinate, and conduct educational and training programs.

An orientation program is planned for each new employee. All new personnel should become familiar with the philosophy, objectives, policies, and procedures of the hospital and patient care services. This general orientation program assists the new employee to adjust to the organization and environment. It is coordinated with an orientation to the duties in the unit to which the employee is assigned.

The in-service coordinator may be a member of the staff development department, the administrative staff, or both. This person is responsible for planning, scheduling, and coordinating the orientation of new staff, including a review of policies and procedures, performance description, and standards specific to the perioperative environment. On the basis of an assessment of individual skills, the new employee is given guidance and supervision for a period of weeks to months until basic competencies are adequate for independent functioning. Head nurses, preceptors, and other experienced staff members assist with the orientation of new personnel.

In-service education programs should be planned to keep the perioperative staff up to date on policies, new techniques, equipment, and patient care practices. Programs that focus on fire prevention, electrical hazards, security measures, and resuscitation training are important to ensure personnel and patient safety and are usually required yearly. Professional and technical programs designed to develop specialized job knowledge, skills, and attitudes that affect patient care are planned and presented. The in-service coordinator is responsible for assessing the educational needs of staff members collectively and individually and then for planning, scheduling, coordinating, and evaluating in-service programs. This individual may also conduct some sessions.

Staff development programs conducted on a continual basis enhance employee performance by maintaining job knowledge and clinical competence. In-service programs may be supplemented by other appropriate continuing education programs held outside the health care facility or presented by qualified people who represent the industry.

Preceptor

The orientation process is facilitated by a one-to-one relationship between the new employee and an experienced staff member. The preceptor teaches, demonstrates, counsels, advises, and encourages until the orientee can function independently. The preceptor is accountable for assessing the orientee's abilities, assigning activities accordingly, and assisting in carrying out duties safely. Learning needs can be assessed through interviews, observation, and a skills checklist.

To ensure consistency in teaching, the preceptor coordinates development of appropriate and measurable behavioral objectives for the orientee with the clinical educator, in-service coordinator, or the management staff. The preceptor should evaluate performance and offer constructive feedback to build the orientee's self-confidence. To be effective, the preceptor should have an interest in teaching and should have acquired the necessary skills and experience with adult learners. Some facilities offer a preceptor class that outlines topics such as communication and setting performance goals to become a successful preceptor. AORN offers a nurse preceptor certificate program with learning modules. A facility may offer a monetary increase for performing in the preceptor role.

Interdepartmental Relationships

The perioperative environment is one of many departments within the total hospital organization. For continuity in patient care, many departments coordinate their efforts through the administration of the formal organizational structure of the hospital.

Every hospital has a governing body that appoints a chief executive officer (CEO), usually with the title of hospital administrator, to provide appropriate physical resources and personnel to meet the needs of patients. Administrative lines of authority, responsibility, and accountability are defined to establish the working relationships among departments and personnel (Fig. 6.1).

A nurse executive, sometimes referred to as vice president of patient care services or director of nursing services, reports to the hospital administrator. The perioperative nurse manager reports to the nurse executive if perioperative services are a division under

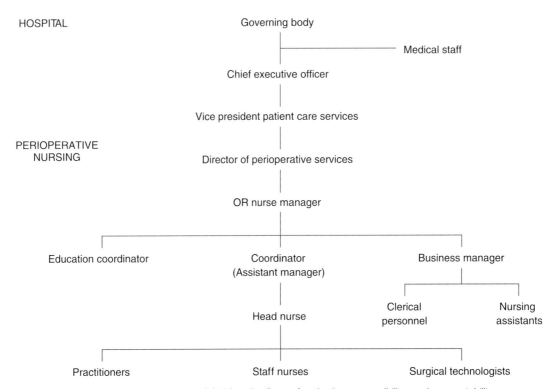

• **Fig. 6.1** Management structure. Administrative lines of authority, responsibility, and accountability are defined to establish working relationships among departments and personnel.

management of the nursing service. In some facilities, perioperative services are an independent unit not managed by the nursing service. The perioperative nurse manager then reports directly to the CEO, an assistant administrator, or the chief of one of the medical services. Through either channel of administration, many activities in the perioperative environment are coordinated with other patient care units and departments within the facility.

Patient Care Departments

Patient Care Division

Patients come to the OR directly from a short-stay or in-house patient care unit, an outpatient ambulatory care area, or the emergency department (ED). Channels of communication should be kept open among perioperative personnel and patient care personnel in other units. Coordination of preoperative preparation and transportation of patients prevents downtime in the perioperative environment. Many facilities use a comprehensive checklist system to ensure adequate preparation of surgical patients in a timely manner. This document accompanies the patient throughout the intraoperative and postoperative periods for continuity of care. An RN or licensed practical nurse/licensed vocational nurse (LPN/LVN) signs or initials each item accomplished. By the time the patient leaves for the patient care unit, all individual patient preparations have been completed along with a detailed handover report.

Emergency Department/Trauma Center

Often, victims of trauma and acutely ill patients are seen initially in the hospital ED. Cardiopulmonary resuscitative and other equipment is available for initiation of prompt triage and treatment. Minor injuries usually can be treated in the ED. Some patients must be scheduled for an emergency surgical procedure. These patients may arrive in the OR before the results of all diagnostic tests are confirmed; therefore communication among the OR, ED, laboratory, and radiology personnel is vital to the success of surgical intervention. OR personnel should be advised as to the nature of the injury or illness to prepare all needed equipment and obtain supplies for the emergency surgical procedure.

Designated regional trauma centers should have teams of surgeons, anesthesia providers, and perioperative personnel who are immediately available in the hospital 24 hours a day. A trauma nurse coordinator is administratively responsible for all personnel and activities to ensure comprehensive trauma care.

Intensive Care Unit

Because surgery has become more specialized and complex, specialized patient care facilities where concentrated treatment can bring the patient to a satisfactory recovery have become a necessity. This care is provided in an intensive care unit (ICU), which is open 24 hours a day, 7 days a week. It is staffed by highly trained and specialized RNs. Critically ill patients who need constant care for several days are admitted directly from the OR, PACU, ED, or other patient care unit. Each bedside is equipped with therapeutic and advanced monitoring equipment.

Depending on the size of the facility and its specialty services, more than one specially designed and equipped surgical intensive care unit (SICU) may be provided. One ICU may admit only cardiovascular surgical patients (coronary care unit [CCU]), and

another may admit only pediatric patients (pediatric intensive care unit [PICU]). In addition to SICUs, most hospitals also have a unit for nonsurgical (medical) patients (medical intensive care unit [MICU] or the neonatal intensive care unit [NICU]). The increased efficiency afforded by these units serves the best interests of both the facility and the patient. They create the most effective use of personnel and equipment and result in lower morbidity and mortality rates.

Movements of patients to and from the SICUs should be closely coordinated with the anesthesia provider, the perioperative nurse, and the PACU personnel. If the surgeon or anesthesia provider anticipates that a patient will need intensive care postoperatively, a SICU bed is reserved at the same time the patient is scheduled for the surgical procedure. The appropriate SICU should be notified promptly when the surgeon determines an unanticipated need for a bed. Sometimes the patient must wait in the OR or PACU for an available bed; occasionally, elective surgical procedures are postponed because sufficient SICU beds or staff are not available.

Obstetric Services

The obstetric unit is divided into three separate areas: labor and delivery (L&D), postpartum care, and newborn nursery. Most L&D units are equipped and staffed for delivery by cesarean section (C-section). However, in other hospitals, patients scheduled for either elective or emergency C-section are brought to the OR. In addition to supplies needed for the surgical procedure, adequate resuscitative equipment must be available for the newborn. Some facilities require the OR personnel to be on call for all C-sections in both the OR and the L&D unit.

The L&D units that staff for C-sections provide their own circulating and scrub nurses. These nurses are eligible for CNOR status. Many departments are staffed with their own RNFAs specific to the role of assisting on C-sections. Certified nurse midwives (CNMs) serve in the first assistant capacity after appropriate training but are not considered RNFAs unless they have completed an RNFA program in accordance with AORN Standards for RNFA Education.

Patient Services Departments

Radiology and Nuclear Medicine Departments

Frequently, personnel from the radiology (x-ray) and nuclear medicine (radiation oncology) departments assist with diagnostic or therapeutic interventional procedures in the OR. For some procedures, perioperative personnel may need to go to the radiology department to assist the surgeon during an interventional procedure that necessitates sterile technique.

Many surgical services departments have an onsite radiologic interventional room for endovascular procedures, such as angioplasty or vascular stenting. Specialized interventional procedure rooms may be located near the main OR in the event an open procedure is necessary.

Large facilities may have a radiology unit in the main OR to perform computed tomography (CT) scans or magnetic resonance imaging (MRI). An emergency plan should be in place for this type of situation to have available staffing, OR, and necessary equipment.

Whenever a diagnostic or surgical procedure is scheduled that will require use of radiology equipment or a radioactive implant, all departments should be notified at least the day before. This facilitates the scheduling of personnel and workload in all departments. Provisions for handling hazardous materials can be made.

Pharmacy

Many drugs are routinely stocked in the OR suite for the anesthesia providers' use, and some are kept for use by the surgeons during surgical procedures. These are obtained via requisition from the pharmacy. Narcotics are always kept under lock, and each dose is recorded as it is dispensed. A satellite pharmacy may be established in the surgical services department to dispense unit doses of medication on a per-case basis.

Pharmacists are resource people who convey drug information to physicians and nurses. They should be responsible for preparing all admixtures, but often the mixing of medications is done by RNs in the preoperative holding area, OR, PACU, and SICU to expedite administration. The pharmacist is responsible for quality control of drug product services throughout the hospital.

Blood Bank

All hospitals have a blood transfusion service or blood bank. This is a highly technical service for collecting, testing, processing, and distributing blood products. If the hospital does not have its own blood bank, blood may be supplied from a regional blood center. Written policies and procedures for blood transfusion services must conform to the standards of the American Association of Blood Banks. These standards include criteria for accepting blood donors, laboratory testing of donor and recipient blood, and preparing and administering blood products for therapeutic purposes. Blood banks dispense whole blood, plasma, packed cells, or platelets only as they are needed.

If in advance of an elective surgical procedure the surgeon anticipates that blood loss replacement may be necessary, the patient may have their own blood (autologous) drawn and stored in the blood bank for autotransfusion—a blood replacement procedure. Blood bank technicians also may participate on autotransfusion teams for collection of patient blood intraoperatively and postoperatively.

If autologous blood is not available or additional units of donor blood (homologous) are needed, a sample of the patient's blood is sent to the blood bank for type and cross-match. In emergency situations this blood sample may be sent from the ED or the OR. The units of blood products ordered by the surgeon or anesthesia provider are prepared and labeled with the patient's name and blood data. Suspected or recognized adverse reactions to blood transfusion must be documented on the patient's chart and reported to the blood bank.

Pathology Department

The pathologist, a physician who specializes in the cause and effect of disease, may be on call at a moment's notice to examine tissue while the patient is anesthetized. This enables the surgeon to proceed immediately with a definitive surgical procedure if malignant tumor cells are found, without subjecting the patient to a second surgical procedure at a later time.

A small laboratory may be located within the perioperative environment with equipment for microscopic tissue examination. This laboratory may be used for other tests and for taking photographs of tissue specimens removed from patients. Routinely, all tissue removed during a surgical procedure is sent to the pathology department for a minimum of gross examination.

Clinical Laboratory

Samples of blood, urine, and body fluids are taken to the clinical laboratory for analysis. Some analyses are routinely performed preoperatively. Others are done during a surgical procedure, such as blood gas analysis. Samples are obtained and immediately sent to the laboratory, or they may be obtained during a surgical procedure for analysis later, such as a culture for determination of the cause of an infection.

Biologic testing of sterile supplies is done routinely. The perioperative environment may undergo biologic testing when a contamination problem is suspected. The bacteriologist, who specializes in the study of microorganisms, may come into the OR suite to collect samples for testing, or OR personnel may collect samples and send them to the laboratory. The results provide a method for evaluating the effectiveness of procedures and the degree of adherence to environmental standards.

Departmental Service Divisions

Medical Records Department

Clinical records include the admitting diagnosis, the patient's chief complaint, complete history and physical examination findings, the results of laboratory examinations, and the physician and nurse care plans. Most hospitals are moving toward electronic medical records accessible to all authorized caregivers via computer and the Internet. Records should state the therapy used, including surgical procedures, and include progress notes, consultation remarks, the patient's condition on discharge, and observations in case of death. A summary of the hospitalization experience should be complete. These records are signed in writing or electronically by the physicians and nurses attending the patient.

The anesthesia record completed during the surgical procedure by the anesthesia provider also becomes part of the patient's record. The circulator should document pertinent remarks regarding the care rendered in the OR and the patient's response on the nurses' note sheets or the progress notes. Documentation is a responsibility of all professional team members who implement direct patient care.

Notes about the surgical procedure should be explicit, dictated promptly after completion of the procedure, and incorporated into the record of each surgical patient. For the surgeons' convenience, many hospitals have dictating machines, a wireless intranet, or a phone hookup with the medical records department installed within the OR suite, usually located in the dressing room or lounge. Voice recognition software can be used to dictate procedural notations in the patient's electronic records. Many surgeons have handheld dictation/transcription devices for immediate use and convenience.

Details of the preoperative and postoperative diagnosis and the surgical procedure itself may have medical and legal significance. Transcription of the surgeon's dictation and maintenance of the patient's chart after discharge from the hospital are responsibilities of the medical records department. The patient's printed chart may be put on microfilm or captured electronically for storage.

Environmental Services

Housekeeping functions are recognized as important preventive measures to eliminate microorganisms from the hospital environment. Each hospital establishes an environmental routine for its particular needs. Usually the environmental services personnel and the perioperative personnel share housekeeping duties in the perioperative environment.

The amount of cleaning done by the perioperative personnel varies from one hospital to another. In many hospitals the members of the environmental services department terminally clean all furniture, flat surfaces, lights, and floors once a day at the end of the surgical schedule. In other facilities, they also clean the furniture and floors before the schedule starts and between each surgical procedure throughout the day. Specific details concerning the care of the perioperative environment can be found in Chapter 12.

Regardless of which plan is followed, environmental services personnel should have a storage area within the OR suite where they keep their equipment and supplies. Equipment used for cleaning in the OR is not taken outside the suite.

The director of environmental services and the perioperative nurse manager plan the division of work. Personnel in each department should understand their responsibilities. The perioperative nurse manager checks the work of the environmental personnel and keeps in touch with the director concerning performance.

The director evaluates and chooses the proper solutions for effective cleaning, sets up a program and standard of performance for personnel, and sees that personnel are properly oriented and taught the appropriate procedures, including procedures for removal and disposal of trash and soiled laundry.

Use of a checklist helps cover all areas to be cleaned and inspected on a routine and preventive maintenance basis, whether it is daily, weekly, or monthly. Weekly or monthly cleaning routines include walls and ceilings, in addition to the daily cleaning schedule within the perioperative environment.

The director impresses on the personnel the importance of the work and the part they play in enabling the perioperative personnel to carry out aseptic technique. The environmental personnel function as members of the team when working with the scrub persons and circulators between surgical procedures.

Facilities Engineering

The facilities engineering department works closely with the OR department by providing a preventive maintenance program. This program includes routine monitoring of ventilation and heating, electrical and lighting systems, emergency warning systems, and water supply. Humidity is recorded every hour in the engineering department. Engineering department personnel should perform a monthly check of all electrical equipment. In addition, the department regularly tests the autonomous emergency power source and maintains a written record of inspection and performance.

The hospital water supply system should not be connected with other piping systems or with fixtures that could allow contamination of the water supply. The hot water supply and steam lines have temperature-control devices and filters regulated by the engineering department personnel. They are cleaned, and filters are changed on a routine schedule, usually weekly, to prevent accumulation of mineral deposits, especially in areas where hard water is used.

Clinical Biomedical Engineering

Competent technical personnel should be available to every area of the hospital to ensure the safe operation of equipment. Nearly every surgical procedure uses some form of powered instrumentation. Because of the variety and complexity of new instrumentation currently in use, most hospitals have a clinical engineer or biomedical equipment technician on staff or at least available. Large facilities may employ multiple engineers and technicians who specialize in medical equipment. This technical support group assists perioperative personnel in evaluating and selecting new equipment as well as installing, operating, and maintaining current equipment.

The clinical engineer is systems and applications oriented. This individual can compare different models and manufacturer specifications and provide recommendations for purchase. The biomedical equipment technician is knowledgeable about the theory of operation, the underlying physiologic principles, and the practical safe clinical applications of biomedical instrumentation. This individual can test, install, calibrate, inspect, service, and repair equipment. Every preventive service or repair is recorded in an instrument history file.

Materials Management

In an effort to control escalating health care costs, many hospitals belong to contract buying groups. This concept has changed the nature of the purchasing function and the management of supplies. The organizational administrative structure varies, but the basic functions of materials management are purchasing, processing, inventorying, maintaining proper function, and distributing supplies and equipment. Several departments are responsible for supplies.

Purchasing Department

The purchasing director coordinates the hospital's acquisition of supplies and equipment. Standardization of products used throughout the hospital fosters quantity purchases, which provides leverage in negotiating prices with vendors. Items that are too expensive to stock in large quantities or that are used infrequently are ordered through the purchasing department as needed. In some hospitals this department is referred to as materials management.

Central Storeroom

The purchasing director or materials manager determines the supplies to be stocked for the hospital. Bulk inventories are received and warehoused in the central storeroom. Each department then requisitions supplies as needed.

Central Processing Department

One area of the hospital is designed specifically for processing, storing, and distributing supplies and equipment used in patient care. This department may be referred to as central service or central supply; central processing; supply, processing, and distribution; or materials management. The functional design and workflow patterns provide for separation of soiled and contaminated supplies from clean and sterile items. Supplies are replenished on the patient care units on a predetermined schedule to maintain standard inventory levels. This may be done by central service with an exchange cart system (i.e., a cart of fresh supplies is exchanged for the one in use).

Control of patient charges for supplies also may be coordinated by central service. Inventory control is computerized in most hospitals. Bar code technology on individual packages may facilitate patient charges and inventory management.

Laundry Services

Many disposable nonwoven fabrics are used. However, some woven fabrics are processed daily for use in the hospital, such as patient gowns, bedding, and towels. Hospitals that do not have laundry facilities as part of their physical plant use a commercial laundry service. An adequate inventory should be maintained for daily use. The manager of laundry services assists in determining appropriate inventories and supervises the laundry processes. Reusable fabrics that must be sterilized before use are packaged and sterilized either in the central service or the sterile processing department.

Human Resources Department

Careful selection of capable, highly motivated people contributes to efficiency and effectiveness. The human resources department helps screen applicants with appropriate qualifications. Those applicants with potential for available positions are referred to the appropriate department head.

Potential employees are processed through human resources before an interview with the perioperative nurse manager is scheduled. The human resources department assists in hiring and terminating all employees. This department also provides resources for employee assistance and assists with progressive discipline.

Human resource departments sometimes use hiring or staffing (recruitment) agencies to find candidates for specific jobs that fit the needs of the facility, such as nursing, managers, and physicians. Online services have made job hunting easier and can reach many people. The use of agencies can reduce the cost of staffing a large full-service human resources department.

Coordination Through Committees

A committee is a group of people delegated to consider, investigate, take specific action on, and report on a matter of mutual concern or interest. Many activities within the facility are coordinated by multidisciplinary committees.

Each committee has a chairperson who conducts the flow of each meeting. A report that includes an attendance roster should be generated to document the activities of the meetings. Each committee member has a special contribution to make in the progress of the work of the group. Each member has a voice in the final outcome charged to the group.

Committee members are usually allotted time during the workday to attend meetings. Other compensation should be made when meetings are scheduled at times when members are not scheduled to work.

Surgical Services Committee

The surgical services committee is composed of the medical staff members who are vital to the management of the perioperative environment. One surgeon is appointed chief or director of the department of surgery. In teaching hospitals a surgeon is

appointed chief of each specialty service (e.g., chief of orthopedics). The anesthesia department also designates a director of that department. These individuals are responsible for professional practice and administrative activities within their respective departments. They should maintain continuing evaluation of the professional performance of all members of the medical staff who have been granted privileges in their specialty. They also serve as liaison representatives between the medical staff and the hospital administrators.

The chief of surgery, the chiefs or representatives of the specialty services, the chief of the anesthesia department, the perioperative nurse manager, the coordinator, and the OR business manager meet at regular intervals to review departmental activities. The hospital administrator and vice president of perioperative services also may be members of this committee or may be invited to attend meetings relevant to their concerns.

The surgical services committee formulates policies and procedures that pertain to use of facilities, a schedule of surgical procedures, and maintenance of a safe environment. Evaluation of techniques and selection of new products may require a review of reports from other departmental surgical services committees, in addition to those prepared by perioperative personnel.

Because this committee determines policies and procedures for efficient functioning within the OR suite, persistent problems are brought before the committee, where recommendations for corrective action are made. For example, if temperature and humidity controls are not being effectively monitored or maintained, the committee may recommend to the hospital administrators that procedures be reviewed and revised by the maintenance department or that new equipment be installed.

If surgeons are repeatedly late in arriving, thus delaying the surgical schedule, a stronger policy may be indicated for the control and better use of facilities. If a new product is purchased, a new procedure may need to be written to specify its use and care.

Through data collection and a problem-solving approach to decision-making, the surgical services committee seeks to improve the working relationships of all members of the OR team and the supportive services concerned with activities within the perioperative environment. Specific areas of concern for the surgical services committee include, but are not limited to, the following topics:
- Setting goals and objectives for the department
- Monitoring policies and procedures
- Planning for growth of services
- Interrelationships between patient care areas within the department and the facility
- Sanctions for noncompliance with policies and procedures
- Review of preparations for the accreditation process
- Resolution of subjects that interfere with the flow of the surgical services department

Policies and associated directives formulated and approved by the committee serve as guidelines for governing the actions of surgeons, anesthesia providers, and the patient care staff while they are in the perioperative environment. The perioperative nurse manager shares with the surgical services committee, hospital administrators, and nursing service the responsibility for clarification, implementation, and day-to-day enforcement of approved policies and procedures.

Operating Room Safety Committees
Radiation Safety Committee

The radiation safety committee reviews the use of radiation exposure monitoring badges. This group sets policies and procedures for maintaining a safe environment where ionizing radiation is present. The committee may establish routines for periodic checking of lead aprons for intactness and for investigating reports of noncompliance with safety practices.

Laser Safety Committee

The laser safety committee establishes policies and procedures, standards, documentation systems, and credentialing criteria for the use of lasers in the health care facility. The laser safety committee also may be responsible for safety equipment and the development of training and continuing education programs for physicians, nurses, and surgical technologists. This committee may be a subcommittee of the surgical services committee. Members should include, but are not limited to, the chief of surgery, the chief of anesthesia, physician representatives from each surgical specialty that uses the laser, the perioperative nurse manager, the laser nurse specialists, a biomedical technician, and a representative of administration.

This committee may delegate safety surveillance duties to a laser safety officer (LSO), who is responsible for identifying problems and safety concerns with the use of lasers. The LSO may be a physician, nurse, or specially trained laser technician. The LSO is given the authority to stop any laser procedure if safety is in question.

Infection Control Committee

The infection control committee investigates hospital-acquired (formerly referred to as nosocomial) infections (HAIs) and seeks to prevent or control them. Membership may vary but should include representatives of the medical staff, hospital administration, and nursing service and the epidemiologist or infection control coordinator. Representatives from other departments attend meetings when the agenda is relevant to their particular concerns.

The committee meets at least quarterly. Members form a defense against HAIs by reviewing environmental factors and by determining whether the hospital is providing a safe environment for patient care. They review all infection reports and investigate HAIs. Committee members also review policies and procedures and scrutinize the entire chain of asepsis in an effort to determine and then eliminate possible sources of infection.

This committee has the authority to approve changes necessary to eliminate any hazardous practices. Included in its jurisdiction is the education of personnel so that they can provide a high standard of patient care. A health care facility has a moral duty to provide a safe environment for its patients. The infection control committee aids the hospital in fulfilling this duty. Surveillance personnel assist in directing infection control policies, procedures, and practices.

Measures are taken to improve postoperative infection prevention by a national quality partnership of hospitals. The list of prevention measures can be found at www.cdc.gov. By adhering to the recommendations, additional costs and length of stay can be reduced by establishing evidence-based practices for prevention of surgical site infections (SSIs). The Center for Medicare & Medicaid Services (CMS) will not reimburse facilities for treatment of

Antibiotic Prophylaxis (Only if Necessary)
One hour before incision—fluoroquinolone (ciprofloxacin)
Two hours before incision—vancomycin (Vancocin) (if indicated)
Antibiotic discontinued within 24 hours postoperatively (48 hours for cardiac patients)

Normothermia
Immediate postoperative body temperature 36° C to 38° C within 1 hour of the surgical procedure

Appropriate Hair Removal
Hair is removed only as necessary with clippers away from the OR.

Urinary Catheters
Urinary catheters are removed within 1 to 2 days of the surgical procedure.

Serum Glucose
Maintain serum glucose between 80 and 110 mg/dL for cardiac patients and <200 mg/dL for other patients. Serum A1C should be <7%.

Oxygenation
Oxygen should be administered and monitored throughout all phases of surgery to promote tissue profusion and optimal wound healing.

Antiseptic Prophylaxis
Selection of antiseptic should be according to facility recommendations.
Use preoperative antiseptic bath with chlorhexidine gluconate (CHG) to reduce SSI risk. Some facilities use a preoperative nasal spray or ointment to minimize the risk of staph infection postoperatively.

infections acquired during the hospitalization period.[6] Best practices associated with SSIs can be found in Box 6.2.

Infection Control Coordinator

An infection surveillance, prevention, and control program uses the services of a strategic person and agent of the infection control committee, the infection control coordinator (ICC). Because this person is often an RN with special training in epidemiology, microbiology, statistics, and research methodology, they may be called an infection control nurse (ICN) or nurse epidemiologist.

The ICC monitors the environment for infections and works closely with the infection control committee. The ICC's duties are as follows:

1. Promptly investigates outbreaks of disease or infection that are over expected levels.
2. Promptly identifies the origin and cause of outbreaks with epidemiologic study.
3. Acquires, correlates, analyzes, and evaluates surveillance data and bacterial colony counts, which includes gathering information to compute and classify specific wound infection rates for all invasive procedures. Rates should be entered in the infection control committee record and be available to the department of surgery.
4. Tracks factors that contribute to infection problems.
5. Consults with directors of critical areas, such as the OR. If an outbreak of SSIs occurs, the ICC confers with the OR nurse manager. They review patient intraoperative records to

determine whether the infected patients had the same procedure or same surgical team or were operated on in the same room.

6. Reviews antiseptic agents used for skin preparation, antibiotics used for intravenous (IV) lines, wound irrigation, and other commonalities in the patient care setting. If a patient develops signs and symptoms of SSI within the immediate postoperative period, a causative factor in the OR is suspect.

7. Coordinates educational programs for personnel who influence infection control. The ICC is a consultant to all hospital personnel and a liaison officer in disseminating information on infection prevention and control.

8. Assists in employee health programs in regard to screening, immunizing, and monitoring the personal health of personnel.

9. Assists in development and implementation of improved patient care procedures.

10. Compares monthly statistics. A significant rise in the monthly reported SSI rate is cause for concern. Reports and data can be helpful in evaluation of aseptic practices if they are brought to the attention of personnel.

11. Reports appropriate diseases to public health authorities.

12. Compares products for effectiveness. The infection control committee approves disinfectants and antiseptics, for example, based on recommendations of the coordinator.

13. Obtains information from surgeons about evidence of infection after discharge and conducts retrospective studies for statistical analysis.

In short, the ICC identifies problems, collects data to find the causes, investigates solutions, and makes recommendations for appropriate hospital policies and procedures to prevent infections. In evaluating infection problems the ICC attempts to find a common denominator, which often leads to the source of the problem. For example, an outbreak of postoperative respiratory infections would lead to an investigation of the cleaning and sterilizing procedures of anesthesia equipment and ventilators. Success of the control program depends in part on the information provided by a conscientious staff, including physicians.

Infection Control Program

An effective infection control program aims to reduce the incidence of infections and to control sources. Information collected through surveillance serves as a basis for corrective action. This information includes written records and reports of known or potential infections among patients and personnel. In 2017 the Healthcare Infection Control Practices Advisory Committee (HICPAC) published the Guideline for the Prevention of Surgical Site Infection. HICPAC is a federal committee that gives advice to the Centers for Disease Control and Prevention (CDC) and Department of Health and Human Services (HHS). The guidelines can be found at www.cdc.gov/HICPAC.

Guidelines and standards for infection control and surveillance are also published by TJC in the *Accreditation Manual for Hospitals* and by the CDC. In general, these standards and guidelines include:

- Establishment of an effective hospital-wide program for surveillance, prevention, and control of infection.
- Establishment of a multidisciplinary committee to oversee the program by reviewing surveillance reports and by approving policies, procedures, and actions to prevent and control infection.

- Assignment of a qualified person to be responsible for management of the infection surveillance, prevention, and control program.
- Provision of written policies and procedures pertinent to infection surveillance, prevention, and control for all patient care departments and supporting services.
- Provision of patient care support services that are adequately prepared to perform all required infection surveillance, prevention, and control functions.

Surveillance

The CDC, an agency of the HSS, is the third largest section of the U.S. Public Health Service. Functioning on both national and international levels, its activities are multifaceted. It carries out a national surveillance of disease incidence and a program, including health education, in prevention of communicable diseases.

Through liaison with state and local health departments, the CDC provides assistance and consultation to health care facilities for specific problem-solving, analysis of surveillance data, and onsite investigation of serious outbreaks of infections. As part of its commitment to the prevention of HAIs, the CDC furnishes information on how to structure an infection-control program.

Continuous Performance Improvement Committee

Members of the performance improvement committee include representatives of both clinical and administrative personnel. This committee monitors routine activities, evaluates clinical outcomes, reviews incident reports, and conducts problem-focused studies in an effort to identify practices deemed substandard.

Actual practices may be in violation of policy or not in compliance with accepted standards or governmental regulations. Noncompliance puts a hospital or ambulatory care facility at risk for legal liability. A productive and efficient committee implements actions designed to eliminate real or potential problems, improve patient care, and reduce financial loss. Because of an emphasis on cost containment, use of facilities and risk management also may be concerns of this committee.

Many facilities employ a quality improvement coordinator or a risk manager to ensure implementation of committee decisions. The primary function of the person in this position is to assess actual practices and evaluate outcomes of patient care. The continuous performance improvement (CPI) coordinator may receive and respond to complaints about patient care or environmental hazards.

Each hospital department and patient care area may have its own quality improvement subcommittee. These unit-based committees monitor performance, identify ways to constructively solve competency problems, and seek opportunities for improvements in practices.

Other interdepartmental subcommittees may focus on specific activities or problems that require input from several disciplines. Reports from these subcommittees are reviewed by the CPI coordinator. Mutual problems are shared with the hospital committee.

Ethics Committee

A multidisciplinary ethics committee should represent the hospital and the community it serves. Representatives include physicians, nurses, social workers, patient relations liaisons, clergy, lawyers, bioethicists, and laypersons from the community. Some facilities have specially trained healthcare ethics consultants (HEC-C) to help with difficult situations.[7] The primary purpose is to educate the staff and the community regarding moral principles and processes of ethical decision-making in the face of diverse populations and subjects that arise in the care of critically and terminally ill patients. They provide consultation to professional staff, patients, and families. This committee recommends policies and guidelines on such subjects as informed consent, research protocols, decision-making, and advance directives.

Perioperative nurses and surgical technologists often are confronted with social, ethical, and legal decisions concerning genetic and reproductive biology, organ transplantation, and death with dignity. The ethics committee can provide a forum for discussion of these subjects. Some hospitals have a nursing bioethics committee in addition to the hospital committee. These committees provide education and consultation and develop policies and procedures. They are not decision-making bodies. They do not get involved in disciplinary matters.

Hospital Safety Committee

Representatives from administration, nursing service, medical staff, infection control, engineering and maintenance departments, environmental/housekeeping services, and the safety director form the nucleus of the hospital safety committee. This group writes policies and procedures designed to enhance safety within the hospital and on hospital grounds. They exchange information with the risk management and quality improvement committees and conduct hazard surveillance programs. They meet at least bimonthly to investigate and evaluate reported incidents. Action is taken when a hazardous condition exists that could result in personal injury or damage to equipment or facilities.

Disaster Planning Committee

Health care facilities should have an organized plan in place to care for mass casualties if a major disaster occurs. External disasters happen outside of the health care facility, such as a terrorist attack, an active shooter, airplane crash, or event of nature (e.g., flood, hurricane, or earthquake).

Internal disasters, such as a fire or an explosion, happen inside the health care facility. In cases such as an active shooter, the disaster can be external or internal. A safety plan should be in place to keep personnel safe, but at the same time triage victims quickly.[8] With the large number of documented cases, facilities need to be prepared and make it part of emergency training. Many resources, tool kits, and emergency preparedness guides are available. The Federal Emergency Management Agency (FEMA) developed a program called The Ready Kids. The program trains individuals and addresses the physical and emotional needs of children during a disaster.[9] Planning by the internal disaster committee includes consultation with local civil authorities and representatives of other medical agencies to establish an effective chain of command and to make appropriate jurisdictional provisions. This planning results in disaster-site triage to separate and distribute patients to ensure the most efficient use of available facilities and services.

Disaster drills are held at least twice a year to test the plans developed by the committee, to seek to improve them, and to familiarize personnel with them. Plans for both types of disasters include the following details:

- *Central command center:* An information center within the hospital to facilitate a unified medical command and the movement of patients.
- *Triage center:* A receiving area for the injured. Severely wounded patients are given emergency care according to their needs and are sent at once to the OR, or to other units as indicated, or transferred to another facility. Ambulatory patients may be treated in the ED for slight injuries and sent home, or admitted to the hospital as indicated.
- *Documentation and communication:* Special disaster medical records or tags that accompany patients at all times to document identification, treatments, medications, destination, and plan of care.
- *A plan of organization of personnel:* As soon as a hospital receives word of a disaster during the evening or night, several strategic people are called. These persons in turn telephone others previously assigned to them, and these call still others, until the full staff has been notified. In cases of disaster, personnel should know where to report if phones or messaging systems are down.
- If the disaster occurs during the day, the full staff is usually on duty, although any off-duty personnel may be called. Other departments are alerted and come on duty as needed, including personnel for the blood bank, laboratory, pharmacy, materials management, radiology department, and patient care units, including the OR, PACU, and ICU. Some laundry and processing personnel also may be alerted. Some strategic maintenance personnel should be available, especially electricians.
- *Written departmental instructions for personnel:* For the perioperative staff, these instructions may include sign-in procedures, checklists of duties, and patient scheduling procedures.

Personnel must know where to report, what to do, and where extra supplies are kept in case of an emergency. Extra supplies are stored in reserve in sufficient quantities to fill possible needs for a minimum of 1 week.

Surgical Services Management

Management of the surgical services department is strategic to the success of this high-cost center within the institution. Power and authority go hand in hand in the roles of administrators and managers. Authority can be bestowed on a person in the role, but power is the ability to influence the outcome in a particular direction. The skillful and effective manager uses both of these attributes to maintain control over the activities and decision-making of the department. Primary managerial activities revolve around safe and efficient patient care, leadership, and budgetary concerns.

Administrative and Management Behaviors
Accreditation

Ongoing policy and procedure updates decrease the need for last-minute compliance documentation necessary for TJC. Most accreditation cycles are 3 years, which is ample time to establish and maintain an accreditation-responsible program. Some managerial considerations for staying in readiness include:

- Set a routine schedule for reviewing and updating policies and procedures. Do not wait until a visit is anticipated to start trying to clean up outdated practices.
- Model each behavior in patient care after the desired outcome. Secure the physicians' support.
- Share information with the staff about the department's progress toward full compliance. Invite some of the surgeons to the meetings. Feature each stride with a report from the achievers during routine staff meetings.
- Keep a copy of the survey questions for the staff to review.
- Establish small groups to tackle small manageable tasks. Collectively this action amounts to a large improvement in participation. Tasks can be delegated to each service.
- Be sure the staff has all the necessary supplies, resources, and support to accomplish the mission.
- With a positive attitude, present each item to be worked. Use the staff's natural talent and creativity. Provide feedback. Coach and encourage.
- Pitch in and help when needed. Make time for the team. Do not micromanage, but take a "hands-on" approach to support the momentum.
- Reward the accomplishments on an ongoing basis, not just for the moment.
- Remain current with evidence-based practices. Dated or unfounded policies and procedures can undermine the authority of the manager in the eyes of the staff and physicians.

Leadership Qualifications and Competency

Leadership is difficult to define, but it is nonexistent without subordinate cooperation. The manager's style, capability, knowledge base, practice reputation, and experience help set the pace for the progress of the department. People skills are very important. Throughout the staff complement, some people show informal leadership abilities that can be positive or negative. Some hallmarks of leadership competency include the following attributes:

- Critical thinking skills
- Objectivity
- Use of credible sources
- Planning ability
- Flexibility
- Creativity
- Self-control
- Negotiation skills

Informal leaders can be harmful if their influence directs the staff away from the main mission of the OR. Winning the support of informal leaders is a significant stride toward better cohesiveness for the staff. Informal leaders can be disruptive when communications break down among the ranks.

The main focus is continual improvement by tempering activities and behaviors of the individual in accordance to the needed productivity of the organization. Each member of the team needs to identify personal strengths and personal relationships with the organization that is working toward becoming a learning organization.

Peter Senge, in his book *The Fifth Discipline*, identified five constructs that are either group or individual relationships with the organization. The process cannot be paced with an exact timeline; however, it can be measured by improved productivity

and personnel in a stable working relationship. The five constructs are simplistically paraphrased as follows:

- *Personal mastery:* Clarify and deepen personal focus.
- *Mental models:* Identify the internal beliefs that cause us to act in a certain way.
- *Shared vision:* Working "on the same page" as the rest of the team. Sometimes this requires more commitment than compliance for growth of the vision, which is where some personnel try to break away and do their own thing.
- *Team learning:* A coordinated group activity in which ideas are receptively expressed in an open dialogue. No judgments are made as would happen in a discussion. Everyone is required to listen and not criticize the ideas of others in the group.
- *Systems thinking:* Discover the root causes of events and fuse the other four constructs together to effect long-range improvement.

Systems thinking is a way to improve the quality of care and help set standards that can be expanded or contracted to meet the needs of the facility and the patient population. When the learning organization has a process of systems thinking in place, the emphasis is on the system, not the individual staff member. Error reduction in the OR can commonly be traced back to a flaw in a system that permitted something to go wrong, such as a retained sponge or a sharps injury. When a decent system is in place and followed by the group, the risk for error is minimized.

Leading by Example

The surgical services staff needs to have respect for the management team. Encouraging the staff to become professionally active on committees or in shared governance, then joining them in professional activities can help cement a sense of pride in accomplishment.

Nurse managers who have no clue about evidence-based practices not only are harmful to the organization but also are less respected by the staff. Failure to keep up with the times makes the nurse manager appear unintelligent and uncaring, especially when the staff attend outside workshops for updates and are met with disdain by the manager. Incompetent managers are a common cause of losing staff to other more progressive facilities.

Perioperative nurse managers should be professionally involved and should be certified as CNORs and possibly certified as administrators.

Although an advanced academic degree is not always necessary, it does make a statement of respect for education and personal growth. Support for line managers and staff who are pursuing baccalaureate degrees is an admirable trait in the management structure.

Rounding up Those "Sacred Cows"

Policies and procedures should have a firm foundation in scientific research and evidence-based practice. Practices that continue despite lack of scientific evidence are referred to as "sacred cows." Managers lose much credibility and look ignorant when they enforce dated practices. The staff respects the manager more when evidence can support the basis for best practice behaviors. Mechanical performance of tasks without knowledge of why is a hazard to patients and the staff. Excuses given by managers commonly include:

- "This is how we do it here."
- "This is how we have always done it."

- "We don't do it that way here" (in reference to the introduction of a newer, more modern approach).
- "The national standards are only voluntary, not mandatory."
- "This is how I was taught. That's good enough for my staff."
- "I did not know that the staff was doing that activity in that manner."
- "Because this is how I want it done."
- "You need to do it this way to save time."

Demanding that the staff perform procedures according to nonexistent rationale is counterproductive. The manager looks incompetent when the staff is required to follow protocols that are not founded in evidence-based practice. Some areas for investigation concerning "sacred cows" in the OR include the following intraoperative behaviors:

- Requiring shoe covers and masks in all areas of the surgical suite
- Cover gowns and laboratory coats worn when leaving the OR
- Forbidding the use of nail polish, including fresh nail polish
- Skin preparations as sterile procedures
- Surgical site hair removal
- Home-laundered versus facility-laundered scrubs
- Timed scrubs, counted brushstroke scrubs, and hand hygiene antisepsis
- Extent of between-case cleaning
- Excessive draping
- Setting time parameters on the sterility of items
- Flash sterilization

Professional Involvement

Managers should be members of their professional organizations and take part in the care and activities that drive their profession. Managers should also be certified with a professional credential.

The administrative and management staff should be knowledgeable about current standards and trends in perioperative patient care. Offering to host professional meetings at the facility or holding open houses for new potential surgical services staff or other departments shows an interest in the departmental growth and insight into the activities behind closed doors.

Meetings

Most management personnel are required to attend and plan a multitude of meetings that pertain to the business of the department and the hospital as a whole. When planning daily activities, they should consider the need to attend these communication sessions. The manager should establish routine meetings within the surgical services department for the dissemination of information as appropriate and adhere to a set time parameter for the proceedings.

Some meetings require the attendance of people from other departments and need to be carefully planned. Offering to hold the meeting in a neutral location can help prevent disruptions by office phones and other distractions.

The chairperson or leader of a meeting should realize the importance of the meeting beginning and ending promptly. Complex topics should be interspersed with simpler group communications. Solicitation of agenda items from attendees in advance helps the chairperson plan and maintain the order of business with minimal digression.

Setting the Agenda

Establishing a time period and content for each meeting is important. Personnel attending meetings should estimate the amount of time they need to plan for attendance. The manager needs to plan a release time for meeting attendees that does not interfere with the daily operation of the surgery department. A meeting agenda should have the following items in its composition:

- Introductions of new personnel and guests
- Short overview of discussion topics
- Old business
- New business
- Special topics
- Delegation of new tasks
- Exchange of information for the good of the group

Minutes of the Meeting

Records of each meeting should be kept at a central location in the department. Personnel in the process of patient care or other shifts may not be able to attend formal staff meetings and need to keep informed about current events in the hospital and department. Secretarial staff or a designated team member should document pertinent facts for the record and verify the accuracy with members of the committee before the group meets for a session.

A loose-leaf notebook with meeting overviews can be maintained in a common area available to all departmental staff members. Some departments set up Internet blog sites where staff members can sign in to participate and communicate ideas. Copies of the minutes can be sent to appropriate people within the facility on a need-to-know basis. The minutes also serve to validate the activities transacted and any resolutions or expectations of future business.

Personnel Management
Motivation and Building a Unified Team

Staff meetings are useful forums for group exchange of ideas, reporting, and concerns. The manager should have regularly scheduled meetings with a formal agenda that has provision for staff input. Allowing the staff to have some ownership of the surgical services department encourages pride in group endeavors.

When the department consists of several areas with specific functions separate from the others, smaller group meetings can be beneficial to work through items not of interest to the entire department. The PACU personnel may have different subjects of interest than the OR team. Collective meetings are useful for consolidating matters that are common to all the areas.

Planning for adequate and appropriate staff to safely and efficiently provide patient care during the implementation of the surgical schedule is a complex task. The AORN Position Statement on Perioperative Safe Staffing and On-Call Practices indicates there should be one RN circulator and one scrub person allotted per case with adequate relief for breaks and meals. The average staffing pattern should be 67% RN to 33% surgical technologists. Orientees are not counted in staffing ratios and are assigned a peer preceptor for the orientation period. The recommendation follows that a staff member should not be assigned to work more than 12 hours in a 24-hour period and no more than 60 hours per work week. Staff should have at least 8 hours of uninterrupted sleep when off-duty. The only situation in which the time elements are prolonged is in the event of a disaster (internal or external). Policies should be formulated to outline staffing in extreme circumstances.

Sometimes managers try to cut corners by stretching the staff numbers to bare-bones teams. Remember that staff efficiency, satisfaction, and retention are not built on working employees to a frazzle. Plans are necessary for break and lunch relief. Consideration should be given to assignments that are emotionally or extremely physically draining. Provision for the relief of an extremely stressed team member is reassuring to the entire staff that they too will not be abandoned by management if the case becomes more complex, lengthy, or emotionally draining than expected. Staff satisfaction is an important part of achieving Magnet status.

Retention of staff is a cost-saving measure. Staffing decisions should not be made based solely on costs. Safety for the patient and the entire team should be foremost in the scheme of planning. The manager should think about the processes associated with hiring, orienting, and maintaining each person on the payroll. Some parameters for staffing newly hired nurses include the following:

- Development or purchase of a perioperative nurse education program
- Recruitment costs
- Duration of orientation
- Preceptor costs
- Materials costs

The cost-effective means for retention is to look for what contributes to staff satisfaction. Giving the staff the opportunity to participate in staffing decisions such as "on-call time" or mandatory overtime can help prevent staff burnout and resignations. Studies show that overworked and exhausted staff frequently cause more human error and increase staff turnover.

Delegation of Duties

When a task is assigned to personnel within the department, the person receiving the instruction should be fully capable and knowledgeable in the action to be taken. The manager should consider the appropriateness of roles and the assignment of duties according to the standards of care and, in some instances, the legality of the role. For example, many states have laws that indicate only an RN may perform the role of circulator. The nurse should understand the laws of delegation in the state of practice. Some states have laws that indicate who may or may not perform in the role of first assistant. Thought should be given to potential consequences of assigning staff to roles that are out of their scope of practice.

Clear instructions should be given, and feedback should be received to indicate understanding. Recognition of a job well done should be freely given. Consequences for poor performance should be moderated appropriately. Competency of each employee should be validated on a regular basis, and incompetent employees should be brought up to speed or put on notice of progressive discipline.

Conflict Management

The OR is a closed environment with a potentially fragile morale. When personnel work closely together for long periods, small disagreements can commonly take place. The manager may need to intervene periodically. Both sides of the disagreement must be heard before any action takes place. Disruptive behavior should not be tolerated; instead it should be managed with firmness and professionalism. Most facilities have developed a "zero-tolerance" policy for unprofessional behavior on the part of surgeons or staff (e.g., humiliation, degradation, harassment, bullying, and so on).

Lateral Violence

Conflicts should not be allowed to fulminate to overstated proportions. Use of the term *violence* indicates the presence of victims. Abuse within the ranks is a form of violence and includes nonverbal innuendos, verbal confrontation, backstabbing, undermining behaviors, sabotage, and gossip.

Personnel have indicated that within their first 6 months they experienced some form of lateral violence. Box 6.3 describes some of the common verbal and nonverbal lateral violence behaviors.

Dissatisfaction among the staff leads to low morale, inadequate performance, and increased personnel turnover.[9] Compromise is a middle-of-the-road approach and should not favor one employee over another. Lateral violence is not a rite of passage in the perioperative environment. The manager needs to identify the problem and address the issue.

The staff should be held accountable for maintaining professional relationships and for preventing the "eating of one's young," as has been the case for many generations. The staff must not be permitted to "dish it out" or be forced to "take it in."[10] The following is a list of behavioral signs of dissatisfied staff and indicate a need to be investigated and managed:

- *Excessive overtime and staff refusal to help:* Cases that run overtime are sometimes caused by staff not performing assigned tasks and failing to prepare appropriately for caseload (foot-dragging).
- *Low productivity:* Turnover between cases is prolonged by staff coming back late from breaks and lunch. Work is unfinished or done poorly.
- *Constant complaining:* The manager needs to listen attentively to find the root cause.
- *High absenteeism and tardiness:* These can be signs that morale is very low.
- *Constant turnover of staff:* Dissatisfied personnel quit or transfer out when resolutions are not sought out or met.
- *Temperaments flare up easily:* Stress can result in acting-out behavior.

Downward Violence

Downward violence is any abusive behavior directed at lower-ranked individuals by higher-ranked individuals and includes abuses by a manager to staff, from a surgeon to manager, or surgeon to staff. Surveys have been conducted for reasons

> **•BOX 6.3 Examples of Verbal and Nonverbal Lateral Violence Behaviors Between Staff Members and Surgeons That Should Not Be Tolerated**
>
> - Eye rolling, eyebrow raising, and tongue clicking
> - Verbal affront: name calling and putdowns
> - Backstabbing and undermining to other staff and surgeons
> - Sabotage and setting up for failure
> - Withholding information or hiding of equipment or supplies
> - Invasion of privacy or broken confidences
> - Gossip or outright lies

concerning transfer requests. OR abuses that resulted in departmental transfers were sparked by management abuse toward staff. Staff may believe that the manager plays favorites and does not assign the workload fairly.

When the disagreement is with a surgeon, the automatic assumption of the staff is that they do not have a fighting chance to say their piece, nor does it matter what they say. This needs to be addressed as soon as possible after an incident.

Verbal abuse by surgeons is not acceptable under any circumstances, regardless of the event, and can cause serious problems in the OR. A surgeon has no right to terrorize the staff. Sometimes, bad behavior is a sign of incompetence and is an attempt to hide or smokescreen personal insecurity. This is true of any person.

Throwing items or other physical displays by the surgeon in the OR are unsafe and should be subject to discipline at the level of the medical staff officers. Failure to attain resolution at that level warrants a report and meeting with the CEO of the facility. Care is taken to follow chain of command; however, the conscientious manager cannot knowingly allow staff or patient endangerment by a surgeon, regardless of the volume of revenue to the facility. Standing up for what is right and just is hard, especially when one is standing alone. The staff will have a sense of respect for the manager who champions the cause of the department fairly and professionally.

Sometimes egos are factors, and a small disagreement gets blown out of proportion. The staff should be assured that many surgeon complaints are not meant on a personal level but rather are directed specifically at a situation. Personal attacks can elicit anger initially and can cause grudges that last months or even years.

The manager, after hearing both sides, has the responsibility to mediate a truce but may have to involve the chief of surgery and the director of nursing service for the facility. Conflicts are costly to the organization in many ways but primarily because of the following factors:

- Staff replacement costs either in orientation of new personnel or in the use of agency workers to fill gaps left in staffing
- Additional staff-hours to complete the schedule at the end of the day; staff frequently take a sick day when feeling overwhelmed and depressed. This is problematic when the person who called off is on call or late that night. Someone else on staff has to pick up the load, causing resentment to grow.
- Refusal to stay overtime because of lack of loyalty
- Increased errors and carelessness
- Legal issues, such as suits for harassment
- Poor productivity and low morale
- Lack of pride in the job can cause injury to the patient

What can the manager do about conflicts or verbal abuse? A few strategies can prove useful when facing this dilemma. The process should be documented in writing. Some ideas are as follows:

- The two people with the disagreement should have a face-to-face meeting away from the OR, perhaps in the manager's office or conference room.
- The manager should be present. Other support may include the chief of surgery, chief of staff, and the director of nursing service. If a physician representative is present, an additional nursing representative also should be present.
- Avoid blaming anyone. Remain objective, and maintain civil tones in all parties.

- Ask each party what would make the situation better on an individual level. Try to reach a compromise with this information. Sometimes a period of working apart allows both parties a chance to cool off.
- The surgeon should not have the right to demand an employee's resignation. Unfounded termination can result in a lawsuit against the facility, the manager, and the surgeon. The surgeon should not have power over an employee's job.
- Praise positive strides for a peaceful resolution. Be aware that some people are overjoyed by being unhappy. Some people have a bad day every day.
- Assure both sides that you will all reach a satisfactory conclusion together. Set some short-term goals and monitor progress.

Documentation

Records of performance reviews should be maintained in the human resources department and in the manager's file. Each employee should have a file that documents attendance, competency, peer review, and practice attributes. Care is taken to document evaluations and anecdotal notes in professional terms because if a staff member files a grievance with higher administration or with a union, the records may be open to scrutiny. Inflammatory comments or slang references could be mistaken for inappropriate labeling of personnel and cause hard feelings.

The manager should evaluate personnel and have them perform self-evaluations in preparation for a face-to-face discussion about performance and performance improvement goals. The contents of the documentation should be the framework for discussion. The staff member should be permitted to retain a copy of all signed performance evaluations for personal records.

Budgeting and Financial Responsibility

For the new nurse manager, preparing a budget for the first time can be intimidating. Before beginning, meet with the facility finance personnel, business manager, and another nurse manager within the facility who may be willing to mentor this process. The materialsmanager can often shed light on the historical use of supplies, and the payroll department can provide information about salaries, performance reviews, and overtime. Computerized records can help with historical department activities and projection of future needs.

A review of previous copies of earlier budgets can be helpful. Most facilities have a specific fiscal year and begin the year with a budget overview meeting, at which time instructional packets are passed out. Computerized methods may include spreadsheets and graphs. Computer literacy and knowledge of financial programs is a must for organization of supplies and records.

After the initial budget is submitted and approved, plans should be underway to begin gathering information for the next fiscal year. Responsibility for the financial affairs of the department includes forecasting needs and growth. The budget in itself is a prime managerial planning tool, not an obstacle to progress.

Day-to-day financial management considerations may include several of the following budgetary factors:

- *Engage the staff in budget dialogue.* Do not use the budget as a weapon or threat, but emphasize the ways the staff can safeguard against waste and promote loss prevention. Include dialogue about first case starts, turnover times, and time management. Understand and discuss what is realistic in terms of safe patient care and efficiency for the type of facility and staffing.

- *Use the operational structure within the facility.* Seek information and advice from other managers, department heads, and purchasing departments. Set up formal and informal meetings to monitor the financial climate of the institution.
- *The cheapest materials may sometimes cost more in the long run.* Establish evaluation groups for new products. Graph the pros and cons of each item tried. Solicit input from other departments that might interface with the product.
- *Encourage planning in ordering of stock.* Keep a standard number of supplies on hand and discourage "squirreling away" of items by staff members. Discourage inventory accumulation in the individual ORs. Staff should be aware of the costs of items used in the OR and not randomly open supplies that may be wasted.
- *Strive for standardization.* Custom packs and routine basic supplies help in this process. It is useful to include the surgeons in planning standardized custom packs. Implantable items such as orthopedic, ophthalmic, or plastic surgery devices could possibly be standardized.
- *Do not skimp on the education of the staff.* The staff needs to know the products and trends associated with the procedures for which they are required to provide patient care. Have regularly scheduled in-service programs, and have specialty leaders demonstrate proper assembly and use of equipment. New machines and supplies can be introduced in an enjoyable atmosphere instead of "on the fly," such as when a new item is foisted on the team in the middle of a procedure, which is an unsafe practice.

Operational Budget

The operating budget directly reflects the department's revenues and expenses. Caseload and staff-hours are the prime considerations during the development of the operational budget. If cases are increasing, so are the numbers of hours and possibly overtime by staff. One method of minimizing the overtime costs is to have staggered staffing shifts. A team that starts later in the day could be assigned to break and lunch relief for the early starting rooms. At the end of the day the late-start team could be available to finish rooms that are still running at the end of the shift. In some facilities this decreases the need for a full second shift crew.

Most facilities provide a monthly departmental summary of expenditures that include the following line items:

- Noncapital purchases (usually less than $500)
- Charges for expenses such as laundry, preventive maintenance contracts, and repairs
- Supply and inventory charges (check the numbers and types of cases each month; are price increases expected? Is there a purchasing contract with a distributor or a buying consortium?)
- Wages and salaries with benefits (holidays and vacation time are calculated, overtime may be projected, and additional full-time equivalents [FTEs] may be needed)
- Educational funds for continuing education, degree-seeking courses, certification, and recertification

Each month the projected amount should be compared with the actual amount of each item. At first the process can seem confusing, but with time this practice becomes second nature. Some vendors charge on a net 30-day basis, and the actual charges

do not appear until 1 to 2 months after the fact. A glance through 3 months at a time to compare and track charging trends is wise. Keep a notebook for observations by the month to help sort out confusing items. Jot down phone numbers, problematic situations, and ongoing questions. Budget software can keep records organized and accurate.

Keeping track of the facility's monthly census may provide some clues as to the accuracy of the figures and whether they will be important for future budget preparation and identification of trends. As these data accumulate, they may demonstrate the need for a change in supplier. Keep good notes of positive and negative encounters with vendors and sales personnel. Always request a business card, and keep it on file for quick contact. A file should be started for each vendor used and notations made if they are associated with a hospital-wide buying contract.

A tablet computer, smart phone, or other portable electronic device is useful for tracking the budget and having portable information for meetings. The device can be synchronized and recharged with a desktop computer, and the information can be kept current at all times. Tablet computers have software that can be used for spreadsheets and document processing. Password protection for all devices is important in case of loss or theft. Some devices contain a global positioning system (GPS) to track their location.

Capital Budget

The capital budget is more concerned with improvements to the physical plant and purchases of large equipment. Patient care devices that are charged per use are considered capital equipment.

Surgeons frequently request equipment for the types of procedures they perform. Some surgeons have the opportunity to preview new equipment at seminars or conferences and then bring the brochures to the manager for future trial use. Sometimes new equipment previewed at medical conferences is discounted for participants of the event. If special capital items are planned for future purchase, it is useful for the manager to attend trade shows and medical conferences where these devices are displayed and demonstrated. New equipment brought in on trial must be checked by the biomedical department before use to validate safety in the OR.

Keeping an ongoing list or file with information about specifications and cost is useful at budget time when preparing requests for capital expenditures. Information that is useful in this process includes the answers to the following questions:

- What is the formal and generic name of the device? Is it available from more than one source?
- Does the device require special hookups or storage? Will we need to modify the physical plant?
- Who will use it and how often? Can it be used by more than one service?
- Who will educate the staff about its use?
- Is software necessary and included with upgrades? Is support available?
- What consumables are necessary, such as disposable leads or parts?
- What is the cost of its use to the facility and the patient? Will we make money on its use? Will we attract surgeons and patients?
- Is use of the device reimbursable by third-party payers?

- Will this device quickly become antiquated? Will we need more than one unit at some point?
- What is currently being used in its place? Are upgrades included?
- Who are the vendors (include contact person, phone number, business card, and email address; date this entry because sales force changes are common)?
- Is it a new project or a replacement (one unit or more)? Is a business plan needed to validate the purchase?
- Is a device available for trial? Is it possible to "rent to buy"? Would renting the device be more cost effective than purchasing it?
- Are any hazards or biologic injury associated with use? Is it approved by the U.S. Food and Drug Administration (FDA)?
- What are the costs (item, installation, PM contract, tax, shipping, maintenance; get a secured price quote)? Sometimes special prices are available if ordered through trade shows. Can you offer to be a demonstration site for a discounted cost?
- What education or credentialing is required to use it? Will dedicated staff be needed to manage the item in the OR?
- What is the warranty and service information?
- What is the delivery and turnaround time for repairs? Is a loaner available if a repair is needed?
- What are the costs of basic repairs and parts?
- Is product support available during the phase-in process?

Outdated or poorly functioning machinery is replaced during this process. The American Hospital Association has prepared a "life expectancy" guideline for most types of devices used in patient care. This resource is valuable in establishing a replacement program for dated items. The manager should project needs and develop plans for growth or improvement for a 5-year cycle of depreciation. Knowledge of current technology is a must to stay on top of new device knowledge. Some surgical services departments include anesthesia and central processing equipment with the OR and PACU capital budget.

New Product and Equipment Evaluation

The user of a product is best qualified to evaluate performance, safety, effectiveness, and efficiency. Before a decision is made to purchase or standardize a particular item, a clinical evaluation should be conducted to solicit feedback from team members whose work is affected by the product. This may involve the surgeons, anesthesia providers, and perioperative nurses and surgical technologists. Instruction should be provided on the correct use of the item before it is evaluated. Vendors and sales representatives may be permitted to assist in the trial of a product in the OR. Although they do not provide direct patient care, they offer suggestions and consult with the users during the product trial. Members of an interdisciplinary product selection committee might include:
- Pharmacists
- Nurse educators
- Biomedical staff
- Wound care team members
- Infection control nurses
- Occupational or physical therapists
- Nurse managers
- Nurses from the postsurgical areas

To be valid, feedback should be an objective evaluation of function, quality, and use. Does it meet a need? Does it solve a problem? Is it cost-effective? Does it improve patient care? How does it compare with other brands? Several brands of the same product may be evaluated to select the most satisfactory one for the intended purpose and to standardize the inventory. Written evaluations are useful for the decision-making process after the trial period.

Many products are used only in the perioperative environment; however, some are also used in other patient care areas. Representatives from all user departments should assist the materialsmanager in selecting products. Most hospitals have a product evaluation committee for this purpose. A representative of the perioperative staff provides this committee with information regarding quality and effectiveness, based on feedback from user staff members.

Once a product has been purchased, the user assumes responsibility for its safety and its proper use for its intended purpose. Problems with medications or patient care items should be reported to the FDA with the MedWatch system. The FDA tracks complaints and orchestrates recalls as appropriate.

Working With Vendors and Sales Representatives

Vendors are important sources of information and support. Each facility should have a policy in place that addresses who has the authority to work with the vendors and under what circumstances they are permitted in the department. The vendor should register at the main information desk in the lobby of the hospital and wear proper identification at all times. They should not cause any disruption or compromise patient privacy in any way.

AORN has established a position statement about vendors in the OR that is useful for determining facility policies and procedures. Vendors should have a basic knowledge of sterile technique and should be able to enter the OR without disruption. The following list provides guidelines for working with vendors:
- The facility should have specific policies in place to govern the activities of credentialed vendors. IDs are worn at all times. Attendance is documented and time-limited.
- Some facilities issue vendors scrub suits that are a different color from those of the staff for identification.
- Meetings are by appointment only. No meetings are to be scheduled with any of the staff without express permission from the manager.
- Physicians may not bring a vendor into the department without going through proper channels.
- Facility security policies are followed at all times. Patient confidentiality is maintained.
- The vendor may not render direct patient care at any time. The patient must have the opportunity to give informed consent to the presence of a vendor.
- Specialized and highly trained manufacturer vendors may have indirect activities, such as calibration of pacemakers and defibrillators, as directed by the surgeon. These personnel should not be scrubbed in at any time.
- Only the products planned for the meeting are presented.
- No fliers or materials are to be distributed without permission of the manager.
- Trial devices are brought in only by request and are examined for safety by the facility's biomedical department.
- Disposable products for trial have appropriate lot numbers for reporting problems or malfunctions.

EVOLVE WEBSITE

http://evolve.elsevier.com/Hornacky/BerryKohn/
- Student Interactive Questions
- Glossary

References

1. www.nursingworld.org. Accessed February 14, 2023.
2. Pintz C, Zhou QP, McLaughlin MK, et al.: National study of nursing research characteristics at Magnet®-designated hospitals, *J Nurs Adm* 48(5):247–258, 2018.
3. Chien L, Slade D, Dahm M, et al.: Improving patient-centered care through a tailored intervention addressing nursing clinical handover communication in its organizational and cultural context, *J Adv Nurs* 78(5):1413–1430, 2022.
4. www.aha.org. Closed-loop communication, *AHA Center for Health Innovation*. Accessed February 23, 2023.
5. Bender M, Veenstra J, Yoon S: Improving interprofessional communication: conceptualizing operationalizing and testing a healthcare improvisation communication workshop, *Nurse Educ Today* 119:105530, 2022.
6. www.cdc.gov. Accessed February 23, 2023.
7. Aaron B, Crites J, Cunnungham T, et al.: Hospital ethics practices: recommendations for improving Joint Commission standards, *Jt Comm J Qual Patient Saf* 48(12):682–685, 2022.
8. Spruce L: Mass causality incidents, *AORN J* 109(1):95–100, 2019.
9. Chin M, Goodman L, Palacios C, et al.: Workplace bullying and the role of voice and ethical leadership. In *Employee voice at work*, 2019, Work, Organization, and Employment, pp 129–146.
10. Edward KL, Ousey K, Warelow P, et al.: Nursing and aggression in the workplace: a systematic review, *Br J Nurs* 23(12):653–659, 2014.

Bibliography

AORN (Association of periOperative Registered Nurses): *Guidelines for perioperative practice*, Denver, CO, 2024, The Association.
AORN: *Position statement on incivility, bullying, and workplace violence.* www.aorn.org.
AORN: *Position statement on perioperative safe staffing and on-call practices.* www.aorn.org.
Northhouse PG: *Leadership: theory and practice*, ed 3, Thousand Oaks, CA, 2004, Sage.
Senge P: *The fifth discipline: the art and practice of the learning organization*, New York, 1990, Currency Doubleday.

7

The Patient: The Reason for Your Existence

CHAPTER OUTLINE

The Patient as an Individual, 99

The Patient With Individualized Needs, 102

The Patient With Cancer, 110

The Patient With Chronic Comorbid Disease, 117

The Patient Who Is a Victim of Crime, 119

End-of-Life Care, 123

Death of a Patient in the Operating Room, 123

CHAPTER OBJECTIVES

After studying this chapter the learner will be able to:

- Describe Maslow's hierarchy of needs.
- Describe some characteristics of diversity in a patient population.
- List the main elements of a patient-centered approach.
- Describe how the patient may perceive care.

KEY TERMS AND DEFINITIONS

Body mass index (BMI) Calculation that divides body weight in kilograms by height in meters squared (kg/m^2).

Comorbidity More than one disease entity in an individual that intersects and requires continual monitoring and treatment.

Domestic violence Abuse perpetrated in the home or living arrangement. Can be physical, psychologic, verbal, or nonverbal.

Homeostasis A balance of biochemical and physiologic systems within a person that sustains life in a disease-free state in the presence of environmental influences.

Paradigm Model used as a foundation for a conceptual framework.

Perception Use of the senses, cognition, and awareness to evaluate the collective stimuli of the environment.

Perpetrator Person who is suspected of committing a crime against another person.

Polypharmacy Use of multiple medications, either prescribed or self-administered.

Stress Internal perception of and response to stimuli in a positive or negative manner.

Victim Person who has been injured by the effects of the environment or suffered abuse by another person.

The Patient as an Individual

Patients are the reason for the existence of the health care team. They look to the perioperative team to fulfill their diverse needs during the preoperative, intraoperative, and postoperative phases of care (Fig. 7.1). The patient is always the center of attention, not just when under the operating room (OR) spotlight. A patient may be defined as an individual recipient of health care services.

Extremes of age (pediatric and geriatric) and comorbid disease entities require individualization of the plan of care. To meet a patient's requirements and expectations effectively, personnel should have knowledge of the patient's needs, problems, and health considerations. From a perioperative perspective it is important to understand the effect a surgical procedure has on a patient's lifestyle. The following are some of the characteristics that individualize patients:

- They are unique with individual needs.
- They respond psychosocially on the basis of personal values, beliefs, gender identity, and ethnocultural background.
- They have the capacity to adapt to internal and external environments.
- They have basic needs that must be met to maintain homeostasis.

Homeostasis is a consistent internal environment maintained by the patient's adaptive capabilities and has a physiologic and a psychologic component. From a physiologic aspect the patient's body strives to maintain equilibrium within normal limits through control mechanisms located in the endocrine glands and in the

• **Fig. 7.1** The OR from the patient's perspective.

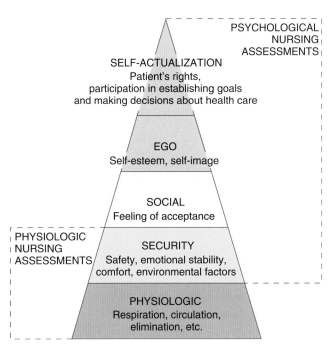

• **Fig. 7.2** Maslow's hierarchy of needs as related to surgical patient needs during perioperative care.

reticular formation in the brainstem. This stability depends partly on the structural integrity of the body, the adequacy of its functions, and environmental influences.

Psychologic homeostasis is based on emotional acceptance and a rational understanding of events that influence health and wellness. Fear and anxiety are common stressors that alter a patient's psychologic response to the health care system.

Patients' Basic Needs

Needs are factors that must be controlled or redirected to restore altered function. Nursing diagnoses are based on knowledge and understanding of a patient's needs and how to fulfill them. The surgical patient faces a threat to the needs identified by humanistic psychologist and motivational theorist Abraham Maslow (1908–1970): physical, security, psychosocial, emotional, and spiritual.[1]

Hierarchy of Needs

Maslow's hierarchy of needs is still an essential part of the surgical patient's perioperative care. In following Maslow's concept of a motivational hierarchy of needs to set priorities for care (Fig. 7.2), the basic lower level (physiologic needs) essential for survival must be met first. Satisfaction of the higher-level needs for safety and security, belonging and acceptance, self-esteem, and self-actualization can then be met. Health care personnel should be concerned with a total picture of the patient's needs and consider meeting all of them. In illness, physiologic and psychologic needs can be influenced by factors such as location of the pathologic condition, type of surgical procedure, and effectiveness of therapy. In addition, priorities may shift with changing situations. Preoperatively, individual needs such as comorbidities, anxiety, nutritional status, safety, comfort, and rehabilitation are addressed. Intraoperatively, the team concentrates on the patient's physiologic needs for oxygen and circulation and the prevention of shock and infection. Postoperatively, team members must prevent complications and encourage patient self-actualization. If the patient's needs are not met satisfactorily, undesirable consequences can occur.

To meet a patient's needs, the health care team should be sensitive to the patient's feelings about the illness. A patient's reactions can influence behavior and the staff's behavioral responses. An understanding of the patient's basic methods of

coping is helpful to the caregiver in developing the plan of care (Table 7.1).

Behavior

Health and human behavior are interdependent and often age dependent. Regardless of age, individuals with physiologic problems experience some emotional change that influences their behavior. Patients react to a new interpersonal environment according to their learned behavioral patterns. The following list includes basic facts about behavior:

- The perception of interaction within the environment creates individual differences in personality, behavior, and needs.
- A person's physical and psychosocial behavior is a response to stimuli in an attempt to maintain homeostasis.
- Behavior is complex. Behavioral acts have multiple causes in addition to a major precipitating one.
- A person functions on many levels simultaneously. Many factors determine an individual's response in a given situation.

Behavior should be evaluated considering the person's specific situation and pertinent social forces, such as family, significant others, culture, and environment. Patients respond to crises or personal threats in different ways. Some persons face suffering and surgical intervention with extreme courage, dignity, and fortitude. Others may revert to extreme fear or helplessness, even when faced with a relatively uncomplicated procedure.

Overt behavior is not necessarily consistent with one's feelings but often reflects them most accurately. Patients often express frustration and fear behaviorally in an effort to cope with environmental stimuli.

Adaptation

In 1984, nursing theorist Sister Callista Roy proposed adaptation as a conceptual model for nursing. Any deviation from a person's normal daily pattern of living necessitates adaptation through innate or acquired defenses. Roy's Adaptation Model (RAM)

TABLE 7.1   Common Coping Mechanisms

Mechanism	Meaning	Objective Assessment	Example
Denial	Rejects responsibility; unable or unwilling to accept the truth	Stammers; may or may not make eye contact; seems to be making excuses	"I do not have lung cancer."
Displacement	Shifts blame to a weaker substitute	Is submissive to power figures but critical and oppressive to subordinates	"My doctor never tells me anything. The laboratory must be wrong."
Identification	Acts like an admired hero or villain	Shows outward signs of indecisiveness and low self-esteem	"My sister and I both feel ill. We both have the same disease, I'll bet."
Projection	Attributes unacceptable behavior to others	Acts suspicious of others; assumes a defensive posture	"The cigarette manufacturer enticed me to smoke."
Rationalization	Justifies behavior with plausible statements	May be defensive or smug; tries to save face; can become hostile	"I became ill only because cancer runs in my family."
Reaction formation	Acts differently than feeling inside	Is confused, irrational; has mood swings; may seem overly conscientious and moral	"These are not tears of sadness; they are tears of joy because I will be dead soon."
Regression	Reverts back to a more primitive state of being	May assume closed, fetal position; has crossed arms and legs; looks downward, cries; has prolonged silences	"I want my mother."
Repression	Blocks unacceptable thoughts and feelings	Has a blank stare, a questioning look; no in-depth discussions	"I don't remember what my diagnosis is. Why am I here?"

involves physiologic or psychologic changes.[2] Her paradigm as it applies to perioperative patient care includes the following factors:

1. The patient takes in stimuli and processes the information to produce a response.
   a. Effective adaptation is exhibited by a favorable response.
   b. Ineffective adaptation is exhibited by an unfavorable response.
2. The environment around and inside the patient is constantly changing. The patient responds either favorably or unfavorably to each change.
3. The health status of the patient integrates the whole person with adaptive changes to internal and external forces.
4. The process of nursing is a science and the application of patient care is an art.

Both the mind and the body must adapt successfully for the patient to recover. Adaptation requires energy, ingenuity, and persistence. The adaptive process includes physiologic or psychologic changes that constitute an attempt to counteract stimuli so the individual can continue to function. If something interferes with this adaptation, the effects can be detrimental. Adaptation to illness includes three stages, as follows:

1. Transition from health: development of symptoms
2. Acceptance: coping and making decisions
3. Convalescence or resolution

Adaptation may be rapid or slow depending on the nature of the stimuli and on the patient's culture, learned responses, and developmental needs. Adaptations may be sensory, motor, or sensorimotor. The extent of adjustment needed is contingent on the type of illness, the magnitude of disability, and the patient's personality. More information about Roy's adaptation theory can be found online at www.currentnursing.com.

Stress

Stress can be defined as a physical, chemical, or emotional factor that causes tension. Stress may be a factor in disease causation. It is the result of a perceived threat and is manifested by changes in physiologic and psychosocial behavior. Stress tolerance depends on the individual and on the stressor—its intensity, duration, and type (either localized or generalized, such as pain).

Stressful factors can originate from within the individual or from the external environment. Intrinsic factors, or those that originate within a patient, include the following:

- Hereditary or genetic factors, such as competency of the hormonal or enzymatic system.
- Nature of the illness or disease process. This may be influenced by nutritional or immunologic status.
- Severity of the illness or the presence of a stigma.
- Previous personal experiences with illness. Chronic illness has a disruptive effect on lifestyle.
- Age can have differences in thoughts and behavior. Children feel threatened, whereas adolescents resent an interruption of activities and are painfully aware of body changes. Older people think about infirmity and death.
- Intellectual capacity. Misconceptions can lead to a knowledge deficit about the disease. Impaired cognitive function creates an inability to understand or comprehend.
- Disturbed sensorium. Hearing or sight loss intensifies a stressful experience.
- General state of personal well-being.

Extrinsic factors originate from external sources and include:

- Environment. The physical and social environment of the hospital is not the same as that of the home.
- Role and status with family and significant others. Expectations and authoritative relationships affect lifestyle, attitudes, and communications.
- Economic or financial situation.
- Religion. Beliefs influence attitudes and values toward life, illness, and death. For example, Jehovah's Witnesses do not permit transfusion of whole blood or blood components. Orthodox Jews must follow dietary laws in any environment. The attitudes derived from some religious beliefs give a person

little control over the environment and can render a patient passive and apathetic.

- Cultural background, education, gender identity, and social class. These factors are closely related to a patient's emotional responses and living habits. Significant cultural elements such as food habits, daily living patterns, hygiene, family organization, child care, and orientation to the past, present, and future should be analyzed in relation to culture. All patients should be asked how they would like to be addressed. This acknowledgment should follow the patient throughout the surgical process.
- An ethnic community is a larger family. Roles taught by a cultural group influence the values, beliefs, and social interactions of its members. Also, responses to pain may vary according to cultural or ethnic background. Some groups commonly show an exaggerated emotional response, whereas other groups believe concealing suffering and feelings is more appropriate.
- Social relationships. Family, significant others, and friends help satisfy the need for reassurance and provide a sense of being cared about.

Stress is both physiologic and psychologic. It can adversely affect appetite and bodily functions such as digestion, metabolism, and fluid and electrolyte balance. The secretion of adrenocortical hormones delays wound healing and decreases resistance to infection. In addition, the patient's emotional needs come to the surface during times of markedly increased stress, which mobilizes defense mechanisms for fight or flight. The patient's ability to adapt depends in part on options and effective intervention.[2]

Anticipatory apprehension, although normal to some degree, may diminish critical thinking and decision-making abilities and may also initiate an exaggerated response. Patients feel vulnerable when threatened with the loss of body parts, bodily function, or life. The assumptions of the OR itself—its noises, odors, and equipment—can be frightening for patients.[3]

Patients' Perceptions of Care

Studies have shown that a patient's perception of high-level care is based on participation in decisions. Patients are better educated and have higher expectations for better care. The patient's belief system defines what is considered to be good care. Perceptions of caring behaviors vary according to the degree of illness, type of procedure, level of cognition, and setting. Most patients believe that proficient and efficient perioperative care includes assistance with pain control, warmth, comfort, and a safe environment. The caregiver is also perceived as a patient advocate and a communication link with the family or significant others.

Research has revealed that preoperatively a patient needs information about the surgical procedure, how it will be performed, and the type of anesthetic to be used. Intraoperatively, the patient assumes a passive role, entrusting care to the perioperative team.

Before administration of the anesthetic the patient may be acutely aware of surroundings and activities. Patients surveyed indicate that during this segment of intraoperative care they want to know what is happening as it takes place and desire reassurance from the circulator at their side. Patients expect the perioperative nurse to remain in physical proximity and act promptly in an emergency. During the check-in and time-out periods of patient identification and verification of the procedure, the patient is included in the dialogue as much as possible. Documentation of the patient's inclusion and responses should be part of the permanent record.

During and after the administration of the anesthetic, the patient places a strong sense of confidence in the team as a whole and has expectations of competence and efficiency. The professional nurse is considered a main source of protection during this period of vulnerability and should not leave the patient's side.

Postoperatively, patients expect the perioperative and perianesthesia nurses to monitor their condition closely and provide pain relief as needed. In continuation of the passive role, patients perceive the nurse as caring, knowledgeable, protective, and efficient. Patients respond favorably to the following scenarios:

- Provision of privacy and dignity
- Sensitivity to the inconvenience of hospitalization
- Frequent updates to family and significant others during the surgical procedure
- Attention to personal and special needs
- Acceptance of personal individuality
- Friendliness
- Accurate and understandable information about tests and treatments

Family and Significant Others

A discussion of the patient is not complete without specific mention of the patient's family or others significant in their life. Illness often creates an emotional and financial burden on the family. They may experience considerable anxiety over the outcomes of surgery, the feelings of isolation, and the disruption of lifestyle. A family's reaction to illness and perception of care is as individualized as the patient.

Families need preoperative instruction to prepare for the postoperative outcomes and rehabilitation. They also need to be kept informed of the patient's progress during the surgical procedure and recovery period. Many surgeons have the circulating nurse call the waiting room when the procedure is started and periodically as the procedure progresses. Some facilities issue pagers so family members may leave the waiting room and not miss any updates. Time passes more slowly during waiting periods, and family members may fear something has gone wrong if the wait is longer than anticipated. Some family members may prefer to wait at home or at work. The surgeon should contact a spouse, family member, or significant other when the surgical procedure is over.

Discussions with anyone other than the patient concerning condition or personal information require the patient's permission as part of the Health Insurance Portability and Accountability Act (HIPAA) requirements concerning patient privacy. Details can be found at www.hhs.gov/hipaa.

The Patient With Individualized Needs

The debilitated, chronically ill, or age-extreme patient has an increased difficulty in combating the stress of surgery and anesthetic agents. Other problems or health considerations that predispose the patient to intraoperative or postoperative complications include substance abuse or other serious subclinical conditions not revealed during the preoperative assessment.

Preoperative diagnostic and laboratory studies assist in establishing diagnoses and in pinpointing areas of deficiency. Surgical intervention is often postponed until one or more physiologic conditions are improved or controlled (e.g., blood work [potassium level, pregnancy]; high blood pressure is lowered; cardiac dysrhythmias are corrected; or anticoagulation is controlled). Patients with more than one physical illness are considered comorbid. Comorbidity and the use of multiple drugs (polypharmacy) for treatment complicate surgery and put the patient at risk during anesthesia and surgical intervention. Preoperative therapy may be indicated to control diabetes, strengthen muscles, reduce obesity, or treat infection to decrease the risk for intraoperative or postoperative complications.

Patients of all ages and stages of development have different needs, and the ways of meeting these needs vary. A family-centered approach to care is valuable. Family cooperation is essential for communication with, interpretation for, and assistance with patients, particularly pediatric and geriatric patients.

The Patient With Sensory Impairment or Physical Challenge

Some patients come to the perioperative environment with conditions unrelated to the surgical problem. Sensory and physically challenged patients commonly have increased anxiety and need a highly individualized plan of care; these patients also have the potential for a problematic postoperative recovery.

Sensory Impairment

Communication is essential to assess adequately the needs of challenged patients and to care for them. Team members should know about and understand the patient's limitations. Patients have a right to know what will happen during the surgical experience and to participate in decisions about their care.

The Rehabilitation Act of 1973 (Rehab Act) states that to receive federal funds an agency "must provide, when necessary, appropriate auxiliary aids to people with impaired sensory, manual or speaking skills to give them an equal opportunity to benefit from services." The Rehab Act prevents discrimination and protects individuals with disabilities. The complexities of each patient's situation should be evaluated and dealt with appropriately.

Language Barrier

A language barrier can be a complex challenge. Anxiety increases in proportion to one's inability to communicate in a stress-producing situation. The inability to understand or to express oneself verbally is frustrating, and the patient's behavior may reflect feelings of inadequacy or insecurity. Offer the patient something to write on, such as paper, an erase board, or a tablet, for communication.

Nonverbal body language through eye contact, pleasant facial expressions, and a gentle touch can comfort the patient who speaks a different language. Every effort should be made to obtain an interpreter to assist the patient and the health care team. Many large hospitals use interpreters for the ethnic groups within the community and for out-of-town visitors.

Some patients are reluctant to share confidential medical information with a relative or friend. The interpreter should be trusted and accepted by the patient and should be sensitive to the needs of the surgeon and caregivers. The patient needs to be adequately informed before giving consent for a surgical procedure and must provide permission for release of information concerning the procedure. The surgeon should make sure the patient fully understands the procedure when working with an interpreter. Confidentiality is stressed throughout the communication process.

Hearing Impairment/Deafness

Hearing impairment varies from inner ear conduction changes that occur during the aging process and affect the distinction of some high-frequency consonant sounds to congenital profound sensorineural deafness. Conductive or sensorineural deafness may result from disease or injury to the ear at any age.

The degree of impairment determines whether the patient communicates through sign language, has a hearing-assistive cochlear implant, wears a hearing aid, or reads lips. Written information is always helpful, provided the patient is literate. Pictograms work well with most patients. An interpreter can assist with patients who use sign language.

The following steps should be observed when communicating with a patient who has a hearing impairment:
1. Make sure the room is quiet and well lit, with minimal distractions. Deaf patients may perceive extraneous sounds as buzzing or air-rushing. Deafness can be manifest in many degrees. Care is taken not to approach so quietly that the patient becomes startled.
2. Greet the patient without wearing a facemask and attract the patient's attention before speaking. Make eye contact.
3. Speak clearly and slowly in a moderate tone of voice, with visible but not exaggerated lip movements. Facial expressions, touch, and body gestures can help communicate feelings and instructions.
4. Be sure the patient understands and responds appropriately to questions.
5. To help explain your actions, show the patient any equipment (e.g., a safety strap) before placement.
6. Allow the patient to wear a hearing aid in the perioperative environment, if possible. Try to know what type of device the patient uses and how to adjust the controls if it should start humming during the procedure. The team should know how to remove and deactivate the device if it could interfere with the planned procedure.

Visual Impairment/Blindness

Like deafness, blindness can be a part of the aging process, a congenital anomaly, or the result of an accident. Cataracts are a common cause of the loss of visual acuity; this condition may be inherited but is more often associated with aging. Vision is affected by the shape of the eye, other structural factors, and diseases and injuries.

Patients who are blind feel insecure in a strange environment; therefore the following steps should be observed when communicating with them:
1. Make some noise as you approach the bed so as not to startle the patient. Address the patient by name in moderate tones and then introduce yourself.
2. Always speak to the patient and explain what will happen before touching them. A gentle word followed by a gentle touch can be comforting.
3. For prevention of a distressful reaction to unexpected noises or sensations, the patient should be told what is going to happen before any physical contact.

4. Guiding the patient's hand helps the patient feel secure, such as when being moved onto the operating bed (OR bed). If this is done, care must be taken not to get fingers pinched between beds.

5. Do not shout; they can still hear. If general anesthesia is given, use the patient's name when waking up so they know they are being spoken too.

A visually impaired patient should be permitted to wear eyeglasses in the perioperative environment as much as possible. If a general anesthetic is used, the eyeglasses should be placed in a container labeled with the patient's name and sent to the post-anesthesia care unit (PACU) so they are available when the patient wakes. Contact lenses and artificial eyelashes must be removed before administration of a general anesthetic because they may dry on the cornea or become dislodged.

Physical Challenge

Patients who are physically challenged need a highly individualized plan of care. Physical problems such as contractures, broken bones, spinal deformity, missing limbs, or pressure sores may make it difficult to position the patient on the OR bed. Patients with spastic muscle motion, as in cerebral palsy, need additional personnel around the OR bed for safety during transfer; otherwise the random body movement could cause the patient to fall.

Creative supports with recommended positioning aids are needed, and additional assistance may be necessary to move the patient safely. Use alternating pressure pads, such as gel pads, as available. Exposure of the surgical site may be difficult to achieve.

Millions of people have some form of arthritis. Children with juvenile rheumatoid arthritis have many systemic problems as a result of the disease process, which continues into adulthood. The onset of this autoimmune disease can occur at any age and may result in stiffness, swelling, and deformity of the joints of the hands, feet, and neck; inflammation of blood vessels; and tissue damage to organ systems. Joints need solid but padded support. Long-term treatment with nonsteroidal antiinflammatory drugs (NSAIDs) or corticosteroid therapy may affect bleeding intraoperatively and wound healing postoperatively.

Paralyzed patients, such as those with spinal cord injuries, are unable to move. Patients with lack of voluntary muscle control must be protected from falls or injuries during transport or transfer. Patients with nerve damage, uncontrollable muscle movements, paralysis, and autoimmune disease may have decreased tactile sensitivity to heat and cold, so they must be protected from burns and hypothermia.

Impairment of Cognitive Function

Communicating with patients who have impaired cognitive function is sometimes difficult. Cognitive functions are based on intelligence and the ability to think, learn, remember, respond, and solve problems.

Explanations about procedures and the environment may seem confusing and frightening to these patients. Verbal communication should be attempted at the patient's level of understanding and response. Simple phrases and soft vocal tones can be reassuring. Some patients benefit from the presence of a family member or significant other.

Patients with an autistic spectral disorder have a variety of cognitive levels. Understanding the individual characteristics of the patient's condition is useful during communications with the patient. Cooperation during the surgical procedure may be hard to

attain, and preoperative sedation may be necessary. More information concerning autistic spectral disorder can be found at www.nichd.nih.gov/health/topics/autism.

The Patient With Alteration of Nutrition

Decreased intake and increased metabolic demands create nutritional problems in surgical patients. Drug therapy and procedure activities affect nutritional status; this should be considered when planning for a patient's nutritional needs. Table 7.2 describes the effects that certain drugs have on nutrition. With so many prescriptions, over-the-counter (OTC) drugs, supplements, and herbal substances on the market, patients should consult a pharmacist about possible side effects, nutritional effects, and long-term medication complications.

The preoperative assessment may reveal risk factors associated with alterations of nutrition. The patient should be asked if any of these categories are taken. Patients may not think supplements or herbs are medication because they are not prescribed by a doctor.

TABLE 7.2 Drugs That Interfere With Nutritional Status

Drug	Effect on Nutrition
Aluminum hydroxide	Binds with other nutrients, causing phosphate malabsorption
Aminoglycosides	Reduce carbohydrate metabolism
Amphetamines	Suppress appetite, causing weight loss
Antacids	Alter gastrointestinal pH
Anticholinergics	Decrease gastrointestinal motility, causing malabsorption
Anticonvulsants	Can cause a decrease in calcium and vitamin D
Antihistamines	Stimulate appetite and can cause weight gain
Antihypertensives	Decrease gastrointestinal motility, causing malabsorption
Antineoplastics	Impair nutrient absorption
Antirheumatoids	Impair nutrient absorption
Benzodiazepines	Stimulate appetite, causing weight gain
Cathartics	Cause calcium and phosphate loss
Chloramphenicol	Inhibits protein binding
Cytotoxic agents	Suppress appetite, causing weight loss
Diuretics	Cause potassium loss (potassium-sparing diuretics are available)
Immunosuppressives	Suppress appetite, causing weight loss
Isoniazid	Causes pyridoxine deficiency
Neomycin	Interferes with bile acids, causing iron, sugar, and triglyceride malabsorption
Phenobarbital	Causes vitamin D deficiency
Phenothiazines	Stimulate appetite, causing weight gain
Phenytoin	Causes osteomalacia
Statins	Lowers CoQ10 enzyme, causing muscle aches, inflammation, low energy, weakness
Steroids	Depletes sodium
Tricyclic antidepressants	Stimulate appetite, causing weight gain

Some patients use cannabis liquid, gummies, or ointments to relieve pain and may not disclose the use. Patients undergoing procedures of the mouth, face, head, and neck may have mechanical difficulty taking adequate nutrition orally. Some patients may have peripheral means of nutrition in place, such as feeding tubes, percutaneous gastric tubes, or central IV lines.

Malnutrition

Malnutrition in the surgical patient is caused by an inadequate intake or use of calories and protein preoperatively and/or postoperatively. The discrepancy between the intake of essential nutrients and the body's demand for them creates a state of impaired functional ability and structural integrity.

Surgical patients are commonly kept without food preoperatively for safe anesthetic administration and postoperatively to prevent nausea and vomiting. Patients who are undernourished have less than 70% to 80% of ideal body weight (IBW) and suffer greatly from the lack of caloric intake. As a result of malnutrition the patient may experience the following side effects:

1. Poor tolerance of anesthetic agents
   a. Decreased metabolism of chemicals by the liver
   b. Inadequate excretion of toxins by the kidneys
   c. Unstable vital signs
   d. Hypothermia
2. Altered wound healing potential
   a. Decreased protein synthesis postoperatively
   b. Increased protein wasting and breakdown of skeletal muscle after severe traumatic injury
   c. Negative nitrogen balance, with a serum albumin value less than 3 g/dL and blood urea nitrogen (BUN) value less than 10 g/dL
3. Decreased serum electrolyte levels associated with anorexia, bulimia, alcoholism, and other chronic metabolic disturbances
   a. Hypokalemia (low potassium level)
   b. Hypomagnesemia (low magnesium level)
   c. Hypocalcemia (low calcium level)
   d. Hyponatremia (low sodium level)
   e. Hypophosphatemia (low phosphate)
4. Increased susceptibility to infection from immunologic incompetence, with a total lymphocyte count less than 1500/mm^3
5. Sequential multisystem organ failure
   a. Dehydration
   b. Abnormalities in glucose regulation
   c. Abnormalities in clotting mechanisms
   d. Renal failure
   e. Cardiopulmonary failure
6. Increased risk for morbidity and mortality

Serum blood tests help determine nutritional status and include total proteins, albumin-to-globulin ratio, and BUN level. Body weight is also significant. The average adult patient needs a minimum of 1500 calories daily to prevent body protein catabolism. Women over 31 years old are recommended to consume 1600 to 2200 calories daily.[4] Men over 31 years old should consume 2200 to 3000 calories daily. Nutritional needs are based on physical activity.

Hypermetabolic states can double that requirement to 3000 calories daily. If caloric intake is less than body requirements, protein is converted into carbohydrates for energy. Protein synthesis then becomes insufficient for restoration of body tissues. Box 7.1 describes conditions that place a patient at risk for protein deficiency and malnutrition. Information about protein and

---

• BOX 7.1   Factors That Increase a Patient's Risk for Protein-Based Nutritional Deficit

- Chronic illness
- Acute illness
- Stress
- Metabolic disease
- Sensory impairment
- Unconsciousness
- Polypharmacy
- Depression
- Immobility
- Edentulousness
- Lack of monetary resources to purchase protein-rich foods

---

dietary guidelines for all age-groups can be found at www.dietaryguidelines.gov.

Depleted reserves of essential elements must be replenished to replace tissue loss and expedite wound healing. Protein deficiency impairs collagen formation, thereby delaying the healing process. Water-soluble vitamins B complex and C are important for tissue repair and nervous system function. The fat-soluble vitamins A, D, E, and K are important for neurovascular activities.

The patient's depleted nutritional status lowers host resistance by impairing lymphocyte and neutrophil production. A definite relationship has been shown between hypoproteinemia and proliferative postoperative infection. Wound healing is impaired.

Metabolism

Metabolism is the phenomenon of synthesizing foodstuffs into complex elements and complex substances into simple ones in the production of energy. It involves two opposing phases:

1. *Anabolism:* The conversion of nutritive material into complex living matter; tissue construction.
2. *Catabolism, or destructive metabolism:* Breaking down or dissolution by the body of complex compounds, often with the release of energy.

Metabolic disorders such as diabetes and the stress response of traumatic injury can complicate the outcome of a surgical intervention. Hormonal responses to physical stress involve both anabolic and catabolic effects on the body, with catabolism being the predominant effect. The degree of metabolic reaction may depend greatly on the body's reserve of labile protein. The patient's preoperative nutritional state, the type and extent of the surgical procedure, and the effect of the surgical procedure on the patient's ability to digest and absorb nutrients affect immediate postoperative metabolism.

Catabolic responses are augmented by preoperative fasting, cathartic preparation, adrenocortical responses to tissue trauma during the procedure, blood loss, hypothermia, and alterations in fluid and electrolyte balance. Patients with burns, traumatic injury, absorptive disorders, or toxemia need careful nutritional replacement because they usually have a severe protein deficit. Hydration and renal function are closely observed and monitored in the perioperative environment.

Drugs also can have an adverse effect on metabolic balance. Broad-spectrum antibiotics limit a disease process, but in association with dietary inadequacy they can cause vitamin K deficiency in older patients by inhibiting the intestinal bacteria that produce that vitamin. Drug detoxification or excretion may be altered in patients with impaired kidney or liver function, leading to possible drug overdose.

Nutritional Supplements

Dietary management is used to correct metabolic and nutritional abnormalities before the surgical procedure. In some patients, special nutritional supplements are indicated to build up or compensate for a permanent metabolic handicap. Enteral feedings help maintain the integrity of the gastrointestinal mucosa. Successful therapy is indicated by weight gain, a rise in plasma albumin, and a positive nitrogen balance. A chemically defined elemental diet may be administered by the following routes:

- Oral intake
- Nasogastric tube for enteral nutrition
- Gastrostomy tube, with or without infusion pump, for enteral nutrition
- IV infusion of protein and dextrose through a peripheral vein for parenteral nutrition
- Central venous cannulation for hyperalimentation for parenteral nutrition

The Patient With Diabetes Mellitus

Diabetes mellitus is an endocrine disorder that affects glucose metabolism and the production of insulin in the beta cells of the pancreas. Insulin is a hormone that helps break down carbohydrates. If insulin is not produced in sufficient quantities or is of poor quality, carbohydrates are not metabolized and are excreted in the urine as glucose. Glucose molecules are large and damage the cellular structure of the renal tubules of the kidneys.

Usually genetic in origin, diabetes mellitus can be triggered in predisposed individuals by environmental stress. Management of the surgical patient with diabetes depends on the type and control of the disorder, which is one of the following types[5]:

1. *Type 1:* Insulin-dependent diabetes mellitus. The pancreas produces little or no insulin, thus necessitating regular administration of insulin via injection. Onset may be at any age but usually occurs in juveniles (adolescents ages 12–16 years) and adults up to age 40 years.
2. *Type 2:* Non–insulin-dependent diabetes mellitus. The pancreas produces varying amounts of insulin. Onset may be at any age but usually occurs after age 40 years in obese persons. Blood glucose levels are controlled by diet, weight loss, exercise, and the administration of oral antihyperglycemics, or injectable noninsulin drugs. In some cases, insulin therapy is necessary to lower blood glucose levels.
3. *Diabetes mellitus associated with other conditions or syndromes:* Impaired glucose tolerance may be the result of pancreatic or hormonal disease, drug or chemical toxicity, abnormal insulin receptors, or other genetic syndromes. Diabetes is also a risk factor for cardiovascular disease (CVD). The diabetes may be latent, asymptomatic, or borderline.
4. *SGLT2 inhibitors:* These drugs are newer to the market and work by preventing the body from reabsorbing sugars through the kidneys. Empagliflozin (Jardiance), dapagliflozin (Farxiga), canagliflozin (Invokana), and ertugliflozin (Steglatro) are examples.
5. *GLP-1 receptors:* This new group of injectable drugs works by lowering blood glucose levels and slows digestion. Examples include semaglutide (Ozempic), exenatide (Byetta), dulaglutide (Trulicity), and liraglutide (Victoza).
6. *GLP-1 and GIP:* Combination drug that activates both receptors to lower blood glucose, slow digestion, and help excrete extra glucose; example: tirzepatide (Mounjaro).

Stress caused by physical and emotional trauma, infection, or fever raises blood glucose levels and stimulates the pituitary and adrenal glands. The pituitary gland secretes adrenocorticotropic hormone (ACTH), which stimulates the production of glucocorticoids. These glucocorticoids in turn increase gluconeogenesis, the formation of glucose by the liver from noncarbohydrate sources. The resultant extra glucose enters the bloodstream.

Coincidentally, the adrenal glands secrete epinephrine, which accelerates the conversion of glycogen in the liver to glucose and also raises the level of blood glucose. More insulin is needed to metabolize this additional blood glucose. The primary goal in controlling diabetes is to maintain a stable internal environment, thereby averting a metabolic crisis. Extreme care must be taken to prevent the following conditions:

1. Hyperglycemia and ketonuria
   a. A rise in blood glucose and ketones can precipitate severe fluid loss, causing dehydration and hyperkalemia from the release of potassium from cells.
   b. Some medications (e.g., cortisone) increase the level of blood glucose and antagonize the effect of insulin.
2. Ketoacidosis and acetonuria
   a. These conditions are caused by insulin insufficiency from natural causes or from a reduced or omitted insulin dosage.
   b. These conditions may result in coma and ultimately death if allowed to progress untreated.
3. Hypoglycemia and hypoglycemic shock
   a. These conditions are caused by too much insulin.
   b. They are of faster onset than ketoacidosis.
   c. Hypoglycemia is especially dangerous. It can occur during major surgical procedures because of the omission or delay of oral intake.
   d. These conditions can cause brain damage and put stress on the cardiovascular system.

Prevention of these states depends on the following factors:

- Physician's treatment of choice for diabetes
- Severity and type of disorder
- Existence of complicating conditions
- Type of surgical procedure
- Blood glucose should be monitored throughout the perioperative care period and maintained between 80 and 180 mg/dL. The optimal preoperative blood glucose A1C should be less than 7%. Surgical procedures for patients with an A1C over 10% should be postponed if possible until the level can be lowered.[6] All diabetic patients undergoing a surgical procedure should discuss NPO (nil per os, nothing by mouth) status, diabetes medication time, and dose amount with the surgeon. Each individual will have a different plan; some patients will be instructed not to take any medication or reduce the dose.
- Patients undergoing general anesthesia may have different intraoperative and postoperative blood glucose numbers. According to the American Diabetes Association (ADA), blood glucose level of 140 to 180 mg/dL is acceptable during the perioperative phase to prevent blood glucose levels dropping below 70 mg/dL (hypoglycemia). Patients had fewer adverse outcomes when blood glucose levels were maintained between 140 and 180 mg/dL for 24 hours or until the patient was stable to resume a presurgical regimen. Patients with blood glucose

levels over 200 mg/dL were at risk for complications and higher mortality rates.[6]

The preoperative assessment of patients with the potential for impaired glucose metabolism includes laboratory testing for fasting and postprandial blood glucose levels, urinalysis, complete blood count, BUN values, and serum electrolyte determinations. A chest x-ray study and electrocardiogram (ECG) also are advisable.

Common Complications

The balance between caloric intake and glucose metabolism is disrupted during the perioperative experience. Patients with type 2 diabetes may be managed easier and withstand a surgical intervention without crisis. Intraoperative metabolic control may be more difficult in patients with type 1 diabetes who have marked unpredictability and greater extremes in blood glucose levels. Lengthy major surgical procedures with extensive tissue trauma present the greatest challenge to regulation. Patients with diabetes are prone to the following conditions:

- Dehydration and electrolyte imbalance
- Infection
- Inadequate circulation from neurovascular disease, which causes deficient tissue perfusion (Fig. 7.3)
- Hypertension and CVD
- Hyperlipidemia that affects both coronary and peripheral arteries; peripheral edema can lead to gangrene
- Delayed wound healing because of increased protein breakdown or compromised circulation; glycogenesis, the breakdown of glycogen to glucose in the liver, diverts protein from tissue regeneration
- Neuropathy or nervous system disorders, which cause motor and sensory deficit
- Nephropathy, which affects small blood vessels in the kidneys
- Retinopathy, which affects small vessels in eyes, and blindness
- Neuropathic musculoskeletal disease; severe bone destruction may cause neuropathic fractures

- Neurogenic bladder, which causes incontinence; urinary tract infections are common
- Hypothermia related to metabolic disorders

Diabetes causes many bodily changes that increase in frequency with duration of the disease. Physiologic dysfunctions, as listed in Table 7.3, make a person with diabetes a potentially high-risk patient.

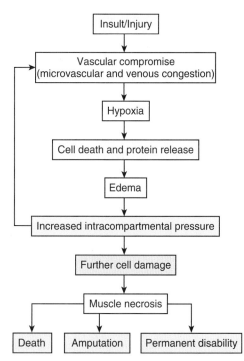

• **Fig. 7.3** Outcomes of tissue injury in the OR.

TABLE 7.3	Physiologic Dysfunctions in Patients at High Risk With Diabetes and Obesity	
Diabetes Mellitus	**Obesity**	
Integumentary System		
Skin that may be dry, itchy	Hirsutism in women	
Loss of fat from adipose tissue	Excess subcuticular fat	
Injuries that heal slowly	Injuries that heal slowly	
Musculoskeletal System		
Neuropathic skeletal disease with bone destruction	Osteoarthritis	
Leg pain, neuropathy	Chronic back pain	
Muscular wasting	Strain on joints and ligaments	
	Joint pain	
	Diminished mobility	
Cardiovascular System		
Increased heart rate	Myocardial hypertrophy	
Predisposition to coronary artery disease	High blood pressure	
Predisposition to thrombophlebitis	Arteriosclerosis	
Peripheral edema	Venous stasis	
	Varicose veins	
Respiratory System		
Predisposition to infection	Shortness of breath	
	Decreased tidal volume	
	Decreased lung expansion	
Renal System		
Nephropathy	Vascular changes in kidneys	
Increased excretion	Decreased intestinal mobility	
Neurogenic bladder	Predisposition to liver and biliary disease	
Gastrointestinal System		
Secretion of glucose by liver		
Neurologic System		
Neuropathy		
Sensory impairment		
Retinopathy and blindness		
Endocrine System		
Poor or nonexistent insulin production	Predisposition to diabetes mellitus	
Poor metabolic control	Pituitary abnormalities	
Increased production of cortisol by adrenal glands under stress	Poor metabolic control	
Electrolyte imbalance	Dysfunctional uterine bleeding	

Special Considerations

Scheduling of elective surgical procedures early in the day for patients with diabetes minimizes the period during which oral intake is restricted. Assessment of these patients can minimize potential risks:

1. Capillary blood should be tested preoperatively for fasting serum glucose. The results provide baseline data for assessment of postoperative control.
2. The preoperative insulin dose may be reduced or eliminated to guard against hypoglycemia or insulin shock during the surgical procedure.
3. Continuous IV access is vital throughout the surgical procedure in case of a metabolic problem. An infusion of dextrose in water may be started to begin administering the daily carbohydrate requirement before the patient comes to the OR.
   a. Optional methods of management for patients who are insulin dependent or who take other glucose-lowering drugs are determined by the severity of the disease, the preoperative control regimen, and the type of surgical procedure. Insulin may be added to the infusion or administered via subcutaneous injection. Amounts are determined by serum glucose levels. Patients with insulin pumps should consult the surgeon and be advised to keep the pump working or disconnect the device. If the pump is disconnected, the anesthesia provider will administer necessary medication.
   b. Adequate hydration must be maintained because a rising blood glucose level upsets osmotic equilibrium. Electrolytes may be added to maintain metabolic status.
   c. Fluid intake and output must be monitored to maintain hydration without fluid overload.
4. A metabolic crisis in an unconscious patient is difficult to detect without frequent blood tests. Therefore during long surgical procedures, blood glucose levels are monitored for hyperglycemia or hypoglycemia. Glucometers accurately measure capillary blood glucose levels. Monitoring is necessary to ascertain the patient's requirements for insulin, glucose, or both.
5. Nasogastric suction may cause acidosis, dehydration, or electrolyte imbalance.
6. Antiembolic stockings are usually worn by the patient during the surgical procedure and postoperatively as a precaution against thrombophlebitis and thromboembolism. Some surgeons use sequential compression leg wraps to prevent deep vein thrombosis during long periods of immobility.
7. Skin integrity must be guarded to avoid breakdown.
   a. Strict aseptic and sterile techniques are extremely important to the infection-prone patient with diabetes.
   b. To protect bony prominences and prevent pressure sores, foam padding or a gel mattress should be placed on the OR bed for surgical procedures expected to take more than 2 hours.
   c. Hyposensitive tape is used to affix dressings.
   d. If an active warming device is used, the patient's skin should be monitored for contact burns.

The Obese Patient

Obesity is prevalent in our society and around the world. More than 75% percent of the adult population in the United States is considered overweight with a body mass index (BMI) over 25 kg/m². Obesity is defined when weight exceeds the ideal weight and the patient's BMI ranges from more than 30 to 39.9 kg/m².[7] The term *extreme obesity* (>40 kg/m²) is now used to describe 100 lbs (45.4 kg) overweight for men and 80 lbs (36.3 kg) for women. BMI is calculated by weight in kilograms divided by the square of height in meters. BMI calculators and formulas can be found on smart devices for easy conversion.

Patients may be offended or embarrassed by use of the term *obese*. In discussing the subject of weight the patient may respond better if kinder terms such as *weight problem* or *weight difficulties* are used. Obesity has serious effects on health and lifestyle, leading to many medical conditions and even early death. It may be of one of two origins:

1. *Endocrine:* Usually associated with biliary, hepatic, or endocrine disease.
2. *Nonendocrine:* Commonly associated with excessive caloric intake.

Common Complications

Surgical patients who are 10% or more overweight have an increased incidence of morbidity and mortality caused by concomitant systemic diseases and physical problems. The degree of morbidity varies with the severity of the obese condition. The physiologic dysfunctions of obesity are listed in Table 7.3.

Obesity predisposes an individual to several conditions, including:

- Increased demand on the heart. Pulse rate, cardiac output, stroke volume, and blood volume increase to meet the metabolic demands of the adipose tissue (fat). Eventually this overload leads to myocardial hypertrophy (enlargement of the heart), and congestive heart failure may result. Coronary artery disease also is common.
- Hypertension (high blood pressure). Vascular changes in the kidneys are associated with hypertension and affect the elimination of protein wastes and the maintenance of fluid and electrolyte balance.
- Varicose veins and edema in the lower extremities. Poor venous return results from pressure on the pelvic veins and the vena cava. Venous stasis can ultimately contribute to thrombophlebitis and thromboembolism. Some surgeons use sequential compression leg wraps or antiembolic stockings to aid venous return and prevent deep vein thrombosis during long periods of immobility.
- Pulmonary function abnormalities. Hypoxemia, or inadequate oxygen in blood, may be associated with decreased tidal volume or poor gas exchange caused by excessive weight on the thoracic cavity. Patients who are obese are susceptible to postoperative pulmonary infection and pulmonary embolism.
- Respiratory compromise sleep apnea is common.
- Diseases of the digestive system, such as liver or gallbladder disease. Diverticulosis is not uncommon.
- Osteoarthritis. This condition may limit mobility of the spine and joints and may in fact contribute to excessive wear on joint cartilage.
- Diabetes mellitus. Type 2 diabetes.
- Malnutrition. Although obese patients are overweight, they may have a protein deficiency or other metabolic disturbance such as hyperlipidemia.

Special Considerations

The physical size of an obese patient presents problems for the OR and PACU teams. Safety precautions against injury to the patient and staff, falls, and burns must be emphasized. Problems include the following situations:

1. Transporting and lifting the patient. Size-appropriate wheelchairs and stretchers should be used. Mechanical patient lifters are desirable. If these are not available, extra people are needed to ensure safety in lifting.

    a. Stretchers and OR beds must be weight appropriate and stabilized. Many standard OR beds cannot support more than 300 to 350 lbs. With the population becoming heavier, facilities are purchasing beds to accommodate obese patients. The manufacturer's instructions should be consulted. OR beds should be tagged with clearly visible weight restrictions. Larger weight loads up to 1000 lbs (453.6 kg) can be borne by beds especially designed for obese patients.

    b. In moving the patient from the stretcher to the OR bed the wheels should be locked and it should be suggested that the patient sit up. The back of the patient's gown should be untied, and the patient should be asked to feel for the side of the OR bed so that they do not move too far and fall over the opposite side. Additional personnel should stand at the opposite side of the bed to prevent falls.

    c. Safety belts should be long enough to provide secure limitation of unwanted mobility. When the patient is supine the circulating nurse should place a small pillow under the patient's knees to relieve low back strain. The safety belt is placed over the thighs 2 to 3 inches above the knees. The safety belt should be placed over blankets. The circulating nurse should be able to slide one hand between the safety belt and the patient to ensure that no pressure is on the patient. A second safety belt may be needed for the lower legs if the patient's calves occupy the spaces closest to the edges of the bed because of the inability to close the legs when supine.

2. Keeping bodily exposure to a minimum as with all patients. Gowns are often small and may cause obese patients to feel self-conscious. Protecting the patient's privacy and dignity is the responsibility of the entire team.

3. Induction, intubation, and maintenance of anesthesia.

    a. On rare occasions, venous cutdown may be necessary to establish an IV line if peripheral veins are difficult to access. Some anesthesia providers may use a central line for better venous access.

    b. Mobility of the cervical spine to hyperextend the neck for intubation may be limited. The anesthesia chapter of this text (see Chapter 24) discusses neck and throat considerations for complex intubation. Some patients may need awake intubation.

    c. Inefficient respiratory muscles, poor lung/chest wall compliance, and increased intraabdominal pressure in the supine position reduce ventilation capability.

    d. Inefficient ventilation lowers the concentration of gases entering the alveoli of the lungs, which prolongs induction time.

    e. Continuous uptake by adipose tissue necessitates higher concentrations of anesthetic agents to maintain anesthesia. Drug dosages are calculated by body weight in kilograms (2.2 lb = 1 kg). The circulating nurse should double-check that the patient's weight is listed in kilograms on the chart for the anesthesia provider.

• **Fig. 7.4** Positioning an obese patient for spinal surgery on an Andrews frame.

    f. The recovery period may be prolonged because adipose tissue retains fat-soluble agents and because the poor blood supply in this tissue eliminates agents slowly.

4. Positioning, prepping, and draping on the OR bed.

    a. Extra personnel may be necessary to assist with positioning.

    b. Massive tissue and pressure areas must be protected. Protuberances must be padded to prevent bruising and pressure injuries (Fig. 7.4). Tissue folds, breasts, and genitalia should not be compressed. Alternating pressure reduction surfaces such as gel pads should be used. Rolled blankets are not appropriate padding because once compressed, they do not disperse the body weight and become a source of localized pressure.

    c. Ventilation and circulation must be ensured.

    d. When an electrosurgical unit is used, the patient's dispersive electrode is applied on a flat, dry, smooth surface and is not surrounded by overlapping skinfolds because tissue could be burned by accumulated radiofrequency energy.

    e. An additional person may need to help hold the legs during Foley catheter insertion in a female patient.

    f. More than one skin prep tray or applicator may be needed to accommodate large body habitus. Great care is taken to be sure that alcohol-based prep solutions do not accumulate in skin folds. This could be a fire hazard because this area will not dry at the same rate as surface areas.

5. Increased operating time because of mechanics of the surgical procedure.

    a. In an open procedure, the accessibility of deep organs (e.g., gallbladder) may be a problem.

    b. Large instrumentation may contribute to surgical trauma and postoperative pain.

6. Thromboembolic complications, which may occur because of venous stasis; erythrocytosis, which increases the viscosity of the blood; and a decrease in fibrinolytic activity. Anticoagulants such as subcutaneous heparin may be given prophylactically.

7. Delayed healing because of poor vascularity of adipose tissue. Obese patients have an increased incidence of postoperative wound infection and disruption caused by dead space in the adipose tissue.

    a. A sterile, closed drainage system is often used to drain accumulated fluid, thereby facilitating healing.

    b. It is harder to eliminate "dead space" in wound closure.

Additional information about working with obese patients, including BMI charts, can be found at www.niddk.nih.gov.

The Patient With Cancer

Oncology is the study of scientific control over neoplastic growth. It concerns the etiology, diagnosis, treatment, and rehabilitation of patients with known or potential neoplasms. A neoplasm is an atypical growth of abnormal cells or tissues that may be a benign or malignant tumor.

Both malignant and benign neoplasms consist of cells that divide and grow uncontrollably at varied rates. The stimulus for growth can be intrinsic (e.g., hormonal) or extrinsic (e.g., exposure to external elements). Neoplastic overgrowth or the invasion of surrounding tissue causes dysfunction and may eventually cause the death of the patient.

Cancer is a broad term that encompasses any malignant tissue change and is potentially curable.[8] Treatment and prognosis are based on the type of cancer and the extent of the disease. Each type differs in its symptoms, behavior, and response to treatment.

The exact cause of cancer is unknown, but it is the second leading cause of death in the United States. Cancerous tumors can be caused by exposure to chemical toxins, ionizing radiation, chronic tissue irritation, tobacco smoke, ultraviolet rays, environmental hazards, viral invasion, and genetic predisposition. Studies have shown that immunosuppression may contribute to the incidence of cancer by altering biochemical metabolism and cellular enzyme production. Other research has shown that dietary influences, such as nitrates, salt-cured or smoked foods, and high-fat diets, may contribute to cancer in certain individuals.

Oncologists study the cause (epidemiology) of cancer and the diagnosis, treatment, and rehabilitation of patients with cancer. Moreover, patients are demanding that their surgeons give attention to the reconstruction of body image and rehabilitation to a useful life. Therefore the treatment of patients with cancer must be accomplished through the efforts of a multidisciplinary team of oncologic surgeons in conjunction with pathologists, radiation oncologists, pharmacists, immunologists, medical oncologists, dieticians, and others. In addition to physical care, nurses in all patient care settings provide psychologic support for cancer patients, families, and significant others.

Cancer Risk Avoidance Behaviors

Patient education should include information about avoiding cancer-causing behaviors and how to minimize the risk for cancer. Behaviors to discuss include the following[8]:

- Avoiding smoking, electronic devices (vaping), and exposure to smoke or vapor. The U.S. Department of Health and Human Services reports that exposure to cigarette smoke is responsible for 87% of all cases of lung cancer. Secondhand smoke, referred to as *environmental tobacco smoke*, has been implicated in the development of cancer in nonsmoking people who are exposed to smoke on a regular basis.
- Increasing dietary intake of fiber and low-fat foods. Antioxidants such as vitamins A and C may reduce an individual's risk for development of cancer. High-fat diets have been implicated in the development of breast, colon, and prostate cancers. According to reports of the American Cancer Society, 35% of cancer deaths are related to dietary causes and are possibly preventable. Hyperglycemia has also been linked to an increase in cancer rates. Information on the risks of diabetes and cancer can be found at www.cancercenter.com. A desirable weight should be maintained, and obesity should be avoided. Excessive alcohol intake also should be avoided.
- Minimizing sun exposure, especially between the hours of 10:00 AM and 4:00 PM.[8] Sun exposure has been shown to be the major cause of skin cancer, especially melanoma. Severe sunburn in childhood may be linked to the development of skin cancer later in life. Certain medications, such as tranquilizers, antidiabetic agents, diuretics, antiinflammatory agents, and antibiotics, can predispose an individual to sunburn. Certain cosmetic products, such as tretinoin (Retin-A) and α-hydroxy acid, are extremely reactive to sunlight and can increase the risk for sunburn within 30 minutes of exposure. Tanning booths also can be hazardous to the skin. A waterproof, broad-spectrum sunscreen with a sun protection factor (SPF) of at least 30 should be applied whenever sun exposure is likely.[8] Sun-blocking products of SPF 30 to 100 are preferred and should provide protection from both ultraviolet A and ultraviolet B (UVA, UVB) rays. (UVA rays can increase the damage caused by UVB rays.) Sunscreen should be applied at least half an hour before going outdoors and reapplied according to the directions. Water-resistant products should have a protection period on the label and be reapplied within those parameters or if wiped off.
- Having regular checkups, especially yearly checkups, after 40 years of age. Family medical history may recommend early screening for cancer. Knowing the warning signs of cancer may promote prompt diagnosis and treatment. Signs to consider in young children include frequent swelling (lymphadenopathy) or bruising, unexplained headaches or fevers, dramatic weight loss or gain, and localized pain.
- Self-examining the skin, breast, and testes may reveal early signs of cancer. These self-examinations should be performed monthly.
- Unsafe sexual practices can lead to disease and higher risk for cancer.

Extent of Disease
Carcinoma in Situ

In carcinoma in situ, normal cells are replaced by anaplastic cells, but the growth disturbance of epithelial surfaces shows no behavioral evidence of invasion and metastasis. This cellular change is noted most often in stratified squamous and glandular epithelium. Carcinoma in situ is also referred to as intraepithelial or preinvasive cancer. Common sites for in situ carcinoma include the following:

- Uterine cervix
- Uterine endometrium
- Vagina
- Anus
- Penis
- Lip
- Buccal mucosa
- Bronchi
- Esophagus
- Eye
- Breast

Localized Cancer

Localized cancer is contained within the organ of its origin.

Regional Cancer

In regional cancer the invaded area extends from the periphery of the organ or tissue of origin to include tumor cells in adjacent organs or tissues (e.g., the regional lymph nodes).

Metastatic Cancer

In metastatic cancer the tumor extends by way of lymphatic or vascular channels to tissues or organs beyond the regional area.

Disseminated Cancer

In disseminated cancer, multiple foci of tumor cells are dispersed throughout the body.

Cancer Treatment Modalities

Cancer is a systemic disease. Therapy is curative if the disease process can be totally eradicated, but the success of therapy depends largely on early diagnosis. Tumors are classified according to location, regional spread, and systemic extension for determination of the most effective therapy. Therapies are customized for each patient. Many drugs and treatment modalities are available. When a cure is not possible, palliative therapy relieves symptoms and improves quality of life; however, it does not cure the disease. Additional information about surgery in patients with cancer can be found at www.cancer.org. This site provides concise descriptions suitable for students and patients and is a useful tool for patient education.

Adjuvant Therapy

Surgical resection, endocrine therapy, radiation therapy, chemotherapy, immunotherapy, hyperthermia, stem cell, targeted therapy, blood transfusion, or combinations of these procedures are used to treat cancer. The surgeon or oncologist determines the most appropriate therapy for each patient. In determination of the most appropriate therapy the following factors are considered:
- Type, site, and extent of tumor and whether lymph nodes are involved
- Type of surrounding normal tissue
- Age and general condition of the patient, including nutritional status and whether other diseases are present
- Whether curative or palliative therapy is possible

Before beginning therapy a patient with cancer undergoes an extensive pretreatment workup. Each form of cancer therapy has certain advantages and limitations. Several factors affect a patient's response to treatment: host factors, clinical stage of malignancy, and type of therapy. The patient is followed carefully to determine the effectiveness of treatment at routine intervals.

Surgical Resection

Surgical resection is a modality to remove most solid tumors. The resection of a malignant tumor is, however, localized therapy for what may be a systemic disease. Each patient is evaluated and treated individually, and the surgical procedure is planned appropriately for the identified stage of disease. Depending on localization, regionalization, and dissemination of the tumor, the surgeon selects either a radical curative surgical procedure or a salvage palliative surgical procedure.

Surgical debulking (cytoreduction), in which the tumor is partially removed, may be the procedure of choice for some types of surgically incurable malignant neoplasms. With surgical debulking the intent is not to cure but to make subsequent therapy with irradiation, drugs, or other palliative measures more effective and thereby extend survival. In planning the surgical procedure the surgeon considers the length of expected survival, the prognosis of surgical intervention, and the effect of concurrent diseases on the postoperative result.

Accessible primary tumors are often treated with excision. An extremely wide resection may be necessary to avoid recurrence of the tumor. The pathologist is able to make judgments about questionable margins by evaluating frozen sections while the surgical procedure is in progress. The pathologist's findings guide the surgeon during resection so residual tumor is not left in the patient. The specimen is also tested after permanent section fixation in the pathology laboratory. Final results are available in 2 to 3 days. Additional discussion about cancer diagnostics is found in Chapter 22.

Many surgical procedures are performed for ablation of tumors with primary resection. In addition, a lymphadenectomy (removal of local lymph nodes) may be performed as a prophylactic measure to inhibit the metastatic spread of tumor cells by lymphatic channels. These nodes are tested to determine the extent of tumor cell spread. Other modalities of therapy may be administered preoperatively, intraoperatively, and/or postoperatively to reduce or prevent a recurrence or metastasis.

Considerations for Intraoperative Care

Malignant tumor cells can be disseminated with manipulation of tissue. Because of their altered nutritional and physiologic status, patients with cancer also may be highly susceptible to the complications of postoperative infection. To minimize these risks the following specific precautions are taken in the surgical treatment of patients with cancer:
1. The skin over the site of a soft tissue tumor should be handled gently during hair removal and antisepsis. Vigorous scrubbing could dislodge underlying tumor cells; this is avoided with the use of "no-touch" techniques. With vascular tumors, manipulation during positioning or skin preparation could cause vascular complications such as emboli or hemorrhage. The no-touch technique means that the tumor is handled as little as possible during its removal.
2. Gowns, gloves, drapes, and instruments may be changed after a biopsy (e.g., a breast biopsy) before incision for a radical resection (e.g., a mastectomy). The tumor is deliberately incised to obtain a biopsy for diagnosis.
3. Instruments placed in direct contact with tumor cells may be isolated in a basin immediately after use. Even when the tumor appears to be localized, most cancers have disseminated to some degree. Therefore some surgeons prefer to use each instrument once and then discard it.
4. Some surgeons prefer to irrigate the surgical site with sterile water instead of sterile normal saline solution to cause the destruction of cancerous cells via lysis. This practice is common during mastectomy.
5. As a prophylactic measure, antibiotics are administered 1 hour preoperatively, with potential redosing intraoperatively for long procedures, and for 24 hours postoperatively to provide an adequate antibacterial level to prevent wound infection.

6. Time-honored precautions such as handling tissue gently, keeping blood loss to a minimum, and avoiding an unduly prolonged surgical procedure influence the outcome for the patient.

During a long surgical procedure the circulating nurse conveys periodic messages to the patient's family members or significant others to reassure them that their loved one is receiving care from a concerned perioperative team. Events to report to the family could include start time, completion of the main surgical procedure, such as tumor removal, and when closure begins. A quick call as the patient leaves the OR for the PACU can be reassuring to the family.

Cancer Therapy

Patients may have many treatments of a varied nature before they come to the OR for formal tumor resection. Many treatments for cancer require surgical implantation of a drug delivery device or tissue preparation before actual therapy can take place. The team should have an understanding of the entire treatment regimen the patient is undergoing in conjunction with surgery. The following methodologies have many different types of effects on the patient's physiology and can alter response patterns during surgical intervention. Some of these treatments require combined chemical, radiation, and multiple surgical procedures to be effective.

Endocrine Therapy

Tumors that arise in organs that are usually under hormonal influence (e.g., breast, ovary, and uterus in female patients; prostate and testes in male patients) may be stimulated by hormones produced in the endocrine glands.

Cellular metabolism is affected by the presence of specific hormone receptors in tumor cells: estrogen or progesterone in females and androgens in males. In some patients, surgical removal of the gonads may be incorporated in the procedure.

Certain breast, endometrial, and prostatic cancers depend on sex hormones for growth and maintenance. Therefore the recurrence or spread of disease may be slowed with therapeutic hormonal manipulation. Endocrine manipulation does not cure, but it can control dissemination of the disease if the tumor progresses beyond the limits of effective surgical resection or radiation therapy.

Hormonal Receptor Site Studies

Identification of the hormonal dependence of the primary tumor through studies of the receptor site is a fairly reliable way of selecting patients who will benefit from preoperative or postoperative endocrine manipulation. After a positive diagnosis of cancer, either with a frozen section biopsy or pathologic permanent sections, the surgeon will probably request a receptor site evaluation of a primary breast, uterine, or prostatic tumor. The tissue specimen removed by surgical resection should be sent to the pathology department fresh or in saline solution. It should not be placed in formalin preservative solution because doing so alters the receptor cells enough to negate the hormonal study.

Endocrine Ablation

Since 1896, surgeons have described positive clinical responses in patients with metastatic breast cancer after treatment with endocrine ablation, the surgical removal of endocrine glands. If the surgeon plans to eliminate endocrine stimulation surgically in a patient with a known hormone-dependent tumor, all sources of the hormone should be ablated chemically, hormonally, or surgically.

- *Bilateral adrenalectomy and oophorectomy.* Both adrenal glands or the ovaries may be resected to prevent the recurrence of endocrine-derived cancer. These may be removed as a one-stage surgical procedure (i.e., bilateral adrenalectomy/oophorectomy). If two separate surgical procedures are preferred, the bilateral oophorectomy precedes the bilateral adrenalectomy except in menopausal women, for whom only the latter surgical procedure may be indicated.
- *Bilateral adrenalectomy and orchiectomy.* After prostatectomy for advanced carcinoma of the prostate, both testes may be removed (i.e., bilateral orchiectomy) to eliminate androgens of testicular origin. Bilateral adrenalectomy also may be indicated.
- *Hormonal therapy.* Hormones administered orally or by injection can alter cell metabolism by changing the systemic hormonal environment of the body. For hormones to be effective, tumor cells must contain receptors. Hormones must bind to these receptors before they can exert an effect on cells.
- *Antiestrogen therapy.* Patients with medical contraindications to endocrine ablation may receive antiestrogen therapy. An estrogen antagonist deprives an estrogen-dependent tumor of the estrogen necessary for its growth. This type of hormone therapy is commonly used for receptor-positive breast cancer. Nafoxidine and tamoxifen (Nolvadex and Soltamox [liquid]) are synthetic nonsteroidal drugs that inhibit the normal intake of estrogen at estrogen receptor sites; they are taken orally. Aromatase inhibitors (AIs) may be given to postmenopausal women to lower the production of estrogen. Examples include letrozole (Femara), anastrozole (Arimidex), and exemestane (Aromasin).
- *Androgen deprivation therapy* (ADT). Patients with prostate cancer may be treated with drugs to lower the level of testosterone production. Luteinizing hormone–releasing hormone (LHRH) agonists such as leuprolide (Lupron), goserelin (Zoladex), or triptorelin (Trelstar) can be implanted or injected to produce hormonal castration without surgical removal of the testicles. LHRH antagonists can also be used to lower testosterone. Drugs such as relugolix (Orgovyx) or degarelix (Firmagon) can be injected under the skin or given in pill form.
- *Immunotherapy.* Immunotherapy is done by giving drugs to stimulate the immune system to target cancer cells and kill them without damaging healthy cells. Treatment is individualized for each patient and type of cancer. It may be used in combination with chemotherapy and surgery.[8]
- *Corticosteroids.* Prednisone, cortisone, hydrocortisone, or some other preparation of corticosteroids may be administered as an antiinflammatory agent, along with the chemotherapeutic agents given to control disseminated disease.

Photodynamic (Laser) Therapy

For photodynamic therapy (also referred to as *photoradiation*), an argon tunable dye laser is used to destroy malignant cells by photochemical reaction. A photosensitive drug such as hematoporphyrin derivative (HPD) from cow's blood (porfimer [Photofrin]), Foscan, or LuTex is absorbed by malignant and reticular endothelial cells. HPD is primarily used in esophageal or endobronchial tumors. This treatment is contraindicated in the presence of esophageal varices.

The photosensitive drug can be taken by mouth, spread on the skin, or injected IV by venipuncture or Hickman catheter 40 to 72 hours before the photodynamic therapy and is taken up by cells to make them fluorescent and photosensitive. It remains longer in malignant cells than in normal cells before being excreted from the body. When exposed to light from an argon laser, the tunable rhodamine B dye laser produces a red beam of approximately 630 nm. An additional laser treatment can be given 96 to 120 hours after initial treatment without the need for further injection. Debridement of initial treatment may be necessary 2 to 4 days after each treatment as necrotic tissue begins to shed.

Other dyes, such as dicyanomethylene, may produce different wavelengths. HPD in cells absorbs the laser light, which leads to a photochemical reaction that causes tissue-oxygen molecules to release cytotoxic singlet oxygen and destroy tumor cells. Depending on tumor site, the laser can be delivered interstitially, endoscopically, externally, or retrobulbarly.

Photodynamic therapy may be used to debulk tumors of the eye, head and neck, breast, esophagus, gastrointestinal tract, bronchus, prostate, and bladder. The tunable dye laser also may be used to diagnose tumor cells. The OR should be darkened or have shades to block outside daylight during the laser treatment.

The patient is cautioned to avoid exposure to sunlight or other sources of UV light both after injection of the dye and postoperatively. Photosensitivity is the primary side effect of the dye and may last 4 to 6 weeks. Patients should be advised to wear sunscreen and sunglasses for at least 30 days posttreatment. Some patients have adverse reactions to bright household lights. Patients with liver impairment may experience photosensitivity for more than 90 days.

Radiation Therapy

Radiation is the emission of electromagnetic waves or atomic particles that result from the disintegration of nuclei of unstable or radioactive elements. The treatment of malignant disease with radiation may be referred to as radiation therapy, brachytherapy, or radiotherapy. Ionizing radiation is used for this type of therapy, which involves the use of high-voltage radiation and other radioactive elements to injure or destroy cells. Like surgical resection and photodynamic therapy, radiation therapy is localized therapy that is applicable for a limited number of specific tumors. Supplemental information on radiation therapy can be found online at https://www.cancer.gov/about-cancer/treatment/types/radiation-therapy.

Ionizing Radiation

Ionization is the physical production of positive and negative ions capable of conducting electricity. Ionizing radiation is radiation with sufficient energy to disrupt the electronic balance of an atom. When disruption occurs in tissue cells or extracellular fluids, the effect can range from minor changes to profound disturbances. Radiation may come from particles of the nuclei of disintegrating atoms or electromagnetic waves that have no mass. Types of ionizing radiation include the following:

- *Alpha particles:* Alpha particles are relatively large particles that have a slight penetrating power. They are stopped by a thin sheet of paper. They have dense ionization but can produce tremendous tissue destruction within a short distance.
- *Beta particles:* Beta particles are relatively small, are electrical, and travel with the speed of light. They have greater penetrating properties than do alpha particles. Their emissions cause tissue

necrosis, and they produce ionization, which has destructive properties. They can be stopped by a thin sheet of plastic or metal.
- *Gamma rays and x-rays:* Gamma rays and x-rays are electromagnetic radiations of short wavelength but high energy and are capable of completely penetrating the body. They affect tumor tissue more rapidly than normal tissue. These types of rays are stopped by a thick lead shield. Protons that omit high amounts of energy are available for the treatment of various cancers based on tumor size and area. Gamma rays are emitted spontaneously from the nucleus of an atom of a radioactive element.

Effects of Radiation on Cells

Cancer cells multiply out of normal body control; they are in a state of active uncontrolled mitosis (the nuclear division of the cytoplasm and nucleus). Radiation affects the metabolic activity of cells. Cells in an active state of mitosis are most susceptible.

Over time, gamma rays and x-rays cause a cessation of cell growth and a regression of the tumor mass. Cells die and are replaced by fibrous tissue.

The sensitivity of a tumor to radiation varies. Some tumors can be destroyed with a small amount of radiation, whereas others require a large amount. The sensitivity of the tumor cells is determined by the sensitivity of the normal cells from which the tumor cells are derived.

The effects of radiation therapy also depend to a large extent on tissue oxygenation. As a tumor grows the periphery is well oxygenated but the central portion becomes necrotic and poorly oxygenated. The number of cells killed with radiation therapy is directly related to the amount of tissue and oxygen within the tumor; therefore the hypoxic effect is a factor in determining the therapeutic dosage of radiation.

Radiation cannot be limited solely to the area being treated. The danger of injuring normal surrounding tissue is a limiting factor in the dosage and selection of the most appropriate type of radiation therapy. A factor in dosage is the ratio of tumor tissue to the surrounding normal tissue. The dosage is computed in roentgen-absorbed doses (rads). A rad is the unit used to measure the absorbed dose of radiation. One rad is the amount of radiation required to deposit 100 ergs of energy per gram of tissue.

Radiophysics or instruments such as Geiger counters or scintillation probes are used to determine the dose of radiation delivered to a specific tissue site; the dose is measured by distance from the source and duration of exposure. Doses are measured in rads to determine whether the dosage is adequate for therapy but not so excessive that it could cause damage to normal tissues.

The penetration of radiation energy is calculated from the rate of decay or disintegration, known as half-life. Half-life is the time necessary for half of the radioactive element to disintegrate and lose half of its activity through decay.

Sources of Radiation

Although the effects of the different types of radiation therapy are similar, their sources and applications do differ. Some sources are implanted into the body in direct contact with tumor tissue, whereas other sources use an external beam to pass the radiation through the body to the tumor.
- *Radium:* Radium is a radioactive metal. Research chemist Marie Curie (1867–1934) and her husband, Pierre (1859–1906), a physicist, discovered and named this metal in 1898. Several years earlier, Mme Curie had been given the task of discovering why pitchblende would record its image

on a photographic plate. She and her husband knew this material emitted more radiation than justified by the known minerals contained in it. It took 6 years of painstakingly difficult work for the Curies to isolate radium as a pure element and to learn of its radioactive properties. Their research eventually led to the use of radium in the treatment of malignant tumors.

- Metallic radium is unstable in air. Radium chloride or bromide salts emit fluorescence and heat. One gram gives off 134 calories per hour. Alpha and beta particles and gamma rays are products of its disintegration. The half-life of radium is approximately 1620 years; half the remaining life is lost in another 1620 years, and so on. The final product is lead.
- Today radiopharmaceutical drugs are combination drugs with a radioactive component to treat cancer. Radium-223 is commonly used for cancer of the bones and lungs.
- *Radon:* Radon is a dense radioactive gas liberated as the first by-product of the disintegration of radium. Mme Curie discovered this gas and first named it *emanation.* Radon is collected by an intricate process in radiopaque glass or gold capillary tubing, and the seeds for implantation are then cut and sealed. The dosage is computed according to the hours of insertion into tissue. It is measured in millicurie-hours. The half-life of radon is 4 days; its total life is approximately 30 days.
- *Radionuclides:* A radionuclide is an element that has been bombarded with radioactive particles in a nuclear reactor. A radionuclide shows radioactive disintegration and emits alpha and beta particles or gamma rays. Radionuclides that emit beta particles and gamma rays are used primarily for treatment of malignant tumors. Therapeutic radionuclides also may be referred to as radiopharmaceuticals. Historically they were known as *radioactive isotopes* or *radioisotopes*; these terms are still found in the literature. Cesium, cobalt, iodine, iridium, lutetium-177, and yttrium are the most used elements for therapy.[9] Radium-223 dichloride (Xofigo) has been approved to treat cancers that have spread into bones.

Radionuclides are controlled by the U.S. Nuclear Regulatory Commission (NRC) and are released only to individuals trained and licensed to use them. Available in liquid or solid forms, they may be ingested orally, infused intravenously, instilled into a body cavity, injected or implanted into a tumor, or applied to the skin externally. The ionizing radiation emitted has an action on tissue similar to that of radium, but radionuclides differ from radium in the following ways:

- The half-life of radionuclides is short. Radionuclides disintegrate at varying rates depending on their type. Each element has a specific half-life that varies from a few hours (e.g., the 6 hours of technetium-99) to 8 days (iodine-131) to 5.3 years (cobalt-60).
- Irradiation with radionuclides does not spread so much into adjoining tissue; therefore a stronger dose can be used in a malignant tumor. Many radionuclides are not absorbed by bone and other normal body tissues. It can be more easily shielded for safe handling. The surgeon and other personnel should take recommended precautions to prevent exposure in placing or removing radionuclides.

Exposure to radionuclides is always potentially dangerous. Radiation may treat cancer, but it can also cause a malignant neoplasm.

Implantation of Radiation Sources

All radiation sources for implantation are prepared in the desired therapeutic dosages by personnel in the nuclear medicine department. Many types of sources are used to deliver maximum radiation to the primary tumor. No single type is ideal for every tumor or anatomic site.

Interstitial Needles. Interstitial needles are hollow sheaths and are usually made of platinum or Monel metal. Radium salts or radionuclides are encased in platinum or platinum-iridium short units or cells, which in turn are sealed in the metal sheath of the needle for implantation into tumor tissue. A needle may contain one or several short units or cells of the radiation source, depending on the length of needle to be used. Needles vary in length from 10 to 60 mm, with a diameter of 1 to 2 mm. The choice of length depends on dosage and on the area involved. Dosage is measured in milligram-hours, which can be converted to rads.

The interstitial needles contain a radiation source specific for the targeted area, such as cesium-137. The needles are implanted in tumors near the body surface or in tissue accessible enough to permit their use (e.g., vagina, cervix, tongue, mouth, neck). In certain patients, stereotactic techniques are used to implant needles for the irradiation of brain tumors.

In the interventional suite or OR these needles are inserted at the periphery of and within the tumor. One end of the needle is pointed, and the other end has an eye for a heavy (size 2) suture. Needles are threaded to prevent loss while in use and to aid in removal. After the surgeon inserts the needles, the ends of the sutures are tied or taped together and then taped to the skin in an adjoining area or secured to buttons. Depending on the anatomic site, a template may be used to position and secure the needles.

A template consists of two acrylic plates separated by rubber O-rings and held together with screws. The plates have holes for insertion of the interstitial needles. The template remains in place until the needles are removed. Depending on the planned dosage to the tumor bed, needles may be left in place for 4 to 7 days.

Interstitial Seeds. Sealed radionuclide seeds may be implanted permanently or temporarily. Because they have a short half-life, gold seeds are permanently implanted, most commonly into the prostate, lungs, or pancreas. Seeds that contain a radiation source such as cesium-137, iridium-192, pallidum-103, or iodine-125 are implanted directly into tumor tissue and removed after the desired exposure.

Seeds are useful in body cavities, in localized areas, and in tumors that are not resectable because of their location near major vessels or the spinal cord. Because they are small, the seeds can be placed to fit a curved area without necessitating immobilization. However, they may move about with much motion.

Radionuclide seeds are 7 mm or less in length, are 0.75 mm in diameter, and have a wall 0.3 mm thick. The length of the seed depends on the desired dosage. Seeds can be inserted with or without an invasive surgical procedure. They may be strung on a strand of suture material or placed in a hollow plastic tube with sealed ends. With a needle attached, the strand or tube is woven or pulled through the tumor. Seeds in a plastic tube may be inserted through a hollow needle, such as a catheter through a trocar. Empty tubes may be inserted in the OR and afterloaded (i.e., the seeds are put into the tube at a later time and place). A microprocessor-controlled machine that pulls wire attached to radioactive material through the tube may be used for remote afterloading.

Brachytherapy

The term *brachytherapy* (also known as internal beam radiation) comes from a Greek term meaning "short-range treatment." Tiny

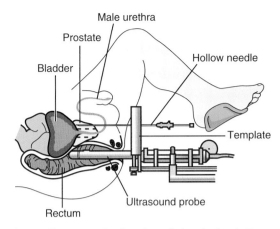

• **Fig. 7.5** Placement of radioactive cylinders for brachytherapy.

*Labels: Male urethra, Prostate, Bladder, Hollow needle, Template, Ultrasound probe, Rectum*

titanium cylinders, capsules, seeds, tubes, balloons, needles, or ribbons that contain a radioactive isotope are implanted to deliver a dose of radiation from the inside out that kills cancer cells while sparing healthy tissue. Brachytherapy is performed for many types of cancers, including breast, uterus, and prostate (Fig. 7.5).

Brachytherapy, an internal application with sealed sources of radionuclides, has almost totally supplanted the use of radium and radon. For example, the gamma rays of cesium-137 have greater penetrating power than radium does.

Brachytherapy is useful for delivering higher cell-killing doses in shorter periods than with conventional radiation treatments. The radionuclides are placed with ultrasound or computed tomography (CT) scan guidance. A rapid delivery system that uses a catheter with a balloon on the tip has been developed to treat breast cancers smaller than 3 cm. The catheter is placed into the breast tissue during tumor excision, and the balloon is expanded with saline. Twice per day for 4 to 5 days a high-dose radiation source is placed inside the catheter to treat the tissue. When the treatment period is complete, the catheter and radiation source are removed.

Patient selection includes those with clear margins of the tumor and with fewer than three affected lymph nodes. Additional information about brachytherapy suitable for students and patients can be found online at www.radiologyinfo.org. The information can be used for patient education.

Intracavitary Capsules. A sealed capsule of radium, cesium-137, iodine-125, yttrium-192, or cobalt-60 may be placed into a body cavity or orifice. The capsule method may be a single tube of radioactive pins fixed in a tandem loader or a group of individual capsules, each of which contains one radioactive pin. Commonly used to treat tumors in the cervix or endometrium of the uterus, a capsule is inserted via the vagina for treatment of the uterine body.

In a patient with cervical cancer an instrument such as an Ernst applicator is used. A metal or plastic tube with radioactive pins is inserted into the uterus. Metal pins are used in conjunction with heat. The tube is attached to two vaginal ovoids, each of which contains a radioactive pin, that are placed in the cul-de-sac around the cervix. This type of application delivers the desired dosage in a pear-shaped volume of tissue, which includes the cervix, corpus, and tissue around the cervix but spares the bladder and rectum from high doses of radiation.

A blunt intracavitary applicator is used to position the parts. The applicator is held securely and remains fixed to ensure proper dosage to the tumor without injuring the normal surrounding

structures. For stabilization the surgeon may suture the applicator to the cervix; vaginal packing is also used. Two different methods of application are used for inserting the radiation source: afterloading techniques and preloading techniques.

Afterloading Techniques. Afterloading techniques afford the greatest safety for OR personnel. In the OR a cold, unloaded, hollow plastic or metal applicator, such as the Fletcher afterloader, is inserted into or adjacent to the tissues that will receive radiation. After x-ray verification of correct placement, the radiation source is loaded into the applicator at the patient's bedside.

Preloading Techniques. Preloading techniques necessitate insertion of the "hot" radiation capsule in the OR by the surgeon. OR personnel should not be permitted in the OR during this procedure. To deliver a uniform dose to the desired area the surgeon inserts an adjustable device designed to hold the radiation source in proper position in the tissues (e.g., the Ernst applicator). The bladder and rectum are held away from the area with packs to avoid undesired irradiation.

For calculation of the necessary dosage, the surgeon uses radiographs of the pelvis to check the position of the radiation source and measure its distance from critical sites.

All preparations for insertion are made by surgical team members before they leave the room. (They wait in the substerile room during insertion.) Preparations include setting the sterile table with vaginal packing, antibiotic cream for packing, radiopaque contrast media for radiographic studies, and a basin of sterile water; placing the x-ray cassette on the OR bed and notifying the radiology technician; obtaining the radiation source; positioning the patient; and putting a radiation notation on the patient's record and a card on the stretcher.

Intracavitary Colloidal Suspensions. Sterile radioactive colloidal suspensions of gold or phosphorus are used as palliative therapy to limit the growth of metastatic tumors in the pleural or peritoneal cavities. Radioactive colloidal gold-198 is most commonly used; it has a half-life of 2.7 days. It also may be instilled within the bladder.

The effect of these suspensions is from the emission of beta particles, which penetrate tissue so slightly that radioactivity is limited to the immediate area in which the colloidal suspension is placed. A trocar and cannula are introduced into the pleural or peritoneal cavity, and the colloidal suspension is injected through the cannula from a lead-shielded syringe. After use, these instruments are stored in a remote area until the decay of radioactivity is complete.

External Beam Radiation Therapy

Ionizing radiation of gamma rays or x-rays generated from machines is used externally to alter tumor cells within the body. This type of radiation therapy is noninvasive.

A maximum dose of radiation is concentrated on the malignant tumor underneath the skin, with a minimum dose to surrounding tissue. A three-dimensional (3D) set of images from CT, magnetic resonance imaging (MRI), or positron emission tomography (PET) scans helps deliver precise beams for the shape of the tumor. The angle of approach is changed a number of times during treatment to spread the amount of radiation to normal tissue over as wide an area as possible. Both orthovoltage equipment (low-voltage equipment that produces 200−500 kV) and megavoltage equipment (e.g., cobalt-60 beams and linear accelerators or betatrons) are used for external beam radiation therapy.

With some cancers, external radiation may be the only therapeutic modality used. Determination of the dosage of radiation that will provide the optimal cure with an acceptable balance of complications is difficult. With the advent of stereotactic techniques and the use of megavoltage equipment, intense rays can deliver cancer cell–killing doses without permanently injuring normal tissue and causing skin irritation. Even so, for many tumors most oncologists recommend a combination of radiation therapy and surgical resection; radiation therapy may be administered preoperatively and/or postoperatively or intraoperatively. External radiation therapy also may be combined with internal sources, such as intracavitary radiation capsules, to build up the dosage to large tumor areas.

Intraoperative Radiation Therapy

During a surgical procedure a single high dose of radiation may be delivered directly to an intraabdominal or intrapelvic tumor or tumor bed to provide an additional palliative or localized means of control. Healthy organs or tissues can be shielded from exposure. Radiation also may be used after resection of the bulk of the tumor.

An orthovoltage unit may be installed in a lead-lined OR for intraoperative radiation therapy. The sterile Lucite cone may be placed directly over the tumor site, or a special mold of plastic or plaster is made to position the head. Marks with colored ink or dots are placed to pinpoint where the beam should be aimed. All team members leave the room during treatment. In some hospitals the patient is transported from the OR to the radiation therapy department. After exposure to a megavoltage electron beam, the wound may be closed in the treatment area or the patient may be returned to the OR for further surgery or wound closure. The open wound is covered with a sterile drape during transport, and sterile technique is used for closure.

Stereotactic Radiosurgery

Gamma knife technology was developed in Sweden in the early 1950s by surgeon Lars Leksell and Borje Larsson, PhD. They experimented with guiding devices and proton beams. Cobalt-60 was found to be most effective in the treatment of brain tumors and was selected as the energy source for the gamma knife. In 1975 the device was used for treatment of brain tumors in humans.

With stereotactic radiosurgery, fiberglass fixation pins are used to apply a base ring (the Leksell head frame) to the patient's head preoperatively. Two small rods are placed in the ear canals to stabilize the head frame during fixation. Care is taken not to injure the ear canal or tympanic membrane during this process. A calibrated ring is affixed to the frame to form X, Y, and Z coordinates to localize the brain lesion. The frame and ring sit within a larger helmet that aims the radiation at the tumor. Newer frames are placed on the skull to prevent any chance of damage to the ear. Thermoplastic masks are now used for custom fit and are more comfortable.

The gamma knife delivers highly concentrated doses of gamma rays to inoperable or deep-seated vascular malformations or brain tumors 1 to 6 cm^3 in size. The localized area is determined with precision stereotaxis. The neurosurgeon places the patient's head, with a head frame and localizing ring, into the collimator helmet so the focusing channels direct 201 pinpointed cobalt-60 beams to the tumor. (The radiation sources are housed in a large spherical chamber within a special room.)

The patient is placed on a sliding bed that accommodates and aligns with the helmet as it enters the spherical chamber. The gamma knife process lasts 1 to 4 hours. During the procedure the patient is in video and voice communication with the perioperative team. All personnel leave the room during treatment because of the intensity of the radiation and its cumulative effects.

Safety Rules for Handling Radiation Sources

The cardinal factors of protection from radiation sources are distance, time, and shielding. For both personnel and patients the following principles of radiation safety apply to handling all types of radioactive materials:

- The intensity of radiation varies inversely with the square of the distance from it (i.e., double the distance equals one-quarter the intensity). Personnel should stay as far from the source as is feasible.
- Radiation sources (e.g., needles, seeds, capsules, suspensions) are prepared by personnel in the nuclear medicine department. Personnel prepare these sources behind a lead screen. Their hands are protected with lead-lined gloves, if possible, or special forceps during handling.
- Radiation sources are transported in a long-handled lead carrier so they are as close to the floor and as far away from the body of the transporter as possible. The lead carrier should be stored away from personnel and patient traffic areas while it is in the OR suite.
- When radiation sources are delivered to the OR, each needle, seed, or capsule is counted by the surgeon with the radiation therapist. This number is recorded.
- All radiation sources are handled with special long, ring-handled forceps from behind a lead protection shield. Radiation sources should never be touched with bare hands or gloves. Radiation sources are never handled with a crushing forceps because the seal of hollow containers can be broken. A groove-tipped forceps designed for this purpose is used.
- Radiation sources are handled as quickly as possible to limit the time that personnel are exposed to radiation.
- All radiation sources are accounted for before and after use, and any loss is immediately reported to the OR nurse manager. Nothing should be removed from the room. To locate a lost radiation source a radiation therapist or nuclear medicine department technician is called to bring a Geiger counter. A Geiger counter has a radiation-sensitive gauge with an indicator that moves and a sound that increases when near radioactive substances. A hazmat team may be summoned.
- A radiation documentation sheet is completed and put in the patient's chart. The surgeon fills in the amount, exact time of insertion, and time the source is to be removed. Each nurse who cares for the patient on the unit signs this sheet just before going off duty, thereby passing responsibility for checking the patient and radiation source to the nurse who relieves. For checking needles, the sutures attached to each needle are counted.
- The patient's bed and door to the room are conspicuously labeled with a radiation-in-use sign.
- The radiation source is removed by the surgeon at the exact time indicated so the patient is not overexposed.
- Radiation is neither seen nor felt; therefore the rules are carefully observed. Exposure is monitored and minimized.

Effects of Radiation Therapy on the Perioperative Patient

The patient may be undergoing several treatment modalities and may experience the specific tissue and systemic effects of each. The perioperative nurse should understand how radiation affects the patient and how it affects the attainment of desired outcomes. The plan of care should include consideration for the potential side effects of radiation therapy.

Chemotherapy

Either alone or in combination, a variety of chemotherapeutic agents are capable of providing measurable palliative remission or regression of primary and metastatic disease, with a decrease in the size of the tumor and no new metastases. In some instances a complete response, with the disappearance of all clinical evidence of the tumor, is achieved.

The trend is toward earlier and greater use of adjuvant chemotherapy. More than one agent may be administered to enhance the action of another cytotoxic or antigenic substance. Adjuvant therapy is designed to maximize the benefits of each agent in the combination while avoiding overlapping toxicities. The following factors are important in determining the ability of tumor cells to respond to chemotherapy:

- *Size and location of the tumor.* The smaller the tumor, the easier it is to reach cells. The mechanism for the passage of drugs into the brain differs from that for other body organs.
- *Type of tumor.* For example, cells of solid tumors in the lung, stomach, colon, and breast may be more resistant than cells in the lymphatic system.
- *Combinations of adjuvant therapy.* In select patients, chemotherapy may be used as an adjunct to all other types of therapies. Precise scheduling of dosages is necessary to attain effective results.
- *Specific biochemical requirements of the tumor.* Agents are selected according to the appropriateness of their structure and function. More than one agent is usually given.
- *State of life cycle of the cancer cells.* Cancer cells and normal cells go through the same life cycle phases. An understanding of this phenomenon is necessary for understanding chemotherapy.

Indications for Chemotherapy

Patients who are at risk for or who have systemic signs of advanced or disseminated disease (generally indicated by extranodal involvement) may be candidates for preoperative, intraoperative, or postoperative chemotherapy.

Preoperative Chemotherapy

The objective of preoperative chemotherapy may be to shrink the tumor sufficiently to permit surgical resection. Adjuvant radiation therapy may be used in combination with chemotherapy to increase tumor regression and necrosis. Agents also may eliminate subclinical microscopic metastatic disease.

Intraoperative Chemotherapy

After the initial incision is made, a Tenckhoff catheter is inserted through the midline abdominal wall for instillation of a heated chemotherapeutic solution suspended in a dextrose-based peritoneal dialysate. Additional active suction drains are inserted in the lower abdomen for drainage of the solution. These drains remain in place for postoperative drainage. A temperature probe is attached to the Tenckhoff catheter, and several liters of

chemotherapeutic solution are infused at 43° C. Because the dialysate causes fluid shifts in the peritoneal cavity, the anesthesia provider closely monitors the patient's urinary output with a Foley catheter. If necessary, medication is given to increase output.

At the conclusion of the instillation, the intended surgical procedure, usually some form of cytoreduction, is performed. The Tenckhoff catheter and the active drains are left in place for future treatments.

Postoperative Chemotherapy

Surgical resection followed by regional chemotherapy often can control local disease to keep a tumor in remission. Residual metastatic disease may be treated with systemic chemotherapy to cure the patient or to prolong life. Multiple doses may be given over a long period (several months to a year or more) to delay or eliminate recurrence of the tumor.

The Patient With Chronic Comorbid Disease

Patients come to the OR for surgical procedures unrelated to a chronic cardiopulmonary or pulmonary disease. Even for unrelated surgeries the presence of these conditions may present a high risk for physiologic complications.

Cardiovascular Disease

The surgeon is particularly concerned about hemostasis and the potential for hemorrhage in a patient who is taking an anticoagulant medication. A patient who takes a daily dose of 81 mg of aspirin prophylactically may be instructed to discontinue its use for 2 weeks preoperatively. Anticoagulation is commonly prescribed for patients who have cardiac stents in place or a history of embolic disease, such as atrial fibrillation, pulmonary embolus, or deep vein thrombosis.

The anesthesia provider regulates the medications of patients who have an unstable blood pressure. Blood pressure is also monitored and maintained with appropriate medications in patients with a history of hypertension or hypotension. Tissue perfusion and oxygenation are critical to wound healing and depend on the circulatory status of the patient.

Pulmonary Disease

Any chronic condition that compromises pulmonary function presents a potential risk for a patient undergoing general inhalation anesthesia. Bronchoconstriction, edema, and excess mucus production cause uneven airway narrowing that creates a ventilation-perfusion mismatch. Severe hypoxemia, an abnormal deficiency of oxygen in arterial blood, can trigger life-threatening dysrhythmias and respiratory failure.

Adequate ventilation is difficult in patients with asthma, chronic bronchitis, and pulmonary emphysema. Chronic obstructive pulmonary disease, which includes these conditions, is characterized by diminished inspiratory and expiratory capacity of the lungs. It is aggravated by cigarette smoking and air pollution. Smokers are advised to stop smoking at least 3 weeks preoperatively and are taught to use a spirometer postoperatively to clear respiratory secretions.

Deep-breathing and coughing exercises may be helpful postoperatively. A mechanical ventilation or intermittent positive pressure breathing apparatus may be necessary postoperatively to assist or control respiration. Patients who have trouble breathing are usually highly anxious and need emotional support.

The Patient With Induced or Acquired Immunosuppression

The immune system creates local barriers and inflammation to protect the body from invasion by pathogenic microorganisms and foreign bodies. Humoral and cell-mediated responses develop if these first-line defenses do not provide adequate protection. The body's natural lines of defense are described in Chapter 14 of this text.

The humoral response produces antibodies to react with specific antigens. The cell-mediated response mobilizes tissue macrophages in the presence of a foreign body. Immunocompetence is the ability of the immune system to mobilize and deploy its antibodies and other responses to stimulation by an antigen. Immunocompetence may be threatened by a disease, age, malnutrition, a virus such as hepatitis B, human immunodeficiency virus (HIV), or an immunosuppressive agent. Patients with immunocompromise have a weakened or deficient immune response with a resultant decreased resistance to infection.

Immunosuppression

Immunosuppressive agents include corticosteroid hormones, which are given to prevent or reduce the inflammation caused by certain diseases. They are often prescribed for patients who have an autoimmune collagen disease (e.g., rheumatoid arthritis, systemic lupus erythematosus, scleroderma) or an autoimmune hemolytic disorder (e.g., idiopathic thrombocytopenic purpura or acquired hemolytic anemia). They also are given to patients with adrenal insufficiency and after organ transplantation to combat rejection. Antineoplastic cytotoxic agents for chemotherapy and radiation therapy, which are used to reduce malignant tumor cells, also may cause immunosuppression.

Common Complications

The manifestations and clinical characteristics of the patient with immunocompromise depend on the specific disease and the affected organ or system. For example, systemic lupus erythematosus can affect every organ system in the body. Adrenal insufficiency, as caused by Addison disease, may be characterized by generalized systemic reaction. In contrast, organ transplantation or a malignant tumor may affect a single organ.

Special Considerations

Many patients with immunocompromise have skin rashes or lesions, painful joints, poor nutrition, and generalized malaise. They need physical and emotional support throughout the perioperative care period. Aseptic and sterile techniques are important considerations for all surgical patients but are especially crucial for individuals with immunosuppression and immunocompromise, who are at high risk for development of a postoperative infection.

Acquired Immunodeficiency Syndrome

Patients with acquired immunodeficiency syndrome (AIDS) test positive for HIV in serum and exhibit one or more signs and symptoms of an opportunistic disease, including pneumonia, fungal or parasitic infection, and malignant neoplasms.

HIV can remain inactive and undetected in the body for many years before seroconverting and causing the immunodeficiency

illness known as AIDS. During this time, no outward signs of HIV infection are noted, but the patient can transmit the virus through blood, body fluids, or sexual contact.

Both males and females, including infants and children, may be HIV positive or diagnosed with AIDS. HIV was once thought to be transmitted only through homosexual behavior among men, IV drug use, or tainted blood transfusions. The virus is now known to be transmitted also through heterosexual contact, and an infected mother may transmit the virus to her fetus.

The diagnosis of HIV infection is confirmed with at least two separate tests. One positive test result is not a conclusive diagnosis, and the test is usually repeated for clarity. Initial testing can be done with an at-home rapid test kit using a fingerstick or an oral fluid test. Lab-drawn tests with the enzyme-linked immunosorbent assay (ELISA) or the nucleic acid test (NAT) are performed to detect the presence of HIV antibodies in the blood. The diagnosis is confirmed with usually two positive tests before a treatment plan is put in place.

If test results are seropositive for HIV infection, the patient does not necessarily have AIDS. HIV invades and destroys T lymphocytes. During this process the patient's immune system is disabled. The normal T lymphocyte level is $1000/mm^3$; the severity of an HIV infection is measured by the level of T lymphocyte cells in the patient's blood. When the T cell level decreases to between 200 and $500/mm^3$, the patient has had seroconversion to an immunodeficient state and is considered to have AIDS.

HIV infection and AIDS have no known cure. Many combination medications are now available to delay seroconversion and keep HIV at undetectable levels and to prolong the life of a patient with seroconversion to AIDS. Pharmacologic therapy may include a combination of broad-spectrum antibiotics, antivirals, antidiarrheals, vitamins, and antineoplastics. HIV was once considered a death sentence, but with early diagnosis and treatment a person can live a long life. Information about HIV can be found at www.cdc.gov/hiv/basics.

Common Complications

A patient with an active HIV infection may have night sweats, unexplained fevers, dry cough, weakness, diarrhea, weight loss, and swollen lymph glands. A patient with seroconversion to AIDS may have multiple opportunistic infections and malignancies concurrently and generalized poor health. Extreme muscle and tissue wasting are common.

Many patients with AIDS have multiple external and internal lesions. The skin may have open wounds with infectious exudate or large, swollen, purple lesions associated with Kaposi sarcoma (a malignant multifocal neoplasm of reticuloendothelial cells that spreads in the skin and metastasizes to the lymph nodes and viscera). Large, painful masses of lymph tissue may be present in the neck, axilla, and groin. Mechanical obstruction caused by Kaposi lesions in the esophagus may prevent swallowing of food. Intestinal lesions may prevent the absorption of nutrients or cause bowel obstruction.

Constant anorexia, nausea, vomiting, and diarrhea may prevent adequate intake by mouth. Nutritional supplementation with hyperalimentation may be indicated to meet a patient's high caloric needs. Hyperalimentation is discussed in Chapter 29.

AIDS causes the body to be susceptible to opportunistic infections because of the lowered resistance of the immune system. Opportunistic infections are caused by microorganisms that normally are nonpathogenic in a healthy individual. The mucous membranes of the mouth and genital areas may have herpesvirus lesions or white patches of candidiasis, a yeastlike fungus. Neurologically, the patient may have recurrent episodes of cryptococcal meningitis or toxoplasmosis, which causes persistent motor dysfunction and mental changes.

The patient with AIDS experiences a continual cycle of acute and chronic respiratory infections. *Pneumocystis jirovecii* pneumonia is the most common lung infection, followed by multiple-drug–resistant tuberculosis. The patient may be in a perpetual state of respiratory distress. Central and peripheral cyanosis may be present. The respiratory effort expends high energy levels, which causes the patient's condition to deteriorate rapidly.

Special Considerations

Patients with AIDS may be in poor physical condition, depending on how the body systems have been affected. Most systems are eventually involved. The plan of perioperative care should incorporate the following considerations:

1. Moving the patient from the transport stretcher to the OR bed may require additional personnel for total lifting. The patient may not be able to move because of weakness or pain in the joints, muscle and tissue wasting, and superficial skin lesions.
2. Bony prominences and areas of decreased muscle mass and devascularized tissue must be protected throughout the positioning process and surgical procedure. Blankets, restraints, monitoring devices, electrosurgical dispersive electrodes, drapes, instruments, and routine care devices may cause inadvertent harm to the patient despite the team's best efforts to protect the patient from injury.
3. IV line insertion, induction of anesthesia, and maintenance of the airway may be difficult. A suitable vein for infusion may be hard to identify because of former IV drug use or large areas of epidermal Kaposi sarcoma. In extreme cases the only IV site may be a central venous catheter. Endotracheal intubation may be contraindicated because of potential hemorrhage from Kaposi lesions in the trachea. Placement of an esophageal stethoscope or rectal temperature probe may rupture other internal Kaposi lesions with the same result.
4. Postoperative wound healing is delayed or absent because of poor nutrition, decreased circulation, poor tissue integrity, and a continued immunodeficient condition.

Patients with AIDS may have been rejected by their families, especially if the virus was transmitted through a route not accepted or understood. The diagnosis of AIDS may be the first time the family is made aware of the patient's alternative lifestyle. Psychologic support systems may consist of a small circle of friends, who also may be infected with HIV or have AIDS. Preoperative consideration should be given to power of attorney, living will, and the potential for future do-not-resuscitate (DNR) status.

Continual counseling should be emphasized in the postoperative discharge plan to include provisions for physiologic care and support. The patient, family, and significant others should be educated about the potential routes of transmission, such as exposure to blood and body fluids through sexual contact or shared IV needles. The virus is also potentially transmissible through shared razors, toothbrushes, and tweezers because of the possibility of blood contamination. Dishes and eating utensils are considered safe when washed in hot soapy water, rinsed, and dried.

Education should include learning about physical activities that do not pose a risk for transmission, such as hugging, shaking hands, and sitting close.

Confidentiality is a concern because of the nature of the routes by which HIV can be transmitted. It is about the patient's right to privacy. Testing for HIV is not a routine preadmission laboratory procedure. If a patient is tested, the results should be placed in the appropriate section of the patient's chart with other laboratory results, not displayed on the front of the chart. Reporting of the results should be governed by institutional policy and treated in the same manner as all patient confidentiality issues.

Dissemination of confidential patient information to inappropriate people is a breach of duty to the patient's privacy and may be subject to legal action. Physicians and nurses may face disciplinary action such as license suspension or revocation by the boards of medicine or nursing, as indicated.

Perioperative patient care personnel should provide care to all patients with equal professionalism, compassion, empathy, and positive regard despite any personal feelings about a patient's lifestyle or disease entity. Nonjudgmental care is essential for the psychologic wellness of patients with AIDS. Immediate caregivers may know the patient's status and put in place a "no touch policy" for sharps to prevent transmission injuries.

The Patient Who Is a Victim of Crime

Violent crime is prevalent in society. As health care professionals we manage the care of victims of crime and sometimes the accused perpetrators. Victims and perpetrators involved in the same incident may present to the same emergency department (ED) within moments of each other. Both are entitled to the same care and legal considerations, including privacy and basic tenets of respect.

The perpetrator is considered innocent until proven guilty in a court of law. Both patients have equal rights to patient advocacy, regardless of the circumstances of their injuries. All members of the health care team need to be in control and aware of subjective feelings and place personal biases and prejudices in proper perspective when caring for these individuals.

Crimes can involve drugs, domestic abuse, shootings, stabbings, gang violence, mugging, sexual assault, and hit-and-run motor vehicle accidents. Injuries can occur to bystanders at a crime scene, such as a robbery, drive-by shooting, or gang fight. All patients who arrive at the ED may provide potential forensic evidence for law enforcement officials and should be carefully processed according the facility policy.

On Arrival to the Emergency Department

Physical assessment is performed immediately on contact with the health care system by paramedics and continued on arrival to the facility by additional medical personnel. The level of consciousness is evaluated and airway, breathing, and circulation are prioritized and stabilized. The first concern is to preserve life, followed closely by the concern to preserve the chain of evidence.

Patients with severe injuries may need to bypass the ED and go directly to the OR.

Notation should be made of psychologic affect. Many crimes are associated with drug abuse, and the administration of medications in the hospital could interact with drugs ingested on the street. The use of street drugs should be carefully ruled out with toxicology screens because they may alter baseline laboratory tests, interfere with lifesaving treatment, and potentiate anesthetics used during emergency surgery.

Unusual odors such as chemicals, alcohol, gasoline, or other volatile substances should be investigated and documented. Chemicals can be hazardous in the OR, where fires can be triggered by electrosurgical devices in the presence of volatile materials.

Baseline vital signs, radiographs, scans, antibiotic prophylaxis, tetanus toxoid, pain control, and hemostasis are some of the prime concerns for stabilization. Facility spokespeople should handle all media interviews, and respect for patient privacy should be provided. Standard precautions are strictly followed at all times concerning all body substances.

Consent for treatment is required and should be obtained as soon as possible. This is important as the chain of evidence is constructed. The chain of evidence incorporates documentation of all material and observational findings associated with the victim, the suspected perpetrator, and the incident. An unconscious person is given full treatment regardless of consent status until family or next of kin can be consulted.

Forensic Evidence in the Operating Room

Forensic evidence is critical for the reconstruction of events in a crime or suspected illegal activity. All forensic evidence is preserved according to institutional policy and procedure and is relinquished only to the appropriate authorities. The documentation of handling and disposition of evidence is referred to as a chain of evidence. This chain is maintained by requiring the signatures of everyone who comes into contact with forensic evidence. The goal is to attempt to validate that the evidence has not been tampered with before reaching the appropriate law enforcement agency.

Any potential evidence discovered during physical assessment should be carefully documented and secured until it can be turned over to appropriate law enforcement authorities. The Fourth Amendment to the Constitution of the United States provides equal protection against unreasonable search and seizure. Items found during intentional searching of a conscious patient without consent may be interpreted as unreasonable search and are potentially not admissible in court.

Illegal substances or weapons discovered during the routine course of assessment that have not been obtained through unreasonable means may be used as evidence in some states. They are packaged dry and in an impervious container to prevent injury. Gloves are worn in handling evidence. Nothing is washed, wiped clean, or discarded. A clear chain of evidence is often difficult to maintain in a crisis, but every attempt is made to document the disposition of evidence and the location from which it was taken.

Assessment and Documentation of the Crime Victim

Data collection begins with emergency medical service and police reports. If a patient with a suspicious injury, such as a gunshot or stab wound, arrives at the ED by some other means, the police should be notified. Critical information about the injury includes where, when, and how the injury occurred and should be documented. Direct quotation of the patient's words is preferred. Differences between accounts of the incident by the patient and other observers should be carefully noted. Variance in reporting by a potential victim may mean that an accused perpetrator is innocent.

Patients who are critically injured may be taken directly to the OR. The perioperative nurse should document physical injury patterning on the OR nurses' notes before evidence, such as bloody handprints, is washed away during the skin preparation process. Most ORs have cameras or photographic staff available. Injuries should be photographed in the lighting of the OR for clarity.

Patients may not be able to communicate vital information, such as when the last meal was eaten, whether they have allergies, or whether medications are taken on a routine basis for some condition. Family may not be available to give a medical or surgical history. It is critical to communicate to the team every detail discovered during the preparation of the patient for surgical intervention. Close observation for responses to treatment and physiologic clues is important for the provision of safe care.

The patient's clothing may provide important information for the police and should be preserved intact if possible. This can be complex if the patient must come to the OR for lifesaving intervention. If clothing must be cut off, care should be taken to avoid cutting through bullet holes or stab wounds.

Keep in mind that the patient may have sharp objects in clothing that could injure a caregiver. If possible, the patient should be placed on a separate bed sheet before clothing is removed and the fabric of the clothing should be cut along the seams. Hairs, carpet fibers, and other environmental information may be contained in folds of fabric and should be left with the clothing for the forensic examiners. The sheet forms a wrapper for the clothing before it is placed in an approved receptacle.

Clothing should not be placed in airtight containers or plastic bags because that may cause degradation of biologic matter. A paper bag may be used, provided the bag has not been used before and the moisture of the clothing is not going to seep through the surface. Contamination of the outer aspect of the paper bag is a hazard to the examining teams and the law officials. Underclothes of sexual assault victims must be carefully preserved in the same manner. Storage and handling of these items should be well documented, and signatures are required when the items are turned over to proper authorities. Some facilities provide tamper-proof evidence tape to seal the package and prevent altering of contents.

The patient's skin is observed for bruising, swelling, and open wounds. Characteristic marks, such as finger-shaped or hand-shaped injuries, tire marks, and repetitive patterning such as stripes, should be documented. The locations of the marks should be indicated on a human-like diagram in the patient's record. Whenever possible, the injuries should be photographed. This may require separate consent.

The study of ballistics is the scientific matching of a particular weapon to its projectile. As a bullet travels down the barrel of a gun, it picks up characteristic markings. Bullets that are removed from a patient should be handled with care so the ballistic markings are not altered. Placement of bullets or metallic evidence in a metal specimen basin could alter the longitudinal design of the identifying marks. Only plastic containers should be used. No solution should be added. Blood evidence could be washed off from either the victim or the perpetrator.

The presence of gunpowder and its distribution pattern around a bullet entrance wound on skin or clothing is important in determination of muzzle-to-body distance. The closeness of the gun barrel determines the amount of skin damage on impact. Small-caliber bullet wounds have a smaller inverted entrance and larger everted exit points. Some bullets are designed to flatten on entry and may exit the body after traveling through several layers of soft tissue or organs. If contact is made with bony structures, the bullet may remain embedded in the body. Fragmentation bullets are designed to burst into tiny pieces as they enter the body and may embolize. Close examination of the victim's back may reveal a gaping bullet exit wound or additional injuries that were initially unnoticed.

Wounds should be copiously irrigated with sterile saline solution. Some surgeons request antibiotic solution. Antibiotic solutions are described in Chapter 14.

Absence of an exit wound may indicate the presence of a nonexploded fragmentation bullet. A retained malfunctioning fragmentation bullet could be deadly during an emergency surgical procedure. The explosive mechanism could inadvertently activate, causing injury to a member of the OR team.

Victims may present with obvious injuries but may also have concealed damage. The initial assault may have been a gunshot or a stab wound, but incidental injury may include blunt trauma caused by falling to the ground. Some victims also have been beaten with fists or solid objects, causing damage to underlying organs and structures. A plain radiograph (i.e., flat plate, scout) of the torso can reveal free air in the abdomen as diagnostic of perforated organs.

Crime victims are at high risk for misdiagnosis of secondary head injury or ruptured viscus. This may be further complicated if the victim is pregnant. Two patients may be affected: the mother and her unborn child. Domestic violence is a leading cause of death for pregnant women. Obstetric-gynecologic staff may need to be included in the surgical team.

Broken bones are misdiagnosed less frequently because of the use of routine radiography. The victim of a hit-and-run driver often suffers a fractured tibia and fibula at the height of the car's bumper. The measurement of the point of impact enables investigators to determine whether the vehicle was traveling at a constant rate of speed or braking at the time of the collision. Thorough head-to-toe assessment is followed by a complete review of all body systems. Every aspect of the physical examination and treatment becomes part of the evidence discovery process.

The Patient Who Is a Victim of Sexual Assault

Patients who have been raped or sexually assaulted begin treatment in the ED. Victims with severe injuries or multiple traumas are treated in the OR. Although frequently used, the term *rape* is a legal conclusion, not a medical diagnosis. Rape is a felony and one of the most underreported crimes. More victims are reporting sexual assaults, rape, and harassment because of the "Me Too Movement" (www.metoomvmt.org). Victims can find local organizations that provide services, support, and safety measures. Sexual offenses include marital rape, sexual battery, felonious sexual penetration, sexual imposition, and corruption of a minor. *Sexual assault* is the appropriate term for both male and female victims.[10]

In reality, 1 of every 3 females is sexually assaulted during her lifetime. Only 1 in 10 ever reports it. One of every 9 males experiences some form of sexual assault. The number of reported assaults is growing with public awareness and safe reporting methods. More than 80% of the assailants are known to their victims.

The rape crisis center should be involved in every aspect of care for both sexes. Female rape trauma victims should always be examined by the gynecology staff, preferably female. Victims of sexual assault may fear examination or physical contact by members of a specific sex. Females may wish to have a female examiner. A male also may prefer a female examiner, especially if his assailant was male. This holds true of the OR team: The patient may have a sexual prejudice that needs to be respected. Sensitivity to the needs of the victim is important, and documentation and preservation of evidence should be maintained. Sexual assault is a crime of violence and power.[10]

Physiologic and psychologic stabilization is critical. Additional physical injuries, such as gunshot or stab wounds, may complicate care related to sexual assault. Medical history, such as current medications, immunizations, and allergies, should be assessed. Douching, bathing, urination, or defecation after an assault may have altered evidence and are taken into consideration. Genital trauma should be closely evaluated. Edema and damage to the genitals of a female may require the use of a pediatric speculum.

Considerations for the Patient With Sexual Trauma

The psychologic affect of a sexual assault victim can range from flat to hyperreactive. The victim should be approached with patience and understanding. Minors may be accompanied by their natural or court-appointed guardians.

Quick, brisk moves by a caregiver can create undue emotional stress. The caregiver should always wear gloves to depersonalize touch and should allow the victim to guide their hands during the physical assessment to provide an element of self-control. Feelings of loss of control and violation increase the victim's anxiety. A calm demeanor can provide a sense of security for any victim of crime, but particularly for a sexual assault victim. The OR should reflect a sense of stability and prevent nonessential noise.

Preoperative assessment of a female sexual assault victim should include past sexual, menstrual, and contraceptive history. The possibility of existing or resultant pregnancy should be considered. A blood test for β-human chorionic gonadotropin should be drawn. Hormonal pregnancy prophylaxis (the "morning-after pill") may be used within 72 hours of the assault to induce menses and is 95% to 98% effective in preventing implantation of a fertilized ovum. Some women may desire the morning-after pill or abortion counseling at a later date. Approximately 1% of sexual assaults result in pregnancy.

During the examination the victim's pubic hair should be combed into a clean white envelope. A few clippings of the victim's pubic hair and the comb should be sealed inside with the examiner's signature, date, and time on the outside. The assailant's hair may be present and is valuable as evidence. Examination with an ultraviolet Wood's lamp should be performed because prostatic secretions and seminal fluid appear fluorescent even when dried. Dried scrapings of blood and secretions from under fingernails and around genitalia should be saved in an appropriate container. Dried semen can be used to verify an assailant's identity by DNA. Toluidine blue dye that stains acidic tissue may be used on the genitals to identify DNA, RNA, or injuries such as tears for both males and females.

A colposcope with a green filter can be used to examine and photograph vaginal tears. The green filter is useful for identification of vascular structures as a direct contrast to reddened or bleeding tissue. Speculum, proctoscopic, or bimanual pelvic examinations are performed with only sterile water as lubrication. Oral, vaginal, or anal mucosal smears, swabs, and washings should be fixed according to laboratory protocol. Maintain the chain of evidence at all times.

Commercial rape-evidence kits are available for the collection of specimens, preservation of evidence, and documentation of physical findings. Baseline blood tests for HIV, hepatitis B virus (HBV), hepatitis C virus (HCV), and syphilis should be performed, with follow-up tests in 4 to 6 months. Cultures for gonococci also should be obtained. Antibiotic prophylaxis may be indicated. Women should be tested for pregnancy that was present before the rape. Treatments can be harmful to the developing embryo or fetus.

The Patient Who Is a Victim of Domestic Violence

Victims of domestic violence may be male or female. Most are female and have a common set of specific injuries. Many beatings go unreported because of fear of retaliation, low self-esteem, and embarrassment over enduring repeated abuse. Other victims claim they love the abuser and want to keep the family together. A battered woman may feel she deserved the beating and may avoid going to the ED unless she experiences symptoms she interprets as life-threatening.

Signs of physical abuse are commonly found around the face and head and consist of multiple abrasions, contusions, chipped teeth, fractured facial bones, epistaxis, and blackened eyes. Often the woman is pregnant for the first time, which is a common theme in 8% to 15% of gravid females suffering abusive treatment. Domestic violence occurs in all socioeconomic groups, but poverty and unemployment may precipitate the event.

The victim of domestic abuse or violence may be afraid to report the event to the police. ED personnel are not bound by law to report domestic violence. Many victims may lie about how the injuries occurred out of fear of future violence. Sometimes the abuser is the person who brought them to the ED and is present. Personnel may ask in private if injuries are caused from violence. Reporting domestic violence in adults depends on the individual case and safety of the victim. ED nurses should completely and accurately document the event and if possible photograph the injuries with the patient's permission. Assure the victim that all information is confidential. Referral can be made to a battered women's shelter as necessary. Most shelters have a 24-hour crisis intervention.

The Patient Who Is a Victim of Child Abuse

Children are the most helpless victims, and more than 1840 die each year as a result of abuse or neglect. Of reported cases of child abuse deaths, 70% are younger than 3 years of age.[11] Child abuse can occur in any socioeconomic group and may take the form of psychologic, physical, or sexual abuse. Other forms of victimization include neglect of physical, psychologic, and medical needs. The National Child Abuse Hotline (1-800) 4-A-Child offers

confidential reporting 24 hours a day, 7 days a week for reporting suspected abuse. Health care workers are mandated to report all forms of child abuse because children cannot help themselves.

Infants and young children are unable to ask for help and are dependent on adults and health care workers to recognize abuse and neglect, treat them for it, and report it. Many injuries and illnesses are characteristic of abuse. However, many forms of abuse are discovered incidentally when a child is brought to the ED, clinic, or physician's office for an unrelated illness. OR personnel may discover signs of abuse when performing simple procedures, such as myringotomy. Health care personnel should be educated to observe for unspoken signals from these helpless victims.

The first signs of child abuse may be discovered while obtaining the child's history from the adult caretaker, parent, or guardian. Clues to look for include discrepancies about injury patterns, visits to multiple hospitals, lack of a consistent medical history, delays in seeking treatment, and visible evidence of old untreated injuries in various stages of healing. Observation of the child's affect can be misleading. Some children may be overcooperative with painful procedures or display extremes of affection.

A child who has known only abuse may show no response to the environment or fail to thrive. The abused child may cling to the abuser or exhibit avoidance behavior. Response patterns can be unpredictable at times. Patient assessment should compare the physical and psychologic development stage of the child with expected normal findings. Further discussion of normal childhood development is found in Chapter 8.

Examples of physiologic developmental discrepancies include long bone fractures in nonwalking infants or head injuries (whiplash-type) associated with violent shaking such as retinal and cerebral hemorrhage.

Violent shaking is a common form of abusive treatment between the ages of 6 weeks and 4 months during episodes of crying. Abusers may feel that shaking a crying infant is more acceptable than actually hitting. Crying may cease during the shaking because of brain edema, and the abuser may repeat the action because it made the baby stop crying. Clinical signs of trauma-induced brain injury are loss of consciousness, seizures, vomiting, and apnea. Brain injury also is caused by nutritional deficit and is manifest by personality change, learning disability, and diminished functional skill.[11]

Visible injuries such as circumferential bruising around wrists or ankles from being held down are sometimes noted. Multiple clusters of similarly shaped discolored skin markings could indicate repeated strikes with a belt or stick. These are sometimes found to be in various stages of healing. Questionable burns may be found on soles of feet, backs of hands, or inside thighs. A scalded stocking pattern may be identified on a child who has been dipped in hot water. Children who accidentally burn themselves by grabbing hot objects usually have burns on the palms of the hands or irregular splash-shaped burns from pulling a pan off the stove. Venereal disease in a child is usually the result of sexual abuse.

Some pathologic conditions commonly mistaken for child abuse include dermatologic conditions, bone diseases, coagulation disorders, infections, skin discoloration (Mongolian spots), and folk healing remedies. Birthmarks can appear bluish and give the impression of bruising in various stages of healing.

Some questionable marks can be caused by clothing dyes or inks. Most of these markings can be removed with rubbing alcohol. Phytodermatosis is a skin discoloration that occurs when lime, lemon, celery, or herbal preparations are rubbed into the skin and exposed to sunlight. These phototoxic reactions can appear like hand marks if an adult was squeezing lemons or limes for summer beverages.

Folk remedies include coining, which involves rubbing a coin over an afflicted area. This sometimes causes striped bruises that resemble strap marks. To avoid erroneous reports of child abuse, the examiner should perform a careful history and physical examination, including appropriate laboratory studies. When in doubt, consult with a specialist who can critically evaluate suspicious injury or illness.

Recognition of child abuse during physical assessment may not be instantly obvious. If the injury or illness does not match the explanation, the child may be a victim of abuse and the incident should be further investigated. In every state a health care worker who suspects child abuse is mandated to report it to child welfare authorities.

Outcomes of Victimization

Regardless of the victim's age or social status, the postassault, postvictimization results can be devastating. Sequelae to victimization may include posttraumatic stress disorder (PTSD), augmented attention-deficit disorder with or without hyperactivity (ADD/ADHD), psychosis, depression, and continued feelings of victimization. Children may experience secondary enuresis and encopresis as a form of regression and display inappropriate sexual behaviors toward adults or other children.

Anger may be projected toward pets and smaller siblings in the form of cruelty and abuse. Abused children may grow up to become abusers. Nightmares are common in all ages. Coping mechanisms become distorted, and conversion reactions can be confused with somatic complaints. Unfortunately, death is sometimes the final outcome of violent crime.

Prevention of violent crime is not always an option. Health care workers become aware of the event after the fact. Referral agencies are available to provide emergency shelter and temporary solace. Encouraging adult victims to report violent acts and follow through with prosecution is equally as important as treating physical injury. The victim who is fearful and unwilling to prosecute is at high risk for being victimized again. Minor victims are helpless and unable to report their injuries without help. Health care workers are required to report confirmed or suspected child abuse to proper authorities. Follow institutional policy and procedure in this regard.

End-of-Life Care

Although perioperative patient care personnel are most often involved with patients who have a favorable prognosis, they also care for patients of all ages who have a catastrophic illness and are undergoing surgery to palliate or relieve a specific problem. The procedure may be palliative rather than curative. Included in this category are patients with the following conditions:
- Malignant diseases that result in severe debilitation and terminal illness
- Severe traumatic disabilities that necessitate lengthy hospitalization, such as after high spinal cord injury or extensive burns
- End-stage renal disease, or patients waiting for an organ transplant
- Patients with a DNR order

Maximum patient comfort and the relief of physiologic disturbances are primary concerns. All these patients need highly individualized care. The manner in which patients are told the diagnosis and prognosis obviously has a great effect on their hope for recovery. Patients who have been thoroughly and considerately informed are easier to talk to, accept therapy more readily, and have greater trust in and communicate more openly with caregivers.

Emphasis is placed on the present, with a focus on the patient's strengths and attributes and how best to use them. Finding hope is difficult when facing a radical, disfiguring procedure. Listening to the patient is particularly important.

Each patient deals with such a diagnosis in their own way. Although it is not always so, many people consider the diagnosis of cancer a death warrant and react accordingly. To be supportive, the caregiver should mentally review Elisabeth Kübler-Ross's (1926–2004) stages of dying: denial, isolation, anger, bargaining, depression, and acceptance. (These stages do not always occur in this sequence.) More information about death and dying can be found at www.ekrfoundation.org/. The National Institute on Aging, National Institutes of Health publishes a 36-page booklet called End-of-Life Care. The booklet can be saved as a PDF document or can be printed. It can be found at https://order.nia.nih.gov (End of Life). The booklet discusses types of care, understanding a loved one's wishes, decision-making, finding care, and how to prepare for difficult situations.

Death of a Patient in the Operating Room

Although it is an uncommon occurrence, a patient may die while on the OR bed or shortly after reaching the PACU or intensive care unit (ICU). When this happens the perioperative manager should be notified immediately. Ideally the family and significant others are informed by the surgeon or the surgeon's designee. It may be appropriate to have organ procurement personnel discuss organ donation with the family if death is imminent and to request permission to proceed with plans for potential organ procurement. If circumstances warrant, an autopsy may be necessary.

In the event of a high-profile accident or event, the facility's public relations personnel should be the contact with the press or news media. Perioperative or perianesthesia personnel should not provide information about any patient to any person not authorized in the patient's care. A breach of confidentiality is a serious ethical consideration and is especially contained in the event of a police investigation or medical malpractice suit.

Coroner's Cases

In some states the body of a patient who dies in the OR or who does not awaken from general anesthesia automatically becomes the property of the coroner. Patients who die as a result of or in the commission of a crime become the property of the coroner. Family consent for autopsy is not necessary in these situations. The coroner must give approval for organ procurement and has the right to overrule the wishes of the family.

Individual state law and institutional policy determine the postmortem care of the patient's body. For example, all drainage tubes, implants, and catheters may need to be left in place for removal and examination at autopsy. All medication vials and IV solution containers should remain with the body.

The body of a patient who dies under these circumstances is also considered the property of the coroner, but postmortem care is more complex. Critical medical-legal issues should be considered if the patient was a suspected victim or perpetrator of violence or was injured in a suspicious manner. All information about the patient's condition, personal effects and attire, and materials discovered during the surgical procedure are considered forensic evidence.

Postmortem Patient Care

A death may occur as a result of shock after extensive traumatic injuries, exsanguination after rupture of an aortic aneurysm, unsuccessful cardiopulmonary resuscitation after cardiac arrest, or other causes. The circulator's responsibilities after intraoperative death include the following:

1. Provide after-death care for the body as appropriate or ensure that forensic protocol is followed before releasing the body to authorities or the morgue.
   a. Follow institutional policy and procedure.
   b. Be sure identification is correct.
   c. Place the patient supine in correct alignment with one pillow under the head. This minimizes pooling fluids in dependent tissue.
   d. Secure the patient's personal effects.
   e. Do not wash the body if it is considered part of forensic evidence.
2. Arrange for transportation of the body from the OR to the morgue, or release it to an appropriate authority.
   a. Release the body from the OR according to institutional policy and procedure.
   b. Avoid exposing other patients, visitors, and family to removal of the body.
   c. If the religious or cultural preference of a patient or family is known, an appropriate member of the clergy or a spiritual adviser may be consulted concerning after-death practices.
3. Complete the intraoperative chart and additional documentation as required by institutional policy.

Policy may allow the family to view a loved one before the body is transported to the morgue. The room in which the viewing takes place should be clean, presentable, and private. The perioperative nurse (or designee) should remain with the family and lend support. Parents may wish to hold a deceased child. Chairs and facial tissues should be available in the room. If forensics are involved, the nurse should not leave the patient's body unattended at any time.

Care is taken not to make statements to the family that sound cliché, such as the following examples:
- "It was God's will" or "God has a plan."
- "Your loved one is in a better place now."
- "God needed an angel."
- "Everything happens for a reason."
- "Things will work out for the best."
- "Time will heal."

- "You have to be strong for your remaining loved ones."
- "Your loved one wouldn't want you to be sad."
- "At least your loved one is not in pain anymore."
- "You shouldn't be so sad. It is for the best."
- "At least your loved one lived a good life."

After a death in the OR, from whatever cause, team members should be given time to express their grief and deal with their feelings about the event. Tears and sadness are normal responses and should not be criticized. The team members should be supportive of each other, including the surgeon and the anesthesia provider.

EVOLVE WEBSITE

http://evolve.elsevier.com/Hornacky/BerryKohn/
- Historical Perspective
- Flashcards
- Self-Assessment Activities
- Glossary

References

1. Karnatovskaia LV, Gajic O, Bienvenu OJ, et al.: A holistic approach to the critically ill and Maslow's hierarchy, *J Crit Care* 30(1):210–211, 2015.
2. Current Nursing: www.currentnursing.com. Accessed February 26, 2023.
3. McLeod S: *Defense mechanisms*, 2020. www.simplypsychology.org/defense-mechanisms.html. Accessed February 26, 2023.
4. Dietary Guidelines for Americans: www.dietaryguidelines.gov. Accessed February 28, 2023.
5. Bays H, Bindlish S, Clayton T: Obesity, diabetes mellitus, and cardiometabolic risk: an Obesity Medicine Association (OMA) Clinical Practice Statement (CPS) 2023, *Obes Pillars* 5:1–25, 2023.
6. Dogra P, Jialal I: Diabetic perioperative management. In *StatPearls*. Updated June 19, 2022. www.ncbi.nlm.nih.gov/books/NBK540965/. Accessed March 7, 2023.
7. Elisha S, Heiner J, Nagelhout J: Obesity and anesthesia practice. In *Nurse anesthesia*, ed 7, St. Louis, 2023, Elsevier, pp 1092–1094.
8. American Cancer Society: www.cancer.org. Accessed March 8, 2023.
9. Elliyanti A: *Radiopharmaceuticals in modern cancer therapy—current research for better diagnosis and therapy*, 2022. www.intechopen.com/chapters/78024. Accessed March 8, 2023.
10. Preventing sexual violence: www.cdc.gov/violenceprevention/sexualviolence/fastfact.html. Accessed March 15, 2023.
11. The issue of child abuse: www.childhelp.org/child-abuse/. Accessed March 15, 2023.

Bibliography

AORN (Association of periOperative Registered Nurses): *Guidelines for perioperative practice*, Denver, CO, 2024, The Association.

8

Perioperative Pediatrics

CHAPTER OUTLINE

Indications for Surgery, 125
Considerations in Perioperative Pediatrics, 126
Perioperative Assessment of the Pediatric Patient, 127
Preoperative Psychologic Preparation of Pediatric Patients, 134

Pediatric Anesthesia, 135
Intraoperative Pediatric Patient Care Considerations, 140
Common Surgical Procedures, 142
Postoperative Pediatric Patient Care, 160

CHAPTER OBJECTIVES

After studying this chapter, the learner will be able to:

- Describe pediatric patient care in terms of developmental stages.
- Identify age-specific considerations in the care of pediatric patients.

- List several procedures that are performed on pediatric patients.

KEY TERMS AND DEFINITIONS

Acholic Stool is pale because of absence of bile pigment.
Atresia Interruption in the continuity of a tubular anatomic structure, such as the trachea or esophagus.
Cloaca Congenital malformation in females in which the vagina, urethra, and anus open into a single orifice from the body.
Congenital Physiologic condition that is present since birth.
Contralateral Opposite side.
Cryptorchidism Testicles fail to descend into the scrotal sac.
Imperforate Opening that failed to form at the terminal end of a natural orifice.
Intussusception Intestinal condition in which the bowel slides backward into itself, causing obstruction, pain, and necrosis.

Ipsilateral Same side.
Neonate Newborn.
Puberty Period of transition between childhood and adulthood when secondary sex characteristics develop. Commonly ages 8 to 13 years for girls and ages 10 to 15 years for boys.
Rule of Tens A measure of neonate physiology in preparation for a surgical procedure: 10 weeks of age, 10 g of hemoglobin, 10 lb of body weight.
Urachus Anatomic connection between the umbilicus and the bladder that usually closes and seals after birth.
Volvulus Kinked segment of midgut that causes bowel obstruction.

The surgical problems peculiar to children from birth to postpuberty are not limited to any one area of the body or to any one surgical specialty. Malformations and diseases affect all body parts and therefore may require the skills of any of the surgical specialists. However, pediatric surgery is a specialty in itself and is not adult surgery scaled down to infant or child size. Indications for surgery include congenital anomalies, acquired disease processes, and trauma. Many of these conditions are treatable or curable with surgical intervention.

Indications for Surgery

Congenital Anomalies

A congenital anomaly is a deviation from normal structure or location in any organ or part of the body that is present from birth. It can alter function or appearance. Multiple anomalies may be present at birth. If an anomaly does not involve vital life functions, surgical intervention may be postponed until the results can be maximized and the risks of the surgical procedure are minimized by growth and development of body systems.

If a newborn has a poor chance of survival without a surgical procedure, the risk is taken within hours or days after birth. Defects in the alimentary tract are the most common indication for an emergency surgical procedure during the newborn period, followed in frequency by cardiac and respiratory system defects.[1] Mortality in the newborn is influenced by three uncontrollable factors: the multiplicity of anomalies, prematurity, and birthweight.

The presence of three or more physical congenital anomalies is referred to as the VACTERL association or syndrome, which includes the following anomalies:

*V*ertebral defect, such as spina bifida or myelomeningocele
*A*nal malformation, such as imperforate anus

*C*ardiac anomaly, such as patent ductus arteriosus or ventricular and atrial septal defects
*T*racheoesophageal fistula
*E*sophageal atresia
*R*enal anomaly, such as horseshoe kidney and renal dysplasia
*L*imb defect, such as short radius syndrome or syndactylism

Another acronym used to describe multiple congenital defects is the CHARGE association or syndrome. These defects may be accompanied by facial clefts and dysphagia. The CHARGE syndrome includes several of the following defects:

*C*oloboma (split iris) defect in the eye
*H*earing impairment caused by structural defects
*A*tresia choanae
*R*etardation or intellectual disabilities caused by brain anomalies
*G*enitourinary defects
*E*sophageal defects

Acquired Disease Processes

Among acquired disease processes, appendicitis is the most common surgically corrected childhood disease. Malignant tumors occur in infants and children but with minimal frequency compared with occurrence rates for adults. Benign lesions are surgically excised, usually without further difficulty to the child.

Trauma

Accidental injury is the leading cause of death in children. In 2022, the Centers for Disease Control and Prevention (CDC) reported that more than 7000 children and teens die of accidents daily throughout the world. In children ages 1 to 5 years, drowning, burns, motor vehicle accidents (MVAs), falls, choking, and poisoning top the list of deaths caused by accidents in all income groups. In the teenaged years, leading causes of death include MVAs, suicide, overdose, homicide, firearm accidents, disease, drowning, childbirth, poisoning, and fire.[2] During the COVID-19 pandemic, there was a 30% increase in poisoning, overdose, suicide, and firearm-related deaths.[3] Males die of accidents more frequently than do females.

The margin for error in diagnosis and treatment of a child is less than that for an adult with a comparable injury. A child's blood volume is low compared with body size, and even a small loss of blood can be critical. Because the child's chest cavity is small, an abdominal or chest injury can be critical. Diagnosis is made quickly, and the patient is sent to the operating room (OR) if indicated. Examples of common injuries include blunt intestinal trauma caused by seatbelt use on small children and head injuries caused by improper use of infant car seats. Other injuries, such as lacerations, fractures, or crushing injuries of hands and arms, may result in nerve, vessel, tendon, bone, and other soft tissue damage.

Considerations in Perioperative Pediatrics

Surgeons who perform pediatric surgery should have knowledge of the embryologic, psychologic, physiologic, and pathologic problems peculiar to the newborn, infant, and child. Knowledge has advanced pediatric surgery in the following ways:
- Recognition of differences between pediatric patients and adults.

- Accurate diagnosis and earlier treatment, which facilitates a more favorable outcome, especially in the fetus and preterm neonate. Neonatology is a growing subspecialty of pediatrics.
- Understanding of preoperative preparation of the patient, family, and significant others.
- Availability of total parenteral nutrition (TPN) and other measures of supportive care for perioperative pediatric management.
- Advances in anesthesiology, including new agents, perfection of techniques of administration, and an understanding of the responses of pediatric patients to anesthetic agents.
- Refinements in surgical procedures and instrumentation.
- Understanding of postoperative care. Larger facilities have neonatal and pediatric intensive care units.

The nursing process is tailored to meet the unique needs of each pediatric patient. Assessment and nursing diagnoses are based on chronologic, psychologic, and physiologic factors specific to each patient. The plan of care should reflect consideration for age and reflect interventions modified according to the child's developmental stage as identified in Table 8.1.

Three developmental theorists, Erikson, Piaget, and Lovinger, emphasized that although the child has reached a certain age or physical size, psychologic growth is the baseline parameter by which communication is measured.[4] Understanding individual differences enables the perioperative team to develop a positive rapport with the patient and caregivers, which facilitates attainment of expected outcomes.

Not every patient of a particular age group meets standardized height and weight criteria; children may be short or tall or thin or heavy for their age. Children approaching puberty have varied growth spurts and physical development. Although norms have been established by age groups, the plan of care should reflect consideration for individual differences.

Chronologic Age

The patient's chronologic age is a primary consideration in the development of the plan of care. An age-related baseline is a useful beginning for effective assessment of pediatric patients. The CDC offers an assortment of information for caregivers, parents, and families regarding childhood milestones, concerns, educational programs, and reference materials. Tools and information can be downloaded from the website (www.cdc.gov).[3] Parents take comfort in knowing their children are being cared for in an age-appropriate manner and not like miniature adults. Use of a pediatric focus with babies and children creates an atmosphere specifically geared toward safety and may minimize risks such as medication dosage errors.

In concert with the care of adult patients and Universal Protocol for patient safety in the OR, a pediatric checklist should be used. No child exactly meets all criteria in chronologic versus emotional age. Authors may vary in small age increments; however, no author can state that all children fit all templates exactly because each is an individual. The following terminology is used to approximately categorize ages of pediatric patients:
1. *Embryo:* Not compatible with life: 1 day to 3 months' gestation
2. *Fetus:* In utero after 3 months' gestation
3. *Newborn infant, referred to as a neonate:*
   a. *Potentially viable:* Gestational age more than 24 weeks; birthweight more than 500 g; capable of sustaining life outside the uterus as defined by the World Health Organization (WHO)

TABLE 8.1   Psychologic Developmental Stage Theories

Chronologic Age Ranges (Approximate)	DEVELOPMENTAL STAGE BY THEORIST			Characteristics of Psychologic Development
	Erikson	Piaget	Loevinger	
Birth–18 months	Trust vs. mistrust	Sensorimotor	Presocial	Learns to view self as being separate from the environment; begins to develop the concept of hope; learns to develop attachments to others; dependent on caregiver for warmth, security, nourishment, nurturing, and stimulation; begins to use sounds and short words to communicate ideas; may view hospitalization as abandonment
19 months–3 years	Autonomy vs. shame/doubt	Preoperational	Symbiotic	Develops a two-way relationship with primary caregiver; suffers separation anxiety when isolated from established relationships; has short trials of independence; personality becomes introverted or extroverted; establishes a sense of will; uses sentences for communication; has fear of immediate threats; does not project thoughts beyond the present situation
4–6 years	Initiative vs. guilt	Preoperational	Impulsive	Asserts a separate identity; begins to have fear of real and imagined situations; senses peer acceptance or rejection; is concerned about disfigurement; may act out feelings; believes that every action has a purpose, either reward or punishment; learns to be self-protective; fears death or nonexistence; death is not always understood as being permanent; develops short-term self-control; uses compound sentences to communicate; mimics terminology used by fantasy characters
7–11 years	Industry vs. inferiority	Concrete operational	Conformist	Imitates actions and attitudes of peers and heroes; is aware of the differences of others and identifies with a particular social group; fears loss of self-control; understands the world in moderate detail; prefers honest explanations and reassurance of safety; does not want to be treated like a baby; strives for competency in daily tasks; can distinguish between fact and fantasy; has a greater understanding of death and its permanence; wants to be accepted as an individual; communicates well verbally and with basic writing skill
12–16 years	Identity vs. role confusion	Formal, operational	Self-aware, conscientious	May change opinion in response to stereotypes; develops close relationships; understands values, rules, and ideals; begins to feel more important as an individual; fears alienation; body image is extremely important; is capable of abstract thought and reasoning; has a sense of aesthetic beauty; can merge sensory information and logic to derive a conclusion; prefers privacy and confidentiality; may question authority; is aware of opposite sex; may explore sexual activity; dreams about future lifestyle; wants to prove self-worth; globally communicates verbally and in writing
17 years–adulthood	Intimacy vs. isolation	Formal, operational	Individualistic	Becomes aware of and accepts the interdependence of humankind; may feel some hostility toward authority; sometimes torn between the desire to be totally independent and dependent; seeks companionship; may be sexually active; refines interpersonal skills; demands privacy and confidentiality; plans for independent lifestyle as approach; refines verbal and written communication skill

b. *True preterm:* Gestational age less than 37 weeks; birthweight 2500 g or less

c. *Large preterm:* Gestational age less than 38 weeks; birthweight more than 2500 g

d. *Term neonate:* Gestational age 38 to 40 weeks; birthweight greater than 2500 g, usually between 3402 and 3629 g (if less than 2500 g, the neonate is considered small for gestational age [SGA])

e. *Postterm:* Gestational age extended by more than 8 weeks

4. *Neonatal period:* First 28 days of extrauterine life
5. *Infant:* 28 days to 18 months
6. *Toddler:* 18 to 30 months
7. *Preschool age:* 2½ to 5 years
8. *School age:* 6 to 12 years
9. *Adolescent:* 13 to 18 years

Perioperative Assessment of the Pediatric Patient

Pediatric Psychosocial Assessment

Assessment of psychologic development is based on age-related criteria (see Table 8.1) but includes assessment of individual differences. Comparison of established norms and assessment data is helpful in developing the plan of care. Environmental and parental influences can cause variance in affect, attitude, and social skills. Environmental influences on psychologic development include ethnic, cultural, and socioeconomic factors.

The age of the patient may indicate the level of involvement with the environment. For example, an infant may have exposure only to immediate family members for external stimuli, but a preschool child may have daily experience with children in preschool and other children. Coping and social skills may be developed, depending on the child's developmental stage.

Parenting practices may directly influence the way the patient responds to caregivers and the perioperative environment. Pediatric patients respond differently in the presence of parents or guardians. Infants may be more cooperative if a parent is present. Conversely, an adolescent may want to show independence by asking the parent to leave the room. These actions may be completely opposite if the child has been abused or neglected. Lack of parental nurturing can cause a global deficit, including poor development of language and cognitive skills. Understanding the patient's level of psychologic development can help the caregiver communicate more effectively with the pediatric patient throughout the perioperative experience. Interaction should be according to the child's individual developmental level regardless of chronologic age.

Pediatric Physical Assessment

The physiologic assessment of pediatric patients is compared with national averages when baseline norms are established. Physiologic development is influenced by genetics, nutrition, health status, and environmental factors. The physical assessment may reveal conditions that can adversely affect the outcome of a surgical procedure. Comparison of the patient's age, size, and psychologic development with established norms may enable the caregiver to assess for deficiencies in size or weight that may indicate a potential health problem.[5]

Unexplained marks or bruises may be signs of physical abuse. Health care personnel are required to report suspected child abuse. Photographs are useful in the documentation of physical findings. Abused children may be afraid of punishment for revealing the origin of an injury. Some physical findings suggestive of abuse discovered during the physical examination or surgical skin preparation may include, but are not limited to, the following:

- Burns and scalding marks
- Genital injuries, such as tears or sexually transmitted diseases
- Human or animal bite marks
- Patterned bruises or skin tears
- Rope-like stricture marks
- Cranial damage or ruptured vessels in eyes

A small, frail child may have a congenital cardiac deformity or a malabsorption syndrome. Abuse or neglect may be manifested as a nutritional deficit. An extremely thin, malnourished adolescent may be intentionally bulimic or anorexic in response to a psychologic body image problem. An obese child may have an endocrine disease or a psychologic disturbance that causes overeating. These issues are important considerations, because most dosages of medications given to pediatric patients are based on body weight in kilograms. Absorption and metabolism of medications are influenced by the same physiologic parameters that govern nutritional status.

Metabolism and Nutritional Considerations

Infants have relatively greater nutritional requirements than do adults for minimizing loss of body protein. The resting metabolic rate of an infant is two to three times that of an adult, which results in rapid metabolic imbalances in infants. Neonates require 110 to 135 calories per kilogram of weight per day to maintain homeostasis. The potential for complications increases proportionately with the duration of fluid restriction because infants are prone to hypovolemia and dehydration.

The neonate's body weight represents 70% to 80% fluid. Fluid weight is directly related to body fat content. Preterm infants have less body fat and consequently lose fluids easily. Other fluid losses are associated with urinary loss, gastrointestinal loss, insensible loss through respiration, and surgical loss by evaporation via the skin and drains. Fluid replacement for babies is calculated according to body weight, as follows:

- *Preterm:* 150 to 50 mL/kg/24 h
- *Term neonates:* 100 mL/kg/24 h
- *Infants more than 10 kg:* 1050 mL/kg/24 h

Procedures performed on infants and toddlers should have priority on the surgical schedule so that these patients can return to a normal fluid and feeding routine as quickly as possible.

Infants may be given regular formula or a varied diet up to 6 hours before anesthesia and clear liquids up to 1 to 2 hours before the surgical procedure. A satisfactory state of hydration is thus maintained, and milk curds are absent from the stomach. Infants may be breastfed up to 4 hours before the surgical procedure. Breast milk has fewer or no curds and empties faster from the stomach than formula. Infants should not miss more than one or two feedings. Oral intake is resumed promptly after the infant recovers from anesthesia.

Toddlers and preschool children may be permitted clear liquids up to 2 to 4 hours preoperatively. Intake of clear oral fluids in small amounts decreases the level of gastric acid contents by stimulating gastric emptying and diminishes the hunger-deprivation response.

Children older than 5 years may have nothing by mouth (nil per os [NPO]) after midnight or 6 hours before induction of anesthesia. Exceptions may be necessary for children with fever, diabetes, or other special problems. For these children, clear liquids with supplemental glucose may be ordered to be given orally up to 2 hours preoperatively. Avoid colored liquids that could be mistaken for blood or other body substance if the child vomits.

Older children may require slower progression of oral dietary intake postoperatively and are maintained with supplemental intravenous (IV) therapy that includes protein and vitamins. Vitamins K and C may be given to patients of any age group.

Fluid and Electrolyte Balance Considerations

The newborn is not dehydrated and withstands major surgical procedures within the first 4 days of life without extensive fluid and electrolyte replacement. The renal system is easily overloaded with the administration of IV fluids. The newborn has a lower glomerular filtration rate and less efficient renal tubular function than does an adult. (Renal function improves during the first 2 months of life and approaches adult levels by age 2 years.) During the time of an average surgical procedure on a newborn, a total of 10 to 30 mL of fluid may be administered. Usually 2.5% to 5% dextrose in half-strength normal saline solution is infused.

Administration of excessive IV dextrose solution is avoided in infants younger than 1 year because they maintain lower glycogen stores. During physiologic stress the patient easily becomes hyperglycemic. Hyperglycemia acts as an osmotic diuretic and causes increased urinary output and dilutional hyponatremia. The increased urine volume can be a false indicator of renal and hemodynamic status. Seizures and neurologic damage may result. Seizures may be clinically undetected while the infant is under general anesthesia because the pharmacologic agents act as anticonvulsants.

Infants have a relatively larger ratio of body surface area to body mass than do adults. When infants become dehydrated, which can occur rapidly, bodily functions are disturbed, as is the acid-base balance. Plasma proteins differ in concentration from those of an adult. Fluid and electrolyte replacements are necessary. In children older than 1 year, isotonic solutions, such as normal saline or lactated Ringer's solution, are given IV per kilogram of body weight.

Urinary output is directly related to body size and age. Neonates can concentrate 400 mOsm/L initially and 500 mOsm/L progressively over the first few days compared with 1200 mOsm/L in the average-size adult. This concentration and excretion of the solute load result in 2 to 4 mL/kg/h urinary output. Older children (toddlers and preschoolers) produce 1 to 2 mL/kg/h of urine when adequately hydrated. Urine measurement in children is difficult to monitor without a Foley catheter.

The hemoglobin level is lowest at 2 to 3 months of age (Table 8.2). The blood volume of the average newborn is 250 mL, approximately 75 to 85 mL/kg of body weight (Table 8.3). A subtle sign of blood loss is a narrowed pulse pressure less than 20 beats per minute. Significant blood loss requires replacement. Blood is typed and crossmatched in readiness. Although blood loss is small in most cases, a loss of 30 mL may represent 10% to 20% of circulating blood volume in an infant. The small margin of safety indicates the need for replacement of blood loss exceeding 10% of circulating blood volume. When replacement exceeds 50% of the estimated blood volume, sodium bicarbonate is infused to minimize metabolic acidosis.

Hypotension in an infant is not apparent until 50% of the circulating volume is lost. Hypotension is usually caused by myocardial depression from anesthetic agents, primarily inhalation anesthesia. The infant's myocardium has fewer contractile muscle fibers and more noncontractile connective tissue than found in an older child or adult and therefore lacks myocardial force to maintain cardiac output. The cardiac output depends on the heart rate. Any decrease in heart rate directly affects blood pressure and body tissue perfusion.

IV infusions should be administered with the following precautions:

- Dehydration should be avoided. Therapy for metabolic acidosis, should it develop, is guided with measurement of pH, blood gas values, and serum electrolyte levels.
- Blood volume loss should be measured as accurately as possible and promptly replaced. In an infant, rapid transfusion of blood may produce transient but severe metabolic acidosis because of citrate added as a preservative.
- IV fluids and blood should be infused through pediatric-size cannulated needles or catheters connected to drip chamber adapters and small solution containers.
- Umbilical vessels may be used for arterial or venous access in newborns less than 24 hours after birth. In extreme circumstances the umbilical vein can be accessed through a small infraumbilical incision and cannulated from inside the peritoneal cavity for rapid infusion. Scalp veins are used frequently on infants.

If venous access cannot be quickly established, intraosseous (IO) infusion may be indicated for fluid replacement or the administration of emergency anesthesia. IO infusion may be indicated when vascular collapse is evident and no other route is available. Most medications, blood, and blood products can be given via this route, but chemotherapy is not advised. Contraindications for IO use are specific to the planned site. IO cannot be used in a fractured limb, a site of previous orthopedic implant, a previously used IO site, or place where there is known infection.

In adults the lateral proximal humerus is used for insertion. In pediatrics the anterior proximal tibia, below the growth plate, is used (Fig. 8.1). The position on the tibia is identified by placing the index finger centrally, below the patella, between the medial and lateral borders. An antiseptic solution of choice is used to cleanse the site before insertion and sterile technique is used. Local anesthetic without preservative may be used. Lidocaine 2% is common.

IO is a direct venous route into the medullary canal for fluid replacement and medication delivery. A specialized power driver is used to insert the stainless steel catheter and stylet at a 90-degree

TABLE 8.3 Pediatric Blood Volume

Age	Blood Volume (mL/kg)
Neonate	75–100
6 weeks–2 years	75–80
2 years–puberty	65–75

TABLE 8.2 Pediatric Hematologic Value Ranges

Age	Hemoglobin (g/dL)	Hematocrit (%)	Leukocytes (mm³)	Platelets (mm³)
Cord blood	13.7–20.1	45–65	9000–30,000	350
2 weeks	13–20	42–46	5000–21,000	260
3 months	9.5–14.5	34–41	6000–18,000	250
6 months–6 years	10.5–14	33–42	6000–15,000	250
7–12 years	11–16	34–40	4500–13,500	250

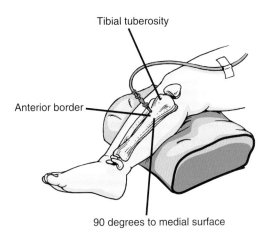

Tibial tuberosity

Anterior border

90 degrees to medial surface

• **Fig. 8.1** Intraosseous Infusion Into Tibia. Insertion site for needle placement is in anterior midline 1 to 3 cm below tibial tuberosity. Note that the needle is perpendicular to the medial surface and that tubing is secured on the thigh.

angle to the bone. After entering the medullary canal, the stylet is removed and the catheter is aspirated to ensure the correct position within the marrow space. Once it is confirmed in the correct location, a plastic hub and stabilizing sheath maintain the position of the delivery device. The plastic hub uses a needleless connector to minimize the risk for needlesticks during the connection of medication lines. A heparin lock (hep lock) device can be used for intermittent infusions. Pressurized pumps can be used, but care is taken to prevent excessive pressure over 250 to 300 mm Hg that will cause the machinery to shut down. Some physicians prefer to use manual pressure bags to regulate flow rates.

Potential complications include, but are not limited to, extravasation of infused fluids, infection caused by contamination, cellulitis, and compartment syndrome (if extravasation occurs). Embolic events are possible, but extremely rare.

A cutdown on an extremity vein, usually the saphenous vein, may be necessary for toddlers and older children. An extremity should be splinted to immobilize it. A 150- or 250-mL solution drip chamber, sometimes referred to as a burette, buretrol, Metriset, or Soluset, is used to help avoid the danger of overhydration. This chamber is available in sizes that range from 50 to 250 mL from multiple manufacturers. Adapters are set for accurate control of the desired flow rate.

Body Temperature Considerations

Temperature regulation is controlled in the anterior hypothalamus. Cooling causes vasoconstriction for the conservation of body heat. Extremes of cooling cause shivering in infants older than 3 months that generates body heat and increases metabolic needs, causing a 200% to 500% increase in oxygen consumption.

Neonates (especially preterm), infants, and children have wider average body temperature variations than do adults. Infants younger than 3 months do not have a shiver response because of immature neurologic development. They are at significant risk for hypothermia. Body temperature in the newborn tends to range from as low as 97° F to 100° F (36.1° C to 37.7° C). Temperature begins to stabilize within this range 12 to 24 hours after birth if the environment is controlled. A relatively high rate of heat loss in proportion to heat production in the infant results from an incompletely developed thermoregulatory mechanism.

The ratio of body fat to lean mass with only a thin layer of subcutaneous brown fat for insulation puts the newborn at risk for hypothermia.

Extensive extracorporeal membrane oxygenation (ECMO) also causes rapid dissipation of heat from the body. A hypothermic newborn or infant metabolizes anesthetic agents more slowly and is susceptible to postoperative respiratory depression and delayed emergence from anesthesia. The first signs of significant hypothermia in a pediatric patient younger than 1 year are a heart rate less than 100 beats per minute, metabolic acidosis, hypoglycemia, hyperkalemia, elevated blood urea nitrogen levels, and oliguria.

Oxygen consumption is at a minimum when abdominal skin temperature is 97° F (36.1° C). A room temperature 5° F (−15° C) cooler than that of abdominal skin produces a 50% increase in oxygen consumption, creating the hazard of acidosis. These factors account for the pediatric patient's susceptibility to environmental changes. The following events can result in heat loss:

- *Evaporation.* When skin becomes wet, evaporative heat loss can occur. Excessive drapes can cause sweating. As sweat evaporates, it elicits a cooling effect.
- *Radiation.* When heat transfers from the body surface to the room atmosphere, radiation heat loss can result.
- *Conduction.* Placement of the pediatric patient on a cold operating bed causes heat transfer from the patient's body to the surface of the bed.
- *Convection.* When air currents pass over skin, heat loss by convection results. Cold, wet diapers and blankets can cause heat loss by conduction.

Neonates, infants, and children are kept warm during the surgical procedure to minimize heat loss and prevent hypothermia. Body temperature tends to decrease in the OR because of cooling from air conditioning and open body cavities. Room temperature should be maintained as warm as 85° F (29.4° C). Continuous core body temperature monitoring should be performed (skin temperature sensors may be sufficient for short procedures). Other precautions should also be taken, as follows:

- A hyperthermia blanket or water mattress may be placed on the OR bed and warmed before the infant or child is positioned. Follow the manufacturer's recommendation before covering a mattress. The temperature is maintained between 95° F and 100° F (35–37.7° C) to prevent skin burns and elevation of body temperature higher than the normal range. Excessive hyperthermia can cause dehydration and convulsions in the anesthetized patient.
- A radiant heat lamp should be placed over the newborn to prevent heat loss through radiation. Warming lights with infrared bulbs may be used if a radiant warmer is not available. These lights should be approximately 27 inches (69 cm) from the infant to prevent burns; the distance should be measured. Halogen bulbs can cause serious burns because of the extreme heat. Plastic wrapping material also provides insulation around the newborn to prevent heat loss by conduction but can cause heat loss by evaporation.
- Wrapping the head (except the face) and extremities in plastic or Webril helps prevent heat loss in infants and small children. An aluminum warming suit or blanket may be used for toddlers and older children. Forced-air warming blankets also are effective in maintaining core temperature. Booties or socks can provide good results.
- Rectal, esophageal, axillary, or tympanic probes are used to measure core temperature. A probe placed into the rectum

should not be inserted more than 1 inch (2 or 3 cm) because trauma to an infant through perforation of the rectum or colon can occur. Urinary catheters with thermistor probes may be useful if urinary catheterization is indicated. Tympanic temperature measurement can be inconsistent with measurements taken elsewhere in the body and should not be the only parameter with which determination of body temperature is made.

- Drapes should permit some evaporative heat loss to maintain equalization of body temperature. An excessive number of drapes, which can retain heat and be heavy on the body, are avoided. Combinations of paper, plastic, and cloth drapes may cause excessive fluid loss through diaphoresis and absorption into the drapes.
- Solutions should be warm when applied to tissues to minimize heat loss by evaporation and conduction. The circulating nurse should pour warm solutions immediately before use. Check the manufacturer's recommendations for warming prep solutions. Some iodine-based solutions become unstable when heated. The concentration of iodine increases when the fluid portion evaporates.

The scrub person moistens sponges in warm saline solution before handing them to the surgeon. Irrigant for urologic procedures should be warmed to body temperature except where contraindicated. Room temperature solutions may be indicated when heated solutions may increase bleeding by vasodilation (i.e., brain).

- Blood and IV solutions can be warmed before transfusion by running tubing through a blood and fluid warmer. Carbon dioxide (CO_2) for insufflation during laparoscopy can be warmed this way. Airway humidification of anesthetic gases can also be warmed.
- Blankets should be warmed to place over the patient immediately after dressings are applied and drapes are removed. The patient should be kept covered whenever possible before and after the surgical procedure to prevent chilling from the air conditioning.

Indicators of Thermoregulatory Status

Hyperthermia (i.e., core temperature of the body over 104° F [40° C]) during the surgical procedure can be caused by fever, dehydration, decrease in sweating from atropine administration, excessive drapes, and drugs that disturb temperature regulation, such as general anesthetics and barbiturates. If the patient is febrile preoperatively, the surgical procedure may be delayed to allow reduction in temperature and to permit fluid administration. If an immediate surgical procedure is necessary and fever persists, anesthesia is induced and external cooling is used. IV fluids may be given at room temperature instead of warmed during administration.

Beginning signs of hypothermia include initial tachycardia and tachypnea as the body tries to compensate by circulating warmed blood throughout the body. As chilling progresses, the pediatric patient becomes bradycardic, with shallow respirations as a result of slowed metabolic processes.

A sudden rise in temperature during the surgical procedure may indicate malignant hyperthermia. Immediate cooling with ice and cool fluids is necessary. More detailed information about malignant hyperthermia is described in Chapter 31.

Cardiopulmonary Status Considerations

The heart rate fluctuates widely among infants, toddlers, and preschool children and varies during activity and at rest (Table 8.4). Infants younger than 1 year tolerate a heart rate between 200 and 250 beats per minute without hemodynamic consequence. Heart rhythm disturbance is uncommon unless a cardiac anomaly is present. Cardiopulmonary complications manifest as respiratory compromise more commonly than as cardiac dysfunction. After age 5 years, cardiopulmonary response to stress resembles that of a young adult.

Cardiac and respiratory rates and sounds are continually monitored in all age groups with precordial or esophageal stethoscopy. Blood pressure, vital signs, electrocardiogram results,

TABLE 8.4	Pediatric Vital Sign Ranges			
Age[a]	Heart Rate/Minute Awake	Heart Rate/Minute Asleep/At Rest	Respirations/Minute Asleep/At Rest	Blood Pressure Systolic (mm Hg)
Newborn				
(2–3 kg)	100–205	80–160	30–60	60–76
Infant				
1–12 months (4–10 kg)	110–180	90–160	30–53	72–104
Toddler				
18–30 months (12–14 kg)	98–140	80–120	22–37	86–106
Preschool				
3–5 years (16–18 kg)	80–120	65–100	20–28	89–112
School Age				
6–9 years (20–32 kg)	75–118	58–90	18–25	97–115
10 years (33 kg)	60–100	60–90	18–22	102–120
Adolescent				
14 years (50 kg)	60–100	50–90	12–20	110–131

[a]Weights from the National Institutes of Health (NIH) represent a combined estimate of weight for girls and boys.
Data from American Heart Association, PALS, Dallas, TX, 2016, The Association.

and other parameters as indicated also are monitored throughout the surgical procedure (see Table 8.4). A pulse oximeter can be placed on the palm of the hand or on the midfoot of a newborn or small infant. Smaller patients experience oxygen desaturation easily. A disadvantage of pulse oximetry is that it cannot detect instantaneous drops in oxygen saturation. It gives readouts of levels that have already occurred. Because of increased carboxyhemoglobin levels, it may be ineffective for patients who have had smoke inhalation or carbon monoxide poisoning. A pulse oximeter reading of 80% is clinically diagnostic of central cyanosis. Hypoxemia can cause bradycardia to decrease oxygen consumption of the myocardium.

Infants are particularly susceptible to respiratory obstruction because of their anatomic structure. They are primarily obligate nasal breathers. They have small nares, a relatively large tongue, lymphoid tissue present, and a small-diameter trachea, which causes disproportionate narrowing of the airway. The pharynx is funnel-shaped and allows secretions to pool and obstruct the airway. A cylindric thorax, poorly developed accessory respiratory muscles, and increased volume of abdominal contents limit diaphragmatic movement. The chest is more compliant and collapses easily.

Pediatric Infection Risk Considerations

Newborns and infants are susceptible to nosocomial infection. Many preterm infants who have respiratory distress and circulatory problems survive because of advances in perinatal medicine, which has increased the population of infants who are at high risk and debilitated with reduced humoral and cellular defenses to infection. Aseptic technique is essential in handling neonates and all other pediatric patients.

An elective surgical procedure should be delayed in the presence of respiratory infection because of the risk for airway obstruction. Intubation of inflamed tissues may cause laryngeal edema. Coryza, inflammation of mucous membranes of the nose, is often a sign of an infectious respiratory disease.

Frequent use of antibiotics may lead to antibiotic resistance in some microorganisms. Many types of antibiotics are used to treat infection; however, prevention via aseptic and sterile techniques is more beneficial to the patient.

Pediatric Pain Management Considerations

Infants and children are sensitive to pain with the same intensity as adults. Their pain may be intense, but infants, toddlers, and preschool children are unable to describe its location and nature with specific terms, although they have some limited pain-descriptive vocabulary around the age of 18 months.

Neonates and infants can be assessed for pain with physiologic parameters such as heart rate and oxygen saturation and with facial expressions such as brow bulge, eye squeeze, and nasolabial furrow, crying, sleep patterns, and body movements. An increase in vital signs can indicate an increase in pain.

Another method of measuring pain is the FLACC behavioral pain assessment scale (*F*ace, *L*egs, *A*ctivity, *C*ry, and *C*onsolability) developed by nurses and physicians at C.S. Mott Children's Hospital at the University of Michigan Health System in Ann Arbor. The chart measures and scores five categories of behavior in pediatric patients ages 2 months to 7 years in relationship to pain (Table 8.5).

School-age children may refer pain to a part of the body not involved in the disease process. Fig. 8.2 describes the Wong-Baker FACES pain rating scale that can be used to determine the severity of pain experienced by a pediatric patient. Insecurity and fear in an older child may be more traumatic than the pain itself. Children should be observed for signs of pain (i.e., vocalizations, facial expressions, crying, body movements, physiologic parameters). Children also differ from adults in their response to pharmacologic agents; the tolerance to analgesic drugs is altered (Table 8.6).

Most pediatric medication errors occur because children vary significantly in body weight. The number of near misses is almost seven times greater in children than in adults. Many errors are as high as 10 times the usual dose because of decimal placement mistakes in calculation. Considerations in pediatric medication should include the following points:

- Children cannot determine and communicate their own responses to drugs with reliable precision.
- Parents or guardians often do not understand drug administration instructions.
- Data are minimal about pediatric responses to medication.
- Few clinical trials are used to support drug use for children, although the drugs are commonly used.

TABLE 8.5 Pain Assessment in Pediatric Patients 2 Months to 7 Years Old: FLACC Behavioral Pain Assessment Scale

Categories[a]	SCORING		
	0	**1**	**2**
Face	No particular expression or smile	Occasional grimace or frown, withdrawn, disinterested	Frequent to constant quivering chin, clenched jaw
Legs	Normal position or relaxed	Uneasy, restless, tense	Kicking or legs drawn up
Activity	Lying quietly, normal position, moves easily	Squirming, shifting back and forth, tense	Arched, rigid, or jerking
Cry	No cry (awake or asleep)	Moans or whimpers; occasional complaint	Crying steadily, screams or sobs, frequent complaints
Consolability	Content, relaxed	Reassured by occasional touching, hugging, or being talked to; distractible	Difficult to console or comfort

[a]Each of the five categories is scored from 0 to 2, resulting in a total score between 0 and 10.
The FLACC scale was developed by Sandra Merkel, MS, RN; Terri Voepel-Lewis, MS, RN; and Shobha Malviya, MD, at C.S. Mott Children's Hospital, University of Michigan Health System, Ann Arbor, MI. Copyright © 2002, The Regents of the University of Michigan.

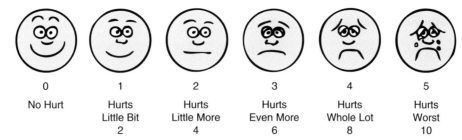

• **Fig. 8.2** Wong-Baker FACES Pain Rating Scale. Explain to the child that each face is for a person who feels happy because they have no pain (hurt) or sad because there is some or a lot of pain. Face 0 is very happy because they do not hurt at all. Face 1 hurts just a little bit. Face 2 hurts a little more. Face 3 hurts even more. Face 4 hurts a whole lot, but Face 5 hurts as much as you can imagine, although you do not have to be crying to feel this bad. Ask the child to choose the face that best describes their own pain. Rating scale is recommended for persons aged 3 years and older. (From Hockenberry MJ, Wilson D: *Wong's essentials of pediatric nursing,* ed 10, St. Louis, 2019, Elsevier. Used with permission.)

TABLE 8.6   Pediatric Sedation and Pain Management

Drug and Dosage	Duration	Considerations in Administration
Acetaminophen		
10–15 mg/kg PO	3–8 hours	Dose dependent
10–20 mg/kg rectally	4–6 hours	Analgesia for minor procedures; antipyretic; absorption is delayed in infants, so dose should not be repeated for 6 hours; no effect on coagulopathy; no respiratory depression; may be combined with narcotic for major procedures
Codeine		
0.5–1 mg/kg PO	3–6 hours	Moderate pain relief; not given IV; can be given with acetaminophen
Diazepam		
0.05–0.03 mg/kg IM or IV	2–4 hours	Sedation and seizure control; can cause respiratory depression, jaundice, and vein irritation at IV site
0.2–0.3 mg/kg PO	4–12 hours	Administer 45–60 minutes before procedure
Not used for continuous infusion: 0.2–0.5 mg/kg rectally		
Fentanyl		
1–2 mcg/kg IM or IV	30–60 minutes	Excellent pain and anxiety relief; metabolized slowly in smaller children and infants; reversible with naloxone; short half-life; can cause respiratory depression, nausea, and vomiting; PO lozenge provides sedation but causes high incidence of preoperative nausea and vomiting
Continuous infusion: 0.5–2 mcg/kg/h		
PO lozenge is available 200 mcg, 400 mcg, 600 mcg, 800 mcg, 1200 mcg, 1600 mg PO buccal/sublingual tablet is available 100 mcg, 200 mcg, 400 mcg, 600 mcg, 800 mcg		Consume over 15 minutes. Check appropriate dose.
Hydromorphone		
0.5–4 mg per dose every 4 hours IM, IV, or PO	4–5 hours	Not used for infants and young children; used for adolescents; side effects include CNS and respiratory depression, hypotension, bradycardia, increased intracranial pressure, and peripheral vascular dilation
Ibuprofen		
4–10 mg/kg PO, IV, or rectally[a]	3–4 hours	Can cause gastrointestinal bleeding; may affect platelet aggregation
Ketamine		
0.5–1.5 mg/kg IV IM 2–5 mg/kg PO 5–10 mg/kg	5–60 minutes 15–90 minutes 30–120 minutes	Can cause respiratory depression, hallucinations, emergence delirium, and behavioral changes

Continued

TABLE 8.6 Pediatric Sedation and Pain Management—cont'd

Drug and Dosage	Duration	Considerations in Administration
Meperidine		
1—1.5 mg/kg IM, IV, PO, or SQ	3—4 hours	Excellent pain relief; reversible with naloxone; can cause respiratory depression, suppression of intestinal motility, and hypotension; may cause nausea and vomiting; not used in increased intracranial pressure; poor sedation; not a good premedication drug. Treats shivering
Continuous IV infusion: titrate up to 0.5—0.7 mg/kg/h		
Midazolam		
0.05—0.1 mg/kg IV	30—60 minutes	Short half-life; may cause respiratory depression; excellent amnesic; sedation of choice for most pediatric patients
0.1—0.15 mg/kg IM	2—6 hours	
0.25—0.75 mg/kg PO		
Intranasal 0.2—0.3 mg/kg		
Continuous infusion: 0.1 mg/kg/h		
Morphine		
0.08—0.1 mg/kg IM, IV, or SQ; not well absorbed PO	4—5 hours	Excellent pain relief; reversible with naloxone; can cause respiratory depression, suppression of intestinal motility, and hypotension; may cause nausea and vomiting; not a good premedication drug
Continuous infusion: 0.25—2 mg/kg/h		
Average dose: 0.06 mg/kg/h		
Sufentanil		
1—2 mcg/kg IV; nasal spray, sublingual	1—2 hours	Is 10 times more potent than fentanyl; very short half-life
Propofol		
125 mcg—2 mg/kg	Maintenance requires constant infusion	Bronchodilator, causes sedation and no analgesia, short acting; contains egg lecithin

[a]Additional values can be found in *Davis's drug guide for nurses*, ed 16, Philadelphia, 2019, F.A. Davis Company.
CNS, Central nervous system; *IM*, intramuscularly; *IV*, intravenously; *PO*, by mouth; *SQ*, subcutaneously.

- Pediatric dosage forms and packaging are not available in all drugs used for children.
- Children have unpredictable disease states and organ responses to drugs.
- Reactions in children may not reflect the responses exhibited by adults.

Prevention of pediatric medication errors should include, but is not limited to, the following activities:

- Be sure the pediatric patient's weight is recorded in grams or kilograms (as appropriate for age and size) on the chart because weight-based dosages require accurate measurement for calculation.
- Do not abbreviate dosages or volumes.
- Clarify any questionable drug, dose, or route.
- Check for allergies. Observe the pediatric patient for new signs of allergy if a new medication is added to the regimen.
- When the drug is measured in decimals, be sure to use a zero at the left of the decimal to signify the fraction (e.g., 0.2 mg rather than .2 mg). Do not use a zero at the right of the decimal (e.g., 5 mg rather than 5.0 mg). Errors happen when someone does not see the decimal.
- Use generic names of drugs as a routine.
- Be sure to have clear signatures and contact numbers for the person prescribing the drug.

- Avoid verbal orders if possible.
- Know the medication and its actions before giving the drug.
- Know the medication delivery devices and be properly trained before using them (e.g., infusion pumps).

Preoperative Psychologic Preparation of Pediatric Patients

The pediatric surgical patient should be considered as a whole person with individual physical and psychosocial needs assessed in relation to the natural stages of development. Equally important are the adjustment and attitude of the parents or guardians toward the child, the illness, and the surgical experience. Parental or guardian anxiety about the impending surgical procedure may be transferred to the child. Emotional support and education of the patient and the parents or guardians are important aspects of preoperative preparation to help them cope.

When an event is threatening, the patient changes cognitive and behavioral responses to deal with the specific demands of the situation. Most adults face stress with more control when fear of the unknown is eliminated. Therefore parents need to be informed of events that will occur and to be taught how to care for their child preoperatively and postoperatively. If children are informed of sensations to be experienced, cognitive control of the event may occur. Children do not differ from adults in this respect. However, understanding varies with age.

The following are general considerations:

1. Correction of a congenital anomaly as soon after birth as possible may be better psychologically for both the infant and the parents. The infant younger than 1 year does not remember the experience. Parents or guardians gain confidence in learning to cope with a residual deformity as the infant learns to compensate for it.

2. Children from 2 to 5 years of age have great sensitivity and a tenuous sense of reality. They live in a world of magic, monsters, and retribution, yet they are aggressive. School-age children have an enhanced sense of reality and value honesty and fairness. Their natural interest and curiosity aid communication. These children need reassurances and explanations in vocabulary compatible with their developmental level. Fear of body mutilation or punishment may be of paramount importance to a preschool or young school-age child. Words should be chosen wisely. Negative connotations should be avoided, and the positive aspects should be stressed. The nurse should talk on the child's level about their interests and concerns.

3. Anxiety in the school-age child may be stimulated by remembrance of a previous experience. Many children undergo two or more staged surgical procedures before the deformity of a congenital anomaly or traumatic injury is cosmetically reconstructed or functionally restored. Familiarity with the nursing staff reassures the child. Ideally the same circulating nurse who was present for the first surgical procedure should visit preoperatively and be with the child during subsequent surgical procedures.

4. Fear of the unknown about general anesthesia may become exaggerated into extreme anxiety with fantasies of death. The school-age child and adolescent need facts and reassurances. General anesthesia should not be referred to as "putting you to sleep." The child may equate this phrase with the euthanasia of a former pet that never returned home. Instead the nurse should say, "You will sleep for a little while" or "You will take a nap." Tell the child about the "nice nurses" who will be in the "wake-up room after your nap." Parents or guardians should be encouraged to also display confidence and cheerfulness to avoid transmitting anxiety.

5. Parents or guardians should be honest with their child but maintain a confident manner. The perioperative nurse should do the same. However, a school-age child should not be given information not asked for; questions should be answered, and misunderstandings should be corrected. The nurse should be especially alert to silent, stoic, noncommunicative children, many of whom have difficult induction and emergence from anesthesia. Children who have lost a sibling or friend to death often fear hospitalization.

6. Some facilities hold tours or get-togethers for children and parents or guardians before or after admission to explain routines and procedures before the surgical experience. At other facilities personnel take children to the OR with their teddy bears so that they can see the different attire, lights, tables, anesthesia machine, and other equipment that might interest them. A child-size anesthesia mask becomes a toy that they are allowed to handle and place on the teddy bear. A clear plastic mask is less psychologically traumatic to a child than is an opaque black rubber mask. An effective method of explaining procedures to children is to use the child's teddy bear and dress it as the child will look postoperatively. For example, a bandage is put on the bear if the child will have one postoperatively.

7. Separation from parents or a trusted guardian is traumatic for infants older than 6 months, toddlers, and preschool children. Infants require cuddling and bonding. Toddlers are only just approaching the autonomy stage, and hospitalization forces them into passive behavior; thus their separation anxiety is greatest. Young children may fear strangers. The parent's or guardian's presence is necessary for the toddler, and they should be encouraged to stay with the hospitalized child as much as possible.

8. The child should be permitted to bring a toy or other security object to the OR suite if a parent or guardian cannot be present. Many anesthesia providers encourage parents or guardians to accompany an infant or child to the OR and to stay through induction if they wish. The presence of a familiar face can significantly reduce anxiety and ease induction. Some facilities allow parents or guardians to accompany the child to the holding area but restrict entrance into the OR. Highly anxious parents or guardians who have difficulty coping with stress may cause an increase in the child's anxiety level.

9. Ambulatory surgery, if feasible, is an advantage because the child enters the facility 1 to 2 hours before the surgical procedure and returns home after recovery from anesthesia. This minimizes the trauma of separation.

10. A preoperative visit by a perioperative nurse should be planned to get to know the child, confirm appropriate consents, and provide emotional support to the family. Parents or guardians should be taught to provide postoperative care, especially before and after an ambulatory procedure. Verbal instructions may be supplemented with a video, coloring book, or storybook to reinforce understanding for both the child and their caregivers.

11. The perioperative nurse should bring the patient to the OR in a crib or on an appropriate-size cart. Carrying a child into the OR presents the risk for dropping or bumping the child. Each situation should be determined by the patient's need. Some facilities use toy wagons for child transport.

Pediatric Anesthesia

Pediatric anesthesia has become increasingly specialized as the many variables in the management of infants and children have become better understood. The anesthesia provider recognizes and respects the small margin for error and the uniqueness of the physiology and responses to drugs of pediatric patients. For example, the high metabolic rate of children causes rapid oxygen consumption. Changes occur rapidly in infants and children.

Preoperative Assessment by the Anesthesia Provider

A preoperative visit by the anesthesia provider to establish rapport and assess the patient is also a vital part of preparation of the pediatric patient. Preferably, this visit is made with the parents or guardians present so that the child considers the anesthesia provider a trustworthy and caring friend. During physical assessment, special attention is given to the heart, lungs, and upper airways. Loose teeth are noted. Possible difficulties are anticipated.

Preoperative care includes correction of dehydration, reduction of excessive fever, compensation for acidosis, and restoration of depleted blood volume. An American Society of Anesthesiologists (ASA) physical status classification is assigned to the pediatric patient. The patient's age, developmental stage, psychologic characteristics, and history are considered to determine the patient's probable response to the anesthesia experience.

Premedication

Psychologic preparation of the child older than 7 years can decrease the need for an anxiolytic (i.e., a sedative or minor tranquilizer to reduce anxiety). Crying greatly increases mucus in the respiratory tract. At the discretion of the anesthesia provider, premedication may be ordered to produce serenity. Some anesthesia providers prefer children to be well medicated; others favor minimal or no sedation. Infants younger than 1 year usually do not require premedication, but pacifiers with medication ports are commercially available for delivery of oral drugs.

Premedication, which is tailored to the individual, varies considerably by age, weight, and health status. Preanesthetic sedation should allow the patient to be taken to the OR lightly asleep or drowsy and should facilitate induction of anesthesia without waking the child. It should also provide some analgesia during the recovery period.

Timing of administration is extremely important. To be effective, slow-absorbing drugs may need to be given 30 to 60 minutes before the surgical procedure. The circulating nurse should check with the anesthesia provider and the surgeon before sending for the patient. If ample time is not available for the appropriate effect of premedication, the anesthesia provider may prefer to omit the medication to avoid precipitation of psychologic trauma. Fast-acting drugs are preferred and may be useful for rapid sedation preoperatively. Narcotics, such as morphine and meperidine (Demerol), are rarely indicated for routine premedication in healthy pediatric patients.

No ideal premedication drug exists, but the following list contains the drugs that are commonly used (see also the comparison of sedatives in Table 8.6):
- Sufentanil (Sufenta) given nasally (i.e., sprayed onto the nasal mucosa) or sublingually facilitates separation from parents by causing relaxation and drowsiness. The child becomes calm and cooperative.
- Fentanyl (Sublimaze) can be incorporated into a lozenge or a flavored hard candy mounted on a stick (i.e., an anesthetic lollipop). When the child licks the candy, the drug is absorbed into the bloodstream through the oral mucosa and produces sedation for 30 to 60 minutes. The correct dose should be double-checked because this form is available in numerous strengths.
- Diazepam (Valium), 0.05 to 0.03 mg/kg administered intramuscularly (IM) or 0.2 to 0.3 mg/kg given orally (PO), causes relaxation for 3 to 4 hours. It can be administered rectally 0.2 to 0.5 mg/kg. This drug has few cardiovascular side effects.
- Midazolam (Versed) administered as a nasal spray (0.2−0.3 mg/kg) is easy and convenient. Oral preparations also work well. The drug can be administered IM (0.01−0.15 mg/kg) 15 minutes before induction and greatly reduces anxiety. This drug is also good for IV conscious

sedation (IVCS) during endoscopy. Doses range between 0.25 and 0.6 mg/kg IV. Cardiovascular stability is good, and ventilation is not depressed.
- Atropine, 0.01 to 0.02 mg/kg, may be administered IM, IV, or subcutaneously (SQ) to inhibit secretions, especially in a child with a severe airway problem, or to counteract bradycardia. Cardiac effects last about 1 hour. Dosage is decreased to 0.004 mg/kg for infants less than 5 kg. It is not given in the presence of fever or glaucoma.
- Glycopyrrolate (Robinul), 0.004 to 0.01 mg/kg administered IM, lowers gastric acidity. It may be given as an alternative to atropine sulfate to reduce secretions. It is contraindicated in the presence of paralytic ileus, urinary tract obstruction, and glaucoma.
- Ketamine can be administered by nasal spray, PO, IM, IV, or rectally. This drug is good for very anxious or uncooperative individuals.

Anesthesia Equipment

Simple lightweight anesthesia equipment is used. Disposable equipment is popular. Facemasks designed for minimal dead space are available to closely fit a child's relatively flat face. Non-rebreathing circuits provide less resistance and valves for fresh flow of gas at higher flow rates relative to a child's metabolism and ventilation. For avoidance of hypothermia, anesthetic gases are warmed and humidified.

Induction

Induction is facilitated with a quiet atmosphere, a soft voice, and a reassuring touch. A parent or guardian may be present if the policies of the facility permit. Children should be told what to expect without precipitating fear. The induction experience can be described as getting on a merry-go-round. Noises will seem louder. To avoid confusion it is best for the child to listen to one person speak. The circulating nurse should remain at the patient's side, maintain a gentle touch, and be alert to the patient's needs and condition.

The considerations for anesthesia induction include the following:
1. Restraints should be loose. Minimal pressure should be applied. If the patient is a newborn, infant, or toddler, restraint straps are omitted while the circulating nurse holds the patient during induction. A toddler or preschool-age child is less frightened when holding on to someone's hands. Restraints can be applied after the patient is asleep.
2. Special scented mask spray, lip balm, or food extract of the child's choosing (e.g., mint, banana, strawberry) can be placed in the facemask. This makes the anesthetic gas more acceptable and gives the patient a sense of control. The scent of anesthetic gas may be compared with the scent of special jet fuel used for airplanes or spaceships.
3. If the child is awake, crying, or struggling, apprehension during induction can be avoided with distraction and rapport. Establishing rapport with young children is not easy. If a parent or guardian is present, the child may be more cooperative. The child's cooperation may be solicited with counting out loud, singing the alphabet song, blowing up a balloon, taking a space trip, or discussing a favorite plaything or television character. The facemask can be held slightly over the face, permitting anesthetic gas to flow by gravity, and lowered

gently as the child becomes drowsy. Some anesthesia providers permit the child to hold the mask. Care is taken to avoid having the parent's or guardian's face too close to the mask when anesthesia gases are flowing. The parent or guardian could be affected and sense altered consciousness.

A child who has been crying may have somewhat edematous tissue in the nose and larynx. Secretions are frequently increased. Swollen tissues in an obligate nose-breather can complicate breathing. Note that the parent or guardian, who may be present, is viewing the child's activities range from animated to lethargic (Fig. 8.3). This gives the appearance of helplessness or death. The parent or guardian may feel emotional and shed tears or feel faint. Reassurance should be given, and they should be escorted to the waiting area before intubation takes place.

4. Induction may be accompanied by regurgitation and aspiration of gastric contents in infants with pyloric stenosis, tracheoesophageal fistula, intestinal obstruction, or food in the stomach. The hazard is minimized with aspiration of gastric contents with a sterile catheter before induction and with the tube left in place for drainage during the surgical procedure. Rapid-sequence induction also may be used. This consists of a sedative or hypnotic agent, muscle relaxant, and intubation with cricoid pressure (Sellick maneuver) applied to close the esophagus and avoid silent regurgitation of food from the stomach. All trauma patients should be considered to have a full stomach.

Types of Induction

Inhalation

If asleep from premedication on arrival in the OR, the child can be anesthetized quickly. If the child is awake, induction may be initiated with inhalant anesthetic. Pregnant caregivers should avoid any anesthetic gases that might escape during mask administration before intubation.

Nitrous oxide may increase peripheral vascular resistance if it is used to maintain general anesthesia for cardiovascular procedures. It may also increase the risk for air embolus because it combines with smaller air bubbles that may enter the system during repair of congenital heart defects. Potent inhalants are absorbed more rapidly in the presence of nitrous oxide and may cause myocardial depression and decrease cardiac output in very young children. Atropine may minimize this effect.

Rectal Induction

Rectal induction is not frequently used. It can be given with foams, creams, gels, suppository, or enema. Given by enema, methohexital (Brevital), 10 to 25 mg/kg of 1% solution, produces

• **Fig. 8.3** Parent sitting with child for administration of general anesthesia.

sleep in 6 to 8 minutes and lasts 45 to 60 minutes. This is a painless method used in the presence of parents for preschoolers or toddlers. The parent may hold the child. It is a good method for short diagnostic procedures. The anesthesia provider remains with the patient.

Once the child is asleep the anesthesia state may be maintained with an inhalant. Gentle assisted ventilation may be needed. This method is tolerated best in children younger than 3 years.

Intravenous Infusion
IV infusion is often preferred for patients older than 9 or 10 years. Induction with a small dose of barbiturate or ketamine is rapid. Studies have shown that IV induction causes less psychologic trauma than do inhalant methods. A mixture of lidocaine and prilocaine in a transdermal cream base is commercially available for application to the site to decrease pain associated with venipuncture.

Care is taken if the child has a central line because infection or thrombosis may result. If the central line is used for anesthetic administration, all residual drug is flushed from the port so that none remains in the tubing after the procedure.

Ketamine, 0.5 to 2 mg/kg IV, is useful in a combative, burned, or hypovolemic patient. If given intranasally, PO, or IM to a healthier child who weighs less than 10 kg, the usual dose is 2 to 10 mg/kg. The pharmacologic predictability of ketamine is a good reason for its use in pediatric sedation. Its onset takes place 1 to 2 minutes after IV administration and 5 minutes if given IM. Either way, the duration of the dose is approximately 45 minutes. Low doses provide sedation and analgesia. Higher doses cause general anesthesia. Ketamine provides a moderate level of general anesthesia and maintains blood pressure, breathing, and airway reflexes. Ketamine offers a safer choice of anesthesia if the patient has a known or potential risk for malignant hyperthermia.

Epidural Block
A caudal epidural block may be used in combination with a general anesthetic for orthopedic, abdominal, and thoracic procedures.

Intubation and Airway Placement
Airway obstruction in infants and children usually occurs early during anesthesia administration, especially if the child has been crying. When anesthesia deepens, oral airway insertion is essential after assisted ventilation with oxygen. Assisted or controlled ventilation reduces the labor of breathing and therefore reduces metabolism. Many anesthesia providers prefer the use of a laryngeal mask airway.

Intubation
Placement of an endotracheal tube in the trachea of a newborn or infant differs from placement in a child or adolescent. Regardless of age, the patient's airway must remain patent. Sterile equipment and gentle manipulation to avoid soft tissue injury are essential for intubation and suctioning. Other considerations include the following:
- Endotracheal intubation is used by some anesthesia providers for all procedures in infants younger than 1 year. It is necessary for intraabdominal, intrathoracic, and neurosurgical procedures; for those in the head or neck areas; and for emergency procedures when contents of the stomach are uncertain. Intubation while the patient is awake may be used in neonates. A

TABLE 8.7 Recommended Endotracheal Tube Sizes

Age	Diameter (mm)
Preterm	2.5–3
Newborn	3
Newborn–6 months	3.5
6–12 months	3.5–4
12 months–2 years	4–4.5
3–4 years	4.5–5
5–6 years	5–5.5
7–8 years	5.5–6
9–10 years	6–6.5
11–12 years	6.5–7
13 years and older	7–7.5

certain amount of jaw tightness (masseter muscle rigidity, trismus) is common in some pediatric patients after the administration of succinylcholine, but this should be observed closely because it also may be a premonitory sign of malignant hyperthermia.
- The size of the endotracheal tube is selected according to the width and length of the trachea (Table 8.7). Endotracheal tubes for children younger than 8 years are not cuffed. The uncuffed tube allows for a slight space around the exterior circumference and a wider internal diameter than a cuffed tube. Soft tissue at the narrowest level of the cricoid cartilage, located just below the vocal cords, forms a loose seal around the tube. The pediatric larynx sits more cephalad (higher) in the throat (C3 in a preterm infant and C4 in the average child compared with C5-6 in an adult).
- The nasotracheal tube may inadvertently dislodge adenoid tissue and carry it into the trachea.
- The head of a newborn or infant is elevated slightly and not hyperextended during placement of the endotracheal tube. A toddler also has a larger occiput and therefore needs little posterior extension of the head. A child with Down syndrome is predisposed to instability of the odontoid articulation at the first cervical vertebra (C1) and is at risk for dislocation if the head is placed in extreme hyperextension.
- A straight blade generally is used on the laryngoscope because the epiglottis must be raised to visualize the glottis during intubation (Fig. 8.4). An infant's epiglottis is long and stiff and projects posteriorly at an angle of 45 degrees above the glottis. The epiglottis of a toddler and a preschool child is short and easily traumatized.
- Intubation and suctioning are preceded and followed by oxygen administration. If the process of introducing the endotracheal tube takes longer than 30 seconds, the patient should be ventilated with 100% oxygen before additional attempts at intubation ensue.
- The length and diameter of the suction catheter should be considered when suctioning oropharyngeal secretions. An oversized catheter may perforate the oropharynx, trachea, bronchus, or esophagus.
- The newborn's head is maintained in a neutral position, midway between full extension and full flexion, while an endotracheal

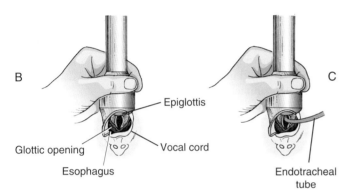

• **Fig. 8.4** Intubation of Infant, Toddler, or Preschool Child. **A,** Straight blade on laryngoscope is advanced to vallecula, space between base of tongue and epiglottis. **B,** Gentle elevation of tip of blade lifts epiglottis to visualize glottic opening between vocal cords. **C,** Endotracheal tube is advanced below the blade and into the trachea.

TABLE 8.8	Local Anesthesia for Pediatric Patients	
Agent		**Maximum Pediatric Dose**
Lidocaine		
Without epinephrine		5 mg/kg
With epinephrine (epinephrine should not exceed 10 mcg/kg)		7 mg/kg
Bupivacaine		3 mg/kg
Tetracaine		3 mg/kg
Ropivacaine		3 mg/kg
Chloroprocaine		10–12 mg/kg
Procaine		12 mg/kg

Data from Davis P, Cladis F: *Smith's anesthesia for infants and children,* ed 10, St. Louis, 2022, Elsevier.

tube is in place. The tip of the tube should be positioned in the mid-trachea. The average distance between the vocal cords and the carina, where the trachea separates into two branches, is only about 2 inches (4–5 cm) in a term neonate and much less in a preterm neonate. If the head shifts, the tube can shift, leading to inadequate oxygenation.

Anesthetic Agents and Maintenance

The following characteristics of anesthetic agents and maintenance of anesthesia are considered:

1. Topical agents are not often used because of the hazard of overdose. Local anesthetic cream (eutectic mixture of local anesthetics [EMLA]) may be used to start an IV access point with minimal risk for toxicity.
2. Inhalation anesthesia, especially with sevoflurane, is popular. Nitrous oxide–oxygen is frequently used in combination with IV agents. Halothane, a volatile agent, and succinylcholine are contraindicated with a family history of malignant hyperthermia because they trigger the condition. Nitrous oxide is used with caution in patients with congenital cardiac defects, particularly cyanotic conditions. Isoflurane (Forane) is irritating and necessitates a slow and more difficult induction to prevent laryngospasm, but it offers the advantage of circulatory support. It is not useful in short procedures. Sevoflurane is less irritating to the airway and is comparable with halothane for induction. Emergence is smooth and rapid. Pain sensation may be immediate after arousal. Analgesia should be administered.

Alveolar concentrations of inhaled anesthetics rise much more rapidly in pediatric patients than in adults because of relatively greater blood flow and smaller functional residual capacity. Children therefore have higher anesthetic requirements than do adults. Increased anesthetic requirement and more rapid induction can cause hypotension and reduced cardiac output in infants and children.

3. Ketamine provides sedation for preschool children during invasive diagnostic procedures. It is a short-acting general anesthetic for short procedures such as burn debridement, tonsillectomy, or circumcision. Because it does not alter pharyngolaryngeal reflexes or skeletal tone, intubation is unnecessary. Cardiovascular and respiratory stimulation is minimal; ketamine may be useful for patients with asthma and other poor-risk patients. It is contraindicated in the patient who has increased intracranial pressure. It is not advised for use with teenagers. Premedication with diazepam counteracts possible emergence delirium.
4. Local anesthesia is commonly used as a supplement to light general anesthesia. Long-acting agents, such as bupivacaine (Marcaine), prolong postoperative analgesia, thus reducing or eliminating the need for narcotics (Table 8.8). Epinephrine added to bupivacaine enhances its duration to a greater extent in children than in adults. Doses of epinephrine up to 10 mg/kg are considered safe.
5. Epidural anesthesia can be administered for sensory blockade intraoperatively. The epidural catheter may be left in place for prolonged postoperative analgesia. A continuous infusion of narcotics provides uninterrupted pain management, as administered to adults to attenuate postoperative stress response.
6. Narcotics are used in situations comparable with adult indications. Nitrous oxide–narcotic relaxant provides stable anesthesia for the very ill patient. Fentanyl has minimal cardiovascular effect.
7. The critically ill neonate does not tolerate anesthesia well. Adequate ventilation and oxygenation are vital, but care is taken to avoid oxygen toxicity with resultant retrolental

fibroplasia; neovascularization of the retina can produce blindness. Neonates and preterm infants less than 34 weeks' gestational age and 1500 g or less body weight are at risk. Adequate blood-gas tension is ensured only with intraoperative invasive measurement.

8. Neuromuscular blockers are used judiciously. Infants younger than 1 year exhibit a lesser degree of blockade from succinylcholine than do older children. Bradycardia and an increase in intraocular tension are more conspicuous in infants. Response decreases with age. The dosage varies. A peripheral nerve stimulator should be used to assess blockade to avoid overdosage. Blockers seldom are needed in infants because of their poorly developed abdominal musculature.

9. Consideration is given for postoperative analgesia. When an inhalation agent is reduced near the end of the surgical procedure, a narcotic may be given. Regional or local infiltration also provides relief of pain (e.g., after circumcision or cleft lip repair).

Emergence and Extubation

Airway problems are the most common concern on emergence from anesthesia and immediately postoperatively. At the conclusion of the surgical procedure, the oropharynx is suctioned. Some anesthesia providers also suction the stomach. All monitors are left in place until the patient is fully awake and extubated.

Reversal with a narcotic antagonist such as naloxone (Narcan) may be used to reverse narcosis, but the drug also has the effect of reversing analgesia. Pain sensation may result in restlessness. The usual dose is 0.01 to 0.1 mg/kg for infants and older children.

Extubation of an infant or child is preceded and followed by oxygen administration and performed either with the patient under deep anesthesia or on return of spontaneous respiration. This is done because laryngospasm is possible between these periods. Heart and breath sounds are monitored after extubation. If spasm occurs, oxygen is given with positive pressure. Airway obstruction, aspiration, and hypothermia are hazards of the recovery period.

Children, particularly in the 2 to 5-year age group, may develop hoarseness and a croupy cough after removal of an endotracheal tube. Racemic epinephrine (Vaponefrin) provides relief; 0.5 mL of 2.25% diluted in 3 mL of sterile water can be delivered through a facemask and nebulizer. Constant observation after extubation is necessary.

The patient should not be taken from the OR with a body temperature less than 95° F (35° C). If this temperature is below this crucial level, the risk for acidosis, hypoglycemia, bradycardia, hypotension, and apnea increases. This metabolic depression and delayed return of activity set the stage for possible sudden cardiac arrest.

Dehydration and low humidity increase the viscosity of secretions. Pediatric patients need close observation for development of laryngeal edema, which is noted by croupy cough, sobbing inspiration, intercostal retraction, tachypnea, or tachycardia. Laryngeal edema greatly reduces the small diameter of the airway of an infant or toddler. Controlled humidity and oxygen are vital.

Intraoperative Pediatric Patient Care Considerations

Basic principles of patient care and OR techniques used for adults apply to pediatric surgery; however, some additional considerations are necessary in the plan of care. The room should be warmed to 78° F (25.5° C) to 85° F (29.4° C) based on age before the pediatric patient is taken to the OR. Heat loss is a serious issue. A warmed blanket should be positioned on the OR bed as an undercover to prevent conduction of the child's body heat into the cooler mattress. A second warmed blanket should be placed over or around the child to prevent heat radiation into the room air. An appropriate-sized safety belt should be placed over the blanket so it is visible at all times.

To differentiate this specialty from care of adult patients, a few points specific to pediatric surgery are mentioned as follows:

1. Hair is not removed with a depilatory or shaved, except for cranial procedures and as ordered by the surgeon. All hair removed should be saved and given to the parents or guardians. Some parents or guardians feel their child's hair is a keepsake.

2. Diagnostic studies may be done in the OR with the patient under local anesthesia before induction of general anesthesia for an open surgical procedure. An infant may be swaddled on a padded (papoose) board to restrain them from moving while radiographs are taken and to permit easy change of position. A pacifier helps comfort and keep the infant quiet. Pacifiers with built-in medication chambers to deliver sedation are commercially available.

3. The patient is protected from injury. An infant or child should never be left alone anywhere in the perioperative environment. Preparation for induction should be made before the child's arrival.
    a. Guard against a fall from a crib or stretcher. Side rails should remain up at all times. An over-bed cage or mesh crib cover on a crib helps confine a toddler without restraint. Children are restrained at all times while on a stretcher or in a specially designed pediatric cart.
    b. Do not place a crib where the patient can reach an electrical outlet or near any article that can be picked up and cause injury.
    c. After the infant is asleep, pad wrists and ankles with several layers of sheet wadding (Webril). Restrain with Kerlix or Kling roller gauze, and secure straps. Sheet wadding prevents possible abrasion of delicate skin by the restraint straps. Care is taken not to restrict circulation.
    d. Small objects are not left within reach of an infant or child.

4. Catheters as small as 6 Fr are available for use as needed in newborns and infants. A plain-tip or whistle-tip catheter is used for a stomach tube. An indwelling Foley catheter with a 3-mL balloon may be used for urinary drainage. Small calibrated drainage containers are connected to permit accurate determination of output.

5. Positioning principles are essentially the same as those described for adults. Fig. 8.5 depicts ideas for positioning small infants. The head of the table or foot section can be lowered to shorten the distance between the team and the patient's body.
    a. Correspondingly smaller pillows, gel pads, and beanbags are used to stabilize anesthetized infants and children. The size of the child or adolescent determines the appropriate supports to maintain the desired position.
    b. A small gel roll or positioning device at each side of the body takes the weight of drapes off the small body of an infant or keeps the patient in a lateral position.

• **Fig. 8.5** Positioning of infant. (From Fortunato N, McCullough SM: *Perioperative nursing series: plastic and reconstructive surgery,* St. Louis, 1998, Mosby.)

• **Fig. 8.6** Upper extremity restraint to splint elbow and hand of infant or toddler. Hand is pronated on armboard.

6. Pediatric-sized drapes are preferred. A disposable drape sheet without a fenestration is sometimes used. The surgeon can cut an opening of the desired size to expose the site of intended incision. Keep in mind that the cut edges of nonwoven drape sheets may shed cellulose fibers into the surgical site that can cause inflammation and stimulate adhesion formation. The use of an adhesive plastic incise sheet over the cut edges before the tissue incision may help minimize fiber shed.

Small towels and nonpiercing towel clips are used with a laparotomy sheet if self-adhering and disposable drapes are not available. A standard opening 3 × 5 inches (7.6 × 12.7 cm) in a pediatric laparotomy sheet is usually too large for a newborn or infant. Part of the fenestration may be covered with a towel. Consider the use of an eye fenestrated drape for tiny incisions.

7. Blood loss on sponges is measured by weighing them while they are still wet. Blood loss on the drapes is estimated, and blood loss through suction is measured. The surgeon and anesthesia provider determine whether blood replacement is necessary, volume for volume, as it is lost. The measurements are calculated in grams. The calculation is 1 g equals 1 mL of blood. Care is taken not to include the weight of the sponge container in the total gram weight. Discussion about weighing sponges is found in Chapter 31.

8. Adhesive tape is abrasive to tender skin and should be avoided when possible. A chemical wound cover such as liquid adhesives or collodion is adequate over a small incision with a subcuticular closure and is especially desirable under diapers unless dressings are needed to absorb drainage. Care is taken that clothing or the blanket does not touch this substance until it is dry. Skin-closure strips may be used instead of a chemical wound cover.

9. Dressings on the face or neck should be protected from vomitus and food particles and from an infant's or a toddler's hands. Elbows should be splinted when the patient potentially may disturb the incision, dressings, or a tube (Fig. 8.6). This is particularly important after eye surgery or cleft lip or palate surgery or when a tracheostomy tube is inserted.

10. A stockinette pulled over dressings on an extremity protects them from becoming soiled and helps keep them in place. This can be changed easily as needed, leaving the dressings in place.

Instrumentation

Gentleness and precision in handling small structures and fragile tissues are essential. Basic or standard instrument sets, sutures, needles, and other items used for surgical procedures on adults are duplicated in miniature for infants and children in each surgical specialty.

The perioperative nurse and surgical technologist should be informed about the patient and then use good judgment in preparing supplies for pediatric surgery. The following principles apply:

- Size and weight are more critical factors than age in the selection of instruments, sutures, needles, and equipment.
- Small instruments are used on the delicate tissues of a newborn, an infant, or a small child.
- Hemostats should have fine points. A mosquito hemostat clamps a superficial vessel but not a major artery.
- Noncrushing vascular clamps permit occlusion of major blood vessels. They also can be placed across the intestine of a newborn or infant rather than a large heavy intestinal clamp.
- Lightweight instruments do not inhibit respiration. Instruments not in use on tissues are never laid on the patient, especially not on the chest. An instrument's weight could restrict respiration or circulation or cause bruises. Return instruments to the Mayo stand or instrument table immediately after use.
- Umbilical tape or vessel loops are used frequently to retract blood vessels and small structures, thereby giving the surgeon greater visibility in a small surgical site and eliminating the weight of retractors.

- Needle holders have fine-pointed jaws to hold small, delicate needles.
- Surgical procedures on an adolescent necessitate adult-size instruments.
- The scrub person closely watches the tissue being dissected and selects the instruments to hand to the surgeon accordingly.

Common Surgical Procedures

General Surgery
Minimally Invasive Surgery

Gastroscopy, colonoscopy, and laparoscopy are performed for diagnosis of complaints of abdominal pain or symptoms of intestinal obstruction or inflammation. Hybrid ORs with advanced technology with three-dimensional imaging, high-definition screens, navigational systems, and single-port systems are being used in pediatric surgery.

The indications for pediatric endoscopic procedures are comparable with those for adults. There are no size or weight restrictions concerning a pediatric patient's suitability to have an endoscopic procedure. Contraindications to pediatric laparoscopy may include, but are not limited to, the following conditions:
- Dense abdominal adhesions
- Hepatosplenomegaly
- Hemodynamic instability
- Coagulopathy or hemorrhagic condition
- Large tumor resection
- Congenital abdominal or diaphragmatic hernia

Preparation of the pediatric patient for laparoscopy should include (1) emptying the bladder by catheterization with a Foley and (2) inserting a nasogastric tube. Small 0° and 30° telescopes are useful. Body size may indicate the use of specialized equipment for unconventional use, such as arthroscopic scopes because of shorter shafts and sheaths.

Keep in mind that the tissues of neonates and tiny infants may be unable to withstand the intraabdominal pressures or the use of steep Trendelenburg position to displace the abdominal organs cephalad. The infant's chest is pliant, and CO_2 pressure may significantly impair diaphragmatic movement and place strain on cardiac motion. The vena cava can be compressed, causing a decrease in preload and cardiac output. Procedures lasting more than 2 hours can cause a decrease in circulating blood volume causing metabolic acidosis. The anesthesia provider may need to use a tiny cuffed endotracheal tube to counteract the need for increased inspiratory pressures. This differs for conventional surgery, in which a noncuffed endotracheal tube is preferred under the age of 8 years.

Insufflated CO_2 for pneumoperitoneum causes a decreased lung capacity up to 30% to 50%. The lung capacity decreases by an additional 20% if the neonate is placed in Trendelenburg position. The peritoneal membrane is highly absorbent of carbon dioxide. The thorax is more absorbent of the gas, and the risk for neurotoxicity is high during thoracoscopic procedures.

The potential for anomalous organ position should be considered with placement of trocars and sheaths. The liver and spleen are proportionately large and difficult to maneuver around, especially in neonates under 3 kg. The open laparoscopic method with a blunt trocar is preferred over the use of a Veress needle for creation of the working space. A risk of the procedure in neonates is creating an access portal near the umbilicus, as it may remain patent resulting in a gas embolus. CO_2 pressures should be kept low, at around 8 to 10 mm Hg, as tolerated until insufflation is complete. Although an open method is preferred for the primary trocar, sharp insertion of the secondary trocars may be performed with direct vision.

Potential for injury to nontarget organs is great. The bowel and adjacent organs are in close proximity and could inadvertently be injured by graspers or electrosurgical instruments. Small injuries can go unnoticed and result in subsequent postoperative bleeding or peritonitis. Renal blood flow can be impaired by increased intraabdominal pressure, causing a decrease in glomerular filtration and urine production. Many neonates and infants temporarily become oliguric or anuric during laparoscopy, and fluid maintenance should not be based on output calculations. Forcing excess fluids at this time could cause fluid overload.

Hypothermia is a serious concern because the CO_2 is cold. The use of heated CO_2 may help in maintaining body temperature. The gas and the light from the laparoscope could be drying to tissues. Gentle irrigation should be used during the procedure. All solutions used in irrigation should be warmed to body temperature and carefully measured for intake and output to prevent fluid overload.

Robotics

Robotics are useful for small spaces and are being used in more endoscopic procedures for pediatric patients, especially urology, cardiac, general, and gastrointestinal procedures. The robot is very large compared with the size of the neonate or small child's body. Most 5-mm instrumentation is made for 8-mm ports, which are too large for the neonate or small child. This increases the difficulty of team maneuverability in the sterile field. Positioning for robotic surgery may be dangerous for circulation and oxygenation for a small child. An increasing number of robotic cases are being done in the larger pediatric and adolescent population. The robot has some benefits such as high (3D) resolution, offering a clear view of small structures with greater magnification, and motion scaling for precise fine hand movement. The use of robotics also has benefits to the patient, including small incisions, less narcotic use, shorter hospital stays, and quicker recovery.[6] Robotic companies are designing specific pediatric instrumentation and systems to accommodate pediatric surgical techniques.

Emergent Procedures

Alimentary tract obstruction in a newborn or young infant is the most frequent cause for an emergency surgical procedure. The common sites of obstruction are in the esophagus, duodenum, ileum, colon, and anus. Atresia, an imperforation or closure of a normal opening, and stenosis, a constriction or narrowing, are the common causes of obstruction. Abnormal fistulas can develop between passages, such as in the tracheoesophageal area. The obstructive lesion is usually resected, and the viable segments of the visceral passages are anastomosed. A temporary or permanent gastrostomy, ileostomy, or colostomy may be necessary.

Intestinal obstruction can develop in infants and children months to years after the newborn period from a predisposing or associated congenital anomaly or acquired disease process. Inflammatory diseases, such as necrotizing enterocolitis, ulcerative colitis, Meckel diverticulum, or Crohn's disease, and other intestinal conditions, such as Hirschsprung disease or familial polyposis (Gardner syndrome), require intestinal resection and anastomosis. An endorectal pull-through (also known as Duhamel procedure) may be the procedure of choice to preserve the rectum.

Biliary Atresia

A form of intrauterine cholangitis that results in progressive fibrotic obliteration of bile ducts, biliary atresia may cause jaundice and acholic stool in the newborn. If untreated, this condition can cause cirrhosis and death within the first year of life. Excision of extrahepatic ducts or hilar dissection with a Kasai (hepatoportoenterostomy) procedure, such as portal hepaticojejunostomy, is performed before the infant is 2 months old to relieve jaundice by improving bile drainage. If liver function becomes progressively impaired, liver transplantation may ultimately be necessary for survival (Fig. 8.7).

Esophageal Atresia

Esophageal atresia (EA), with or without tracheoesophageal fistula (TEF), is an acute congenital anomaly characterized by esophageal

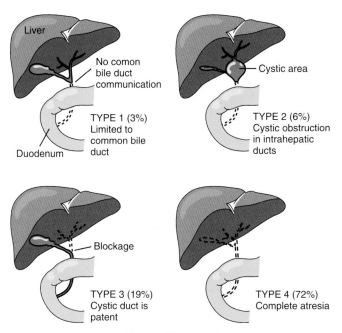

• **Fig. 8.7** Biliary atresia.

obstruction, accumulation of secretions, gastric reflux, and respiratory complications (Fig. 8.8). The incidence is approximately 1 in 2500 live births and the presence of polyhydramnios. The goal of repair is to obtain an end-to-end esophageal anastomosis and closure of any tracheal fistula. The timing and technique to accomplish this goal depend on the specific type of anomaly, degree of prematurity, birthweight, and extent of other associated anomalies.

Repair may be either primary or staged. Gastrostomy (either open or endoscopic) is performed initially to establish a conduit for feeding the newborn weighing less than 1200 g. Percutaneous placement of the gastrostomy tube (percutaneous endoscopic gastrostomy [PEG] tube) is commonly performed (Fig. 8.9).

Open repair includes division of the tracheoesophageal fistula, if present, and anastomosis of the esophageal pouches. Submucosal myotomies and lengthening of the upper pouch permit primary anastomosis to establish alimentary tract continuity. This may be delayed to allow the esophagus to grow as the infant grows so that the gap between the pouches shortens. A transthoracic or retrosternal interposition colon graft may be necessary for esophageal replacement if the gap between the proximal and distal segments is too large for a primary esophageal anastomosis. Usually an extrapleural approach is used for these procedures.

Imperforate Anus

Anorectal malformation generally occurs during the 4th to 12th week of fetal development. The incidence of anal malformations is 1 in 4000 live births. More males have the condition than females. Imperforate anus (IA) is classified as high or low in relation to the levator muscles. Males have more high-level IA incidence and manifest fistulas between the colon and bladder. Females may have more low-level IA incidence with vestibular-vaginal fistulas but also can have a fusion of the anogenital tract referred to as a cloaca, a single opening for the urethra, rectum, and vagina.

If the anus remains closed (i.e., imperforate) during fetal development, the intestinal tract is opened surgically soon after birth. A posterior sagittal anorectoplasty or an abdominoperineal pull-through procedure may be done for primary management with a temporary colostomy. Some children experience fecal incontinence or chronic constipation as they grow into their teens after repair procedures for high IA in infancy. Various secondary

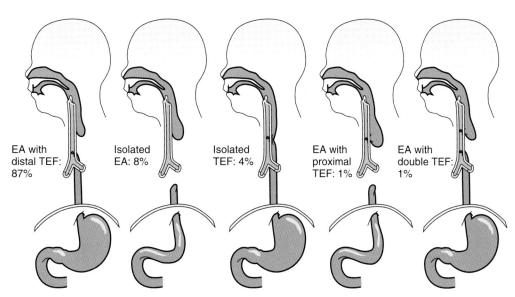

• **Fig. 8.8** Esophageal atresia.

• **Fig. 8.9** Percutaneous endoscopic gastrostomy tube placement.

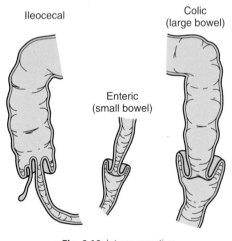

• **Fig. 8.10** Intussusception.

procedures are performed, most frequently an endorectal pull-through procedure or gracilis muscle transplant for reconstruction of the rectal sphincter.

Intussusception

Intussusception occurs when a portion of bowel slides into another segment and causes obstruction (Fig. 8.10). The most common site is the ileocolic junction. The motion is like a telescope. The ileum moves into the cecum. The ileum can twist causing volvulus (a twisted obstruction). The bowel becomes inflamed, hemorrhagic, and necrotic. Most cases are diagnosed between 5 months and 1 year, and the incidence ranges from 1 to 4 in 1000 live births. This is the most common surgical emergency for children younger than 2 years and occurs primarily in the spring and fall months. The condition may be accompanied by Meckel diverticulum.

Theories about the cause include lingering viral infection that causes inflammation of the lymph glands (Peyer patch) in the lumen of the bowel that develop hypertrophied adhesions. These adhesions cause the bowel to stick together during peristaltic motion stimulated by digestion. Other theories indicate that when a baby is weaned from the bottle or breast and new foods are introduced into the diet, the digestive tract has not yet adjusted to the change. Intussusception occurs more frequently in males than in females.

The symptoms range from intense pain to nausea and vomiting. A sausage-shaped curve is sometimes apparent across the abdomen over the location of the intussusception. The baby may have bloody, jelly-like stool.

Treatment can range from hydrostatic reduction with a barium enema to open laparotomy through a right lower quadrant incision. Some surgeons use oxygen as a gas enema to insufflate the colon and small bowel (at the ileum) for intussusception less than 12 hours in duration and with no signs of obstruction or bleeding. The flow rate is maintained around 2 L/min without exceeding 80 mm Hg in pressure until fluoroscopy shows small bowel insufflation and its return to a natural anatomic position. Parents are advised to observe for signs of recurrence during convalescence. If open laparotomy is required, a transverse incision is made in the right lower quadrant and the overriding bowel is "milked" into the correct anatomic position. A cecopexy is done. If Meckel diverticulum is present, it is resected. A patent urachus may be closed, and an appendectomy is also performed.

Pyloromyotomy

Pyloric stenosis is a congenital obstructive lesion in the pylorus of the stomach. The opening becomes hypertrophic and prevents food from entering the intestine. It occurs in 3 in 1000 live births. Symptoms include progressive vomiting after every meal. The onset of symptoms usually occurs between the third and eighth weeks of life and is more common in males. The stenosis is relieved with modified pyloromyotomy, also known as a Fredet-Ramstedt procedure. After the serosa is cut through, the muscle layers of the pylorus are divided. Pyloromyotomy can be performed endoscopically. Feeding in small amounts can resume 8 to 10 hours postoperatively.

Herniorrhaphy

Herniorrhaphy (i.e., hernia repair) is the most frequently performed elective surgical procedure in infants and children by general surgeons. Of the four types of hernias seen in pediatric patients, indirect inguinal hernia is the most common; it occurs much more frequently in male patients than in female patients and appears during the first 10 years of life. Inguinal hernia is found in 3% of all live births. Female patients who have an inguinal hernia also may have a prolapsed ovary in the hernia sac.

A risk of an untreated hernia is migration of bowel loops into the hernia sac. If bowel enters the sac, it can become twisted and incarcerated (i.e., entrapped). The first line of treatment is to reduce the bowel back into the abdomen. If the loop reincarcerates, surgery is performed as an urgent procedure. Strangulated bowel can become ischemic and necrotic, causing peritonitis and sepsis. The child will be in extreme pain.

Male pediatric patients with an inguinal hernia may also have a hydrocele. A hydrocele is more common on the right side and is a collection of fluid between the layers of the tunica vaginalis that extends into the scrotum. Diagnosis can be made by transillumination of the scrotum with a flashlight and confirmed by ultrasound. Some hydroceles resolve without surgical intervention by age 2 years. Aspiration of the fluid should not be attempted. Hydroceles that accompany hernias can be surgically repaired at the same time as the herniorrhaphy procedure. Laparoscopy can be used to repair the hernia and permits the surgeon to inspect the contralateral inguinal ring for potential hernia. Postoperatively the child can resume normal activity as tolerated without restrictions.

Although frequently seen, most umbilical hernias do not always need surgical intervention. Femoral hernias need surgical correction but are rarely acute problems in childhood.

A hiatal hernia is a surgical emergency in the newborn if abdominal contents are in the chest and cause acute respiratory distress (Fig. 8.11). Diaphragmatic hernias in infants and children are caused by congenital weakness in the fascia, abdominal wall, or diaphragm. They are more common in males and manifest by respiratory distress and cyanosis within a few minutes to hours after birth.

Diaphragmatic hernias are more common in the left chest, and radiographs show the intestines in the chest. If the defect is large, the liver or spleen may be shifted cephalad. Pulmonary hypertension caused by poor lung development is usually present. The patient should be immediately intubated and a nasogastric tube inserted to decompress the bowel. ECMO can be used. The surgical approach is abdominal, and the repair is made with mesh. In most cases, 70% of infants will survive but may have health issues such as breathing difficulty and poor growth and

Intestine protruding through hole in diaphragm

• **Fig. 8.11** Diaphragmatic hernia.

development. Unfortunately, prenatal diagnosis before 25 weeks has a high mortality rate close to 60% despite the best care.

Advances with intrauterine fetal surgery have allowed surgeons to correct birth defects that would normally lead to physical disabilities or death. The first intrauterine fetal surgery took place in 1981 at the University of California at San Francisco to correct a urinary obstruction. More facilities are offering this option. Criteria for the procedure include (1) no risk to the life of the mother or her future reproductive capacity, (2) tocolytic treatment to forestall labor postoperatively, and (3) the premise that no other treatment is an option. If the hernia involves the liver and partial resection, the risk to the umbilical circulation could cause fetal demise.

Two types of congenital diaphragmatic hernias are possible based on the location of the defect. The Bochdalek hernia is the most common. It is located in the posterolateral aspect of the diaphragm. The Morgagni hernia is a retrosternal defect.

Other correctable surgical procedures include urinary tract obstruction, myelomeningocele (spina bifida), sacrococcygeal teratoma, and twin-to-twin transfusion syndrome. More information about intrauterine fetal surgery can be found in Chapter 34 of the text.

Omphalocele and Gastroschisis

Failure of abdominal viscera to become encapsulated within the peritoneal cavity during fetal development results in herniation through a 4 to 10-cm defect in the abdominal wall at the right paraumbilical area (Fig. 8.12). The intestines, liver, and spleen can be within the sac. The sac containing the protruding organs consists of chorion, Wharton jelly, and peritoneum. The normal size of the intraabdominal cavity is reduced because the organs have been displaced from within. Surgical repair is done in stages to allow the abdominal cavity to accommodate the placement of the organs.

Diagnosis is usually made with ultrasound before the 20th week of pregnancy. If routine prenatal blood work shows an elevated α-fetoprotein (AFP) level, a transvaginal ultrasound may reveal the condition as early as 12 weeks' gestation. When the condition is discovered the physician usually performs echocardiography and genetic studies to rule out heart or inherited problems, including genitourinary defects. Plans are made for preterm surgical delivery between 37 and 38 weeks' gestation.

• **Fig. 8.12** Omphalocele.

The contents of the sac are surgically reduced back into the peritoneal cavity. The method of closure depends on the extent of the defect. Skin may be closed primarily if the defect is small. More commonly, primary closure of the abdominal wall is facilitated by tissue expanders in the abdominal wall and reduction of organs from the sac. Closure is performed without undue tension or compartment syndrome can develop. Synthetic mesh or sheeting may be used.

For large defects, closure of the abdominal wall usually is staged over a period of weeks or months, with implantation of a silicone silo or tissue expansion prosthesis to reduce intestines at the first stage, followed by removal of the device and abdominal wall closure at the second stage. Fluid management and temperature regulation are important because the exposed viscera can dry out and become cool, thus lowering the infant's body temperature. The bowel was exposed to amniotic fluid in utero, which caused tissue damage and loss of peristalsis. Other defects may be present, such as intestinal atresia. Nutritional status is supported parenterally, and an ostomy may be necessary for elimination. Necrotizing enterocolitis requires bowel resection.

Appendectomy

Appendicitis, an acute inflammation of the appendix, is the most common cause for an abdominal surgical procedure in the child aged 5 to 10 years. Appendectomy may be performed with laparoscopy or open laparotomy. Appendectomy was one of the earliest procedures performed endoscopically on pediatric patients.

Gangrene or rupture may occur before diagnosis or surgical intervention. A questionable diagnosis may be confirmed or ruled out with laparoscopy. Endoscopic approaches are associated with fewer postoperative complications, such as paralytic ileus and wound infection, except in the case of a ruptured appendix.

Splenectomy

Removal of the spleen may be indicated to correct hypersplenic disease, either congenital or acquired. Emergency splenectomy is necessary after rupture of the spleen, usually from blunt trauma. An attempt is made to salvage as much of the organ as possible to minimize future susceptibility to infection.

Bezoars

Intestinal obstruction can be caused by ingested matter that forms a foreign body and accumulates in the stomach, possibly even extending into the small bowel. The foreign body consists of hair (tricho-), vegetable matter (phyto-), or milk curd (lacto-) and is commonly associated with strange appetite compulsions (trichophagia) and emotional disturbances. Removal can be done endoscopically with hydrodissection or with open laparotomy. Shockwave therapy is sometimes successful in fragmenting the bezoar mass for endoscopic removal.

Genitourinary Surgery

Pediatric urology basically concerns the diagnosis and treatment of infections and congenital anomalies within the genitourinary tract. Some type of anomaly of the genitourinary system may be found in 10% to 15% of newborns. Secondary infections are frequently associated with congenital anomalies; chronic diseases are frequently associated with infections. Pediatric and adolescent gynecology is discussed in Chapter 34. The following surgical procedures include those most performed by pediatric urologists.

Cystoscopy

Diagnostic evaluation and therapeutic removal of obstructions within the structures of the genitourinary tract may be performed through an infant-size or child-size cystoscope. Cystoscopes from 9.5 Fr through 16 Fr are used for infants and children. A 3-Fr ureteral catheter can be introduced through the smallest cystoscope. Hypothermia can occur when the fluid used to expand the bladder is cooler than body temperature.

Nephrectomy, Nephrostomy, or Pyeloureteroplasty

Hydronephrosis, congenital or acquired, may necessitate surgical intervention. Nephrectomy is indicated only if severe disease is unilateral, with a contralateral kidney capable of life-sustaining function. More conservative nephrostomy or pyeloureteroplasty is indicated for bilateral or moderate to mild kidney disease.

Wilms Tumor

Wilms tumor is a malignant solid renal tumor that develops rapidly in a child usually younger than 5 years. Nephrectomy is necessary to resect the tumor. If the adrenal gland is intimately connected to the tumor in the upper pole of the kidney, the gland is resected en bloc with the renal mass. Vascular extension of the tumor into the suprahepatic vena cava may necessitate a cardiopulmonary bypass to ligate all tumor vessels. Ipsilateral periaortic lymph node dissection often is performed to stage the extension of cancerous cells.

Neurogenic Bladder

Defective bladder function may be a result of a central nervous system lesion such as a myelomeningocele or spinal cord trauma. For preservation of renal function and achievement of urinary continence in the presence of a neurogenic bladder, an enterocystoplasty may be performed. This procedure retains an intact urinary tract. An artificial urinary sphincter can be implanted to achieve dryness in the child who has sufficient dexterity to operate the pump.

Exstrophy of the Bladder

In exstrophy of the bladder, a congenital anomaly, the bladder herniates through the lower abdominal wall in the suprapubic region. Repair requires reconstruction of the lower abdominal wall and external genitalia, which usually can be accomplished in one surgical procedure on a female infant but requires two or more staged procedures on a male infant. A gastrocystoplasty may be the procedure of choice. If urinary continence cannot be established, urinary diversion through ureteral reimplantation may become necessary.

Ureteral Reimplantation

Repositioning the ureters (i.e., ureteral reimplantation) may be performed to correct either congenital or acquired total urinary incontinence or vesicoureteral reflux.

Incontinence causes parents to seek help for an infant or child. Incontinence is usually not caused by a single factor. The urologist plans the procedure based on an accurate assessment of anatomic and physiologic causes. Creation of a tubularized trigonal muscle, when reconstructed into a new bladder neck, acts as a sphincter to maintain continence. With ureters in the normal position, this muscular tube in the bladder wall cannot be constructed. Therefore the ureters are reimplanted superiorly into the bladder through a created tunnel. Care is taken that the ureters are not hooked or angled but follow a smooth curve into the bladder.

Vesicoureteral reflux is the most common reason for reimplantation of ureters in pediatric patients.

Chronic reflux, regurgitation of urine from the bladder into the ureters, can lead to pyelonephritis and hydronephrosis. Ureteral reimplantation may be necessary to prevent kidney damage. The objective of the surgical procedure is to position a segment of the ureters at a higher level within the bladder wall so the level of urine is below the orifices and intravesical pressure prevents reflux.

When ureters cannot be reimplanted in the bladder, a urinary diversion procedure may be necessary. Ureters are usually anastomosed to a nonrefluxing colon conduit.

Urethral Repair

The external opening (meatus) of the urethra may be displaced at birth. Hypospadias is an anomaly in the male in which the urethra terminates on the underside of the penis or on the perineum (Fig. 8.13); in the female with hypospadias the urethra opens into

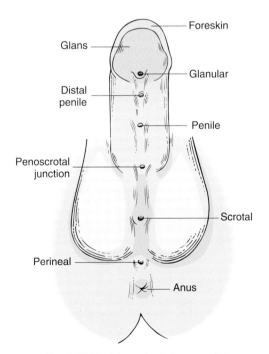

• **Fig. 8.13** Meatal opening in hypospadias.

the vagina. With epispadias in the male the urethra terminates on the dorsum of the penis; in the female it terminates above the clitoris. Hypospadias has a familial association and occurs in approximately 1 in 250 newborn males.

Multistage procedures are usually necessary to correct these anomalies. The goal is to center the meatus at the tip of the glans penis of the male. This may be accomplished in a one-stage procedure with a transverse island flap derived from prepuce or with a vertical-incision/horizontal-closure technique for distal coronal or subglandular hypospadias.

Some surgeons use androgen treatment briefly preoperatively to cause enlargement of the penis to facilitate handling during the procedure. The androgens are discontinued after the procedure and have no known lasting adverse effects. Tissue grafts from the inner mouth mucosa can be used to span structural gaps. Oral mucosa grafts well in the moist environment of the urethra.

Females with meatal anomalies may need multistage procedures to approximate normal anatomic position. In addition to general anesthesia, a caudal or epidural is commonly used to manage postoperative pain. A Foley catheter is used for several days to a week. This procedure is usually performed between ages 6 and 12 months.

Orchiopexy

One or both testicles that failed to descend the inguinal canal during fetal development can be brought into the scrotum and stabilized with a traction suture until healing takes place before the age of 2 years. Upon abdominal exploration the testes can be located along a pathway between the inguinal ring and the hilum of the kidney. Most undescended testes are on the right side; however, 25% of cases can be bilateral. The most important consideration is to reposition the testicles before the Leydig cells degenerate. The risk for seminoma in undescended testes is higher in these patients than other males in the population. Although malignancy is uncommon, it is the highest form of cancer in the 15 to 35-year age range. Cryptorchidism (undescended testicles) may be present in males with hypospadias.

In the two-stage Torek operation the testicle and supporting structures are dissected free from the inguinal region. An adequate length of spermatic vessels is released to permit the testicle to reach the scrotal sac. After it is pulled down through the scrotum, the testicle is sutured to fascia of the thigh. At the second-stage procedure, 2 to 3 months later, the testicle is freed from the fascia and embedded into the scrotum.

If one or both testicles are absent, silicone prostheses may be inserted into the scrotum for cosmetic appearance. Psychologically for the child and parents, absence (agenesis) of testicles is cosmetically repaired at age 5 or 6 years, before the boy begins school.

Circumcision

Excision of the foreskin of the penis (circumcision) may be done to prevent phimosis, in which the foreskin becomes tightly wrapped around the tip of the glans penis, or to remove redundant foreskin. Complications can ensue if the phimotic foreskin strangulates around the erect penis.

Circumcision is the most performed pediatric surgical procedure but is not necessary in all male babies. Some physicians perform the procedure on newborns without anesthetic. Local anesthesia without epinephrine additive can be safely used to avoid pain and discomfort during the procedure (Fig. 8.14).

• **Fig. 8.14** Circumcision.

• **Fig. 8.15** Hip abduction splint for congenital dislocation of the hip.

Circumcision, as an elective procedure, is contraindicated if an abnormality of the glans penis or urethral meatus is present. Urethral repair can require the use of foreskin tissue as graft tissue.

Orthopedic and Spinal Surgery

Pediatric orthopedic surgery is principally elective and reconstructive for correction of deformities of the musculoskeletal system. These deformities may be congenital, idiopathic, pathologic, or traumatic. Traumatic injuries do not always manifest on conventional radiographs. Magnetic resonance imaging is used to disclose injuries that could be missed. The extent of the anomalies and functional disorders often involves prolonged immobilization and hospitalization. Many patients need a series of corrective procedures.

Some of the conditions most seen in the OR include those discussed in the following sections.

Fractures

Fractures that occur in infants and children generally are treated as they are in adults. Fixation devices are not well tolerated by children and often prevent uniting of the fracture. Closed reduction of long-bone fractures is preferable.

Tendon Repair

Tendons may be lengthened, shortened, or transferred to correct congenital deformities of the hand or foot. Lacerated tendons are repaired to restore function. A tourniquet is used to control bleeding. The tourniquet cuff size should be appropriate for the size of the infant or child. Padding under the cuff is applied smoothly. Sheet wadding may be used under an infant cuff to protect delicate skin. The cuff should be tight but should not restrict circulation before inflation. The time of inflation is closely watched to prevent ischemia. The surgeon may ask the circulating nurse to release the pressure every 30 minutes on an infant or up to every 1 to 2 hours for an older child, depending on age. Tendon procedures are often lengthy.

Congenital Dislocated Hip

Displacement (dysplasia) of the femoral head from its normal position in the acetabulum can be present at birth, either unilaterally or bilaterally. If dysplasia is diagnosed early in infancy, closed reduction with immobilization usually corrects the dislocation without residual deformity (Fig. 8.15). If dysplasia is not diagnosed until after the child has begun to walk, open reduction of the hip with an osteotomy to stabilize the joint may be necessary.

Leg Length Discrepancies

The epiphyseal cartilaginous growth lines progressively close as the child matures. Bones lengthen from the activity of the epiphyses. The absolute physiologic criterion for completion of childhood is when this cartilage becomes a part of bone. A discrepancy in activity of an epiphyseal line may retard or over-stimulate growth of a bone in one extremity and not in its contralateral counterpart. When this occurs in one femur, legs become unequal in length.

The orthopedic surgeon may correct leg length discrepancies, usually more than 1 inch (2.5 cm), with epiphyseal arrest (i.e., stopping growth of the bone). This is done in the contralateral leg to let the shorter extremity catch up. The longer leg may be shortened with a closed intramedullary procedure. With use of fluoroscopy, a reamer is inserted into the medullary canal of the femur through a small incision high on the hip. After the reamer widens the canal, a rotating saw is manipulated to cut a section from the bone. The bone ends are aligned and fixed with a flexible intramedullary rod.

Slipping of the upper femoral epiphysis causes displacement of the femoral head, which can occur because of traumatic injury or as a chronic disability usually seen in obese adolescents. Fusion of the epiphysis to the femoral neck may be necessary to prevent slipping and shortening of the leg.

Many limb deformities in children are a complex combination of angulation and shortening because of trauma, infection, metabolic bone disease, congenital deformity, and developmental problems. The Ilizarov external fixator technique provides an alternative treatment option.[7] Thin strong wires are transfixed through bones and attached to rings under tension. The rings, which encircle a leg or arm, are held firmly in place with threaded rods. Bolts on the rods are turned several times a day to pull cut ends of bone apart. Corticotomy, performed through a small skin incision after wires are inserted, preserves periosteal and endosteal blood supply to bone. This promotes rapid healing to regenerate new bone that fills in the gap.

New technology offers hybrid and hexapod fixators that are controlled by special software. Motorized internal lengthening plates and nails reduce the need for multiple surgical procedures.[7]

Talipes Deformities

Combinations of various types of deformities of the foot, especially those of congenital origin, are referred to as *talipes*; the addition of the medical term is used to describe whether the forefoot is inverted (*varus*) or everted (*valgus*) and whether the calcaneal tendon is shortened or lengthened.

• **Fig. 8.16** Denis Browne splint for clubfoot deformity.

Talipes Varus

Talipes varus, known as clubfoot, is the most common of the talipes deformities; it may be unilateral or bilateral. The forefoot is inverted and rotated, accompanied by shortening of the calcaneal tendon and contracture of the plantar fascia. Conservative treatment with casting or a brace during infancy usually corrects a mild postural deformity before the infant bears weight on the foot (Fig. 8.16). A wedge cast with turnbuckles may be applied to an older child to allow gradual manipulation. If conservative treatment is unsuccessful, an open surgical procedure may be necessary.

Talipes Equinovarus

Talipes equinovarus, an idiopathic true clubfoot deformity, almost always necessitates surgical intervention for correction. In varying degrees, talipes equinovarus includes an incomplete dislocation (subluxation) of the talocalcaneonavicular joint with deformed talus and calcaneus bones, a shortened calcaneal tendon, and soft tissue contractures. As a result the forefoot curls toward the heel (adduction, supination), the midfoot points downward (equinus), and the hindfoot turns inward (varus). The orthopedic surgeon uses a sequential-release approach to obtain maximum correction of all contractures and realigns bones in the ankle joint. Pins are inserted, and the extremity is put in a cast to maintain alignment of the foot and ankle.

Scoliosis

Scoliosis is a lateral curvature and rotation of the spine, most frequently seen in rapidly growing school-age (older than 10 years) or adolescent females (Fig. 8.17). Treatment depends on the degree and flexibility of the curvature, chronologic and skeletal age of the child, and preference of the surgeon. The child may be fitted with a Milwaukee brace (Fig. 8.18), immobilized in a cast, or stretched with traction. As an alternative to these techniques, an electrical device may be applied with an underarm brace to stimulate muscle contraction on the convex side of the curvature.

If untreated at an early stage, scoliosis produces secondary changes in vertebral bodies and in the rib cage. Spinal fusion is ultimately performed if the curvature has become severe (40% or more) or must be stabilized after corrections. Government-mandated screening programs in schools have reduced the need for surgical correction in many children. Surgical techniques using technology that grows with the child are being used for early-onset scoliosis, along with other minimally invasive techniques. Surgical correction for scoliosis is described in Chapter 38.

The following procedures are examples of treatments used for the correction of scoliosis:

1. A wedge body jacket or Minerva jacket may be applied. Turnbuckles may be incorporated. Turnbuckles are adjustable metal rods placed along the edges of the wedge of the cast.

• **Fig. 8.17** Scoliosis.

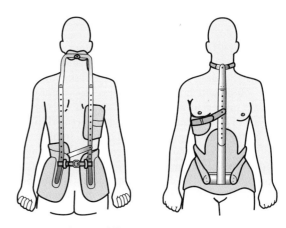

• **Fig. 8.18** Milwaukee brace for scoliosis.

Gradual opening of the turnbuckles by the surgeon as tolerated by the patient corrects the lateral curvature of the spine.
2. A Sayre sling, an appliance used for head traction, is sometimes used when applying a body jacket to correct slight scoliosis. Traction is obtained by means of pulleys and a rope suspended from the ceiling or an arm of the fracture table.
3. Halo traction is used to stretch the spine in some patients in whom the spine is too rigid to be straightened in a cast. A metal band is applied to the skull by means of four pins inserted into the cortex of the skull. A Steinmann pin is inserted into the distal end of each femur. A traction bow is put on each pin. Weights, usually equal, are put on the halo and Steinmann pins and gradually increased as tolerated. When radiographs show maximum correction, a spinal fusion is done. Traction may be continued until healing has taken place to the degree that there will be no loss of correction; a plaster jacket is then applied.
4. A Risser jacket is applied a few days before posterior spinal fusion to gain as much correction as possible. The orthopedic table is used. Traction is applied with a chin strap, similar to a Sayre sling, and countertraction is applied with a pelvic girdle. The spine is straightened as much as possible, and the body and head are encased in plaster.

Posterior spinal fusion may be performed as a two-stage procedure: vertebral body wedge resection at the first stage and

• **Fig. 8.19** Harrington rods.

insertion of Cotrel-Dubousset or Harrington rods (Fig. 8.19) with fusion at the second stage. Bone fragments removed during the first stage may be saved for the second-stage fusion or sent to the bone bank. Rods and hooks are stainless steel; appropriate instruments are needed to insert them. Two rods are inserted, one on either side of the curvature. These rods are secured to the spine and force it into a more nearly normal position. Implanted on the outside of the vertebral column, the rods apply a longitudinal force on the spine. The spine is then fused.

The procedure may be done through a window in the Risser jacket, but usually the cast is bivalved and the patient lies in the anterior section. If the procedure is done through a window, an electric cast cutter should be at hand to bivalve the cast if the patient has any respiratory difficulties. After the procedure, the bivalved posterior part is put in place and the jacket is fastened together with several rounds of plaster or with webbing straps with buckles. The patient is in the Risser jacket for a year. Progress is checked with radiographs.

5. Segmental spinal fixation with Luque rods may be the procedure of choice to stabilize the spine after fusion. Two L-shaped rods are placed next to the spinous processes and held by wires threaded under the lamina of each vertebra to be fused. Transverse traction internally on each vertebra stabilizes the spine without the need for a postoperative cast.
6. Anterior spinal (nonfusion) tethering method, done through an endoscopic transthoracic approach, is performed as a one-stage procedure to correct severe curvatures in growing children. Titanium staples are fitted over vertebral bodies on the convex side of the curve. Each staple is held in place by one or two titanium screws. A polyethylene terephthalate cable, threaded through the heads of the screws, is tightened to compress the vertebrae and straighten the curve. Staples and screws are secured the full extent of the curvature. The compressed cable corrects the curve immediately. A plaster body jacket may be applied after the procedure to immobilize the back until the fusion is healed. The patient is then ambulatory.
7. For adolescents who are done growing, a minimally invasive nonfusion device with three screws and one rod is placed through a posterior approach.

Ophthalmologic Surgery

Congenital Obstruction of the Nasolacrimal Duct

An obstruction, usually at the lower end of the nasolacrimal duct that enters the inferior meatus of the nose, often results in dilation and infection of the lacrimal sac. Treatment consists of passing a malleable probe from the lid punctum through the nasolacrimal passages to push out the obstructing plug of tissue.

Oculoplastic Procedures on the Eyelids

Congenital malformations such as ptosis (drooping of the upper or lower eyelid) are corrected with extraocular procedures. Ptosis repair is indicated when the levator is inadequate. In the levator resection procedure, which shortens the muscle and gives a more physiologic result, the levator muscle may be approached through the skin (Berke method) or the conjunctiva (Iliff method). A fascial sling procedure to support the lid consists of attaching the upper lid margin to the frontalis muscle. Materials used include autogenous fascia from the thigh, homograft fascia, and synthetic nonabsorbable suture material. The Fasanella-Servat operation is a simpler procedure for obtaining only a small amount of lid elevation.

Extraocular Muscle Procedures

Surgical procedures on extraocular muscles to correct strabismus or squint are the third most performed pediatric procedures on patients between ages 6 months and 6 years. The trend is to correct the congenital type during infancy and the acquired type in preschool years. Patterns of using two eyes together are more flexible and adaptable in a young child.

These procedures on extraocular muscles are done to correct muscle imbalance and promote coordination either by strengthening a weak muscle or by weakening an overactive one. The mechanical strength of a weak muscle can be increased by the following factors:

- *Tucking:* A tuck is sutured in the muscle to shorten it, thereby increasing its effective power.
- *Advancement:* The attachment point of the muscle is freed and reattached closer to the cornea, thereby increasing its leverage.
- *Resection:* Part of the muscle is removed to shorten it, and cut ends are sutured together.
An overactive muscle can be weakened by the following factors:
- *Tenotomy:* The point of attachment of the muscle is severed, and the muscle is dropped back, held by ligaments only.
- *Recession:* The muscle is detached from the eyeball and reattached farther back to decrease its action.
- *Myotomy:* The fibers of a section of the muscle are divided to diminish muscle action.
- *Myectomy:* A section of the muscle belly is excised.
- The Faden procedure: The muscle belly is sutured to the posterior sclera, thereby restricting muscle action considerably, producing a super-weakening effect.

Congenital Cataract Extraction

Under the operating microscope, with use of irrigation-aspiration and cutting instruments, the cataract and often the posterior capsule and a portion of the anterior vitreous are removed at one time. This procedure obtains a clear optical zone so that a contact lens can be fitted on the infant's eye within a few days postoperatively. The goal is to avoid intractable amblyopia (lazy eye) by correcting the defect during the first few weeks of life. An intraocular lens may be implanted. More commonly, epikeratophakia is performed to reshape the cornea.

Keratoplasty may be performed on children with Fuchs dystrophy. The corneal endothelial cells degenerate, causing reduction in vision and corneal edema. The cornea is removed and replaced with a donor corneal graft.

Goniotomy

Although congenital glaucoma is rare, early surgical intervention is urgent to prevent blindness. Goniotomy is a microsurgical procedure that involves dividing a congenital layer of abnormal tissue that covers the drainage angle of the anterior chamber. It is performed with use of a special operative contact lens placed on the eye that permits visualization of the angle. An incision is made through an opening in the contact lens.

Otorhinolaryngologic Surgery
Foreign Body Removal

Although often instructed not to put objects in their mouths, children continue to do so. They often swallow small objects or insert them into the nose or ears. Foreign objects placed in the nose can be removed using a pediatric nasal speculum and bayonet forceps. Care is taken not to advance the object further into the cavity. Many small swallowed items can be allowed to pass naturally through the gastrointestinal tract. The child is carefully observed for signs of pain, abdominal distention, constipation, or lack of appetite that could signal bowel obstruction. Prompt evaluation at a medical facility is necessary.

Aspiration of tiny parts of toys is a common occurrence. It is possible to cough or sneeze when holding an item in the mouth and cause it to be inhaled into the bronchus of the lung. Emergent rigid bronchoscopy under general anesthesia is necessary for removal. The object usually enters the right main bronchus because it is straighter than the left and is a direct line from the trachea.

Larger objects, such as coins, can become lodged in the esophagus or trachea. A radiograph or fluoroscope can confirm the size and location of the item. One technique for removal uses a small 12 to 14-Fr Foley catheter inserted in the passage past the occluding item. The retention balloon is inflated distally and slowly drawn toward the mouth. The balloon can elevate the foreign object to a point at which it can be grasped with forceps. Other instrumentation, such as stone basket snares from urology, can be useful.

Ingestion of coin-sized batteries or multiple magnets can cause serious damage if not removed promptly. Batteries can degrade and discharge their contents, causing necrosis or poisoning. Magnets can cause bowel obstruction by attracting each other internally. Loops of bowel can twist in response to the magnetism, causing ischemia and necrosis. Multiple magnets can stack internally and appear as one piece on radiographs, then later separate and disperse. Deaths have been reported in the literature. Use of stainless steel instruments can complicate removal because they may increase the magnetic attraction. Titanium, plastic, or nonferrous instruments are useful because they do not have magnetic properties. Removal by endoscopy can be difficult. Exploratory laparotomy may be necessary, especially if multiple magnets have been swallowed. A single magnet may pass from the body naturally, and patients are advised to avoid wearing apparel with metallic buttons, zippers, studs, or buckles that might cause

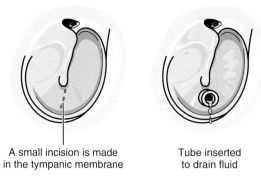

A small incision is made in the tympanic membrane

Tube inserted to drain fluid

• **Fig. 8.20** Myringotomy with peri-eustachian tube.

the magnet to stop moving toward the rectum. Serial radiographs are commonly performed to monitor progress.

Myringotomy

Secretory otitis media is the most common chronic condition of childhood. Fluid accumulates in the middle ear from eustachian tube obstruction. This condition is corrected with myringotomy, an incision in the tympanic membrane (eardrum) for drainage (Fig. 8.20). Through aspiration of fluid and pus, pressure is released, pain is relieved, and hearing is restored and preserved. Ear tube placement can now be done as an office procedure with a topical anesthetic. A handheld instrument containing a cutting device can make the incision, then deploy an ear tube in one step.[8] This new device eliminates general anesthesia and trauma for the patient. Myringotomy is done to prevent perforation of the eardrum and possible erosion of middle ear ossicles. When exudate is especially viscid, the patient has "glue ear," or mucoid otitis media.

Tympanostomy is commonly performed bilaterally in association with myringotomy. A self-cleaning, plastic pressure-equalizing tube is placed through an incision in the tympanic membrane, bypassing the eustachian tube, to facilitate aeration of the middle ear space and prevent reformation of serous otitis media. The tube usually extrudes spontaneously. Premature extrusion before normal eustachian tube function resumes may necessitate replacement of the tube.

Middle Ear Tympanoplasty

Congenital fused ossicles in the middle ear often are associated with stenosis or absence of an external auditory canal. Depending on the deformity, tympanoplasty may be performed with a temporalis fascia graft. If mobilization or ossiculoplasty is impossible, a total or partial ossicular prosthesis may be implanted to replace one or more ossicles. Congenital or acquired conductive deafness may be helped with tympanoplastic surgical techniques. Single-channel cochlear implants, approved for children, may be helpful for the profoundly deaf child.

Correction of Choanal Atresia

Newborns are obligate nose breathers and may die at birth if choanal atresia (congenital closure of nasal passages) is undiagnosed. They are unable to breathe and feed properly without an adequate nasal airway. Bone or fibrous tissue blocking the posterior choanae usually is excised via a transseptal approach to create an opening into the nasopharynx. A CO_2 laser may be used to develop appropriate apertures.

Adenoidectomy

Abnormally enlarged lymphoid tissue or infected adenoids can obstruct breathing. A child usually is at least 2 years old before adenoid tissue in the nasopharynx is removed, but they can undergo an adenoidectomy at an earlier age. Removal of adenoids can positively influence the outcome of otitis media with effusion in childhood. Adenoidectomy is usually performed in conjunction with tonsillectomy.

Tonsillectomy

Tonsillectomy, the excision of hypertrophied or chronically infected tonsils, is not generally advised before the child is 3 years of age (Fig. 8.21). General anesthesia is used for patients up to about 14 years of age. Tonsillectomy and adenoidectomy frequently are performed together; the procedure appears on the surgical schedule as T&A. Sterile technique is carried out throughout the procedure because the patient's vascular system is encountered. Precautions during the surgical procedure include control of bleeding and prevention of aspiration of blood or tissue.

Esophageal Dilation

Children, usually of preschool age, may ingest caustic agents that cause chemical burns of the mouth, lips, and pharynx and corrosive esophagitis. Long-term gradual esophageal dilation with balloon catheters or bougies (pronounced *boogee*) may be necessary to restore adequate oral intake of food after the acute phase of traumatic injury. When all attempts at dilation fail, the esophagus is replaced. The most successful source of esophageal replacement is the colon.

Laryngeal Papillomas

Recurrent respiratory papillomatosis is localized in the larynx of children. Laryngeal papillomas are benign wartlike lesions caused by the human papillomavirus (HPV). HPV can be transmitted during passage through an infected mother's birth canal. Hoarseness is an early symptom; airway obstruction is a later, life-threatening sign. Ablation with the CO_2 laser, manipulated through the operating microscope, preserves underlying laryngeal muscles and ligaments while vaporizing papillomas located on vocal cords.

• **Fig. 8.21** Tonsillectomy.

Laser ablation is not a cure; recurrence often necessitates repeated procedures to maintain a patent airway. HPV is a common cause of throat cancer later in life.

Tracheal or Laryngeal Stenosis

Some accidental injuries result in a narrowing (i.e., stenosis) of the trachea or larynx. Of greater concern are the injuries that result from therapy for respiratory problems, especially in newborns. Prolonged endotracheal intubation can lead to injury from tubes that are too large for the lumen, are too long, or move too much. These injuries may necessitate balloon dilation or endoscopic resection of the stenotic area. Most infants then need an intraluminal stent to maintain patency of the airway.

In the presence of severe circumferential intraluminal scarring with involvement of the cartilages, surgical reconstruction becomes necessary. Laryngotracheoplasty widens the stenosed cartilaginous framework of the airway in the midline anteriorly and posteriorly and reconstructs the mucosal lining. Free or composite rib cartilage grafts are taken with mucosal tissue of the perichondrium for lining the airway. A stent assembly with a tracheostomy tube supports the reconstructed airway during healing. It can then be removed and the tracheostomy closed.

Tracheotomy

Tracheotomy, incision into the trachea and insertion of a tracheostomy tube, is advisable in cases of severe inflammatory glottic diseases, when endotracheal intubation is needed for longer than 72 hours, and when respiratory support is necessary for more than 24 to 48 hours to treat respiratory problems. Prolonged endotracheal intubation can lead to tracheal malacia, or softening, which in turn destroys the tracheal integrity.

Appropriate sizes and types of tracheostomy tubes for infants and children should be available. Tubes that are too large, too rigid, or too long or that have an improper curve can produce ulceration and scarring at pressure points. Strictures that develop at the site of the tracheotomy may necessitate resection to relieve airway obstruction after decannulation. Infants have a shorter neck and are prone to distal displacement of the tracheostomy tube from the intratracheal insertion point. Head motion causes the tube to shift superiorly if it is not secured in position by ties.

Plastic and Reconstructive Surgery

Except for burns and other traumatic tissue injuries, most plastic and reconstructive surgery performed on infants and children is to correct congenital anomalies. The most common of these surgeries include those discussed in the following sections.

Cleft Lip

Lack of fusion of the soft tissues of the upper lip creates a cleft or fissure. The degree of cleft lips varies from simple notching of the lip to extension into the floor of the nose (Fig. 8.22). The cleft may be unilateral or bilateral. The number of procedures necessary for correction depends on the severity of the deformity. Some plastic surgeons do a primary cheiloplasty, closure of the cleft lip, within the first few days after birth to facilitate feeding and minimize psychologic trauma of parents. Surgeons who prefer to wait until the infant is older follow the "Rule of Tens": 10 weeks of age, 10 g of hemoglobin, 10 lbs of body weight.

To relieve tension on the incision postoperatively, a Logan bow (a small, curved metal frame) may be applied over the area of the incision and held in place with narrow adhesive strips to splint the

• **Fig. 8.22** Cleft lip and palate.

lip. Skin closure strips may be used. Arm or elbow restraints are used to prevent the infant from removing the bow or strips and injuring the repaired lip. These restraints are applied in the OR.

Cleft Palate

Failure of tissues of the palate to fuse creates a fissure through the roof of the mouth. Palatal clefts may be a defect only in the soft palate or may extend through both hard and soft palates into the nose and include the alveolar ridge of the maxilla. Cleft palate is often associated with cleft lip; however, the two deformities are closed separately. Palatoplasty, closure of the soft palate, is done before speech begins, to avoid speech defects. A mouth gag is used during the surgical procedure to permit access to the palate without obstructing the airway. General anesthesia is administered via an endotracheal tube. This may be supplemented with infiltration of a local anesthetic agent. When epinephrine is used by the surgeon to minimize bleeding, the anesthesia provider is informed. Epinephrine can increase the patient's heart rate as it vasoconstricts the surgical site.

In patients with bilateral and, frequently, unilateral clefts an additional surgical procedure is performed to elevate the tip of the nose and correct asymmetry before the child is 4 years of age.

Hemangioma

Hemangiomas are the most common of all human congenital anomalies. A hemangioma is a benign tumor (angioma) made up of blood vessels that may pigment or appear as a growth on the skin. All hemangiomas have abnormal patterns of hemodynamics, which is the effect of blood flow through tissues. Variations in vessel size distinguish the different types of these tumors. Argon or tunable dye laser or surgical excision in combination with a skin graft or pedicle flap repair is the treatment of choice for intradermal capillary hemangiomas (port-wine stain). Cryosurgery, surgical excision, or steroid therapy may be used for some other cavernous-type tumors.

Otoplasty

Abnormally small or absent external ears can be reconstructed in several surgical stages. An autogenous rib cartilage graft with the perichondrium intact or a silicone or porous polyethylene prosthesis is used for the supporting framework to produce an anatomic contour. Usually necessitated by microtia, a congenital anomaly, reconstruction of the external ear can follow traumatic injury with loss of all or part of the pinna. Free flaps of temporoparietal fascia are used to secure a prosthesis or may be used to cover a carved cartilage armature procured from the patient's rib or other site for secondary reconstruction.

Otoplasty procedures to correct protruding or excessively large ears are performed more frequently than are procedures for

Before   After

Z-plasty incisions

• **Fig. 8.23** Syndactyly.

microtia. These procedures often are done on preschool-age children, usually boys, to prevent psychologic harm from teasing.

Syndactyly

Syndactyly is a congenital anomaly characterized by fusion of two or more fingers or toes. Webbing between fingers is the most common congenital hand deformity (Fig. 8.23). Tissue that is holding digits together is cut to separate the fingers if phalangeal bones are present. Separation of webbed digits almost always necessitates skin grafts to achieve good functional results.

Polydactyly

Polydactyly is a congenital anomaly characterized by the presence of more than the normal number of fingers or toes. A supernumerary digit may be alongside a thumb or little finger on one or both hands (Fig. 8.24). Extra digits on the feet are less common. Skin and tissue resemble a rudimentary digit. Some supernumerary digits contain bone, ligament, and tendon. Excision is recommended at an early age. If the excised digit contains rudimentary bone, multistage procedures may be necessary to enhance function of the remaining digits of the affected extremity.

Neurologic Surgery

Children of all ages sustain head injuries with hematomas that must be evacuated. Although brain tumors occur in children, the more commonly performed pediatric neurosurgical procedures are related to correction of congenital anomalies.

Craniosynostosis

If one or more of the suture lines in the skull, normally open in infancy (Fig. 8.25), fuses prematurely (craniosynostosis), the skull cannot expand during normal brain growth.

A newborn with multiple-suture involvement may need surgical intervention because of increased intracranial pressure. Even

• **Fig. 8.24** Polydactyly.

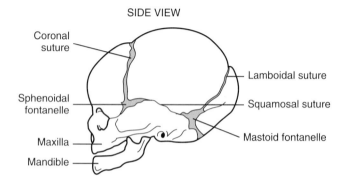

SIDE VIEW

Coronal suture

Lamboidal suture

Sphenoidal fontanelle

Squamosal suture

Maxilla

Mastoid fontanelle

Mandible

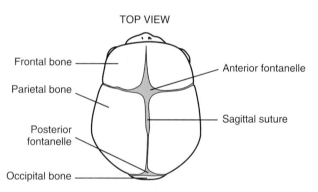

TOP VIEW

Frontal bone

Anterior fontanelle

Parietal bone

Posterior fontanelle

Sagittal suture

Occipital bone

• **Fig. 8.25** Craniosynostosis.

fusion of a single suture puts a newborn at risk for altered cranial capacity and brain damage. The surgeon performs a craniectomy to remove the fused bone and to reopen the suture line. A strip of polyethylene or Silastic film may be inserted to cover bone edges on each side.

In an older infant or child, more extensive freeing of other bones may be necessary to achieve decompression of frontal lobes and orbital contents. The standard procedure takes 8 hours or more to perform.

Craniofacial microsomia with severe facial asymmetry and the dysostosis of Apert syndrome and Crouzon disease also are associated with multiple skull and facial deformities. Congenital malformations of the skull are described in Chapter 41.

Craniofacial surgery, performed by a multidisciplinary team, involves repositioning and reshaping of skull and facial bones and a variety of soft tissue reconstructive techniques.[5] Microplating systems may be used for rigid fixation of bones. The skull may provide a donor site without creating a deformity if bone grafts are necessary. Demineralized cadaver bone powder may be used to stimulate bone growth.

Endoscopic techniques have been developed that enable the surgeon to separate the dura from the skull and snip away stenosed suture lines to free up the skull segments. The whole procedure takes less than 1 hour. The child then wears a skull-molding helmet for several months. Blood loss has been minimized, and the maximum hospital stay is 3 days. The endoscopic procedure is preferred for infants younger than 3 months; however, infants younger than 6 months can still be cared for with this method. The most commonly stenosed suture lines are the sagittal, coronal, metopic, and lambdoid. Older children are treated with the more extensive form of surgery because they have more stenotic areas.

Encephalocele

Encephalocele is the herniation of brain and neural tissue through a defect in the skull. This is present at birth as a sac of tissue on the head. Usually these lesions can be removed 6 to 12 weeks after birth unless the condition is complicated by hydrocephalus.

Hydrocephalus

Usually a congenital condition, hydrocephalus occurs when the passages between the ventricles are blocked and are dilated by accumulated cerebrospinal fluid. Failure of the absorptive mechanisms also can produce impairment in the normal circulation of cerebrospinal fluid and cause excess fluid to accumulate in the ventricles. The intracranial pressure created causes enlargement of the infant's head if the condition develops before fusion of cranial bones and often causes brain damage.

Hydrocephalus may be diagnosed in utero with an ultrasound scan. Cephalocentesis can be performed, and a ventriculoamniotic shunt may be inserted to drain the ventricles. After birth, surgical treatment involves establishment of a mechanism for transporting excess fluid from the ventricles to maintain an intracranial pressure close to normal. This may be done with implantation of a shunt, which carries fluid from the lateral ventricle to the peritoneal cavity (ventriculoperitoneal shunt) or to the right atrium of the heart (ventriculoatrial shunt; Fig. 8.26). Ventriculoatrial shunts are more commonly associated with infection, pleural effusion, and cardiac dysrhythmia. Other types of shunts are used, but less commonly, to bypass localized obstructions.

One end of the shunt catheter is put into the ventricle; the other end may connect to a one-way valve, which in turn is connected to the catheter that drains fluid distally from the head. An endoscopic technique may be used for catheter placement in the ventricle. Shunt malformation is usually caused by obstruction by the choroid plexus or debris. This complication can be reduced by positioning the shunt catheter tip opposite the foramen of Monro visually via a miniature fiberoptic pediatric neuroendoscope.

Catheters are made of silicone. An antithrombotic coating may be incorporated into the distal end. Some valves are regulated to open for drainage when predetermined pressure in the ventricle is reached. Other valves are designed as flushing devices to keep the distal catheter patent; the skin over the device is manually depressed to flush the system. For each patient the surgeon chooses the shunt mechanism that is safest for the type of hydrocephalus being treated. Follow-up minor revisions are sometimes necessary, generally because of growth of the child.

As an alternative to a shunt procedure a ventriculostomy can relieve intracranial pressure. A rigid neuroendoscope is introduced into the third ventricle. The contact fiber of a

• **Fig. 8.26** Hydrocephalus.

• **Fig. 8.27** Spina bifida.

neodymium:yttrium-aluminum-garnet (Nd:YAG) laser, inserted through the scope, blanches and perforates the floor of the third ventricle at several points to establish circulation of cerebrospinal fluid into the subarachnoid space.

Myelomeningocele

A saclike protrusion may bulge through a defect in a portion of the vertebral column that failed to fuse in fetal development. If the nerves of the spinal cord remain within the vertebral column and only the meninges protrude into the sac, the congenital anomaly is a meningocele. However, if the sac also contains a portion of the spinal cord, it is a myelomeningocele, with associated permanent nerve damage. The degree of impairment depends on the level and extent of the defect.

Clubfeet (talipes deformities), dislocated hips, hydrocephalus, neurogenic bladder, paralysis, and other congenital disorders often accompany a myelomeningocele.

Each patient is evaluated and treated individually according to their needs. In general it is best to delay the surgical procedure to repair a myelomeningocele until danger of development of hydrocephalus has passed or cerebrospinal fluid has been shunted. If the sac is covered with a thin membrane, meningitis is an imminent danger. The defect is repaired soon after birth, usually within the first 48 hours, to close cutaneous, muscular, and dural defects.

Spina Bifida

Spina bifida, incomplete closure of the paired vertebral arches in the midline of the vertebral column, may occur without herniation of the meninges (Fig. 8.27). A spina bifida may be covered by intact skin and can occur at different levels of the spine (Fig. 8.28), causing various types of disability. Laminectomy may be indicated to repair the underlying defect.

Spastic Cerebral Palsy

Selective posterior rhizotomy can improve muscle tone and function of school-age children with spastic cerebral palsy. The procedure involves division of lumbar and sacral posterior nerve roots associated with an abnormal motor response as identified by nerve stimulation.

Thoracic Surgery

Aspiration of a foreign body can seriously compromise a child's respiratory status. Bronchoscopy with the child under general anesthesia may be necessary to remove the object. Bronchoscopy is also performed to diagnose tracheobronchial compression by an innominate artery, a vascular ring, or some other pathologic condition causing obstruction, stridor, or apnea. Thoracoscopy provides visualization of the chest wall and visceral pleura for diagnosis of diffuse or localized pulmonary disease. An intrathoracic biopsy can be obtained via a thoracoscope.

Pectus Excavatum

Pectus excavatum, a congenital malformation of the chest wall, is characterized by a pronounced funnel-shaped concave depression over the lower end of the sternum beginning at the angle of Lewis and extending to the xyphoid. Cardiopulmonary impairment can result from extreme pectus excavatum during the pubertal growth period. Children with moderate to severe forms have displacement of the heart and lung tissue, which results in exercise intolerance and chest pain. Pectus is more common in males than females.

Minimally invasive procedures have been developed that require a curved metal bar to be slid under the ribs to elevate the sunken part (Fig. 8.29). No ribs or cartilage are removed. Thoracoscopic vision is used to guide the metal bar through two incisions made in the bilateral chest at the level of T4-5 interspace. The bar is secured to the ribs on each side to maintain the elevation of the deformity. Each bar is individually tailored to the recipient. The patient remains in the hospital for 2 to 3 days to be monitored for complications and frequently has a thoracic epidural for pain management. Movement is restricted during convalescence. The child must remain supine with a small pillow under the head. Side lying or twisting can cause a shift in the bar. The child can return to school within 2 weeks.

The Nuss procedure, developed in 1987 by Dr. Donald Nuss, is less complicated in younger children because the cartilage is softer and less calcified. Teens and young adults can have the procedure performed successfully, but their osseous tissue is less flexible. The bar is removed after 2 to 3 years as an outpatient procedure.

The deformity can be corrected during an open procedure with resection of lower intercostal cartilages and substernal ligaments to free up the sternum in a procedure referred to as the Ravitch repair. The sternum is elevated, and the cartilages are fitted to the sides of the sternum. Some pediatric surgeons believe that endoscopic approaches minimize chest wall scarring that could minimize physical motion.

Care is taken to try to avoid extreme positioning of the arm in abduction by suspending the arm rather than exceeding a 90-degree angle of shoulder-arm positioning. Occasionally a pediatric patient has transient postoperative brachial plexus injury

7 Neck bones
(cervical vertebrae)

12 Back bones
(thoracic vertebrae)

5 Waist bones
(lumbar vertebrae)

5 Joined bones
at the seat
(sacrum)

• **Fig. 8.28** Levels of spina bifida.

Metal bar

• **Fig. 8.29** Pectus excavatum.

caused by extremes of arm positioning during the procedure for the insertion of the bar and the camera.

Risks of the Nuss procedure include bleeding, cardiac perforation, pericardial effusion, pneumothorax, and dysrhythmias. Chest asymmetry in older children may necessitate surgical adjustment and the insertion of double chest bars and side stabilizers.

Pectus Carinatum

Pectus carinatum is a protrusion of the breastbone. The cartilage buckles and causes pain. The condition progresses during periods of growth. The chest is rigid and stationary in a full inspiration position. Respiratory effort is compromised and uses the diaphragm and accessory muscles instead of the normal processes. Pulmonary function is diminished, and emphysema can develop. The condition may be genetically mediated and increases in severity with age.

Pectus carinatum is seen in combination with some connective tissue disorders such as Marfan syndrome or Ehlers-Danlos syndrome. Some cases have scoliosis and mitral valve prolapse. Other vascular disease is sometimes present.

In mild cases the patient wears a brace across the chest for 12 to 18 months. In moderate to severe cases a transverse incision is made across the chest for an open correction. Bilateral wedges are removed from the ribs, and excess cartilage over the sternum is removed to correct the condition. The perichondrium is left in place to grow over the excised area. The patient needs to remain hospitalized for several days. Outcomes are usually excellent.

Cardiovascular Surgery

Congenital cardiovascular defects are the result of abnormal embryologic development of the heart or major vessels. During fetal life, blood bypasses the lungs through the foramen ovale and the ductus arteriosus to the placenta. From the placenta the blood bypasses the liver through the ductus venosus. The right ventricle (RV) pumps 66% of the circulation, and the left ventricle (LV) pumps 34%. At birth the pulmonary ventilation is established during the first breath and the increasing atmospheric pressure causes increased left atrial force that in turn causes the foramen ovale to close. The right atrial pressure drops, causing the blood flow to reverse. The ductus arteriosus usually closes after 15 hours. Some neonates have a delay of 1 to 3 weeks for complete closure of the ductus.

Most cardiovascular defects are diagnosed before birth or in infancy, often when symptoms of congestive heart failure develop within the first few days or months after birth.[9] Corrective or palliative procedures are necessary to sustain or prolong the life of these infants. Many of these cardiovascular procedures are enhanced by or are made possible with the use of hypothermia and cardiopulmonary bypass. However, significant brain damage may be associated with a cardiovascular bypass in infants. Bypass perfusion time should not exceed 40 minutes between periods of temporary normal circulatory perfusion.

The use of robotics has revolutionized the field of pediatric cardiac surgery because the dexterity of the surgeon is enhanced in a small, confined space. Implantable materials such as grafts and valves have reduced the rate of reoperation. Congenital cardiovascular defects in infants or children that are amenable to conventional or endoscopic surgical intervention include, but are not limited to, the conditions covered in the following sections.

Anomalous Venous Return

Failure of any one pulmonary vein or a combination of these veins to return blood to the left atrium precludes the full complement of oxygenated blood from entering the systemic circulation. The anomalous pulmonary vein or veins are transferred and anastomosed to the left atrium.

Coarctation of the Aorta

A coarctation is a narrowing or stricture in a vessel. This is one of the more common congenital cardiovascular defects; it usually occurs in the aortic arch. It may cause hypertension in the upper extremities above the obstruction and hypotension in the lower extremities from slowed circulation below the coarctation. For correction of the defect the coarctation is resected and the aorta may be anastomosed end to end. An aortic patch graft may be necessary when the length of the coarctation prevents anastomosis. A subclavian flap angioplasty capable of growth in length and width is referred to as the Waldhausen procedure.

Patent Ductus Arteriosus

During fetal life the ductus arteriosus carries blood from the pulmonary artery to the aorta to bypass the lungs. Normally this vessel closes in the first 24 hours after birth to prevent recirculation of arterial blood through the body. If closure does not occur, blood flow may be reversed by aortic pressure, which causes respiratory distress (Fig. 8.30).

Signs of patent ductus arteriosus (PDA) include widening pulse pressure and a characteristic murmur. The incidence of PDA is 10% of all congenital cardiac defects; PDA is usually diagnosed by 1 month of age. Surgical intervention is indicated, in lieu of prolonged ventilatory support, to prevent development of chronic pulmonary changes. The PDA can be clamped and ligated with ligating clips or suture in an open procedure or occluded with a coil using a transcatheter approach or endoscopically with a thoracoscope.

Septal Defects

An open-heart procedure with cardiopulmonary bypass is necessary to close abnormal openings in the walls (septa) separating the chambers within the heart.

Atrial Septal Defect

An opening in the septum between the right and left atria may be sufficiently large to allow oxygenated blood to shunt from left to right and return to the lungs (Fig. 8.31). An atrial septal defect (ASD) can increase pulmonary blood flow, with resultant pulmonary hypertension, if the defect is not closed. The incidence of ASD is 8% to 14% of all congenital heart defects; the defect can remain asymptomatic until adulthood. Signs include acyanosis, thin body stature, and decreased tolerance to exercise. ASD is more common in females than in males (4:1). If the defect cannot be closed with sutures, a patch graft is inserted.

Ventricular Septal Defect

A ventricular septal defect (VSD) is usually located in the membranous portion of the septum between the right and left ventricles (Fig. 8.32). It is the most common of the congenital heart anomalies (25–30% of all congenital cardiac defects). Signs include alternation between cyanosis and acyanosis.

Patients with small defects are relatively asymptomatic, and repair may be unnecessary. One-third of the small defects spontaneously close by age 2 years. Large defects with left-to-right shunting of oxygenated blood back to the lungs, which increases pulmonary hypertension, become symptomatic by age 2 months. A patch graft may be necessary to close the defect.

Atrioventricular Canal Defect

An atrioventricular canal defect is present if the atrioventricular canal of connective tissue that normally divides the heart into four

• **Fig. 8.31** Atrial septal defect.

• **Fig. 8.30** Patent ductus arteriosus.

• **Fig. 8.32** Ventricular septal defect.

chambers has failed to develop. Deficiencies are present in the lower portion of the interatrial septum, upper portion of the interventricular septum, and tricuspid and mitral valves. The result is a large central canal that permits blood flow between any of the four chambers of the heart.

A corrective procedure referred to as the Rastelli procedure involves repair of mitral and tricuspid valves and patch grafts to close septal defects. Creation of a competent mitral valve is of utmost importance to relieve pulmonary hypertension.

Tetralogy of Fallot

Tetralogy of Fallot is a combination of four defects (Fig. 8.33):
1. VSD (large)
2. Stenosis or atresia of the pulmonary valve or outflow tract into the pulmonary artery
3. Hypertrophy of the right ventricle
4. Dextroposition (displacement) of the aorta to the right so that it receives blood from both ventricles

Often referred to as "blue babies," infants with tetralogy of Fallot are cyanotic because insufficient oxygen circulates to body tissues. The incidence is 8% of all congenital cardiac defects; the defect is commonly associated with Down syndrome.[9] Total correction of the multiple anomalies is difficult. Assessment of the technical ease of correction is generally the dominant consideration. If cyanosis is severe, one of the following palliative shunt procedures may be performed during infancy to increase pulmonary blood flow:

- *Blalock-Taussig procedure:* The right subclavian artery is anastomosed, end to side, with the corresponding pulmonary artery (Fig. 8.34). Mixed arteriovenous blood from the aorta flows through the shunt to the pulmonary artery and into the lungs for oxygenation. A modification of this includes the use of a conduit graft, such as Gore-Tex.
- *Potts-Smith-Gibson procedure:* The descending aorta is anastomosed, side to side, with the left pulmonary artery (Fig. 8.35). The shunt enlarges as the child grows, but it is more difficult to reconstruct than a Blalock-Taussig shunt later, when a corrective procedure is performed.
- *Glenn procedure:* The superior vena cava is anastomosed with the right pulmonary artery. Modern versions are bidirectional and allow flow to the right and left pulmonary arteries.
- *Waterston procedure:* The ascending aorta is anastomosed with the right pulmonary artery (Fig. 8.36). The anastomosis is placed on the posterior aspect of the aorta to provide perfusion to both pulmonary arteries.

With cardiopulmonary bypass and hypothermia, the VSD is closed with a patch graft that also corrects the abnormal communication between the right ventricle and the aorta. Then the obstruction to pulmonary blood flow is relieved. This may include enlarging the pulmonary valve or widening the outflow tract. Resection of obstructing cardiac muscle may be necessary with insertion of a prosthetic outflow patch.

An aortic allograft that contains the aortic valve with the septal leaflet of the mitral valve and the ascending aorta attached may be inserted. The septal leaflet of the mitral valve is used as a portion of the right ventricular outflow patch. All or part of the aortic

• **Fig. 8.34** Blalock-Taussig repair.

• **Fig. 8.35** Potts-Smith-Gibson repair.

• **Fig. 8.33** Tetralogy of Fallot.

• **Fig. 8.36** Waterston procedure.

valve and ascending aorta is used as a new conduit with the pulmonary artery or as a patch graft.

Transposition of the Great Vessels

In a transposition the aorta arises from the right ventricle and the pulmonary artery arises from the left ventricle (Fig. 8.37). This creates essentially two separate circulatory systems, one systemic and the other pulmonary, but they are not interconnected as in normal anatomy. Life depends on the presence or creation of associated defects to permit exchange of blood between the two systems.

The incidence of complete transposition of the great vessels is 10% of all cardiovascular defects. Males are affected more than females (2:1). A palliative procedure, such as one of the following, is performed in the newborn to improve oxygenation and sustain life until the infant grows enough to tolerate a corrective procedure:

- *Rashkind procedure, or balloon septostomy:* In the cardiac catheterization laboratory, with fluoroscopy, a balloon catheter (deflated) is advanced into the right atrium, through the foramen ovale, and into the left atrium. The balloon is inflated and pulled backward out of the left atrium across the atrial septum to enlarge the foramen ovale, thus creating an ASD.
- *Park procedure:* In the cardiac catheterization laboratory, with fluoroscopy, a catheter with a knife tip is passed through the right atrium to enlarge the opening of the foramen ovale.
- *Blalock-Hanlon procedure:* Atrial septectomy is done to create an ASD. A segment of the right atrium is excised.
- *Pulmonary artery banding:* The pulmonary artery is constricted in the presence of a large VSD to prevent irreversible pulmonary vascular obstructive changes from developing.

A corrective procedure, such as one of the following, is usually performed when the child is between 18 and 36 months of age:

- *Mustard procedure, atrial switch:* An intraatrial baffle made of pericardial tissue is sutured between the pulmonary veins and the mitral valve and between the mitral and tricuspid valves. The baffle directs systemic venous return into the left ventricle and lungs and allows pulmonary venous return to enter the right ventricle and aorta.
- *Senning procedure, atrial switch:* Flaps of the intraatrial septum and right atrial wall form new venous channels to divert pulmonary venous blood flow. Any atrial or septal defects are closed.

- *Jatene procedure, atrial switch:* The aorta and pulmonary artery are anatomically switched (i.e., transposed). This procedure is useful in infants with a VSD or a large PDA in addition to transposition of the great arteries.

Tricuspid Atresia

The absence (atresia) of a tricuspid valve between the right atrium and ventricle prevents normal blood flow through the chambers of the heart. Blood flows through an ASD, into an enlarged left ventricle, and through a small rudimentary right ventricle to the pulmonary artery. Anastomosis of the superior vena cava with the right pulmonary artery or an aorticopulmonic artery shunt may be created as a palliative procedure to increase pulmonary blood flow in infancy. When the child is 3 or 4 years old, the corrective reconstructive Fontan procedure is performed. This procedure involves direct anastomosis of the pulmonary artery to the right atrium to create a connection between the pulmonary and systemic venous circulation.

Truncus Arteriosus

In truncus arteriosus a single great artery carries blood directly from the heart (with a large associated VSD) to the coronary, pulmonary, and systemic circulatory systems. A single tricuspid valve is present with two to six cusps. Initial palliative banding of the pulmonary arteries, as close to their origins off the truncus as possible, decreases pulmonary blood flow in an infant with congestive heart failure. At a later stage a corrective procedure can be performed to close the VSD and insert a conduit with an ascending aortic graft and aortic valve. Correction in infancy necessitates replacement of the conduit as the child grows. Incidence of this defect is 1% of all congenital cardiovascular defects.

Valvular Stenosis

Congenital aortic or pulmonary valve stenosis necessitates valvotomy, which is also referred to as the Brock procedure. An incision is made into the valve to open the narrowed or constrictive area obstructing blood flow.

Hypoplastic Left Heart Syndrome

Hypoplastic left heart syndrome is the most common cause of cardiac death in the first week of life. The left ventricle is severely underdeveloped (Fig. 8.38). The severity of the situation can vary according to the multitude of defects that can be present. The

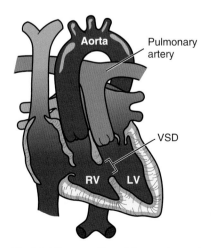

• **Fig. 8.37** Transposition of the great vessels.

• **Fig. 8.38** Hypoplastic left heart syndrome.

systemic perfusion of the aorta is entirely through a patent ductus arteriosus. The right ventricle is overloaded, and the patient is extremely dusky. The patient is in complete heart failure within 28 hours of life. The only real immediate treatment is cardiac transplant. Hearts available for neonatal transplant are few.

Postoperative Pediatric Patient Care

The patient is taken to a postanesthesia care unit (PACU) for observation. Larger facilities have a PACU specifically designed to accommodate phase I and II pediatric patients. Parents or guardians are typically permitted in the pediatric PACU. The patient usually finds comfort in the presence of parents or guardians. The pediatric patient is never to be left unattended.

The PACU nurse receives the postanesthesia report from the anesthesia provider and a postprocedure report from the perioperative nurse. Vital signs are taken and include temperature, pulse, respirations, and blood pressure. The objective signs found in the head-to-toe assessment are compared with preoperative baseline values. Cardiac monitoring and pulse oximetry are done. Physical assessment is performed and compared with other data obtained about the patient. Fluid intake and output are evaluated. The surgical site is inspected. Specific physician orders pertaining to treatments and laboratory work are carried out.

The patient's recovery is evaluated at 5 to 15-minute intervals as the patient emerges from anesthesia to a more alert state. Each evaluation is documented in the patient's record per facility policy. The patient is discharged from the PACU when specific physiologic parameters are reached according to departmental policy. The anesthesia provider is responsible for the patient in the PACU and is responsible for release criteria.

The parents or guardians are instructed in postoperative home care and are informed about signs and symptoms that should be reported to the physician. The instructions should be given verbally and in writing with the appropriate emergency phone consult numbers included. Directions for prescription medications such as antibiotics or analgesics should be explained to the parents or guardians by the PACU nurse. Pediatric patients who are of an age of reason and understanding should be addressed directly and given the opportunity to ask questions.

Within 24 to 48 hours after discharge a postoperative phone call should be made as a follow-up to care. Pertinent information should be exchanged about the care of the patient and progress in recovery. The caller should be qualified to answer questions about the procedure and the recovery phase. Patient and family satisfaction should be evaluated. Some facilities ask the parent to call in during the evening hours to give an update to the PACU nurse.

ⓔ EVOLVE WEBSITE

http://evolve.elsevier.com/Hornacky/BerryKohn/

- Student Interactive Questions
- Glossary

References

1. de Beaufort C, van den Akker A, Kuijper C, et al.: The importance of screening for additional anomalies in patients with anorectal malformations: a retrospective cohort study, *J Pediatr Surg* 58(9):1699–1707, 2023.
2. Goldstick J, Cunningham R, Carter P, et al.: Current causes of death in children and adolescents in the United States, *N Engl J Med* 386(20):1955–1956, 2022.
3. Centers for Disease Control and Prevention: CDC Wonder. www.wonder.cdc.gov. Accessed April 3, 2023.
4. Saracho ON: Theories of child development and their impact on early childhood education and care, *Early Child Educ J* 51(15–30), 2023.
5. Resnick C, Ball J, Dains J, et al: Age-specific examination: infants, children, and adolescents, *Seidel's physical examination handbook*, ed 10, St. Louis, 2023, Elsevier, pp 269–296.
6. Lombardo A, Gundeti M: Review of robot-assisted laparoscopic surgery in management of infant congenital urology: advances and limitations in utilization and learning, *Int J Urol* 30(3):250–257, 2022.
7. Malkova T, Borzunov D: International recognition of the Ilizarov bone reconstruction techniques: current practice and research (dedicated to 100th birthday of G.A. Ilizarov), *World J Orthop* 12(8):515–533, 2021.
8. Kosko J, Nimmons G, Raisen J: In-office insertion tympanostomy tubes in children using single-pass device, *Laryngoscope Investig Otolaryngol* 6(2):325–331, 2021.
9. American Heart Association: www.heart.org. Accessed April 12, 2023.

Perioperative Geriatrics

CHAPTER OUTLINE

Perspectives on Aging, 161

Perioperative Assessment of the Geriatric Patient, 164

Intraoperative Considerations, 174

Postoperative Considerations, 175

CHAPTER OBJECTIVES

After studying this chapter the learner will be able to:

- Discuss the theories of aging.
- Describe how comorbidity influences the care of geriatric patients.
- List the effects of aging on four body systems.
- Identify the effects of surgery on the geriatric patient.

KEY TERMS AND DEFINITIONS

Aged Social and legislative policies define aged as 65 years. Physiologic evaluation terms incorporate aged as 75 years.

Caregiver Any person who provides physical and emotional care and help with activities of daily living for another individual.

Comorbidity Two or more medical conditions in addition to current diagnosis.

Frailty syndrome Age-related decline in skeletal muscle that may predict the risk for postoperative complications.

Gerontology The study of aging and the older adult in all phases of life: sociologic, biologic, psychologic, and physiologic.

Life cycle The span of time and events from birth to death.

Longevity The condition of living a prolonged life span.

Sarcopenia Loss of skeletal muscle mass, quality, and function caused by inactivity or altered metabolism that can be a predictor of postoperative complications.

Senescence The process of growing old.

Senile The state or process of aging. Derived from the Latin word *senex*, meaning "old man" or "old age." Aging takes place at all biologic levels.

Perspectives on Aging

The process of aging is an orderly transformation of the body and mind that begins with birth and concludes with death. Gerontology is the study of elderly people. People older than 65 years are often considered old or elderly. In actuality, persons with advanced age may maintain functional capabilities throughout their lifetime until adaptation to biologic, psychologic, or social influences is no longer sufficient to sustain the independent activities of daily living (ADLs). The main influences on the aging process are genetics, environment, and lifestyle.

Data about the changes that occur as the result of natural processes and environmental exposure are inconclusive because the only data available are those derived from comparisons among existing generations. The experiences and exposures of these generations have been vastly different and widely influenced by the period of the life span and senescence.[1] No normal measurements are available on which to base the parameters of the aging process.

Life expectancy increased steadily over the years with major advancements in the study of disease processes, prevention, and treatment. According to the U.S. Social Security Life Expectancy Calculator 2022, males born in 2023 might expect to live to age 83 years and females might expect to live to age 86.9 years. With the increasing age of the "baby boomer" population (those born between the years of 1946 and 1964), over 78 million people will be over the age of 65 by 2035. These ages do not account for lifestyle or comorbidity. The increase in life expectancy and the decrease in mortality mean that the largest patient population will be geriatric patients—the fastest-growing segment of the population.

There will be more than 95 million geriatric patients by 2060. The U.S. Census Bureau calculated that more than 38 million people over the age of 50 were living alone.[2] The statistics indicate a problem because research is seeing an increase in loneliness, mental health problems, isolation, and conditions that lead to higher comorbidities, thus increasing the need for medical and housing resources. The United Nations have declared the years

2021 to 2030 the Decade of Healthy Ageing. Many programs, public awareness campaigns, and resources are available at www.who.int to help the elderly population live independent lives.

As the life expectancy of the geriatric population increases, so does the incidence of comorbidity. Comorbidity is the existence of two or more disease processes in a single individual (e.g., coronary artery disease in a patient who has osteoporosis and also may be hypertensive and diabetic). It is the most common negative influence on the health status and functional ability of geriatric patients. A chronic condition affects recovery after surgical intervention, and many geriatric patients have multiple chronic or debilitating health problems. Comorbidity is also a major consideration in the attainment of expected outcomes; all medical diagnoses should be considered in the development of the plan of care.

Another consideration is the frailty syndrome, which is a natural process that accompanies aging. The frailty syndrome is a collection of physiologic changes that affects organ systems and older adult patients' reserves, leading to increased morbidity and loss of independence.[3] In combination with comorbidity, frailty can predispose patients to unfavorable outcomes in the perioperative environment. Clinical frailty scales are available to assess the needs of the patient and put plans in place to achieve better surgical outcomes and return to daily activities. Sarcopenia is a loss of muscular strength and function that significantly increases after 70 years of age. Body mass index (BMI) shifts because of weight loss, but it can shift in obese patients, who maintain a high BMI with decreased muscle mass. Sarcopenia can be a factor leading to weakness, falls, or permanent disability.

Aging is viewed from many perspectives, some positive and some negative. The positive aspects involve respect for maturity and the wealth of knowledge gleaned from experiences. The negative aspects involve the debilitation, pervading weaknesses, and dependence that can occur during the closure of life. Philosophers tend to focus on the positive inner peace derived from the wisdom acquired over many years. The view of aging adopted by individuals is based in part on the view of aging created by their cultural background. Geographic, financial, educational, religious, and subjective influences shape the prototype of the older adult's place in society.

Cultural Considerations

Positive views of aging are found in many cultures that can trace their heritage back for many generations. Repetitious storytelling and historical accounts support the cultural growth of an individual from youth to old age. Many cultures appreciate, honor, and respect their older members for experience and maturity. Growing old with dignity is not feared or deemed repulsive. A positive view of aging may be observed in an individual who is a first-generation immigrant to a new land because they may not have assimilated the value systems of the new environment. The individual may have retained many time-honored beliefs of the country of origin; the values are held dear and are deeply ingrained.

Negative views of aging may be generated by cultures that are primarily youth-oriented. Most members of these societies are second- and third-generation descendants of immigrants. They have developed value systems that do not reflect their country of origin. In a close community, values are supported within the belief structure of the group as a whole.

A culture is a set of structured social behaviors and personal beliefs that enable an individual to respond to social situations and relationships within a close community. The foundation of human relationships in a culture is more than ethnicity or race. Specific cultural practices such as dietary habits, lifestyle, and hygiene should be of concern to the perioperative nurse. For example, a patient's physical condition may be a direct result of a traditional activity, such as fasting during holy days. A geriatric patient who has been fasting may appear dehydrated, malnourished, or confused.

The perioperative nurse also should be aware of gender identity. Some patients may have significant others of the same sex and hide the information because it is "taboo" or prohibited within the culture or portrayed as a younger person's lifestyle. Same-sex relationships may have been legally sanctioned like a marriage. Spousal relationships are treated equally.

The psychologic assessment may reflect a high risk for an alteration in self-image because although patients may feel comfortable in their culture, they may have had a negative interaction with societal influences. For example, the media glorify young bodies and degrade the natural aging process, with advertisers using models that reflect the desirable aspects of youth and beauty. Cultural climate has a direct effect on the geriatric patient. The expected outcomes of the geriatric patient undergoing a surgical intervention are influenced by cultural views of aging and those of society as a whole.

Theories of Aging

Biologic, psychologic, and ethnocultural factors influence the way an individual ages. The extrinsic influences surrounding the physical and psychosocial components depend on the interaction of persons with the environment and their view of health and wellness. Many older people tend to optimistically overstate their actual health status and minimize or dismiss symptoms as age-related. The intrinsic influences on the aging process are also interdependent, but to a less controllable degree. Certain inherited traits, such as pathologic conditions, are continued through the generations.

Each aged individual is unique. Perioperative nurses should understand the distinct aspects of each geriatric patient before developing a plan of care. Generic care plans do not address the specific problems, needs, and health considerations of the individual. Understanding the theories of the aging process enables the perioperative nurse to provide care throughout the surgical experience that optimizes the attainment of identified expected outcomes. The following theories explain aging and the life cycle as they are defined by science and research.

Wear-and-Tear Theory

The wear-and-tear theory suggests that the body loses its ability to keep pace with life processes. The sustenance of life suffers because the body begins to deteriorate in a natural wearing-down process. The body continually tries to maintain homeostasis but degenerates over time because of cellular loss and destruction caused by interactions with the environment. During this process the body becomes increasingly vulnerable to injury and disease. If a disease state occurs, the body is less able to maintain normal homeostasis and even less able to tolerate the assault of illness. Eventually the body is unable to support life and ceases to function. Examples of wear and tear include, but are not limited to, the following scenarios:

- Prolonged exposure to the sun and other external sources can cause breakdown of the skin. Thinning of the skin makes bedridden or inactive people vulnerable to pressure sores.
- Turbulent blood flow in the areas of bifurcation of blood vessels may cause rupture if the vessels are weakened by arteriosclerosis.
- Abuse of chemical substances and alcohol can damage liver and brain cells. Nicotine is responsible for many effects of smoking. Although these effects are self-induced rather than the result of natural wear and tear, they do affect health status.
- Wearing of muscles and joints can lead to risk for falls. Fracturing a hip, head injuries, or broken bones can lead to immobility.

Genetic Mutation Theory

DNA has been a target for age-related changes because it preserves the ongoing genetic message for cell replication and organism maintenance. DNA is a template, or coding mechanism, for the preservation of the life processes of cellular structures. Various agents damage DNA codes through physical, chemical, or biologic interactions. An alteration in the structure of DNA can cause an organism to change. This alteration can occur within the cell itself or be caused by a force in the environment. Mutated DNA cannot perform the processes necessary for normal cell activities. A cell containing wrongly coded DNA continues to replicate itself in the wrong patterns. It does not return to normal.

In the aging process, DNA may mutate for a variety of reasons and continues to produce the wrong types of cells during replication. For example, skin cells may be deficient in collagen or in the elastic properties associated with supple tissue. As a result, the skin replication process may yield drier, less elastic skin. This is characteristic of the skin of an older person. In certain circumstances the mutated DNA could cause tumor production or other pathologic conditions, such as skin cancers.

Major organ systems affected by these changes are the central nervous system, the musculoskeletal system, and the cardiovascular system. Other systems affected include the gastrointestinal, genitourinary, endocrine, and integumentary systems. Essentially, all body systems change during the aging process as part of the frailty syndrome.

Viral Theory

Researchers have approached the concept that viruses may invade human cells and remain inactive until the body loses its ability to suppress them. This theory is closely linked to the genetic mutation theory because the virus can hide undetected in the DNA for many years. The replication process of the virus is comparable to the replication of DNA. Some viruses are able to use genetic materials as a disguise to fool the body's immune system. The body does not recognize the virus as an invader or foreign substance.

The mechanism of viral activation is unknown but is very injurious to the body. Major targets include the endocrine, nervous, and immune systems. The incubation period may be several decades. Because the viral theory has no proof, a treatment or cure is unknown.

Environmental Theory

Exposure to natural and synthetic elements in the environment may accelerate the aging process. Although climate is often blamed for an increased rate of aging, studies indicate that the natural flow of the aging process is comparable among different geographic regions. Tropical climates are cited most often as areas of premature aging. Studies of tropical populations show that aging is not accelerated by the temperature, although mortality in these areas is affected by poor nutrition, parasites, and tropical diseases.

Extremes of climate do not seem to accelerate the aging process. Cold environments may cause a reduction in body temperature and metabolic rates, which could slow the aging process. Studies involving Eskimo populations have shown that despite the difficult conditions of their lifestyles, blood pressure and cholesterol measurements do not vary significantly between the ages of 20 and 54 years. Mortality is affected by the harshness of the cold climate and the risk for physical injury or death associated with hunting and lifestyle practices. The Centers for Disease Control and Prevention (CDC) provide tables of life expectancy based on census data collected. Individuals in certain areas showed longevity, especially in colder climates.

Altitude has not been shown to accelerate the aging process. Results of studies performed among indigenous people of Peru have shown stable blood pressures in a range lower than that of people living at sea level. The incidence of ischemic heart disease is lower at higher altitudes. In several documented communities of mountain-dwelling people, many residents were older than 100 years.

Ionizing radiation has been targeted as a cause of environmentally accelerated aging, but studies have not shown this to be true. Relevant evidence has shown that exposure to ionizing radiation does accelerate disease processes and pathologic conditions such as skin cancer, blood dyscrasias, and reproductive anomalies. Populations living in areas where nuclear tests frequently occurred have not shown signs of rapid aging compared with control groups in nuclear-free areas. The most significant finding was an increase in leukemia and skin tumors.

Pollution causes many physiologic changes in the body. Chemicals in air, food, and water supplies have been shown to increase the incidence of health decline and disability. Exposure to many different pollutants throughout the life span can dramatically shorten an individual's life expectancy through pathologic processes such as chronic lead poisoning, pesticides, water pollution, and lung cancer.

Physical Factor Theory

Free radicals are being investigated as a potential cause of premature aging. Free radicals represent imbalances between the production and the elimination of unstable chemical compounds in the body. More research is needed to prove or disprove this theory.

Low-calorie diets do not alter the aging process in humans. In populations studied for dietary habits no increase in the life span is evident between control groups and groups that have a low calorie intake. The most remarkable factor is the lack of increase in body weight after 30 years of age. A low-calorie diet may range between 1500 and 2500 kcal per day depending on body size and sex. Notably, low-calorie diets are usually deficient in animal protein. Aged individuals who have low-calorie diets generally have lower blood pressure and lower serum cholesterol levels, with no significant change throughout the aging process. Subcutaneous fat deposits do not increase with age.

High-calorie diets that exceed 3200 kcal per day for men and 2200 kcal per day for women have the opposite effect on aging.

An increase in caloric intake is accompanied by an increase in body mass that causes the individual to decrease body mobility. This is particularly evident in Euro-American populations, who often show a steady increase in weight up to the age of 60 years. Women in particular experience a thickening in fat deposits as they mature. Blood pressure and serum cholesterol levels steadily increase. The most significant elevations begin at age 50 years, with the development of coronary artery heart disease and atherosclerosis.

Animal fat content and excess calories are not the only considerations in the dietary aspect of aging and health. Vegetarians do not always follow a low-calorie pattern. They also can have a diet rich in fats, particularly if they consume saturated fats in the form of coconut oil. Salt is another consideration in the aging of the cardiovascular system. Diets high in sodium tend to increase circulating blood volume, thereby increasing systolic blood pressure. Studies have shown that an increase in systolic blood pressure significantly increases the risk for heart disease and stroke.

Exercise plays an important role in the health of the aging individual. Most populations studied have an exercise regimen linked to their ADLs. People in cultures characterized by many intrinsic diseases, parasites, malnutrition, poor hygiene, and harsh living conditions have remarkable physical fitness because of the amount of exercise they must perform to sustain life. People in societies in which the inhabitants are overfed and underexercised do not enjoy good health in the same manner as the moderately fed and highly exercised residents of less advantaged societies.

As the body ages, the endocrine system declines and the hormones responsible for the regulation of many interrelated body systems decrease in volume. Beta cells of the pancreas, thyroid, ovaries (in females), and testes (in males) exhibit less activity, which affects many other organ systems. For example:

- A decrease in estrogen production can increase the risk for osteoporosis and heart disease in women.
- A decrease in thyroid activity decreases the basal metabolic rate and increases weight gain.
- A decrease in the efficiency of insulin production decreases the efficiency of glucose metabolism.
- A decrease in testosterone production may decrease the libido in men.

Myths About Aging

Many misconceptions and myths surround the process of aging. Myths are stories created to explain the practices or beliefs of unknown origin regarding a person, place, or event. The creation of a myth about aging may be based on an isolated incident or a single observation and may not apply to all older adults.

Some myths have a small basis in fact, but most are unfounded and have a harmful effect on social policy and interpersonal relationships. Myths about the aging process may result in negative stereotypes, and a belief in negative stereotypes results in discrimination and improper treatment of the aging individual. Abnormal signs, symptoms, or behaviors exhibited by a geriatric patient usually indicate the presence of a pathologic process and should not be discounted as normal expectations of the aging process. Some of the negative myths about aging are as follows:

- *Myth:* Older adults are senile. *Truth:* If mental processes decline, a contributing factor, such as stroke, carotid insufficiency, or Alzheimer disease, is usually the cause.
- *Myth:* Older adults do not engage in sexual behavior. *Truth:* Sexual desire remains throughout the life span. Sexual activity may decline because of decreased physical mobility, circulatory impairment, or the unavailability of a partner. Self-gratification may be the only outlet.
- *Myth:* Older adults always decline in health after a surgical procedure. *Truth:* The identification of problems, needs, and health considerations during the assessment phase of the nursing process decreases the probability of unmet expected outcomes.
- *Myth:* Older adults should not drive. They cause more accidents. *Truth:* Teenage drivers between the ages of 16 and 19 years have the highest rates for car accidents. They are also the group with the highest death-related accidents according to the CDC. Older individuals must keep a current driver's license through renewal, pass the eye examination, and retake a road test if safety is a question. After the age of 70, an application for renewal must be completed around every 3 years or as determined by each individual state.
- *Myth:* Older adults are not capable of using technology. *Truth:* A 2020 study found that 60% of adults over 65 years old are using technology daily.[4] The use of computers, smartphones, tablets, and smartwatches have given seniors more independence to pay bills online, order groceries and other items, get daily news, call or video chat with friends and family, monitor medical conditions, play games, read, and engage in social media. Technology users were happier, less lonely, and felt safer and more independent.

Myths and stereotypes should not be allowed to influence the assessment of geriatric patients. Every aspect of the physical, psychosocial, and ethnocultural data should be assessed as unique to each individual and not as a generic group expectation. Reaching the age of 65 years does not instantly transform individuals into being old and debilitated.

As people grow older, they may experience more developmental aging before they experience physical aging. Some people become frail as they age, but this is not true of everyone. Age alone does not make individuals less productive members of society. Limitations and disabilities may be decreased because of scientific advances and a better understanding of the aging process and health-promotion activities.

Perioperative Assessment of the Geriatric Patient

The patient's ability to adapt to aging should be assessed by the perioperative nurse as part of the nursing process. With the exception of nursing diagnoses directly associated with the anticipated surgical procedure, specific nursing diagnoses should be associated with the patient's adaptation to the aging process. If positive adaptation has not been met, the risk is high for an augmentation of existing health conditions, such as a cardiovascular incident (e.g., stroke, myocardial infarction, hypertensive crisis). Comorbidity is a leading cause of death among older adults. More than 80% of all geriatric patients have more than one medical diagnosis capable of causing death; therefore recognition of potential problems in the attainment of expected outcomes is as important as identification of actual problems.[5]

Geriatric patients may present to the perioperative environment for urgent or emergent surgery because of the clinical signs and symptoms associated with a life-threatening illness. Common urgent problems include intestinal obstruction, ruptured diverticula, and orthopedic fractures. Vascular incidents such as a ruptured aneurysm or bleeding from the gastrointestinal tract necessitate immediate surgery. Sudden arterial occlusion that is unresponsive to chemical treatment is also considered emergent.

The postoperative phase of care is important to the well-being of the geriatric patient. Maintaining or improving the preoperative level of wellness should be considered a primary expected outcome. A preoperative functional assessment is the foundation of the plan of care. Baseline parameters vary to a high degree among individuals, and all patients do not age at the same rate. Some patients are very young at 70 years of age, and some are very old. The difference should be assessed, and optimal outcomes should be identified for each geriatric patient. Influences on the level of functioning include physical ability, psychosocial support and resources, and environmental interactions.

Functional Assessment

Functional assessment can serve multiple purposes. In the preoperative phase the plan of care includes the patient's unique differences, involvement of family and significant others, resources, and level of independence. Many of these data are obtained with observation, interview, and lifestyle questionnaires. The information may be obtained from the patient, family, or significant others. Gathering accurate information is important because many individuals do not like to admit any deficiencies.

Many aspects of the patient's unique nature are easily discerned during the preoperative interview. Adequate time should be allowed for the interview so the patient has time to reflect and respond. Reaction time slows with age. The nurse should listen for subtle modifications or inconsistencies in the patient's information regarding health status. Sensory deficits should be considered, and the environment should be modified as needed during the interview. The nurse should establish rapport and have respect for the patient's dignity.

During the intraoperative phase, the functional assessment may allow for anticipation of needed supplies or additional help to accommodate the patient's needs. The patient's physical capabilities allow some independence in self-care. Patients tend to regress when they are not permitted to do things for themselves. A self-care deficit takes place when a patient feels the loss of independence while restrained on an operating room (OR) bed. The freedom to assist with the transfer as able from the transport stretcher to the OR bed gives patients a sense of participation in their own care. Maintaining a high level of self-esteem and value enables patients to prevent emotional regression or loss of control.

Activities of Daily Living

During the course of a normal day an individual performs self-maintenance tasks and interacts with the environment. The ability to perform these ADLs is influenced by health status, emotions, mental clarity, and mobility. Limitations in performing these activities may be permanent or temporary, and many of the temporary limitations can be eliminated with medical or surgical treatment.

The perioperative nurse should assess the activity level of the geriatric patient. Advance preparations may need to be considered before the patient can undergo a surgical procedure. Because of identified physical limitations, special positioning or additional padding may be needed in combination with some form of communication assistance at the time the surgical procedure is performed. The functional baseline is the patient's capacity to perform self-care (e.g., feeding, bathing, toileting). Any deviation

from the baseline assessment in the postoperative phase should be recorded and reported to the patient's physician.

Functional Activities

The activity patterns of geriatric patients reflect many aspects of their daily lives. Their ability to feed, bathe, and toilet themselves is one way to measure physical and psychologic wellness. Basic daily activities such as grooming and dressing may be indicators of the level of the patient's involvement with personal care.

The range of self-care activities depends on various factors, such as whether the patient is active and mobile enough to shop for food and prepare meals or is living in assisted housing where these services are provided. The ability to provide self-care should be assessed preoperatively to evaluate the outcome in the postoperative phase (i.e., resumption of activity level).

Functional Capacity

A basic assessment of physical strength and endurance indicates whether the patient will be able to move from the transport stretcher to the OR bed. A patient who is weak or disabled by arthritis will need assistance or a total lift device. A patient who is visually impaired also may need assistance.

Communication through speech and hearing is vital to establishing the cognitive baseline. A hearing deficit or aphasia could be mistaken for a cognitive impairment. The patient who uses a hearing-assist device should be permitted to wear it to the OR and, if possible, throughout the surgical procedure. It should be in place during emergence from anesthesia so the patient can hear requests to deep breathe or move extremities.

The patient's sensory ability should be assessed. Tactile sensation dulls with age, and a patient's inability to feel external stimuli may lead to an inadvertent injury. Any sensory deficit, including a visual or hearing impairment, should be documented in the plan of care. The administration of a general anesthetic alters the tactile assessment parameter during the intraoperative phase of care.

As the patient emerges from anesthesia the postanesthesia recovery, nurses use the baseline assessment to measure the progress of the patient in the postoperative phase. Because of the interdependent aspects of the central nervous system with other vital physiologic systems, the evaluation of expected outcomes should include a sensory assessment.

Cognitive ability also should be assessed. The patient may be required to comprehend a command that is vital to the perioperative experience. A cognitive deficit may be of organic origin or result from a language barrier. Regardless of the reason, an inability to understand can cause anxiety for the patient and the caregiver. Alertness, short-term memory, capabilities to concentrate and problem-solve, and motivation toward self-care are areas of cognition that influence the ability of the geriatric patient to adapt to illness and recovery. A patient who is cognitively impaired experiences disorientation and responds inappropriately to the environment. The impairment may be temporary but often is prolonged after anesthesia. Cognitive impairment also may be a permanent or chronic condition.

The patient's psychologic state should be assessed preoperatively; a change in mood or temperament may indicate an unexpected outcome caused by an injury or a physical problem resulting from the surgical procedure. Dementia, delirium, and emotional depression are common in older adults. Sudden withdrawal or a change in affect should be investigated promptly.

External Interactions

The manner in which an individual experiences illness depends on external forces and the number of barriers that may interfere with the attainment of outcomes. The nursing diagnoses may include self-care deficit or impaired mobility. These diagnoses factor significantly in the postoperative phase and should be considered and placed in the plan of care. The reaction of patients to either one of these nursing diagnoses depends on interactions with the external environment, the availability of resources, and the presence of barriers.

Resources

The level of independence exercised by the geriatric patient may depend on the resources available. The type of housing may depend on self-care ability and financial security. In developing the plan of care the perioperative nurse should consider how the patient will meet postoperative needs at home. Will help be available or will arrangements for a visiting nurse or a family/significant other caregiver be needed? The patient's possible need for transportation to and from the surgeon's office for postoperative checkups should be considered. With age comes the need for assistance, especially after a surgical procedure. Many resources are available for home health care, transportation, nutrition, legal advice, learning, and discount programs. A variety of information can be found on the Internet, government agencies for the aging, local libraries, and health care facilities. Additional information is available on the following websites:

- www.ssa.gov
- www.americangeriatrics.org
- www.eldercare.acl.gov
- www.aarp.org
- www.noca.org (National Council on Aging)
- www.nia.nih.gov (National Institute on Aging)

Barriers

The type of housing may be a problem for the postoperative geriatric patient. If the patient lives alone in a multilevel dwelling, using the stairs may pose a significant problem. The location of the bathroom or kitchen may complicate the self-care process. Financial constraints may limit the number of home health care visits by an independent agency. The inability to drive may prevent the individual from getting necessary medication and food. The unavailability of family members may necessitate planning for institutionalization, which may be temporary but may become permanent.

The perioperative nurse should be aware of possible signs of elder abuse. According to the National Institute on Aging, some signs to look for include the following:

- Physical: bed sores, burns, bruises, malnutrition, trouble sleeping
- Emotional: agitation, depression, afraid
- Neglect: unbathed, body odor, dirty clothes
- Financial: the patient may be forced to sign over all assets to another person, a lawyer may have the patient sign papers before a mental evaluation is completed.

Psychosocial Assessment

Gathering data about geriatric patients should begin with the assessment of how the individuals view other aged people and their own progression through the aging process. The assessment

of a patient's self-concept may be an important indicator of a decline in the status of psychologic health. A patient's views of health and normative activity are influenced by culture and affect the attainment of outcomes.

If patients believe that older people are helpless, they may see the role of the aging process as one of helplessness. Although capable of many independent activities, individuals may adapt to an illness by becoming helpless. Even needing help temporarily may cause an older patient to believe that the condition is permanent. The perioperative nurse should be aware that the geriatric patient might experience a temporary period of helplessness. By establishing a functional baseline and stressing the temporary nature of postoperative recovery, the nurse can help patients return to their routine.

The geriatric patient may feel rejected, unsupported, and worthless. Geriatric patients experience higher rates of depression and an alteration in self-image. Depression is not part of the aging process. The physical decline may be rapid when psychologic well-being is threatened. The perioperative nurse should be aware that the geriatric patient who is depressed and lonely needs additional emotional support throughout the surgical experience.

Perioperative nurses should be aware of their own subjective views of aging and cultural attitudes and should not allow personal feelings to influence the assessment process. When assessing the geriatric patient the nurse should consider the culture of origin, the cultural influence of the patient's current residence, and the patient's subjective perception of wellness and illness.

Self-perception has a great influence on how well the geriatric patient adapts to aging. The nursing diagnoses should reflect the patient's adaptation because adaptation affects the attainment of the expected outcomes. The perioperative plan of care should reflect the need for ongoing evaluation by postoperative caregivers.

Adaptation to the Aging Process

An individual should make many adjustments during the aging process. The adaptation to aging is unique for each individual and is influenced by physical condition, psychologic strengths and weaknesses, family and significant others, social support systems, financial resources, and functional ability. The geriatric patient develops a belief system about life expectations primarily on the basis of subjective feelings.

If the patient's condition is in decline, the outlook is usually negative. Outcome can be based on how the patient feels at a particular time. If the patient is feeling well and able-bodied, the outlook is usually positive, which helps delay the patient's fear of declining health outside the expected parameters of aging.

The prevention of decline not related to normative aging is an important factor in avoiding health deficits. The patient who can postpone health problems caused by factors that include avoidable health considerations—accidents, poor nutrition, inactivity, depression, and the effects of loneliness, smoking, substance abuse, and obesity—enjoys a higher quality of life in the later years.

Self-Perception of Health

The patient's view of personal health plays an important role in the actual health status. If the patient perceives health as important, preventive health maintenance should be a priority. Patients who feel well perform ADLs to the best of their ability. Minor interruptions in health status do not cause a major problem in the long-term prognosis of the patient's return to baseline parameters.

Physical Assessment

The nurse should have the knowledge and understanding of the geriatric examination.[6] The physical assessment of the geriatric patient begins with general appearance. The perioperative nurse should first observe the patient from head to toe. The basic picture or image the patient creates can provide information about the health status. The patient should be assessed for posture, mobility, gait, rising or sitting, dexterity, body height and weight, abdominal girth, body odors, psychologic affect, communication, and comprehension of surroundings. The perioperative nurse should perform an assessment of the total patient by each body system. A summary of the physiologic changes associated with the normal aging process is provided in Table 9.1.

Any medications the patient takes on a routine or periodic basis should be listed on the chart, with the last dosages itemized. The patient should be encouraged to discuss all medications, including vitamins, cannabis, and topical ointments. Recreational drugs (e.g., street drugs, narcotics) should not be excluded from consideration just because the patient is older. Glomerular function and metabolism can cause drugs to remain in the patient's system for prolonged times, thereby increasing the circulating serum concentration when the next dose is taken.

Many medications can alter the results of blood work and the findings of the physical assessment. Patients with multiple physicians may have prescriptions for drugs that interact with each other. Drugs such as aspirin can alter blood tests for clotting times. Pain medications can alter sensorium.

Smoking and alcohol use are important assessments because they can affect many body systems. All assessment data should be recorded in the chart. The perioperative nurse should read the physician's medical history and physical examination report and review laboratory reports to discern the medical diagnoses. Any additional abnormal findings should be reported to the surgeon and the anesthesia provider.

Integumentary System

Establishing a preoperative baseline for the condition of the skin facilitates evaluation of the expected outcome (i.e., no injury to the skin as a result of surgical intervention). Assessment of the integumentary system includes the skin, fingernails and toenails, and all hair patterns of the body, face, and scalp. The nurse should ask the patient whether any skin changes have taken place within the past several months.

The skin is inspected for color, temperature, sensation, texture, turgor, thickness, and amount of subcutaneous tissue. The geriatric patient has a decreased number of sweat glands and an increased sensitivity to external temperature. The patient may have skin dryness, itching, and flaking.

The surface of the body should be inspected for sores, ulcers, and moles that have exhibited change over time. Broken or injured skin areas may indicate a pathologic condition such as skin cancer or diabetes. Skin rashes may indicate an allergy. Skin color can indicate liver disease or problems with other body systems (e.g., cardiovascular, respiratory). Bruises or abrasions may indicate a recent fall or possible elder abuse.[7]

Careful assessment of the body surface can reveal pertinent data about the patient's health status, but differentiating normal from abnormal skin conditions may be difficult. Skin is often wrinkled as a result of changes in connective tissue. Pigmentation and skin tags can be normal lesions in the aging process.

The nails and nailbeds of the fingers and toes should be observed for their presence or absence, texture, growth pattern, cleanliness, infection, and color. Clubbing and cyanosis of the fingertips and nailbeds may indicate cardiovascular disease. Extreme overgrowth and deformity of the toenails may indicate decreased circulation to the feet and legs. An accumulation of soil and debris under the nails may indicate an inability to wash properly. Twisted and gnarled digits may be painful to the touch, which should be considered when planning positions for the surgical procedure (Fig. 9.1). The perioperative nurse should be aware that even the weight of the surgical drapes might create enough pressure to cause discomfort on the toenails.

Hair patterns on the scalp may show areas of thinning or loss. The nurse should note the condition of the hair, such as cleanliness, hair dye, and grooming. The condition of the hair may indicate the patient's level of interest or ability in performing self-care. A lack of care may be caused by inability or disinterest caused by depression. A patient with dementia may be unaware that the hair is dirty or uncombed.

Body hair patterns may be sparsely distributed in geriatric patients, with areas of thinning or absence. For this reason, hair removal from the surgical site is not routinely indicated.

The extremities should be observed for patterns of hair growth or its absence. The lower legs may not have much hair because of circulatory changes. The color of the legs should be observed at this time; duskiness and mottling may indicate a problem with arterial blood flow, whereas ruddiness may indicate a venous blood flow problem and possible deep vein thrombosis risk. The shape, size, and equality of the lower legs should be checked for edema or ulceration. The condition of the extremities may have implications for positioning during the surgical procedure and may indicate the need for further systemic testing.

Musculoskeletal System

Assessment of the musculoskeletal system includes muscles, bones, posture, and gait. Muscle mass is usually decreased because muscle fibers atrophy, decrease in strength, and are fewer in number as noted in sarcopenia. Fibrous tissue replaces the lost mass. With less exercise and motion, muscle strength is compromised. Tendons become hardened, and range of motion decreases. Muscle cramps are common.

The patient may report a decrease in height. This is caused by demineralization of the bones, kyphosis, and narrowing of disk spaces in the vertebral column. The long bones do not decrease in length but become thin and brittle (osteoporosis), especially in older women; 80% of all patients older than 70 years have some degree of osteoporosis that is complicated by osteoarthritis (Fig. 9.2).[8] An osteoporosis assessment should be done to identify those at risk for fractures. The Fracture Risk Assessment Tool (FRAX) uses a questioner and the results of a bone density test can estimate an individual's 10-year risk factor. This can be valuable information to reduce osteoporosis and begin early treatment. Estrogen supplements after menopause may decrease the occurrence of brittle bones. However, fractures in the hips, vertebrae, wrists, and ends of long bones are common in older adults (Fig. 9.3).

Assistance with moving or total lifting may be necessary to help the geriatric patient move from the transport stretcher to the OR bed for the surgical procedure. The plan of care should include lifting help or devices and adequate positioning supplies. Care must be taken not to injure bony structures that may be weakened

TABLE 9 1 Physiologic Changes Associated With Normal Aging Processes in the Geriatric Patient

Age-Related Factors	Assessment Factors
Integumentary System	
Decreased subcutaneous fat, decreased turgor (elasticity)	Thin dry skin, wrinkles
Diminished sweat glands, dulled tactile sensation	Poor thermoregulation, heat and cold sensitivity
Thickened connective tissue	Keratosis (patchy overgrowths of dermis), warts, skin tags (especially on face and neck)
Increased fat deposits over abdomen and hips	Poor excretion of fat-soluble drugs
Diminished capillary blood flow, reduced vascularity, capillary fragility	Pressure sores, delayed wound healing, purpura or lentigo (liver spots), bruises
Dry mucous membranes, decreased salivation and secretions	Dry mouth and vagina
Musculoskeletal System	
Diminished protein synthesis in muscle cells, decreased muscle mass and tone	Muscle weakness, reduced strength, muscle wasting
Erosion of cartilage, thickened synovial fluid, fibrosed synovial membranes	Joint pain, swelling, stiffness, diminished range of motion
Diminished mobility, flexibility, and balance	Poor gait, poor posture, risk for falling
Increased porosity and demineralization of bone, thinning of intervertebral disks, decreased height	Ankylosing spondylosis, kyphosis, osteoporosis
Respiratory System	
Atrophied respiratory muscles, kyphosis or other postural changes, ribcage rigidity	Chest wall limitations
Reduced vital capacity	Dyspnea
Risk for pneumonia	Ineffective cough
Cardiovascular System	
Decreased cardiac output and stroke volume	Chronic fatigue and dyspnea, orthostatic hypotension
Myocardial irritability and stiffness, decreased size of sinoatrial and atrioventricular nodes	Slow heart rate and circulation, dysrhythmias and murmurs
Increased vascular resistance, rigidity in arteries	Hypertension
Thickening and dilation of veins	Venous insufficiency, varicosities
Decline in renal blood flow	Edema in tissues
Gastrointestinal System	
Decreased esophageal peristalsis, slowed emptying of stomach	Indigestion, frequent antacid use
Diminished saliva production, which slows breakdown of carbohydrates; reduced gastric secretion of hydrochloric acid, which impairs absorption of vitamins and minerals; hepatic insufficiency, which affects absorption of fats	Malnutrition
Loss of perineal and anal sphincter tone	Diarrhea, fecal incontinence
Decreased intestinal peristalsis, loss of abdominal muscle turgor, reduced mucosal secretions in intestines	Constipation, frequent laxative use
Endocrine System	
Reduced hormonal activity, decreased physical activity	Slowed basal metabolic rate, subnormal temperature
Slowed release of insulin from pancreas	Impaired glucose metabolism
Reduced thyroid hormone production	Dry skin, temperature intolerance, poor appetite, lethargy, memory lapse
Disturbed fluid and electrolyte balance	Hydration status
Genitourinary System	
Decreased renal blood flow, reduced number of glomeruli, reduced glomerular filtration rate, decreased excretory ability	Diminished renal function, risk of acid-base imbalance and drug toxicity
	Urinary frequency, urgency, and nocturia
Loss of elasticity and muscle tone in ureters, bladder, and urethra	Stress incontinence
Decreased bladder muscle and sphincter tone, estrogen deficiency in female	Urinary retention
Enlarged prostate in male	
Reduced testosterone levels, hypertrophied prostate, sclerosis of penile arteries and veins	Male: slow erection and ejaculation
Reduced estrogen levels; atrophied vulva, clitoris, and vagina	Female: sagging breasts, painful intercourse
Nervous System	
Decreased number of brain cells, reduced cerebral blood flow, reduced oxygen supply to brain	Cognitive deficits: delirium, temporary state of confusion, forgetfulness, disorientation, irritability, and insomnia; dementia, a permanent state of cognitive impairment
Decreased neurons	Paresthesia, akinesia, diminished pain perception
Diminished neurotransmitters, decreased neurons	Tremors, head nodding, and other repetitive movements
Degeneration of myelin sheath, which lessens motor neuron conduction	Slowed reflexes and reaction time
Reduced sound transmission as eardrum thickens, decreased hair cells and neurons, reduced blood supply to cochlea	Auditory impairment
Weakened lens muscles; hardening of lens; flattening of cornea; reduced blood supply, which leads to macular deterioration; increased rigidity of iris; reduced pupil size	Visual impairment: decreased acuity, poor perception of light and color, poor peripheral vision

Rheumatoid arthritis   Hammertoes

• **Fig. 9.1** Deformities of the hands and feet.

• **Fig. 9.2** Areas of the body commonly affected by osteoarthritis.

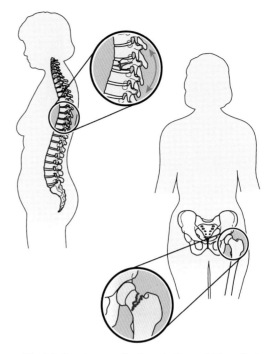

• **Fig. 9.3** Spontaneous fractures in the geriatric patient.

Wedged upper vertebrae

Crushed lower vertebrae

Young woman   Elderly woman

• **Fig. 9.4** The effects of osteoporosis.

by osteoporosis. Care is taken when log rolling by placing the hands at the shoulder and hips rather than grasping the ribcage. Ribs are easily fractured and vertebrae can break when twisted.

Ankylosing spondylosis, a chronic inflammatory disease characterized by the fixation or fusion of a vertebral joint, often causes age-related postures. The body of the geriatric patient assumes an altered shape with an increased forward thoracic curvature (kyphosis) and a flattening of the lumbar curvature, particularly common in patients with osteoporosis (Fig. 9.4). The patient may not be able to lie flat on the OR bed. Supine positioning may be painful unless the upper back and neck are supported. Fractures or subluxation of the cervical spine is possible if the ankylosed neck is allowed to fall back with the weight of the head. Twisting and forceful flexion can cause permanent damage to the vertebral column or contribute to rupture of the vertebral arteries.

Anteroposterior angles of the chest may be increased because of respiratory disease. Respiratory effort and chest excursion should be considered in planning positioning. In the preoperative assessment the flexibility of the patient's spine and the presence of any deformity or associated disease should be noted. Flexion at the hip may be painful when the legs are maintained in a straight position. Placement of a safety belt over the thighs may exert counterpressure on the thighs and cause the legs to forcefully straighten against the flattened lumbar curvature. Modified positioning may include a small pillow under the knees to allow the

natural flexion angle of the hips. Care in the placement of a safety belt or other restraint should include circulatory checks throughout the surgical procedure. The blankets should not exert pressure on the toenails, which can be painful.

The hands and feet may have painful deformities that should be considered when moving the patient to the OR bed and during positioning. Joints may be affected by arthritis, thickened synovium, and crystalloid formation in the synovial fluid. Patients may have osteoarthritis (Fig. 9.5) caused by cartilage degeneration, or they may have rheumatoid arthritis (Fig. 9.6) caused by the attack

• **Fig. 9.5** Osteoarthritis.

• **Fig. 9.6** Rheumatoid arthritis.

of the autoimmune system on joint lining. Either type of arthritis can cause pain on motion and positioning difficulties.

The patient may have a long history of taking herbal preparations, nonsteroidal antiinflammatory medications, corticosteroids, salicylates, and analgesics. The preoperative assessment should include an evaluation for the side effects associated with long-term use of these medications. In reality, several herbs used by older people to improve memory and circulation are forms of anticoagulants. Gastrointestinal bleeding, prolonged clotting times, renal insufficiency, liver changes, loss of appetite, and alteration in mental status are common side effects that could adversely affect the desired outcomes of the surgical procedure.

The patient's center of gravity is altered by multiple changes in body shape. Postural imbalance caused by impaired mobility is often the cause of falls that result in fractures. Some geriatric patients limit attempts at ambulation because they fear the possibility of falling. The risk for falls is further increased by complicating conditions such as sedation, electrolyte imbalance, impaired vision, and altered proprioception (muscular stimulation). Orthostatic hypotension contributes to the potential for falling when the geriatric patient rises from a sitting position and experiences a sudden drop in blood pressure. A fall may be symptomatic of a health problem or a systemic illness.

Cardiopulmonary System

Assessment of the lungs, heart, and circulation provides a good source of information about the general health of the patient. The cardiovascular and respiratory systems are closely interrelated. For assessment of the lungs the nurse should ask the patient to describe how breathing is affected by exertion. The nurse can assess difficulty or inefficiency in breathing by observing the patient's physical activity, respiratory effort, chest shape, and lip color for circumoral cyanosis. The nurse should palpate the trachea to determine whether it is in midline. A deviation to the right

or left may indicate the presence of a tumor. Tracheal position is an important consideration in the maintenance of an airway during a surgical procedure.

By listening to lung sounds with a stethoscope over the intercostal spaces, the nurse can refine the assessment to include specific sounds found in identified areas of each lobe. Percussion of the posterior chest wall tends to produce resonance, except in very thin older adults in whom tone is hyperresonant. The normal sound is hollow and moderately loud, with a low pitch and long duration; the sound flattens over the rib bones. If the patient slumps forward and rounds the shoulders, the intercostal spaces widen for better percussion.

Establishment of a preoperative respiratory system baseline is important. Intraoperative breathing difficulties may be avoided by adapting a position to accommodate the needs of the patient. Postoperative problems may be diagnosed and treated more efficiently if the patient's original respiratory condition has been assessed. Lung disease may affect the ability to clear secretions from the bronchial tree with coughing. Pneumonia is a common postoperative complication in geriatric patients. Coughing and deep-breathing exercises should be taught preoperatively.

The heart and systemic circulation are assessed as separate units and together as a system. The patient should be asked whether dizziness, fainting, palpitations, or other abnormal subjective symptoms are experienced. The perioperative nurse should listen to heart sounds with a stethoscope.

Dysrhythmias unrelated to heart disease are not uncommon in the geriatric patient, and many have systolic murmurs caused by aortic stenosis. The sinoatrial and atrioventricular nodes decrease in size with age, and signal interruption may occur. Clicks, murmurs, and abnormal sounds should be recorded in the assessment data. The apical pulse should be counted and compared with the peripheral pulses of the radial, popliteal, posterior tibial, and dorsalis pedis arteries. A difference between the apical and the peripheral pulse may indicate an obstruction in a major artery. The jugular veins should be observed for distention. Veins in the lower extremities should be inspected for varicosities. Leg pain caused by circulatory impairment is common in older adults.

The carotid arteries should be auscultated with a stethoscope. Bruits and systolic murmurs, which are abnormal sounds, may indicate an evolving blockage (Fig. 9.7). Dizziness or cognitive impairment may be caused by carotid insufficiency. Care must be taken not to exert pressure over the carotid area because manipulation of a plaque could cause an embolus to break loose and travel to the brain. Sudden changes in mental status during a surgical procedure performed with a local anesthetic could be the result of an arterial occlusion caused by a plaque embolus.

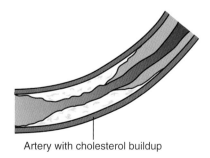

Artery with cholesterol buildup

• **Fig. 9.7** Atherosclerosis and plaque of the carotid artery.

The geriatric patient usually has decreased or slowed circulation to all areas of the body. This should be considered with administration of local anesthetics because absorption of the medication takes longer and the effects are delayed. The surgical site should be tested for the effects of the anesthetic before the incision is made. Vasoconstrictive additives, such as epinephrine, may have an exaggerated effect. Postoperative dressings should not be applied too tightly because healing is affected by circulatory efficiency.

Blood pressure should be assessed with the patient in the sitting and lying positions and measured in both arms. Elevated systolic and diastolic blood pressures caused by arteriosclerosis are a common finding in the geriatric patient population.

Assessment of laboratory blood values is important. Anemia is common among older adults and is often overlooked as a potential cause of cerebral ischemia. Both men and women will have slight normal decreases in hemoglobin and hematocrit levels because the blood-forming mechanisms lose efficiency with age. In men the decrease in androgen production may cause a noticeable decrease in hemoglobin.

Extreme decreases in hemoglobin and hematocrit values are significant in the diagnosis of pathologic conditions in major organ systems, especially the gastrointestinal or genitourinary system. Anemic conditions also can be caused by a nutritional deficit. In the absence of any other confirmed pathologic condition, hemoglobin or hematocrit levels less than the lower limit of altitude-adjusted normal values (at sea level: hemoglobin 12 g/dL, hematocrit 35%) may signal anemia caused by malnutrition.

The white blood cells do not decrease in number, but they do decrease in effectiveness. Inflammatory responses may be decreased or absent in the geriatric patient. This natural body response to injury may leave the patient more vulnerable to infection. The febrile response to infection may be diminished and therefore may not be a good indicator of a disease process. Older adults often have a subnormal baseline temperature.

Gastrointestinal System

Assessment of the gastrointestinal system should begin with observation for the visual signs of nutritional status, such as body weight, muscle wasting, bloating, and generalized weakness. Postoperative healing is profoundly affected by the ability of the cells to repair themselves. Both adequate nutrition and the ability to handle the necessary nutrients in the gastrointestinal system are essential for tissue restoration.

Many socioeconomic, psychologic, and physiologic factors influence the nutritional status of the geriatric patient. Living on a fixed income may limit the amount of nutritious food a patient can purchase. An adequate diet should include at least 1 g of protein per kilogram of desirable body weight, with an emphasis on a decreased number of calories. According to the Dietary Guidelines for Americans, the average daily caloric intake of an older woman should range between 1600 and 2000 calories; for an older man the average daily caloric intake should range between 2000 and 2600 calories.[9]

The perioperative nurse should keep in mind that actual caloric needs are unique for each patient and may vary in the presence of diabetes or other disease processes. A rapid weight gain or loss may indicate a serious pathologic condition and not an increase in body fat. Dietary control should focus on the quality, not the quantity, of food. Weight should be considered a vital sign in older adults and should be recorded in both pounds and kilograms because many medications are prescribed according to body weight in kilograms.

Psychologically, the patient may feel that food does not taste right and may refuse to eat. Many psychologic reasons for malnutrition are rooted in a physiologic cause. The geriatric patient's appetite may be decreased because of fewer taste receptors in the mouth. Nutrition in the older adult can be affected by physiologic anorexia associated with aging. Alterations in taste and smell can affect the desire to eat. Men are affected more often than women. Nutritional status should be assessed when planning to keep the patient on nothing by mouth status in anticipation of a planned surgical procedure. The patient's teeth may be in disrepair. Some patients are totally edentulous (toothless). The inability to taste, chew, and swallow discourages eating. Saliva production decreases and makes swallowing more difficult. Loose or missing teeth must be assessed because of the danger of aspirating a tooth during the surgical procedure. Patients with dentures, bridges, or partials may need to remove them just before general anesthesia. If dental appliances are removed in the OR, they must be placed in a labeled cup and placed with the patient's belongings. The anesthesia provider may want dentures left in the patient's mouth to have a better fit of a facemask for oxygen. Many patients are embarrassed and do not want to be seen without their teeth. In 2016, the Older Americans Act added funding for oral health because research shows periodontal disease can lead to disease in several body systems, such as the cardiac, pulmonary, and musculoskeletal systems.

During the preoperative assessment the perioperative nurse may find that a decreased ability to taste salty and sweet foods may cause the patient to increase the amount of salt and sugar in the diet. Increased salt intake may predispose the patient to congestive heart failure and fluid retention. Added sugar in the diet may cause an increase in unwanted body fat in proportion to muscle mass and difficult management of blood glucose.

The geriatric patient undergoing general anesthesia may receive stimulants and depressants; many of these are fat soluble. The fat-soluble drugs absorb faster but are excreted more slowly because of lower levels of intracellular fluid. Medications are unevenly distributed in the body, and the anticipated actions are unpredictable because fewer receptor sites react to the presence of the drug.

Digestion can be assessed by questioning the patient about food intake and the effects of the presence of food in the stomach. Older adults have decreased stomach motility, decreased gastric secretions, and slower stomach emptying time. Food may remain in the esophagus for longer periods. The esophagus and lower stomach lose muscular tone and dilate slightly. This phenomenon is referred to as "antral stretch" and simulates fullness and satiety.

The perioperative nurse should ask the patient about the use of antacids and laxatives. Frequent use of antacids may indicate swallowing or stomach problems that should be investigated. Esophageal reflux in the presence of a hiatal hernia may need to be assessed preoperatively to prevent aspiration of gastric secretions. The inability to lie flat with food in the stomach may be the first symptom of a high-risk situation. Positioning and rapid-sequence induction of anesthesia may be considerations. Cricoid pressure (Sellick maneuver) or awake intubation may be necessary to prevent aspiration.

The geriatric patient may use laxatives to maintain bowel regularity. Constipation is caused by decreased motility, lowered intake of bulk and fluids, and inactivity. Oil-based laxatives can lead to malabsorption of the fat-soluble vitamins A, D, E, and K, which further impairs nutritional and general health status. The absorption of nutrients is impaired naturally in older adults as a process of aging because intestinal blood flow is reduced and the absorptive cells lining the intestines are decreased. Diverticulosis and diverticulitis are common (Fig. 9.8). Fiber is an important dietary additive but should be used with caution because it can cause bowel obstruction or diarrhea. Diarrhea in the geriatric patient causes a serious threat to well-being because it may lead to dehydration.

The minimum oral fluid intake should be 1500 mL/day. Some geriatric patients have limited fluid intake. A patient may fear incontinence, have altered sensorium and cognition, be unable to drink fluids independently, or have a decreased thirst sensation as part of the aging process. The serious nature of fluid balance in older adults is reflected in unstable electrolyte values and their direct effect on cardiac status.

The perioperative nurse should perform a preoperative assessment of hydration. Signs of dehydration are dry tongue, sunken cheeks and eyes, severe loss of skin turgor, concentrated urine, and in some instances mental confusion. Blood tests may show a urea level greater than 60 mg/dL. A geriatric patient who is dehydrated should receive preoperative intravenous (IV) fluids to prevent complications.

Endocrine System

The endocrine system interfaces with all major systems of the body. The assessment of endocrine functioning is complicated by the normal age-related changes in other body systems. The endocrine system consists of the thyroid gland; the parathyroid gland; the pancreas; the adrenal, pituitary, and pineal glands; and the ovaries or testes (Fig. 9.9).

Thyroid hormone production decreases by age 60 years in men, whereas women experience decreased production by age 70 years. By 80 years of age the thyroid gland reduces thyroid hormone production by 50%. The effects of this decreased production may be dry skin, memory lapse, temperature intolerance, lethargy, and appetite disturbance. Many signs and symptoms of thyroid disease may be confused with the normal aging process.

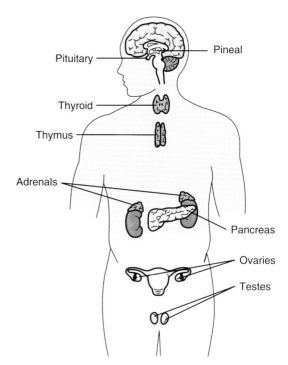
• **Fig. 9.9** Endocrine glands.

Comorbidity may lead to abnormal laboratory test results in a patient with normal thyroid function.

Insulin is produced by the beta cells in the pancreas and affects the metabolism and storage of glucose. In healthy patients, glucose levels in the blood cause the pancreas to release insulin. The response of the pancreas is slowed in older adults, and the release of insulin may not be triggered by the same stimulus. More than 33% of the adult population over 65 has diabetes mellitus with impaired glucose metabolism.[10]

A precursor to diabetes is metabolic syndrome, characterized by elevated triglycerides, low high-density lipoprotein, hypertension, high uric acid levels, and high blood glucose. The patient has a larger abdomen-to-hip ratio caused by fatty deposits on the abdominal viscera fat buildup in the skeletal muscles. Males are affected more than females. Increased exercise and an appropriate diet can forestall conversion to diabetes in geriatric patients.

Diabetes mellitus may be caused by deficient insulin production, insensitive insulin receptors, altered insulin release mechanisms, or inactivation of circulating insulin. An imbalance in blood glucose levels during the surgical procedure may predispose the patient to an unwanted outcome. Patients with diabetes mellitus often experience more postoperative infections and complications than do patients without diabetes.[10] Uncontrolled blood glucose metabolism has negative implications for all major body systems. Therefore ongoing assessment is important to attain expected outcomes.

Genitourinary System

Assessment of the genitourinary system includes the bladder, urethra, ureters, kidneys, reproductive history, and genitalia. The first noticeable sign of a problem with the genitourinary system may be the odor of urine on clothing. The odor may be caused by lack of cleanliness but is usually from incontinence. More than 30% of the older population experience some form of urinary incontinence, but many are reluctant to discuss this problem and

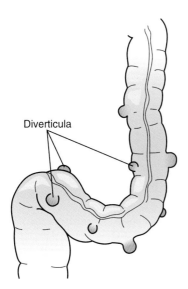
• **Fig. 9.8** Diverticulosis.

Diverticula

may try to avoid it. The problem may stem from stress incontinence, confusion, neurologic disorders, urinary tract infection, or immobility that prevents the patient from getting to the bathroom quickly.

The geriatric patient may fear loss of bladder control during the surgical procedure. Previous bladder or prostate gland surgery may predispose a patient to involuntary urine release. The perioperative nurse should include this situation in the plan of care. The problem may be minimized during the surgical procedure if the patient has an opportunity to empty the bladder preoperatively. The nursing diagnoses should reflect not only urinary incontinence but also the associated anxiety level of the patient.

Assessment of the genital area should include observation of the perineum for redness and excoriation. The bladder should be palpated with the patient in the supine position. The presence of a distended bladder after the patient has voided may indicate urinary retention with an overflow condition. This condition should be checked preoperatively before the patient is catheterized in the OR. The urethra could be inadvertently traumatized if an obstruction (e.g., tumor, enlarged prostate gland) is present.

The effectiveness of the kidneys decreases as the patient ages. By the time a person reaches 50 years of age, renal blood flow and glomerular filtration rate decrease by as much as 50%. Although no overt signs of a disease process may be found, the perioperative nurse should be aware that the older patient is at increased risk for renal insufficiency and is highly susceptible to fluid overload, dehydration, and renal failure.

The perioperative nurse should make a baseline assessment of intake and output. During the surgical procedure, urinary output may be used to monitor the renal status of the patient. Renal impairment may delay the excretion of drugs by the kidneys and further complicate fluid balance. The urine should be assessed for color, concentration, presence of particulate matter, and odor. Urinary output during the procedure should be at least 30 mL/h; more urine may be produced if the patient is taking diuretics or medications for blood pressure or cardiac control. Monitoring urinary output is difficult if the patient does not have an indwelling catheter or experiences urinary incontinence during the procedure. Postoperative care should include emptying the bladder to evaluate the expected outcome of adequate urinary output.

The reproductive assessment consists of the number of pregnancies a woman had during her childbearing years. Data about the method of birth should be included. Childbirth via cesarean section or a previous gynecologic surgery may indicate the possibility of pelvic adhesions that may be encountered if the planned surgical procedure includes entering the peritoneal cavity. Multiple vaginal births may cause uterine and bladder prolapse.

Pessaries are sometimes used for conservative treatment of prolapsed pelvic organs. Some women use a pessary to minimize urinary incontinence. Patients are taught to remove the device for cleaning before bedtime and replace it in the morning. Pessaries are useful for the patient who cannot withstand a surgical procedure for prolapse, cystourethrocele, or rectocele. The presence of an intravaginal pessary for uterine or bladder elevation should be noted (Fig. 9.10).

Female patients scheduled for surgery to obliterate the vagina to support pelvic organs should be counseled concerning the inability for coital function postoperatively. Surgical closure of the vagina is referred to as *vaginal colpocleisis* or *LeFort procedure* and involves strengthening the levator muscles and high

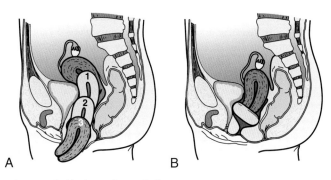

• **Fig. 9.10 A,** Uterine prolapse. **B,** Donut pessary in place for correction of uterine prolapse.

perineorrhaphy. The patient's physiologic condition dictates whether full or partial colpocleisis is performed. This method is not the first choice for pelvic organ support but may be the best option in a very ill patient who is no longer sexually active.

The use of estrogen replacement therapy should be documented with the current dosage and the last doses taken. The possibility of osteoporosis and heart disease is greater in older women who have not had estrogen replacement after menopause.

The breasts of both male and female patients should be palpated for masses. The male patient may exhibit gynecomastia, which is an increase of breast tissue caused by decreased production of testosterone. Previous mammograms should be available if breast surgery is planned. Any hormonal therapy should be noted in the assessment. If a biopsy of the breast is performed, the specimen may be tested for estrogen receptor sites. The loss of fibrous breast tissue in the woman is normal. The main palpable finding is the terminal milk ducts, which feel like strands or spindles. Masses are not a common finding and should be investigated.

Nulliparous women and those with a history of hormone replacement therapy may be predisposed to breast cancer. Nipple discharge or retraction may indicate a serious condition. The breasts of the older adult woman may be pendulous and flaccid. Prepping and draping may be slightly more difficult because of sagging skin and lack of muscle tone.

In males, size of the genitalia may be diminished. The penis may be smaller, and the testes descend lower into the scrotum because the rugae are decreased or absent. Pubic hair may be sparse, pale, and coarse. The ability to achieve an erection may be decreased or absent, and the ability to ejaculate may be diminished. Orgasm may still be possible without the presence of an erection. The ejaculate may flow retrograde into the bladder. Assessment should include the use of erectile dysfunction drugs, both prescribed and over-the-counter "male enhancement" forms. These drugs affect the cardiovascular system and may have an effect on the anesthetic process.

The prostate may be enlarged, and the incidence of prostate cancer increases with age. The male geriatric patient may experience embarrassment during a prostate examination; all efforts should be made to preserve his dignity.

Positioning for this examination may be difficult because of inflexible joints. The patient can be placed in a lateral, modified jackknife or a modified dorsal recumbent position. The presence of stool may hinder the palpation.

For many prostate biopsies, transrectal ultrasound and needle aspiration are used. Rectal sphincter tone should be assessed in the patient who is undergoing a transrectal procedure. Anal tears, hemorrhoids, fissures, and defects in the musculature should be documented in the assessment data. Any stool present on the examiner's gloved finger should be tested for occult blood to establish the baseline; otherwise, postoperative bleeding could be wrongly assessed as a problem caused by the surgical procedure. Baseline data may help resolve the situation. Keep in mind that inserting a urinary catheter into the urethra may be impeded by an enlarged prostate gland. If difficulties are encountered, the surgeon should be consulted and a stylet used.

The female genitalia should be assessed both externally and internally. The patient should be placed supine in a modified lithotomy position. Spinal curvature or respiratory difficulty may prevent the patient from lying flat, and arthritic joints make lithotomy positioning painful. Care should be exercised not to create embarrassment during the examination. The vulvar area should be inspected. The mons and labia appear smaller and looser because of the loss of subcutaneous fat pads and the decrease in estrogen production. Lesions and discolorations should be noted. The skin of the perineum may be shiny, atrophic, and dry. The prepuce and clitoris may be atrophied, but orgasm is still possible. The vaginal opening may appear small, dry, and inelastic. A previous history of gynecologic surgery, such as hysterectomy or oophorectomy, should be obtained. The absence of the uterus or ovaries does not preclude examination of the vaginal vault. The anus should be inspected for tears, fissures, and hemorrhoids.

The internal assessment of the female genitalia includes a gentle examination that involves insertion of a gloved, well-lubricated finger into the vagina. The vagina may feel shortened. The position of the bladder, rectum, and cervix should be ascertained. Protrusion of the bladder, rectum, or cervix may be present because the patient experiences a loss of muscle tone with age. The abdomen is palpated as the uterus is carefully elevated. The uterus atrophies as part of the aging process; enlargement is caused by disease. The endometrium still responds to the stimulation of hormonal therapy, causing uterine bleeding. The adnexa are identified, and no masses should be palpable.

The use of a smaller, prewarmed, well-lubricated speculum is usually necessary for visualization of the cervix and for obtaining a Papanicolaou (Pap) smear. Pediatric instrumentation may be needed. The vaginal lining looks thin, smooth, dry, and atrophied. Care is essential to prevent trauma when fingers or instruments are inserted into the vagina. Discharge and foul odors are abnormal and should be reported. Vaginal bleeding is a sign of a pathologic condition in the older, postmenopausal woman.

Sexuality in older adults is an often overlooked and ignored reality. The activity between geriatric sex partners may vary in performance, but sexual pleasure is not abandoned because of advancing age. Intercourse may not take place in the same way as when the partners were young, but sexual contact and mutual gratification remain pleasurable. Many geriatric patients have been forced to deny their sexuality because of the loss of their sex partner. Self-gratification may be practiced but is not openly discussed because of the personal nature of the act.

The subject of sexuality should be approached gently, without jokes or condemnation. Dislocations of total hip joint prosthetics can occur during sexual intercourse. A surgical procedure—such as colpocleisis, orchiectomy, or vulvectomy—that may alter sexual habits can be devastating. Empathy is critical to the patient's adjustment to a change of lifestyle. Counseling may be necessary

to assist the patient and the sex partner in expressing concerns. The perioperative nurse should be prepared to answer questions and listen to patients as they express a sense of loss. When appropriate, the plan of care should reflect the nursing diagnosis of sexual dysfunction or ineffective sexuality patterns.

Nervous System

Assessment of the nervous system includes the brain, spinal cord, peripheral nerves, and sensory organs. The nervous system is uniquely interdependent with every system of the body. Age-related changes in the brain consist of a decreased number of neurons, a decreased rate of impulse transmission, an increased reflex response time, and a decreased brain mass.

The perioperative nurse should assess the geriatric patient and establish a baseline of neurologic function. Any deviation from baseline during the surgical procedure may indicate the presence of an additional or new pathologic condition involving the brain (e.g., stroke). Postoperatively, the ongoing assessment monitors the risk for a postprocedure deficit caused by medication or a pathologic condition.

The spinal cord and peripheral nerves are assessed together. During the functional assessment the patient is observed ambulating, sitting, standing, maintaining posture, making intentional hand motions, and performing cooperative and purposeful actions such as writing. The perioperative nurse is able to observe for tremor, gait disturbance, shuffling of feet, unilateral weakness, or an alteration in mobility caused by a neurologic deficit. An assessment of the medications taken at home is important to determine the presence of transient nervous system side effects such as shaking and intention tremor. Smoking can cause a temporary decrease in cerebral blood flow and result in dizziness that may mimic a neurologic problem.

The sensory changes associated with aging involve decreased pressure and pain perception, difficulty differentiating between hot and cold, hearing loss, decreased visual acuity, and alterations in the senses of smell and taste and in spatial perception during locomotion. Preoperative assessment of tactile sensory conditions enables the nurse to develop a plan of care that reflects the need for protection of bony pressure points and for caution during the use of heat-producing or cold-producing equipment such as a hypothermia or hyperthermia mattress.

If a patient has sensory impairments such as a visual disturbance, a hearing loss, or altered spatial perception, there is a high risk for injury caused by falls. Patients with cataracts may be sensitive to the glare from bright OR lights. Allowing patients to wear hearing aids and eyeglasses to the OR helps them adapt to the surgical environment. Unexpected outcomes caused by sensory alteration can be prevented with a plan of care that considers the combined baseline abilities and sensory needs of the patient. For example, an assessment of hearing ability dictates the need to facilitate communication.

Intraoperative Considerations

Special precautions are indicated in caring for geriatric patients in the OR. The following factors should be considered:

- *Hypothermia:* Geriatric patients are at risk when their core body temperature falls below 96.8° F (36° C). A decreased basal metabolic rate, limited cardiovascular reserves, thinning of the skin, and reduced muscle mass affect the production and conservation of body heat. Measures must be taken to prevent inadvertent hypothermia caused by environmental factors. Precautionary measures include raising room temperature; using warm blankets and devices to circulate warmed air over body surfaces not included in the surgical site; warming anesthetic gases, solutions, and IV fluids; and covering the patient's head.

- *Positioning:* Patients should be lifted, not pulled, during transfer to and from the OR bed and during positioning on the OR bed. Skin is sensitive to abrasion because of decreased dermal thickness and turgor (elasticity). Joints may be stiff or painful because of calcification or degenerative osteoarthritis. Support of the back and neck prevents discomfort from osteoporosis, kyphosis, or rheumatoid arthritis. Hyperextension of the neck during thyroidectomy can cause damage to the vertebral artery or bony structures. Padding and air supports protect pressure points and bony prominences. Circulation and respiration must not be further compromised. Decreased cardiac output, arteriosclerosis, venous stasis, reduced vital lung capacity, and reduced tissue oxygenation are characteristic changes in older adults.
- *Antiembolic measures:* Slow circulation and hypotension predispose older adults to thrombus formation and emboli. Antiembolic stockings or a sequential compression device on the legs help decrease this risk.
- *Monitoring:* A decrease in renal circulation and excretory ability affects electrolyte balance and the excretion of drugs. Fluid and blood losses are not well tolerated, and hypovolemia can progress rapidly. Blood loss and urinary output must be monitored. Blood gases and electrolytes may need to be monitored, depending on the type of surgical procedure and the patient's preoperative condition. The reaction to any anesthetic agents and drugs is closely monitored in all patients. Fluctuations in cardiac rate and rhythm may portend an impending crisis.

Anesthesia Considerations

Geriatric patients present a special challenge to the anesthesia provider. Physiologic function gradually deteriorates with age but not in a predictable progression. The aging process is not a disease but a fundamental biologic alteration. In geriatric patients, disease is superimposed on senescent changes. Older individuals are prone to multiple organ system failure. Changes in the central nervous system produce effects on other body systems.

Reactivity to stimuli decreases with advancing years. These patients therefore experience an altered response to stress, which is exemplified by a high pain threshold. They are more susceptible to the action of all drugs. Abnormal sleeping and breathing patterns, with the production of apnea by hyperventilation, are accentuated by opioids. These phenomena translate to a need for lower doses of anesthetics and opioids for analgesia; the minimum anesthetic concentration required declines progressively with advanced age.

In older adults, oxygen masks may be difficult to fit because of the loss of teeth or bony substance in the jaw. Induction may be prolonged and ventilation made difficult because of chronic obstructive pulmonary disease such as emphysema. With a rapid fall in blood pressure, patients are susceptible to hypoxia, stroke, renal failure, and the development of myocardial infarction. The problems of anesthetization are augmented because surgical procedures tend to be major and take longer; some procedures pertain to malignant tumors, with additional surgery necessary.

A decrease in muscle mass, including the myocardium, with a corresponding increase in body fat takes place in the aging process; most anesthetics are fat soluble. Cardiac output and pulmonary capacity also diminish with age, with a decline in maximal oxygen uptake. In addition, anesthetics may reduce oxygen to the heart, kidneys, and brain, and geriatric patients are prone to hypotension, hypothermia, cerebral edema, and hypoxemia postoperatively. These fundamental physiologic changes necessitate a reduction of anesthetic dosages in geriatric patients.

Surgical mortality is higher in older adults than in the general population, especially if the surgery is an emergency procedure that does not allow sufficient time for a thorough preoperative evaluation and preparation. Complications related to the cardiovascular system and cerebral circulation often are followed by respiratory problems, aspiration, and infection. Surgical morbidity can be reduced, however, with skillful anesthesia management. Terminally ill patients with do-not-resuscitate (DNR) or allow-natural-death (AND) orders should have a discussion with the anesthesia provider and the surgeon. The patient has the right to keep the DNR or AND order in effect for the OR. Everyone must be on the same page and honor the patient's wishes if resuscitation is questioned.

Postoperative Considerations

The health status of geriatric patients is compromised by the interaction of drugs and anesthetics and by the surgical procedure itself. The following situations must be monitored postoperatively:

- *Drug interactions:* Tolerance may be poor and detoxification is slow. Drugs metabolize slowly in the liver and are excreted slowly by the kidneys. Fat-soluble drugs have a prolonged duration because they are absorbed by body fat, which increases with aging. Many anesthetic agents are fat soluble and are myocardial and respiratory depressants. Narcotics, opioids, and sedatives interact with anesthetics. Patients must be monitored for hypoxia because oxygenation to the heart, kidneys, and brain is less efficient. General anesthetics and some drugs cause transient mental dysfunction.
- *Aspiration:* Older adults may have difficulty swallowing because of dry mucous membranes, reduced salivation, and reduced esophageal peristalsis. Coughing is less productive because of muscular atrophy in the chest and rigidity of the ribcage. Patients must be watched for aspiration.
- *Infection:* Respiratory, urinary, or gastrointestinal tract infections may develop because of immunodeficiency. Pneumonia can be fatal. Poor dental hygiene may be the source of systemic infection. Healing is further delayed if an infection develops in a wound already compromised by a reduced vascular supply. The fever associated with infection in younger patients may not be as obvious in geriatric patients. Elevation of white blood cell count may be a better indicator if the patient is not immunocompromised as the result of some other disease.
- *Catheterization:* A Foley catheter may be needed for some time to monitor fluid input and output. Use of a Foley will be determined by the surgeon or anesthesia provider based on the length of the surgical procedure.

Geriatric patients need a thorough preoperative assessment, an experienced anesthesia provider, considerate and knowledgeable caregivers, meticulous aseptic and sterile techniques, and careful postoperative management. Patients and their family or significant others should be included in the development of the postoperative discharge plan. Planning should incorporate follow-up care with the surgeon.

EVOLVE WEBSITE

http://evolve.elsevier.com/Hornacky/BerryKohn/

- Historical Perspective
- Student Interactive Questions
- Glossary

References

1. Benbow E: Ageing and death. In Cross S, editor: *Underwood's pathology*, ed 7, St. Louis, 2019, Elsevier, pp 219–228.
2. U.S. Census Bureau: www.census.gov. Accessed March 20, 2023.
3. Viswanath M, Clinch D, Ceresoli M, et al.: Perceptions and practices surrounding the perioperative management of frail emergency surgery patients: a WSES-endorsed cross-sectional qualitative survey, *World J Emerg Surg* 18(7), 2023.
4. Technology for Seniors: www.seniorliving.org. Accessed March 21, 2023.
5. National Council on Aging: *Get the facts on healthy aging*. www.ncoa.org. Accessed March 22, 2023.
6. Ball J, Dains J, Flynn J, et al.: Age-specific examination: special populations and older adults. In *Seidel's physical examination handbook*, ed 10, St. Louis, 2023, Elsevier.
7. National Center on Elder Abuse: www.ncea.acl.gov. Accessed March 22, 2023.
8. Siris E: *Bone health basics: get the facts*. www.bonehealthandosteoporosis.org. Accessed March 24, 2023.
9. Dietary Guidelines for Americans: www.dietaryguidelines.gov. Accessed March 24, 2023.
10. Endocrine Society: *Diabetes and older adults*. www.endocrine.org. Accessed March 24, 2023.

10

Physical Facilities

CHAPTER OUTLINE

Physical Layout of the Surgical Suite, 178

Transition Zones, 179

Peripheral Support Areas, 180

Operating Room, 183

Special Procedure Rooms, 193

Construction or Renovation of the Surgical Suite, 194

CHAPTER OBJECTIVES

After studying this chapter, the learner will be able to:

- Identify specific areas within the surgical suite in which attire and behaviors affect the manner of care delivery.
- Discuss how environmental layout contributes to aseptic technique.
- Describe methods of environmental controls that contribute to an aseptic environment.
- Describe the specialty rooms used for endoscopy, minimally invasive procedures, and urology.

KEY TERMS AND DEFINITIONS

Cesarean delivery The birth of a baby via an abdominal incision.

Control desk Authorized personnel use this centralized area in the surgical suite to facilitate surgical procedures, organize patient flow, disseminate information, and arrange departmental activities. Located in the unrestricted area, it commonly borders the semirestricted corridors.

Displacement ventilation The rate of positive pressure air exchanges to fresh air displacement in an OR related to the size of the room where anesthesia is delivered. Procedure rooms (formerly class A ORs) are 15:3; larger rooms up to 600 ft^2 are 20:4.

Endoscopic procedures Surgical procedures that use natural body orifices or percutaneous techniques with fiber-optic lighting to use with cameras and long specialized instruments during tissue manipulation and invasive intervention (e.g., colonoscopy, bronchoscopy).

HVAC The system for controlling environmental temperature and humidity. This is an acronym for heating, ventilation, and air conditioning.

Hybrid operating room An operating room with permanently installed equipment for imaging during the surgical procedure.

Interventional radiographic procedure A specialized surgical procedure that permits the use of radiologic imaging during tissue manipulation and invasive intervention through small incisional portals.

Laminar airflow A unidirectional flow of clean air from a higher plane to lower exhaust grilles. The uninterrupted flow permits higher air changes per hour (ACH) for a cleaner environment around the sterile field.

Minimally invasive surgical (MIS) procedure Surgical procedures that use small incisions and fiber-optic lighting with cameras and long specialized instruments during tissue manipulation and invasive intervention (e.g., laparoscopy or mediastinoscopy).

Operating room (OR) A specially equipped room where many types of surgical procedures are performed. This room is one part of the restricted area of the surgical suite.

Procedure room A room designated for a specific collection of surgical procedures that may not require the same equipment and supplies as the main ORs. This room is one part of the unrestricted area of the surgical suite and may border the semirestricted area. Formerly known as class A ORs.

Restricted surgical suite Areas where scrub suits, hair covers, OR-specific closed-in shoes, and masks are worn. Can be accessed only through a semirestricted area.

Semirestricted surgical suite Areas where scrub suits, hair covers, and OR-specific closed-in shoes are worn.

Sterile core A special room within the suite where sterile supplies are stored for ease of use. This room is one part of the restricted area of the surgical suite.

Substerile room A room with a double sink separated from the OR by a door and where select clean and contaminated activities take place during the surgical procedure. Some substerile rooms have warming cabinets for solutions or blankets and a steam autoclave. A disposal sink for contaminated fluids might be in here (e.g., hopper). This room is one part of the restricted area of the surgical suite.

Suite A collection of rooms that are used interactively during a surgical procedure in which each room has a specific purpose (e.g., OR, substerile room, scrub sink room, and sterile storage core).

Thermal plume An invisible layer of heat emanating from the equipment, team members, and the patient that can change the airflow and particulate distribution in the presence of laminar air diffusers.

Unrestricted surgical suite Areas where street clothes and shoes are permitted.

Physical Layout of the Surgical Suite

Efficient use of the physical facilities is important. The design of the surgical suite offers a challenge to the planning team to optimize efficiency by creating realistic traffic and workflow patterns for patients, visitors, personnel, and supplies. The design also should allow for flexibility and future expansion. Architects consult surgeons, perioperative nurses, and surgical services administrative personnel before designating functional space within the surgical suite.

Type of Physical Plant Design

Most surgical suites are constructed according to a variation of one or more of four basic designs:
1. Central corridor, or hotel style (Fig. 10.1).
2. Central core, or clean core plan with peripheral corridor (Fig. 10.2).
3. Combination central core and peripheral corridor, or racetrack plan (Fig. 10.3).
4. Grouping, or cluster plan with peripheral and central corridor (Fig. 10.4).

Each design has its advantages and disadvantages. Efficiency is affected if corridor distances are too long in proportion to other space, if illogical relationships exist between space and function, and if inadequate consideration was given to storage space, material handling, and personnel areas.

Location

The surgical suite is usually located in an area accessible to the critical care surgical patient areas and the supporting service departments, the central service or sterile processing department, the pathology department, and the radiology department. The size of the hospital is a determining factor because locating every desirable unit or department immediately adjacent to the surgical suite is complex.

A terminal location is preferred to prevent unrelated traffic from passing through the suite. A location on a top floor is not necessary for microbial control because all air is specially filtered to control dust. Traffic noises may be less evident above the ground floor. Artificial lighting is controllable, so the need for daylight is not a factor; in fact, daylight may be a distraction during the use of video equipment and other procedures that require a darkened environment. Most surgical suites have solid walls without windows. However, some ambulatory surgery rooms have windows to create an ambiance of openness in the suite.

Space Allocation and Traffic Patterns

Space is allocated within the surgical suite to provide for the work to be done, with consideration given to the efficiency with which it can be accomplished. The surgical suite should be large enough to allow for correct technique yet small enough to minimize the movement of patients, personnel, and supplies.

Provision must be made for traffic control. The type of design predetermines traffic patterns. Everyone—staff, patients, and visitors—should follow the delineated patterns in appropriate attire. Signs should be posted that clearly indicate the attire and environmental controls required (Table 10.1). The surgical suite is divided into three geographic areas that are designated by the physical activities performed in each area.

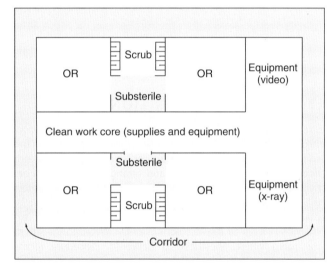

• **Fig. 10.2** Central core, peripheral corridor style.

• **Fig. 10.1** Central corridor, hotel style.

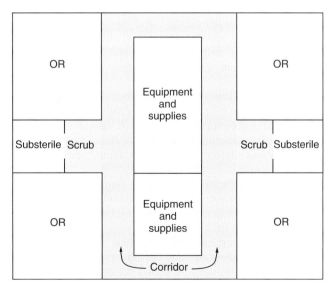

• **Fig. 10.3** Central corridor, racetrack style.

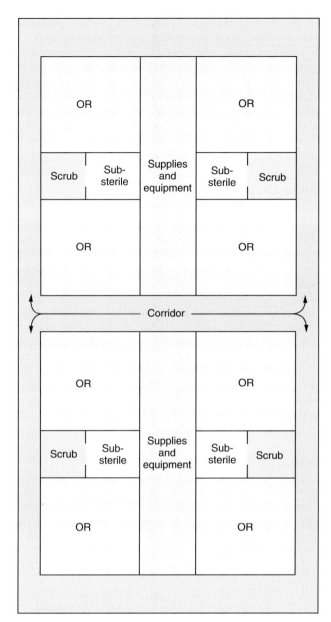

• **Fig. 10.4** Cluster combination, peripheral and central corridor style.

Unrestricted Area

In the unrestricted surgical area street clothes are permitted. A corridor on the periphery accommodates traffic from outside, including patients. This area is isolated by doors from the main hospital corridor and elevators and from other areas of the surgical suite. It serves as an outside-to-inside access area (i.e., a transition zone). Traffic, although not limited, is monitored at a central location. The control desk is accessible from the unrestricted area.

Semirestricted Area

In the semirestricted surgical area traffic is limited to properly attired, authorized personnel. Scrub suits and head/beard coverings are required attire. This area includes peripheral support areas, central processing, and access corridors to the operating rooms (ORs). The patient's hair is also covered. Bald heads are covered to prevent distribution of dead skin cells and dander that carry microorganisms.

Restricted Area

In the restricted surgical area masks are required to supplement OR attire where open sterile supplies and scrubbed personnel are located. Sterile procedures are carried out in the OR and procedure rooms. There are also scrub sink areas and substerile rooms or clean core areas where unwrapped supplies are sterilized. Personnel entering this area for short periods, such as laboratory technicians, accompanied patient support personnel, and maintenance personnel, may wear clean surgical cover gowns or jumpsuits to cover street clothes. Hair, head, and beard covering is worn, and masks are donned as appropriate.

Transition Zones

Both patients and personnel enter the semirestricted and restricted areas of the surgical suite through a transition zone. This transition zone, inside the entrance to the surgical suite, separates the semirestricted OR corridors from the rest of the facility. Masks, caps, shoe covers, and cover gowns (or jumpsuits) may be located on a cart near transition zones adjacent to restricted areas. Nonsurgical personnel who need to enter the restricted zone can don a cover gown or jumpsuit, cap, shoe covers, and mask before proceeding to the designated OR.

TABLE 10.1 Environmental Controls in the Surgical Suite

Environmental Controls	Class A OR (Procedure Room)	Class B and C OR	Cesarean Delivery Room	Storage Room	PACU
Pressure	Positive	Positive	Positive	Positive	N/A
ACH	15	20	20	4	6
OA	3	4	4	2	2
Humidity[a] (%)	20–60	20–60	20–60	20–60	20–60
Temperature (° F)	70–75	68–75	68–73	60–73	70–75

[a]Note: Humidity is expected to decrease as low as 20% by the 2018 edition of the AIA Guidelines. The rationale is that the old 30% to 60% is based on the use of flammable anesthetics and the risk for fire by static spark, which is not a consideration in modern times.

ACH, Air changes per hour; N/A, ventilated fresh air; OA, outside air; PACU, postanesthesia care unit.

Modified from the Facility Guidelines Institute: Guidelines for design and construction of health care facilities, Chicago, 2018, The Institute. www.fgiguidelines.org.

Preoperative Admission and Holding Unit

A designated unit in the unrestricted zone should be available for preoperative patients to change from street clothes into a gown and wait with their families and significant others before their surgical procedure. The decor should create a feeling of warmth and security. Lockers should be provided for safeguarding patient personal items. The location of the area should shield the patient and others from potentially distressing sights and sounds. Lavatory facilities and handwashing stations must be available. Alcohol-based hand-rub dispensers should be conveniently located in each patient care cubicle.

The area must ensure privacy and offer a minimum of 80 ft^2 per patient of space to accommodate a transport cart.[a] It may be compartmentalized with individual cubicles or be an open area with curtains. Curtains do not deflect sound and offer little privacy when the nurse is performing the assessment and having conversations with the patient. Curtains also accumulate dust and particulate and should be laundered on a regular basis.

Insertion of intravenous (IV) lines may be done here. In some cases, nerve blockades for pain management may be done in the holding area as ambulatory procedures. These procedures require good lighting. Each cubicle is equipped with oxygen, suction, and devices for monitoring blood pressure. A crash cart should be easily accessible for emergencies.

A nurses' station within the area provides close patient observation and computer access to patient electronic medical records (EMRs), such as laboratory reports. Many facilities have portable rolling computer carts for documentation that can be done at the patient's bedside. Medication dispensers or medication storage rooms are strategically placed for quick and easy access. Care is taken not to have loud conversations at the nurses' station. Private information may be overheard by patients and others.

Assignment and scheduling boards should not be within view of the patients to avoid breaching privacy standards. When wipe-off boards are used for daily scheduling, care is taken not to use patient names. Coordination of the holding room staff and the personnel managing the surgical schedule is essential to prevent delays. More information about preoperative patient care areas is available in Chapter 21.

Some preoperative holding units serve as ambulatory care areas after the surgical procedure. Patients who are admitted in the morning are brought back to the holding unit to recover. They can go home a few hours after the surgical procedure when their health status is stable.

Induction Room

Some surgical suites have an induction room within the restricted area adjacent to a group of ORs, where the patient is prepared for anesthesia administration preoperatively and before actual induction of general anesthesia and airway management. Families and significant others of patients are not permitted in this area. Appropriate surgical attire is required, including a mask.

Peripheral IV lines, central lines, and invasive arterial monitoring lines are inserted, and regional anesthesia (e.g., epidural catheter for postoperative pain management) may be placed in the induction room. Performing these procedures in an induction room saves actual OR time, which is more costly. Induction rooms are more common in larger facilities, where procedures such as open-heart surgery or transplantation are performed.

In some induction rooms (not all), patients are premedicated and stabilized on the same OR bed that will be used for the procedure. The OR bed is used as the transport vehicle to the OR, where it is connected and locked to a base unit permanently mounted in the floor. This minimizes the number of times critically ill patients are moved from one surface to another. These rooms are usually larger to accommodate emergency equipment and staff.

Postanesthesia Care Unit

The postanesthesia care unit (PACU) may be outside the surgical suite, or it may be adjacent to the suite so that it may be incorporated into the unrestricted area with access from both the semirestricted area and an unrestricted corridor. In the latter design, the PACU becomes a transition zone for the departure of patients. Space allotted should equal a minimum of 1.5 beds per OR.

Hospitals and ambulatory care facilities accommodate patients and their families and significant others during the perioperative waiting period. Some facilities have small private conference rooms where the surgeon can meet to discuss postoperative care with families/significant others. A designated waiting area is provided near the PACU. Some facilities permit certain family members and significant others to sit with recovering patients when they are stable but not ready for release. More information about the PACU can be found in Chapter 30.

Peripheral Support Areas

Adequate space must be allocated to accommodate the needs of OR personnel and support services. The need for equipment, supply, and utility rooms and housekeeping determines support space requirements. Equipment and supply rooms should be decentralized and placed near the appropriate ORs.

Control Desk

From a central control point, traffic in and out of the surgical suite may be observed. This area usually is within the unrestricted area but adjacent to the semirestricted corridor. The clerk-receptionist is located at the control desk to coordinate communications. A pass-through window may be used to stop unauthorized people, to schedule surgical procedures with surgeons, and to receive drugs, blood, and various small supplies. A computerized pneumatic tube system within the hospital can speed the delivery of small items and paperwork, thus eliminating some courier services, such as from the pharmacy to the control desk. Tissue specimens and blood samples also can be sent to the laboratory through some tube systems. The tubes used to send items should be periodically cleaned with an approved disinfectant solution.

Computers and printers may be located in the control area. Information systems and computers assist in financial management, statistical recording and analysis, scheduling of patients and personnel, materials management, and other functions that evaluate the use of facilities. An integrated computer system interfaces with other hospital departments, such as the laboratory, pathology, or patient care divisions. It may have an intranet connection that allows surgeons to schedule surgical procedures directly from their offices.

---

[a]The *Guidelines for Design and Construction of Health Care Facilities* by the Facility Guidelines Institute is available online at www.fgiguidelines.org.

Retrieval for review of patient records gives the perioperative nurse manager the opportunity to evaluate the patient care given and documented by nurses. Personnel records can be maintained. Other essential records can be stored in and retrieved from computer databases on a password-controlled basis. The central processing unit for the OR computer system usually is located in or near the control desk. A fax and/or scanner machine may be available for the electronic transfer of documents, records, and patient care orders between the OR, pharmacy, or surgeons' offices.

Security systems usually can be monitored from the control desk. Alarms are incorporated into electrical and piped-in systems to alert personnel to the location of a system failure. A centralized emergency call system facilitates summoning help. Some facilities have a panic button to summon the security department. Narcotics, opioids, and prescription pads are kept in locked cabinets, rooms, or dispensing machines and can be signed out only by appropriate personnel.

Access to exchange areas, offices, and storage areas may be limited during evening and night hours and on weekends. Doors may be locked. Some hospitals use alarm systems, video surveillance in hallways and ORs, and electronic metal detection devices to control intruders and prevent theft or vandalism. Computers and records must be secured to protect patient confidentiality.

Offices

Offices for the administrative patient care personnel and the anesthesia department should be located with access to both unrestricted and semirestricted areas. Most administrative offices are located near the control desk. The administration staff frequently needs to confer with outside people (e.g., vendors/sales representatives) and needs to be kept informed of activities within all areas of the surgical suite.

Locker Rooms and Lounges

Dressing rooms with secure lockers are provided for both male and female personnel to change from street clothes into OR attire before entering the semirestricted area and vice versa. The area should be secure from unauthorized personnel. Doors separate this area from lavatory facilities and adjacent lounges.

Walls in the lounge areas should have an aesthetically pleasing color or combination of colors to foster a calming atmosphere. A window view of the outdoors is psychologically desirable because many staff members arrive for the day shift when it is still dark outside. Affect is enhanced by natural sunlight. Some personnel bring a meal, so a refrigerator designated only for food should be located in this room. A routine refrigerator cleaning schedule should be established. Some lounges have televisions, coffeemakers, and microwaves for employee use. All appliances must be approved for use. Antiseptic hand-rub dispensers should be conveniently located at the entrance and near all food storage areas.

Dictating equipment, computers, and telephones should be available for surgeons in the physicians' lounge or in an adjacent semirestricted area.

Conference Room/Classroom

Ideally, a conference room or a classroom is located within the semirestricted area with entrance and exit doors to unrestricted areas. This room is used for patient care staff in-service educational programs and is used by the surgical staff for teaching. Closed-circuit television and video equipment also may be

available for self-study. The departmental reference library may be housed here. Tables and chairs for staff should be sturdy and easily cleanable. Shoe covers and masks should not be worn in this room. Antiseptic hand-rub dispensers should be conveniently located at the entrance.

Some facilities permit covered beverages and small snacks during meetings. Departmental holiday parties or special event celebrations may be set up in here.

Consultation Room

Some surgical suites have small meeting rooms where a surgeon can have a private conversation with the patient's family and significant others. These are usually located in the unrestricted area near the PACU.

Support Services

The size of the health care facility and the types of services provided determine whether laboratory and radiology equipment are needed within the surgical suite.

Laboratory

A small laboratory where the pathologist can examine tissue specimens and perform frozen sections expedites the decisions that the surgeon must make during a surgical procedure when a diagnosis is questionable. A designated refrigerator for storing blood for transfusions also may be located in this room. Tissue specimens may be tested here by frozen section before they are delivered to the pathology department for permanent section.

Radiology Services

Special procedure rooms may be outfitted with x-ray and other imaging equipment for diagnostic and invasive radiologic procedures or insertion of catheters, pacemakers, internal defibrillators, and other devices. The walls of these rooms contain lead shields to confine radiation. Although most facilities have converted to digital imaging, a darkroom for processing x-ray films usually is available within the surgical suite for immediate processing of scout films or contrast dye studies of organ systems.

Work and Storage Areas

Clean and sterile supplies and equipment are separated from soiled items and trash. If the surgical suite has a clean core area, only clean or sterile items are stored there. The air handlers are set to positive pressure as in the restricted area, so the doors should always remain closed when traffic is not entering or leaving.

Soiled items are taken to the decontamination area for processing before being stored, or they are taken to the disposal area. The air handlers in the contaminated areas are set to negative pressure as in the corridors, so the doors should remain closed when personnel are not entering or leaving. Ventilation should be six air exchanges with two fresh per hour. Work and storage areas are provided for handling all types of supplies and equipment, whether clean or contaminated.

Anesthesia Work and Storage Areas

Space must be provided for storing anesthesia equipment and supplies. Gas tanks are stored in a well-ventilated (a minimum of eight air exchanges per hour), negative-pressure area separated from other supplies. Care is taken not to allow tanks or cylinders to be knocked over or damaged. They should stand upright in a secure stable base for safety. Full and empty gas tanks should be stored in separate areas to prevent confusion about supplies.

Nondisposable items must be thoroughly decontaminated and cleaned after use in an area separate from sterile supplies. A separate workroom usually is provided for care and processing of anesthesia equipment. Dirty and clean supplies must be kept separated.

The storage area includes a secured space for anesthetic drugs and agents. Most facilities have drug-dispensing machines that require positive identification to obtain medications for patient use. Larger facilities have a pharmaceutical station where a pharmacist dispenses drugs on a per-case basis. Signatures are required for controlled substances. Unused drugs are returned to the pharmacist for accountability.

Housekeeping Storage Areas

Cleaning supplies and equipment need to be stored; the equipment used within the restricted area is kept separate from that used to clean the other areas. Therefore more than one storage area may be provided for housekeeping purposes, depending on the design and size of the surgical suite. Sinks are provided, as are shelves for supplies. Trash and soiled laundry receptacles should not be allowed to accumulate in the same room where clean supplies are kept; separate areas should be provided for these. Conveyors or designated elevators may be provided for prompt removal of bags of soiled laundry and trash from the suite. The ventilation is set to negative pressure with 10 air exchanges per hour with 2 of fresh air.

Central Processing Area

Conveyors, dumbwaiters, or elevators connect the surgical suite with a central processing area on another floor of the hospital. If efficient material flow can be accomplished, support functions can be removed from the surgical suite. Effective communications and a reliable transportation system must be established. Some ORs send all the instruments and supplies to the sterile processing department for cleaning, packaging, sterilizing, and storing. This system eliminates the need for some work and storage areas within the surgical suite, but exchange areas must be provided for carts. The movement of clean and sterile supplies must be kept separate from that of contaminated items and waste by means of space and traffic patterns. The ventilation is set to positive pressure with four air exchanges per hour with two of fresh air.

Utility Room

Some hospitals use a closed-cart system and take contaminated instruments to a central area outside the surgical suite for cleanup. This room contains a washer-sterilizer, sinks, cabinets, and all necessary aids for cleaning. If the washer-sterilizer is a pass-through unit, it opens also into the general workroom, which eliminates the task of physically moving instruments from one room to another.

General Workroom

The general work area should be as centrally located in the surgical suite as possible to keep contamination to a minimum. The work area may be divided into a cleaning area and a preparation area. If instruments and equipment from the utility room are received from the pass-through washer-sterilizer into this room, an ultrasonic cleaner should be available here for cleaning instruments that the washer-sterilizer has not adequately cleaned. Otherwise, the ultrasonic cleaner may be in the utility room.

Instrument sets, basin sets, trays, and other supplies are wrapped for sterilization here. Internal biologic and external chemical indicators are used. The preparation and sterilization of instrument trays and sets in a central room ensures control. This room also contains the stock supply of other items that are packaged for sterilization. The sterilizers that are used in this room may also open into the next room, the sterile supply room. This arrangement helps eliminate the possibility of mixing sterile and nonsterile items.

Storage

Technology nearly tripled the need for storage space in the 21st century. Many older surgical suites have inadequate facilities for storage of sterile supplies, instruments, and bulky equipment. Those responsible for calculating adequate storage space for instruments, sterile and unsterile supplies, and mobile equipment, such as special OR beds, specialty carts, and equipment, should consider the size of the entire surgical suite. American Institute of Architects (AIA) Guidelines state that a minimum of 150 ft^2 or 50 ft^2 per OR, whichever is greater, should be dedicated to equipment storage to prevent accumulation of machines and supplies in hallways. Blocked hallways prevent rapid transfer of crash carts and emergency equipment. Particulate can accumulate on machinery.

The OR storage space does not include additional storage space needed for postanesthesia equipment. Anesthesia storage should be considered separately. Use of a case cart system may slightly decrease the amount of instrument space needed. Plans should include accommodation for the size of each type of case cart used and the numbers that will be in the suite at a given point in the daily surgical schedule.

Sterile Supply Room

Most hospitals keep a supply of sterile drapes, sponges, gloves, gowns, and other sterile items ready for use in a sterile supply room within the surgical suite. As many shelves as possible should be freestanding from the walls, which permits supplies to be put into one side and removed from the other; thus older packages are always used first. However, small items must be contained in boxes or bins to prevent them from falling to the floor. Inventory levels should be large enough to prevent running out of supplies, yet overstocking of sterile supplies should be avoided. Storage should be arranged to facilitate stock rotation. Consideration is given to items that have an expiration date. Unstable elements, such as sutures or chemically treated supplies, will expire and be unsuitable for patient use if not rotated during stocking.

The sterile storage should be as close as possible to the sterile processing area and should be under positive pressure with four total air exchanges per hour with two exchanges of fresh air. Access to the sterile storage area should be limited; it should be separated from high-traffic areas and the doors should be closed. Humidity (20–60%) and temperature (72–75° F [22–23.9° C]) should be controlled. Humidity over 70% causes concern for condensation within sterile packages and may permit microorganism transfer by capillary action.

Instrument Room

Most hospitals have a separate room or a section of the general workroom designated for storing nonsterile instruments. The instrument room contains cupboards in which all clean and decontaminated instruments are stored when not in use. Instruments usually are segregated on shelves according to surgical specialty services.

Sets of basic instruments are usually cleaned, assembled, and sterilized after each use. Special instruments such as intestinal clamps, kidney forceps, and bone instruments may be wrapped separately or incorporated into specialty sets. Some surgeons have trays designated for personal use and are labeled with their names. These are stored with the specialty instruments.

Scrub Room

An enclosed area for preoperative cleansing of hands and arms should be provided adjacent to each OR. Scrub solutions, soaps, and scrub brushes are located near the sinks. Water spills and drips on the floor are particularly hazardous. Skid-proof mats should be in place in front of each scrub sink. An enclosed scrub room is a restricted area within the surgical suite. Paper towel dispensers and mirrors should be located in this area. Trash receptacles, limited to only those items used within this room, should be emptied several times per day. Some facilities have boxes of additional caps, masks, shoe covers, and eye protection in the event of biologic contamination requiring a change of these items during a procedure. The contaminated item should be discarded in the biohazard trash bin in the OR after changing.

Operating Room

Each OR, regardless of size, is a restricted area because of the need to maintain a controlled environment with minimal traffic for sterile and aseptic techniques (Fig. 10.5).

Categories of Operating Rooms

The American College of Surgeons (ACS) describes OR facilities based on the types of procedures performed therein. The AIA

• **Fig. 10.5** Basic OR. (Courtesy Grey McVicar. In Lewis SL, et al: *Medical-surgical nursing: assessment and management of clinical problems,* ed 8, St. Louis, 2011, Mosby.)

Guidelines in cooperation with the ACS use specific criteria when determining safe environmental factors for surgical facilities and include provision for all types of surgical interventions and the use of anesthetic agents. The criteria include minimal floor space, types of anesthetics used, and circumferential clearance around the OR bed. The types of ORs with minimal floor space are as follows:

- *Procedure room:* 160-ft^2 floor area with 12-ft minimum clear dimensions at the head, sides, and foot of the OR bed. Local anesthesia used here.
- *General OR:* 270 to 400-ft^2 floor area with 15 to 20-ft minimum clear dimensions at the head, sides, and foot of the OR bed. Local, general, and regional anesthesia used here.

Other ORs range in size from 600 to 800 ft^2 with a 24 to 25-ft width or larger to accommodate multiple ceiling-mounted booms, monitors, and high-technology equipment such as robotics and controlling consoles.

Size Determinations

The size of individual ORs varies according to use. Procedure rooms are commonly used for smaller operations performed with topical, local, or limited regional blocks that have minimal equipment needs. Many ambulatory centers have procedure rooms that fit this usage.

General ORs are better suited for procedures in which the patient may be sedated and physiologically supported with IV medication. General anesthesia and spinal or epidural blocks can be used. Intermediate to complex procedures are performed in these rooms. Additional space is appropriate where the potential for larger equipment and longer procedures is possible.

It is desirable to have the ORs in a hospital setting the same size so that they can be used interchangeably to accommodate elective and emergency surgical procedures. Large general ORs provide adequate space for typical surgeries with at least 400 ft^2 of clear floor space. Approximately 20 ft^2 of space should be planned between fixed cabinets and shelves on two opposing walls if possible. A specialized room, such as one equipped for cardiopulmonary bypass, trauma, or transplant surgeries, may require as much as 600 to 800 ft^2 of useful space.[1]

A room may be designed for a specialty service if use by that service will be high. The room must accommodate equipment, such as lasers, microscopes, or video equipment, either fixed (permanently installed as in hybrid operating room) or portable (movable). Portable equipment requires more floor space.

Some rooms are designated for special procedures, such as gastrointestinal endoscopy, interventional radiologic procedures and studies, or the application of casts. Other rooms have adjacent areas used for specific purposes, such as visitor viewing galleries, or for installing special equipment, such as monitors or x-ray devices for imaging.

Operating Room Humidity

An air-conditioning system controls humidity via the heating, ventilation, and air-conditioning (HVAC) system. High relative humidity (weight of water vapor present) should be maintained between 20% and 60%. Moisture provides a conductive medium and allows a static charge to flow to ground as fast as a spark is generated. Humidity over 70% can permit condensation inside sterile packaging.

Operating Room Temperature

OR temperature is maintained within a range of 68° F to 75° F (20–24° C). A thermostat to control room temperature can be advantageous to meet patient needs; for example, the temperature can be increased to prevent hypothermia in pediatric, geriatric, and burn patients. Overmanipulation of controls can result in calibration problems. Controls should not be adjusted solely for the comfort of team members; patient normothermia is a strong consideration. Only the maintenance department can regulate temperature in some surgical suites; this department should be called early enough to reset the temperature for patients at risk for hypothermia, such as pediatric, geriatric, or burn patients.

Substerile Room

A group of two, three, or four ORs may be clustered around a central scrub area, work area, and a small substerile room. Only if the latter room is immediately adjacent to the OR and separated from the scrub area is it considered the substerile room throughout this text.

A substerile room adjacent to the OR contains enclosed storage cupboards, a sink, a warming cabinet, and a steam sterilizer. Most warming cabinets have two chambers—one for blankets and one for solutions. The blanket chamber should not be set to heat greater than 130° F (54° C). The solution warming chamber should be set to 110° F (43.3° C) to prevent thermal burns to patients. Each manufacturer of patient-use irrigation and IV solutions sets parameters for the temperature and duration of heating permitted for their products. Any warmed solution taken out of the warming cabinet and allowed to reach room temperature cannot be returned for reheating. Solutions should be labeled with the date for removal from the cabinet as an expired product.

The AORN (Association of periOperative Registered Nurses) guidelines for 2024 recommend that immediate-use steam sterilization (IUSS; i.e., flashing) is used only if there is no other option. Although cleaning and sterilizing facilities are centralized, either inside or outside of the surgical suite, a substerile room with this equipment offers the following options:

- The circulating nurse can do emergency cleaning and sterilization of small items here, which reduces waiting time for the surgeon and reduces anesthesia time for the patient. The circulating nurse, or scrub person if necessary, can lift sterile articles directly from the sterilizer onto the sterile instrument table without transporting them through a corridor or another area. IUSS closed containers can be used.
- It allows the circulating nurse to stay within the room.

Rooms adjacent to orthopedic or cast rooms should have a sink with a plaster trap for disposal of casting solutions.

The substerile room also usually contains a combination blanket, solution warmer, printer, and cabinets for storage. Empty sterile specimen containers and labels may be conveniently stored in this room. Slips for charges or other records may be kept here. Individual hospitals may find it convenient to keep other items in this room to allow the circulating nurse to remain in or immediately adjacent to the OR during the surgical procedure.

Doors

Doors should be 4 ft wide or larger for ease in moving patients on carts and in beds. Ideally, sliding doors should be used exclusively in the OR for the main corridor. They eliminate the air currents caused by swinging doors. Microorganisms that have previously settled in the room are disturbed with each swing of the door. The microbial count is usually at its peak at the time of the skin incision because this follows disturbance of air from gowning, draping, movement of personnel, and opening and closing of doors.

Sliding doors should not recede into the wall like pocket styles but should be of the surface-sliding type. Fire regulations mandate that sliding doors for ORs can be swung open if necessary. Doors do not remain open either during or between surgical procedures. The room air handlers generate higher pressure than in the halls to minimize the amount of dust and debris pulled in toward the sterile field. Closed doors decrease the mixing of air within the OR with that in the corridors, which may contain higher microbial counts. Air pressure in the room also is disrupted if the doors remain open.

When construction or renovation is in process, always keeping the doors closed when not transporting patients is important because the ORs are ventilated with positive pressure. The air-handling systems are strained because of the disrupted processes and are further compromised when the airflow is allowed to equalize. This causes unstable temperature and humidity control. The desired temperature should be between 68° F and 75° F, with a relative humidity of 20% to 60%.

The door to the substerile area is usually a swinging style door with a small window. These doors are not used for moving patients in and out of the OR and should remain closed. During the surgical procedure, the microbial count rises every time doors swing open from either direction. Also, swinging doors may touch a sterile table or person. The risk for catching hands, equipment cords, or other supplies is increased. Always look through the window before opening this door to prevent contamination or injury.

Ventilation

The OR ventilation system must ensure a controlled supply of filtered air under positive pressure. The primary concerns for flow of ventilation include how the air is distributed, filtered, and exhausted. Air changes per hour (ACH) is an important concern based on the size of the individual OR. HVAC manufacturers continually study the best ways to ventilate ORs and provide ventilation systems compatible with the needs of the sterile team for aseptic air quality.

Air changes and circulation provide fresh air and prevent accumulation of anesthetic gases and microbiologic particles in the room.[2] Concentration of gases depends solely on the proportion of pure air entering the air system to the air being recirculated through the system using displacement ventilation. Fifteen ACH with three exchanges of outside air (OA; 15:3) is recommended for procedure rooms. General ORs and cesarean delivery suites require 20 ACH with 4 OA exchanges (20:4) according to the AIA Guidelines for Design and Construction of Health Care Facilities.[b] A gas scavenger system is used to prevent the buildup of waste anesthetic gases where general inhalation anesthesia is used. The scavenger attaches directly to the outflow of the anesthesia machine.

Various types of scavengers, vacuum systems, and smoke evacuators are used throughout the OR to minimize air pollutants

---

[b] The *Guidelines for Design and Construction of Health Care Facilities* by the Facility Guidelines Institute is available in its entirety online at www.fgiguidelines.org.

that are health risks for patients and perioperative team members. The American Society of Heating, Refrigeration, and Air-conditioning Engineers (ASHRAE) sets the standard for safe ventilation.

If new air ducts are installed, they should be thoroughly cleaned before activation to prevent the dispersal of particulate material into the air. The risk for airborne contaminants is significantly increased.

PROS/CONS

OR Ventilation and Foot Traffic

Pros

- Laminar airflow ventilation systems are designed to reduce airborne contaminates. The systems have a unidirectional flow of clean air from a higher plane to lower exhaust grilles.
- Uninterrupted laminar airflow permits higher air exchanges, which relates to cleaner air and fewer airborne contaminates. Fewer contaminates in the air may result in fewer surgical site infections (SSIs).
- Internal OR ventilation systems (HVAC) are set at positive pressure and the hallways are set to negative pressure to minimize the amount of air moving into the room as the door is opened.
- OR doors must be kept always closed unless absolutely necessary and foot traffic kept to a minimum for the ventilation system to work properly.
- Foot traffic can be described by the amount of movement around the room, personnel in and out of the room, and how many persons are in the room at one time.
- The Joint Commission is promoting a reduction in OR traffic as an effective practice to reduce SSIs.
- Common reasons for door movement and heavy foot traffic are gathering supplies or information, communication, employee breaks, vendors, change of personnel, and social visits.
- Education about facility ventilation systems and how foot traffic and opening and closing doors can decrease the rate of SSIs.

Cons

- Maintaining proper airflow is a problem for every OR. Airflow can be interrupted by foot traffic and opening and closing of OR doors.
- Propping OR doors open causes the airflow to equalize and prevents the positive pressure in the room from moving potential contaminates away from the field.
- Door movement and foot traffic cause air turbulence that sends contaminates from the floor into the air. This can disperse contaminates leading to a possible SSI.
- Research has identified that elevated airborne bacterial counts were higher when OR doors were opened and closed more often and foot traffic was excessive.
- Foot traffic can be kept to a minimum by having PRN items in the room, such as supplies and implants. Post "Do not enter" signs. Use the phone for communication and discourage social visits during surgical procedures.
- Health care staff should be monitored to keep foot traffic to a minimum.

References

1. Carr D: Reducing OR traffic, *AORN J* 116(6):570–576, 2022.
2. Khankari K: Hospital operating room ventilation systems. www.ashrae.org. Accessed April 14, 2023.
3. Wang Q, Xu C, Goswami K, et al.: Association of laminar airflow during primary total joint arthroplasty with periprosthetic joint infection, *JAMA Netw Open* 3(10), 2020.
3. Hamilton W, Balkam C, Purcell, et al.: Operating room traffic in total joint arthroplasty: identifying patterns and training the team to keep the door shut, *Am J Infect Control* 6(6):633–636, 2018.

Ultraclean laminar airflow is installed in some ORs to combat airborne particulate contamination by providing 70 to 160 ACH. Laminar airflow is a high-pressure, unidirectional air-moving diffuser housed in a cluster in a wall or ceiling enclosure. It is designed to flow uninterrupted from the cleanest area to the less clean area into air return grilles in the lower sidewalls. Cool air from the laminar diffuser travels more quickly than isothermic air. Care is taken to continually monitor the patient's temperature for any hypothermic effect. Hypothermia can support the development of a surgical site infection (SSI).[2] Laminar airflow systems are expensive to install and maintain.

The airflow is divided into tiny linear columns of cool clean air that generates little velocity and blowing as it courses toward the sterile field. Objects that emit thermal plume, such as spotlights, persons, or equipment, cause the air currents to move in a different direction.[3] *Horizontal airflow* passes from the wall diffuser to an opposite lower return grille. Objects in the air pathway shed particulate into the clean airstream (Fig. 10.6). *Vertical airflow* styles have fewer obstacles to the line of direction of the air.

Vertical downward airflow is designed to flow from the top of the room; flow over the patient, lights, and equipment; and continue downward, forming a canopy toward the lower corners of the room where the air return grilles are located. Studies have shown an 89% reduction in colony-forming units when vertical laminar airflow is used appropriately. This includes making sure that the open instrument tables are well within the confines of the airflow canopy.[3] One additional consideration is when the surgeon and team are directly over the patient to view the surgical site. Particulate from the nonsterile head/cap/mask and neck are passed directly into the sterile field depositing cells into the patient. Wearing skull caps rather than the bouffant-style hats permits additional shed when hair extends at the nape of the neck.

• **Fig. 10.6** Human thermal plume pattern that can alter laminar airflow.

In contemporary ORs that use laminar airflow, three styles of vertical downward-directed airflow originate in the ceiling directly clustered over the field with slightly different effects.

1. Standard vertical laminar flow provides a narrow boundary of operating space that begins at the ceiling and interfaces with the field, personnel, and ambient room air before it is exhausted through air return grilles (Fig. 10.7).
2. Air curtained vertical flow uses a peripheral secondary airflow at a higher velocity to widen and frame the primary laminar flow from the ceiling to the lower pressure air return grilles in the base of the walls (Figs. 10.8 and 10.9).
3. Physical curtained vertical flow uses air foils hanging from the ceiling on four sides to maintain the downward direction of airflow. The air funnels down toward the field, flowing around and behind the team (Fig. 10.10).

Obstacles to Laminar Airflow Effectiveness

Objects that pass between the flow of clean air and the sterile field around the patient shed particles that can contaminate the surgical site. Heat emanating and rising from the team members, the patient, and equipment—referred to as the *thermal plume*—changes the course of the laminar flow (Fig. 10.11). Several physical barriers and events that interrupt airflow and return include the following:

- Spotlights over the field
- Ceiling booms with surgical machinery and equipment
- Mayo stands over the patient
- Microscopes, articulated laser arm, and C-arm
- Personnel and patient thermal plume
- Opening and closing the OR door (sliding and swinging doors; proportionally higher with swinging doors)

Laminar airflow was first trialed during hip replacement surgery by Sir John Charnley in Great Britain in the 1950s. Charnley believed that if particulate could be removed from the air, the 7% infection rate could drop. His studies showed that the infection rate did fall to less than 2%. Although the laminar system contributes to removing particulates, the improvements in sterile technique and appropriate antibiotic therapy overall may have a larger effect on infection rate.

Research has shown that the particulate dispersal is proportionate to the number of personnel in the room, the opening and closing of doors (and their type), placement of instrument tables, and attire worn.

Other types of filtered air-delivery systems that have a high rate of airflow are as effective in controlling airborne contamination. Filtration through high-efficiency particulate air (HEPA) filters can be 99.7% efficient in removing particles that are larger than 0.3 mm. These microbial filters in ducts filter the air, practically eliminating all dust particles. The ventilating system in the surgical suite is separate from the hospital's general system and is to be cleaned, inspected, and maintained on a preventive maintenance (PM) schedule.

Positive air pressure in each OR is greater than that in corridors, scrub areas, storage, and substerile rooms. Positive pressure forces air from the room. The air enters at the ceiling and leaves through the grilles at floor level. Microorganisms and particulate in the air can enter the room unless positive pressure is maintained.

• **Fig. 10.7** Horizontal airflow pattern.

• **Fig. 10.8** Vertical airflow pattern with no air curtain.

• **Fig. 10.9** Vertical airflow pattern with downdraft air curtain.

• **Fig. 10.10** Ceiling view of vertical airflow diffusers with air curtain vents around periphery.

Closed doors maintain this environment and prevent equalization of air pressure. The recommended parameters include a dual filtration system with two filters in succession. The first filter should be at least 30% efficient, and the second filter should be at least 90%. Filter changes and duct cleaning should be on a PM schedule with OR maintenance.

Floors

In the past, floors were conductive enough to dissipate static from equipment and personnel but not enough to endanger personnel from shock or cause explosions from flammable anesthetic gases. Conductivity is not a prime concern in contemporary OR design because explosive anesthetic gases are no longer used.

The most common flooring used is seamless polyvinyl chloride that is continued up the sides of the wall for 5 or 6 inches and welded into place. These materials should not degrade or stain with age and cleaning. Metal oxides can be incorporated to decrease the slipperiness of the surface when wet.

A variety of hard plastic, seamless materials are used for minor procedure room floors. The surface of all floors should not be porous but suitably hard for cleaning with the flooding, wet-vacuuming technique. Personnel fatigue may be related to the type of flooring, which can be too hard or too soft. Cushioned flooring is available. The floor should be slip-proof when wet, because surgical hand cleansing causes splashes and spills around the scrub sink and drips into the OR, where the hands are dried.

Many of the glues and adhesives used in the installation of the flooring are malodorous and potentially toxic. During construction or renovation, care is taken to vent any fumes from the area. A minimum of 2 weeks may be needed to fully rid the area of the smell before it can be safely used for patient care.

Floors in older buildings may need reinforcement to support larger and more sophisticated equipment. Some of the wiring may be run in conduits under the floor.

Walls and Ceiling

Finishes of all surface materials should be hard, nonporous, fire-resistant, waterproof, stain-proof, seamless, nonreflective, and easy to clean. The ceiling should be a minimum of 10 ft high and have seamless construction. The height of the ceiling depends on the amount and types of ceiling-mounted equipment. The ceiling color should be white to reflect at least 90% of the light in even dispersion.

Walls should be painted a calming light color. Paneling should be made of hard vinyl material that is easy to clean and maintain. Seams should be sealed with a silicone sealant. Laminated polyester or smooth painted plaster provides a seamless wall; epoxy paint tends to flake or chip. Dust and microorganisms can collect between tiles because the mortar between them is not smooth. Most grout lines, including those made of latex, are porous

• **Fig. 10.11** Vertical airflow pattern with short physical barrier as air director.

enough to harbor microorganisms even after cleaning. Tiles can also crack and break. A material that can withstand considerable impact also may have some value in noise control. Stainless steel cuffs at collision corners help prevent damage.

Walls and ceilings often are used to mount devices, utilities, and equipment to reduce clutter on the floor. The ceilings should be reinforced with steel beams to support the load. In addition to the overhead operating light, the ceiling may be used for mounting an anesthesia service boom, operating microscope, x-ray image intensifier, electronic monitor, and a variety of hooks, poles, and tubes. Demands for ceiling-mounted equipment are diversified.

Suspended track mounts are not recommended because they engender fallout of dust-carrying microorganisms each time they are moved. If movable or track ceiling devices are installed, they should not be mounted directly over the OR bed but away from the center of the room and preferably recessed into the ceiling to minimize the possibility of dust accumulation and fallout.

Piped-in Gases, Computer Lines, and Electrical Systems

Vacuum for suction, anesthetic gas evacuation, compressed air, oxygen, and nitrous oxide may be piped into the OR. For safety, the hoses used to pipe in the gases and evacuate waste anesthetic gas are color coded (Fig. 10.12). The pin-index safety outlets may be located on the wall or suspended from the ceiling in either a fixed rotating boom or a retractable column. The anesthesia provider needs at least two outlets for oxygen and suction and one for nitrous oxide. The pin-index safety connectors that fit into the outlets have different shapes to prevent placing the wrong gas supply to the anesthesia machine (Fig. 10.13). To protect other rooms, the supply of oxygen and nitrous oxide to any room can be shut off at control panels in the corridor should trouble occur in a particular line. A panel light comes on, and a buzzer sounds in the room and in the maintenance department. The buzzer can be turned off, but the panel light stays on until the problem is

corrected. The buzzer should be tested on a routine schedule and should always remain active. Turning off the sound could lead to unsafe operating conditions.

Computers are widely used in the OR. They are commonly located adjacent to the anesthesia machine and the circulating nurse's desk. Most facilities have wireless access to the Internet and the in-house intranet. Both the circulating nurse and the anesthesia provider can document patient care and supply charges in the medical record. Additional computers can be used in specialties such as neurosurgery or orthopedics to display computed tomography (CT) images during the intraoperative care period. Digital radiographs can be displayed directly from the radiology department. Care is taken not to use the keyboard with soiled hands or soiled examination gloves. The keyboard should be of a design that permits adequate cleaning between patients. Seamless touch keypads or keyboard covers are easiest to maintain and clean.

Electrical outlets are grounded and must meet the requirements of the equipment that will be used. Some machines require 220-V power lines; others operate on 110 V. Electrical receptacles are color coded to show usability during a power outage. The white or ivory outlets are for general use. The red outlets are designed to work through the emergency power system's generator (Fig. 10.14). All equipment used for patient physiologic maintenance should be plugged into the red outlets.

Permanently mounted fixtures, such as a clock and radiograph view boxes, can be recessed into walls and wired in rather than plugged into outlets. Electrical cords that extend down the wall or across the floor are hazardous. Ceiling-mounted booms are strategically placed for bringing piped-in gases, vacuum lines, and electrical outlets close to the OR bed. They eliminate the hazard of tripping over cords.

Multiple electrical outlets should be available from separate circuits. This minimizes the possibility of a blown fuse or a faulty circuit shutting off all electricity at a critical moment. All personnel must be aware that the use of electricity introduces the hazards of electric shock, power failure, and fire. Faulty electrical equipment may cause a short circuit or the electrocution of

Instrument Air

Oxygen (O_2)

Medical Air

Carbon Dioxide (CO_2)

Nitrous Oxide (NO_2)

Helium (He)

Waste Anesthesia Gas

Nitrogen

• **Fig. 10.12** Color-coded hoses for the anesthesia gas machine.

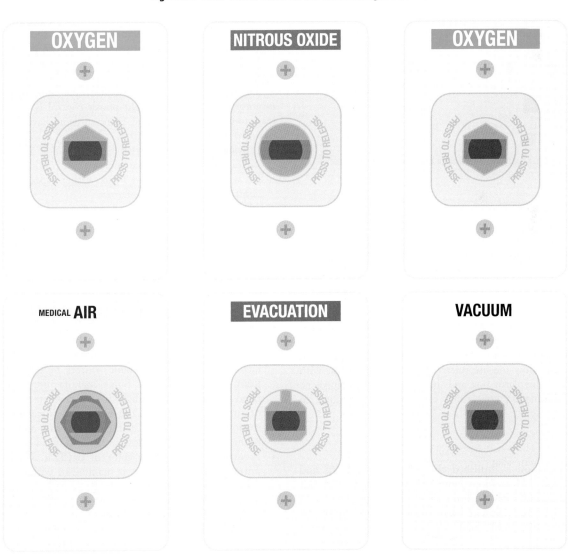

• **Fig. 10.13** Outlets for anesthetic hose connections. Each portal has a different shape to prevent error during connection.

• **Fig. 10.14** Electrical receptacles are color coded—red for emergency use and white/ivory for general use.

patients or personnel. These hazards can be prevented by taking the following precautions:

1. Use only electrical equipment designed and approved for use in the OR. Equipment must have cords of adequate length and adequate current-carrying capacity to avoid overloading.
2. Test portable equipment immediately before use.
3. Discontinue use immediately if any malfunction takes place, and report any faulty electrical equipment.
4. If a ground fault buzzer sounds, unplug the last device engaged and remove it from service.

Fire safety systems are installed throughout the hospital. All personnel must know the fire rules. They must be familiar with the location of the alarm box and the use of fire extinguishers. Additional information concerning OR fires can be found in Chapter 13.

Lighting

General illumination is furnished with static ceiling lights and mobile spotlights. Most room lights are white fluorescent, but they may be incandescent. Lighting should be evenly distributed throughout the room without harsh shadows, especially in the working area of the sterile field. The anesthesia provider must have sufficient light, at least 200 foot-candles, to adequately

evaluate the patient's color. Intraoperatively, the lighting should not cause the organs to appear discolored.

For minimized eye fatigue, the ratio of intensity of general room lighting to that at the surgical site should not exceed 1:5, preferably 1:3. This contrast should be maintained in corridors and scrub areas, and in the room itself, so the surgeon becomes accustomed to the light before entering the sterile field. Color and hue of the lights also should be consistent. Some facilities use a green light system to balance the color.

Illumination of the surgical site depends on the quality of light from an overhead spotlight source and the reflection from the drapes and tissues. Drapes should be blue, green, or gray to avoid eye fatigue. White glistening tissues need less light than dull dark tissues. Endoscopic cameras have a built-in white-balancing feature to facilitate a natural color of the organs visualized. Light, either endoscopic or in open procedures, must be of such quality that the pathologic conditions are recognizable. Some lighting systems have video cameras installed that can be connected to monitors for observation by nonsterile personnel outside the field. The view is close to the same field of vision of the surgeon and first assistant.

The overhead operating light must:
• Make an intense light, within a range of 3700 to 15,000 foot-candles (40,000−160,000 lux), into the incision without glare on the surface. It must give contrast to the depth and relationship of all anatomic structures. The light should be equipped with an intensity control with a minimum of four brightness levels. The surgeon asks for more light when needed. A reserve light should be available.

Lighting needs differ when endoscopic equipment with video monitors is used. Lower light power control is beneficial to the team to minimize eye fatigue. Some surgeons have the room lights dimmed for certain procedures.
• Provide a light pattern that has a diameter and focus appropriate for the size of the incision. An optical prism system has a fixed diameter and focus. Other types have adjustable controls mounted on the fixture.

Most fixtures provide focused depth by refracting light to illuminate both the body cavity and the general operating field. The focal point is where illumination is greatest. It should not create a dark center at the surgical site. A 10 to 12-inch (25−30-cm) depth of focus allows the intensity to be relatively equal at both the surface and the depth of the incision.

To avoid glare, a circular field of 20 inches (50 cm) in diameter provides a 2-inch (5-cm) zone of maximum intensity in the center of the field with 20% intensity at the periphery.
• Be shadowless. Multiple light sources and reflectors decrease shadows. In some units, the relationship is fixed; other units have separately maneuverable sources to direct light beams from converging angles. Some manufacturers have incorporated sensors in the spotlight to detect when the first assistant or surgeon's head is in the beam and threatening to cast a shadow. The lights sense the obstruction and decrease the beam, preventing a shadow over the surgical site.
• Produce the blue-white color of daylight. Color quality of normal or diseased tissues is maintained within a spectral energy range of 3500° K to 6700° K. Most surgeons prefer a color temperature of about 5000° K, which approximates the white light of a cloudless sky at noon.
• Be freely adjustable to any position or angle with either a vertical or a horizontal range of motion. Most overhead operating

lights are ceiling mounted on mobile fixtures. Some have dual lights or dual tracks with sources on each track. These are designed for both lights to be used simultaneously to provide adequate intensity and minimize shadows in a single incision. Many fixtures are adapted so the surgeon can direct the beam by manipulating sterile handles attached to the lamp or by remote control at the sterile field. Automatic positioning facilitates adjustment, and braking mechanisms prevent drift (i.e., a movement away from the desired position).

Fixtures should be manipulated as little as possible to minimize dispersion of dust over the sterile field. For the best illumination in the shortest time, the first spotlight should be positioned at the surgical site, followed by the second. Ideally, the light can be maneuvered in a 360-degree rotation as needed, quickly and without effort. Smaller lights commonly are restricted because of wiring bundles.

- Produce a minimum of heat to prevent injuring and drying exposed tissues. Most overhead lights dissipate heat into the room, where it is cooled by the air-conditioning system. Halogen bulbs generate more light and heat than do other types but do not last as long. Prolonged exposure to halogen light can be drying to the patient's tissues. The average halogen bulb lasts 1000 to 3000 hours. The risk for fire from a halogen bulb is significant, and the hot bulb should not be permitted to come in contact with any flammable material or a person's skin.

Lamps should produce less than 25,000 mW/cm of radiant energy. If multiple light sources are used, collectively they must not exceed this limit at a single site. Beyond this range, the radiant energy produced by infrared rays changes to heat at or near the surface of exposed tissues. A filter globe absorbs some infrared and heat waves over the light bulb or with an infrared cylindric absorption filter of a prism optical system. Nonfiltered lights, particularly halogen, can burn tissue from a distance.

- Be easily cleaned and maintained. Tracks recessed within the ceiling virtually eliminate dust accumulation. Suspension-mounted tracks or a centrally mounted fixture must have smooth surfaces that are easily accessible for cleaning. Light bulbs should have a reasonably long life. Light-emitting diode (LED) lights are semiconductors. LED lights last longer than halogen bulbs and do not generate heat. The average LED light lasts 20,000 hours, and more advanced LED lights last 60,000 hours. New LED fixtures can last a facility up to 10 years.

Changing the bulb should not require additional tools because time may be an issue in a critical part of a surgical procedure. The bulb is usually too hot to touch with the bare hand. Many styles are available that contain several bulbs that provide backup light when one bulb burns out.

A supplemental surgical task light may be needed for a secondary surgical site, such as for the legs or arms during conduit procurement for cardiovascular procedures. Some hospitals have portable explosion-proof lights. These lights should have a wide base and should be tip-proof. Others have satellite units that are part of the overhead lighting fixture. These should be used only for secondary sites unless the manufacturer states that the additional intensity is within safe radiant energy levels when used in conjunction with the main light source. The use of multiple teams in complex multidisciplinary procedures requires adequate lighting for each operating surgeon.

A source of light from a circuit separate from the usual supply must be available for use in case of power failure. This may require a separate emergency spotlight. It is best if the operating light is

equipped so that an automatic switch can be made to the emergency source of lighting when the usual power fails. The International Electrotechnical Commission (IEC) requires that new lighting must have the capability to restore power within 5 seconds after shutdown. Flashlights with fresh batteries should always be immediately available.

Some surgeons prefer to work in a darkened room with only indirect illumination on the surgical site during minimally invasive procedures. This is particularly true of surgeons working with endoscopic instruments and the operating microscope. If the room has windows to the hall or substerile room, lightproof shades may be drawn to darken the room when this equipment is in use. Because of the hazard of dust fallout from shades, the windows may have blinds contained between two panes of glass with a handle to open or close the louvers in rooms where this equipment is routinely used.

Although the surgeon may prefer the room darkened, the circulating nurse or anesthesia provider must be able to see adequately to observe the patient's color and to monitor the patient's condition. One dim spotlight can be aimed away from the field in the direction of the anesthesia provider. In some circumstances, the radiograph view box can be turned on for additional illumination.

Some surgeons wear an adjustable headlight designed to focus a light beam on a specific area, usually in a recessed body cavity (14–20 inches) such as the nasopharynx. Avoid using the headlamp at distances less than 10 inches. Too much heat and drying can harm tissues. The surgeon will don the headlamp and aim the beam before scrubbing. Fiber-optic headlights produce a cool-colored light and reduce shadows. Both the surgeon and first assistant may wear a headlight. The fiber-optic light cable should be clipped to the back of the surgeon's gown and enough length should be provided to prevent pulling on the light source when the surgeon moves. The cable should not be kinked or folded because the glass fibers will break and stop transmitting light. When not in use the cable should be loosely coiled.

Alternatively, a light source that is an integral part of a sterile instrument, such as a lighted retractor or fiber-optic cable, may be used to illuminate deep cavities or tissues difficult to see with only the overhead operating light. Fiber-optic cables should not be permitted to become detached from the instrument and shine directly on the drape for a prolonged period because a fire may ignite. During operation, do not permit blockage of the cooling vents by drapes or other equipment. Avoid looking directly into the beam because it may cause eye injury. The light source intensity setting should be completely at zero before disconnecting the cable for processing. Care is taken not to touch the connector until it is completely cooled. Refer to the manufacturer's recommendations for cleaning and servicing.

Monitoring Screens

Monitors and computers are designed to keep the OR team aware of the physiologic functions of the patient throughout the surgical procedure and to record patient data. The anesthesia provider or a perioperative nurse uses monitoring devices as an added means to ensure safety for the patient during the surgical procedure.

The screens may be built into portable carts or attached to articulated arms or ceiling booms. They may be plasma or liquid crystal display (LCD) and measure 20 to 22 inches, and in some facilities up to 42 inches. Plasma screens are heavier and do not last as long as LCD versions. Newer screens with surface-conduction electron emitter displays (SEDs) will likely replace LCD and plasma screens in the future. LED screens use light-emitting diodes as pixels and offer clear, bright color pictures. These screens are popular in the OR setting for a detailed image.

More commonly, video monitors serve several useful purposes for the surgeon within the OR. They are widely used for teaching surgical techniques. This minimizes the number of visitors in the OR, which, in the interest of sterile technique, is advantageous. In addition, monitors provide a better view for more people to see the surgical procedure from a remote area or through a microscope or endoscope. They can also be used for recordkeeping and documentation for legal purposes for the surgeon. Video recording is possible for this purpose. If video recording is done while patients are in the rooms, each patient should have the opportunity to sign a permission form.

As an aid to diagnosis, an audiovisual hookup between the OR and the radiology department permits digital radiographs to be viewed on the monitor in the OR without having to be transported into the OR and mounted on view boxes. With such a hookup, the surgeon gains the advantage of remote interpretive consultation when desired.

A two-way audiovisual system between the pathology laboratory and the OR enables the surgeon to examine the microscopic slide by video in consultation with the pathologist without leaving the OR bed. The pathologist can view the site of the pathologic lesion without entering the OR.

Radiograph Screens or View Boxes

Many facilities have changed from plain film viewing to digital computer monitors. The monitors may be on articulated arms that extend from the wall or ceiling. In this circumstance, lighted view boxes are still useful in the event old films are brought from the archives for comparison with the patient's new digital images. The view boxes also can be used as indirect lighting during low-light procedures.

Radiograph view boxes can be recessed into the wall. The viewing surface should accommodate a minimum of four standard-size films. The best location is in the line of vision of the surgeon standing at the OR bed. Lights for view boxes should be of high intensity. A film-holding basket should be placed within reach of each view box station.

Clocks

Two clocks should be in each OR. A standard clock, analog or digital, for basic time observation should be visible from the field. A time-elapsed clock, which incorporates a warning signal, is useful for indicating that one or more predetermined time periods have passed. This may be used during surgical procedures for total arterial occlusion, with use of perfusion techniques or a pneumatic tourniquet, or during cardiac arrest. Start, stop, and reset buttons should be within reach of the anesthesia provider and the circulating nurse.

Cabinets or Carts

Each OR may be supplied with closed-in stationary cabinetry unless a cart system or pass-through entry is used. Supplies for the types of surgical procedures done in that room are stocked, or every OR may be stocked with a standard number and type of supplies.

Having these basic supplies saves steps for the circulating nurse and helps eliminate traffic in and out of the OR. Glass shelves and sliding doors provide ease in finding and removing items.

Many cabinets are made of stainless steel or hard plastic. Wire shelving minimizes dust accumulation. Cabinets should be easy to clean. One cabinet in the room may have a pegboard at the back to hang items, such as table appliances. Gloves used in patient care should be removed when opening the cabinet and removing supplies.

Pass-through cabinets that circulate clean air through them while maintaining positive air room pressure allow transfer of supplies from outside the OR to inside it. They help ensure the rotation of supplies in storage or can be used only for passing supplies as needed from a clean center core. Some pass-through cabinets between the OR and a corridor accommodate supply carts directly from the sterile core, which are easily removable for restocking.

In lieu of or as an adjunct to cabinets, some hospitals stock carts with special sutures, instruments, drugs, and other items for some or all surgical specialties. The appropriate cart is brought to the room for a specific surgical procedure.

Furniture and Other Equipment

Stainless steel furniture is plain, durable, and easily cleaned. Each OR is equipped with these basic items:

- OR bed with a mattress covered with an impervious surface, foam or gel construction, attachments for positioning the patient, and armboards.
- Instrument tables. These are commonly called *back tables*, although they are at the side of the scrub person during the surgical procedure. Some rooms use over-bed tables such as Phelan or Mayfield style.
- Mayo stand. The Mayo stand is a frame with a removable rectangular stainless steel tray. The footplate of the frame slides under the OR bed and the support that holds the tray positions over the sterile field. The Mayo tray is supplied with immediate-need instruments and supplies. The height is adjustable.
- Small tables for gowns and gloves and the patient's skin preparation equipment and catheterization supplies.
- Ring stand for basins. This is optional because most ORs do not use splash basins.
- Anesthesia machine and table for anesthesia provider's equipment.
- Sitting stools and standing platforms that safely stack to give additional height to the user.
- IV poles for IV solution bags. The anesthesia provider may clip the upper drapes to the IV poles.
- Suction canisters, preferably portable on a wheeled base or waste management system that suctions fluids and surgical plume.
- Laundry hamper frame.
- Kick buckets in wheeled bases. Commonly called *sponge buckets.*
- Wastebasket near the circulating nurse's desk, biohazard red trash bins, and clean trash bins.
- Writing surface. This may be a wall-mounted stainless steel desk or an area built into a cabinet for the circulating nurse.
- Computer station. This may be permanently affixed to a hard-wired station or mobile wireless. The keyboard should be positioned so the circulating nurse can observe the sterile field. A scanning device may be incorporated for bar-coded drugs and supplies.

Communication Systems

A communication system is a vital link to summon routine or emergency assistance or to relay information to and from the OR team. Many surgical suites are equipped with telephones, intercoms, call lights, video equipment, and computers. These communication systems may connect the OR with the clerk-receptionist's desk, the nurse manager's office, the holding area, the waiting room, the PACU, the pathology and radiology departments, the blood bank, and the sterile processing department. These systems make instantaneous consultation possible through direct communication.

Voice Intercommunication System

Telephone and intercom systems are useful for the OR team to communicate with the control desk. Sounds are distorted to the patient in early stages of general anesthesia. Incoming calls over an intercom should not be permitted to disturb the patient at this time. Also, an awake patient should not overhear information about a pathologic diagnosis (e.g., from a voice coming through an intercom speaker box after a biopsy has been performed). Installation of any type of intercom equipment either in the adjacent substerile room or scrub area rather than in the OR helps eliminate sounds that could disturb both the patient and the surgeon.

Call-Light System

This system is used to summon assistance from the anesthesia staff, pathologist, patient care staff, and housekeeping personnel. It is activated in the OR with a hand-operated switch; a light alerts personnel at a central point in the suite or displays at several receiving points simultaneously.

Closed-Circuit Television

Television surveillance is an easy way for the nurse manager to keep abreast of activities in each OR. By means of a video camera with a wide-angle lens mounted high in the corner of each OR, managers may make rounds simply by switching from one room to another by pushing buttons at the desk and viewing a monitor in the office. Signs should be posted to indicate that video surveillance is in process, and the patient should be made aware that this is happening.

Computers

A computer in each OR affords access to EMR information and allows data input by the circulating nurse. The types of hardware and software programs available dictate the capabilities of the automated information system. A keyboard, light pen, or barcode scanner may be used for input. The computer processes and stores information for retrieval on the viewing monitor and by printout from a central processing unit.

The computer system should be wireless for fast transmission of data and should require a password for each user in the system for security. The staff should be encouraged to log on and log off, but the system has idle time parameters, so if inactive for a time, the system automatically logs off the user. Failed password attempts lock out the user for a designated period or may require the system administrator to assign a new password.

The computer database and EMRs help the circulating nurse obtain and enter information that may include the following:

- Schedule, including the patient's name, surgeon, procedure, special or unusual equipment requirements, wound classification, and whether procedure is elective, urgent, or emergency
- Patient EMR, preoperative patient assessment data, nursing diagnoses, expected outcomes, and plan of care
- Results of laboratory and diagnostic tests
- Surgeon's preference card with capability to update
- Inventory of supplies and equipment provided and used
- Charges for direct patient billing
- Intraoperative nursing interventions
- Timing parameters, including all staff activity, procedure, and room turnover
- Incident reports
- Postoperative care in the PACU

The computerized patient information generated in the OR may interface with the hospital-wide computer system.

Caution: The printer should not be in direct patient care areas. Printers use toner powder that can become airborne in the OR and cause contamination. According to the Safety Data Sheets (SDSs) for printer toner, the primary routes of entry of toner powder are via direct contact and inhalation.[c] Chronic lung exposure can cause irritation and lung fibrosis. Toner is combustible, and the powder has explosive qualities. It should be kept away from heat and flame. Personal protective goggles, gloves, and mask (PPE) should be worn if toner spills. A HEPA filter should be used if vacuuming the material. The Occupational Safety and Health Administration (OSHA) has not set permissible exposure limits at this time.

Special Procedure Rooms

Certain procedures or outpatient treatments may indicate the need for rooms designed for a specific purpose, such as interventional radiology, endoscopy, or cystoscopy. These rooms are designed with equipment for performing the specific interventional procedures, including specialized radiologic and monitoring devices. An interventional radiologist, cardiologist, and several endoscopists should be consulted when planning these types of facilities.

Interventional Radiography Room

Endovascular stenting, balloon angioplasty, cardiac catheterization, and other interventions that require fluoroscopy can be performed in a room with fixed x-ray equipment and specialized radiographic beds (Fig. 10.15). The endovascular instrument table may be double the average length because the aortic guidewires and deployment devices are extremely long. Proximity to the OR is important in case of an emergency that necessitates an open procedure. Many interventional rooms have doors that open into the semirestricted area of the surgical services department. Some interventional rooms double as minimally invasive rooms.

Cardiac catheterization (angioplasty and stenting) may be performed within the surgical suite in a room equipped for fluoroscopy. Imaging screens are located near the head of the OR bed or on articulated arms directly across the OR bed to allow the surgeon and the team to visualize the coronary arteries during the procedure. Monitors, suction, oxygen, and cardiopulmonary resuscitation equipment are available in this room for each cardiac catheterization procedure. The team must be alert for emergency situations, such as a perforated coronary artery, and be prepared for an emergency thoracotomy or transfer to an OR for an open procedure.

[c] See www.ehso.com for details per each manufacturer.

• **Fig. 10.15** Hybrid interventional OR has permanently installed imaging equipment.

• **Fig. 10.16** Cesarean delivery room. (Courtesy Michael S. Clement, MD.)

Minimally Invasive Surgery Room

Some rooms are equipped specifically for laparoscopic procedures, with ceiling booms in four quadrants of the room for endoscopic light sources, camera boxes, insufflators, electrosurgical generators, and video monitors. A dedicated minimally invasive surgery (MIS) procedure room has all the equipment for puncture and natural orifice endoscopy located on a large cart or a ceiling-mounted boom. The use of booms in these rooms helps minimize the amount of equipment spread around the room.

Several video monitors are located around the room on articulated arms or on the booms for ergonomic viewing of the surgical field by the surgical team. These rooms should have the capability of immediately converting to an open procedure in the event of an untoward event such as arterial or organ puncture.

Endoscopy Room

Many surgical suites have a designated class A size room in which natural orifice flexible or rigid endoscopic procedures, such as bronchoscopy, gastroscopy, sigmoidoscopy, or colonoscopy, are performed. Most are equipped for the use of lasers and electrosurgery. Some endoscopy rooms have x-ray and video capabilities. Equipment for natural orifice endoscopy is usually affixed to mobile carts so they can easily be transported to a regular OR for intraoperative bronchoscopy, gastroscopy, or colonoscopy added to a major surgical procedure.

Cystoscopy Room

A cystoscopy room (cysto room) may be available for a urologic examination or procedure. Ideally, the room should be a class A or class B size located in the restricted area of the OR. Waste fluids are collected in special canisters or waste management suction devices and are disposed of like other biologically contaminated fluids. Older cystoscopy rooms may be equipped with special floor drains for the disposal of fluids during the procedure. The drain cover must be removable for cleaning. Modern styles have eliminated this drain for infection control reasons.

A cystoscopy room is also equipped with x-ray and fluoroscopy machines because many procedures require the use of IV or ureteral contrast media to visualize the kidneys, ureters, and bladder. Radiographic digital screens should be adjacent to the OR bed, and view boxes should accommodate a minimum of four still films simultaneously. Imaging screens are located in the room, either freestanding or mounted on articulated arms, to allow the urologist to visualize the urologic structures during fluoroscopy. Some urologists use ultrasonic equipment, lasers, and electrosurgery to perform minimally invasive procedures.

A portable cystoscopy cart should be available for dispatch from the cystoscopy room when a procedure in the main OR requires placement of ureteral catheters, stents, or a cystoscopic examination. The cart should be equipped with a light source, sterile camera, video monitor, sterile cystoscopes (0° and 30°) and light cord, bridges and sheaths, an assortment of ureteral catheters in pairs, Foley catheters, urinary drainage bags, and lubricant.

Cesarean Delivery Room

Most facilities that have obstetric departments have a self-contained OR within the delivery suite (Fig. 10.16). This is a restricted room with an attached substerile room and scrub sink area. The purpose of this room is to provide equipment and supplies in support of a surgical birth of the baby through the mother's abdomen (cesarean section) instead of a vaginal birth.

A few differences of the cesarean delivery room include resuscitation supplies and equipment for the newborn and a specialized warming bed that can be used to transport the baby to the special care nursery.

Construction or Renovation of the Surgical Suite

Considerations for Planning and Design

The planning and design of the new perioperative environment generally entail both renovation and new construction. Most facilities cannot shut down for the construction process and must continue with patient care services. Adequate planning and projection of needs during the process take some of the stress out of running the department around construction obstacles.

Infection Control Issues
- Are walls and doors adequately sealed against particulates?
- Are potential sites of vermin entry sealed?
- Is ductwork free from material transferred from unclean areas?
- Are waterlines secured and leak free?
- Is a designated trash collection path identified?
- Is the environmental services need established?

Safety Concerns
- Are rerouted entrances and exits clearly marked? Will patient traffic change?
- Are fire alert mechanisms in place? Is a fire walkthrough necessary?
- Is life-saving equipment in an accessible location? Any Code Blue changes necessary?
- Is a backup power source immediately available?
- Is a backup water supply immediately available?
- Will other departments be directly affected?
- Is the project boss immediately available to halt the work crew in the event of a critical event or emergency?

The AIA Guidelines require a preconstruction risk analysis in a consultative format. The Infection Control Risk Assessment (ICRA) is determined, with all parties offering multidisciplinary input about features such as water temperature between 105° F (40.6° C) and 120° F (48.9° C), electric safety, ventilation air changes, and containing potential contamination. Box 10.1 describes additional preconstruction assessment factors to consider.

Goals to strive for include (1) timing of construction phases, (2) precision of work done, and (3) staying within the budget. Generating a concurrent plan for maintaining patient flow and expanding/renovating the department requires a multidisciplinary team, which may include the following members:
- Department director, nurse manager, and senior perioperative nursing personnel
- Physicians (surgeon, anesthesiologist, pathologist)
- Infection control, risk management, and environmental services personnel
- Maintenance and biomedical personnel
- Project manager (may be in-house personnel or a consultant), architect, equipment vendor, and purchasing personnel; a collaboration between the architect and equipment vendor can generate three-dimensional drawings that can offer a preview of the area
- Communications and information technology personnel (e.g., computers, telephone, intercom, emergency call)
- Support services (e.g., laboratory, radiology, pharmacy) personnel
- City or municipality planning personnel
- Interior decorator

No one construction or renovation plan suits all hospitals or surgical centers; each plan is individually designed to meet projected specific future needs. Visiting other hospitals where building and reconstruction have taken place is beneficial. Ask about the good and bad points.

The number of ORs, storage areas, and immediate perioperative patient care areas required depends on the following:
- Number, type, and length of the surgical procedures to be performed. This determines the class of OR size to build.
- Type and distribution by specialties of the surgical staff and equipment for each. Some specialties may use the same room most of the time and use mounted equipment such as booms, microscopes, imaging equipment, and endoscopy.
- Proportion of elective inpatient and emergency surgical procedures to ambulatory patient and minimally invasive procedures.
- Scheduling policies related to the number of hours per day and days per week the suite will be in use and staffing needs.
- Systems and procedures established for the efficient flow of patients, personnel, and supplies.
- Consideration of volume changes and need for future expansion capabilities.
- Technology to be implemented and plans for potential technology to be developed.
- Safety of staff, patients, and other personnel during construction or renovation.
- Infection control procedures.

Principles in Construction or Renovation Planning

The universal problem of environmental control to prevent wound infection exerts a great influence on the design of the surgical suite and the plans for construction or renovation. Surgical suites older than 20 years do not have the capability of supporting newer technology with renovation for space and technologic, HVAC, and electrical capabilities.

Architects, administrators, and surgical suite designers follow several concepts in planning the physical layout and construction of a surgical suite, as follows:
1. Strategic planning
   a. Avoid as much inconvenience to facility personnel as possible.
   b. Include facility personnel in the planning phase as much as possible.
   c. Expedite completion as fast as possible without compromising safety of patients, staff, and construction personnel.
   d. Keep costs down by planning ahead. Do not substitute cheap materials for durable materials. They only cost more to replace later. Always follow manufacturer and blueprint specifications.
   e. Plan the project in steps, or phases, completing each area before starting the next. After each phase, have a group of committee members walk through to evaluate the work and the effectiveness of the design.
   f. Minimize the ordering of supplies for patient use to only those items needed for immediate procedures. Inventory storage is an issue as the project unfolds.
   g. Resolve replacement issues for current equipment in use. Sometimes it is financially better to buy units in a lot than to replace one at a time. Deals can be made regarding pricing when planning equipment for the new rooms. It is better to install equipment from scratch than to add later at an added construction/installation cost.
   h. Plan for the closing of rooms without too much disruption if they are to be updated.
   i. Determine the balance of fixed equipment versus mobile equipment for use in several rooms.
   j. Determine the need for dedicated rooms, such as for endoscopy, cystoscopy, orthopedic, minimally invasive procedures, interventional radiology, and cardiac procedures.

2. Plans for problems or emergencies
   a. Power, communications, medical gases, vacuum system, waste gas scavenger, air handlers, water, and sewage cannot be interrupted. A plan should be in place to counter any accidental cutting of lines by construction personnel. *Legionella* bacteria have grown in standing water lines during phases of construction. *Aspergillus* spores have been isolated and transmitted to patients.
   b. Plan for capability of construction work stoppage at a moment's notice if requested by a surgeon during a critical phase of surgery.
3. Exclusion of contamination from outside the suite with sensible traffic patterns to and from the suite
   a. A sealed barrier must be in place between working ORs and the portion of the suite under construction. Wood or drywall panels as temporary walls sealed over all edges with duct tape can keep dust and fungal spores from entering the suite. Plastic sheeting is not sturdy and can be easily punctured.
   b. Negative pressure must be maintained in halls with exhaust filtered to the outside of the building.
   c. Traffic patterns must be unobstructed for debris removal. Asbestos may be present and will require special handling of all materials removed. Toileting and hand-cleansing areas must be available to construction workers.
   d. Traffic patterns must be unobstructed for bringing in construction supplies and materials. Walk-off sticky mats can be placed on the floors at entrances and exits to attract particulate matter from the shoes of the workers. The sticky mats have tear-off sheets that can be removed as they become soiled, revealing a fresh sticky mat.
4. Separation of clean areas from contaminated areas within the suite during the building phase
   a. Patient traffic should be separated from construction traffic.
   b. Clean supplies are transferred in an area separate from construction supplies.
   c. Biologic decontamination and processing areas remain functional at all times.
5. Noise control
   a. Noise pollution should be kept at a minimum when surgical procedures are in process or the general patient population in the hospital is sleeping.
   b. Vibrations from powered equipment and jackhammers can disrupt microscopic or other procedures.

Physical plant design and construction/renovation planning of a surgical suite should include detailed consideration for the activities of patients, caregivers, and environmental maintenance.

ⓔ EVOLVE WEBSITE

http://evolve.elsevier.com/Hornacky/BerryKohn/

- Historical Perspective
- Student Interactive Questions
- Glossary

References

1. Fassbinder M, Abernathy J: Redesigning the operating room, *Handbook of perioperative and procedural patient safety*, St. Louis, 2024, Elsevier.
2. Wagner J, Vosik D, Eller M, et al.: Untended perioperative hypothermia and surgical site infection in children, *J Surg Res* 276:235–241, 2022.
3. Wang Q, Xu C, Goswami K, et al.: Association of laminar airflow during primary total joint arthroplasty with periprosthetic joint infection, *JAMA Netw Open* 3(10), 2020.

Bibliography

AORN (Association of periOperative Registered Nurses): *Guidelines for perioperative practice*, Denver, 2024, The Association.
Hornacky A, Phillips NM: *CNOR pass*, St. Louis, 2019, Elsevier.
The Facility Guidelines Institute: *Guidelines for design and construction of health care facilities, Chicago*. Available at: www.fgiguidelines.org/.

11

Ambulatory Surgery Centers and Alternative Surgical Locations

CHAPTER OUTLINE

Ambulatory Surgical Setting, 197

Alternative Sites Where Surgery Is Performed, 206

CHAPTER OBJECTIVES

After studying this chapter, the learner will be able to:

- Compare the differences between hospital-based services and ambulatory surgery centers.
- Distinguish between activities in fixed and mobile surgery locations.

- Describe key elements of human versus veterinary surgery.

KEY TERMS AND DEFINITIONS

Ambulatory care Care delivered to a patient who is not confined to bed or in need of formal admission to a facility for a prolonged period.

Deployment A term that refers to sending one or more active duty soldiers forward into an area where medical war support is needed.

DEPMEDS A system of mobile military hospital components that are assembled and dismantled close to the location of military activity.

Monitoring Clinical observation of a patient's condition through continuous interpretation of vital signs, activities, and responses.

PAT center Area of a facility designated for patient assessment and preprocedural examination.

Telehealth A term used for the activities of health care with the use of computers, mobile health applications, live video conferencing, monitoring systems, and electronic records. All aspects of health can be covered, such as health information, digital records, provider contact, medical care, and education.

Ambulatory Surgical Setting

Ambulatory surgery can be defined as surgical patient care performed with general, regional, or local anesthesia without overnight hospitalization. Some ambulatory surgery centers (ASCs) offer diagnostic testing and radiologic examinations, such as mammography and magnetic resonance imaging (MRI).

The following are organizations specifically for professional ambulatory surgical nurses:

- American Society of PeriAnesthesia Nurses (ASPAN); www.aspan.org
- American Academy of Ambulatory Care Nurses (AAACN); www.aaacn.org
- Ambulatory Surgery Center Association (ASCA); www.ascassociation.org
- AORN (Association of periOperative Registered Nurses); www.aorn.org

AORN has established a specialty assembly for nurses who practice in the ambulatory setting. AORN's website has an Ambulatory Surgery Center Solutions Guide for ASC leaders. It contains information on leadership, risk management, anesthesia monitoring, infection prevention, specific details for ambulatory facility practice, sterilization, nursing education modules, an administrator course, and a career center at www.aorn.org.

Ambulatory Surgery Programs

Various terms are used to describe *ambulatory care* facilities, including *outpatient surgery, same-day surgical unit, day surgery,* and *ambulatory surgery center.* Conceptually, an ambulatory facility has the following:

- Preprocedural testing and assessment area (PAT center)
- Admitting area
- Changing and dressing room with lockers and toilets
- Preoperative holding/preparation area
- Operating room (OR)
- Postanesthesia care unit (PACU) or access to a PACU
- Waiting room

The decor of the ambulatory facility should be pleasing to enhance relaxation of the patient, family, and significant others. Recliners are commonly available for postprocedure recovery. Many facilities have televisions, reading material, and may offer a children's play area and beverages for waiting individuals. Figure 11.1 depicts a sample floor plan that shows the various areas within an ASC. Priority patient parking areas should be conveniently located near the entrance to the facility, with parking spaces for disabled patients located nearest the entrance.

Many hospital-based ASCs offer valet parking. The convenience of dropping off and picking up patients should be accommodated in the design of the facility. Studies have shown that this is a point of patient satisfaction. Newer facilities have a drive-up area that is covered overhead from the weather for convenient drop-off and pickup. Space requirements for parking areas are determined by the numbers and types of surgical procedures to be performed.

The location of an ASC may vary. Government laws indicate that a true ASC is not dependent on the main hospital and is physically independent in services, such as ORs, postprocedure care, and central service. ASCs are not designed to take emergency patients and typically employ fewer than 20 employees.

The future of ambulatory surgery is on the rise. More procedures are shifting to ambulatory surgery centers.[1] The Centers for Medicare & Medicaid Services (CMS) plan to remove procedures from the hospital-only pay list. The removals of in-hospital—only procedures are expected to shift into the ambulatory setting. According to Fortune Business Insights, the ambulatory surgery market could increase to over $58 billion by 2028. New large freestanding facilities or hybrid facilities are

• **Fig. 11.1** Schematic of ambulatory surgery floor plan. (Reprinted with permission Herman Miller, Inc.)

opening that offer state-of-the-art technology in a comfortable and convenient setting. Some facilities specialize in only one service, such as orthopedic, spine, or cardiac. Patients have access to surgeon appointments, diagnostic and preoperative testing, and surgery with the availability of extended stay in one building. These new facilities employ more than 20 employees and operate like a small hospital. Examples of outpatient surgery departments include the following:

- *Hospital-based dedicated unit.* Patients come to a self-contained unit that is located within or attached to the hospital but physically separate from the inpatient OR suite.
- *Hospital-based integrated unit.* Ambulatory patients share the same OR suite and other hospital facilities with inpatients. The preoperative admission and holding area is shared. Ambulatory patients usually return to the same admission area for discharge after the procedure.
- *Office-based center.* Patients come to a physician's office that is equipped for surgery. Many private surgeons, dermatologists, periodontists, and podiatrists perform surgical procedures in their offices with a local or moderate sedation anesthetic. An anesthesia provider is employed to administer sedation drugs. This office-based center may accommodate one or more surgeons in the same specialty, or it may be a multiphysician, interdisciplinary clinic. Although these are not always attached to a hospital, they are not considered an ASC. Examples of ASCs by the definition of ASCA are the following:
- *Hospital-affiliated satellite surgery center.* Patients come to an ASC that is owned and operated by a larger facility but geographically separate from it.
- *Freestanding or hybrid ASC.* Patients come to a completely independent facility. Many of these facilities are owned and operated by physicians or a business. Facilities must follow approved construction guidelines.

Accreditation of Ambulatory Facilities

The ASC should comply with standards set by the Accreditation Association for Ambulatory Health Care (AAAHC; www.aaahc.org), The Joint Commission (TJC; www.jointcommission.org), the Ambulatory Surgery Center Association (www.ascassociation.org), and the American Osteopathic Association (AOA; www.osteopathic.org). These patient advocacy and consumer groups advise patients to select facilities carefully and to look for accreditation and credentialing by professional and governmental agencies. The ASC should be certified by the CMS.[2] The AAAHC is one organization that is authorized by the CMS to conduct surveys of health care facilities for compliance with the standards.

The updates for Ambulatory Health Care and Office-Based Surgery National Patient Safety Goals (www.jointcommission.org) include the following[3]:

- *Improve the accuracy of patient identification:* Use a minimum of two patient identifiers (name and date of birth) when administering pharmacologic agents or blood, taking blood samples or specimens, or providing any treatments or procedures.
- *Improve communications among caregivers:* All verbal orders or results should be read back to the person delivering the information. Standardize a list of all abbreviations, acronyms, and symbols that are not to be used within the organization. Improve the timeliness of information exchange between the reporter and receiver regarding test results and values.

Standardize the handover report of patient care to qualified personnel between phases of care.

- *Improve medication safety:* Standardize the numbers and concentrations of drugs within the facility, identify sound-alike/look-alike medications and limit the use to prevent error, and label all containers and delivery devices with the name and concentration of the drug. Discard any unlabeled medication containers. Medications should be verified by two individuals. Visual identification of the original container and confirmation with verbal read back.
- *Determine the patient's medication history and be sure there are no potential drug interactions during the course of care:* Take care with patients who routinely take blood-thinning medications. Provide adequate education concerning postoperative home-going drugs by providing drug name, dose, frequency, route, and contact information in case of reaction.
- *Reduce the risk for health care—related infections:* Comply with Centers for Disease Control and Prevention (CDC) recommendations for hand hygiene. All deaths or permanent injuries associated with health care—related infection are treated as sentinel events and reported to the accrediting agency.
- *Reduce the risk for surgical fires:* Staff education should include spark, fuel, and ignition sources, including oxygen concentration under drapes and fumes from alcohol prep solutions, as a source of surgical fire.
- *Prevent mistakes in surgery:* The surgeon should mark the surgical site. A "time out" is performed to confirm the correct patient, procedure, supplies, implants, and pertinent health information (e.g., allergies) with the team. Include the patient in the confirmation as possible.
- *Implement Revised Pain Assessment and Management Standards:* This revision requires education for employees and patients, prescribing requirements for narcotics and opioid monitoring, treatment, and resources. This revision is the result of the opioid crisis in an effort to reduce patient dependency.

ASCs should be licensed by the state wherein they are established. Requirements for licensure are similar to those for accreditation. Inspection visits are scheduled on a routine basis. Ambulatory centers are highly regulated by governmental agencies. Medicare and Medicaid certification is required for reimbursement. Accreditation and credentialing of an ambulatory facility can be attained by, but is not limited to, the following:

- Compliance with structural standards
- Establishment of policies and procedures that support competent standards of care
- Appropriate credentialing of personnel
- Emergency preparedness
- Appropriateness of procedures performed at the facility

According to statistics compiled by the CDC, approximately two-thirds of all surgical procedures performed are done on an ambulatory or outpatient basis safely and without complications. Some smaller facilities limit the use of ambulatory surgery to procedures that can be performed with local or regional block anesthetics. Facilities with PACU capability allow surgeons to perform procedures with the patient under general anesthesia.

Although procedures performed in an ambulatory care facility are usually of short duration (15—90 minutes), the appropriate selection and evaluation of patients are essential. Patient care and anesthesia management are crucial factors in the experience of the ambulatory surgical patient.

Some facilities are prohibited from performing complicated laparoscopy because of the risk for injury to the patient. More ASCs are doing bariatric, total joint replacement, spine, and palliative care procedures. (More information can be found at the ASCA website at (www.ascassociation.org.)

Patient Selection for Ambulatory Surgery

After a surgical procedure, patients may prefer to recuperate at home rather than in the hospital. These patients may be candidates for ambulatory surgery, depending on the nature and extent of the surgical procedure and on the patient's ability to follow instructions or to receive adequate care at home. Consideration is given to the duration and complexity of the surgical procedure, the risks of anesthesia, and the probability of postoperative complications.

Patients are carefully screened before being considered safe candidates for ambulatory surgery. The following are some of the criteria considered:

1. General health status. Acceptable patients are in class I, II, or stable III of the physical status classification of the American Society of Anesthesiologists (ASA).[4] Patients are evaluated physically and emotionally to determine the possibility of complications during or after the surgical procedure. CMS regulations require three separate health assessments before a patient is placed on the OR bed. The three assessments include:
   a. A complete medical history and physical examination (H&P) no earlier than 30 days before the intended surgical procedure. The H&P must be redone if 30 days have passed.
   b. A physical assessment on arrival at the surgery center to validate that no changes have occurred since the H&P was performed. Care is taken when discussing private information in the ASC cubicles. Other patients can overhear conversation through the divider curtains.
   c. A preanesthesia evaluation to assess the safety of administration of anesthesia before the patient enters the OR.
2. Results of preoperative tests. Patients may have tests on admission the morning of the surgical procedure, but preferably these tests are performed before the scheduled surgery date so the results can be evaluated. This prevents cancellation on the day of surgery if test results are unsatisfactory. Test results are documented in the medical record before the patient is brought to the OR. Preoperative tests may include the following:
   a. Complete blood count (CBC) and urinalysis (usually included in basic laboratory tests)
   b. Pregnancy test, unless patient previously had a hysterectomy or oophorectomy
   c. Multichemistry profile for patients at higher risk
   d. Chest radiograph (may be required if clinically indicated)
   e. Electrocardiogram (may be required before general anesthesia for patients older than 35 years)
3. Willingness and psychologic acceptance by patient and significant others. The patient should be willing and able to recuperate at home. Some patients lack adequate home care and may need other arrangements.

Each patient is individually assessed. Provision is made for competent care at home by either an agency or the patient's family and significant others. Compliance with preoperative and postoperative instructions by the patient and the availability of a responsible adult support person are essential. Other factors to consider when screening a patient for possible ambulatory surgery include the following:

- *Recovery period:* The surgeon should anticipate minimal or no postoperative complications. Patients in whom a prolonged period of nausea and vomiting is anticipated or in whom pain will not be relieved with oral analgesics are not ideal candidates for ambulatory surgery.
- *Reimbursement sources:* Most third-party payers prefer less costly ambulatory surgery whenever a procedure can be safely performed in this setting. Patient safety and quality of care depend on patient screening and support systems.

PROS/CONS

Selecting an Ambulatory Surgery Center (ASC)

Pros
- Can the surgical procedure be done safely without complications?
- Accredited surgical centers offer convenience for preoperative testing, parking, and easy access.
- Accreditation requires the facility to follow set standards, performance measures, and site visits for compliance.
- Same-day surgery allows the patient to recover at home.
- Wait times may be shorter because a schedule is followed without interruption of emergencies.
- Reduced infection rates. Orthopedic surgery centers are becoming popular because the patient does not have exposure to hospital-acquired infections.
- Patients may be able to shop around for procedure prices and reduce out-of-pocket expenses.
- Medicare patients can download the "What's Covered" application on Google Play or the Apple store to see which procedures are covered.

Cons
- Patients with high-risk factors or certain ages may not qualify to have a procedure at an ASC.
- Complex procedures or procedures with risk for complications cannot be performed at an ASC.
- If an emergency occurs, the patient must be transferred to the nearest hospital.
- No overnight stay. Some facilities may offer a 23-hour stay.
- Some insurance companies will not cover certain outpatient facilities.
- Some patients may be transferred to a rehabilitation facility for recovery.

References
1. American Society of Anesthesiologists: *Guidelines for ambulatory anesthesia and surgery.* www.asahq.org. Accessed March 28, 2023.
2. Centers for Medicare & Medicaid Services: *New app displays what original Medicare covers.* www.medicare.gov. Accessed March 28, 2023.
3. Accreditation Association for Ambulatory Health Care: www.aaahc.org. Accessed March 28, 2023.

Preoperative Patient Care

Written instructions for both preoperative and postoperative care are given to the patient by the surgeon during an office visit or by the nurse during a preadmission visit to the ambulatory care facility. These instructions describe the admission, preoperative, intraoperative, recovery, and discharge procedures, and they should be written in a language the patient can understand.

For the protection of both the surgeon and the facility, the patient should sign for receipt of these instructions and should sign that informed consent has been given to the surgeon for the intended surgical procedure. Instructions should include the following:

1. Preoperative instructions
   a. Make an appointment for preadmission assessment and testing.
   b. Take nothing by mouth (NPO) after midnight (or other specified hour) before admission unless ordered to do so by the surgeon. This includes medications, unless ordered.
   c. Perform any necessary physical preparation such as bathing with antimicrobial soap as ordered.
   d. Arrive at the facility (facility address or suite) by ____ AM/PM. (Time depends on the scheduled time for the surgical procedure. A minimal wait at the facility helps reduce preoperative anxiety. Patients are usually admitted at least 1 hour before the scheduled time of their surgical procedure. Figure 11.2 shows an ambulatory preoperative holding area.)
   e. Notify the surgeon immediately of a change in physical condition, such as a cold or fever.
   f. Wear loose and comfortable clothing, leave jewelry (including face, tongue, and body piercings) and valuables at home, and remove contact lenses, artificial eyelashes, makeup, and nail polish. (This may include the removal of acrylic fingernails for some procedures if affixing the pulse oximeter to another location, such as the toe, is not an option.)

2. Postoperative instructions
   a. Arrange for a responsible adult support person to take you home. (After most procedures, the patient may not be permitted to drive or leave unattended.)
   b. Do not ingest alcoholic beverages, drive a car, cook, or operate machinery for 24 hours if a sedative or general anesthetic has been administered.
   c. Delay important decision-making until full recovery is attained.
   d. Take medications only as prescribed and maintain as regular a diet as tolerated.
   e. Shower or bathe daily unless instructed otherwise. This helps relieve muscle tension and discomfort and keeps the wound clean.
   f. Call the surgeon if postoperative problems arise.

Preoperative Holding

Patients arriving for surgical procedures are held in this area until the appropriate operating room is ready.

Patients will change into hospital attire in dressing cubicles before entering the preoperative holding area. An area should be available to store patients' clothing and personal belongings.

This area also may be called preanesthesia as patients may be given medications or intravenous fluids under close observation of the nursing staff.

A nurses control station and medication preparation area are often an integral part of this area.

Movable Modular Casework Applications
A preoperative holding area can be planned using movable modular casework and may include

- Small workstation.
- Locker to hold patient care supplies.
- L cart, procedure/supply cart, or rail-hung C-frame storage unit placed near each stretcher.
- Procedure/supply carts.
- Extra-deep modular shelving units.
- Sink unit.
- Med prep area.

Plan View of a Preoperative Holding Area
A preoperative holding area will range in size from 350 to 800 square feet.

    8 linear feet work surface
    6 linear feet overhead storage
    40 filing inches
    1 locker for medications
    1 locker for IVs
    2 lockers for supplies
    1 C-frame storage unit per bed
504 square feet

• **Fig. 11.2** Preoperative holding area. This area is used for patients before surgery and can be used after surgery. If a local anesthetic has been used, the patient returns directly from the OR. If more complex anesthesia is used, the patient returns here after postanesthesia care unit discharge. (Reprinted with permission Herman Miller, Inc.)

g. Report to the nearest emergency department if your condition deteriorates.

h. Keep follow-up appointment with the surgeon.

The patient should be reminded that the postoperative information will be reinforced and possibly updated at the time of discharge. The patient's level of understanding of the preoperative instructions (NPO reminder or medication modification) and planned procedure is assessed with a telephone call from the perioperative nurse to the patient the day before surgery; at this time, the scheduled date and arrival time are also verified. Patients should be reassured that they will be given a set of written instructions before discharge from the facility. The nurse should document patient instructions and responses in the record.

Intraoperative Patient Care

Intraoperatively, the same precautions are observed by all team members as for any surgical procedure. These include strict adherence to the principles of aseptic and sterile techniques and other OR routines. Consideration for patient privacy and avoidance of embarrassment are essential. The general layout of the OR is similar to that of larger facilities but on a smaller scale (Fig. 11.3).

The careful selection of patients, preoperative evaluation, and instructions helps prevent complications from the anesthetic. Premedication, if given, is minimal. The surgical procedure should be less than 90 minutes in duration for general anesthesia and less than 3 hours for regional block. Local anesthesia or a regional block is preferable if appropriate. Spinal anesthesia is seldom used.

Scrub Area
Scrub areas are placed strategically outside operating rooms. Surgical scrub sinks are generally ceramic or stainless steel with foot or knee controls. It is helpful to place shelves above the sink to hold scrub brushes and masks.

Movable Modular Casework Applications
Depending on the design of the scrub area, scrub brushes and masks can be housed in modular shelving hung on rail, on wall strips above the sinks, or in rail-hung C-frame storage units with drawers beside the sinks.

Plan View of a Scrub Area
8 linear feet overhead storage (2 feet per sink)
50 square feet

A

Operating Room
An operating room is the area where surgical procedures are performed under strict sterile techniques.

For sanitization purposes, operating rooms should contain little or no built-in casework. Supplies and equipment are moved in and out as needed. Rather than using wall strips, horizontally mounted rail with rail-hung components are appropriate for hanging work surfaces for documenting/charting. Rail-hung shelves or CST units are suitable for overhead storage.

Plan View of an Operating Room

An operating room will range in size from 300 to 800 square feet.

4 linear feet work surface

4 linear feet overhead storage

3 lockers for supplies

1 L cart

1 anesthesia cart case carts as required

336 square feet

Movable Modular Casework Applications

An operating room can be planned using movable modular casework and may include

L carts or procedure/supply carts used for
- Anesthesia supplies and equipment.
- Suction and cautery equipment.
- Monitoring equipment.
- Prep and dressing.

Stainless steel case carts, which can also be used as a back table.

Lockers used for
- General supply storage.
- Backup supplies.
- Specialty procedure carts.

Process tables used as
- Administrative/computer workstations.
- Back table for instruments.

B

• **Fig. 11.3** A, Scrub area. **B,** OR layout. (Reprinted with permission Herman Miller, Inc.)

Cardiopulmonary resuscitation (CPR) equipment and nurses certified in CPR at a minimal level of basic cardiac life support (BCLS) should be available during the procedure (certification in advanced cardiac life support [ACLS] is preferred). Perioperative nurses who specialize in the care of pediatric patients should have certification in pediatric advanced life support (PALS).

Patients who undergo general anesthesia or moderate sedation are scheduled for surgery early in the day to allow for a maximum recovery time. Rapidly dissipating agents are administered, and various combinations of agents and drugs are used. Drugs associated with prolonged recovery are avoided unless there is a specific indication for their use. Doses of intravenous (IV) agents, such as narcotics and barbiturates, may be reduced to avoid delayed emergence.

Technologic monitoring, including bispectral analysis (BIS monitoring), allows the anesthesia provider to administer minimal amounts of an agent based on the patient's level of consciousness and sensorium. Anesthetic techniques should provide adequate depth of anesthesia but with minimal cardiopulmonary changes and side effects. Indications for endotracheal intubation are the same as for inpatients.

The patient who is undergoing local anesthesia is monitored continuously for any reaction to the medications or change in physiologic status. If an anesthesia provider is not in attendance, a qualified perioperative nurse should be assigned to monitor the patient for behavioral and physiologic changes. This nurse should have a basic knowledge of the function and use of monitoring equipment and should not be assigned other duties while monitoring the patient's condition.

The monitoring perioperative nurse measures and records the patient's vital signs before the injection of a local or regional block anesthetic or analgesic and every 15 minutes thereafter; monitors physiologic status according to written policy and procedure; and institutes emergency measures if an adverse reaction occurs.

The perioperative nurse should be responsible for interpreting, identifying, and reporting abnormal readings to the surgeon. Additional functions of this nurse may include starting oxygen, administering IV therapy, and giving medications when clinically indicated. The perioperative nurse should have periodic competency reviews for the departmental files. These may be examined by accreditation officials during a site visit. Suggested noninvasive intraoperative monitoring methods for patients undergoing local anesthesia are listed in Box 11.1. Each OR must have a cardiac monitor, pulse oximeter, blood pressure apparatus, and oxygen delivery equipment. Each OR should have immediate access to a crash cart in the case of an emergency.

The policies and procedures for monitoring patients undergoing local anesthesia should include patient risk criteria, the type of monitoring to be used, documentation of vital signs and medications administered, and interventions within the scope of nursing practice. All pertinent data and therapy are documented according to the policies of the facility.

•BOX 11.1 **Noninvasive Monitoring Equipment Used for Patients Under Local Anesthesia**

- Electrocardiograph
- Pulse oximeter
- Blood pressure apparatus

The awake and alert patient needs to receive physical and emotional comfort throughout the surgical procedure. The field of vision may be small while the patient is draped, and tactile and other stimuli come as a surprise if the patient is not forewarned. The patient should be told what is about to occur (e.g., "You will feel a needle sting"), what to expect (e.g., "You will have a burning sensation"), and what is expected (e.g., "Tell us if you feel pain"). The patient's questions should be answered truthfully and realistically. The patient should be reassured that appropriate amounts of the anesthetic will be administered as needed.

Conversation by team members should be appropriate and kept to a minimum. The use of an intercom system should be avoided. Hand signals between the surgeon and scrub person are more useful than a verbal request for instruments. However, the surgeon may request a No. 10 or 15 rather than a knife, or a Mayo or Metz rather than scissors. Strange noises and smells should be explained to the patient (e.g., the sound of suction to remove an irrigating solution; the sound of the electrosurgical unit [ESU] and odor of ESU plume).

Background music of the patient's choice may help with relaxation and distraction. Headsets are one option for this purpose and help block out other noises. Although headsets can distract the patient from the ambient room noise, they can also distract the patient from following necessary directions during the procedure; therefore cautious use is suggested.

Traffic in and out of the room should be kept to a minimum. A sign should be placed on the outside of the door to indicate the type of anesthesia being used (e.g., "Patient awake, local anesthesia").

Postoperative Patient Care

Patients who have received a local anesthetic are returned to the ambulatory unit for assessment and discharge. Patients who have undergone general anesthesia or moderate sedation or who need postoperative pain management are taken to the PACU for stabilization and observation (Fig. 11.4). Medications may be given IV in small dosages; oral medications may cause nausea and vomiting that may prolong the length of stay. Routine orders may be established by policy for these analgesics and antiemetics.

Consciousness, rational behavior, and ambulation do not imply full recovery. Blood pressure and pulse rate may return to the normal range while residual myocardial depression continues. Patients may lapse back into sleep or drowsiness as the drugs used for general anesthesia are metabolized. Patients are always under observation in the PACU. Although the Aldrete Scoring System (Table 11.1) is commonly used for establishing postoperative discharge criteria, this method should not be used to replace patient assessment data in determining suitability for discharge.[4]

A hospital short-stay unit may provide postoperative care for observation and pain control for up to a 23-hour stay. When all discharge criteria are met, patients are discharged on written order of the anesthesia provider or surgeon according to policy. Discharge is contingent on the patient's generalized condition. Vital signs are measured and compared with baseline, and the condition of the surgical site is documented before the patient leaves the premises. Patients who have questionable vital signs or an unstable physiology should be seen by a physician before discharge.

Patients are not allowed to drive home if a general or regional anesthetic has been administered. The patient should leave the facility via an appropriate mode of transportation and

Postanesthesia Care Unit (PACU/Recovery Room)

This area is adjacent to the operating room. Patients are brought to this area after surgery to recover from anesthesia and regain stable vital signs. After the patients are stable, they are moved to secondary recovery before being discharged.

The space is usually in an open area with patients separated with cubicle curtains. Those patients who need to be isolated are kept in a separate isolation recovery room. The isolation room also can be used for pediatric patients.

The layout of this space usually includes a nurse control station with a medication preparation area, a physicians' dictation area, an area for supplies and equipment, hand-washing sinks, and a patient toilet.

Plan View of a Postanesthesia Care Unit

A PACU will range in size from 2000 to 4000 square feet.

```
26  linear feet work surface
18  linear feet overhead storage
80  filing inches
 8  lockers for supplies
 1  locker for medications
 1  L cart for supplies
 1  I cart for isolation cart
 1  emergency cart
 1  C-frame storage unit per bed
    Dictation area
2126 square feet
```

Movable Modular Casework Applications

Movable modular casework components appropriate for use in the PACU include

- Nurses control station.
- L cart or rail-hung C-frame storage units with drawers for supplies for each patient.
- Lockers for linen and medical supplies.
- Cantilevered sink units.
- Dictation area.

• **Fig. 11.4** Postanesthesia care unit. (Reprinted with permission Herman Miller, Inc.)

TABLE 11.1 Aldrete Postanesthesia Scoring System

			Admission	15 min	30 min	45 min	60 min
Activity	Able to move voluntarily on command	4 Extremities	2	2	2	2	2
		2 Extremities	1	1	1	1	1
		0 Extremities	0	0	0	0	0
Respiration	Able to breathe deeply, cough freely		2	2	2	2	2
	Dyspnea or limited breathing		1	1	1	1	1
	Apnea		0	0	0	0	0
Circulation	BP + 20 of preanesthesia level		2	2	2	2	2
	BP + 20–50 of preanesthesia level		1	1	1	1	1
	BP + 50 of preanesthesia level		0	0	0	0	0
Consciousness	Fully awake		2	2	2	2	2
	Arousable on calling		1	1	1	1	1
	Not responding		0	0	0	0	0
O_2 saturation	Able to maintain O_2 saturation >92% on room air		2	2	2	2	2
	Needs O_2 inhalation to maintain O_2 saturation >90%		1	1	1	1	1
	O_2 saturation <90% even with O_2 supplementation		0	0	0	0	0

BP, Blood pressure.
Modified from Aldrete A, Wright A: Revised Aldrete score for discharge, Postanesthesia Care Practice Considerations, American Association of Nurse Anesthesiology. www.aana.com. Accessed March 29, 2023.

accompanied by a responsible adult. Select patients who have undergone local anesthesia without sedation may be permitted to drive home if an order is written by the surgeon. The means of the patient's discharge, regardless of transportation, should be documented.

Patient education is an essential element of ambulatory surgical care. Written discharge instructions are verbally reviewed with the patient and a responsible adult. The perioperative nurse should document how the patient or the representative signified understanding of the instruction. Some patients can verbalize or perform a return demonstration as confirmation.

The patient is instructed when to arrange for a follow-up visit with the surgeon. Appropriate phone numbers for the surgeon, ambulatory center, and emergency help should be listed on the discharge instruction sheet. If problems occur after discharge, the patient is encouraged to contact the surgeon or surgeon's designee.

Recovery Centers

Freestanding recovery care centers have been developed to accommodate a 24 to 48-hour uncomplicated postanesthesia recovery period. Although they occur infrequently, the most common reasons for admission to a freestanding recovery care center or hospital after ambulatory surgery are pain, nausea and vomiting, urinary retention, and concern for wound integrity. Several types of homelike or hotel-like facilities provide care for up to 72 hours after surgery. Many new facilities performing complicated procedures are offering extended care. For select ambulatory surgery patients, arrangements for postoperative care can be made with a private home health agency.

Interfacility Transfer Management

If complications develop (e.g., adverse reactions to an anesthetic or cardiac changes), the patient may need to be admitted to a hospital for intensive care monitoring. Therefore freestanding ASCs and office-based centers need to have a patient transfer/admission agreement with a nearby hospital. Accredited facilities have guidelines and policies for patient emergency transfers. Surgeons may have admitting privileges at the nearest hospital. The team in the room should notify the nurse in charge and arrange for transport. Smaller facilities use the emergency number 911 to request emergency medical services (EMS) personnel for the physical transport of the patient to the hospital.

The doorways of office-based practices should be wide enough to accommodate the EMS stretcher. A registered nurse (RN) may be designated to travel with the patient. The plans for emergency transfer of a patient should be reviewed with the entire staff on a routine basis.

Accrediting bodies require the ASC staff to have drills on patient emergency management, such as malignant hyperthermia, cardiac arrest, or other crisis events. Emergency supplies and equipment must be immediately available and tested on a regular schedule.

Follow-up Phone Calls and Technology

Most complications occur within the first 48 hours after surgery. Therefore an RN or a qualified medical provider should call to check on the patient's progress and to reiterate postoperative instructions the next day or, at most, within 2 days of discharge. The nurse or provider reminds the patient to keep the follow-up appointment with the surgeon. Some facilities ask several survey questions for quality improvement during this call. Other forms of communication are used to communicate with patients after surgery such as text messaging, medical applications, telehealth,

and email. Follow-up methods should be standardized, but the nurse should document any barriers to communication such as literacy, language barriers, or other conditions that can lead to poor communication. The follow-up method should be clear and easy for the patient to communicate.

Patients who plan to return to work within 1 or 2 days after surgery may be asked to phone, text message, or email the nurse themselves because they may not be home when the nurse makes routine calls during the day. Patient satisfaction can be surveyed with technologic methods of postoperative contact.

PROS/CONS

Follow-up Communication

Pros

- Follow-up communication after surgery or hospital discharge is usually done within 48 hours. The patient may have a choice of communication method.
- A telephone call from a specially trained health care provider discusses patient progress and complaints, confirms discharge and medication instructions, and confirms physician follow-up appointments.
- Follow-up telephone calls reduce hospital readmissions by recognizing lack of patient knowledge and preventing medical problems.
- Telephone calls to postoperative patients have proved to be cost saving to the health care facility.
- Patient satisfaction was higher when follow-up telephone calls or messaging was done.
- Some surgeons give out a personal cell phone number to receive text messages if problems arise from patients.
- Medical applications are being used to have patients answer questions at a convenient time about symptoms. An immediate call can be made to the patient if symptoms are concerning. Educational material also can be put onto the app.
- For patients who live far from a health care facility, telehealth can be used to video chat with the patient. The surgeon can see the incision, and the patient saves a trip to the office. Some insurance companies are now paying for telehealth.
- Many patients like to use technology because it is fast, user friendly, and can provide a personal response from the nurse or surgeon.

Cons

- Failure to follow up with patients after surgery or hospital discharge increased hospital readmission rates.
- Hospital readmission within 30 days is attributed to poor communication and education.
- Hospital readmission or health problems are costly to the health care system.
- Patients were less likely to follow discharge instructions and follow up with their physician without a follow-up telephone call or other form of communication.
- If a computer system or an Internet connection is lost, communication can be obstructed.
- Literacy, language barriers, or other issues can cause communication barriers.

References

1. Liu T, Tokita H, Simon B: An enhanced ambulatory surgery experience for patients with cancer through end-to-end patient engagement, *Adv Anesth* 40(1), 2022.
2. Hedge S, Nagaraj M, Gonzalez-Guardiola G, et al.: Overcoming health literacy barriers by developing standardized surgical discharge instructions, *J Surg Res* 278:386—394, 2022.
3. Billings K, Bhushan B, Berkowitz R, et al.: Outcomes of a postoperative day one call to families after adenotonsillectomy in children, *Laryngoscope Investig Otolaryngol* 7(4):1200—1205, 2022.

Documentation of Ambulatory Procedures

The development, implementation, and evaluation of the plan of care should be documented in the patient's medical record. Documentation should include, but is not limited to, the following:

1. Preoperative care
   a. Preanesthetic evaluation by the anesthesia provider if a general, regional, or local anesthetic with sedation is to be given
   b. Nursing assessment data, nursing diagnoses, expected outcomes, plan of care, and preoperative teaching by the perioperative nurse
   c. Medical history and physical examination
   d. Laboratory reports and results of other tests
   e. Informed consent for the surgical procedure
2. Intraoperative care
   a. Anesthetic and medications administered
   b. Vital signs and intraoperative monitoring data
   c. Intraoperative implementation of the plan of care
   d. Surgical procedure note by the surgeon
   e. Wound classification at the end of the procedure
   f. Any unexpected outcomes
3. Postoperative care
   a. Postanesthesia care, including monitoring of patient responses and medications
   b. Discharge instructions, including follow-up appointment with the surgeon and signs and symptoms of potential complications that require immediate medical attention
   c. Radiology, pathology, and any other medical reports
   d. Physical and psychologic status at the time of discharge
   e. Attainment of expected outcomes
   f. Mode of transport from the facility and destination, including relationship to the accompanying support person
4. Remote postoperative care
   a. Follow-up phone call or confirmed use of technology method within 24 to 48 hours to assess the patient's progress
   b. Follow-up phone call or communication within 6 weeks to assess the patient's satisfaction with outcomes and services (for continuous quality improvement data)
   c. Patient follow-up with the surgeon

Most patients who undergo ambulatory surgery are satisfied with their care. Studies have shown that if further surgery is indicated, most patients choose to have the new procedure performed in an ambulatory setting. Fewer incidents of postoperative complications have been documented, as have lower costs of treatment for the patient. Preoperative teaching is beneficial in helping patients attain the expected outcomes. Careful patient evaluation and planning can make the ambulatory surgery a successful and positive experience for the patient, family, significant others, and caregivers.

Alternative Sites Where Surgery Is Performed

Mobile Army Military Hospital

Military medical personnel can be categorized as active duty or reserves. Several branches of military service personnel operate hospitals in the time of war or disaster. Colonel Michael Ellis DeBakey, MD (1908–2008), was integral in the initial design of the Mobile Army Surgical Hospital (MASH) and received the Legion of Merit Award in the early 1940s. This section discusses the Army Nurse Corps and the activities associated with mobilization of a mobile surgical hospital in the second millennium. (Additional information can be found online at www.defense.gov.)

Active duty personnel can be stationed in their homeland or abroad for a particular tour of duty. Wherever they are located, there are medical facilities for the care and health maintenance of the troops in times of peace, war, or disaster. In a war zone or natural disaster such as a hurricane, flood, or earthquake, military hospitals care for injured civilians as well. Nurses and other supporting personnel provide care according to the same standards followed by health care personnel located in main hospitals in civilian locations. Nurses and other medical support personnel are deployed to the duty area in the same manner regardless of active duty or reservist status. Many surgical personnel employed by civilian hospitals are members of reserve units and could be called for active duty. The civilian surgical knowledge and skill are valuable attributes when caring for battlefield or disaster casualties.

Reservists who are called to active duty for any augmentation or supporting role first go through mobilization activities to prepare for deployment. During the mobilization period, which can be several days or weeks, the soldiers are prepared for the specific area where they will be stationed for active duty. Activities include creating family care plans, immunization updates, physical examination, overview of geographic location, briefing on local native customs and language, and military-specific roles. Family care plan considerations are finalized by providing support for dependents and confirming childcare arrangements for single parents. During the Persian Gulf War, 16,337 single parents were called to active duty.

Nursing and medical support personnel are considered soldiers and train with weapons and bioprotective gear (i.e., gas masks, hazmat attire [mission-oriented protective posture, or MOPP, gear]). Field-grade officers and chief nurses wear a side arm pistol (e.g., M17- Sig Sauer P320) and carry extra rounds at all times in defense of the mobile hospital and its patients. The ammunition is loaded into clips but not inserted into the pistol unless under imminent threat. Weapon chambers are always cleared before entering the medical facility. Only security troops' weapons always remain loaded. Additional weapons (M16 rifles) are stored in a centralized location for personnel to use in case of an attack.

All personnel are responsible for erecting the hospital and support structures for the deployment period (Fig. 11.5). Teams specially trained in setting up mobile medical facilities construct patient care wards, intensive care units, emergency triage tentage, supply areas, and ORs. Additional service structures, such as soldier sleeping quarters, dining tent (mess tent), laboratory, radiology, and pharmacy units, are set up as well. All services and structures are self-supporting in terms of electricity, water supply, sanitation, laundry, showers, food service, and communications.

Deployable Medical Systems

Deployable medical systems (DEPMEDS), developed in the 1980s, are essentially mobile hospital units (Fig. 11.6). One type, the combat support hospital (CSH), consists of special tents, known as *TEMPER tents* (Tent Expandable Modular PERsonnel), measuring 64 × 20 ft or larger, which are designed to be used in all climates (Fig. 11.7). The U.S. military is now using lightweight TEMPER air-supported tents that are faster to construct and

• **Fig. 11.5 A,** Hospital being moved into position. **B,** Hospital under construction. **C,** Teamwork setup.

• **Fig. 11.6** Aerial view.

require fewer personnel.[5] They are used in combination with large rooms destined to be ORs or laboratories fashioned from fold-out aluminum box rooms referred to as International Standards Operations containers (ISOs; Fig. 11.8). The ISOs and tentage are transported to the site by cargo planes, helicopters, or large trucks. All personnel are specially trained to erect the DEPMEDS facility. Fort McCoy in Wisconsin is one training center where specialized training takes place.

Some of the ISOs open out to create a protected environment double or triple its compacted size. ISOs are used to create environments for laboratory, radiology, pharmacy, sterile processing, and ORs. TEMPER tents are used to house patients and auxiliary work areas. Some DEPMEDS facilities can house up to 1000 hospital beds. Chemically protected types of ISOs and TEMPERs are used in areas where nuclear, chemical, or biologic terrorism threat exists.

The OR ISO is designed to provide a surgical setting for two patients at once with two OR beds (Fig. 11.9). In severe situations, two surgical teams can work in the same room simultaneously. Each half of the ISO has complete OR usage with two independent anesthesia stations placed in opposite ends of the structure.

Passages made of canvas, referred to as *vestibules*, connect the TEMPER tents and ISOs to form the working environment of the hospital in a series of connecting hallways complete with flooring and climate control (heating and air conditioning) for all weather (Fig. 11.10). The completed structure is reasonably comfortable and efficient.

The grounds on which the mobile hospital is built are surveyed and cleared of hazards. Some dangers to look for during war are unexploded landmines, poisonous plants and animals, disease-carrying insects, and human-made booby traps. Snipers are always a threat until the perimeter is secure. A specialized administrative team inspects the grounds and marks off each site for the layout to the exact inch. If the team miscalculates the plan, the TEMPERs and the ISOs do not line up correctly when the connecting vestibules are attached.

• **Fig. 11.7 A,** TEMPER tent frame. **B,** TEMPER tent setup for patient care area.

• **Fig. 11.8 A,** Fold-out ISO with door open. **B,** Completed ISO setup from outside.

• **Fig. 11.9 A,** Duplicate sets for the OR ISO. **B,** One side of OR ISO.

The integrity of each structure is inspected daily for stability in all types of weather. Desert areas are subject to sandstorms. Rainwater, mud, hurricanes, and earthquake aftershocks can cause dramatic shifts. The team checks the ISOs daily with a level device for any shift in balance. Delicate equipment (e.g., scanners) does not work correctly on uneven ground. Jacks on the corners of the ISOs are used to shift the baseline to balance the unit.

In a hostile environment, the functionality of the hospital depends on the maintenance of the physical plant. Security patrols continually monitor the perimeter of the area and diligently

• **Fig. 11.10** Vestibule connects ISO and TEMPER.

protect the hospital from sabotage by the enemy. Power generators and water supplies are prime targets for disabling the effectiveness of the mobile hospital's mission. The constant threat of chemical and biologic weapons is also a consideration. All personnel carry a protective mask in a holder attached at the belt. The personnel are trained to respond to a warning (e.g., the sound of banging metal against metal) by donning the mask and providing protection for the patients. The personnel of the hospital must be prepared to dismantle the hospital and move to a new location on short notice.

Patient care in the mobile hospital is based on returning the soldier to duty as soon as possible. Studies have shown that soldiers who are separated from their units for prolonged periods because of war-inflicted injury suffer increased duration of traumatic stress. A wounded soldier who can be saved with available resources is triaged and treated according to the type of injury or injuries incurred. After stabilization, the wounded can be evacuated to a larger hospital away from the war zone.

Surgery in a Mobile Hospital Setting

Injured soldiers or civilians who can be treated with a surgical procedure are taken to a presurgical holding area, where their conditions are stabilized for surgery. The surgical procedures are performed by two separate teams who maintain individual sterile fields for both patients. Although the OR ISO is designed to accommodate two surgical procedures at the same time, great care is given to maintain sterile and aseptic techniques.

Postoperatively, the patients are taken to the postsurgical recovery area. The ISO is cleaned and set up for two more patients. The OR must always be prepared. The instrumentation is taken to an adjoining tent or processing ISO for cleaning and sterilization to prepare for subsequent surgical procedures. The processing area is referred to as the *central materials service* (CMS).

Each type of injury is carefully evaluated in a mass casualty scenario. This activity is used in civilian areas when terrorist attacks or natural disasters take place in nonmilitarized zones. Each patient is triaged according to the amount of care needed. If chemical, biologic, or radiation contamination has been used in the attack, the patient is taken to a decontamination area before going to the patient care area. Clothing and personal effects are removed. Clothing is discarded appropriately, but personal effects (e.g., jewelry) are bagged and marked for decontamination later.

The patients are tagged with colored tags to indicate where they will be taken within the hospital according to the type of injury (Table 11.2). The decontamination team is specially trained for this task. They also decontaminate the area and dispose of contaminated materials before the next patient is brought into the area for processing. Deceased contaminated personnel must be decontaminated before delivery to the morgue.

Wounded soldiers or other personnel who need extraordinary surgical procedures and are not likely to survive are transferred to an expectant ward, where they receive comfort measures until they expire. Expectant patients are protected from the view of other patients. This is extremely stressful to the nursing and medical staff because in the civilian sector resources are frequently expended in the care of expectant patients, regardless of survivability. In a CSH environment, standard operating procedures mandate the type of care given to patients who are treated onsite, patients who are shipped out, and those who are beyond treatment. Some examples of expectant categories include open head wound with exposed brain in an unconscious-unresponsive patient, radiation exposure greater than 500 rads and signs of advanced radiation sickness, or totally absent pulses and no spontaneous breathing with airway support.

Consideration is given to the injured enemy prisoners of war (EPW). A separate hospital facility is set up to accommodate EPW care. Security is complex, and additional training is required to manage patient care. Interpreters should be available. EPW are allocated resources according to need per the Geneva Convention.

Service animals, such as mine-sniffing or search and rescue dogs, may need surgical treatment. A separate surgical tent is set up for their care. Instrumentation and other sterile supplies are processed separately from items used in human care. A separate sterilizer may be set up for the sterilization of instruments used in animal surgery.

The living quarters of the mobile hospital personnel consist mainly of tents capable of housing 20 or more people. During field training exercises, smaller two-person tents are used to conserve space and expedite setup. Personal belongings are limited to what can be packed into two duffel bags and carried by one person. Equipment, such as protective masks, pistol belts, Kevlar helmets, and other survival gear, leaves little room for personal belongings. Uniformity in attire is part of the unity of the group.

TABLE 11.2	Patient Classification With Tags for Mass Casualty	
Color Tag	**Definition**	**Explanation**
Green	Minimal care needed; ambulatory	Minor injuries. Return to duty as soon as possible
Yellow	Need urgent care, but can be delayed; not ambulatory	Not in immediate life threat
Red	Need immediate care; in critical condition and treatment may save life	Cannot be delayed
Black	Expectant or expired; unconscious and no available treatment can save life	Nonresponsive, but all available measures for comfort are given until all vital signs cease

Individuality is not stressed. The standard clothing worn by all army personnel is referred to as an *all-climate uniform* (ACU). Helmets are always worn when not in the confines of the hospital.

The workday is 12 hours long. Every soldier is expected to perform the manual labor necessary to keep the hospital running 24 hours. Physical preparedness includes remaining strong through proper exercise and diet. A regular routine of workouts and running keeps the soldiers in condition. Periodic physical testing (sit-ups, push-ups, and running 2 miles) is performed to assess each soldier's readiness status. The intensity of the testing is determined by age and sex. Each person is required to be qualified in weapons use according to rank. Although hospital attacks are not common because of perimeter guards, the need to be prepared to protect the hospital is always foremost in the minds of all medical personnel.

Stress of combat and treating injured people during natural disasters is unavoidable. Although nurses, technologists, and physicians are healers, not warriors, they suffer the same levels of combat stress as fighting soldiers. The personnel are exposed to horrific injuries not commonly seen in civilian hospitals. The treatment for a nurse or other caregiver suffering from post-traumatic stress disorder (PTSD) is the same as that for a combat soldier. After a war or disaster, caregivers with PTSD may experience intense intrusive thoughts, such as flashbacks or nightmares, and may have many personal issues to resolve. Psychologic counseling is usually indicated. Specific categories of military caregivers are designated for the psychologic care and well-being of military personnel. Support groups are available when discharged from duty.

Much preparation goes into the readiness for war and disaster. Medical personnel learn the same soldiering skills as the fighting force in combination with remaining current in health care knowledge. In February 2023, military troops were deployed to Turkey to aid in the aftermath of the devastating earthquake. The military constructed a 100-patient bed field hospital to treat causality victims.

Veterinary Surgical Facilities

Animals have been the companions of humans since the beginning of time. They serve as a physical source of medication, food, and other by-products that we encounter every day. Service animals have a special place in our society because they are used to protect humans from harmful substances and items with their keen sense of smell; they serve as part of search and rescue teams, guides, and transportation; and they also serve as diagnosticians by sensing seizures and sniffing cancer cells. Specialized facilities, such as veterinary clinics, provide health services to this unique segment of society. Animal health insurance is becoming a popular concept for animal health care.

Scrub personnel are sometimes employed in a facility where investigational procedures are performed on animals or employed by veterinary clinics for the treatment of domestic animals. This specialized role requires knowledge in sterile and aseptic techniques; instrumentation; and modifications of positioning, prepping, and draping according to the size and body habitus of the veterinary patient.

The setting for performance of surgical procedures on animals should be treated with the same sterile and aseptic techniques as used for human surgery. The outcomes directly reflect the care given by the absence of infection and freedom from other untoward injury. Microbial carriage of an animal undergoing a surgical procedure can be minimized by containment of contaminated fur, fins, and feathers with adequate cleansing and draping practices. Precautions are taken for personnel with sensitivities to animal dander. Antiseptic preparations can reduce the microbial load of the skin in the same way they render human skin surgically clean.

Instrumentation is decontaminated and sterilized with the same methods as implements used in human care. Some hospitals have animal laboratories and clinics for research purposes within a separate section of the facility. Care is taken to isolate and process animal care instrumentation and supplies in a location that does not intermix with instruments and supplies intended for surgical procedures on humans. The risk for inadvertent transmission of infectious material, such as prions, between species is significantly increased when instrumentation used for susceptible animals is mixed with instrumentation used for other animals.

The physical plant is similar to ORs used for humans except for specialized beds and positioning devices for extremely large animals, such as horses, or for small animals, such as birds or rodents. Postanesthesia care areas for large standing animals, such as horses, should have padded walls and floors and minimal equipment to prevent an animal's self-inflicted injury.

Institutional animal care is accredited by the Association for Assessment and Accreditation of Laboratory Animal Care (AAALAC). Policies and procedures are specifically designed to meet the needs of animals in laboratory settings. Funding and grants for research commonly include provisions for the care and use of animal subjects. Humane treatment is stressed. Documentation of housing, bedding, feeding, and watering is required as part of the accreditation process.

Regulation of hazardous materials and infection control is required for the safety of human handlers and the welfare of the animals in their care. Waste disposal and sanitation is monitored. Animals involved in investigational studies are tagged for identification and sometimes quarantined as part of the study.

EVOLVE WEBSITE

http://evolve.elsevier.com/Hornacky/BerryKohn/

- Historical Perspective
- Student Interactive Questions
- Glossary

References

1. Morse S: *Ambulatory surgery centers compete with hospitals for outpatient dollars.* www.healthcarefinancenews.com. Accessed April 1, 2023.
2. The Accreditation Association for Ambulatory Health Care: www.ascassociation.org. Accessed March 28, 2023.
3. The Joint Commission: Facts about ambulatory care accreditation. www.jointcommission.org. Accessed March 28, 2023.
4. Fridman J, Meta T, Nguyen J: Optimal discharge strategy. In *Evidence-based practice of anesthesiology*, ed 4, St. Louis, 2023, Elsevier.
5. Crown E: *Army updating medical tents with lighter, easier air-supported shelters.* www.mrdc.health.mil. Accessed April 1, 2023.
6. Porta CR: The hidden war: humanitarian surgery in a combat zone, *Am J Surg* 207(5):766–772, 2014.

12

Care of the Perioperative Environment

CHAPTER OUTLINE

Guidelines for Cleanliness in the Surgical Environment, 211

Establishing the Surgical Environment, 211

Room Turnover Between Patients, 212

Daily Terminal Cleaning, 216

CHAPTER OBJECTIVES

After studying this chapter, the learner will be able to:

- Describe how a room is prepared for the first case of the day.
- Describe how a room is cleaned and prepared between patients.
- Describe how a room is terminally cleaned at the end of the day.
- Discuss environmental responsibility.

KEY TERMS AND DEFINITIONS

Between-case cleanup Cleaning that takes place at the end of one case to prepare the environment for the next case of the day. Also referred to as turnover.

Case cart system Computerized method of selecting and delivering instrument sets and supplies to the perioperative environment. Some models include provision for the return of instruments and contaminated items to the appropriate decontamination area.

Contamination Potentially pathogenic material that must be contained.

Custom packs Prepackaged disposable supplies standardized and assembled into packages and sterilized by the manufacturer or distributor according to specific instructions and requests by a particular service at a facility.

Decontamination Cleaning reusable items with an approved sporicidal disinfectant to render the item safe for handling.

Fomite Inanimate objects that can harbor and transmit infectious material.

Iatrogenic Condition that results during or from the process of treatment or care that has unfavorable results.

Terminal cleaning Thorough cleaning and disinfection of the perioperative environment at the end of daily use.

Turnover Cleaning and preparation of the OR between cases for the next patient's arrival. Areas are cleaned according to level of need.

Guidelines for Cleanliness in the Surgical Environment

AORN (Association of periOperative Registered Nurses) has established guidelines and recommended practices for cleaning and maintaining optimal cleanliness in the perioperative environment. The recommendations include, but are not limited to, the following:

1. All patients are entitled to a clean environment for their surgical procedures.
2. Any contamination encountered during a surgical procedure should be contained and confined. Cleaning starts at the cleanest area and works toward the dirtiest area and works from the top down.
3. Between-case cleanup should reestablish the cleanest environment possible for the next patient.
4. Procedure rooms, processing areas, and utility areas should be cleaned daily.
5. A schedule should be in place for routine cleaning of all areas and equipment in the surgical department.
6. All environmental sanitation processes should be defined by a multidisciplinary team and supported by facility policy and procedure.

Establishing the Surgical Environment

The duties of the scrub person and circulating nurse are many and varied as they prepare for the arrival of the patient in the OR. They are responsible for the cleanliness of the environment preoperatively, intraoperatively, and postoperatively so that the potential for contamination of the patient is kept to a minimum. They prepare the room and maintain the sterile field, work within it, and then break it down for terminal cleaning at the end of the day. These activities are performed in specific steps to minimize the risk for infection and maximize the use of time and supplies. Standardization is in the best interest of the patient and the personnel performing the cleanup.

Preliminary Preparations

Preliminary preparations of the operating room (OR) are completed by the circulating nurse and scrub person before each patient enters the OR. Assistance is provided by educated environmental service personnel. It is a cooperative effort. Clean, organized surroundings are part of total patient care.

A visual inspection of the room and its contents should be performed by the team before bringing in supplies for a case. Keep in mind that the human eye cannot see microscopic contamination. The environmental sanitation activities described in this chapter are for the benefit of the patient's protection in the spirit of surgical conscience and should not be taken for granted as an unnecessary inconvenience for the staff. Preparation for the start of the day requires making sure the room is as clean as it can be.

Basic room contents should include the OR bed, anesthesia machine and supplies, electrosurgical unit (ESU), instrument table, prep table, Mayo stand, suction apparatus, receptacles for biohazard and regular trash, and a linen hamper for reusable woven fabrics (Fig. 12.1). Other tables and equipment are added as needed. According to the Centers for Disease Control and Prevention (CDC), anything brought into the room for the procedure must be wiped down with an Environmental Protection Agency (EPA)—registered intermediate sporicidal disinfectant before used by the team.[1]

Before the First Surgical Procedure of the Day

The following housekeeping duties should be done before bringing sterile surgical supplies into the room for the first case of the day:

1. Remove unnecessary tables and equipment from the room. Arrange the appropriate furniture in an organized manner away from the traffic pattern. Some head and neck procedures require the OR bed to be oriented in a sideways direction to provide working space for the team. The anesthesia provider might be positioned at the patient's side.
2. Damp-dust from the top down (with a facility-approved sporicidal disinfectant solution and lint-free cloth) the overhead operating light, articulated arms, furniture, flat surfaces, and all portable or mounted equipment.[2] Avoid dry-dusting because this sets dust aloft. Start at higher surfaces and work down to lower levels because dust may fall from higher areas. "High touch" areas such as knobs, handles, and keyboards must be cleaned after every patient.
3. Damp-dust the tops and rims of the sterilizer and/or washer-sterilizer and the countertops in the substerile room adjacent to the OR.
4. Visually inspect the room for dirt and debris. The floor may need to be damp-mopped.

Room Turnover Between Patients

Physical facilities influence the flow of supplies and equipment after the surgical procedure. However, basic principles of aseptic technique dictate the procedures to be performed immediately after a surgical procedure is completed and prepare the OR for the next patient. Every patient has the right to the same degree of safety in the environment. In addition, personnel working in surgical services should be protected.

Personnel cleaning the room between patients should wear personal protective equipment (PPE) appropriate for the cleaning task. Gloves worn for cleaning should be durable in the presence of cleaning agents. Vinyl gloves are not reliable and may not protect the wearer from environmental contamination in the presence of degradation caused by cleaning agents.

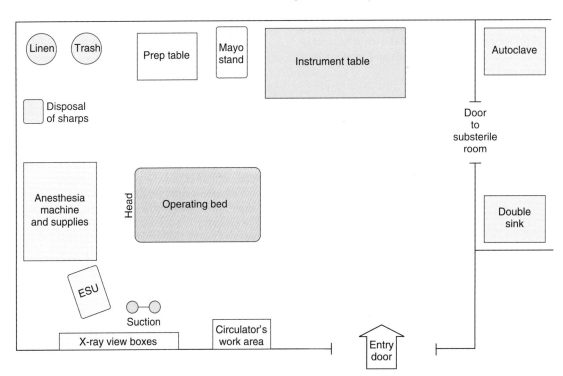

• **Fig. 12.1** Layout of basic OR and substerile room. The traffic pattern from the doors should not interfere with the setup of the sterile tables or the transfer of the patient to the OR bed.

PROS/CONS

Damp Dusting

Pros

- Cleaning the OR is a collaborative effort between the environmental services personnel and the OR staff.
- Specific cleaning procedures and schedules should be in place to keep room contaminants to a minimum and provide the patient with a clean, safe environment.
- Environmental services personnel are responsible for the cleaning of the OR after the last procedure of the day. Terminal cleaning is done with high-level disinfectants.
- All hospital cleaning chemicals are registered and rated by the Environmental Protection Agency (EPA). They are rated from high-level disinfectants to low-level disinfectants.
- Health care providers should be educated on the correct procedure of damp-dusting and which chemicals are accepted for use, how to safely use them on equipment and surfaces, and personal protective equipment (PPE) requirements.
- Keeping the OR clean is the responsibility of every staff member. The OR should be inspected for cleanliness before any surgical equipment is brought into the room.
- The process of damp-dusting should take place before the first procedure of the day. All horizontal surfaces such as surgical lights, furniture, booms, tables, and beds are wiped with a damp cloth starting from top to bottom.
- The purpose of damp-dusting is to remove any dust that has settled on surfaces after terminal cleaning and disinfection have taken place.
- Dust can become airborne and eventually settle on surfaces. Dust is known to contain particles from numerous sources such as skin, bacteria, mold, fibers from supplies, insect parts, and many more contaminants.
- Damp-dusting is done with low-linting cloths moistened with an EPA-approved hospital-grade disinfectant. The damp cloth prevents the dust from becoming airborne, which could contaminate supplies or a surgical wound.
- Surfaces that were damp dusted with a hospital-grade cleaner and allowed to dry retain the ability to kill microorganisms that come into contact with the surface.
- All chemicals used in the perioperative setting must have a Safety Data Sheet (SDS) available containing all information about the chemical and steps to take if exposure occurs.

- Any chemical removed from its original container must be labeled with the chemical name, expiration date, and concentration.

Cons

- Some health care providers do not think it is their responsibility to do any cleaning because specific staff is hired at the facility to do the job. They may skip the damp-dusting process.
- Areas that are not easily reached, such as OR surgical lights, are commonly skipped and disperse dust particles when moved during a surgical procedure, exposing the patient to microorganisms.
- Some ambulatory facilities depend on the OR staff to do all the cleaning between cases. Staff may be rushed to complete cases and may skip the damp-dusting process and do a poor job of cleaning the OR between cases.
- Damp-dusting is not performed to disinfect surfaces when tap water is used.
- Environmental cleaning chemicals should not be used from a spray bottle; this method can aerosolize the dust and cleaning solution.
- Many health care workers do not wear PPE while performing the damp-dusting process, which exposes them to any aerosolized dust or chemical particles.
- Alcohol should not be used as a damp-dust cleaner because it does not remove soil and it is not registered by the EPA for that purpose. Alcohol is a fire hazard.
- Lack of knowledge about the damp-dust process and purpose puts patients and employees at risk for contamination from microorganisms that were once airborne.

References

1. Centers for Disease Control and Prevention: *Guidelines for environmental infection control in health-care facilities.* www.cdc.gov. Accessed April 16, 2023.
2. AORN: Environmental cleaning. In *Guidelines for perioperative practice*, Denver, CO, 2024, The Association.
3. Environmental Infection Control: www.guidelinecentral.com. Accessed April 16, 2023.

Some patients have known pathogenic microorganisms; others have unknown infectious organisms. Therefore every patient should be considered a potential contaminant in the environment. Cleanup procedures should be rigidly followed to contain and confine contamination, known or unknown. Some examples of conditions that require special consideration are the following:

1. Patients with known respiratory-borne disease (e.g., Covid, rubeola, varicella, tuberculosis) may deposit microorganisms in the environment. They should be wearing a high-efficiency particulate air (HEPA) mask during transit and in the room as much as possible. In addition to routine environmental decontamination after they leave the room, the air exchanges should be 99% complete before the next patient is brought into the room. This may take 20 to 30 minutes on a 15 to 20 air change per hour cycle. Staff should wear appropriate filtration masks during room cleaning.

2. Patients with known endospore-forming bacterial contamination (e.g., *Clostridia* or *Bacillus*) may deposit bacterial endospores in the environment on inanimate objects, known as fomites. These endospores have been shown to survive in the environment for 5 months and have been cultured in ORs 40 days after the patient has used the room. AORN-recommended practices state that an approved sporicidal disinfectant should be used for cleaning the environment.

3. Patients with known or suspected transmissible spongiform encephalopathies such as Creutzfeldt-Jakob disease (CJD) and new variant CJD may deposit prions in the environment. Prions are nonliving proteins found in neurologic tissue and fluids that cause fatal neurodegenerative diseases in humans and animals.[3] Iatrogenic introduction of prion disease can happen if the patient is exposed to the protein during the surgical procedure by instrumentation or the environment. Prions are nonliving proteins that persist on surfaces and require special cleaning solutions. Disposable equipment, instruments, linens, and supplies should be used in the presence of known or suspected prion diseases. All environmental

surfaces should be covered with disposable impervious material during the surgical procedure.

The routine cleanup procedure can be accomplished expeditiously by the circulating nurse and scrub person working cooperatively. While the circulating nurse secures the outer layer of dressing and prepares the patient for transport from the OR, the scrub person begins to dismantle the sterile field before removing gown and gloves.

All instruments, supplies, and equipment should be decontaminated, disinfected, terminally sterilized, or contained for disposal as appropriate before being handled by other personnel.

After a patient leaves the room, the immediate environment is cleaned with an approved sporicidal disinfectant and all surfaces must dry completely. Room cleanup between patients is directed at the prevention of cross-contamination. The cycle of contamination is from patient to environment and from environment to OR personnel and subsequent patients.

Exposure to infectious waste is a hazard to everyone who encounters it. After each surgical procedure the environment should be made safe for the next patient to follow in that room. Institutional policies and procedures for routine room cleanup should be designed to minimize the OR team's exposure to contamination during the cleaning process.

Room Turnover Activities by the Scrub Person

The patient should be thought of as the center, or focal point. The surrounding sterile field and all areas that have come in contact with blood or body fluids are considered contaminated. The primary principles of cleaning procedures are to confine and contain contamination and physically remove microorganisms as quickly as possible.

Do not contaminate the table or Mayo stand until the patient has left the room if there is a question of patient stability, especially during trauma, cardiac, vascular, and neurologic procedures. Remain sterile until the patient leaves the room.

When the patient leaves the room, the sterile field is broken down by the scrub person, who remains protected with the gown, gloves, a mask, protective eyewear, and a cap during the dismantling procedure. Contaminated instruments, basins, and other reusable items are collected by the scrub person and placed in the case cart for decontamination, packaging, and sterilization in the processing department.

The following are activities and responsibilities of the scrub person at the end of the case:

1. Push the Mayo stand and instrument table away from the OR bed as soon as the dressing is applied and the drapes are removed. Roll drapes off the patient from head to foot to prevent airborne contamination; do not pull them off.
2. Check drapes for towel clips, instruments, and other items. Be sure that no equipment is discarded with disposable drapes or sent to the laundry.
   Disposable drapes are placed in a red biohazard container for disposal. Soiled drapes, whether disposable or reusable, should be handled as little as possible and with minimum agitation to prevent gross microbial contamination of air by dispersal of lint and debris.
3. Discard soiled sponges, other biologically contaminated waste, and disposable items in red biohazard containers. Discard unused sponges, nonwoven drapes, and other disposable waste into the main trash.

4. Dispose of sharp items safely. Special care should be taken in handling all knife blades, trocars, sharp instruments such as hooks or rakes, burrs and bits, surgical needles, and needles used for injection or aspiration. Remove the tip from the ESU handle (pencil). A self-closing adhesive pad or box designed for this purpose is the safest device to use. A safe disposal procedure should be implemented and sustained. Place these items in an appropriate rigid, puncture-resistant container for safe disposal to prevent injury and potential risk for contamination.
   The primary cause of accidental cuts and punctures to personnel, both inside and outside the OR, is disposal of surgical sharps at the end of the surgical procedure. Adherence to standardized systems designed specifically for safe handling and disposal of sharps prevents virtually all accidental cuts, punctures, and lacerations. Unused suture packets are discarded.
5. Basins and trays too large for the case cart are put into plastic bags for transport to the decontamination area. The Mayo tray may be included at some facilities. Place these on the lower shelf of the case cart. Some cases require a second cart for dirty instrumentation.
6. The instruments are opened completely and placed into the wire mesh basket with all box locks spread apart. Blood, tissue, bone, and any other gross debris are removed from instruments during the case as much as possible. All instruments, used and unused, must be decontaminated, terminally sterilized, or undergo high-level disinfection (as appropriate) before they are processed for reuse. Instruments should be presoaked and/or prerinsed before processing in a washer-sterilizer or decontaminator. Some facilities have the scrub person spray enzymatic foam over the instruments to start the cleaning process.
   Any biologic material remaining on instruments is more difficult to remove if left to dry or after the instruments have been heat-sterilized because the material becomes baked on them. The biologic debris inhibits sterilization and disinfection processes.
7. Remove knife blades from handles using a heavy hemostat; never use fingers. Using a needle holder can cause the jaws of the instrument to become misaligned. Point the blade toward the table and away from the field and other people in the area so that if it breaks or slips it will not fly across the room.
   a. Unloaded scalpel handles and other instruments with sharp tips or edges, such as scissors, should be placed in a container separate from the other instruments so they can be easily identified by the processing personnel.
   b. Do not put knife handles in an instrument tray with blades left on them. Other instruments designed for replaceable cutting blades, such as dermatomes, should have blades removed and discarded; thereafter the device may be handled with other instruments.
   c. Place reusable surgical needles, either on a needle rack or loose, into a perforated stainless steel box to be decontaminated and sterilized with the instruments.
8. Dispose of solutions and suction bottle contents according to facility policy. The facility must follow all state and federal regulations for disposal of contaminated fluids.[2] If a flush hopper is used, it should go into a sanitary sewer system.

Wear PPE to protect from splashes. Some facilities have closed-system liquid waste disposal units that empty suction canisters and decontaminate the contents. Disposable suction units simplify disposal. Commercial substances can be added to liquid in the disposable canister to solidify or gel contents for solid waste disposal.

9. The scrub person removes gown and gloves before taking the case cart to the processing area. The gown is removed first before removing gloves. The circulating nurse unfastens neck and back closures. Protect arms and scrub clothes from the contaminated outside of the gown. The gown is turned inside out as it is removed to prevent contamination of the scrub suit. Discard the gown in a laundry hamper if it is reusable or in a trash receptacle if it is disposable.

To remove gloves, use a glove-to-glove and then skin-to-skin technique to protect the hands from the contaminated outside of gloves. Turn gloves inside out as they are removed to contain the biologic contamination, and then discard them into a trash receptacle. Wash hands after removing gloves. Clean examination gloves are worn to transport all items to the processing area. Wash hands after removing gloves.

10. Instruments should be placed in leakproof containers. Contaminated items should be placed in labeled or color-coded containers for easy identification. The case cart should be totally enclosed or covered in plastic before taking it to the decontamination and processing area. Fresh examination gloves are worn when transporting the case cart.

Room Turnover Activities by the Team

After the patient leaves, the environmental service personnel should be available to perform room cleaning. Regardless of which member of the team performs them, specific functions should be performed to complete the between-case room cleanup. The following personnel and areas are considered contaminated during and after the surgical procedure:

- Members of the sterile team, until they have discarded their gowns, gloves, caps, masks, and shoe covers. These items remain in the contaminated area; scrub clothes are changed if they are wet or contaminated.
- All furniture, equipment, and the floor within and around the perimeter of the sterile field. If accidental spillage has occurred in other parts of the room, these areas are also considered contaminated.
- All anesthesia equipment.
- Stretchers used to transport patients and patient-moving devices. These should be cleaned after each patient use.

Clean examination gloves are worn to complete the room cleanup. Decontamination of the environment includes the following tasks starting at the highest point and working down:

- *Overhead operating light.* Wipe overhead lights with a clean cloth that has been wetted with sporicidal disinfectant solution specifically intended to prevent clouding of the surface that can cause dullness and glare. Lights and overhead tracks become contaminated quickly and present a possible hazard from fallout of dust particles onto sterile surfaces or into wounds during surgical procedures.
- *Furniture.* Wash horizontal surfaces of all tables and equipment, including the anesthesia machine, with a sporicidal disinfectant. Apply disinfectant from a squeeze-bottle

dispenser, and wipe with a clean cloth or a disposable wipe that is changed frequently. Spray bottles can cause particles to become aerosolized and should be avoided.[2]

All surfaces of mattress, pads, and screw connections of the OR bed are included. Safety straps should be cleaned between patients. Velcro straps can be laundered according to the manufacturer's recommendations. Mobile furniture can be pushed through sporicidal disinfectant solution used for floor care to clean casters. Excess strands of loose suture should be removed from the wheels.

Knobs, machine controls, keyboards, cabinet handles, and other frequently touched surfaces must be cleaned with sporicidal disinfectant between patients.

- *Anesthesia equipment.* Most masks and anesthesia tubing are disposable. Any reusable anesthesia masks and tubing are cleaned and sterilized between patient uses. Reusable equipment is processed according to the manufacturer's recommendations. Some items can be steam or chemically sterilized.
- *Laryngoscope blades and handles* should be disassembled, thoroughly decontaminated, and disinfected. Any parts that can tolerate a sterilization process should be terminally sterilized.
- *Noncritical items,* such as blood pressure cuffs, should be cleaned with an approved sporicidal disinfectant between patient uses.
- *Laundry.* After all cleaning procedures have been completed, discard cleaning cloths or put into a laundry bag if they are not disposable. When all reusable woven fabric items, used and unused, have been placed inside the laundry bag, close it securely. To help protect laundry personnel, an alginate bag that dissolves in hot water may be used as the primary laundry bag or as a liner within a cloth bag. Transport reusable woven fabrics soiled with blood or body fluids in leakproof bags.
- *Trash.* Collect all trash in plastic or impervious bags, including disposable drapes and kick bucket and wastebasket liners. Bags should be sturdy to resist bursting or tearing during transport. Trash is separated into biohazardous waste, noninfectious trash, and recyclable items. Separate receptacles for each type of trash should be available. Disposition of potentially infectious waste must comply with local, state, and/or federal leakproof regulations for contamination control measures. Use appropriately labeled and color-coded bags for infectious waste, and use puncture-resistant containers for sharps.
- *Floors.* Clean a perimeter of 3 to 4 ft in circumference of the surgical field between cases. This perimeter expands from the clean area to dirty area—in the direction of visible soilage. Hot water may hasten the biocidal/sporicidal action of the disinfectant agent but may also soften tile adhesive. Floors are always considered contaminated. Standing platforms (stepstools) are considered part of the floor and should be cleaned between cases. Sticky or tacky mats with adhesive surfaces are not recommended because they have not proved to reduce the contaminants on OR shoes. They may be used in areas of new construction where workers come in and out of areas from the outside.
- *Mops.* Clean mops are used with fresh EPA-registered sporicidal disinfectant solution. The floor is flooded with fresh detergent-disinfectant solution. A clean mop is used to apply solution and used to take up solution beginning in the cleanest area and working toward the dirtiest areas. After one-time use, remove mop heads and place in a laundry hamper with other contaminated reusable woven fabrics. Mop handles should be

cleaned with disinfectant after use and stored in the house-keeping storage area until they are needed again. Use clean mops and sporicidal disinfectant solution for each cleanup procedure.

- *Wet vacs* can be used to clean the OR flooring. The wet vac unit should be cleaned and disinfected between uses.
- *Walls.* If walls are splashed with blood or organic debris during the surgical procedure, wash those areas. Otherwise, walls are not considered contaminated and need not be washed between surgical procedures.

Cart System Cleanup

All contaminated reusable instruments and basins are put on or inside the case cart. The cart is covered or closed and taken to the central decontamination area outside surgical services for cleanup. The case cart with contaminated supplies should be removed from surgical services via the outer corridor if this is the design of the suite. If dumbwaiters or elevators are used, a separate one is provided for contaminated carts. Even when the cart is covered, the person returning the cart to the processing area must wear examination gloves.

The instrument-processing personnel will unload the contaminated cart in the workroom. The instruments will be managed in the following manner:

1. The instrument-washing tray is loaded with heavy instruments in the bottom. All hinged instruments are fully opened to expose maximum surface area, including box locks. Instruments designed to be disassembled are taken apart. The instruments are spaced apart to prevent contact of sharp edges or points with other instruments. Small basins and solution cups are inverted in a tray. Concave surfaces are turned down.
2. Glass syringes, medicine glasses, and other glassware, including those used by the anesthesia provider, are placed in a separate tray. Reusable syringe plungers are removed from the barrels.
3. Detergent-disinfectant solution is suctioned through the lumen of reusable suction tips. The lumen is difficult to clean if biologic debris dries. Disposable suction tips and tubing are recommended.
4. The cart is designed to go through an automatic steam cart washer or a manual power wash for terminal decontamination after it is emptied and before it is restocked with clean and sterile supplies.

Getting the Room Ready for the Next Patient

The cleaning procedures described provide adequate decontamination and terminal sterilization after any surgical procedure. With a well-coordinated team, minimal turnover time between surgical procedures can be accomplished. In an average time of 10 to 15 minutes, the room will be ready for the next patient. The turnover time includes cleaning up after one procedure and setting up for the next procedure. Additional equipment brought into the room for the next patient should be damp-dusted with sporicidal disinfectant before entering the OR where sterile supplies are opened.

Individual Patient Setups

Each patient has a right to individual supplies prepared just for their surgery. Sterile supplies should not be opened until they are ready to be used. Case cart systems and the use of custom packs eliminate the need for preparing the sterile field several hours ahead of the patient's arrival. The scrub person, working with an efficient circulating nurse, should have time to set up the instrument table immediately before each surgical procedure. There is no arbitrary life span of a setup table once it is open and prepared as a sterile field for a patient. Sterility is event related, not time related. The sterile table must be under in-room surveillance at all times.

Unless it is under constant surveillance, sterility of any setup cannot be guaranteed. If a scheduled surgical procedure is delayed and a sterile setup has not been contaminated by the patient's presence in the room, the setup may remain open, under surveillance by someone in the room, with the doors closed. The setup should be used as close to the time of preparation as possible.

If a patient is taken into the OR and for some reason the surgical procedure is canceled before the procedure has begun, the tables are torn down and the room cleaned as if the surgical procedure had taken place. The setup is considered potentially contaminated and may not be saved for another patient. Disposable items may be useful for the clinical educator in the department during orientation and education sessions.

Daily Terminal Cleaning

In the Operating Room

At completion of the day's schedule, each OR, whether or not it was used that day, should be terminally cleaned. Additional and more rigorous cleaning is done in all areas already discussed for cleanup between surgical procedures. At the end of the day's schedule, the following routine should be followed:

- Ceiling- and wall-mounted fixtures and tracks are cleaned on all surfaces.
- Furniture is thoroughly scrubbed, using mechanical friction in addition to chemical disinfection. Special attention to high-use items such as computer keyboards, telephones, intercom buttons, and cabinet handles is important.
- Casters and wheels should be cleaned and kept free of suture ends and debris.
- Equipment such as ESUs and lasers should be cleaned with care so as not to saturate surfaces to the degree that disinfectant solution runs into the mechanism, causing malfunction and requiring repairs.
- Kick buckets, laundry hamper frames, and other waste receptacles are decontaminated and disinfected.
- Floors are thoroughly wet-mopped with a clean mophead and sporicidal disinfectant solution. A wet vac may be used.
- Walls and ceilings should be checked for soil spots and cleaned as necessary.
- Cabinets and doors should be cleaned, especially around handles or push plates, where contamination is common. Clean all knobs, machine controls, and keyboards.
- Air-intake grilles, ducts, and filter covers should be cleaned.
- Some facilities use automated ultraviolet C (UVC) band lighting to disinfect surfaces. The UVC light deactivates the DNA in bacteria to prevent replication within 30 to 60 minutes.[4]
- Some facilities use hydrogen peroxide misting systems as an adjunct to routine terminal cleaning practices. The vapor is effective against multidrug-resistant bacteria and endospores.

Outside the Operating Room

- Countertops and sinks in the substerile room are cleaned. The outer surface of the sterilizer, including the top, is washed.
- Scrub sinks and spray heads on faucets undergo thorough cleaning daily. A mild abrasive on sinks removes the oily film residue left by scrub antiseptics. Spray heads, faucet aerators, or sprinklers should be removed and disassembled, if possible, for thorough cleaning and sterilization of parts. Tap water is not sterile and can deposit microorganisms on the skin. Contaminated faucet aerators and sprinklers can transfer accumulated organisms directly to hands or items washed under them. Scrub sinks should not be used for routine cleaning purposes or disposal of waste solutions.
- Soap dispensers should be disassembled, cleaned, and terminally sterilized, if possible, before they are refilled with antiseptic solution. These dispensers can become reservoirs for microorganisms.
- Walls around scrub sinks should receive daily attention. Spray and splash from scrubbing cause buildup of antiseptic soap film around the sink. This film should be removed daily.
- Transportation and storage carts need to be cleaned, with specific attention given to wheels and casters.
- Cleaning equipment must be disassembled, cleaned, and dried before storage.

Weekly or Monthly Cleaning

A weekly or monthly cleaning routine is set up, in addition to the daily cleaning schedule, by the director of environmental/housekeeping services and the OR manager. Any routines for housekeeping are based on the physical construction of the department. However, if specific schedules are not established, some areas could be inadvertently missed. Areas to be considered are the following:

- *Walls.* Walls should be cleaned when they become visibly soiled. If they are painted or tiled with wide porous grouting, these factors should be considered in planning cleaning routines. Washing walls in the OR and throughout the suite once a week is reasonable, but less frequent time intervals for cleaning may be acceptable if spot disinfection is performed daily. This requires adequate continuous supervision.
- *Ceilings.* Ceilings may require regular special cleaning techniques because of mounted tracks, air diffusers, and lighting fixtures. Specialized ceiling mounts for microscopes and booms for suspended equipment should be included in this plan. The types of fixtures are considered in planning cleaning routines.
- *Floors.* Floors throughout surgical services should be machine-scrubbed periodically to remove accumulated deposits and films. Rounded corners and edges facilitate cleaning.
- *Air-conditioning grilles.* The exterior of air-conditioning grilles should be vacuumed at least weekly. Additional cleaning is necessary when filters are checked and changed. Debris can be discharged into the room when the filter is changed. In-room air handlers are positive pressure. The filters should be changed on an off-shift or on the weekend. The room should be terminally cleaned after changing the filters.
- *Storage shelves.* Storage cabinets have been replaced in many OR suites by portable storage carts or pass-through shelving to a sterile core. Storage areas should be cleaned at least weekly or more often, if necessary, to control accumulation of dust, especially in sterile storage areas.

- *Sterilizers.* All types of sterilizers should be cleaned regularly and tested as recommended by the manufacturer.
- *Transfer zones.* Walls, ceilings, floors, air-conditioning grilles, lockers, cabinets, and furniture should be cleaned on a regular schedule.

Greening of the OR: Environmental Responsibility

Many surgical supplies are recyclable. Recycling reduces not only air pollution and the amount of waste in landfills but also the amount of virgin resources consumed.[5] Paper wrappers and many plastic items that are noninfectious, nonregulated trash can and should be recycled. Recycling in the OR should be an integral part of the overall recycling and sustainment program of the health care facility. Consideration of recycling potential can be part of the evaluation process in selecting products. OR personnel should be taught how to recycle and what items are disposable or reusable. A definition of the different waste products should be defined as follows:

Clinical waste. Waste contaminated with blood, bodily fluids, or pharmaceuticals is placed in biohazard bags. These bags or containers are usually red.

Recycled items. Noncontaminated wrappers, plastic, paper, and packaging from sterile items are placed in regular trash bags for recycling.

Reusable instruments. Reusable instruments should be placed in a labeled container and sent to the proper destination for reprocessing.

OR personnel should also think about the energy cost to run the facility. Energy efficiency plans should be in place to turn off lights and equipment when not in use.

The OR team should not use more consumable product than necessary. Overfilling prep basins with antiseptic solution and then disposing of it in the sanitary sewer exposes the environment to risk for resistant microorganisms and pollution. The Green Guide for Health Care is one organization that gives ideas on how to reduce waste in the health care setting.

ⓔ EVOLVE WEBSITE

http://evolve.elsevier.com/Hornacky/BerryKohn/

- Historical Perspective
- Student Interactive Questions
- Glossary

References

1. Centers for Disease Control and Prevention: *Guidelines for environmental infection control in health-care facilities.* www.cdc.gov. Accessed April 16, 2023.
2. AORN: Environmental cleaning. In *Guidelines for perioperative practice*, Denver, CO, 2024, The Association.
3. Swire E, Colchester A: Out of sight, out of mind? BSE 30 years on: continuing environmental risks to human health, *Land Use Policy* 126:106521, 2023.
4. Demeersseman N, Saegeman V, Cossey V, et al.: Shedding a light on ultraviolet-C technologies in the hospital environment, *J Hosp Infect* 132(3):85–92, 2023.
5. Hayley J, Petit BS, Reiter A, et al: Going green in operating rooms reduces cost and improves environmental impact. www.facs.org. Accessed April 16, 2023.

13

Potential Sources of Injury to the Caregiver and the Patient

CHAPTER OUTLINE

Environmental Hazards, 218

Physical Hazards and Safeguards, 219

Chemical Hazards and Safeguards, 231

Biologic Hazards and Safeguards, 233

Risk Management, 236

CHAPTER OBJECTIVES

After studying this chapter the learner will be able to:

- Identify potential environmental sources of injury to patients and personnel in the perioperative environment.
- Discuss the prevention of injury through proper testing and use of equipment in the operating room.
- Discuss the importance of fire and disaster drills.

KEY TERMS AND DEFINITIONS

Anaphylaxis An acute, life-threatening physical condition resulting from exposure to an allergen that affects two or more organ systems (e.g., respiratory and cardiovascular); fatal if untreated promptly.

Ergonomics The study of people's efficiency in their working environment. It is concerned with how people arrange and design equipment to maximize productivity and reduce fatigue and injury.

Fire triangle Three conditions, when in combination, cause a fire. Fuel—Ignition—Oxidation. Practicing safety at the sterile field can prevent a fire.

Ionizing radiation Sufficient radiant energy to yield ions from the disintegration of the nuclei of unstable or radioactive elements. This radiation occurs naturally from cosmic rays, and these ions disrupt the electronic balance of atoms. Synthetic x-rays and

nuclear power are capable of modifying molecules within body cells as they pass through tissue. They can be mutagenic (i.e., cause mutations of DNA) in somatic body cells, predisposing a person to cancer, and in germ cells, predisposing a person to spontaneous abortion or congenital malformations.

Nonionizing radiation Radiant energy that does not produce ions but can produce hyperthermic conditions that are harmful to the skin and eyes. With the possible exception of ultraviolet rays, wavelengths from the electromagnetic spectrum do not alter DNA in body cells.

Urticaria A rash resulting from exposure to an allergen or other irritant. Urticaria is also known as hives and can appear as itchy, erythematous wheals.

Environmental Hazards

The perioperative environment poses many hazards for both patients and personnel. The potential for physical injury from electric shock, burns, fire, explosion, exposure to bloodborne pathogens, and inhalation of toxic substances is ever present. Therefore it is important that staff have knowledge of the hazards involved in equipment use, the causes of accidental injury, and the sources of health risks. Faulty equipment or improper usage increases the hazards of potential risk factors. The health care facility should be made as safe as possible.

Potential hazards should be identified and safe practices established. The facility's risk management personnel are charged with the responsibility of tracking issues of safety and potential injury. The recommendations that arise from these data are established to guide personnel in corrective actions. Patients and caregivers are never completely free from risks, but the risks can be minimized.

Safety refers to conditions that will not cause injury or harm to the employee, the patient, and other people in the health care facility. Safety goes hand in hand with knowledge, skill, and competency. Some equipment, such as lasers, x-ray equipment, and chemical sterilizers, can cause long-range injury if personnel are lax in safety and protective practices. The education and training of personnel are essential to create an awareness of the potential hazards. No one should be permitted to use equipment until properly instructed in its correct use and care.

Each caregiver should seek instruction when needed and follow the safety and control measures established by facility policies and procedures. Failure to use equipment and devices safely places both the caregiver and the patient at risk for injury.

Competency in using equipment should be tested periodically because technology changes frequently, and the knowledge and skill associated with one piece of equipment may not apply to a newer model. In some instances the technology may become safer, but this is not always the case.

Classification of Hazards

Injuries can be caused by faulty equipment, using equipment improperly, exposing oneself or others to toxic or irritating agents, or coming into contact with harmful agents. Hazards in the operating room (OR) environment can be classified as follows:

- *Physical*, including back injury, falls, noise pollution, irradiation, electricity, and fire
- *Chemical*, including anesthetic gases, toxic fumes from gases and liquids, cytotoxic drugs, and cleaning agents
- *Biologic*, including the patient (as a host for, or source of, pathogenic microorganisms), infectious waste, cuts or needlestick injuries, surgical plume, and latex sensitivity

Regulation of Hazards

Standards, guidelines, and recommended practices have been developed by many professional associations, such as the AORN (Association of periOperative Registered Nurses), and governmental agencies, such as the Department of Health and Human Services (HHS). The policies and procedures of the health care facility should be developed and enforced in compliance with local, state, and federal regulations. Others include, but are not limited to, the following agencies:

- The American Conference of Governmental Industrial Hygienists (ACGIH; www.acgih.org) sets standards for threshold limits for exposure to toxic materials.
- The American National Standards Institute (ANSI; www.ansi.org) sets standards to limit exposure to devices that emit light or sound, such as lasers, ultraviolet light, and nonionizing radiation.
- The National Fire Protection Association (NFPA; www.nfpa.org) sets standards for electrical codes and fire safety.
- The Joint Commission (TJC; www.jointcommission.org) sets standards of patient care for accreditation.
- The Centers for Disease Control and Prevention (CDC; www.cdc.gov) sets standards for infection control.
- The National Institute for Occupational Safety and Health (NIOSH; www.cdc.gov) sets standards for ventilation systems and environmental protection in the workplace.
- The Environmental Protection Agency (EPA; www.epa.gov) sets standards for the disposal of infectious and hazardous waste.
- The U.S. Food and Drug Administration (FDA; www.fda.gov) sets standards and controls for the use of drugs, biologics, devices, and chemicals in patient care.

- An FDA organization, the Center for Devices and Radiologic Health (CDRH; www.fda.gov) sets standards for the management and monitoring of radiation in patient care.
- The National Patient Safety Foundation (NPSF; https://psnet.ahrq.gov) sets goals for patient safety in health care organizations.

In 1970, the Occupational Safety and Health Administration (OSHA) was created within the U.S. Department of Labor. Initially OSHA adopted preexisting federal and national consensus standards and guidelines for environmental, patient, and personnel safety. Since its inception, OSHA has issued new standards and amended others, such as permissible exposure limits (PELs) to various occupational health and safety hazards. OSHA is authorized by law to enforce its standards, which may require employers to measure and monitor exposure to toxic or harmful agents, notify employees of overexposure and provide medical consultation or care, and maintain records of corrective actions. OSHA inspects health care facilities for compliance with standards. (More information can be found at www.osha.gov.)

The CDC oversees the activities of NIOSH. The research branch of NIOSH is the National Occupational Research Agenda (NORA).

Physical Hazards and Safeguards

The architectural design of the perioperative environment affects its overall efficiency and productivity. The physical facility is designed to control traffic patterns, decrease contamination, facilitate the handling of equipment and supplies, and provide a comfortable working environment.

Environment Factors

Several factors contribute to providing a safe, comfortable working environment: temperature control, ventilation, lighting, color, and noise. Temperature control should provide physical comfort, 68° F to 75° F (20−24° C) (i.e., it should not be too warm or too cool).

The heating, ventilation, and air conditioning (HVAC) system in the OR usually evacuates odors fairly quickly by exchanging air 20 times per hour, with 4 exchanges of fresh air. The ventilating system should help remove toxic fumes and anesthetic gas waste that is not picked up by the scavenger system on the anesthesia machine. Perfume and other odors can cause headaches, nausea, or respiratory congestion in people with sensitivities to smells. Heavy perfume can also have an annoying, lingering effect; therefore people in the perioperative environment should avoid wearing it.

Lighting should be adequate, but excessive glare causes fatigue. Illumination is the product of the light and the reflectance of the target. A bright, highly polished mirror finish on an instrument tends to reflect light and can restrict vision. Satin- or dull-finished instruments eliminate glare and lessen eyestrain. These instruments are made with varying degrees of dullness depending on the manufacturer. Lightly tinted or polarized eyewear may save sterile team members from visual fatigue but should not distort the color of tissues. For drapes and walls, soft, cool colors, especially blues and greens, are less reflective than white. Drapes with blue, gray, or green tones help reduce the contrast between most tissues and the surrounding field.

Environmental design is specific to ventilation, lighting, color, and auditory effects. Some facilities have piped-in music in waiting areas. Music can be stimulating for personnel and relaxing for patients who are awaiting surgery or undergoing a surgical procedure under local anesthesia. The selection of music should be appropriate for the intended listener. Music with a low volume, moderate rhythm, and bright tone can motivate muscular activity and increase levels of efficiency of OR personnel. However, this type of music would not be conducive to relaxation for the patient who is awaiting surgery. On the other hand, music can be a distraction and an annoyance, especially for the anesthesia provider, who may depend on auscultation when monitoring the patient. Music should be turned off at the request of the patient, surgeon, or anesthesia provider.

Extreme noise from drills, fan motors in equipment, and other sources can be annoying and potentially dangerous to patients and personnel. The noise can become intense enough to increase blood pressure and provoke peripheral vasoconstriction, dilation of the pupils, and other subtle physiologic effects. It also can interfere with necessary communication and thereby provoke irritation. The EPA recommends that noise levels in hospitals not exceed 45 decibels during daytime hours.

The OR should be as quiet as possible except for the essential sounds of communication among team members directly concerned with the patient's care. Excessive noise and distractions in communication are directly linked to medical errors, injuries, and even patient death.[1] Nurses have an obligation for patient safety; noise and unnecessary tasks must be discontinued during critical situations and communication. Any necessary talking should be done in a low voice. Counts or requests for supplies should be done quietly or by hand signals. Conversation unrelated to the surgical procedure is out of place. Even during the deep stages of anesthesia, a patient may perceive and remember noise that occurs during the surgical procedure. This phenomenon is referred to as anesthesia awareness.

If a regional or local anesthetic is used, the patient can hear the conversation. Because patients interpret anything they hear in terms of themselves, all words should be guarded.

Major sources of noise in the OR involve paper, gloves, objects wheeled across the floor, instruments striking one another, monitors, and high-pitched power instruments, including suction. The scrub person should keep in mind the sources and the effects of this noise. The clattering of instruments should be avoided. Except while in actual use, suction tubing can be clamped or kinked to minimize noise. Paper wrappings should not be crushed. Monitors with necessary audible signals should be placed as far away from the patient's ears as possible; continuous monitor beeps also can distract the surgeon and anesthesia provider but should never be turned off. The circulating nurse should keep the doors to the OR closed to shut out the noise of the corridors, water running in the scrub room, or the sterilizer operating in the substerile room. Aside from blocking noise, the doors should remain shut to maintain the proper functioning of the air-handling system in the OR.

Working in a pleasantly quiet environment is less fatiguing, produces fewer psychologic and physiologic adverse effects, and allows for greater efficiency on behalf of the patient.

Body Mechanics

Backache is a leading cause of work-related lost time, second only to upper respiratory tract infections. Standing for prolonged periods, often in an awkward position, is a common cause of low back pain. Tiring body motions or an awkward or strained body posture should be avoided. Weight-bearing on only one foot causes additional strain. When the feet are placed together while standing, constant muscular effort is required by the thigh muscles to maintain an erect posture. In contrast, when the feet are apart the ligaments of the hips and knees support the body with less effort. Therefore maintaining a wide stance, with knees periodically slightly flexed while standing at the OR bed for prolonged periods will be less fatiguing for the scrub person.

While in a location to observe both the surgical procedure and the instrument table, the circulating nurse can stand with the upper and lower extremities in a resting position. In this standing position the arms are clasped behind the back and the feet are in a wide stance.

Shoes should be considered for comfort and safety. Nonporous canvas or leather athletic shoes that tie or secure with Velcro provide adequate, nonskid support for the foot. OSHA requires all OR personnel to wear impervious closed-in shoes. If running is required during an emergency, these shoes will be more secure than clog varieties with open backs. Soft shoes do not afford protection from dropped items.

The OR bed is adjusted to the best working height for the tallest person on the sterile team. The reach potential of the entire team should be considered when planning where each individual team member will stand (Fig. 13.1). Team members should be able to stand erect with their arms comfortably relaxed from the shoulders, without stooping, and they should not need to raise their hands above the level of their elbows for the majority of their work motions. Standing platforms (stepstools, referred to as *steps*) may be needed to elevate the scrub person and/or the assistant to a feasible working height. These platforms should be long enough and wide enough to allow a wide stance. A shorter surgeon can stand on steps to allow the team to have the OR bed at a comfortable working height.

Correct posture while in the sitting position is equally important. The back is strongest when it is straight. When seated, team members should sit far back in the chair or on the stool with the body straight from hips to neck. They should lean forward from the hips, not the shoulders or waist. This position puts the least strain on muscles, ligaments, and internal organs. Before and after the surgical procedure the circulating nurse and scrub person(s) should rest in a sitting position between long periods of standing. If work is done in a sitting position, the stool or chair should be adjusted to the correct height for the working surface. Sterile persons should not change the height of the sterile field by sitting while dressed in sterile attire.

First assistants may develop carpal tunnel syndrome as a result of holding retractors in one position for prolonged periods. Carpal tunnel syndrome is a form of repetitive stress injury caused by tenosynovitis that places pressure on the median nerve of the hand. Consequently, the thumb, index, and ring fingers tingle and feel swollen. Self-retaining retractors help relieve some of this strain.

Sprains and strains are common injuries sustained to the back, arms, or shoulders as a result of lifting patients or moving

• **Fig. 13.1** Work motion of each sterile team member should be ergonomically safe and comfortable.

equipment. The following principles of body mechanics should be observed to minimize physical injury[2]:

- While maintaining a straight back, keep the body as close as possible to the person or equipment to be lifted or moved.
- Lift with the large muscle groups of the legs and abdominal muscles, not the back.
- Bend the knees to get body weight under the load, and then straighten the legs to lift with the heels flat on the floor.
- Lift with a slow, even motion, keeping pressure off the lumbar (lower back) area.
- Push, do not pull, stretchers, tables, and heavy equipment on wheels or casters.
- Use large body muscles to maneuver the base of portable equipment such as laser equipment or microscopes.
- If standing for prolonged periods, stand in a wide stance with the heels apart so the ligaments of the hips and knees can support the body without effort.
- Distribute weight evenly on both feet, but shift the body occasionally during prolonged periods of standing. Do not stiffen the legs at the knee. A slight flex at the knees is less stressful.
- Sit with the back straight from the hips to the neck, and lean forward from the hips.
- Align the head and neck with the body when standing or sitting, maintaining the lumbar curve.
- Change position, stretch, or walk around occasionally if possible.
- Pivot the entire body to avoid twisting at the waist.
- Bend forward with hip flexion and hand support.
- Avoid overhead reaching or overstretching; keep materials in the chest-to-knee range if possible; use steps as appropriate.

A lifting frame, sliding board, air mattress, or Davis roller helps relieve the potential strain of moving unconscious or obese

• **Fig. 13.2** Four surgical personnel using a patient roller correctly to move the patient from one surface to another.

patients (Fig. 13.2). A clean draw sheet must always be used to protect the patient from contact with the moving device. A minimum of four persons is required to move an unconscious patient. If one caregiver attempts to move these patients alone, it can cause injury to the patient or the caregiver. Assistance is also needed to position patients on the OR bed. Physical therapy department personnel or the occupational health director can be a resource for teaching the patient care staff the proper techniques for lifting, bending, reaching, and pivoting.

Body Mechanics

Pros

- Body mechanics plays a major role in the perioperative workplace. The perioperative setting is a physically demanding area in which there is a high risk for musculoskeletal injuries.
- The perioperative setting requires staff to push, pull, and lift patients, heavy equipment, and supplies.
- The National Institute for Occupational Safety and Health (NIOSH) offers a Musculoskeletal Health Program to improve workplace efficiency and prevent musculoskeletal injuries.
- Ergonomics is the study of people's efficiency in their working environment. It is concerned with how people arrange and design equipment to maximize productivity and reduce fatigue and injury.
- OSHA has a General Duty Clause that employers must provide a safe working environment for all personnel, patients, and visitors. It offers guidelines for safety and training programs for employees.
- AORN offers a Safe Patient Handling Tool Kit. It recognizes high-risk activities uniquely acquired from working in the perioperative setting. These tools include Lateral Transfer from Stretcher to and from the OR Bed, Positioning and Repositioning the Patient on the OR Bed, Lifting and Prepping Head and Limbs, Prolonged Standing, Retraction, Lifting and Carrying Supplies and Equipment, and Pushing and Pulling Equipment on Wheels.
- The Ergonomic Tools give recommendations on how to safely complete each task and the rationale for each. It also incorporates the NIOSH lifting equation, which recommends how much weight an individual can lift and still be considered safe. It also explains the proper lift technique: lift with the legs, bend the knees, get under the object, and lift slowly and evenly.
- Assistive devices are available, such as a Davis roller or air-assisted mattresses, for patients to move from a stretcher, instead of manual labor.
- Posture while standing or sitting is fundamental in preventing injury because the back is stronger in a straight position.
- OR equipment should be in good working condition to reduce the force necessary to push or pull.
- Perioperative education on body mechanics has been shown to reduce the amount of lost time from work-related injuries.

Cons

- The perioperative setting requires staff to lift patients, heavy equipment, and supplies. These actions also require pushing and pulling movements that can put staff at risk for injury.
- Many health care workers leave the profession because of the high physical demand and occupational injury such as back injuries and muscular pains and strains. Back injuries are one of the most common injuries among health care workers.
- Lifting and moving patients can cause injury to workers if they do not use assistive devices or the correct amount of people necessary to properly move a patient.
- Lifting limbs during skin prep can cause a sprain or strain to a worker if the weight of the limb is too heavy or held for a longer period.
- Standing in one position for a long time is common and can cause fatigue and pain. Standing on both feet with a wider stance may help relieve some fatigue.
- Standing or holding retractors in awkward positions may result in poor posture, thus causing fatigue, back pain, neck pain, or carpal tunnel syndrome. The height of the OR bed should be at a safe working level to prevent awkward positions.
- If one person cannot safely move equipment, then staff help should be available when necessary.
- Lack of knowledge about proper body mechanics is the leading cause of work-related injuries.

References

1. Garbarino C: The importance of ergonomic education in preventing perioperative musculoskeletal disorders, *AORN J* 115(4):365–369, 2023.
2. National Institute for Occupational Safety and Health: *Ergonomics and musculoskeletal disorders.* www.cdc.gov. Accessed April 17, 2023.
3. Smith C: Workplace issues and staff safety. In Rothrock JC, editor: *Alexander's care of the patient in surgery*, ed 17, St. Louis, 2023, Mosby, pp 39–43.
4. AORN: Guidance statement: safe patient handling and movement in the perioperative setting. In *Guidelines for perioperative practice*, Denver, CO, 2024, The Association.

Ionizing Radiation

Radiation cannot be seen or felt. Ionizing radiation produces positively and negatively charged particles that can change the electrical charge of some atoms and molecules in cells. These changes can alter enzymes, proteins, cell membranes, and genetic material. This can cause the death of cancer cells when radiation is used in therapeutic doses; however, exposure to radiation also can cause cancer, cataracts, bone marrow injury, burns, tissue necrosis, genetic mutations, spontaneous abortion, and congenital anomalies. When radiation is in use, warning signs should be prominently displayed (Fig. 13.3).

Perioperative patient care personnel may assist with invasive x-rays. If personnel are unprotected, they are exposed to scatter radiation from the patient during intraoperative and interventional procedures when radiographs are taken or fluoroscopes and image intensifiers are used. Team members are also exposed during the implantation or removal of radioactive elements. Patients exposed to radioactivity for therapeutic purposes or by accident may emit radiation.

• **Fig. 13.3** Radiation warning sign.

• **Fig. 13.4** C-arm keeps image intensifier and x-ray tube in alignment to amplify fluoroscopic optical image.

Intraoperative radiographs may be taken during, but are not limited to, procedures, urologic examinations, biliary tree visualization, angiography, or orthopedic bone alignments. The sterile team should be wearing lead protective garments under the sterile gown or should step behind a lead screen when the image is made. The x-ray cassette (if one is used) may need to be draped or encased in a sterile cover, and the surgical incision may need to be protected with a sterile drape to prevent contamination by the x-ray machine. When a C-arm image intensifier is used, a large, specialized, sterile, clear plastic tubular drape is slid over the entire machine (Fig. 13.4).

The effect of radiation is directly related to the amount and length of time of exposure. Exposure is cumulative, and because there is an extended latency period, the effects may not be evident for years. Therefore constant vigilance for personal safety is essential to avoid excessive exposure to ionizing radiation. Protection implies understanding the basic terms and adhering to strict policies and procedures.

Safety Considerations in the Use of Ionizing Radiation

Because of the adverse and cumulative effects of ionizing radiation on body tissues, safety precautions are taken to protect patients and personnel from the potential hazards. Box 13.1 lists safe radiation exposure limits according to the area of the body. Monitoring badges must be worn if radiation devices are in use.

Patient Safety

A patient can be exposed to the primary beam of x-rays, the radioactivity of implants, and scatter radiation. Any exposure to radiation has biologic risks; therefore the exposure should be as

•**BOX 13.1** **Permissible Doses of Radiation as Established by the National Council on Radiation Protection and Measurements**

Permissible doses of radiation are based on units of an equivalent dose quantity that express all radiations on a common scale for the purpose of calculating their biologic effects. The maximum permissible doses per year for occupationally exposed people older than 18 years of age varies by body parts:
- Whole body, including blood-forming organs, bone marrow, and gonads: 5 rem, 50 mSv
- Lenses of eyes: 15 rem, 150 mSv
- Other organs and tissues: 50 rem, 500 mSv
- Fetus in utero: 0.5 rem, 5 mSv; no more than 50 mR, 0.5 mSv in any 1 month of gestation during pregnancy
- Exposure should not exceed 100 mR, 1 mSv per week

low as possible. To reduce the amount of radiation exposure, the following precautions should be taken:
1. The fluoroscope should be turned off when not in use. The patient is continuously exposed to radiation during fluoroscopy. Keep in mind that the radiation emanates from the part of the C-arm that is under the OR bed.
2. Every effort should be made to reconcile an incorrect sponge, sharps, or instrument count. A radiograph should be made only as a last resort to locate a missing item.
3. Body areas should be shielded from scatter radiation or the focused beam whenever possible. A lead shield can be positioned between the patient and radiation source if it will not interfere with the sterile field or visualization for the x-ray study. The shield is placed before the patient is draped. A shadow shield connected to the x-ray tube may be a preferable alternative if a lead shield cannot be used.
   a. Lymphatic tissue, the thyroid gland, and the bone marrow of the sternum are especially sensitive to radiation. Therefore a thyroid/sternal shield should be used during x-rays or fluoroscopy of the head, upper extremities, and chest.
   b. To protect the testes or ovaries, a gonad shield should be used during x-rays or fluoroscopy of the hips and thighs.
   c. A lead shield always should be used to protect the fetus of a pregnant patient. Even low levels of scatter radiation may be harmful to the fetus. Therefore radiographs of the abdomen and pelvis are avoided if possible, especially during the first trimester.

Intraoperative documentation should include the anatomic location of the direct x-rays or fluoroscopy, the types and locations of radioactive implants, and shielding measures to protect the patient from scatter radiation. The FDA and AORN have a list of facility requirements that must be followed for personnel safety in the perioperative setting.[3,4] Safety requirements include the following:
- The amount of radiation used should be as low as reasonably achievable (ALARA).
- A safety program must be in place and run by an experienced radiation expert or physicist.
- Personnel training programs must include proper wearing of protective devices such as lead aprons, dosimeter placement, thyroid shields, eye protection, and protective measures for patients.
- Documentation for patients includes the type of radiation and protection measures.
- Any radioactive tissue, bodily fluids, or radiation implants must be disposed of by a trained individual in the correct manner.

- According to the Centers for Medicare & Medicaid Services, equipment must be checked regularly and run by trained individuals.
- Safety program must pass annual safety inspections.

Personnel Safety

Safety precautions should be taken to protect team members from the potential hazards of ionizing radiation. Three vital factors must always be remembered: time, distance, and shielding.

Time

Overexposure and unnecessary exposure should be avoided in everyone, and especially in those of childbearing age. Changes may occur in the reproductive cells as a result of radiation, leading to potential genetic defects. The following precautions should be used to limit the length of exposure to radiation:

- Patient care personnel should rotate assignments on procedures that involve radiation.
- Staff members may request relief from exposure during pregnancy. If this is not possible, a pregnant staff member should leave the room or be adequately shielded when x-rays are made or fluoroscopy is used.
- Radiation from an x-ray tube, fluoroscope, and image intensifier is present only as long as the machine is energized. These machines should be turned off when not in use.
- Radioactive elements should remain in lead-lined containers until ready for implantation. Trained personnel should handle the radioactive elements as quickly as possible and always with special forceps. A careful accounting of how many items are present and used should be made.
- A patient who has received radioactive substances for diagnostic studies may emit up to 2 milliroentgens (mR)/h. If possible, the surgical procedure should be delayed for at least 24 hours after the test.
- Personnel should limit the time spent in proximity to a patient who has had a diagnostic study with or an implantation of radioactive elements until disintegration reaches a low level.
- Body tissues and fluids removed from patients with radioactive emissions should be contained quickly.

Distance

Automatic or manual collimators, which confine the x-ray beam to the precise size of the image or fluoroscopic screen, are required for all equipment. Most image intensifiers have a lead shield as part of the installation. A single-frame computerized recording device incorporated into the fluoroscopy system also helps reduce exposure. Fluoroscopy produces more scatter radiation than do direct x-ray beams. Personnel should distance themselves as far as possible from the source of radiation, as demonstrated by the following procedures:

- Unsterile team members who can safely do so should leave the room or stand behind lead shields during each single x-ray.
- Inanimate holding devices should be used to maintain the position of the x-ray and patient.
- Sterile team members and others who cannot leave the room should stand 6 ft (2 m) or more from the patient, if possible, and out of the direct beam during exposure. Team members should remember the inverse square law of distance: double the distance equals one-fourth the intensity.
- If possible, team members should stand behind or at a right angle to the beam on the side of the patient where the beam enters, not exits.
- Lateral or oblique x-ray increases scatter radiation. Positioning the beam in a plane vertical to the pelvis or thighs helps reduce scatter. For supine and upright x-rays, the beam should be directed at the floor or walls.

Shielding

Lead that is at least 0.5 mm thick offers the most effective protection against gamma rays and x-rays to halt and absorb radiation scatter. Alpha and beta particles do not require shielding. The following guidelines for shielding should be observed:

1. The walls of rooms with fixed radiation equipment are usually lined with lead. Gamma rays can penetrate lead to a depth of 12 inches (30.5 cm). X-rays can be stopped with lead or thick concrete.
2. Portable lead screens should be available.
   a. Sterile team members and others who cannot leave the room should stand behind a lead screen while x-rays are taken or the patient is exposed to intraoperative radiation therapy. The screen(s) should be positioned behind a portable machine.
   b. When a lateral exposure is taken, the screen should be positioned behind the x-ray cassette to absorb rays that penetrate through or scatter from the cassette.
   c. People preparing radioactive implants that emit gamma rays should do so from behind a lead screen that is up to 12 inches (30.5 cm) thick. A sterile drape can be put over the screen so the scrub person or other sterile team member can stand behind the screen and reach around it.
3. Sterile and unsterile team members should wear intact lead aprons (Fig. 13.5).

• **Fig. 13.5** Lead apron.

a. The lead apron is worn under the sterile gown. Lead aprons that bear the total weight from the shoulders can cause fatigue and back strain. Lead protective attire can be worn like a vest and skirt to distribute the total lead weight.

b. If the apron does not wrap around the body, team members should face the radiation source so the apron provides protection between the source and the body.

c. To protect against beam and scatter radiation, team members should wear aprons during fluoroscopy and for lateral or oblique x-rays. Levels of scatter radiation are greater at lateral and oblique angles, and exposure time is prolonged during fluoroscopy.

d. Lead aprons should be hung or laid flat when not in use. They should not be folded. Folding can crack the lead, making the shield ineffective. The aprons should be examined under x-rays periodically to determine intactness. A policy should be in place concerning lead apron testing.

4. Lead-impregnated rubber gloves can attenuate (reduce the intensity of) rays by 15% to 25%.

a. Sterile team members should wear sterile gloves over lead-impregnated gloves when the hands will be in direct exposure (e.g., during fluoroscopy), when injecting radioactive dyes or elements, and while handling radioactive implants.

b. If it is necessary to hold a cassette in position for a single x-ray exposure, lead gloves should be worn.

c. Lead gloves may be supplied sterile or sterilized by the appropriate method for reuse. The rubber should allow adequate aeration to avoid skin irritation of the wearer. Latex-sensitive individuals should wear latex-free gloves under the rubber lead gloves.

5. Lead thyroid/sternal collars or shields should be worn during fluoroscopy and exposure to oblique-angle x-rays. Personnel within 6 ft (2 m) of the radiation source, including the anesthesia provider, risk exposure of the head and neck (Fig. 13.6).

6. Leaded glasses may be worn to protect the eyes from cataract formation during fluoroscopy.

Lead shields should be tested routinely by the radiology department every 6 months and whenever damage is suspected. Defects may not be visually detected.

Monitoring Radiation Exposure

All personnel exposed to ionizing radiation with any frequency or during prolonged procedures should wear a monitoring device. The purpose of the device is to measure the total rems of accumulated exposure. Therefore the monitor is worn only by the person to whom it is issued and at all times of exposure for the designated period. Exposure data on the monitor are recorded for each individual either monthly or weekly, depending on the type of monitor.

Film badges (dosimeters) are the most widely used monitors. These monitors contain small pieces of photographic film that are sensitive to different types of radiation: beta rays, gamma rays, and x-rays. Thermoluminescent badges and pocket dosimeters also are available. When only a single monitor is used, it is worn outside the lead apron along the neckline.

Two dosimeters may be worn. One monitor should be worn external to the lead apron at the level of the neck to measure exposure of the head and neck, especially during fluoroscopy. The second monitor should be worn on the scrub suit under the lead apron to measure exposure of the whole body and gonads (Fig. 13.7). A double monitoring system validates the effectiveness of the lead apron when exposed to ionizing radiation.

Nonionizing Radiation

Radiant energy in the form of heat and/or light is emitted from radio waves, microwaves, televisions, computers, radiant warmers, and light sources. For example, overhead lights in the OR produce heat. Fiberoptic light cables are cool, but the light transmitted is intense and can produce heat. Radiation from these sources is nonionizing (except for ultraviolet lights, which can produce radiant energy in wavelengths and intensity sufficient to alter DNA in cells, burn tissue, and damage the eyes). Nonionizing

• **Fig. 13.6** Lead thyroid shield.

"Double-Badging" for Fluoroscopy

Wear one badge (Red) at the collar outside of the apron (or any other lead PPE).

Wear the second badge (Yellow) underneath the lead apron.

• **Fig. 13.7** Placement of radiation dosimeter monitors.

• **Fig. 13.8** Laser warning sign.

radiation does not accumulate in the body and therefore does not require monitoring. Nonionizing radiation per se is not hazardous when properly controlled.

Lasers, one form of nonionizing radiation, concentrate very high-energy light beams within a small circumference to produce intense heat. (*Laser* is an acronym for *l*ight *a*mplification by *s*timulated *e*mission of *r*adiation.) Laser equipment should be used in accordance with established regulatory standards and guidelines and the manufacturer's instructions for laser safety. Lasers can vaporize, cut, or coagulate tissues directly exposed to the beams. They can cause thermal burns from indirect exposure.

Fire, explosion, eye and skin exposure, and laser plume (smoke) also are potential hazards for patients and personnel. Eyewear of the correct optical density is required, and reflective surfaces should be covered. Safety measures should be taken. A laser warning sign is prominently displayed outside the door where a laser is in use (Fig. 13.8). Correct eyewear should be available outside the door in case authorized personnel must enter the room when the laser is active. Lasers are described in more detail in Chapter 20.

PROS/CONS

Eyewear: Does It Need to Be Worn at All Times?

Pros

- Eyewear is part of the personal protective equipment (PPE) required by the Occupational Safety and Health Administration (OSHA) according to their Bloodborne Pathogens Standard. Eyewear must be provided by the facility to protect the mucous membranes of the eyes.
- Eyewear is necessary to protect the wearer against chemical, mechanical, radiologic, environmental, and biologic hazards and irritants. Liquid and chemical hazards can be from splashes, splatter, vapor, mist, fumes, dust, and airborne particles. Contaminated eyewear should be decontaminated or replaced with a clean pair. X-ray personnel can wear eye protection made of leaded glass.
- All employees should be trained about PPE. Eyewear is provided by the facility because it must meet certain standards to provide adequate protection. If employees would like to purchase their own eyewear, it must pass the facility standards and be cleaned after each use.
- Eyewear comes in a variety of styles such as disposable goggles, glasses with side shields, face shields, antifog goggles, surgical masks with attached visors, laser eyewear, and full-face respirators. All eyewear must be wide enough to protect the eyes in front as well as have side shields to protect from splashes entering at the side of the face. Some procedures require specific eyewear for protection.
- Eyewear should be put on and secured before performing the surgical scrub and worn throughout the procedure and during cleanup. It should be worn when handling dirty instruments or during patient care if there is a risk for coming into contact with bodily fluids. Goggles provide the best circumferential protection.
- Protective eyewear is specifically manufactured for use with lasers. There is protective eyewear with specific optical density lenses for each laser. They prevent the energy or wavelength from reaching the lens or retina of the eye. Eyes are vulnerable to injury from scattered, reflected, or diffused laser beams.
- The eyes of the patient also must be protected with eyewear that prevents exposure from all angles. The direction of the hazard differs because the patient is lying down. Moist eye pads secured over the patient's eyes can be used during general anesthesia.
- Signs must be placed on the outside of the surgical suite warning other staff members that a laser is in use, and special eyewear is to be donned before entering the room. Specific eyewear should be available outside the door for personnel who may need to enter the room during a procedure in progress.
- Eyewear with a small digital video camera can now be used as an educational tool. The glasses are lightweight, wrap around the sides of the face for protection, and are cable free. They contain a battery and a secure digital (SD) card.

Cons

- Many health care workers do not wear eye protection. They forget to put it on or think they are not at risk for contamination.
- Any health care worker who does not follow the policy for wearing eyewear may receive a verbal or written warning. OSHA or other regulatory agencies may conduct an unannounced visit. The facility could be fined for each breach by a government agency if they are not enforcing mandatory policies.
- Many health care workers do not put on eyewear while scrubbing, setting up a sterile table, prepping a patient, intubating or extubating a patient, cleaning up after a procedure, cleaning a room, and washing their hands after the procedure. All of these are examples of activities that put them at risk for eye contamination.
- Personal eyeglasses are not a substitute for proper eyewear. Even if side shields are applied to eyeglasses, they may not provide protection from splashes. Health care workers may wear their eyeglasses under a full-face shield.
- Many health care workers do not wear the appropriate type of eyewear for the procedure. For example, if a health care worker is doing an orthopedic procedure, a full-face shield or large goggles should be worn to prevent splatter from power equipment or irrigation devices.

References

1. Rothrock JC: *Alexander's care of the patient in surgery*, ed 17, St. Louis, 2023, Mosby.
2. AORN: Guideline for surgical attire. In *Guidelines for perioperative practice*, Denver, CO, 2024, The Association.
3. Association of Surgical Technologists: *Guideline I: eye protection*. www.ast.org. Accessed April 17, 2023.
4. Centers for Disease Control and Prevention: www.cdc.gov. Accessed April 18, 2023.

Magnetic Resonance Imaging

The first human testing of magnetic imaging took place in 1977 and took more than 5 hours to accomplish. Today this technology is a diagnostic and interventional standard. Some larger facilities have interventional suites with high-tech surgical equipment for real-time magnetic imaging during a surgical procedure that creates three-dimensional maps of the patient's body with radio waves. Noise from the magnetic resonance imaging (MRI) machine is shielded from the patient's ears by earplugs or headphones.

Patients with implanted stainless steel clips and other components, such as older style pacemakers, can suffer injury in the presence of MRI.[5] Implanted clips may be attached to intracranial vessels or other structures that could be injured if exposed to extreme magnetic forces. Patients with retained ferromagnetic bullet fragments or armor-piercing munitions (e.g., victims of a crime or a suspected perpetrator) are at risk. These bullet-type or shrapnel materials may be present in hospitalized military or law enforcement personnel from previous duty-related injuries. A careful history must be taken before MRI testing.[5,6]

Patients with stimulator leads are at risk because the metal in the leads will become superheated, causing tissue injury. Examples of implanted stimulators include pacer wires, spinal or neurologic stimulators, and internal defibrillator wires. Patients with extreme black ferrous tattooing may experience burns. Many radiologists used to refuse MRI to patients with tattoo eyeliner. The U.S. Food and Drug Administration (FDA) does not regulate tattoo ink or the practices of permanent makeup.[5,6] If a doctor recommends an MRI, precautions such as cold compresses or ice packs can be applied to the area of concern.

No magnetic metal object can be used within the MRI environment. Items have been pulled from caregivers' pockets, including scissors. Instrument tables, intravenous (IV) poles, oxygen tanks, instrumentation, and OR furniture cannot be composed of any magnetic substance. Titanium or plastic is commonly used in this environment because it is inert and nonmagnetic. Most patients are required to change into facility attire because some personal clothing can contain metal such as buttons or metal fibers.

The floor of the hybrid MRI OR is marked with safe distance positions referred to as *gauss lines*. Special equipment, such as anesthesia machines, can be positioned outside the gauss line marked "5-G." A sudden shutdown for an emergency cutoff of the magnet causes a release of helium into the OR, which can be harmful to personnel. Safety precautions include having oxygen masks available for all persons in the room in case of an emergency shutdown of the MRI. The emergency shut-off panel (referred to as the *quench button*) is in the control booth of the MRI suite.

Electricity

The appropriate use of electronic devices is a prime concern of health care providers and industry personnel who seek safer patient care. Underlying this concern is the rapidly expanding use of electronic equipment. The marketing and safety standards of medical electronic devices used in the perioperative environment are federally regulated. The standards and practices recommended by the Association for the Advancement of Medical Instrumentation (AAMI) are helpful to both manufacturers and users. Standards set by TJC also should be met for facility accreditation. Inadequately trained personnel or the malfunctioning of devices such as electrosurgical units (ESUs), defibrillators, and x-ray machines are responsible for the fatalities and near-fatalities that occur. Facilities must also be up to date on safety

codes for electrical systems. The Health Care Facilities Code NFPA99 has special standards for the OR to prevent electrocution, especially for procedures that use large amounts of water that can end up on the floor.[7]

Parameters of Electricity

Electricity is the flow of electrons along a path. It consists of three basic parameters: voltage, resistance, and current.

Voltage

Voltage forces electrons to move through material in one direction and causes current to flow. It is measured in volts. The greater the number of volts, the more direct the path of the current.

Resistance

Resistance is the measurement of opposition to the flow of electrons through material. It is measured in ohms. Electricity flows easily through conductors (e.g., metals, carbon, water); flow is minimized by insulators (e.g., rubber, plastic, glass) that prevent the flow of electricity. The resistance of the human body is more comparable to a conductor than an insulator.

Current

Current is the rate of flow of electrons through a conductor. It is measured in amperes—the number of electrons passing a given point each second. Current flow is proportional to voltage and inversely proportional to resistance. Current may be one of the following two types:

1. Direct current (DC), as from a battery. This is a low-voltage current.
2. Alternating current (AC), as from a 110 or 220-volt line. This type of current has an alternating directional flow. AC is considered low voltage, but it is three times more powerful than low-voltage DC.

Grounding

The grounding of all electrical equipment is essential for safety and prevention of stray current leakage. Grounding systems are designed to discharge any harmful electricity directly to the ground without including the patient in the circuit. This prevents the inadvertent passage of electric current through the patient, thereby preventing shock or burn.

ESUs are grounded. When using a monopolar ESU a return electrode or dispersive electrode is positioned on the patient to disperse the electrical energy and return it to the generator. The pad itself is not a ground, but a path for the current to return back to the machine. ESUs are described in more detail in Chapter 20.

Electrical power is supplied through two wires—hot and neutral—that transmit current to the three-wire outlets in the building. The third wire is the ground wire. When the cord from an electrical device is plugged into an outlet, the hot and neutral wires deliver the current. The ground wire is attached to a copper pipe that is driven into the ground at the point where power enters the building. An electrical connection to the ground provides a means for current to flow through the ground wire (or any other conductive surface) to the ground rather than going to the neutral wire. The copper ground wire is used to prevent the metal housings of electrical equipment from becoming electrically "hot." The ground wire within the three-wire power plug and cord connects the equipment (instrument) housing to the ground contact in the receptacle (wall outlet). This provides a constantly available return path for current to the electrical source.

When an instrument is grounded, leakage current returns through the ground wire to earth, causing no damage. However, if the ground path is absent or broken, leakage current will seek another path to ground. For example, if the insulation on wires is defective (e.g., broken or frayed cords or plugs), some current will leak or flow to other nearby conductors, such as the equipment housing. The same is true of endoscopic instrumentation with fractured insulation. The current will pass into the patient's tissues, causing an inadvertent injury.

Equipotential Grounding System

Current flows between points only when a voltage difference exists between them. Therefore electric shock can be minimized by eliminating voltage differences. One system designed to do this is the equipotential grounding system, which maintains an equal potential or voltage between all conductive surfaces near the patient. To achieve equipotential grounding, all exposed conductive surfaces within 6 ft (2 m) of the patient are electrically connected to a single point that is itself connected by a copper conductor to the ground tie point at the electrical distribution center serving the area. Consequently, all exposed metal surfaces are electrically tied together and to the ground.

Isolation Power System

Isolated power systems are used in hazardous locations such as ORs. An isolation transformer isolates the OR electrical circuits from grounded circuits in the power mains. Thus the isolated circuit does not include the ground in its pathway; the current seeks to flow only from one isolated line to the other. As a result, accidental grounding of people in contact with the hot wire does not cause current to flow through the individual.

A line isolation monitor checks the degree of isolation maintained by an isolated power system by continually measuring the resistance and capacitance between the two isolated lines and the ground. This measurement is called the hazard index. The monitor, a wall-mounted meter, has an alarm that is activated at the 2-milliampere (mA) level. This warning system indicates when inadvertent grounding of isolated circuits has occurred and alerts personnel to a dangerous situation. Because grounding can take place only when faulty equipment is plugged into ungrounded circuits, maximum safety is afforded by use of the isolation transformer. Ungrounded circuits fed through isolation transformers are required in OR and obstetric suites. Permanently installed overhead OR lights and receptacles in anesthetizing locations should be supplied by ungrounded electrical circuits.

The following steps should be taken in the event that the line isolation monitor alarm is activated during a surgical procedure:
1. Unplug the last piece of electrical equipment that was plugged into the power system.
2. Continue to unplug all equipment in the OR to identify the faulty equipment. A battery-operated backup system may be needed.
3. Close the OR until a biomedical engineer can check for current leakage.

Electric Shock

Electrocution occurs when an individual becomes the component that closes a circuit through which a lethal current may flow. Lethal levels may be attained by currents through the intact body via the skin or by currents applied directly to the heart. Electric shock occurs when a current is large enough to stimulate the nervous system or large muscle masses (e.g., when the body becomes the connecting link between two points of an electrical system that are at different potentials).

The physiologic effect of shock may range from a mere tingling sensation to tissue necrosis, ventricular fibrillation, or death. This effect is an electrical response of sensory cells, nerves, or muscles to electrical stimuli that originate either intrinsically (within the body) or extrinsically (outside the body). The severity of shock depends on the magnitude of the current flow and the path taken through the body. There are two types of shock: macroshock and microshock:

1. *Macroshock.* Macroshock occurs when current flows through a relatively large surface of skin. It usually results from inadvertent contact with moderately high-voltage sources, expressed in milliamperes (1/1000 ampere). A current intensity of 1 to 5 mA through the chest can cause severe burn at the point of contact. If the cardiac conduction system is involved, a current intensity of 50 to 100 mA through the chest can cause ventricular fibrillation because the heartbeat is electrically controlled.

Macroshock occurs through the trunk of the body, with the current following many paths; each path carries a fraction of the current. It may or may not be harmful, depending on how much current flows through a susceptible heart along its path. Common sources of macroshock are electrical wiring failures that allow skin contact with a live wire or surface at full voltage. The victim, instrument, or surface should never be touched with bare hands in a case of shock. The power supply should be disconnected, or an insulating material should be used to push the victim away from the source of electricity.

2. *Microshock.* Microshock occurs when current is applied to a very small contact area of skin. The development of medical techniques that permit the application of electrical impulses directly to the heart muscle has raised awareness of the extreme danger of microshock to an electrically sensitive patient. Cardiac microshock is a potential hazard of indwelling catheters filled with conductive fluid, probes inserted into the great vessels, and electrodes implanted around the heart. These devices multiply the potential for electrocution because they can be conductors of electricity.

The external portion of a cardiac catheter generally consists of two parts: an inner conductor(s) of wires or conductive fluid and an outer insulating sheath. When there is a highly conductive pathway from outside the body to the great vessels and heart, small electric currents may cause ventricular fibrillation and cardiac arrest. When a shock has an internal route to the heart, it takes only one thousandth as much electricity to be fatal as when the shock is transmitted through the surface of the skin. Microshock occurs only if current from an exterior source flows through the cardiac catheter or conductor. Conductive intravascular catheters that disperse current at skin level diminish the risk for microshock. The most important precaution is to protect the exposed end of the cardiac conductor from contact with conductive surfaces, including the body. Rubber or plastic gloves should always be worn when handling the external end of a cardiac catheter or conductor.

Safeguards

Although the value of electronic devices is unquestionable, their use must not be allowed to cause electric shock or electrocution.

Cardiac fibrillation and arrest may occur if a patient encounters an excess of accumulated small currents while connected to the ground through implanted electronic devices or by contact with other grounded objects, such as electrocardiograph (ECG) leads. Faulty electrical equipment may cause a short circuit or electric shock or can cause severe sparks that may be a source of ignition. The following safeguards should be used when working with electrical equipment[8]:

- Care should be used when operating high-voltage equipment such as x-ray machines, ESUs, lasers, and electronic monitoring devices. These machines should be checked for frayed or broken power cords, properly functioning power switches, and grounding.
- Power cables should not be stretched taut or across traffic lanes.
- Liquids should never be placed on an electrical unit. A spill could cause an internal short circuit.
- Electrosurgical and laser units may interfere with the operation of other equipment. Therefore they should be located on the operator's side of the table and as far as possible from the monitoring equipment. Preferably these units are plugged into separate circuits to avoid overloading powerlines. They should not be plugged into extension cords.
- Equipment should be properly grounded to prevent small extraneous current leaks.
- Machines should be turned off when plugging or unplugging them from the power receptacle and when attaching cords to the machine.
- Power cords should be unplugged by pulling on the plugs, never the cords; this prevents breakage of wires.
- All electrical equipment, including a surgeon's personal property, should be inspected by the biomedical engineering department before its initial use. Every piece must meet Underwriters Laboratory (UL) standards or other electrical safety requirements. All equipment should be inspected, preferably monthly but at least quarterly, and verified as safe for use. Equipment should be used according to the manufacturer's instructions.

Electrical and Thermal Burns

Monitors and all high-powered equipment are hazardous. Electrical energy is converted into thermal energy, and therefore the electricity supplied by a defective system may cause burns. The amount of heat produced depends on current density, contact time, and tissue resistance. As little as 300 mA of current for 20 seconds can produce enough heat (113° F [45° C]) to burn intact skin. Current that is concentrated or has a high density at the point of contact can result in an electrical burn severe enough to require debridement.

ESUs generate high-frequency current. In these units current flows to an active electrode that is used to cut or coagulate tissue. The use of a dispersive electrode (also known as a return electrode or Bovie pad) protects the patient. This provides the high-frequency current present at the active electrode with a low-current density pathway back to the generator. This is not the same as a ground. Proper connections from the dispersive electrode to the patient and the unit are essential to prevent burns. Deep-tissue burns can occur at the site of a dispersive electrode if it does not have adequate surface contact with skin or body tissue. Burns also can occur at the site of rings, piercings, or other metal jewelry, ECG electrodes, or other low-resistance points from invasive monitor probes (e.g., temperature probes) if the current diverts to an alternative path.

Conductive surfaces should be capable of providing a return path for current other than through the OR bed or its attachments. If the return circuit of high-frequency equipment is faulty, the circuit may be completed through inadvertent contact with metal parts or attachments of the OR bed. If the pathway for the current is small, the current passing through the exposed area of skin contact will be relatively intense, causing a deep burn to the patient. For example, one such contact point may be the thigh touching the leg stirrup when the patient is in the lithotomy position.

Surface burns can occur when battery-operated equipment, such as a peripheral nerve stimulator, is used with external electrodes. Tetanic stimuli should be limited to 1 or 2 seconds. Handheld battery-operated cautery pencils can cause pinpoint burns when the tip remains hot after use. The heat from this tip can cause ignition to drapes or dry sponges.

Other potential sources of burns include malfunctioning controls on heat-generating devices that are in contact with the patient, such as radiofrequency diathermy or hypothermia/hyperthermia machines. Individual reactions to electrical hazards are influenced by factors such as the patient's nutritional state, the amount of body fat that acts as insulation, and the circulation in the body part in contact with the device.

Static Electricity

Static electricity consists of current of high voltage and low ampere. An electrostatic spark develops from friction and accumulates on physical objects. When two static-bearing objects come into contact, the one bearing the higher potential discharges to the one with the lower potential. Air is a nonconductor, but a high enough potential can overcome air resistance and jump the gap to a lower potential object. This causes an arc across air gaps, which are seen as spark(s) from the heat thus generated. These sparks can ignite flammable materials or gases.

Objects accumulate static in inverse proportion to their conductivity. A spark between two objects can occur only when an electrical path of good conductivity does not exist between them. Because earth has a zero potential, a charge is discharged to the ground if it is brought into contact with earth directly or indirectly through a conductor. The aim is to provide adequate channels for the dissipation of static. Moderate conductivity has a tendency for the gradual spread of charge over both objects so they come to the same potential. The generation of static electricity cannot be prevented absolutely because its intrinsic origins are present at every interface. For static electricity to be a source of ignition, the following situations must be present:

- An effective means of static generation
- A means of accumulating the separate charges and maintaining a suitable difference of electrical potential
- A discharge of energy adequate to make a spark in an ignitable mixture

Fire and Explosion

Fire should be a matter of prime concern in the OR. Fires in an oxygen-enriched atmosphere (OEA) are fundamentally different in character from those occurring in a normal atmosphere. The fire severity potential should be regarded as serious, with the potential for extensive damage and endangerment to lives of patients and personnel. The presence of flammable and combustible liquids, vapors, and gases in an OEA can result in the ultrarapid combustion of surrounding materials with explosive violence (Fig. 13.9).

Anesthesia providers have discontinued the use of highly flammable anesthetic agents (e.g., cyclopropane, ether) in favor of halogenated agents. These noncombustible agents are mixed with medical air, oxygen, or nitrous oxide.

• **Fig. 13.9** Fire triangle.

Critically ill patients brought to the OR from an intensive care unit in beds with powered dynamic air mattresses are sometimes surgically treated in their bed while in the OR. The mattress is electrically powered to maintain an alternating pressure surface during the procedure. Occasionally, a tracheotomy or another invasive procedure is performed. The possibility of a puncture in the air mattress could release air under the drapes, causing a fire in the presence of a spark.

Although oxygen and nitrous oxide are nonflammable gases, they do support and accelerate combustion. A fire or explosion is the result of a combination of these factors, known as the fire triangle:

- **Fuel:** A flammable gas, vapor, or liquid (e.g., ethylene oxide, alcohol, ether, methane from the bowel, collodion). Dry sponges are flammable. Alcohol-based prep solutions can ignite if not permitted to dry before draping.
- **Ignition:** A source of ignition (e.g., laser, electrosurgery, fiberoptic light cord)
- **Oxidizer:** Oxygen (pure or in medical air with greater than 21% oxygen) or some other substance that provides oxygen, such as nitrous oxide gas or medical air. Oxygen can build up under the drapes and cause ignition when the cautery is used.

Safeguards

Standards of the NFPA and AAMI are evaluated by TJC to safeguard against fire and explosion in anesthetizing locations. Requirements are less stringent when only nonflammable inhalation agents are used. For example, nonconductive flooring and footwear are acceptable when a nonexplosive anesthetic is used. The factors that can cause fire should be controlled.

Flammable Agents

Spontaneous combustion can occur when flammable or combustible agents are exposed to an ignition source in the presence of oxygen. The following safeguards help prevent spontaneous combustion:

- Anesthesia machines, cylinders of compressed gas, and flammable liquid containers should be kept away from any source of heat and must not touch one another. A mixture of gases under high pressure is hazardous.
- Oil or grease is not used on oxygen valves or on parts of anesthesia machines. Oil or grease should not contact any cylinders, including those containing ethylene oxide, compressed air, or nitrogen.
- Flammable antiseptics containing alcohol and fat solvents are used with care for preoperative skin preparation before laser or electrosurgery. Vapors under drapes or pooled material on or around the skin can ignite if the prep solution is not completely dry before draping. Common pooling areas include the umbilicus and the sternal notch. The patient's hair should be coated with a water-soluble gel to decrease the risk for fire.
- Petroleum products used on the skin can ignite in the presence of an ESU or a laser. Water-soluble jelly can be used to coat eyebrows and lashes to render them less likely to ignite.
- Bowel gases (methane) are flammable. The rectum should be packed with a moist radiopaque sponge before using an ESU or laser near the perineum.
- Other flammables include collodion, benzoin, paraffin, and white wax (bone wax).

Ignition Sources

The minimum ignition temperatures of combustible materials in an OEA are lower than in air.

The following list contains precautions to use when working with combustible materials:

1. Thermal devices and other heated objects can cause a fire or an explosion.
   a. Precautions should be taken to prevent a laser beam, either directly or indirectly, igniting drapes, sponges, and gowns or melting an endotracheal tube. Place damp towels around the surgical site when using a carbon dioxide laser.
   b. ESUs should not be used on the neck, trachea, nasopharynx, and adjacent areas. Oxygen can cause a fire if the endotracheal tube is ignited or leaks into the field. Avoid using pieces of red rubber catheter as electrode insulation.
   c. Inadvertent activation of laser and ESUs should be avoided. When not in use, handpieces should be placed in a holder on the sterile field, not left loose. Handpieces are hot after activation. Laser units should be on standby or turned off as appropriate.
   d. Beams from fiberoptic light carriers should not be directed onto a drape. Heat can build up until sufficient to produce burning or smoldering.
   e. Lights and sources of heat should be kept at least 4 ft (more than 1 m) away from the anesthesia machine and cylinders.
   f. Heat-generating equipment, such as the operating microscope and the projection lamp for fiberoptic lighting, must not be completely enclosed. Heat can build up under the covering.
   g. The hypothermia/hyperthermia machine should be at least 3 ft (1 m) away from the anesthesia machine, and both should be adequately grounded.
   h. Only approved photographic lighting equipment with suitable enclosures can be used. Strobe lamps are preferred.

i. High-speed burrs and drills create extreme heat and can cause ignition.
2. An electrostatic (incendiary) spark can be an ignition source.
   a. The relative humidity (weight of water vapor present) in the perioperative environment should be maintained between 50% and 60%. Moisture provides a relatively conductive medium, allowing static electricity to leak to earth as fast as it is generated. Sparks form more readily in low humidity.
   b. Explosion-proof electrical receptacles or locking Hubble plugs cannot be pulled apart accidentally. Grounding adapter plugs, multiple-outlet plugs, and extension cords are prohibited.
   c. Power cords should be rubber coated, and switches should be explosion-proof. Electrical equipment should be plugged into the power receptacle before the anesthetic is administered and before the power switch is turned on.
   d. Motion should be minimal in the area around the anesthesia equipment and the patient's head. Friction on the reservoir bag should be avoided. Team members should watch that drapes do not touch the bag or cover the anesthesia machine.
   e. Patients are covered with cotton blankets. Woolen or synthetic blankets are prone to producing static electricity.
   f. The hair of patients, personnel, and visitors is covered to avoid static discharge.
   g. Antistatic outer garments are worn. Hose and undergarments in close contact with the skin may be made of synthetic material.
   h. Antistatic liners in kick buckets are handled with caution.
   i. Metals should not make contact with a force sufficient to produce percussion sparks.
   j. Anesthesia is discontinued as soon as possible if the ground monitoring system indicates a warning. After completion of the surgical procedure the room is not used until the electrical defect is corrected.

Fire Safety

All health care facilities have fire warning and safety systems. Staff members should be familiar with the location and operation of fire alarms and fire extinguishers as well as with evacuation routes and procedures. Fire drills should be scheduled routinely and be part of competency testing. Personnel should know the uses of fire extinguishers, be able to distinguish among the three main classes of them, and know how to operate them:

- *Class A* (pressurized water for combustibles such as paper, cloth, wood). A picture of a trashcan or campfire may be on the side. The "A" is imprinted within a triangle.
- *Class B* (carbon dioxide or dry chemical to smother flammable liquids, oil, gas). A picture of a gas can may be on the side. The "B" is imprinted inside a square. A number may precede the B. This number represents the distance in feet the spray will reach.
- *Class C* (halon [bromochlorodifluoromethane halogenated compressed gas] to smother an electrical or a laser fire without leaving a residue on equipment). A picture of an electrical plug may appear on the side. The "C" is imprinted in a circle.

When a fire extinguisher is used, the mnemonic **PASS** may aid in remembering how to operate the device:

*P*ull the safety ring out of the handle.
*A*im the nozzle.
*S*queeze the handle.
*S*weep the spray over the base of the fire.

If fire should occur in the OR during a surgical procedure, the first concern is for the safety of the patient and personnel. To prevent an explosion, the burning article is removed immediately from the proximity of the oxygen source and the anesthesia machine or outlet of piped-in gases. The fire on the field is smothered with wet towels, and burning drapes are removed from the patient. The shut-off valves for piped-in gases are turned off, and electrical power cords are unplugged.

The mnemonic **RACE** may aid in preventing panic and should enable the team to act quickly in the event of fire anywhere within the perioperative environment:

*R*escue anyone who is in immediate danger.
*A*ctivate the fire alarm.
*C*ontain the fire if possible.
*E*vacuate the area. (Some facilities use the term *Extinguish.*)

The patient should be removed immediately from any danger, and the fire should be extinguished in the room, if possible. The anesthetized patient is evacuated on the OR bed to a distant location on the same floor. Lateral evacuation is when the team movement from the fire is creating a distance from danger on the same floor. Anesthesia personnel should be assisted with life-support equipment, such as breathing bags (Ambu bags) and tubing. Keep in mind that oxygen will support the fire.

Pack the surgical site with saline-moistened lap tapes, and cover with a sterile towel or drape. Although attempts are made to prevent infection, this is a secondary thought to the loss of life. All fires, no matter how small, must be reported to the facilities risk management department. Team members should refer to the departmental policy and procedure manual for evacuation and safety protocols specific to the facility.

Fires within the patient's body are usually small, but deadly. The most common type is an endotracheal fire. The cause is usually laser or ESU contact with a flammable endotracheal tube. In the event of an endotracheal fire, immediately withdraw the burning tube and pinch the nose and mouth shut to extinguish the fire (this removes the fuel and oxygen). Flush the airway with sterile saline if necessary, but have the suction immediately available. The anesthesia provider must immediately reintubate with a smaller, uncuffed tube and reoxygenate the patient. A cuffed tube would increase pressure on the damaged tissue.

Chemical Hazards and Safeguards

Health care providers are exposed to many hazardous chemicals daily. The hazards of these chemicals include irritation of the eyes or mucous membranes, contact dermatitis or burns, toxicity that causes renal or liver disease, and exposure to carcinogens or mutagens. These or other effects may be immediate, delayed, or chronic. Hazardous chemicals in the workplace are controlled by government regulations, such as those of OSHA and the EPA in the United States or those of the Control of Substances Hazardous to Health (COSHH) in Great Britain.

Chemicals should be labeled by the manufacturer with the identity of the agent(s) and appropriate warnings of hazards. The latter may be symbolic; that is, pictures added to words. Labels must not be removed or defaced. Employees should read the labels and understand procedures for safe handling and use. OSHA has incorporated right-to-know regulations in its standards. One part of this Hazard Communication Standard requires that employees have access to the safety data sheet (SDS), formerly known as the material safety data sheet (MSDS), supplied by the manufacturer for each hazardous chemical in the workplace. A SDS specifies the following information:

- Composition and common names of the chemical
- Chemical and physical properties
- Known acute and chronic health effects, such as carcinogenic, mutagenic, or allergenic
- Exposure limits
- Protective measures
- Antidote or first-aid measures

OSHA standards are legally enforceable. Although not legally enforceable, NIOSH and ACGIH recommendations for exposure limits to hazardous gases and vapors in ambient air should be adopted for the safety of personnel.

Anesthetic Gases

Air conditioning or ventilating systems help prevent pockets of anesthetic gases in the OR, although concentrations around the anesthesia machine and the patient's head may not be remarkably reduced. Substantial amounts of gases can escape during surgical procedures. The patient's exhalations also can pollute the air in the OR and the postanesthesia care unit (PACU). Heavy gas can accumulate and channel along the floor as far as 50 ft (15 m). Confining agents by using a closed carbon dioxide absorption technique tends to restrict gases from getting into airstreams.

Waste anesthetic gases and vapors can escape from the anesthesia machine and its hoses and connections, from around the facemask on the patient, and from the patient's expirations. Although not conclusive, data indicate that personnel may incur health hazards if chronically exposed to waste anesthetic gas. Stress, long working hours, and other unknown related factors may contribute to this occupational risk. Possible health hazards include the risk for spontaneous abortion, congenital abnormalities in the offspring of male and female personnel, cancer, and hepatic and renal disease. Significant behavioral changes have been observed and include decreased perception, cognition, and manual dexterity. Personnel also may complain of fatigue or headache.

Studies of the retention of anesthetic agents in anesthesia providers after the administration of clinical anesthesia have demonstrated traces of gas in expired air for varying lengths of time—from 7 hours after nitrous oxide administration to 64 hours after halothane administration. It has been shown that high doses of nitrous oxide block the metabolism of vitamin B12. Chronic exposure to trace levels of nitrous oxide may also lead to neurologic problems or neuropathy.

Because millions of inhalation anesthetics are administered annually, a substantial number of OR staff are occupationally exposed to these gases. OSHA enforces the NIOSH recommendations that room air not be contaminated by more than 0.5 parts per million (ppm) of halogenated agents per hour when used in combination with nitrous oxide or more than 2 ppm/hr when used alone. Nitrous oxide should be controlled to less than 25 ppm during an 8-hour time-weighted exposure.

The use of scavenging equipment and procedures is strongly recommended. Scavenging involves the removal of waste anesthetic gases, mainly by trapping them at the site of overflow on the breathing circuit; this is followed by disposal to the outside atmosphere, where the gases are safely diluted. The rate of removal of gases by the disposal system depends on the rate at which fresh air enters the OR and the patterns taken by air currents as they circulate through the room.

The proper use of vacuum scavenging equipment attached to the anesthesia machine can reduce exposure to trace concentrations of gas by 90% to 95%. Personnel exposure should be reduced to the lowest practicable limits by reducing waste gas to the most technically feasible level. Waste gas is vacuumed with a purple hose connected to the rear of the anesthesia machine. When setting up the room for the day, make sure that the hose is connected. A waste-gas control program to ensure the continuing purity of environmental air includes the following measures:

1. Good work practices of anesthesia providers. The major source of waste gas in the OR is the intentional outflow of gases from the anesthesia breathing system. The quantity of gases discharged varies depending on the type of breathing system, the gas flow rate, and gas concentration.
2. Use of a well-designed, well-maintained scavenging system. Inexpensive, practical, and effective exhaust systems are available. The gas evacuation system should be attached to every anesthesia machine and ventilator to scavenge excess gases directly into a vacuum line with a minimum flow rate of 440 ppm.
3. Use of proper anesthesia technique:
   a. Different techniques of administration result in different exposure levels. Some leakage is uncontrollable.
   b. All components of the breathing system should fit well. Masks should fit facial contours to ensure a good seal. An oral or nasal airway may reduce the escape of gas from around the mask.
   c. Liquid halogenated agents should not be spilled. The gas flow should not be turned on until the mask is in place or the patient is intubated and the endotracheal tube is connected to the breathing circuit.
   d. Masks, tubing, reservoir bags, and endotracheal tubes should be inspected after each cleaning for leaks, holes, and abnormalities. Disposable equipment is preferable to recycled equipment.
4. Proper maintenance of anesthesia equipment through the following measures:
   a. Daily routine checking of anesthesia machines for leaks. NIOSH recommends that the total leak rate of each machine not exceed 100 mL/min at 30 cm of water pressure. Leaks can be detected with a gas analyzer or bubble test.
   b. Periodic preventive maintenance of all machines and fittings by a manufacturer's representative every 6 months, with in-house monitoring at least quarterly.
5. Maintenance of a high flow rate of fresh air into the air conditioning system through engineering control procedures. A good ventilating system (preferably not a recirculating one) is also important in the PACU. The ventilation system should comply with the minimum requirements of 20 air changes per hour to minimize the risk to PACU personnel.
6. Use of an OR atmospheric monitoring program to record trace anesthetic levels and determine the effectiveness of the previous measures. Specialized monitoring equipment, such as an infrared analyzer, is the only way to detect leaks. Dosimeters are available for each individual to wear to indicate exposure.

Sterilizing Agents

The chemical agents used to sterilize heat-sensitive items can be toxic or can vaporize to emit noxious fumes that are irritating to the eyes and nasal passages, even at low levels of exposure.

Ethylene Oxide

Ethylene oxide (EO) is used in a gaseous form for sterilization and is a known mutagen and carcinogen. The residual products can be toxic if there is direct contact with the skin or the gas is inhaled. Exposure can cause dizziness, nausea, and vomiting. Ethylene glycol and ethylene chlorohydrin are by-products of a reaction with moisture, such as on the hands. All porous items sterilized with EO should be aerated to dissipate the gas. The PELs for EO are 5 ppm for a short-term exposure of 15 minutes and 1 ppm time-weighted average (TWA) over 8 hours.

Formaldehyde

Formaldehyde may be used in a gaseous or liquid form. The vapors are toxic to the respiratory tract. Formaldehyde is a potent allergen, mutagen, and carcinogen, and it can cause liver toxicity. The PEL is 1 ppm TWA (NIOSH recommendation) to 2 ppm for short-term exposure of 15 minutes and 0.75 ppm TWA (OSHA standard) over 8 hours. Automated dispensing systems are available that can dispense formalin without the risk of breathing in any fumes or splashes.

Glutaraldehyde

Glutaraldehyde is the least toxic of the three sterilizing agents, but the fumes from the liquid form may be irritating to the eyes, nose, and throat. Contact dermatitis and hives have been reported. The PEL is 0.2 ppm per exposure. Glutaraldehyde should be used only in a closed container and in a well-ventilated area. PPE should be worn. A dosimeter is available to determine the airborne concentration of fumes.

Disinfectants

Some of the disinfectants used to clean or decontaminate equipment and furniture can be irritating to the skin and eyes. Gloves and goggles should be worn when using these chemicals, and the agents should be used in proper dilution. The fumes from some agents can irritate the nasal passages. The following substances can cause gloves to degrade:
- Isopropyl alcohol
- Phenol
- Sodium hypochlorite
- Glutaraldehyde
- Hydrogen peroxide
- Quaternary amines
- Povidone iodine

More information on sterilizing agents can be found in Chapter 18.

Methyl Methacrylate

Commonly referred to as *bone cement*, polymethylmethacrylate (PMMA) is a mixture of liquid and powder polymers. Some brands are mixed with antibiotic powder, and it is important to double-check patient allergies before use. It should be mixed at the sterile field just before use. The vapors released during mixing are irritating to the eyes and can damage gas-permeable contact lenses. The monomer vapors are also irritating to the respiratory tract, and they can cause drowsiness. The fumes are flammable. PMMA mixing devices with vacuum attachments are commercially available.

Patients may experience adverse reactions during or immediately after the placement of PMMA. The patient can become hypotensive within a few moments of use and continue a hypotensive state for up to 5 minutes. The FDA reports that some asystolic events have occurred. Continuous monitoring is critical for the well-being of the patient.

PMMA may be a mutagen, a carcinogen, or toxic to the liver. The liquid solvent can cause corneal burns if it splashes into the eyes. It also can diffuse through latex gloves to cause an allergic dermatitis; gloves that are impermeable to this solvent are available. Gloves should be changed after handling the doughy mixture. PMMA has an exothermic effect. A scavenging system should be used to collect the vapors during mixing and to exhaust it to the outside air or absorb it through activated charcoal. The PEL for methyl methacrylate has been established at 100 ppm TWA. PMMA is considered a hazardous waste and must be disposed of according to facility and government policies.

Drugs and Other Chemicals

Antineoplastic cytotoxic drugs used for chemotherapy can be hazardous, as can laser dyes and other pharmaceuticals. All chemical agents should be prepared and administered to minimize unnecessary exposures for both patients and personnel. Chemicals should be combined or mixed with diluents only when this is known to be a safe practice, as specified by the manufacturer.

Intraperitoneal chemotherapy can be administered in the OR during laparotomy. The surgeon can use the Coliseum technique in which the chemical is introduced via a Tenckhoff catheter and a roller pump with a heat exchanger set at 111.2° F (44° C). The solution remains in the patient's abdomen for 90 minutes. The surgeon, wearing two sets of sterile gloves, continually manipulates the intraabdominal organs to evenly distribute the heated chemical as it continually circulates through the cavity and is removed through several abdominal drains. The air is continually filtered through activated charcoal and a smoke evacuator to protect the OR environment from aerosolization of the drug.

Safe Handling of Cytotoxic Agents

Antineoplastic cytotoxic agents have carcinogenic and mutagenic properties, and most can cause local and/or allergic reactions. Personnel should avoid inadvertent direct contact with skin or eyes, inhalation, and ingestion during handling.

Written precautions and procedures for handling, preparing, administering, and disposing of cytotoxic agents should be followed. Basic guidelines for the use of cytotoxic agents include the following:
1. Protect self from skin and respiratory contact. Preferably, prepare agents under a vertical laminar flow hood. Regardless of whether a containment hood is available, wear thick gloves, a mask, eye protection, and a gown.
2. Wash hands after handling cytotoxic agents and all items that have been in contact with them, including those used for administration.
3. Place all cytotoxic waste in sealed leakproof bags or containers. Incineration is recommended for all materials used in preparing and administering cytotoxic agents.

Biologic Hazards and Safeguards

The transmission of infection and disease within the health care facility is a concern of both consumers and providers. Biologic hazards do exist in the environment, and every effort should be made by health care providers to protect their patients and themselves. Standard precautions are a necessity (i.e., treating all body fluids and materials as infectious). Employers must ensure that the appropriate protective equipment is available and that employees are trained to wear and use it.

Surfaces such as door handles and computer keyboards have been found to harbor active vancomycin-resistant *Enterococcus* (VRE), methicillin-resistant *Staphylococcus aureus* (MRSA), and *Pseudomonas aeruginosa* for prolonged periods. Endospore-forming clostridia (i.e., *Clostridium difficile* [*C. diff*]) can persist for months.

Simple handwashing is becoming less effective in adequately removing these microorganisms. Antiseptic gel hand hygiene is recommended after handwashing. Cleaning contaminated surfaces such as computer keyboards may be unreliable because these surfaces were not designed for exposure to disinfectant solutions. Some chemicals and solutions can damage the equipment. The surface of the keyboard can be covered with a plastic cover that is easier to clean.

Infectious Waste

Infectious medical waste is an environmental concern both within and outside the health care facility. The EPA defines infectious waste as waste-containing pathogens with enough virulence and quantity that exposure to them could result in an infectious disease in a susceptible host. The disposal of potentially infectious waste generated in health care facilities is regulated by governmental mandates. Although regulated medical waste refers to the portion of waste that has the potential to transmit infectious disease, a uniform definition of what constitutes regulated medical waste has not been universally adopted. Consider the following factors when deciding if something is infectious waste:

- The presence of pathogenic organisms in sufficient numbers to be capable of causing infection in living beings. Many microorganisms are incapable of causing infection.
- The presence of a portal of entry into a susceptible host. A cut, needlestick, puncture wound, or skin lesion provides a portal of entry, but not all living beings are susceptible hosts to infectious diseases.

These two factors permit the regulation of medical waste that poses a risk to public health and the environment and creates aesthetic concerns for the public. Potentially infectious waste is considered to be blood and blood products, pathologic waste, microbiologic waste, and contaminated sharps. This includes items contaminated by blood, such as sponges, drapes, gowns, and gloves. These items should be segregated from general waste, such as wrappers.

Infectious waste is placed in leakproof containers or bags strong enough to maintain integrity during transport. These bags should be closed and either labeled or color coded. For example, red bags may be used to indicate infectious waste. Needles and sharps should be put in puncture-resistant containers. If the outside of the container is contaminated, double-bagging is necessary for safe handling during transport to the disposal area. Waste can be steam sterilized or decontaminated with microwaves before compaction and disposal in a landfill, or it can be incinerated. Federal, state, and local regulations should be followed for disposal.

Biohazards

All patients are potential sources of infection. OSHA defines occupational exposure as reasonably anticipated skin, eye, mucous membrane, or parenteral contact with blood or other potentially infectious materials during the course of duty. This contact includes blood, tissues and organs, and all body fluids. Careful handling of and adequate protection from potentially contaminated equipment also are important. Personnel, such as radiologists who handle tissue as part of the diagnostic process, are at risk not only from biologic exposure but also from marker wires used in needle localization. Handwashing is a must after every patient contact or glove removal. Personal exposure should be a concern of all team members.

To be compliant with OSHA standards, every health care facility must develop a written exposure control plan that includes procedures for evaluating an incident and determining when exposure has occurred. Engineering controls include safety devices or equipment designed to minimize or eliminate a biohazard. Likewise, restrictions or changes in work practices should ensure the safety of all patients and personnel in the environment. For example, food must not be stored in the same refrigerator as blood products or specimens. Eating, drinking, and applying lip balm are prohibited in areas where contact with blood or other potentially hazardous material is possible. Eating or drinking should never be allowed at any time in the OR during a surgical procedure.

Punctures and Needlesticks

A penetrating injury (e.g., needlestick, cut) or a splash (e.g., into the eye, onto mucous membranes) with fluid contaminated with blood or body fluids must not be ignored. Hepatitis, human immunodeficiency virus (HIV), and other bloodborne pathogens can be transmitted through breaks in the skin or contact with mucous membranes. The hepatitis B vaccine is recommended for all high-risk health care workers.

If exposure to blood or body fluid occurs, the following procedures should be performed:
1. Stop activity immediately and step back from the point of contamination. Remove glove.
2. Squeeze the skin around the needlestick or cut to expel blood and contaminants.
3. Cleanse the puncture site or flush the eye with cool water. Flush cut or puncture with alcohol or iodine preparation. Continue to squeeze blood until coagulation takes place.
4. Report the incident according to facility policy and procedure and seek medical attention promptly. Baseline blood may be drawn from the patient and injured person for determination of risk for transmission of disease. The patient should be informed.
5. Follow the particular protocol established by the facility for follow-up.

If a needlestick is involved, most facilities will draw a baseline blood sample from the patient and the injured caregiver. Periodic blood samples are drawn over a period of months to make sure results remain clear. Caregivers who have been contaminated by a high-risk patient or a patient known to have hepatitis B or to be positive for HIV should be prophylactically treated with the appropriate drugs and followed by the employee health department. Additional information about postexposure prophylaxis and guidelines for treatment can be found at www.cdc.gov.

Surgical Plume

Plume (surgical smoke) is generated by the thermal destruction of tissue or bone. Bloodborne pathogens, mutagens, carcinogens, and other toxic substances can be aerosolized by lasers, electrosurgery, and powered surgical instruments.[9] Twenty air exchanges with four fresh, clean air duct filters, and positive room pressure help minimize buildup of plume in the OR atmosphere. Masks capable of filtering particles at least as small as 0.1 μm (high filtration) are recommended to prevent inhalation of plume particulate. Face shields, goggles, or eyeglasses with side shields should be worn to protect the eyes.

A smoke evacuator should be used to suction laser and electrosurgical plumes. The evacuator has a filtration system that incorporates a prefilter to trap particles, an ultralow penetrating air filter for particles in the 0.1-μm range, and a charcoal filter to absorb odor and hydrocarbons. The vacuum nozzle should be held close to the surgical site. Wall suction only filters 5 ft^3 per minute and is not recommended for large volumes of smoke evacuation. An inline filter is necessary to avoid clogging the department vacuum system.

OR personnel can change the filters in some evacuators, whereas others require maintenance by a biomedical technician. Filters are contaminated with biohazardous material and should be disposed of in the same manner as items contaminated with blood and body fluids. Complete PPE, such as gloves, masks, and protective eyewear, should be worn when changing filters because the connecting couplers have been contaminated with plume and the material may be released into the air when the connection is disengaged.

Reproductive Hazards
Male Reproductive Health Implications
Chemical, radiologic, and physical exposures can cause abnormalities in sperm numbers, shapes, and motility. The reaction experienced by an individual will depend on the agent, duration of exposure, and other health status considerations. Chemicals such as ethylene varieties can accumulate in the epididymis, seminal vesicles, or prostate, causing decreased sperm production and decreased ability to fertilize an ovum.

Some chemicals can affect a man's ability to perform sexually because of impotence or decreased libido. Chromosomal DNA can be affected because sperm are produced every 72 days and are stored in the epididymis for 15 to 25 days, where they mature and begin to swim. These changes can cause fetal abnormality if fertilization takes place.

According to NORA, more than 1000 workplace chemicals can cause reproductive effects in animals. Many chemicals have never been tested and also may be implicated in birth defects. Additional information is available at www.cdc.gov.

Female Reproductive Health Implications
Excessive exposure to ionizing radiation, waste anesthetic gases, and ethylene oxide during pregnancy may cause a spontaneous abortion or a congenital fetal anomaly. Pregnant employees may be more susceptible to fatigue from standing for prolonged periods, lifting heavy items, and eating and taking breaks at irregular intervals. Exposure to infectious diseases also is a hazard. The health care facility should have a policy for pregnant employees, which may include transferring a pregnant employee from a hazardous area such as the OR. For the safety of the fetus, assignments should limit exposures whenever possible. For example, a pregnant woman should not assist with the implantation of radioactive elements or be exposed to fumes from bone cement.

An employee who is pregnant is responsible for her own welfare and the safety of her fetus. Immunizations should be current, especially for hepatitis B and rubella, and she should follow the safeguards described in this chapter to limit her exposures to the lowest possible levels. Ultimately the employee should decide whether she wishes to continue working in the perioperative environment.

Latex Sensitivity/Allergy
Many items used in the OR, such as surgical gloves, catheters, drains, medication vial stoppers, tubing, anesthesia breathing circuits, endotracheal tubes, breathing bags, and syringe plungers, contain natural rubber latex (Table 13.1). Some synthetic products are referred to as latex but do not contain the protein that causes reaction. Natural rubber latex is manufactured from the milky sap obtained from rubber trees (*Hevea brasiliensis*). A water-soluble protein in natural latex contains an antigen that can cause a fatal allergic response.

Two types of responses have been identified: local and systemic.[10] Local reactions are less severe and occur when latex comes into contact with the skin, causing skin rash, itching (urticaria), redness, and burning that usually subside within 24 hours.

A patient may have a systemic reaction when a latex product comes into contact with the mucous membranes, serosa, or peritoneum during a surgical procedure. This reaction is more severe, causing anaphylactic shock or death. The signs of severe anaphylaxis are hypotension, tachycardia, bronchospasm, and generalized erythema. Treatment of choice is adrenaline and IV fluids, either crystalloid or colloid, to manage hypotension associated with anaphylaxis.

FDA studies have shown that 6% to 7% of direct patient care personnel and surgeons are sensitive to natural rubber latex. Health care personnel who are frequently exposed to latex products can become sensitized. Several items used in the OR contain latex but are not identified as having natural rubber latex as its content (e.g., the elastic bands on caps and shoe covers or mattress and pillow covers). The manufacturer should be consulted to determine whether a product in use contains latex and whether a latex-free substitute is available.

Latex proteins can contaminate the starch on prepowdered gloves, thus providing a potential route of airborne exposure to allergens during donning. Sterile surgical nonlatex gloves are available commercially but are more expensive. They should be used only when an allergy is confirmed or is highly suspected in the user or in a patient receiving care.

Testing procedures are available for the detection of a latex allergy. Testing all personnel and patients would be a costly endeavor, but testing people suspected of having a latex sensitivity should be considered. According to the World Allergy Organization, 15% of all health care personnel are sensitive compared with 1% to 7.6% of the general population. Surgeons, dentists, and nurses can have sensitivity as high as 25% to 50%.[10] Patients should be asked preoperatively if they have a known sensitivity (e.g., a history of a reaction after handling a toy balloon or wearing rubber gloves). Children with spina bifida, people with constant latex exposure, and those with multiple allergies are known to be prone to latex allergy. Allergies to certain foods, such as avocados, potatoes, bananas, tomatoes, chestnuts, kiwifruit, and papaya, may be implicated in natural latex allergies per NIOSH.

TABLE 13.1   Care of the Latex-Sensitive Patient

Commonly Used Latex Products	Latex-Free Alternatives	Patient Teaching	Considerations
Anesthesia breathing circuit, endotracheal tube, Ambu breathing bag	Disposable plastic breathing circuits and endotracheal tubes	NA (not applicable)	Dispose of used equipment
Bite blocks for oral surgery	Dental rolls, rolled gauze squares, silicone blocks	NA	Avoid using counted radiopaque sponges
Catheters, enema tips, and drains	Silicone catheters and drains	Instruct patient to report irritation or discomfort in area of drain or catheter	Patients rarely have silicone sensitivity; check product for content in manufacturer's enclosed literature
Electrocardiogram (ECG) leads, dispersive electrodes, pulse oximeter leads	Nonlatex gel pads	Instruct patient to report irritation at application site	Patient may have sensitivity to conductive gel; may need to use water-soluble lubricant
Elastic bandages, antiembolism stockings	White cotton bandages	Instruct patient to report any sensory changes in bandaged part, such as tingling, pain, or loss of sensation	Nonelastic bandages or stockings may restrict movement and have less expansion properties; circulation may become impaired if applied too tightly
Elastic and adhesive tape	Plastic, paper, or silk tape	Instruct patient to report irritation around or under area of tape	Some patients have sensitivity to adhesive rather than tape backing
Elastic bands on surgical caps, shoe covers, urinary catheter leg bags, plastic pants, disposable diapers	Cloth towel or paper caps with ties to cover hair; cloth hook and loop leg bands, cloth diapers	Instruct patient to report irritation around hairline or leg(s)	Cloth diapers will not be impervious to leaks; cloth hook and loop bands may impair circulation to leg
Embolectomy catheters	Silicone catheters	NA	Check composition of entire catheter and balloon
Hypothermia/hyperthermia blanket, hot water bottle, heating pad, mattress cover	Disposable plastic warming blankets and pads	Instruct patient to report irritation or discomfort	Observe for temperature control of device to avoid skin injury
Latex gloves, finger cots	Plastic or other nonlatex gloves	Instruct patient that utility gloves used at home may contain latex	Use nonlatex sterile gloves; vinyl utility gloves for nonsterile activities
Positioning devices, such as egg crate–type, donuts, wedges, rolls	Silicone rolls	NA	Silicone gel pads can be rolled around bolsters for added height
Rubber shods	Silicone catheter or plastic tubes	NA	Should be radiopaque; plastic shods are not as pliable
Syringe plungers in plastic syringes	Glass syringes	Instruct patient that plungers in plastic syringes used for self-administered injectable medications contain latex	Air-powered autoinjector device or implantable medication-dispensing mechanism is an option at home
Tubing as on blood pressure cuffs and endoscopic insufflators	Disposable plastic tubing and cuff covers	NA	Wrap limb with cotton sheet wadding to avoid contact

Risk Management

The perioperative environment is a high-risk environment. The risks can be minimized by adhering to the many safeguards discussed in this chapter. An effective risk management program continually seeks to provide working conditions that will not jeopardize the health and safety of employees. Such a program has at least four essential elements:

1. Administration
   a. Regulations, recommendations, guidelines, and laws should be enforced to prevent disastrous consequences of occupational hazards.
   b. Policies and procedures should be written, reviewed periodically, and updated as appropriate. All employees should have access to them.
   c. Protective attire and safety equipment should be made available to employees, as appropriate.
   d. Monitoring devices should be used in all hazardous locations as recommended by regulatory agencies.
   e. Employee health services should be provided for immunizations and in the event of injury.
2. Prevention
   a. Regular in-service programs should be conducted to keep employees informed about hazards and safeguards.

b. Employees should be taught how to use and care for new equipment before it is put into service.

c. Employees must know the location and use of emergency equipment, such as fire extinguishers and shutoff valves.

d. Employees must wear protective attire, as appropriate.

e. Routine preventive maintenance should be provided for all potentially hazardous equipment.

3. Correction

a. Faulty or malfunctioning equipment should be taken out of service immediately.

b. Any injury should be reported, with medical attention sought as soon as possible.

c. Unsafe conditions should be reported.

4. Documentation

a. Records of preemployment medical examinations and periodic examinations for the surveillance and early detection of disease should be maintained for each employee. These records should be retained in a permanent file after termination of employment in case there is a future health problem.

b. At the time of employment, new employees may be given a letter explaining the occupational risks.

c. Accident reports regarding injuries to personnel and patients should be filed with the administration of the facility.

The prevention of injuries is vital to maintaining a safe environment. It is everyone's responsibility.

EVOLVE WEBSITE

http://evolve.elsevier.com/Hornacky/BerryKohn/

- Historical Perspective
- Student Interactive Questions
- Glossary

References

1. Nasri BN, Mitchell JD, Jackson C, et al.: Distractions in the operating room: a survey of the healthcare team, *Surg Endosc* 37(3):216–235, 2023.
2. Letvak S, Apple B, Jenkins M, et al.: At risk safety behaviors of the perioperative nursing team: a direct observational study, *Healthcare (Basel)* 11(5):698, 2023.
3. AORN: Radiation safety. In *Guidelines for perioperative practice*, Denver, CO, 2024, The Association.
4. U.S. Food and Drug Administration: *Facility guidelines and personnel qualifications*. www.fda.gov. Accessed April 17, 2023.
5. MRI safety. www.radiologyinfo.org. Accessed April 17, 2023.
6. U.S. Food and Drug Administration: *Tattoos, temporary tattoos, and permanent makeup*. www.fda.gov . Accessed April, 2023.
7. Mizrahi J: *How operating room designs avoid the shock of electrical system accidents*. www.csemag.com. Accessed April 17, 2023.
8. AORN: Environment of care. In *Guidelines for perioperative practice*, Denver, CO, 2024, The Association.
9. Bouchat-Friedman D: The secrets of a successful surgical smoke evacuation program, *Outpatient Surgery*. www.aorn.org. Accessed April 17, 2023.
10. Parisi C, Kelly K, Ansotegui I, et al.: Update on latex allergy: new insights into an old problem, *World Allergy Organ J* 14(8):100569, 2021.

14

Surgical Microbiology and Antimicrobial Therapy

CHAPTER OUTLINE

Microorganisms: Nonpathogens Versus Pathogens, 239

Types of Pathogenic Microorganisms, 244

Antimicrobial Therapy, 255

CHAPTER OBJECTIVES

After studying this chapter the learner will be able to:

- Differentiate between microorganisms.
- Describe the natural lines of defense of the human body.
- Identify several favorable living characteristics of microorganisms.

- Describe how disease is spread.

KEY TERMS AND DEFINITIONS

Aerobic Microorganism that requires air or the presence of oxygen for maintenance of life.

Anaerobic Microorganism that grows best in an oxygen-free environment or one that cannot tolerate oxygen (e.g., *Clostridium* species that causes gas gangrene).

Antibiotics Substances, natural or synthetic, that inhibit growth of or destroy microorganisms. Used as therapeutic agents against infectious diseases; some are selective for a specific organism; some are broad-spectrum antibiotics.

Antimicrobial agent Chemical or pharmaceutical agent that destroys or inhibits growth of microorganisms.

Biofilm Three-dimensional layers of living bacteria embedded in a sticky matrix that persist on the surface of tissues and implanted medical devices. Commonly the cause of chronic infections, such as otitis media and rhinitis.

Bioterrorism Covert event involving introduction of microbial contamination and infection of humans or animals.

Community-acquired infection (CAI) Infectious disease process that developed or was incubating before the patient entered the health care facility.

Cross-contamination Transmission of microorganisms from patient to patient and from inanimate objects to patients, and vice versa.

Endospore Forms of bacterial classes clostridia and bacillus that are generated when living conditions are not favorable. Protective capsule that forms inside specific bacterial species encircles and protects the genetic matter to resist destructive forces, such as disinfection or sterilization.

Epidemiology Study of occurrence and distribution of disease; the sum of all factors controlling the presence or absence of a disease.

Florae Bacteria and fungi normally inhabiting the body, resident or transient.

Hospital- (or health care–) acquired infection (HAI) An infection that was not present when the patient was admitted to the health care facility. Infection may occur at the surgical site or as a complication unrelated to the surgical site (formerly known as nosocomial infection).

Infection Invasion of the body by pathogenic microorganisms and the reaction of tissues to their presence and to toxins generated by the organisms.

Logs of bacterial growth Colonies of bacterial microorganisms grow at doubling rates exponentially (binary fission). The rate of growth is measured by the number of bacterial logs. Before the log phase begins the bacteria adapt to the environment and are in a lag phase in which they are preparing to double in number. When the environment changes in nutrients, temperature, or basic living conditions, the bacteria begin to die at the same rate they are "born" and they enter a stationary phase that precedes the final death stage.

Microorganisms Living organisms, invisible to the naked eye, including bacteria, fungi, viruses, protozoa, yeasts, and molds.

Opportunists Microorganisms that do not normally invade tissue but are capable of causing infection or disease if introduced into the body mechanically through injury, such as tetanus bacillus, or when resistance of the host may be lowered, as by human immunodeficiency virus infection. Opportunistic infection.

Pathogenic Producing or capable of producing disease.

Prion Protein that contains no genetic material and in its pathologic form causes fatal neurodegenerative disease. Difficult to inactivate. Requires special handling. Three types of disease transmission: sporadic, familial, and iatrogenic.

Sepsis Severe toxic febrile state resulting from infection with pyogenic microorganisms, with or without associated septicemia. Septicemia is a clinical syndrome characterized by significant invasion into the bloodstream of microorganisms from a focus of infection in tissues. Microorganisms may multiply in the blood. Infection of bacterial origin carried through the bloodstream is sometimes referred to as bacteremia.

Standard Precautions Procedures followed to protect personnel from contact with blood and body fluids of all patients (formerly referred to as universal precautions).

Superinfection Secondary subsequent infection caused by a different microorganism that develops during or after antibiotic therapy.

Surgical site infection (SSI) An infectious process that develops in one or more surgical sites.

Microorganisms: Nonpathogens Versus Pathogens

Specific numbers of microorganisms with plantlike or animal-like characteristics are considered nonpathogenic in the human if they are not transferred to a different location in the body. Nonpathogenic microorganisms do not pose a particular threat to health if they remain constant in microbial numbers (logarithms: referred to as logs [logs of bacterial growth]). Natural resident florae can be found in the reproductive tract secretions, gastrointestinal tract, nasopharyngeal mucus, respiratory passages, and any superficial ductal opening, such as sweat and oil glands.

Resident florae have specific roles in their natural location. Some resident florae of the large intestine aid in the synthesis of vitamin K, vitamin B12, and folic acid, but can cause an infection if they are relocated to a surgical incision.

The term infection is used when nonresident florae invade a susceptible area. The term superinfection is used when resident florae are out of balance and the increased number causes a pathogenic condition. If the count of microbial colonies increases over what is considered normal or the colonies grow in an area where they are not usually found, an infection results and the microorganisms are considered pathogenic. They can invade healthy tissue through some power of their own or can injure tissue by producing a toxin. Pathogenic microorganisms can cause sepsis—a severe toxic febrile state, leading to organ failure or death.[1]

In a healthy state, body fluids such as urine and cerebrospinal fluid do not normally contain microorganisms and are considered sterile. Other fluids that under normal circumstances do not contain microorganisms include blood, peritoneal fluid, synovial fluid, amniotic fluid, tears, semen, and breast milk. Because microorganisms are not visible on gross inspection, exposure to any body substance, including respiratory exhalations, should be considered contaminated and treated accordingly.

Identification of Microorganisms

Microorganisms, with the exception of viruses, have intracellular DNA. The DNA is either enclosed in a nuclear membrane (eukaryotic) or loose in the cytoplasm (prokaryotic). Bacteria and blue-green algae are the only prokaryotic microorganisms. Bacteria remain in a primitive state unchanged by evolution. All other microorganisms are eukaryotic and have changed many times on an evolutionary scale.

Specimens and cultures of tissues or body fluids may be sent to the microbiology laboratory for identification. Treatment is prescribed according to the type of microorganism present in the body. The type of substance taken from the body for testing may be a clue as to the type of microorganism.

Accurate identification of the microorganism is critical to the selection of the appropriate therapy. The following criteria are used by laboratory personnel to identify the type of microorganism:
- Cell morphology
- Mobility or motility
- Presence or absence of spores
- Native pigment
- Gram stain reaction
- Growth factors (optimal growth conditions, speed of replication/reproduction, and how it grows in various media)
- How it colonizes (log phase)
- Antibody detection in the host
- Metabolism and atmosphere requirements
- Biochemical activity (endotoxin or exotoxin)
- Sensitivity to exogenous chemicals or substances

Viability of Microorganisms

Any microorganism can become a pathogen when transferred from one place to another. Each type of microorganism has its own method of duplicating itself. Epidemiology is the study of how microorganisms multiply and spread.

Bacteria pass through four phases during their colonization/duplication/reproductive stage:
1. *Lag phase:* The microorganism adjusts to the new environment.
2. *Log phase (logarithm, exponential) growth phase:* This is characterized by a maximum and constant rate of multiplication. If conditions are favorable, *Escherichia coli* can double in 20 minutes. *Mycobacterium tuberculosis* (tubercle bacillus) may require 5 hours.
3. *Stationary phase:* The multiplication rate and death of microbes equalize and balance. This period can last several days.
4. *Death:* The rate of microbial death exceeds the rate of multiplication. A few living cells can linger for several days or months but not at the same level as the growth phase.

The rate of bacterial growth is depicted in Fig. 14.1. The population of microbes will double during the log phase at a predictable interval referred to as *generation time* or *doubling time*. Changes in temperature, moisture, illumination, nutrients, and pH can influence the rate at which any microbe passes through doubling time. If all favorable living conditions are met, the microbe can proliferate into disease state. Bacteria secrete a slime that accumulates in layers known as biofilm.

Any change in the favorable conditions can alter the amount of time it takes for the microbe to pass through any one of the four

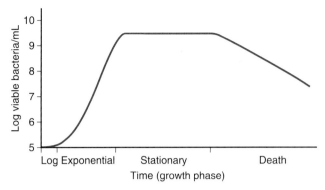

• **Fig. 14.1** Logarithmic growth of a bacterium.

•BOX 14.1 **Favorable Living Conditions for Microorganisms**

• Can live with oxygen (aerobic) or without oxygen (anaerobic). Some require no special gaseous environment (facultative).
• Can live with or without moisture. Some can completely dry out and be reconstituted.
• Can live with or without light. Some like complete darkness.
• Can live in a neutral or an alkaline pH. Most will die in an acidic environment.
• Can live with or without warmth. Some can grow in the freezer compartment of the refrigerator.
• Can get nourishment from a living host or decayed matter. Some can absorb nutrients from the environment of the host.

---

phases. Box 14.1 describes the favorable living conditions associated with the proliferation of microorganisms.

The essential element in preventing pathogenic disease is to understand the microorganism's mode of transmission, life cycle, and favorable living conditions. Interference with the viability, doubling, and survival of pathogenic microorganisms can minimize the risk for infection.

Three Lines of Defense

The human body is remarkable in its ability to protect itself by intact barriers, membranes, and bacteriostatic secretions. Three lines of defense are particularly important for prevention of disease.

The first line of defense involves generalized good health and incorporates natural biochemical, mechanical, and anatomic protection through the following features:
• *Skin:* Stratified epithelium contains sweat (sudoriferous) and oil (sebaceous) glands, which are bactericidal. Natural florae inhibit each other. The epithelium must remain intact to afford protection. Desquamation and low pH impede bacterial colonization.
• *Mucous membranes:* An effective barrier when intact, these line all natural body orifices except the ears, which secrete cerumen (earwax). Mucous membranes have bactericidal properties and a slightly acidic pH.
• *Reflexes:* Examples include vomiting, gagging, and blinking.
• *Sneezes:* Mucociliary escalator of the respiratory tree moves mucus and debris from the respiratory tract.

• *Genitourinary/reproductive tracts:* Immunoglobulin A (IgA), found in mucus, and enzymes are produced; these have a slightly acidic pH. Peristalsis is unidirectional.
• *Eyes:* Enzymes and IgA protect the conjunctiva and structures of the eye.
• *Cellular level:* Interferon is naturally formed in the cell to fight against viral attack.
• *Stomach acid:* Acid kills most pathogens.
• *Muscular closure of orifices:* Muscular closure provides a mechanical barrier against orifices such as the cervix and sphincters.

The second line of defense involves the collaborative effort of several body systems to prevent the proliferation of pathogenic microorganisms. These provide secondary protection if the microorganism breaks through the first line of defense. The second line of defense includes the following factors:
• *Inflammatory response:* This can be localized or systemic; biochemical, mechanical, and anatomic activities fight invading microorganisms and lay the groundwork for healing.
• *Antibody production:* Production is stimulated by the presence of an antigen. Some antibodies can be replicated for future exposures to the same microorganism.
• *Temperature elevation:* This can be localized or systemic. Some microorganisms are destroyed or repelled by heat.

The third line of defense can be acquired naturally or induced therapeutically. It requires actual exposure to the pathogen in some form during which temporary or quasipermanent resistance is attained. Methods include the following:
• *Passive immunity:* A "preformed" immunoglobulin (antibody) is introduced into the body. No memory for replication of the protective antibodies remains in the body.
• *Active immunity:* The body can develop a memory for production of antibodies in response to specific antigens. Live, dead, or attenuated microorganisms trigger the response. Some exposures require a booster injection to spark the memory and maintain immunity.

Pathogenic Invasion

Pathogenic microorganisms initially invade and aggregate in a body system or at a localized site, such as an abscess. The proliferation of infectious material is easily supported by warmth, chemical composition, moisture, and other components of the body.

Local spread is supported by the surface of the wound, necrosis of tissue, diminished or ineffective inflammatory response, and absence of anatomic barriers. Other pathways of infection include any body orifice, duct, or lumen of a broken blood vessel.

Veins are particularly vulnerable because they are often associated with venous sinuses and have low pressure. Venous stasis permits the growth of microbial colonies. The central nervous system shares a similar risk for infection because the cerebrospinal fluid is under lowered pressure and has components that are rich in nutrients. As microbial colonies increase in number, infection may be carried through the body in the lymphatic system and may eventually become bloodborne. Major organ systems can become involved and can result in multisystem organ failure and death. Any body fluid or substance is a potential carrier of pathogens (Box 14.2).

•BOX 14.2 Body Fluids and Substances That May Transmit Pathogens

- Amniotic fluid
- Any exudate or transudate
- Any open wound
- Aqueous humor
- Bile
- Blood
- Breast milk
- Carbon dioxide gas from deflation
- Cerebrospinal fluid
- Cerumen
- Feces
- Irrigation solution
- Nasal secretions
- Pericardial fluid
- Peritoneal fluid
- Plume from electrosurgery or laser
- Respiratory secretions and exhalations
- Saliva
- Sebum
- Semen
- Smegma
- Synovial fluid
- Tears
- Tissue
- Unfixed tissue specimen
- Urine
- Vaginal secretions
- Vitreous humor

According to the Centers for Disease Control and Prevention (CDC), 1 in 31 patients acquire one or more health care–acquired infections (HAIs). The full report can be accessed at www.cdc.gov. A surgical site infection (SSI) increases the length of stay and increases the cost of care.[2]

Knowledge of how the cycle of infection works is the most important element of prevention. Considerations include, but are not limited to, the following:
- Identifying the reservoir of the pathogen
- Identifying the portal of exit of the pathogen from the reservoir
- Identifying how pathogens are transmitted
- Identifying the portal of entry into a susceptible host
- Identifying the invasion of the susceptible host

Infectious Processes in the Body

Clinical infection is the product of the introduction, metabolic activities, and pathophysiologic effects of microorganisms in living tissue. It can develop in the surgical patient as a preoperative complication after an injury, known as a community-acquired infection (CAI), or as a postoperative complication acquired in the hospital, which is referred to as an HAI.

A localized HAI infection may begin at the surgical site between the fourth and eighth postoperative days. Infection, usually bacterial in origin, develops as a diffuse, inflammatory process, known as *cellulitis,* and is characterized by pain, redness, and swelling. This inflammatory response is the body's second line of defense directed toward localization and containment of the infecting organism after it has passed through the first line of defense.

Red blood cells, leukocytes, and macrophages infiltrate the affected area, with pus formation (suppuration) often ensuing. An abscess forms as a result of tissue liquefaction with pus formation, supported by bacterial proteolytic enzymes that break down protein and aid in the spread of infection. Fibrinolysin, for example, an enzyme produced by hemolytic streptococcus, may dissolve fibrin and delay surgical-site healing.

The body attempts to wall off an abscess by means of a membrane that produces surrounding induration (hardened tissue) and heat. Localized pus should be drained promptly.

If localization is inadequate and does not contain the infectious process, spreading and extension occur, causing regional infection. Microorganisms and their metabolic products are carried from the primary invasion site into the lymphatic system, spreading along anatomic planes and causing lymphangitis. Failure of the lymph nodes to hold the infection results in uncontrolled cellulitis. Subsequently, regional and/or systemic infection may develop, characterized by chills, fever, and signs of toxicity.

Septic emboli may enter the circulatory system from septic thrombophlebitis of regional veins communicating with local infections. These emboli and pathogenic microorganisms in the blood seed invasive infection and abscess formation in remote tissues.

Sepsis elevates the patient's metabolic rate 30% to 40% above average, imposing additional stress on the vital systems. For example, cardiac output is about 60% higher than normal resting value. The body's defenses and ability to meet the stress govern whether the infectious process progresses to systemic infection or septic shock. Multiple infection sites, the presence of shock, and inappropriate antibiotic therapy result in a poor prognosis.

Obviously the strategy to avoiding infection is prevention. However, if an infection begins, the next most important step is to identify the microorganism and treat it appropriately. More than one microorganism may be present; therefore treatment is highly individualized. Diagnosis of systemic infection may include any two of the following:
- Temperature more than 100.4° F (38° C) or less than 96.8° F (36° C) (late sign)
- Heart rate more than 90 beats/min
- Respiratory rate more than 20 to 22 breaths/min
- White blood cell count more than 12,000/mm^3 or less than 4000/mm^3

Septic shock may include decreased urinary output (less than 30 mL/hr), altered mental state, and hypoxemia. The patient usually becomes very hypotensive (low blood pressure) and has signs of blood-clotting defects, such as bruising.

The ultimate resolution of infection depends on immunologic and inflammatory responses capable of overcoming the infectious process. This is associated with drainage and removal of foreign material, including debris of bacteria and cells, lysis (breakdown) of microorganisms, resorption of pus, and sloughing of necrotic tissue. Healing then ensues.

Who Is at Risk for Exposure?

Perioperative personnel who provide direct and indirect patient care are at risk for exposure to potentially harmful microorganisms. Wearing personal protective equipment (PPE), such as masks, gowns, gloves, and eyewear with side shields, decreases the risk but does not eliminate it. The risk for exposure is proportionate to the proximity to the patient in the operating room (OR).

PROS/CONS

Laboratory Coats

Pros

- Laboratory coats are a symbol of professionalism and identification in rank.
- White laboratory coats favorably influence trust and increase confidence during patient contact.
- Laboratory coats are also associated with an increased perception of a provider's competency.
- They are designed to be a barrier to protect the clothing under the laboratory coat from pathogens.
- They provide additional pocket space for personal items.
- They provide additional identity information when embroidered with name and position.

Cons

- White laboratory coats and long neck ties were identified as unhygienic by health care workers because they are not regularly laundered.
- Patients and health care providers have a different opinion of wearing laboratory coats. Health care workers have a negative attitude because the placement of personal items in the pockets is a risk for infection.
- Old laboratory coats with stains may potentially be a risk for transmission of microorganisms because microorganisms can harbor in the stain.
- Laboratory coats should not be worn outdoors or from facility to facility because they can carry pathogens with them.
- Methicillin-resistant *Staphylococcus aureus* (MRSA) and *Clostridium difficile* (an endospore) have been cultured on laboratory coats. They can be transmitted between individuals who have touched any object contaminated with these organisms.

- Storing contaminated laboratory coats in a personal locker encourages microbial growth and transfers the microbes to other items that may be taken home.
- Laboratory coats worn over scrubs need to be clean, buttoned closed, and laundered in an accredited laundry facility after each wear to effectively decrease contamination.
- If a laboratory coat is worn outdoors, it should be exchanged for a clean coat to prevent bringing any risk for infection into the facility.
- The cuffs of the sleeves and pockets were the areas most contaminated based on what was touched and what was placed into the pockets.
- Staff may have inadequate knowledge of the principles of infection control.
- Unauthorized personnel can assume the identity of the person whose name may be embroidered on the front of the laboratory coat.

References

1. Chan C, Lam T, Mohanavel L, et al.: Development and validation of the knowledge, attitude and practice questionnaire (LAUNDERKAP) regarding white coat use among medical students during clinical practice, *Am J Infect Control* 50(12):1374–1380, 2022.
2. Goyal S, Khot S, Ramachandran V, et al.: Bacterial contamination of medical providers' white coats and surgical scrubs: a systemic review, *Am J Infect Control* 48(3):994–1001, 2019.
3. AORN: Guideline summary: surgical attire. In *Guidelines for perioperative practice*, Denver CO, 2024, The Association.

PROS/CONS

Wearing Scrub Jackets

Pros

- A long-sleeved cover jacket or scrub jacket should be worn by all nonscrubbed staff members.
- Scrub jackets are designed to cover the bare arms and help prevent shedding skin cells from dropping onto surfaces and/or becoming airborne.
- Scrub jackets should be provided by the facility and laundered daily because microorganisms can survive on fabric from 1 to 90 days.
- Studies have shown that microorganisms from skin cells dispersed into the air can be transferred to a patient, putting them at risk for a surgical site infection (SSI).
- A long-sleeved scrub jacket should be worn during the surgical prep to prevent skin shedding over the surgical area.
- Scrub jackets should be made of low-linting, stain-resistant, durable, and tightly woven material.
- The proper size scrub jacket and how it is worn is important. The jacket should fit close to the body and arms and come down to the wrists. It should be completely closed with buttons or snaps to prevent the jacket material from coming into contact with a sterile area.
- Policies and procedures with recommended wear of surgical attire must be established by each health care facility. Policies should include proper attire when leaving the restricted and semirestricted areas.
- Some facilities offer disposable scrub jackets.

Cons

- Many health care providers do not wear the correct size jacket or do not change them daily because of the lack of facility supply.
- Some health care providers wear their jackets multiple times and store them in their lockers, thereby putting themselves and patients at risk for infection.
- Oversized jackets can drag along contaminated surfaces and transfer microorganisms to the wearer or a patient.
- Scrub jackets with pockets can get contaminated from any personal item such as scissors, papers, or cell phones.
- Health care personnel's lack of knowledge and policy awareness puts everyone at risk for transferring microorganisms.
- Nonenforcement of surgical attire policies can lead to increased SSIs within a facility.

References

1. Phillips NM, Hornacky A: *Pass CNOR*, St. Louis, 2019, Elsevier.
2. AORN: Guideline summary: surgical attire. In *Guidelines for perioperative practice*, Denver, CO, 2024, The Association.
3. Rothrock JC: *Alexander's care of the patient in surgery*, St. Louis, 2023, Elsevier.

The closer to the surgical field (source of blood and/or body substance) one is, the higher is the risk for exposure. The surgeon, assistants, and scrub persons have a higher risk by role and proximity. They share an increased incidence of needlesticks and puncture wounds.[3] The circulating nurse, environmental services personnel, and instrument processors are also at increased risk for body substance exposure because of specimen handling, cleaning processes, and other contaminants in the environment. The Occupational Safety and Health Administration (OSHA) has provided guidelines for immediate treatment of a needlestick at www.osha.gov.

Exposure rates to blood and body substances for OR personnel must be reported. Sharps were responsible for 3 in 100 reported exposures. Of glove tears reported, most were in single-gloved caregivers who revealed a blood exposure. In double-gloved individuals who had a glove puncture, only a few individuals reported an inner-glove puncture. Double-gloving does not ensure avoidance of a puncture in the event of a needlestick. Most reported injuries with sharps were self-inflicted by carelessness. Individuals should act quickly, notify the supervisor, and follow the needlestick protocol for the facility.

The patient is also at risk. If a needlestick occurs, the needle may come into contact with the patient after penetrating the caregiver, thereby exposing the patient. Some patients have health conditions that predispose them to vulnerability for infection. Considerations related to higher risk include immunosuppression, an immature immune system (preterm and term infants), radiation therapy, burns, diabetes, nutritional depletion, smoking, chemotherapy for cancer, older patients, steroid use, sickle cell disease, alcoholism, liver and kidney disease, and preexisting infection being treated with antibiotic therapy (superinfection/opportunistic infection may ensue).

Biofilm

Biofilm forms when one or more species of bacteria, fungi, and other microorganisms adhere in layers to moistened surfaces, such as biologic tissue, implantable metals, and plastics (Box 14.3). The slimy matrix that binds the microorganisms together creates a barrier against antibiotic treatment that results in a persistent disease state. Plaques can break off and attach elsewhere, causing a separate biofilm colony.

Biofilm can form on any biologic tissue surface or on inert devices implanted in the body, such as catheters, artificial joints, and mechanical heart valves. The biofilm begins as a single cell layer that attaches to a surface and multiplies and thickens rapidly (Fig. 14.2). Research has shown that biofilm is a genetically mediated process in which bacteria exchange intercellular information that gives rise to newly formed biofilm in a process known as *quorum sensing*.[4]

Persistent bacterial cells contain a gene (*HipA*) that codes for a toxic protein, which puts the cell into hibernation until the effects of a specific antibiotic have worn off. Antibiotics work only on growing, animated cells. When the antibiotic ceases to work, the cells reanimate and repopulate the site. Deleting or deactivating the *HipA* gene could end the ongoing battle with biofilm.

A biofilm infection may linger for months, years, or even a lifetime, regardless of the state of the patient's intact immune system. Bacteria in biofilm can be difficult to eliminate. The National Institutes of Health (NIH) points out that most of human chronic infections are attributed to biofilm. An infected implant may need to be explanted.

Mandatory Reporting of Health Care—Acquired Infections

The Healthcare Infection Control Practices Advisory Committee (HICPAC) of the CDC published updates on reporting HAIs; updates can be found at www.cdc.gov. Infections to be reported include a wide range of patient-related infections that are traceable to health care intervention. Examples include, but are not limited to, the following infections:
- Indwelling catheter infections
- SSIs
- Ventilator-associated pneumonia
- Central line infections
- Communicable diseases
- Septicemia

Methodology and surveillance activities are described by HICPAC in the recommendations to the CDC. The pros include public reporting of infection rates; cons include a potential for misunderstanding by the general lay population and misrepresentation of published data.

•BOX 14.3 Examples of Microbiologic Biofilms Associated With Chronic and Resistant Infections

Bacteria
- *Pseudomonas aeruginosa*
- *Staphylococcus aureus*
- *Streptococcus pneumoniae*
- *Haemophilus influenzae*
- *Moraxella catarrhalis*

Fungi
- *Candida albicans*
- *Cryptococcus*
- *Pneumocystis*
- *Aspergillus*
- *Coccidioides*

• Fig. 14.2 Biofilm Life Cycle. The process can be broken down into conditioning film formation and initial attachment of the organism to the surface, growth, and development of the biofilm, and organism detachment and dispersal. (From P. Dirckx, Montana State University Center for Biofilm Engineering, Bozeman, MT. Reproduced with permission.)

Types of Pathogenic Microorganisms

Infections may be caused by one microorganism or a combination of them. Each type of microorganism has a specific set of characteristics that promotes survival and proliferation. Knowing the specific needs for microbial life aids in the prevention of infection. In this chapter each type of microorganism is described according to structure, life cycle, and mode of transmission. Examples of each type of microorganism are provided in Table 14.1.

Bacteria

Bacteria are unicellular microbes essential to human life. We depend on many of their metabolic processes. Many antibiotics are derived from bacteria, such as erythromycin, chloramphenicol, streptomyces, and kanamycin. Some photosynthesizing types convert carbon dioxide to water and oxygen.

More than 5000 species of bacteria have been named, and many unidentified species exist. Most of the morphologic differences in bacteria are found in metabolism, chemical composition, or resultant effect on the host. Unfortunately, many varieties of bacteria are pathogenic or are capable of becoming pathogenic (Fig. 14.3).

Bacteria can survive in diverse environments. For example, *Thermoplasma acidophilum* is found in the hot springs of Yellowstone National Park and is capable of living in a 140° F (60° C) environment with an acidic pH of 1 to 2. *Geobacillus stearothermophilus* endospores (formerly known as *Bacillus stearothermophilus*) are used to test steam sterilizers because they can

withstand temperatures up to 140° F. *Bacillus atrophaeus* endospores are used to test dry heat and low-temperature hydrogen peroxide sterilizers because they are destroyed at a lower temperature of 98.6° F (37° C).

Characteristics

1. *Structure:* Most bacteria are microscopic, single-cell structures (1–10 μm). Two billion bacteria can be contained in a single drop of water. Bacteria have DNA but no formal nucleus (prokaryotic) and no membrane-bound organelles.
   a. Cocci are round. Examples include strains of *Staphylococcus* and *Streptococcus*. Diseases include impetigo and gonorrhea.
   b. Bacilli are rod shaped, and some can form endospores. They are the most common types of bacteria. Examples include *Bacillus, Clostridium, Escherichia, Proteus,* and *Pseudomonas* species.
   c. Spirochetes are spiral shaped. Diseases include syphilis, leptospirosis, and Lyme disease. In the later stages of illness, syphilis and Lyme disease can have fatal neurologic effects known as *neurosyphilis* and *neuroborreliosis* (Lyme).
   d. Pleomorphs can change shape from rod to round, making positive identification difficult. Diseases include mycoplasmal infection, typhus, rickettsial infection, chlamydia, psittacosis, and Rocky Mountain spotted fever. Rickettsia and chlamydia organisms must live in a host cell. They are intracellular parasites.
2. *Life cycle:* Bacteria can be aerobic, anaerobic, facultative, or microaerophilic. They can reproduce asexually by binary fission (split into equal halves). Some studies have shown that some genes may be transferred between bacterial species during viral infection (plasmid transfer).
3. *Communication:* Some bacteria can communicate that conditions are adequate for reproduction and colonization. The process of cells gathering and communicating is known as *quorum*

TABLE 14.1	Common Microorganisms in an OR Environment	
Microorganism	**Usual Environment**	**Mode of Transmission**
Staphylococci	Skin, hair	Direct contact
	Upper respiratory tract	Airborne
Escherichia coli	Intestinal tract	Feces, urine
	Urinary tract	Direct contact
Streptococci	Oronasopharynx	Airborne
	Skin, perianal area	Direct contact
Mycobacterium tuberculosis	Respiratory tract	Airborne, droplet
	Urinary tract	Direct contact
Pseudomonas	Urinary tract	Direct contact
	Intestinal tract	Urine, feces
	Water	Water
Serratia marcescens	Urinary tract	Direct contact
	Respiratory tract	Water
Clostridium	Intestinal tract	Direct contact
Fungi	Dust, soil	Airborne
	Inanimate objects	Direct contact
Hepatitis virus	Blood	Bloodborne
	Body fluids	Direct contact

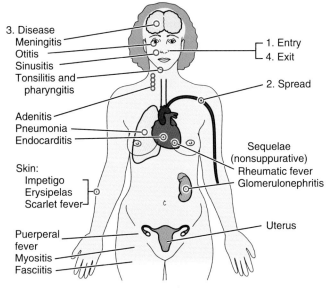

3. Disease
Meningitis
Otitis
Sinusitis
Tonsilitis and
pharyngitis

Adenitis
Pneumonia
Endocarditis

Skin:
Impetigo
Erysipelas
Scarlet fever

Puerperal
fever
Myositis
Fasciitis

1. Entry
4. Exit

2. Spread

Sequelae
(nonsuppurative)
Rheumatic fever
Glomerulonephritis

Uterus

• **Fig. 14.3** *Streptococcus* infection.

sensing. When the cells have populated an area to a sufficient degree, the process of formal infection takes place. Quorum sensing is commonly found in biofilm accumulations. Some bacteria can actually pass on DNA to their offspring asexually, producing two identical daughter cells. These cells can multiply the same way, causing infection.

Studies have shown that engineered nanofactories show promise in the disruption of this form of communication between cells, thus decreasing the need for antibiotic administration. This works by allowing the bacteria to think there are enough cells in the area to cause infection. In reality the bacterial presence triggers immune response and there are not enough bacterial cells to combat the body's white cell activity. This may prove useful when antibiotic resistance is present because antibiotics do not play a role.

4. *Transmission:* Infection is passed along by direct contact or through animal or insect bites.
5. *Encapsulation:* Some bacteria are enclosed within a thick wall, which is a defense mechanism against phagocytic activity of leukocytes. These bacteria may be ingested by white blood cells, but instead of being killed and digested they remain within the phagocyte for a time and are then extruded in a viable condition. The presence of a capsule is associated with virulence among pathogenic bacteria. This is not to be confused with endospore formation, which is discussed in later paragraphs.

Differentiation of Bacterial Types

Gram Stain

A universal way to determine the differences in bacteria is to stain the cell. Danish physician Christian Gram (1853−1938) developed a method of applying a solution of crystal violet and iodine (gentian violet) to the cell wall (bacterial coat) followed by exposure to 95% alcohol and acetone. Gram-positive bacteria retain a stain of dark purple-blue. Gram-negative bacteria retain only a stain of light pink after the rinsing process (Table 14.2).

Gram stain is also used to identify nonbacterial substances such as trophocysts (helminth eggs) and larvae.

Endospores

Endospores are the resting, protective stage of about 150 species of gram-positive rod-shaped bacilli, specifically *Clostridium* and *Bacillus*. Gram-negative bacilli do not form endospores. The endospores encapsulate and protect their internal genetic matter (DNA and ribosomes) for future reproduction during exposure to a threatening environment. The process of forming an endospore is called *sporulation*. When conditions are suitable for survival, the endospore reverts back to its original bacterial cellular structure for active germination and outgrowth (Fig. 14.4). In the vegetative or active growth state, endospore-forming bacilli are no more difficult to kill than non—endospore-forming bacteria.

Endospore positioning within the bacterium is how the pathology department differentiates species of endospore-forming bacteria. Examples of locations include central *(Bacillus cereus)*,

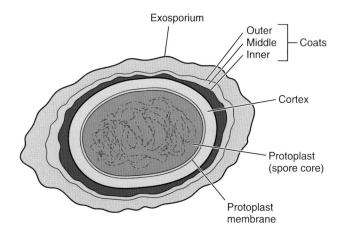

• **Fig. 14.4** Bacterial endospore.

<table>
<tr><td colspan="2">**TABLE 14.2**</td><td colspan="4">**Bacterial Gram Stain Chart**</td></tr>
<tr><td></td><td></td><td>Gram-Positive Cocci</td><td>Gram-Negative Cocci</td><td>Gram-Positive Rods</td><td>Gram-Negative Rods</td></tr>
<tr><td>Aerobic</td><td></td><td>*Staphylococcus aureus*
Staphylococcus epidermidis
Streptococcus pneumoniae
Streptococcus pyogenes
Streptococcus viridans
Enterococcus faecalis
Enterococcus faecium</td><td>*Neisseria gonorrhoeae*
Neisseria meningitides
Moraxella catarrhalis</td><td>*Listeria monocytogenes*
Bacillus anthracis
Corynebacterium diphtheriae</td><td>*Escherichia coli*
Klebsiella pneumoniae
Proteus mirabilis
Serratia marcescens
Pseudomonas aeruginosa
Enterobacter
Haemophilus influenzae
Legionella pneumophila
Salmonella
Shigella
Brucella
Bordetella
Campylobacter</td></tr>
<tr><td>Anaerobic</td><td></td><td>*Peptostreptococcus*
Peptococcus</td><td></td><td>*Clostridium difficile*
Clostridium perfringens
Clostridium tetani
Actinomyces</td><td>*Bacteroides fragilis*
Fusobacterium</td></tr>
</table>

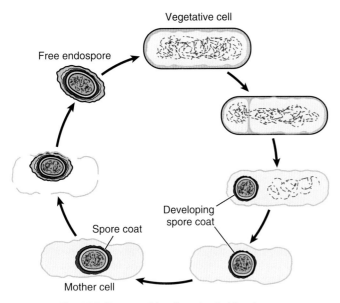

Free endospore

Vegetative cell

Developing spore coat

Spore coat

Mother cell

• **Fig. 14.5** Process of forming a bacterial endospore.

lateral *(Bacillus subtilis)*, and at either terminal polar end *(Clostridium tetani)*. Stains and dyes on the exterior wall of the bacteria can make definitive identification of the endospore difficult. In its natural state the endospore itself is clear. Stains have been developed to tint the endospore within the bacterial coat for visualization.

Most other microorganisms are killed easily by the processes of sterilization and disinfection, but bacterial endospores are not. Nonpathogenic varieties of the bacillus endospore-forming microorganisms are used in sterilizers to test for efficacy and by brewers for fermentation of spirits (e.g., *B. subtilis*). *Clostridium* is exceptionally pathogenic, being the cause of *C. difficile*, tetanus, anthrax, botulism, and gangrene (Fig. 14.5) The strain of *C. difficile* known as ribotype 027 produces stronger toxins of A and B and is becoming resistant to vancomycin.

Bacterial Toxicity

Pathogenic microorganisms produce substances that on invasion adversely affect the host locally and/or systemically. Toxic substances affecting tissues, cells, and possibly enzyme systems diffuse from the microbial cells. The cellular substance of a wide variety of organisms is toxic also. In addition, harmful effects may be produced indirectly by activation of tissue enzymes by bacteria. The following list includes toxic substances:

1. *Exotoxins:* These classic bacterial toxins are the most potent toxins known. As little as 7 ounces (200 mL) of crystalline botulism type A toxin is said to be able to kill the world's entire population. Exotoxins appear to be proteins, are denatured by heat, and are destroyed by proteolytic enzymes, which break down protein. These bacteria are typically gram-positive and form spores. Examples of diseases are tuberculosis (TB), clostridia, diphtheria, anthrax, and leprosy.
2. *Endotoxins:* These toxins are contained within the cell wall of bacteria and are released when the cell wall is broken. They are heat stable and are not digested by proteolytic enzymes. On parenteral inoculation, they cause a rise in body temperature

and are known as *bacterial pyrogens.* They increase capillary permeability with the resultant production of local hemorrhage.

Endotoxins cause injury to body cells at the site of infection, but more importantly they cause serious, often lethal, effects by systemic dissemination and widespread injury to many tissues throughout the body. Endotoxic shock may occur in bacteremia caused by gram-negative bacteria. Examples of diseases are typhoid, shigellosis infection, and plague. Microorganisms include *E. coli, Salmonella,* and *Pseudomonas.*

3. *Heterogeneous substances:* Microorganisms also form a variety of other heterogeneous (dissimilar) toxic substances, which may contribute to the disease process directly or facilitate the establishment of foci of infection. Toxins that diffuse from the intact microbial cell have the following various effects:
   a. Cytotoxic effect (leukocidin) destroys white blood cells (e.g., causing leukopenia, or reduction of the number of leukocytes below what is considered normal).
   b. Kinase effect interferes with the clotting mechanism of blood.
   c. Enzymatic effect causes bacterial hemolysins to dissolve red blood cells or fibrin, thereby inhibiting clot formation. Coagulase, an enzymatic substance of bacterial origin, is causally related to thrombus formation. Coagulase-positive *Staphylococcus, B. subtilis, E. coli,* and *Serratia marcescens* accelerate clotting of blood and induce intravascular clotting.

Toxic Shock Syndrome

Toxic shock syndrome (TSS) is an acute condition caused by exotoxins secreted by strains of *S. aureus.* The pathogen can invade any part of the body. TSS is characterized by fever with temperature over 102° F (38.9° C), hypotension, erythematous rash, and injury to multiple organ systems. Diagnosis is based on the presence of abnormal clinical and laboratory findings. Prompt supportive treatment and antibiotic therapy are crucial. Desquamation, peeling of skin (usually from the palms of the hands and soles of the feet), occurs 1 to 2 weeks after onset.

Recovery is usually complete, but TSS is potentially fatal if untreated. It can originate from a surgical wound, burn, postpartum infection, or septic abortion infected or colonized with the implicated toxin. TSS can afflict any age-group of either sex (Fig. 14.6).

Septic Shock

Septic shock is a state of widely disseminated infection, often borne in the bloodstream (i.e., septicemia). Early septic shock may begin with fever, restlessness, sudden unexplained hypotension, confusion, hypoxia, tachycardia, tachypnea, and/or oliguria. One or more of these signs and symptoms may be present. Toxic or metabolic by-products increase capillary permeability, permitting loss of circulating fluid into the interstitial fluid. Endotoxins released by bacteria promote vasodilation and hypotension.

Septic shock is most frequently produced by gram-negative bacteria. As shock progresses the patient develops cold, clammy skin; sharply diminished urinary output; respiratory insufficiency; cardiac decompensation; disseminated intravascular coagulation; and metabolic acidosis. The high-risk category comprises patients

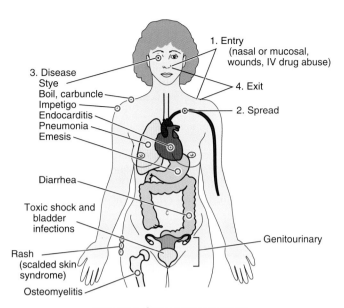

1. Entry
(nasal or mucosal,
wounds, IV drug abuse)

3. Disease
Stye
Boil, carbuncle
Impetigo
Endocarditis
Pneumonia
Emesis

4. Exit

2. Spread

Diarrhea

Toxic shock and
bladder
infections

Genitourinary

Rash
(scaled skin
syndrome)

Osteomyelitis

• **Fig. 14.6** *Staphylococcus aureus.*

with severe infection (e.g., peritonitis), trauma, burns, impaired immunologic status, diabetes mellitus, or extreme age, as well as patients who have undergone an extensive invasive procedure.

Treatment consists of control of the infectious process, early administration of antibiotics, fluid-volume replacement, and oxygen. Diuretics, sodium bicarbonate, vasoconstrictors, vasodilators, inotropic agents, or heparin also may be indicated. Corticosteroids may be used, but their use is controversial. A monoclonal antibody may be administered to reduce endotoxins.

Tuberculosis

TB is caused by the acid-fast gram-positive bacterium *M. tuberculosis*. Tubercle bacilli can remain dormant in the body, encased in a tough shell, for years after exposure.[5] This is not to be confused with endospore formation. The caseous coat of TB is a tough form of cell wall.

Tubercle bacilli usually infect the lungs (pulmonary TB), but they may be present in joints, kidneys, ovaries, or other organs. Acute miliary TB may be seen in an abdominal procedure as generalized peritonitis. *M. tuberculosis* is an opportunistic organism. Individuals at high risk for TB include those immunosuppressed from human immunodeficiency virus (HIV) infection, corticosteroid therapy, chemotherapy, or malnutrition. Persons with diabetes mellitus, cirrhosis, alcoholism, silicosis or other lung disease, or who have had prolonged contact with an actively infected person are also at risk.

Because TB may become airborne by droplets from the respiratory tract, the disease must be monitored and controlled to prevent cross-infection. Unsuspected active cases and inactive carriers represent a particular hazard. Patients with acute disease are isolated and placed on respiratory secretion precautions for approximately 2 weeks after initiation of treatment.

Therapy is long term (usually 4–12 months of drug therapy). Isoniazid (INH) and rifampin most effectively kill reactive bacilli and prevent reactivation. Clinicians note that widespread use of rifampin has resulted in multidrug-resistant TB (MDR-TB).[6]

Pyrazinamide, ethambutol, and streptomycin also may be used for multidrug therapy; some other drugs that are less effective and have more side effects may be indicated. *M. tuberculosis* mutates and may become resistant to any single-drug or multidrug therapy regimen. MDR-TB and extensively drug-resistant TB (XDR-TB) can be fatal, especially in those infected with HIV.[6] The drugs bedaquiline fumarate and pretomanid are used when other drugs have been ineffective. Bedaquiline must be taken for 24 weeks and can have multiple side effects. It is given in combination with other TB drugs. Patients with active TB should be isolated from the public and follow the medication regimen. TB medications are recommended to be given with observation by another person to keep to the scheduled plan.[6]

The following recommendations should be used in the care of surgical patients who have active TB:
- Postpone elective surgical procedures, if possible, until the patient shows a response to drug therapy (i.e., is no longer infectious as confirmed by a negative sputum smear).
- Use disposable anesthesia equipment to the extent possible. Reusable equipment must be sterilized immediately after use. A bacterial filter on the endotracheal tube or at the expiratory side of the breathing circuit may be useful in reducing the risk for contamination of anesthesia equipment or the discharge of tubercle bacilli into ambient air.
- Use respiratory isolation precautions for patients with TB-positive sputum culture. OR team members should wear face-fitting masks that filter particles of 1 μm at a 95% efficiency level (i.e., a disposable high-efficiency particulate air [HEPA] filtered mask, valveless dust-mist respirator, or dust-fume-mist filtered respirator). This includes putting a HEPA mask on the patient during transport to the OR. The transporter also wears a HEPA mask.
- Perform the surgical procedure at a time when other patients and a minimum number of staff members are present in the OR suite (i.e., at the end of the day's schedule, if possible). Keep OR doors closed and traffic to a minimum.
- Sterilize critical items (i.e., those entering the bloodstream or body cavity); semicritical items (i.e., those in contact with mucous membranes only) may be sterilized or undergo high-level disinfection with a tuberculocide.
- Move the patient into an isolation room that has negative pressure ventilation with a local exhaust and HEPA air filtration and/or ultraviolet radiation lamps.
- Screen high-risk patients and test personnel at least annually. Testing includes a chest radiograph and a Mantoux one- or two-step TB skin test. Exposed personnel should be retested every 6 months.
- A single blood test called interferon-γ release assay (IGRA) is also available for the diagnosis of TB.

TB is the leading fatal infectious disease in the world. In many facilities, yearly TB testing of all OR personnel is mandatory. The most accurate test is the Mantoux test, which is administered by injecting 0.1 mL of purified protein derivative (PPD) of tubercle bacillus subcutaneously in the forearm to form a small wheal under the skin. The site is examined in 24 to 72 hours. Redness, itching, and induration of 8 to 10 mm at the site of injection are considered a positive or a significant reaction. Many facilities have adopted the two-step method testing that involves performing the Mantoux test twice in succession 1 week apart.

Further testing and chest radiographs may be performed before treatment can begin. Reaction of less than 8 mm at the site of injection is considered an insignificant or negative reading, and no further action is needed. Any acute lung disease or symptoms should include TB in the differential diagnosis.

Sexually Transmitted Diseases

Any sexually active person who has multiple partners is at risk for acquiring a sexually transmitted disease. In addition to those previously discussed (hepatitis B virus [HBV], HIV, and herpes simplex virus [HSV] infections), gonorrhea, syphilis, and chlamydia are transmitted by sexual contact or by contact with infectious material containing the microorganisms. Splashes with infectious material to the face and eyes or transmission through broken skin during a surgical procedure can expose a caregiver to infection. According to the CDC, cases of gonorrhea, syphilis, and chlamydia have increased, with the highest rate reported in 2021.[7]

Gonorrhea

Neisseria gonorrhoeae most often infects the genitourinary tract, but it may infect the rectum, pharynx, or conjunctiva. Burning, itching, and pain around the vaginal or urethral orifice with purulent discharge are characteristic symptoms. If untreated, the infection can spread to cause septicemia and inflammation within the peritoneal cavity. Disseminated infection is more common in women than men. Gonorrhea is treated with penicillinase-inhibiting antibiotics. In 2022, the CDC updated its guidelines recommending dual treatment with ceftriaxone and azithromycin. A strain of antibiotic-resistant gonorrhea has been reported and has shown resistance to ceftriaxone.[7] Generally patients should be treated simultaneously for presumptive chlamydial infections.

As a prophylactic measure the CDC recommends a one-time instillation of erythromycin 0.5% ophthalmic ointment within 1 hour after birth to protect the neonate's eyes against potential contamination by vaginal secretions of an infected mother. Single-use tubes or ampules are preferable to multiple-use tubes to prevent cross-contamination between newborns. A newborn with a known gonorrheal infection will need further antibiotic treatment.

Syphilis

Routine screening for syphilis in hospitalized patients and couples applying for marriage licenses is a thing of the past. However, the incidence of syphilis is on the increase again. *Treponema pallidum* is a bloodborne spirochete that may infect any organ system. Syphilis is characterized by three distinct stages of effects over a period of years if it is untreated by antibiotics. Congenital syphilis results from prenatal infection unless the infected mother is treated within the first 4 months of pregnancy.

In the first stage (primary syphilis) a lesion on the skin or mucous membrane, most commonly around the anogenital region, quickly forms a chancre. This is a painless ulceration that exudes fluid laden with spirochetes. The chancre heals spontaneously within 40 days. During the second stage (secondary syphilis), spirochetes migrate from the chancre throughout the bloodstream. The disease can remain contagious for as long as 2 years during this stage.

The third stage (tertiary syphilis) may not develop for many years. When it does, secondary lesions may damage or destroy tissues and body structures, including the heart and central nervous system, with ensuing mental disability or death.

Chlamydia

Chlamydial infection is caused by *Chlamydia trachomatis* (bacteria). It is the most prevalent sexually transmitted disease—more common than gonorrhea and syphilis. It is transmitted only by person-to-person contact. It occurs more often in men than in women, but women are more frequently asymptomatic than are men.

Chlamydia can cause epithelial tissue inflammation, ulceration, and scarring of the urethra and rectum, as well as damage to reproductive organs. Pelvic inflammatory disease (PID) is a serious complication in women. Asymptomatic salpingitis is a major cause of tubal infertility or ectopic pregnancy. Exposure of infants to *C. trachomatis* in the birth canal can cause neonatal conjunctivitis and pneumonia.

Viruses

A virus is not an independent cell unit and is incapable of autonomous metabolism. It is an obligate intracellular parasite that is confined to living in a host cell, such as a somatic cell, or a bacterium. As a bacteriophage, a virus can attach itself to a bacterium and create an opening. While still attached, the nucleic acid of the viral capsule enters the bacteria. The empty capsule remains attached to the bacteria.

Once the virus is inside the host cell, regardless of the cell type, it uses the cell's genetic contents and metabolic machinery for replication. New viruses are passed out the cell membrane, and they in turn attach to other cells to repeat the replication process. Some viruses engorge the cell, causing it to rupture and disperse the virus into the host's body.

During viral infection the host cell reacts to invasion by producing an inflammatory response, antibodies, and interferon to slow the progression of viral replication. Some cellular immunity is developed (e.g., in mumps, chickenpox). Some viruses can attach to nerve cells and undergo activation, deactivation, and reactivation cycles, such as in herpes simplex types I and II (HSV). Some of the nerve cells destroyed by viral invasion include motor neurons, which when damaged cannot be repaired or replaced, such as in polio.

Until the discovery of viruses as a separate entity by Dmitri Ivanovsky (1864–1920) in 1892, viruses were identified only by the diseases they caused. Martinus Beijerinck (1851–1931) made significant contributions to scientific knowledge by expanding the knowledge of viruses. The virus species can usually be identified by the specific alterations in structure and function effected in the host cell as seen under electron microscopy. Other diagnostics include detection of viral antigen, nucleic acid, or antiviral antibody in the serum.

Characteristics

- *Structure:* Viruses are composed of a protein capsule but have no true cellular components other than nucleic acid. They are categorized by the morphologic core structure of their nucleic material—either DNA or ribonucleic acid (RNA) (not both)—and the presence or absence of an envelope. They can mutate. Viruses are extremely small and are visible only by electron microscope.
- *Life cycle:* A virus must have a living biologic host cell. The virus enters a host cell and uses the host's genetic and other cellular protein material for replication.

- *Transmission:* Infection can be transmitted through blood and body fluids of animals and humans. Some viruses can be transmitted by insect bites, such as ticks or mosquitoes; other viruses are transmitted by the fecal-oral route. Direct contact of virus with nonintact skin or mucous membranes can allow entry.

Viral Disease Examples

Hepatitis Infection

Viruses can produce several types of acute and chronic inflammation of the liver. The pathogens causing viral hepatitis create an occupational hazard to health care providers. A patient may be in an acute stage of the infection but more commonly is an unknown carrier of one and occasionally two of the viruses that can cause hepatitis.

Hepatitis A. Hepatitis A virus (HAV) infection is an acute illness that is usually brief but can last for several months. It is spread by oral ingestion of contaminated water and food, especially shellfish, and by fecal contaminants. It is most infectious during the 2 weeks before the onset of symptoms and until after the first week of jaundice. The incubation period is 14 to 90 days, with an average of 28 days. Immune globulin may be effective if given within 2 weeks of exposure.

HAV infection is the most common type of viral hepatitis and causes critical disease if it occurs in combination with other types of hepatitis. HAV infection as a single entity is not a health care–associated problem because it does not have a chronic carrier state. It is usually self-limiting and does not typically cause chronic liver damage. A vaccine is available for areas where HAV is endemic.

Hepatitis B. Hepatitis B virus (HBV) infection is a major health care–associated problem. Carriers are a main source of cross-infection. Hepatitis B surface antigen is the carrier state of HBV. This can be harbored for prolonged periods of up to 15 years and has been found in practically all body fluids of infected persons. It is transmitted percutaneously or permucosally by blood, saliva, semen, and other body fluids. It is not found in feces or urine, according to the U.S. Department of Health and Human Services.

HBV can be transmitted by fomites, through sexual intercourse, and from an infected mother to a neonate during birth. The incubation period is 60 to 90 days before mild to severe symptoms become apparent. Chronic hepatitis, cirrhosis, or liver carcinoma may develop. A liver transplant may be necessary.

Serologic tests are used to diagnose infection, detect carriers, and monitor high-risk persons. Patients who have undiagnosed hepatitis, fail to reveal that they have chronic hepatitis, or are asymptomatic carriers can transmit the virus to health care providers. Perioperative, emergency department, blood bank, laboratory, and hemodialysis unit personnel are especially at risk. HBV surface antigen is easily transmitted by direct contact with blood and body fluids via a needlestick or break in the skin, such as a minor cut or hangnail, or via a splash into the mucosa of the eye, nose, or mouth.

Preexposure immunization over a period of 6 months through a series of three injections of 10 mg (1 mL) of recombinant vaccine against HBV is recommended for all persons at risk. The injections are given in the deltoid muscle because injection in the gluteal muscle has been shown to not produce immunity. After exposure, such as after an accidental needlestick, both the vaccine and hepatitis B immune globulin are given.

Since 1991, OSHA has mandated that health care facilities make these immunizations available to personnel. The series may need to be repeated in 7 years if the titer falls below a detectable level in the serum.

Hepatitis C. Hepatitis C virus (HCV) is a bloodborne RNA virus. Recipients of multiple transfusions or chronic hemodialysis, intravenous (IV) drug users, persons with tattoos or piercings, and health care workers are at risk. Persons with acute HCV infection are asymptomatic but have a higher mortality if they are simultaneously exposed to HAV. A screening test detects the presence of antibodies in the blood. Incubation varies from 2 weeks to 6 months. The infection may progress insidiously in a carrier for as long as 25 years. Immediate HCV postexposure treatment consists of immune globulin injections.

Persons who become infected with HCV have a 40% to 60% chance of becoming chronic carriers. Newer treatments approved by the U.S. Food and Drug Administration (FDA) can cure hepatitis in 8 to 12 weeks with antiviral agents. With awareness and treatment, 95% of people can be cured. The Infectious Diseases Society of America (IDSA) has guidelines for treatment, information, and new medications for providers at www.hcvguidelines.org. There are a group of antivirals, such as elbasvir, daclatasvir, glecaprevir, sofosbuvir, and ledipasvir, for treatment. Many of these medications are combination drugs and are very expensive. Medication selection is based on serologic testing.[8] Women should avoid becoming pregnant while taking these drugs.

HCV infection can precipitate chronic hepatitis, cirrhosis, and liver cancer if untreated. A liver transplant may be needed. Mortality rates associated with HCV infection exceed 10,000 deaths per year. This form of hepatitis may surpass HIV infection in the number of new cases reported each year. An estimated 5 million persons in the United States have HCV infection.

Hepatitis D. Hepatitis D virus (HDV) infection coexists with HBV infection or superinfects an HBV carrier. A defective RNA virus, HDV requires HBV for its survival and replication in both acute and chronic forms. HDV infection is communicable during all phases of active infection. It can lead to necrotizing liver disease and death. Most patients developing this complication of HBV infection are IV drug abusers who used contaminated needles. Immunization against HBV will also prevent hepatitis D.

Hepatitis E. Hepatitis E virus (HEV) infection is common in Asia, Africa, and Mexico. The incubation period is 15 to 64 days, with an average of 25 to 42 days in different epidemics. The characteristics of HEV are comparable with those of HAV, and there are no specific serologic tests for HEV currently. HEV infection is spread via the fecal-oral route through contaminated water or food or from poor sanitation conditions. Current immunoglobulins do not provide protection. HEV infection has no known chronic carrier state, and full recovery in infected persons usually can be expected. The best protection is proper handwashing.

Hepatitis G. Hepatitis G virus (HGV) infection is rare (2000 cases diagnosed per year). Most infected persons have no clear symptoms. It is transmitted by infected blood, and exposure to HCV increases mortality associated with the disease.

Herpes Infection

Related DNA viruses that form eosinophilic intranuclear inclusion bodies are collectively called herpesviruses. The viral infections they cause may be acute and highly contagious, or they may remain latent for many years, even if antibodies are in circulation.

Herpes Simplex Infection. HSV is the pathogen of herpes simplex infections. These cutaneous infections may cause localized eruptions, comparable to blisters, on the border of the lips or external nares, in the mouth, or in the genital or anal region. Transmission is by direct contact with vesicle fluid from lesions or with saliva. The infection may be transmitted to the neonate during passage through an infected birth canal. HSV also can cause cutaneous eczema, acute stomatitis, keratoconjunctivitis, acute retinal necrosis, and meningoencephalitis. Herpes simplex infections are common in HIV-infected and other immunocompromised patients.

Patients who have a history of HSV infection may be treated with oral acyclovir, famciclovir, and valacyclovir preoperatively to prevent an outbreak in the surgical wound. This prophylaxis is particularly important for patients who are having facial procedures, such as a chemical peel or facelift.

Herpetic Whitlow. Herpetic whitlow, a herpesvirus infection of the fingers, is transmitted by direct contact with oral secretions from a person with active herpesvirus or from an asymptomatic carrier. Entry of the virus into the host is via a cut or break in the skin or in nail folds. Herpetic whitlow is an occupational hazard to nurses, physicians, dentists, and anesthesia providers.

Cytomegalovirus Infection

Cytomegalovirus (CMV) may infect salivary glands or viscera, causing enlargement of cells. Transmission can be by direct contact with body fluids, secretions, and excretions. CMV infection usually is asymptomatic in a healthy person, but it is an opportunistic pathogen in immunosuppressed patients with HIV infection or acquired immunodeficiency syndrome (AIDS). Lymphadenopathy, enteritis, and pneumonitis may persist. Chorioretinitis and blindness may result in the end stage of infection. CMV infection also may be associated with hepatitis. CMV may infect arterial smooth muscle cells, stimulating them to proliferate, which can contribute to the formation of atherosclerotic plaque.

CMV is the most common cause of congenital viral infection; it may be transmitted from an asymptomatic mother during pregnancy. A CMV-infected infant may develop neurologic problems. Latent CMV may become reactivated after organ transplantation. The incidence of primary and reactivated CMV infection is fairly high after renal, cardiac, and bone marrow transplantation.

Human Papillomavirus Infection

Condylomata (venereal warts) are caused by the human papillomavirus (HPV) and are transmitted through skin-to-skin contact during vaginal, anal, or oral-genital sexual acts. Condoms offer little protection because HPV is not dependent on the exchange of body fluids. Warts manifest within 3 months of exposure; however, they can be latent for years. Even with seemingly effective treatment, the recurrence rate is high.

The infectious process appears as accumulations of warts over the perineal and/or anogenital surface. HPV infection in women can lead to cervical carcinoma. More than 100 types have been identified via DNA testing, with 40 varieties specifically targeting mucosal surfaces such as in the perineal and oral mucosa. HPV types 6 and 11 are rarely associated with cancer. Types 16 and 18 are considered high risk for causing cervical cancer. HPV is not

diagnosed via culture or blood test but is differentiated by the types of epithelial cells affected and DNA markers. HPV is associated with 90% of anal cancer; 40% of vulvar, vaginal, and penile cancers; and 70% of oral and pharyngeal cancers.

Some patients are infected simultaneously with multiple varieties of both carcinogenic and noncarcinogenic HPV. Administration of an HPV vaccine is recommended by the CDC as routine prophylaxis for boys and girls as young as 9 years of age and all sexually active individuals up to age 26 years. Individuals 27 to 45 years old may request to be vaccinated. The process is a series of three injections comparable to the administration of the hepatitis B vaccine.

HPV-positive individuals should be vaccinated as prevention of acquisition of additional varieties of the virus. The vaccine has no effect on infections present before injection. The vaccine is not recommended for use during pregnancy; however, there are no restrictions concerning breastfeeding during the series of vaccine injections. The HPV vaccines are contraindicated for patients with sensitivity to components of the drug. Some types are manufactured using baker's yeast. Some of the prefilled syringes have latex plungers and can stimulate reactions in patients who are allergic or sensitive to latex.

Venereal Warts. Treatment for venereal warts from HPV includes cryotherapy with liquid nitrogen, electrosurgical removal, carbon dioxide laser ablation, chemical peel with trichloroacetic acid (TCA), and/or topical application of medication (podophyllum 10−25% in a benzoin tincture, podofilox 0.5% solution or gel, or imiquimod 5% cream). Patients with wart accumulations of 0.5 to 1 cm^2 respond to topical applications. Patients with larger areas greater than 10 cm^2 may require staged surgical intervention. Not all HPV warts are easily visible or pigmented for surgical treatment. A weak 1% to 3% solution of acetic acid (white vinegar) can be swabbed over the affected area to cause the warts to become erect and visible.

Some infections are extensive, and the treatment may leave the patient with chronic reflexive neurologic pain, such as vulvodynia. Patients should be advised that their sexual partners also need to be evaluated for venereal warts.

Pregnancy complicates treatment because the lowered immune response accelerates wart growth. Cesarean section is indicated to prevent exposure of the fetus during passage through the birth canal. Infants exposed to the infected vaginal environment risk development of laryngeal papillomatosis. Most of the topical medications have not been approved for safe use during pregnancy.

Studies have shown longer range issues associated with HPV infection. Increased incidence of head and neck cancer has been demonstrated by laryngeal biopsy and laryngectomy specimens.

Human Immunodeficiency Virus Infection

HIV was a deadly worldwide threat to public health until recently. Since HIV was introduced into the United States in the late 1970s, the resultant infection was spread at an alarming rate via contaminated blood and infected persons. Clinical problems in seropositive patients began appearing in 1978. Because of its effect on the immune system and its unknown origin when first reported in 1981, this infection became known as acquired immunodeficiency syndrome (AIDS).

In 1983, researchers at the Institut Pasteur in Paris isolated the lymphadenopathy-associated virus (LAV). In 1984, a similar retrovirus called human T-cell lymphotropic virus type III (HTLV-III) was reported by the National Institutes of Health in Bethesda, Maryland. Since 1986, LAV and HTLV retroviruses causing AIDS or related illnesses have been known collectively as HIV.

Retroviruses synthesize DNA from RNA, a reversal of the usual process. As a result of this reversal process, there is a rapid rate of mutation, making resistance to antiviral drugs a major problem. Normally when a virus enters the body, helper T lymphocytes (T cells) release proteins that activate the immune system to produce antibodies against the virus and macrophages to attack the virus. HIV is different from other viruses in that it attacks the cell membrane of these white blood cells. When the virus penetrates the T-cell membrane, the viral RNA and enzyme are released into the T-cell cytoplasm and converted into DNA. This newly formed DNA penetrates the T-cell nucleus, causing replication of the HIV virus. The cell dies and the virus is released into the bloodstream to attack other helper T lymphocytes and macrophages, thus compromising the immune system.

HIV can live and reproduce in macrophages without stimulating the production of antibodies because the viral composition resembles the host cell. HIV will survive in blood and any body fluid that contains white blood cells. The primary routes of transmission are through sexual intercourse and direct contact with blood and blood products. HIV may be transmitted to the fetus by the blood of an infected mother or to the neonate via breast milk. HIV is not transmitted by casual contact with an infected person. The virus is relatively fragile and easily destroyed outside the body.

After exposure, antibodies may not be identified through serologic testing for 6 to 12 weeks, and detection can be delayed for up to 18 months or longer. Enzyme immunoassays (EIAs) and antibody and antigen analysis are used to test for the presence of antibodies. Blood banks test donor blood for HIV antibodies. Transplant donors also are tested. Blood screening for HIV has been routine in the United States since 1985, thus decreasing the potential for transmission by blood transfusion. Seropositive blood is destroyed, and the donor is notified.

The incubation period before symptoms of infection develop ranges from 6 months to 5 years or longer. Persons in whom the antibody is identified are considered infected and infective. They are classified by physical findings.

Acute Infection. The acute stage of HIV infection lasts 2 to 3 weeks. Signs and symptoms may be specific to an opportunistic infection or disease, but marked fatigue, prolonged diarrhea, weight loss, dry cough, enlarged lymph nodes, fever, and night sweats are striking features. Infections are primarily viral, mycobacterial, and fungal in origin. Oral candidiasis lesions (thrush) may be the first observable symptom. *Pneumocystis jirovecii* (formerly known as *Pneumocystis carinii*) pneumonia, an unusual lung infection caused by a fungal parasite, is a common occurrence.

Other common infections are CMV, HSV, cryptococcosis, and *Mycobacterium avium-intracellulare* complex disease. The patient may survive one infection only to succumb to another. Prophylactic drug therapy aims to prevent or delay the onset of infections. Malignancies and lymphomas also may develop.

Acquired Immunodeficiency Syndrome. As the HIV infection progresses, the cell-mediated immune system is irreversibly compromised. As concentration of the virus gradually increases, the patient becomes symptomatic for clinical manifestations of AIDS. Clinical diagnosis of AIDS requires a positive test for HIV antibodies, any one of the specified opportunistic infections, and a lowered T-cell count. AIDS is not a well-defined disease but rather a state of immune dysfunction.

AIDS causes persistent destruction of the helper T lymphocytes (white blood cells that stimulate production of antibodies), resulting in profound immunosuppression (diminished resistance to infection and disease). The acronym AIDS helps define the disease process:

- *Acquired:* HIV has passed from one person to another by blood or body fluid in direct cell-to-cell contact. Infection is not hereditary except through transplacental transfer from an infected mother to a fetus.
- *Immune:* The normal defense system protects the body against certain diseases and opportunistic infections. Immunity depends on the production of antibodies.
- *Deficiency:* The immune system becomes compromised (i.e., immunosuppressed against opportunists). The host is unable to protect the person with no previous history of immunodeficiency against opportunists.
- *Syndrome:* A group of symptoms or laboratory evidence indicates the presence of a particular disease, abnormality, or infection. Seroconversion is positive for HIV antibodies. *P. jirovecii* pneumonia is the most common opportunistic respiratory infection. *M. avium-intracellulare* complex, the most common AIDS-related bacterial infection, is a leading cause of the wasting syndrome (i.e., loss of body fat and weight). Kaposi sarcoma, a vascular tumor, is the most common malignancy. HPV and HSV infection may be present. Neurologic disease may cause dementia. Lymphomas and opportunistic infections of the brain, spinal cord, and peripheral nerves are not uncommon.

Asymptomatic Infection. The patient may be completely asymptomatic of infection yet test seropositive for HIV antibodies, which confirms the presence of virus in the body.

Persistent Generalized Lymphadenopathy. Swelling or enlargement of lymph nodes suggests cellular immune dysfunction. Prolonged infection with HIV may occur without the formation of HIV antibodies.

HIV-Related Clinical Manifestations. Originally referred to as AIDS-related complexes, a variety of health conditions suggest an impaired immune system. The patient who does not have one of the specific opportunistic infections but is seropositive for HIV antibodies does not technically have AIDS. An infectious disease such as TB and some cancers may be a result of a deteriorating immune system. AIDS may develop within a year of seroconversion.

A patient may be infected with HIV but may not yet test positive. Health care providers who have a valid reason to be concerned that they may have been infected may request to be tested. Few health care providers seroconvert from a single needlestick or splash of blood on mucous membranes. Handling all needles and sharp instruments carefully and using barriers to avoid direct contact with blood and body fluids are the best measures to prevent work-related transmission of HIV. An HIV inhibitor or postexposure prophylaxis (PEP) such as zidovudine, Truvada, or Descovy may be given immediately after exposure. Early treatment can reduce the risk of disease by 74% to 99%. A vaccine has not been developed for immunization. Antiviral agents interfere with the life cycle of the virus, reducing the viral load. Immune-modulating agents stimulate function of the suppressed immune system. Multiple medications are needed to prevent secondary infections.

HIV can now be undetectable in the blood with regular treatment. Many people who are at high risk for contracting HIV take daily medication such as Cabenuva, Biktarvy, Dovate, or Symtuza to lower their risk of exposure. Information can be found at https://hivinfo.nih.gov.

COVID-19

In 2020, the world witnessed a major pandemic from a virus of an unknown source. The SARS-CoV-2 virus (coronavirus) spread throughout the world with deadly consequences, killing more than 3.3 million people worldwide according to the World Health Organization (WHO). The virus is spread quickly and easily by the respiratory system from droplets and aerosolized particles from the mouth and nose. It can be spread by talking, coughing, sneezing, breathing, and singing close to others. The virus is so small (0.07–0.09 μm) that particles can remain in the air and droplets can remain on hard surfaces.[9] Many people spread the virus before becoming symptomatic.

Symptoms. COVID-19 can present within 2 to 10 days as a mild respiratory infection or severe respiratory failure requiring mechanical ventilation, or even death. Symptoms may include:

- Headache
- Body aches
- Sore throat
- Fever and chills
- Congestion and cough
- Fatigue
- Diarrhea or vomiting
- Loss of taste or smell
- Difficulty breathing
- Pneumonia
- Chest pain
- Confusion
- Sleepiness
- Blood clots
- Multiorgan failure

Risk Factors. Older adults and individuals with chronic health problems have a higher risk of getting severe symptoms from COVID-19. The following can lead to a greater risk of severe illness:

- Immunocompromised or weakened immune system because of cancer, use of steroids, kidney disease, or HIV
- Heart diseases
- Obesity
- Lung diseases such as chronic obstructive pulmonary disease, history of smoking, cystic fibrosis, and asthma
- Endocrine disorders like diabetes
- Sedentary lifestyle
- Neurologic and mental health conditions
- Disabilities such as Down syndrome, cerebral palsy, or birth defects

Testing. Testing for COVID-19 is the best way to prevent spreading the virus. Antibody serology blood tests can detect the virus but are done in a lab or hospital. A polymerase chain reaction (PCR) test or nucleic acid amplification test (NAAT) done with a nasal swab can identify whether there is any genetic material or RNA from the virus present. These tests can be more accurate than others because they can detect small amounts of the virus before symptoms appear. Home test kits or antigen tests can give an inaccurate result if there is an insufficient virus load, but the person can still be positive for the virus. If someone tests positive for COVID-19, they should isolate themselves and

contact their physician if they have risk factors or worsening symptoms. Antiviral medications such as Paxlovid, remdesivir, and molnupiravir must be taken within 7 days of infection. Hospitalized patients need specialized care with multiple medications. Most people can recover at home.

Prevention. Preventive measures should be taken to reduce the risk of contracting COVID-19. The CDC recommends handwashing or the use of hand sanitizer, sanitizing surfaces, avoiding crowds, limiting exposure time with others, gathering outdoors or providing ventilation, and keeping a physical distance of at least 3 feet; high-risk individuals can wear a face covering or mask. Health care employees should follow facility guidelines for wearing PPE and caring for patients with COVID-19, especially when general anesthesia is used. For more information about COVID-19, visit www.cdc.gov.

Prions

Stanley Prusiner created the term prion from the official scientific name *proteinaceous infectious particle that lacks nucleic acid*. Prions are natural protein-based helical structures with various gene encoding that can change or evolve. Prions are not alive and therefore cannot be "killed." Prions are resistant to deactivation or destruction by heat, chemicals, radiation, freezing, drying, and conventional detergents. Special handling is required when pathogenic prions are known or suspected.

Studies have shown that prions do not need RNA or DNA to change to another form in an evolutionary sense. The natural prion proteins in the body can change form when exposed to stimulus from a diseased prion.

Prions become infectious and cause disease when they sporadically mutate or are transmitted via direct tissue contact. Other modes of prion transmission include familial inheritance and, in some forms, oral consumption.

In pathologic prion disease the encoded helix converts from α-helical PrP^{Sc} to β-helical PrP^{Sc}. When diseased, prions fold over on themselves, causing vacuoles in the surrounding brain tissue that look like holes in a sponge. The term *spongiform* is used when referring to prion diseases. Clumps of plaques known as *amyloids* form and disrupt nerve signals in the brain. Because the patient's own tissue is changed, there is no inflammatory response to signal infection or disease.

Transmissible spongiform encephalopathy (TSE) is a family of prion-mediated diseases that cause fatal neurologic disorders. Known forms of TSE that affect humans and animals include the following diseases:

- Human forms:
  - Creutzfeldt-Jakob disease (CJD). CJD can be sporadic, familial, or iatrogenically introduced by contaminated instruments, blood transfusion, growth hormone, or exposure to neurologic tissue.
  - New variant Creutzfeldt-Jakob disease (vCJD). Not known to science before 1994, suspected to be transmitted by eating infected cattle.
- Animal forms:
  - Bovine spongiform encephalopathy (BSE) (cattle)
  - Scrapie (sheep and goats)

Creutzfeldt-Jakob Disease

Although rare, CJD is a progressive, fatal neurodegenerative disease characterized by dementia, myoclonus (muscle spasms), and multifocal neurologic signs and symptoms. It cannot be diagnosed by blood tests. The only definitive diagnosis is from neurologic tissue samples positive for protein prion folding and amyloid plaque formation. CJD is not the same as vCJD or BSE. Autopsies of the brains of patients with suspected Alzheimer disease revealed that 13% had undiagnosed CJD, and the tissue sampled resembled that of other TSE-infected mammals.

CJD was first described in 1920 by German psychiatrists Hans Gerhard Creutzfeldt and Alphonse Maria Jakob. Thought to be associated with genetic factors that influence susceptibility to the formation of abnormal neurologic protein, the condition may be dormant for more than 30 years before the onset of symptoms around the age of 65 years. The disease then progresses rapidly, leading to coma and death, usually within 2 to 5 years after onset of symptoms.

Studies have shown that items contaminated with prions can cause infection many years after initial contamination. One study demonstrated that brain probes caused CJD in an animal subject 2 years after being used in a contaminated patient.

Managing Pathogenic Prion-Contaminated Instruments

Adequate cleaning, soaking in deactivator, and sterilization can render noncomplicated instruments safe for use. Allowing the instruments to dry before processing makes decontamination difficult. Disposable instruments are preferred when working with a suspected prion infection. Flashing instrumentation for immediate use is never appropriate. Persons processing instrumentation should always wear PPE. Current literature, WHO, and AORN (Association of periOperative Registered Nurses) recommend the following procedures for deactivating prions before handling contaminated items for processing:

1. Keep the instruments moist until they can be cleaned.
2. Wearing appropriate PPE, clean separately from other instruments with an alkaline detergent.
3. Soak contaminated items in sodium hydroxide (NaOH [lye]) or sodium hypochlorite (NaClO [bleach]) for 1 hour. Rinse well. Review the safety data sheets (SDSs) before using these solutions:
   a. *Sodium hydroxide (NaOH):* Available as a commercially prepared solution. Very caustic. Terminology concerning the premixed concentration of the NaOH solution is 1 mole or 1 normal. This means 40 grams of solid NaOH is mixed into 1 liter of water. The container will read "1 molar solution."
   b. *Sodium hypochlorite solution:* 1 part bleach to 5 parts water.
4. Terminally steam-sterilize instruments after rinsing for 1 hour at 274° F (134° C) for 18 minutes in a prevacuum sterilizer or at 272° F (132° C) in a gravity displacement sterilizer for 60 minutes before handling.
5. The Joint Commission recommends quarantine of the instrument tray until the patient has been officially declared pathogenic prion free.
6. Environmental surfaces can be cleaned with 1:5 or 1:10 solution of sodium hypochlorite or sodium hydroxide with a contact time of 15 minutes. This includes the instrument tray and sinks used for instrument cleaning. The internal aspect of the washer-sterilizer should be cleaned before using for routine set cleaning resumes.

The process of soaking instruments in sodium hydroxide followed by steam autoclaving is deleterious to surgical instruments and the autoclave, according to the CDC. Autoclaving an instrument immersed in the chemical without a sealed lid can release a gaseous form of sodium hydroxide that may be harmful to humans.

Transmission of Prion Disease

Standard precautions for prevention of bloodborne exposure must be strictly observed. A bloodborne source has been confirmed in the United Kingdom. At least four confirmed cases of vCJD transmission through blood transfusion have been identified. There have been no known cases to date in the United States. Human illness has been demonstrated after ingestion of beef from BSE-contaminated cattle.

Contaminated neurologic tissue sources include dural grafts, corneal transplants, and human growth hormone. Prion contamination has been found in tonsil tissue, lymphatics, Peyer patches in the bowel, and the spleen. Suction canister contents and used cleaning solutions should not be disposed of in the sanitary sewer system. Solidifiers may be an alternative disposal method. Incineration is the preferred method for destroying prion contamination.

Postexposure Prophylaxis for Transmissible Spongiform Encephalopathy

Any percutaneous exposure to known or suspected TSE-infected central nervous system tissue should be irrigated with 0.5% sodium hypochlorite (bleach solution). Skin exposure requires a thorough handwash with sodium hydroxide. Mucous membrane exposure should be followed by cleansing with soap and water. To date, no known direct transmission from patient to OR personnel has been reported in the literature.

Fungi

More than 100,000 species of fungi have been identified. Not all fungi are pathogenic (causing mycosis). A *Penicillium* variety is used to make the antibiotic penicillin and give flavor to Roquefort cheese. The blue color of the cheese is caused by collections of spores.

The body responds with an inflammatory response to tissue invasion by a fungus. Respiratory responses include hypersensitivity reaction to fungal antigens. According to statistics compiled by the CDC, the number of health care–associated fungal (mycotic) infections doubled between 2020 and 2021.[10] Fungal infections are classified according to the degree of tissue involvement and mode of transmission.

Characteristics

- *Structure:* Fungi are plantlike structures that lack chlorophyll and therefore are unable to photosynthesize. True fungi are nonmotile. Fungi are eukaryotic and range in size from microscopic to large mushroom forms. Yeast species are single cell but cling together with similar cells. Fungi are aerobic. Molds are multicellular and reproduce by airborne spores that can be inhaled.
- *Life cycle:* A fungus grows as a mold (filamentous, spore forming) or a yeast (round, budlike cells). Molds can reproduce sexually and asexually by forming spore sacs. Yeasts produce buds. A parasitic saprophyte that thrives in a dark, damp, aerobic, warm environment, a fungus lives on decaying material. It can produce toxins referred to as *aflatoxins* and *mycotoxins,* which are found in moldy foodstuffs.

- *Transmission:* Infection can be transmitted by spores in direct contact with the respiratory system, nonintact skin, or mucous membranes.

Fungal Disease Examples

- *Superficial:* Dermatophytes such as tinea (ringworm). Localized to skin, hair, and nails; *Candida albicans* (thrush and vaginitis), athlete's foot.
- *Subcutaneous:* Confined to the dermis and subcutaneous tissue.
- *Systemic:* Infections of internal organs can gain entry via intestinal tract, IV line, or lungs. Respiratory fungal diseases include aspergillosis *(Aspergillus fumigatus)*, histoplasmosis *(Histoplasma capsulatum,* commonly found in bat and bird excreta), cryptococcosis *(Cryptococcus neoformans,* found in pigeon excreta).
- *Opportunistic: Pneumocystis* pneumonia *(P. jirovecii,* which was originally thought to be a protozoan. DNA and RNA studies showed it was a red yeast fungus possibly carried on dogs).

Protozoa

Although microscopic, protozoa are relatively large. They grasp and ingest food particles and are motile. Protozoa have many diverse pathogenic mechanisms, although most types are not harmful to healthy humans. Protozoa become pathogenic as a result of opportunistic infection. Each species has a distinct reproductive cycle. Some parasitic protozoa reproduce only in a living host, such as in a female mosquito of the genus *Anopheles* (e.g., *Plasmodium malariae*).

Other species of protozoa living free in watery environments split by binary fission to form two daughter cells. Cryptosporidiosis *(Cryptosporidium parvum* from calves) and toxoplasmosis *(Toxoplasma gondii* from domestic cats) are examples of parasitic diseases that currently cause diseases in humans living in contemporary cities.

Characteristics

- *Structure:* Protozoa are animal-like parasites that are single-cell microorganisms without a morphologically distinct cell wall. They are eukaryotic with chromosomes and aerobic.
- *Life cycle:* Protozoa reproduce sexually (in a sanguineous host) or by binary fission (free in nature). They can wall off and resist drying out by becoming cystic. They can be reactivated by moisture and prefer to live in a watery environment. Larger and more complex than bacteria, they ingest decaying organic matter. They have some diffusion through the cell membrane.
- *Transmission:* Contact is through ingestion of a cyst in soil or water, the fecal-oral route, or more commonly a bug bite. Dissemination is commonly bloodborne directly to major organs. There may be direct contact with the organism through mucous secretions from the genitourinary tract.

Protozoan Disease Examples

Intracellular

- Bloodborne protozoa passed by insect vectors include *P. malariae* that is found in red blood cells and liver cells.
- A localized parasitic infestation passed by the sandfly is leishmaniasis (nonhealing skin lesions; the *Leishmania* organism lives in macrophages).
- A parasite from cats is *T. gondii.*

Extracellular

- Intestinal protozoa acquired free in nature include *Giardia lamblia* (enteritis), which is commonly misdiagnosed because symptoms mimic colitis.
- Genitourinary protozoa include *Trichomonas vaginalis.* Vulvovaginitis or urethritis can be transmitted through sexual contact or fomites.
- Amebic dysentery protozoa include *Sarcodina* and *Entamoeba* species.
- *Trypanosoma cruzi* (South American: Chagas disease can be extracellular and intracellular; lives in macrophages and muscle cells) and *Trypanosoma rhodesiense* (African sleeping sickness; parasite lives freely in blood).

Helminths

Adult helminths (worms) are not true microorganisms but are considered parasites in humans and animals. Most adult worms are visible to the naked eye, but the eggs and larvae are microscopic. Symptoms are increased as the number of worms increases. The host responds by increasing immunoglobulin E (IgE) and macrophage levels in the blood to fight the invasion. The eggs and larvae are very irritating to tissues, causing intense granulomatous inflammation.

Large volumes of invading worms can cause mechanical obstruction of lumens, such as in the gastrointestinal tract, or tunnel through organs, such as the heart or lungs. Many intestinal varieties cause nutritional and/or hematologic depletion of the host. If a worm dies while in the host's tissue, it becomes encased in inflammatory exudate. Helminths may be found in immigrant communities or in populations living in rural farmlands with feces in the soil. Young children may acquire pinworms through fecal-oral ingestion in daycare or school settings.

Characteristics

- *Structure:* Morphologically more complex than protozoa, helminths can be round and tubular (nematodes), flat (cestodes), or flat and large (trematodes).
- *Life cycle:* Helminths are hermaphrodites. Eggs are laid in a host and are passed through excreta. Eggs hatch, becoming larvae and reentering a host by penetration or introduction through a vector. Larvae mature in the host, becoming adults capable of self-reproduction. They can become bloodborne and lymph-borne.
- *Transmission:* Introduced by insect bites, some can self-penetrate host tissues and skin, and some are acquired by ingesting undercooked flesh from an infected animal or shellfish. Fecal-oral route transmission of eggs and/or larvae is common. Wading in contaminated water permits penetration of skin by active larvae.

Helminth Disease Examples

- Nematode diseases include intestinal pinworms and hookworms, and trichinosis in skeletal muscle of pigs. Filarial worms cause filariasis (elephantiasis), which is transmitted by fly or mosquito bites and becomes bloodborne.
- Cestode diseases include intestinal tapeworms.
- Trematode diseases include bloodborne flukes.

Antimicrobial Therapy

Antimicrobial drugs or agents are adjuvants to—not substitutes for—strict adherence to aseptic and sterile techniques. Perioperative patients receive antibiotics or antimicrobials in several ways in the OR. Routes for administration include the following:

- Oral (PO) administration preoperatively or postoperatively
- IV administration
- Irrigation and lavage
- Implantable disks, powder, or timed-release base (e.g., bone cement with timed-release beads)
- Topical solutions or ointments
- Surgical skin prep antiseptics

Antibiotics

Antibiotics act by killing bacteria (bactericidal) or inhibiting the growth of bacteria (bacteriostatic). Antibiotics do not attack other body cells because a higher-order cell wall and advanced synthesis are not recognized by the drug.

To be effective, the bacteria must be sensitive to the activity of the antibiotic. Some antibiotic classes are broad spectrum and attack many aerobic and anaerobic bacteria; others selectively destroy specific species. Antibiotics do not affect viruses and many fungi and yeasts. Antibiotics can be used alone or in combination with other antimicrobial drugs. The main actions that enable antibiotics to work include inhibiting cell wall synthesis, inhibiting protein synthesis, or inhibiting genetic activity. These actions can be bactericidal (killing) or bacteriostatic (stopping). Antibiotic categories that inhibit cell wall synthesis are listed in Table 14.3. Antibiotic categories that inhibit protein synthesis are listed in Table 14.4. Antibiotic categories that alter genetic activity are listed in Table 14.5.

The incidence of allergic reactions to antibiotics is relatively high. Patients should be questioned about allergies and known reactions before any drug is administered and should be closely watched for signs of toxicity as evidenced by skin rash, gastrointestinal disturbance, renal disorder, fever, or blood dyscrasias.

The efficacy of antibiotics is greatly reduced when multiple organisms are involved in an infection and if a biofilm has formed. Antibiotics are usually given as follows:

1. Therapeutically to eliminate sensitive viable organisms during a clinical course of infection and in grossly contaminated and traumatic wounds. The choice of antibiotic and the duration of therapy should be determined by clinical factors (i.e., pathogen, severity and site of infection, and clinical response). A broad-spectrum drug may be given while awaiting results of culture and sensitivity tests.

TABLE 14.3 Antibiotics That Inhibit Cell Wall Synthesis in Bacteria

Categories	Drug Name Examples	Mechanism	Action	Generation	Gram Stain	Considerations and Cautions
Penicillins (PCN) β-Lactam antibiotics	Amoxicillin Ampicillin Augmentin Carbenicillin Piperacillin Ticarcillin Timentin	Inhibition of cell-wall synthesis	Bactericidal		Pos	Narrow spectrum Safe in pregnancy Hypersensitivity reaction hemolytic anemia, interstitial nephritis Interacts with allopurinol, warfarin, and methotrexate
Cephalosporins β-lactam antibiotics	(see Generations)		Bactericidal	1st Cephalexin 2nd Cefuroxime 3rd Rocephin 4th Cefepime	Pos Neg	Broad spectrum Surgical prophylaxis Safe in pregnancy Renal excretion 10% cross-link to penicillin Colitis
Carbapenems	Doripenem Ertapenem Imipenem Meropenem		Bactericidal		Pos Neg	Broad spectrum Good for anaerobes Given IV Renal excretion
Glycopeptides	Vancomycin		Bactericidal		Pos	Narrow Treat *Clostridium difficile*, endocarditis Ototoxic, nephrotoxic Interacts with cyclosporin, aminoglycosides, diuretics
Monobactams	Aztreonam		Bactericidal		Neg	Found in breast milk and crosses the placenta Hepatotoxic, bone marrow depression
Polypeptides	Bacitracin Polymyxin B Colistin Neomycin		Bactericidal		Pos Neg	Topical prophylaxis for skin infection

TABLE 14.4   Antibiotics That Inhibit Protein Synthesis in Bacteria

Categories	Drug Name Example	Mechanism	Action	Gram Stain	Considerations and Cautions

Macrolides	Erythromycin
	Azithromycin
	Clindamycin
	Ketolide:
	  Telithromycin
	  Cethromycin
		Inhibition of protein synthesis	Bacteriostatic	Pos	Broad spectrum, penicillin alternative
					Ketolide used in anthrax and lung infection
					Jaundice, hepatitis, prolonged cardiac QT, found in breast milk
					Interacts with antiarrhythmics, warfarin, statins

Tetracyclines	Doxycycline Minocycline Eravacycline		Bacteriostatic	Pos Neg	Broad spectrum. Not used in pregnancy. Discolors teeth and bones of children younger than 8 years, nephrotoxicity Malaria prophylaxis Treats acne Interacts with warfarin, phenytoin, and carbamazepine
	Gentamycin Streptomycin Tobramycin Neomycin Kanamycin Amikacin		Bactericidal	Pos Neg	Broad spectrum. Not used for anaerobes. IV use for treating septicemia, meningitis. Can be used with other antibiotic treatment Nephrotoxic, ototoxic, aggravates myasthenia gravis Interacts with methotrexate, digoxin, diuretics, and other antibiotics
Chloramphenicols	Chloromycetin		Bacteriostatic	Pos Neg	Broad spectrum. Treats conjunctivitis Not safe in pregnancy or lactation. IV treatment of typhoid Marrow suppression, aplastic anemia. Interacts with anticoagulants, phenytoin, and oral hypoglycemic
Lincosamide	Clindamycin		Bacteriostatic	Pos	Broad spectrum for anaerobes; weaker for aerobes. Excellent bone penetration Treats protozoa, toxoplasmosis, osteomyelitis, intraabdominal sepsis, malaria, and toxic shock. Decreased effectiveness of estrogen contraceptives
Oxazolidinones	Linezolid		Bacteriostatic	Pos	Treats VRE Bone marrow suppression, low platelet count
Glycylcycline	Tigecycline		Bacteriostatic	Pos Neg	Broad spectrum for gram positive. Given IV for intraabdominal and complicated skin infections. Related to tetracycline

IV, Intravenously; *VRE,* vancomycin-resistant *Enterococcus.*

2. Prophylactically to prevent the development of infection. Prophylaxis implies that the microorganism is attacked by the antimicrobial agent when it harbors in tissue before colonization takes place. A prophylactic antibiotic is given 30 minutes to 1 hour before the surgical incision and continued for 24 hours postoperatively. These agents are effective as supplements to host defense mechanisms in selected patients. Antibiotic prophylaxis is commonly used as follows:

a. For procedures associated with brief exposure to possible infection; evidence indicates that antibiotics can reduce infection (e.g., cystoscopy after cystitis).

b. Since 2010 the CDC recommends using erythromycin ophthalmic ointment 0.5% for neonatal ophthalmic prophylaxis immediately after birth either vaginally or by cesarean section.

c. For procedures not frequently associated with infection but when occurrence would have disastrous or life-threatening consequences (e.g., clean wounds; insertion of a prosthetic implant such as a heart valve, vascular graft, or total joint replacement).

d. For procedures associated with a high risk for infection. Organisms are predictable and susceptible to antibiotics (e.g., clean-contaminated wounds such as a biliary tract with obstruction or transection of the colon).

e. Intraoperative irrigation to minimize bacterial colonization; for example, some surgeons use bacitracin 50,000 units/mL of sterile 0.9% sodium chloride, lactated Ringer's solution, or sterile water. Although bacitracin is absorbed by the peritoneal and mediastinal membranes, it is most effective against gram-positive bacteria. It is slowly excreted through the renal system and is contraindicated in patients with renal failure. The irrigation decreases the surface tension of the wound and may decrease the development of biofilm.

The probability of infection is determined in the first few hours after bacterial invasion, when capillary permeability and host inflammatory response are at a peak immediately after bacterial contamination. Therefore timing and duration of drug administration are crucial. To be effective the prophylactic antibiotic must be present in adequate concentration in tissues at the time of wound creation or contamination.

TABLE 14.5   Antibiotics That Inhibit Nucleic Acid Synthesis and Replication in Bacteria

Categories	Drug Name Example	Mechanism	Action	Generation	Gram Stain	Considerations and Cautions
Ansamycin	Rifampin	Inhibition of nucleic acid synthesis	Bactericidal		Pos Neg	Effective for TB, leprosy, and osteomyelitis. Taken with other antimicrobials. Taken on empty stomach. May cause discolored (red-orange) body fluids when taken with clofazimine (dye-based). May need to increase the dose of warfarin. Reduces the effectiveness of hormonal contraceptives. Excreted in breast milk and may cause skin pigmentation in infant. Hepatotoxic
Fluoroquinolones	Clinafloxacin		Bactericidal	1st Cinoxacin 2nd Ciprofloxacin 3rd Levofloxacin 4th Trovafloxacin, delafloxacin	Pos	Renal excretion. Phototoxicity Interacts with seizure drugs, theophylline, glyburide, and warfarin. May impair bone healing by interfering with chondrocytes
Quinolones	Ciprofloxacin Norfloxacin		Bactericidal		Pos Neg	Broad spectrum. Treats anthrax, salmonella, campylobacter. Central nervous system toxicity. Interacts with phenytoin, NSAIDS, thyroxin, and warfarin Contraindicated in lactation
Sulfonamides	Sulfadoxine Triple sulfa Bactrim Septra Gantrisin		Bacteriostatic		Pos	Treats urinary infections Can cause blood dyscrasia. Avoid in third trimester of pregnancy
Nitroimidazoles	Metronidazole		Bactericidal		Pos Neg	Narrow spectrum. Good with anaerobes. Treats *Clostridium difficile*, trichomoniasis, giardia, should not be used during lactation or 1st trimester of pregnancy (mutagenic). Peripheral neuropathy, intolerance to alcohol Interacts with warfarin and cytotoxics
Nitrofurantoin	Macrobid		Bactericidal		Pos Neg	Treats urinary tract infection, found in breast milk
Other synthesis inhibitors	Isoniazid		Mycobacterial inhibitor		N/A	Treats tuberculosis by inhibiting mycolic acid synthesis
Antifolates	Pyrimethamine		Antimalarial		N/A	Treats malaria by blocking folic acid synthesis
Combination drugs	Artesunate-amodiaquine, artemether-lumefantrine, atovaquone-proguanil					Treats malaria by disrupting the metabolism of the infected cells

NSAIDs, Nonsteroidal antiinflammatory drugs.

Studies are underway in the prevention of biofilm formation on implants and the potential for disrupting biofilm in situ. Antibiotic hydrogel coatings are being tested on the surfaces of several types of implantable medical and surgical devices. The mechanism is not merely a timed release but a stimulated release in response to ultrasonic waves. Unnecessary antibiotic exposure is avoided but is there if needed. This provides a more controlled distribution in the site of implantation.

Selection of the appropriate drug and early use are pertinent factors (Box 14.4). The antibiotic regimen is governed by the site of the surgical procedure, potential pathogens to be found, and the patient's history of drug sensitivities. The metabolism and excretion of the drug should be considered, as well as any inherent toxicities. The CDC recommends the following regimen:
- Except for cesarean section, parenteral antibiotic prophylaxis should be started within 1 to 2 hours before a surgical

Resistance can be inherent or acquired. Mechanisms by which bacteria resist antibiotic action include, but are not limited to, the following:

1. Inherent resistance
   a. Bacterium does not absorb the antibiotic by forming an impermeable biofilm membrane. The bacterial cell can coat its molecules or the molecules of the antibiotic with protein to prevent binding between the cell wall and the antibiotic.
   b. Bacterium can physically expel, or pump out, the antibiotic. This process is referred to as *efflux.*
   c. Bacterium can render the antibiotic ineffective by chemical or enzymatic means. The action of the antibiotic is changed by material synthesized by the bacterial cell.
   d. Bacterium can alter the molecular or ribosomal target of the antibiotic. A bacterium can physically alter itself, making interaction between the antibiotic and the bacterial cell harmless.
2. Acquired resistance
   a. *Vertical evolution:* A bacterium spontaneously mutates and imparts a chromosome to a member of its own bacterial population.
   b. *Horizontal evolution:* A bacterium with a resistant gene releases that resistant gene to a different bacterial type.

procedure to produce a therapeutic level during the surgery and should not be continued for more than 48 hours. A 12-hour limit is desirable for most types of wounds. Parenteral use for more than 24 hours increases the risk for antibiotic toxicity and development of resistant strains of bacteria or superinfection and does not further reduce the risk for infection.

- For cesarean section, prophylaxis may be given intraoperatively after the umbilical cord is clamped.
- Oral absorbable prophylactic antibiotics should not be used to supplement or extend parenteral prophylaxis. They should be limited to 24 hours before the surgical procedure when used prophylactically in colorectal operations.
- Topical antimicrobial products used in the wound should be limited to agents that will not cause serious local or systemic side effects.

Resistance to Antibiotic Therapy

Antibiotic resistance is a serious problem costing more than $30 billion annually in the United States. A drastic change in the pattern of life-threatening infections has occurred since the advent of broad-spectrum antibiotics and penicillinase-resistant penicillins. Many of the products used in health care end up in the water supply, causing conditions supportive of an increased antibiotic resistance in environmental microorganisms. A new group of antibiotics are in the testing phase and look promising to treat multidrug-resistant bacteria.[11]

Gram-negative bacilli, both aerobic and anaerobic, deeply concern clinicians because the incidence of infections by bacteria of supposedly low virulence (e.g., *Serratia* and *E. coli* organisms) is increasing. These microorganisms can cause deep, latent infections, rapidly colonize, and are transferred among individuals by hands or equipment.

Many of these organisms develop plasmid-mediated resistance to antibiotics. This means that a bacterium carrying genetic particles (plasmids) that allow it to replicate will be resistant to it.

Methicillin-Resistant Staphylococcus aureus

MRSA is not plasmid mediated. However, it is resistant not just to methicillin, a penicillin, but to other categories of antibiotics as well. This resistance has probably developed because of overuse of these broad-spectrum agents. Clinically MRSA poses an important health care–associated problem, whether by infection of patients or colonization in health care workers. Some patients arrive at the hospital already colonized with community-acquired MRSA. Preoperative bathing with chlorhexidine and/or intranasal mupirocin can prevent the patient from developing an infection with MRSA postoperatively.

Vancomycin-resistant enterococci (VRE) have flourished since 1989. Studies have shown that VRE genes can be passed on to other gram-positive cocci, such as vancomycin-resistant *Streptococcus pneumoniae* and *S. aureus* (VRSA). Cases of VRSA have been reported in Japan. The CDC is currently compiling statistics on gram-positive vancomycin resistance. Previous treatment with vancomycin or treatment with multiple antimicrobial therapies increases the risk for VRE. The greatest routes for spread of VRE are the hands of caregivers and contaminated equipment. According to the CDC, prevention of VRE includes, but is not limited to, the following guidelines:

- Education of the staff
- Prevention of transmission by isolating known colonized or infected patients
- Early detection of colonization or infection with VRE
- Screening of all enterococci isolated from blood and body substances (except urine) for vancomycin resistance
- Prudent use of vancomycin

Approved antimicrobial agents have been shown to be effective for the cleaning and disinfection of medical devices and environmental surfaces used in the care of antibiotic-resistant patients. The CDC has not issued timelines for periods of isolation or contact precautions for VRE-infected patients, but three successive negative cultures, 1 or more weeks apart, is one possible guideline that has been used by some institutions.

Antifungal and Antiviral Drugs

Fungal and viral infections can be problematic. Topical antifungal drugs usually control fungus. *C. albicans*, for example, can lead to a fatal opportunistic systemic infection. Candicidin is a specific fungicide for this organism.

Viruses are not usually a risk to a healthy patient undergoing an elective procedure. Hepatitis and HIV present a unique challenge because they are potential threats to the caregiver. Knowledge of the medication and the disease it treats may be required for perioperative patient education. Dosages will vary. Multiple antiviral drug classes are available depending on the stage of the HIV virus.[12] Combination drugs are now available for convenience. Examples of available antiviral agents include, but are not limited to, the following medications[12]:

- Ribavirin for respiratory syncytial virus infection
- Zidovudine/dideoxyinosine for HIV infection
- Ganciclovir for CMV infection
- Acyclovir/famciclovir/valacyclovir, tenofovir for HSV infection
- Rimantadine/amantadine for influenza
- Trogarzo, didanosine for retrovirus infection
- Lamivudine, efavirenz for retrovirus infection
- Many combination antiretrovirals: Atripla, Biktarvy, Genvoya, Stribild, Cimduo, Combivir, Truvada, Cabenuva, Dovato

Microorganisms in Mass Casualty and Bioterrorism

Health care workers should have a basic familiarity with microorganisms associated with bioterrorism. Many terrorist acts against populated areas have resulted in mass casualties that enter the hospital systems. In many circumstances the hospital system will be the first agency to recognize clusters of infections that signal a biologic terrorist attack. Each facility should have a response and reporting plan in place as a first responder to bioterrorism. Agents used in bioterrorism are listed in Box 14.5.

> **•BOX 14.5 Microbiologic Agents Used in Bioterrorism**
>
> - Anthrax
> - Arenavirus
> - Botulism
> - Brucellosis
> - Cholera
> - Ebola
> - Glanders
> - Lassa fever
> - Melioidosis
> - Plague
> - Psittacosis
> - Q fever
> - Ricin toxin
> - Shigella
> - Smallpox
> - Tularemia
> - Typhus

Perioperative personnel should be aware that in the event of a mass casualty, patients may arrive at the facility in a biologically contaminated state. The facility should have a plan for decontamination of these patients before permitting them to enter the general patient population. (Additional information is available at www.ahrq.gov under the search term *mass casualty* and at www.cdc.gov under the search term *bioterrorism*.)

EVOLVE WEBSITE

http://evolve.elsevier.com/Hornacky/BerryKohn/
- Historical Perspective
- Student Interactive Questions
- Glossary

References

1. Pak T, Rhee C, Klompas M, et al.: Timing and spectrum of antibiotic treatment for suspected sepsis and septic shock, *Infect Dis Clin North Am* 36(4):719–733, 2022.
2. Centers for Disease Control and Prevention: *Healthcare-associated infections (HAIs)*. www.cdc.gov. Accessed April 27, 2023.
3. King K, Strony R: *Needlestick*. www.ncbi.nlm.nih.gov. Accessed April 27, 2023.
4. Ledwoch K, Dancer S, Otter J, et al.: Beware biofilm! Dry biofilms containing bacterial pathogens on multiple healthcare surfaces; a multicenter study, *J Hosp Infect* 100(3):47–56, 2018.
5. Carr W, Kurbatova E, Starks A, et al.: CDC interim guidance: 4-month rifapentine-moxifloxacin regimen for the treatment of drug-susceptible pulmonary tuberculosis—United States 2022, *MMWR Morbid Mortal Wkly Rep* 71(8), 2022.
6. Mase S, Chorba M: Treatment of drug-resistant tuberculosis, *Clin Chest Med* 40(4):775–795, 2019.
7. Evan C, Ewers MD, Curtain J, et al.: Challenges in managing gonorrhea and new advances in prevention, *Infect Dis Clin North Am* 37(2):223–243, 2023.
8. Kim A, Hepatitis C. In Kellerman RD, Rakel DP, editors: *Conn's current therapy*, Philadelphia, 2019, Elsevier, pp 222–224.
9. Lee B: Minimum sizes of respiratory particles carrying SARS-CoV-2 and the possibility of aerosol generation, *Int J Environ Res Public Health* 17(19):6960, 2020.
10. Gold J, Ahmed F, Cisewski J, et al.: Increased deaths from fungal infections during the coronavirus disease 2019: pandemic—national vital statistics system, United States, January 2020–December 2021, *Clin Infect Dis* 76(3):255–262, 2023.
11. Terreni M, Taccani M, Pregnolato M: New antibiotics for multidrug-resistant bacterial strains: latest research developments and future perspectives, *Molecules* 26(9):2671, 2021.
12. Understanding HIV/AIDS. https://hivinfo.nih.gov. Accessed January 22, 2024.

15

Principles of Aseptic and Sterile Techniques

CHAPTER OUTLINE

What Is the Difference Between Aseptic and Sterile Techniques?, 261

Transmission of Microorganisms, 262

Human-Borne Sources of Contamination, 262

Nonhuman Factors in Contamination, 263

Sources of Infection, 264

Environmental Controls, 264

Standard Precautions, 267

Principles of Sterile Technique, 269

No Compromise of Sterility, 274

CHAPTER OBJECTIVES

After studying this chapter the learner will be able to:

- Define aseptic technique.
- Define sterile technique.
- Describe the transmission of microorganisms.

- List several principles of Standard Precautions.
- Discuss the obligation of the team to practice aseptic and sterile techniques.

KEY TERMS AND DEFINITIONS

Aerosol Dispersion of fine mist, droplets, or particulate matter into air (transitive verb: aerosolize, to become airborne).

Antisepsis Prevention of sepsis by the exclusion, destruction, or inhibition of growth or multiplication of microorganisms from body tissues and fluids.

Antiseptics Inorganic chemical compounds that combat sepsis by inhibiting the growth of microorganisms without necessarily killing them. They are used on skin and tissue to arrest the growth of endogenous microorganisms (resident flora), and they must not destroy tissue.

Asepsis Absence of microorganisms that cause disease; freedom from infection; exclusion of microorganisms. Not the same as sterile.

Aseptic technique Methods by which contamination with microorganisms is prevented (alternative term: *aseptic practice, to maintain asepsis*).

Barrier Material used to reduce or inhibit the migration or transmission of microorganisms in the environment. Barriers include attire of personnel, drapes over furniture and patients, packaging of supplies, and filters in ventilating system.

Carrier Person who has potentially pathogenic microorganisms on or in their body and disperses them into the environment without becoming ill from the pathogen.

Contaminated Soiled or infected by microorganisms.

Cross-contamination Transmission of microorganisms from patient to patient and from inanimate objects to patients, and vice versa.

Decontamination Cleaning and disinfecting or sterilizing processes carried out to make contaminated items safe to handle.

Disinfection Chemical or mechanical destruction of most pathogens rendering an object safe to handle.

Fomite Inanimate object that may be contaminated with infectious organisms and that serves to transmit disease.

Irreducible minimum Microbial burden cannot get any lower. Object is sterile to its highest degree.

Isolation Special precautions taken to prevent the transmission of microorganisms from specific body substances.

Pathogenic Producing or capable of producing disease.

Pathogenic microorganisms Microorganisms that cause infectious disease. They can invade healthy tissue through some power of their own or can injure tissue by a toxin they produce.

Sepsis Severe toxic febrile state resulting from infection with pyogenic microorganisms, with or without associated septicemia.

Spatial relationships An awareness of sterile, unsterile, clean, and contaminated areas and their proximity to each other. This includes the height of scrubbed team members in relation to each other and the sterile field. The circulating nurse must be aware of closeness to the sterile field and the appropriate means to control environmental contaminants.

Standard Precautions Procedures followed to protect personnel from contact with the blood and body fluids of all patients (formerly referred to as Universal Precautions).

Sterile Free of living microorganisms, including all spores.

Sterile field Area around the site of incision into tissue or site of introduction of an instrument into a body orifice that has been prepared for the use of sterile supplies and equipment. This area includes all furniture covered with sterile drapes and all personnel who are properly attired in sterile garb.

Sterile technique Methods by which contamination with microorganisms is prevented to maintain sterility throughout the surgical procedure.

Terminal sterilization and terminal disinfection Procedures carried out for the destruction of pathogens at the end of the surgical procedure in the operating room or other areas of patient contact (e.g., postanesthesia care unit [PACU], intensive care unit [ICU], nursing unit).

Unsterile Inanimate object that has not been subjected to a sterilization process; the outside wrapping of a package containing a sterile item; a person who has not prepared to enter the sterile field (synonym: nonsterile).

What Is the Difference Between Aseptic and Sterile Techniques?

The terms *aseptic* and sterile are not synonymous, although aspects of both are closely related. An object can be aseptic without being sterile. Asepsis literally means "without dirt," and it implies the absence of pathogenic microorganisms that cause infection. Aseptic technique and sterile technique are based on sound scientific principles and are carried out primarily to prevent the transmission of microorganisms that can cause infection. The degree of processing, whether disinfected or sterile, depends on the importance of the item's use in patient care.

Spaulding's Levels of Importance of Patient Care Items

Depending on their intended purpose and body contact, the items and equipment for patient care are classified into the following categories described by Spaulding according to the level of sterility necessary for safe patient care use:

- *Critical:* Any item entering the bloodstream, body tissues underlying the skin, and mucous membranes must be sterile (i.e., free of microorganisms, including endospores). Items include invasive devices, implants, surgical instrumentation, endoscopes, and instrumentation that can come in contact with the vascular system.[1] Critical items must go through the sterilization process, with biologic indicators confirming sterility. These items are handled using sterile technique to maintain sterility.
- *Semicritical:* Semicritical items require high-level disinfection.[1] These items are clean and safe to handle with bare hands (i.e., mechanically cleaned and disinfected to reduce microorganisms, but unsterile). Some items are disinfected immediately before use and are handled using aseptic technique to prevent contamination before use. Other items are terminally sterilized between uses on different patients, but sterility is not maintained during storage or use. Examples include vaginal probes, respiratory and anesthesia equipment.
- *Noncritical:* Items that will come into contact with only intact skin or mucous membranes in an area remote from the surgical site may be cleaned, terminally disinfected, and stored unsterile between patient uses. Items include tourniquets, blood pressure cuffs, linens, and positioning devices. No special technique in handling is observed.

Surgical procedures are performed under sterile conditions; contamination with microorganisms is prevented to maintain sterility throughout the procedure. A sterile field is created around the site of incision into tissues or the site of introduction of sterile instruments into a body orifice. Conversely all materials and equipment used during a surgical procedure are terminally decontaminated and sterilized after use with the assumption that every patient is a potential source of infection for other persons.

It is essential that all members of the perioperative team know the common sources and mechanisms of contamination by microorganisms in the perioperative environment. The practices of sterile and aseptic techniques are the responsibility of everyone caring for the patient in the operating room (OR). All members of the OR team must be vigilant in safeguarding the sterility of the sterile field because any contamination must be remedied immediately.

Aseptic Technique

It is impossible to exclude all microorganisms from the environment, but for the safety of both patients and personnel, every effort is made to minimize and control these microorganisms. Microorganisms are present in the air and on animate and inanimate objects at all times. To effectively apply the principles of asepsis, environmental control, and sterile techniques discussed in this chapter, the meaning of terms related to aseptic technique must first be understood. Therefore the basis of prevention is the knowledge of causative agents and their control, as well as the principles of aseptic and sterile techniques.[2]

The methods by which microbial contamination is contained in the environment are referred to as *aseptic technique.* The OR in the restricted area is aseptic at best because the room and air cannot ever be 100% free of microbial content. Some key elements of asepsis include the following facts:

- Aseptic technique is sometimes referred to as *clean technique.*
- Items have been cleaned and decontaminated so they are safe to handle with clean, bare hands.
- Items in use in patient care are handled with examination gloves for the protection of both the caregiver and the patient.
- Items have been cleaned, decontaminated, disinfected, or terminally sterilized, and stored in a clean, dry place.
- Items may start out sterile but are not maintained or used under sterile conditions. Skin preps may be packaged sterile, but skin cannot be sterilized. The process is aseptic.
- Contamination is contained. Extraneous contamination is avoided.
- Items are set up on clean towels or drapes and used with examination gloves.
- Items are not sterile or maintained sterile during use. Extraneous contamination is avoided.
- Disposable items are not cleaned and reused for another patient.

- Items are classified as *semicritical* or *noncritical* by Spaulding's classification of the importance of patient care items.
- Items can be used outside the confines of the restricted area.
- Items are used on intact skin or mucous membranes.
- Items are not used when the patient's vascular system will be entered.

Sterile Technique

Sterile technique incorporates many processes associated with asepsis but to a higher, more controlled degree. In sterile technique all microorganisms must be maintained at an irreducible minimum, meaning as low as absolutely possible.

Keep in mind that a sealed sterile package must be opened at some point during patient care to use the contents. That means opening the package to the room air. Even in the restricted area the room air has a microbial count that we cannot eliminate. We try as hard as possible to minimize the room traffic and maintain environmental controls to maintain the sterile field. Essential elements of sterile technique include the following factors:

- Items are used only in a sterile field in the restricted area.
- Items are used by sterile team members wearing appropriate sterile attire.
- Items are used in areas of the patient's body where the site has been prepped.
- Items may be used in invasive surgery.
- Items may be used in body areas with nonintact skin and membranes and may enter the patient's vascular system.
- Items are classified as *critical* according to Spaulding's level of importance of patient care items.
- Items have been cleaned, decontaminated, and packaged before sterilization.
- Items processed by sterilization are stored wrapped and remain so until use by a sterile team member.
- Items are for individual patient use only. Reusable items can be reprocessed and resterilized for use with another patient. Disposable items are discarded after use. If opened and unused, disposable items are discarded.
- Items that become contaminated are discarded and replaced immediately.

Transmission of Microorganisms

People remain the major source of microorganisms in the environment. In the OR the surgical team is the most common source of transmission, followed by contaminated instrumentation. Everything on or around a human being is contaminated by the body in some way. The action and interaction of personnel and patients also contribute to the prevalence and dispersion of microorganisms.

There are many sources of contamination in the OR environment. Transmission-based precautions should be implemented in the perioperative environment and in any area with the potential to transmit potentially pathogenic microorganisms. Transmission-based precautions are described in Box 15.1. Perioperative personnel are concerned primarily with protecting the environment of the OR suite because surgical procedures should be performed under optimal conditions.

Most microorganisms grow in a warm, moist host, but some aerobic bacteria, yeasts, and fungi can remain viable in the air and on inanimate objects. Because the OR can provide only an aseptic

environment, infection control practices for the minimization of microbial counts include the following options:

- OR ventilation, humidity, and temperature controls
- Decontamination, disinfection, and sterilization methods
- Improved barriers, such as impervious drapes between sterile, clean, and contaminated surfaces
- Surgical technique and tissue handling
- Antimicrobial prophylaxis is used only as appropriate

Despite advances, surgical site infections (SSIs) continue to cause significant morbidity and mortality in surgical patients. Emergence of resistant microorganisms is complicated by patients with comorbid disease and the increasing numbers of implants and transplants. Microbiologic considerations and specific microorganisms that concern the perioperative team are described in Chapter 14.

Factors to consider when evaluating the reasons for the emergence of antibiotic-resistant microorganisms include the following:

- Inadequate or inappropriate uses of antibiotic
- Overuse of antimicrobials and antiseptics shed into the waterways and environment
- Sequestered microorganisms in biofilm or retained foreign body
- Inadequate infection control practices

Human-Borne Sources of Contamination

Skin

The skin of patients, OR team members, and visitors constitutes a microbiologic hazard. Sebaceous (oil) and sudoriferous (sweat) glands contain abundant resident microbial flora, many of which have the potential to become pathogenic if colonized in greater than average numbers or if colonized on a weakened host. In an average individual an estimated 4000 to 10,000 viable contaminated

---

•BOX 15.1 **Transmission-Based Precautions**

Airborne
The use of special air handlers and ventilation and respiratory protection is recommended for susceptible people. Contaminated air currents can settle on or be inhaled by those who are susceptible.
Particles smaller than 5 μm may carry airborne droplet nuclei. Examples of airborne diseases include COVID-19, varicella, tuberculosis, and rubeola.

Droplet
A distance of more than 3 ft from the source patient is recommended. Masks should be worn by those closer than 3 ft and should be worn by the source patient during transport. Droplet particles are larger than 5 μm and are disseminated during coughs, sneezes, and talking. Droplets do not travel more than 3 ft and are not suspended in the air. Examples of droplet diseases include diphtheria, mumps, pertussis, and influenza.

Contact
The use of gloves when coming into contact with items contaminated with blood or body substances is recommended. Gowns are recommended if there is a potential for contamination of clothing.
Cleaning and disinfecting patient care equipment after use protects other patients.

Data from U.S. Department of Health and Human Services: www.hhs.gov; and Centers for Disease Control and Prevention: www.cdc.gov.

particles are shed by the skin each minute. Some disperse up to 30,000 particles per minute; these individuals are referred to as *shedders*. Shedders are densely populated with virulent organisms, such as *Staphylococcus aureus*, and shed contaminated skin cells into the environment.

Patients who are shedders have a much higher incidence of infection at the surgical site. On all individuals the major areas of microbial shedding include the head, neck, axillae, hands, groin, perineum, legs, and feet. Cosmetic detritus and body powders are also laden with potential pathogens. Microbial shedding is contained effectively by appropriate antiseptic cleansing and maximum skin coverage.

The following list includes vital points for all personnel entering the OR:
- Bathe daily with soap and water.
- Wash hands before entering the OR suite and after every patient contact to prevent infection and cross-infection. Hands should be washed before donning gloves and after removing them because gloves are not 100% impervious. Handwashing technique involves vigorously rubbing together all surfaces of well-lathered, soapy hands, followed by rinsing under a stream of water.
- Don clean OR attire for each entry into the OR suite. Unsterile team members should wear long-sleeved warm-up jackets that are fully buttoned.
- Cover any cuts and abrasions. Open wounds on the skin are portals for infection, and infected wounds can disseminate microorganisms.
- Wear gloves when handling blood, body fluids, or tissue specimens, and wash hands after removing sterile and unsterile gloves.

Hair

Hair is a gross contaminant and a major source of staphylococci. The extent to which the microbial population is attracted to and shed from hair is directly related to the length and cleanliness of the hair. Hair follicles and filaments harbor resident and transient flora. Hair can become a mechanical irritant in wound healing and cause a foreign body tissue reaction. Hair should be shampooed frequently. Clean caps or hoods are worn to cover the scalp, all hair, including facial hair.[3] The nape of the neck and ears should be covered. Surgeon's skullcap styles do not enclose the hair at the nape of the neck and do not cover the ears. Hair should be contained at all times in semirestricted and restricted environments.

Microorganisms forcibly expelled by talking, coughing, or sneezing give rise to bacteria-laden dust and lint as droplets settle on surfaces and skin. Carriers harbor many organisms, most notably group A streptococci and *S. aureus*, without experiencing the harmful physical effects of infection. Surgeons and anesthesia providers may be carriers more so than other caregivers because of their intimate contact with patients' respiratory tracts.

Shedders and carriers may be identified through nasopharyngeal culturing. Some departments, such as obstetrics and the newborn nursery, may require routine periodic nasal cultures as a condition of employment. Positive nasal carriers can be treated with antimicrobial nasal spray or ointment. When multiple patients develop the same or comparable postoperative infections, infection control teams at the facility actively seek the source of the infection.

Masks are worn in all restricted areas to cover the nose and mouth and should be changed after caring for each patient. Masks protect the wearer and the patient. Coughing and sneezing explode droplets into the environment, and therefore people with a respiratory infection should not be permitted in the OR suite. Talking should be kept to a minimum. The contaminated mask should be handled only by the ties and not by the facial portion for disposal.

Human Error

Direct person-to-person contact is the most common route of transmission. Human error is an exogenous source of contamination, and it is not to be underestimated. Failure to follow the principles and applications of sterile and aseptic techniques places the patient and personnel at risk—a risk that could be prevented. Errors should be readily admitted and corrected.

Cross-Infection

Every patient in the OR should be considered a potential source of infection. Standard Precautions and routine aseptic techniques are observed regardless of whether a patient is known to have an infectious condition. All patients should be treated as though they have a known infection. Care, caution, and conscientiousness on the part of all team members are essential at all times. Thorough handwashing after every patient contact is important.

Nonhuman Factors in Contamination

Fomites

Fomites are contaminated particles present in the dust that rests on inanimate objects such as furniture, OR surfaces (e.g., walls, floors, cabinet shelves), equipment, computer keyboards, cabinet handles, supplies, and fabrics. Covert contamination may result from improper handling of equipment such as anesthesia apparatus or intravenous (IV) lines and fluids. Contamination also may result from the administration of unsterile medications or the use of unsterile water to rinse sterile items. Any unsterile item placed within the sterile field causes contamination and increases the risk for infection.

In maintaining an aseptic environment, the following points should be considered:
- Prompt disinfection and decontamination of used equipment and reusable supplies.
- Prompt disinfection of OR surfaces (e.g., disinfecting furniture, lights, and floors, disposing of waste and laundry).
- Separation of clean and soiled items. Sterile storage areas are physically separated from decontamination areas.
- Proper packaging and storing of supplies. External shipping cartons should be removed before bringing supplies beyond the unrestricted area in the OR suite. Insects and rodents can gain entrance to the suite in corrugated cartons.
- Placement of dust covers over sterile items during transport and while in prolonged storage.
- Dispensing medication to the sterile field in the correct form and with the recommended device.

Air

The perioperative environment contains thousands of particles per cubic foot of air. During a long surgical procedure the particle count can rise to more than 1 million particles per cubic foot. Air and dust are vehicles for transporting particles laden with microorganisms. Heat rises, and therefore the lights and other heat-generating equipment of the OR produce convective up-currents referred to as thermal plume.

Personnel walking about the room can generate airborne contamination; every movement increases the potential for infection of the surgical site. Traffic should be kept to an absolute minimum. Particulates bearing microorganisms become airborne and settle in an open wound.

Between 80% and 90% of the microbial contaminations found in an open surgical site come from ambient (room) air. β-He-molytic streptococci have been directly traced from contaminated personnel and contamination of a patient. The actual microorganism was recovered from the room air.

Microorganisms have an affinity for horizontal surfaces, of which the floor is the largest. From the floor, microorganisms are projected into the air. Endogenous flora from the patient's skin, oropharynx, tracheobronchial tree, and gastrointestinal tract, as well as exogenous flora, also are significant. Microorganisms from patients or carriers settle on equipment and flat surfaces and then become airborne. Airborne particles increase significantly during the activity before incision and after wound closure. Relief personnel create significant air currents. The potential for contamination increases each time the door to the OR opens and closes.

An effective ventilation system is essential to prevent patients and personnel from breathing potentially contaminated air, which can predispose them to infection.

Sources of Infection

The incidence and types of infections that occur in surgical patients may be the result of a preexisting localized infectious process, a systemic communicable disease, or an acquired perioperative complication.

Community-Acquired Infection

Community-acquired infections are natural disease processes that developed or were incubating before a patient's admission to the hospital or ambulatory care facility. Patients known to be carriers of nasal microorganisms can be treated preoperatively to minimize some of the risk.

Communicable Infection

Systemic bacterial, viral, or fungal infections may be transmitted from one person to another. These infections are discussed in detail in Chapter 14.

Spontaneous Infection

Examples of localized infections that require surgical diagnosis and treatment for management or that occur as an adjuvant to medical therapy include acute appendicitis, cholecystitis, and bowel perforation with peritonitis. Therapy consists of identification of the infection site and causative microorganism, excision or drainage, prevention of further contamination, and augmentation of host resistance.

Health Care–Acquired Infection

An infection is considered health care acquired (HAI; formerly referred to as *nosocomial*) during the course of health care if it was

neither present nor incubating when the patient was admitted. The nurse admitting the patient must document anything that was present on admission or the assumption is that the patient became infected at the facility. This is grounds for Medicare to deny payment.

Approximately 20% of all *S. aureus* HAIs develop in surgical patients.[4] They may occur as complications of surgical or other procedures performed on uninfected patients. They also may occur as complicating infections in organs unrelated to the surgical procedure that occur with or as a result of postoperative care. The majority of HAIs are related to instrumentation of the urinary and respiratory tracts. Microbial colonization is the primary component of HAI. The potential for SSIs can be conceptualized in the following equation:

$$\frac{\text{Dose of contamination} \times \text{virulence}}{\text{Resistance of the host}} = \text{Risk for SSI}$$

The following list includes examples of HAIs:
- Urinary tract and respiratory tract infections
- Infected pressure and stasis ulcers
- Cellulitis and abscess formations in pressure sores
- Thrombophlebitis, which is a regional extension of postoperative IV infection
- Bacteremia and septicemia, the postoperative systemic infections that result from dissemination of microorganisms into the bloodstream from a distributing focus
- Septicemia caused by intravascular catheters
- Persistent infections at the site of surgical implants

Exogenous

An exogenous HAI is acquired from sources outside the body such as personnel or the environment. Cross-contamination occurs when organisms are transferred to the patient from another individual or inanimate object.

Endogenous

An endogenous infection develops from sources within the body. Most postoperative wound infections result from seeding by endogenous microorganisms. Disruption of the balance between potentially pathogenic organisms and host defenses permits the invasion of microorganisms for which the patient is the primary reservoir. For example, abdominal sepsis may result from enteric flora if the intestine is perforated or transected.

Criteria for Defining a Surgical Site Infection

According to the Centers for Disease Control and Prevention (CDC), an SSI is the most common type of infection reported. For example, the hospital stay was significantly increased, thereby exposing the weakened patient to increased risk for additional infections. A synopsis of the criteria for defining an SSI as described by the CDC is presented in Table 15.1.

Environmental Controls

Control of the environment is a necessary part of overall infection prevention. The inanimate and animate environment of the OR suite presents a risk for the transmission of microorganisms. The aim of a microbiologically controlled environment is to keep contamination to a minimum. The key to controlling microorganisms lies in the knowledge of their favorable living conditions.

TABLE 15.1   Criteria for Defining a Surgical Site Infection (SSI)

Superficial Incisional SSI	Deep Incisional SSI	Organ/Space SSI

Infection occurs within 30 days of the surgical procedure. Infection involves only skin or subcutaneous tissue of the incision and at least one of the following symptoms from the superficial incision unless the wound is culture negative:
1. Purulent drainage from the incision, x-ray with or without laboratory confirmation
2. Organisms isolated from an aseptically obtained culture of fluid or tissue
3. At least one of the following signs or symptoms of infection:
  a. Pain or tenderness
  b. Localized swelling
  c. Redness or heat
  d. Surgeon deliberately opens the incision
4. Diagnosis of superficial incisional SSI by the surgeon or physician
Do not report the following conditions as superficial SSI:
1. Stitch abscess (minimal inflammation and discharge) confined to the points of suture penetration
2. Infection of episiotomy or newborn circumcision site (these have separate criteria)
3. Localized stab wound
4. Cellulitis (by itself)
	Infection occurs within 30–90 days after the procedure. Infection involves deep soft tissues (e.g., fascial and muscle layers) of the incision and at least one of the following symptoms unless the site is culture negative:
	1. Purulent drainage from the deep aspects of the incision but not the organs or compartments
	2. A deep incision spontaneously dehisces or deliberately opened by the surgeon because of:
	  a. Fever >100.4° F (38° C)
	  b. Localized pain
	3. Diagnosis of deep SSI by physician or surgeon
	Additional factors:
	1. Report combined superficial and deep infections as deep SSI
	2. Report organ space or deep infection that drains through the incision as deep SSI
		Infection occurs within 30–90 days after the procedure. Infection involves any part of the anatomy (e.g., organs or spaces) other than the incision that was opened or manipulated during an operation and at least one of the following symptoms:
		1. Purulent drainage from a drain that is placed through a stab wound into the organ or space
		2. Organisms that are isolated from an aseptically obtained culture of fluid or tissue in the organ or space
		3. An abscess or other evidence of infection involving the organ or space that is found by direct examination or by radiograph

From the Centers for Disease Control and Prevention: NHSN Surgical site infection (SSI) checklist, 2023. www.cdc.gov. Accessed April 18, 2023.

Best practices in asepsis should be rooted in prevention of proliferation and spread of microorganisms.

All health care facilities should incorporate into their policies and procedures the recommendations for infection control from the CDC/Healthcare Infection Control Practices Advisory Committee (HICPAC) Core Practices, as well as the regulations for the prevention of exposure to bloodborne pathogens from the Occupational Safety and Health Administration (OSHA).[4,5]

The perioperative environment is designed to optimize function and safety and to protect patients from sources of contamination. The surgical suite includes specific areas for traffic, support systems, administration, communication, and storage, as described in Chapter 10.

Traffic patterns are designed to flow smoothly and prevent backtrack and crossover traffic. Clean and soiled activities, areas, and personnel and sterile and unsterile supplies should be distinctly separated.

Impervious barriers such as sterile drapes, gowns, and gloves protect sterile areas, isolate surgical sites, and keep the number of microorganisms to an *irreducible minimum*. These barriers must remain impervious to the passage of microorganisms under ordinary operating conditions. Procedures are established to use barriers effectively against microorganisms from any potential source of contamination.

Environmental Services/Housekeeping

Housekeeping practices that use the most effective supplies, techniques, and equipment available are an important aspect of infection control. Policies and procedures for cleaning should be in place. Employees should be educated in the spread of

pathogens and special disinfection products. Proper training and cleaning procedures are mandatory requirements. Housekeeping procedures include cleaning and disinfecting the perioperative environment, handling soiled laundry, and disposing of solid waste. Disinfectants are used in combination with thorough mechanical cleaning. These procedures are performed by environmental service personnel under supervision and are carried out according to established practices, policies, and schedules, as described in Chapter 12. Of primary concern are locations that by design or construction are difficult to clean (e.g., lavatories, workrooms) and areas that may be touched by patients or personnel.

Any equipment requiring water in its operation can support microbial growth, especially if the water is not changed frequently. Unsterile water, the universal solvent and transporter, can support, maintain, and protect almost every contaminant produced by humans. Water especially supports the growth of gram-negative bacilli, including *Serratia* and *Pseudomonas*.

Airborne aerosolized particles produced during hand scrubs can contaminate the area around the scrub sink. Disinfectants reduce the contamination potential of unsterile cleaning water.

The following housekeeping points are especially relevant to infection control and the prevention of cross-infection and are listed to emphasize the importance of aseptic environmental control:
- The faucet head should be of a type that does not hold water and should be removed for *terminal sterilization*. Containers for antiseptic hand hygiene agents should be disassembled, cleaned, and terminally sterilized before refilling.
- No surface should remain wet, which would support microbial growth and the formation of biofilm.

- Organic debris should be promptly removed from walls and other surfaces with a disinfectant to prevent drying and airborne contamination.
- Lights should be cleaned after every procedure. Overhead tracks should be cleaned upon completion of the day's schedule.
- The entrance to the OR suite and the floors in corridors and rooms should be cleaned at the end of the day's schedule.
- Housekeeping equipment should be cleaned and dried for storage. Moisture and darkness are conducive to microbial growth.
- Disposable trash should be separated into infectious and noninfectious waste and put in impervious receptacles.
- Service elevators rather than chutes should be used to remove soiled laundry and waste/trash from the OR suite. Chutes become grossly contaminated with airborne particles and are a fire hazard.
- Waste should be contained at the source of origin to prevent aerosol generation during handling. Contaminated waste is decontaminated and/or sterilized before compaction or disposal in the general environment. Incineration is the most effective means of waste disposal, especially of infectious wastes. However, health care facilities must comply with local, state, and federal regulations for contamination control and waste disposal.
- Adequate time must be allowed between patients for proper terminal disinfection of the OR. A patient must not be assigned to an inadequately cleaned OR, which could be a source of an SSI.
- All areas and equipment throughout the perioperative environment should be cleaned on a scheduled basis as defined by institutional policy. These areas include the grilles, vents, and filters of the air conditioning system; storage shelves and cabinets; lighting fixtures; walls; and other areas in offices, lounges, dressing rooms, storage areas, workrooms, and corridors. Handles of cabinets and push plates of doors should be cleaned several times daily.

Control of Airborne Contamination

Air currents and movement in the OR should be kept to a minimum to prevent airborne contamination. Viable microorganisms from the air settle on horizontal surfaces. Proper cleaning of these surfaces helps control this contamination. The ventilating system and efforts to minimize air turbulence and contaminants also are important factors. Doors to the OR should remain closed during the procedure to maintain a positive pressure atmosphere.

When properly designed, installed, and maintained, a conventional air conditioning system effectively reduces the number of airborne organisms by removing dust and aerosol particles. Air contaminated by dust and lint is removed as fresh, clean outside air is supplied. Recirculation of filtered air at a minimum rate of 20 volume exchanges per hour, at least 4 of which are fresh air, is considered safe and economical as recommended by the American Institute of Architects in collaboration with the Facility Guidelines Institute *Guidelines for Design and Construction*. However, fire codes in some states require 100% outside fresh air. All air, whether recirculated or fresh, is filtered before entering the OR. The system uses high-efficiency particulate air (HEPA) filters to remove particles larger than 0.3 μm.

Air enters from a ceiling vent, is diluted, and passes through vents at floor level. Filters are located downstream from the air-processing equipment so microorganisms will not be drawn into

the room. The system maintains a positive pressure if the doors to the room remain closed.

Laminar Air System

Often referred to as ultraclean airflow, a special air-handling system for the filtration, dilution, and distribution of air may be installed in one or more ORs. High-risk procedures such as total joint replacement, cardiac surgery, and organ transplantation are performed in this environment. Laminar airflow is a controlled, unidirectional, positive-pressure stream of air. More information about laminar airflow is found in Chapter 10.

Doors

The doors to the OR should be kept closed except as necessary for passage of the patient and personnel and supplies and equipment. If the door is left open, the positive air pressure in the room equalizes with the negative air pressure in the hallway. Disrupted pressurization mixes the clean air of the OR with the corridor air, which has a higher microbial count. Cabinet doors should also remain closed.

Traffic and Movement

Traffic in and out of the OR is kept to a minimum. Only essential personnel should be allowed inside the OR. The amount of activity in the room increases as the number of people present increases. This in turn increases the potential for contamination as a result of the shedding and air turbulence that carries microbes to the wound. Movement in the OR should be reduced to a minimum.

Lint

Agents are added to the final rinse during laundering to minimize the lint that results from the friction of woven fibers against each other. Disintegrated paper from disposable nonwoven products is another source of lint on fabrics. Therefore paper products should not be discarded in the same receptacle as soiled reusable woven fabrics.

Isolation Precautions

The isolation of patients by diagnosis or body substance is related to the mode of transmission of pathogenic microorganisms (i.e., air, droplet, contact). A patient with a communicable disease could need emergency surgery, and perioperative personnel should know about appropriate patient handling and exposure precautions. A communicable disease such as tuberculosis (TB) or COVID-19 could be diagnosed via bronchoscopy.

Isolation precautions and guidelines are discussed in detail in hospital procedure books and in the CDC's *Guidelines for Isolation Precautions in Hospitals* and at http://www.osha.gov/. There are different methods of the isolation technique, as follows[4,5]:

- Category-specific isolation precautions for patients with suspected or confirmed communicable disease transmitted either by droplets via the airborne route (e.g., TB or COVID-19) or by enteric excretions, drainage, or secretions
- Disease-specific isolation precautions for contact with patients known to be infected with specific pathogens
- Body-substance isolation precautions incorporating Standard Precautions for contact with all body substances of all patients, regardless of the diagnosis (all patients are considered contaminated)
- Protective isolation for immunosuppressed patients

The purpose of these precautions is to prevent the transmission of pathogenic microorganisms. Isolation and barrier techniques protect both personnel and other patients. Each hospital may incorporate into its procedures whichever methods are most appropriate for its particular needs and patient population.

The perioperative staff should be informed that a patient requires isolation precautions before that patient comes to the OR. Some situations, such as pulmonary TB or COVID-19, require the use of HEPA masks for the staff and the patient.

For most patients the same precautions apply in the OR as on the patient care unit, and a commonsense approach is used. In all types of isolation the most important infection control measure is thorough handwashing before and after close patient contact; after handling contaminated objects, body fluids, and excretions; and between patients.

Isolation techniques must not be implemented in a way that causes the patient to feel ostracized. Patients should be educated to understand that the isolation protects them as well as the caregiver and that they must comply with the regimen.

Standard Precautions

As established by the CDC and enforced by OSHA, Standard Precautions protect health care workers from contact with blood and body fluids of all patients. Standard Precautions include the following considerations:
- All body fluids
- Handwashing
- Barrier clothing
- Handling of used patient care equipment and linen
- Occupational exposure to bloodborne pathogens
- Patient placement and management

Recommendations for Standard Precautions have been modified to reflect routes of transmission. The format for the CDC's identification of routes of transmission includes airborne, droplet, and contact precautions.[4] The potential for becoming infected through skin exposure depends on colonization, duration of contact, the presence of skin lesions on the hands, and immune status.

Standard Precautions supplement other recommended practices for environmental controls and are the minimum precautions for all invasive procedures. An invasive procedure involves any entry into body tissues or cavities in any procedural environment. Standard Precautions are in effect for any procedure during which bleeding occurs or for which the potential for bleeding or exposure to body substances exists. The following list involves Standard Precautions[5]:
1. *Protective barriers and personal protective equipment (PPE):* Appropriate barriers, such as PPE, prevent contact of the skin and mucous membranes with blood and body substances. PPE and other barrier materials must prevent blood and other fluids from passing through or reaching the wearer's clothing or body. The type of PPE used depends on the task and the degree of anticipated exposure. Examples include gloves, eyewear, gowns, hair covers, and masks.
   a. Gloves reduce contamination of hands. Intact gloves, both sterile and unsterile, are used. Latex, vinyl, and other materials are used in the manufacturing of these gloves. Care is taken to avoid natural rubber latex when either the patient or the caregiver has a latex sensitivity. Vinyl may be more permeable to some viruses than is latex.
      (1) Sterile gloves are worn for procedures that involve the invasion of body tissues when a sterile field is created.
         (a) Double-gloving does not prevent puncture wounds but may be appropriate for procedures in which the risk for glove tears is high.
         (b) Sterile glove liners may provide protection from glove tears and skin cuts, particularly when working with heavy orthopedic equipment. Double-gloving also may substantially reduce the risk for exposure from the seepage of blood and fluid through gloves onto hands during long procedures or in the presence of voluminous blood loss. No glove is 100% impervious.
      (2) Unsterile latex or vinyl examination gloves are worn for procedures that do not require a sterile field, such as handling specimens, placentas, newborns, and contaminated items (e.g., sponges). Powdered gloves leave a residue that may carry latex particles.
      (3) General-purpose utility gloves are worn for cleaning instruments and for decontaminating and housekeeping procedures involving potential blood contact. These heavy-duty gloves may be decontaminated and reused.
      (4) Gloves are changed after every contact with patients or contaminated items. Latex and vinyl gloves are discarded. Washing gloves between patient contacts is not an acceptable practice.
      (5) Hands are washed immediately after glove removal. All gloves have microscopic holes and may be permeable to certain substances or microorganisms. The mechanical and chemical actions of handwashing significantly decrease the risk associated with the permeability of glove materials.
   b. Masks protect personnel from aerosols and patients from droplets. They are worn for all invasive procedures. Specialty masks to filter laser plume are commercially available. The mask should be changed immediately if grossly contaminated by a splash of blood or body fluid. Patients with a known infectious process such as COVID-19, varicella, TB, or rubeola should wear a HEPA mask during transport to and from the OR.
   c. Eyewear with side shields protects the mucous membranes of the eyes, and full face shields protect the mucous membranes of the eyes, nose, and mouth. They are worn for procedures in which blood, bone chips, amniotic fluid, and the aerosol of other body fluids may splash or be projected into the eyes. Goggles with enclosed sides and chin-length face shields offer better protection than do simple eyeglasses.
   d. Gowns or aprons made of fluid-resistant material protect the wearer from a splash with blood and body fluids. A plastic apron may be worn under a woven fabric gown. Impervious gowns offer better protection. Disposable impervious gowns are preferred.
   e. Shoe covers or boots protect the wearer when gross contamination on the floor can be anticipated. Grossly soiled shoe covers or knee-high disposable boots are removed before the wearer leaves the room.
2. *Prevention of puncture injuries:* Needles, knife blades, and sharp instruments present a potential hazard for the handler

and user. Skin may be punctured or cut if caution is not taken. Specific recommendations for handling disposable surgical needles, syringes and needles, and knife blades (collectively referred to as *sharps*) include the following guidelines:

 a. Do not manipulate sharps by hand. Use an instrument such as a heavy hemostat to attach and remove the scalpel blade. Arm the needle directly from the suture packet when possible. Do not bend or break an injection needle. Pass needles in a needle holder or use a "neutral zone" to transfer sharps on the field. Sharp instruments and needles may be passed on a puncture-resistant tray or magnetic mat for a hands-free technique rather than from hand to hand. Remove instruments from the surgical field after use, and return them to the Mayo stand or instrument table promptly.

 b. Do not recap used injection needles by hand except with a recapping safety device. Use a one-handed technique in the sterile field.

 c. Do not remove the needle from a disposable syringe by hand after use. Use a hemostat or other instrument to exchange or remove a hypodermic needle from the syringe.

 d. Place all used sharps in a puncture-resistant container for disposal.

3. *Management of puncture injuries:* If a glove is torn or punctured, remove the puncturing sharp or instrument from the sterile field immediately and change the glove promptly, using the open-glove method. If the skin is punctured or cut, remove both gloves immediately. If both gloves are not removed, the risk for introducing microorganisms from the remaining contaminated glove is increased. Squeeze the skin to release blood. Wash out contaminants under running water with an antiseptic; then irrigate the wound with a virucidal disinfectant such as an iodophor, bleach, or hydrogen peroxide.

Report the incident immediately, and document all actions on the appropriate forms. Baseline testing may be necessary for both the punctured individual and the patient. These actions are necessary to protect the employee and the patient should either party seroconvert to a positive status at a later date. OSHA has provided guidelines for immediate treatment of a needlestick at www.osha.gov.[5]

4. *Oral procedures:* Contact with blood-contaminated saliva and gingival fluid is expected during dental and surgical procedures in the oropharyngeal cavity. Mouth protection, Ambu bags, and/or other ventilation devices should be available for emergency airway resuscitation. Respiratory secretions coughed up during endotracheal procedures are often infectious.

5. *Care of specimens:* All specimens and cultures of blood, body fluids, and tissues should be contained in a puncture-resistant container to prevent leaking during transport to the laboratory. The outside of the container should be clean and enclosed within a biohazard-labeled plastic bag. Care is taken not to get blood and body fluids on the pathology requisition slip.

6. *Decontamination:* All instruments are thoroughly decontaminated and cleaned before sterilization or high-level disinfection. The surfaces of furniture and floors are cleaned and decontaminated with a detergent-disinfectant. Blood or body fluids that have spilled on the floor during a procedure should be wiped up immediately and the area decontaminated. Gloves, masks, and eyewear are worn for cleaning procedures.

7. *Laundry:* Soiled woven fabrics should be handled as little as possible and are transported to the laundry in leakproof bags. Unused, folded linens should be completely opened before placing in the linen hamper. All laundry is considered contaminated and should be handled only by gloved hands. Laundry should be washed in water at 160° F (71.1° C) or higher with 50 to 150 parts per million (ppm) of chlorine bleach. Temperatures lower than 160° F can be used for washing laundry if the appropriate antimicrobial detergent is used.

Commercial dry cleaning uses chemicals that reduce the transmission of pathogens. Home laundering of surgical scrub suits may not consistently meet parameters for adequate disinfection.[6]

8. *Waste:* Blood and suctioned fluids may be safely poured down a drain connected to a sanitary sewer. A solidifying agent can be added to disposable suction containers to disinfect the contents and convert it into solid waste. Trash is disposed of by incineration or sent to a sanitary landfill in sealed containers as required by local ordinances or state regulations. Trash bags must be leakproof and of sufficient thickness and strength to ensure integrity during transport. For disposal purposes, waste may be differentiated as either infectious or noninfectious. Bags are either color-coded (e.g., red for infectious waste) or labeled as biohazard.

9. *Handwashing:* Thorough handwashing with an approved antimicrobial agent after every contact with a patient, contaminated items, or suspected contamination protects both the patient and personnel and cannot be overemphasized. Hands should be washed after removing contaminated gloves because gloves are not 100% impervious.

10. *No touching of mucous membranes:* Eating and drinking are prohibited in any area where there is a risk for exposure. Applying lip balm or cosmetics or adjusting contact lenses in the perioperative environment significantly increases the risk for exposure. Hand-to-mouth and hand-to-eye contact can contribute to microbial transmission.

11. *Prophylaxis:* Perioperative personnel are encouraged to know their human immunodeficiency virus (HIV), hepatitis B virus (HBV), and hepatitis C virus (HCV) antibody status. The disclosure of a positive status to the appropriate facility is recommended. Personnel who participate in invasive procedures are at risk for bloodborne exposure and should have the HBV immunization series. Some facilities require personnel to get vaccinated or prove immunity by having titers drawn before being hired. Personnel who choose not to have the immunization series because of a past allergic reaction or special circumstance need documentation and should sign a release stating the declination. The CDC offers a recommended adult immunization schedule. Individuals should consult a physician about necessary immunizations.

For personal protection and the safety of patients, all health care providers should be familiar with policies and procedures and must understand the need for Standard Precautions. A health care provider should report a blood or body fluid exposure as defined by policy. The surgeon and first assistant usually are at greatest risk. Comparably a patient should be informed of any incident in which they are exposed to the blood of a health care provider.

Principles of Sterile Technique

Sterile technique is the foundation of modern surgery. The patient is the center of the sterile field, which includes the personnel wearing sterile attire and the areas of the patient, operating bed, and furniture that are covered with sterile drapes. The level of the surgical site is the central focus of the level of the sterile field. Strict adherence to the recommended practices of sterile technique reflects the surgical conscience of the perioperative team and is mandatory for the safety of the patient and personnel in the environment. The principles of sterile technique are applied under the following conditions:

- In preparation for an invasive procedure by sterilization of necessary materials and supplies
- In preparation of the sterile team to handle sterile supplies and intimately contact the surgical site by scrubbing, gowning, and gloving
- In the creation and maintenance of the sterile field, including skin preparation and draping of the patient
- In the maintenance of sterility throughout the entire surgical procedure; breaches in sterility are remedied immediately
- In terminal decontamination, disinfection, and sterilization at the conclusion of the surgical procedure

Only Sterile Items Are Used Within the Sterile Field

Items such as sterile instrument sets, drapes, sponges, and basins are obtained from the sterile core. Only if absolutely necessary, items such as unwrapped instruments may be steam sterilized immediately before the surgical procedure and taken directly from the sterilizer to the sterile field. This rapid steam sterilization method is referred to as *flashing* and must be used only if no other alternative is available. Facilities must keep a record of each time flashing is used and the items, parameters, and individuals involved.

Every person who dispenses a sterile item to the field must be sure of its initial and continued sterility until used. Proper packaging, sterilizing, delivery to the field, and handling should provide such assurance. If there is any doubt about the sterility of any item, it should be considered unsterile and therefore should not be used. The phrase "when in doubt, throw it out" applies to this situation. Examples of questionably sterile items include, but are not limited to, the following situations:

- If a sterilized package is found in a contaminated area (e.g., the general unsterile workroom, the locker room).
- If uncertain about the actual timing or operation of the sterilizer. Items processed in a suspect load are considered unsterile. Other items processed in that load may need to be recalled to the processing department for reprocessing (e.g., the external process monitor has irregular color changes).
- If the instruments are still assembled, are clamped closed, or contain debris.
- If an unsterile person or object comes into close contact with a sterile table, and vice versa.
- If a sterile table or unwrapped sterile items are not under constant observation (e.g., a sterile field under a table cover is not directly visible).
- If the packaging material is not intact.

- If a sterile package wrapped in a material other than plastic or another moisture-resistant barrier becomes damp or wet. Humidity in the storage area or moisture on hands may seep into the package.
- If a sterile package wrapped in a pervious woven material drops to the floor or other area of questionable cleanliness. These materials allow the implosion of air into the package. A dropped package is considered contaminated on the outside. If the wrapper is impervious and the area of contact is dry and intact, the outer wrapper is removed and item may be transferred to the sterile field. Packages that have been dropped on the floor should not be put back into sterile storage.

Sterile Personnel Are Gowned and Gloved

- Gowns are considered sterile only from the chest to the level of the sterile field in the front, and from 2 inches above the elbows to the cuffs on the sleeves (Fig. 15.1). When wearing a gown, only the area that can be seen in front down to the level of the sterile field should be considered sterile. Keep in mind that the level of the patient's surgical site establishes the level of the sterile field (Fig. 15.2). Usually this does not extend below waist level. The following practices are observed:
- Self-gowning and gloving should be done from a separate sterile surface to avoid dripping water or skin cells onto sterile supplies or a sterile table. Closed gloving technique is preferred for the person who is establishing the sterile field and gowning and gloving others.

• **Fig. 15.1** Zones of Sterility on Front of Gown. The zones of sterility can change based on position of draped patient and sterile team.

• **Fig. 15.2** Zones of sterility when standing at sterile field with patient as the baseline for the level of the sterile field.

- The stockinette cuffs of the gown are enclosed beneath sterile gloves. The stockinette is absorbent and retains moisture; therefore this part of the gown does not provide a microbial barrier and permits the transfer of microorganisms. Once the cuff has been contained within the closed glove, it should not be pulled back over the hand for any regloving procedure because it is contaminated. Regloving should be performed using the open-assisted gloving technique. Another sterile team member can assist with this process as necessary.
- Sterile people must keep their hands in sight at all times and at or above waist level or the level of the sterile field (Fig. 15.3).
- Hands are kept away from the face, and the elbows are kept close to the sides. The hands are never folded under the arms because of perspiration in the axillary region. The neckline, shoulders, and back also may become contaminated with perspiration. The back of the gown is not under constant observation and therefore is considered contaminated.
- Sterile people are aware of the height of team members in relation to each other and the sterile field. Changing levels at the sterile field is avoided. All team members must be aware of spatial relationships at all times. The gown is considered sterile only down to the highest level of the sterile working field. If a sterile person must stand on a platform to reach the surgical site, the standing platform should be positioned before this person steps up to the draped area. Sterile personnel should sit only when the entire procedure will be performed at this level. If one person on the team sits, the entire team should be seated (Fig. 15.4).

Tables Are Sterile Only at Table Level

Because tables are sterile only at table level, OR personnel must adhere to the following procedures:
- Only the top of a sterile, draped table is considered sterile. The edges and sides of the drape extending below table level are considered contaminated. The Mayo stand, when covered by a sterile drape, may be placed over the sterile field. Minimal contact is had with the underside of the Mayo drape.

• **Fig. 15.3** Sterile personnel keep hands in sight at or above waist or level of sterile field. Gowns are considered sterile only in front from the chest to the level of the sterile field, and the sleeves from above the elbows to the cuffs.

- Anything falling or extending over the table or OR bed edge, such as a piece of suture or suction tip, is contaminated. The scrub person does not touch the part hanging below the level of the established sterile field.
- When unfolding or applying a sterile drape, it is unfolded away from the sterile person and the part that drops below the table surface is not brought back up to table level. Once placed, the drape is not moved or shifted.
- Cords, tubing, and other materials are secured on the sterile field with a nonperforating clip to prevent them from sliding over the edge of the operating bed.

Sterile Personnel Touch Only Sterile Items or Areas; Unsterile Personnel Touch Only Unsterile Items or Areas

- Sterile team members maintain contact with the sterile field by means of sterile gowns and gloves.
- The unsterile circulating nurse does not directly contact the sterile field.
- Supplies are brought to sterile team members and opened by the circulating nurse using aseptic technique. The circulating nurse ensures a sterile transfer to the sterile field. Only sterile items touch sterile surfaces.

Unsterile Personnel Avoid Reaching Over the Sterile Field; Sterile Personnel Avoid Leaning Over an Unsterile Area

- The unsterile circulating nurse never reaches over a sterile field to transfer sterile items.
- The circulating nurse holds only the lip of the bottle over the basin when pouring solution into a sterile basin to avoid reaching over a sterile area (Fig. 15.5). They should avoid making contact with the bottle and the basin and avoid splashing solutions. The entire contents of the bottle should be dispensed in one pouring motion. If some of the solution is not poured, it is considered contaminated and may not be recapped for later use or dispensed to another sterile basin. Once the cap is off, the solution is considered contaminated.
- The unsterile solution may be saved for cleaning the patient's skin after the incision is dressed and the surgical site is undraped.
- The scrub person sets basins or medicine cups to be filled at the edge of the sterile table; the circulating nurse stands a safe

• **Fig. 15.4** Seated Team for Upper Extremity Procedure. The zones of sterility change based on the placement of the team in relation to the type of surgical procedure.

• **Fig. 15.5** Circulating Nurse Pouring Sterile Solution Into Sterile Basin. Note that only the lip of bottle is over the basin. The unsterile person avoids reaching over the sterile field.

• **Fig. 15.6** Sterile Scrub Person Draping a Small Table. Sterile personnel avoid reaching over the unsterile field. The scrub person therefore drapes an unsterile table first toward themself, then away. Gown is protected by distance, and hands are protected by cuffing drape over them.

distance away from the edge of the table to fill them. Medications are drawn up in a syringe, the needle is removed, and the drug is dispensed to the cup without aerosolization. It is unsafe to draw up a drug if another person is holding the bottle. This is no different from recapping a needle by hand. It is not advised to dispense the drug via syringe and needle because the needle could cause an aerosolization of a drug to which a team member might be sensitive.

• The team uses sterile light handles for manipulation and adjustment of the surgical lights. Light handles should not be placed until after the patient is fully draped.

• The surgeon or team member steps away from the sterile field to have perspiration removed from the brow by the circulating nurse.

• The scrub person drapes an unsterile table by:
  • Unfolded drape. Placing the drape over the unsterile surface nearest to themself first and carefully completing the coverage of the far side. This protects the front of the gown from coming into contact with the unsterile surface being covered. Gloved hands are protected by cuffing a drape over them (Fig. 15.6).
  • Folded drape. Unfolding toward themself first to protect the gown when working with a folded drape (Figs. 15.7 to 15.9). When completing the coverage, the rest of the drape is unfolded away from themself.
  • The scrub person stands back from the unsterile table when draping it to avoid leaning over an unsterile area.

The Edges of Anything That Encloses Sterile Contents Are Considered Unsterile

The boundaries between sterile and unsterile areas are not always rigidly defined (e.g., the edges of wrappers on sterile packages and the caps on solution bottles). The following precautions should be taken:

• When opening sterile packages, a margin of safety is always maintained. The inside of a wrapper is considered sterile to within 1 inch of the edges. The circulating nurse opens the top flap away from themself and then turns the sides under. The ends of the flaps are secured in the hand so they do not dangle loosely. The last flap is pulled toward the person opening the package, thereby exposing the package contents away from the unsterile hand.

• Sterile personnel lift contents from packages by reaching down and lifting them straight up, holding their elbows high.

• **Fig. 15.7** Draping Large Unsterile Table. Scrub person holds sterile fan-folded table drape high and drops it on center of table, standing back from table to protect gown.

• **Fig. 15.8** Scrub Person Unfolding Sterile Table Drape. Scrub person stands back from unsterile table and unfolds drape first toward themself. Note that hands are inside sterile cover to protect them.

• The flaps on peel-open packages should be pulled back, not torn, to expose the sterile contents. The contents should not be permitted to slide over the edges. The inner edge of the heat seal is considered the line of demarcation between sterile and unsterile. The sterile item should be presented to the scrub person. Flipping can cause air turbulence, and the item may miss its mark and fall to an unsterile area. Staplers and comparable devices should not be flipped because they may be damaged by impact with the table and may misfire when used.

• **Fig. 15.9** Scrub Person Continuing to Unfold Sterile Table Drape. Note that the hands are inside sterile cover for protection. Scrub person may now move closer to table because the first part of unfolded drape now protects gown.

- If a sterile wrapper is used as a table cover, it should amply cover the entire table surface. Only the interior and surface levels of the cover are considered sterile.
- After a bottle of sterile solution is opened, the contents are either used or discarded. The cap cannot be replaced without contaminating the pouring edges.
- Steam reaches only the area within the gasket of a sterilizer. Instrument trays should not touch the edge of the sterilizer outside the gasket when being removed after flash sterilization.
- When using a rigid closed container system with an inner sterile basket, the edges of the rigid outer container are not sterile. The inner basket is carefully lifted out by the scrub person and set on the sterile field. Sterile items should never be dispensed into the rigid container because of the high risk for contamination by the edges.

The Sterile Field Is Created as Close as Possible to the Time of Use

The degree of contamination is proportionate to the length of time that sterile items are exposed to the environment. Precautions must be taken as follows:

- Sterile tables are set up just before the surgical procedure. There is not an established time period or duration wherein the table is considered sterile or unsterile. Setting up as close to the time of use is in the best interest of the patient.
- If a table is not used immediately after setup, it may be covered by a sterile drape placed halfway with a cuffed edge horizontally. A second sterile cuffed drape is placed from the opposite side completely overlapping the first cuff. When removing the drapes to uncover the table, the top drape is removed first without touching the second drape. The hands must remain under the cuffed edge as each drape is removed in succession. None of the edges that overhang the edges may be brought over the sterile surface when being removed.
- A transparent drape with a seam that separates in the middle is made for covering tables.[7]
- Covering sterile tables prepared earlier for later use is not recommended as a general practice.

- It is not appropriate to set up a room and leave it unattended. Taping the door shut is not a guarantee of continued sterility.

Sterile Areas Are Continuously Kept in View

Inadvertent contamination of sterile areas must be readily visible. To ensure this principle, the following steps must be taken for uncovered sterile setups:

- Sterile personnel face sterile areas.
- Someone must remain in the room to maintain vigilance when sterile packs are opened in a room or a sterile field is set up. Sterility cannot be ensured without direct observation. An unguarded sterile field should be considered contaminated.

PROS/CONS

Covering a Sterile Table

Pros
- Sterility is event related, and a cover can help prevent contamination.
- The sterile field can be preserved if the case is delayed. If a sterile field needs to be covered, it should be done by a person in sterile attire using sterile technique.
- A sterile field can be covered using two cuffed drapes placed horizontally over the sterile surface. The second drape should completely overlap the cuff of the first drape.
- A single transparent drape made specifically to cover set-up tables is acceptable. It separates in the middle for removal.
- The drapes should be removed sequentially, with the last drape being removed first.

Cons
- Avoiding contamination of the sterile field cannot be guaranteed regardless of the method used.
- Nonwoven paper drapes can become airborne and shift as personnel walk by.
- The proper technique of drape placement or removal is not always followed or known by staff. A single drape must never be used because nothing should pass over the open sterile field during covering or uncovering.
- The covered field should be continuously monitored.
- Some organizations recommend never covering tables because of contamination risk.
- Traffic patterns can cause contamination even if a table is covered.
- Tables should be set up as close to the case time as possible.
- "When in doubt, throw it out."
- Staff should know the rationale and timing for covering a table.
- The table should not be set up, covered, and moved to another area in the department.

References

1. Qvistgaard M, Almerud-Osterberg S, Lovebo J: Covering surgical instruments with single- or double-layer drape pending surgery: an experimental study in a perioperative setting, *J Infect Prev* 22:126–131, 2021.
2. Markel T, Gormley T, Greeley D, et al.: Covering the instrument table decreases bacterial bioburden: an evaluation of environmental quality indicators, *Am J Infect Control* 46(10):1127–1133, 2018.

Bibliography

AORN: Guideline for sterile technique. In *Guidelines for perioperative practice*, Denver, CO, 2024, The Association.

Sterile Personnel Keep Well Within the Sterile Area

Sterile persons allow a wide margin of safety when passing unsterile areas and observe the following rules:

- Sterile personnel stand back at a safe distance from the OR bed when draping the patient.
- Sterile personnel pass each other back to back at a 360-degree turn (Fig. 15.10).
- Sterile personnel turn their backs to an unsterile person or area when passing.
- Sterile personnel face a sterile area to pass it.
- Sterile personnel ask an unsterile individual to step aside rather than risk contamination.
- Sterile personnel stay within the sterile field. They do not walk around or go outside the room.
- Use shielding devices during x-ray to prevent leaving the room or stepping away from the sterile field.
- Movement within and around a sterile area is kept to a minimum to avoid contamination of sterile items or personnel.

Sterile Personnel Keep Contact With Sterile Areas to a Minimum

To keep contact with the sterile areas to a minimum, sterile personnel observe the following rules:

- Sterile personnel do not lean on sterile tables or the draped patient. Leaning on the patient can cause injury to tissues and structures.
- Sitting or leaning against an unsterile surface is a break in technique. If the sterile team sits to operate, they do so without proximity to unsterile areas.

Unsterile Personnel Avoid Sterile Areas

Unsterile personnel maintain an awareness of sterile, unsterile, clean, and contaminated areas and their proximity to each. They must be aware of their closeness to the sterile field. A wide margin of safety must be maintained when passing sterile areas by observing the following rules:

- Unsterile personnel maintain a distance of at least 1 foot (30 cm) from any area of the sterile field.
- Unsterile personnel face and observe a sterile area when passing it to be sure they do not touch it.

- Unsterile personnel never walk between two sterile areas (e.g., between sterile instrument tables).
- The circulating nurse restricts to a minimum all activity near the sterile field.

Destruction of the Integrity of Microbial Barriers Results in Contamination

The integrity of a sterile package or sterile drape is destroyed by perforation, puncture, or strike-through. Strike-through is the soaking of moisture through unsterile layers to sterile layers, or vice versa. Ideal barrier materials are resistant to abrasion and impervious to permeation by the fluids or dust that transports microorganisms. The integrity of a sterile package and the appearance of the process monitor must be checked for sterility just before opening.

To ensure sterility, the following precautions should be taken:

- Sterile packages are laid on only dry surfaces.
- If a sterile package wrapped in absorbent material becomes damp or wet, it is discarded or wrapped in fresh wrappers and resterilized. The package is considered unsterile if any part of it comes into contact with moisture.
- Drapes are placed on a dry field.
- If solution soaks through a sterile drape to an unsterile area, the wet area is covered with impervious sterile drapes or towels.
- Packages wrapped in woven fabric or paper should cool after being removed from the sterilizer and before being placed on a cold surface; this prevents steam condensation and the resultant contamination.
- Sterile items are stored in clean, dry areas.
- Sterile packages are handled with clean, dry hands.
- Undue pressure on sterile packs is avoided to prevent forcing sterile air out and pulling unsterile air into the pack. Peel packs should be stored on their sides to prevent pressure that could rupture the integrity of the package.

Microorganisms Must Be Kept to an Irreducible Minimum

Sterile technique in the surgical site is an ideal to be approached; it is not absolute. All microorganisms in the environment cannot be eliminated, but this does not obviate the necessity for strict sterile technique. There is general agreement about the following guidelines:

• **Fig. 15.10** Sequence of One Sterile Person Going Around Another. *They pass each other back to back, keeping well within the sterile area and allowing a margin of safety between them.*

- Skin cannot be sterilized. Skin is a potential source of contamination in every invasive procedure. Inherent body defenses usually can overcome the relatively few organisms remaining after preparation of the patient's skin. Microorganisms on the face, neck, hair, hands, and arms of the OR team and patient are a hazard. All possible means are used to prevent the entrance of microorganisms into the wound. Preventive measures include the following techniques:
  - Mechanical washing and chemical antisepsis is used to remove or inactivate transient and resident flora from the skin around the surgical site of the patient and from the hands and arms of sterile team members.
  - Gowning and gloving of the OR team is accomplished without contamination of the sterile exterior of gowns and gloves.
  - Sterile, gloved hands do not directly touch the skin and then touch deeper tissues. Instruments used in contact with skin are discarded and not reused.
- If a glove is torn or punctured by a needle or instrument, it is changed immediately. The puncturing needle or instrument is removed from the sterile field.
- A sterile dressing should be applied to the surgical site before the drapes are removed to reduce the risk for the incision being touched by contaminated hands or objects.
- Some areas cannot be scrubbed. When the surgical site includes the mouth, nose, throat, or anus, the number of microorganisms present is great. Various parts of the body, such as the gastrointestinal tract and vagina, usually are resistant to infection by the flora that normally inhabit these parts. However, the following steps may be taken to reduce the number of microorganisms in these areas and prevent them from scattering:
  - The surgeon makes an effort to use a sponge only once and then discards it.
  - The gastrointestinal tract (especially the colon) is contaminated, and measures are used to prevent spreading this contamination.
  - Irrigation and suction may be used to remove gross debris.
  - Aseptic technique is generally used when these mucous membranes are intact, but if the vascular system of the patient is entered, the items in use should be sterile. No case should ever be considered "dirty" when the vascular system is entered.
- Infected areas are grossly contaminated. The team avoids disseminating the contamination.
- Air is contaminated by dust, droplets, and shedding. The following environmental control measures are used:
  - Drapes placed over the anesthesia screen or attached to IV poles at the head of the bed separate the anesthesia area from the sterile field.
  - Movement around the sterile field is kept to a minimum to avoid air turbulence.
  - To avoid the dispersion of lint and dust, drapes are not flipped, fanned, or shaken.
  - Talking is kept to a minimum in the OR. Moisture droplets are expelled with force into the mask during the process of articulating words.

- OR attire is worn properly: The mask covers the nose and mouth; the scalp and hair are completely covered, with long or loose pieces tucked into the cap; and body covers are close fitting. Unsterile personnel should wear long-sleeved warm-up jackets with knitted cuffs. Fronts of jackets should be completely buttoned.

No Compromise of Sterility

There is no compromise with sterility. In clinical practice an item is considered either sterile or unsterile. Team members should always be as certain of sterility as possible. That certainty rests on the fact that the necessary conditions have been met and that all factors in the sterilization process have been observed. Obviously it is impossible to prove that every package is free from bacteria, but a single break in technique can compromise the life of a patient.

OR personnel must maintain the high standards of sterile technique that they know are essential. Every individual is accountable for their own role in infection control. The patient should be considered an extension of the caregiver's own body. The patient completely trusts the team to provide safe care and protection from infection. This is a solemn obligation, with moral implications.

ⓔ EVOLVE WEBSITE

http://evolve.elsevier.com/Hornacky/BerryKohn/

- Historical Perspective
- Student Interactive Questions
- Glossary

References

1. Phillips NM, Hornacky A: *CNOR pass*, St. Louis, 2019, Elsevier.
2. Kyle E: Sterile technique, *AORN J* 117(1):64−69, 2023.
3. American Society of Anesthesiologists: *Statement on surgical attire*. www.asahq.org. Accessed April 17, 2023.
4. Centers for Disease Control and Prevention: *Guidelines for isolation precautions*. www.cdc.gov. Accessed April 18, 2023.
5. Occupational and Safety Health Administration: www.osha.gov. Accessed April 18, 2023.
6. Guideline for surgical attire, periop briefing, *AORN J* 117(4):P12, 2023.
7. Zarei M, Babajani V: The safety of a novel single-drape cover for sterile back tables in the operating room compared to the standard two-drape method: an experimental study, *Patient Saf Surg* 16(1), 2022.

Bibliography

AORN: *Guidelines for perioperative practice*, Denver, CO, 2024, The Association.
Rothrock JC: *Alexander's care of the patient in surgery*, ed 17, Philadelphia, 2023, Elsevier.

16

Appropriate Attire, Surgical Hand Hygiene, and Gowning and Gloving

CHAPTER OUTLINE

Appropriate Operating Room Attire, 276

Surgical Hand Hygiene, 285

Gowning and Gloving, 288

CHAPTER OBJECTIVES

After studying this chapter the learner will be able to:

- Identify the components of appropriate operating room attire worn in specific areas of the surgical suite.
- Identify the components of personal protective equipment donned before performing surgical hand cleansing.
- Identify the sterile parameters of a surgical gown.
- Demonstrate the correct method of gowning and gloving before establishing the sterile field.
- Demonstrate the appropriate method of changing a contaminated glove during a surgical procedure.
- Demonstrate the proper method for removing a contaminated gown and gloves.

KEY TERMS AND DEFINITIONS

Antimicrobial agent Antiseptic soap or cleanser used for cleaning the skin of patients and caregivers; has a fast-acting, broad-spectrum action to reduce the count of microorganisms before a surgical procedure.

Attire Appropriate operating room attire consists of body covers such as a two-piece pantsuit, head cover, mask, and shoe covers (shoe covers are used as appropriate).

Barrier Physical or mechanical obstacle between a person and a hazardous substance or microorganism.

Closed-assisted gloving Method for applying sterile gloves to another person who has their hands enclosed within the cuffs of a sterile gown.

Closed-gloving Method of self-applying gloves while the hands are concealed within the cuffs of a sterile gown.

Double-gloving The wearer applies two pairs of sterile gloves. The inner gloves should be a half-size larger than the outer glove to create a comfortable air cushion. The inner glove can be a different color to help detect a tear in the outer glove. Wearing two gloves of the same size can cause compression of the median nerve and aggravate carpal tunnel syndrome in some susceptible people.

Gloving Applying or donning gloves using one of several methods.

Gowning Applying a sterile gown to oneself or another member of the sterile team.

Hand hygiene Scrubbing the hands with a brush, water, and antiseptic agent or brushless antiseptic gel hand rub.

Indicator gloves Specialized sterile colored gloves worn under a pair of sterile surgical gloves that reveal color, commonly green or blue, when the outer glove is punctured.

Open-assisted gloving Method for applying sterile gloves to another person who has their hands exposed through the cuffs of a sterile gown

Open-gloving Method of self-applying gloves while the hands are exposed with or without a sterile gown. This is how gloves are reapplied after a contaminated glove is removed by the circulating nurse. The cuffs are not pulled back over the hands because they are absorbent and considered contaminated.

Personal protective equipment (PPE) Eyewear, mask, hair cover, shoe covers, gown, apron, and/or gloves worn to prevent airborne, droplet, or contact-based transmission of potentially hazardous substances or microorganisms between caregiver and patient.

Scrub suit Appropriate attire intended for wear in the operating room. Consists of a shirt, pants, and fully buttoned long-sleeved jacket. Attire should be laundered within the facility to prevent transmission of infectious material.

Sterile attire Consists of basic appropriate attire for the operating room with the addition of sterile gown and sterile gloves for entering the sterile field.

Subungual Under the fingernails.

Surgical hand hygiene (surgical scrub) Process by which the hands and arms of the team are rendered clean by mechanical and chemical action before a surgical procedure.

Appropriate Operating Room Attire

Purpose of Appropriate Attire

Sebaceous and sweat glands in and around hair follicles over the entire surface of the body contain microorganisms that are continually shed into the environment. The purpose of operating room (OR) attire is to provide effective barriers that both prevent the dissemination of microorganisms to patients and protect personnel from blood and body substances of patients. OR attire has been shown to reduce microbial shedding and prevent contamination of the surgical site and sterile field by direct contact.

Definition

OR attire consists of body covers such as a two-piece pantsuit, head cover, mask, and shoe covers, as appropriate. Each cover has a purpose to combat sources of contamination exogenous (external) to the patient. A sterile gown and gloves are added to this basic attire for sterile team members at the sterile field. Appropriate attire is a part of aseptic environmental control that also protects personnel against exposure to communicable diseases and hazardous materials. Personal protective equipment (PPE) such as eyewear and other protective items are worn by personnel as appropriate for anticipated exposure to blood and body fluids. Box 16.1 describes attire for the OR according to specific areas.

Considerations for Appropriate Attire

The OR should have specific written policies and procedures for proper attire to be worn within the semirestricted and restricted areas of the OR suite. The dress code should include aspects of personal hygiene important to environmental control. Protocol is strictly monitored so everyone conforms to established policy, such as the following rules:

1. Dressing rooms located in the unrestricted area adjacent to the semirestricted area of the OR suite are reached through the outer unrestricted corridor. Street clothes are not worn beyond the unrestricted area.
2. Only approved, freshly laundered attire intended for use in the OR is worn within the semirestricted and restricted areas. This policy applies to everyone entering the OR suite, both professional and nonprofessional personnel and visitors. Home laundering of scrub suits may cause cross-contamination between hospital and home microflorae. Laundry conditions at home

are not controlled for temperature and cleaning products and may not consistently take microbial counts to an irreducible minimum.[1]
   a. Clean, fresh attire is donned each time on arrival in the OR suite and as necessary at other times if the attire becomes wet or grossly soiled. Bloodstained or soiled attire, including shoe covers, is not only unattractive but also can be a source of cross-contamination. Soiled attire is not worn outside the OR suite.
   b. An adequate supply of clean scrub suits should always be available and laundered daily, preferably in the hospital's laundry facilities. These suits should not be taken home for laundering because standardized sanitation processes may not be followed. The risk for contamination of family members might be increased if clothing were contaminated with resistant microorganisms (e.g., prions causing Creutzfeldt-Jakob disease or *Mycobacterium tuberculosis* causing tuberculosis [TB]).[2]
   c. Masks should be changed between patients and whenever wet or soiled.
3. OR attire should not be worn outside the OR suite or outdoors. This protects the OR environment from microorganisms inherent in the outside environment and protects the outside from contamination normally associated with the OR. Before leaving the OR suite, everyone should change to street clothes. Surgeons who wear scrubs back and forth to the office place patients at risk for exposure, not to mention that their appearance is unprofessional.
   a. On occasion, such as for lunch breaks, a single-use cover gown or other jacket may be worn over OR attire outside the suite. The practice of wearing cover gowns is not encouraged. After a gown is worn it should be placed in a laundry hamper or it should be discarded if it is disposable. Some hospitals provide laboratory coats. These are completely buttoned and worn only once.
   b. OR attire should not be hung or put in a locker for wearing a second time. It should be discarded in the trash if disposable or put in a laundry hamper after one use, as appropriate. Shoes should be stored in an area that prevents contamination of street clothes.
4. Impeccable personal hygiene is emphasized. Each person should bathe daily with an antimicrobial product and apply deodorant as appropriate. Body odor is the result of microorganisms in the hair-bearing areas of the body. This becomes unpleasant when confined to an OR while wearing a gown and gloves under hot lights. This is augmented when working with pediatric or geriatric patients where the room temperature has been intentionally elevated for patient care.
   a. A person with an acute infection, such as a cold or sore throat, should not be permitted within the OR suite. Personnel with cuts, burns, or skin lesions should not scrub or handle sterile supplies because serum, a bacterial medium, may seep from the eroded area. An open skin lesion may be a portal of entry for cutaneous contact with bloodborne pathogens.
   b. Some sterile team members who are known carriers of pathogenic microorganisms should be treated with appropriate medications, until nasopharyngeal culture findings are negative.
   c. Fingernails should be kept short (i.e., should not extend past the fingertips). Routine manicures prevent cracked

---

•BOX 16.1 Attire in the Specific Surgical Suite Areas

Appropriate Attire for the Unrestricted Area
- Street clothes
- Basic scrub attire: scrub suit

Appropriate Attire for the Semirestricted Area
- Basic scrub attire: scrub suit, hair cover

Appropriate Attire for the Restricted Area
- Basic scrub attire: scrub suit, warm-up jacket, hair cover, and mask
- Sterile attire for scrubbed person: scrub suit, hair cover, mask, sterile gown, sterile gloves, and protective eyewear. Shoe covers are added if necessary.

cuticles and hangnails. Subungual areas harbor the majority of microorganisms on hands. Fresh nail polish, lacquers, or gels on short, healthy nails may not alter the microbial count on fingernails. Polish, lacquers, and gels may seal crevices. Gel-based polishes need ultraviolet (UV) light to cure and are less resistant to chipping. However, damaged nails and chipped or peeling polish may provide a harbor for microorganisms. Studies have shown that artificial nails and other enhancers harbor organisms, especially fungi and gram-negative bacilli.

d. Jewelry, including rings and watches, should be removed before entering semirestricted and restricted areas. Organisms may be harbored under rings, thus preventing effective handwashing. Necklaces or chains can grate on the skin, increasing desquamation. They might break and fall into a wound or contaminate a sterile field. Pierced-ear studs should be confined within the head cover. Dangling earrings are inappropriate in the OR.

e. Facial makeup should be minimal.

f. Eyewear or eyeglasses should be wiped with a cleaning solution before each surgical procedure and secured to the face with a head strap to prevent slippage.

g. External apparel that does not serve a functional purpose should not be worn. Identification badges should be secured to prevent their contact with the sterile field or equipment used for patient care. Lanyards are a source of microbial carriage.

h. Hands are washed frequently and thoroughly to remove bioburden.[3] Hand hygiene should be performed before and after every patient contact, before and after wearing gloves, before and after eating, before and after using the restroom, and before leaving the facility.[3] Clean hands are the first-line defense against transmitting microorganisms.

Using hand cream regularly helps prevent chapped, dry skin. Bacteriostatic varieties may help reduce microbial counts on the skin. Hand sanitizer can be of benefit in reducing flora.

5. Comfortable, supportive, skid-proof shoes should be worn to minimize fatigue and for personal safety. Shoes should have enclosed toes and heels. Clogs may not provide a safe surface for fast walking or running during an emergency, especially while pushing a crash cart. Cloth shoes do not offer protection against spilled fluids or sharp items that may be dropped or kicked. Shoes are cleaned frequently, regardless of whether shoe covers are worn.

PROS/CONS

Wearing Jewelry

Pros
- Jewelry is a way to express personality and wealth.
- It can have sentimental meaning, such as a wedding ring.
- Cultural artifacts can define a certain religion or custom.
- Jewelry that can be contained under clothing and head covering may be permitted according to facility policy.
- Lanyards are worn in the clinical setting to hold an identification badge.
- Jewelry should be removed and placed in a locker or attached to clothing for safekeeping.

Cons
- A wedding ring may be acceptable if it is worn for religious or cultural purposes. It is, however, not recommended in high-risk areas such as the OR.
- Bacteria and fungi are carried on or under jewelry. Jewelry worn below the elbow such as bracelets, watches, and rings are barriers for appropriate handwashing or hand hygiene.
- Ringed hands carry a significantly higher colony of gram-negative bacilli than ringless hands and provide an ideal environment for microbial growth because they trap moisture, build up irritants underneath, and cause contact dermatitis.
- Long earrings that stick out of the head covering should be removed because they are a shedding risk and can be dislodged. A patient may become restless and catch on a hanging earring, tearing through the earlobe of the wearer.
- Dislodged jewelry may become lost or fall into the sterile field, thereby contaminating it.
- Lanyards and necklaces are a risk for infection because they are not routinely cleaned and frictional forces increase bacterial fallout.
- Rings may have sharp edges that can tear gloves.
- Inability to remove a tight ring may lead to long-term carriage of pathogenic bacteria that are not easily removed with routine handwashing.
- Body piercings and jewelry must be removed from patients before surgery because electrical burns can occur with the use of electrocautery. A sterile plastic intravenous catheter may be placed through the patient's pierced area to keep the subcutaneous tract open after the skin prep.
- Visible facial piercings above the mask line, such as eyebrow rings or nasal bridge bars, can cause distrust of the caregiver by the patient.
- Jewelry can cause injury to the wearer or patient because it may be caught on patient-moving devices or appliances used in patient care. Jewelry on the hands or wrists can cause skin abrasions.
- Jewelry should not be worn in restricted areas and the OR for safety reasons.
- Policies restricting jewelry are not often enforced.

References
1. Association of Surgical Technologists: *AST guidelines for best practices for wearing jewelry.* http://www.ast.org/. Accessed April 24, 2023.
2. Blumenstein N, Wickemeyer J, Rubenfeld A: Bringing to light the risk of burns from retained metal jewelry piercings during electrosurgery—torching the myth, *JAMA Surg* 157(5):455–456, 2022.
3. AORN: Guideline for surgical attire. In *Guidelines for perioperative practice*, Denver, CO, 2024, The Association.

Home Laundered Scrubs

Pros

- Home laundering is economic for the facility.
- Facilities save on hiring staff, washing machines, and chemicals.
- Active barrier textiles repel fluids from uniforms.
- Tightly woven scrub attire material reduces microbes.
- Some materials are treated with antimicrobials.
- Low-linting materials prevent transfer of microbes.
- Durable stain-resistant materials reduce pathogen transmission.
- Detergent of choice can minimize skin sensitivity.

Cons

- Health care workers may wear uniforms multiple times before laundering.
- Microorganisms can be transferred during transport of soiled clothes to home.
- Dirty scrubs can contaminate tote bags, electronic devices, cars, or any personal item.
- Microbes, organisms, and endospores can contaminate washing machines.
- Water temperature at facilities reaches 160° F; water temperature at home reaches 110° F.

- Facilities monitor water quality, correct measurement of cleaning chemicals, water temperature, mechanical action, duration of cycle, and drying temperature and time.
- Healthcare Laundry Accreditation Council and Centers for Disease Control and Prevention follow state standards.
- Laundered uniforms worn from home into a facility can harbor microorganisms and pet dander.
- Fragrance from home detergent can cause sensitivity in others.

References

1. The Joint Commission: *Laundering attire, including surgical attire and uniforms.* http://www.jointcommission.org/. Accessed April 20, 2023.
2. Association of Surgical Technologists: *AST guidelines for best practices for laundering scrub attire.* www.ast.org. Accessed April 22, 2023.
3. Centers for Disease Control and Prevention: *Protect your family: reduce contamination at home.* http://www.cdc.gov/. Accessed April 20, 2023.

Bibliography

AORN: Guideline for surgical attire. In *Guidelines for perioperative practice*, Denver, CO, 2024, The Association.

Components of Appropriate Attire

Each item of OR attire is a specific means for containment of or protection against the potential sources of environmental contamination, including skin, hair, and nasopharyngeal flora and microorganisms in air, blood, and body substances. Scrub suits and head covers are worn by all personnel in the semirestricted areas of the OR suite (Fig. 16.1). Masks also are worn in the restricted areas. Additional items, such as protective eyewear, gloves, and shoe covers, are worn during a surgical procedure and for protection during hazardous exposure.

Body Cover

Everyone dons attire intended for use within a semirestricted or restricted area (e.g., scrub suit). A variety of scrub suits—two-piece pantsuits or one-piece coveralls—are available in either a solid color or an attractive print. All should fit the body snugly. Pantsuits confine organisms shed from the perineal region and legs more effectively than do dresses; 90% of bacterial dissemination originates from the perineum. Pantyhose do not contain this shedding and may in fact increase it by constant friction.

Shirt and waistline drawstrings are tucked inside pants to avoid their touching sterile areas. Microorganisms multiply more rapidly beneath a covered area. A tunic top that fits snugly may be worn on the outside of pants. The scrub suit should be changed as soon as possible whenever it becomes wet or visibly soiled.

Those who will not be sterile team members should wear long-sleeved jackets with front closures over a scrub suit. The sleeves help contain shedding from axillae and arms and help protect from biologic contamination caused by splashes. The jacket should be closed to prevent a bellows effect and the possibility of brushing against the sterile field during movement.

A one-piece coverall, head cover, mask, and shoe covers are convenient garb for a visitor whose presence in the OR will be brief (e.g., pathologist, laboratory personnel). These coveralls are usually made of white or gray, disposable, tear-resistant material and resemble jumpsuits with a zipper down the front.

• **Fig. 16.1** Appropriate attire for the restricted area in preparation for scrubbing.

Head Cover

Because hair is a gross contaminant, a cap or hood is put on before the scrub suit to protect the garment from contamination by hair. Hair should not be combed while one is wearing a scrub suit. Bald heads should be covered to prevent the shed and dispersal of scalp dander.

All facial and head hair is completely covered in the semirestricted and restricted areas. Various types of lightweight caps and hoods are available. Most of them are made of disposable, lint-free, nonporous, nonwoven fabrics. If hair is long, a bouffant-style hat or

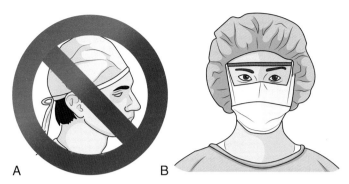

• **Fig. 16.2** **A,** Skull cap does not cover all hair and should not be worn. **B,** All hair must be covered.

hood is worn to cover the neck area. Skullcaps do not cover the entire head, and hair can shed from the inferior edges. Headgear should fit well so that it confines and prevents escape of any hair (Fig. 16.2).

Some facilities permit the wearing of reusable cloth bouffant-style caps. These should be freshly laundered daily. Many facilities require the use of a disposable bouffant cap over a cloth hat. Personnel wearing turbans for cultural or religious reasons should completely cover the headwear with a bouffant cap. Anyone with a scalp infection should be excluded from the OR and treated.

PROS/CONS

Wearing Cloth Surgical Caps

Pros

• Head coverings function to contain the outflow or shedding of organisms from the hair and scalp. Wearing appropriate headgear can reduce the number of bacteria in the air. A clean surgical head cover or hood should contain the ears; all hair, including sideburns; and hair on the nape of the neck. The head cover should be put on before the scrub suit to keep it free from shedding. At the end of the day the scrub top should be removed before the cap to protect the hair from contamination by the clothing.

• Cloth surgical caps are reusable caps that are purchased from a store or sewn by employees. They are usually the bouffant style, skull cap, or hood. The cloth caps can be made from material with any pattern that may reflect the wearer's personality, emotion, hobby, favorite colors or pattern, sports team, college, favorite animals, or whatever pattern makes them feel good. It is usually the only piece of surgical attire that may be different from the rest of the staff.

• If a cloth cap is allowed, it must be made of a tight-woven, low-linting material. The cap should be washed daily; the preferred method is for the cap to be washed by an accredited laundry facility.

• Hair spray has been shown to diminish bacterial counts for all types of head covers.

Cons

• Allowing the use of cloth caps differs from facility to facility. It is recommended that reusable cloth caps NOT be worn because surgical site infections have been traced to bacteria from hair, scalp, and skin. This is to protect the wearer and patient from cross-contamination of pathogens.

• Most health care workers who wear cloth caps wear them for a whole day and do not change them after every procedure. This puts the wearer and patient at risk for cross-contamination. Contamination can come from the hands when removing the cap when leaving restricted areas, placing it in a locker or pocket, and putting the cap back on when returning to restricted areas.

• Proper attire is not something that is usually on a health care worker's mind; it is usually a habit. Health care workers usually have several cloth caps in their locker and have a habit of taking their cap off at the end of the day and placing it back into their locker and donning a new pattern the next day.

• Many workers have a habit of laundering the caps after they have been worn several times. Some studies have shown that 25% to 40% of surgical personnel were colonized with *Staphylococcus aureus.*

• Most facilities do not wash personnel's cloth caps. If caps are taken home to be laundered, staff must follow the facility policy for home laundering. AORN (Association of periOperative Registered Nurses), Association of Surgical Technologists (AST), and the CDC do not recommend home laundering for any attire worn in surgery.

• If a cloth cap gets soiled, it must be immediately removed and laundered. The health care worker may take home a bloody soiled cap and transport it in a tote bag or purse. This leads to possibly contaminating themselves, their washing machine, or family with pathogens.

• Every health care facility should have policies in place regarding wearing proper attire and staff compliance. Health care facilities need to address wearing of head covers and the rationale behind each type of cover. Some facilities permit cloth caps if covered with a disposable bouffant head cover.

References

1. Farach S, Kelly K, Farkas R, et al.: Have recent modifications of operating room attire policies decreased surgical site infection? An American College of Surgeons NSQIP review of 6,517 patients, *J Am Coll Surg* 226(5):804–813, 2018.
2. Stern V: Are surgical caps on the verge of a comeback? www.anesthesiologynews.com. Accessed April 19, 2023.

Bibliography

AORN: Guideline for surgical attire. In *Guidelines for perioperative practice*, Denver, CO, 2024, The Association.

PROS/CONS

Wearing Skull Caps

Pros

• Each facility offers a variety of head covers.
• Skull caps can be markers of individuality and status of each surgeon.
• Skulls caps are comfortable.
• Positive emotion and self-esteem.
• Personal preference.
• Male surgeons find skull caps more masculine than the bouffant cap.

Cons

• Skull caps do not cover all the hair, ears, facial hair, sideburns, and nape of the neck.
• Folding the edges of the skull cap into a cuff for a better fit shortens the coverage around the head and ears.
• Bouffant caps offer more complete coverage.
• Hair, scalp, and skin shedding are sources of infection because they harbor bacteria. *Staphylococcus aureus* and *Staphylococcus epidermidis* adhere to hair and are not completely removed with routine shampooing.
• Skull caps can become contaminated with sweat, especially on the forehead.
• Staff may not have adequate knowledge of infection control principles.
• Skull caps may not be changed after every case.

References

1. Rios-Diaz A, Chevrollier G, Witmer H, et al.: The art and science of surgery: do the data support the banning of surgical caps? *Surgery* 164:921–925, 2018.

PROS/CONS—cont'd

Wearing Skull Caps

2. Gologorsky Y: Bouffant versus skull cap: does operating room headwear really matter? *World Neurosurg* 119:437, 2018.
3. Cotton M: Operating room attire, *J Am Coll Surg* 228(2):209—210, 2019.

Bibliography

AORN: Guideline for surgical attire. In *Guidelines for perioperative practice*, Denver, CO, 2024, The Association.

Shoe Covers

Shoe covers may be worn in the semirestricted and restricted areas as needed to protect from blood and fluid. Knee-high impervious styles will protect the wearer from spills into or onto shoes during procedures wherein extensive fluid irrigation and/or blood loss can be anticipated. Some surgeons wear plastic or rubber boots. The legs of scrub pants are tucked into the boots.

Studies have not shown a significant correlation between footwear and wound infection. However, the flow of traffic is one critical factor in airborne dispersal of microbes from the floor. Unprotected street shoes can increase floor contamination and conversely carry biologic material home from the OR. Shoes restricted to wear in the OR are preferable in reducing microbial transfer from the outside into the OR suite.

Protective gloves should be worn to change shoe covers whenever they become wet, soiled, or torn. Shoe covers can inadvertently become soiled and harbor microorganisms. They should be removed before entering the dressing room area and must be removed before leaving the OR suite.

PROS/CONS

OR-Specific Shoes or Shoe Covers: Do They Really Make a Difference?

Pros

- Shoe covers are provided by the facility to protect the footwear and feet from the exposure of blood and bodily fluids. Shoe covers are kept close to semirestricted areas for easy access. OSHA requires that shoe covers or knee-high boots be worn in a situation in which gross contamination can be anticipated.
- Knee-high boots made of an impervious material are recommended if a large amount of irrigation fluid will be used or there is an anticipation of contact with blood or other body fluids. They also protect the bottoms of the scrub pants from getting wet and contaminated.
- Disposable shoe covers are made to be worn in the restricted and semirestricted areas. Shoe covers are not designed to be worn outside the surgical department.
- Shoe covers are also disposable so that they can be changed after every procedure or if soiled during a procedure.
- Facilities have policies about wearing OR-specific shoes so that health care workers do not bring microorganisms in from the outside or take them home.
- OR-specific shoes should be made of rubber or leather; be comfortable, breathable, and supportive; have nonskid bottoms; provide protection; and be easily cleaned. Shoes should remain intact and impermeable to prevent foot contamination. OSHA requires shoes to be enclosed with no opened backs.

Cons

- Many health care workers do not wear shoe covers because they wear a specific OR shoe such as a closed back clog that can be wiped off if soiled. This type of footwear is designed specifically for the OR and should not be worn outside of the surgery department.
- Shoes made of soft permeable material, open toe shoes, sandals, and high heels do not meet the standards for health care facilities.
- Many health care workers do not change their shoe covers unless visibly soiled. Shoe covers might be soiled with blood, have holes in them, or be worn outside of the restricted areas, such as to the cafeteria, locker room, or outdoors. Shoe covers must be changed daily or if wet or soiled. They should be removed with gloves in the OR suite before leaving it and disposed in the appropriate trash receptacle, and then hand hygiene should be performed.
- Contamination of the hands was a bigger concern when studying shoe covers. Studies found that the bacterial counts of staff that just put on or took off shoe covers had a higher bacterial count on their hands. This transferred organisms from the floor, to staff hands, and directly to patients if hand hygiene was not performed.
- Shoe covers must not be worn outside of the surgical suite to avoid tracking any contaminants in or out of the department. It is recommended that clean shoe covers be donned when returning from outside the department.
- Studies have been inconclusive about shoe covers. Shoe covers are not considered infection prevention but rather a protective barrier. The wearing of shoe covers has not proven to decrease the bacterial counts on operating room floors. Some studies have proved that room traffic is responsible for some surgical site infections because the microorganisms from the floor may become airborne.
- Studies are conflicting about OR-specific shoes and transfer of microorganisms. OR-specific shoes are recommended to prevent bringing in pathogens from the outside and taking pathogens back outside. Outdoor shoes have been shown to harbor more bacteria than OR-specific shoes.
- Every facility has a policy regarding shoe covers and OR-specific shoes. It is recommended that shoe covers be removed before leaving the restricted area. OR-specific shoes worn without shoe covers must not be worn outside the department. Recommended standards are the responsibility of the health care facility to establish policies and procedures for surgical attire. These policies and procedures should be reinforced to protect everyone.

References

1. Hafiani E, Cassier P, Aho S, et al.: Guidelines for clothing in the operating theatre, 2021, *Anaesth Crit Care Pain Med* 41(3), 2022.
2. Clesham K, Ryan PR, Murphy CG: Assessment of theatre shoe contamination in an orthopaedic theatre, *J Hosp Infect* 99(3):299—302, 2018.
3. Pyrek KM: *Shoe sole and floor contamination: a new consideration in the environmental hygiene challenge for hospitals 2018.* http://www.infectioncontroltoday.com/. Accessed March 3, 2019.
4. Association of Surgical Technologists: *Recommended standards of practice for shoe cover rationale.* http://www.ast.org/. Accessed April 22, 2023.

Bibliography

AORN: Guideline for surgical attire. In *Guidelines for perioperative practice*, Denver, CO, 2024, The Association.

Mask

A single mask is worn in the restricted area to hold and filter droplets containing microorganisms expelled from the mouth and naso-pharynx during breathing, talking, sneezing, and coughing. Some tight-fitting masks also effectively reduce exposure to submicron particles by filtration of inhaled air. Many masks filter approximately 99% of particulate matter larger than 5 μm in diameter but only approximately 45% to 60% of particles 0.3 μm in diameter.

Aerosolized particles and viruses dispersed in laser and electrosurgical plume or by power instruments may be this small. Masks provide some protection to the sterile team members from bloodborne pathogens that may splash or spray toward the nose or mouth. Wearing double masks forms a barrier instead of a filter and may actually cause expulsion of airborne particles to escape from the cheek folds.

Reusable cotton masks are obsolete; they filter ineffectively as soon as they become moist. Contemporary disposable masks of soft, cloth-like material in very fine synthetic fiber materials fulfill the following essential criteria:

- They are at least 95% efficient in filtering microbes from droplet particles in exhalations and also filter inhalations. A fluid-resistant mask is advantageous.
- They are cool, comfortable, and nonobstructive to respiration.
- They are nonirritating to the skin. Disposable masks are made of polypropylene, polyester, or rayon fibers. Some have fiberglass filters. Sensitive persons should try another brand.
- Mask styles include rectangle shapes with four strings or cup-shaped, formed masks with an elastic band that fits around the head.
- High-efficiency particulate air (HEPA) filtration masks are cup shaped and are worn when working with patients who have COVID-19 or TB. Employers should have each employee fitted so the size worn will be known. The patient should wear a mask during transport as well.
- Laser masks are high-filtration masks worn when plume from a laser or electrosurgical unit is in the environment. These masks filter airborne viruses.

Some experts believe that masks should be worn to protect team members, rather than patients, from moisture droplets. However, current practice recommendations of AORN are that masks be worn at all times in the restricted area of the OR suite, areas where sterile supplies will be opened and scrubbed personnel may be present, and areas where scrub sinks are located.

Masks should always be worn in the OR, regardless of whether a surgical procedure is in progress. Masks are worn on entering the room before, during, and after the surgical procedure (i.e., from setup through cleanup). This includes terminal cleaning at the end of the day and restocking of supplies. The policy in some OR suites may be less restrictive. All team members, departmental staff, and visitors should follow the institution's policy.

To be effective, a mask filters inhalations and exhalations. Therefore it is worn over both the nose and the mouth. Air must pass only through the filtering system; thus the mask must conform to facial contours to prevent leakage of expired air. Venting, the drawing of air back and forth, can occur along the sides, top, and bottom of the mask. The inside of the mask is covered with droplets from the mouth and nose and should not be touched with the hands.

Masks are designed with pleats or are conical, like a cup, for a close fit, but improper application can negate their efficiency. The strings should be tied tightly, if this is the method of securing the mask, to prevent the strings from coming loose during the surgical procedure. The upper strings are tied at the back of the head; the lower strings are tied behind the neck (Fig. 16.3). The strings are never crossed over the head because this distorts the contours of the mask along the cheeks.

Masks have a pliable strip that can be bent to contour the mask over the bridge of the nose. A close-fitting mask or a small strip of nonallergenic tape over the nosepiece also helps avoid fogging of eyewear. To prevent cross-infection, personnel should follow these steps:

1. Handle the mask only by the strings, thereby keeping the facial area of a fresh mask clean and the hands uncontaminated

• **Fig. 16.3** Mask covers nose and mouth and conforms to the facial contours. Upper strings are tied at back of head; lower strings are tied behind neck.

by a soiled mask. Do not handle the mask excessively. Hand hygiene should be performed any time the mask is handled.
2. Never lower the mask to hang loosely around the neck, never place the mask on top of the head, and never place the mask in a pocket. Avoid disseminating microorganisms.
3. Promptly discard the mask into the proper receptacle on removal. Remask with a fresh mask between patients.
4. Change the mask frequently. Do not permit the mask to become wet. Limit talking to a minimum.

If a sneeze is imminent, one should step back and away from the field and sneeze into the mask without turning the head sideways. Expelled air will be forced out the sides of the mask and directly into the sterile field through the vent if the head is sideways. The purpose of the mask is to filter air through the filtration material. Ideally, stepping away from the field and turning the head 180 degrees with the back of the head to the field may minimize exposure of the field. It may be necessary to remove the gown, gloves, and mask.

The hands should be washed with antimicrobial soap before and after cleaning the nose and applying a new mask. The hands should be rescrubbed before donning a sterile gown and gloves.

PROS/CONS

Wearing Masks in the Restricted Area

Pros
- Masks are worn as a barrier to protect the wearer from fluid, blood, smoke particulate, and microorganisms that contaminate the air. They also protect the patient against any pathogen from the caregiver.
- Masks are part of the standard respiratory-based precautions. A surgical mask should cover the mouth and nose and prevent venting of air from the sides of the mask.
- Health care facilities must provide personal protective equipment (PPE) according to federal laws. PPE includes masks, gloves, gowns, eye protection, shoe covers, and any other special protection device.
- Special fitted masks for airborne droplet precautions are individually fitted for face size and features. They are tested with the caregiver performing certain maneuvers. If a patient has a respiratory disease such as COVID-19 or tuberculosis (TB), a caregiver must wear a special fitted mask such as a HEPA or an N95, N99, or N100. This is an OSHA standard, and only caregivers following these policies can provide direct patient care. These masks may be referred to as respirators because they filter aerosolized particles and viruses. These special masks may be given to patients to wear when not in isolation or to visitors. Signs must be posted when entering a respiratory protection room so proper precautions can be taken.

PROS/CONS—cont'd

Wearing Masks in the Restricted Area

- A respiratory protection program must be in place that trains employees how and when to use their special masks, conducts fit testing, inspects and maintains respirators, and instructs how to dispose of contaminated items.
- Masks come in many styles and shapes. Most facilities offer a selection to employees to protect them and also provide comfort.
- New technology may be a solution to PPE shortages. Reusable high-filtration respirators have been produced with the use of a 3D printer.
- Masks should always be worn in the restricted areas. They should be put on before entering the OR, during the procedure, and during cleanup.

Cons

- Not every caregiver changes their mask after each procedure. A fresh mask should be donned before each new procedure and changed if it gets wet from personal excretions or soiled from a patient's fluids. Contaminated masks should be placed in the appropriate trash receptacle.
- Masks are easily contaminated. Masks should never dangle around the neck, be placed on the top of the head, or placed into a pocket because they can be contaminated by the area it touches. Many caregivers go in and out of OR rooms and never change their masks. They pull down their masks and let them dangle around their neck, thus contaminating them with their hands and droplets from their mouth and nose. This puts patients at risk for cross-contamination.
- Some caregivers cover only their mouth with their mask. This is unacceptable because it exposes the patient to microorganisms from the nose.
- A mask should be removed by the ties after each procedure to prevent contaminating the hands with droplets from the mouth and nose. Hand hygiene should follow immediately after mask removal.
- PPE should be donned within 3 ft of the patient's head especially when the patient is intubated or extubated. Many caregivers remove their masks, eyewear, and gowns before the patient is awake. This puts them at risk for contamination with bodily fluids.
- The clinical use of masks is so much a part of health care that proper studies are not conducted on their usefulness. Some studies have concluded that staff not directly in the vicinity of a surgical procedure do not pose a risk for infection to the patient.
- Current practices of AORN recommend that masks always be worn in restrictive areas. PPE is the responsibility of all health care workers. All staff members should reeducate themselves on their institution's policy.

References

1. Sokolove P, Moulin A: Standard precautions and infectious exposure management. In Roberts JR, Custalow CB, Thomsen TW, et al., editors: *Roberts and Hedges' clinical procedures in emergency medicine and acute care*, ed 7, Philadelphia, 2019, Elsevier, pp 1470–1480.
2. Centers for Disease Control and Prevention: *Guidance for the selection and use of personal protective equipment (PPE) in the healthcare settings.* http://www.cdc.gov/. Accessed April 24, 2023.
3. AORN: Guideline for surgical attire. In *Guidelines for perioperative practice*, Denver, CO, 2024, The Association.
4. Levine M: A more fitting approach to mask policy, *Am J Med* 135(11):1280–1281, 2022.

Personal Protective Equipment

Personnel should be protected from hazardous conditions in the semirestricted and restricted areas. Depending on the exposure that will be encountered, PPE should be worn. The types and characteristics of this attire depend on the task and degree of exposure anticipated. Protective attire does not allow blood or other potentially injurious materials to reach the inner clothing, skin, or eyes. Other considerations concerning protective attire are as follows:

1. Aprons
   a. A decontamination apron worn over the scrub suit protects against liquids and cleaning agents during cleaning procedures. It should be a full-front barrier. These are usually disposable plastic.
   b. When extensive blood loss or irrigation is anticipated, sterile team members wear fluid-proof aprons under their permeable, reusable sterile gowns. They should be lightweight and full front. These are usually disposable plastic.
   c. Lead aprons worn under sterile gowns protect against radiation exposure during procedures performed under fluoroscopy or image intensification or when personnel are exposed to radioactive implants. Lead aprons may be full front, full circumferential body cover, or vest and skirt style.
2. Eyewear and eye protection
   a. Eyewear or a face shield is worn whenever a risk exists of blood or body substances from the patient splashing into the eyes of sterile team members (Fig. 16.4). Bone chips and splatter can be projected from bone-cutting instruments. Several styles of goggles and eyeglasses with top and side shields fit securely against the face. Antifog goggles fit over prescription eyeglasses.

   A combination surgical mask with a visor eye shield or a chin-length face shield is another option. Care is taken that

• **Fig. 16.4** Face shield with hood.

the lower edge of the face shield does not touch the front of the gown. Side shields applied to eyeglasses may not be adequate protection for random splashes.

b. Laser eyewear is worn for eye protection from laser beams. Lenses of the proper optical density for each type of laser should be available and worn. An extra pair should be placed on the outer door for personnel who may need to enter the room during the procedure. The color of the glasses has no bearing on which laser light is blocked. Many manufacturers have tried to create clear lenses to minimize visual distortion.

c. Protective eyewear, preferably a face shield, should be worn by personnel handling or washing instruments when this activity could result in a splash, spray, or splatter to the eyes or face. Eyewear should be worn when cleaning the room to avoid splashing chemical germicides into eyes during mopping or cleaning. Surgical hand and arm scrubbing and patient skin prepping can release aerosolized antiseptic solution into the air. Protective eyewear should always be worn when working with detergent-based prep solution.

d. Eyewear or a face shield that becomes contaminated should be decontaminated or discarded promptly.

3. Gloves

a. Nonsterile latex or vinyl gloves are worn to handle any material or items contaminated by blood and body substances. Gloves should be worn only during the period of contact, not continuously. Gloves are never washed between patient contacts; they are discarded. Clean objects and sterile packages should not be handled with contaminated gloves. Avoid opening cupboard doors, using a keyboard, or adjusting monitor settings while wearing soiled gloves.

b. Sterile gloves are worn by sterile team members and for all invasive procedures. Sterile Kevlar-woven glove liners may be worn over or under gloves to protect the hands from cuts caused by heavy instrumentation. Liners can be worn between two layers of gloves and should be a half-size larger to prevent constriction. If double-gloving, the first pair of gloves can be colored to serve as an indicator glove. If the outer glove is punctured, the color shows through to make the perforation visible.

c. Lead and radiation protective gloves may be needed for protection from scatter during ionizing radiation exposure for diagnostic and therapeutic procedures that use real-time imaging. The surgeon may wear natural rubber gloves impregnated with lead for procedures performed under fluoroscopy. The lead is not in direct contact with skin.

When evaluating radiation protective gloves, be sure to note whether they are protective when used in direct radiation beams or if they are intended for use as protection from scatter. Not all radiation protective gloves are intended for use in direct beams. Radiation protective gloves without lead are commercially available.

d. Utility gloves are worn for cleaning and housekeeping duties. Sterile and nonsterile single-use, disposable latex and vinyl gloves are discarded after use. They should not be washed and reused. Soaps and surfactants decrease the surface tension of the gloves and increase the risk for wicking through microscopic holes in the gloves. Hands are washed after gloves are removed.

Surgical Gown

A sterile gown is worn over the scrub suit, a component of sterile attire to permit the wearer to enter the sterile field. It prevents contamination between the wearer and the field and differentiates sterile from nonsterile team members (Fig. 16.5). The gown should provide a protective barrier from strike-through (i.e., migration of moisture-borne microorganisms from the skin and scrub suit of the wearer to the sterile field and the patient, and penetration of blood and body substances from the patient to the scrub suit and skin of the wearer).

Both reusable and disposable gowns, in a variety of styles, are available. Although the entire gown is sterilized, the back is not considered sterile nor is any area below the level of the sterile field once the gown is donned. Wraparound sterile gowns that provide coverage to the back by a generous overlap are recommended. These gowns are secured at the neck and waist before the sterile flap is brought over the back and secured by ties at the side or front.

A separate sterile vest put on over the gown covers any exposed back area of scrub attire but does not render the back sterile. The back is never in view of the team, so it cannot be guaranteed to be sterile.

The cuffs of gowns are knitted stockinette to snugly fit wrists and are not fluid impervious. The material and weave absorb the wearer's body sweat, rendering the cuffs contaminated. Sterile gloves must cover the cuffs of the gown completely to prevent contamination of the sterile field (Fig. 16.6).

Changing a contaminated glove by pulling the cuff back down over the hand and using the closed gloving method to reglove contaminates the fresh glove's sterile surface with the wearer's sweat in the process.

• **Fig. 16.5** Appropriate Attire for the Sterile Scrubbed Person in the Restricted Area. The gown and gloves are worn over the scrub suit. Hair cover, protective eyewear, and mask are worn.

A   B

• **Fig. 16.6** Knitted cuffs are not impervious and should never be pulled back down over the hands to reglove by the closed method. Cuffs must be covered at all times when wearing gloves. **A,** Covered cuffs. **B,** Uncovered cuffs.

• **Fig. 16.7** Orthopedic Sterile Scrub Attire Used by Some Orthopedic Surgeons and Teams. No mask is required. The suit has a small air compressor to provide fresh air within the enclosed headgear.

Gowns should be resistant to penetration by fluids and blood and should be comfortable without producing excessive heat buildup. Most single-use disposable gowns are made of spun fibers or nonwoven, moisture-repellent materials. Some of these are reinforced with plastic on the forearms and front.

Sterile team members may not need a reinforced barrier gown for every procedure; the scrub person usually can safely wear a single-layer impervious gown. The surgeon and first assistant are at greatest risk during procedures when blood loss will be more than 20 mL or when the time will exceed 2 hours. The amount of blood and fluid on the outside of the gown is a critical factor in strike-through by wicking. Bloodborne pathogens can penetrate fabric without visible strike-through. The forearms are the most frequently contaminated areas. Therefore the surgeon and first assistant should wear a gown with at least reinforced or plastic-coated sleeves for these procedures.

Reusable woven textile gowns should be made of a densely woven, moisture-repellent material. Some reusable gowns are a cotton-polyester or Gore-Tex blend. Tightly woven 100% polyester gowns are impervious to moisture. Seams of the gowns should be constructed to prevent penetration of fluids. Monitoring the number of uses and washings is necessary to remove the gown from rotation when it is no longer an effective barrier.

All woven and some nonwoven gowns are not flame retardant. Fire-resistant gowns should be worn for laser surgery and preferably when electrosurgery is used.

Special attire often is worn with ultraclean laminar airflow systems (Fig. 16.7). (See Chapter 10 for more information concerning laminar airflow systems.) A body exhaust gown with helmet envelops the wearer from the top of the head to within about 16 inches (40 cm) of the floor. If a gown that fits closely at the neck is used, a clear, rigid face shield or helmet is worn. A standard surgical mask is not necessary under this helmet. With both types of gowns, an exhaust system is attached for body cooling and airflow. Powered coolant vests for wear under scrub attire are commercially available.

Surgical Gloves

Sterile gloves complete the attire for sterile team members. They are worn to permit the wearer to handle sterile supplies and tissues of the surgical site. Surgical gloves are made of natural rubber latex, synthetic rubber, thermoplastic elastomers, neoprene, vinyl, or polyethylene. Disposable synthetic gloves are worn most frequently. Latex is a polymeric membrane of natural rubber; most facilities are limiting or not allowing the use of latex gloves

for allergic reasons. However, latex provides a better barrier than vinyl, which may allow permeation of blood and fluids over prolonged exposure. Selection of surgical gloves worn during specific procedures depends on the following parameters:

- Length of surgical procedure
- Type of surgical procedure
- Need to double-glove
- Stresses to which the glove is exposed
- Chemical exposure to the gloves during surgical procedure
- Caregiver and patient sensitivity
- Individual preference

Latex gloves of varying thickness, with a minimum of 0.1 mm, can be chosen to meet the needs of the surgeon for tactile sensation. Latex contains protein antigen and is cured with agents that may cause a localized dermatitis or systemic anaphylaxis. Hypoallergenic milled gloves that do not contain these sensitizers are available. However, latex gloves labeled "hypoallergenic" do not always prevent reaction in a highly sensitive person. In 2017 the U.S. Food and Drug Administration (FDA) banned the use of powdered (cornstarch) surgical gloves because of the risks to patients and employees. Risks included airway problems from the inhalation of the powder, formation of granulomas, adhesions, inflammation, and immune reactions.

Several varieties of synthetic nonlatex sterile gloves (e.g., those made of neoprene) are available commercially. Sterile team members should not wear latex gloves if the patient has a known latex sensitivity or allergy.

Gloves are packaged in pairs with an everted cuff on each to protect the sterile outer surface of the glove during donning. The inner sterile paper wrap of the disposable glove package protects the sterility of the gloves when they are removed from the peel-pack outer wrap. Before opening, the package should be inspected for damage or wetness, which indicates contamination. When the inner paper is unfolded, the wearer finds the right glove to the right and the left glove to the left, both with palm sides up and thumbs on the outside edge (Fig. 16.8).

Most health care facilities have replaced latex and powder-containing gloves for safety reasons. Gloves coated on the inside with a hydrogel lubricant allows smooth donning of gloves.

One study demonstrated that surgeons puncture their gloves most often on the index finger of the nondominant hand. Glove

• **Fig. 16.8** Gloves on unfolded open wrapper: right glove to right, and left glove to left, palm sides up.

puncture and miniscule holes in gloves are hazardous to both patients and team members and can go unnoticed by the wearer. Seepage under the glove poses a threat to a team member if their skin is not intact. The risk for blood contamination of the fingers increases the longer the glove is worn. If a sterile glove is punctured or torn, it should be changed immediately to prevent escape of microorganisms from the wearer's skin and seepage of blood and body substances from the patient into the glove.

The scrub person should not be intimidated by politely informing the surgeon or any sterile team member of having a potentially contaminated glove. This is an important part of surgical conscience. The circulating nurse will obtain new gloves and dispense them to the sterile field. The circulator should don nonsterile gloves to remove contaminated gloves from a sterile team member.

Double-gloving is recommended for all sterile team members. The gloves do not need to be of the same variety or composition, but they both need to be sterile. The inner pair of sterile gloves should be applied using the closed-gloving method and should be a half-size larger than the outside glove to create a cushion of air. The outer sterile glove should be the wearer's normal size and can be applied using any sterile method. If available, the inner glove should be colored (i.e., blue or green) to serve as an indicator glove. The rationale is that if the outer glove gets punctured, the hole would be easier to see if color in that area were visible. Wearing two pairs of gloves in the same size can cause compression on the median nerve, resulting in carpal tunnel syndrome in susceptible people.

High-molecular-weight polyethylene orthopedic gloves resist punctures and tears. Some sterile team members wear sterile glove liners for protection from scalpel cuts or instrument tears. These do not protect the hands from needlesticks. Liners are usually worn between two pairs of sterile surgical gloves, usually a half-size larger than normal so they will not cause constriction. The liners may be made of polymer fibers or a Kevlar metal mesh. Some are disposable; others may be reprocessed and sterilized with steam or ethylene oxide.

Petrolatum-based lotions or lubricants should not be used on the hands before donning latex gloves. Hydrocarbons will penetrate latex, causing a change in its physical characteristics, including tear resistance.

Criteria for Surgical Attire

Surgical attire should be as follows:
• An effective barrier to microorganisms. Both reusable woven and disposable nonwoven materials are used. The design and composition should minimize microbial shedding.

• Made of closely woven material void of dangerous electrostatic properties. The garment should meet National Fire Protection Association standards (NFPA-56A), including resistance to flame.
• Resistant to blood, fluids, and abrasion to prevent penetration by microorganisms.
• Designed for maximum skin coverage.
• Hypoallergenic, cool, and comfortable.
• Nongenerative of lint. Lint can increase the particle count of contaminants in the OR.
• Made of a pliable material to permit freedom of movement for the practice of sterile technique.
• Able to transmit heat and water vapor to protect the wearer.
• Colored to reduce glare under lights. Various types of clothes in colorful prints that fulfill the necessary criteria are both attractive and functional.
• Easy to don and remove.

Surgical Hand Hygiene

Surgical hand hygiene (also called the surgical scrub) is the process of removing as many microorganisms as possible from the skin of the hands and arms before donning sterile surgical attire. Despite the antimicrobial component of the hand- and arm-cleansing process, skin is never rendered sterile. Consider that the tap water used in the rinse is from the public water system. This water is not sterile and can in itself grow microbial cultures. The process of surgical scrubbing is not a sterile procedure.

The scrub room is adjacent to the OR for safety and convenience. Scrub sinks with automatic sensor controls or foot- or knee-operated faucets are preferred to eliminate the hazard of contaminating the hands after hand and arm washing. Protective eyewear should be worn when performing a surgical scrub. Aerosolization from the scrub brush can cause chemicals to be dispersed into the user's eyes.

The sink should be deep, wide, and low enough to prevent splashes. Aerated faucets prevent splatter. A sterile gown cannot be donned over damp scrub attire without resultant contamination.

Scrub sinks should be used only for scrubbing or handwashing. They should not be used to clean or rinse contaminated instruments or equipment. Bioburden could inadvertently be transferred to personnel who scrub in the vicinity.

Microbiology of the Skin

The skin is inhabited by the following list of organisms:
• Transient organisms acquired by direct contact. Usually loosely attached to the skin surface, they are almost completely mechanically removed by thorough washing with soap and water.
• Resident organisms below the skin surface in hair follicles and sebaceous and sweat glands. They are more adherent and therefore more resistant to removal. Their growth is inhibited by the chemical phase of the surgical hand-cleansing process. Resident skin flora represents the microorganisms present in the hospital environment. Prolonged exposure of skin to contaminants yields a more pathogenic resident population (i.e., capable of causing infection).

Purpose of Specialized Hand Hygiene

The purpose of surgical hand and arm hygiene is to remove or deactivate soil, debris, natural skin oils, hand lotions, and transient microorganisms from the hands and forearms of sterile team members. More specifically, the purposes are as follows:

- To decrease the number of resident microorganisms on skin to an irreducible minimum
- To keep the population of microorganisms minimal during the surgical procedure by suppression of growth
- To reduce the hazard of microbial contamination of the surgical wound by skin flora

Antimicrobial Skin-Cleansing Agents

Various antimicrobial soaps are used for surgical hand cleansing. The same antiseptic agents are used for the patient's skin prep. The desirable characteristics of antimicrobial agents are as follows:

- Broad spectrum
- Fast acting and effective
- Nonirritating and nonsensitizing
- Prolonged action (i.e., leaves an antimicrobial residue on the skin to temporarily prevent growth of microorganisms)
- Independent of cumulative action

Variables in effectiveness of the antimicrobial cleansing process are bioburden, mechanical factors, chemical factors, and individual differences in skin flora. Antiseptics alter the physical or chemical properties of the cell membrane of microorganisms, thus destroying or inhibiting cellular function. Skin-cleansing agents selected by a facility should be approved by the FDA for effectiveness and safety. Many products are currently under review or have been removed or banned. More than one FDA-approved antimicrobial agent is available in the scrub room for personnel who are allergic or sensitive to a particular agent.

Chlorhexidine Gluconate

A 4% aqueous concentration of chlorhexidine gluconate (CHG) in a soap base or 0.5% in alcohol exerts an antimicrobial effect against gram-positive and gram-negative, fungal, and viral microorganisms. It reacts poorly against TB microorganisms. Antimicrobial residues bind with the stratum corneum with repeated use and produce a prolonged effect. This agent produces effective, intermediate action and cumulative reductions of resident and transient flora for more than 6 hours.

CHG is rarely irritating to the skin, but it is highly ototoxic and will irritate if splashed in the eye. It can cause permanent corneal damage. Caution should be used when scrubbing with this agent. It is an ingredient in several of the antiseptic hand gels. The alcohol-based chlorhexidine preparation is effective if the hands are coated in the solution for 20 to 30 seconds after mechanical cleansing.[4] The alcohol evaporates rapidly and has minimal odor. Personnel with reactive airway conditions should be aware of minor volatile qualities when using this product. Allow the product to dry thoroughly before donning gowns and gloves.

Iodophors

A povidone-iodine complex in detergent fulfills the criteria for an effective surgical scrub. It is available in concentrations of 10%, 7.5%, 2%, and 0.5%. Iodophors are intermediate-acting antimicrobial agents against gram-positive and gram-negative, TB, fungal, and viral microorganisms. Iodophors have minimal residual effect. Iodophors can be irritating to the skin.

Triclosan

A solution of 1% triclosan is a nonirritating, intermediate antimicrobial agent that inhibits growth of a wide range of gram-positive

and gram-negative and TB microorganisms by interruption of hormonal activity within the cell. Triclosan does not work as well against fungi. Antiviral action is unknown. It develops a prolonged cumulative suppressive action when used routinely. The agent is blended with lanolin cholesterols and petrolatum into a creamy, mild detergent. It may be used by personnel sensitive to other antiseptics, although it can be absorbed through intact skin. In 2017 the FDA banned the use of triclosan for safety reasons.[5]

It was found in many daily-use products, such as toothpaste, shampoo, and dish soap, and consequently ends up in the nation's water supply. It may play a role in antibiotic resistance. It has been found in urine and breast milk. Triclosan is no longer available in the health care setting and has been removed from consumer products. More information can be found at http://www.fda.gov/.

Alcohol

Ethyl or isopropyl alcohol (70–91.3%) is rapidly antimicrobial against all microorganisms. It is volatile and does not have residual activity. Many facilities have banned its use in the OR because it is flammable. It is nontoxic but has a drying effect on skin. Alcohol preparations, usually in foam, contain emollients to minimize drying. If dispensers are used, they must be away from the sterile field or any ignition source. If other agents cannot be used because of skin sensitivity, mechanical cleansing with soap to remove transient organisms may be followed by cleansing with an alcohol-based skin cleanser.

Parachlorometaxylenol

Used in a concentration of 1% to 3.75%, parachlorometaxylenol (PCMX) does not substantially reduce microorganisms immediately. It does not produce sustained residual activity. Its antimicrobial activity can be altered significantly by the composition of the antiseptic product. Efficacy data should be reviewed before these products are used for surgical scrubs.

Opening the Gown and Gloves

The scrub person wears all the appropriate attire for the restricted area before entering the OR (i.e., scrub suit, head cover, eye protection, and mask). The gown and gloves must be opened before performing surgical hand hygiene. The double-wrapped gown package contains one sterile folded gown and towel. The outer wrap is a peel pouch, and the inner wrap is envelope style. The gown is folded inside out to facilitate donning. The folded gown resembles a thick book with the main fold as its binding. A folded woven fabric or disposable paper towel for drying the hands is packed on top of the gown. The towel is folded into a square or rectangle with one corner turned down for ease of grasping without disturbing the entire gown-towel assembly.

The gown package is opened before the glove package on a separate surface from the main sterile field. The gown inner wrapper is removed from the peel pouch and is used to create a temporary sterile field of its own. It is inappropriate for the scrub person establishing the sterile field to gown and glove off the main sterile field.

The gloves are double-wrapped in a peel pouch and folded paper. The peel pouch is opened and the paper-wrapped gloves can be dispensed to the side of the gown on the inner aspect of the sterile gown wrapper. Do not dispense on top of the towel. The glove wrapper can be contaminated when reaching for the towel with wet hands. Ideally, if another surface is available, the glove wrapper can be opened in its entirety to fashion a temporary sterile area for the purpose of donning the gloves.

Preparations Immediately Before Surgical Hand Hygiene

1. The skin and nails should be kept clean and in good condition, and the cuticles should be uncut. If hand lotion is used to protect the skin, a non–oil-based product is recommended. Oil can weaken the integrity of gloves.
2. Fingernails should not reach beyond the fingertips to avoid glove puncture.
3. Fingernail polishes, gels, lacquers, and UV-cured polishes should not be chipped or cracked. More studies on UV-cured polishes and gels need to be done to determine if they can withstand the surgical scrub. Freshly applied polish may be worn if permitted by facility policy.
4. Artificial nails and decals harbor microorganisms such as bacteria and fungi and are inappropriate for scrub personnel.
5. All jewelry is removed from the fingers, wrists, and neck. Jewelry harbors microorganisms.
6. All hair should be covered by headwear. Pierced-ear studs should be contained by the head cover because they are a potential foreign body in the surgical site. A quick look in the mirror by the scrub sink to be sure all hair is secured helps prevent infection.
7. Adjust the disposable mask snugly and comfortably over the nose and mouth.
8. Clean your eyeglasses if they are to be worn. Adjust and secure protective eyewear or the face shield comfortably in relation to the mask and eyeglasses.
9. Adjust water to a comfortable temperature. Cooler water helps minimize dry skin. Hot water can increase chafing by degreasing the skin.

Surgical Hand and Arm Scrub With a Brush

When arriving in the surgical department for the day, the first hand cleansing should be a brush scrub, either timed or a counted brushstroke method. When an individual scrubs with a brush and antimicrobial agent the soap decreases the surface tension of the skin, thus permitting the shed cells to be rinsed away with the tap water. Care is taken to avoid scrubbing longer than 3 to 5 minutes because skin can become abraded and release microorganisms from hair follicles.

In surgical scrubbing with a brush, antiseptic soap, and water the skin is cleansed of microorganisms using the following two properties:
1. *Mechanical:* The mechanical properties remove soil and transient organisms with friction. Nails are cleaned under running water with a nail pick.
2. *Chemical:* The chemical properties reduce resident flora and inactivate microorganisms with an antimicrobial or antiseptic agent.

Debris should be removed from the subungual area of each finger. Single-use disposable products are a brush-sponge combination with an enclosed nail-cleaning pick. Some brushes are individually packaged and impregnated with antiseptic-detergent agents. Additional antiseptic solution is dispensed onto the brush or sponge by a foot pedal from a container adjacent to the sink. Six drops (approximately 2–3 mL) of solution is sufficient to generate a lather for the scrub procedure. Waste of antiseptic solution should be avoided.

A timed or counted brushstroke method can be used to scrub the hands and arms. A vigorous 2 to 5-minute scrub with a reliable agent is effective. A counted brushstroke method is equally effective in decreasing the microbial count on the skin. Prolonged scrubbing raises resident microbes from deep dermal layers and is therefore counterproductive. Care should be taken not to abrade the skin during the scrub process. Denuded areas allow the entry of microorganisms. Too short a scrub may be equally ineffectual.

Every member of the surgical team should scrub according to a standardized written procedure. The time required may be based on the manufacturer's recommendations for the agent used and documentation of the product's efficacy in the scientific literature. A copy of the procedure should be posted in every scrub room.

Subsequent scrubs should follow the same procedure as the initial scrub of the day. When gloves are removed at the end of the surgical procedure, the hands are considered contaminated and should be immediately washed with soap and water. Resident microorganisms multiply rapidly in the warm, moist environment under the gloves.

Personnel who scrub should think of their fingers, hands, and arms as having four sides or surfaces. Both methods (timed and counted brushstroke) follow an anatomic pattern of scrubbing: the four surfaces of each finger, beginning with the thumb and moving from one finger to the next, down the outer edge of the fifth finger, over the dorsal (back) surface of the hand, then the palmar (palm) surface of the hand, or vice versa, from the small finger to the thumb, over the wrists and up the arm, in thirds, ending 2 inches (5 cm) above the elbow. Because the hands are in most direct contact with the sterile field, all steps of the scrub procedure begin with cleaning the fingernails and hands and end above the elbows.

During and after scrubbing, keep the hands higher than the elbows to allow water and suds to flow from the cleanest area—the hands—to the marginal area of the upper arms. Take care not to slip in water that may have dripped to the floor during the process. A waterproof mat is suggested in front of the sink.

Surgical Hand Hygiene With Antiseptic Rub

In an antiseptic hand rub method the antimicrobial chemical properties of the agent kill microorganisms. Antiseptic hand gels, lotions, and foams do not use mechanical action or friction. There is no water rinse to physically remove microorganisms; the main action is chemical. The antiseptic does not remove debris from under the nails and hands.

That is why a simple handwashing and drying is recommended by AORN to remove gross soil before using a surgical hand cleansing agent.

Many rub-type surgical skin cleansers have a lasting antimicrobial effect for several hours after application. The coating of the antiseptic agent on the skin should be rubbed in evenly without clumps in the crook of the elbows or between the fingers. The agent is alcohol based and should be completely dry before donning the sterile gown and gloves. The material should not be wiped off the skin, and the hands and arms should not be waved through the air in a drying motion. Air currents cause particulates in the environment to disperse throughout the restricted area.

Most brushless cleansing agents have an alcohol base with an antimicrobial ingredient such as CHG. Care is taken to allow the agent to completely dry before donning the sterile gown and gloves. All products of this nature should be used as directed by the manufacturer. Each product has a specific application process and drying protocol.

Gowning and Gloving

The sterile gown is put on after drying the hands and arms with a sterile towel, immediately after the surgical hand and arm hygiene. The hands and arms must be dry before donning the sterile gown. The sterile gloves are put on immediately after gowning using the closed-glove technique described in the next section.

Purpose

A sterile gown and gloves are worn to exclude skin as a possible contaminant and create a barrier between the sterile and nonsterile areas. The gown protects the patient and the wearer from cross-contamination.

General Considerations

1. The scrub person gowns and gloves from a surface separate from the main sterile field using the closed-gloving method and then gowns and gloves the surgeon and the rest of the sterile team using the open-assisted or closed-assisted gloving method.
2. Gown packages preferably are opened on a separate table from other packages to avoid any chance of contamination from dripping water.
3. Splashing water on scrub attire during the surgical scrub should be avoided because moisture may contaminate the sterile gown.

Drying the Hands and Arms

The hands and arms are dried as follows:
1. Reach down to the opened sterile gown package and pick up the towel with one hand by one corner. Be careful not to drip water onto the pack because contamination may occur. Be sure no one is within arm's reach (Fig. 16.9). Be aware of the environment to prevent contamination.
2. Grasp the opposing corner of the towel with the other hand and open the towel full length. Use one end of the towel to dry one hand and arm. Use a circumferential motion to rub in one direction from hand to upper arm. Do not rub back and forth (Fig. 16.10). Bend slightly forward to avoid letting the towel touch the attire.
3. To dry the second arm, hold the dry, clean end of the towel in the opposite hand and use a circumferential motion to dry the hand and all areas of the arm to the elbow.

4. Discard the towel with the hand that is currently holding it without letting it touch the scrub suit. Do not wad the used towel and toss it across the room to the laundry hamper or trash.

Gowning and Gloving Techniques

The scrub person will don the gown before the gloves. The scrub person may don gloves in one of two ways: by the closed-gloving technique or by the open-gloving technique. The closed-gloving method is preferred for establishing the initial sterile field by the scrub person. Properly executed, the closed-gloving method ensures against contamination when donning gloves; no bare skin is exposed in the process because the bare hands do not extend through the cuffs of the gown.

The open-gloving method is used when changing a glove during a surgical procedure or when donning gloves for procedures not requiring gowns. The assisted open-gloving technique is used by the scrub person to help other sterile team members don gowns and gloves before entering the sterile field.

Gowning Self

1. Reach down to the sterile pack and lift the folded gown directly upward (Fig. 16.11). This is like picking up a book by its binding. Take care not to touch the sterile gown

• **Fig. 16.10** Scrub person, holding towel away from body, dries only scrubbed areas, starting with hands. They avoid contaminating hands on areas proximal to elbows and then discard towel.

• **Fig. 16.9** Scrub person preparing to gown removes the hand towel on top of gown from open package.

• **Fig. 16.11** Scrub person, picking up gown below neck edge, lifts it directly upward and steps away to avoid touching the edge of the wrapper. Note that inside of wrapper covers the table. Gown is folded inside out.

wrapper because the sterile gloves will be opened completely on this surface after the gown is donned.

2. Step back and away from the table into an unobstructed area to provide a wide margin of safety while gowning to prevent contamination.

3. Holding the folded gown like a book by its binding, carefully locate the neckline and the armholes.

4. Holding the inside front of the gown just at the armholes with both hands, let the gown unfold, keeping the inside of the gown toward the body and the hands in the armholes. Do not touch the outside of the gown with bare hands. If the top of the gown drops downward inadvertently, discard the gown as contaminated. Never reverse a sterile gown if the wrong end is dropped toward the floor.

5. Extend both arms into the armholes simultaneously as the gown and its sleeves unfold (Fig. 16.12).

6. The circulating nurse, standing behind the scrub, brings the gown over the shoulders by reaching inside to the shoulder and arm seams. The gown is pulled on, leaving the cuffs of the sleeves extended over the hands. Do not push the hands through the cuffs. The back of the gown is securely tied at the waist first, followed by the neckline. The circulating nurse takes care not to pull the gown so snug that the cuffs are pulled back and expose the hands (Fig. 16.13).

If the gown is wraparound style, the sterile flap to cover the back is not touched until the scrub person has donned the gloves. A sterile gown may be wrapped around for a "tie-in" in various ways:

1. *Reusable gown:* The wraparound ties are secured to the front of the gown by a single hitch knot. With sterile gloved hands, pull the knot open. Take the longer right tie in the right hand and the shorter left tie in the left hand. Hold onto the left tie. Hand the long right tie to a sterile team member who remains stationary.

Allowing a margin of safety, turn around toward the left, thereby completely covering the back with the extended flap of the gown. Take the long right tie from the sterile person and tie it to the short left tie on the left side of the gown. Do not place the long right tie under an object on the sterile field to tie yourself in. This causes the back to be turned to the field. It is best to have a sterile person tie you in.

2. *Disposable gown:* The ends of the wraparound ties are covered by a disposable paper tag. Disengage the left short tie from the tag with the left hand. Hold onto the left tie. The tag will remain attached to the long right tie. Hand the tag with the right tie still attached to the circulating nurse, taking care to protect the hands and not disconnect the tag (Fig. 16.14). Turn toward the left, closing the gown flap in the back. Grasp the long right tie about 4 to 6 inches from the tag that the circulating nurse is holding, and pull the tie out of the paper tag. The circulating nurse discards the tag. Tie the long right tie to the short left tie at the side of the gown.

Do not have the circulating nurse walk in front of the gown to wrap around. Do not turn the back to the sterile field.

3. If either of the ties drops at any time, the circulating nurse retrieves both ties and secures them behind the scrubbed person's back because the dropped tie has fallen below the level of the sterile field and is contaminated.

Closed-Gloving Technique

During the closed-gloving process the scrub person keeps the hands inside the cuffs of the sterile gown. At first this seems tricky, but with practice the technique will become more refined and quick. Remember to keep the hands inside the cuffs at all times. In this explanation the left hand is gloved first. This is a mirror

• **Fig. 16.12** Scrub person, putting on gown, gently allows the gown to unfold away from body and then slips arms into sleeves without touching sterile outside of the gown with bare hands.

• **Fig. 16.13** Circulating nurse ties the inner waist ties of the sterile gown.

• **Fig. 16.14** The circulating nurse ties in the sterile scrub person. The scrub person hands the paper tag that holds the long right wraparound tie to the circulating nurse while holding the shorter left tie. The nurse walks behind the scrub person and passes the long sterile tie to the scrub person without touching anything but the removable paper tag.

image of the instructor's demonstration. Either hand can be gloved first when establishing the sterile field.

1. If the gloves are still in the folded inner paper wrapper, they need to be opened. Using the cuff-covered hands, place the wrapper in front of you like a book. Open the two sides. There is an inner fold to the glove wrapper. With two cuff-covered hands grasp the lower inner corners of the bottom fold. Lift both corners open and fold under at the same time. When this method is used the wrapper will remain open and not fall closed during the gloving process (Fig. 16.15).

2. Extend the left forearm with the palm upward (supinated).
3. With the cuff-covered right hand, pick up the left glove from the inner wrap of the glove package by grasping the fingers, lifting straight up, and placing the glove on the left palm thumb side down. The glove fingers will be pointing toward the body (Fig. 16.16, *A*).
4. Grasp the edges of the glove cuff with the cuffed right hand and the opposite edge with the cuffed left hand. Peel the glove over the left cuffed hand, over the end of the left sleeve, and wiggle the fingers to extend them into the glove-covered left

• **Fig. 16.15** Closed Gloving. The scrub person opens the glove wrapper on a sterile field with hands contained inside sleeves and cuffs. **A,** Primary one-fourth fold. **B,** Secondary one-half fold. **C,** Open folded wrapper is labeled "right" and "left." Gently pull lower wrapper flap down. **D,** Grasp inner corner of the wrapper and pull open. **E,** Fold bottom flap under the glove wrapper to hold the paper open.

• **Fig. 16.16** Closed Gloving. The hands remain within the cuffs at all times. **A,** Grasp the fingers of the first glove with the opposite cuffed hand and flip directly over onto the wrist of the supinated hand. **B,** Grasp the upper side and undersides of the glove cuff and begin to pull the glove over the first cuffed hand. Work the fingers into the glove until it is fully on the hand. The white part of the first cuff must be completely covered. **C,** With the sterile gloved hand grasp the fingers of the second glove and directly flip it onto the second cuffed hand. **D,** Grasp the upper and undersides of the glove and pull it up and over the second cuff.

hand (Fig. 16.16, *B*). The cuff of the left glove is now over the stockinette cuff of the gown, with the hand still inside the sleeve.

5. Grasp the cuff of the left glove and underlying left gown sleeve with the covered right hand. Pull the glove on over the extended left fingers until it completely covers the stockinette cuff.

6. Glove the right hand in the same manner, reversing hands. Use the sterile gloved left hand to grasp the fingers of the right glove and position the glove on the right forearm (Fig. 16.16, *C*). Be sure that the entire cuff of each sleeve is contained within the sterile glove (Fig. 16.16, *D*).

Open-Gloving Technique

Gowning for the open-gloving method is the same as for the closed-gloving method. The only difference is that the scrubbed person extends the hands all the way through the cuffs and sleeves. The hands are totally exposed outside the cuffs (Fig. 16.17). This method is not preferred for the person establishing the sterile field but is used when changing a contaminated glove. In this explanation the left hand is gloved first. This is a mirror image of the instructor's demonstration. Either hand can be gloved first.

• **Fig. 16.17** Open Gloving. The scrub person's hands are exposed through the cuffs. The circulating nurse ties the inner back of the gown.

The open-gloving method uses a skin-to-skin, glove-to-glove technique. The hand, although scrubbed, is not sterile and must not contact the exterior of the sterile gloves. The everted cuff on the gloves exposes the inner surfaces. The first glove is put on with the skin-to-skin technique, bare hand to inside cuff. The sterile fingers of that gloved hand then may touch the sterile exterior of the second glove (i.e., glove-to-glove technique).

The procedure is as follows:

1. With the right hand, grasp the inner edge of the cuff of the left glove and lift from the wrapper (Fig. 16.18, *A*). Take care not to touch the inner aspect of the wrapper or the sterile exterior portions of the glove.
2. Align the fingers of the left hand and insert the hand into the glove, pulling it on, leaving the cuff turned well down over the hand. Be sure to keep the thumb adducted into the palm of the hand until it is well inside the confines of the glove. Do not adjust the cuff. This will be done as a last step.
3. Slip the fingers of the sterile gloved left hand under the everted right cuff, on the sterile side of the right glove (Fig 16.18, *B*). Pick up the glove, then step back.
4. Align the fingers of the right hand and insert the hand into the right glove, keeping the thumb adducted until well inside the glove. Pull the right glove on all the way, unfolding the cuff, and enclosing the knitted right cuff at the wrist (Fig 16.18, *C*).
5. With the sterile gloved fingers of the right hand, pull the cuff of the left glove up and over the knitted cuff of the sleeve. Avoid touching the bare wrist. Sterile surfaces may touch only sterile surfaces (Fig 16.18, *D*).

Assisted Gowning and Gloving of a Team Member

A team member in sterile gown and gloves, usually the scrub person, may assist the surgeon or another team member in gowning and gloving by taking the following steps:

1. Open the hand towel and lay one end on the freshly scrubbed team member's right hand, being careful not to touch the hand.

Do not hand a towel from a bloody back table or hand a towel with contaminated gloves or any instrument from the active sterile field. The biologic contamination is a hazard. The circulating nurse can open a separate gown and towel package for additional persons who need to enter the sterile field. Each person can pick up their own towel from the opened package. The scrub person can help with the remaining gowning and gloving procedure without touching any surface of the gown or gloves that would come in contact with the wearer's skin or clothing.

2. Lift the gown and unfold it carefully with the sterile outside toward you and the unsterile inside toward the person being gowned, holding it open at the shoulders and neckline by cuffing over the hands (Fig. 16.19).

• **Fig. 16.18** Open Gloving. **A,** The wrapper is opened without touching the inner surface. The first inner glove cuff is grasped without touching the sterile surface and slid over the first hand. The first cuff remains folded. **B,** The first gloved hand is slid into the second cuff on the sterile surface. **C,** The second glove is applied all the way up and over the knitted cuff. **D,** The first cuff is now pulled over the knitted cuff.

• **Fig. 16.19** Gowning a team member by holding the armholes open and protecting hands inside sterile surface of the gown.

Do not hand a gown from a back table when the case is in progress. The drapes and gowns on the field in progress are considered biologically contaminated and could contaminate the wearer.

3. Keeping your hands on the sterile side of the gown under a protective cuff of the neck and shoulder area, offer the inside of the gown for the team member to don. They slip their arms into the sleeves. Take care not to let the sleeves make contact with unsterile areas.
4. Release the gown when it is secured by the person being gowned. The team member holds arms outstretched while the circulating nurse pulls the gown onto the shoulders and adjusts the sleeves so that the cuffs are properly slid back to expose the hands for open-assisted gloving. If the closed-assisted method is preferred, the person being gowned will keep the hands within the knitted cuffs. The circulating nurse touches only the inside of the gown at the seams and secures the gown at the back.

Gloving a Team Member

1. Offer the right glove first. Pick up the right glove, grasping it firmly with the fingers of both hands under the everted cuff on the sterile side. Hold the palm of the glove toward the person being gloved.
2. Stretch the cuff sufficiently open to allow for passage of the right hand. Avoid touching the hand by holding your thumbs out (abducted) (Fig. 16.20).
3. Exert upward pressure as the person slides the hand into the glove. Do not allow the hand to drop below the level of the sterile field.
4. Pull the glove cuff up and over the knitted cuff of the right sleeve. Enclose the entire cuff.
5. Repeat for the left hand. The person being gloved can facilitate the process by supinating the gloved right hand and flexing the fingers like a hook to hold open the cuff of the glove being donned.
6. If a sterile vest is needed, hold it for the surgeon to slip the hands into the armholes. Be careful not to contaminate the gloves at the neck level. If the gown is a wraparound, assist the person to tie it. Remember that the back of the gown is not considered sterile even if a sterile vest is worn. The back is not considered sterile because it is not in the field of vision of the sterile team.

• **Fig. 16.20** Gloving a team member by open-assisted method.

• **Fig. 16.21** Sequence of Scrub Person Removing Soiled Gown at End of Surgical Procedure. The gown is removed before the gloves. Clean arms and scrub suit are protected from contamination outside of gown. Do not reach behind the gown to untie the back strings. Have someone untie the back. **A,** With gloves on, grasp the front shoulder of gown and pull forward. **B,** In pulling gown off arms, make sure that gown sleeve is turned inside out to prevent contamination of scrub attire. **C,** The other shoulder is grasped with the other hand, and the gown is removed entirely by pulling it off inside out and rolling it away from body.

Removing or Changing Contaminated Gown and Gloves

Occasionally a contaminated gown must be changed during a surgical procedure. This means that both gown and gloves must be removed and changed. The circulating nurse obtains sterile gowns and gloves for personnel needing to change. The gown is always removed first, followed by the gloves. The contaminated team member steps away from the field and unties the wrap-around tie, and the circulating nurse unfastens the neck and the inner back tie of the soiled gown. The contaminated person grasps the front of the gown at the shoulders below the neckline (Fig. 16.21, *A*). The gown is pulled off inside out by the wearer and rolled off away from the body (Fig. 16.21, *B and C*).

The gloves are removed using a glove-to-glove and then skin-to-skin technique. The cuffs of the gloves usually turn down as the gown is pulled off the arms. A glove-to-glove and then skin-to-skin technique is used to protect the clean hands from the contaminated outside of the gloves, which bear blood and body fluid of the patient (Fig. 16.22). The gloves are removed as follows:

1. Grasp the cuff of the left glove with the gloved fingers of the right hand, and pull it completely off inside out.

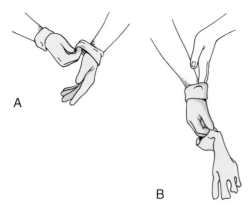

• **Fig. 16.22** Scrub person removing the contaminated gloves.

2. Slip the ungloved fingers of the left hand under the cuff of the right glove, and slip it off inside out.
3. Both gloves will be inside out to contain the contamination. Discard the gloves in a biohazard trash receptacle.
4. Wash hands. Gloves are never 100% impervious.

This is the same manner in which a gown and gloves are removed at completion of the surgical procedure. Contaminated gowns and gloves are disposed of immediately in the appropriate biohazard receptacle.

When a sterile team member becomes contaminated during a case, rescrubbing is not necessary to regown and reglove to reenter the sterile field. If only a sleeve is contaminated, a sterile sleeve may be put on over the contaminated one. If the person is not planning to reenter the sterile field, they should wash their hands immediately after removing the gloves.

Managing Contaminated Gloves or Objects During the Surgical Procedure

Contamination of the gown and gloves depends on the nature of contamination and whether the scrub person is double gloved. Any puncture of a glove requires a complete glove change, even if double gloved. The puncturing instrument is passed off to the circulating nurse.

Contamination When Wearing Two Sets of Gloves

The contaminated outer glove can be removed, leaving the sterile under glove intact. A new second pair of gloves can be applied over the remaining gloves. If the nature of the contamination is a puncture, both sets of gloves are considered contaminated and must be removed. Regloving is accomplished by the open-gloving method.

Contamination When Wearing a Single Set of Gloves

A second glove can be applied over the top of a superficially contaminated glove by using the open-gloving method. If covering with a second glove is not possible, the contaminated glove must be changed immediately. If stepping away immediately is not feasible, the contaminated hand and any object involved in the contamination should be held away from the sterile field for the circulating nurse to remove.

The glove is changed as follows:

1. Turn away from the sterile field and request a new pair of sterile gloves from the circulating nurse. Regloving should take place on a surface separate from the main sterile field.
2. Extend the contaminated hand to the circulating nurse who, wearing protective gloves, grasps the contaminated objects and sets them aside. The circulating nurse then grasps the outside of the contaminated glove cuff about 2 inches (5 cm) below the top of the glove, closer toward the palm, and pulls off the glove inside out. The scrubbed person can scrunch the palm of the hand to make grabbing the glove easier for the circulating nurse. Care is taken not to snap the glove, creating an aerosol. If the nurse tries to grasp the cuff of the glove, the gown can be contaminated.
3. Preferably, a sterile team member gloves another. If this is not possible, step aside and glove the hand using the open-gloving technique.

The closed-gloving technique is inappropriate for a glove change during a surgical procedure because contamination of the new glove by the porous cuff of a gown in use is inevitable. The hand will be contaminated by the knitted cuff of the gown, which has absorbed body sweat. The contaminated cuff may not be pulled down over the hand because the cuff is contaminated by shed skin cells. Using the cuff to perform closed gloving will contaminate the fresh gloves.

The only way closed gloving is acceptable is for the scrub person to remove both the contaminated gown and gloves and another sterile gown is donned before regloving using the closed-gloving method. The scrub person should change their own gloves before gowning and gloving another team member to avoid exposing the team member to contamination.

ⓔ EVOLVE WEBSITE

http://evolve.elsevier.com/Hornacky/BerryKohn/
- Historical Perspective
- Student Interactive Questions
- Glossary

References

1. AORN: Periop briefing: laundering scrubs outside the home, *J AORN* 12, 2023.
2. Centers for Disease Control and Prevention: *Protect your family: reduce contamination at home.* www.cdc.gov. Accessed April 20, 2023.
3. Lucero S, Dryden M: Antisepsis, asepsis and skin preparation, *Surgery* 37(1):45–50, 2019.
4. Centers for Disease Control and Prevention: *Hand hygiene in the health care setting.* www.cdc.gov. Accessed April 23, 2023.
5. U.S. Food and Drug Administration: *Safety and effectiveness of health care antiseptics; topical antimicrobial drug products for over-the-counter human use.* (A rule by the FDA, 2017). www.fda.gov. Accessed April 24, 2023.

Bibliography

AORN: *Guidelines for perioperative practice,* Denver, CO, 2024, The Association.
Phillips NM, Hornacky A: *Pass CNOR,* St. Louis, 2019, Elsevier.

17

Decontamination and Disinfection

CHAPTER OUTLINE

Central Processing Department, 296

Central Service Personnel, 296

Instrument Cleaning and Decontamination, 297

Disinfection of Items Used in Patient Care, 301

Methods of Disinfection, 302

Disposable Products, 309

CHAPTER OBJECTIVES

After studying this chapter the learner will be able to:

- Describe the steps in decontamination.
- List Spaulding's classifications of patient care items.
- Compare and contrast the three levels of disinfection.

- Discuss how an instrument is rendered safe for handling.
- Identify three safety issues associated with the use of chemical disinfectants.

KEY TERMS AND DEFINITIONS

Bactericide Kills gram-negative and gram-positive bacteria unless specifically stated to the contrary (adj: bactericidal). Action may be specific to a species of bacteria.

Bacteriostatic Inhibits growth of bacteria.

Bioburden Degree of microbial load on an item before sterilization.

Biofilm Microbial load attached to a surface in a fluid environment. Microbes in slime adhere to surfaces of all kinds of moist material, such as implantable metals, plastics, and tissue, causing antibiotic resistance. Difficult to remove.

Decontamination Process by which chemical or physical agents are used to clean inanimate, noncritical surfaces. A specific contact time is not specified. A low-level disinfectant is commonly used for this purpose. If a known organism, such as hepatitis B virus (HBV), *Mycobacterium tuberculosis* (TB), or human immunodeficiency virus (HIV), is present on the surface, an intermediate-level disinfectant should be used.

Deionized water Water that has been processed through synthetic cation-anion resins to remove the positively or negatively charged ions.

Disinfection Chemical or physical process of destroying most forms of pathogenic microorganisms except bacterial endospores; used for inanimate objects but not on tissue. The degree of disinfection depends primarily on the strength of the agent, the nature of the contamination, and the purpose for the process.

Distilled water The process of evaporating water and creating condensation from the steam that is collected for future use.

Endospore Protective capsule that forms inside specific bacterial species (class Clostridia and genus *Bacillus*) to protect the genetic matter from destructive forces, such as disinfection or sterilization.

Enzymatic cleaner Protease product used to remove organic protein material from surgical instruments before disinfection.

Fungicide Kills fungi.

High-level disinfection Process that destroys all microorganisms except high numbers of bacterial endospores.

Intermediate-level disinfection Process that inactivates vegetative bacteria, including *M. tuberculosis*, and most fungi and viruses but does not kill bacterial endospores.

Low-level disinfection Process that kills most bacteria, some viruses, and some fungi but does not destroy resistant microorganisms such as *M. tuberculosis* or bacterial endospores.

Pasteurization Not a method of sterilization. This heating process kills many pathogenic microorganisms that are found in biosubstances such as milk or wine.

Sporicide Kills endospores.

Virucide Kills viruses.

Central Processing Department

Workflow in the Processing Areas

The central service (CS) personnel work within confined areas in a specialized department. Each CS worker has a specified set of duties based on infection control parameters of the facility. The surgical services central processing department (CPD or SPD) is located close to the main surgical suite to minimize the potential for cross-contamination between soiled and clean instruments and supplies. The CPD is composed of the decontamination area, set assembly room, sterile processing, sterile storage, and case cart packing room.

The CPD is set up to receive soiled instruments through one entrance, the decontamination room. The soiled instruments are delivered by the surgical personnel to the CPD covered and contained to prevent dispersal of microorganisms along the traffic pattern. Some facilities use elevators or dumbwaiters to transport soiled instrumentation.

CS personnel, wearing the appropriate personal protective equipment (PPE), are responsible for cleaning instruments and equipment in the decontamination area and do not enter areas where cleaned instruments are stored, packaged, or sterilized. Care is taken to ensure that sharps and contaminated disposables are discarded into the proper puncture-proof containers per facility policy.

The CS decontamination personnel have specialized training in cleaning many types of instruments using several methods, as described later in this chapter. The decontamination process renders soiled instruments safe for handling but not safe for patient use. After decontamination the cleaned instruments are transferred via a pass-through door to the instrument set assembly room. Some facilities have a conveyor system that automatically sends the cleaned items to the clean assembly area after passing through the washer.

The CS personnel in the clean set assembly room organize the instruments into standardized trays according to tray inventory sheets. Some assembly rooms have computerized scanning equipment to track instruments through bar codes and validate set contents. Most facilities have computerized instrument count sheets that correspond to the contents of the tray. A copy of the count sheet accompanies the assembled tray as it is wrapped or packed into a closed container for sterilization. CS personnel in the clean area also operate the sterilizers and place the sterilized trays in the sterile storage area until they are needed for use.

When a tray is needed for a surgical procedure, other CS personnel in the sterile storage area pack a case cart with the necessary sterile tray and supplies for the surgical team. The case cart exits the CPD through a separate door that has no communication with the decontamination area. Detailed information concerning sterilization is found in Chapter 18.

Central Service Personnel

CS personnel entrusted with the care, cleaning, assembly, and processing of patient care equipment to the appropriate degree of safety require specific training and credentialing. Training entails learning about thousands of surgical instruments and their care. CS personnel need to know and understand all methods of instrument processing such as decontamination, disinfection, and sterilization. The role of the CS technician requires attention to detail.

Credentialing of Central Service Personnel

New Jersey, New York, Connecticut, and Tennessee require certification for CS personnel. Personnel currently holding positions in CS are required to become certified. New hires will have 2 years from the date of hire to attain the credential as recommended by the Association for the Advancement of Medical Instrumentation (AAMI). Training programs take between 6 and 12 months to complete. There are two recognized organizations for CS certification. AAMI sets the standards for instrument processing in the United States and recognizes both certifying bodies.

The Healthcare Sterile Processing Association (HSPA), formerly known as the International Association of Healthcare Central Service Material Management (IAHCSMM), is driving the effort to require mandatory standardization of education and certification of all CS personnel. Information about CS certification requirements via HSPA can be found at http://www.myhspa.org/.[1]

Certification signifies that an individual professional has attained specific knowledge and skill in a specific professional practice. It sets a standard for performance and raises the bar for expectations in the profession. Successful passage of the certification examination is represented by the certified registered central service technician (CRCST) designation after the name of the CS employee. HSPA offers short-term 1-year certification at four levels: (1) technician, (2) instrument processing, (3) leadership, and (4) vendor certification.[1]

The Certification Board of Sterile Processing and Distribution (CBSPD) is an international sterile processing certification examination program accredited by the National Commission for Certifying Agencies (NCCA) offered four times per year. The examination is offered only in English. CBSPD offers six levels of certification: (1) technician, (2) supervisor and manager, (3) flexible endoscope reprocessor, (4) surgical instrument processor, (5) ambulatory surgery, and (6) surgical instrument specialist.

CBSPD certification eligibility requires one of the following: 12 months of employment in the role or completion of a formal central processing course with a passing grade of 70% or higher. Successful candidates earn the certified sterile processing and distribution technician (CSPDT) credential. Certification is valid for 5 years and can be renewed through reexamination or by continuing education, attaining 100 to 150 points through education or work experience. Information about certification of CS personnel can be found at www.cbspd.net.

Becoming certified encourages individuals to seek additional training that exemplifies certification-level knowledge. Periodic competency testing should be incorporated into performance assessment. (An example of CS personnel competency testing can be found at http://www.apic.org/.)

Coordination of Central Service Staff and Operating Room Staff

The relationship between CS staff and operating room (OR) staff is complex and synergistic. The OR staff relies on the CS staff to provide complete instrumentation processed to the appropriate degree of safety for patient use. The CS staff relies on the OR staff to return used sets in a safe-to-process condition without concealed blades or other sharps that pose a risk for injury during preparation for processing. Each person has a stake in the intricate coordination of preparing for a surgical procedure. Mutual respect and cooperation between the two specialty areas is in the best interest of safe and efficient patient care.

Instrument Cleaning and Decontamination

Decontamination of instrumentation is performed in a designated area by specially trained personnel immediately after completion of the surgical procedure. The scrub person can facilitate the instrument decontamination process by wiping instruments as they are used on the sterile field and then opening the instruments completely before placing in a tray for return to the processing area. This is referred to as *point-of-use cleaning*. An approved enzymatic cleaner such as a foam or solution can be applied to the instruments to prevent debris drying during transport to the CS area. All instruments on the table during a surgical procedure require decontamination before processing to the required level of safety for patient use. The processing of endoscopes is discussed in Chapter 32.

Decontamination combines mechanical or manual cleaning and a physical or chemical microbicidal process. Prerinsing, washing, rinsing, and disinfecting/sterilizing are done in the processing department to render the instrumentation safe for handling by CS personnel. This part of the process is referred to as *thorough cleaning* or *return-to-use cleaning*.

After the formal decontamination process, instrumentation is assembled into sets by the CS technician and processed either by sterilization or disinfection (high level, intermediate level, or low level) for use by the OR staff in patient care. Methods and procedures for decontamination and disinfection vary according to the item to be processed and the recommended agent used in processing. Personal protective equipment (PPE) should be worn while using chemical disinfecting agents.

Prerinsing/Presoaking

The purpose of prerinsing or presoaking is to prevent blood and debris from drying on instruments or to soften and remove dried blood and debris. The circulating nurse can prepare a basin or plastic bin (with a cover) of enzymatic solution for the scrub person. For a short immersion period, instruments may be presoaked in the following list of agents and solutions:

- A triple proteolytic enzymatic detergent. Proteolytic enzymes dissolve blood and debris, and the detergent removes dissolved particulate from the surfaces of instruments, including otherwise inaccessible areas such as lumens.
- An enzymatic agent diluted per manufacturer's instructions.
- Water with a low-sudsing, near-neutral detergent. The detergent should be compatible with the local water supply.
- Plain, clean, demineralized distilled water.
- Sodium hypochlorite (chlorine bleach) is corrosive; however, it is used as a presoak in suspected or potential prion disease such as transmissible spongiform encephalopathy (TSE). Instruments should not be soaked in any chlorine compound for more than 1 hour and should not be autoclaved with chlorine solution because of the formation of toxic chlorine gas.
- Soaking in a phenolic or sodium hydroxide is an alternative, but chlorine bleach is the most reliable in reducing the prion titer within 1 hour. These chemicals are extremely corrosive and are not appropriate for use on endoscopes.

Prerinsing or presoaking instruments with an enzymatic solution in the OR can make further processing more efficient. The soaking solution should be disposed of, if possible, before transport to eliminate the possibility of spillage and contamination. Instruments should not be cleaned in scrub sinks or utility sinks in the substerile room. Instruments transported in an enzymatic soak solution should be transported to the processing department in a covered container that is leak and puncture proof. The container should be labeled biohazard and easily identified.

Manual Cleaning

If a washer-sterilizer or washer-decontaminator is not available, instruments are washed by hand in the processing area. The purpose of manual cleaning is to remove residual blood and debris before terminal sterilization or high-level disinfection.

Delicate and sharp instruments should be handled separately and processed according to the manufacturer's instructions. Complex instruments require complete disassembly before cleaning. Other instruments require special care. For example, the outside surfaces of powered instruments must be cleaned, but these instruments cannot be immersed in liquid. Some powered equipment requires lubrication as part of the cleaning process.

Personnel in the processing area wear PPE such as caps, gloves, waterproof aprons, shoe coverings, and face shields to prevent accidental spray from contaminated body fluids and chemical cleaning solutions.

The following steps should be observed when cleaning instruments manually:
1. Fill the washing sink with clean, warm water to which a noncorrosive, neutral pH, low-sudsing, free-rinsing detergent has been added.
   a. Detergent should be compatible with the local water supply. The mineral content of water varies from one region to another; a water softener may be used in the system routinely to minimize mineral deposits. Regardless of the water content, the detergent should be anionic or nonionic and have a pH as close to neutral as possible. An alkaline detergent (pH more than 8.5) can stain instruments; an acidic detergent (pH less than 6) can corrode or pit them.
   b. Proteolytic enzymatic detergents dissolve blood and protein and remove dissolved debris from crevices. These detergents are effective in a wide range of water qualities.
   c. Liquid detergents are preferable because they disperse more completely than do solids. Dilute the concentration before contact with instruments to avoid corrosion and staining. Do not pour liquid or put solid detergents directly on instruments.
2. Wash instruments carefully to guard against splashing and creating aerosols.
   a. Use a soft brush to clean serrations and box locks. A soft-bristle toothbrush may be used to clean ophthalmic, microsurgical, and other delicate instruments. Keep instruments totally submerged while brushing to minimize aerosolizing microorganisms and chemicals.
   b. Use a soft cloth to wipe surfaces. A nonfibrous cellulose sponge will prevent damage to delicate tips.
   c. Remove bone, tissue, and other debris from cutting instruments.
   d. Never scrub surfaces with abrasive agents such as steel wool, wire brushes, scouring pads, or powders. These agents will scratch and may remove the protective finish on metal, thus increasing the likelihood of corrosion. The

finish on stainless steel instruments protects the base metal from oxidation.

    e. Instruments that contain lumens should be soaked vertically in solution, brushed inside, and flushed with cleaning solution. Some lumens can be flushed with 70% to 90% alcohol before processing.

3. Rinse instruments thoroughly in distilled water or deionized water at the temperature recommended by the manufacturer. All facility water is tested regularly for contaminants. Some enzymes can be inactivated by extreme temperatures. The water should not exceed 140° F (60° C) to prevent burns of the skin. Inadequate rinsing can leave a surface residue that can stain instruments.

4. Load instruments into the appropriate trays for terminal sterilization or containers for high-level disinfection.

    a. Put instruments back into sterilization racks or replace the protective guards as appropriate.

    b. Arrange instruments that can be steam-sterilized in sterilizer trays for the washer-sterilizer or washer-decontaminator. The unwrapped tray is terminally steam-sterilized to make it safe for handling.

    c. Unless an automatic cleaning, disinfecting, and sterilizing machine is available, immerse lensed instruments that are heat sensitive in a high-level disinfectant after manual cleaning.

    d. Follow the manufacturer's instructions for the proper decontamination, cleaning, lubrication, and terminal sterilization of powered instruments.

Washer-Sterilizer/Washer-Decontaminator

Mechanical cleaning and terminal sterilization/decontamination can be accomplished in an automated washer-sterilizer or washer-decontaminator. Precleaning takes place before instruments are placed in any automated machine.

A washer-sterilizer requires instruments to be prewashed by hand in germicidal solution at 110° F (43.3° C) before being placed in the machine. All bioburden must be removed for the washer-sterilizer cycle to be effective. The temperature of the washer-sterilizer ranges from 250° F to 280° F (121−138° C) and would cause coagulation and crusting of protein. The instruments should be thoroughly rinsed. At the end of the cycle the instruments may be safely handled without gloves. The sets can be assembled and prepared for routine sterilization. A cycle in a washer-sterilizer makes the instruments safe to handle with the bare hands, but it does not render instruments safe for immediate patient use or sterile storage.

A washer-decontaminator cleans with a spray-force action. It is comparable to the washer-sterilizer in that the cycle includes a cold-water prerinse to loosen blood and protein, an alkaline low-sudsing detergent wash, a neutral rinse, and finally steam and heat. A washer-decontaminator does not reach the same temperature as a washer-sterilizer. It cleans at a maximum temperature of 140° F to 180° F (60−82° C), rendering the instrument safe to handle without gloves at the end of the cycle. Some models incorporate ultrasonic capabilities and lubrication for select loads. The sets can be assembled and prepared for routine sterilization when the process is complete.

An indexed washer-decontaminator has several chambers. The instrument tray automatically passes from chamber to chamber like a car wash. It is indexed for the prerinse, ultrasonic cleaning, wash, rinse and lubrication, and drying cycles. The multiple

chambers of the indexed washer-decontaminator can process several trays simultaneously.

Instruments should be arranged in perforated trays for processing in the washer-sterilizer or washer-decontaminator. The following steps should be observed when arranging the instruments:

1. Place heavy instruments in a separate tray or in the bottom of a tray, with smaller, lightweight instruments on top.

2. Turn instruments with concave surfaces, such as curettes and rongeurs, with the bowl side down; this facilitates drainage of the concave surface. Be certain that bone and tissue are removed from these surfaces during precleaning.

3. Open the box locks and pivots of hinged instruments to expose maximum surface area.

4. Disassemble complex instruments that can be taken apart without tools (e.g., stapling devices).

5. Position sharp or pointed instruments carefully on top of other instruments to prevent contacts that could damage the cutting edges or surfaces of other instruments. An alternative is to either place sharp instruments in a separate tray or terminally sterilize them after manual cleaning. Fine, delicate instruments should be put in a washer-sterilizer or washer-decontaminator according to the manufacturer's instructions.

6. Always arrange instruments neatly. They should not be randomly piled on top of one another.

Ultrasonic Cleaning

Surgical instruments vary in configuration from smooth surfaces, which respond to most types of cleaning, to complicated devices that contain box locks, serrations, grooves, blind holes, and interstices that are difficult to clean. Using high-frequency sound waves, ultrasonic energy thoroughly cleans by a process of cavitation. These sound waves generate tiny bubbles in the solution of the ultrasonic cleaner. The bubbles are small enough to get into the serrations, box locks, and crevices of instruments that are impossible to clean by other methods. The bubbles expand until they become unstable and collapse in on themselves. This implosion generates minute vacuum areas that dislodge, dissolve, or disperse soil.

For ultrasonic cleaning, precleaned and decontaminated instruments are completely immersed in the cleaning solution. The tank should be filled to a level of 1 inch (2.5 cm) above the top of the instrument tray. Suitable detergent, as specified by the manufacturer, is added. The temperature of the water should be between 100° F and 140° F (37.7−60° C) to enhance the effectiveness of the detergent, but it should not be extremely hot, which would coagulate protein material on instruments. Instrument trays should be designed for maximum transmission of sonic energy. An important relationship exists among wire gauge, opening size, and sonic frequency. A large mesh of small wire size transmits more energy than heavy wire with narrow spacing.

The solution is degassed by the ultrasonic energy. Gas, which is present in most tap water, impedes the transmission of sonic energy. An electrical generator supplies electrical energy to a transducer. The transducer converts the electrical energy into mechanical energy in the form of vibrating sound waves of such high frequency that they are not audible to the human ear. The presence of excess gas prevents the cleaning process from being fully effective because the cavitation bubbles fill with gas and the energy released during implosion is reduced. Tap water should be degassed for 5 minutes or longer each time it is changed.

The solution should be changed at least once per shift and whenever the detergent solution is visibly soiled. The inside of the tank should be cleaned between fillings.

An ultrasonic cleaner is not a sterilizer like the washer-sterilizer. The ultrasonic process uses mechanical and chemical action to process the instrumentation, but the instrument does not go through a sterilization process that renders the item safe for handling. The terminal sterilization function is performed separately in a different machine after rinsing the cleaning solution from the instruments.

Most surgical instruments, including ophthalmic instruments, microinstruments, glassware, rubber goods, and thermoplastics, can be definitively cleaned by this method to remove the tiniest particles of debris from crevices. The manufacturer's instructions must be carefully followed. In general, these instructions include:

1. Arrange heavy instruments at the bottom of the tray and light-weight instruments on top.
2. Open the box locks and pivots of hinged instruments. Disassemble instruments as appropriate.
3. Protect cutting edges from other instruments. Fine, delicate microsurgical and ophthalmic instruments may be damaged by vibrations or contact with each other. Some small units may be suitable for delicate instruments.
4. Separate dissimilar metals. Do not mix stainless steel instruments with other metals because electrolysis with resultant etching may occur.
5. Do not clean plated instruments in an ultrasonic cleaner. Cavitation will accelerate the rupture and flaking of plating. Plated instruments are not suitable for use in surgery. The surface coating of the instrument could potentially flake or peel during use and leave particles in the patient's tissues. Plated instruments will rust if the coating is removed.
6. Rinse instruments thoroughly in hot deionized water after the cleaning cycle to remove any surface debris and detergent residue.
7. Dry instruments promptly and completely before reassembling or storing. Instruments will corrode, spot, or stain if they are stored with trapped moisture.

Many facilities have large ultrasonic cleaning systems that are automated. The systems have sonic or high-pressure flow irrigation to clean lumens or cannulated items. The system may have automatic chemical and water delivery and measurement, temperature regulation, set time parameters, and digital readings.

Lubrication

All instruments with moving parts should be lubricated after cleaning. This is particularly important after ultrasonic cleaning because the sonic energy removes all lubricant. Instruments are immersed in steam-penetrable antimicrobial water-soluble lubricant that is sometimes referred to as *instrument milk*. The antimicrobial properties help prevent microbial growth in the lubricant bath, which can be reused for up to 7 days. A water-soluble lubricant deposits a thin film deep in box locks, hinges, and crevices but does not interfere with sterilization. Some lubricants also contain a rust inhibitor to prevent electrolytic mineral deposits.

Mineral oil, silicones, and machine oils are not used to lubricate instruments because they leave a residue that interferes with steam or ethylene oxide sterilization. Oiling any surgical instrument constitutes a break in technique by introducing a nonsterile item into a sterile field during its use in patient care. Oil deposits can be left in a patient's tissues.

The lubricant should be used according to the manufacturer's instructions for dilution, effectiveness, and exposure. To use most lubricants, instruments are completely immersed for 30 to 45 seconds; they are dipped and then allowed to drain dry. The solution is not rinsed or wiped off; excess solution can be shaken off. The thin film will evaporate during steam sterilization. This process is sometimes referred to as *milking* the instrument because the solution is white and opaque like milk.

Inspecting and Testing

Each instrument must be critically inspected after each cleaning. Instruments with movable parts should be inspected and tested after lubrication. Each instrument should be completely clean to ensure effective sterilization, and each should be inspected for proper function. The following essential points should be observed when inspecting an instrument after cleaning:

- Check hinged instruments for stiffness. Box locks and joints should work smoothly. Stiff joints are usually caused by inadequate cleaning. Lubrication eases stiffness temporarily. If box locks are frozen, leave the instruments in a water-soluble lubricant bath overnight, then gently work the jaws back and forth. Reinspect the instrument for cleanliness and function.
- Test forceps for alignment. A forceps that is out of alignment can break during use. Close the jaws of the forceps slightly; if they overlap, they are out of alignment. The teeth of forceps with serrated jaws should mesh perfectly. Hold the shanks in each hand with the forceps open and try to wiggle them. If the box lock has considerable play or is very loose, the forceps will not hold tissue securely. If a surgeon continues to use it, jaw misalignment will occur and impair the effectiveness of the forceps.
- Check the ratchet teeth. Ratchet teeth are subject to friction and metal-to-metal wear by the constant strain of closing and opening. Ratchets should close easily and hold firmly. To check this, clamp the forceps on the first tooth only. Hold the instrument at the box lock and tap the ratchet teeth lightly against a solid object. If the forceps springs open, it is faulty and should be repaired. A forceps that springs open when clamped on a blood vessel or duct is hazardous to the patient and is an annoyance to the surgeon. The ratchets must hold.
- Check the tension between the shanks. When the jaws touch, a clearance of 1/16 to 1/8 inch (1.5–3 mm) should be visible between the ratchet teeth of each shank. This clearance provides adequate tension at the jaws when closed. The misalignment of hinged instruments is a common problem that occurs primarily because of misuse. The instrument needs to be repaired or replaced if the teeth or serrations do not mesh perfectly or the jaws overlap.
- Test needle holders for needle security and precision. Clamp an appropriate-size needle in the jaws of the needle holder and lock it on the second tooth of the ratchet. If the needle can be turned easily by hand, the needle holder needs repair or replacement. Using a needle holder for placement of a blade on a scalpel handle can cause the jaws of a needle holder to loosen. Needle holders are designed for holding needles and should not be used for any other purpose.
- Test scissors for correctly ground and properly set blades. The blades should cut on the tips and glide over each other

smoothly. Use tissue/operating scissors to cut through four layers of gauze at the tip of the blades (or through two layers if the scissors are less than 4 inches [10 cm] long). The scissors should cut with a fine, smooth feel and a minimum of pressure. Tissue scissors should not be used to cut dressings or tape.

- Electrical insulation should be intact on all reusable electrosurgical equipment. Split insulation can cause inadvertent tissue damage during use.
- Inspect the edges of sharp and semisharp instruments such as trocars, needles, chisels, osteotomes, rongeurs, and adenotomes for sharpness, chips or dents, and alignment. Remove any questionable items from service, and send for repair or replacement. Shards of metal could be deposited in the patient's tissue during use.
- Inspect microsurgical instruments under a magnifying glass, microscope, or borescope to check alignment and detect burrs on tips and nicks on cutting edges. The exact alignment of teeth on fine-tooth forceps is an absolute necessity. Microscopic teeth are very easily bent. Be certain that these instruments are thoroughly dry. A chamois is useful for drying delicate tips.
- Check pins and screws of reusable staplers to be sure they are secure and intact. They can become loose or fall out during ultrasonic cleaning as a result of vibration.
- Flatten or straighten malleable instruments such as retractors and probes. Weakened or cracked items should be immediately replaced.
- Self-retaining retractors should provide free motion and sliding of the retracting blades. They should attach, slide, and detach easily. The tilts and ratchets should slide and hold as appropriate. All screws, wing nuts, and removable parts should be inspected for stripped threads.
- Demagnetize instruments by passing them back through a magnetic field. Although this is not a common occurrence, instruments can become magnetized when magnetic sheets are used in the OR.
- Unclean or questionable instruments should be returned to the cleaning area for ultrasonic cleaning. Instruments in poor working condition should be removed from the processing area. A place is usually designated in the OR suite or the CS department for the collection of instruments for repair. A defective instrument should be tagged as unsafe for use and not be allowed to remain in circulation. These instruments are good for use in a teaching environment.

Instrument Marking for Identification

New instruments may be marked for identification before they are put in service. Some manufacturers will imprint identification numbers or bar codes with a laser when their instruments are purchased. The surface of the instrument should not be etched or engraved by personnel in the department. Etching and engraving cause destruction of the instrument surface that permits trapped microorganisms and endospores.

Some facilities affix specialized heat-stable tape to instruments to color code them by sets or specialty. These tapes must withstand cleaning and sterilizing without peeling. They must be replaced if they loosen. The tape is wrapped around the circumference of the handle but should not overlap. The edges should just meet. The presence of marking tape allows debris to accumulate in the folds. Worn or peeling tape leaves an adhesive residue on the instrument that is hard to remove and attracts debris. The tape manufacturers have commercial tape-removal

systems available for purchase. The kits include a tape cutter and solvent that is safe for use on instruments. Other instruments may have a laser-etched code or barcode system that uses electronic tracking.

Instrument processing departments may find that a loose-leaf binder containing pictures and descriptions of each instrument is useful for the identification of specialty set contents. This process can be cumbersome and time-consuming because manufacturers use different numbers and names for like devices.

Repairing or Restoring Versus Replacing Instruments

Instruments in poor working condition inhibit the surgeon and create a serious hazard for the patient. Instruments should be repaired at the first sign of damage or malfunction. If an instrument breaks during a procedure, all pieces should be accounted for in their entirety. A lighted magnifying lens is a useful CS tool for examining instrumentation.

Repair

Even with normal usage the blades of scissors and the edges of other cutting instruments become dull over time, just as kitchen knives do at home. Steam sterilization causes the softening of the metal that in turn dulls the edge. Cutting instruments must be sharp. For this reason, scalpel blades are disposed of after a single patient use. Osteotomes, chisels, gouges, and meniscotomes can be sharpened by specialty companies that use handheld hones or a honing machine designed for this purpose. Some specialty instrument repair companies will come to the facility in a mobile van fully equipped with all the machines and tools needed to recondition and repair surgical instruments. Scissors, curettes, rongeurs, and reamers should be frequently rotated for sharpening. OR and CS personnel are not qualified to sharpen or repair surgical instruments.

Drill bits and saw blades should be single-use items. Reuse and processing cause the cutting edges to rip tissue instead of cutting. Stiff joints or frozen box locks are the result of inadequate cleaning or corrosion caused by trapped moisture or a corrosive substance. The instrument should be repaired before the box lock cracks and the instrument must be replaced.

After repeated use, instruments eventually wear, misalign, and stiffen. Parts such as inserts, screws, or springs may need to be replaced. The life of many instruments can be extended by preventive maintenance or prompt repair.

Restoration and Resurfacing

Instruments may become spotted, stained, corroded, pitted, or rusted. Some surface discoloration will appear with normal use, but the unusual or severe buildup of deposits may impair function or sterilization. The color of a stain may help identify a problem that needs to be corrected, such as the following examples:

- Light or dark water spots (from mineral content in tap water or condensate in sterilizer; caused by inadequate drying)
- Rust-colored film (from iron content or softening agents in steam pipes)
- Bluish-gray stain (from some chemical sterilizing or disinfecting solutions)
- Brownish stain (from polyphosphate cleaning compounds that are incompatible with local water supply, leaving a chromic oxide film on instruments)

- Purplish-black stain (from detergents that contain ammonia or from amines in steam lines)
- Rust deposits (from inadequate cleaning or drying, agents not thoroughly rinsed, electrolytic deposits from exposed metal under chipped chrome plating onto stainless steel, or residues in textile wrappers; avoid the use of plated instruments in surgery; these are not surgical-grade instruments)

Blood, saline solution, and detergents that contain chloride can cause pitting if they are not rinsed promptly and thoroughly. Detergents with high or low pH can destroy the protective chromium oxide layer on stainless steel.

If an instrument has been damaged, the surface can be repolished and passivated by the manufacturer to restore the integrity of the finish.

Replacement

Broken instruments must be replaced if they are beyond repair or restoration. With normal use, good-quality surgical instruments have an expected life of at least 10 years. Using these precise tools for only their intended purpose cannot be overemphasized. Misuse and abuse are the most common causes of instrument breakage. Use of a lightweight instrument on heavy tissue causes the jaws to bend or "spring." Using a needle holder to load and disarm knife blades can damage the jaws. A heavier clamp should be used for this purpose.

Instrument counts, electronic tracking, and accountability activities in the OR help prevent instruments from being discarded into the trash or sent to the laundry. Replacing instruments that have been needlessly damaged is an unnecessary expense for the OR. Repairing the laundry equipment can be an additional expense. Personnel could be injured by instruments that protrude through trash bags and puncture the skin. Some facilities, having had extreme instrument losses, have installed metal detectors in the trash room. These are valid reinforcements for accountability for instrumentation in the OR.

Disinfection of Items Used in Patient Care

Disinfection differs from sterilization by its lack of sporicidal power. Theoretically, all items used in the sterile field must be sterilized. Surfaces of items that will penetrate or separate tissue or invade the intravascular system must be sterile to prevent the introduction of potentially harmful microorganisms into the patient's body. Items that cannot be sterilized by conventional sterilization methods discussed in Chapter 18 are disinfected to eliminate as many microorganisms as possible.

Some specialized instruments and equipment cannot be sterilized between each patient use or will not withstand a sterilization process. Disinfection may be the only alternative. Disinfection can be accomplished with chemical and physical agents. The application and selection of disinfecting agents depend on the level of importance of the item as used in patient care, risk for exposure to biologic material, or environmental contamination.[2]

Chemical agents used for disinfection of the environment or instrumentation are prepared and maintained for use according to the manufacturer's recommendations. Care is taken not to overdilute the solution by immersing wet items. Anything placed into the solution must be absolutely dry to prevent inactivity of the chemical properties. Dipsticks are commercially available to test the concentration and efficacy of the solution before use.

Care is taken to note the correct use and shelf life of mixed solutions. A reconstituted chemical container should be labeled with the date of mixing and date of expiration. It should always remain covered to minimize evaporation, and PPE should be worn any time the solution is used. Disposal of used or expired solution may be subject to special handling to meet federal environmental guidelines.

Spaulding's Classification of Patient Care Items

Earle H. Spaulding, a well-known microbiologist, developed a classification system in 1968 to determine the appropriate method to attain the desired level of processing required for safety in patient care items. This system was adopted and later modified by the Centers for Disease Control and Prevention (CDC). Spaulding's classifications of the importance of patient care items are still applicable in the 21st century.

- *Critical items* must be sterile because they enter sterile tissue, break the mucosal barrier, or come into contact with the vascular system. Examples include surgical instruments, endoscopes, endoscopic accessories that cut tissue, catheters, implants, and needles.[3] Sterilization is required for all critical items. High-level chemical disinfection should not be confused with chemical sterilization. Some of the same chemicals used for disinfection are used for longer times in higher concentrations to cause sterilization.
- *Semicritical items* come into contact with intact skin and mucous membranes and require high-level disinfection, although they also may be sterilized. Examples include respiratory therapy equipment, anesthesia equipment, and vaginal probes.
- *Noncritical items* are used in contact only with intact skin. Intermediate- or low-level disinfection is adequate. Examples include blood pressure cuffs, furniture, linens, bedpans, and eating utensils.

Levels of Disinfection

Disinfection is the process of destroying or inhibiting growth of pathogenic microorganisms on inanimate objects. It reduces the risk for microbial contamination but does not provide the same level of assurance as sterilization because all endospores are not killed. Disinfection levels are classified by the effectiveness of the process (i.e., the ability of the agent to kill microorganisms) as follows:

- **High-level disinfection**: Kills all bacteria, viruses, and fungi. The process may kill endospores if contact time is sufficient and other conditions are met. A high-level disinfectant should be used if a semicritical item is disinfected rather than sterilized. Some chemicals used in high-level disinfection can produce sterilization if they are allowed to remain in contact with the surface of the item for the time specified by the manufacturer. Chemicals used in the high-level disinfection process must be approved by the U.S. Food and Drug Administration (FDA) and disposed of according to local, state, and federal agencies.

Note: High-level disinfection is not effective against Creutzfeldt-Jakob disease (CJD; also including new variant CJD, which is a transmissible spongiform encephalopathy (TSE). The biologic material that causes CJD is not a living microorganism like a bacteria or virus. It is a protein, referred to as a prion, that is extremely difficult to remove and inactivate. Prions and other specific microorganisms are discussed in detail in Chapter 14.

- **Intermediate-level disinfection**: Kills most bacteria, viruses, and fungi on noncritical items. The process does not attack endospores. It inactivates tuberculosis (TB).
- **Low-level disinfection**: Kills most vegetative bacteria (bactericide, bactericidal), fungi, and the least resistant viruses on noncritical items, including human immunodeficiency virus (HIV).

A record of the agent, concentration, and time of exposure should be maintained for semicritical items that have undergone high-level disinfection (Fig. 17.1). The level of disinfection that can be achieved depends on the type and concentration of the agent, contact time, and bioburden. Items that are disinfected are patient safe for their intended uses to minimize risks for infection for the patient. An all-purpose disinfectant does not exist. The best housekeeping agents are not the best disinfectants and vice versa.

Methods of Disinfection

Methods of disinfection include manual wiping with a chemical-impregnated cloth or sponge, soaking by total immersion, and processing by flush-through machinery. The method used depends on the desired level of disinfection.

Chemical Disinfectants

Chemical agents for disinfection are registered with the Pesticide Regulation Division of the Environmental Protection Agency (EPA) to be sold in interstate commerce. An EPA registration number is granted only when requirements of laboratory test data, toxicity data, product formula, and label copy are approved. Any chemical agent accepted for use by a facility must be FDA approved and have a copy of the safety data sheet (SDS) readily available in the event of a spill or exposure as required by the Occupational Safety and Health Administration (OSHA).

Disinfectants are labeled with the chemical properties and appropriate warnings of precautions. The labels must be read, and directions for dilution and/or use must be followed. The product label should indicate several salient points important to the selection of the appropriate agent for the desired task. The user should read the label before use. Sample labeling information is listed in Box 17.1. Isopropyl alcohol, sodium hypochlorite, formaldehyde, glutaraldehyde, and phenol are considered hazardous chemicals. Some other chemicals can cause contact dermatitis. Gloves and eyewear should be worn when handling all chemical agents. Avoid neoprene and polyvinylchloride gloves because they can absorb some chemicals.

To be labeled for hospital use a chemical disinfectant should be proved effective against *Staphylococcus aureus* (gram-positive), *Salmonella enterica* (gram-negative), and *Pseudomonas aeruginosa* (gram-negative); these are the most resistant gram-positive and gram-negative organisms. The agent can be classified as a hospital disinfectant without being pseudomonacidal, but the label is required to say whether it is effective against *Pseudomonas* organisms. Influences on efficacy of the solution can be found in Box 17.2.

The EPA defines a disinfectant as an agent that kills growing or vegetative forms of bacteria. The terms *germicide* and *bactericide* may be used synonymously with the term *disinfectant* according to this definition. However, *Mycobacterium tuberculosis* has a waxy envelope that makes it comparatively resistant to aqueous germicides. Effective agents against *M. tuberculosis* should be labeled "tuberculocidal." Agents also are labeled regarding whether they kill fungi (fungicide), viruses (virucide), and/or endospores (sporicide).

• BOX 17.1 Information to Look for on a Disinfectant Label

Information About Active Ingredient
- Trade and generic name
- Concentration or strength
- Environmental Protection Agency (EPA) registration number

Warnings
- Toxicity alert
- Cautionary statement
- Treatment for untoward exposure
- Poison control listing
- Hotline number

Instructions for Use
- Dilution information
- Personal protective equipment (PPE) requirements
- Intended use
- Surfaces safe for use
- Method of application
- Duration of necessary contact

Intended Action
- Antimicrobial activity
- Residual action (if any)

Aftercare
- Of equipment
- Of treated surface
- Of cleaning supplies
- Disposal or storage of unused product
- Biodegradability and effects in the natural environment

Date:

Solution:

   Type/agent _____

   Strength _____

   Activation date _____

   Expiration date _____

   Temperature _____

   Immersion:

      Time in _____

      Time out _____

Load:

   Control number _____

   Location _____

   Contents _____

• Fig. 17.1 Record for sterilization or high-level disinfection with chemical solutions.

- Concentration of the solution
- Temperature of the solution
- Shelf life and storage of the solution
- Compounded agents in the solution
- Precleaning and drying of item before immersion
- Degree of bioburden and biofilm on the surface of the item
- Composition and surface texture of the item
- Duration of contact with the agent
- Humidity of the environment
- Temperature of the environment
- pH and mineral content of the diluent

Agents effective enough to be labeled as tuberculocidal will kill HIV. Those that meet the EPA testing requirements may be labeled specifically as HIV virucides. HBV cannot be adapted to laboratory testing, but it is known to survive exposure to many disinfectants.

The most common liquid chemical disinfectants used in the perioperative environment are listed in Table 17.1. With few exceptions, most liquid chemical disinfectants are not sporicides. Analysis of the label statements helps determine whether a product is appropriate for a specific purpose in the OR. Items disinfected by chemical agents for patient care require removal of the agent before the item is safe for use on a patient. Items need to be rinsed with clear water until the chemical is removed. The sterility of the rinse water depends on the intended use of the item. Sterile and high-level disinfected items will require the use of sterile water as a rinse. Noncritical items can be rinsed with tap water.

Factors to be considered in the selection of an agent include the following:

1. Microorganisms, particularly endospore-forming bacteria and certain viruses, differ markedly in their resistance to liquid chemical disinfectants. Factors influencing the microbial response include the structure and design of the item to be disinfected, the active ingredient of the chemical, pH, hardness of the water, exposure time, and extent of precleaning before processing. Resistance levels of select microorganisms are described in Table 17.2.

2. Disinfectants differ widely in the level of microbicidal action they produce and mechanisms involved. All are protoplasmic poisons that can coagulate or denature cell protein, oxidize or bind enzymes, or alter cell membranes. In-use culture testing must determine the number of viable microorganisms after an agent is used for the intended purpose.

3. The nature of the microbial contamination influences the results of chemical disinfection. Bacteria, spores, fungi, and viruses are present in air and on surfaces throughout the environment. However, organic soil such as blood, plasma, pus, feces, and tissue absorbs germicidal molecules and inactivates some chemicals. Therefore good physical precleaning before disinfection helps reduce the number of microorganisms and maintain the effectiveness of the disinfectant.

4. Requirements of the chemical agent vary.
   a. Housekeeping products should be detergent-disinfectants that meet the following requirements for both cleaning and disinfection:
      (1) They must be effective against a broad spectrum of microorganisms, including *P. aeruginosa* and *M. tuberculosis*, preferably in the presence of organic soil.
      (2) They must be compatible with tap water for dilution.
      (3) They must be low-foaming and prevent waterborne deposits.
      (4) They must rinse easily and not leave a residual film that could affect electrical conductivity or transfer to the patient.
      (5) They should be nontoxic and nonirritating to patients and personnel.
      (6) They should be virtually odorless.
   b. Instrument and equipment disinfectants should be registered by the EPA and should kill as many species of microorganisms as possible to decontaminate items effectively for handling by personnel or for preparing items for patient use, such as stethoscopes and monitors.

5. The kill time is correlated with the concentration of the agent and the number of microorganisms present. Most disinfectant chemicals are used in aqueous solution. Water brings the chemical and microorganisms together. Without this water reaction, the process stops. Increasing the concentration of the chemical may shorten exposure time but not necessarily.
   a. All tap water contains *Pseudomonas* bacteria. The pH, calcium, and magnesium in hard tap water can inactivate disinfectants. Therefore deionized water may be recommended for use in dilution.
   b. The temperature of hot water may make chemical agents unstable.
   c. Disinfectants should be premixed in required concentrations and stored in properly labeled containers to ensure personnel use the product in the correct concentration.
   d. Instruments are completely submerged for the maximum time recommended by the manufacturer of the product used.
   e. All instruments should be clean and dry when put into solution. Wet items will dilute the solution and change the concentration of the chemical agent.

6. The composition of items to be disinfected varies. Nonporous items, such as metal instruments, are more easily disinfected than are porous materials. Items must be stable in a wet environment.

7. The method of application influences the effectiveness of the chemical agent.
   a. Direct application of a liquid disinfectant, either by mechanical action for housekeeping purposes or immersion for instrument disinfection, is the most effective method of applying chemicals to the surface of inanimate objects.
   b. Aerosol spray from a pressurized container is an effective method of spot disinfection on smooth surfaces and into crevices not otherwise accessible. Care is taken not to disperse the aerosol in the room environment. Spray bottles are not appropriate for surface disinfection in the OR.

8. Disinfection should be done immediately before and after use or contamination. All patients are considered to be potential carriers of microbial contamination. Therefore adequate bactericidal and virucidal disinfection is needed before and after every invasive procedure.

9. The shelf life and safe storage after reconstitution are other factors to be considered. Room temperature and exposure to lighting may be factors in efficacy. The chemical manufacturer provides information about storage methods and duration of efficacy.

TABLE 17.1 Common Liquid Chemical Disinfectants

Disinfectant Agent	Level of Disinfection	Timing	Virucidal	Fungicidal	Sporicidal	Mycobacterium (Tuberculocidal)	Hazards	Notes
Alcohol, 70–95%								
Ethyl	Intermediate level	10–30 min for both	Yes, but not all lipid viruses, HAV	Yes	No	Yes	All forms are flammable.	Bactericidal but not bacteriostatic. Ineffective against spores. Noncorrosive.
Isopropyl	Intermediate level		Yes, but not enteroviruses	Yes	No	Yes		Denatures proteins. Harms rubber and plastic. Combined with other disinfectants to form a tincture that can extend the bactericidal action. Rapid evaporation. Used in skin antisepsis.
Aldehyde							Toxic: skin, eye, and respiratory irritant.	
Aqueous acidic 2%	High level	20–90 min at 68–77°F (20–25°C)	Yes	Yes	No	Yes; very slow	OSHA exposure limit is 0.05 ppm. Can cause respiratory irritation. Carcinogenic.	Excellent materials compatibility. Local regulations may restrict disposal of used product. Inexpensive to use. Use in well-ventilated area. Reduced effect in detergent.
Glutaraldehyde								
Banicide 3.5%	Sterile	10 hr at 77°F (25°C)	Yes	Yes	Yes	Yes		30-day reuse period. Absorbed by neoprene or PVC gloves.
	High level	45 min at 77°F (25°C)						
Cidex activated alkaline 2.4% dialdehyde	Sterile	10 hr at 77°F (25°C)	Yes	Yes	Yes	Yes		Coagulates blood and tissue. Activated alkaline form has shelf life of 14–30 days.
	High level	45 min at 77°F (25°C)	Yes	Yes	Some	Yes		Concentration level must be monitored.
Cidex OPA (0.55%) ortho-phthalaldehyde	High level	12 min at 68°F (20°C)	Yes	Yes	Some, but improves when the pH is increased to 8	Yes; superior action	No known irritations.	Requires no activation and remains more stable over a wide range of pH (3–9). Stains protein gray; 14-day reuse period.
					Scopes pass sporicidal test at 32 hr at 20°C			Concentration level must be monitored.
Cidex OPA (5.75%) ortho-phthalaldehyde concentrate	High level	5 min at 122°F (50°C)			Scopes pass sporicidal test at 32 hr at 122°F (50°C)			Used in an automated endoscope high-level disinfector.
Phenol Compound								
1.6% with 0.95% glutaraldehyde (Sporicidin)	Sterile	12 hr at 77°F (25°C)	Yes	Yes	Yes	Yes	Skin and eye irritant. Carcinogenic. Toxic to animals.	Effective in presence of organic matter. Leaves an active residue. Effective in detergents.
	High level	20 min at 77°F (25°C)	Yes, but limited	Yes	No	Yes		Maximum reuse period of 7 days.

Agent	Level	Contact time					Precautions	Comments
Quaternary Ammonium Compounds (Quats)								
CO.1–2% concentration	Low	10 min	Limited; lipophilic only	Yes	No	No	No odor and low toxicity.	Easily inactivated by organic debris. Effective in temperatures up to 212° F (100° C). Most effective in alkaline solution. Neutralized by detergents and hard water. Nonirritating and noncorrosive. Inexpensive. Inactivated by use with gauze pads. Surface disinfection.
Halogens								
Chlorine and chlorine compounds such as sodium hypochlorite	Low to high based on concentration and pH	10–30 min	Yes	Yes	Limited	Yes	Toxic and corrosive. Do not autoclave chlorine solutions; will vaporize and cause free chlorine gas inhalation hazard. Dangerous gas forms if mixed with ammonia.	Ethyl alcohol 60% can be added to increase kill potential. Oxidizes metallic objects. 1:10 dilution of 6% chlorine bleach (household bleach) contains 6000 ppm available chlorine. Combines with protein and decreases in effectiveness. Premixed solution can be stored in cool place in a light-proof container.
Iodophors (Wescodyne)	Low at a wide range of pH	10–30 min	Yes	Yes	No	Yes		Alcohol can be added to extend effectiveness in a solution of 1:10 in 50% ethyl alcohol. Vaporizes in hot water (120–125° F [48–51.6° C]). Reduced action in presence of protein. Inactivated iodophor loses brown-yellow color. Becomes clear when deactivated.
Peracetic Acid								
STERIS 0.2%	Sterile	12–30 min at 122–133° F (50–56° C)	Yes	Yes	Yes	Yes	Wear PPE if risk for contact to skin, eyes, or mucous membranes.	Used in STERIS processing as a single-use liquid chemical sterilant. No residue. Uses filtered tap water for rinse. Can corrode metallics. Approximately $6 per cycle. No special disposal requirements. Protect from light and heat.
Sporox Hydrogen Peroxide								
7.5%	Sterile	6 hr at 68° F (20° C)	Yes	Yes	Yes	Yes	Wear PPE to protect eyes.	Requires no activation. Has no special disposal instructions.
	High level	30 min at 68° F (20° C)	Yes	Yes	Some	Yes		Must monitor minimal effective concentration. Maximum reuse period of 21 days. May enhance removal of organic debris. Not effective as a disinfectant in presence of organic matter.

HAV, Hepatitis A virus; *OSHA,* Occupational Safety and Health Administration; *PPE,* personal protective equipment; *ppm,* parts per million.

TABLE 17.2 Resistance Levels of Select Microorganisms		
MINIMAL RESISTANCE	**INTERMEDIATE RESISTANCE**	**HIGH RESISTANCE**
Lipid Viruses	**Nonlipid Viruses (Hydrophilic)**	**Bacterial Endospores**
Influenza	Echovirus	Gram positive
Rubeola	Parvovirus	*Bacillus subtilis*
Cytomegalovirus (CMV)	Hepatitis A virus	*Bacillus stearothermophilus*
Human immunodeficiency virus (HIV)	Rhinovirus	*Clostridium tetani*
Herpes simplex virus types 1 and 2 (HSV)	Poliovirus	*Bacillus anthracis*
Hepatitis B virus (HBV)	Coxsackievirus	*Clostridium botulinum*
Hepatitis C virus (HCV)	*Clostridium perfringens*	
Respiratory syncytial virus (RSV)	*Clostridium difficile*	
Epstein-Barr virus (EBV)	Gram negative	
	Coxiella burnetii	
Vegetative Lipid-Coated Bacteria	**Fungi**	**Mycobacteria**
Non–Endospore Forming		
Gram Positive	*Trichophyton* species	*Mycobacterium bovis*
Staphylococcus aureus	*Cryptococcus* species	*Mycobacterium tuberculosis*
Staphylococcus epidermidis	*Candida* species	*Mycobacterium leprae*
Streptococcus groups A and B		
Pseudomonas aeruginosa		
Salmonella enterica		
Corynebacterium diphtheriae		
Gram Negative		
Haemophilus influenzae		
Helicobacter pylori		

Knowledge of microbial resistance to decontamination, disinfection, and sterilization is important in selecting which method to use during reprocessing.

Alcohol

Ethyl or isopropyl alcohol, 70% to 95%, kills microorganisms by coagulation of cell proteins.

Effectiveness

- It may be used as a housekeeping disinfectant for damp-dusting furniture and lights or wiping electrical cords without leaving a residue on treated surfaces. It is nonstaining.
- It can disinfect semicritical instruments. To prevent corrosion of metal, 0.2% sodium nitrite is added.
- It is bactericidal, pseudomonacidal, and fungicidal in a minimum of 10 minutes' exposure by total immersion. It is not sporicidal.
- It is tuberculocidal and virucidal for most viruses (except hydrophilic viruses), including HIV, in a minimum of 15 minutes' exposure. It is effective against HBV.

Precautions

- The pattern of effectiveness of 95% isopropyl alcohol on HBV is irregular because it evaporates rapidly and does not have prolonged moist contact with the microorganism. It should not be used for cleaning up blood or body fluid spills because it is inactivated in the presence of biologic matter.
- It is volatile; it will act only as long as it is in solution. Alcohol becomes ineffective as soon as it evaporates, and it loses its microbicidal activity in concentrations below 50%; it should be discarded at frequent intervals.
- It is inactive in the presence of organic soil. It does not penetrate skin oil that lodges on instruments through handling.
- It will blanch asphalt floor tiles.
- It cannot be used on lensed instruments with cement mountings because it dissolves cement.
- With long exposure, it will harden and swell plastic tubing and items, including polyethylene.
- It is flammable, so it is stored in a cool, well-ventilated area. Many ORs are banning alcohol-based products because of increased fire risk.
- It is a skin irritant.

Chlorine Compounds

Inorganic chlorine is valuable for the disinfection of water. Chlorine compounds kill microorganisms by the oxidation of enzymes. Sodium hypochlorite (household bleach), 1:10 dilution of 5.25%, is a low-level disinfectant. Concentration may range up to 1:100, or 500 parts per million (ppm). Sodium dichloroisocyanurate (Presept disinfectant tablet) has a lowered pH, which enhances its microbicidal action.

Effectiveness

- Chlorine compounds are housekeeping disinfectants for spot cleaning of blood and body fluid spills and for cleaning of floors and furniture.
- They are bactericidal, fungicidal, and tuberculocidal and have a virucidal effect on HIV, HBV, and other viruses.

Precautions

- Sodium hypochlorite is unstable and dissipates rapidly in the presence of organic soil. A dilution is prepared daily.
- The odor may be objectionable. It can be a respiratory irritant.
- Chlorine is corrosive to metal; it cannot be used for instrument disinfection and decontamination.
- Chlorine compounds are potentially carcinogenic if combined with formaldehyde.
- Do not combine with ammonia because a toxic gas is emitted.
- Do not autoclave instruments saturated in a chlorine compound because a toxic gas is released.

Formaldehyde

Formaldehyde kills microorganisms by coagulation of protein in cells. The solution may be 37% formaldehyde in water (Formalin) or 8% formaldehyde in 70% isopropyl alcohol. Formaldehyde is not commonly used for housekeeping purposes as a surface disinfectant.

Precautions

- Formaldehyde fumes are irritating to the eyes and mucous membranes.
- Fumes are potentially carcinogenic; it is toxic to tissue.
- Formalin 10% may be used for permanent section specimens.
- Formaldehyde should be stored in an area with adequate ventilation.
- PPE is required when handling.
- Exposure protocols should be followed for medical monitoring.

Glutaraldehyde

An aqueous solution of glutaraldehyde kills microorganisms by denaturation of protein. It is most used in an activated 2.0% to 2.4% solution that can be reused for the specified period of activation. Both alkaline and acid solutions are available for high-level disinfection of critical and semicritical items that cannot be steam-sterilized. A 1:16 dilution is not considered a high-level disinfectant; a 2% solution is. Glutaraldehyde is not used for housekeeping purposes.

Effectiveness

- It is a noncorrosive high-level disinfectant for endoscopes and lensed instruments.
- It is safe as a high-level disinfectant for most plastic, rubber, and heat-sensitive items.
- It is bactericidal, pseudomonacidal, fungicidal, and virucidal, including against HIV and HBV, in a minimum of 10 minutes' exposure at a temperature between 68° F and 86° F (20–30° C).

- It is tuberculocidal. Variations in formulations of products available affect the exposure time and temperature of the solution, especially after reuse. A 2% solution at 77° F or 86° F (25° C or 30° C) may be 100% tuberculocidal in 45 to 90 minutes, depending on the formulation. Label instructions of the manufacturer should be followed.
- Most of the products labeled as cold sterilants are sporicidal in a minimum of 10 hours' exposure at room temperature.
- Some products can be reused in closed containers or in an automatic machine for a period of activation specified by the manufacturer.
- It remains active in the presence of organic matter; it does not coagulate protein material.

Precautions

- Thorough and careful cleaning in a mild detergent is essential to remove organic debris and reduce microbial contamination. Detergent is rinsed off, and the item is dried before immersion.
- Items are completely immersed and lumens are filled with glutaraldehyde solution for no longer than 24 hours.
- Items are thoroughly rinsed before use.
- Odor and fumes may be irritating to the eyes, throat, and nasal passages. The solution should be kept covered and used in a well-ventilated area.
- Shelf life of glutaraldehyde is limited after activation.
- Proper training, PPE, and knowledge are required before handling.

Iodophors

A complex of free iodine with detergent kills microorganisms through a process of oxidation of essential enzymes. An iodophor is an effective low- to intermediate-level disinfectant. The iodine-detergent complex enhances the microbicidal activity of free iodine and renders it nontoxic, nonirritating, and nonstaining when used as directed. The concentration varies among the products available. The manufacturer's instructions for use should be followed.

Effectiveness

- Iodophors are commonly used as surgical scrubs and preoperative skin preps in the surgical setting. Iodine is effective as long as it is wet. An aqueous solution is more effective for cleaning than is an alcohol solution because it dries more slowly.
- An iodophor can be used as an instrument disinfectant if no other agent is available. To prevent corrosion of metal, 0.2% sodium nitrite is added.
- Iodophors are bactericidal, pseudomonacidal, and fungicidal in a minimum of 10 minutes' exposure in a concentration of 450 ppm of iodine or a minimum of 20 minutes' exposure in a concentration of 100 ppm of iodine.
- They are tuberculocidal and virucidal, including against HIV and HBV, in a minimum of 20 minutes' exposure with a minimum concentration of 450 ppm of iodine. They are not sporicidal.

Precautions

- Some iodophors are unstable in the presence of hard water or heat and are inactivated by organic soil.
- Iodine stains fabrics and tissue; however, this is reduced or is temporary when iodine is used as an iodophor.

Phenolic Compounds

Derivatives of pure phenol kill microorganisms mainly by coagulation of protein. Depending on the phenol coefficient and species of organisms, phenolic compounds may cause rapid lysis of cells, leakage of cell constituents without lysis, or death by denaturing enzymes. Pure phenol, obtained from coal tar, is an extremely caustic agent and dangerous to tissue, causing painless burns and blanching. Derivatives are used as low-level disinfectants, usually with a minimum of a 2% phenolic compound in an aqueous or detergent solution. Phenolic compounds are used primarily for housekeeping purposes.

Effectiveness

- Phenolic compounds may be used as housekeeping disinfectants for cleaning surfaces such as floors, furniture, and walls. Phenolics retain a safe level of activity in the presence of heavy organic soil.
- They are the disinfectants of choice when dealing with fecal contamination. They have good stability and remain active after mild heating and prolonged drying. Subsequent application of moisture to dry surfaces can redissolve the chemical so that it becomes bactericidal again.
- They are tuberculocidal.

Precautions

- Tissue irritation precludes use for semicritical instruments that will come into contact with skin and mucous membranes (e.g., anesthesia equipment).
- Personnel should wear gloves when cleaning with these products to avoid skin irritation.
- Rubber and plastics may absorb phenol derivatives.
- The product may have an unpleasant odor.
- Pure phenol is inactivated by the application of alcohol. Phenol is solid at room temperature and liquefies when warm.

Quaternary Ammonium Compounds

"Quats," as these compounds are often called, cause gradual alteration of cell membranes to produce leakage of protoplasm of some microorganisms, primarily vegetative bacteria. These compounds possess detergent properties and are used to sanitize noncritical surfaces. Benzalkonium chloride, one of the most widely used of these compounds, should be used in a concentration of 1:750.

Effectiveness

- They are rarely used as housekeeping disinfectants for surfaces such as floors, furniture, and walls.
- For low-level, noncritical instrument disinfection, 0.2% sodium nitrite is added to the solution to prevent corrosion of metal.
- They are bactericidal, pseudomonacidal, fungicidal, and lipid virucidal in a minimum of 10 minutes' exposure. They are nonirritating to skin.
- There is no buildup on surfaces. They are not inactivated by hard water.

Precautions

- The microbicidal effect can be reversed by adding a neutralizer such as soap.
- They are not effective against TB or hydrophilic viruses, such as poliovirus.

- The active agent can be selectively absorbed by fabrics, thus reducing the strength perhaps to an ineffectively low level. Gauze or a towel must not be put in the basin used for immersing instruments.
- Compounds are inactivated in the presence of organic soil.

Hydrogen Peroxide
Effectiveness

- It is rapidly bactericidal, virucidal, fungicidal, and tuberculocidal.
- It is useful for disinfection of noncritical items.
- Hydrogen peroxide is used in some room fogging devices for disinfection of surfaces.
- Hydrogen peroxide can be used for sterilization when turned into a gas or vapor (see Chapter 18).

Precaution

- It is inactivated by blood.

Physical Disinfectants
Boiling Water

Boiling water cannot be depended on to kill endospores. Heat-resistant bacterial endospores will withstand water boiling at 212° F (100° C) for many hours of continuous exposure. Inactivation of some viruses, such as those associated with hepatitis, is uncertain.

If no other method of sterilization or disinfection is available, boiling water can be rendered more effective by adding sodium carbonate to make a 2% solution, which reduces the hydrogen-ion concentration. At sea level the recommended boiling time for disinfection is 15 minutes. Rubber goods and glassware must not be boiled in sodium carbonate because it is destructive to both. If sodium carbonate is not used, the minimum boiling period is 30 minutes. At high altitudes the boiling time is increased to compensate for the lower temperature of boiling water.

Pasteurization

A high-level disinfection process, sometimes referred to as pasteurization, can be used for items such as reusable respiratory devices and anesthesia breathing circuits to render them safe for patient use.

Pasteurization is a method of hot water decontamination/disinfection performed with chlorine detergents at low temperatures. Although not a sterilization process, exposure to hot water (140−180° F [60−82° C]) for 30 minutes kills microorganisms without killing endospores.

Anesthesia hoses, masks, and fluted breathing bags are positioned in the pasteurization unit on special pegs and hooks that permit total immersion and full-surface contact of the sprayer arms. Time and temperature are closely monitored to provide high-level disinfection. The pasteurization process takes approximately 1 hour to complete, followed by air-drying in a specially filtered cabinet. The items must be completely dry before being placed in storage. The average pasteurization unit can process up to 10 complete anesthesia circuits in one cycle.

Ultraviolet Irradiation

Ultraviolet (UV) rays at wavelengths of 240 to 480 nm photochemically transform nucleic acid bases to denature DNA and proteins. Generated by low-pressure mercury vapor bulbs, UV lights produce nonionizing radiant energy in sufficient wavelengths and intensity for low-level disinfection. The rays can kill select vegetative bacteria, fungi, and lipoprotein viruses on contact in air or water.

The practical usefulness of UV irradiation is still being studied, however, because the rays must make direct contact with the organisms and may actually support life for some varieties. Current studies show promise in effectiveness of killing 99.8% of *Clostridium difficile*. Microorganisms are in a constant state of motion in the air currents of the ventilating system and in water. Moving across the ray of UV light, pathogens may be exposed for too short a time for effective contact with the radiant energy.

Three types of UV systems are used: UV rays with mercury lamps, UV light-emitting diodes or UV-C machines with wavelengths between 250 and 280 nm, and pulsed xenon lights with wavelengths around 230 nm.[4] Effectiveness is determined on how close the light is to an object, size of the area, time setting, and placement of the machine. Fixed UV light systems are built into the room and require no positioning and are set for room size and dose-intensity delivery.

UV lights are used to augment surface disinfection after terminal cleaning in some surgical environments. Only surfaces in contact with the UV system are disinfected.

UV rays can cause skin burns, comparable to sunburn, and conjunctivitis. These lights may be turned on only when the room is unoccupied to reduce airborne and surface contamination.[4]

UV irradiation is used in conjunction with activated carbon 5-μm filters for water purification. UV irradiation kills bacteria but does not remove impurities. The filtration process is followed by exposing water flowing at a constant rate and temperature to a 5-watt UV lamp. This produces purified, not sterile, water. UV irradiation is not sporicidal, and HBV can survive exposure.

Disposable Products

Disposable products can be useful in the OR. It is sometimes easier to discard a contaminated item after use than to clean and process it. The use of disposable products has become popular, but consideration of the logistics of using them includes determination of the benefits and/or consequences of their use and reuse.

The production of disposable products often involves the use of natural resources and potential industrial damage to the Earth's environment. Disposal of the contaminated item by incineration or in landfills can pose comparable problems. Many issues concerning economy, including labor costs, storage, and delivery, need to be evaluated on an individual basis. Economy may be shown with the use of disposable products.

Considerations for the Use of Disposable Products

A disposable product is used once with reasonable assurance of safety and effectiveness. Most disposables are patient-charge items (i.e., the cost of these items is added to the patient's bill). Use of patient-charge items requires specific and accurate recordkeeping.

Most surgical computer systems send all the estimated items into a case cart system with an estimated charge sheet. The case cart usually contains only the items needed for a routine procedure. If the total complement of items is used during the procedure, the disposables are already charged in the system. This saves personnel time and money by having much of the paperwork done in advance. This process facilitates flat-rate costing by procedure.

If a disposable item remains completely intact (is not opened or contaminated in any way), it can be returned to stock. The cost of the item is then removed from the patient's charge sheet in the computer, using a process referred to as *charging by exception*. The cost is removed by personnel in the stock room, and the patient is not charged. The item is then electronically credited to stock for future use in the departmental inventory.

Barcode technology is very useful for inventory tracking. Many manufacturers have included a barcode on their packaging. Items can be scanned as used and the computer automatically charges it to the patient. Examples include staplers, single-use instrumentation, and implants.

Conversely, taking an item from the stock room without accounting for it in the computer system will leave an inaccurate number of items available for actual use. Planning for other cases depends on having correct numbers of disposables available for use. The system will know when an item is really available only if the records are complete and up to date.

Advantages

- When a sterile item is required, proper packaging and sterility must be ensured. Sterility is guaranteed by reliable manufacturers as long as the integrity of their packages is maintained. Industry conforms to far more rigid standards of quality control than onsite conditions permit. All sterilized products are tested for sterility before they are distributed to purchasers.
- Single-use items, such as urinary and suction catheters, are esthetically more acceptable to patients. More important, disposable products eliminate a potential source of cross-contamination.
- Items such as needles and disposable trocars ensure more comfort for the patient because they are always new and sharp. Proper function is thus ensured.
- Standardized service at reduced cost per unit may be provided. Sponges are precounted and sterilized, for example. Packs and trays become standardized and can be customized.
- Loss and breakage in reprocessing reusable items are eliminated.
- Labor costs of processing supplies are reduced, particularly in the tedious, meticulous cleaning and packaging.
- The need for expensive mechanical cleaning equipment is eliminated.
- Contaminated used items can be contained for safe disposal. Handling is minimal, and processing is eliminated.

Disadvantages

- Costly waste occurs if sterile items are contaminated by carelessness or are unnecessarily opened. Extreme care is needed in opening packages to maintain sterility. Handling should not compromise the integrity of wrappings and pose a threat to the maintenance of sterility.
- Flexibility in complying with requests of individual physicians for special setups can be complicated. No allowance is made for deviation from custom packs. Procedures need to be standardized to conform to available items and sets.
- If a defect is found in one package, it may extend throughout the total lot, requiring replacement of the total supply on hand.

Each lot is numbered for identification and recall if a problem arises.

- The circulating nurse may have to open an increased number of individually packaged items if the custom pack is not adequate.
- In the event of a sudden increase in use, adequate inventory may not be readily available.
- Potentially unstable products, such as some disposable trays containing medications, may carry an expiration date. Unless oldest products are used first, unnecessary costs are incurred if a product must be discarded because its time of reliability has expired. All dated products should be routinely checked for expiration.
- Environmental ecology may be affected by incineration or disposal in landfills. Some medical waste is regulated by local and federal laws.

Other Considerations

Other considerations regarding the use of disposable products include the following:

- Some hospitals have saved money by reducing their labor force through conversion to as many totally disposable systems as possible, such as intravenous therapy, drapes, and special procedure trays. In some geographic areas where efficient labor may be readily available at minimum wage, disposable products are more costly than labor. However, if professional personnel are being used for reprocessing supplies, use of disposable products will enable them to spend more time giving more care to patients and less time on processing supplies.
- Proper and safe storage facilities should be provided. More storage space or more frequent deliveries may be required to maintain adequate inventories of disposable products.
- Disposal may be an ecologic problem. Used items are taken to an incinerator, compactor, or other safe waste-disposal area. Waste should not be allowed to accumulate in the OR suite or in other hospital areas.
- Disposables opened but unused or exposed to patients in any way can be set aside for orientation or practice sessions or donated to nursing schools. Care is taken not to use anything from a sterile field that has been used in a surgical procedure. Cases that are set up and immediately canceled are ideal for salvaging items for learning situations.

Reusing/Reprocessing Disposable Single-Use Products/Devices

Manufacturers use extensive controls and testing procedures to ensure cleanliness, nontoxicity, nonpyrogenicity, biocompatibility, sterility, and function of disposable products. All items must be safe and effective for their intended patient uses. The manufacturer guarantees product stability and sterility for a single use only. A single-use device (SUD) must be labeled for one-time use and may not withstand reprocessing.

In this era of cost containment, salvage of undamaged disposable items may be attempted. The risks of salvaging items should be evaluated seriously. The health care facility assumes legal responsibility for items it chooses to reuse, reprocess, and resterilize. The manufacturer cannot be held liable for the efficacy of a disposable product or one intended for single use if the user chooses to reprocess it. The burden of liability rests with the processor.

Reuse

A used, disposable, single-use item requires cleaning, packaging, and sterilizing if it will be reused as a sterile item. Some products degrade with use. Many manufacturers have not tested their products for more than one use. For a product to be reused, it should be tested to validate patient safety. Patients have the right to know they are being treated with a reused single-use product. They should not be charged the cost of a new item.

Reprocessing

Repackaging and resterilizing unused sterile disposable items may be hazardous. These are items that were opened and not needed, or they are clean but have been contaminated in some way (i.e., the original packaging is not intact). Many of these items are very expensive, and salvage seems to be an acceptable alternative.

The manufacturer must provide written instructions for resterilization of unused but contaminated items by onsite personnel. Many of these items are heat sensitive. Services that reprocess and resterilize some types of clean, unused, and undamaged products are available. Such services must guarantee product stability and sterility. The FDA regulates reprocessing and requires specific guidelines and tracking of reprocessed items.[5] Third-party reprocessing facilities must be approved by the FDA.

Resterilization

The sterilization process must not alter the characteristics of any part of the product, regardless of whether it is intended to be disposable or reusable. Some products are labeled "do not resterilize." This instruction means that the product will be damaged or rendered ineffective in the process of resterilization. The manufacturer's recommendations should be followed if any reprocessing is performed.

Safety Considerations

Patient safety should be the prime concern in the decision to reuse, reprocess, or resterilize a disposable item. The following questions should be answered:

- Is the item a noncritical/noninvasive device? Critical items, particularly those that will enter or be in contact with the bloodstream or mucous membranes, present the greatest risks for adverse effects. Disposables of this type should not be reprocessed.
- Is the item really clean? Many porous materials cannot be thoroughly cleaned after use. If these are not adequately cleaned, microbial growth can predispose patients to infection. Lumens of catheters and tubing are especially difficult to clean. Biologic debris interferes with the sterilization process. Many items cannot be disassembled for adequate cleaning.
- Is the item nontoxic or nonpyrogenic after cleaning and reprocessing? Residues from some cleaning compounds and sterilizing processes are toxic. Chemicals can be retained by the item during reprocessing.
- Is the item truly sterile? The sterilization method should be appropriate for materials in the item and in the packaging.

The packaging material should allow penetration of the sterilant to all surfaces of the item and should prevent contamination during storage. Sterility should be verified by biologic testing for each type of product that is resterilized.

- Is the integrity of the product maintained? Physical and/or chemical characteristics may be altered by cleaning agents, the cleaning process, or resterilization. Some materials deteriorate or become brittle, which can affect function.
- Is the number of times an item has been reprocessed tracked and controlled? The manufacturer's written instructions should include the number of times the product may safely be reused or sterilized if the item can be reprocessed. The user should ensure that this number is not exceeded. The manufacturer has no control after a product leaves the factory. If the item is not in its original package, pertinent product information may not be immediately available.
- Is the item traceable? Reprocessing of any implantable item, such as synthetic mesh or graft material, should be controlled by lot numbers. The lot number on the product when first obtained from the manufacturer corresponds only with the processes at the point of controlled production.

If the product is reprocessed onsite, the lot number is no longer valid because the same controls are not in place for subsequent sterilization. Many variables can alter the safety of the product for reuse. Any patient receiving this implantable material after reprocessing is not getting the same level of care as the first patient for whom it was opened.

- Is the item being charged for twice? How are charges determined? Charging full price for a used item is not ethical.

If in doubt about the appropriateness of a reprocessed item, it should not be reused. With or without written instructions from the manufacturer, the health care facility is liable for product safety, stability, and sterility of any item it processes and sterilizes.

EVOLVE WEBSITE

http://evolve.elsevier.com/Hornacky/BerryKohn/

- Student Interactive Questions
- Glossary

References

1. The Healthcare Sterile Processing Association: *Certification*. www.myhspa.org. Accessed April 28, 2023.
2. Garcia R, Barnes S, Boukidjian, et al.: Recommendations for change in infection prevention programs and practice, *Am J Infect Control* 50(12):1281−1295, 2022.
3. AORN: *Guidelines for perioperative practice*, Denver, CO, 2024, The Association.
4. Ploydoeng M, Rajatanavin N, Rattanakaemakorn P: UV-C light: a powerful technique for inactivating microorganisms and the related side effects to the skin, *Photodermatol Photoimmunol Photomed* 37(1):12−19, 2020.
5. The Joint Commission: *Ensuring critical instruments and devices are appropriate for reuse, Quick Safety Issue 64*, 2022. www.jointcommission.org.

Bibliography

Phillips NM, Hornacky A: *Pass CNOR*, St. Louis, 2019, Elsevier.

18

Sterilization

CHAPTER OUTLINE

Sterilization Versus Disinfection, 313

Sterilization, 313

Assembly of Instrument Sets, 315

Packaging Instruments and Other Items for Sterilization, 316

Thermal Sterilization, 320

Chemical Sterilization, 326

Radiation Sterilization, 333

Control Measures, 333

Custom Packs, 335

CHAPTER OBJECTIVES

After studying this chapter, the learner will be able to:

- Define the term *sterilization*.
- List three methods of sterilization.
- Describe the process for preparing an item for sterilization.
- Identify the primary hazards associated with each type of sterilization.

- Discuss sterilization process monitors.
- Discuss the use of a case cart system.

KEY TERMS AND DEFINITIONS

Aeration Warm circulating air is used to remove ethylene oxide sterilant gas from packages in a special chamber for a specified time.

Bowie-Dick test Class 2 chemical indicator used in a prevacuum sterilizer to test the efficacy of the air removal cycle.

Capillary action Moisture penetrates through a permeable surface and carries with it microbial material.

Case cart System of gathering and delivering instruments and supplies to the perioperative environment. Some models include provision for the return of instruments and contaminated items to the appropriate decontamination area after the surgical or interventional procedure.

Custom packs Prepackaged collections of disposable supplies, drapes, sponges, and containers prepared by the manufacturer or the distributor according to specific instructions and requests by a particular service at a facility.

Flash sterilization A rapid method of steam sterilizing properly prepared instruments for immediate use. These instruments are not wrapped. Flash sterilization is not the preferred method of sterilization.

Gravity displacement sterilizer A steam sterilizer that uses steam in a downward motion to remove air from the sterilizing chamber. Air exits near the front lower drain. Can be high speed or pulsing.

Indicator Devices inserted into a packed set and attached to the outside of the wrapper/container used by health care personnel to monitor sterilization exposure conditions. Biologic indicators are the best indicators that parameters are adequate to kill microorganisms. Chemical indicators are not proof of

sterility, but they signify that the item was exposed to the parameters necessary for sterilization. Autoclave tape is a class 1–type indicator.

Integrator A chemical device inserted into a packed set that changes in response to the time, temperature, and steam penetration to demonstrate visually that parameters necessary for sterilization have been met. An integrator mimics the conditions required of a biologic monitor.

Prevacuum sterilizer A faster steam sterilizer that removes air by a vacuum before filling the chamber with steam. Also known as dynamic air removal steam sterilization.

Process challenge pack/process challenge device (PCD) A prepackaged unit consisting of dense materials and sterilization indicators or integrators used to test the effectiveness of the sterilization process.

Rigid container An instrument case that seals and locks. Instruments are placed in a rigid container for sterilization.

Sterile Microorganisms are at an irreducible minimum. No viable microbes.

Sterilization Processes by which all pathogenic and nonpathogenic microorganisms, including endospores, are killed. This term refers only to a validated process capable of destroying all forms of microbial life, including endospores. The sterilizer is a piece of equipment used to attain either physical or chemical sterilization. The agent used must be capable of killing all forms of microorganisms.

Strike-through Moisture or other substance penetrates through a sterile drape or wrapper to an unsterile surface. Strike-through provides a pathway for capillary action.

Terminal cleaning Thorough cleaning and disinfection of the perioperative environment at the end of use.

Terminal sterilization Procedures carried out for the destruction of pathogens on instruments at the end of the surgical procedure in the operating room or in other areas of patient contact (e.g., postanesthesia care unit [PACU], intensive care unit [ICU], patient care unit).

Turnover Activity geared toward cleaning and preparation of the operating room between cases for the next patient's arrival.

Wet pack Internal aspect of the sterile package remains moist or damp after passing through all sterilization parameters. Indicates a nonsterile item.

Wicking Passage of fluids through a material by passive action. Also referred to as capillary action or strike-through.

Sterilization Versus Disinfection

Pathogenic microorganisms, as well as those that do not normally invade healthy tissue, can cause infection if introduced mechanically into the body. Standardized procedures that are based on accepted principles and practices are necessary for the sterilization or disinfection of all supplies and equipment used for patient care in the perioperative environment.[1] Following established protocols for instrument processing helps minimize the patient's risk for infection of the surgical site.

A sterile item has been exposed to a sterilization process to render it free of all living microorganisms, including endospores. As long as sterility is maintained, this process renders items safe for contact with nonintact tissue and for exposure to the vascular system without transmitting infection. The sterilization process should provide assurance that an item can be expected to be free of known viable pathogenic and nonpathogenic microorganisms, including endospores. For items and materials that cannot be sterilized, disinfectants are used to kill as many microorganisms in the environment as possible. (Decontamination and disinfection are described in Chapter 17.)

Sterilization

Bacterial endospores (e.g., *Clostridia* and *Bacillus*) are the most resistant of all living organisms because of their capacity to withstand external destructive agents. Although the physical or chemical process by which all pathogenic and nonpathogenic microorganisms (including endospores) are destroyed is not absolute, supplies and equipment are considered sterile when all parameters have been met during a sterilization process.

Reliability Parameters for Sterilization

Two types of parameters are considered for the reliability of sterilizing methods: product-associated parameters and process-associated parameters.

Product-Associated Parameters

- *Bioburden:* The degree of contamination with microorganisms and organic debris
- *Bioresistance:* Factors such as heat and/or moisture sensitivities and product stability
- *Biostate:* The nutritional, physical, and/or reproductive phase of microorganisms
- *Bioshielding:* Characteristics of the packaging materials
- *Density:* Factors affecting penetration and evacuation of the agent

Process-Associated Parameters

- Temperature
- Humidity/moisture/hydration
- Time
- Purity of the agent and air, and the residual effects or residues
- Saturation/penetration
- Capacity of the sterilizer and the position of items within the chamber

Methods of Sterilization

Reliable sterilization depends on the contact of the sterilizing agent with all surfaces of the item to be sterilized. Selection of the agent used to achieve sterility depends primarily on the nature of the item to be sterilized. The time required to kill endospores in the available equipment then becomes critical. Sterilization processes are either physical or chemical, and each method has its advantages and disadvantages. The following are available sterilizing agents (sterilants)[2]:

1. Thermal (physical)
   a. Steam under pressure/moist heat
   b. Hot air/dry heat
2. Chemical
   a. Ethylene oxide gas
   b. Hydrogen peroxide plasma/vapor
   c. Ozone gas
   d. Acetic acid solution
   e. Glutaraldehyde solution
   f. Peracetic acid 0.2% solution
   g. Hypochlorous acid (electrochemical conversion process)
3. Radiation (physical)
   a. Microwave (nonionizing)
   b. X-ray (ionizing)

Sterilization Cycle

The time required to achieve sterilization is referred to as the process cycle, which includes the following:
- Heat up and/or penetration of the agent
- Kill time (i.e., exposure to the agent)
- Safety factor for bioburden
- Evacuation or dissipation of the agent

Monitoring the Sterilization Cycle

To ensure that instruments and supplies are sterile when used, it is essential that the sterilization process be monitored. Care is taken to ensure that testing products such as chemical and biologic indicator strips and packs have not expired before use. The accuracy of monitoring depends on the systems in place for the task.

Appropriate care and maintenance of mechanical equipment plays a large part in accurate readouts and documentation of processing cycles performed. The general considerations are mentioned in the following sections. Specific tests are discussed later in this chapter with each method of sterilization.

Administrative Monitoring

Work practices are supervised. Written policies and procedures are strictly followed by all personnel responsible for sterilizing and handling sterile supplies. If sterility cannot be achieved or maintained, the system has failed. Policies and procedures pertain to the following:

- Decontaminating, terminally sterilizing, and cleaning all reusable items; disposing of disposable items in the appropriate manner
- Packaging and labeling items
- Loading and unloading the sterilizer
- Operating the sterilizer and checking its efficacy
- Monitoring and maintaining the records of each cycle
- Adhering to safety precautions and preventive maintenance (PM) protocol
- Transporting sterile packages to the sterile storage room. Cart should be enclosed and have a solid bottom
- Storing sterile items
- Handling sterile items ready for use
- Making a sterile transfer to a sterile field at the point of use
- Tracking and recalling items if an item in a particular load is not safe for use

Mechanical Indicators

Sterilizers have gauges, thermometers, timers, recorders, and/or other devices that monitor their functions. Most sterilizers have automatic controls and locking devices, and some have alarm systems that are activated if the sterilizer fails to operate correctly. Records are reviewed and maintained for each cycle. Test packs or special diagnostics are run at least daily, as appropriate for the type of sterilizer, to monitor the functions of each sterilizer. Such tests can identify processing errors.

The manufacturer of the sterilizer provides a manual for the comprehensive care and maintenance of the sterilizing device. Reliable operation depends on the following:

- Routine maintenance that consists of daily inspections and scheduled cleanings per the manufacturer's recommendation. All gaskets, gauges, graph pens, drain screens, paper rolls, ink cartridges, and charting devices should be repaired or replaced by qualified personnel as needed.
- PM that includes periodic calibration, lubrication, and function checks by qualified personnel on a scheduled basis should be documented.

Chemical Indicators

External indicators such as tape, labels, or paper strips should be clearly visible on the outside of every package to differentiate between sterilized and unsterilized items. The indicator helps monitor the physical conditions within the sterilizer to alert personnel to malfunctions, human errors in packaging, or improper loading of the sterilizer.

An internal indicator/integrator is placed inside a package in a position most likely to be difficult for the sterilant to penetrate. If a chemical reaction of the indicator does not show the expected results, the item should not be used. Indicators do not establish the sterility of an item; they indicate only that process parameters have been met.

Chemical indicators are categorized into classes according to the type of process measurement they perform.

- *Class 1:* Immediate visual indicator on the exterior of the processed pack, such as striped tape or a tab that changes color in response to the sterilizer.
- *Class 2:* Autoclave test packs used to test for air removal during the cycle.
- *Class 3:* Single-variable indicator of one of the parameters of sterilization.
- *Class 4:* Multivariable monitor strip that displays two or more changes in response to sterilization. Commonly used in a dry heat cycle.
- *Class 5:* Chemical integrator strip that reacts in the same way as a biologic indicator in the presence of time, temperature, and steam penetration.
- *Class 6:* Emulating indicator responds to all critical variables during the use of a sterilization process challenge pack/process challenge device (PCD).

Biologic Indicators

Positive assurance that sterilization conditions have been achieved can be obtained only through a biologic control test. A biologic indicator is a preparation of living endospores that are resistant to the sterilizing agent. The preparation may be supplied in a self-contained system (e.g., dry endospore strips) or in sealed vials, discs, or ampules of endospores in suspension.

To perform the test, a biologic unit that has been exposed to the sterilant and an unprocessed biologic unit (control) from the same lot number are incubated for the same time period. If sterilization has occurred, the processed biologic unit will not grow any microorganisms. The unprocessed biologic control unit will grow microorganisms and display a change in color. If the unprocessed biologic unit fails to grow microorganisms, its endospores have been inactivated. In such a case, the processed unit also may have been inactive before processing; thus the biologic test is rendered invalid. The entire load is considered unsterile when either the test indicator or the control is in question. Test indicators and controls should be interpreted by qualified personnel.

Each sterilization process requires biologic testing at regular intervals. Consecutive biologic monitors should be run each time the sterilizer is calibrated, repaired, or relocated. Biologic testing involves incubation according to the manufacturer's recommendations. The gram-positive bacterial endospores used for biologic monitoring and testing intervals include the following:

- *Geobacillus stearothermophilus* at 131° F to 140° F (55–60° C) tests steam under pressure daily and with each load of implants.
- *Bacillus atrophaeus* at 95° F to 98.6° F (35–37° C) tests dry heat and ethylene oxide (EO) with every load.
- *B. atrophaeus* testing is performed daily for low-temperature hydrogen peroxide plasma.
- Peracetic acid sterilizers are tested according to the manufacturer's recommendations. The user can employ commercial endospore strips for use during the cycle but may want to test rinse water as a secondary measure.

A rapid-readout biologic indicator specifically for monitoring a high-speed pressure steam sterilizer with a gravity displacement cycle is based on the fluorometric detection of a *G. stearothermophilus*–bound enzyme rather than on endospore growth. The enzyme becomes fluorescent yellow within 60 minutes as the endospores are killed.

Biologic indicators need to conform to the testing standards of the United States Pharmacopeia (USP). A control test is performed at least weekly in each sterilizer (Table 18.1). Many hospitals monitor daily; others test each cycle. Every load of implantable devices is monitored, and the implant should not be used until negative test results are known. All test results are filed in a permanent record for each sterilizer.

Assembly of Instrument Sets

The weight of instruments and density of metal mass are distributed in the tray to allow steam penetration for sterilizing and revaporization for drying. A large tray distributes instruments so they make minimum contact with one another.

The size, design, and density of instruments are more important than their weight. The conditions necessary for steam sterilization are difficult to achieve in exceedingly heavy sets. Trays should not be overloaded. Closed container instrument sets should not weigh more than 25 pounds. Consideration is given to the personnel who must lift and move the packed sets when determining the presterilization weight. To assemble instrument sets for sterilization, the following steps should be performed:

TABLE 18.1   Guidelines for the Use of Chemical and Biologic Indicators[a]

AAMI	AHA	AORN	CDC	TJC
Chemical				
Purpose: To indicate items exposed to the sterilization process; to monitor one or more sterilization parameters; to detect failures in packaging, loading, or sterilizer function. Indicators do not verify sterility.				
Placement				
External: on all packages except if internal indicator is visible	With each package; can be used inside or on outside	External: visible on every package	External: attached to each package	With each package, no designation to inside or outside
Internal: in center or area least accessible to sterilant within each package		Internal: inside each package	Internal: inside large pack	
Biologic				
Purpose: To document efficacy of sterilization process by killing resistant endospores; to ensure that all process parameters are met; to detect nonsterilizing conditions in sterilizer.				
Steam				
Frequency: at least weekly, preferably daily	Frequency: once a day	Frequency: at least once a week, preferably daily, and with each load of implants	Frequency: at least once a week, and with each load of implants	Frequency: at least weekly (daily is recommended), or with each load if sterilization activities are performed less frequently or if load contains implantable or intravascular material
Placement: positioned in cold point in process challenge test pack, normally bottom front of sterilizer				
Ethylene Oxide				
Frequency: every load	Frequency: every load	Frequency: every load	Frequency: at least once a week, and with each load of implants	Frequency: at least weekly (daily is recommended), or with each load if sterilization activities are performed less frequently or if load contains implantable or intravascular material
Placement: inside pack in geometric center of load				

[a]All organizations require that indicators and integrators be used routinely.

AAMI, Association for the Advancement of Medical Instrumentation; *AHA*, American Hospital Association; *AORN*, Association of periOperative Registered Nurses; *CDC*, Centers for Disease Control and Prevention; *TJC*, The Joint Commission.

1. Make sure the instruments are thoroughly dry. All instruments belonging to each set must have passed through terminal cleaning and terminal sterilization before they are safe to handle.

2. Unless contraindicated, place an absorbent towel or foam in the bottom of the tray to absorb condensate, as for a rigid container with vacuum valves. Include a biologic indicator or chemical integrator in the tray.

3. Count instruments as they are placed in the tray, and record the number of each type. A preprinted form is often used for this purpose. This form might be placed in the tray before wrapping and sterilization so the circulating nurse and scrub person can verify the baseline count. The form can be folded in half and placed in a paper peel pouch without a plastic coating to prevent printer toner from transferring to the instruments during processing. Concerns for toner particulate transfer to the instruments during the cycle are under study. The best choice may be to affix the tray inventory count sheet to the outside of the package.

4. Arrange the instruments in a definite pattern to protect them from damage and to facilitate removal for counting and use. Follow the instrument book or other listing of instruments to be included.

5. Place heavy instruments, such as retractors, in the bottom of the tray.

6. Open the hinges and box locks on all hinged instruments.

7. Place ring-handled instruments on stringers or holders designed for this purpose. The curved jaws of hemostatic forceps and clamps should point in the same direction from smallest to largest. Instruments should be grouped by style and classification (e.g., six straight hemostats, six curved hemostats). Do not band with rubber bands. The metal under the band will not sterilize adequately.

8. Place sharp and delicate instruments on top of other instruments. They can be separated with an absorbent material or left in a sterilizing rack with the blades and tips suspended. The blades of scissors, other cutting edges, and delicate tips should not touch other instruments. If the instrument has a protective guard, leave it on. Tip-protecting covers or instrument-protecting plastic sleeves should be made of material that is steam-permeable and does not melt or deform with heat.

9. Place concave or cupped instruments with the cupped surfaces down so that water condensate does not collect in them during steam sterilization and drying.

10. Disassemble all detachable parts. Some parts, such as screws and springs, can be put in a peel pouch that is left open. Sealed pouches may not process correctly during the sterilization process.

11. Separate dissimilar metals. For example, brass knife handles and malleable retractors should be separated from stainless steel instruments. Preferably, put each metal in a separate tray, or separate metals with absorbent material.

12. Place instruments with a lumen, such as a suction tip, in as near a horizontal position as possible. These instruments should be tilted as little as possible to prevent trapped air or the pooling of water condensate.

13. Distribute weight as evenly as possible in the tray. Some trays have dividers, clips, and pins that attach to the bottom, which help prevent instruments from shifting and keep them in alignment.

14. Wrap the tray or place it in a rigid container. Check woven textile wrappers for holes or abrasion. Sequentially double-wrap in a woven or nonwoven material, or use a double-thickness wrap in a single-fold configuration.

15. Place a chemical indicator tab or tape on the outside wrapper or container for proof that the package has been through the parameters necessary for sterilization.

16. Label the sets appropriately with their intended use (e.g., basic set), the date sterilized, and the process lot control number.

Packaging Instruments and Other Items for Sterilization

To be effective, the sterilizing agent must come into direct contact with all surfaces of every instrument. Therefore instruments must be packaged (individually or in sets) in such a way to allow adequate exposure to the sterilant, prevent air from being trapped and moisture from being retained during the sterilization process, and ensure sterile transfer to the sterile field.

Most surgical instruments are made of stainless steel and can be sterilized by steam under pressure. Effective steam sterilization involves the direct contact of all surfaces with steam and the revaporization of water condensate to produce a dry, sterile instrument.

Instrument Packaging

For sterilizing and transporting, instruments are put in a closed container or wrapped individually. Instruments placed in open trays are wrapped as sets. Instruments may be prepared in advance as for a case cart or may be retained in sterile core storage until needed.

Packaging Considerations

The packaging materials for all methods of sterilization should do the following:

- Permit penetration of the sterilizing agent to achieve sterilization of all items in the package.
- Allow the release of the sterilizing agent at the end of the exposure period and allow adequate drying or aerating.
- Withstand the physical conditions of the sterilizing process.
- Maintain integrity of the package at varying atmospheric and humidity levels. In dry climates or at high altitudes, some packaging materials are susceptible to rupture during sterilization or dry out and crack in storage.
- Provide an impermeable barrier to microorganisms, dust particles, and moisture after sterilization. Items must remain sterile from the time they are removed from the sterilizer until they are used.
- Cover items completely and easily and fasten securely with adhesive strip or a heat seal that cannot be resealed after opening. Seal integrity should be tamperproof. A margin of at least 1 inch (2.5 cm) is considered a standard for safety on all sealed packages. Scissors should not be used to cut off the end of a package. Contents cannot be drawn out over this cut end because the contents would be contaminated by the edge of the packaging material. For the same reason, packages are never torn open below a seal.
- Resist tears and punctures in handling. If accidental tears and holes do occur, they must be visible.

- Identification of the contents and the chemical indicator evidence of exposure to a sterilizing agent should be placed on a label that is visible on the outside of the package.
- Be free of toxic ingredients and nonfast dyes.
- Be lint-free or low-linting.
- Protect the contents from physical damage.
- Permit easy removal of the contents with transfer to the sterile field without contamination or delamination (separation into layers).
- Be economical.

Packages should be wrapped far enough away from sterile storage areas so that mixing sterile and nonsterile packages is not possible. Cabinets that contain nonsterile items should be labeled conspicuously. A procedure for sending items to and receiving items from the sterilizer should be set up so sterile and nonsterile packages can never be confused en route. This procedure must be understood by everyone.

Packages may be wrapped with nonwoven or woven materials sequentially in two layers. Double-thickness wrapping in one layer without using the sequential method is also acceptable. The wrappers can be stitched around the edges or bonded/fused together. Aseptic presentation to the sterile field is the prime consideration. Each facility should determine which method and material is best suited to the clinical environment.

Items are enclosed with all corners of the wrapper folded in. Either a square or an envelope fold may be used (Figs. 18.1 and 18.2).

- *Sequential wrapping with two wrappers:* An item is wrapped in one wrapper; the package is wrapped in a second wrapper. A cuff turned back on the first fold of each wrapper provides a margin of safety to prevent contamination when opening after sterilization. Packages can be fastened securely with chemical indicator tape.
- *Single wrap:* An item is wrapped in a single wrap that is of double thickness. The package is sealed with chemical indicator tape.

Packaging Materials and Methods

Packaging materials must be compatible with the sterilization process. The following materials may be safely used to wrap items for steam sterilization because they permit steam penetration, adequate air removal, and adequate drying.

Woven Fabrics

Reusable woven fabrics are commonly referred to as *muslin* or *linen*. When no other alternative is available, a 140-thread count, carded, 100% cotton muslin is used. Steam sterilizer cycles are based on a time-temperature profile of 140-thread count muslin. This type of fabric is not moisture resistant and is used in a double thickness. Two pieces are sewn together on the edges only, with a blind hem and without cross-stitching, so the wrapper is free of holes.

This wrapper should withstand between 50 and 75 launderings before becoming too worn to be a microbial barrier. A laundering mark-off system is helpful to monitor the number of times a wrapper has been used. The manufacturer should provide information about the number of launderings and sterilization cycles the wrapper can withstand.

Before resterilization, woven fabrics are laundered to rehydrate them. The moisture content of the woven material affects steam penetration and prevents superheating during the sterilization

process. The fabric should be stored in an area with controlled room temperature and humidity, according to the manufacturer's instructions. Before use, the woven fabric is inspected for holes and patched with vulcanized patches if necessary. Check manufacturer's recommendation with the use of vulcanized patches because some sterilants may not penetrate the patches. Fabric may create free-floating lint in the OR.

Nonwoven Fabrics

Nonwoven fabrics are a combination of cellulose and rayon with strands of nylon randomly oriented through it, or they are a combination of other natural and synthetic fibers bonded by a method other than weaving. These fabrics have the flexibility and handling qualities of woven materials and are available in several weights. Lightweight is used in four thicknesses; medium weight is the most economical for wrapping items in two thicknesses; and heavy-duty weight is used when a single wrap is used for wrapping supplies for sterilization.

Packages are wrapped in the same manner as woven fabrics. Nonwoven fabrics provide an excellent barrier against microorganisms and moisture during storage after sterilization. They are disposable and virtually lint free. Some manufacturers provide a recycling service for nonwoven wrappers.

Peel Packs or Pouches

Peel pouches and tubes made of a combination of paper on one side and clear plastic film on the other are satisfactory for wrapping single instruments, odd-shaped items, and small items. Double-sided paper pouches are commercially available. For sterile presentation, a peel-open seal may be preformed on one end. The open end is either heat sealed or closed with indicator tape after the item is inserted. All air is expressed from the package before sealing. Self-sealing pouches with adhesive flaps that do not require heat sealing also are available.

The sequential packaging of supplies in a smaller pouch into a larger pouch is not routinely necessary. However, this method may be useful for keeping multiple small items together, such as a set of bone screws. The aseptic presentation of tiny parts to the sterile field without dropping items on the floor can be accomplished with sequential packaging. The manufacturer's instructions should be consulted if sequential peel pouches will be used.[3]

A peel pouch should not be processed flat but rather positioned on its side. The plastic side of the pouch can impede the flow of steam penetration through the package. Inclusion of plastic-sided pouches within an instrument set can impair the process of steam through a tray. Obstruction of the steam flow can compromise the entire load. After processing, the peel pouch should be stored on its side to maintain integrity of the packaging.

Sealants and Labeling

Chemical indicator tape is used to seal packages such as peel pouches and wrapped items. Steam-sensitive tape resembles tan masking tape and reveals dark stripes when exposed to steam sterilizing conditions. Gas-sensitive tape is light green and reveals dark stripes after exposure to gas sterilizing conditions.

Peel pouches are usually heat-sealed or self-sealing and have an indicator area or dot that changes color in response to steam or gas exposure.[3] They may be sealed with steam- or gas-sensitive tape. These sealants are not indicators of sterility but are a visual means by which to validate exposure to sterilant conditions. Labels or

1. Place items assembled for pack in center of two sheets of wrapping material.

2. Fan-fold open end away from you over items. Cuff top layer.

3. Repeat same procedure with end toward you, lining up cuff directly on top of first cuff.

4. Miter left end and fold neatly up and over top of pack.

5. Repeat with right side of pack.

6. Repeat step 2.

7. Repeat step 3.

8. Repeat step 4.

9. Repeat step 5 and securely affix with pressure-sensitive indicator tape over end.

• **Fig. 18.1** Square fold for wrapping item for sterilization. Single-layer (double-thickness) heavy wrap may be applied in a nonsequential manner. (Modified from the Association for the Advancement of Medical Instrumentation: *Good hospital practice: steam sterilization and sterility assurance,* ANSI/AAMI ST46, Arlington, VA, 2009, American National Standards Institute.)

writing should be applied on the plastic side of the peel pouch to allow the sterilant to penetrate the paper side without transferring the ink to the instrument.

The sealing tape on the outside of the package should be labeled with a dark marker that is nontoxic and resistant to moisture, bleed-through, or smearing. Preprinted labels may be used instead. The date of processing and a load number should be attached to each package. These forms of identification are helpful in tracking and locating items that have been processed in batches. A recall of items may be necessary if the sterility of a particular load is in doubt.

Wrapped Trays

To allow steam penetration around instruments and prevent air from being trapped in the tray, trays cannot be solid. Therefore instruments are placed in open trays with mesh or perforated bottoms. Absorbent towels or foam may be placed in the bottom of the tray and over instruments to absorb condensate and protect instruments from snagging in the perforations. Trays are sequentially double-wrapped in woven or nonwoven wrappers. They must be allowed to cool and dry at the end of the sterilizing cycle before they are handled. Hot packages should not be placed on cool surfaces. Condensation under the tray can generate strike-through,

1. Place two wrappers on flat surface with one point toward you. Place item to be wrapped in center of wrapper with its length parallel to you.

2. Fold corner nearest you over item until it is completely covered. Fold corner back toward you 2 to 3 inches.

3. Fold left side of wrapper over and parallel to item. Fold end of corner back 2 to 3 inches.

4. Repeat with right side. Lap center folds at least 1/2 inch.

5. Tuck in side edges of remaining corner to eliminate any direct opening to item. Bring top corner down to bottom edges and tuck in, leaving point for opening.

6. Repeat step 2.

7. Repeat step 3.

8. Repeat step 4.

9. Bring point of wrapper completely around package and seal with appropriate tape.

• **Fig. 18.2** Envelope fold for wrapping item for sterilization. Single-layer (double-thickness) heavy wrap may be applied in a nonsequential manner. (Modified from the Association for the Advancement of Medical Instrumentation: *Good hospital practice: steam sterilization and sterility assurance,* ANSI/AAMI ST46, Arlington, VA, 2009, American National Standards Institute.)

promoting capillary action of moisture between the warm sterilized tray and the shelving. The moisture can carry microorganisms to the inside of the package.

Rigid Closed Containers

A metal or plastic rigid closed container system may be used for sterilizing instruments singly or in sets. A stainless steel mesh or perforated basket lined with foam porous padding nests in the rigid container. The lid is affixed to the container base by metal snap locks. Plastic breakaway shrink bands secure the flip locks and act as chemical external indicators by changing color. The body of the container is labeled with the contents. A load-identifying label is affixed to the container before processing.

Most styles of closed containers have single-use unidirectional air filters in the lid and bottom. These filters are changed each time the container is processed. The closed container is placed into the steam sterilizer so the steam can penetrate through the bottom and lid. Some containers do not have vents in the bottom. The manufacturer of the closed container system should establish the processing temperature and time.

After the sterilization process is complete, the container is placed on a firm, dry surface adjacent to the sterile table. The circulating nurse breaks the shrink band seal by flipping open the locks and then lifts the lid toward them. The outer rigid container is not considered sterile. The scrub person carefully reaches into the container without touching it and grasps the handles of the sterile inner basket, lifting it straight up and out. The sterile basket containing the instruments can be placed on the sterile back table.

Sterile supplies are not to be opened into the rigid container because the edges are not considered sterile. Condensate in the bottom of the nonvented closed container is considered sterile because it is not permeable to the capillary action associated with other packaging methods.

Specialized Tray Sets

A manufacturer may supply a fitted case or rack for a set of instruments or implants, such as orthopedic devices. These cases or racks help protect the instruments and keep them separated for sterilization and use. These cases or racks are double-wrapped before sterilization; they are not the same as rigid closed containers.

Count Sheets

Count sheets are sometimes packed inside the instrument set for use in counting instruments in the OR. The inks and toner pose a questionable risk for depositing foreign matter inside the patient during the surgical procedure. Toner in the printer cartridge is fused to the paper by heat. The transfer of the toner from the paper to the instruments is of concern during thermal sterilization. Although no data exist to demonstrate harm from toner on count sheets, no data are available to prove that toner is harmless. It may contribute to the formation of adhesions in the same way any foreign body can stimulate an inflammatory response.

Some facilities place the count sheet in a peel pouch. The plastic side of the pouch can obstruct the flow of steam if placed flat in the tray. A paper peel pouch is preferred. Another option is to place the count sheet in a separate labeled peel pouch and process it separately from the packed tray.

Thermal Sterilization

Heat is a dependable physical agent for the destruction of all forms of microbial life, including endospores. It may be used moist or dry. The most reliable and commonly used method of sterilization is steam under pressure.

Steam Under Pressure (Moist Heat Sterilization)

Heat destroys microorganisms, and this process is hastened by the addition of moisture. Steam alone is inadequate for sterilization. Pressure that is greater than atmospheric pressure is necessary to increase the temperature of steam for the thermal destruction of microbial life. Moist heat in the form of steam under pressure causes the denaturation and coagulation of protein or the enzyme-protein system within cells.

Direct saturated steam contact is the basis of the steam sterilization process. For a specified time and at a required temperature, the steam must penetrate every fiber and reach every surface of the items to be sterilized. When steam enters the sterilizer chamber under pressure, it condenses on contact with cold items. This condensation liberates heat, simultaneously heating and wetting all items in the load and thereby providing the two requisites: moisture and heat. This sterilization process is spoken of in terms of degrees of temperature and time of exposure—not in terms of pounds of pressure. Pressure increases the boiling temperature of water but alone has no significant effect on microorganisms or steam penetration.

Exposure time depends on the size and contents of the load and the temperature within the sterilizer. At the end of the cycle, reevaporation of water condensate must effectively dry contents of the load to maintain sterility; the water is dried from the sterilized pack or item.

The vegetative forms of most microorganisms are killed in a few minutes at temperatures ranging from 130° F to 150° F (54–65° C); however, bacterial endospores will withstand a temperature of 240° F (115° C) for more than 3 hours. No living thing can survive direct exposure to saturated steam at 250° F (121° C) for longer than 15 minutes. As the temperature of the steam is increased, the time of exposure may be decreased. A minimum temperature-time relationship is maintained throughout all portions of the load to accomplish effective sterilization.

Special Circumstances

Prions (pronounced pree-ons) such as those that cause Creutzfeldt-Jakob disease (CJD) are not a living plant, animal, or virus. They are infectious protein material, and the instruments used must be steam-sterilized for a minimum of 1 hour at 270° F (132° C) after soaking in sodium hydroxide (bleach) or sodium hypochlorite at room temperature for 1 hour, then rinsed. This solution should be solidified and incinerated after use.

If a **prevacuum sterilizer** is used, the item can be safe to handle if processed for 18 minutes at 274° F (134° C) after the 1-hour exposure to sodium hydroxide. If a **gravity displacement sterilizer** is used, the processing time increases to 1 hour. After the soaking and steam sterilizing procedures, the instruments can be processed through the routine washer-sterilizer procedure like other instruments.

Prion material becomes resistant to removal methods if left to dry. Instruments should be kept moist until they can be decontaminated and processed. Drapes and gowns should be disposable and incinerated because prions are not deactivated by laundry procedures used on woven material. The use of disposable instruments and supplies is highly recommended.

Eye instrumentation that is improperly cleaned and processed can subject the patient to toxic anterior segment syndrome (TASS). An inflammatory response in the anterior chamber of the eye causes permanent damage to intraocular tissues and predisposes the patient to secondary glaucoma. Eye instruments should be cleaned separately from other instruments and sterilized according to the manufacturer's instructions.

Advantages of Steam Sterilization
- Steam sterilization is the easiest, safest, and surest method of onsite sterilization. Heat- and moisture-stable items that can be steam-sterilized without damage should be processed with this method.
- Steam is the fastest method; its total time cycle is the shortest.
- Steam is the least expensive and most easily supplied agent. It is piped in from the facility's boiler room. An automatic, electrically powered steam generator can be mounted beneath the sterilizer for emergency standby when steam pressure is low.
- Most sterilizers have automatic controls and recording devices that eliminate the human factor from the sterilization process as much as possible when operated and cared for according to the recommendations of the manufacturer.
- Steam leaves no harmful residue. Many items such as stainless steel instruments withstand repeated processing without damage.

Disadvantages of Steam Sterilization

- Precautions must be used in preparing and packaging items, loading and operating the sterilizer, and drying the load.

- Items need to be clean, free of grease and oil, and not sensitive to heat.
- Steam must have direct contact with all areas of an item. It must be able to penetrate packaging material, but the material must be able to maintain sterility.
- The timing of the cycle is adjusted for differences in materials and sizes of loads; these variables are subject to human error.
- Steam may not be pure. Steam purity refers to the amount of solid, liquid, or vapor contamination in steam. Impurities can cause wet or stained packs and stained instruments.

Types of Steam Sterilizers

Sterilizers that are designed to use steam under pressure are often referred to as *autoclaves* to distinguish them from sterilizers that use other agents. Personnel charged with the responsibility of operating steam sterilizers must fully understand the principles and operation of each type. They must be aware of the problems that cause malfunction, which include attaining the sterilization temperature and maintaining it for the required time, trapped air, and dirty traps.

Gravity Displacement Sterilizer

The metal construction of the gravity displacement sterilizer contains two shells that form a jacket and a chamber. Steam fills the jacket that surrounds the chamber. After the door is tightly closed, steam enters the chamber at the back, near the top, and is deflected upward. Air is more than twice as heavy as steam. Thus, by gravity, air goes to the bottom and steam floats on top. Steam entering under pressure and remaining above the air displaces air downward (both in the chamber and in the wrapped items) and forces it out through a discharge outlet at the bottom front. The air passes through a filtering screen to a waste line.

A thermometer located at this outlet below the screen measures the temperature in the chamber. When steam has filled the chamber, it begins to flow past the thermometer (Fig. 18.3). The timing of the sterilizing period starts only when the thermometer reaches the desired temperature.

When air is trapped in the chamber or in wrapped items, the killing power of steam is decreased in direct proportion to the amount of air present. Because the vital discharge of air from the load always occurs in a downward direction, never sideways, all supplies are prepared and arranged to present the least possible resistance to the passage of steam downward through the load from the top of the chamber. Air and steam discharge lines are kept free of dirt, sediment, and lint.

Many gravity displacement steam sterilizers operate on a standard cycle of 250° F to 254° F (121–123° C) at a pressure of 15 to 18 pounds per square inch (psi). The size and contents of the chamber determine the exposure period; the average exposure time is 30 minutes for wrapped instruments. Exposure time may vary if a closed sterilization container system is used. Some air-powered instruments may require longer exposure periods at different temperatures. The manufacturer's instructions included with the instrumentation should be consulted for the recommended times and settings for steam sterilization.

Prevacuum Sterilizer (Dynamic Air Removal)

In this high-vacuum sterilizer, air is almost completely evacuated from the chamber before the sterilizing steam is admitted. The desired degree of vacuum is achieved by means of a pump and a steam-injector system.

• **Fig. 18.3** Schematic cross-section of steam-under-pressure sterilizer. Steam enters at top of chamber to displace air or enters after air is withdrawn by vacuum. Air and steam are evacuated at bottom of chamber. Temperature of steam is measured in air-steam drain line near vent.

A prevacuum period of 8 to 10 minutes effectively removes the air to minimize the steam penetration time. The steam injector preconditions the load and helps eliminate air from the packages. As a result, the sterilizing steam almost instantly penetrates to the center of the packages when admitted to the chamber because the air has been vacuum-pumped out. If the items in the load are easily penetrable and the sterilizer is functioning properly, there is no demonstrable time difference between complete steam penetration of large or small and tight or loose packages. Therefore the maximum capacity of the sterilizer can be used.

A postvacuum cycle draws moisture from the load to shorten the drying time. The Bowie-Dick test is performed daily to ensure that the air vacuum pump is functioning properly.

Temperatures in the prevacuum sterilizer are controlled at 270° F to 276° F (132–135.5° C) at a pressure of 27 psi. Some prevacuum sterilizers with computer-controlled pulsing air evacuation systems reach temperatures between 275° F and 286° F (135–141° C). All items are exposed to a temperature of at least 270° F (132° C) for a minimum of 4 minutes. A complete cycle takes approximately 15 to 30 minutes, depending on sterilizer capacity.

Immediate-Use/"Flash" Sterilization

A flash/high-speed pressure sterilizer may have either a gravity displacement or a prevacuum cycle for immediate-use sterilization (IUSS), formerly referred to as flash sterilization (Table 18.2). The high-speed pressure sterilizer operates at a pressure of 27 psi at sea level (or a maximum of 22 psi at 5000 feet above sea level) to increase the temperature in the chamber to between 270° F and 275° F (132–135° C).

TABLE 18.2 IUSS Unwrapped Instruments for Immediate Use After Cleaning With Approved Instrument Cleanser

Item	Gravity Displacement	Prevacuum	Notes
Stainless steel	3 minutes at 270° F (132° C)	3 minutes at 270° F (132°C)	Items must be clean, disassembled, open box locks; 30 psi
Nonporous			Use chemical indicator
No lumens			
Porous lumens	10 minutes at 270° F (132° C)	4 minutes at 270° F (132° C)	Items must be clean, disassembled, open box locks; 30 psi
Mixed loads			Lumen should be flushed with water and sterilized wet
			Use chemical indicator
Complex device	Follow steam and dry times	Follow steam and dry times	Refer to manufacturer's recommendations
Saws or drills	Most require longer times at temperatures between 120° F and 132° F (48.9–55.6° C)	Most require shorter steam exposure and longer dry times at temperatures between 120° F and 132° F (48.9–55.6° C)	Use chemical indicator

The minimum exposure time at this temperature is 3 minutes for unwrapped, nonporous, uncomplicated stainless steel items without lumens. When porous items or instruments with instrument marking tape or lumens are included in the load, timing is increased to 4 minutes or longer in a prevacuum sterilizer and to 10 minutes or longer in a gravity displacement sterilizer.

With these cycles, the entire time for starting, sterilizing, and opening the sterilizer is a minimum of 6 to 7 minutes. The process should be documented for the record (Box 18.1). Steam should be maintained in the jacket at all times.

IUSS should not be used for routine sterilization of complete instrument sets and should be used only in urgent, unplanned, or emergency situations (e.g., individual items inadvertently dropped or forgotten) for which no alternative method exists.

AORN indicates that one or more steps in the decontamination and sterilization processes may be skipped when IUSS is used, leading to surgical site infection, and that all instruments should be thoroughly washed and dried before processing. Closed container IUSS pans/trays should be used if flashing is unavoidable.

Specially designed surgical suites with in-room sterilizers may provide an emergency form of IUSS sterilization if needed. Items to be permanently implanted in the body are not sterilized for immediate use unless the results of biologic monitoring are immediately available. Sterility is not ensured without the results of biologic test indicators.

Closed container systems are available for flash sterilization to protect items during transfer from the sterilizer to the sterile field.

•BOX 18.1 Content of Flash Sterilization Record

- Date
- Time
- Patient name or number
- Load contents
- Sterilizer identification number
- Cycle parameters (time, temperature, pressure)
- Indicator verification (chemical and/or biologic)

The manufacturer of the container should provide scientific evidence of its suitability for the sterilizer in use.

A high-speed pressure sterilizer used for the flash sterilization of unwrapped instruments is physically located in or immediately adjacent to the OR (e.g., the substerile room). A sterile transfer is made from the sterilizer to the sterile field. Transferring the sterilized item to the sterile field without contaminating it is difficult.

Closed varieties are commercially available that allow an item to be flash-sterilized in a covered container. The outside is considered contaminated, but the inside is considered sterile. The circulating nurse removes the lid toward them, touching only the edges. The scrub person reaches inside to remove the sterile item without touching the sides of the outer container.

Precautions

With all types of steam sterilizers, the following precautions are taken to ensure safe operation:

Note: Most steam sterilizers are automatically ready for immediate use. Older models are described for facilities that need additional instruction.

1. Turn on the valve for steam in the jacket before use. Steam may be kept in the jacket throughout the day. (It may be turned off at the end of the surgical schedule if departmental policy indicates this practice.) The jacket maintains heat, so do not touch the inside of the chamber when loading. Check the sterilizer; not all of them have a steam jacket.
2. Never put heat-sensitive items into a steam sterilizer of any type; they will be destroyed.
3. Close the door tightly before activating either the automatic or the manual controls.
4. Unless it is an automatically controlled device, do not set a manually operated timer until the desired temperature registers on the thermometer and recording graphic chart. Thermometers, not pressure gauges, are the guides for sterilization.
5. Open the door only when the exhaust valve registers zero. Stand behind the door and open it slowly to avoid the steam that may escape around the door.

6. Cleaning of the unit should be done by a trained individual. Wash the inside of the chamber according to the manufacturer's directions and with manufacturer-approved solution, rinse it with tap water, and dry it with a lint-free cloth every day. Remove and clean the filtering screen daily. Flush the discharge lines weekly with a recommended solution. Some manufacturers offer a cleaning service for their systems.
7. Wipe the gasket daily with a lint-free cloth, and check for signs of wear and defects.
8. Provide routine PM, including the evaluation of steam and air purity. The amount of solid, liquid, or vapor contamination in the steam is minimal. An ineffective air filter may contaminate a load when air is drawn into the chamber at the end of the cycle. A defective steam trap or clogged exhaust line can cause malfunction. Make sure the thermometer is correctly calibrated.

Preparing Surgical Instruments for Steam Sterilization

Most instruments are made of metal, but many are difficult to clean. For effective steam sterilization, organic material and debris are first removed. Items that come apart should be totally disassembled and all instruments with box locks opened. Heavy instruments should be placed on the bottom levels of the tray, with lighter instruments on top. The tray contents should be evenly distributed and not exceed the weight set forth by the manufacturer. Items are thoroughly rinsed and dried after cleaning and before sterilization.

Manuals (which often contain photographs) or index file cards are available in the room in which supplies are packaged; these materials provide ready reference during preparation and for wrapping single items, packs, or trays. Instructions are strictly followed to ensure safety in sterilizing items.

Powered Equipment

Powered equipment should be placed in the cases provided by the manufacturer after appropriate decontamination and lubrication. Powered equipment requires special cleaning, decontamination, and sterilization. Follow the manufacturer's instructions for sterilization to prevent damage to the equipment.

Basin Sets

If they are nested (placed one inside another), basins and solid utensils are separated ½ inch by porous material, such as toweling. This permits the permeation of steam via wicking around all surfaces and the condensation of steam from the inside during sterilization. Sponges and drapes are not packaged in basins because steam could be deflected from penetrating fabrics. Basin sets should not exceed 7 pounds (3.15 kg).

Drape Packs

Freshly laundered woven fabric drapes and gowns are fan-folded or rolled loosely to provide the least possible resistance to the penetration of steam through each layer of material. Packs must not exceed a maximum size of 12 × 12 × 20 inches (30 × 30 × 50 cm) and must not weigh more than 12 pounds (5.5 kg).

Drapes are loosely crisscrossed so they do not form a dense, impermeable mass. Pack density should not exceed 7.2 lb/ft (see Box 18.2 for the calculation of density). The inner aspect of the outside wrapper becomes the temporary sterile field when the

• BOX 18.2 Calculation of Density of Drape Pack

$$\frac{\text{Size of pack (inches)}}{1728(\text{in}/\text{ft}^2)} = \text{Cubic feet of pack}$$

$$\frac{\text{Weight of pack(lb)}}{\text{Cubic feet of pack}} = \text{Density factor}(\text{lb}/\text{ft}^3)$$

Example:

$$\frac{12'' \times 12'' \times 12''}{1728(\text{in}/\text{ft}^2)} = 1.666\ \text{ft}^3$$

$$\frac{12\ \text{lb}}{1.666\ \text{ft}^3} = 7.2\ \text{lb}/\text{ft}^3\ (\text{maximum density})$$

pack is opened. An impervious sterile barrier drape should be placed on the instrument table before the sterile field is established for the procedure. The drapes are transferred to the table covered with the impervious barrier drape.

Rubber Goods and Thermoplastics

A rubber or Silastic sheet or any other impervious material should not be folded for sterilization because steam can neither penetrate it nor displace air from the folds. It should be covered with a piece of gauze fabric or toweling of the same size, loosely rolled, and then wrapped. For example, a layer of roller gauze is rolled between layers of an Esmarch bandage.

The mechanical cleaning of tubing, including catheters and drains, is a factor in reducing the microbial count inside the lumen. A residual of distilled water should be left in the lumen of any tubing that is to be steam-sterilized by gravity displacement. The residual becomes steam as the temperature rises, which helps displace air in the lumen and increase the temperature within it. (This is not necessary in a prevacuum sterilizer.) The tubing should be coiled without kinks. Keep in mind that disposable tubing is generally preferred because of the complexities associated with cleaning tubing.

Detachable rubber or plastic parts should be removed from instruments and syringes for cleaning and sterilizing. Rubber surfaces should not touch metal, glassware, or each other during sterilization; this prevents melting or sticking and permits steam to reach all surfaces. Rubber bands should not be used around solid items because steam cannot penetrate through or under rubber.

Wood Products

During sterilization, lignocellulose resin (lignin) is driven out of wood by heat. This resin may condense onto other items in the sterilizer and cause reactions if it gets into the tissues of a patient. Therefore wooden items are individually wrapped and separated from other items in the sterilizer.

Repeated sterilization dries wood so that during sterilization it absorbs moisture from the saturated steam. Cracks in the wood could harbor microorganisms. As the water content of the saturated steam decreases, the steam becomes superheated and loses some of its sterilizing power. Because of this problem, the use of wood products that require steam sterilization should be minimized and their repeated sterilization is avoided.

Loading the Sterilizer

All packages are positioned in the chamber to allow free circulation, steam penetration, and prevent the entrapment of air or water. A gravity displacement sterilizer is loaded so steam can displace air downward and out through the discharge line. Wire mesh or perforated metal shelves separate layers of packages. Shelves may be contained within the chamber on sliding racks or a transfer carriage. The shelves are loaded and rolled into the sterilizer. Floor loaders are easier to manage than off-floor carriage racks. Steam sterilizers should be loaded as follows:

1. Flat packages of textiles are placed on the shelf on edge so flat surfaces are vertical, as shown in Fig. 18.4. Instrument trays and closed container systems with perforated bottoms may be laid flat.
2. Large packs are placed 2 to 4 inches apart in one layer only on a shelf. Small packages may be placed on the shelf above with 1 or 2 inches between them. If small packages are placed one on top of another, they should be crisscrossed.
3. Packages must not touch the chamber walls, floor, or ceiling.
4. Rubber goods are placed on edge, loosely arranged, and in one layer to a shelf; this allows free steam circulation and penetration. No other articles should be with the rubber goods.
5. Basins and solid containers are placed on their sides to allow air to flow out of them. They should be placed so that if they contained water all of it would flow out. If being sterilized in a combined load with fabrics, basins and containers should be placed on the lowest shelf.

Timing the Load

The timing of a sterilization cycle begins when the desired temperature is reached throughout the chamber. Materials that need different lengths of exposure to ensure sterilization in a gravity displacement sterilizer should not be combined in the same load if the maximum time needed will be destructive to some items. The minimum time standards, which are calculated after effective steam penetration of porous materials and the rate of heat transfer through wrapping materials, are listed in Table 18.3.

Most sterilizers are equipped with a graphic recorder and automatic electromechanical or microcomputer time-temperature controls. Some sterilizers print out a computer record to document each load. The time and temperature for each load are recorded for a 24-hour period. The record of each load should be

• **Fig. 18.4** Proper loading of gravity displacement steam sterilizer; packs should be placed on edge, and the rack should not be overloaded. Steam must completely surround and penetrate every package in all sterilizers.

checked before unloading to be certain that the desired temperature was achieved. Also, the temperature being recorded should be checked daily against the thermometer to see that the recording arm is working properly.

Drying the Load

After the sterilizer door is opened, the load of wrapped packages is left untouched to dry for 15 to 60 minutes. The time required for drying depends on the type of sterilizer and the types of supplies in a load. Large packages require a longer time than small ones. The packages are then unloaded onto a table or cart containing wire mesh shelves padded with absorbent material. Warm packages laid on a solid, cold surface become damp from steam condensation and thus contaminated by strike-through (capillary action).

Packages are observed for water droplets on the exterior or interior and for absorbed moisture in the package. Packs wrapped in moisture-permeable materials that have water droplets on the outside or inside are unsafe for use because the moisture can be a pathway for microbial migration into the package via capillary action. A package should be considered contaminated if it is wet when opened for use. Packages should be completely dry after cooling at a room temperature of 68° F to 75° F (20−24° C) for a minimum of 1 hour.

Biologic Testing of the Steam Sterilizer

Biologic test packs with *Geobacillus stearothermophilus* for steam sterilizers vary according to the type of sterilizer being tested. Each steam sterilizer is tested at least weekly for routine monitoring and as needed for a process challenge test. Many hospitals test sterilizers daily. Because of the variations in sterilizers, the appropriate test is used for each type of sterilizer.

Gravity Displacement Sterilizer

With a gravity displacement sterilizer, a test pack/PCD is placed on edge in the lower front of the load. This is the coldest area and therefore represents the greatest challenge in sterilization. The chamber is fully loaded. Most facilities use commercial test packs, but one can be made if a commercial pack is unavailable. The contents of the test pack may be any of the following:

- The equivalent of 3 woven fabric gowns, 12 towels, 30 gauze sponges (4 × 4 inches), 5 laparotomy tapes/sponges (12 × 12 inches), and 1 woven fabric drape sheet. Two biologic indicators are placed in the center of the pack, with a chemical indicator placed one towel above or below them. The pack is double-wrapped. It should be approximately 12 × 12 × 20 inches (30 × 30 × 50 cm) and should weigh 10 to 12 pounds.
- The equivalent of 16 freshly laundered reusable huck towels or absorbent towels in good condition, each approximately 16 × 26 inches (40 × 66 cm), folded 9 × 9 inches (23 × 23 cm), and stacked with a biologic indicator in the center. The pack is taped to provide a density of 12 lb/ft^3, and it should weigh 3 pounds.
- An equivalent commercial test pack.

Prevacuum Sterilizer

With a prevacuum sterilizer, the contents of the test pack/PCD with biologic indicators can be the same as for a gravity

TABLE 18.3	Minimum Exposure Time Standards for Steam Sterilization After Effective Steam Penetration and Heat Transfer		
	GRAVITY DISPLACEMENT		PREVACUUM
Materials	250° F (121° C)	270° F (132° C)	270° F (132° C)
Basin sets, wrapped	20 minutes	Not applicable	4 minutes
Basins, glassware, and utensils, unwrapped	15 minutes	Not recommended	3 minutes
Instruments, with or without other items, wrapped as set in double-thickness wrappers	30 minutes	Not applicable	4 minutes
Instruments, unwrapped but with other items, including towel in bottom of tray or cover over them	20 minutes	10 minutes	4 minutes
Instruments, completely unwrapped	15 minutes	3 minutes	3 minutes
Drape packs, 12 × 12 × 20 inches (30 × 30 × 50 cm) maximum size, 12 lb (5.5 kg) maximum weight	30 minutes[a]	Not applicable	4 minutes
Fabrics, single items wrapped	30 minutes[a]	Not applicable	4 minutes
Rubber and thermoplastics, including small items and gloves but excluding tubing, wrapped	20 minutes[a]	Not applicable	4 minutes
Tubing, wrapped	30 minutes	Not applicable	4 minutes
Tubing, unwrapped	20 minutes	Not applicable	4 minutes
Sponges and dressings, wrapped	30 minutes	Not applicable	4 minutes
Solutions, flask	(Slow exhaust)	Not applicable	Automatic selector determines correct temperature and exposure period for solutions
75-mL flask	20 minutes		
250-mL flask	25 minutes		
500-mL flask	30 minutes		
1000-mL flask	35 minutes		
1500-mL flask	45 minutes		
2000-mL flask	45 minutes		

[a]Fabrics and rubber deteriorate more rapidly with repeated sterilization for prolonged periods in gravity displacement sterilizer.

displacement sterilizer. In addition, a Bowie-Dick test is conducted daily, usually on the first run of the day, to check for air entrapment in the prevacuum sterilizer. A biologic indicator may be put into this test pack. The test pack is placed horizontally on the bottom shelf at the front, near the door, and over the drain of an empty prevacuum chamber. The test pack consists of the following:

- Between 24 and 44 absorbent towels folded in a stack no smaller than 9 × 12 × 11 inches (23 × 30 × 28 cm)
- One Bowie-Dick test sheet placed in the center of the stack
- One double-thickness wrapper

Dry Heat Sterilization

Dry heat in the form of hot air is used primarily to sterilize anhydrous oils, petroleum products, and talc, which steam and EO gas cannot penetrate. The destruction of microbial life by dry heat is a physical oxidation or slow burning process that involves coagulating the protein in cells. Higher temperatures are required in the absence of moisture because the microorganisms are destroyed through a very slow process of heat absorption by conduction. Dry heat sterilizers are not commonly

found in the OR processing areas. Dry heat is commonly used in dental suites.

Advantages of Dry Heat Sterilization

- Hot air penetrates certain substances that cannot be sterilized by steam sterilization or another method.
- Dry heat is a protective method of sterilizing some delicate, sharp, or cutting-edge instruments. Steam may erode or corrode cutting edges.

Disadvantages of Dry Heat Sterilization

- A long exposure period is required because hot air penetrates slowly and possibly unevenly.
- The time and temperature required will vary for different substances.
- Overexposure may ruin some substances.

Types of Dry Heat Sterilizers

Mechanical Convection Oven

The most efficient and reliable dry heat sterilizer is an electrically heated, mechanical convection hot air oven. A blower forces hot air in motion around items in the load to hasten the heating of substances and ensure a uniform temperature in all areas of the oven.

Early models operated at 320° F to 340° F (160–171° C) for 1 to 2 hours. Faster portable tabletop models are available; these run at 375° F to 400° F (190.5–204° C), with total cycle times of 6 minutes for unwrapped items and 12 minutes for wrapped ones. Optional cooling chambers are also available.

Gravity Convection Oven

A conventional gravity displacement steam sterilizer chamber can be used for dry heat sterilization. Heat is provided by steam in the jacket only; this heat may not be evenly distributed throughout the chamber. The hot air rises initially and by gravity displaces cooler air at the bottom of the chamber. The maximum temperature that can be obtained is 250° F (121° C) or 270° F (132° C) in a high-pressure gravity displacement sterilizer. To ensure adequate heat conduction through all items, the exposure period is a minimum of 6 hours and preferably overnight.

Preparing Items for Dry Heat Sterilization
Oils

The amount of oil—including mineral oil and lubricating oil for electrically powered or air-powered instruments—put into a container should not exceed 1 ounce (30 mL). The depth of the oil is preferably not more than ¼ inch (6.35 mm). The greater the depth, the longer the exposure period.

Talc

A maximum of 5 g to 1 ounce of talc may be spread out in a glass container so the depth of the layer does not exceed ¼ inch (6.25 mm). The lid is secured, with the cap screwed tightly on the bottle or jar, and a dry heat process chemical indicator is affixed to the bottle. The sterilizing cycle for a gravity convection oven (steam sterilizer with steam in the jacket only) should be a minimum of 9 hours at 250° F (121° C) or 6 hours at 270° F (132° C).

An average quantity of 2 to 3 g of talc is usually needed as an intrapleural sclerosing agent for poudrage. This smaller quantity may be evenly distributed inside a sealed glassine envelope or peel pouch, which is then inserted into a second envelope or pouch. The talc should not accumulate into a mass exceeding ¼ inch (6.25 mm); the package should lie flat in the sterilizer. Prepackaged sterile talc is commercially available and is preferred.

Packaging Materials for Dry Heat Sterilization
Glass

Petri dishes, ointment jars, flasks, small bottles, or test tubes can be used for dry heat sterilization. Caps or lids are affixed or screwed tightly onto containers.

Stainless Steel Boats or Trays

Covers must fit tightly. They can be held in place with indicator tape. The heat causes the adhesive to stick to the surface of the container and is hard to remove.

Aluminum Foil

Foil conducts heat rapidly.

Woven Fabric and Peel Pouches

These materials can be used for wrapping instruments if the temperature in the chamber will not exceed 400° F (204° C). Powders and talc can be put in double glassine envelopes.

Loading the Sterilizer

When loading a dry heat sterilizer, it is necessary to allow space between the items and along the chamber walls so the hot air can circulate freely. The chamber is never loaded to full capacity.

Timing the Load

The time of exposure in a dry heat sterilizer varies depending on the characteristics of individual items, the layer depth in containers, and the temperature in the sterilizer. The timing of exposure begins when the thermometer registers the desired temperature. Items are exposed for the following minimum periods, assuming the amount in each container is kept to a minimum and the sterilizer is loaded according to the manufacturer's recommendations:

- 6 minutes at 400° F (204° C), unwrapped
- 12 minutes at 375° F (190.5° C), wrapped
- 1 hour at 340° F (171° C), wrapped or unwrapped
- 2 hours at 320° F (160° C), wrapped or unwrapped
- 3 hours at 285° F (140.5° C), wrapped or unwrapped
- 6 hours at 250° F (121° C), wrapped or unwrapped

Biologic Testing of the Dry Heat Sterilizer

Biologic indicators with endospores of *Bacillus atrophaeus* are used to monitor the dry heat process. Commercially prepared endospore strips in glassine envelopes should be used. Each load should be tested and the items quarantined until negative results are confirmed.

Chemical Sterilization

The only chemicals used for sterilization are those that are registered as a sterilant by the Environmental Protection Agency (EPA). They may be approved for use in a gaseous, plasma, or liquid state.

Ethylene Oxide Gas Sterilization

EO gas is used to sterilize items that are sensitive to heat or moisture. EO or EtO is a chemical alkylating agent that kills microorganisms (including endospores) by interfering with the normal metabolism of protein and reproductive processes, resulting in cell death. Used in the gaseous state, EO must have direct contact with microorganisms on or in the items to be sterilized. EO is the most regulated sterilization process in the United States. Strict monitoring, safety for long-term exposure, and reduction of emissions have been updated by the EPA.[4]

EO is highly flammable and explosive in air and therefore must be used in an explosion-proof sterilizing chamber in a controlled environment. The machine is equipped with alarms and will automatically lock if a malfunction occurs.

When handled properly, EO is reliable and safe for sterilization, but the toxic emissions and residues of EO present health hazards to personnel and patients. Therefore the environment in which EO is used is constantly monitored for unsafe exposure levels. Employee exposure records are required by law to be retained for 30 years.

EO gas sterilization depends on four parameters, each of which may be varied. Consequently EO sterilization is a complex, multiparameter process. Each variable affects the other dependent parameters:

1. *Concentration of EO gas:* Liquefied EO is supplied in high-pressure metal cylinders, tanks, and disposable cartridges. In the sterilization process, air is withdrawn from the chamber and the EO enters as gas under pressure. The only means for controlling EO concentration is to operate the sterilizer according to the manufacturer's instructions. The operating pressure of the cycle influences the rate of gas diffusion through the items to be sterilized. The absorbency of the items and packaging materials influences the concentration of the gas.[5] EO gas may be diluted or used in pure form:
   a. *100% EO:* Unit-dose cartridges of 67 g or 134 g pure EO are used in small self-contained sterilizers. Because pure EO is highly flammable, only a small number of cartridges are kept in inventory.
   b. *EO/CO_2, referred to as 10/90:* This is a mixture of 10% EO in 90% carbon dioxide. Because of the great pressure differential between EO and carbon dioxide, maintaining a uniform mix is difficult. A high-pressure cycle must be used; therefore not all devices can be sterilized safely in this mixture.
2. *Temperature:* Temperature influences the destruction of microorganisms and affects the permeability of EO through cell walls and packaging materials. Higher density items and loads require a longer heat-up time. As temperature is increased, exposure time can be decreased. Gas sterilizers operate at temperatures ranging from 85° F to 145° F (29−63° C). The uppermost limit for many heat-sensitive plastic materials is 140° F (60° C). The temperature in the chamber is raised by the injection of saturated steam.
3. *Humidity:* Moisture is essential in achieving sterility with EO gas. Desiccated or highly dried bacterial endospores are resistant to EO gas; they must be hydrated. The moisture content of the immediately surrounding atmosphere and the water content within organisms are important to the action of EO gas. Therefore to hydrate the items during preparation, the relative humidity of the room in which the items are packaged and held for sterilization should be at least 50% and must not be less than 30%. The ability of the item and packaging material to absorb moisture affects the humidification and diffusion of gas during the sterilization process. A humidity level of 30% to 80% is maintained throughout the cycle; excessive moisture will inhibit sterilization. Saturated steam provides the necessary humidity.
4. *Time.* The time required for the complete destruction of microorganisms is related primarily to the concentration and temperature of the gas. The cleanliness of items, types of materials, arrangement of load, and rate of penetration also influence exposure time. Drawing an initial vacuum at the start of the cycle aids in penetration of the gas.

Advantages of EO Gas Sterilization

1. EO gas is an effective substitute agent to use with most items that cannot be sterilized by heat, such as plastics with low melting points.
2. EO gas provides an effective method of sterilization for items that steam and moisture may erode; it is noncorrosive and does not damage items.
3. EO gas completely permeates all porous materials; it does not penetrate metal, glass, and petroleum-based lubricants. EO gas sterilization is not recommended for oils, liquids, and powder (including talc).

   Solutions in glass ampules can be sterilized in EO because the gas does not penetrate glass. But a glass vial with a rubber stopper must not be put in the sterilizer because the gas will penetrate the rubber and may react with the drugs in solution, causing a potentially harmful chemical reaction.
4. Automatic controls preclude human error by establishing proper levels of pressure, temperature, humidity, and gas concentration. The sterilizer is operated according to the manufacturer's instructions.
5. EO gas leaves no film on items.
6. EO gas sterilization is used extensively in the preparation of commercially available, packaged, presterilized items because packaging materials that prolong storage life can be used.

Disadvantages of EO Gas Sterilization

1. EO gas sterilization is a complicated and long process that is carefully monitored.
   a. An item that can be safely steam-sterilized should never be gas-sterilized.
   b. Biologic indicator (*B. atrophaeus*), external chemical indicators, sterilizer operation, and maintenance records should be reviewed to verify the adequacy of every cycle.
   c. Implants should not be used until the results of biologic testing are known.
   d. Items are completely aerated before use to eliminate harmful residues.
2. EO sterilization takes longer than steam sterilization; it is a long, slow process.
3. EO gas requires special, expensive equipment. Gas is somewhat expensive per cycle.
4. Items that absorb EO gas during sterilization, such as rubber, polyethylene, or silicone, require an aeration period (Table 18.4). Air admitted to the sterilizer at the end of the cycle only partially aerates the load.
5. Toxic by-products can be formed in the presence of moisture droplets during the exposure of some plastics, particularly polyvinyl chloride.
6. Repeated sterilization can increase the concentration of the total EO residues in porous items. These increased levels can be hazardous unless the gas can be dissipated.[5]
7. EO is a vesicant when in contact with skin and mucous membranes.
   a. Liquid EO may cause serious burns if not removed immediately by thorough washing.
   b. Gloves made of neoprene, polyvinyl fluoride, nitryl or butyl rubber, or other material known to be impermeable to EO penetration should be worn for handling sterilized packages before aeration. If thick cotton gloves are worn, they should be placed in the aerator between uses.
   c. Personnel who wear contact lenses, especially soft lenses, should wear protective goggles when working around EO sterilizers to avoid eye irritation.
8. Inhaled EO gas can be irritating to mucous membranes. It is a colorless gas, but its presence is easily detectable by odor.

TABLE 18.4 Minimum Aeration Times After Ethylene Oxide Sterilization at Different Temperatures

Materials	AMBIENT ROOM AIR 65° F to 72° F (18–22° C)	MECHANICAL AERATOR 122° F (50° C)	MECHANICAL AERATOR 140° F (60° C)
Metal and glass			
Unwrapped	May be used immediately		
Wrapped	2 hours	2 hours	2 hours
Rubber for external use—not sealed in plastic	24 hours	8 hours	5 hours
Polyethylene and polypropylene for external use—not sealed in plastic	48 hours	12 hours	8 hours
Plastics except polyvinyl chloride items—not sealed in plastic	96 hours (4 days)	12 hours	8 hours
Polyvinyl chloride	168 hours (7 days)	12 hours	8 hours
Plastic and rubber items—those sealed in plastic and/or those that will come in contact with body tissues	168 hours (7 days)	12 hours	8 hours
Internal pacemaker	504 hours (21 days)	32 hours	24 hours

Overexposure causes nasal and throat irritation. Prolonged exposure may result in nausea, vomiting, dizziness, difficulty breathing, and peripheral paralysis.

a. Immediately after the completion of each cycle, the sterilizer door should be opened approximately 2 inches and the area cleared of all personnel for 15 minutes before unloading.

b. Loading carts should be pulled, not pushed, from the sterilizer to the aerator. Air currents flowing over the load may accumulate a residual gas that could be inhaled.

9. Long-term exposure to EO is known to be a potential occupational carcinogen, causing leukemia. It is also a mutagen, causing spontaneous abortion, genetic defects, chromosomal damage, and neurologic dysfunction.

a. The standards of the Occupational Safety and Health Administration (OSHA) limit an employee's exposure to EO to 1 part per million (ppm) of air averaged over an 8-hour period to an active level of 0.5 ppm, and to a short-term limit of 5 ppm averaged over a 15-minute period. These exposure limits are referred to as permissible exposure limits (PELs).

The short-term limit addresses exposure to bursts of gas, such as when opening a sterilizer. Breathing zone sampling is performed daily throughout an 8-hour shift on at least one employee for each job classification of exposed personnel. Passive dosimeter badges are the most popular monitoring devices for personnel. Chromatographs and other types of detectors are used for continuous gas analysis of the environment.

b. EO gas is vented from the sterilizer to the outside atmosphere to avoid personnel exposure. Audible and visual alarm systems should be installed to indicate a failure in the ventilation system. Most sterilizers have an exhaust hood over the sterilizer door.

c. The sterilizer door has locking and sealing mechanisms. The integrity of the seals is checked regularly. Automatic controls must function properly so the door cannot be opened until the gas is evacuated from the chamber.

Types of EO Gas Sterilizers

The capacity of EO chambers varies from approximately 2 ft (57.5 L) in a tabletop size of 12 × 12 × 24 inches (30 × 30 × 60 cm) to very large floor-loading units that are 28 × 67 × 78 inches (72 × 180 × 198 cm). These chambers automatically control gas concentration, temperature, humidity, and time. Most models have vacuum pumps to evacuate air from the chamber and steam ejectors to humidify and increase temperature. Microcomputer controls and digital printouts of cycle parameters provide evidence of proper operation.

A purge cycle follows the timed gas-exposure cycle to vent the chamber of airborne residual gas. Some chambers are a combination sterilizer/aerator, which eliminates the need for personnel to handle the load immediately after sterilization; the load is removed only after aeration.

Preparing Items for EO Gas Sterilization

All Items

All items to be sterilized with EO gas are thoroughly cleaned and dried. Detachable parts are disassembled, and syringes are separated. Impermeable items such as caps, plugs, and stylets are removed. All items must be completely dry.

Lumens

Any tubing or other item with a lumen should be blown out with air to force it dry before packaging because water combines with EO gas to form ethylene glycol, a harmful acid that causes hemolysis of red blood cells in the patient.

Lensed Instruments

Endoscopes with cemented optical lenses require special cement for EO gas sterilization.

Lubricated Instruments

All traces of lubricant, especially petroleum-based lubricants, should be removed before sterilization. EO cannot permeate the film of the lubricant.

Cameras

As a permanent record or teaching aid, photographs are sometimes taken at the surgical site. Digital cameras are frequently used in the OR. A digital camera may be designated for the department, and a qualified individual may take pictures at the surgeon's request.

Some cameras and film can be sterilized with EO gas. The film is loaded before packaging for sterilization.

Packaging Materials for EO Gas Sterilization

The type and thickness of the wrapper, the size and shape of the package, and the porosity of the contents used influence the time it takes for the EO gas to penetrate. Items wrapped for EO gas sterilization should be tagged for gas to prevent them from being inadvertently steam-sterilized and damaged. Materials used for wrapping items are permeable to EO gas and water vapor and allow effective aeration. The materials discussed in the following sections are acceptable.

Woven Fabric

Reusable double-thickness woven fabrics are used as they are for steam, with the same advantages and disadvantages.

Nonwoven Fabric

Tyvek spun-bonded olefin and other high-density polyethylene fabrics are highly permeable to EO and moisture. These single-use disposable wrappers offer the same advantages as the nonwoven fabrics described for use in steam, but not all of them can be used interchangeably; the cellulose/nylon/rayon combination should be used only for steam sterilization. Packages should be sequentially single- or double-wrapped or the material used according to the manufacturer's recommendations.

Peel Packs and Pouches

Double-wrapping may not allow adequate penetration of the gas and moisture. Peel pouches with either coated or uncoated paper on one side and coated Mylar on the other are generally acceptable for most gas sterilizers, and they allow visualization of contents.

Materials not to be used for EO sterilization because of inadequate permeability include nylon, polyvinyl chloride film (Saran), polyester, polyvinyl alcohol, cellophane, and aluminum foil. Combinations of materials that make a package insufficiently permeable for adequate humidification, gas penetration, and aeration are avoided.

Loading the Sterilizer

All packages are positioned in the chamber to allow free circulation and penetration of gas. Overloading creates conditions that can slow the penetration of EO gas, moisture, and heat. Air space should be provided between the chamber ceiling and the uppermost packages in the load, and packages should not touch the chamber walls and floor. Packages should not be stacked tightly; space is allowed between them. If paper or plastic pouches are used, the packages are placed on edge, with the plastic side of one facing the paper side of another.

Timing the Load

The timing of the EO cycle varies depending on the size of the chamber, the contents of the load, gas concentration, temperature, and humidity. For example, a cool cycle at 99° F (37° C) may require more than 5 hours, whereas the same load at 131° F (55° C) may take less than 3 hours. The instructions provided by the manufacturer of the sterilizer should be followed closely.

Aerating Items After EO Gas Sterilization

EO gas exerts toxic effects on living tissue. Therefore after EO gas sterilization, adequate aeration is absolutely essential for all absorbent materials that will come into contact with skin or tissues, either directly or indirectly. Residual products after sterilization can include the following:

1. *Ethylene oxide:* Porous materials, such as plastic, silicone, rubber, wood, and leather, absorb a certain amount of gas that must be removed. The thicker the walls of items, the longer the aeration time required. Residual EO gas in plastic tubing or in parts of a heart-lung pump oxygenator causes hemolysis of blood. Rubber gloves or shoes worn immediately after exposure can cause irritation or burns on skin. The following are acceptable limits for residual EO:
   a. 25 ppm for blood dialysis units, blood oxygenators, heart-lung machines, and all implants
   b. 250 ppm for all topical medical devices
2. *Ethylene glycol:* Ethylene glycol is formed by a reaction of EO gas with water or moisture; this reaction leaves a clear or brownish oily film on exposed surfaces. This substance causes hemolysis of the red blood cells. It also can cause irritation to the mucous membranes if left on plastic or rubber endotracheal tubes or airways. The following are acceptable limits of ethylene glycol:
   a. 250 ppm for blood dialysis units, blood oxygenators, heart-lung machines, and all implants
   b. 1000 ppm for all topical medical devices
3. *Ethylene chlorohydrin:* This by-product is formed when a chloride ion is present to combine with EO, such as in polyvinyl chloride plastic. Rubber, soft nylon, and polyethylene items that have been in contact with saline solution or blood can retain enough chloride ions to cause this reaction in the presence of moisture. To avoid this hazard, disposable products should be discarded after use. The following are acceptable limits of ethylene chlorohydrin:
   a. 25 ppm for blood dialysis units, blood oxygenators, heart-lung machines, and all implants
   b. 250 ppm for all topical medical devices

Residuals are expressed as the weight of EO gas remaining in the item divided by the weight of the item. For example, 25 ppm in a device weighing 2500 g (approximately 5.5 lb) equals 0.01 mg of EO. Residues cannot be removed by rinsing items in water or liquids.

To purge residual gas, air is admitted into the chamber at the end of the sterilization cycle. In sterilizers with a pulse-purge cycle, the air is admitted and immediately removed as many as six times in 30 minutes. Additional aeration is required for all wrapped and porous items. Aeration to diffuse any residual products may be accomplished with ambient (room) air or preferably with an aerator chamber designed for this purpose.

Manufacturers of products suitable for EO sterilization should provide written instructions for the sterilizing cycle and for aerating. The available recommendations are followed. Polyvinyl chloride is one of the most difficult materials to aerate. If the composition of an item is not known, the minimum time for polyvinyl chloride should be followed (see Table 18.4). Aeration time depends on the following:

- Composition, density, porosity, weight, and configuration of the item
- Packaging material
- Sterilizing conditions, such as the size of the load, the nature of the items in it, and variable required factors
- Aeration conditions, such as ambient versus mechanical airflow and temperature
- Acceptable limits of residual products for the intended use of the item, such as external application or internal implantation

Aeration at an elevated temperature enhances the dissipation rate of absorbed gas, which results in faster removal. The entire load on the sterilizer carriage can be transferred into an aerator. A blower system draws air in from the outside to the heater in the upper part of the chamber to maintain a minimum rate of four air exchanges per minute. The aerator is vented to the outside atmosphere. Items cannot be safely used until they have been completely aerated.

All materials remain in the aerator for 8 hours at 140° F (60° C) to 12 hours at 120° F (49° C) or longer, depending on temperature and the instructions of the manufacturer of the aerator or item. In a combination sterilizer/aerator, aeration time varies according to temperature and airflow (e.g., 12 hours at 130° F [54° C] or 32 hours at 100° F [38° C]).

If an aerator is not available, packages may be moved on a cart or in a basket from the sterilizer into a well-ventilated clean storage area that has at least 10 air exchanges per hour. The cart should be pulled, not pushed, to this area to avoid being downwind of the EO gas adhering to the wrappers. Aeration time is prominently noted on the cart or basket. At a room temperature controlled between 65° F and 72° F (18–22° C), a minimum aeration time of 168 hours (7 days) is required for polyvinyl chloride and plastic and rubber items sealed in plastic packages and for porous items that:

1. Come into direct contact with blood
2. Are implanted, inserted, or applied to body tissues
3. Are used for assisted respiration

Unwrapped, nonporous metal and glass may be handled immediately. Wrapped metal should be aerated for at least 2 hours. Intravenous (IV) or irrigation fluids in plastic containers must not be stored in a room where gas-sterilized items are aerating because the residual diffusing gas could be absorbed through the plastic.

Biologic Testing of the EO Gas Sterilizer

Biologic indicators carrying endospores of *B. atrophaeus* are used to monitor EO gas sterilizers. Each sterilizer is tested in each load. Every load containing implantable devices should be tested. An implant should not be used until the test results are negative. The manufacturer's recommendations should be followed for the use of biologic test packs for EO gas sterilizers.

Hydrogen Peroxide Plasma Sterilization

Hydrogen peroxide (H_2O_2) can be activated to create a reactive plasma. Plasma has been described as the fourth state of matter, being not a liquid, gas, or solid. It can be produced through the action of either a strong electrical or magnetic field, somewhat like a neon light. The cloud of plasma created consists of ions, electrons, and neutral atomic particles that produce a visible pink glow. Free radicals of the hydrogen peroxide in the cloud interact with cell membranes, enzymes, or nucleic acids to disrupt the life functions of microorganisms. The processing time ranges between 35 and 75 minutes. The user must know the parameters necessary for the sterilization of items processed by this method.

The plasma and vapor phases of hydrogen peroxide are highly sporicidal, even at a low concentration and temperature. The sterilizer chambers are simple in design, but the process of the sterilization cycle differs with the method used to convert hydrogen peroxide into plasma or vapor. Plasma technology uses an oxidation process that can be corrosive to some polymers and adhesives. This can cause problems with some lensed instruments.

This method is used for sterilization of metal and nonmetal surgical devices at low temperatures in a dry environment. This method works well for instruments that have diffusion-restricted spaces, such as box locks on clamps. Instruments with lumens have specific requirements:

- Metallic or nonmetallic instruments with lumens of 6 mm or larger and lengths of 310 mm or shorter can be processed.
- Stainless steel lumens larger than 3 mm and shorter than 400 mm are safely processed.

Advantages of Hydrogen Peroxide Sterilization

- The process is dry and nontoxic.
- The by-products of oxygen and water vapor are safely evacuated into the room atmosphere.
- Aeration is not necessary.
- A low temperature allows the safe sterilization of some heat-sensitive items.
- Plasma has significantly less effect on metal than does steam sterilization; corrosion does not occur on moisture-sensitive microsurgical and powered instruments.
- The sterilizer is simple in design and connects to standard electrical outlets.

Disadvantages of Hydrogen Peroxide Sterilization

- Metal trays block radiofrequency waves and cannot be used.
- Hydrogen peroxide is not compatible with cellulose (i.e., woven textiles with cotton fibers and paper products). This causes a decrease in the sterilant concentration by absorbing the vapors. This method cannot be used with liquids.
- Nylon becomes brittle after repeated exposure to hydrogen peroxide sterilization.
- This method is not approved in the United States for use with flexible endoscopes with lumens.

Low-Temperature Gas Plasma Sterilizers

STERRAD by Advanced Sterilization Products

The STERRAD sterilizer connects to a standard electrical outlet. The supplies are placed in the chamber, and a strong vacuum is created. A solution of water and 58% hydrogen peroxide is vaporized by radiofrequency energy to create a pink, glowing reactive plasma. The reactive particles in the plasma are maintained at 104° F (40° C) and sterilize the heat- and moisture-sensitive load in approximately 1 hour.

No aeration is necessary because the by-product is primarily oxygen and water. The cycle will automatically abort if the sterilant concentration is not adequate. Users must wear PPE if handling items from an aborted load or when changing the sterilant cartridge.

Vapor Phase Sterilizer

A vacuum is created in the chamber for delivery of a cold vapor of hydrogen peroxide at 39° F to 46° F (4–8° C). A vacuum exhausts vapor at the end of the cycle.

Considerations for Hydrogen Peroxide Sterilization

- All items are thoroughly clean, free of organic debris, and dry.
- Items are wrapped in nonwoven polypropylene. Tyvek peel pouches may be used.
- Trays are placed flat on the shelf for penetration. Peel pouches are stood on the side. Nothing should rest on the walls of the chamber.
- The timing of the cycle varies with the process, capacity of the chamber, and contents of the load. The manufacturer's instructions are followed. May take more than 75 minutes to run a load.
- Biologic indicators with endospores of *G. stearothermophilus* with adjusted pH are used to monitor the hydrogen peroxide process daily. Monitoring with each load is preferred.

Ozone Gas Sterilization

Ozone sterilizes by oxidation, a process that destroys organic and inorganic matter. It penetrates the membrane of cells, causing them to explode. Ozone has been used to purify water since the early 20th century. Ozone is a metastable gas that can be generated easily from oxygen and water at the point of use. No special outlet or water supply is required. No special cartridges or canisters of a chemical are needed. This is a low-temperature method of sterilization that has been in use in industry for more than 100 years.

Safety of ozone gas exposure is measured in PELs. OSHA has set limits as 0.1 ppm per 8-hour period. The PEL is not to exceed 0.3 ppm/15 minutes. Severe pulmonary edema will result at levels of 0.3 ppm exposure for 30 minutes. Personnel using ozone sterilization do not encounter the gas in its intact state. The gas is converted back to water and oxygen at the end of the cycle before the unit can be opened. There is only one setting for all cycles, so the risk for error in operating the machine is minimized. The process takes approximately 1 hour.

The ozone sterilizer is used for plastic, metal, titanium, polypropylene, and some rigid lumens. Cellulose packaging cannot be used. Nonwoven pouches or vented closed container systems are used for instrumentation in ozone sterilizers.

The ozone sterilizer works in four phases over a period of 4.5 hours:

- Cold water vapor is humidified. About 75 mL per load. Oxygen is electrically charged to create ozone (O_3). Ozone has a bluish color.
- The water vapor and ozone combine in the chamber. One oxygen atom is released from the O_3 molecule to combine with and deactivate microorganisms.
- The water vapor, ozone, and free oxygen molecule are vented into a catalytic converter that separates out the water and oxygen (H_2O and O_2) for discharge into the drain and room air.

Advantages of Ozone Gas Sterilization

- The sterilizer generates its own agent using hospital-grade oxygen, water, and the electrical supply. It is simple and inexpensive to operate.

- Ozone gas sterilization provides an alternative to EO gas sterilization of many heat- and moisture-sensitive items.
- Ozone gas sterilization does not affect anodized aluminum, titanium, chromium, silicone, neoprene, and Teflon.
- Aeration is not necessary; ozone leaves no residue and converts to oxygen in a short time.
- Low temperature is safer for heat-sensitive instrumentation.

Disadvantages of Ozone Gas Sterilization

- Ozone can be corrosive. It will oxidize steel, iron, brass, bronze, zinc, nickel, and copper.
- It destroys natural rubber, such as latex, natural fibers, and some plastics.
- Not used to sterilize implants or flexible endoscopes at this time.
- Not used to sterilize sealed glass ampules.
- Each cycle takes 4.5 hours.
- Pure ozone damages proteins and fatty acids and is harmful if inhaled in its intact state.

Considerations for Ozone Sterilization

Preparing items, packaging, loading the sterilizer, and timing the cycle are done according to the instructions provided by the manufacturer of the sterilizer. *G. stearothermophilus* biologic indicator process challenge packs are used to monitor the process and are recommended for each cycle.

Chemical Sterilants in Solution

Liquid chemical agents registered as sterilants by the EPA provide an alternative method for sterilizing minimally invasive heat-sensitive items if a gas or plasma sterilizer is not available or the aeration period makes EO gas sterilization impractical. Items processed for patient care are categorized as critical, semicritical, and noncritical according to the Spaulding classification system. Items that enter tissue or the vascular system are considered critical and must be sterile.

Items are sterilized with a liquid sterilant by immersing them in solution for the required time specified by the manufacturer to be sporicidal (i.e., to kill endospores). All chemical solutions have advantages and disadvantages, and each sterilant has specific assets and limitations. (Additional information is available at www.fda.gov.) Policies and procedures should be in place to regulate and guide the use of chemical sterilants in solution. PPE should be worn, and eyewash stations should be conveniently located near the point of use.

Advantages of Chemical Sterilants

- The solution has a low surface tension; it penetrates crevices and is readily rinsed from items.
- It is noncorrosive, nonstaining, and safe for instruments that can be immersed in a chemical solution.
- It does not damage lenses or cement on lensed endoscopes.
- It is not absorbed by rubber or plastic.
- It has low volatility and is stable for the time specified by the manufacturer.

Disadvantages of Chemical Sterilants

- Prolonged exposure to a chemical sterilant may be necessary for sterilization.

- Some chemical sterilants have hazardous effects associated with exposure.
- Even if a chemical has low toxicity and irritation, items must be thoroughly rinsed in sterile distilled water before use.
- Failure to adequately rinse an endoscope can cause a chemically induced colitis.
- Sterile transfer is difficult because items are wet.
- Chemically sterilized items cannot be held in long-term sterile storage. They must be processed for immediate use.
- The solution can become diluted during use if an item is wet when placed in it.

Types of Chemical Sterilants

In addition to EPA registration, chemical sterilants are approved by the FDA as a method of sterilization for critical items that are heat sensitive and can be immersed. The manufacturer is responsible for providing processing instructions on the container label, and the user is obligated to follow the instructions. All solutions should be tested before use with an appropriate test strip to validate the concentration of the sterilant. This is the only way to know if the chemical will be effective.

Acetic Acid

Acetic acid mixed with peracetic acid and hydrogen peroxide kills microorganisms by a process of oxidation to denature proteins in a process that takes 5 to 6 hours at a room temperature of 77° F (25° C). The solution is commonly used as a sterilant for dialysis machines. It is biodegradable and leaves no residue.

Glutaraldehyde

According to the FDA, a 2.4%, 2.5%, or 3.4% aqueous solution of activated buffered alkaline glutaraldehyde kills microorganisms by the denaturation of protein in cells. The solution is activated by adding a powdered buffer to the liquid. Alkaline glutaraldehyde solution changes pH and gradually loses its effectiveness after the date of activation. The expiration date specified by the manufacturer is marked on the container when activated (e.g., 14 days for aqueous Cidex-activated dialdehyde solution). The solution is reusable until this date, after which it is discarded according to EPA requirements. In most locales it may be discarded into the sanitary sewer, where it is bioxidized by sewer microorganisms into glutaric acid and then into carbon dioxide and water.

Most manufacturers claim that glutaraldehyde is a sterilant at 10 hours and a high-level disinfectant at 20 to 30 minutes, although the long-life varieties require 90 minutes to attain the same level of disinfection. These solutions are effective at room temperature.

Glutaraldehyde vaporizes rapidly and must remain covered to retain its concentration parameters. The fumes may have a mild odor and can be irritating to the eyes, nose, and throat. OSHA has established an exposure limit of 0.2 ppm in room air averaged over 8 hours. A glutaraldehyde exposure monitor should be worn by personnel who are at risk. Nitrile or butyl rubber or polyethylene gloves are worn to prevent skin sensitivity and contact dermatitis. Double-gloving with latex provides protection. Neoprene and polyvinyl chloride gloves are not protective.

The concentration of glutaraldehyde in solution should be monitored. A test strip or kit of reagents is used for testing the concentration before and after each use. If the solution has become diluted below 1.5%, it is ineffective and should be discarded.

Peracetic Acid

A proprietary chemical formulation of 35% peracetic acid, hydrogen peroxide, and water inactivates critical microbial cell systems. Peracetic acid is an acetic acid plus an extra oxygen atom that reacts with most cellular components to cause cell death. The mechanism may vary with each type of cell (e.g., vegetative bacterial endospores, mycobacterium). The sterilant is supplied in unit doses for each cycle and is diluted during the sterilization process to 0.2% peracetic acid solution. During the 23-minute sterilization process, the solution is heated to 122° F to 131° F (50−55° C) as it passes through the self-contained processing chamber. All items and internal components of the STERIS unit are submerged in the heated sterilant.

On completion of the sterilizing cycle, the sterilant is discharged into the sanitary drain. The used chemical is not considered a hazardous material by the EPA. The instruments are automatically rinsed in tap water that is passed through ultraviolet light, filtered through two external prefilters and two 0.1-μm internal microfiltration systems. The smallest known bacterium, *Pseudomonas diminuta*, is unable to pass through the pores in this filter system. (This is the same method used by pharmaceutical manufacturers to make sterile injectable medications.)

The STERIS unit uses a standard tap water supply, a sanitary drain, and a 110-V electrical connection. This tabletop unit has a printout to document each cycle. Periodic maintenance includes filter changes based on the chemical components of the external water supply. Biologic monitoring according to the manufacturer's recommendation is performed daily with a commercially prepared endospore strip containing *G. stearothermophilus*.

Hypochlorous Acid

Hypochlorous acid is derived from electrochemical activation of a brine solution. Although technically a high-level disinfectant, it kills many endospores.

Hypochlorous acid is nontoxic and environmentally safe. This chemical is a nonaldehyde oxidation material that kills endospores. No special handling or precautions are required.

Containers for Chemical Sterilant in Solution

A large bin with a perforated inner tray (nested) and lid is used with chemical sterilant solutions at room temperature. With chemical sterilization, items are completely immersed and the lumens filled with sterilant solution. The outside of the bin is labeled with the product name, date of activation, date of expiration, and initials of the person who mixed the solution. The inside of the bin, inner tray, and its lid should be kept sterile throughout the duration of use of that batch of solution. The lid should remain on the bin to prevent evaporation of the solution and to minimize vaporization of the solution. Evaporation changes the concentration of the mix and will alter the sterilant properties.

Preparing Items for Sterilization by Chemical Immersion

Items should be clean and free of organic debris and blood. Items should be washed thoroughly in a nonfilming soapy solution, rinsed, and thoroughly dried before placing them in the chemical sterilant. Lumens should be dried with jets of forced air. The solution will become diluted and lose effectiveness if other solutions such as water are added. No biologic material should be permitted to contaminate the solution.

Timing the Immersion Cycle

The time required for sterilization varies with the sporicidal activity of the chemical agent. The FDA has published a chart with brand names and timetables on the Internet. Below is an example of chemical sterilants and time ranges:

- *Acetic acid:* 20 minutes at 77° F (25° C) in a processing unit
- *Glutaraldehyde:* 10 to 12 hours at 77° F (25° C); concentrations of 1.12% to 3.4%; specialized processors using glutaraldehyde 2.5% take 7 hours and 40 minutes at 95° F (35° C)
- *Hydrogen peroxide:* 1% to 7.5% (3–8 hours at 68° F [20° C])
- *Peracetic acid:* 12 minutes at 122° F to 132° F (50–56° C)

A load control record of the items sterilized in solution is kept as for other methods of sterilization (see the sample record in Box 18.1).

Rinsing After Immersion

At the completion of the exposure period, all items are thoroughly rinsed in sterile distilled water before use. This step is automatic with the STERIS unit and other automatic endoscope processors. Sterile gloves are worn to transfer items from the chemical sterilant solution bin to a second sterile bin for rinsing. Items should then be dried with a sterile towel before being transferred to or placed on a sterile field. Items being terminally sterilized should be completely dry before placing in storage. Flexible endoscopes should be hung from a rack so the lumens are in a straight configuration, not coiled.

Radiation Sterilization

Microwave Sterilization

The nonionizing radiation of microwaves produces hyperthermic conditions that disrupt life processes. This heating action affects water molecules and interferes with cell membranes. Microwave sterilization uses low-pressure steam with the nonionizing radiation to produce the localized heat that kills microorganisms. The temperature is lower than conventional steam, and the cycle is faster—as short as 30 seconds. Metal instruments can be sterilized if placed under a partial vacuum in a glass container. Small tabletop units may be useful for rapid sterilization of a single instrument or a small number of instruments. Current models have a small chamber size—1 to 3 ft^3.

Gamma Ray and Beta Particle Sterilization

Some commercially available products are sterilized by irradiation. Ionizing radiation produces ions by knocking electrons out of atoms. These electrons are knocked out so violently that they strike an adjacent atom and either attach themselves to it or dislodge an electron from the second atom. The ionic energy that results becomes converted to thermal and chemical energy. This energy kills microorganisms by disrupting the DNA molecule, thus preventing cellular division and the propagation of biologic life.

The principal sources of ionizing radiation are beta particles and gamma rays. Beta particles are free electrons and are transmitted through a high-voltage electron beam from a linear accelerator. These high-energy free electrons penetrate matter before being stopped by collisions with other atoms. Thus their usefulness in sterilizing an object is limited by the density and thickness of the object and the energy of the electrons. They produce their effect by ionizing the atoms they hit, producing secondary electrons that in turn produce lethal effects on microorganisms.

Cobalt-60 is a radioactive isotope capable of disintegrating to produce gamma rays and is the most used source for irradiation sterilization. Gamma rays are electromagnetic waves and have the capability of penetrating to a much greater distance than do beta particles before losing their energy from collisions. Because they travel at the speed of light, they must pass through a thickness of several feet before making sufficient collisions to lose all their energy.

Irradiation sterilization with beta particles or gamma rays is limited to industrial use. Depending on the strength of the source, the product is exposed to radiation for 10 to 20 hours. Ionizing radiation penetrates most materials to sterilize reliably. However, the physical properties of some materials are altered by exposure to ionizing radiation, thus limiting its use. Irradiation can be used to sterilize heat- and moisture-sensitive items because the rays have a very low temperature effect on materials and because the process is dry. Because gamma rays can penetrate large bulky objects, cartons ready for shipment can be sterilized in the cobalt-60 irradiator; this is cost-effective for the manufacturer.

Ionizing radiation is the most effective sterilization method. No residual radiation is generated. The process may be monitored with biologic indicators using *Bacillus pumilus*. However, products can be released for use based on dosimetry (measurements of radiation dose) without the quarantine periods required for biologic testing. It is commonly used for commercially prepared single-use, prepackaged disposable items such as drug products, catheters, syringes, IV sets, and gloves.

Control Measures

Except for items sterilized in a high-speed pressure flash steam sterilizer for immediate use or by immersion in a chemical solution, all items are wrapped before sterilization. The integrity of the packaging material is maintained before use and during storage. Packages are labeled so the contents are known (unless they are visible through the packaging material). The label also includes the conditions of sterilization. A chemical indicator on the exterior of each package verifies exposure to a sterilization process.

Load Control Number

Whether sterilized onsite or offsite, a load control number should be imprinted on or be part of the label on every package of sterile items. This number designates the sterilization equipment used, the cycle, and the sterilization date. For sterilizers with microcomputer processor printouts, a label gun correlates the same control number for every package put in the load. Load control numbers are used to facilitate the identification and retrieval of supplies, if necessary, in the event of a sterilization failure. A load control number also should be assigned to items immersed in a chemical sterilant.

The sterilization date can be recorded as a Julian date (day 1 through 365) or as a Georgian date (month, day, year). The package may be stamped with the date of sterilization as it is removed from the sterilizer. The date also may be written or affixed on the package when it is wrapped. Monthly, color-coded machine-labeling systems may be used. Peel-off barcode labels also help control inventory and patient charges for items.

Wet Packs

All sterilizing methods in which humidity, usually steam, is a parameter of the process potentially present the hazard of producing wet packages. Microorganisms migrate easily through moisture when a pathway is provided from outside to inside a package. Water droplets may be visible on the outside or inside, or absorbed moisture may be seen or felt. Unless the wrapper is completely impermeable to water, a pack should be considered unsterile and unacceptable for use if it is wet. A stain on a wrapper may indicate that moisture was present and has dried. The cause of the wet pack is investigated and promptly corrected. Reprocessing is necessary for a wet package or a load with one or more wet or suspect packages.

Closed container systems with nonvented bottoms may have some retained condensate after processing. This retained moisture within the closed tray is not considered contamination because the container is sealed and impermeable to capillary action. The condensate is considered sterile.

Causes/Conditions of Wet Packs

Excessive moisture may be related to the steam itself, to the load, or to the sterilizer.

Wet Steam

If the steam is abnormally wet, water droplets may form on the outside or inside of packages, and absorbent materials will become soaked with moisture. At the boiling point, water becomes steam. Saturated steam contains as much water in the vapor state as physically possible (98%) and minimal liquid water (2% water droplets). In a steam sterilizer, pressure increases the temperature to raise the boiling point to 250° F (121° C) or above at a pressure of 15 pounds or more above atmospheric pressure at sea level. The temperature of steam does not increase above the boiling point at normal atmospheric pressure in other types of sterilizers. If steam loses water vapor, it can achieve a higher temperature at the same pressure, thus becoming superheated. In steam sterilization, superheating decreases the effectiveness of steam to kill microorganisms.

The dryness (purity) of steam depends on the amount of water in the vapor state in proportion to the amount of solid, liquid, or vapor contamination. This contamination can come from particles in the boiler, steam lines, or sterilizer; chemical additives in the water; or moisture in the load. When steam contacts cold surfaces, a lowering of its temperature reverts steam to water, producing condensation on surfaces and raising the temperature of the remaining vapor, which causes superheating of the steam. Dry, dehydrated textiles and other porous materials will absorb water from steam, which changes the proportion of the water content of steam and causes superheating. The water content of steam should not fall below 97% during the sterilization cycle. Below this level items in the load can become supersaturated with water and subsequent drying will be inadequate.

Characteristics of the Load

Many factors affect the penetration of the sterilant through the load. The following characteristics are reiterated for emphasis:
1. Items are cleaned before they are packaged. Nonporous items must be dry. Porous materials, such as woven fabrics, are hydrated (i.e., humidified) but not wet.
2. Basins are separated by absorbent material and positioned on the side rim so the water condensate will drain out.

3. Heat penetrates different materials at different rates. For even heating of the load, it is preferable not to mix materials. For example, a load may contain only instrument sets and metals or only packs of fabrics.
4. The density of a pack must allow the circulation of air, moisture, and sterilant within the pack. Porous items should not be wrapped tightly.
5. The permeability of packaging materials varies. A water droplet on an impermeable wrapper may not be a problem, but it can be absorbed by an adjacent package with a permeable wrapper.
6. Because condensation diffuses at different rates, the drying and cooling cycle depends on the materials in the load. Packages should not be handled until this cycle is complete.

Sterilizer Malfunctions

Clogged drains, steam traps, and air filters; inoperable control valves; worn gaskets; and a dirty chamber can cause the sterilizer to malfunction. Routine cleaning and PM techniques are imperative. Malfunctioning equipment requires the recall of the entire load.

Reprocessing Wet Packs

Wet packs are disassembled and the items properly dried and repackaged before resterilization. Reusable woven fabrics should be sent to the laundry and relaundered before use. Damp or wet fabrics will cause superheating during steam sterilization.

Shelf Life

Sterility is event related; it is not time related unless the package contains unstable components such as drugs or chemicals. Storage conditions are established to maintain the integrity of the package. An item is considered sterile based on the following events:
- Handling of the package during transport and storage (i.e., the prevention of contamination and physical damage)
- Integrity, type, and configuration of packaging material
- Conditions of storage

Specific written policies should address the handling and storage of all stored sterile supplies. Expiration dates should be placed on a tray that contains medications or other unstable supplies. Most commercially sterilized products are considered sterile indefinitely or as long as the integrity of the package is maintained. An expiration date put on the label by the manufacturer indicates the maximum time the manufacturer can guarantee product stability and sterility based on test data approved by the FDA.

Integrity of Packaging Material and Handling

The method of sterilization establishes the type of packaging material that may be used. Shelf life is affected by the permeability and density of the material, the type of closure used, and the method by which the package is handled. The following are considerations regarding the integrity of packaging materials:
1. An item is no longer considered sterile after an accidental puncture, tear, or rupture of the package. Paper may become brittle and crack.
2. Squeezing or crushing a package may force air out and draw unsterile air in, thus contaminating the contents. Packages wrapped in woven fabrics should be handled carefully and not packed tightly together for storage.

3. The accidental wetting of a package contaminates the contents. It is necessary to avoid the following:
   a. Handling the package with moist or wet hands
   b. Handling the package with soiled gloves
   c. Placing the package on a wet surface
4. The density of nonwoven fabrics and plastic materials protects the integrity of the package.
5. Heat- or self-sealed pouches protect the contents from dust.
6. Commercially packaged sterilized items are usually considered sterile until the package is opened or damaged or the stability of the product becomes outdated.

Dust Cover

A sealed, airtight plastic bag protects a sterile package from dust, dirt, lint, moisture, and vermin during storage. After sterilization and immediately after aerating or cooling to room temperature, infrequently used items may be sealed in plastic 2 to 3 mil thick (1 mil = one-thousandth of an inch or 0.001 inch). A dust cover will protect the integrity of the package.

Storage Conditions

The maintenance of sterility is related to the event and is not based on time. How sterile packages are handled and stored is as important as how long they can remain sterile. The following guidelines are helpful in maintaining the sterility of a package during storage:

1. Storage areas are clean and free of dust, lint, dirt, and vermin. Routine cleaning procedures are followed for all areas in the perioperative environment. Shipping containers and cardboard boxes should not be brought into the storage room. They can be sources of vermin and dust.
2. All sterile items should be stored under conditions that protect them from the extremes of temperature and humidity. Prolonged storage in a warm environment at high humidity can cause moisture to condense inside packages and thus destroy the microbial barrier of some packaging materials. Ventilating and air-conditioning systems with filtered air should maintain a temperature below 75° F (24° C) and a relative humidity between 20% and 60%. Four air exchanges per hour are recommended by the Association for the Advancement of Medical Instrumentation (AAMI).
3. Packages should be allowed to cool to room temperature before being put into storage to avoid condensation inside the package.
4. Peel pouches should be stored on their sides to minimize the pressure from items stacked on top of them.
5. For open shelving, the highest shelf should be at least 18 inches (46 cm) below the ceiling or sprinkler heads and the lowest shelf 8 to 10 inches (20–25 cm) above the floor. Shelving should be at least 2 inches away from the wall. Closed cupboards are preferred.
6. Sterile storage areas should have controlled traffic patterns that do not pass by open shelving storage.

Rotation of Supplies

When the standard number of packages kept sterile is adjusted according to daily needs, packages seldom need to be held for prolonged storage periods. In the interest of economy and good management, a stock supply of day-to-day items should be regulated to have enough for the busiest day, with used items replenished daily.

Many items are seldom used, yet several are always kept sterile. These supplies should be sterilized, or commercially sterilized items ordered, only in quantities sufficient to ensure prompt use and rapid turnover.

Sterile supplies should be checked daily for the integrity of the packages. Some items deteriorate with repeated sterilization or prolonged storage (e.g., latex items). Any sterile packages that become contaminated are reprocessed and resterilized. Older supplies always should be used first to minimize storage. The acronym FIFO (first in/first out) is helpful to remember for the rotation of supplies—particularly sterile supplies.

Loaner Instrumentation

Instrumentation brought to the facility by vendor/sales representatives should be covered by a specific set of policies and procedures for safe use. When the instruments are brought to the department, they should be inventoried and processed according to the same protocol as any instrument set used in patient care. All loaner sets should be considered contaminated until processed according to the guidelines set forth by facility policy and the manufacturer's recommendations.

The request for a loaner set should be made in enough time to deliver, process, and sterilize the instruments before the scheduled procedure. IUSS should not be used to process these items. Loaner sets should be processed with a class 5 chemical indicator and a biologic indicator, particularly those with implantables (e.g., screws, plates, and joints), appropriate for the method of processing used.

After using the set it should be decontaminated, inventoried, and processed according to policy. Documentation of each step is required. The department could use a loaner log that indicates receipt, inventorying, processing, use in the field, decontamination, return to owner, and documentation procedures. The names of personnel receiving, using, and returning the loaner set should be recorded.

Custom Packs

A custom pack is a preassembled collection of disposable supplies sterilized as a single unit. The components are specified by the user (i.e., the OR's specifications) for a particular procedure or specialty or a surgeon's preferences. These components are assembled and sterilized by a custom pack supplier or the manufacturer. A pack assembled by a manufacturer will have an assortment of products in a specific category, such as a kit of sutures, ligating clips, and skin staplers or a custom pack of disposable drapes. Many custom packs have approximately 100 diversified items needed for a specific type of surgical procedure, such as a pack for an open-heart procedure. Care should be taken in handling packs because damage to or contamination of a custom pack may waste many sterile items.

The assembler sterilizes packs with either EO gas or gamma radiation. All components of the pack must be compatible with the sterilization method. The assembler must adhere to government manufacturing regulations for testing to guarantee product stability and sterility and package integrity. Using custom packs may be cost-effective for the health care facility, and the following indirect savings are shared by the materials management department and the OR:

1. Personnel time (labor costs) for handling supplies is reduced.
   a. It reduces turnover time between procedures by saving time spent gathering and opening supplies. The circulating nurse has more time for direct patient care activities.
   b. It reduces setup time for the scrub person. Items can be prearranged in order of use and with components in proximity, such as suction tubing with a tip.
   c. It facilitates transport of supplies into storage or into a case cart system.
2. Storage space requirements are consolidated by storing supplies in bulk rather than individually.
3. Inventory control is facilitated.
   a. It simplifies listing of items in inventory. The supplier may maintain a computerized information system of usage and inventory levels.
   b. It reduces inventory. A minimal backup of supplies can be maintained.
   c. It reduces lost patient charges. The circulating nurse can process one charge for the custom pack rather than itemizing items.
4. Standardization is encouraged by incorporating the basic items routinely used by surgeon(s) into custom packs. This helps standardize preparations.
5. The infection rate may be decreased. The physical activity of opening supplies can disperse lint and dust into the air. Opening fewer packages decreases this potential environmental hazard.
6. Less environmental waste is generated by packaging material. Fewer disposable wrappers are used.

Many custom pack processors have addressed the problem of changes in surgeons' preferences by offering to supply the packs in small quantities. Changes are incorporated into new stock, thus decreasing the number of pack contents that may not be used. Some manufacturers will replace older or damaged packs for new stock. Evaluation of pack usefulness is ongoing and may change as the types and complexity of surgical procedures change.

Case Cart System

Most facilities use a surgery case cart system to gather and deliver supplies for each surgical procedure. These sterile and nonsterile supplies are selected according to standard routines and the individual surgeon's preferences. For the system to be efficient, good communication must exist among the staff in the OR and the central processing department (CPD). The surgeon's preference data should be current in the computer. Personnel in CPD prepare the case carts with the required supplies and instrument sets according to computerized schedules, preference cards, and case cart pull sheets (Fig. 18.5). Designated clean elevators connect these respective areas in the two departments if they are not located on the same floor.

Most of the drapes and disposables will be contained within the custom pack that is on the cart as designated by the facility. This saves time in opening supplies for the case. The items on the cart are patient charge items. Inventory lists that are supplied with the carts may be used for patient charges and inventory control. A barcode or other computer label system may be used to facilitate these functions. Any items not used or opened during the

• **Fig. 18.5** Surgery case cart being loaded for transport to the OR.

procedure are returned to stock and credited to the patient's account. Some carts are designed to serve as the instrument table during the surgical procedure.

After use, the cart is loaded with the contaminated instrument sets and taken back to the decontamination area. Unopened sterile supplies are not placed on the contaminated cart. They are returned separately. The cart and its contaminated supplies are enclosed during transport to the decontamination area. Usually the decontamination and reprocessing of OR instruments and equipment are done in areas separated from supplies used in other hospital departments. This prevents mixing expensive surgical instruments with those of hospital grade supplied to other units.

The personnel assigned to the surgery case cart areas should be familiar with the supplies needed for each surgical procedure, how surgical instruments are used, and the proper method of cleaning and sterilizing each. Surgical technologists frequently are assigned to sterile processing because of their technical background.

ⓔ EVOLVE WEBSITE

http://evolve.elsevier.com/Hornacky/BerryKohn/

- Historical Perspective
- Student Interactive Questions
- Glossary

References

1. Solon J, Killeen S: Decontamination and sterilization, *Surgery* 37(1):51–57, 2019.
2. Centers for Disease Control and Prevention: *Guideline for disinfection and sterilization in healthcare facilities*, 2019. www.cdc.gov. Accessed 12 March 2023.
3. Spruce L: Back to basics: packaging systems, *AORN J* 107(5):602–610, 2018.

4. Environmental Protection Agency: *Hazardous air pollutants: ethylene oxide*. www.epa.gov. Accessed April 30, 2023.

5. McEvoy B, Wiehle S, Gordon K, et al.: Advancing the sustainable use of ethylene oxide through process validation, *Biomed Instrum Techol* 55(3):35–44, 2021.

Bibliography

AORN: *Guidelines for perioperative practice*, Denver, CO, 2024, The Association.

Phillips NM, Hornacky A: *Pass CNOR*, St. Louis, 2019, Elsevier.

19

Surgical Instrumentation

CHAPTER OUTLINE

Fabrication of Metal Instruments, 338

Classification of Instruments, 339

Handling Instruments, 356

CHAPTER OBJECTIVES

After studying this chapter, the learner will be able to:

- Identify the use and function of each type of surgical instrument.
- Demonstrate the appropriate methods for passing each type of instrument.

- Understand the rationale and methods of decontamination of instrumentation.
- Demonstrate the assembly and passing of sharps.

KEY TERMS AND DEFINITIONS

Alloy A mixture of metals or of substances with metallic properties.

Anodized Dull blackened surface. The instrument is exposed to conditions that cause an oxide coating that is relatively impenetrable to atmospheric oxygen. Instruments can be anodized to reduce reflections. Tints and dyes can be added during the process.

Approximating Bringing edges together.

Atraumatic Without injury.

Crushing Destructive effects of specific instruments. Some procedures require the use of crushing clamps.

Cutting Separating with a sharp instrument or device.

Debulking Decrease in mass or volume using an instrument or device.

Dilation Enlarging an opening in a progressive manner.

Dissection Process of separating tissues through anatomic planes by using sharp or blunt instrumentation.

Evacuating Emptying a cavity or space.

Grasping Holding in a traumatic or an atraumatic manner.

Instillation Fluid is slowly introduced into a cavity or space.

Metallurgy The study of metals.

Occlusion Closing a lumen for the purpose of the procedure. The closure can be permanent or temporary.

Percutaneous Enter directly through the skin; without incision.

Retraction Stabilizing a tissue layer in a safe position for exposure of a part. A retractor can be manual or self-retaining.

Sharp Instrument with a cutting edge or pointed tip(s) that is used to cut or dissect tissue. These items include blades, scissors, needles, and other dissection devices.

Traumatic Causing injury by penetration or crushing.

Trocar A device used for penetration of tissue layers. It is commonly used for percutaneous endoscopy. It is used as a temporary pathway for gases, fluids, other instrumentation, or the removal of an organ or substance.

Fabrication of Metal Instruments

Metallurgy is the study of metals and their properties. This science enhanced the development of surgical instruments over the centuries. Although some surgical instruments are made of titanium, cobalt-based alloy (Vitallium), or other metals, the vast majority are made of stainless steel. The alloys used must have specific properties to make them resistant to corrosion when exposed to blood and body fluids, cleaning solutions, sterilization, and the atmosphere. The manufacturer chooses the alloy for its durability, functional capacity, and ease of fabrication for the intended purpose.

Stainless Steel

Stainless steel is an alloy of iron, chromium, and carbon. It may also contain nickel, manganese, silicon, molybdenum, sulfur, and other elements to prevent corrosion or add tensile strength. The formulation of the steel plus the heat treatment and finishing processes determine the qualities of the instrument. Chromium in the steel makes it resistant to corrosion. Carbon is necessary to give steel its hardness, but it also reduces the corrosion-resistant effects of chromium. Iron alloys in the 400 series (low in chromium and high in carbon) are most commonly used for the fabrication of surgical instruments.

Steel is milled into blanks that are forged, spun, drawn, die cast, molded, or machined into component shapes and sizes. These components are assembled by hand, then heat-hardened (tempered) and buffed. X-ray and/or fluoroscopy techniques are used to detect any defects that may occur as a result of the forging or machining operations. The stress and tension must be in balance; that is, the instrument must have the flexibility to withstand the stresses of normal use. The temper of the steel determines this balance.

The instrument is then subjected to processes that protect its surfaces and minimize corrosion. Oxidation of the surface chromium by a process called *passivation* forms a hard chromium oxide layer. Nitric acid removes carbon particles and promotes the formation of this surface coating. Polishing creates a smooth surface for the continuous layer of chromium oxide. Passivation continues to form this layer when the instrument is exposed to the atmosphere and oxidizing agents in cleaning solutions. The term *stainless* is a misnomer. Steel does not tarnish, rust, or corrode easily, but some staining and spotting will occur with normal use and prolonged exposure to corrosive agents.

Stainless steel instruments are fabricated with one of three types of finishes before passivation:
1. A mirror finish is shiny and reflects light. This highly polished finish tends to resist surface corrosion, but the glare can be a distraction for the surgeon or an obstruction to visibility.
2. An anodized finish, sometimes referred to as a *satin finish*, is dull and nonreflective. Protective coatings of chromium and nickel are deposited electrolytically and reduce glare. This type of finish is somewhat more susceptible to surface corrosion than is a highly polished surface, but the corrosion is usually easily removed.
3. An ebonized finish is dull black, which eliminates glare. The surface is darkened by a process of chemical oxidation. Instruments with an ebony finish are used in laser surgery to prevent beam reflection. In other surgical procedures, instruments with an ebony finish may offer the surgeon better color contrast because they do not reflect the color of tissues.

Titanium

Compared with stainless steel, the metallurgic properties of titanium alloy developed in 1950 are excellent for the manufacture of microsurgical instruments. Titanium is nonmagnetic and inert. Titanium alloy is harder, stronger, lighter in weight, and more resistant to corrosion than is stainless steel. A blue anodized finish of titanium oxide reduces glare. Titanium can be used in magnetic resonance imaging (MRI) procedures.

Vitallium

Vitallium is the trade name for an alloy of cobalt, chromium, and molybdenum developed in 1937. This inert alloy has the strength and corrosion-resistant properties suitable for some orthopedic devices and dental and maxillofacial implants. Vitallium contains no nickel or beryllium and causes less metal allergy than alloys with these components. Instruments made of Vitallium must be used when these devices are implanted. In an electrolytic environment such as body tissues, metals of different potentials can cause corrosion if they come into contact with each other. Therefore an implant of a cobalt-based alloy is not compatible with instruments that are iron-based alloys (stainless steel) and vice versa. Vitallium implants demonstrate three times the artifact scatter in radiography as titanium.

Other Materials

Although most instruments are made of steel alloys, other materials are used. Some instruments are fabricated from brass, silver, aluminum, or medical-grade plastics (e.g., polyarylamide, polyphenylsulfone). Tungsten carbide is an exceptionally hard metal used for laminating some cutting blades or as inserts on the functional tips or jaws of some instruments. Silver and copper are known to have antimicrobial properties. Ancient Egyptians stored water in copper jugs to decontaminate enteric microbes found in river water. Studies have validated microbial destruction in water when stored in copper containers. It has been suggested that the use of copper in the surface of touch pads in health care settings could decrease microbial transfer on high-touch surfaces. Medical-grade plastics are being used for single-use instruments, reusable instruments, and 3D printing. The U.S. Food and Drug Administration (FDA) has guidelines for the use of 3D printing for implanted devices.[1]

Plated Instruments

A shiny finish can be put on a basic forging or tooling of an iron alloy. Chromium, nickel, cadmium, silver, and copper are used for coating or flash-plating. When deposited directly on the steel, any of these metals is prone to rupturing, chipping, and spontaneous peeling. It is difficult to keep plated instruments from corroding, and rust can form beneath the plating. Plated instruments are used infrequently today.

Classification of Instruments

Various basic maneuvers are common to all surgical procedures. The surgeon dissects, resects, or alters tissues and/or organs to restore or repair bodily functions or body parts. Bleeding must be controlled during the process. Surgical instruments are designed to provide the tools the surgeon needs for each maneuver. Whether they are small or large, short or long, straight or curved, sharp or blunt, all instruments can be classified by their function. Because the nomenclature is not standardized, the names of specific instruments must be learned in the clinical practice setting. All instruments should be used only for their intended purpose, and they should not be abused.

Dissecting and Cutting Instruments

Dissection instruments have sharp edges. They are used to cut, incise, separate, or excise tissues. There are two types of dissecting instruments: sharp and blunt.

Sharp dissecting instruments should be kept separate from other instruments, and the sharp edges should be protected during cleaning, sterilizing, and storing. Specialized tip protectors may be placed on sharp instruments before the sterilization process and removed before use. To prevent injury to the handler and damage to the sharp edges, proper precautions are necessary to take during the handling or disposing of all sharps, blades, or scalpels.

• **Fig. 19.1** **A,** Disposable blades: Ten series for the no. 3 scalpel. Blade sizes 10, 11, 12, and 15. **B,** Twenty series for the no. 4 scalpel. Blade sizes 20, 21, 22, 23, 24, and 25.

Blunt dissection instruments are used to push or peel soft tissue away from another surface. Examples are Penfield or Freer elevators used to strip muscle and periosteum from bony surfaces.

Scalpels

The type of scalpel most used has a reusable handle with a disposable blade. Most handles are made of brass; the blades may be made of carbon steel. Blades vary by size and shape (Fig. 19.1); handles vary by width and length (Fig. 19.2). Blades with a numeric prefix of "1" as in a "10" series (e.g., 10, 11, 12, and 15) fit handle size number 3 or 7. Blades with a numeric prefix of "2" as in "20" series (e.g., 20, 22, or 25) fit handle size number 4. Disposable scalpels also are available but are not weighted the same as metal handles. Most surgeons prefer reusable metal scalpel handles.

The blade is attached to a reusable handle by slipping the blade into the grooves on the narrow edge of the handle. An instrument, never the fingers, is used to attach and detach the blade; this instrument, usually a heavy hemostat or Kelly clamp, should not touch the cutting edge. Needle holders are not designed to load scalpel blades, and the jaws can become misaligned by excess torque. The following are descriptions of blade and scalpel combinations:

- Number 10 blades are rounded toward the tip and are often used to open the skin.
- Number 11 blades have a linear edge with a sharp tip. Can be used to make the initial skin puncture for tiny deep incisions.
- Number 12 blades have a curved cutting surface like a hook. Commonly used for tonsillectomy.
- Number 15 blades have a short, rounded edge for shallow, short, controlled incisions.
- Number 20 blades are shaped like number 10 blades but larger.
- An assortment of blades with angulations and configurations for specific uses, such as a Beaver blade, also are used (Fig. 19.3). These blades insert into a special universal handle that secures by turning a screw-in collar (Fig. 19.4).

• **Fig. 19.2** Most common scalpels: 4, 3, and 7.

• **Fig. 19.3** Beaver scalpel blades.

• **Fig. 19.4** Beaver scalpel handle.

Knives

Knives come in various sizes and configurations. Like a kitchen paring knife, they usually have a blade at one end that may have one or two cutting edges. The knives are designed for very specific purposes (e.g., cataract knife). Other types of knives have detachable and replaceable blades (e.g., dermatome). A knife blade may be incorporated into a multifunctional instrument, such as a gastrointestinal anastomosis (GIA) or an end-to-end anastomosis (EEA) stapler that cuts and staples tissue simultaneously.

Scissors

The blades of scissors may be straight, angled, or curved, as well as serrated, wedge-shaped, sharp, blunt, or combined sharp-blunt tips (Fig. 19.5). The handles may be long or short. Some

• **Fig. 19.5** Surgical scissors. **A,** Tissue scissors. Blades may be straight or curved, and either tip can be sharp or blunt. **B,** Suture scissors. **C,** Wire suture scissors. **D,** Joseph nasal scissors. **E,** Potts angled scissors. **F,** Lister bandage scissors. **G,** Tenotomy scissors.

scissors are used only to cut or dissect tissues; others are used to cut other materials. To maintain sharpness of the cutting edges and proper alignment of the blades, scissors should be used only for their intended purpose:
- Tissue/dissecting scissors have sharp or blunt tips. The type and location of tissue to be cut determine which scissors the surgeon will use. Blades needed to cut tough tissues are heavier than those needed to cut fine, delicate structures. Curved or angled blades are needed to reach under or around structures.
- Tissue scissors with blunt tips can be used to bluntly dissect between individual planes before sharply dissecting. Handles to reach deep into body cavities are longer than those needed for superficial tissues (Fig. 19.5, A).
- Suture scissors have sharp-blunt points to prevent structures close to the suture from being cut. The scrub person may use scissors to cut sutures during preparation if needed (Fig. 19.5, B).
- Wire scissors have short, heavy serrated blades. Wire scissors are used instead of suture scissors to cut stainless steel sutures (Fig. 19.5, C). Heavy wire cutters are used to cut bone fixation wires.
- Short-jaw, sharp-tipped scissors are used for deep, confined areas such as the nasal cavity (Fig. 19.5, D).
- Sharp-tipped angled scissors with short jaws are used for vascular surgery (Fig. 19.5, E).
- Dressing/bandage scissors are used to cut drains and dressings and to open items such as plastic packets (Fig. 19.5, F). The protective tip prevents cutting into concealed structures.
- Small scissors with special wedge-shaped tips, such as tenotomy scissors, are used for blunt and sharp dissection (Fig. 19.5, G)

Bone Cutters and Saws

Many types of instruments have cutting edges suitable for cutting into or through bone and cartilage. Some have moving parts, such as rib cutters. Others, such as drills, saws, and reamers, are powered by air or electricity and have disposable tips and blades.

Blunt Dissectors

Friable tissues or tissue planes can be separated by blunt dissection. The scalpel handle, the blunt sides of tissue scissor blades, and dissecting sponges may be used for this purpose (Fig. 19.6). Elevators, strippers, and dissectors can be used to remove adherent tissue such as periosteum from bone or dura from the inner aspect of the skull.

Debulking Instruments

Debulking instruments include curettes, chisels, osteotomes, gouges, rasps, and files (Fig. 19.7). The purpose of these instruments is to decrease the bulk of firm tissue and not necessarily cut along defined tissue planes.
- *Biopsy forceps and punches.* A small piece of tissue for pathologic examination may be removed with a biopsy forceps or punch. These instruments may be used through an endoscope (Fig. 19.8).
- *Curettes.* Soft tissue or bone is removed by scraping with the sharp edge of the loop, ring, or scoop on the end of a curette (Fig. 19.9). Blunt curettes are designed to strip away layers without damage to underlying structures. Thomas uterine curettes are blunt and are used for debulking friable postpartum endometrium.

• **Fig. 19.6** Blunt dissectors. **A,** Penfield blunt dissectors and tamps. **B,** Periosteal elevators.

• **Fig. 19.7** **A,** Osteotomes. **B,** Rasps.

• **Fig. 19.8** Punch biopsy instrument.

• *Snares.* A loop of wire may be put around a pedicle to dissect tissue such as a tonsil or a polyp. The wire cuts the pedicle as it retracts into the instrument. The wire is discarded and replaced with a new one after use (Fig. 19.10).

Grasping and Holding Instruments

Tissues should be grasped atraumatically and held in position so the surgeon can perform the desired maneuver, such as dissecting or suturing (approximating), without injuring the surrounding subcutaneous tissues or perforating the skin (Fig. 19.11). Forceps without ring handles are commonly referred to as *pick-ups.*

Delicate Forceps

Fine tissues such as eye tissue are held with delicate forceps (Fig. 19.11, *A*). They can be toothed or smooth, straight, or angled.

Adson Forceps

Forceps are used to pick up or hold soft tissues in approximation during closure (Fig. 19.11, *B*). They can be toothed or smooth.

Bayonet Forceps

Forceps are angled like a bayonet to prevent the user's hand from occluding vision in a small space (Fig. 19.11, *C*). They can be toothed or smooth.

Smooth Tissue Forceps

Also referred to as *thumb forceps* or *pick-ups,* smooth forceps resemble tweezers. They are tapered and have serrations (grooves) at the tip. They may be straight or bayonet (angled), short or long, and delicate or heavy. Smooth forceps are atraumatic and will not injure delicate structures (Fig. 19.11, *D*).

Toothed Tissue Forceps

Toothed forceps differ from smooth forceps at the tip. Rather than being serrated, they have a single tooth on one side that fits between two teeth on the opposing side, or they have a row of multiple teeth at the tip. Heavy types are sometimes referred to as *rat-toothed forceps.* Toothed forceps provide a firm hold on tough tissues, including skin. Finer versions have delicate teeth for holding more delicate tissue (Fig. 19.11, *E*). Care is taken not to perforate the epidermis or dermis when holding tissue.

Allis Forceps

Allis forceps have ringed handles and lock with ratchets. Each jaw curves slightly inward, and there is a row of teeth at the end. The teeth grasp tissue edges securely (Fig. 19.12, *A*). Allis forceps can be short or long. Some of the long forceps have a slight curve, such as those used with a hemorrhoid band ligator.

• **Fig. 19.9** Tissue curettes. **A,** Soft and compact tissue curettes. **B,** Uterine curettes.

• **Fig. 19.10** Surgical snare (tonsil snare).

Babcock Forceps

Babcock forceps have ringed handles and lock with ratchets. The end of each jaw of a Babcock forceps is rounded to fit around a tubular structure (e.g., fallopian tube) or to grasp tissue without injury. This rounded section is circumferentially fenestrated (Fig. 19.12, *B*). Babcock forceps are straight and can be short or long; they are not occlusive or crushing.

Lahey Forceps

Lahey forceps have ringed handles and lock with ratchets. The jaws of the Lahey forceps have sharp apposing points for grasping

tough organs or tumors during excision (Fig. 19.12, *C*). They are not occlusive or crushing.

Stone Forceps

Either curved or straight forceps are used to grasp polyps or calculi such as kidney stones or gallstones. Stone forceps have blunt loops or cups at the end of the jaws and do not have ratchets.

Tenaculums

Tenaculums have ringed handles and lock with ratchets and may have a single tooth or multiple teeth, such as a Jacob tenaculum (Fig. 19.13). The curved or angled points on the ends of the jaws of tenaculums penetrate tissue to grasp firmly, such as when a uterine tenaculum is attached to the cervix and used to manipulate the uterus during laparoscopy.

Some uterine tenaculums have a built-in uterine cannula or probe elevator tip, such as a Hulka tenaculum (Fig. 19.14). A uterine cannula, or probe, can be used during laparoscopy to raise the uterus into the visual field (Fig. 19.15). The cannula tip is inserted into the cervical os as the tenaculum is clamped on the anterior aspect of the cervix. Dye or contrast media can be instilled through the cannula into the uterine cavity to visualize tubal patency or the inner configuration of the uterine cavity. Some styles have a tenaculum stabilizer tip attached.

Bone Holders

Grasping forceps, vise-grip pliers, and other types of heavy holding forceps stabilize bone (Fig. 19.16). Some styles have ring handles and locking ratchets. Others have compression grips and do not lock.

Clamping and Occluding Instruments

Instruments that clamp and occlude are used to apply pressure. Some clamps are designed to crush the structure as the instrument is applied and are considered traumatic. The clamped crushed structure is usually sewn, clipped, or electrocoagulated and then removed. Other clamps are noncrushing (atraumatic) and are used to occlude or secure tissue, which is restored to patency at some point during the surgical procedure.

Hemostatic Clamps

Most clamps used for occluding blood vessels have two opposing jaws (with or without serrations or fine teeth), ringed handles, and lock with ratchets. Most ring-handled clamps have a common design (Fig. 19.17). The length and shape of the shanks or jaws may vary according to the intended function of the instrument.

Hemostats

Hemostats are the most commonly used surgical instruments and are used primarily to clamp blood vessels. They have a crushing action. Hemostats have either straight or curved slender jaws that taper to a fine point. The serrations are longitudinal or horizontal inside the jaws (Fig. 19.18).

Crushing Clamps

Many variations of hemostatic forceps are used to crush tissues or clamp blood vessels. The jaws may be straight, curved, or angled, and the serrations may be horizontal, diagonal, or longitudinal. The tip may be pointed or rounded or have a tooth along the jaw such as on a Heaney clamp or hysterectomy clamps (Fig. 19.19). The length of the jaws and handles varies. Many forceps are

• **Fig. 19.11** Tissue forceps. **A,** Bishop eye or forceps. **B,** Adson forceps. **C,** Bayonet forceps. **D,** Smooth forceps. **E,** Forceps with teeth.

• **Fig. 19.12** Ring-handled forceps used for grasping. **A,** Allis forceps. **B,** Babcock forceps. **C,** Lahey forceps.

• **Fig. 19.14** Hulka uterine elevator and tenaculum.

• **Fig. 19.13** Uterine cervix graspers. **A,** Single-tooth uterine tenaculum. **B,** Jacob multitooth uterine tenaculum.

• **Fig. 19.15** Kahn uterine cannula and manipulator.

• **Fig. 19.16** Lambotte bone holding forceps.

Serrated jaws

Box lock

Shank

Ratchets

Ring handle

• **Fig. 19.17** Anatomy of a ring-handled clamp.

• **Fig. 19.18** Crushing clamps. Jaws may be straight or curved. Tips may be pointed or rounded. Serrations may be horizontal or longitudinal. Jaws and handles may be long or short.

named for the surgeon who designed the style, such as the Kocher and the Ochsner clamps (Fig. 19.20).

Some instruments are designed to be used on specific organs. The features of the instrument will determine its use. Fine tips are needed for small vessels and structures. Longer and sturdier jaws are needed for larger vessels, dense structures, and thick tissue.

• **Fig. 19.19** Hemostatic uterine clamps. **A,** Heaney clamp with teeth along crosshatched jaw. **B,** Hysterectomy clamp with longitudinal jaw and crosshatched tips.

• **Fig. 19.20** Kocher or Ochsner clamp tips.

Longer shanks are needed to reach structures deep in body cavities. Tissue that has been crushed is usually sutured or stapled.

Noncrushing Clamps

Noncrushing clamps are used to occlude bowel or major blood vessels temporarily, which minimizes tissue trauma. The jaws of these types of clamps have opposing rows of fine serrations but have a softer hold on tissues. The jaws may be straight, curved, angled, or S-shaped (Fig. 19.21).

Retracting and Exposing Instruments

Soft tissues, muscles, and other structures should be pulled aside for exposure of the intended surgical site.

Manual Retractors

Most handheld retractors have an ergonomic handle and blade (Fig. 19.22). The term *blade* should not be confused with scalpel. The blades vary in width and length to correspond to the size and

• **Fig. 19.21** Noncrushing vascular clamp.

• **Fig. 19.22** Manual retractors. **A,** Solid blade appendiceal retractor. **B,** Volkmann rake retractors (tips can be sharp or blunt). **C,** Double-ended Army-Navy retractor.

• **Fig. 19.23** Manual specialty retractors. **A,** Freeman facelift retractor. **B,** Harrington Sweetheart liver retractor. **C,** Double-ended Eastman retractor. **D,** Mayo retractor.

depth of the incision. The curved or angled blade may be solid for body wall retraction (e.g., Mayo, Richardson, or Kelly retractors), fenestrated like a wire whisk for delicate tissue retraction (e.g., lung retractor), or pronged like a rake for raising tissue edges (e.g., Freeman facelift retractor). The prongs on the blades of a rake can be dull or sharp.

Some retractors have different sized blades at both ends with a handle in the middle (Fig. 19.23). Other retractors have traction grooves or serrations for slippery surfaces such as the tongue (Fig. 19.24). Manual retractors are often used in pairs, and they are held by the first or second assistant.

Malleable Retractors

A malleable retractor is a flat length of low-carbon stainless steel, silver, or silver-plated copper that may be bent to the desired angle and depth for retraction (Fig. 19.25). Referred to as ribbon retractors, they can be found in assorted widths from ½ inch to 4 inches. Some malleable blades attach into self-retaining or bed-mounted retractors.

Hooks

Single, double, or multiple very fine hooks with sharp points are used to retract delicate structures. Hooks are commonly used to retract skin edges during a wide-flap dissection such as a facelift or mastectomy (Fig. 19.23, *A*). Some styles of hooks have ball tips,

• **Fig. 19.24** Tongue retractor.

which cause less trauma to tissues (Fig. 19.26). Some hook styles have elastic attachments that are mounted into a preformed frame over the incision. Care is taken not to perforate the epidermis or dermis when using a hook retractor. Only the subcutaneous tissue is held back.

Self-Retaining Retractors

Holding devices with two or more flat or hooked blades can be inserted to spread the edges of an incision and hold them apart (Fig. 19.27). For example, a rib spreader holds the chest open

• **Fig. 19.25** Malleable "ribbon" retractor bends to the shape of the body part to be retracted. Widths vary.

• **Fig. 19.26** Double skin hooks depicted as sharp and ball-tipped.

during a thoracic or cardiac procedure with flat blades. A self-retaining retractor may have shallow or deep blades. Some retractors have ratchets or spring locks to keep the device open; others have wing nuts to secure the blades. Some self-retaining retractors have interchangeable blades of different sizes. Each part of the self-retaining retractor is accounted for at the end of the surgical procedure. Detachable blades or wing nuts can be lost during closure.

Bed-Mounted Retractors

Some self-retaining retractors can be attached to the operating room (OR) bed for stability when a long surgical incision is planned (Fig. 19.28). A bed-mounted retractor is packaged and sterilized separately in one or two trays because of the numerous blades and attachments. All the parts are counted items.

The component parts include an assortment of blades, connecting ratchets, a mounting frame for the blades (which can be an assortment of shape and sizes from round to oval), and an upright post that attaches to the side rail of the OR bed at the level of the mattress. The scrub person passes the attaching end of the upright post to the circulating nurse, who securely connects the post to the OR bed frame with a screw-bolt. The attached end touched by the circulating nurse is no longer sterile.

The upright part of the post remains sterile, and the mounting frame is attached by the surgeon at the working height desired. The individual blades and ratchets are placed by the surgeon and the first assistant to attain the exposure needed to perform the surgical procedure. Bed-mounted retractors are useful in preventing fatigue of the team for long procedures. Care is taken to prevent the upright post from resting against the patient's body. Permanent nerve injury can result from prolonged pressure of an immobile post against a nerve during the surgical procedure.

Closure and Approximation Instruments

Suture materials, surgical needles, and surgical staples are discussed in detail in Chapter 28. Only the instruments required for suture or staple placement are mentioned here.

Needle Holders

Most needle holders have ring handles and locking ratchets. They are used to grasp and hold curved surgical needles. Most needle holders resemble hemostatic forceps; the basic difference is the shortness of the jaws (Fig. 19.29). A needle holder has short, sturdy jaws for grasping a needle without damaging it or the suture material. The jaws are usually straight, but they may be curved or angled. The inner surfaces of the jaws also may differ such as crosshatched, serrated, or have a central notch for stability. The size of the needle holder should match the size of the needle (i.e., heavy jaws for large needles and slim jaws for small needles) (Fig. 19.30).

Needle holders can be constructed of various lengths and weights. Heavy snub-nosed needle holders are useful for stainless steel sutures. Long-handled needle holders facilitate needle placement in surgical sites such as the pelvis or chest. Short needle holders are used superficially on the skin or subcuticular tissue.

Specialty needle holders may have spring handles with or without locks. The jaws of the micro needle holders used for ophthalmic surgery and microsurgery may be either diamond-cut or crosshatched. They can be curved, angled, or straight. A needle holder should not be placed on a magnetic pad because it may become magnetized and cause needle release problems when suturing.

Tungsten Carbide Jaws

Tungsten carbide is a hard metal. Jaws with an insert of solid tungsten carbide with diamond-cut precision teeth are designed specifically to eliminate the twisting and turning of the needle in the needle holder (Fig. 19.31). These diamond-jaw needle holders can be identified by the gold plating on the handles.

Crosshatched Jaws

The serrations on the inside surface of the jaws are crisscrossed rather than grooved. Crosshatching provides a smoother surface and prevents damage to the needle.

• **Fig. 19.27** Self-retaining retractors. **A,** Weitlaner. **B,** Gelpi. **C,** Balfour. **D,** O'Sullivan-O'Connor.

Upright post attaches to OR bed

• **Fig. 19.28** Bookwalter bed-mounted self-retaining retractor. **A,** Bookwalter retractor assembled. **B,** Bookwalter retractor disassembled.

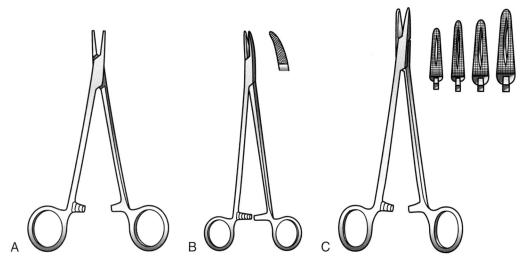

• **Fig. 19.29** Standard needle holders. **A,** Crile needle holder. **B,** Heaney needle holder. **C,** Mayo Hegar needle holder.

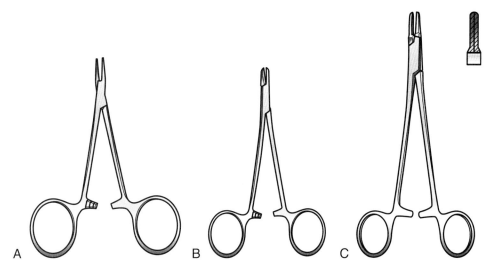

• **Fig. 19.30** Standard small needle holders. **A,** Webster smooth jaw needle holder. **B,** Derf snub-jaw needle holder. **C,** Ryder narrow tip needle holder.

• **Fig. 19.31** Tungsten carbide insert in jaws of needle holder, with diamond-cut teeth, is designed to eliminate needle twisting and turning.

Smooth Jaws

Some surgeons prefer needle holders that have jaws without serrations. These needle holders are used with small needles, such as those used for plastic surgery.

Staplers

Whether reusable or disposable, all surgical staplers are bulky, heavy instruments. Reusable staplers have many moving parts and are assembled at the sterile field before use. Sterile, single-use disposable staplers that are completely assembled eliminate the many problems associated with reusable instruments. The staples are usually made from titanium, stainless steel, or absorbable material. Staplers are mechanical instruments that should never be flipped to the sterile field. The impact of the stapler when it hits the field can cause misalignment of the preloaded staples, causing a misfire or put a hole in the table cover. In 2021, the FDA reclassified staplers for internal use from Class I to Class II devices. The change to Class II falls under the special control category. Internal staplers must go through a premarket review that evaluates them for effectiveness and safety after numerous complaints of the devices causing harm to patients.[2] The FDA also has a list of recommendations for the use of staplers for health care providers. More information can be found at www.fda.gov.

Clip Appliers

Individual staples can be placed with a preloaded or single clip applier. These clips are used to mark tissue and occlude vessels or

• **Fig. 19.32** Clip applier.

• **Fig. 19.33** Internal staplers. **A,** Terminal end stapler. **B,** Internal anastomosis stapler. **C,** End-to-end stapler.

small lumens of tubes (Fig. 19.32). Powered or manual styles are available. Endoscopic clip appliers have been used for many years with laparoscopic tubal occlusion for reproductive sterilization. Some varieties can ligate and divide tissue simultaneously, which can expedite removal of large organs from multiple vascular attachments quickly, such as bowel.

Terminal End Staplers

Terminal end staplers are designed for closing the end of a hollow or large organ (e.g., bowel, stomach) with a double staggered line of staples.[2] The stapler is L-shaped and is positioned across the end of the hollow organ to be closed or the tissue to be amputated. A pin is positioned in the stapler head to contain the tissue neatly, and the instrument is closed and fired with a pistol grip handle. A scalpel is used to trim the tissue extruding from the end of the closed instrument. The stapler is opened, and the staple line is inspected for integrity. Some types of terminal end staplers have articulating ends for placement across hard-to-reach areas, such as the vaginal cuff during a hysterectomy (Fig. 19.33, *A*).

Internal Anastomosis Staplers

Internal anastomosis staplers are designed to connect hollow organ segments to fashion a larger pouch or reservoir.[3] Two tube-shaped organs are aligned side by side, and one fork of the two-forked stapler is positioned in each opening. The instrument is fired, and the tubes are stapled along the adjoining lengths. An internal knife blade cuts between the two sets of double staple lines, creating a longitudinal opening on the inside of the anastomosed organ segments. Intestinal pouches can be fashioned in this manner. Some styles of side-to-side staplers do not have a self-contained knife. Endoscopic styles are available (Fig. 19.33, *B*).

End-to-End Circular Staplers

End-to-end circular staplers are designed to staple two hollow, tubular organs end to end to create a continuous circuit. These staplers are commonly used for bowel anastomosis after resection. The instrument can be inserted via the rectum or inserted through a small incision in the wall of one limb of the tubes to be anastomosed.

The ends of the tubes are positioned over the distal and proximal tips of the stapler and are secured with circumferential purse string sutures. The send of the stapler is closed, with the tissue of the tied ends completely enclosed in the stapler head.

When the instrument is fired, a double row of staples is placed in a circle, and a circular knife automatically trims the excess rim from the joined tubes.

When the instrument is opened, the trimmed rims (donuts) are removed from the stapler head and examined for circular integrity. These trimmed rims should be carefully separated and identified as proximal and distal tissue for the pathologist; the margins may be examined for the presence or absence of cancer cells. End-to-end staplers may be curved or straight (Fig. 19.33, *C*).

Viewing Instruments

Surgeons can examine the interior of body cavities, hollow organs, or structures with viewing instruments and can perform many procedures through them. Endoscopic telescopes have a fixed lens and attach to an external light source to illuminate the interior aspect. Hollow tubes, such as sigmoidoscopes do not have a fixed lens. A small light pipe with a fiberoptic cable provides lighting through the lumen of the bowel.

Speculums

The hinged, blunt blades of a speculum enlarge and hold open a canal (e.g., vagina, rectum [Fig. 19.34]) or a cavity (e.g., nose [Fig. 19.35]). Disposable speculums are available. An ear speculum is like a funnel (Fig. 19.36).

Endoscopes

The round or oval sheath of an endoscope is inserted into a body orifice (rigid or flexible) or through a small percutaneous skin incision guided by a trocar assembly (rigid). Each type of endoscope is designed for viewing in a specific anatomic location. Many accessory instruments and robotics are used through endoscopes. Endoscopes are illuminated through a separate light

• **Fig. 19.36** Ear speculum.

• **Fig. 19.37** Rigid sheaths and lensed endoscope.

• **Fig. 19.34** Speculums and anoscopes. **A,** Auvard vaginal speculum. **B,** Graves vaginal speculum. **C,** Hirschman anoscope. **D,** Brinckerhoff anoscope.

Hollow Endoscopes

In a hollow endoscope, the rigid hollow sheath permits viewing in a forward direction through the endoscope in a natural body orifice (e.g., bronchoscope, esophagoscope, or sigmoidoscope). The sheath is made of layered polymers, stainless steel, or plastic. A light carrier supplied by a fiberoptic cable provides illumination. A working space is created by manual insufflation of air.

Lensed Endoscopes

Lensed endoscopes have either rigid or flexible sheaths, and they have an eyepiece with a telescopic lens system for viewing in several directions. Some endoscopes have motor-driven lenses with optical zoom technology for high-magnification images. Lighting is provided through a fiberoptic cable and an electric light source with extremely bright lamps. Used in combination with video-assisted technology, computerization permits recording action videos and still digital photography. Many flexible endoscopes have working channels for performing specialized procedures such as biopsies. Lensed instruments are complex and require careful handling to avoid damage (Fig. 19.37).

Aspiration, Instillation, and Irrigation Instruments

Blood, body fluids, tissue, and irrigating solution may be removed by mechanical suction or manual aspiration. Reusable suction tips and aspiration devices have lumens that are difficult to terminally clean and sterilize. Most of these items are available in disposable models.

Aspiration

Aspiration, or suction, involves the application of negative pressure (less than atmospheric pressure) for evacuating blood or fluids, usually for visibility at the surgical site. An appropriate style tip is attached to sterile tubing; many tips are disposable. The style of the suction tip depends on where it is to be used and the surgeon's preference (Fig. 19.38). Disposable styles are preferred because the inner lumen is difficult to clean.

Blood, body fluid, or tissue may be aspirated manually to obtain a specimen for laboratory examination or to obtain bone

• **Fig. 19.35** Nasal speculum.

source using an electric power source. Care is taken not to allow an illuminated light cable or instrument to rest on the drapes to prevent a potential fire.[4] A discussion of endoscopic and robotic principles is found in Chapter 32 of this text.

• **Fig. 19.38** Tips of suction tubes. **A,** Poole abdominal tip. **B,** Frazier tip. **C,** Yankauer tip.

marrow for transplantation. Suction is often performed with a needle and syringe.

Poole Abdominal Tip

The Poole abdominal suction tip is a straight hollow tube with a perforated outer filter shield. It is used during abdominal laparotomy or within any cavity in which copious amounts of fluid or pus are encountered. The outer filter shield prevents the adjacent tissues from being pulled into the suction apparatus. This outer shield is completely removable.

Frazier Tip

The Frazier tip is a right-angle tube with a small diameter. It is used when encountering little or no fluid except capillary bleeding and irrigating fluid, such as in brain, spinal, plastic, or orthopedic procedures. The Frazier tip keeps the field dry without the need for sponging. One model has a connection for an electrosurgical unit, and the tip can be used for fulguration. A fiberoptic cable can be attached to another model. The vacuum exerted by the suction is controlled by a small hole that is covered by the thumb in the handgrip of the Frazier. Disposable right-angled suction tips are supplied with a stylet that can be inserted into the lumen to dislodge tissue or clots that could interfere with the suction quality.

Yankauer Tip

The Yankauer tip is a hollow tube that has an angled shaft and a perforated round-ball tip. This suction tip is also referred to as tonsil suction. Large quantities of blood and fluid can be suctioned quickly with a Yankauer tip, which is useful for visualization during ruptured aneurysms. Reusable Yankauer suction tips may be metal and have a removable end cap that screws in place. This must be accounted for at the end of the procedure. It is easily lost in a patient. Disposable plastic models are constructed in one piece with no removable tip.

• **Fig. 19.39** Ochsner gallbladder trocar.

Autotransfusion

A double-lumen suction tip is used to remove blood for autotransfusion. Only blood intended for reuse is suctioned into the autotransfusion machine. Great care is taken not to suction other material into this suction line. Hemostatic material and solutions can cause serious damage to the patient if reinfused into the patient.

Trocar

A trocar assembly may be needed to cut through tissues for access to fluid or a body cavity. A trocar has two parts—a sharp obturator and a sheath or a blunt obturator and sheath. The sharp obturator with the sheath is used to perforate the tissues. When the trocar assembly is in place the obturator is removed, leaving the sheath in position and creating a stented tunnel for drainage of fluids, introduction of instrumentation, or instillation of medication. Some trocars have suction ports, such as is used for draining the gallbladder (Fig. 19.39).

Endoscopic instruments may be manipulated through special trocars that have valves for insufflation, irrigation, and aspiration. Endoscopy and the eight essentials associated with endoscopic procedures are described in detail in Chapter 32.

Cannula

A cannula with a blunt end and perforations around the tip may be used to aspirate fluid without cutting into tissue. Cannulas also are used to open blocked vessels or ducts for drainage or to shunt blood flow from the surgical site.

Dilating and Probing Instruments

Malleable copper and brass dilators and probes can be plated with chromium or silver. A set of Hank, Hawkins, Pratt, or Hegar dilators are used to dilate the uterine cervix (Fig. 19.40). A probe is used to explore a path in the structure or to locate an obstruction. Probes are used to explore the depth of a wound or trace the path of a fistula. Probes and dilation instruments used as tunneling devices can make a passage under the skin for a vascular graft or shunt.

• **Fig. 19.40** **A,** Uterine sound. **B,** Hegar uterine dilators.

• **Fig. 19.41** Calipers.

Measuring Instruments

Rulers, depth gauges, templates, and trial sizers are used to measure parts of the patient's body (Fig. 19.41). Some of these devices are used to determine the precise size needed for an implant, such as a joint or breast prosthesis.

Accessory Instruments

Many accessories are used in addition to the basic instruments previously discussed. For example, a mallet may be needed to drive a cutting instrument into bone (Fig. 19.42).

Screwdrivers are used to affix screws into bone. Each surgical specialty has its own accessories, many of which are described in the specialty chapters. One example is the Hudson brace that is used to manually drill through the cranium (Fig. 19.43).

Of the thousands of instruments available, surgeons choose those that are most suitable to meet their needs. Differences in the size, curvature, or angulation of jaws or blades; in the length of handles; and in the weight and shape of the instruments can simplify, improve, and even shorten surgical time, which

• **Fig. 19.42** Mallet.

• **Fig. 19.43** Hudson brace for manual drilling into skull.

ultimately benefits the patient. Instruments should be maintained to provide the specific function each has been designed to do.

Microinstrumentation

Improved outcomes of surgical intervention using microsurgical techniques are, to a great extent, the result of the miniaturized precision instrumentation developed in association with the performance of these delicate procedures. The instruments are extremely fine, delicate, and miniature enough to handle in very small working areas, such as the eye, spine, brain, or other body parts requiring microsurgery. Manipulation becomes more difficult with increased size or bulk and weight.

As with techniques, instruments are constantly being improved. Surgeons work with manufacturers to develop appropriate instruments, suture materials, and needles. Many surgeons purchase the instruments of their choice. Whether owned by the surgeon or the facility, microinstruments require exacting care to maintain desired function.

Instruments are designed to conform to hand movements under the microscope. They must permit secure grasp, ease of holding and manipulation, and fulfillment of their intended purpose. They are shaped to not obscure the limited field of view. Although these factors are important criteria for any instrument, they are especially vital for microinstruments. Everyone assisting in or setting up for microsurgical procedures must know the identification and functions of these unique instruments. Design is coincident to function.

Material and Surface

Microinstruments are made of stainless steel or titanium. Titanium alloy is considerably stronger yet lighter weight than stainless steel. Some microinstruments are malleable for desired angling. Some are disposable. All are extremely vulnerable to abuse.

Finishes of at least the portions of instruments exposed to light in the surgical field are deliberately dulled during manufacture to reduce glare under the microscope, which is both annoying and tiring to the surgeon. Titanium microinstruments have a dull blue finish.

Shape and Tips

Microinstruments are shorter than standard instruments and often are angulated for convenience of approach and avoidance of obstruction of the surgical field.

Instrument tips have minimal separation, which is compatible with their function. Finger pressure and movement necessary to close wide tips are undesirable because they may induce tremor.

Handles

Handles are designed for a secure and comfortable grasp, with a diameter comparable to that of a pen or pencil. Minimal diameter between fingers facilitates feel and accuracy of manipulation. Double-handled instruments (scissors, needle holders) have a slightly larger diameter than single-handled ones (razor knife). The shape of the handle is also important for manipulation. For example, instruments that are rotated between fingers when in use, such as forceps, must be turned easily. Their handles therefore are rounded or have six sides like a pencil (Fig. 19.44). Those that are not rotated have finger grips or are flattened. Ring-handled instruments are not practical in microsurgery.

Many instruments, particularly scissors and some needle holders, have spring handles that return tips to the open position between cutting or grasping functions (Fig. 19.45). The distance

from hinge to tip will vary according to function. Proper spring tension can be easily ruined by mishandling.

Handles should be long enough for comfort in the working position but must not extend beyond the working distance to contact the unsterile objective of the microscope. The maximum length of most microinstruments is about 4 inches (100 mm). Gripping surfaces should be functionally located to prevent fingers from slipping during manipulation. These surfaces serve as a guide to accurate finger positioning. The gripping area may have a six-sided, round, knurled, or flat and serrated surface. Tactile sense is important to the procedure so the surgeon does not have to look at the instrument to use it.

Primary Uses

Appropriate instrumentation is used for specific types of procedures. Although all surgical instruments are structured for a definitive use, the function of microinstruments is even more restricted. Tissue can be severely injured by use of an improper or imperfect instrument. Instruments, too, can be damaged by use on inappropriate tissue. Primary use includes cutting (knives, scissors, saws), exposure (spatulas, retractors), gross and fine fixation (forceps, clamps), and suture and needle manipulation (needle holders). Instruments must not be used for manipulations other than the intended purpose.

Knives

Edges of razor, diamond, and dissecting knives have different degrees of sharpness and thickness of blades that are appropriate to the cutting function of each (e.g., to make penetrating or slicing incisions). A clean cut is desired to minimize trauma and tissue destruction. Disposable micro knives are preferred to get a clean sharp cut each procedure.

Scissors

Like knives, scissors are designed to make a specific type of incision related both to the plane and to thickness. Incisions are vertical, horizontal, or of a special configuration, such as curved or two-planed. Use is governed by hinging and blade relationship.

1-mm
straight

1-mm
ring tips

• **Fig. 19.44** Microsurgical forceps.

• **Fig. 19.45** Microsurgical instruments with spring handles. **A,** Scissors. **B,** Needle holder.

Scissors are hinged to cut vertically or obliquely. Cutting is usually done by the distal part of blades for better control. Some scissors come in pairs with right and left curves. Often a part number inscribed by the manufacturer on the handle will be an even number for a right-handed instrument and an odd number for a left-handed one. Blades may be sharp or blunt, long or short, and straight or angulated. Available with straight or curved blades, microsurgical scissors have a spring-type handle (Fig. 19.45, *A*).

Powered Instruments

Microsurgical air-powered drills and saws vary in sizes and shapes. They have a fingertip control; some have an optional foot control. Only the operator of the powered instrument should control a foot pedal to prevent premature activation of the device. It is unsafe to allow any powered instrument to rest on the patient's body when not in use.

Spatulas and Retractors

Spatulas and retractors are used to draw tissue back for better exposure or protection. Nerve hooks and elevators also are used for these purposes. These instruments are available in many shapes and sizes for individual tissue types and organs.

Forceps

Straight and curved forceps may be toothed or smooth. They have light spring action and minimal tip separation. Teeth of some tissue forceps may be as small as 1/250 inch (0.03 mm) in diameter. Therefore many tips are barely visible to the unaided eye. Toothed forceps are used for grasping tissue but never for grasping needles or sutures. Smooth forceps are used for tying delicate ligatures and sutures. For stability of grasp and avoidance of injury to the suture strand, the tips of the forceps should be absolutely parallel and have perfect apposition of grasping surfaces. Sutures should be grasped firmly but without trauma, often from a slippery surface. Other smooth forceps are used on friable tissues. Bipolar forceps are used for electrocoagulation.

Clamps

Mosquito hemostats and various clamps are used for vascular occlusion and for approximation of edges of tissues such as nerves and vessels. Crushing of vessels should be avoided.

Needle Holders

Microsurgical needle holders should be used to hold only minute microsurgical needles so as not to alter alignment. Handles are round to permit easy rotation between fingers. Some have spring handles. Although a lock on a needle holder may cause tips to jerk when engaged or released, some have a holding catch for use in deep wounds to prevent loss of small needles (Fig. 19.45, *B*). Needle holders held closed by finger pressure, rather than by a catch, firmly hold a needle shaft yet permit easy adjustment of the needle position. The tips can be curved or straight.

Powered Surgical Instruments

Most surgical instruments have movable parts that are manipulated by the surgeon. Some instruments are pneumatically powered by compressed air or nitrogen or are electrically powered by a battery or alternating current. Powered surgical instruments are complex assemblies of gears, rotating shafts, and seals. They require special handling during preparation and use and special considerations for cleaning and sterilizing.

Powered instruments are used primarily for precision drilling, cutting, shaping, and beveling bone. They also may be used for skin grafts and to abrade skin. Powered instruments increase speed and decrease the fatigue caused by manually driven drills, saws, and reamers. The instrument may have rotary, reciprocating, or oscillating action. Rotary movement is used to drill holes or insert screws, wires, or pins. Reciprocating movement (a cutting action from front to back) and oscillating movement (a cutting action from side to side) are used to cut or remove bone or skin. Some instruments have a combination of movements and can be changed from one to another by adjusting controls.

Depending on the function desired, the surgeon chooses a drill, burr, blade, reamer, or abrader of appropriate size. These accessories attach securely into the handpiece. Small drill bits, burrs, cutting blades, and abraders may be disposable.

The heat generated by powered instruments can damage bone cells. The site is irrigated during the use of powered equipment. Blood loss from bone is reduced by the tiny particles that these high-speed instruments pack into the cut surfaces. The speed of these instruments may disperse a fine mist of blood and bone cells. For this reason, the Occupational Safety and Health Administration (OSHA), Centers for Disease Control and Prevention (CDC), and American Academy of Orthopaedic Surgeons recommend wearing protective eyewear; a face shield or hood-type headgear should be considered if splatter is anticipated.

Unless the instrument is carefully controlled, tissue can be unintentionally caught in a rapidly spinning drill or oscillating saw, or the instrument may cut more than desired. When a powered instrument is being used, particularly one with a rotating movement, all team members must be very careful to keep their hands away from the blade. Most powered instruments have a safety mechanism on the handpiece. Some are operated by foot pedals.

Power Sources

The type of power used by an instrument determines the accessories needed to operate the instrument.

Air-Powered Instruments

Air-powered instruments are small, lightweight, free of vibration, and easy to handle for pinpoint accuracy at high speeds. Compared with electrical instruments, they cause minimal heating of bone because they operate at a faster and higher speed.

In operating air-powered instruments, medical-grade compressed air or pure (99.97%) dry nitrogen is either piped into the OR or supplied from a black cylinder tank on a stable carrier. The pressure must be set and monitored by the operating pressure gauges of the regulator. The correct pounds per square inch (psi), as determined by the manufacturer, is set after the instrument is assembled and turned on. The operating pressure is usually within a range of 70 to 160 psi, and storage pressure in the cylinder is at least 500 psi. Excessive pressure can damage the instrument and the hose that connects it to the regulator. A broken air hose under pressure can whip out of control and injure personnel or the patient.

Electrically Powered Instruments

Electrically powered instruments such as saws, drills, dermatomes, and nerve stimulators are potential explosion hazards in the OR. Most of the motors are designed to be explosion-proof. All must have spark-proof connections.

Because of the heat generated when using electrical instruments, the surgeon usually has the assistant use a bulb syringe to drip saline solution on the area to cool the bone and wash away particles. Care must be taken so the syringe does not touch the blade.

Battery Power

Some battery-operated instruments are cordless and have rechargeable batteries in the handpiece. Rechargeable batteries are placed in a battery charger, which is plugged into an electrical outlet. The batteries are charged, and some can be sterilized for use on the sterile field. Batteries that cannot be sterilized are charged and dropped into a cordless instrument by the circulating nurse using a sterile transfer device provided by the scrub person. The scrub person should not send these batteries for sterilization because they can be damaged.

Alternating Current

Power switches should be off before cords are plugged into electrical outlets. The power supply cord should be connected to the outlet before anesthetic gases are administered and should not be disconnected during anesthesia administration. The anesthesia provider should be alerted that electrical equipment will be used. The scrub person may be able to disconnect the instrument from its power source when it is not in use so a team member cannot inadvertently activate it. Many of these instruments are activated by foot pedals. The circulating nurse can move the foot pedal away from the surgeon until it is needed.

Sonic Energy

Some instruments are activated by sonic energy to move cutting edges in a linear direction. This is a power assist without the rotary motion and high speed of other electrically powered instruments.

Handling Powered Instruments

Before any new or repaired powered instrument is put into use, the biomedical technician should verify that the instrument is functioning according to the manufacturer's specifications. Powered instruments are not without some inherent dangers. Key points in handling powered instruments include the following:
1. Set the instrument and attachments alone on a small sterile table or Mayo stand with the safety switch on when they are not in use. This provides added protection from inadvertent activation.
2. Handle and store the air hose or electrical power cord with care. A broken air hose can whip out of control. A broken electrical cord can short-circuit the instrument. Always inspect the hose and cord for cracks and breaks.
3. To prevent inadvertent activation, assemble the appropriate handpiece, attachments (e.g., blades, drills, reamers), and power source with the safety mechanism in position. Always be certain that attachments are completely seated and locked in the handpiece.
4. Test whether the instrument is in working condition before the surgeon is ready to use it and before it is applied to the patient. To prevent inadvertent activation, the safety mechanism must be set in position until ready to use and when changing attachments.
5. When changing sharp attachments, a sterile towel or sponge may help remove slippery attachments and prevent puncturing gloves.

Cleaning and Sterilizing Powered Instruments

Powered instruments should always be operated, cleaned, and sterilized according to the manufacturer's directions for use and care. Each instrument has different cleaning, lubricating, packaging, and sterilizing requirements because of its various component parts. The bioburden is determined by the size, design, complexity, and condition of the instrument; the degree of contamination during use; and subsequent decontaminating and cleaning procedures. Microorganisms can become entrapped around the seals on rotating shafts. For instruments with a specific biologic challenge, manufacturers test in the area most difficult to sterilize and recommend sterilization cycles accordingly. The following general guidelines apply to the care of all powered instruments:
1. Clean and decontaminate the instrument immediately after use to maintain optimal function.
   a. During the surgical procedure, the scrub person should wipe off any organic debris between uses.
   b. The accessories are disassembled for cleaning. Do not process the powered instrument with a bit, burr, or blade in place. The metal against metal prevents sterilization of the unit. If the blade, burr, or bit needs to be changed during the procedure, the exposed unsterile surfaces will contaminate the field.
   c. The air hose and electrical cord should be wiped with detergent, a damp cloth, and a dry towel.
   d. The motor is not immersed in liquid. The power mechanism cannot be cleaned in a basin of solution or put in a washer-sterilizer, a washer-decontaminator, or an ultrasonic cleaner. The surface of the instrument is wiped with a mild detergent, and caution is used to prevent solution from entering the internal mechanism. The detergent is wiped off with a damp cloth, and the mechanism is dried with a lint-free towel.
2. Lubricate the instrument as recommended by the manufacturer.

Handling Instruments

Surgical instruments are expensive and represent a major investment. Surgical procedures have become more complicated and intricate, and as a result, instruments have become more complex, more precise in design, and more delicate in structure. Abuse, misuse, inadequate cleaning or processing, or rough handling can damage and reduce the life expectancy of even the most durable instrument, and the cost of repair or replacement becomes unnecessarily high. Instruments do deteriorate from normal use, but with proper care an instrument should have a life of 10 years or more.

Setting Up the Instrument Table

Standardized basic sets of sterile instruments are selected for each specific surgical procedure. A set is a group of instruments that may include all appropriate classifications of instruments or the instruments needed for a specific part of the procedure (e.g., a gallbladder set). The surgeon may prefer some specific instruments that are wrapped separately or added to the instrument set.

Instruments are usually prepared, wrapped, and sterilized several hours or days before the surgical procedure so they are dry and cool for safe handling. Instruments are sometimes steam-sterilized immediately before use if there is no other alternative, but this method is not recommended as a routine practice. Key elements of decontamination and processing might be skipped, leaving the instruments unready for sterilization.

The scrub person counts all instruments, sponges, and sharps with the circulating nurse. Some sets will have printed count sheets enclosed. Observe for incidental transfer of toner from the count sheet to the instruments during steam sterilization. Instruments with fused-on toner should not be used in patient care. Essential points in handling instruments before the surgical procedure include the following:

1. Handle loose instruments separately to prevent interlocking or crushing.
   a. Instruments are never piled one on top of another on an instrument table; they are laid side by side on a rolled sterile towel. Close the box locks on the instrument to avoid entanglement when placed on the Mayo stand.
   b. Microsurgical, ophthalmic, and other delicate instruments are vulnerable to damage through rough handling. Tip protectors are removed and discarded during setup.
   c. Metal-to-metal contact should be avoided or minimized. Scalpel blades should not be set in a metal basin. The edges can become dull, and small chips of metal can become dislodged and inadvertently transferred to the patient during irrigation.
2. Inspect instruments such as scissors and forceps for alignment, imperfections, cleanliness, and working condition. Unclean instruments render the entire set contaminated. Remove any malfunctioning instrument from the set. It should be labeled and sent for repair. Replace it in the set with a correctly functioning instrument before processing. If the procedure is in process, the circulating nurse can obtain a sterile replacement and tag the instrument for repair. Be sure to reconcile the count sheet.
   a. Scalpel blades should be properly set in handles using a heavy instrument, not fingers.
   b. Teeth and serrations should align exactly.
   c. Tips should be straight and in alignment.
   d. Scissors should be snug and sharp in action.
   e. Cannulas should be clear and without obstruction. Stylets should be removed.
3. Sort instruments neatly by classifications.
4. Keep ring-handled instruments together with the curvatures and angles pointed in the same direction positioned smallest to largest. Do not permit the instruments to become tangled on the towel roll.
   a. Hang ring handles over a rolled towel or over the edge of the instrument tray or container within the sterile field. Instruments hanging over the back of an instrument tray could be contaminated by someone walking past the table.
   b. Remove instrument stringers or holders if used to keep box locks open during processing.
   c. Close box locks on the first ratchet as the setup progresses.
5. Leave retractors and other heavy instruments in a tray or container, or lay them out on a flat surface of the table. Do not permit any instrument to hang over the edge of the sterile field. Everything on the field should be within 1 inch of the edge and not extend beyond the sterile field.
6. Protect sharp blades, edges, and tips. They should not touch anything. Take care not to perforate the sterile table cover.

Place items so they do not get caught on gown sleeves and fall off the table.
   a. Sets of instruments, such as osteotomes or microsurgical instruments, may be in sterilization racks so that the blades and tips are suspended. These instruments can remain in racks during the initial table setup and until they are needed during the surgical procedure.
   b. Tip-protecting covers or instrument-protecting plastic sleeves should be removed and discarded before the instruments are used on the patient. Most covers and sleeves are not radiopaque and could become a retained foreign body.
   c. If they are not in a rack, handles should be supported on a rolled towel or gauze sponge. This keeps the blades and tips of microinstruments suspended in midair for easy visualization.

Handling Instruments During the Surgical Procedure

Efficient instrument handling throughout the surgical procedure is the hallmark of an efficient scrub person. Key points in handling instruments during the surgical procedure include the following:

1. Know the name and appropriate use of each instrument. Using fine instruments for heavy tissue damages the instrument.
2. Handle instruments individually. Tangled instruments are hard to separate in an emergency. Instruments on the Mayo stand should be closed to minimize fumbling for the correct item.
   a. If several instruments of the same type will be needed in rapid succession (e.g., hemostats to clamp subcutaneous vessels), three or four may be picked up at one time, but they are closed and passed individually to the surgeon and/or first assistant.
   b. Instruments with sharp edges and fine tips are more susceptible to damage than are standard instruments. The edges are easily dulled, and the tips are easily bent or broken. Extreme caution is necessary to prevent catching the tips of microinstruments on any object that could bend them.
3. Hand the surgeon or assistant the correct instrument for each particular task. Remember the following principle: Use for the intended purpose only.
   a. Avoid placing fingers in the instrument rings as the instrument is passed. The instrument may inadvertently drop or snag on drapes, causing an untoward injury to the patient or a team member. The instrument may fall to the floor, thus becoming damaged and contaminated.
   b. Many surgeons use hand signals to indicate the type of instrument needed. An understanding of what is taking place at the surgical site makes these signals meaningful.
   c. Select instruments appropriate to the location of the surgical site; short instruments are used for superficial work, and long ones are used for work deep in a body cavity. Experience will facilitate instrument selection according to the surgeon's preference and need.
   d. Many instruments are used in pairs or in sequence. When the surgeon clamps and/or cuts tissue, they will usually request suture. To use suture, the surgeon will need to grasp the tissue with a pick-up for stabilization. After using suture, the surgeon or assistant will need scissors to cut or a hemostat to hold the end of the strand as a tag.

e. Hand instruments around the incisional area, not directly over it, to prevent possible injury.

f. Knowledge of anatomy is useful for determining which instrument is needed.

4. Pass instruments decisively and firmly. When the surgeon extends their hand, the instrument should be placed firmly into their palm in the proper position for use. In general, when passing a curved instrument, the curve of the instrument aligns with the direction of the curve of the surgeon's hand. The following points should be remembered when passing an instrument to the surgeon:

a. If the surgeon is on the opposite side of the OR bed, pass across right hand to right hand (or with the left hand to a left-handed surgeon). The curve of the instrument should match the curve of the surgeon's hand.

b. If the surgeon or assistant is on the same side of the OR bed and to the right, pass with your left hand; if the surgeon or assistant is to your left, pass with your right hand.

c. Ring-handled instruments are held near the box lock by the scrub person and passed by rotating the wrist clockwise to place the handle directly into the surgeon's waiting hand (Fig. 19.46).

d. Clip appliers are held between the fingers by the hinged joint during loading and passing. Placing fingers in the rings may cause the clip to be discharged unintentionally. The loaded applier is passed so the rings automatically pass over the surgeon's finger in a position of function for rapid use.

e. Sharp and delicate instruments may be placed on a flat surface for the surgeon to pick up (e.g., "no touch zone"). This technique avoids potential contact with items such as cutting blades, sharp points, and needles in hand-to-hand transfer. Always protect the hands when manipulating sharp instruments. Some surgeons prefer to have all instruments passed directly, so great care is taken to place the instrument in the waiting hand without causing the surgeon to look up away from the field. This is common in microsurgery.

5. Watch the sterile field for loose instruments. After use, wipe the blood from the surface and place them promptly on the Mayo stand or instrument table in a position of function. The weight of instruments can injure the patient or cause postoperative discomfort. Keeping instruments off the field also decreases the possibility of their falling to the floor.

6. With a moist sponge, wipe blood and organic debris from instruments promptly after each use. This is referred to as point-of-use cleaning.

• **Fig. 19.46** Passing an instrument. Tip is visible; hand is free. Handle is placed directly into waiting hand. Avoid placing fingers in the rings as the instrument is passed.

a. Demineralized, sterile distilled water should be used to wipe instruments. Saline, blood, and other solutions can damage surfaces, causing corrosion and, ultimately, pitting.

b. Blood and debris that are allowed to dry on surfaces, in box locks, and in crevices increase the bioburden that could be carried into the surgical site. Dried material is harder to remove during processing.

c. A nonfibrous sponge should be used to wipe off microsurgical, ophthalmic, and other delicate tips. This type of sponge prevents the snagging and breaking of delicate tips, and the potential for lint is decreased. Commercial microsurgical instrument wipes are available.

7. Flush the suction tip and tubing with sterile distilled water periodically to keep the lumens patent. Use only a few milliliters of solution if using irrigating fluids from the surgical field. Keep a tally of the amount used to clear the suction line, and deduct this amount from the total used to irrigate the surgical site. Accurate accounting of the solutions used for patient irrigation is necessary when determining the amount of blood lost during the surgical procedure.

8. Remove debris from electrosurgical unit (ESU) tips to ensure electrical contact. Disposable abrasive tip cleaners are helpful for maintaining the conductivity and effectiveness of the surface of the tip. Do not use an abrasive tip cleaner on Teflon-coated ESU tips. Avoid using a scalpel blade to clean electrosurgical tips because the debris may become airborne and contaminate the surgical field.

9. Place used instruments that will not be needed again (except sharp, cutting, delicate, or powered instruments) back in their original position and into a tray or basin at the end of the surgical procedure. Instruments should be organized for easy counting.

a. Blood and gross debris are removed at the point of use before cleaning and decontamination in the processing area.

b. Carelessly dropping, tossing, or throwing instruments into a basin causes damage.

c. Instruments that have been wiped can be immersed in a basin of sterile demineralized distilled water, not saline solution. The sodium chloride in saline solution and in blood is corrosive and can damage instrument surfaces. Bloody instruments should not soak in a basin of solution for a prolonged period.

d. Heavy instruments such as retractors should not be placed on top of tissue and hemostatic forceps and other clamps. Place them in a separate tray.

e. Reusable sharps should be kept separate from other instruments of the same or similar size to prevent injury to instrument processing personnel.

f. Keep instruments accessible for final counts.

Dismantling the Instrument Table

The scrub person breaks down the instrument table at the end of the surgical procedure while wearing the gown and full personal protective equipment (PPE). This process may be delayed and the scrub person and instrument table maintained as sterile for a short time if the patient is in critical condition. The breakdown should not be started until a critical patient is out of the OR and admitted to the postanesthesia care unit (PACU). Some examples of when to wait before breakdown include cardiac, vascular, some neurologic, multiple trauma, or other procedures or patient condition that could precipitate expedient return to the OR for immediate surgical reopening.

When the scrub person is assured that the patient will not return to the OR, the table breakdown can begin. Whether used or unused, all instruments on the instrument table are considered contaminated and must be promptly and properly decontaminated/cleaned, inspected, terminally sterilized, and prepared for subsequent use. Wearing gloves, a gown, a mask, and protective eyewear, the scrub person prepares instruments for the cleaning process. Instruments are cleaned in a designated instrument processing area, not in the OR. Key points in handling instruments when dismantling the instrument table include the following[5]:

1. Check drapes, towels, and table covers to be sure that instruments do not go to the laundry or into the trash. A final quick count is a safeguard.
2. Collect instruments from the Mayo stand and any other small tables, and collect those that may have been dropped or passed off the sterile field.
3. Separate delicate, small instruments and those with sharp or semisharp edges for special handling.
4. Disassemble all instruments with removable parts to expose all surfaces for cleaning.
5. Open all hinged instruments to expose box locks and serrations.
6. Separate instruments of dissimilar metals. Instruments of each type of metal should be cleaned separately to prevent electrolytic deposition of other metals.
7. Flush cold, distilled water through hollow instruments or channels, such as suction tips or endoscopes, to prevent organic debris from drying.
8. Rinse off blood and debris with demineralized distilled water or an enzymatic detergent solution or foam.

Small facilities have the same methods to process, decontaminate, and sterilize instruments. Follow the manufacturer's recommended procedures for preparing each instrument for decontamination or terminal sterilization. Procedures vary depending on the type of instrument and its components and on the equipment available and its location.

Key points for preparing for sterilization:

1. Some air-powered instruments can be lubricated with a sterile lubricant after sterilization and immediately before use.
2. Some manufacturers supply lubricant (usually a silicone-based oil).
3. Some instruments must be run after lubrication to disperse the lubricant through the mechanism.
4. Wrap the instrument for sterilization.
5. Most manufacturers supply sterilizing cases for powered equipment. These cases can be wrapped in woven or nonwoven material.
6. The instrument must be disassembled.
7. The sharp edges of accessories must be protected.
8. Hoses or cords should be loosely coiled.
9. Sterilize the instrument in steam unless contraindicated by the manufacturer.
   a. A prevacuum sterilizer removes entrapped air and allows steam to access the internal mechanism; this type of sterilizer is therefore preferred to a gravity displacement sterilizer.
   b. Exposure time depends on the type of sterilizer, the design and complexity of the instrument, and packaging. In a gravity displacement sterilizer at 250° F (121° C), exposure time may be as long as 1 hour.
   c. Sterilization of an unwrapped instrument in a gravity displacement sterilizer at 270° F (132° C) must provide exposure that is long enough to sterilize the internal mechanism (usually at least 15 minutes).
   d. Ethylene oxide gas sterilization should be used only if the instrument cannot withstand the heat or moisture of steam sterilization. The instrument must be free of all traces of lubricant. The manufacturer should specify the aeration time.

EVOLVE WEBSITE

http://evolve.elsevier.com/Hornacky/BerryKohn/

- Historical Perspective
- Student Interactive Questions
- Glossary

References

1. Kabra A, Mehta N, Garg B: 3D printing in spine care: a review of current practices, *J Clin Orthop Trauma* 35:102044, 2022.
2. Mezher M: *FDA reclassifies surgical staplers, staples after review links devices to injuries and deaths.* www.raps.org. Accessed May 4, 2023.
3. Zivanovic O, Sonoda Y: Small bowel and large bowel resection and anastomosis. In Ramirez P, Frumovitz M, Abu-Rustum N, editors: *Principals of gynecologic oncology surgery*, Philadelphia, 2019, Elsevier, pp 227–244.
4. Kohl D, Baillie J: How endoscopes work. In Chandrasekhara V, Elmunzer B, Kashab M, Muthusamy VR, editors: *Clinical gastrointestinal endoscopy*, ed 3, Philadelphia, 2019, Elsevier, pp 24–31.
5. AORN guideline quick view: instrument cleaning, *AORN J* 108(1):106–109, 2018.

Bibliography

AORN: *Guidelines for perioperative practice*, Denver, CO, 2024, The Association.
Phillips NM: *Surgical instrumentation*, ed 3, Boston, 2024, Cengage.

20

Specialized Surgical Equipment

CHAPTER OUTLINE

Using Specialized Equipment in Surgery, 361

Electrosurgery, 361

Laser Surgery, 365

Microsurgery, 372

Ultrasonosurgery, 377

Integrated Technologies, 377

CHAPTER OBJECTIVES

After studying this chapter, the learner will be able to:

- Distinguish between monopolar and bipolar electrosurgical units and applications.
- List the basic elements of electrosurgical safety.
- Identify three basic types of lasers.

- Describe the tissue effects of the different types of laser light in vivo.
- Identify potential safety hazards associated with high technology in patient care.

KEY TERMS AND DEFINITIONS

Active electrode Apparatus used to deliver electric current to the surgical site.

Beam splitter Attachment to the microscope that splits light; one part is reflected laterally, and the other part is relayed upward to the binocular tube; the percentage can be 50/50 or 30/70. The greater portion may be directed to a camera or video system.

Binocular Using two eyes to see in stereoscopic vision.

Bipolar electrosurgery Current is delivered to the surgical site and returned to the generator by forceps. One side of the forceps is active; the other side is inactive. The current passes only between the tips of the forceps.

Blended current Current that divides tissue and controls some bleeding.

Coaxial illumination The light path follows the same direction as the visual image.

Coagulating current Current that passes intense heat through the active electrode used to sear vessels and control bleeding.

Contraves stand Series of weights used to balance some microscopes.

Current Flow of electrical energy.

Cutting current Current that arcs between tissue and the active electrode to divide tissue without coagulation.

Depth of field Distance of focus.

Diopter Power of the lens to assist vision by refractive correction of reflected light.

Electrosurgical unit (ESU) Generator, foot pedal, cords, active electrode, and inactive dispersive return electrode designed to safely deliver electric current through tissue.

Emissions Surgical lasers emit nonionizing radiation, heat, and debris.

Focal length Distance between the lens and the object in focus.

Generator Machine that produces electric current by generating high-frequency radio waves.

Ground Conducting connection among the generator, the patient, and the earth.

Inactive dispersive return electrode Apparatus used to return current from the patient back to the generator; also referred to as inactive electrode, return electrode, or patient plate.

Laser Acronym for *l*ight *a*mplification by *s*timulated *e*mission of *r*adiation. Light, concentrated and focused, stimulates atoms to emit radiant energy when activated.

Laser beam Light beams, either pulsed or continuous, go through a medium to produce a lasing effect. The beam has three distinct characteristics: coherent, collimated, and monochromatic. Coherent light beams are sustained over space and time because electromagnetic waves are in the same frequency and energy phase with each other. Collimated light beams are parallel. Monochromatic refers to a light beam being one color because waves are all the same length in the electromagnetic spectrum.

Laser plume Carbonized cell fragments, toxic hydrocarbons, viruses, and noxious fumes can be dispersed from tissues exposed to the laser beam. Vaporization converts solid tissue to smoke and gas. This plume (smoke) is evacuated to maintain visibility and also to minimize the hazard of inhalation by personnel.

Medium Gases, synthetic crystals, glass rods, liquid dyes, free electrons, and semiconductors are used to produce the lasing effect.

Microscope Equipment that uses a series of lenses to magnify very small objects.

Monocular Using one eye for vision. Depth of field is absent; the image is two-dimensional.

Monopolar electrosurgery Current flows from the generator to the active electrode, through the patient to the inactive dispersive return electrode, and returns to the generator.

Objective Power of the lens that determines the focal distance of vision.

Ocular Eyepiece lens that multiplies the basic magnification of the microscope.

Power All lasers have a combination of duration, intensity, and output of radiation when wavelengths are activated.

Pupillary distance Measurement between the pupils of the eyes; used to position the binocular eyepieces.

Source Power to energize the light beam; this may be electrical, radiofrequency, or optical.

Stereopsis Vision with two eyes that enables objects to appear three-dimensional.

Wavelength Electromagnetic waves transfer energy progressively from point to point through a medium. The wavelength is the distance traveled along the electromagnetic spectrum. Radiation penetration differs at different wavelengths. Each laser has a different wavelength and color, depending on the medium the light beam passes through.

Working distance Physical space between the objective lens of the microscope and the surgical field.

Zoom To change the range of focus in continuous magnification; the change can be closer or more distant.

Using Specialized Equipment in Surgery

Advances in technology have made possible the complex surgical techniques of the present. Technology may be defined as the branch of knowledge that deals with the creation and use of technical means for scientific purposes. In the context of surgery, *technology* refers to a system that uses devices as well as people to perform specific tasks. Continuing research will further enhance technology. New devices are usually adjuncts to or extensions of devices or techniques already in use. To enhance the use of new devices in patient care, perioperative team members constantly need to learn about new equipment and its applications.

The focus of technology used in patient care is improvement of care beyond human capability. Users of multiple technologic devices in the operating room (OR) need to be acutely aware of safety.[1] One aspect of safety in this environment is paying attention to the patient as a physical being as well as to the devices used in care. Equipment used in concert with patient care includes, but is not limited to, the following:
- Anesthesia machine
- Defibrillators
- Monitors
- Sterilizing machinery
- Warming and cooling devices
- Surgical headlights
- Pressurized fluid delivery systems

Before handling new equipment, patient care personnel on the perioperative team should be knowledgeable about its care and use. Some surgical procedures use more than one of these technologies (e.g., laser surgery through an attachment to the operating microscope).

Preparing and handling these expensive pieces of equipment are major responsibilities of perioperative nurses and surgical technologists. In addition, all OR personnel should be aware of and safeguard against hazards associated with equipment.[1] The perioperative environment should be safe for patients and personnel.

The following are safety points to consider when using equipment in the OR:
- Has the equipment been serviced on a routine schedule?
- Has the equipment had calibration testing?
- Has the equipment been cleaned or processed to the degree of safety for patient use?
- Are the cords and attachments connected properly?
- Are foot pedals in a secure position for safe use?
- Are reusable components in serviceable condition?
- Are disposable components in stock in the appropriate sizes?
- Are adjunct devices and machines in proper working order?
- Are alarms in working order?
- Are power sources available?
- Is the team knowledgeable about the correct sequence for powering up, settings, and using the equipment?
- Have policies and procedures for equipment use been developed and provided to the OR team?
- Has the OR team had formal training on the new equipment?

All equipment in the OR has an individual asset tag number. The asset number is a combination of alphanumeric figures used to identify the unit. When documenting the use of equipment in the OR, the identifying number is placed in the patient's record. Some departments log all asset tags in a master log and assign a simple unit-identifying number or letter that corresponds to the equipment in use. This simplifies documentation.

If any equipment is not in good working order, it must be taken out of service immediately and tagged for repair. It should not be put back into service until the biomedical engineering department clears it for use. Some manufacturers will provide loaners when equipment is out for repair. All loaner equipment must be checked by the biomedical engineering department before use in the OR. Information on the service tag of malfunctioning equipment should include the following:
- Name of person reporting
- Date of report
- Description of the problem
- Any other information that may be pertinent

Electrosurgery

Principles of Electrosurgery

Electrosurgery is used to a greater or lesser extent in all surgical specialties. Personnel should be familiar with the manufacturer's detailed manual of operating instructions for each type used.

Electric current can be used to cut or coagulate most tissues. Attempts to coagulate large vessels can result in an extensive burn and necrosis. Excess charring and devitalized tissue create a barrier for wound healing and may provide a medium for infection.

The initial incision is made by a scalpel. The electrosurgical unit (ESU) is not used to incise the skin. Electrosurgery can be used on fat, fascia, muscle, internal organs, and vessels. ESUs operate at frequencies between 100,000 Hz and 10,000,000 Hz. This current can be passed through tissue without causing stimulation of muscles or nerves.

New smart generator technology has been introduced into the market. The technology uses high radiofrequencies to produce heat for accurate results. The system uses software to analyze and recognize all types of tissue. The system automatically adjusts for constant power at lower levels. It can be used for monopolar, bipolar, argon coagulator, and smoke evacuation systems. This technology is also available for other coagulation devices.

Electrosurgery differs from electrocautery. Electrocautery is the use of a unidirectional current generated by a self-contained battery-operated disposable instrument with a wire at the tip. The wire heats when activated and coagulates the tissue. The energy does not enter the patient's body. The ESU uses an alternating current that passes through the patient's tissues and returns to the generator. Two forms of ESU generators are commonly used in surgery: monopolar and bipolar. Each type has specific uses and considerations.

Monopolar Electrosurgery

With monopolar ESUs the electric current flows from the generator to the active electrode, through the patient to a return electrode, and returns to the generator (Fig. 20.1). The generator returns the current to ground. Any break in the current flow from the generator and back again causes the machine to shut down and sound an alarm as a safety feature.

The surgeon selects the type of current and power setting. The circulating nurse verbally confirms and documents the power settings before the generator is activated. It is seldom necessary to use full-power settings. A safe general rule is to start with the lowest setting of current that accomplishes the desired effect, and then increase the current at the surgeon's request.

ESU Generator

The generator produces the electrical current in three forms. The generator is mounted on a portable rolling stand. Nothing should be set on the machine. Each machine has an asset number that should be recorded in the patient's records. The machine can be set to one or a combination of the three currents[2]:

1. *Coagulating current:* Intense heat is produced to seal small to moderate vessels on contact. The current is continuous but diminishes for short gaps of time.
2. *Cutting current:* The current is a constant flow of high energy output without gaps of time. The continuous flow of current causes the tissues to separate before high levels of heat build up.
3. *Blended current:* Both coagulating and cutting currents are produced at the same time in modified cycles. Small vessels are sealed as the tissue divides. Settings can be selected that have varied degrees of coagulation and cutting.

Active Electrode

The sterile active electrode directs flow of current to the surgical site. The style of the electrode tip (e.g., blade, loop, ball, or needle) will be determined by the type of surgical procedure and current to be used. It is attached to a conductor cord, which is connected to the generator. The active electrode tip may be in a pencil-shaped handpiece operated by a rocker switch, or it may be incorporated into a tissue forceps or suction tip operated by a foot pedal. Only the user of the active electrode should activate the current with the pedal to prevent accidental discharge of electricity into the field.

The end of the cord for the active electrode is passed off the field by the scrub person and attached to the generator by the circulating nurse. The sterile part of the cord should not be secured to the field by a metal instrument because cracks in the cord could permit conduction of electrical energy sufficient to cause a fire or severe burns. When not in use, the handpiece and active tip should be kept clean and housed in a holder designed for this purpose. Standard active electrodes are cleaned with an abrasive tip polisher. Teflon-coated tips are wiped clean with a dampened sponge. A crusty tip prevents the current from effectively passing into tissues. Do not scrape off the char with a scalpel. This causes debris to be discharged into the room atmosphere.

When in use, the generator emits a buzzing sound as the handpiece is activated. There are two pitches to the sound. One sound signifies the use of the coagulating current, and the other sound indicates activation of the cutting current. The alarm system has a volume control. It should never be set to "off."

The surgeon places the active electrode tip on the tissue and then activates the foot switch or hand control to transfer electric current from the generator to the tissue. Some hand switches are color-coded to identify coagulating and cutting functions. Rather than placing the tip directly on tissue, bleeding vessels may be clamped with a hemostat or smooth-tipped tissue forceps. As little extraneous tissue as possible should be clamped to minimize damage to adjacent tissue. Vessels are coagulated when any part of the metal instrument is touched with the active electrode; this is frequently referred to as *buzzing*.

To avoid arcing, the active electrode should be in contact with the instrument before electric current is applied. The person holding it should have a firm grip on as large an area of instrument as possible and avoid touching the patient. The active current should not be applied for more than 3 seconds. Inadvertent patient injury can occur if the metal instrument is in contact with retractors or other instrumentation placed in the surgical field. Low-voltage cutting current should be used. Current can burn through surgical gloves if these precautions are not taken.

The active electrode handpiece and cord are disposable. Reusable active monopolar forceps and cords should be inspected for damage before reprocessing and before use at the sterile field.

• **Fig. 20.1** Monopolar current path.

Patient Return Electrode (Inactive Dispersive Electrode)

When using monopolar electrosurgery, the current is returned to the generator through an inactive return electrode attached to the patient. The active tip sends the current through the patient's tissues. The current returns to the generator through the inactive return electrode attached to the patient.

The current's path from the generator to the patient and from the patient to the return electrode and back to the generator completes a circuit. If the circuit is broken, the current will find an alternative route back to ground, such as through metal in contact with a body. An isolated generator offers the advantage of a non–ground-seeking circuit. The flow of current is isolated and restricted to active and dispersive return electrodes, and the current returns directly back to the generator. With an isolated generator, if the circuit is broken, the generator shuts down.

One form of a patient return electrode adhesive pad is placed in direct contact with skin (Fig. 20.2). The contact area must exceed 100 mm^2 and have a diameter greater than 1.2 cm. The adhesive return electrodes are flexible to mold to the appropriate body surface.

MEGADYNE manufactures a reusable capacitive return electrode that does not adhere to the patient's body.[3] This large gel pad is placed underneath the patient on the OR bed. The patient makes contact with the pad over most of the contact surface through the bed sheet. The pad comes in adult and pediatric sizes. This style of return electrode is useful when there is not a suitable site for a disposable return electrode, such as on a burn patient. A positioning chart is available from the manufacturer. The pad is compatible with most electrosurgical generators, radiolucent, and can be reused up to 2 years. The cord attaches to the generator in the patient return electrode socket.

Electrosurgery causes more patient injuries than any other electrical device used in the OR. Most incidents are caused by user error. When a return electrode is used, the following safeguards must be followed[4]:

1. The return electrode should be as close as possible to the site where the active electrode will be used to minimize current through the body.
2. The patient should be in the desired position before the adhesive return electrode is applied to prevent it from becoming dislodged or buckled during patient positioning. Do not remove or reposition the disposable return electrode because the integrity of the adhesive will be altered. A new electrode is used each time.
3. The return electrode should never be cut to fit.
4. The return electrode should cover as large an area of the patient's skin as possible in an area free of hair or scar tissue, both of which tend to act as insulation. An area may need to be dry shaved. The surface area affects heat buildup and dissipation.

• **Fig. 20.2** Placement of ESU patient return electrode.

Avoid areas where bony prominences might result in pressure points, which in turn can cause current concentration. Place the pad on a clean, dry skin surface over or under as large a muscle mass area as possible. The gel conduction material on the pad is cold and sticky to the touch; a patient who is awake should be forewarned of its application.

5. Any area that overlies an implant is a former surgical site and is not suitable for placement of a return electrode. The surgical scar tissue will not disperse the current. The return electrode should not be placed on skin over a metal implant, such as a hip prosthesis, because current could be diverted to the implant and generate excessive heat.
6. The integrity of the package of a disposable return electrode should be inspected before use. Do not use the electrode if the package is damaged or has been previously opened.
7. Special care should be taken to ensure that the cord does not become dislodged. Do not put a safety belt over the electrode or cord. The connector should not create a pressure point on the patient's skin.
8. The connection between the return electrode and generator should be secure and made with compatible attachments. If the return circuit is faulty, the ground circuit may be completed through inadvertent contact with the metal OR bed or its attachments. This is referred to as an *alternative pathway* for the current.

If the return pad surface area is too small, current passing through an exposed area of skin in contact with metal will create intense heat. For example, one such contact point could be the thigh touching a leg stirrup while the patient is in the lithotomy position. A serious full-thickness burn can occur.

The circulating nurse should record on the patient's chart the type and/or location of the dispersive return electrode, the condition of the patient's skin before and after electrosurgery, the generator identification number, and the settings used. Some institutions also require documentation of the dispersive return electrode lot number.

Argon Beam Coagulator

Argon gas can be incorporated into a monopolar ESU to create a path between the tissue and the active electrode handpiece. The gas is inert and noncombustible and is easily ionized by the electrical current. Argon is heavier than air and creates less plume. The argon-enhanced ESU tip is held at a 60-degree angle and does not contact the tissue during coagulation, thereby causing less tissue damage. The depth of penetration is less than with other forms of monopolar energy.

The active ESU tip and gas stream are passed over tissue to evenly coagulate larger areas. The gas displaces the bleeding over the surface of the target organ. The argon beam coagulator is used for cases that may encounter excessive bleeding. Care is taken not to cause the gas to enter large open vessels because of the risk for gas embolism. Argon-enhanced electrosurgery is a form of monopolar ESU and requires the use of a patient return electrode.

Argon-enhanced electrosurgery is used with caution during laparoscopy. The argon gas adds to the cumulative effect of pneumoperitoneum and overpressurization. Argon is less soluble in blood than CO_2 and could persist long enough to pass to the heart in the form of a gas embolus. One port should be available for venting gases between extended uses of the argon to prevent buildup of the gas.

• **Fig. 20.3** Bipolar current path. No patient return electrode is used.

Bipolar Electrosurgery

With bipolar electrosurgery the current is directed from the generator to a special forceps with one active tip and one inactive tip. The current flows from the generator to the active tip and returns to the generator through the inactive tip (Fig. 20.3). The energy does not flow through the patient's body as in monopolar electrosurgery. No return electrode is used. Output voltage is relatively low. This provides extremely precise control of the coagulated area.

Bipolar electrosurgery is safe to use in cases in which electrical current passing through the body could cause disruption in implantable devices such as pacemakers or internal defibrillators. Because the current does not pass beyond the tines of the forceps, the function of peripheral devices remains uninterrupted.

Other bipolar energized devices include the *LigaSure* instrument designed to permanently divide and fuse vessels and tissue of up to 7 mm. The grasper tip dissects and holds securely. The generator has an activation sound when operating and an alarm if the device is not working properly. Each application should last no longer than 1 minute for the best tissue effects.

Coblation

Coblators use high-frequency bipolar energy in a conductive medium to create a highly focused plasma field. The energy is passed through a flow of saline irrigation to cause a field of highly charged electrons to break the molecular bonds of the target tissue while preserving the integrity of surrounding healthy tissue. The saline is conductive, causing a vaporized plasma field the thickness of a sheet of paper. The temperature does not need to reach extremes of thermal effect as with other coagulation devices to separate the tissues. The average temperature is only 68° F to 158° F (20–70° C).

The tip of the wand instrument is 1 to 2.5 mm wide and has two tiny electrodes through which the saline is passed over the target area. Coblation was originally designed for use in arthroscopy but later found favor with otorhinolaryngologists for nasal and tonsil procedures. In oral and nasal tissue procedures the greatest limitation is in sinus procedures, in which a bony obstruction may be encountered. Plastic surgeons have been working with coblation as a tool for skin resurfacing for deep acne scars and facial wrinkles. Coblation offers an alternative to chemical peels and laser surface modifications.

Generalized Safety Factors for the Use of Electrosurgery

Electrical burn through the patient's skin is the greatest hazard of electrosurgery. These burns are usually deeper than flame burns,

causing widespread tissue necrosis and deep thrombosis to the extent that debridement and grafting may be required. Not all deep thermal injury is immediately apparent.

In addition to the precautions noted for preparing the ESU and for positioning the dispersive return electrode used with monopolar units, other precautions should be taken as follows:

1. Electrosurgery (monopolar and bipolar) should not be used in the mouth, trachea, around the head, or in the pleural cavity when high concentrations of oxygen or nitrous oxide are used. During some procedures, such as eye surgery, oxygen is administered via nasal cannula or mask. Oxygen builds up under the drapes and sets the stage for a combustible situation. Flame-retardant drapes can conceal a fire in a confined space. The anesthesia provider is advised to administer medical air instead of oxygen to minimize the risk for fire. Safety regulations for use with all inhalation anesthetic agents are followed.

2. Electrocardiogram electrodes should be placed as far away from the surgical site as possible. Burns can occur at the site of electrocardiogram electrodes and other low-impedance points from invasive monitor probes if the current diverts to an alternative path of least resistance. Metallic electromyographic or neurologic monitoring needles should not be used.

3. Rings and other jewelry should be removed. Metallic jewelry, including those used in body piercings, presents a potential risk for burn in the patient from diverted currents from the monopolar unit with either an isolated or ground-referenced output.

4. Flammable agents containing alcohol should be used with great care in skin preparation. If they are used, the skin surface should be completely dry before draping. Volatile fumes and vapors may collect in drapes and ignite when the electrosurgical or cautery unit is used.

5. If another piece of electrical equipment is used in direct contact with the patient at the same time as the ESU, connect it to a different source of current if possible. The cutting current of the ESU may not work if another piece of electrical equipment is on the same circuit. The ESU may interfere with the operation of some equipment, such as older models of cardiac monitors. The isolated power system of solid-state generators may prevent these problems.

6. New models of cardiac pacemakers are unaffected by monopolar ESU generators. Other implanted electrical devices such as defibrillators could malfunction. Check with the device manufacturer regarding compatibility.

The bipolar ESU may be used because the current does not pass through the patient's body and return to the generator. The patient is continuously monitored. A defibrillator should be on standby in the OR.

7. Connection of a bipolar active electrode to a monopolar receptacle may activate current, causing a short circuit. Plugs on cords should be differentiated to prevent misconnections of active and inactive electrodes.

8. Secure the active electrode handle in an insulated holster/container when not in use. Do not immerse an active electrode in liquid.

9. To prevent fire, only moist sponges should be permitted on the sterile field while the ESU is in use. This includes using moist sponges during the use of battery-operated electrocautery. Dry sponges can ignite.

10. Investigate a repeated request by the surgeon for more current. The dispersive return electrode or connecting cord may be at fault and should be checked first, followed by the handpiece connection. Shock to those touching the patient may result. The patient may be burned at the dispersive return electrode site.

11. For safety of the patient and personnel, follow instructions for use and care; these appear on the machine or in the manual provided by the manufacturer that accompanies each ESU. Grasp and pull only the plugs, not cords, when disconnecting attachments from the generator or the power source. Position the power cord away from the team to avoid tripping team members. Avoid rolling equipment over the power cord. Disposable cords should not be cut with scissors.

12. Any malfunctioning ESU should be labeled with the problem and taken out of service until cleared for use by biomedical engineering department personnel.

13. The patient and personnel should be protected from inhaling plume (smoke) generated during electrosurgery. A suction evacuator device should be placed as close to the source of plume as possible to maximize evacuation of smoke and enhance visibility at the surgical site.

14. Electrosurgery devices are available with combined suction systems for removal of surgical plume and fluid.

15. Inspect insulated instruments for breaks in the insulation covering. Current can leak from fractures in the insulation and create a thermal burn.

Laser Surgery

The term laser is an acronym for *l*ight *a*mplification by *s*timulated *e*mission of *r*adiation.

Physical Properties of Lasers

The laser focuses light on atoms to stimulate them to a high point of excitation. The resulting radiation is then amplified and metamorphosed into the wavelengths of laser light. This light beam is monochromatic (one color) because all the electromagnetic waves are the same length and collimated or parallel to each other. The light is totally concentrated and easily focused. Unlike conventional light waves, which spread and dissipate electromagnetic radiation by many different wavelengths, the coherence of the laser beam is sustained over space and time with wavelengths in the same frequency and energy phase.

Lasers may produce energy in brief, repeating emissions that have a duration of only an extremely small fraction of a second; these are pulsed laser systems. Or they can produce continuous light beams; these are continuous-wave lasers. All lasers have a combination of duration, level, and output wavelengths of radiation emitted when activated. Power density, the irradiance, is the amount of power per unit surface area during a single pulse or exposure. This is expressed as watts per centimeter squared. Regardless of beam characteristics, components of a laser system are the same (Fig. 20.4). These components include the following:

- An active medium to produce a lasing effect of the stimulated emission. Gases, solids or crystals, liquid dyes, and free electrons are used. Each produces a different wavelength, color, and effect.
- An excitation power source to create population inversion by pumping energy into the active medium. This may be electrical

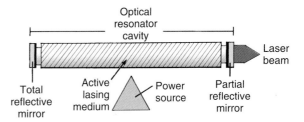

• **Fig. 20.4** Basic laser components.

or radiofrequency power or an optical power source such as a xenon flash lamp or another laser.

- An amplification mechanism to change random directional movement of stimulated emissions to a parallel direction. This occurs within an optical resonator or laser cavity, which is a tube with mirrors at each end. As photons traveling the length of the resonator reflect back through the medium, they stimulate more atoms to release photons, thus amplifying the lasing effect. The power density of the beam determines the laser's capacity to cut, coagulate, or vaporize tissue.
- Wave guides to aim and control the direction of the laser beam. The optical resonator has a small opening in one end that permits transmission of a small beam of laser light. The smaller the beam, the higher its power density will be. Fiberoptic wave guides or a series of rhodium reflecting mirrors then direct the beam to tissue. The wave mode may be continuous, pulsed, or a Q-switched single pulse of high energy.
- Backstops to stop the laser beam from penetrating beyond the expected impact site and affecting nontargeted tissue. Quartz titanium or polycarbonate sheets will stop the beam.

Types of Lasers

Lasers use argon, carbon dioxide, holmium, krypton, neodymium, phosphate, ruby, glass, or xenon as their active medium. When delivered to tissues, laser light can be absorbed, reflected, transmitted, or scattered, depending on the characteristics of the laser and the type of tissue. Only absorbed light produces thermal effects in tissue. Thermal penetration varies according to the ratio of absorption versus scattering. Energy absorbed at the surface will destroy superficial cells; further penetration extends cell destruction in surrounding tissues.

The wavelength of the laser light, power density, rate of delivery of energy, and exposure time will vary the effects on tissue. Energy density is based on the laser's wattage, beam or spot size, and time of exposure. The spot size depends on the laser fiber size and distance of the tip from tissue; it increases and becomes defocused as fiber is moved farther from tissue. Variables in tissue reaction are listed in Box 20.1.

•BOX 20.1 **Factors Associated With Tissue Reaction to Laser Light**

- Type of laser (wavelength)
- Intensity of laser focus
- Duration of application
- Depth of penetration
- Type of tissue (color and composition)

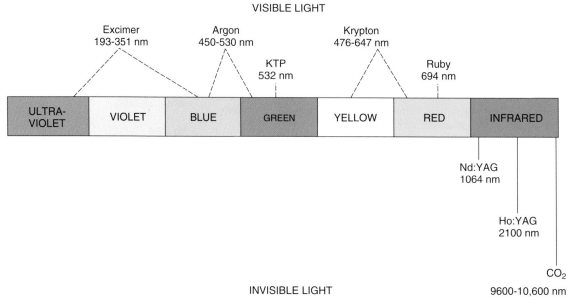

• **Fig. 20.5** Electromagnetic spectrum of laser light beams at wavelengths in nanometers (nm). *CO₂*, Carbon dioxide; *Ho:YAG*, holmium:yttrium aluminum garnet; *KTP*, potassium titanyl phosphate; *Nd:YAG*, neodymium:yttrium aluminum garnet.

Laser beams cut, vaporize, or coagulate tissue. Coagulative effect causes collagen bonding and welding of tissue surfaces. Each laser has selective uses. Laser light colors vary from the visible, near-ultraviolet range to the invisible, far-infrared range of the electromagnetic spectrum (Fig. 20.5). Wavelengths also vary, providing different radiation penetration depths. Lasers are commonly used in conjunction with the operating microscope and/or an endoscope. The surgeon selects the appropriate laser for the tissue to be incised, excised, or coagulated.[4]

Argon Laser

Argon ion gas emits a blue-green light beam in the visible electromagnetic spectrum at wavelengths of 450 and 514 nm. This wavelength passes through water and clear fluid, such as cerebrospinal fluid, with minimal absorption. It is intensely absorbed by the brown-red pigment of hemoglobin in blood or melanin in pigmented tissue and converted into heat. Thermal radiation penetrates to a depth of 1 or 2 mm in most tissue.

The argon laser operates from electrical power. A water-cooling system is often required to dissipate heat generated in the argon medium. The argon laser beam usually is transmitted through a (tube) wave guide. This can be directed to a handpiece or through an endoscope or operating microscope. Most argon laser machines deliver a nonfocused beam that vaporizes tissue poorly and scatters more radiation than other types of lasers. Irradiance may vary from less than 1 watt to 20 watts, depending on the model.

Argon lasers coagulate bleeding points or lesions involving many small superficial vessels, such as a port-wine stain. They are used primarily to destroy specific cutaneous lesions while sparing adjacent tissue and minimizing scarring. Argon lasers may be used to treat vascular lesions and remove plaque and to coagulate superficial vessels in mucosa, such as in the gastrointestinal tract. They are also used in ophthalmology, otolaryngology, gynecology, urology, neurosurgery, and dermatology.

Carbon Dioxide Laser

Using a mixture of carbon dioxide (CO_2), nitrogen, and helium molecular gases, the CO_2 laser emits an invisible beam from the mid- to far-infrared range of the electromagnetic spectrum at wavelengths of 9600 and 10,600 nm. This wavelength is intensely absorbed by water. It raises water temperature in cells to the flash boiling point, thus vaporizing tissue. Vaporization is the conversion of solid tissue to smoke and gas. This plume should be evacuated or suctioned through a filter device from the site of lasing. The intense heat of the CO_2 laser also coagulates vessels as it cuts through them. It penetrates the surface to a depth of 0.1 to 0.2 mm per application to tissue, with minimal thermal effect to surrounding tissue.

The CO_2 laser operates from electrical power. The machine has a self-contained cooling system. The CO_2 laser beam should be delivered in a direct line of vision. It can be directed through a rigid endoscope, but it cannot be transmitted through a fiberoptic wave guide because its longer wavelength prevents conduction through crystal fibers. It is transmitted through an operating microscope or an articulating arm with a series of mirrors. The articulating arm allows precise focus and direction of the beam to a pencil-like handpiece.

CO_2 lasers have a helium-neon (HeNe) laser coaxial target beam that superimposes the invisible CO_2 beam to provide a visible red aiming light. The wave generated may be continuous or pulsed. Irradiance can vary from less than 1 watt to up to 300 watts. A portable handheld laser tube with a hollow needle to deliver the CO_2 beam is available for use in vascular surgery and microsurgery.

The vaporization and hemostatic actions of the CO_2 laser are of value to the surgeon in treating soft tissue and vascular lesions. Large or small masses of tissue can be removed rapidly and efficiently. The CO_2 laser cannot be used in a fluid environment. The peritoneal cavity is insufflated with gas to create a working space before the beam is directed through an endoscope.[5] This laser is used primarily in otolaryngology, gynecology, plastic surgery, dermatology, neurosurgery, orthopedics, and cardiovascular and general surgery.

Excimer Laser

When organic molecular bonds are broken up by a photochemical reaction, cool laser energy is emitted. Short wavelengths in the ultraviolet to visible blue-green spectrum are produced by gas used in the excimer laser combining with a halide medium. Argon fluoride produces a wavelength of 193 nm; krypton fluoride, 248 nm; xenon chloride, 308 nm; and xenon fluoride, 351 nm. These gases are extremely toxic. The beams they produce offer precision in cutting and coagulating without thermal damage to adjacent tissue. Excimer lasers have been developed for use in ophthalmology, peripheral and coronary angioplasty, orthopedics (to cut bone), and neurosurgery.

Free Electron Laser

Free electrons, which are not bound to a specific atom, pass from a particle accelerator through a series of magnets to create a light beam. The beam can be tuned anywhere within the electromagnetic spectrum from ultraviolet to infrared. The free electron laser (FEL) produces light waves as a series of rapid superpulses of high energy and short duration, with minimal thermal damage. These light waves can fragment calculi. The FEL can be used for precise cutting of tissues.

Holmium:Yttrium Aluminum Garnet (Ho:YAG) Laser

A crystal that contains holmium, thulium, and chromium elements increases the wavelength of YAG laser energy to 2100 nm. This invisible beam in the midinfrared range of the electromagnetic spectrum is absorbed by tissues containing water. Combined with high-energy pulsed delivery, it penetrates less deeply into tissue than does the neodymium (Nd:YAG) laser for more precise cutting and less generalized heating of tissue. It may be used percutaneously through a laser fiber threaded through a hollow needle or can be delivered through a fine fiberoptic fiber. It may be used in a fluid medium. It acts on water in cells without char or extensive tissue damage.

Approved for use in all joints except the spine, the Ho:YAG laser is useful in orthopedics to cut, shape, and sculpt cartilage and bone and to ablate soft tissues. Holmium lasers are also used in urology for prostate surgery and kidney stone lithotripsy.[5]

Krypton Laser

The krypton ion gas laser emits a red-yellow light beam in the visible electromagnetic spectrum at wavelengths of 476.2 to 647.1 nm. It is intensely absorbed by pigment in blood and retinal epithelium. The krypton laser resembles the argon laser in construction and use. It operates from electrical power and is water cooled. Used in ophthalmology, it is more versatile than the argon laser in selective photocoagulation of the retina.

Neodymium:Yttrium Aluminum Garnet (Nd:YAG) Laser

Neodymium, yttrium, aluminum, and garnet (Nd:YAG) constitute the solid-state crystal medium from which the light beam of this laser emanates. This invisible beam in the near-infrared range of the electromagnetic spectrum has a wavelength of 1064 nm. It is poorly absorbed by hemoglobin and water but is intensely absorbed by tissue protein. The wavelength penetrates to a depth of 3 to 7 mm to denature protein by thermal coagulation and shrinkage of tissue beneath the surface.

The Nd:YAG laser operates from electric current through the optical power source of xenon flash lamps. It must have an air, a carbon dioxide, or water cooling system.

The Nd:YAG laser beam can be transmitted through a flexible quartz fiber which passes through a rigid endoscope. It also can be transmitted through a fiberoptic wave guide to a handpiece or a flexible endoscope or be focused through an operating microscope. An aiming light of blue xenon or red neon-helium may be used in conjunction with the Nd:YAG beam. Sapphire or ceramic tips allow direct contact with tissue for cutting and vaporizing without diffuse coagulation, using less than 25 watts of power. These tips are available on handheld scalpels or to fit on the ends of fibers for endoscopic use. Many of these tips are reusable; some are for single use only.

The Nd:YAG laser has the most powerful coagulating action of all the surgical lasers. Its continuous or pulsed wave penetrates deeper into tissues than do other lasers (i.e., up to 2 cm) and will coagulate large vessels (up to 4 mm). It is used to coagulate and vaporize large volumes of tissue. This versatile laser has applications in rhinolaryngology, urology, gynecology, neurosurgery, orthopedics, and thoracic and general surgery.

For ophthalmology, the Nd:YAG laser uses a Q-switching mode to store energy in a resonator during pumping action, followed by release of a single short pulse of high energy. This does not burn tissue but disrupts it with minute shock waves.

Potassium Titanyl Phosphate Laser

The solid-state potassium titanyl phosphate (KTP) crystal emits a visible green light at a wavelength of 532 nm. This laser produces less power than CO_2 or Nd:YAG lasers but can be focused to a smaller diameter for precision work, such as in the middle ear. KTP absorbs most effectively into red or black tissue for coagulation. The beam can be directed by a handpiece at or in contact with tissue or through a rigid or flexible fiberoptic fiber or micromanipulator. The beam cuts, vaporizes, or coagulates tissue with minimal lateral thermal damage and plume. Cooling gases are not necessary, but the system should be water cooled. Instruments are available that provide both KTP and Nd:YAG wavelengths selected by a button on the control panel or that pass the Nd:YAG beam through the KTP crystal. Many accessories are available for specific applications in all surgical specialties. The KTP laser has good cutting properties.

Ruby Laser

The ruby solid-state crystal laser emits a visible red light at a wavelength of 694 nm. A synthetically machined crystal rod is placed in a resonator cavity with a xenon flash lamp that when activated creates the optical pumping to produce the ruby laser beam. Blood vessels and transparent substances do not absorb this beam. A pulsed system, the ruby laser can generate large fields of energy on impact. This shock wave effect can injure internal tissues and bone. Irradiance is 1 watt. Originally used in ophthalmology, the ruby laser currently is used primarily to eradicate port-wine stain lesions of the skin.[6]

Tunable Dye Laser

Fluorescent liquid dyes or vapors can produce lasing energy. When exposed to intense laser light, usually an argon beam, dye absorbs light and fluoresces over a broad spectrum from ultraviolet to the far-infrared range. The laser may be delivered interstitially, endoscopically, externally, or retrobulbarly. A tunable prism can adjust the laser wavelength from 400 to 1000 nm, in either continuous or pulsed mode, for the specific dye in use.

The argon tunable dye laser system emits a blue-green beam at a wavelength of 430 to 530 nm from an argon laser that pumps a rhodamine B dye laser to produce a red laser beam at a wavelength of approximately 630 nm for selective destruction of malignant tumor cells. A dye laser tuned to 577 nm can be used on vascular lesions. Other wavelengths, such as through copper vapor, may be used to treat skin lesions or superficial tumors, such as of the bladder wall. The site can be repeatedly treated as long as cells remain photosensitive. This tunable dye laser is used most for photodynamic therapy.

Photodynamic Therapy

For photodynamic therapy, the patient is injected 24 to 48 hours before laser therapy with a photosensitive drug that is absorbed by normal and malignant tissue. Normal tissue gradually releases the drug, but abnormal tissue retains it. The abnormal photosensitive tissue is destroyed when exposed to the laser beam. Normal adjacent tissue appears sunburned but is not permanently damaged. All dyes used with tunable dye lasers are potentially toxic and are handled with caution.

Safety Factors

All surgical lasers present hazards to patients and to the OR team. This equipment should be used in accordance with established regulations, standards and recommended practices, manufacturer's recommendations, and institutional policies. Laser safety is based on knowledge of the specific laser to be used, its instrumentation, its mode of operation, its power densities, its action in tissues, and its risks.

Regulatory Agencies

Lasers are classified as medical devices and are subject to regulation. The Code of Federal Regulations' Performance Standards for Light-Emitting Products provides specifications for manufacturers of medical laser systems.

The Center for Devices and Radiological Health

The Center for Devices and Radiological Health (CDRH) is the regulatory section of the U.S. Food and Drug Administration (FDA) in the Department of Health and Human Services (HHS). More than 250 types of lasers are regulated by the FDA. Those intended for medical and surgical use come under the jurisdiction of medical device regulations. They are categorized as class III, subdivision class 4, because lasers are potentially hazardous (Box 20.2).

With the increased demand for laser surgery and new products, manufacturers must verify that their products meet all safety requirements of the federal standard. They must receive approval from the CDRH to market or test a laser for a particular clinical application or use, and they must comply with labeling requirements.

American National Standards Institute

The American National Standards Institute (ANSI) is a voluntary organization of experts who determine industry consensus standards in technical fields. The standard developed specifically for

---

• BOX 20.2   Medical Device Regulations

FDA Classification of Medical Devices

Medical devices were classified in 1976 by the FDA according to their safety factors.

Class I

Subject to general controls

Class II

Devices for which general controls are not enough

Class III

Implants and life support devices

Classification of Lasers

Lasers are classified according to potential hazard of exposure.

Class 1

Enclosed system, considered safe based on current medical knowledge; no light emission escapes the enclosure.

Class 2

Limited to visible light (400–710 nm). Output power is 1 mW or less. Momentary viewing (0.25-second maximum permissible exposure) is not considered hazardous. Staring into the beam is not recommended; it is hazardous long term. Protective eyewear of the correct optical density should be worn.

Class 3A

Emitted laser viewed directly through collecting optics would cause permanent eye damage. Output power is 0.5 mW or less. Protective eyewear of the correct optical density should be worn.

Class 3B

Continuous laser light with 0.5-watt or less output can cause permanent eye damage. Exposure to the beam should be avoided; it can cause skin and eye damage. Protective eyewear of the correct optical density should be worn.

Class 4

Laser light produced is hazardous to skin and eyes. Strict control measures are enforced. Scatter and reflection can cause skin and eye damage. Protective eyewear of the correct optical density should be worn.

FDA, U.S. Food and Drug Administration.

---

laser safety in health care facilities is intended for all users. Existing federal legislation and state laser safety regulations are based on the ANSI standard. Simply stated, this standard implies that every health care facility that uses surgical lasers must establish and maintain an adequate program for control of laser hazards. This program shall include provisions for the following:

- *Laser safety officer:* This person should have authority to suspend, restrict, or terminate operation of a laser system if hazard controls are inadequate. A laser safety committee, often a subcommittee of the OR committee, may appoint this surveillance officer.
- *Education of users:* A safety training program must ensure that all users, including surgeons, perioperative nurses, surgical technologists, and biomedical engineers and technicians, are knowledgeable of correct operation, potential hazards, and control measures.
- *Protective measures:* Protective measures are for patients, personnel, and the environment.

- *Management of accidents:* Management includes reporting accidents and developing plans of action to prevent a future occurrence.

Occupational Safety and Health Administration

The Occupational Safety and Health Administration (OSHA) is concerned primarily with the safety of health care workers. The agency can enforce ANSI standards.

State and Local Agencies

State regulations and local ordinances vary. Knowledge of and compliance with any requirements should be established.

Policies and Procedures

Specific policies and procedures related to use of lasers should be written by the laser safety committee before a laser program is instituted. These policies and procedures will need to be revised or updated when new equipment is installed. Applicable policies include, but are not limited to, the following:

1. Credentialing and clinical practice privileges of medical staff. Physicians authorized to use a laser should be required to complete a postgraduate laser course in their specialties.[7] Hands-on experience and a preceptorship with a qualified user also should be required. The physician must have training for each type and wavelength of laser. A list of approved physicians should be available to the perioperative staff. Scheduling privileges should be denied to those surgeons who are not appropriately credentialed.
2. Initial and ongoing educational laser use and safety programs for perioperative personnel. Perioperative personnel should have thorough knowledge and understanding of laser equipment, laser physics, tissue reactions, applications, and safety precautions.
3. Continuous quality improvement. A program of continuous quality improvement includes appropriate care, use, and maintenance of equipment and prevention of laser-related accidents.
4. Documentation. The surgeon, procedure, type of laser used, length of use, and wattage should be recorded in the patient's medical record. This information, plus the patient's name, also should be recorded in the OR log.

Patient Safety

The surgeon must explain laser surgery and its potential complications to the patient before obtaining written consent. Some lasers are considered investigational devices by the FDA. The patient must sign a specific consent form permitting experimental use and data collection. With all lasers, appropriate precautions (including protection of the patient's eyes, skin, respiratory tract, and tissue surrounding the target area from thermal burns) are taken to ensure patient safety, as follows:

1. The eyes and eyelids should be adequately protected from the specific laser beam in use.
   a. Patients who are awake must wear the same types of safety glasses or goggles with side shields of the correct optical density as those worn by the laser team.
   b. The eyelids can be taped shut on patients who are under general anesthesia.
   c. Eye pads moistened with saline solution should be taped securely in place for procedures around the head and neck, except for ophthalmic procedures and those using

the Nd:YAG laser. Nonflammable material, such as aluminum foil with the reflective side down, can be taped over the eyes for Nd:YAG laser procedures. Moistened eye pads will not stop a laser beam.
   d. Protective shields should be used on the eyes during ophthalmic procedures. Corneal eye shields can be applied directly onto anesthetized eyes to protect corneal tissue.
2. Antiseptics used for skin preparation should be nonflammable.
   a. Aqueous solutions are safest, but they can retain laser heat if they are allowed to pool on or around skin. The skin should be thoroughly dry before the laser is activated.
   b. Alcohol and tinctures are flammable and volatile when wet. Vapors must not accumulate under drapes because they can ignite.
3. The immediate area around the incision and/or tissue surrounding the target site should be protected from thermal injury. Hair is flammable and should be completely covered with wet sponges or coated with water-soluble jelly. Flammable materials are avoided or safeguarded to prevent fire.
   a. Flame or fire-resistant drapes should be used. Metallic foil and polypropylene laser-retardant and ignition-resistant drapes are available. Polypropylene and plastic incise drapes can melt if a laser beam strikes them. Woven and nonwoven fabrics can ignite.
   b. Woven textile or cellulose-based absorbent nonwoven towels saturated with sterile normal saline solution or water should be placed over fabric drapes around the incision before the laser is used.
   c. The laser handpiece should be laid on a moistened surface. The laser tip is extremely hot and may shatter if placed in contact with a cold surface.
   d. Moistened sponges, towels, or compressed patties should be placed around target tissue except when the Nd:YAG laser is used. Sponges and other material should be removed from tissue near the target site of the Nd:YAG laser because wetting will not stop this beam and they could be ignited.
   e. The rectum should be packed with a moistened sponge to prevent methane gas, which is potentially explosive, from escaping from the intestinal tract during use of a laser in the perineal area. Placement of the sponge in the anal orifice and removal of the rectal packing should be recorded as part of the sponge count.
4. Anesthetic agents should be noncombustible. Nonflammable anesthetics and oxygen mixed with nonflammable agents are administered in a closed system.
   a. Oxygen and nitrous oxide concentrations around the head should be as low as possible during use of a laser in the aerodigestive tract (i.e., oral, laryngeal, bronchial, or esophageal procedures).
   b. Flexible metallic or insulated silicone endotracheal tubes are preferred for aerodigestive tract procedures. Laser-approved varieties are commercially available. If used, red rubber tubes are wrapped with reflective aluminum or copper tape to prevent ignition. Polyvinyl chloride endotracheal tubes should not be used because they ignite easily. The endotracheal tube cuff should be inflated with saline solution, which may be tinted with methylene blue to facilitate detection of a leak.
5. The teeth should be covered during oropharyngeal procedures to protect against reflective radiation.

6. Patients who are awake may wear a protective high-filtration mask during CO_2 laser ablation, such as of condylomata (venereal warts), to prevent inhaling airborne material into the lungs. An intubated patient is not considered at risk for respiratory contamination.
7. Postoperative instructions should include care of a healing thermal skin wound.

Personnel Safety

Exposure to nonionizing laser radiation can be hazardous for personnel. Precautions are taken to avoid eye and skin exposure to direct or scattered radiation and inhalation of plume. Some facilities require laser personnel to have baseline retinal screening performed before working in the laser unit.

Eye Protection

The eye is the organ most susceptible to laser injury. Different laser wavelengths affect eyes differently: argon and Nd:YAG lasers will be absorbed by the retina, and the CO_2 laser will be absorbed by the cornea. Therefore safety glasses or goggles of the correct optical density are always worn while the laser is in use. Optical density is the ability of the lens to absorb a specific wavelength (Table 20.1). The color of the lens is not the protective feature of the eyewear. Each type of wavelength requires protective eyewear of a specific optical density as recommended by the manufacturer of the laser. The following considerations apply to eye protection:
1. Protective eyewear is available outside the room near posted signs designating the specific type of laser in use. Only people with appropriate eye protection are admitted in the room while the laser is in use.
   a. All protective eyewear (i.e., safety glasses, goggles) must shield the wearer's eyes from the top, bottom, and sides of the visual field.
   b. Goggles will fit over eyeglasses, or prescription lenses of the correct optical density can be obtained. Contact lenses do not provide eye protection.
   c. Scratches on the lens or breaks in the frame can negate eye protection.
2. Lens covers with filter caps are available for optical eyepieces of endoscopes and operating microscopes. Their use does not eliminate the need for the entire team to wear eye protection.

<table>
<tr><td colspan="2">**TABLE 20.1**   **Optical Density Necessary for Protective Eyewear**</td></tr>
<tr><td>**Optical Density**</td><td>**Transmission of Light (% of Wavelength)**</td></tr>
<tr><td>0</td><td>1</td></tr>
<tr><td>1</td><td>0.1</td></tr>
<tr><td>2</td><td>0.01</td></tr>
<tr><td>3</td><td>0.001</td></tr>
<tr><td>4</td><td>0.0001</td></tr>
<tr><td>5</td><td>0.00001</td></tr>
<tr><td>6</td><td>0.000001</td></tr>
</table>

Light transmission is measured with a spectrophotometer to calculate the optical density needed for protective eyewear.

Skin Protection

Skin sensitivities can develop from overexposure to ultraviolet radiation. Skin also can be burned from exposure to direct or reflected laser energy. These hazards are minimized if personnel are alert to precautions for environmental safety. Other personnel safety precautions reduce risks and include the following:
- Metallic jewelry should not be worn. It could absorb heat or reflect the beam.
- Fire-resistant gowns may be worn.

Laser Plume

Toxic substances, including carcinogens and viruses, may become airborne from vaporization of tissues, especially from CO_2 and Nd:YAG lasers. The smoke produced, referred to as laser plume, contains water, carbonized particles, mutated DNA, and intact cells. It may have a distinct odor.

Laser plume should not be inhaled. One gram of plume is equivalent to smoking six cigarettes. Smoke evacuation from the site of lasing and high-filtration masks prevent personnel from inhaling plume. Removal of plume also enhances visibility at the target site for the surgeon. Plume can bend or refract the beam, thus inadvertently causing injury to adjacent tissues. The following precautions should be taken:
1. A mechanical smoke evacuator or suction with a high-efficiency filter should be turned on before or at the same time as the laser and should be run during activation and for 20 to 30 seconds after the laser is deactivated. The tip should be placed as close as possible, at least within 2 inches (5 cm), to the lasing site of tissue vaporization.
   a. Several types of mechanical smoke evacuators are available. Many systems have charcoal filters.
   b. Charcoal filters in most evacuators are changed regularly. Gloves, eyewear, and a mask (personnel protective equipment [PPE]) are worn when handling contaminated filters.
2. Masks should be tight fitting and should filter particles as small as 0.1 μm.

Environmental Safety

Only properly trained personnel are authorized to participate in laser surgery. Others should be made aware of its hazards. The following considerations apply to environmental safety[7]:
1. Warning signs (e.g., Laser Surgery in Progress) should be posted on the outside of all OR doors when the laser is in use. The design, symbols, and wording on the warning sign should be specific for the type of laser in use.
2. Walls and ceilings should have nonreflective surfaces. Glass, as in windows, cabinet doors, and/or the x-ray viewing box, should be covered with nonreflective material to stop reflective beams. CO_2 laser beams do not penetrate glass and plastic but can bounce off reflective surfaces.
3. Warning labels on the machine, affixed by the manufacturer, must indicate points of danger to avoid personnel exposure to laser radiation.
4. The machine should be prepared, checked, and tested before the patient is brought into the room. A preoperative checklist is helpful. Any malfunction should be reported immediately, and the equipment should not be used until it is in proper working order.
5. When not in use, the machine should be kept on the "standby" setting with the beam terminated in a beam stop of highly absorbent, nonreflecting, fire-resistant material to

avoid accidental activation. It should be turned off and locked with a key when left unattended. Only authorized personnel should have access to the key.

6. The foot switch should be operated by the surgeon who delivers the laser energy to the tissue. The foot pedal can be covered when not in use so that the surgeon will not inadvertently activate the laser. Foot pedals for other equipment should be moved away while the laser is in use. The laser pedal can then be removed after use.

7. Nonreflective instruments should be used in or near the beam. These instruments may be of a dull blue titanium alloy or an ebonized or anodized stainless steel. These finishes defocus and disperse the laser beam. Reflective instruments can cause burns or start fires.

8. Fire is a potential hazard that must not be underestimated. Personnel should be aware of fire safeguards and adhere to precautions for their own and the patient's safety.
   a. A basin of sterile water or normal saline solution should be readily available at the sterile field.
   b. A halon fire extinguisher should be available.
   c. Oxygen concentration in the room should be as low as possible. Oxygen leaking from the side of a patient's facemask can be ignited by the laser beam. The anesthesia provider should be knowledgeable about flash points and fire retardation when the laser is in use.
   d. Liquids should not be placed on the machine. A spill could act as a conductor and short-circuit the mechanism.

9. Electrical codes and standards should be enforced to avoid electrical hazards. An isolation transformer is recommended for a high-power laser power source to avoid dangerous overload of the existing OR power system. Electrical circuitry must provide adequate amperage for power requirements. Preferably, the laser should have its own dedicated circuit.

10. The manufacturer's instructions for operation, care, handling, and sterilization of the laser system should be followed. Proper care of lasers and accessory equipment is essential to patient, personnel, and environmental safety.

Laser Team

A laser team should be designated to carry out the duties that are different from those of the traditional OR team. This team may include the following personnel:

1. *Clinical laser nurse:* The responsibilities of the clinical laser nurse are different from those of the circulating nurse. Duties include the following:
   a. Preparing and teaching the patient preoperatively, intraoperatively, and postoperatively.
   b. Bringing laser equipment to the OR and checking it. The chassis and the floor around it should be inspected for water leak. Using sterile technique, the clinical laser nurse and scrub person calibrate the laser as appropriate.
   c. Covering windows, posting signs, and distributing appropriate protective eyewear.
   d. Covering the patient's eyes.
   e. Positioning the laser foot pedal for the surgeon's convenience and removing it after use.
   f. Operating the key switch and monitoring activation of the laser. The wattage and exposure time are set according to the surgeon's orders. These should be repeated before and after adjusting controls.

   g. Cleaning and checking laser fibers after use and preparing them for sterilization.
   h. Completing the laser log.
   i. Collaborating with the laser safety officer and biomedical engineer and/or technician to ensure safe use of laser equipment.

2. *Biomedical technician:* The biomedical technician provides preventive maintenance and handles minor problems with the laser system. A log of laser use and maintenance is maintained.

3. *Camera operator:* Endoscopic procedures performed under video control may require an additional sterile team member to operate the camera attached to the endoscope while the surgeon controls the laser.

Advantages of Laser Surgery

Surgical lasers emit nonionizing radiation. This radiation is selectively absorbed by different tissues with resultant penetration and destruction at the focal point but with differential thermal protection of surrounding tissues. Lasers offer the surgeon and the patient many advantages over other surgical techniques, including the following:

- Precise control for accurate incision, excision, or ablation of tissue. The laser beam is precisely focused for localized tissue destruction. The depth of radiation penetration is precisely regulated by the duration of focus, power density, and type of tissue.
- Access to areas inaccessible to other surgical instruments through minimally invasive techniques. The beam can be directed through endoscopes or deflected off rhodium reflector mirrors.
- An unobstructed view of the surgical site. The laser beam comes in contact with tissue to be cut, coagulated, or vaporized. It can be directed through the operating microscope.
- Minimal handling of and trauma to tissues. Traction on target tissue is unnecessary.
- A dry, bloodless surgical field. The laser beam simultaneously cuts and coagulates blood vessels, thus providing hemostasis in vascular areas.
- Minimal thermal effect on surrounding tissue. Essentially no permanent thermal necrosis of tissue occurs beyond 100 mm from the edge of the area incised. This minimizes postoperative pain.
- Reduced risk for contamination or infection. The laser beam vaporizes microorganisms, thus essentially sterilizing the contact area.
- Prompt healing with minimal postoperative edema, sloughing of tissue, pain, and scarring.
- Reduced operating time. Because procedures can be done more quickly, both anesthesia time and operating time are shorter. Many procedures can be done without general anesthesia. Many are done in ambulatory care facilities.

Disadvantages of Laser Surgery

- The costs to start and maintain a program are high. Equipment, instrumentation, supplies, and staff education are expensive initial investments. Most aspects need frequent updates and maintenance.
- Decisions should be made about the use of disposable versus reusable supplies and the effect on patient care. Most reusable supplies are fragile and should be replaced on a regular basis.

- Liability may increase as the number of users increases. Specific credentialing and continuing education require planning and are time-consuming.

Microsurgery

The simplest magnifying instrument consists of a single lens with relatively high magnification (e.g., a magnifying glass or a jeweler's lens). Surgeons requiring less magnification than that provided by the microscope use operating loupes. Loupes magnify approximately two times the diopter power of the native lens in the surgeon's eye. Loupes attach to a headband or to the surgeon's eyeglasses like binoculars. The use of loupes in surgery terminates where microsurgery begins. From loupe surgery and refinements of the binocular microscope, microsurgery has evolved.

Technique of Microsurgery

Performance of surgical procedures while directly viewing the surgical field under magnification affords surgeons greater visual acuity of small structures. The microscope provides a more limited, although more readily visible, surgical field. All things look considerably different under magnification. Tissues not otherwise visible can be manipulated.

Use of microsurgical instrumentation and techniques is not simply a matter of adapting formerly learned conventional methods for use under the microscope. The techniques themselves for handling instruments, sutures, and tissues are different and infinitely more complex, precise, and time-consuming because of the meticulous skill involved. Coordination must be adapted to working with minute materials in a field of altered perception and position.

Proficiency and facility in using the operating microscope entail laboratory practice in movements and manipulation of instruments and suture materials under various magnifications.

Divergence from tactile-manual to vision-oriented techniques requires that the surgeon and assistants pay maximum attention to detail. The most common maneuvers for placing and manipulating instruments, making an incision with scissors, and tying sutures involve a combination of several basic movements:

- *Compression-decompression:* To close scissors and forceps
- *Rotation:* To insert a needle, to cut, to extract, to engage or disengage
- *Push-pull, direct,* or *linear:* To incise with a razor knife

The surgeon also must be able to maintain a steady, stationary position during remote activation of equipment such as a laser beam. It is advisable that surgeons and assistants do no manual labor for at least a day before operating. Caffeinated drinks such as coffee the morning of surgery may decrease steadiness in some individuals. Very little tremor is tolerable in microsurgery.

Advantages of Microsurgery

Microsurgery provides unique advantages in the restoration of wholeness and function of the body, such as restitution of hearing, vision, tactile sensation, circulation, and/or motion. It is used in many surgical specialties to improve precision of already-established surgical procedures and permit successful performance of procedures previously not possible. For example, blood vessels less than 3 mm in exterior diameter can be sutured. Nerves can be anastomosed.

Replantation of amputated parts and some reconstructive surgeries are possible only under magnification. In general, microsurgery allows the following:

- Dissection and repair of fine structures through better visualization
- Adaptation of surgical procedures to individual patient requirements (variation in anatomic landmarks is more distinct with magnification)
- Diminution of surgical trauma and complications because of safer dissection
- Superior focal lighting of the surgical field, particularly in deep areas

Operating Microscope

Compound microscopes use two or more lens systems or several lenses grouped in one unit. The operating microscope is a compound binocular instrument. Single-eye viewing with a monocular lens does not provide the depth of field necessary for surgical procedures. Interchangeable objective lenses combined with interchangeable binocular eyepieces allow a wide range of magnification and working distances adjustable to the surgeon's needs.

The operating microscope uses light waves for illumination. These waves are bent as they pass through the microscope, causing the image seen by the viewer's eye to be magnified.

The users must understand the parts and their functions. Basically, all operating microscopes incorporate the same essential components: an optical lens system and controls for magnification and focus, an illumination system, a mounting system for stability, an electrical system, and accessories.

Optical Lens System

The ability to enlarge an image is known as magnifying power. This is the ratio of the size of the image produced on the viewer's retina by magnification to the size of the retinal image when the object is viewed without optical aid. To create a distinct image, adjacent images must be separated. An indistinct image remains unclear no matter how many times it is magnified. The ability to discern detail is known as resolving power.

Components

The heart of the optical system is the body, which contains the objective lens (lens closest to the object). The head or binocular oculars (eyepieces) through which the surgeon looks are physically and optically attached to the body. The optical combination of the objective lens and the oculars determines the magnification of the microscope (Fig. 20.6).

Objective lenses are available in various focal lengths ranging from 100 to 400 mm, with intervening increases by 25-mm increments. The 400-mm lens provides the greatest magnification. The designation of the objective lens enumerates the working distance (the distance from the lens to the surgical field). Distances vary from 6 to 10 inches (15–25 cm). For example, a 200-mm lens will be in focus at a working distance of 200 mm, or approximately 8 inches (20 cm).

The oculars serve as magnifying glasses used to examine the real image formed by the objective. Most objectives are achromatic so the true color of tissues can be viewed in sharp detail. The binocular arrangement provides stereoscopic viewing. Stereopsis is basically achieved through binocular viewing, wherein each eye

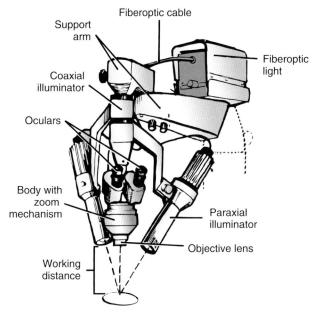

• **Fig. 20.6** Microscope body in detail.

has a slightly different positional view of the object under examination.

The observer's brain then combines the two dissimilar images taken from points of view a little distance apart, thus producing a perception of a single three-dimensional image. If the user is wearing corrective lenses, the eyepieces are set to zero. If the user needs corrective lenses but is not wearing them, they should preset the eyepieces to a position of visual comfort, pupillary distance, and acuity before draping the microscope. Detachable rubber eyecups for the eyepieces are commercially available for the user's comfort.

Magnification

The ability of the microscope to magnify depends on the design and quality of the parts in addition to the resolving power. The total magnification is computed by multiplying the enlarging power of the objective lens by that of the lenses of the oculars. The depth of the field, which is the vertical dimension within which objects are seen in clear focus, decreases with increases in magnification of power. Likewise, the width of the field of view narrows as the power of magnification increases.

Vertical viewing of the surgical field is extremely important, particularly in higher magnification ranges. It allows the surgeon more effective use of the increasingly limited depth of field.

In more complex microscopes, a third set of lenses is interposed between the oculars and the objective lens to provide additional magnification in variable degrees as desired by the surgeon. A continuously variable system of magnification for increasing or decreasing images is possible with a zoom lens. Most surgeons prefer a faster, easier-to-handle zoom lens to a simpler turret magnifier that manually changes magnification by fixed increments.

The zoom lens is usually operated by a foot control that permits the surgeon to change magnification without removing their hands from the surgical field. The popular range of magnification in the zoom microscope is from 3.5× to 20× magnification. At 3.5× magnification, the depth of the field is about 0.10 inch

(2.5 mm); at 20× magnification, the depth is about ½ inch (12.7 mm). Some microscopes magnify to 50 times.

Focus

Focusing is accomplished manually or by a foot-controlled motor that raises and lowers the body of the microscope to the desired distance from the object to be viewed. Some microscopes divide the focus into gross and fine. The focus of the ocular lens usually is set at zero; the surgeon adjusts the focus as desired.

Illumination System

Illumination of the operating microscope uses light waves. The shorter the wavelength, the greater the resolving power. The intensity of illumination can be varied by controls mounted on the support arm of the body. The operating microscope has two basic sources of illumination: paraxial and coaxial.

Paraxial Illuminators

One or more light tubes (paraxial illuminators) contain tungsten or halogen bulbs and focusing lenses. The illuminators are attached to the mounting of the body of the microscope in a position to illuminate the field of view. Light is focused to coincide with the working distance of the microscope.

One of the paraxial illuminators may be equipped with a diaphragm containing a variable-width slit aperture. This device permits a narrow beam of light to be brought into focus on the objective field. This slit image assists the surgeon in defining depth perception (i.e., in ascertaining the relative distance of objects within the field—which are closer, which are farther).

Coaxial Illuminators

In fiberoptic coaxial illumination, light is transmitted through the optical system of the microscope body. This type of illumination is called coaxial because it illuminates the same area in the same focus as the viewing, or objective, field of the microscope. The fiberoptic system provides intense, though cool, light that protects the patient's tissues and the optics of the microscope from excessive heat. The light intensity ranges from 600 to 2250 footcandles without creating shadows. Reflected glare may be a problem. Frequent wound irrigation with a cool solution is necessary to avoid tissue damage from radiant energy during long procedures.

If a fiberoptic system is not used for coaxial illumination, a heat-absorbing filter must be interposed in the illumination system. Direct heat from a high-intensity source can damage and even burn tissues. Tungsten and halogen bulbs are used in some housings.

Another type of optical prism assembly provides a larger area of coaxial illumination with a brighter light than that obtained with fiberoptic light bundles. Known as *liquid light,* it uses ionic, inorganic saline solution with quartz glass inserts inside a flexible aluminum spiral tube insulated with a polyvinyl chloride coating. Light is conducted throughout the cross-section of the liquid, unlike the light provided by a fiberoptic bundle.

Mounting Systems

The stability of the microscope is of paramount importance. The body, the optical portion, is mounted on a vertical column that may be supported by the floor, ceiling, or wall or by attachment to the OR bed. The body of the microscope is attached to the column by a hinged arm and a central pivot. The mounting permits positioning as desired. It may be adjusted horizontally or vertically, rotated on its axis, and tilted at different angles. The microscope can be aimed in any direction. The objective is aimed at the principal surgical site.

Floor and ceiling mounting systems are the most popular and versatile. All microscopes must have a locking mechanism to immobilize the microscope body over the surgical field.

Floor Mount

The base of the vertical support, which rests on the floor, has retractable casters for ease in moving the entire instrument. When the base is lowered to working position, it is locked into position (Fig. 20.7).

The base should be properly positioned in relation to the OR bed before the anesthetic is administered or the patient is prepped. To maintain balance and control, one should gently push (not pull) the microscope when moving it. Jarring or banging the scope should be avoided because the lenses may dislocate and obscure vision. The brake should be released or casters activated before the microscope is moved. The arms should be folded close to the column, with all the attachments locked into place. Cords should be out of the way. Observation tubes should not be used as handles. Force should never be used in moving the microscope or in applying attachments; one should look for the problem instead. A floor-based microscope with column support is placed to the left of a right-handed surgeon. The base should not interfere with foot controls or power cables. It should be clear of any table attachments.

Some microscopes use a Contraves stand. This is a counterbalanced weight system used to position the operating microscope

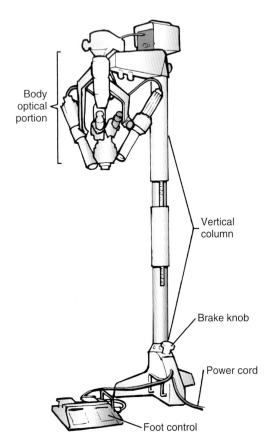

Body optical portion

Vertical column

Brake knob

Power cord

Foot control

• **Fig. 20.7** Floor-mounted operating microscope.

in a suspended position over the surgical field. The weights are set and locked according to the types of attachments on the body of the microscope. The balance is set before activating the power switch.

As a safety factor, the base must not be moved when the microscope is positioned over the patient because it is top-heavy. Gross adjustments, such as height in relation to the surgical field and focus, are made with the microscope swung away from the patient. The OR bed height, chair, and armrest heights are adjusted when gross adjustments are made. Fine focusing and adjustments are done after the microscope is in position for the surgical procedure. The assistant's microscope is adjusted to the same focus as that of the surgeon. During prepping and draping, the microscope is rotated out of position and then brought over the surgical field for the procedure.

Ceiling Mount

A ceiling mount, either a fixed or track-mounted model, provides more floor space for placement of foot pedals. The fixed unit is suspended from a telescoping column attached directly to the ceiling. Vertical support of a track-mounted unit is suspended from a ceiling rail. It can be moved out of the way when not in use (Fig. 20.8). The microscope is positioned and focused after the patient is anesthetized. A ceiling-mounted instrument is operated by a control panel on a wall (on-off switch) and by foot controls for focusing, magnifying, raising, and lowering.

A ceiling mount is generally very stable, but it is only as stable as the supporting ceiling. Mechanical devices adjacent to the OR, such as air conditioning units, may cause vibration. The microscope should be vibration free. A ceiling mount permits the same flexibility of positioning as a floor mount. Care is taken to ensure that the mounting track is dust free. Flecks of dust falling into the field can cause serious problems with infection and adhesions.

The vertical support has a memory stop mechanism that can be preset for a preselected OR bed height. This setting should be checked and adjusted for each OR bed position change. The mechanism is a safety factor to prevent accidental lowering of the microscope at high speed too close to the patient. High-speed lowering should be done away from the patient until the memory stop is reached. As with the floor-mounted instrument, gross adjustments are never made over the patient. Fine adjustment and focusing are done after the microscope is positioned over the surgical field.

• **Fig. 20.8** Ceiling track-mounted microscope.

Wall Mount

The microscope is bracketed by a flexible arm to a stable wall. The swing-arm extension permits proper positioning.

Operating Bed Mount

Smaller microscopes may be mounted on the framework of the OR bed. This system has many disadvantages and thus is not popular.

Electrical System

The same precautions are observed with the operating microscope as with any electrical equipment in the OR. Switches and wall interlocks should be explosion proof. Circuits are protected from overload by breaker relays and fuses. All light controls should be in the off position when the power plug is inserted or removed from the wall outlet to avoid short-circuiting or sparking. A red pilot light illuminates on the control panel when the electrical power is on.

Accessories

Several accessories are available to enhance the versatility of microsurgery. The value of a good microscope is negated without proper ancillary equipment.

Assistant's Binoculars

A separate optical body with a nonmotorized, hand-controlled zoom lens can be attached to the main microscope body for use by the assistant (Fig. 20.9). This mechanism can be focused on the same plane as the surgeon's oculars. Its field of view may not coincide exactly with that of the surgeon. This can be rectified by using a beam splitter, which takes the image from one of the surgeon's oculars and transmits it through an observer tube, thereby providing the assistant with an identical image of the surgeon's view (see Fig. 20.8). This is particularly important in critical areas where a difference of 1 or 2 mm is crucial.

The assistant's binocular co-observer tubes can be placed on the body of the microscope so that the assistant can work and observe from the same side of the OR bed as, at a right angle to, or directly opposite the surgeon. Binocular tubes (tiltable, straight, or inclined) can be attached on the right or left side of the body of the microscope. A dual viewing bridge, the quadroscope, is attached when the surgeon and assistant sit opposite each other. They have exactly the same view of the field with this accessory. Binoculars should be appropriately placed on the microscope body before the surgical procedure begins.

Broadfield Viewing Lens

A low-power magnifying glass is used for grasping needles or for getting an overall view of the field adjacent to the objective. This lens attaches to the front of the body of the surgeon's ocular (see Fig. 20.9).

Couplings

Couplings allow versatility in positioning the microscope for specific applications. An automated mechanism, the X-Y attachment, provides precision in controlling small movements of the microscope in the field of view. A coupling piece lets surgeons change the angle for side-to-side or front-to-back viewing. A universal tilt coupling can be integrated into the X-Y coupling.

Cameras

Still photographic, motion picture, video, and television cameras may be attached to the beam splitter, permitting filming of the surgical procedure (Fig. 20.10). The camera unit should be in the upright position when connected to the operating microscope. It may require the use of a stronger illumination source. Check to ensure film is in the camera if it is not digital. The patient's and surgeon's names, the date, and the time are documented on the film or video cartridge to prevent mixing recorded images among patients. The use of recording equipment may require special patient consent in some institutions. The recorded procedure is useful in assisting, teaching, and research.

Laser Microadapter

Laser beams can be directed through the operating microscope. The microscope and laser head couplings should be perfectly aligned in the grooves and protrusions on the metal adapters. A screw and locking pin secure the coupling. In the operating position, the laser head is at approximately a 60-degree angle to the microscope. It will not fire in a horizontal or upside-down position.

The microadapter must have a compatible lens with a focal length of 200, 300, or 400 mm so that the surgeon can properly adjust the focal point of the laser beam. A CO_2 laser with electronic components that delivers milliwatt energy may be used to vaporize tissues or weld tissues together. Colposcopes can be used for laser ablation of the uterine cervix. The laser is directed using a joystick.

Other types of lasers are directed through fiberoptics. To protect the surgeon's eyes, filter caps over optics should be the appropriate optical density for the wavelength of the laser being used. The entire team and patient must wear eye protection of the appropriate optical density when the laser is in use.

Remote Foot Controls

Simple microscopes are manually operated. It is more convenient for the surgeon to use motorized foot controls for functions such as focus, zoom, and tilt. Foot controls may be activated by switches of the pushbutton type, heel-to-toe, or side-to-side motion. The number of switches corresponds to the number of

• **Fig. 20.9** Surgeon's microscope on right with assistant's binoculars attached on left.

• **Fig. 20.10** Microscope accessories.

motor-controlled functions. There may be additional foot switches for the camera or for other non—microscope-associated equipment, such as cryosurgical, bipolar electrosurgical, or laser units.

Switches may be separated by a vertical bar to prevent inadvertent contact. The bar also serves as a footrest for the surgeon. Because the surgeon and assistant usually are seated during microsurgical procedures, the height of the OR bed must permit them adequate knee room to operate foot controls.

Microscope Drape

The entire working mechanism and support arm of the microscope are encased in a sterile drape. Draping the entire microscope permits it to be brought into the sterile field so that the surgeon can position the body and adjust the optics. Disposable drapes that are heat resistant, lint-free, nonreflective, transparent, and quiet are available to fit the configuration of all microscopes and attachments. The scrub person slides the drape over the body of the microscope, with hands protected as for draping a Mayo stand. The circulating nurse helps guide the drape toward the vertical column and secures it. The scrub person secures the drape to the oculars. Sterile lens covers or rubber bands may be supplied with the drape for this purpose.

If it is not heat resistant, a plastic drape may cause heat buildup beneath it that can damage the microscope. A heat guard may be applied over the light source, or heat may be evacuated through an opening in the top of the drape.

Care of the Microscope

Persons responsible for the microscope should consult the manufacturer's manual. Any malfunction should be reported to the OR manager or appropriate person who can arrange for repair service. A checklist to verify care and functioning of various parts before the surgical procedure is helpful. Everyone who assists with microsurgery must know how to set up, position, and otherwise care for the microscope as follows:

1. The microscope should be damp-dusted before use.
   a. External surfaces, except the lenses, are wiped with a clean cloth saturated with detergent-disinfectant solution.
   b. Casters or wheels should be clean to reduce contamination and prevent interference with mobility.
2. Lenses should be cleaned according to the manufacturer's recommendations only, to avoid scratching or damage to antireflective lens coating. Most manufacturers recommend sterile distilled water and lens paper. Lenses must not be soaked in any solution.
3. The circulating nurse should prepare the microscope.
   a. When changing oculars, do not drop or fingerprint lenses. Avoid stripping the threads of screw mounts by seating the optics and turning in a counterclockwise direction until the threads align. Proceed by turning in a clockwise motion until secure. Take care not to overtighten. Right turns tighten; left turns loosen.
   b. Both hands should be used for attaching observation tubes, which are heavy.
   c. Extra lamp bulbs and fuses should be on hand. The circulating nurse must know where they are stored and how to change them. It is advisable to check bulbs periodically to avoid the necessity of replacing them during a procedure. New bulbs should be inserted if a long procedure is anticipated. Bulbs should be changed with the power off.

   d. Check electrical connections for proper fit or wire fraying. Take special care of power cables to prevent accidental breakage from heavy equipment rolling over them.
   e. Check that all knobs are secured after the microscope is in the operating position.
   f. Place foot controls in a convenient position so the surgeon does not have to search for them.
4. The microscope and accessories should be properly stored. Store away from traffic but close to areas where used.
   a. Openings into the microscope body for attachment of accessory devices, such as the observer tube, should be closed with covers provided by the manufacturer when not in use to prevent accumulation of dust.
   b. Lenses and viewing tubes should be protected.
   c. The microscope and attachments should be enclosed in an antistatic plastic cover when not in use to keep them free from dust.
   d. Power cords should be neatly coiled for storage.

General Considerations in Microsurgery

Patient

The patient is prepared for the surgical procedure according to the location of the surgical site. They should be positioned comfortably and safely with the OR bed locked in position. The surgical site is immobilized if possible.

Anesthesia

If a general anesthetic is to be administered, the anesthesia provider should be informed in advance of the surgeon's intention to use the microscope. This is especially pertinent in procedures in which patient movements under light anesthesia could result in disaster. In addition, the anesthesia provider's position in relation to the patient should be considered to allow room for the microscope. The anesthesia provider should be aware that microsurgical procedures will take somewhat longer.

With local anesthesia, the patient should be instructed to lie quietly and tell the anesthesia provider or circulating nurse of a desire to move. Many patients sleep during the procedure. A startle reflex on awakening or unexpected movement is especially hazardous in microsurgery, wherein the surgeon's mobility and field of view are limited. If the patient jerks or turns, they literally may move out of the surgeon's hands and often out of view of the microsurgical field. Therefore the patient should be closely monitored.

Stability of the Surgical Field

A vital factor for successful microsurgery is stability of the surgical field, microscope, and surgeon's hands. The complete microsurgical unit consists of the OR bed with the patient, the microscope, and the surgeon's position. These should be functionally positioned in relation to each other so that major adjustments need not be made during the surgical procedure. The surgeon and circulating nurse should check that all components are properly placed before the incision is made.

Armrests and Chair

It is important that the surgeon's hands be adequately supported because a shift of even ½ inch (12.7 mm) can alter the precision of motion, particularly at high magnifications. Support of the surgeon's arm should be continuous from shoulder to hand to give stability and to minimize tremor, especially in fine finger movements. A detachable, sterile, padded wrist support may be affixed to the OR bed for eye procedures.

If the surgeon is seated, a chair with hydraulic foot controls for raising or lowering provides the necessary forearm support by means of attached armrests. These armrests are individually draped. Mayo stand covers are convenient. Armrests can be moved independently to a variety of levels and positions. They are secured in the desired position. The surgeon should be in a comfortable position to work.

Duties of the Scrub Person

Although a stabilized situation is crucial, a second fundamental necessity is for the surgeon and assistant to always keep their eyes on the field of view through the microscope. Looking away from the field requires readjustment of vision to the field. Cooperation and coordination by the scrub person in carrying out the following duties will prevent the surgeon's distraction from the surgical site:

1. Set up the Mayo stand and instrument table without touching the tips of instruments. Holders are available to keep instrument tips in the air and to keep them separated. Microinstruments are handled individually. They are more susceptible to damage than are standard instruments. Edges are easily dulled, and fine tips are easily bent or broken. Extreme caution is necessary not to catch tips on any object that could bend them.
2. Place instruments on the Mayo stand in anticipated order of use. Place the Mayo stand and instrument table conveniently, so the surgeon does not have to look around the microscope.
3. Pass instruments by placing them in the surgeon's hand in position for use, and guide the hand toward the surgical field so that the surgeon and assistant can keep their eyes on the field.
4. Keep debris (e.g., blood, mucus, suture ends) from the tips of instruments by wiping them gently on a nonfibrous sponge or lint-free gauze. Replace them in their original position on the Mayo stand, not touching each other.
5. Assist efficiently but never put hands in the surgical field unless requested to do so.
6. Understand the need for slow dissection at times. Do not let attention stray or make excessive movements; observe the video monitor if one is available. Noise should be kept to a minimum during critical times to avoid distraction.

The increased time needed for use of the operating microscope can be minimized by adequate preparation and efficient assistance. Each team member should thoroughly understand the microscope and every aspect of microsurgical techniques.

Team members can be kept up to date by in-service explanation of new instruments and demonstration of the microscope. It is extremely helpful and contributory to understanding for the surgeon to show perioperative team members anatomic structures and instruments through the microscope. A comparison of microinstruments with standard instruments under the microscope is always a revelation.

A monitor is advantageous in providing the scrub person and anesthesia provider continuous observation of the surgical procedure. All members should be completely familiar with instrumentation. Not only are instruments properly cared for, but even more important, surgical time is reduced.

Ultrasonosurgery

Ultrasonosurgery, also referred to as cytoreductive debulking surgery, is useful in removing or reducing tumors in highly vascular, delicate tissue such as the brain, liver, kidney, and spleen. The original prototypes of ultrasonic equipment were developed in 1967 to fragment and aspirate cataracts. An ultrasonic aspirator, such as the Cavitron, simultaneously fragments, irrigates, and aspirates tissue.[8] During the fragmentation process, sterile fluid passes through the handpiece to emulsify target tissue. The emulsified tissue is aspirated and collected in a closed-container system. This method is infrequently used because tumor cells can remain in the body and disseminate.

A transducer in the handpiece converts electrical energy into mechanical motion. Ultrahigh-frequency sound waves produce vibrations at the tip. These vibrations are of the same physical nature as sound but with frequencies above the range of human hearing. Ultrasound has a frequency greater than 30,000 Hz. The vibrating tip of the ultrasonic aspirator fragments tissues at the cellular level. When the tip contacts tissue, vapor pockets within high-water-content cells cause cell walls to separate and collapse. The ultrasonic aspirator is used to disrupt tissues, or tracts, particularly in the central nervous system. It is also used to emulsify tumors with minimal mechanical trauma to surrounding nerves and blood vessels. A device that combines electrosurgery with ultrasonic dissection also allows coagulation during resection and aspiration of a tumor mass.

An ultrasonic probe can be inserted through an endoscope to fragment renal or ureteral calculi (i.e., kidney stones). A suction channel is incorporated into the probe to aspirate fragments as stone is pulverized by ultrasonic energy.

Ultrasonic Blade and Scissors

The harmonic scalpel is a handpiece that receives electrical energy from a generator activated by a foot pedal or finger control but does not function as an ESU. The bipolar energy is converted into mechanical vibrations at the rate of 55,000 waves per minute. The instrument cuts and spot-coagulates protein molecules by ultrasonic vibration with minimal thermal effects. The tissue dissolves on contact and coagulates in response to the protein denaturation.

The working end of the handpiece accommodates scissors or a blade tip. The tip should be kept clean with a moist sponge during the procedure and the team should avoid contact with any byproducts of the protein molecule destruction such as steam or plume. Although heat production is minimal, the risk for burning nontarget tissue is possible until the tip cools. Do not place the hot tip on a wet towel over the patient because the heat will transfer to the patient's tissues via the moisture and cause a burn. When activated, the generator emits a humming sound.

Integrated Technologies

As mentioned, several technologies may be used for minimally invasive surgical procedures. Video-assisted laser endoscopy allows the surgeon to remove organs and tumors and ablate or repair tissues without making a major incision. An endoscope is introduced into a body cavity through a small incision. The viewing area from the telescopic lens of the scope is magnified from a video camera to a video screen. While viewing the screen, the surgeon can direct a laser beam through the endoscope to the target tissue. (Endoscopy is described in detail in Chapter 32.)

Other instrumentation may be introduced through adjacent small incisions for dissection, ligation, and suturing. These instruments can be manipulated while the surgeon looks through the endoscope or at a monitor. Manipulations may be observed with use of fluoroscopy or a video camera. Ultrasonic and thermal probes, electrosurgical electrodes, and laser beams can be directed through endoscopes.

Laser beams also can be directed through the operating microscope. Lasers and microscopes may be controlled by computerized systems. Computers can automatically scan tissues to select target tissue for the laser beam. Operating microscopes may contain voice-activated minicomputers that manipulate controls for fine adjustments, thus eliminating foot and hand switches.

EVOLVE WEBSITE

http://evolve.elsevier.com/Hornacky/BerryKohn/

- Historical Perspective
- Student Interactive Questions
- Glossary

References

1. Etheridge J, Moyal-Smith R, Lim S, et al.: Utility of a device briefing tool to improve surgical safety, *J Surg Res* 280:218−225, 2022.
2. Benias P, Carr-Locke D: Principles of electrosurgery. In Baron T, Kozarek R, Carr-Locke D, editors: *ERCP*, ed 3, St. Louis, 2019, Elsevier, pp 86−92.
3. Borgmeier P, Ricketts C, Clymer J, et al.: A review of capacitive return electrode in electrosurgery, *J Sci* 9(1):31−35, 2021.
4. U.S. Food and Drug Administration: *Compliance guide for laser products*. www.fda.gov. Accessed May 5, 2023.
5. Morris M, Hwang JH: Electrosurgery in therapeutic endoscopy. In *Clinical gastrointestinal endoscopy*, ed 3, St. Louis, 2019, Elsevier, pp 69−80.
6. Sakamoto F, Avram M, Anderson R: Lasers and other energy-based technologies: principals and skin interactions. In *Dermatology*, ed 4, St. Louis, 2018, Elsevier, pp 2354−2364.
7. Occupational Safety and Health Administration: *Laser hazards*. www.osha.gov. Accessed May 5, 2023.
8. Pio L, Guerin F, Martucci C, et al.: The use of Cavitron ultrasonic surgical aspirator for high-risk neuroblastoma with image-defined risk factors in children, *Children* 10:89, 2023.

Bibliography

AORN: *Guidelines for perioperative practice*, Denver, CO, 2024, The Association.

21

Preoperative Preparation of the Patient

CHAPTER OUTLINE

Hospitalized Patient, 379

Preoperative Preparation of All Patients, 379

Transportation to the Operating Room Suite, 390

Admission to the Operating Room Suite, 390

CHAPTER OBJECTIVES

After studying this chapter the learner will be able to:

- Discuss the importance of preoperative preparation.
- Describe the content of preoperative patient teaching.
- List several preoperative assessment factors relevant to all presurgical patients.

- Identify the key elements in a successful preoperative interview.

KEY TERMS AND DEFINITIONS

Anxiety Emotional state characterized by subjective feelings of tension, apprehension, and/or worry. The autonomic nervous system is activated.

Electronic medical record (EMR) Patient charts are primarily electronic and require password access. Paper documentation is not used in all facilities.

Preadmission testing (PAT) Preadmission testing area where preoperative patients are assessed and instructed.

Presurgical holding area Area within the perioperative environment where the patient waits immediately before entering the operating room.

Hospitalized Patient

Regardless of the physical setting in which an invasive or surgical procedure will be performed, each patient should be adequately assessed and prepared so the effects and potential risks of the surgical intervention are minimized. This involves both physical and emotional preparation. Perioperative caregivers should establish a baseline for the patient's preoperative condition, so changes occurring during the perioperative/perianesthesia care period can be easily recognized.

Although most patients undergoing a surgical procedure are admitted the day of surgery, some are admitted to the hospital one or more days before the scheduled procedure. The acuity of illness or the patient's general health status, as well as the surgical procedure to be performed, will influence whether the patient should be admitted to the hospital preoperatively or can arrive the day of the procedure. Radiologic, endoscopic, or other diagnostic studies may be performed to confirm the medical diagnosis. Systemic disease or chronic illness, such as diabetes or heart disease, should be under control to the extent possible preoperatively. A procedure may be rescheduled if a patient has an abnormal test result or needs cardiac clearance from a cardiologist for safety.

Most patients who will remain in the hospital postoperatively are admitted the day of the surgical procedure. Often referred to as

AM or morning admission, to come in (TCI), or to be admitted (TBA), these patients may be prepared for the procedure in a same-day admission unit before transferring to the operating room (OR) suite. (Some facilities have a preoperative check-in area within the OR suite.) From the OR, some patients may go to the postanesthesia care unit (PACU) to recover from anesthesia before being transferred to a patient care unit; others are transferred directly from the OR to the intensive care unit (ICU). The magnitude of the surgical procedure and the patient's postoperative needs for complex care will determine when the patient can be discharged safely.

Preoperative Preparation of All Patients

Specific activities such as the preoperative history and physical examination are completed and documented before the patient arrives in the OR. This process can be performed before admission to the hospital or ambulatory care facility; other activities are performed when the patient arrives in the preadmission testing (PAT) area. The preoperative physical preparation is designed to help all patients overcome the stresses of anesthesia, pain, fluid and blood loss, immobilization, and tissue trauma. Preparation often begins before the patient's hospital admission, with the institution of nutritional or drug therapy. An attempt is made to bring all patients to their best possible physical status before surgery. Appropriate consultations, such as a cardiac workup, weight loss, or physical therapy, are sought when necessary. Some facilities offer programs that include preoperative and postoperative therapies for total joint, cardiac rehabilitation, and bariatric surgeries.

Preadmission Procedures

Some preoperative preparations can be performed in the surgeon's office. Patients are then referred to the preoperative testing center of the hospital or ambulatory care facility. Tests and records should be completed and available before the patient is admitted the day of the surgical procedure. PATs are scheduled according to the guidelines of each facility. Some tests are acceptable for up to a 30-day period or are repeated before admission. The type of testing performed depends on the patient's known or suspected condition, type of anesthesia, and the complexity of the surgical procedure. The preoperative preparations include the following[1]:

1. *Medical history and physical examination:* These are performed and documented by a physician, nurse practitioner, physician assistant (PA), or the registered nurse first assistant (RNFA). A list of medications and herbal supplements should be documented, and any allergies and sensitivities should be noted. The preoperative nurse establishes the baseline for the patient's vital signs (Fig. 21.1).

2. *Laboratory tests:* Testing should be based on specific clinical indicators or risk factors that could affect surgical management or anesthesia. Tests include age, sex, preexisting disease, magnitude of surgical procedure, and type of anesthesia. Ideally these tests should be completed 24 hours before admission so the results are available for review. Some facilities perform laboratory studies the morning of the procedure.
   a. Hemoglobin, hematocrit, blood urea nitrogen, and blood glucose may be routinely tested for patients.
   b. Hematocrit is usually ordered for women before the administration of a general anesthetic.
   c. Complete blood count and blood chemistry profile may be indicated. Differential, platelet count, activated partial thromboplastin time, and prothrombin time tests also may be ordered.
   d. Urinalysis may be indicated by the type of surgical procedure, medical history, and/or physical examination.
   e. A pregnancy test may be required for females of childbearing age who have not had a hysterectomy.

3. *Blood type and crossmatch:* If a transfusion is anticipated, the patient's blood is typed and crossmatched. Many patients prefer to have their own blood drawn and stored for autotransfusion. Patients should be advised that blood banks charge an additional fee to store and preserve autologous blood for personal use.

Even if the patient is to have an autotransfusion, their blood should still be typed and crossmatched in the event that additional transfusions are needed. If the patient refuses to accept blood transfusions, the appropriate documentation of refusal should be completed according to the policies and procedures of the facility.

4. *Chest radiograph:* A preoperative chest x-ray study is not routinely required for all patients. It may be required by facility policy or medically indicated as an adjunct to the clinical evaluation of patients with cardiac or pulmonary disease and for smokers, patients aged 60 years or older, and cancer patients.

5. *Electrocardiogram (ECG):* If the patient has known or suspected cardiac disease, an ECG is mandatory. Depending on the policy of the facility, an ECG may be routine for patients ages 40 years or older.

6. *Diagnostic procedures:* Special diagnostic procedures are performed when specifically indicated (e.g., Doppler studies for vascular surgery).

7. *Written instructions:* The patient should receive written preoperative instructions to follow before admission for the surgical procedure. The written literature should be written with the patient's literacy level in mind. Additional methods of instruction should be made available for patients with special needs. Do not use abbreviations or acronyms because they can be confused and misunderstood. Web-based videos can be helpful for patients who cannot read. These instructions should be reviewed with the patient in the surgeon's office or in the preoperative testing center (Fig. 21.2).
   a. To prevent regurgitation or emesis and aspiration of gastric contents, the patient should not ingest solid foods before the surgical procedure. These instructions are usually stated as *NPO* (NPO is the Latin abbreviation for nil per os, or nothing by mouth). Solid foods empty from the stomach after changing to a liquid state, which may take up to 12 hours. The patient should be given an NPO time based on the time of surgery.

   Clear fluids may be unrestricted until 2 to 3 hours before the surgical procedure, but only at the discretion of the surgeon or anesthesia provider in selected patients. NPO time usually is reduced for infants, small children, patients with diabetes, and older adults prone to dehydration.

   b. The physician may want the patient to continue any essential medications. These can be taken as prescribed with a minimal fluid intake (a few sips of water) up to 1 hour before the surgical procedure. Diabetic patients may be asked to hold

• **Fig. 21.1** Performance of the preoperative assessment is important to establish a health baseline. Vital signs, height in centimeters, weight in kilograms, and review of systems should be done.

GETBETTER HOSPITAL

PREOPERATIVE INSTRUCTIONS

Your doctor has scheduled your surgery to be performed at Getbetter Hospital on _____ (day) _____ (date) at _____ AM/PM. Please arrive at _____ AM/PM.

If you develop a cold, flu, or illness before surgery or cannot keep your surgery appointment, please call your surgeon.

DIETARY RESTRICTIONS

- Avoid alcoholic beverages and cigarette smoking for at least 24 hours before surgery.
- Finish dinner the evening before surgery no later than 8 PM.
- Nothing to eat or drink after midnight the night before surgery.
  (This includes candy, gum, mints, Lifesavers, ice chips, and water.)
- Eating or drinking may result in the delay or cancellation of surgery.
- Medications to be taken the day of surgery _____ with sip (1 ounce) of water.
- Medications *not* to be taken the day of surgery _____ .

FOR YOUR SAFETY AND COMFORT

- No makeup—it may cause eye irritation or corneal abrasions while under anesthesia.
- Remove nail polish and artificial nails from at least one finger on each hand—oxygen is measured by placing a sensor on your fingertip.
- Do not bring valuables or jewelry—jewelry must be removed before surgery.
- Dress simply in loose-fitting clothes (sweatsuits or yoga attire are ideal).

UPON YOUR ARRIVAL

- Report to Main Lobby Admissions Desk.

AFTER YOUR SURGERY

- No driving, operating of heavy machinery, heavy physical activity, or decision making for 24 hours after receiving an anesthetic.
- If you are returning home on the same day as your surgery, make arrangements for a responsible adult to accompany you. Your operation cannot be performed if a responsible adult is not with you.
- Call your surgeon for postoperative appointments.

If you have any questions, do not hesitate to call the <u>Preadmission Testing Unit</u> at xxx-xxx-xxxx or <u>The Department of Anesthesia</u> at xxx-xxx-xxxx.

Patient signature: _____

RN signature: _____

• **Fig. 21.2** Sample of written preoperative instructions for the patient.

medications the day of surgery. Patients taking anticoagulants or steroids may be asked to stop the medication for a specific number of days before the procedure.

c. The skin should be cleansed to prepare the surgical site. Many surgeons want patients to clean the surgical area with an antimicrobial soap or wipes preoperatively. The patient may be instructed to shower with an antimicrobial soap, commonly chlorhexidine, for several days before and the morning of surgery.[2] Patients should be told not to allow the soap to get in the eyes or ears. Chlorhexidine preparations can harm the corneas and tympanic membranes. Patients who will undergo a surgical procedure on the face, ear, or neck are advised to shampoo their hair before admission because this may not be permitted again for a few days or weeks after the procedure.

d. Nail polish and acrylic nails should be removed to permit observation of and access to the nailbed during the surgical procedure. The patient should be advised to uncover at least one fingernail if the anesthesia provider will use these monitoring devices during the procedure. Either the finger or toe can be used when a digit is desired, but the finger is usually more accessible.

Some sensors are adhesive and can be placed on an earlobe or across the bridge of the nose. The nailbed is a vascular area, and the color of the nailbed is one indicator of peripheral oxygenation and circulation. The Oxisensor (optode) of a pulse oximeter may be attached to the nailbed to monitor oxygen saturation and pulse rate. A finger cuff may be used for continuous blood pressure monitoring. Nail polish or acrylic nails inhibit contact between these devices and the vascular bed.

  e. Jewelry and valuables should be left at home to ensure safekeeping. If electrosurgery will be used, patients should be informed that all metal jewelry, including wedding bands, religious artifacts, and piercings should be removed to prevent possible burns. Loss prevention is a consideration as well.
  f. Patients should be given other special instructions about what is expected, such as when to arrive at the surgical facility. A responsible adult should be available to take the patient home if the procedure, medication, or anesthetic agent renders the patient incapable of driving. Family members or significant others should know where to wait and where the patient will be taken after the surgical procedure.
8. *Informed consent:* The physician should obtain informed consent from the patient or legal designee. After explaining the surgical procedure and its risks, benefits, and alternatives, the surgeon should document the process and have the patient sign the consent form. This documentation becomes part of the permanent record and accompanies the patient to the OR. Policy and state laws dictate the parameters for ascertaining an informed consent.
9. *Nurse interview:* A perioperative/perianesthesia nurse should meet with the patient to make a preoperative assessment. Through physiologic and psychosocial assessments the nurse collects data for the nursing diagnoses, expected outcomes, and plan of care.

From the assessment data and nursing diagnoses, the nurse establishes expected outcomes with the patient. The nurse develops the plan of care, which becomes a part of the patient's record. The nurse reviews the written preoperative instructions and consent form with the patient to assess the patient's knowledge and understanding. The nurse also provides emotional support and teaches the patient in preparation for postoperative recovery. Educational information and instruction may be given with a list of additional resources.

10. *Anesthesia assessment:* An anesthesia history and physical assessment are performed before a general or regional anesthetic is administered. The history may be obtained by the surgeon, and/or the patient may be asked to complete a questionnaire for the anesthesia provider in the surgeon's office or in the preoperative testing center.

An interview by an anesthesia provider or nurse anesthetist may be conducted before admission if the patient has a complex medical history, is high risk, or has a high degree of anxiety. All patients should understand the risks of and alternatives to the type of anesthetic to be administered. After discussion with the anesthesia provider, the patient should sign an anesthesia consent form.

A preoperative phone call by a perioperative nurse to the patient several days in advance of the scheduled surgical procedure may prevent cancellation because of inadequate preoperative testing. Testing requirements are reviewed with the patient, and arrangements for additional tests can be made as needed. The importance of preoperative preparations (such as colon prep) is reiterated, especially NPO status, when to take medications, and the availability of a responsible adult for transportation home after the surgical procedure (if having ambulatory surgery).

Before an Elective Surgical Procedure

In addition to the preadmission procedures described, the surgeon may write specific orders for other appropriate preoperative preparations.[3] All preadmission assessment and testing procedures may be performed after the patient is admitted to a surgical unit before the surgical procedure. Some patients may have the following requirements:
1. Bowel preparation: "Enemas till clear" may be ordered when it is advantageous to have the bowel and rectum empty (e.g., gastrointestinal procedures such as bowel resection or endoscopy, and surgical procedures in the pelvic, perineal, or perianal areas). An intestinal lavage with an oral solution that induces diarrhea may be ordered to clear the intestine of feces. Solutions such as GoLYTELY or Colyte normally will clear the bowel in 4 to 6 hours. Because potassium is lost during diarrhea, serum potassium levels should be checked before the surgical procedure. Geriatric, underweight, and malnourished patients are prone to other electrolyte disturbances from intestinal lavage.
2. Bedtime sedation for sleep in select circumstances for in-house patients.
3. The patient may be sent to the radiology department for x-rays or placement of a J-wire before breast biopsy surgery.

Preoperative Visit by the Perioperative/Perianesthesia Nurse

The patient should be assessed preoperatively. Every effort should be made through supportive measures to minimize the potential hazards of adverse psychosocial distress. Ideally this assessment takes place before the day of the surgical procedure; its purpose is to alleviate anxiety and fears. Factual information and clarification of misunderstandings will be helpful in this regard, as will the opportunity for the patient to express their feelings.

The broadened scope of perioperative nursing encompasses the phases of preoperative and postoperative care that contribute to the continuity of patient care. Preoperative visits to patients are made by RNFAs or perioperative/perianesthesia nurses skilled in interviewing and assessment. The interview provides the nurse an opportunity to learn about the patient, establish rapport, and develop a plan of care before the patient is brought to the perioperative environment.

Pros of Preoperative Visits

Preoperative visits with patients include the following list of advantages:
1. An experienced perioperative/perianesthesia nurse is well qualified to discuss a patient's OR experience. The nurse can

orient and prepare the patient and family/significant others for the procedure and the postoperative period.

2. The perioperative/perianesthesia nurse can review critical data before the procedure and assess the patient before planning care. The surgical site is marked with initials by the surgeon or surgeon's designee. An X is never used to mark the surgical site. Some surgical sites cannot be marked. The facility should have a policy and procedure for identifying surgical sites that cannot be easily marked, such as perineal regions, teeth, pharyngeal, intracranial, and other areas of the body not readily seen and initialed.

3. Visits improve and individualize intraoperative care and efficiency and prevent needless delays in the OR.

4. Visits foster a meaningful nurse-patient relationship. Some patients are reluctant to reveal feelings and needs to someone in a short-term relationship.

5. Visits make intraoperative observations more meaningful by establishing a baseline for the measurement of patient outcomes.

6. Visits contribute to patient cooperation and involvement by facilitating communication. Mutual goals and expected outcomes are more easily developed.

7. Visits enhance the positive self-image of the perioperative nurse and contribute to job satisfaction, which in turn reduce job turnover and are thus benefits to the hospital. Because of increased patient contact, visits make perioperative and perianesthesia nursing more attractive to those who enjoy patient proximity and teaching.

Cons of Preoperative Visits

The disadvantages associated with preoperative visits include the following:

1. Cost-containment measures may not provide adequate qualified staffing or allow time to visit patients.

2. The admission of patients on the day of the surgical procedure or late the day before the procedure makes the timing of visits difficult.

3. Visits may produce friction among different patient care divisions if the preoperative visit program is not well planned and performed.

4. Repetitious use of interviewing terminology may lead to a lack of enthusiasm and spontaneity on the part of nurse interviewers.

5. If the nurse's interviewing skills are not practiced, patients may feel their privacy is being invaded. This could foster mistrust of the health care personnel.

6. Barriers to visits may arise from the perioperative nurse's inability to do the following functions:
   a. Verbalize and communicate effectively.
   b. Handle or accept a patient's illness.
   c. Handle emotionally stressed persons.
   d. Understand cultural, ethnic, and value system differences.
   e. Function efficiently outside of their customary environment.
   f. Recognize how personal beliefs and biases can influence objectivity.

Interviewing Skills

Interviewing is a form of verbal interaction and is a valuable tool for obtaining information. The interview can be directive and structured with predetermined questions in a specific, predetermined

order that limits responses. An example of a directive question is "Have you had a surgical procedure before?" A nondirective interview gives the patient more of an opportunity to respond openly. An example of a nondirective question is "Can you tell me about your previous surgical experience?" The choice of technique depends on the information desired.

Determine the level of patient understanding about the surgical procedure. One method is to ask "Can you tell me what we will be doing for you during your surgical procedure?" Some patients will not be able to articulate the terms or adequately describe the procedure. Direct inquiry about specific procedures may be necessary, but give the patient plenty of opportunities to describe the anticipated procedure in their own words. Nonverbal patients may be able to point to a body region.

A structured interview is valuable in learning about an individual's health history. The unstructured interview gives a portrait of the patient's emotional reactions, concerns, and personality. An effective preoperative interview usually includes questions about both facts and feelings. The informal observation of nonverbal behavior is an essential component of the interview. The setting should be conducive to communication, and all questions should be relevant. The interviewer should be able to handle the situation with spontaneity, judgment, and tact. The interview should be meaningful to both the patient and the nurse.

Structured Preoperative Visits

1. Review the patient's chart and electronic medical records (EMRs). Focus on medical and nursing diagnoses and the surgical procedure to be performed. Collect any information relevant to planning care in the OR. If the patient is admitted to the hospital, discuss the assessment data and the plan of care with the unit nurses before visiting the patient.

Consideration is given to the patient who is a health care professional. Nurses, surgeons, technologists, and others may need surgical intervention. They may have extended knowledge of what will be done in the procedure and the potential for complications beyond what the average patient may possess. It is suggested that these patients be treated with respect for their knowledge, but still treated as patients. Do not assume they know everything about what will happen. Elicit feedback as the visit progresses to determine where to fill in or hold back on explanations. Never discuss personal information concerning the patient who is a health care professional with colleagues unless it is a need-to-know situation involving direct care. Privacy is a serious ethical concern.

The perioperative nurse should not do the preoperative visit for a family member, neighbor, or friend. This visit should be deferred to another nurse, who is unknown to the patient.

Nursing data include the following pertinent information; these baseline parameters are essential for accurate intraoperative and postoperative assessment.

a. Biographic information (name, age, sex, family status, ethnic background, educational level, literacy, patterns of living, previous hospitalization and surgical procedures, religion).

b. Physical findings (vital signs; height; weight; skin integrity; allergies; the presence of pain, drainage, or bleeding; state of consciousness and orientation; sensory or physical deficits; assistive aids or prosthetics).

c. Special therapy (tracheostomy, inhalation therapy, hyperalimentation).

d. Emotional status (understanding, expectations, specific problems concerning comfort, safety, language barrier, and other concerns).

2. Choose an optimal time and place without interruptions. Handwashing should be done before and after the visit.

a. Patients who will be admitted on the day of the surgical procedure may be interviewed in the preoperative testing center several days before the surgical procedure. If this is not feasible, a telephone call to the patient may provide an alternative means of contact.

b. Patients who have been admitted to the hospital may be visited in a patient care unit the day before the surgical procedure.

c. Allow adequate time for the interview, usually 10 to 20 minutes unless the patient has complex problems or special needs that require more time. Give the patient time to think and respond and to ask questions.

d. If the patient is in acute physical or psychologic distress, offer support and consider rescheduling the visit. The visit may need to be canceled or conducted through a family member or significant other. An emergency surgical patient may be assessed in the preoperative holding area.

e. Do not conduct the interview on the morning of the procedure unless there is no other option. Patients are not psychologically receptive to preoperative teaching at this time. Premedicated patients may be susceptible to suggestions such as "You will have minimal discomfort after the surgical procedure."

3. Greet the patient by introducing yourself and explaining the purpose of the visit. Tell the patient that the visit is a routine part of care so that they do not feel singled out because of their medical diagnosis. Unless specifically requested to use a first name, always show respect by addressing the patient by their last name, preceded by Mr., Mrs., or Ms. Terms such as "honey," "dear," or "sweetheart" are unacceptable. Children are usually addressed by their given first name unless asked to use a nickname.

a. Put the patient at ease. Sit close enough so the patient can easily see and hear you. Avoid standing over the patient. Sitting will make the patient feel that there is no hurry.

b. Secure the patient's attention and cooperation. Establish eye contact.

c. Speak first with the patient alone (unless the patient is a small child, an individual who needs an interpreter, or an individual who is mentally impaired). This affords the patient privacy and encourages them to talk freely. Then, if the patient is willing, the family and significant others may be invited to participate and ask questions. They should also be present during the preoperative teaching to learn how to assist the patient postoperatively.

d. Allow the patient to maintain self-respect and dignity.

e. Instill confidence in the patient by having a neat appearance and a positive attitude. Establish rapport by demonstrating warmth and genuine interest. Avoid displaying an authoritative manner.

f. Use language at the patient's level of development, understanding, and education.[4]

Gathering Information

1. Obtain information by asking about the patient's understanding of the surgical procedure. Disfiguring or palliative procedures can be stressful to the patient. Psychologic counseling may be indicated.

a. Assess the patient's level of information and understanding and check its accuracy to determine whether further instruction or clarification is needed. Ask questions such as "What has your surgeon told you about the surgical procedure?" Correct any misconceptions about the surgical procedure as appropriate within the scope of nursing.

b. Permit the patient to talk openly. The objective is to gather data that will generate the plan of care to be implemented by the perioperative team.

c. Direct questions should be used with caution and are not suitable for collecting all objective data. Construct open-ended questions to elicit information more detailed than one-word answers.

d. Listen attentively. To preserve self-esteem the patient may tell you what they think you want to hear. A patient's statement that ends in a question may be either a request for more information or an expression of a feeling or attitude.

2. Orient the patient to the environment of the OR suite and interpret policies and routines.

a. Tell the patient the scheduled time of the surgical procedure, the approximate length of the procedure, and the probable length of stay in the PACU. Explain the procedures that will be performed in the preoperative holding area before the surgery if this is the routine.

b. Ask the patient who will be at the facility during the surgical procedure. They should be informed how early to be there to see the patient before sedation is given. Direct them to the waiting room.

c. Tell the patient that family and significant others will be updated on the progress of the surgical procedure and informed when they arrive in the PACU if this is hospital policy. Communicating the progress of the procedure, especially if it is prolonged, provides emotional support and decreases anxiety. Some facilities use smart boards for tracking patient progress.

3. Review the preoperative preparations that the patient will experience.

a. Familiarize the patient with whom and what will be seen in the perioperative environment. Many perioperative nurses wear OR attire and cover jackets with displayed name tag when they visit patients; attire can familiarize patients with the way they will see personnel the next day.

b. Use discretion regarding how much the patient should know and wants to know. Use words that do not evoke an anxiety-inducing state of mind. Do not use words with unpleasant associations, such as *knife, needle,* or *nausea.*

c. Postoperative recovery begins with preoperative teaching, but keep the explanations short and simple. Excessive detail can increase patient anxiety, which reduces the attention span.

d. Give practical information about what the patient should expect, such as withholding fluids, drowsiness, and/or dry mouth caused by preoperative medications; transportation to the OR and the holding area; and where they will be taken after the surgical procedure. Instruct the patient not to hesitate to ask for assistance at any time. Explain any other relevant special precautions.

e. Give the basic reasons for procedures and regulations; this reduces patient anxiety. With children and older adults, the nurse may have to repeat information as reinforcement.

f. Explain only the procedures of which the patient will be aware.

g. If the patient will be going to the ICU after the procedure, prepare family and significant others what they will see and hear, such as monitors and machines.

4. Tell the patient that an anesthesia provider will visit to discuss specific questions relative to anesthesia if this is routine.

5. Answer the patient's questions about the surgical procedure in general terms. Refer specific questions to the surgeon.

a. Be honest and responsible in communications about a proposed diagnostic or surgical procedure. Complement, but do not overlap, the surgeon's area of responsibility. Do not be unrealistic, falsify the truth, or give false reassurances. Do not say things such as "It will be alright" or "Everything will be fine." Better to express, "We will take very good care of you."

b. Be extremely cautious about spelling out specific details of the treatment, procedure, and postoperative care unless you have been thoroughly briefed by the surgeon in charge. Surgeons individualize and tailor the plan of care to their own techniques and the patient's needs, and certain forms of therapy may be controversial. Continual interdisciplinary communication is essential.

c. If unable or unprepared to answer a legitimate question, tell the patient that the concern will be answered by the appropriate personnel. For example, say, "I don't know, but I'll get that information for you." Then be certain to follow up with an answer.

6. Encourage the patient, family, and significant others to discuss their feelings or anxieties regarding the surgical procedure and anticipated results.

a. Motivate and assist the patient, family, and significant others to gain perspective, objectivity, awareness, and insight. A skilled professional nurse will know how to discourage wishful thinking for miraculous cures while also communicating an understanding of fears and wishes for an uncomplicated, fast recovery.

b. Observe emotional reactions.

Addressing Patient Needs

1. As an interviewer, be objective about personal feelings. Listen to what the patient is asking without feeling threatened. Do not superimpose personal feelings onto what the patient is expressing. Empathy is appropriate in this environment.

a. Acknowledge the effect of the procedure on the patient's sexuality if appropriate. Allow the patient to express personal feelings without evoking shame or guilt. Address the needs of a transgender or diverse patient if necessary.[5] Include family or significant others as the patient desires. Adolescent patients may not want to talk about personal issues in front of parents.

b. Try to help the patient solve their own problems when possible. Ask open-ended questions that help explore a subject or feelings, but do not probe to elicit specific responses. Do not destroy the patient's coping mechanism; encourage

an appropriate one. The visit is not a structured psychiatric counseling session.

c. Listen to the anxieties of the patient, family, or significant others in a realistic time frame, and get others to follow through as necessary. Do not attempt too full an agenda, but sort out what is legitimate. You cannot solve all problems in 20 minutes. For example, say, "I'll share this information with someone who can help you with this problem." Use a colleague's expertise to assist you or to make a proper referral.

d. Comfort the patient and convey a sense of security and trust. Use touch as appropriate. Touch has a positive effect on physiologic parameters, such as respiration and circulation, and it can lower heart rate and blood pressure. Its calming effect can improve perceptual and cognitive abilities. It establishes rapport, provides reassurance, and conveys warmth, empathy, encouragement, and support. Touch should be comfortable. A perceptive nurse can tell when a patient resents being touched; respect the patient's feelings. Patients with decreased visual acuity appreciate the assurance that touch can give, but always speak first to avoid startling the patient. Remember to wash hands after the visit.

e. Reassure the patient that they will not be alone but will be constantly attended by competent perioperative team members. Try to increase the patient's trust and confidence in the team.

f. Allow time to deal with the patient's questions or concerns. Ask the patient, "Do you have any other concerns?" Never bring a patient's feelings into the open and then cut off the conversation. Do not interrupt, interrogate, or belittle an expressed fear or seemingly irrelevant topic. All questions are significant to the patient. Answer the questions honestly, and try to resolve concerns.

2. Identify any special needs of the patient that will alter the plan for intraoperative care. The preoperative visit is the time for a total assessment to guard against a traumatic experience for the patient.

a. Observe any physical characteristics of the patient that might affect positioning or require special setups. The plan of care will include considerations for extra tall, obese, or left-handed patients. For example, an intravenous (IV) infusion should be started in the right arm of a left-handed person to minimize the limitation of manual dexterity unless contraindicated.

b. Observe the patient for physical limitations such as pain on moving, an amputated extremity, paralysis, or sensory loss. This information enables the circulating nurse to anticipate how much cooperation to expect from the patient and how much additional help may be needed. A pad of paper and pencil may be needed to communicate with a patient who is unable to speak or hear. In certain instances an interpreter may be needed.

c. Ask the patient whether they wear any type of prosthetic device. Explain, per accepted hospital policy, that the device should be removed before the surgical procedure, either at the bedside or in the OR. Explain that contact lenses, jewelry, or removable eyelashes should be removed to prevent damage or loss. Peripheral swelling of fingers can be complicated by the wearing of rings. Piercings could cause alternative pathway burns when cautery is used and could interfere with the surgical site.

d. Determine how a preexisting medical condition should be managed in the OR. For example, it is important that the circulating nurse know about the presence of an implanted pacemaker or defibrillator. A monopolar electrosurgery unit (ESU) could cause certain models of implanted devices to malfunction; therefore monopolar ESU would be contraindicated, and bipolar ESU should be used instead.

e. Know the patient's special requests. Placing a note on the front of the chart or in a special section of the EMR is one method of relaying temporary information about a patient's special requests. These notes are not part of the permanent record.

3. Use educational materials to supplement the interview, if available and appropriate.

a. Written instructions with photographs or drawings are useful for explaining procedures and equipment. These can be presented in a booklet, coloring book for children, or pamphlet that the patient can keep and share with family members or significant others.

b. Use of smart devices, videos, slide/taped programs, or DVDs helps reinforce the preoperative teaching.

Preoperative Teaching

Teaching is a function of perioperative nursing practice and embraces perception, thought, feeling, and performance. During the preoperative visit the perioperative nurse supplements the instructions of the other perioperative team members and gives information unique to the patient's specific surgical procedure. Care is taken not to use jargon and explanations the patient does not understand.

The perioperative nurse teaches patients how to participate in their own postoperative recovery. Patients must have a readiness to learn. Preoperative teaching should take place at three levels:

1. *Information:* Explanations of procedures, patient care activities, and physical feelings that the patient may encounter during the perioperative experience help the patient identify what is happening and what to expect. Such explanations also enhance patient satisfaction with care.

2. *Psychosocial support:* Interactions enhance coping mechanisms to deal with anxiety and fears and provide emotional comfort.

3. *Skill training:* Guided practice of specific tasks to be performed by the patient in the postoperative period can decrease anxiety, hasten recovery, and help prevent complications.

Effective Teaching

Patient teaching involves emotional energy on the part of the nurse. It can produce behavioral changes in patients as they become better prepared, both physically and emotionally, for the surgical procedure. They also learn how to use the health care system. Learning self-help has a positive effect. Discharge planning begins during preoperative teaching. The patient knows what to expect and where to go for help after discharge if needed, such as a support group.

Patient teaching may be conducted in an informal, individual manner or in a formal, group instructional setting. In conjunction with other team members the nurse-instructor should first formulate attainable learning objectives with the patient's input. The development of learning objectives is based on the assessed level of the patient's emotional receptivity and mental capacity.

The nurse also assesses, by observation and elicited response, factors such as the patient's developmental level, sight, hearing,

and acceptance of patient problems. Before beginning an explanation, the nurse should verify what the patient already knows, needs to know, and wants to know. An understanding relationship with the patient facilitates the teaching/learning experience.

The nurse assists family and significant others in coping with the situation to the extent of their ability. The success or failure of treatment often depends on what happens after the patient leaves the hospital. Knowledge and understanding of the patient's needs, coping skills, and their willingness to help are important factors in recovery. Teaching should be presented at the level of resources and knowledge base. Other points to consider include:

1. Arrange the environment so that a teaching/learning exchange can take place. A quiet, undisturbed environment and proper timing are important.

2. Language is the fundamental tool for education. Use understandable terms. Do not equate intelligence level with educational level. The nurse is accountable for what is taught.

3. Set priorities and teach what is significant and appropriate to the patient's particular needs.

a. Break down instructions into manageable steps; for example, instruct the patient to breathe deeply and then cough while splinting the site of the surgical incision with a pillow.

b. Put content into a logical sequence of activities to facilitate learning. For example, to avoid the possibility of an inappropriate dosage, instruct the patient to write down the time medication is taken when at home.

c. Give the reasons for and the benefits of specific activities. For example, the movement of legs and toes and ambulation postoperatively, unless contraindicated, aid circulation and prevent venous stasis.

d. Adapt the teaching method and timing to the specific situation. The patient may reject teaching not relevant to the immediate present. For example, a patient about to have a heart procedure may listen to instructions but may be concentrating on the fact that their heart is going to be cut open.

e. Do not overburden the patient with a multitude of facts.

4. Recognize the patient's need to know. This recognition, not pressure, should be the motivating factor in learning.

5. To evaluate understanding, ask the patient to repeat in their own words what has been explained during the instructional session and to demonstrate deep breathing and leg exercises.

6. Written information is helpful in reviewing verbal instruction. Go over the material with the patient, and test their comprehension by asking questions. A patient who is experiencing pain or anxiety or who is under the influence of medication may not fully understand verbal communication.

7. As the resource person, be consistent, concise, and organized. Repeat instructions to help the patient retain them.

Patients who receive preoperative instructions from and interact with the perioperative nurse may experience less apprehension, better tolerate the surgical procedure, and seem more secure and comfortable postoperatively. Patients usually remember what has been taught. They react more positively to their perioperative experience than do patients who have not been given the benefit of this interaction.

At the end of the preoperative assessment and teaching session the perioperative nurse should not depart from the patient abruptly but should briefly summarize the events that have taken place. The nurse should give the patient time for any questions before leaving. The patient should be left with the understanding that a postoperative visit may be made after the procedure if this is the policy.

Preoperative Visit by the Anesthesia Provider

The anesthesia provider is knowledgeable in the pathophysiology of disease as it pertains to anesthetic agents. Participation in the patient's preoperative preparation can reduce intraoperative complications. If the patient has been admitted the evening before the surgical procedure, the anesthesia provider usually assesses the patient if anesthesia is scheduled. Otherwise the patient may be seen before admission in the preoperative testing center, in the same-day procedures unit, or in the preoperative holding area. All patients should be evaluated before any anesthetic is administered.

Judgment and skill are important in the selection of agents and the administration of anesthesia, but firsthand knowledge of the patient is extremely valuable. The anesthesia provider visits the patient to seek information and establish rapport, inspire confidence and trust, and alleviate fear. Preparation for anesthesia begins with this visit.

Before meeting the patient, the anesthesia provider reviews the patient's past and present medical records. If recent laboratory or other test reports are not in the chart, all decisions and the surgical procedure are delayed until all essential information is available. Special attention is given to past surgical procedures and any disease or complicating processes, especially those involving vital organs or administration of anesthesia drugs.

After introduction to the patient, the anesthesia provider performs the following tasks:

1. Obtains a history pertinent to the administration of anesthetic agents by questioning the patient about past anesthetic experiences, allergies, adverse reactions to drugs, and habitual drug usage (Fig. 21.3). Tranquilizers, cortisone, heart and blood pressure medications, alcohol, herbal preparations, and recreational drugs, for example, influence the course of anesthesia. Smoking habits, genetic and metabolic problems, and reactions to previous blood transfusions also influence the choice of anesthetic.

Patients are advised to report all herbal supplements because they can cause serious complications such as bleeding (Table 21.1

• **Fig. 21.3** The anesthesia provider assesses the patient and plans the anesthetic for the surgical procedure.

describes common herbs and dietary supplements). The American Society of Anesthesiologists (ASA) cautions about herbal remedies and the serious complications that can ensue.

2. Evaluates the patient's physical, mental, and emotional status to determine the most appropriate type and amount of anesthetic agent(s).
   a. Examines the patient as necessary to obtain the information desired, with particular interest in the heart and lungs.
   b. Palpates the needle insertion site and observes for skin infection if a regional block anesthesia is contemplated.
   c. Assesses the patient's mental state and cognitive ability subjectively and observes for signs of anxiety.
3. Investigates the patient's cardiac reserve and observes for signs of dyspnea or claudication.
4. Asks the patient about their teeth, and loose or removable dental work such as dentures or bridges. If indicated, explains that dental work may be damaged inadvertently during airway insertion.
5. Evaluates the patient's physique for possible technical difficulties in the administration of the anesthetic. The patient will be asked to move their head and neck in a natural range of motion. The oropharynx will be assessed.
   a. A short, stout neck may cause respiratory problems or difficult intubation. A stiff neck or unstable cervical spine such as from rheumatoid arthritis can make intubation difficult or dangerous, especially in a geriatric patient. Fiberoptic laryngoscope and/or awake intubation may be necessary.
   b. Active athletic and obese patients require more anesthetic than do inactive patients.
   c. The patient's accurate weight should be known in both kilograms and pounds because the dosage of medications is calculated from body weight. Most dosages are calculated in milligrams per kilogram.
6. Explains preference of anesthetic, pending the surgeon's approval, and informs the patient what to expect concerning anesthesia. The patient's wishes are considered, if expressed.
7. Tells the patient or asks about restricted or prohibited oral intake before anesthesia, and gives the reasons for these restrictions. IV therapy is explained.
8. Discusses preoperative sedation in relation to the time the surgical procedure is scheduled to begin. Antibiotic administration is discussed if indicated 1 hour before the incision is made.
9. Reassures the patient that constant observation will be maintained during the surgical procedure and in the immediate postoperative period. Also explains the methods of monitoring vital functions.
10. Explains the risks of anesthesia without causing the patient undue stress.
11. Answers the patient's questions and allays fears related to anesthesia.

Anesthesia Plan of Care

After this visit with the patient, the anesthesia provider performs the following list of steps:
1. Estimates the effect of the necessary positioning during the surgical procedure on the patient's physiologic processes.
2. Records preliminary data on the anesthesia chart.

TABLE
21.1   **Examples of Common Herbal and Dietary Supplements and Potential Complications**

Herbal or Dietary Supplement	Action and Potential Complications	Notes on Patient Usage
St. John's wort	Prolonged sedative effect, photosensitivity, peripheral neuropathy, interferes with metabolism of some antibiotics, calcium channel blockers, and warfarin	Antidepressant, antiinflammatory, possibly antiviral
Ginkgo biloba	Bleeding, anticoagulant	Improves circulation and memory
Ginseng	Hypertension and tachycardia, hypoglycemia, bleeding	Boosts vitality, stimulant, enhances sexuality
Vitamin E	Bleeding, slows wound healing and collagen repair	Prevents heart disease
Vitamin A (beta carotene converts to vitamin A in the body)	Can cause complications in pregnancy	Reverses the adverse effects on wound healing caused by steroid use, enhances healing, boosts immune system, fights infection, fights inflammation
Vitamin C	Potential for kidney stones and anemia in toxic state; can interfere with vitamin B12; water-soluble; excreted readily via kidneys	Enhances wound healing
Garlic	Bleeding, hypotension, hypoglycemia, antithrombotic, antiplatelet	Lowers cholesterol, prevents heart disease, fights infection
Fish oil	Bleeding, hypotension	Prevents heart disease
Bromelain (found in pineapple stems)	No known complications	Antiinflammatory, digestive aid
Echinacea	Liver complications, interferes with immunosuppression, can cause transplant rejection	Antiinfective, fights common cold, enhances wound healing
Ephedra (also known as ma huang)	Cardiovascular instability, palpitations, hypertension, seizures	Appetite suppressant, respiratory treatment, boosts energy
Kava	Prolonged sedative effect, liver toxicity	Sedative, antiepileptic
Valerian	Prolonged sedative effect, can go through withdrawal, potentiated by alcohol, nausea	Sedative, sleep aid, muscle relaxant
Black cohosh	Bradycardia, peripheral dilation, hypotension	Alternative to estrogen replacement
Ginger	Bradycardia, bleeding, hypotension	Antiemetic, digestive aid, cough suppressant, relieves menstrual cramps
Licorice	Hypokalemia and dysrhythmia, hypertension, bleeding, can affect electrolytes, edema	Digestive aid
Dong quai	Can increase the risk for bleeding	Used to treat menstrual issues
Green tea	Can increase the risk for bleeding, may elevate heart rate and blood pressure	Stimulant
Saw palmetto	Can increase the risk for bleeding	Used to treat urinary retention in men with benign prostatic hypertrophy and hair loss
Chaparral	Liver complications	Alternative anticancer therapy
Chamomile	Potential allergy, bleeding, can affect electrolytes	Digestive aid, antiinflammatory, antiinfective

3. Writes preanesthesia orders, including times for medication administration.
4. Writes a summary of the visit and the proposed anesthetic management of the patient on the physicians' progress note. This summary has medicolegal value if a problem subsequently develops, and it is also necessary for regulatory accreditation, such as for the state or The Joint Commission (TJC).
5. Assigns the patient a physical status classification for the purpose of anesthesia, as per the taxonomy adopted by the ASA.
   a. Class I theoretically includes relatively healthy patients with localized pathologic processes. An emergency surgical procedure, designated E, signifies additional risk. For example, a hernia that becomes incarcerated changes the patient's status to Class I-E.
   b. Class II includes patients with mild systemic disease (e.g., type 2 diabetes controlled by oral hypoglycemic agents or diet).
   c. Class III includes patients with severe systemic disease that limits activity but is not totally incapacitating (e.g., chronic obstructive pulmonary disease or severe hypertension).
   d. Class IV includes patients with an incapacitating disease that is a constant threat to life (e.g., cardiovascular or renal disease).
   e. Class V includes moribund patients who are not expected to survive 24 hours with or without the surgical procedure. They are operated on in an attempt to save their life; the surgical procedure is a resuscitative measure, as in a massive pulmonary embolus. The patient may or may not survive the surgical procedure.

f. Class VI includes patients who have been declared brain dead but whose organs will be removed for donor purposes. Mechanical ventilation and life support systems are maintained until the organs are procured.

6. Consults with the surgeon and other physicians (e.g., cardiologist) about a patient who has been assigned a Class III, IV, or V status. Considers the critical nature of the surgical procedure in relation to the risks of anesthesia.
   a. In elective situations, the surgical procedure is postponed until anesthesia will be less hazardous (e.g., after acute respiratory infection or cardiac decompensation).
   b. In emergency situations, ideal practices may be altered or disregarded to meet the exigencies of the situation. For example, if a patient is hemorrhaging, there is no time to wait to replace a low red blood cell count. A multiple trauma victim with a full stomach may need a nasogastric tube inserted and suction applied, an endotracheal intubation while awake, or spinal anesthesia as applicable, and may undergo a surgical procedure despite food ingestion.

In addition to the preoperative assessment of the patient and the administration and maintenance of the intraoperative anesthetic, the anesthesia provider may see the patient postoperatively. The anesthesia provider has a responsibility to inform the patient of any unfavorable reaction to a medication or agent so that the patient is forewarned and can report these reactions to other physicians and anesthesia providers in future experiences.

Before Taking the Patient to the Operating Room

Before the patient goes to the OR suite, their physical and emotional status and vital signs should be assessed and recorded by the nurse on the surgical unit or in the same-day admission unit. Any untoward signs and symptoms and extreme apprehension are reported to the surgeon because they could affect the patient's intraoperative course. The following list outlines the preparations:

1. The patient puts on a clean hospital gown. The surgeon permits some patients to wear underpants or pajama pants if the lower body segment is not part of the surgical site. This is helpful in adolescents and patients who are embarrassed and uncomfortable. Any clothing removed in the OR should be placed in a clear plastic bag and labeled with the patient's name, date, and surgeon's name.

Menstruating patients should use a sanitary napkin if they will be under general anesthesia for more than 2 hours. Tampons can be used if they will not remain in place for more than a few hours total. The presence of a tampon should be clearly noted in the chart, so it is not forgotten if the surgery becomes more extensive and longer in duration. The circulating nurse should be informed verbally about the patient's menses, so confusion does not arise if vaginal bleeding is noted.

2. Jewelry is removed for safekeeping. If a wedding ring cannot be removed, it is taped loosely or tied securely to prevent loss. The patient may be permitted to keep a religious symbol, but the patient should understand that it may be removed during the surgical procedure. Document the personal items and their disposition in the chart before, during, and after the procedure.
3. Unless otherwise ordered, dentures and removable bridges are removed before the administration of the general anesthetic

to safeguard them and prevent them from obstructing respiration. Dentures are permitted during local anesthesia, especially if the patient can breathe more easily with them in place.

Some anesthesia providers prefer that securely fitting dentures be left in place to facilitate the airway maintenance. Dentures are necessary to retain facial contours for some plastic surgery procedures. Dentures removed in the OR should be labeled and taken to PACU for placement in the patient's mouth during the postprocedure period.

4. All removable prostheses (e.g., eye, extremity, contact lenses, hearing aids, eyeglasses) are removed for safekeeping. In some instances the patient may be permitted to wear eyeglasses or a hearing aid to the OR. The circulating nurse safeguards them and sends them to the PACU with the patient. Contact lenses and removable eyelashes are removed before the administration of a general anesthetic because they may become dry, cause corneal abrasions, or dislodge.

The patient's personal property is safeguarded to prevent loss or damage. Jewelry and valuables can be given to family and significant others or sent to the hospital security department and locked in a safe. The clothing of ambulatory surgery patients can be stored in a locker. The clothing of TCI patients can be sent to the room or unit where the patient will be admitted postoperatively. Be sure that all items are bagged and clearly marked with the patient's name and date. Document the disposition of all patient belongings.

5. Long hair may be braided. Wigs should be removed or, in special cases, covered with a surgical cap. Hairpins are removed to prevent scalp injury.
6. Antiembolic stockings may be ordered for the lower extremities to prevent embolic phenomena. The stockings are applied before abdominal or pelvic procedures; for patients who have varicosities, are prone to thrombus formation, or have a history of emboli; and for some geriatric patients. They also are often applied for long procedures.
7. The patient voids to prevent overdistention of the bladder or incontinence during unconsciousness. This is especially important for abdominal or pelvic procedures in which a large bladder may be traumatized or may interfere with adequate exposure of the abdominal contents. The time of voiding is recorded. Double-check that a urine specimen is not needed before having the patient void. When indicated, an indwelling Foley catheter is inserted in the OR after the patient has been anesthetized. Some urologic procedures require a full bladder, such as urodynamics with cystometrography, or electromyography; therefore the patient should not void preoperatively.
8. If ordered, an antibiotic may be given 1 hour preoperatively to establish and reach a therapeutic blood level of antibiotic prophylaxis intraoperatively. This may be a one-time dose or may be continued into the postoperative period. If cultures or specimens are obtained during the surgical procedure, a notation should be made on the pathology specimen sheet to indicate antibiotic use.
9. Preanesthesia medications are given as ordered. Their purpose is to eliminate apprehension by making the patient calm, drowsy, and comfortable. Patients who receive a preanesthesia medication should be cautioned to remain in bed.

Many of the drugs cause drowsiness, vertigo, or postural hypotension. Therefore the side rails on the bed should be raised and the call bell placed within the patient's reach.

10. The patient, bed, and chart are accurately identified, and identifications are fastened securely in place. Allergies should be prominently noted on the chart and patient's wristband.

A preoperative checklist helps ensure the patient has been properly prepared. If preparation is inadequate, the surgical procedure may be canceled. All essential records, including the plan of care, must accompany the patient.

Emotional Preparation

By fulfilling spiritual and psychosocial needs, the caregiver helps provide the preoperative patient with as much peace of mind as possible. Understandably, the patient's tension level rises as the time for the surgical procedure approaches. An emotionally prepared patient will have a smoother postoperative course. If the patient has not seen their personal cleric or the hospital chaplain and makes such a request, the nurse should make every effort to contact that person for the patient.

Family members or significant others should be permitted to stay with the patient until it is time to go to the OR suite. Some hospitals permit parents to accompany infants and children into the OR suite. After leaving the patient, the family or guardian should be escorted by transport staff to the waiting area.

Transportation to the Operating Room Suite

Patients may be taken to the OR suite via a transport stretcher or wheelchair. If a stretcher is used, it should be pushed from the head end so the patient's feet go first. Rapid movements through corridors and around corners may cause dizziness and nausea, especially if the patient has been medicated. The attendant at the head end can observe for vomiting or respiratory distress. The patient may be more comfortable if the head end of the stretcher is raised.

If transporting by wheelchair, the patient should be instructed not to help with door opening and to keep hands on the lap. A blanket or sheet should be placed on the seat of the chair and a cover over the lap for modesty. It is inappropriate for bare buttocks to be seated on the uncovered surface of the wheelchair. Take care with tubing such as IV lines or catheters so they do not get tangled in the wheels. Urinary drainage bags should be maintained below the level of the bladder to prevent reflux infection.

Some ambulatory patients may be permitted to walk to the OR. They are given foot protection such as slippers to prevent injury. The slippers should be skid-proof on the bottom. Paper slippers may be unsafe. They do not protect from injury or slippage. The slippers may need to be removed for the procedure but should be retained until the end of the procedure and returned to the patient for use within the facility.

Ideally certain elevators are designated "For OR Use Only," which ensures privacy and minimizes microbial contamination. The patient should be comfortable, warm, and safe during transport. Side rails are raised and restraint straps are applied if necessary. The patient should be instructed to keep arms, hands, and fingers inside the side rails during transport to avoid injury when going through doorways.

IV solution bags hung on poles during transportation are attached securely and placed at the foot of the bed away from the patient's head; this minimizes the danger of injury to the patient if the container should fall. Gentle handling is indicated to prevent dislodging IV needles or indwelling catheters.

Parent(s) sometimes are permitted to accompany a child. If the patient has a language barrier or is profoundly deaf, an interpreter may accompany them to the OR and stay until the induction of anesthesia. Persons accompanying the patient should be appropriately attired in cap, mask, and scrubs or jumpsuit before entering the OR suite.

Admission to the Operating Room Suite

Presurgical Holding Area

The patient is brought through the outer corridor to the presurgical holding area by transport personnel 30 to 45 minutes before the scheduled time of the surgical procedure, where they remain until taken to the OR. In some facilities this holding area is in the PACU in a designated space on one end of the unit that is not occupied by patients who are recovering from anesthesia. This can be an advantage because many of the nurses in the holding area also perform patient care in the PACU area. This can promote familiarity between the patient and the nurse.

Some conditions justify bringing patients to the OR suite in their beds. Such conditions include patients on pressure-reducing air mattresses, patients in traction, or cardiac patients who cannot be moved until transferred to the OR bed. The surgeon chooses the course that best benefits the individual patient.

Personnel stabilize beds, stretchers, and frames by locking the wheels when a patient is moved or is permitted to move from one surface to another. Mattresses also should be stabilized. An adequate number of personnel and a transfer device should be available to ensure patient safety during transfer between surfaces. The patient's head, arms, and legs are protected. When using a transfer roller or other device, a minimum of four people is required to control the head, foot, and both sides of the patient.

Some hospitals have individual rooms for anesthesia induction. The patient waits in this room and is administered an anesthetic before being taken into the OR.

Admission to the Presurgical Holding Area

The holding area nurse greets the patient by name and introduces themself. The nurse stands next to the midsection of the stretcher so the patient can comfortably see them. The holding area nurse performs the following steps and documents them on the surgical checklist:

1. Places a warm blanket on the patient, verifies patient identification (checking wrist band information) by name and date of birth, and notifies the individual at the surgery control desk that the patient is in the holding area.
2. Verifies the surgical procedure, site, and surgeon verbally with the patient and/or others, as appropriate. The surgical site is validated by observing the indelible ink of the surgeon's initials. Hospital policy is followed for identification of surgical sites that cannot be marked.
3. Reviews the patient's chart and EMR for completeness (Fig. 21.4).
   a. Medical history and physical examination
   b. Laboratory reports
   c. Consent forms and documentation of consents
      (1) Informed consent data
      (2) General consent to treat

• **Fig. 21.4** The holding room nurse reviews the patient's chart for completeness.

(3) Anesthesia consent
(4) Blood or blood products consent
(5) Living will and DNR order
4. Measures the vital signs and blood pressure.
5. Verifies allergies, sensitivities, and medication history.
6. Checks skin tone and integrity.
7. Verifies physical limitations.
8. Notes the patient's mental state.
9. Puts a cap on the patient to protect their hair, for purposes of asepsis, and to help minimize hypothermia. Patients who are bald are required to wear a head covering to prevent heat loss and scalp dander shed.
10. Notifies the individual at the surgery control desk when the patient and surgical team are ready for transport to the OR. The patient is under constant observation by the patient care staff until transported from the surgical department to another patient care unit or discharged.

The holding area nurse records pertinent findings in the perioperative patient care record and on the surgical checklist. If a perioperative patient assessment has not been performed, the holding area nurse will assess the patient, formulate the nursing diagnoses and expected outcomes, and prepare an individualized plan of care.

Preanesthesia Preparations

The anesthesia provider or surgeon may wish to talk with the patient before sedation is given. The patient should be informed about all procedures before they are initiated. The following list of procedures may need to be completed before the induction of anesthesia; some or all of these procedures can be performed in the preoperative holding area if there are adequate facilities for patient privacy:
• Removal of body hair, if ordered.
• Marking of surgical incision sites such as for plastic surgery of the face and torso.
• Insertion of IV access. Be sure the placement does not interfere with the surgical site. Avoid the operative side of the body if possible.
• Insertion of invasive hemodynamic monitoring lines, as appropriate.

• Administration of the preanesthesia medication and other drugs, such as preoperative antibiotics, as ordered. The preanesthesia medication can precipitate respiratory depression and hypotension, and the perioperative nurse should be alert and take prompt action for airway maintenance if necessary. The holding area should be equipped for cardiopulmonary resuscitation. An emergency or code blue button should always be accessible to summon help.

The anesthesia provider may perform regional blocks in the holding area. All procedures performed in the holding area are documented on the patient's record.

Despite the activities around them, patients may feel more alone in a holding area than in any other location. Time passes slowly, causing a possible increase in anxiety. An anxious patient looks to the nurse for comfort, reassurance, and attention. A compassionate expression in the eyes and voice and a reassuring touch of the hand can convey concern and understanding to the patient.

If the patient is drowsy, unnecessary conversation should be avoided. The nurse should answer questions and see to the patient's comfort. The patient should be kept warm, or the blanket should be turned down if they are too warm. An extra pillow should be placed under the patient's head or under the knees. Dry lips should be moistened, if appropriate. Any delay or unusual circumstances should be explained to the patient, family, and significant others.

A quiet, restful atmosphere enables the patient to gain full advantage of the premedication. Some holding areas and ORs have piped-in recorded music, which diverts attention from the many other sounds in the environment. Music with a slow, easy rhythm and a low volume is most conducive to relaxation. Familiar music is more pleasing and relaxing because the patient can associate it with pleasant experiences. Some facilities provide earphones or headsets so patients can listen to the music of their choice. Earphones also muffle extraneous noises and conversations. Ideally the patient should have a choice in selecting the music or in having no music at all; this is the advantage of individual headsets over piped-in systems.

Transfer to the Operating Room

When the OR is ready, the circulating nurse comes to the holding area for the patient. A handover report is given by the holding room nurse to the circulating nurse. The surgical checklist is one way to ensure an accurate exchange of information is given as patient care changes hands. The circulating nurse will in turn continue documenting on the checklist for continuity and relay the information to the PACU nurse after the surgical procedure is completed and patient care is transferred for postanesthesia recovery.

It is advantageous if the circulator is the perioperative nurse who made the preoperative visit; the patient will appreciate seeing a familiar face. Before transporting the patient into the OR, the circulating nurse has several important duties to fulfill:
1. Greet the patient and validate their identity (Fig. 21.5).
   a. The circulating nurse should introduce themself if not previously done. The patient should be addressed as Mr., Mrs., or Ms.—not by the first name. The patient should be asked to state and/or spell their full name and date of birth.
   b. When the patient arrives at the facility, an identifying wristband is put on in the admitting area. The holding

• **Fig. 21.5** The circulating nurse greets and identifies the patient.

room nurse checks the band before the patient leaves for the OR. The circulating nurse compares the information on the wristband, including the identification number, with the information on the medical record and with the information on the surgical schedule: name, anticipated surgical procedure, time, and surgeon. An allergy band and other notification band (e.g., Do Not Resuscitate [DNR]) should be checked at the same time. A discussion of the order should take place between the surgeon, anesthesia provider, and patient if requested.

c. Identification on the stretcher or bed ensures the patient's return to the same stretcher or bed after surgery, if this is the procedure. If the patient is an infant or a child, the identification bracelet may be on the ankle. Any tag on the crib should be out of reach. Always validate the identity of a child with a parent or legal guardian. Ask what procedure is being performed. Validate the surgical site marking as appropriate.

d. Verification of the surgical procedure, site, and surgeon with the patient provides reassurance that this is the correct patient. The patient's own words should be documented on the chart. The circulating nurse should note the presence of the surgeon's identifying mark on the surgical site. If the patient is heavily sedated or confused, the surgeon may be asked to help identify the patient.

2. Check the side rails, restraining straps, IV infusions, and indwelling catheters.

3. Observe the patient for any reaction to the medication.

4. Observe the patient's anxiety level.

5. Check the history and physical data, laboratory tests, x-ray reports, and consent form(s) or documentation in the patient's medical record.

6. Review the plan of care and the surgical checklist.
   a. Pay particular attention to allergies and any previous unfavorable reactions to anesthesia or blood transfusions.
   b. Become familiar with this patient's unique and individual needs.

The patient is taken into the OR after the surgeon visit and the anesthesia provider is ready to receive the patient. The main preparations for the procedure should be complete so the circulating nurse can devote undivided attention to the patient.

Before the Induction of Anesthesia

The anesthesia provider also has immediate preanesthesia duties, such as the following:[6]

1. Checking and assembling equipment before the patient enters the room. Airways, endotracheal tubes, laryngoscopes, suction catheters, labeled prefilled medication syringes, and other items are arranged on a cart or table.

2. Reviewing the preoperative physical examination, history, and laboratory reports in the chart.

3. Making certain that the patient is comfortable and secure on the OR bed.

4. Checking for denture removal or any loose teeth.

5. Checking to be certain that contact lenses have been removed.

6. Asking the patient when they last took anything by mouth, including medications.

7. Checking the patient's pulse, respiration, and blood pressure to obtain a baseline for the subsequent assessment of vital signs while the patient is anesthetized.

8. Listening to the heart and lungs and then connecting ECG monitor leads and attaching the pulse oximeter and other monitoring devices (Fig. 21.6).

• **Fig. 21.6** The anesthesia provider prepares for induction of anesthesia.

9. Starting the IV access. This may be done in the holding area or an induction room. Some patients arrive with an IV line in place.
10. Preparing for and explaining the induction procedure to the patient. If properly premedicated, the patient should be able to respond to simple instructions.

Circulating Nurse's Role During Induction

The patient's welfare and individual needs take priority over all other activities before and during the induction of anesthesia. The patient is the most important person in the OR. If the circulating nurse gives more attention to the equipment than to the patient, the patient may feel abandoned. In addition, the monitoring equipment is not the best indicator of patient condition. At this time of stress the patient wants the physical presence of a trusted, competent, and compassionate person.

The patient expects the circulating nurse to be cognizant of their problems and conditions and willing to help relieve them. The patient will perceive the circulating nurse's attitude as one of either acceptance or rejection. Consequently, the behavior of the circulating nurse affects the patient in either a positive or a negative way. Positive actions include staying close to the patient, paying attention to the patient's needs and comfort, looking directly at the patient when they speak, touching the patient with kindness, and appearing poised, confident, and professional.

Humans react through their senses. The positive effect of touch is a helpful nonverbal communication in establishing nurse-patient rapport within a short time. Touch communicates caring. A gentle touch can bridge a language barrier by establishing human contact. Holding a patient's hand warmly or laying a hand on an arm during the induction of anesthesia or a painful procedure can do much to alleviate anxiety and elicit trust.

A smile has been called the universal language. Even though the circulating nurse is wearing a mask, their eyes can convey a smile or hope. Likewise they can reveal anger or hostility. Physiognomy, the ancient Chinese art of discovering qualities of the mind and temperament from the expression of facial features, still has relevance. Facial expressions, eye contact, and body movements have either a positive or a negative effect on the patient. Warmth and caring can be conveyed by a pleasant manner and the expression of the eyes.

Although routine procedures for care and teaching have been established, each patient deserves personalized care in the face of a disruptive life experience. The circulating nurse should not become insensitive to patients because of depersonalized procedures and routines or their own prejudices.

The patient must not be treated as inanimate or anonymous or categorized by the disease or surgical procedure. The patient is a living, feeling person, not "Dr. Brown's hysterectomy," "the cardiac in Room 4," or "the arthritic I need help to move." Jargon such as this is depersonalizing, demoralizing, offensive, and unacceptable. The goal of perioperative patient care is to combine efficiency with caring.

The protection of modesty, dignity, and privacy is essential regardless of whether the patient is conscious or unconscious. Unnecessary exposure should be avoided. The gown and cotton blanket protect modesty and keep the patient warm. The OR door should be kept closed for privacy; this is also important in terms of aseptic technique. Surgical procedures may be viewed only by authorized personnel who have a definite function. All privileged information is kept confidential.

Patients are unnerved by stimuli such as strange odors and disturbing sights. A used, unclean OR, with its soiled linen, instruments, equipment, unconscious patients, and bright lights, can be frightening. Patients feel isolation amid the hustle and bustle of activity, and a lack of team preparedness increases the patient's stress level. The patient may feel embarrassment from body exposure, and loud noises such as voices, inappropriate conversation, staff disagreements, clattering instruments, crumpling paper, and sterilizer noises contribute to the atmosphere of fear perceived by the patient.

Anxiety and preoperative sedation tend to alter the patient's ability to interpret events objectively. The patient may relate everything heard to themselves, even though they may not actually be the subject of the conversation, and they may misinterpret or react unfavorably. Hearing is the last sense lost when becoming unconscious. It is not known at precisely what moment a person can no longer hear and interpret what is said, but it is known that patients remain aware of their environment much longer than their seemingly unconscious state would indicate.

A lack of consideration can destroy the patient's confidence in the team. An overheard thoughtless comment can create a lasting traumatic memory and fear. Negative recall can induce anxiety in similar future experiences. Therefore team members should think before speaking and should not converse near the patient while excluding them from the conversation. Sedation does not imply exclusion. The patient may be aware of conversation, even if they appear to be asleep! Out of the patient's hearing, conversation should pertain only to the work at hand. The OR is not the place for social discourse.

Time is of the essence to keep anesthesia and procedure time to a minimum, and it is a protective factor to provide as little disturbance to physiologic homeostasis as possible. However, efficiency and safety must not be sacrificed for speed. Safety is the prime concern.

The OR imposes a high degree of vulnerability on patients and the entire staff. Patients lack the power to defend and protect themselves during a surgical intervention; therefore the circulating nurses are their advocates and protectors. They provide supportive care and safeguard patients from emotional and physical harm by maintaining constant vigilance. Circulating nurses can minimize the potential hazards in the following manner:

- *Never leave a sedated patient unguarded.* In addition to causing mental anguish from a feeling of abandonment, an unattended patient may fall or be injured by equipment.
- *Correctly identify patients, surgical sites, and medications.* An incorrect surgical procedure on a patient or an error in medication is usually the result of inadequate identification. Validation of the planned procedure is signified by a time out wherein the patient's identity is confirmed along with the surgical site, physiologic conditions (allergies), and the presence of necessary equipment, scans, implants, and materials for

the procedure. The patient is included in the time out as condition permits. The time out is documented on the surgical checklist.

- *Create, maintain, and control an optimally therapeutic environment in the OR.* This involves control of the physical environment, such as temperature, humidity, and personnel. Traffic flow in and out of the room should be kept to a minimum. The more movement and talking, the greater the microbial count in the room. The OR should be kept quiet once the patient is there so the effects of sedation are not counteracted. A tranquil, relaxed atmosphere is conducive to team concentration and orderly functioning so all can go well. The standards of ethical conduct should be strictly enforced.

The effect inherent in any type of surgical intervention can be reconciled when the patient has hope and confidence in the caregivers. Nurses are the central figures in patient care and can do much to relieve fear and provide security. Preoperative preparations can influence the outcome of the surgical procedure.

Ⓔ EVOLVE WEBSITE

http://evolve.elsevier.com/Hornacky/BerryKohn/

- Historical Perspective
- Student Interactive Questions
- Glossary

References

1. Metz A, Berlin N, Yost M, et al.: Comprehensive history and physicals are common before low-risk surgery and associated with preoperative test overuse, *J Surg Res* 283:93–101, 2022.
2. Wilson E, Marra A, Ward M, et al.: Patient's experiences and compliance with preoperative screening and decolonization, *Am J Infect Control* 51(1):78–82, 2023.
3. Shah B: How to deliver safer and effective patient care: tips for team leaders and educators, *Gastroenterology* 156(4):852–855, 2019.
4. Tomlinson S, Carney M, Wolf M: Advances in medical education and implications for the emergency department, *Pediatr Clin North Am* 65(6):1221–1227, 2018.
5. Neira P, Bowman RL: Improving perioperative nursing care for transgender and gender-diverse patients, *AORN J* 116(5):404–415, 2022.
6. Krombach J, Zucher C, Simon S, et al.: Persisting high rates of omissions during anesthesia induction are decreased by utilization of a pre- & post-induction checklist, *Anaesth Crit Care Pain* 42(2): 101186, 2023.

Bibliography

AORN: *Guidelines for perioperative practice*, Denver, CO, 2024, The Association.

Phillips NM, Hornacky A: *Pass CNOR!*, St. Louis, 2019, Elsevier.

22

Diagnostics, Specimens, and Oncologic Considerations

CHAPTER OUTLINE

Diagnosing Pathology, 396

Specimens and Pathologic Examination, 396

Radiologic Examination, 399

Magnetic Resonance Imaging, 404

Nuclear Medicine Studies, 405

Ultrasonography, 406

Doppler Studies, 406

Sensory Evoked Potential, 407

Plethysmography, 408

Endoscopy, 408

The Patient With Cancer, 408

CHAPTER OBJECTIVES

After studying this chapter the learner will be able to:

- List several invasive diagnostic tests.
- List several noninvasive diagnostic tests.
- List several interventional procedures that incorporate diagnostics.

- Describe several aspects of patient care associated with diagnostic testing.
- Discuss the role of diagnostics in oncology.

KEY TERMS AND DEFINITIONS

Anaplasia Change in cellular differentiation and orientation that causes a more primitive structural appearance and function. Anaplastic cell changes are characteristic of malignancy.

Benign tumor Aggregation of cells that closely resemble those of the parent tissue of origin. The tumor usually grows slowly by expansion, is localized, and is surrounded by a capsule of fibrous tissue.

Biopsy Procedure for obtaining a representative tissue sample for gross and/or microscopic examination. The specimen can be obtained surgically or by other means.

Brachytherapy Placement of radioactive material inside of or close to a tumor. Radioactive elements are introduced through catheters inserted into the tumor.

Cancer Broad term that describes any malignant tumor within a large class of diseases. More than 100 different forms of cancer are known to exist, each with histologic variations. Cancerous tumors are divided into two broad groups, benign and malignant.

Carcinoma Malignant tumor of epithelial origin that affects glandular organs, viscera, and skin.

Chemotherapy Use of chemical or pharmacologic agents to treat diseases, such as cancer.

Contrast medium Use of a substance in the creation of density on a radiographic imaging device; radiopaque contrast injected or instilled to outline an organ or a structure. A radiolucent

substance, such as air, can help define a hollow space, such as a ventricle of the brain.

Cytoreductive surgery Mechanical reduction in cell volume at the tumor site by sharp or blunt tissue dissection. Vessel- and nerve-sparing procedures include the use of an ultrasonic aspirator and hydrostatic pulsed lavage.

Immunotherapy Use of agents that stimulate or activate the body's own host defense immune system to combat disease.

Interventional radiology Invasive procedures performed under radiologic control. Examples include balloon angioplasty, coronary artery stent placement, and inferior vena cava filter placement.

Malignant tumor Progressively growing tumor that originates from a specialized organ such as the lung, breast, or brain, or a tumor localized to a specific body system such as bone, skin, lymph nodes, or blood vessels.

Neoplasm Atypical new growth of abnormal cells or tissues, which may be malignant or benign.

-oma Suffix denoting a tumor or neoplasm.

Palliation Measures taken to decrease the negative effects of a terminal or moribund condition. This is not considered a cure, but rather a temporary solution to a problematic situation. Examples include removing an obstruction or attempts to preserve fertility in the face of cancer.

Pathologic examination Series of tests and examinations conducted by a pathologist to determine the cause of changes in the structure or function of a body part or tissue.

Percutaneous Directed through the skin and tissues of the external body surface. Diagnostics, treatments, or tissue removal can be performed by direct percutaneous routes.

Plethysmography Procedure to determine variations in blood flow between parts.

Sarcoma Malignant tumor of mesenchymal origin that affects bones, muscles, and soft tissue.

Scintigraphy Recording of the emissions of radiologic substances as they are collected or secreted by tissues and/or organs in the body.

Smear Sample of tissue cells or fluid aspirated or scraped from a mucous membrane or a potentially pathologic site. The material is stained and studied for cellular components to make a diagnosis.

Stereotaxis Computerized localization of a lesion.

Tomography Computerized method of imaging a structure in layers.

Tumor Any neoplasm in which cells are permanently altered but have the capability of growth and reproduction. A tumor consists of two elements the tumor cells themselves and a supporting framework of connective tissue and vascular supply.

Diagnosing Pathology

Diagnosis of a pathologic disease, anomaly, or traumatic injury is established before a surgical procedure is undertaken. Many modalities and techniques help surgeons assess each individual patient problem, guide them through the surgical procedure, and help them verify the results of surgical intervention. The term *diagnosis* refers to the art or the act of determining the nature of a patient's disease. Diagnostic procedures can be classified as follows:

- *Noninvasive:* Noninvasive techniques use equipment placed on or near the patient's skin but outside body tissues.
- *Invasive:* Invasive techniques use equipment placed into a body cavity or vessel and/or use substances injected into body structures.
- *Interventional:* Interventional techniques involve invasive diagnostics and procedures performed in a specialty department, such as in radiology.

Perioperative nurses and surgical technologists should be familiar with the modalities and equipment necessary to assist with diagnostic procedures in the operating room (OR) and interventional departments.

Patient Care Considerations for Diagnostic Procedures

1. Patients should be assessed for their physical condition and any metal implants, pacemakers, infusion pumps, sensitivities, and allergies. Patients who will be administered contrast media should be evaluated for kidney function before testing.
2. Clear instructions should be given verbally and in writing before the test is performed.
3. Preprocedure preparations should be confirmed before the patient begins testing. A "time out" process that includes the pertinent patient and procedure information should be conducted by the team.
4. Explanations of procedures should be given to patients to allay fears and ensure their understanding of the value of the procedure in making a diagnosis. Before the procedure begins, an explanation should be given of the equipment being used.
5. Sterile and aseptic techniques of invasive procedures are strictly observed.

Specimens and Pathologic Examination

Clinical pathology is the use of laboratory methods to establish a clinical diagnosis of a disease by examining body fluid, tissue, and organs. Surgical pathology is the study of alterations in body tissues removed by surgical intervention.

Cultures and Smears
Cultures

Aerobic or anaerobic cultures may be obtained before or during the surgical procedure. If obtained before the procedure, the culture must be done before the skin prep. Cultures should be refrigerated or sent to the laboratory immediately. The culture tube and plastic transport bag should be labeled with the patient's identification (two identifiers), date, and site of culture. A paper requisition usually accompanies all specimens with patient, surgeon, and specimen details.

The sterile culture tube and swab are prepackaged in a peel pouch and are dispensed to the sterile field. The culture tube has a small, sealed plastic media chamber at the bottom that preserves the material obtained from the patient on the swab. Nothing other than the fluid or tissue to be cultured should touch the sterile swab.

The sterile swab is withdrawn from the tube by the sterile team member and dipped into the area to be cultured. The swab is replaced into the culture tube and seated tightly. The media chamber at the bottom of the tube is crushed to release the culture media and immerse the tip of the swab. The scrub person can drop the closed culture tube into a small plastic bag held by the gloved circulating nurse, who will affix the patient's identification label and biohazard sticker.

Cultures for suspected anaerobic microorganisms require immediate attention. Exposure to room air may kill anaerobes in a few minutes. The purulent material can be aspirated into a sterile disposable syringe through a disposable needle. This needle is removed with a hemostat and placed with counted sharps on the instrument table. The aspirated material may be transferred into a sterile specimen cup and sent immediately to the laboratory in a plastic bag with a biohazard sticker affixed to the outside.

Smears

Cells and small pieces of tissue are suspended in liquid and smeared on glass microscope slides. The specimen is "fixed" by being sprayed with fixative or immersed in liquid. The fixed slide is then stained and examined under a microscope by the pathologist or specially trained technician. This technique is useful for the examination of fine-needle aspirate or scrapings. Smears can be examined within minutes after they have been obtained from the patient. Instant diagnosis is possible in many cases.

Biopsies

The removal of tissue or fluid for diagnosis is referred to as a biopsy. Biopsy specimens can be obtained by several invasive methods. The pathologist determines and/or confirms the diagnosis by histologic examination (the study of tissue) and cytologic analysis (the study of cells).

Aspiration Biopsy

In an aspiration biopsy, fluid is aspirated through a 22 to 25-gauge needle placed in a lesion, such as a cyst or abscess, or in a joint or body cavity. Fine-needle aspiration biopsies are done most commonly to obtain cells from solid lesions in the breast, thyroid, neck, lymph nodes, or soft tissues. The needle is manipulated in the mass while suction is placed on the syringe. Several hundred cells are drawn into the syringe. The cells can be chemically fixed and then examined under the microscope. Aspiration biopsies can be performed under computed tomography (CT) or ultrasonic guidance with minimal local anesthesia.

Bone Marrow Biopsy

For a bone marrow biopsy a trocar puncture needle or aspiration needle is placed into bone, through a small skin incision or percutaneous puncture. The sternum and iliac crest are common sites for bone marrow aspiration. Patients with abnormal blood counts or unusual blood morphology can benefit from cytologic studies of bone marrow.

Local anesthesia to the level of the periosteum is necessary. In obese patients a spinal needle may be needed to reach this depth. After satisfactory anesthesia, a larger bore needle is introduced into the marrow space and the specimen is aspirated. The aspiration may feel painful to the patient because the bone is not numb. A core sample of bone may be obtained at this time for pathologic examination.

Percutaneous Needle Biopsy

With percutaneous needle biopsy, tissue is obtained from an internal organ or solid mass by means of a hollow needle inserted through the body wall. Percutaneous puncture into a lesion may be guided by fluoroscopy under image intensification, by ultrasound, or by CT scanning.[1] Special needles are used; some types are disposable.

Punch Biopsy

For a punch biopsy, an instrument with a 3 to 4-mm circular, sharp, hollow tip is used to sample skin lesions in a cookie-cutter manner. The plug of tissue is sent for pathologic study. Dermatologists or plastic surgeons use this method for skin biopsy.

Brush Biopsy

In brush biopsy, stiff brushes of nylon or steel are passed through an endoscope to the interior of the respiratory tree or urinary tract. Tissue samples are collected as the brush rubs against the target organ. Smears are made on glass slides; the tip of the brush is then cut off and placed in formalin for a minimum of 1 hour for fixation. The slides and fixed tissue are subjected to histologic studies for diagnosis.

Excisional Biopsy

A mass or entire structure is cut from the body in an excisional biopsy. The advent of fine-needle aspiration has decreased the need for full excisional biopsy except for a friable organ or a breast mass. In cases of suspected lymphoma an entire lymph node is necessary for adequate diagnosis. Some excisional biopsies can be performed endoscopically (Fig. 22.1).

Incisional Biopsy

A portion of a mass is removed during incisional biopsy. Soft tissue masses incised for diagnosis include muscle, fat, or other connective tissue (see Fig. 22.1).

Frozen Section

Special preparation and examination of tissue can determine whether it is malignant and whether regional nodes are involved. When the surgeon removes a piece of tissue and wants an immediate diagnosis, it is placed in a basin or specimen container without any added preservative, such as formalin or normal saline solution.[2] Formalin or normal saline solution will alter the freezing process used in the specialized pathologic study. The circulating nurse should alert the pathologist that a frozen section will be sent. When the tissue examination is complete, the pathologist will report the results directly to the surgeon in the OR.

The patient's level of consciousness should be considered during report of pathologic results, especially if the patient is awake. The use of speakerphones should be avoided for patient confidentiality. If a malignant lesion is present and the individual situation calls for it, the surgeon proceeds with a radical resection of the affected organ or body area. In some situations, additional tissue is needed for diagnosis.

Permanent Section

The specimen is placed in fixative, commonly formalin, for several hours to cause the cells to become firm. The fixed specimen is placed in a machine that removes all the water from the tissues, replacing it with paraffin. When this process is complete, the specimen is embedded into a block of wax. It is placed in a microtome and is sliced tissue-paper thin and floated in a water bath. The slices are placed on glass slides, where the paraffin is dissolved with solvent and the water is restored to the tissue on the slide. The slices readily accept dyes and stains used for diagnosis. Permanent section is the best diagnostic biopsy tool. Box 22.1 lists several tissue dyes and stains used in diagnostic procedures.

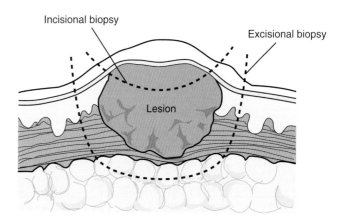

• **Fig. 22.1** Comparison between incisional and excisional tissue biopsies.

•BOX 22.1 Surgical Dyes and Tissue Stains

Dyes

Blue
- Trypan blue
- Isosulfan blue
- Methylene blue
- Indigo carmine
- Cyanosine

Green
- Brilliant green
- Indocyanine green

Red
- Congo red
- Carmine

Yellow
- Fluorescein sodium

Purple
- Crystal violet
- Gentian violet

Black
- India ink

Stains

Brown-yellow
- Lugol (iodine)
- Monsel (ferric)

Collecting Surgical Specimens

All tissue removed during the surgical procedure is sent to the pathology laboratory for verification of the diagnosis. Any unidentifiable or unusual item removed from a patient should be sent for identification by the pathology department. Some examples include removal of retained surgical items, such as instruments, sponges, and towels. Any questionable item should be sent to the laboratory and documented by the circulating nurse. Facility policy and procedure should delineate disposition of all surgical specimens.

Tissue specimens may be stored in a refrigerator in the laboratory or some other location within the OR suite until they are taken to the pathology department at the end of each day's schedule of surgical procedures or at intervals during the day.

Correct solutions for storage and correct labeling of specimens are critical for accurate diagnosis. Table 22.1 lists types of specimens for pathologic study.

Specimen containers may be plastic containers, waxed cardboard cartons, or glass jars with preservative solution. AORN (Association of periOperative Registered Nurses) recommends that the specimen container be leak-proof, puncture-resistant, and labeled accordingly. The closed, labeled container is placed into a plastic bag or additional container with a biohazard sticker for transport to the laboratory. The double-packaged specimen should be handled while wearing gloves.

The handling of specimens should be kept to a minimum and only while wearing gloves and appropriate personal protective equipment (PPE). Use care to avoid contaminating the outside of a specimen container. If it is contaminated, wipe it with an antiseptic solution. Always wash hands thoroughly after removing gloves that have been worn to handle specimens. If instruments are used for handling, be careful not to tear, crush, or damage tissue. The routine care for each type of tissue specimen may vary, as follows:

- Pathology tissue specimens should not be allowed to dry out. Saline or a solution of aqueous formaldehyde (10% formalin) is commonly used as the fixative until the specimen is processed further in the laboratory. Formalin is flammable and should not be stored in the OR. The formalin is added after the specimen is in the container. Dropping the specimen into a prefilled container can cause a splash. Some facilities have a closed system formalin dispenser to prevent splashes and inhalation of fumes.

TABLE 22.1 Specimen Types and Considerations for Handling

Specimen Type	Test	Preparation	Example
Fluid	Bacteriology	Anaerobic or aerobic on culture swab in sterile tube	Exudate
	Virology	Fresh, in sterile container	Cerebrospinal fluid
	Cytology	Fresh or added solution of pathologist's choice in sterile container	Cell washings, urine
	Genetic studies	Fresh, in sterile container	Amniotic fluid
	Cell count	Fresh, in sterile container	Semen for infertility study
Tissue	Permanent section	Fresh or added solution of pathologist's choice in sterile container	Diseased organ
	Frozen section	Fresh, in sterile container; no saline	Margin of malignant lesion
	Biopsy	Fresh or solution of pathologist's choice in sterile container	Suspicious lesion
	Hormonal assay	Fresh, in sterile container	Breast tissue
	Donor tissue	Fresh or added solution of pathologist's choice	Cadaver skin
	Calculi	Dry, in sterile container	Gallstone
	Ova	Fresh or added solution of surgeon's choice	Human egg for preservation
	Muscle	Fresh, extended in special clamp in sterile container	Test for malignant hyperthermia
Nonbiologic specimen	Foreign body Projectile from crime scene	Fresh, in sterile container Dry, in nonmetallic container	Glass fragments Bullet
	Clothing of crime or accident victim	Dry, in porous paper	Underclothes of rape victim
	Explanted prosthesis	Dry, in sterile container	Orthopedic screws or plates

- Some pathology laboratories prefer moistening the specimen with sterile normal saline. Check for the preference of the laboratory that will be examining the specimen.
- Fresh tissue and frozen sections are not placed in preservative solution or saline unless instructed otherwise by the laboratory personnel.
- Stones are placed in a dry container so they will not dissolve. Organs containing stones, such as the gallbladder, may be placed in saline or formalin.
- Foreign bodies should be sent for accession according to policy, and a record is kept for legal purposes. The description and the disposition of the object are recorded. A foreign body may be given to the police, surgeon, or patient, depending on legal implications, policy, or the surgeon's wishes. A chain of specimen custody slip should be signed by all persons handling the specimen.
- Forensic evidence, such as bullets or knife blades, should be placed in a dry plastic container. Do not allow the item to contact metallic basins, because ballistic evidence could be altered. Chain of custody documentation should always accompany the specimen to protect the evidence.
- Amputated extremities are wrapped in plastic before sending them to a refrigerator in the laboratory or morgue. Avoid placing the amputated limb in the patient's field of vision. Most patients needing amputation have spinal or epidural anesthesia for the procedure. The sight of the body part may cause emotional distress in the patient. The patient may request that an amputated extremity be sent to a mortuary for preservation for burial with their body after death. This request must be noted on the requisition sent to the laboratory. Refer to institutional policy and procedure for the care of amputated limbs.

Radiologic Examination

An x-ray is a high-energy electromagnetic wave capable of penetrating various thicknesses of solid substances and affecting photographic plates. X-rays are generated on a vacuum tube when high-velocity electrons from a heated filament strike a metal target (anode), causing it to emit x-rays.

The image obtained using x-rays may be referred to as an x-ray, roentgenogram, radiograph, or other -gram or -graph name associated either with the specific technique used to obtain the photograph or the anatomic structures identified (e.g., mammogram, x-ray, or radiograph). Most facilities have eliminated the use of x-ray film and have changed to a digital viewing format. Digital imaging does not need processing, and the image is viewed immediately on a screen.

X-rays are also used for diagnostic imaging with fluoroscopy, CT, and digital radiography.[3] Computerized radiologic images may be stored on disks, picture archiving and communication systems (PACS), or external hard drives.

Types of Radiologic Equipment and Accessories

Many hospitals have one or more rooms within the OR suite that are equipped for diagnostic as well as intraoperative radiologic procedures. In some facilities, OR personnel are cross-trained to assist with diagnostic and interventional procedures in the radiology department.

Contrast Media

Agents composed of nonmetallic compounds or heavy metallic salts that do not permit the passage of radiant energy are radiopaque. When exposed to x-rays, the lumen of a body structure filled with these agents appears as a dense area. Radiopaque contrast media frequently used for the procedures to be described are listed in Box 22.2.

Patients with renal disease are given contrast media if necessary at the lowest possible dose.[4] Studies have shown that contrast agents are excreted in breast milk in small amounts. Contrast agents cross the placenta and are excreted by the fetal kidneys into the amniotic fluid. Sensitization of the infant has not been shown. The contrast is cleared by the mother's circulation within 24 hours. She may wish to abstain from breastfeeding during that period. Refer to the product package insert for specific information.

Some contrast agents are fluorescent dyes. Most contain iodine, either bound or unbound. The contrast media is designated low osmolarity or high osmolarity. Low osmolarity is associated with fewer reactions to contrast. Few patients have an immediate reaction; however, a small population of patients may react several hours later. Known reactors may be given prednisone and Benadryl (diphenhydramine) several hours before the anticipated use of any contrast agents.

A history of systemic sensitivity to substances that contain iodine, such as shellfish, or other allergies is obtained before these agents are injected. True shellfish allergies are not related to iodine but to specific proteins in the fish. True allergy is not a common event. Studies have shown that other allergies, such as milk and egg, both high in protein, may play a role. Precautionary administration

---

•BOX 22.2   Radiopaque Contrast Media

Barium sulfate for gastrointestinal studies
- Diatrizoate meglumine, injectable:
  - Cardiografin for angiography and aortography
  - Hypaque-M, 30%, for urography and computed tomography (CT)
  - Hypaque-M, 60%, for urography, cerebral and peripheral angiography, aortography, venography, cholangiography, hysterosalpingography, and splenoportography
- Diatrizoate sodium, injectable:
  - Hypaque sodium, 25%, for urography and CT
  - Hypaque sodium, 40%, same uses as for Hypaque-M, 60%
- Diatrizoic acid, injectable, used as meglumine and sodium salts:
  - Hypaque-M for angiocardiography, angiography, aortography, and urography
  - Renografin for cerebral angiography, peripheral arteriography and venography, cholangiography, splenoportography, arthrography, discography, urography, and CT
  - Renovist for aortography, angiocardiography, peripheral arteriography and venography, venacavography, and urography
Ethiodized oil for splenoportography and CT
- Iodipamide meglumine, injectable:
  - Cholografin meglumine for cholangiography and cholecystography
  - Renovue for IV excretory urography
  - Sinografin for hysterosalpingography
- Iohexol (Omnipaque) for CT
- Gadolinium-based contrast for MRI
- Ioversol (Optiray) for arteriography and CT
- Metrizamide for myelography and CT
- Propyliodone (Dionosil) for bronchography
- Sodium iothalamate (Angio-Conray) for arteriography

of prednisone and Benadryl minimizes the risk. The use of low-osmolarity contrast helps decrease reactions.

Iodine allergy information may be unreliable because studies have shown that immediate reactions to contrast are non-immunologic. This means that the adverse reaction is not caused by allergy. The patient's immunoglobulin E (IgE) is not activated. True allergic reactions to any contrast agent ingredient stimulate IgE, and the patient can exhibit hives, angioedema, respiratory difficulty, and cardiovascular collapse.

A test dose of 1 or 2 mL may be given before the dose required for x-ray study to rule out a potential reaction. The patient should be observed for symptoms of reaction throughout the procedure. Signs of reaction may include the following:

- Red rash over face and chest
- Extreme agitation
- Sudden elevation of body temperature
- Complaints of muscle, joint, and back pain
- Respiratory distress
- Tachycardia
- Hypotension
- Blood-tinged urine
- Convulsions
- Loss of consciousness
- Cardiac arrest

Radiolucent Gases

Filtered room air, oxygen, nitrogen, carbon dioxide, or a combination of gases may be injected into body spaces or structures that normally contain fluid other than blood. Gases are radiolucent (i.e., transparent to x-rays). Thus gas-filled spaces appear less dense on x-rays than do surrounding tissues.

Radiologic Table

The tabletop the patient lies on is made of acrylic or some other radiolucent material (Fig. 22.2). Some OR beds have a Bakelite top that fits over the length of the table and permits insertion of the x-ray cassette at any area. For fluoroscopy with image intensification, the entire top must be radiolucent, because the image intensifier is positioned underneath the table. If the entire OR bed is not radiolucent, the foot section can be lowered and a radiolucent extension attached that will accommodate specialized x-ray machinery.

A

B

• **Fig. 22.2** Pedestal Bases. **A,** Central. **B,** Eccentric for C-arm image intensifier placement.

Cassette

The lightproof holder for x-ray film is referred to as a *cassette*. The patient is positioned between the x-ray tube and the cassette. Holders for cassettes may be built into or attached to the OR bed. Intraoperative x-rays may require the use of a sterile disposable cassette cover. If a sterile cover is unavailable, a sterile Mayo stand cover may be substituted. In some circumstances a cassette may be slid under a patient on the OR table. Care is taken not to contaminate the sterile drapes. Many facilities have discontinued the use of x-ray film and have converted to a digital viewing format.

Processing Equipment

Conventional x-ray equipment projects a black-and-white image on x-ray film that is developed by a chemical process. Some OR suites have a darkroom where x-ray film is developed after exposure so that the surgeon can see results of the study without excessive delay. An automatic processor in which film can be developed within 90 seconds to 3 minutes may be available.

Fixed X-Ray Equipment

A fixed overhead x-ray tube with housing may be mounted on a ceiling track for unrestricted movement of the x-ray beam into the desired position over the patient. When not in use, it can be moved against a wall and retracted toward the ceiling. Some units are fixed to specially designed tables, such as the urologic table for cystoscopic examinations. The controls are in an adjacent room or behind a lead shield and are activated by the radiologist or radiology technician.

Portable X-Ray Machine

An x-ray tube mounted on a portable electric- or battery-powered generator of a nonexplosive design may be moved from one room to another in the OR suite and postanesthesia care unit (PACU). A portable x-ray machine offers the advantages of flexibility in scheduling procedures and availability for when and where it is needed.

Portable x-ray machines can be a source for cross-contamination. All portable equipment should be thoroughly disinfected before being brought into the OR/PACU and again after use. It should be stored within the perioperative environment between uses. Portable x-ray machines are used for intraoperative angiography, cholangiography, orthopedic localization, and urologic contrast procedures.

Intraoperative images require the x-ray machine to be in proximity to the sterile field and could cause contamination. A few options to prevent contamination include draping the machine with a specialized drape or temporarily placing a sterile towel over the site to be imaged. Extreme care is taken to prevent contamination when the towel is removed. Reasons for intraoperative x-ray imaging include performing diagnostic examinations with contrast media or looking for a lost surgical object.

In the PACU the portable x-ray machine is used for immediate (stat) chest and kidney, ureter, and bladder (KUB)/flat plate films. X-ray films can be used to check the location of implants and delayed passage of contrast medium through an organ system.

Fluoroscope

Similar to an x-ray generator, a fluoroscope has an additional screen, composed of fluorescent crystals, which lies in contact with a photocathode. When an x-ray beam passes through this screen, it fluoresces. Fluorescent light sets electrons free from an adjacent photocathode to produce an electron image. Rather than this image of body structures being photographed on x-ray film, it is reproduced as a digital image on a luminescent screen. Known as fluoroscopy, examination under a fluoroscope allows visualization of both form and movement of internal body structures. Fluoroscopy is used frequently for both preoperative and intraoperative procedures.

It is an invasive technique because a fluorescent substance must be injected or a radiopaque device inserted. When exposure time is prolonged to perform a procedure with visual fluoroscopic control (e.g., cardiac catheterization), fluoroscopy exposes the patient and personnel to radiation at higher levels than do conventional x-rays. Personnel must wear lead aprons during fluoroscopy, even though a lead shield is part of the installation. Patients in the vicinity should be protected with gonad and thyroid shields.

Image Intensifier

The image intensifier is used with the fluoroscope. It amplifies the image onto a monitor screen. The surgeon activates the image intensifier with a foot pedal. Clarity of the image is an aid in diagnosis, particularly of vascular, urologic, neurologic, and bone disorders. The surgeon can observe the progression of an injected fluorescent substance as it moves through internal structures or the placement of a device, such as a catheter, into the body. When connected to other closed-circuit television facilities, the image can be transmitted to other rooms for teaching purposes. In addition, the image can be videoed for a permanent record and teaching. The monitoring screen may be mounted on the ceiling and positioned over the OR bed to save space in the OR, or it may be portable.

C-Arm Image Intensifier

Designed primarily for orthopedic procedures, foreign body and calculi localization, and catheter placement, mobile image intensifiers offer the same advantages and disadvantages of portable x-ray machines. The C-arm, so named because of its shape (see Fig. 13.4), keeps the image intensifier and x-ray tube in alignment; the intensifier is directly under the tube. It can be moved from an anterior to a lateral position. Utility of the mobile C-arm image intensifier is enhanced when the system can make electronic x-rays for permanent records. An additional formatting device is required for this function.

Computerized Digital Subtraction Processor

After intravenous (IV) injection of a radiopaque contrast medium, the computerized digital subtraction x-ray imaging system visually records perfusion within the cardiovascular system (e.g., extracranial and intracranial vessels). The procedure is known as digital subtraction angiography (DSA).

Initially, before contrast medium is injected, fluoroscopic body images are converted to digital data for storage in a memory unit in the processor. Termed the *mask image*, these digitized data are integrated into single or multiple video frames. The video signal is logarithmically amplified and digitized. The mask image is electronically subtracted from subsequent images with the contrast medium. This process removes unwanted background, thus providing optimal visualization of vessels with contrast density that cannot be achieved by other image intensifiers. The resultant images (digital x-rays) are displayed on a video screen and can be recorded on CD or other peripheral media.

Radiologic Diagnostic Procedures
Chest X-ray

Most surgeons consider a chest x-ray film as an extension of the patient's history and physical examination if it is clinically necessary. An x-ray study of the chest may be part of the admission procedure for elective surgical patients to rule out unsuspected pulmonary disease that could be communicable or would contraindicate the use of inhalation anesthetics.

This procedure may be routine for patients older than 40 years. It is always a part of the diagnostic workup in patients with suspected or symptomatic pulmonary abnormalities if they will be undergoing general anesthesia.

X-ray Studies for Trauma

In addition to being an aid in determining the extent of traumatic injury, x-ray films and scans may be entered as legal evidence in a court of law to establish injuries sustained by the patient or to justify medical care given. Conventional noninvasive x-ray images will show the following features:

- Bone fractures
- Presence and location of some types of foreign bodies (e.g., bullets)
- Air or blood in the pleural cavity
- Gas or fluid in the abdominal cavity
- Outline of abdominal and chest organs and any deviation from normal size or location

Mammography

A technique for projecting an x-ray image of soft tissue of the breast, mammography is the most effective screening method for early diagnosis of small, nonpalpable breast tumors.[5] Mammography may be performed in conjunction with ultrasonography if the woman has fibrocystic breasts and difficult-to-palpate masses less than ¼ inch (0.5 cm) in diameter. Patients with a family history of breast cancer may have a genetic blood test for a mutation in the *BRCA1* or *BRCA2* gene. This genetic defect may contribute to the risk for ovarian cancer.

Three views of each breast are exposed to conventional x-rays and developed on film. The use of three-dimensional technology (3D breast tomosynthesis [DBT] mammography) takes pictures from the front and side angles of the breast, and the digital images are viewed on a computer screen. The images can be enlarged on a computer screen for better viewing, especially for dense breast tissue. Images can be electronically sent to a health care provider and easily stored in the computer. The procedure may be somewhat painful for the woman because compression is needed for radiologic imaging. Tumors appear on the mammogram as opaque spiculated (star-shaped) areas or, occasionally, as areas of calcification. The radiologist places a small, BB-like radiolucent bead with crosshairs over a suspicious area. Another x-ray view of this area is obtained. Fine-needle aspiration may be performed under ultrasonic guidance to gather cells for cytologic study. If more information is needed for diagnosis, magnetic resonance imaging (MRI) may be ordered.

Patient Teaching

The American Cancer Society recommends that women 40 years of age have a baseline screening mammogram. Between the ages of 45 and 54 years, they should have additional screening x-rays yearly or as recommended by their physician. After age 55, women should have a mammogram every 2 years. Women with a family history of breast cancer may be recommended to have a mammogram before the age of 30. The use of MRI may be suggested along with mammography.

Mammography is not contraindicated in women with breast implants. The technician obtaining the x-ray should be informed of previous breast surgeries, hormone replacement therapy, and augmentation mammoplasty. Special breast-imaging techniques are used to displace an implant or obtain an x-ray view of extremely dense breast tissue.

Men with suspicious breast lesions or pronounced gynecomastia should have mammographic screening to rule out cancerous tissue.

Every patient should be taught breast self-examination and practice it every month as a baseline diagnostic test. Early diagnosis is the best chance for a cure. Fig. 22.3 depicts the average sizes of masses discovered in patients who do and do not practice breast self-examination.

Stereotactic Core Breast Tissue Biopsy

A needle biopsy device may be used in conjunction with mammography to obtain a tissue specimen from a lesion seen on the mammogram. The patient is positioned prone on a special table with her breasts placed through a biopsy porthole. Stereotactic imaging equipment is used to isolate breast lesions that may not be palpable. Percutaneous needle biopsies are performed with the patient under local anesthesia.

Computed Tomography

In CT, special complex and expensive equipment uses an x-ray in conjunction with a computer. Because the x-ray beam moves back and forth across the body to project cross-sectional images, the technique is referred to as computed tomography, computed axial tomography (CAT), or, simply, scanning. It produces a highly contrasted, detailed study of normal and pathologic anatomy.

The x-ray tube and photomultiplier detectors rotate slowly around the patient's head, chest, or body for 180 degrees in a linear fashion along the vertical axis. The computer processes the data and constructs a two- or three-dimensional picture on a black-and-white monitor or in colors that correspond to the

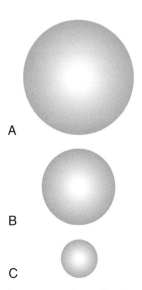

• **Fig. 22.3** Average-Size Lumps Found by Breast Self-Examination (BSE). **A,** Woman not practicing BSE. **B,** Woman practicing occasional BSE. **C,** Woman practicing monthly BSE. (From Fortunato NM, McCullough SM: *Plastic and reconstructive surgery,* St. Louis, 1998, Mosby.)

density of tissue. Structures are identified by differences in density. This picture is photographed for a permanent record. The computer also prints out on a magnetic disk the numerical density values related to the radiation-absorption coefficients of substances in the area scanned. The radiologist uses this printout to determine whether a substance is fluid, blood, normal tissue, bone, air, or a pathologic lesion. The exact size and location of lesions in the brain, mediastinum, and abdominal organs are identified.

CT becomes an invasive procedure when a radiopaque contrast medium is injected IV to enhance visualization of the vascular and renal systems. Oral diluted barium contrast can be used to examine the gastrointestinal tract when a perforated organ is not suspected. Tissue biopsy can be performed under CT guidance. Needle aspiration can be performed under direct CT visualization.

CT exposes the patient to ionizing radiation and a potential allergic reaction to contrast medium, if used. To ensure proper use of this complex equipment, as well as to protect the patient from excessive or unnecessary radiation, the procedure is done under the supervision of a qualified radiologist.

Ventriculography

Ventriculography is the x-ray study of the ventricles after injection of gas, radionuclide, or contrast medium directly into the lateral ventricles of the brain. It may be used to evaluate a patient with signs of increased intracranial pressure as a result of blockage of cerebrospinal fluid circulation. Ventricular needles or catheters are inserted into one or both lateral ventricles through holes made in the skull. The ventricular needle has a blunt, tapered point that prevents injury to the brain as it is inserted into the ventricle. Openings on the side near the point permit removal of spinal fluid and injection of agent. If the patient is an infant whose suture lines in the skull are not yet closed, needles are inserted through these.

The entire ventriculographic procedure may be done in the OR. Otherwise the holes are drilled and the ventricular needles or an intraventricular catheter is inserted, and the patient is then transferred to the radiology department or an interventional room within the OR suite. If a lesion is identified, the diagnostic procedure may be followed immediately by a surgical procedure because of the possibility of a further increase in intracranial pressure. If the patient is returned to the unit after the procedure, sterile ventricular needles should accompany the patient. If intracranial pressure becomes too great after injection, a needle can be inserted to remove the gas, radionuclide, or contrast media.

Arthrography

Arthrography is the study of a joint after the injection of gas or contrast medium into it. Conventional x-ray views show only the bony structure of a joint. Through injection of a dye or gas, injury to cartilage and ligaments may be visualized. A double-contrast study uses both gas and contrast, which is particularly useful in knee arthrograms.

Angiography and Arteriography

Angiography is a comprehensive term for studies of the circulatory system after injection of a radiopaque substance to permit visualization of the venous blood vessel system. These procedures are useful in the differential diagnosis of arteriovenous malformations, aneurysms, tumors, vascular accidents, or other circulatory abnormalities caused by traumatic injury or an acquired structural disease.

Intraoperative studies often are essential to assess the results of vascular reconstruction. Angiography is one method of assessment to confirm the position and patency of an arterial or venous graft or the quality of a restored vessel lumen. Intraoperative angiography frequently is indicated for these assessments in the peripheral vessels of extremities. After insertion of a bypass graft or endarterectomy, patency of the graft or vessel is checked by pulsations, arteriography, or ultrasound to examine the arterial blood vessels of the circulatory system.

Angiography is also used at the time of the surgical procedure to identify vascularity or the exact location of some types of lesions in the extremities, brain, and thoracic and abdominal cavities. After venous injection of radiopaque contrast medium, radiologic studies are done. Techniques and equipment to be used will vary according to the specific procedure, but all types of angiography have the following list of features in common:

1. Access to the vessel (either an artery or vein) to be injected with a radiopaque contrast medium may be made by a percutaneous puncture or a cutdown.
   a. Cannulated needles with or without a radiopaque plastic catheter, similar to those used for IV infusions, may be used for a percutaneous puncture to penetrate an artery or vein. To prevent backflow of blood, cannulated needles have an obturator that remains in place until the contrast medium is injected. Long catheters have a guidewire to assist threading through the vessel.
   b. A Seldinger (18-gauge) needle has a sharply beveled inner cannula and a blunt outer cannula. The blunt end of the outer cannula prevents trauma to the vessel. After insertion, the inner cannula is replaced with a guidewire and the outer cannula is removed. A 20-cm vessel dilator sheath (which is approximately 8 inches long) is threaded over the guidewire to create a track for a radiopaque catheter.

   After the dilator sheath is removed, the catheter is positioned and the guidewire is withdrawn. This method is generally preferred for angiography because blood vessels other than the one punctured can be injected with contrast medium.

   c. A Cournand needle has a curved, flanged guard that contours to the body. It is particularly useful in carotid arteriography to hold the needle in position in the neck during injection.
   d. A Robb cannula is blunt, with a large lumen and a stopcock at the hub. It is inserted via a cutdown and is used with a Robb syringe that has a large opening in the tip for fast injection.
   e. A Sheldon needle has an occluded point with an opening at 90 degrees to the lumen. When the vertebral artery is entered, a right-angle injection is made into the lumen of the artery.
2. The amounts of radiopaque contrast substances injected into blood vessels are computed for infants and children according to weight. In adults the amount is measured so that it can be repeated safely for more exposures if necessary.

Aortic imaging may require the use of full-strength contrast media because of the size of the structure. Radiopaque agents dissipate very rapidly in the bloodstream.

3. Radiopaque contrast material should be warmed to body temperature to prevent precipitation and reduce viscosity. Cold contrast is thicker and requires more pressure to infuse into smaller vessels. The risk for extravasation exists if the vessel perforates.
4. If awake, the patient should be told to expect a warm feeling and possibly a burning sensation when the contrast medium is injected. Procedures may be done with the patient under local anesthesia.
5. Sterile plastic tubing, 30 inches (76 cm) long with a syringe on one end and an adapter on the other, is connected to the needle or catheter in the vessel to prevent jarring from the pressure of injection and to keep the hands of the operator out of the x-ray beam.
6. An automatic injector may be used instead of injecting contrast medium by hand. This device correlates injection and x-ray exposure. When an automatic injector is used, special high-pressure nylon tubing is used that does not pull apart with pressure. When this tubing is used, a stopcock is placed on the end for closing it off at the syringe connection because nylon tubing cannot be clamped.

The consistency of pressure associated with a power injector minimizes the risk for air bubbles in the line and possibly air embolization. In the event of air embolus, the patient should be immediately placed in a left lateral position. Large quantities of air may need to be removed through a catheter inserted into the right atrium of the heart. Removing the air from the heart is known as the Durant procedure. The anesthesia provider can perform this procedure. Some patients respond well to hyperbaric oxygen treatments.

7. Automatic radiologic equipment takes rapid multiple exposures while the contrast medium is in sufficient concentration to visualize the vessels. It can be set at 0.5 to 2-second intervals to take multiple pictures in succession.
8. Digital subtraction angiography converts the x-ray beam into a video screen image. A small amount of contrast medium is injected IV. Vessel catheterization is unnecessary, and less contrast medium is used. This procedure may be done on an ambulatory basis.

Cholangiography

In addition to preoperative diagnostic x-ray studies, some surgeons routinely request radiologic studies in conjunction with cholecystectomy or cholelithotomy to identify gallstones in the biliary tract. Other surgeons selectively include cholangiography at the time of the surgical procedure in patients in whom they suspect stones might be present or retained in the bile ducts. Conventional x-ray equipment or an image intensifier may be used for these intraoperative studies.

The basic difference between preoperative and intraoperative cholangiography is the site of administration of the radiopaque contrast medium. For preoperative invasive cholangiography, the contrast medium injected IV through percutaneous venipuncture is excreted by the liver into the bile ducts. During open surgical procedures, the medium is injected directly into bile ducts.

Gastrointestinal X-ray Studies

Studies are performed to identify lesions in the mucosa of the gastrointestinal tract, such as an ulcer, a stricture, or a tumor. Inflammatory lesions and partial or complete obstructions also may be identified. Barium sulfate is either swallowed by the patient or instilled by enema to outline the lumen of segments of the tract to be studied if the bowel is intact, not perforated. These studies are done in the radiology department, but surgeons often refer to views during the surgical procedure. Care is taken not to use natural latex rubber enema tubing for this procedure if the patient is sensitive to latex.

Myelography

Lesions in the spinal canal are studied by myelography. It is helpful to localize a filling defect, spinal cord tumor, or herniated nucleus pulposus. Most surgeons do not rely entirely on this method of diagnosis; the patient's symptoms and signs are important in making a final diagnosis. Arachnoiditis is a potential complication of intrathecal injection of iophendylate (Pantopaque). Therefore a water-based contrast medium may be preferred.

Urography

Urography is a comprehensive term for radiologic studies of the urinary tract. Most procedures are performed in the radiology department, but some are done in conjunction with cystoscopic examinations. Urographic studies are described as follows:

- *Cystography:* The study of the bladder after instillation of a contrast medium. It is valuable in detecting ureterovesical reflux, a malfunction of the sphincter valves.
- *Cystourethrography:* The study of the bladder and urethra to determine whether there is an obstruction or abnormality in contour or position. X-ray views may be taken as contrast medium is injected into the bladder or when the patient voids the material.
- *Intravenous pyelography (IVP):* The study of the structures of the urinary tract and kidney function. Contrast medium is introduced into the circulatory system by rapid IV injection or slow IV infusion drip. It is excreted through the kidneys. X-ray views are taken at carefully timed intervals. If the medium is poorly excreted through the kidneys, the last view may be taken as late as 24 hours after injection. Tomograms also may be taken while the contrast material is still in the urinary tract. These procedures are done in the radiology department rather than in the cystoscopy room.
- *Retrograde pyelography:* The study of the patency, shape, and position of the kidneys and ureters. Contrast medium is injected through catheters placed in each ureter. This procedure is used to visualize the renal pelves and calyces.
- *Voiding cystourethrography:* The study of the contour and patency of the urethra. Contrast medium may be instilled into the bladder. X-ray views are taken as the patient voids. The medium must flow well but be viscous enough to distend the urethra and provide good detail on the x-ray view. If the patient is anesthetized, a very viscous contrast medium is injected into the urethra and then views are taken. Because the female urethra is rather short, the latter technique is of little value in female patients.

Incidental X-ray

An unanticipated need for an x-ray view occurs when a sponge, needle, or instrument is unaccounted for at the time the final count is taken during wound closure. An x-ray view will confirm whether the item is still inside the patient. Unless the patient's condition demands immediate wound closure, an x-ray should be taken before closure is completed.

A simple, noncontrast x-ray of the abdomen is referred to as a flat plate. Another name for a flat plate is KUB, which stands for kidneys, ureters, and bladder.

Interventional Radiology

The radiologist may work in collaboration with the surgeon to insert catheters for infusion of cytotoxic and pharmacologic drugs, dilation, or embolization of vessels or organs. Cardiac catheterization, angioplasty, and stent placement are performed in an interventional radiology department. Biopsies may be performed percutaneously under radiologic C-arm control. Foreign bodies and thrombi may be extracted.

Interventional radiologic procedures are performed with the patient positioned on a fluoroscopic table equipped with an image intensifier for x-ray visualization of anatomic structures as the surgical procedure progresses. Positioning aids should be used as compatible with the machinery.

The x-ray equipment that will extend over the surgical site should be free from dust. It should be damp-dusted with a disinfectant solution before the patient arrives and the surgical procedure begins. It may be covered with a sterile drape or sleeve before it is moved over the sterile field.

Time, distance, and shielding are the key factors in minimizing ionizing radiation exposure. Personnel should stand at least 6 ft (2 m) away from the radiation source and wear lead aprons with thyroid, sternal, and gonad shields. Patients should be protected with gonad shields if possible. C-arm imaging sends the ionizing radiation from under the patient's body; therefore the shielding should be placed under the patient for adequate protection.

A stock of routine supplies should be kept on a portable cart if procedures are done in the radiology department or other interventional area. In general the following list of items should be readily available:

1. Sterile tray for the specific procedure (e.g., micropuncture kit)
2. Skin preparation tray and solutions
3. IV administration sets and solutions
4. Local anesthetic agents, needles, and syringes
5. Radiopaque contrast material
6. Guidewires, catheters, sheaths, and trocars
7. Sterile gowns, gloves, drapes, and dressings

The following list of emergency equipment should be readily available:

1. Cardiac resuscitation equipment, including a defibrillator and emergency medications
2. Oxygen supply, Ambu bag, endotracheal tubes, and tubing

Patients should be carefully observed and monitored during all procedures for any change in condition. If a procedure is done with the patient under local anesthesia, a qualified registered nurse should monitor the patient's vital signs. A standby anesthesia provider should be available to check the patient's physiologic status as needed.

Magnetic Resonance Imaging

MRI was introduced in U.S. hospitals in 1981. Unlike CT scanning, MRI does not use radiation. The patient lies flat inside a large electromagnet. In this static magnetic field the patient is exposed to bursts of alternating radiofrequency energy waves. The magnetic nuclei of hydrogen atoms in the water of body cells are stimulated from their state of equilibrium. As nuclei return to their original state, they emit radiofrequency signals. These signals are converted by a digital computer into two-dimensional color images displayed on a monitor and recorded on video. Cross-sectional views of the head and all body soft tissue planes can be obtained. A computer software system is also available that produces three-dimensional images.

MRI is based on the magnetic properties of hydrogen in the body rather than on the radiodensity of calcium, which is the basis of radiology. MRI looks at both the body's structure and function. It defines soft tissues in relationship to bony and neurovascular structures. It distinguishes among fat, muscle, compact bone and bone marrow, brain and spinal cord, fluid-filled cavities, ligaments and tendons, and blood vessels. The major applications of MRI are detection of tumors, inflammatory diseases, infections, and abscesses and evaluation of functions of the cardiovascular and central nervous systems and other organs.

MRI paramagnetic IV contrast media, such as gadopentetate, gadoterate, or gadoteridol, are used to localize tumors in the central nervous system. The U.S. Food and Drug Administration (FDA) approved gadopiclenol in 2022; it requires half the dose of other contrast agents and produces the same clear images. These media do not contain iodine, and allergic reactions are rare. All metals can cause artifacts that distort MRI scans—some more so than others. Titanium ligating clips, for example, create less distortion than do ferromagnetic (iron) or stainless steel clips. Iron-containing (ferrous) pigments used in tattoos and permanent eyeliner can alter the image produced and generate heat. The magnetic field can cause ferromagnetic components of implants, such as pacemakers and cochlear implants, to malfunction. The magnetic field will also disable metallic devices in the area, such as cardiac monitors, infusion pumps, and wristwatches.

Some patients feel a sense of claustrophobia in a conventional MRI machine (Fig. 22.4). The procedure lasts from 30 to 90 minutes, and the patient must remain still. As the magnets switch on and off, a banging noise echoes through the chamber. The use of ear plugs and headphones helps reduce the sound. Open MRI technology has decreased the feeling of being closed in and has decreased the noise level caused by the scanning (Fig. 22.5).

MRI is used during select neurosurgical procedures since the advent of open units. Dedicated MRI interventional rooms permit the use of MRI during the actual surgical procedure. It is critical to prevent any magnetic metallic equipment or instrumentation from being used in the vicinity of the MRI. Severe patient injury can be caused by metal objects such as an oxygen tank being

• **Fig. 22.4** Conventional closed magnetic resonance imaging.

• **Fig. 22.5** Open magnetic resonance imaging.

pulled into the field by the powerful magnets. Patients are screened for metal implanted in their body such as plates, screws, wires, and shrapnel. Facilities also require patients change into a facility-approved gown to prevent injuries from metal buttons or items in pockets. Some types of fabrics contain copper or other metals that can cause burns.

Nuclear Medicine Studies

Radionuclides

Radioactive isotopes used in nuclear medicine studies are referred to as *radionuclides*. A nuclide is a stable nucleus of a chemical element, such as iodine, plus its orbiting electrons. A nuclide bombarded with radioactive particles becomes unstable and emits radiant energy; it becomes a radionuclide.

Radionuclides that emit electromagnetic energy are used for diagnostic studies to trace the function and structure of most organs of the body. They may be given by the oral, intracavitary, or IV route, including slow IV infusion. These agents may be used to visualize specific areas rather than radiopaque contrast media in some of the procedures previously described. They are particularly useful in studies of the bone marrow, liver, spleen, biliary tract, thyroid, brain, urinary tract, and peripheral vascular system. Because they provide better quantification of arrival times for vascular perfusion above and below lesions, radionuclides may be a more accurate index of the functional significance of a lesion than are other radiopaque contrast media.

Total-Body Scanning

Total-body scanning does not refer to CT but to a radiologic scanning procedure after IV injection of a radionuclide material. Uptake of the radionuclide within the tissues depends on blood flow. Therefore the imaging procedure may be delayed for several hours after the dose is given—not because it takes long for the material to localize in a tumor or inflammatory lesion, where the uptake is high, but because differentiation is achieved after washout from normal structures.

Scanning may include the whole body or only areas of specific interest. Total-body scanning includes identification of structures in the skeletal and vascular systems for diagnosis of a pathologic process such as metastatic bone tumors or thrombotic vascular disease. The scanner can be angled for many views of the same structure.

Scintigraphy and Lymph Node Mapping

Distribution of gamma radioactivity, such as from gallium-67 citrate or radiotracer, may be determined by an external scintillation detector. This is referred to as scintigraphy; the record produced is a scintigram or scintiscan. A sterile probe may be used intraoperatively to count gamma emissions from cancer cells. A radionuclide, such as technetium-99m, and specific antibodies for antigen-producing tumors are injected approximately 2 to 4 hours before the surgical procedure. The computerized display unit emits an auditory signal when the probe detects radioactivity in tissue.

Lymphoscintigraphy (Sentinel Node Sampling)

Spread of cancer from the primary tumor starts with cells entering an adjacent lymph node, referred to as the sentinel lymph node. Some patients have multiple sentinel nodes in some areas of the body. The degree of tumor progression is measured, and the prognostics of the disease can be predicted by evaluating the findings in the sentinel node(s). It is possible to detect spread to other nodes in the area. If the sentinel node is disease free, it can be assumed that the cancer has not spread to other nodes in the area.

Lymphoscintigraphy uses technetium-99m sulfur colloid, which is an isotope that emits gamma rays as it spontaneously degrades. The isotope is injected around the primary tumor and taken up by the lymphatics. A high-resolution gamma camera follows the isotope's path. Images are captured on digital media until the sentinel node is visualized. An excisional biopsy is performed in the OR.

Some surgeons prefer to use isosulfan blue dye, which is selectively picked up by lymphatic vessels, to visually observe the location of the sentinel node. The dye is injected 1 hour before the excisional biopsy. Care is taken not to transect the lymphatic vessels that carry the dye because nontarget tissue could be stained and the location of the node in question would be obscured. The excised specimen is sent to the laboratory for fixation or frozen section. Before permanent slides are made, the specimen is stored in the nuclear medicine department for 2 or 3 days until the isotope has degraded to normal. At this point the permanent slide is sent to the pathology department for further diagnosis.

Positron Emission Tomography

Positron emission tomography (PET) is a form of nuclear imaging that combines elements of CT scanning and nuclear scanning to create a picture representing the brain or other organ structure. The radioisotopes used emit positrons that cause pairs of gamma rays to be discharged. The rays are detected by the scanner and are relayed to a computer that converts them into cross-sectional, three-dimensional color images. PET studies provide detailed measurements of biochemistry and physiologic activity. They are used to study blood flow and metabolic functions, primarily in the brain and heart. Higher metabolic activity appears red, lesser activity appears yellow, still lesser activity appears green, and the least activity appears blue.

A PET scan can be used with fludeoxyglucose-F18 to identify and localize lymph node activity. Metastasis can be detected, and/or the patient's response to therapy can be assessed. This method is costly because the radioisotopes have a short half-life. The patient is placed on a table that slides into a tube-like opening. A similar form of scan is the single-photon emission computed tomography (SPECT) scan, which is done with a rotating gamma camera and is commonly used in brain, liver, and cardiac imaging.

Ultrasonography

Ultrasonography uses vibrating high-frequency sound waves in the frequency of 20,000 to 10 billion cycles per second—beyond the hearing capability of human ears—to detect alterations in anatomic structures or hemodynamic properties within the body. The basic component of any diagnostic ultrasound system is its specialized transducer, which is a piezoelectric crystal. The transducer converts electrical impulses to ultrasonic waves at a frequency greater than 1 million cycles per second. These ultrasonic frequencies are transmitted into tissues through a transducer placed on the skin.

A water-soluble gel is applied to the skin to maintain airtight contact between the skin and the transducer because ultrasonic waves do not travel well through air. A portion of the transmitted ultrasonic waves is reflected back as real-time images to a receiving crystal. The transducer, connected to a microprocessing computer, is held on the skin long enough to obtain a graphic recording of the reflected high-frequency sound waves. Uniform imaging of a wide range of body tissues is possible. Ultrasound is not effective in the presence of bone or gases in the gastrointestinal tract.

Whether used as a preoperative or intraoperative diagnostic technique, ultrasonography is a rapid, painless, noninvasive procedure that distinguishes between fluid-filled and solid masses.

Ultrasonic frequencies are reflected when the beam reaches target anatomic structures of different densities and acoustic impedance. The reflected signal is picked up by the transducer/receiver as an echo. The intensity of the returning echo is determined not only by the angle formed between the ultrasound beam and the reflecting surface of the anatomic structure but also by the acoustic properties of that surface. The resulting echo is described in terms of time and intensity and displayed on a computerized monitor for immediate interpretation of movements and dimensions of structures.

The image can be recorded on video or printed to provide a permanent record known as an *echogram* or a *sonogram*. Sonograms can be obtained on multiple planes. Ultrasonography is a useful adjunct in the diagnosis of the following conditions:

- *Space-occupying lesions in the neonatal brain:* The echoencephalogram will show a shift of the brain caused by tumor.
- *Lesions in the breast, thyroid, and parathyroid glands and in abdominal and pelvic organs:* Ultrasound can distinguish between a cystic and a solid tumor mass in the kidney, pancreas, liver, ovary, and testis. It is the best imaging method in patients with gallbladder disease.
- *Emboli (air, blood, or fat):* Ultrasonography is particularly useful in the early diagnosis of pulmonary embolism. Fat embolus syndrome can develop after long bone fractures.
- *Fetal maturation:* Fetal head size is an aid in the determination of fetal maturation. This can be measured by ultrasound before an elective cesarean section (C-section) or to determine the need for a C-section if the head is too large for vaginal delivery. Ultrasonography is also used to determine the position of the fetus and placenta, identify sex, and detect fetal abnormalities.
- *Cardiac defects:* Structural defects, insufficient valvular movement, and blood flow volumes within the heart chambers and myocardium can be detected. This diagnostic technique is known as *echocardiography*. The echo probe is inserted into the esophagus to obtain a transesophageal echocardiogram (TEE) or placed over the chest for a two-dimensional effect. The esophageal method is useful during open-heart surgery.

Doppler Studies

Blood flow velocity and pressure measurements are possible with ultrasound because moving blood cells produce a sufficient interface with surrounding vessels to independently reflect high-frequency sound waves. The Doppler ultrasonic velocity detector emits a beam of 5 to 10 megahertz (MHz) that is directed through the skin into the bloodstream. A portion of the transmitted ultrasound is reflected from moving particles in the blood. Known as the Doppler effect, the reflected sound wave changes in frequency because the source of the sound is in motion. This shift in frequency is proportional to the velocity of the blood flow.

Originally introduced for use in detecting obstruction in arterial blood flow, the Doppler instrument is used extensively to locate and evaluate blood flow patterns in peripheral arterial and venous diseases or defects, such as the following:

- *Arterial disease:* Detection of altered hemodynamics in arterial flow is significant in diagnosis of obstructive or occlusive arterial lesions. For example, the Doppler will indicate regions in the neck where carotid artery blood flow to the brain is obstructed by atherosclerosis.
- *Obstruction, ischemia, and aneurysms:* A surgical procedure can be performed to remove or bypass the obstruction to prevent the patient suffering a cerebrovascular accident (stroke/brain attack). It also may help the surgeon determine the appropriate level of lower extremity amputation for ischemia caused by peripheral arterial occlusive disease. It is useful in diagnosis of aortoiliac aneurysms.
- *Venous disease:* Occlusion of superficial or deep veins and the presence of incompetent valves can be located and identified by sounds made by the flow of blood through the peripheral venous system. This qualitative information of abnormal venous hemodynamics in patients with varicose veins and thrombotic disease helps the surgeon plan surgical intervention.

Intraoperative Ultrasonography

A sterile ultrasound transducer probe or scan head may be placed on tissue to evaluate vascularity or density. A pathologic condition can be diagnosed or localized. The handheld transducer must make an acoustic coupling with tissue. Tissues are moistened with sterile normal saline solution, sterile water-soluble jelly, sterile acoustic gel, or peritoneal fluid (if the transducer is placed on the abdomen). The flexible transducer cable is attached to the ultrasound machine, which has a visible display screen.

Permanent recordings of images may be immediately printed or saved on a CD incorporated into the machine. The sound waves may be either continuous or pulsed. A transducer can range from 2 to 15 MHz. A three-dimensional transducer has a frequency between 7.5 and 11 MHz. Ultrasonography is less time-consuming and requires less tissue manipulation than do other intraoperative diagnostic procedures and does not expose the patient to radiation and contrast medium.

Hemodynamics

Ultrasound imaging is used to evaluate the adequacy or restoration of blood flow during vascular reconstruction procedures, such as of peripheral vessels in the lower extremities, hepatic and portal shunts, and carotid arteries. A transesophageal echocardiogram (TEE) may be obtained during coronary revascularization by placing the transducer in the esophagus. Doppler instruments are frequently used to assess blood flow through reconstructive tissue flaps and grafts and microvascular anastomoses.

Air Embolus

The Doppler instrument can be used to monitor patients during neurosurgery, open-heart surgery, or procedures on the great vessels in the chest to detect the escape of air into the circulation. Whenever the surgical site is higher than the right atrium, the risk for venous air embolism is possible. Air entering an artery to the brain (cerebral air embolism) or venous system may cause anoxic brain damage or death. A venous air embolus of 50 mL causes

severe cardiac dysrhythmias by blocking blood flow through the right atrium of the heart; however, 300 mL can be fatal. If an air embolus is detected at the time it occurs, the Durant procedure to evacuate the air can be initiated immediately by the anesthesia provider.

In the Durant procedure the right atrial air embolus is treated by placing the patient's head lower than the heart in steep Trendelenburg position and elevating the right side of the table or rolling the patient into left lateral position. A multilumen right atrial catheter is inserted through a central venous line into the superior vena cava and into the right atrium of the heart. The air can be manually removed by the anesthesia provider with a large syringe.

Localization of Lesions

Ultrasound imaging is used for intraoperative localization of subcortical brain lesions, spinal cord lesions, pancreatic and hepatic tumors, pelvic masses, and lesions in other soft tissues to determine whether the lesion is resectable. The exact location of gallbladder and kidney stones also can be identified.

Percutaneous Puncture

The direction and depth of needle punctures to locate lesions in various abdominal organs, such as a pancreatic cyst, can be determined by following the ultrasound that is continuously visualized on the monitor. The echo from the tip of the needle is easily visible on the scope when the lesion is entered. These procedures are performed to aspirate cytologic specimens for diagnosis.

Sensory Evoked Potential

Sensory evoked potential (SEP) measures neural pathways and involves placement of multiple recording electrodes over peripheral nerves or the scalp and ears. The evoked potentials generated in response to stimulation are recorded. Components of the computerized system provide sensory stimulation; acquisition, amplification, and filtering of electrophysiologic signals; signal processing; and display, measurement, and storage of SEP waveforms. These noninvasive measurements may be taken preoperatively to assist in the diagnosis of a pathologic condition, such as acoustic neuroma. The techniques also may be used for intraoperative monitoring to assess the status of the central nervous system. Multimodality evoked potentials aid in assessment of patients with trauma. Three modalities are used:

1. *Somatosensory evoked potential (SSEP):* An objective evaluation of peripheral and central neural pathways. Pairs of surface or needle skin or scalp electrodes are placed in desired patterns over the appropriate peripheral nerves and areas of the spinal cord and cerebral cortex. These electrodes record somatosensory responses elicited on application of electrical stimuli, such as to the peroneal peripheral nerve at the knee or from over the spinal column or scalp. These impulses along neural pathways are charted to determine whether the nerve is functioning properly or a lesion is impeding impulses to the brain. Testing time can range from 45 minutes to 4 hours, depending on the number of peripheral nerves stimulated and sites necessary to assess neural pathways.
2. *Auditory brainstem evoked potential:* A test of the eighth cranial nerve and the auditory pathway to the cerebral cortex. The

patient, wearing headphones or earphones, responds to auditory clicks or tones. Multiple electrodes on the scalp and ears record responses. This study is used to assess the physiologic condition of the brainstem and the patient's hearing threshold.

3. *Visual evoked potential:* A test of responses to visual pattern-reversal stimulation of the optic nerve and its associated pathways to the cerebral cortex. The patient receives stimuli via a television monitor or special eye goggles. Multiple electrodes on the scalp and ears record the evoked potentials.

Plethysmography

In plethysmography, pressure-sensitive instruments placed on an organ or around an extremity record variations in volume and pressure of blood passing through tissues. Pen-recorded tracings reflect pulse wave impulses transmitted from moving currents within arteries and veins. These impulses may be measured, computed by electronic circuits, and displayed as digitized data. Plethysmography does not identify the exact anatomic location, extent, or characteristics of vascular disease. It will quantitatively measure the rate of blood flow or degree of vascular obstruction. The following four techniques are used:

1. *Oculoplethysmography:* A technique for determining hemodynamically significant carotid artery stenosis or cerebrovascular obstruction. The instrument is placed on each eyeball to record pulse waves emanating from the cerebrovascular system.

2. *Strain-gauge plethysmography:* A technique to evaluate altered venous hemodynamics in deep venous thrombosis and varicose veins. Two pneumatic cuffs are placed on the leg snugly around the thigh and calf or the ankle and great toe. A mercury strain gauge attached to the plethysmograph is secured around the leg or foot between the two cuffs. Cuffs are inflated sequentially for distal arterial occlusion and proximal venous occlusion. Changes in blood flow volume are measured as the gauge detects changes in the circumference of the calf or foot caused by sequential inflation and deflation of the pneumatic cuffs.

3. *Venous impedance plethysmography:* A technique to measure venous reflux in the lower extremity. Impedance electrodes are attached to the calf under a pneumatic boot. As the boot is inflated, blood is forced proximally out of the veins. Tissues are compressed, causing a concomitant increase in impedance and decrease in calf volume.

4. *Cutaneous pressure photoplethysmography:* A technique to identify peripheral arterial occlusive disease. An infrared light source in a handheld photoplethysmograph probe is applied to the skin with increasing pressure until the pulse is occluded. Infrared light is absorbed by blood. The intensity of the reflected light changes as the volume of blood increases as pressure is released. The probe measures the ability of the vascular system to force arterial blood into skin tissue.

Endoscopy

Direct visualization within body cavities and structures aids in determination of the appropriate course of therapy for many conditions. Diagnostic endoscopy frequently is performed in conjunction with radiologic studies or to obtain specimens for pathologic examination. A tissue-staining dye and/or radiopaque contrast material may be injected through the endoscope or an accessory before radiologic studies. Fluid and secretions may be withdrawn for culture or chemical analysis. Biopsy specimens are frequently obtained.

Direct visualization alone may confirm the presence or absence of a suspected lesion or abnormal condition. This may be enhanced by an ultrasonic transducer at the end of a flexible fiberoptic scope. Endoscopic diagnosis often provides the information necessary to proceed with an open procedure or to cancel an anticipated surgical procedure. Small video capsules can be swallowed to allow visualization of the small intestine.

Endoscopy is described in detail in Chapter 32, and specific endoscopic procedures are discussed in subsequent chapters when they are pertinent to diagnostic and surgical procedures in the appropriate surgical specialties.

The Patient With Cancer

Oncology is the study of scientific control over neoplastic growth. It concerns the etiology, diagnosis, treatment, and rehabilitation of patients with known or potential neoplasms. A neoplasm is an atypical growth of abnormal cells or tissues that may be a benign or malignant tumor.

Cancer is a broad term that encompasses any malignant tissue change. The exact cause of cancer is unknown. Cancerous tumors can be caused by exposure to chemical toxins, ionizing radiation, chronic tissue irritation, tobacco smoke, ultraviolet rays, viral invasion, and genetic predisposition. Studies have shown that immunosuppression may contribute to the incidence of cancer by altering biochemical metabolism and cellular enzyme production. Other research has shown that dietary influences, such as nitrates, salt-cured or smoked foods, and high-fat diets, may contribute to cancer in certain individuals.

Both malignant and benign neoplasms consist of cells that divide and grow uncontrollably at varied rates. The stimulus for growth can be intrinsic (e.g., hormonal) or extrinsic (e.g., exposure to external elements). Neoplastic overgrowth or the invasion of surrounding tissue causes dysfunction and may eventually cause the death of the patient.

Table 22.2 compares the characteristics and effects of benign and malignant tumors. Four characteristics distinguish malignant

TABLE 22.2 Comparison of Benign and Malignant Tumors

Benign	Malignant
Characteristics	
Expansive	Invasive
Localized	Spreads to distant sites
Encapsulated	No capsule
Slow growth	Rapid growth
Resembles parent tissue	Varied differentiation
Normal cell reproduction	Disorganized cell reproduction
Organized mitoses	Abnormal mitoses
Effect on Patient	
Pain uncommon	Severe pain common
Little nutritional effect unless mechanical obstruction is involved	Cachexia, nausea, and vomiting

from benign tumors, with a malignant tumor having characteristics as follows:

- It is anaplastic. Cancer cells resemble normal cell forms but are morphologically and functionally differentiated from the normal tissue of origin. They vary in size, shape, and texture.
- It infiltrates and destroys adjacent normal tissue.
- It grows in a disorganized, uncontrolled, and irregular manner, usually increasing in size both rapidly and perceptibly within weeks or months.
- It has the power to metastasize. Cancer cells migrate from the primary focus to another single focus or to multiple foci in distant tissues or organs via lymphatic or vascular channels.

Clinical Signs and Symptoms of Cancer

According to the American Cancer Society, the following are the clinical signs and symptoms of cancer:

- Palpable mass or abnormal thickening of tissue
- Abnormal bleeding or discharge
- Obvious change in a wart or mole
- Lesion that does not heal
- Steady decrease in weight, appetite, and energy
- Chronic cough
- Change in bowel or bladder habits

Potential Causes of Cancer

The early detection of cancer decreases the incidence of morbidity and mortality. A screening examination may identify a neoplasm before clinical symptoms develop. Recommended cancer screening examinations are listed in Table 22.3. (More screening information can be found on the American Cancer Society website at http://www.cancer.org/.[6])

Risk-Related Factors

Risk factors for cancer include the following:

- Age, sex, racial, genetic, or hereditary predisposition. Table 22.4 identifies neoplasms associated with familial cancer syndromes.
- Exposure to carcinogens (cancer-producing agents) such as tobacco smoke, coal tar, ionizing radiation, ultraviolet rays, and chemicals. Table 22.5 lists examples of chemical carcinogens.
- Predisposition from specific environmental conditions or acquired conditions or diseases. Table 22.6 gives examples of viral-mediated carcinogens.

Extent of Disease

Carcinoma In Situ

In carcinoma in situ, normal cells are replaced by anaplastic cells but the growth disturbance of epithelial surfaces shows no behavioral evidence of invasion and metastasis. This cellular change is noted most often in stratified squamous and glandular epithelium. Carcinoma in situ is also referred to as *intraepithelial* or *preinvasive cancer*. Common sites for in situ carcinoma include the following:

- Uterine cervix
- Uterine endometrium
- Vagina
- Anus
- Penis
- Lip
- Buccal mucosa
- Bronchi
- Esophagus
- Eye
- Breast

Localized Cancer

Localized cancer is contained within the organ of its origin.

Regional Cancer

In regional cancer the invaded area extends from the periphery of the organ or tissue of origin to include tumor cells in adjacent organs or tissues (e.g., the regional lymph nodes).

Metastatic Cancer

In metastatic cancer the tumor extends by way of lymphatic or vascular channels to tissues or organs beyond the regional area. The cancer cells multiply erratically (anaplasia) and move to other areas of the body. Anaplasia implies that the cancer cells have taken on unusual shapes and reproduce in unpredictable patterns.

Disseminated Cancer

In disseminated cancer, multiple foci of tumor cells are dispersed throughout the body.

Tumor Identification System (TNM)

A standardized tumor identification system, which includes classification and staging, is essential for establishing treatment protocols and evaluating the end result of therapy. Hospitals maintain a tumor registry of patients to evaluate therapeutic approaches to specific types of tumors. Classification includes the anatomic and histologic description of a tumor, whereas staging refers to the extent of the tumor. There are three basic categories of the tumor identification system:

- Primary **T**umor
- Regional **N**odes
- Distant **M**etastases

The TNM categories are identified by pretreatment clinical diagnosis, tissue biopsy, and/or histopathologic examination after surgical resection of the tumor. Numeric and alphabetic characters are used to describe the findings; for example, bronchogenic carcinoma T1 N0 M0 means a primary tumor in the lung without positive regional nodes or distant metastases. If a positive lymph node is identified in the area, it is indicated in an abbreviated sequence (e.g., T1 N1 M0). If a metastatic site also is diagnosed, it too is indicated in the same format (e.g., T1 N1 M1).

The numeric and alphabetic sequence corresponds to the number of separate tumors at the identified primary site, positive lymph nodes, or metastatic sites (Box 22.3). Other staging systems are referred to in the literature as stages I, II, III, and IV. After treatment, the estimation of residual tumor volume is indicated by the letter R.

Monitoring Tumor Markers

Tumor markers are serum studies used to measure specific enzymes emitted by tumor cells. Elevated tumor markers in the patient's blood and tissues can help determine the patient's treatment and prognosis. Table 22.7 describes common blood tests for serum tumor markers and their implication in cancer prognostication.

TABLE
22.3 **Cancer Screening Examinations**

Sex	Age	Frequency of Examination
Pelvic Examination by Palpation and Inspection		
Female	25 years	Every 3 years (PAP, cytology)
	Ages 25 and up	Every 5 years (HPV)
Pelvic Examination by Palpation and Inspection, Including Pap Smear and HPV Testing		
Female	25–65 years. Screening every 3 years. HPV minimum of every 5 years	Frequency performed on advice of physician
Endometrial Tissue Sample		
Female	At menopause or sooner at recommendation of physician	Sample for baseline in high-risk patient
Breast Self-Examination		
Female and male	No recommendations. Individuals should report any changes to their physician	*Female:* monthly after menses or at same time each month after menopause *Male:* monthly
Clinical Breast Examination		
Female	No recommendations	Corresponds with pelvic examination sequence unless patient has a previous history of breast disease or is at high risk for breast disease
Mammography		
Female	Baseline at age 40, yearly ages 40–54 55 and older, every 2 years High risk at age 30 years	Frequency after baseline is individualized according to age, health, and risk factor analysis by physician; mammography, when performed, should precede clinical breast examination so that data analysis will be complete
Testicular Self-Examination by Palpation and Inspection		
Male	Throughout life span	Monthly
Prostate		
Male	More than age 50; start at age 40 for men at high risk	Yearly, prostate-specific antigen (PSA) blood test
Digital Rectal Examination		
Male and female	Over age 50; start at age 45 for risk factors	Yearly; frequency may vary according to individual risk factors or the recommendation of physician
Stool Guaiac Examination		
Male and female	Over age 45	Yearly; age and frequency may vary according to symptoms and the recommendation of physician
Sigmoidoscopy or Colonoscopy		
Male and female	Over age 45	Every 5–10 years or according to the advice of physician; age and frequency may vary in the presence of risk factors or individual symptoms; colonoscopy may be advised according to risk factors
Generalized Physical With Health Counseling		
Includes palpation of thyroid, gonads, and lymphatics, as well as inspection of oral mucosa		
Male and female	Over age 20	Every 2–3 years
Male and female	Over age 30–40 Over 50	Every other year Yearly

HPV, Human papillomavirus.

TABLE 22.4 Familial Cancer Syndromes	
Syndrome	Associated Neoplasm
Autosomal Dominant Gene	
Familial polyposis coli	Adenocarcinoma of colon, adenomatous polyps
Gardner syndrome	Adenocarcinoma of colon, musculoaponeurotic tumors
Peutz-Jeghers syndrome	Adenocarcinoma of small intestine, colon, ovary
Neurofibromatosis	Neurofibroma, neurogenic sarcoma, pheochromocytoma
Multiple endocrine neoplasia (MEN type I), or Wermer syndrome	Pituitary, pancreatic islet cells, parathyroid glands
Multiple endocrine neoplasia (MEN type IIA), or Sipple syndrome	Thyroid, parathyroid glands, pheochromocytoma
Multiple endocrine neoplasia (MEN type IIB)	Thyroid, parathyroid, pheochromocytoma, mucosa ganglioneuromas
Autosomal Recessive Gene	
Xeroderma pigmentosum	Basal and squamous cell carcinoma of skin, malignant melanoma
Ataxia-telangiectasia	Acute leukemia, lymphoma, some gastric cancers

TABLE 22.5 Examples of Chemical Carcinogenesis	
Chemical	Site of Neoplasm
Alkylating Agents	
Nitrogen mustard, cyclophosphamide, chlorambucil	Leukemia, urinary bladder
Vinyl chloride	Angiosarcoma of liver
Polycyclic Hydrocarbons	
Tar, soot, oils	Skin, lung
Aromatic Amines and Azo Dyes	
α-Naphthylamine, benzidine	Urinary bladder
Food Products	
Saccharin	Urinary bladder
Aflatoxin (mold on peanuts)	Liver
Betel nuts	Oral mucosa
Medication	
Androgenic metabolic steroids	Liver
Diethylstilbestrol	Vagina
Phenacetin	Renal pelvis
Inorganic Compounds	
Chromium	Lung
Nickel	Lung, nasal sinuses
Asbestos	Serosal membranes, lung
Arsenic	Skin
Mercury Pesticides and insecticides Non-Hodgkin's Lymphoma, multiple cancer types	Fetal growth and development abnormalities

Cancer Treatment

Cancer is a systemic disease and is treated based on location and cell type. Therapy is curative if the disease process can be totally eradicated, but the success of therapy depends largely on early diagnosis. Tumors are classified to determine the most effective therapy. When a cure is not possible, palliative therapy relieves symptoms and improves quality of life but does not cure the disease.

Before beginning therapy a patient with cancer undergoes an extensive pretreatment workup. Each form of cancer therapy has certain advantages and limitations. Several factors affect a patient's response to treatment: host factors, clinical stage of malignancy, and type of therapy. The patient is followed carefully to determine the effectiveness of treatment at routine intervals. Each type of cancer is treated with a customized plan of drugs, surgery, or combination. In 2022, the FDA approved two drugs (durvalumab, tremelimumab) for unresectable liver cancer.

Adjuvant Therapy

Surgical resection, ablation, endocrine therapy, radiation therapy, chemotherapy, immunotherapy, hyperthermia, or combinations of these procedures are used in the treatment of cancer. The surgeon or oncologist determines the most appropriate therapy for each patient. When determining the most appropriate therapy, the following parameters are considered:
- Type, site, and extent of tumor and whether lymph nodes are involved

TABLE 22.6 Viral-Mediated Carcinogenesis	
Viral Family	Type of Neoplasm
DNA-Associated	
Papilloma (condyloma)	Squamous papilloma and squamous cell carcinoma
Hepatitis B	Hepatocellular carcinoma
Herpesvirus	
Epstein-Barr	Burkitt lymphoma, nasopharyngeal carcinoma
Cytomegalovirus	Kaposi sarcoma
Herpes simplex type II	Uterine cervical carcinoma
RNA-Dependent	
Human T cell lymphotropic type 1 (retrovirus C)	T cell leukemia, lymphoma

DNA, Deoxyribonucleic acid; *RNA,* ribonucleic acid.

• BOX 22.3 Tumor Identification Scale

Primary Tumor
TX Primary tumor discovered by the detection of malignant cells in secretions or cell washings but not directly visualized
T0 No evidence of primary tumor
Tis Tumor (carcinoma) in situ
T1 Tumor is 2 cm or less at largest dimension
T2 Tumor is larger than 2 cm at largest dimension
T3 Tumor directly invades surrounding tissue
T4 Tumor invades surrounding tissue and adjacent structures, such as blood vessels or bone

Regional Lymph Nodes
NX Unable to assess nodes
N0 No regional lymph node metastasis
N1 Metastasis to ipsilateral nodes or direct extension to nodes
N2 Metastasis to contralateral nodes

Distant Metastasis
MX Distant metastasis cannot be assessed
M0 No distant metastasis
M1 Distant metastasis confirmed

Posttreatment Residual Tumor
RX Unable to assess residual tumor
R0 No residual tumor
R1 Microscopic residual tumor
R2 Macroscopic residual tumor

TABLE 22.7 Common Serum Tumor Markers

Test	Value	Indication
Carcinoembryonic antigen (CEA)	0–2.5 ng/mL	Colorectal
Alpha-fetoprotein (AFP)	10 ng/mL	Testicular, liver
Ca-125	<35 U/mL	Ovarian
Human chorionic gonadotropin (HCG)	0–1 ng/mL	Choriocarcinoma testicular
Prostate-specific antigen (PSA)	0–4.0 ng/m/L (>40 years)	Prostate

• BOX 22.4 Palliative Oncologic Surgical Procedures

- Reduction of tumor to prevent obstruction (debulking)
- Reduction of tumor cells to aid effectiveness of chemotherapy
- Treatment of oncologic emergencies such as hemorrhage or compression
- Removal of enlarged organs such as the spleen
- Repair of perforations in irradiated parts such as the rectum
- Removal of a hormone-producing part such as a gonad or other gland
- Removal of a diseased organ such as the uterus, prostate, or breast
- Insertion of a nutritional support device such as a feeding gastrostomy or total parenteral alimentation line
- Pain control such as nerve blocks or the severing of a neural pathway or receptor site

- Type of surrounding normal tissue
- Age and general condition of the patient, including nutritional status and whether other diseases are present
- Whether curative or palliative therapy is possible

Surgical Resection and Palliation

Surgical resection is the modality of choice to remove solid tumors. The resection of a malignant tumor is, however, localized therapy for what may be a systemic disease. Each patient is evaluated and treated individually, and the surgical procedure is planned appropriately for the identified stage of disease. Depending on localization, regionalization, and dissemination of the tumor, the surgeon selects either a radical curative surgical procedure or a salvage palliative surgical procedure.

Surgical debulking or cytoreductive surgery, in which the tumor is partially removed, may be the procedure of choice for some types of surgically incurable malignant neoplasms. With surgical debulking the intent is not to cure but to make subsequent therapy with irradiation, drugs, or other palliative measures more effective and thereby extend survival. In planning the surgical procedure the surgeon considers the length of expected survival, the prognosis of surgical intervention, and the effect of concurrent diseases on the postoperative result.

Accessible primary tumors are often treated by excision. An extremely wide resection may be necessary to avoid recurrence of the tumor. The pathologist can make judgments about questionable margins by evaluating frozen sections while the surgical procedure is in progress. The pathologist's findings guide the surgeon during resection so that residual tumor is not left in the patient. The specimen is also tested after permanent section fixation in the pathology laboratory. Results are available in 2 to 3 days.

Many surgical procedures are performed for ablation of tumors by primary resection. In addition, a lymphadenectomy (removal of local lymph nodes) may be performed as a prophylactic measure to inhibit the metastatic spread of tumor cells via lymphatic channels. These nodes are tested to determine the extent of tumor cell spread. Other modalities of therapy may be administered preoperatively, intraoperatively, and/or postoperatively to reduce or prevent a recurrence or metastasis.

Preservation of Reproductive System

Females and males of reproductive age with cancer who are facing radiation therapy are at risk for becoming sterile as a result of treatment. Gonadal shields are used whenever possible. Males can donate sperm for cryopreservation and later use it for in vitro fertilization or artificial insemination. In some circumstances females can have a laparoscopic procedure to relocate their ovaries to a deeper or medial location in the pelvis where they will experience little or no exposure to radiation. Other palliative surgical interventions are described in Box 22.4.

Endocrine Therapy

Tumors arising in organs that are usually under hormonal influence (e.g., breast, ovary, and uterus in female patients; prostate and testes in male patients) may be stimulated by hormones produced in the endocrine glands. Cellular metabolism is affected by the presence of specific hormone receptors in tumor cells: estrogen and/or progesterone in females and androgens in males.

Certain breast, endometrial, and prostatic cancers depend on sex hormones for growth and maintenance. Therefore the recurrence or spread of disease may be slowed by therapeutic hormonal manipulation. Endocrine manipulation does not cure, but it can control dissemination of the disease if the tumor progresses beyond the limits of effective surgical resection or radiation therapy.

Hormonal Receptor Site Studies

Identifying the hormonal dependence of the primary tumor through studies of the receptor site is a fairly reliable way of selecting patients who will benefit from preoperative or postoperative endocrine manipulation. After a positive diagnosis of cancer, either by a frozen section biopsy or pathologic permanent sections, the surgeon will probably request a receptor site evaluation of a primary breast, uterine, or prostatic tumor.

The tissue specimen removed by surgical resection should be sent fresh or in saline. It should not be placed in formalin preservative solution because doing so will alter the receptor cells enough to negate the hormonal study.

Endocrine Ablation

Since 1896, surgeons have described positive clinical responses in patients with metastatic breast cancer after treatment by endocrine ablation—the surgical removal of endocrine glands. If the surgeon plans to eliminate endocrine stimulation surgically in a patient with a known hormone-dependent tumor, all sources of the hormone should be ablated chemically, hormonally, or surgically.

- *Bilateral adrenalectomy and oophorectomy.* Both adrenal glands and/or ovaries may be resected to prevent the recurrence of endocrine-derived cancer. These may be removed as a one-stage surgical procedure (i.e., bilateral adrenalectomy/oophorectomy). If two separate surgical procedures are preferred, the bilateral oophorectomy precedes the bilateral adrenalectomy, except in menopausal women in whom only the latter surgical procedure may be indicated.
- *Bilateral adrenalectomy and orchiectomy.* After prostatectomy for advanced carcinoma of the prostate, both testes may be removed (i.e., bilateral orchiectomy) to eliminate androgens of testicular origin. Bilateral adrenalectomy also may be indicated.

Hormonal Therapy

Hormones administered orally or via injection can alter cell metabolism by changing the systemic hormonal environment of the body. For hormones to be effective, tumor cells must contain receptors. Hormones must bind to these receptors before they can exert an effect on cells.

- *Antiestrogen therapy:* Patients with medical contraindications to endocrine ablation may receive antiestrogen therapy. An estrogen antagonist deprives an estrogen-dependent tumor of the estrogen necessary for its growth. Nafoxidine, tamoxifen (Nolvadex), and abemaciclib (Verzenio) are synthetic nonsteroidal drugs that inhibit the normal intake of estrogen at estrogen receptor sites; they are taken orally.
- *Corticosteroids:* Prednisone, cortisone, hydrocortisone, or some other preparation of corticosteroids may be administered as an

antiinflammatory agent along with the chemotherapeutic agents given to control disseminated disease.

Photodynamic (Laser) Therapy

For photodynamic therapy (also referred to as *photoradiation*), an argon tunable dye laser is used to destroy malignant cells by photochemical reaction. A photosensitive drug, either hematoporphyrin derivative (HPD) from bovine blood (porfimer [Photofrin]) or purified dihematoporphyrin ether, is absorbed by malignant and reticular endothelial cells.

The photosensitive drug is injected intravenously via venipuncture or Hickman catheter 24 to 48 hours before the photodynamic therapy and is taken up by cells to make them fluorescent and photosensitive. It remains longer in malignant cells than in normal cells before being excreted from the body. When exposed to light from an argon laser, the tunable rhodamine B dye laser produces a red beam of approximately 630 nm. Other dyes, such as dicyanomethylene, may produce different wavelengths.

HPD in cells absorbs the laser light, which leads to a photochemical reaction that causes tissue-oxygen molecules to release cytotoxic singlet oxygen and destroy tumor cells. Depending on tumor site, the laser can be delivered interstitially, endoscopically, externally, or retrobulbarly.

Photodynamic therapy may be used to debulk tumors of the eye, head and neck, breast, esophagus, gastrointestinal tract, bronchus, and bladder. The tunable dye laser also may be used to diagnose tumor cells. The OR should be darkened or have shades to block outside daylight during the laser treatment. The patient is cautioned to avoid exposure to sunlight or other sources of ultraviolet light both after injection of the dye and postoperatively. Photosensitivity is the primary side effect of the dye and may last 4 to 6 weeks.

Radiation Therapy

Radiation is the emission of electromagnetic waves or atomic particles that result from the disintegration of nuclei of unstable or radioactive elements. The treatment of malignant disease with radiation may be referred to as radiation therapy, brachytherapy, or radiotherapy. Ionizing radiation is used for this type of therapy, which involves the use of high-voltage radiation and other radioactive elements to injure or destroy cells. Like surgical resection and photodynamic therapy, radiation therapy is localized therapy that is applicable for a limited number of specific tumors.

Ionizing Radiation

Ionization is the physical production of positive and negative ions capable of conducting electricity. Ionizing radiation is radiation with sufficient energy to disrupt the electronic balance of an atom. When disruption occurs in tissue cells or extracellular fluids, the effect can range from minor changes to profound disturbances. Radiation may come either from particles of the nuclei of disintegrating atoms or from electromagnetic waves that have no mass. Types of ionizing radiation include the following:

- *Alpha particles:* Alpha particles are relatively large particles that have a very slight penetrating power. They are stopped by a thin sheet of paper. They have dense ionization but can produce tremendous tissue destruction within a short distance.
- *Beta particles:* Beta particles are relatively small, are electrical, and travel with the speed of light. They have greater penetrating properties than do alpha particles. Their emissions cause

tissue necrosis, and they produce ionization, which has destructive properties.

- *Gamma rays and x-rays:* Gamma rays and x-rays are electromagnetic radiations of short wavelength but high energy, and they are capable of completely penetrating the body. They affect tumor tissue more rapidly than normal tissue. These types of rays are stopped by a thick lead shield. Protons ranging in energy from 30 kilovolts (kV) to 35 million electron volts (eV) are available for the treatment of various cancers. Gamma rays are emitted spontaneously from the nucleus of an atom of a radioactive element.

Implantation of Radiation Sources

All radiation sources for implantation are prepared in the desired therapeutic dosages by personnel in the nuclear medicine department. Many types of sources are used to deliver maximum radiation to the primary tumor. No single type is ideal for every tumor or anatomic site.

Interstitial Needles. Interstitial needles are hollow sheaths that are usually made of platinum or Monel metal. Radium salts or radionuclides are encased in platinum or platinum-iridium short units or cells, which in turn are sealed in the metal sheath of the needle for implantation into tumor tissue. A needle may contain one or several short units or cells of the radiation source, depending on the length of needle to be used. Needles vary in length from 10 to 60 mm, with a diameter of 1 to 2 mm. The choice of length depends on dosage and on the area involved. Dosage is measured in milligram-hours, which can be converted to rads.

The interstitial needles, which usually contain cesium-137, are implanted in tumors near the body surface or in tissue accessible enough to permit their use (e.g., vagina, cervix, tongue, mouth, neck). In certain patients, stereotactic techniques are used to implant needles for the irradiation of brain tumors.

In the OR these needles are inserted at the periphery of and within the tumor. One end of the needle is pointed, and the other end has an eye for a heavy (size 2) suture. Needles are threaded to prevent loss while in use and to aid in removal. After the surgeon inserts the needles, the ends of the sutures are tied or taped together and are taped to the skin in an adjoining area or secured to buttons.

Depending on the anatomic site, a template may be used to position and secure the needles. A template consists of two acrylic plates separated by rubber O-rings and held together with screws. The plates have holes for insertion of the interstitial needles. The template remains in place until the needles are removed. Depending on the planned dosage to the tumor bed, needles are usually left in place for hours to several days.

Interstitial Seeds. Sealed radionuclide seeds may be implanted permanently or temporarily. Because they have a short half-life, gold seeds are permanently implanted, most commonly into the prostate, lungs, or pancreas. Seeds containing cesium-137, iridium-192, or iodine-125 implanted directly into tumor tissue are removed after the desired exposure.

Seeds are useful in body cavities, localized areas, and tumors that are not resectable because of their location near major vessels or the spinal cord. Because they are small, the seeds can be placed to fit a curved area without requiring immobilization. However, they may move about if there is much motion.

Radionuclide seeds are 7 mm or less in length, are 0.75 mm in diameter, and have a wall 0.3 mm thick. The length of the seed depends on the desired dosage. Seeds can be inserted with or without an invasive surgical procedure. They may be strung on a strand of suture material or placed in a hollow plastic tube with sealed ends. With a needle attached, the strand or tube is woven or pulled through the tumor.

Seeds in a plastic tube may be inserted through a hollow needle, such as a catheter through a trocar. Empty tubes may be inserted in the OR and afterloaded (i.e., the seeds are put into the tube at a later time and place). A microprocessor-controlled machine that pulls wire attached to radioactive material through the tube may be used for remote afterloading.

Brachytherapy. The term brachytherapy comes from a Greek term meaning "short-range treatment." Tiny titanium cylinders that contain a radioactive isotope are implanted to deliver a dose of radiation from the inside out that kills cancer cells while sparing healthy tissue. Brachytherapy is performed for many types of cancers, including breast and prostate (see Fig. 7.5).

Brachytherapy is useful for delivering higher cell-killing doses in shorter periods than conventional radiation treatments. The capsules are placed under ultrasound guidance. A rapid delivery system that uses a catheter with a balloon on the tip has been developed to treat breast cancer smaller than 3 cm. The catheter is placed into the breast tissue during tumor excision, and the balloon is expanded with water. Twice per day for 4 to 5 days a high-dose radiation pellet is placed inside the catheter to treat the tissue. When the treatment period is complete, the catheter and pellet are removed. Patient selection includes those with clear tumor margins and with fewer than three affected lymph nodes.

Intracavitary Capsules. A sealed capsule of radium, cesium-137, iodine-125, yttrium-192, or cobalt-60 may be placed into a body cavity or orifice. The capsule may be a single tube of radioactive pins fixed in a tandem loader or a group of individual capsules, each of which contains one radioactive pin. Commonly used to treat tumors in the cervix or endometrium of the uterus, a capsule is inserted via the vagina for treatment of the uterine body.

In a patient with cervical cancer an instrument such as an Ernst applicator is used. A metal or plastic tube with radioactive pins is inserted in the uterus. Metal pins are used in conjunction with heat. The tube is attached to two vaginal ovoids, each of which contains a radioactive pin, that are placed in the cul-de-sac around the cervix. This type of application delivers the desired dosage in a pear-shaped volume of tissue, which includes the cervix, corpus, and tissue around the cervix but spares the bladder and rectum from high doses of radiation.

A blunt intracavitary applicator is used to position the parts. The applicator is held securely and remains fixed to ensure proper dosage to the tumor without injuring the normal surrounding structures. For stabilization, the surgeon may suture the applicator to the cervix, and vaginal packing also is used. Two different methods of application are used for inserting the radiation source: afterloading techniques and preloading techniques.

Afterloading Techniques. Afterloading techniques afford the greatest safety for OR personnel. In the OR a cold, unloaded, hollow plastic or metal applicator, such as the Fletcher afterloader, is inserted into or adjacent to the tissues that will receive radiation. After x-ray verification of correct placement, the radiation source is loaded into the applicator at the patient's bedside.

Preloading Techniques. Preloading techniques require insertion of the "hot" radiation capsule in the OR by the surgeon. OR personnel should not be permitted in the OR during this procedure. To deliver a uniform dose to the desired area, the surgeon inserts an adjustable device designed to hold the radiation source in proper position in the tissues (e.g., the Ernst applicator). The bladder and rectum are held away from the area with packs to avoid undesired irradiation. To calculate the necessary dosage, the surgeon uses x-ray views of the pelvis to check the position of the radiation source and measure its distance from critical sites.

All preparations for insertion are made by nursing team members before they leave the room. (They wait in the substerile room during insertion.) Preparations include setting the sterile table with vaginal packing, antibiotic cream for packing, radiopaque solutions for x-ray studies, and a basin of sterile water; placing the x-ray cassette on the OR bed and notifying the radiology technician; obtaining the radiation source; positioning the patient; and putting a radiation sheet on the patient's chart and a card on the stretcher.

Intracavitary Colloidal Suspensions. Sterile radioactive colloidal suspensions of gold or phosphorus are used as palliative therapy to limit the growth of metastatic tumors in the pleural or peritoneal cavities. Radioactive colloidal gold-198 is most commonly used; it has a half-life of 2.7 days. It also may be instilled within the bladder. The effect of these suspensions is caused by the emission of beta particles that penetrate tissue so slightly that radioactivity is limited to the immediate area in which the colloidal suspension is placed. A trocar and cannula are introduced into the pleural or peritoneal cavity, and the colloidal suspension is injected through the cannula from a lead-shielded syringe. After use, these instruments are stored in a remote area until the decay of radioactivity is complete.

Intraoperative Radiation Therapy

During a surgical procedure, a single high dose of radiation may be delivered directly to an intraabdominal or intrapelvic tumor or tumor bed to provide an additional palliative or localized means of control. Normal organs or tissues can be shielded from exposure. Radiation also may be used after resection of the bulk of the tumor.

An orthovoltage unit may be installed in a lead-lined OR for performing intraoperative radiation therapy. The sterile Lucite cone is placed directly over the tumor site. All team members leave the room during treatment. In some hospitals the patient is transported from the OR to the radiation therapy department. After exposure to a megavoltage electron beam, the wound may be closed in the treatment area or the patient may be returned to the OR for further surgery and/or wound closure. The open wound is covered with a sterile drape during transport, and sterile technique is used for closure.

Stereotactic Radiosurgery

Gamma knife technology was developed in Sweden in the early 1950s by surgeon Lars Leksell and Börje Larsson, MD, a radiobiologist. They experimented with guiding devices and proton beams. Cobalt-60 was found to be most effective in the treatment of brain tumors and was selected as the energy source for the gamma knife. In 1975, the device was used to treat brain tumors in humans.

With stereotactic radiosurgery, fiberglass fixation pins are used to apply a base ring (the Leksell head frame) to the patient's head preoperatively. Two small rods are placed in the ear canals to stabilize the head frame during fixation. Care is taken not to injure the ear canal or tympanic membrane during this process. A calibrated ring is affixed to the frame to form X, Y, and Z coordinates

to localize the brain lesion. The frame and ring sit within a larger helmet that aims the radiation at the tumor.

The gamma knife delivers highly concentrated doses of gamma rays to inoperable or deep-seated vascular malformations or brain tumors 1 to 10 cm^3 in size. The localized area is determined by precision stereotaxis. The neurosurgeon places the patient's head, with the Leksell head frame and localizing ring, into the collimator helmet so that the focusing channels direct 201 pinpointed cobalt-60 beams to the tumor. (The radiation sources are located in a large spherical chamber that is located within a special room.) Other styles of frames are available that attach in the front and back of the head or use markers to pinpoint the direction of gamma rays.

The patient is placed on a sliding bed that accommodates and aligns with the helmet as it enters the spherical chamber. The gamma knife process lasts 3 to 4 hours. During the procedure the patient is in video and voice communication with the perioperative team. All personnel leave the room during treatment because of the intensity of the radiation and its cumulative effects.

Effects of Radiation Therapy on the Perioperative Patient

The patient may be undergoing several treatment modalities and may experience the specific tissue and systemic effects of each. The perioperative nurse should understand how radiation affects the patient and how it affects the attainment of desired outcomes. The plan of care should include consideration for the potential side effects of radiation therapy. Box 22.5 describes the patient's responses to the physiologic effects of radiation.

Chemotherapy

Either alone or in combination, a variety of chemotherapeutic agents can provide measurable palliative remission or regression of

---

• BOX 22.5   Physiologic Effects of Radiation Therapy

External Beam
- Gastroenteritis
- Nausea and vomiting
- Diarrhea
- Menstrual irregularities
- Miscarriage
- Sexual dysfunction
- Fatigue
- Cystitis
- Erythema
- Skin desquamation
- Headache
- Decreased circulation

Internal Implants
- Bleeding tendency
- Increased infections
- Sexual dysfunction

Intracavitary Implants
- Bleeding
- Infection
- Sexual dysfunction

Intraoperative Radiation
- Anorexia
- Nausea and vomiting

primary and metastatic disease, with a decrease in the size of the tumor and no new metastases. In some instances a complete response, with the disappearance of all clinical evidence of the tumor, is achieved.

The trend is toward earlier and greater use of adjuvant chemotherapy. More than one agent may be administered to enhance the action of another cytotoxic or antigenic substance. Adjuvant therapy is designed to maximize the benefits of each agent in the combination while avoiding overlapping toxicities. The following factors are important in determining the ability of tumor cells to respond to chemotherapy:

- *Size and location of the tumor:* The smaller the tumor, the easier it will be to reach cells. The mechanism for the passage of drugs into the brain differs from that for other body organs.
- *Type of tumor:* For example, cells of solid tumors in the lung, stomach, colon, and breast may be more resistant than cells in the lymphatic system.
- *Combinations of adjuvant therapy:* In select patients, chemotherapy may be used as an adjunct to all other types of therapies. Precise scheduling of dosages is necessary to attain effective results.
- *Specific biochemical requirements of the tumor:* Agents are selected according to the appropriateness of their structure and function. More than one agent is usually given.
- *State of life cycle of the cancer cells:* Cancer cells and normal cells go through the same life-cycle phases. An understanding of this phenomenon is necessary for understanding chemotherapy.

Indications for Chemotherapy

Patients who are at risk for or who have systemic signs of advanced or disseminated disease (generally indicated by extranodal involvement) may be candidates for preoperative, intraoperative, or postoperative chemotherapy.

Preoperative Chemotherapy. The objective of preoperative chemotherapy may be to shrink the tumor sufficiently to permit surgical resection. Adjuvant radiation therapy may be used in combination with chemotherapy to increase tumor regression and necrosis. Agents may also eliminate subclinical microscopic metastatic disease.

Intraoperative Chemotherapy. Chemotherapeutic agents can be instilled during a surgical procedure. The agent may be heated to encourage absorption by the tissues. Care is taken during the process because chemotherapeutic agents are considered hazardous materials.

Postoperative Chemotherapy. Surgical resection followed by regional chemotherapy often can control local disease to keep a tumor in remission. Residual metastatic disease may be treated with systemic chemotherapy to cure the patient or to prolong life. Multiple doses may be given over a long period (several months to a year or more) to delay or eliminate recurrence of the tumor.

Delivery Devices for Chemotherapeutic Agents

The method of chemotherapy administration depends on the extent of dissemination or localization of the tumor cells and on the agent or combination of agents selected. Agents can be instilled locally into a target site by continuous infusion, injected intramuscularly (IM) or intrathecally, infused by IV push or drip, or ingested orally (PO).

A patient with widely disseminated metastatic disease usually receives systemic chemotherapy via the IV, IM, or PO route. Agents may be infused regionally for patients whose tumor cannot

be removed because of its location (e.g., a primary or metastatic tumor in the liver). The patient may come to the OR for insertion of an indwelling catheter or implantable infusion pump of the brain.

Infusion Catheters. An indwelling infusion catheter may be placed percutaneously or directly into a vein, artery, or body cavity. Continuous or intermittent infusion of the chemotherapeutic agent can be maintained by means of a portable infusion pump attached to the catheter, or the catheter may be used on an intermittent basis.

Central Venous Catheter. Under local anesthesia, a long-term Hickman, Quinton, Groshong, or other central venous catheter is inserted percutaneously through a particular blood vessel and into the right atrium of the heart. The catheter also may be used for hyperalimentation. Varieties include single-, double-, and triple-lumen styles and require heparinized saline flushes between uses (Fig. 22.6). Groshong catheters have a self-closing distal tip, do not require heparinization, and are available in single-, double-, and triple-lumen styles. Therefore the Groshong catheter can be used for patients with bleeding tendencies without the same risk associated with added heparinization. Sterile normal saline for injection is used to flush the line between uses.

Short-term subclavian catheters in double- and triple-lumen styles can be used for the administration of chemotherapeutic agents and total parenteral nutrition (TPN). These types of catheters require heparin flushes between uses.

Hepatic Artery Catheter. Hepatic artery catheterization may be performed to establish regional chemotherapy to treat primary or metastatic disease of the liver. With the use of a local anesthetic

• **Fig. 22.6** Intravenous Catheters for Long-Term Intravascular Access. **A,** Hickman and Broviac single-lumen catheter for intravenous (IV) fluids or total parenteral nutrition (TPN). **B,** Hickman and Leonard multipurpose dual-lumen catheter for IV fluids or blood sampling. **C,** Hickman triple-lumen catheter for IV fluids, TPN, and blood administration.

the catheter may be inserted percutaneously into the left axillary artery and threaded into the common hepatic artery. This technique eliminates the need for a laparotomy to cannulate the hepatic arteries. However, some patients have variant anatomy that requires a dual-catheter delivery system.

Vascular reconstruction, ligation, and/or occlusion of an artery may be necessary for local or regional perfusion. Regardless of the method of catheterization, an infusion pump is attached to the catheter(s) to deliver the cytotoxic agent to the tumor.

Intraperitoneal Catheter. Intraperitoneal chemotherapy permits the delivery of high concentrations of an agent to an ovarian or colorectal tumor without exposing normal tissues systemically. With the use of a local anesthetic, a Tenckhoff catheter is inserted into the peritoneal cavity. An incision in the anterior abdominal wall is usually located just lateral to the right or left of the rectus abdominis muscle at the level of the umbilicus. The anterior rectus sheath is incised to allow a Verres needle to penetrate the peritoneum. To prevent the catheter from kinking, air is injected before the catheter is placed in the peritoneal cavity. A subcutaneous tunnel is made between the initial incision and stab wound to secure the catheter. A Dacron cuff is embedded in the subcutaneous tissue to anchor the catheter in place. The agent exits the peritoneal cavity via the portal circulation.

Infusion Devices

Devices with reservoirs for the chemotherapeutic agent are implanted into body tissues.

Subcutaneous Infusion Port. With the use of a local anesthetic a venous access device is implanted subcutaneously for continuous or intermittent injections of cytotoxic agent(s), TPN, or blood products. Depending on the manufacturer, the device consists of a plastic or silicone rubber self-sealing port on a plastic or stainless steel reservoir (Fig. 22.7). The catheter attached to the reservoir is inserted into a central vein, hepatic artery, peritoneal cavity, or epidural space. A tunnel is created from the point at which the catheter enters the vessel, cavity, or space to a subcutaneous pocket (Fig. 22.8). The pocket is made wherever necessary to stabilize the port.

The reservoir is sutured to the underlying fascia. A Huber needle with a 90-degree-angle tip is used to enter the port for heparinizing and infusing agents (Fig. 22.9). Extension tubing may connect the needle to an infusion pump for continuous infusion. After use, the port is flushed with 10 mL of sterile normal saline followed by 3 to 10 mL of heparinized saline (100 units/mL). Thrombosis and infection are potential complications of long-term venous access devices and catheters.

Implantable Infusion Pump. With the patient under local, regional, or general anesthesia, an infusion catheter is placed into an artery, vein, body space, spine, or ventricle for localized chemotherapy to a tumor in the liver, head, neck, or brain. The infusion pump device is implanted in a subcutaneous pocket created in the abdominal wall, beneath the clavicle, or under the scalp.

The titanium, stainless steel, and silicone rubber device resembles a hockey puck and delivers the agent by means of a bellows device or by radio signals. The inner reservoir is filled with the cytotoxic agent. When the reservoir is collapsed by pressure, the agent is infused into the catheter. The pump is warmed initially to activate the fluorocarbon propellant in the chamber around the reservoir. It is placed over a bony prominence for support when refilling. Insulin, heparin, or morphine is infused, respectively.

The drug is replenished periodically by percutaneous injection. A bolus can be administered through a side port on the pump. These implanted infusion devices also are used to control severe systemic conditions such as diabetes, thromboembolic disease, or pain from a malignancy. Smart technology pumps can be programmed to delivery an exact amount of medication at a programmed rate or time.

Perioperative Care of the Patient With Cancer

Malignant tumor cells can be disseminated by manipulation of tissue. Because of their altered nutritional and physiologic status, patients with cancer also may be highly susceptible to the complications of postoperative infection. To minimize these risks, the following specific precautions are taken in the surgical management of patients with cancer:

1. The skin over the site of a soft tissue tumor should be handled gently during hair removal and antisepsis. Vigorous scrubbing could dislodge underlying tumor cells; this is avoided by using "no-touch" techniques. With vascular tumors, manipulation during positioning or skin preparation could cause vascular complications such as emboli or hemorrhage. The no-touch technique means that the tumor is handled as little as possible during its removal. Radiated skin is very fragile.
2. Gowns, gloves, drapes, and instruments may be changed after a biopsy (e.g., a breast biopsy) before incision for a radical resection (e.g., a mastectomy). The tumor is deliberately incised to obtain a biopsy for diagnosis.
3. Instruments placed in direct contact with tumor cells may be discarded immediately after use. Even when the tumor appears to be localized, most cancers have disseminated to some degree. Therefore some surgeons prefer to use each instrument once and then discard it.
4. Some surgeons prefer to irrigate the surgical site with sterile water instead of sterile normal saline solution, which causes the destruction of cancerous cells by crenation. This practice is common during mastectomy.
5. As a prophylactic measure, antibiotics are administered preoperatively, intraoperatively, and postoperatively to provide an adequate antibacterial level to prevent wound infection.
6. Time-honored precautions such as handling tissue gently, keeping blood loss to a minimum, and avoiding an unduly prolonged surgical procedure influence the outcome for the patient.

During a long surgical procedure, messages should be conveyed periodically to the patient's anxiously waiting family members or significant others to reassure them that the patient is receiving care from a concerned perioperative team.

Self-sealing rubber diaphragm

Metal chamber

• **Fig. 22.7** Implantable subcutaneous infusion port.

Peel-away
introducer

Subclavian
vein

Infusion port

• **Fig. 22.8** Placement of an implantable subcutaneous infusion port.

• **Fig. 22.9** Huber needle with a 90-degree-angle tip.

Teaching Patients Risk-Avoidance Behaviors

Patient education should include information about avoiding cancer-causing behaviors and how to minimize the risk for cancer. Behaviors to discuss include:

- *Avoiding smoking and exposure to smoke.* The American Cancer Society reports that exposure to cigarette smoke is responsible for 80% of all cases of lung cancer. More than 480,000 people die each year from smoking. Secondhand smoke, referred to as *environmental tobacco smoke,* has been implicated in the development of cancer in nonsmoking people who are exposed to smoke on a regular basis. The use of E-cigarettes and vaping has been on the rise in teens and young adults. Serious respiratory illness and even death have been linked to vaping. The FDA has rules for retailers who sell tobacco and electronic delivery systems (ENDS). Regulatory requirements and purchasing age are controlled. The purchasing age is 21 years or older. The FDA has banned fruit flavor and mint products popular with teens.

- *Increasing dietary intake of fiber and low-fat foods.* Antioxidants such as vitamins C and A may reduce an individual's risk for developing cancer. High-fat diets have been implicated in the development of breast, colon, and prostate cancers. According to reports of the American Cancer Society, 30% to 40% of cancer deaths are related to dietary causes and are possibly preventable.

A desirable weight should be maintained, and obesity should be avoided. Excessive alcohol intake should be avoided.

- *Minimizing sun exposure, especially between the hours of 10:00 AM and 4:00 PM.* Sun exposure has been shown to be the major cause of skin cancer, especially melanoma. Severe sunburn in childhood may be linked to the development of skin cancer later in life. Certain medications, such as tranquilizers, antidiabetic agents, diuretics, antiinflammatory agents, and antibiotics, can predispose an individual to sunburn. Certain cosmetic products, such as tretinoin (Retin-A) and alphahydroxy acid, are extremely reactive to sunlight and can increase the risk for sunburn within 30 minutes of exposure. Tanning booths and sun lamps can be hazardous to the skin.

- *Using a water-resistant sunscreen lotion with a sun-protection factor (SPF) of at least 30.* Water-resistant sunscreen should be applied whenever sun exposure is likely. Sun-blocking products of SPF 30 to 70 are preferred. The sun-blocking product should provide protection from both ultraviolet A and ultraviolet B (UVA, UVB) rays. (UVA rays can increase the damage caused by UVB rays.) Sunscreen should be applied at least 30 minutes before going outdoors and then reapplied every two hours thereafter.

- *Scheduling regular checkups, especially yearly checkups after 40 years of age.* Knowing the warning signs of cancer may promote prompt diagnosis and treatment. Signs to consider in young children include frequent swelling (lymphadenopathy) or bruising, unexplained headaches or fevers, dramatic weight loss or gain, and localized pain.

- *Self-examining the skin, breast, and testes.* Examining these areas on a routine monthly basis may reveal an early sign of cancer.

ⓔ EVOLVE WEBSITE

http://evolve.elsevier.com/Hornacky/BerryKohn/

- Historical Perspective
- Student Interactive Questions
- Glossary

References

1. Yang H, Xiao M, Zheng W, et al.: Ultrasound-guided core needle biopsy for accessing laryngeal masses with unsatisfactory laryngoscopy and biopsy results, *Am J Otolaryngol Head Neck Med Surg* 44(2):103716, 2022.
2. Association of Surgical Technologists (AST): *Standards of practice for handling and care of surgical specimens.* www.ast.org. Accessed May 9, 2023.
3. RadiologyInfo.org: *Diagnostic techniques.* www.radiologyinfo.org. Accessed May 9, 2023.
4. Harisinghani M, Chen J, Weissleder R: Contrast agents. In *Primer of diagnostic imaging*, ed 6, St. Louis, 2019, Elsevier, pp 729–738.
5. American Cancer Society: *Mammograms.* www.cancer.org. Accessed May 8, 2023.
6. American Cancer Society: *Screening guidelines.* www.cancer.org. Accessed May 9, 2023.

Bibliography

AORN: Guidelines *for perioperative practice*, Denver, CO, 2024, The Association.
Ball J, Dains J, Flynn J, et al. In *Seidel's physical examination handbook*, ed 10, 2023.
Chang X, Lu X, Guo J, et al.: Interventional therapy combined with immune checkpoint inhibitors: emerging opportunities for cancer treatment in the era of immunotherapy, *Cancer Treat Rev* 74:49–60, 2018.
Ibrahim MA, Hazhirkarzar B, Dubliu AB: Gadolinium magnetic resonance imaging. In *Stat Pearls*. www.ncbi.nlm.nih.gov. Accessed May 9, 2023.

23

Surgical Pharmacology

CHAPTER OUTLINE

Pharmacology Baselines, 421

Considerations in Surgical Pharmacology, 424

Surgical Drug and Pharmaceutical Sources, 426

Pharmacologic Forms Used in Surgery, 428

Potential Complications Caused by Pharmaceuticals and
  Herbal Medicine, 430

CHAPTER OBJECTIVES

After studying this chapter the learner will be able to:

- Calculate drug dosages in the perioperative environment.
- List common drugs used in surgery.

- Identify drug sources and their effects on patient use.
- Demonstrate drug handling in a sterile environment.

KEY TERMS AND DEFINITIONS

Absorption Drug is taken in by the cells of the body.

Ampule Sealed glass tube containing a drug. Tip is scored for removal by snapping off. Drug is removed by a sterile syringe and filter needle to prevent aspiration of glass shards.

Antagonist One drug is used to alter or stop the effect of another drug.

Contrast medium Radiopaque solution used during radiography or fluoroscopy to define structures on film or digital media.

Conversion Standard scale of equivalents used to measure between metric, English, and apothecary units.

Diagnostic chemical Used to perform a medical test or confirm a pathogenic condition.

Diluent Liquid used to decrease the concentration of a substance.

Distribution Drug is evenly absorbed by the entire body.

Dye Colored solution used to identify structures with gross vision.

Excretion Drug is released from the body in naturally excreted substances.

Gas Nonsolid, nonliquid form of a chemical.

Generic Chemically equivalent drugs formulated as substitutes for brand-name products.

Hypodermic Below the skin; subdermal.

Infusion Flow of a drug directly into the circulatory system.

Inhalant Drug that is taken in like a breath, then absorbed through the respiratory tract.

Injection Insertion of a drug directly into the tissues using a syringe and needle.

Loading dose First dose of a series given in a larger quantity than the subsequent doses.

Localized drug effect Physiologic response to a drug is in a select area of the body and not carried to other regions in an effective form.

Metabolism Drug is used throughout the body and broken down by major organs.

Pharmacokinetics Actions and disposition of a chemical in the body. These include absorption, distribution, metabolism, and excretion.

Placebo Inert substance given to a patient to stimulate the power of suggestion of effectiveness. Commonly used as a control in experimental medicine.

Polypharmacy Term used to describe when a patient has multiple prescription medications from one or multiple prescribers.

Potentiation Synergistic action of one drug against another to cause an increased response by the body.

Preventive drug Chemical or biologic preparation given with the intent of avoiding a disease state.

Reaction Physiologic response of the body when exposed to a drug. The response can be positive or negative. Sensitivity refers to when physiologic mechanisms are triggered by exposure to small doses of a given drug. Allergy refers to when physiologic defense mechanisms are triggered by exposure to a drug or chemical, causing a potentially life-threatening response. Anaphylaxis refers to a severe physiologic response to exposure to a drug or chemical, causing a definite threat to the patient's life.

Receptor site Location in the body that acts in response to a chemical stimulus. Some drugs act by blocking a receptor site and prevent naturally produced chemicals from bonding.

Side effect Secondary reaction that occurs in response to administration of a drug.

Stain Chemical used in solution to tint cellular structures for microscopic study.

Systemic effect Physiologic response to a drug is manifest in the entire body.

Tolerance Physiologic response caused by prolonged use of large quantities of a drug that makes average doses ineffective.

Toxic Level of any given drug that causes a negative or possibly fatal physiologic response.

Vial Vacuum-sealed glass or plastic container of medication that is sealed by a rubber stopper. The drug is removed by a sterile syringe and needle.

Pharmacology Baselines

The main purpose of this chapter is to highlight information concerning the drugs specifically used in perioperative patient care. It is not intended to be an all-inclusive pharmacologic resource. Drugs used in diagnostics, surgical procedures, anesthesia, and emergencies in the operating room (OR) are described in more depth in the corresponding subsequent chapters.

Many drugs and pharmaceutical substances require special preparation and handling in the surgical environment. Some of these pharmaceuticals are found only in the OR, and their proper use is based on sterile technique, precise actions, and extreme caution. Correct dosing, mixing, and delivery to the sterile field are important for the safety of the patient and the team.

Safe drug and pharmaceutical administration in the OR is practiced according to the seven rights of medication administration in any setting:
- Right patient
- Right drug
- Right timing (cements/glues, antibiotics)
- Right dose
- Right route
- Right reason
- Right documentation

Patient assessment will provide information about the patient's health and general condition. Knowledge of how a drug acts in the body should be compared with the patient's assessment and current vital sign trend. The patient's weight should be documented in kilograms because many dosages are calculated according to milligrams per kilograms. The patient's history or body size may require a change in the plan of care involving medications for the intraoperative care period. Allergies are assessed and documented, and adverse reactions are prevented.

Prescription items in the OR are more than drugs and medications. The effectiveness of surgical drugs and chemicals depends on the desired localized drug effect and the specific targeted receptor sites. Some drugs are used to decrease consciousness; others are used to alleviate pain. Many drugs cause amnesia. Some drugs are given as a preventive measure against a possible complication. The physiologic drugs have systemic effects and are given in larger loading doses to induce the desired effect and titrated to maintenance doses to keep the patient's body relaxed and pain-free during the surgical procedure. The patient is carefully monitored for side effects and toxic levels.

Surgical pharmacology encompasses many chemicals ranging from dyes to adhesives, most of which are not used in any other patient care area. All the specialized items require specific handling within the confines of the sterile field. Other items used in the OR include gaseous materials and surgical-site closure materials.

Avoiding Pharmaceutical Error

Every patient population is at risk for errors during the use of pharmaceutical materials in the perioperative environment. Known and unknown allergies and sensitivities can lead to serious illness or death. Constant patient monitoring can identify signs and symptoms of evolving reactions and permit time to effect treatment. Always investigate when patients report unusual feelings when a drug has been given.

Dosage error can affect any patient, but pediatric and geriatric patients or those with impaired body systems are particularly at risk. Pediatric error is usually related to doses greater than their bodies can tolerate. Geriatric and system-impaired patients metabolize medications at a slower rate. Any drug in their systems can be augmented by additional drugs in a subsequent dose. The result can be unintentional overdosage. Anticoagulants, antibiotics, and steroidal compounds are the pharmaceuticals most frequently identified as the source of such problems.

Key points in avoiding error include double-checking labels for drug, dose, and method of delivery. The patient should be identified at least twice by name and other identifier approved by facility policy. Allergy and sensitivity alerts should be clear in the record and on the patient's identification wristband.

The risk for pharmaceutical error is high when patients take prescribed or unprescribed medications at home. A patient may use an inhaler for asthma and forget to report its use before surgery. Dietary supplements, herbs, home remedies, and over-the-counter (OTC) drugs are not considered "medication" to some patients, and they may neglect to report their use.

Some patients may hide the fact that they are using additional medications at home for fear of angering the physician. Patients using recreational drugs may hide the fact for fear of punishment. Most facilities do not routinely test for illegal drugs unless prompted by the situation or by a patient who acts suspicious when queried concerning their use. Not only does the use of drugs (legal and illegal) and supplements alter the course of treatment, but they can potentially interact adversely with many forms of anesthesia and physiologic stabilization drugs during surgery or emergency treatment.

Pregnancy, Lactation, and Reproductive Considerations

The safe administration of any drug to a pregnant or lactating woman requires knowledge of how the drug might affect a developing fetus or a breastfed infant. The risks should be identified before any drug is administered to a pregnant or possibly pregnant woman. Previously the U.S. Food and Drug Administration (FDA) had a lettering system concerning safety of a drug during pregnancy. In 2015, the FDA discontinued the use of the lettering system for labeling drugs. The FDA requirements for drug labeling include all persons of reproductive age regardless of sex. The labels should include information about infertility safety and contraception if necessary. Additional information about this required labeling change can be found at www.fda.gov. The labeling requirements for all prescription drugs have been changed as follows:
- *Pregnancy:* Includes labor and delivery
- *Lactation:* Includes nursing mothers
- *Females and males of reproductive potential:* Indicates the need for pregnancy testing, advice about contraception during therapy, and information concerning the potential for infertility

A breastfeeding mother and her infant are at risk if a drug given is transferred by breast milk. Antidepressants, antibiotics, antihypertensives, narcotics, opioids, cardiac drugs, salicylates, psychotropics, some anesthetics, and anticholesterol drugs are examples of some drugs passed in breast milk that can affect the infant. A mother can be advised to pump and store milk preoperatively if a potentially harmful drug will be used in her procedure. The physician will advise when it is safe to resume regular breastfeeding. The mother should be instructed what to look for in her infant after feeding.

The labeling of OTC drugs must contain descriptive drug information and dosing on the outside of the container that is easily readable.

Drug Development

New drugs take many years to become available for patient use. According to the Center for Drug Evaluation and Research (CDER), it takes almost 12 years for a drug to be discovered and placed into use. Safety and efficacy testing on animals and laboratory simulation takes an average of 3.5 years to complete. It is estimated that only 1 in 1000 compounds is tested in human trials. Each potential drug is filed with the FDA in an Investigational New Drug (IND) application. The detailed application must include information on animal testing studies, toxicity, side effects, manufacturer and investigational information, clinical study plan, and any prior human studies. The FDA has 30 days for a board of experts to approve or disapprove the application. A series of clinical trials are performed on humans who have given informed consent, as follows:

- *Phase I clinical trial:* 20 to 80 healthy individuals for a period of 1 year. The drug is studied for safety in dosage, duration of action, absorption, distribution, metabolism, and excretion.
- *Phase II clinical trial:* 100 to 300 people with actual disease for which the drug is proposed treatment for a period of up to 2 years. The drug is studied for dose, effectiveness, and tolerability. Adverse reactions are monitored.
- *Phase III clinical trial:* 300 to 3000 patients in multiple health care settings participate. The drug is monitored to validate effectiveness and safety. The trial phase can take 1 to 4 years.
- *Phase VI postmarket surveillance:* After the drug is on the market, the manufacturer monitors the users for therapeutic and nontherapeutic effects and reports to the FDA.

Clinical trial results are reported yearly to the FDA. Only one in four drugs ever completes the process of the three clinical trials. The long period needed for the clinical trials permits the researchers to observe for long-term effects of the compound. On completion of the clinical trial phases, the drug manufacturer submits a New Drug Application (NDA). Once approved by the FDA, the new drug is made available for physicians to prescribe. The approval process takes between 6 and 10 months to complete.

Expedited Drug Approval

The Office of Oncologic Diseases (OOD) has had numerous drugs approved under the accelerated drug program.[1] The program looks at the data for drugs and therapies that look promising for life-threatening diseases or with no known cure. Multiple drugs for aggressive cancers, bone marrow stimulants, and drug treatment for neuroblastoma have been approved. The drugs must go through extensive review while treating patients with life-threatening conditions. More information can be found at www.fda.gov.

Drug Names

Drugs have three names. The first name is the chemical name and describes the chemical components such as molecular and atomic structure of the drug. It is not commonly used when referencing the drug.

The second name is the official name, referred to as generic, and given to the compound by the initial manufacturer. The generic name is derived from the chemical name and is not capitalized. The drugs are listed in the United States Pharmacopeia (USP) and the National Formulary (NF) according to the generic names. The first letter of a generic drug name is written lowercased.

The third name is given when the drug company who sells the drug assigns a copyrighted trade name, or a brand name, which is proprietary. The trade name is capitalized and designated by a registration mark ($^{®}$).

Mathematic Baselines
Decimals

Numbers to the left of the decimal are whole numbers. Numbers to the right of the decimal are decimal fractions and are read according to their place value, as follows:

0.1	one tenth
0.01	one hundredth
0.001	one thousandth
0.0001	one ten thousandth

Addition of Decimals

1. Write numbers in a column with the decimals vertically aligned.
2. Place the decimal in the answer beneath the decimal in the problem.
   Example: Add 1.33, 4.0, 2.146, and 0.03

$$\begin{array}{r} 1.33 \\ 4.0 \\ 2.146 \\ + 0.03 \\ \hline 7.506 \end{array}$$

Subtraction of Decimals

1. Write numbers in column with the decimals vertically aligned.
2. Subtract and place the decimal in the answer beneath the decimal in the problem.
   Example: Subtract 0.025 from 15.838

$$\begin{array}{r} 15.838 \\ - 0.025 \\ \hline 15.813 \end{array}$$

Multiplication of Decimals

1. Find the product of the numbers.
2. Total the number of decimal places in the multiplicand and in the multiplier.
3. Mark off the total decimal places in the product and insert a decimal.
   Example: Multiply 2.05 by 0.2

$$\begin{array}{rl} 2.05 & \text{(multiplicand)} \\ \times\ 0.2 & \text{(multiplier)} \\ \hline 0.410 & \text{(product with three decimal places marked off [answer])} \end{array}$$

When the number of decimal places to be marked off goes beyond the numbers in the product, add a zero in each place.

To multiply a decimal by 100, 1000, or 10,000, move the decimal to the right as many places as there are zeros in the multiplier.

Example: Multiply 0.25 by 100. There are two zeros, so move the decimal two places to the right: 025., or 25.

To multiply a decimal by 0.1, 0.01, 0.001, move the decimal to the left as many places as there are decimal places in the multiplier.

Example: Multiply 0.25 by 0.1. There is one decimal place, so move the decimal one place to the left: 0.025.

If the decimal must be moved farther than there are numbers, add a zero for each decimal place.

Division of Decimals

To divide a decimal by a whole number:

1. Write the problem.
2. Place a decimal in the quotient directly above the decimal in the dividend.
3. Solve the quotient.

Example: Divide 0.1 by 50

$$\text{(divisor) } 50\overline{)0.100} \quad \text{(dividend)}$$
$$0.002$$

To divide a whole number or decimal by a decimal:

1. Move the decimal in the divisor to the right until the divisor is a whole number.
2. Move the decimal in the dividend to the right as many places as you moved the decimal in the divisor.
3. Place the decimal in the quotient directly above the (moved) decimal in the dividend.
4. Solve the quotient.

Example: Divide 0.225 by 0.5

$$0.5\overline{)0.225}$$
$$0.450$$

To divide a decimal by 10, 100, 1000, and so on, move the decimal to the left as many places as there are zeros in the divisor.

Example: Divide 0.25 by 1000. There are three zeros, so move the decimal three places to the left: 0.00025.

To divide a decimal by 0.1, 0.01, 0.001, and so on, move the decimal to the right as many places as there are decimal places in the divisor.

Example: Divide 0.25 by 0.1. There is one decimal place, so move the decimal one place to the right: 02.5, or 2.5.

Percent

The word *percent* means part of 100. Twenty-five percent (25%) means 25 parts of 100, or 25/100; it can also be written as the decimal 0.25. Percent indicates a fraction in which the denominator is 100.

Fractions

A fraction represents a part of a whole number. If a circle is divided into four equal parts, each part is ¼ of the circle, as seen in Fig. 23.1. The numerator is 1 and the denominator is 4. The line between 1 and 4 means *divide*.

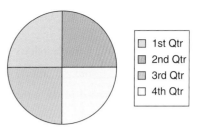

• **Fig. 23.1** Parts of the whole (fractions).

Common Denominator

Unlike denominators cannot be added or subtracted. Common denominator means the fractions have the same denominator.

Reduce a Fraction to Lowest Terms

Determine the largest number that divides evenly into both numbers; when the fraction cannot be reduced any further, it is in its lowest terms.

Example: Reduce to lowest terms: 20/80

Both numbers are divisible evenly by 20: 20 ÷ 20 = 1, and 80 ÷ 20 = 4

Therefore the lowest terms of 20/80 are ¼.

Improper Fraction

⁵⁄₄ is an improper fraction; when reduced to its lowest terms, it becomes 1¼, a mixed number.

Ratio and Proportion

Ratio

We use ratios to compare two things. If we have six hemostats and four scissors, the ratio is termed 6:4 (stated six to four). Any two sets of quantified items (numbers of things) can be put into ratio format for comparison. The ratio concept can be expressed with "to," a colon, or a fraction.

Example:

$$6:4$$
$$6 \text{ to } 4$$
$$6/4 \text{ (six divided by four)}$$

In pharmacology the use of a ratio is expressed in relatively equal terms. For example, 1 ounce of medicine is the same as 30 mL of medicine. It is expressed as (1 oz is to 30 mL) and written as 1 oz : 30 mL. A ratio is one way of saying that 1 oz is equal to 30 mL.

Proportion

When we compare two ratios or need to solve for an unknown quantity to make the ratios balance, the process uses the following format:

$$1 \text{ oz} : 30 \text{ mL} = 2 \text{ oz} : x \text{ mL} \text{ (stated: 1 ounce is to}$$
$$30 \text{ milliliters as 2 ounces is to } x \text{ milliliters.)}$$

The outer numbers are referred to as the *extremes* and the inner numbers are referred to as the *means*. The problem is solved by equalizing the formula. That is why an equal sign connects the two ratios.

Notice that the order of the formula follows ____oz:

$$\_\_\_\_mL = \_\_\_\_oz: \_\_\_\_mL.$$

The quantities must be expressed in the same order on both sides of the equation.

Here is one method of using ratios and proportions. (1) Multiply the extremes. (2) Multiply the means. (3) Divide the left side by the right side with x. (Note: Think of the phrase "x goes into" because the number next to the x goes into the number on the other side of the equal sign to get the answer.)

1 oz : 30 mL = 2 oz : x mL	Multiply the extremes.
1 × x = 2 × 30	Multiply the means.
1x = 60	Divide the number on the
x = 60	right side by the number
Therefore:	on the left side with the x.
1 oz : 30 mL = 2 oz : 60 mL	The product is 60.

Using ratio and proportion is a good way to solve most medication problems for mixing solutions in the OR; however, several measurements from the conversion chart must be known to complete the formula. For example, knowing that 1 oz is the same as 30 mL is important to finding out that 2 oz is 60 mL.

If the ratio is x mL : 2 pints (stated as x milliliters is to 2 pints) the problem is to solve for x or the number of milliliters in 1 pint. This is how to use ratio and proportion to solve this problem. Knowing the baseline conversion of 500 mL : 1 pint is the key to solving for x. Here is how to set up the formula:

$$500 \text{ mL} : 1 \text{ pint} = x \text{ mL} : 2 \text{ pints}$$

$$1000 = 1x$$

(remember the phrase "x goes into") (1000 is divided by 1)

$$1000 = x$$

Answer: 500 mL : 1 pint = 1000 mL : 2 pints

Pharmacologic Conversions

Medications are measured in metric, English/household, or apothecary equivalents. Each unit of measure has a designated accepted abbreviation. Standardization of abbreviations is important for prevention of errors in dosage caused by misinterpretation (Table 23.1).

Accepted Abbreviations
Documentation of medication in the OR is done by using a series of abbreviations and symbols. Standardization of the abbreviations used is important for accuracy. Most of these are expressed in Latin terminology. Abbreviations should be used according to facility policy.

Weights and Measures
Converting dosages between metric, English/household, or apothecary systems is done by calculating with a standard set of measures (Table 23.2). Tables are commonly used for conversions of units between systems.

TABLE 23.1 Abbreviations for Measurement and Administration of Medications

Measurement	Abbreviation
Centimeter	cm
Dram	dr
Drops	gt or gtt
Foot/feet	ft
Gallon	gal
Grains	gr
Gram	g
Inch	in
Kilogram	kg
Liter	L
Meter	m
Microgram	mcg
Micron	μ
Milligram	mg
Milliliter	mL
Millimeter	mm
Ounce	oz
Pint	pt
Pound	lb
Quart	qt
Tablespoon	tbsp
Teaspoon	tsp

Administration	Measurement
After meals	pc
As desired	ad lib
As needed	prn
Before meals	ac
By mouth	PO
Drop	gt
Four times per day	qid
Nothing by mouth	NPO
Quantity sufficient	qs
Three times per day	tid
Twice per day	bid

Considerations in Surgical Pharmacology

Pharmaceuticals used in the OR are not limited to medicines in the ordinary concept of medication. Sources for surgical pharmaceuticals can be living matter from a biologic source or compounded from some other natural or synthetic mixture. Some surgical pharmacologic materials remain inside the body permanently (e.g., an implant), whereas others are systemically absorbed.

Items procured from the pharmacy require special handling within the sterile field. Care is taken not to expose the patient or surgical staff to an allergen or any substance that can cause a sensitivity reaction.

TABLE 23.2	Basic Weights and Measures in Pharmacology		
Metric	**Household/English**	**Apothecary**	
Fluid Measure			
4 L/4000 mL	1 gal	1 gal	
1 L/1000 mL	1 qt/32 oz/2 pt	32 oz (no plural for pints)	
500 mL	1 pt/16 oz/2 cups	16 oz	
250 mL	1 cup/8 oz	8 oz	
30 mL	1 oz	1 oz/8 dr	
15 mL	1 tbsp/3 tsp	225 gtt	
5 mL	1 tsp	75 gtt	
1 mL		15 gtt	
0.0667 mL		1 gtt	
Mass Weight			
1 mg/1000 mcg		1/60 gr	
60 mg		1 gr	
1 g		15 gr	
4 g		60 gr	
1000 g/1 kg	2.2 lb		
	16 oz/1 lb	12 oz	
Measure of Size			
1 m/1000 mm	3.281 ft		
10 mm/1 cm			
2.54 cm	1 in		
	12 in/1 ft		
	3 ft/1 yd		

• **Fig. 23.2** Drug vial with rubber stopper and plastic cap in place.

- Solutions in plastic bottles should be kept in a warmer no longer than 2 weeks between 104° F and 110° F (40–43° C). While in the warmer, the bottle expands. Allowing the solution to reach room temperature after removing from the warmer causes the plastic bottle to contract.
- Replacing the cooled bottle into the warmer causes the plastic to expand. Several manufacturers advise against allowing the bottle to cool and rewarm because of the potential for contamination via expansion and contraction of micropores on the surface of the bottle that can allow microorganisms to enter.
- Intravenous (IV) solutions are dispensed to the sterile field for use in expandable implants and vascular cases. The IV bag is emptied in its entirety by the circulating nurse into a sterile basin using a bag decanter device.

The main difference between irrigation solutions and IV solutions is the method of filtering microparticulates. Both solutions used in surgery are sterile. Baxter Corporation prepares irrigation and IV solutions with the same filtration process rendering the bag and bottle contents identical. The main difference is the packaging.

- Products in peel packs may be dispensed directly to the field, or the scrub person can take the item with a forceps from the opened package as it is held open by the circulating nurse. Remember that the edges of the peel pack are not sterile.
- Drugs in vials (Fig. 23.2) for injection should be removed from the vial by the circulating nurse, using a syringe (Fig. 23.3) and an 18 or a 19-gauge hypodermic needle (Fig. 23.4). The scrub person should place a sterile glass or plastic medicine cup near the edge of the table. Metal medicine cups are not advised for some drugs because they may chemically bind with the metallic substance. Popping off the cap of the vial contaminates the lip, and pouring over that lip renders the drug contaminated.
  - After the circulating nurse withdraws the drug from the vial with the syringe and needle, the needle is removed and the drug is carefully delivered from the syringe into the medicine cup. The needle is removed because dispensing via the needle creates an aerosol that can cause exposure to an allergen.
  - The scrub person should not use a needle and syringe to pierce the rubber stopper on the bottle as the circulating nurse holds it over the field. This places the nurse at risk for needlestick injury. This is an unsafe practice that parallels recapping needles by hand.
  - The circulating nurse should use a filter needle when withdrawing drugs from a glass ampule (Fig. 23.5). Shards of glass can get into the solution and inadvertently be injected into a patient.

Handling Drugs and Pharmacologic Materials in Surgery

Drugs and pharmaceuticals are given to the scrub person for use in the field by a physician, physician assistant, or circulating nurse who is a registered nurse (RN). The surgeon requests a drug or pharmaceutical either verbally or in writing for use during surgery, and the circulating nurse obtains it from the pharmacy or stock. The circulating nurse validates the integrity of the package or container, checks the expiration date, checks for patient allergy or contraindication, and shows the complete label to the scrub person for verification. Administration routes in the field include injection, instillation, irrigation, topical, and spray.

As the drug is dispensed to the field, the circulating nurse should say the drug name and concentration out loud. The drug or material is dispensed to the sterile field in one of the following ways:

- Solutions for irrigation are poured in their entirety into a sterile basin. If the contents are not completely dispensed, the bottle is not recapped and saved for later use. Once the bottle is opened, the lip of the bottle has rendered the contents unsterile as soon as pouring has started. Do not splash or create an aerosol. Aerosolization can cause anaphylaxis in susceptible patients or staff.

• **Fig. 23.3** Anatomy of a syringe.

• **Fig. 23.4** Anatomy of a hypodermic needle.

• **Fig. 23.5** Drug ampule.

• **Fig. 23.6 A,** Control syringe. **B,** One-milliliter syringe used for insulin or tuberculosis (TB) testing. **C,** Standard syringe.

into the wrong cup. The container and the syringe/delivery device (Fig. 23.6) should be clearly marked with the name and concentration of the drug. Sterile labels and sterile marking pens are commercially available and come packed in many custom packs. Some facilities have sterile preprinted labels available. If these types of labels are not used in the facility, wound closure strips, such as Steri-Strips, and a sterile marking pen can be used. All containers of drugs and solutions must be labeled; this includes basins of sterile water and sterile saline.

According to The Joint Commission (TJC), the content of the sterile field drug label should include the first three items on the following list and all five if prepared for use and not yet dispensed to the sterile field:

1. Drug name
2. Strength
3. Amount if not apparent by markings on the container
4. Expiration date if not used within 24 hours
5. Expiration date if expiration occurs within 24 hours

Some facilities require additional labeling on all solutions and drugs such as date, time, and initials of the accepting scrub person. Only facility-approved abbreviations should be used, if abbreviations are used at all. The scrub person should say the name and strength of the drug as the syringe is handed to the surgeon. The circulating nurse documents the delivery of the drug to the sterile field and its usage. The scrub person reports the actual dose given to the patient and recorded on the OR record. The actual dosage is relayed to the anesthesia provider to avoid any incompatibility with medicines given during anesthesia.

Some patients arrive in the OR with peripheral IV access lines in place. These are different from central lines. The circulating nurse takes great care in the access of double- or triple-lumen central venous lines. Some of the connectors can be misconnected to a harmful infusion if universal adapters are used. Intravascular catheters should not be compatible with other infusion devices.

Surgical Drug and Pharmaceutical Sources

Biologic Sources

Biologic sources for drugs can be found in glands, body fluids, organs, fats, and cells of living entities.

• Ointments and creams should be purchased in unit-dose tubes. Multidose tubes are easily contaminated. If a multidose tube is used, ½ inch of the ointment or cream should be squeezed out into the trash before any is used for the current patient. The sterility is questionable. The drug can be dispensed onto a sponge or other sterile surface. It should be labeled immediately.

The drug or pharmaceutical should be labeled as soon as it is received into the sterile field. Labeling the cup or basin before the drug is dispensed could allow for error if the wrong drug is poured

Animal Sources

Animals are used for the manufacturing of drugs. Examples of animals used in the production of pharmaceuticals are found in Box 23.1.

Plant Sources

All portions of plants are used for the manufacturing of drugs. In addition to the anatomic parts of the plant, gums, oils, and bases are used as vehicles for drug administration. Cannabis is an example of an old plant grown for new uses. The cannabis plant (marijuana) is legal in some states and can be purchased in small amounts for recreational use. Cannabis can be purchased legally for medical reasons with a prescription from a doctor. Medical marijuana is grown in a controlled environment, harvested, and processed with the removal of tetrahydrocannabinol (THC), known as the psychoactive component. It is prescribed to relieve pain, reduce seizures, treat anxiety, and reduce inflammation. Examples of plant usage are found in Box 23.2.

Mineral Sources

Many minerals such as calcium, potassium, and chlorides are used intraoperatively. Fibrinogen can be mixed with calcium preparations to form an adhesive that acts as both a sealant and a hemostatic material. Potassium is mixed with other minerals and chemicals to form a cell-protectant cardioplegia solution during cardiac surgery when the heart is not beating (Box 23.3).

Synthetic and Semisynthetic Sources
Chemical Sources

Replication of natural drugs from synthetic sources is common. Narcotic pain medications resembling the action of opioids are used for postoperative patients.

Engineered Protein From Plant, Animal, and Chemical Combinations

Skin substitute, pharmaceuticals, and blood products have been manufactured using biologic material as their base. Skin has been

---

• BOX 23.2   Plant Sources of Drugs

- Leaves (atropine from belladonna leaves, indigo carmine, cannabis)
- Blossoms (opium poppy, colchicine from crocus)
- Seeds (arabic, cannabis)
- Fruit (cranberry)
- Tubers/roots (ginseng) and rhizomes (valerian, gentian)
- Oils (camphor, eucalyptus)
- Sap (aloe, gum arabic preservative)
- Bark (aspirin, quinine, cascara)
- Wood extract
- Resin (benzoin)
- Fungi (some antibiotics)
- Herbs (tranquilizers, anticoagulants)
- Cellulose fibers (hemostatic)

• BOX 23.1   Animal and Biologic Sources of Drugs

Bovine (Beef Cattle)
- Hemostatic agent
- Blood-based oxygen carrier (Hemopure)
- Insulin
- Serum albumin
- Heparin

Porcine (Pigs)
- Hemostatic agent
- Biologic dressing
- Insulin
- Heparin
- Pancreatic enzymes
- Pericardial implant

Equine (Horse)
- Serum vaccine
- Hormones (estrogen)
- Pericardial implant

Ovine (Sheep)
- Suture
- Lanolin
- Hyaluronidase ophthalmic

Rodents (Hamster)
- Protein used in recombinant thrombin

Avian (Birds)
- Viscoat for eye surgery

Microbes (Fungi and Bacteria)
- Antibiotics

Marine Animals
Snails
- Ziconotide (Prialt) for neuropathy

Fish
- Protamine

Reptilian (Snakes and Lizards)
- Antivenom (antivenin)
- Ancrod
- Exenatide (Byetta)
- Blood pressure drugs (Captopril)

Human
- Blood
- Blood fraction
- Insulin from DNA technology
- Tissue
  - Reconstruction
  - Biologic dressing
- Semen
- Hormones (growth hormone and insulin)
- Human source extraction
  - Human skin equivalent
- Hemoglobin-based oxygen carrier (PolyHeme)

Insects and Arachnids
- Bee's wax: hemostasis as bone wax
- Spider antivenom

- Multivitamins contain calcium, iron, copper, magnesium, selenium, and zinc.
- Potassium is replaced after diuretic administration.
- Iodine is used in contrast media and radioactive markers.
- Zinc is used for wound healing.
- Fluoride strengthens teeth.
- Gold salts are used to treat rheumatoid conditions.
- Silver is used for antimicrobial action.
- Iron helps treat anemia.
- Copper is necessary for the use of iron in red cell formation.
- Sulfur found in protein is used for cartilage production.
- Tungsten compounds treat AIDS.
- Lithium is used for bipolar disorder.
- Sodium and chloride balance body fluids.
- Talc is powdered magnesium silicate. Used for sclerosis in pleurodesis.

cultured for use in wound repair. Blood cells from bovine and human sources have been engineered for use in humans as an oxygen-carrying medium. An oxygen-carrying medium is not intended to replace blood but aims to provide a source of oxygen distribution in the vascular system of the body.

Pharmacologic Forms Used in Surgery

Table 23.3 gives examples of select surgical medications. Drugs used in surgery are found in many forms, ranging from liquids to solids. Routes of drug administration can be found in Box 23.4.

Liquids

A variety of solutions and liquids are used within the sterile field and nonsterile fields before, during, and after the surgical

TABLE 23.3 Examples of Drugs Used in Surgery

Drug Category	Drug Classifications	Individual Drugs
Anticoagulants and Coagulants		
Antiplatelet agents	Anticoagulant	Aspirin Ticlopidine
Anticoagulants	Anticoagulant	Enoxaparin Heparin Protamine Warfarin
Coagulant hemostatics	Coagulant	Thrombin
Thrombolytics	Thrombolytic Streptokinase Urokinase	Alteplase Streptase Kinlytic
Antiinfectives and Antibiotics		
	Aminoglycosides	Gentamicin Kanamycin Neomycin Streptomycin Tobramycin
	Cephalosporins	Cefazolin Cefonicid Cefotaxime
	Lipopeptides	Daptomycin
	Macrolides	Erythromycin
	Oxazolidinones	Ketolides Linezolid Telithromycin
	Penicillins	Amoxicillin Ampicillin Carbenicillin Mezlocillin Penicillin G potassium Ticarcillin
	Quinolones	Ciprofloxacin
	Sulfonamide antimicrobials	Glycylcycline Sulfamethoxazole Tygacil
	Tetracyclines	Doxycycline Tetracycline

TABLE 23.3   Examples of Drugs Used in Surgery—cont'd

Drug Category	Drug Classifications	Individual Drugs
Autonomic Nervous System Agents		
Adrenergic agonists	α- and β-Adrenergic agents	Epinephrine
Adrenergic antagonists	Antidysrhythmics	Isoproterenol
		Propranolol
Anticholinergics	Muscarinics	Atropine sulfate
		Glycopyrrolate
		Scopolamine
Benzodiazepines		
Antianxiety medications	Sedative	Diazepam
		Lorazepam
		Midazolam
Central Nervous System Agents		
Analgesic agents	Narcotics	Fentanyl
		Meperidine
		Morphine
Surgical Dyes, Contrast Media, Stains		
Dyes		Bismarck brown
		Brilliant green
		Congo red
		Gentian violet
		Indian ink
		Indigo carmine
		Indocyanine green (florescent)
		Isosulfan blue (radioisotopes)
		Methylene blue
		Trypan blue
Contrast media		Diatrizoate meglumine
		Iohexol
		Vasovist MRI contrast
Tissue stains		Lugol iodine solution (Schiller solution)
		Monsel ferric solution

• BOX 23.4   Routes for Administration of Drugs

- Oral
- Sublingual
- Nasogastric
- Gastric tube
- Rectal
- Vaginal
- Topical
- Transdermal
- Inhalation
- Parenteral
- Subcutaneous
- Intramuscular
- Intravenous
- Intraarticular
- Endotracheal
- Intraarterial
- Intracardiac
- Intradermal
- Intraperitoneal
- Intraosseous
- Intrathecal
- Irrigation and instillation
- Umbilical artery or vein

procedure. Many of these can be used topically or as an injection. Uses of solutions include the following:

- *Irrigations:* Lactated Ringer's solution, saline, water. The patient can be at risk for fluid overload if the solution accumulates in the body and is resorbed.
- *Diluents:* Commonly saline or water (with or without preservative). If large quantities are used, take care to use only preservative-free fluids; the quantity of preservative can pose toxicity in the patient's system.
- *Additives to injections or irrigations:* Vasoconstrictors, anticoagulants, and buffers.
- *Antineoplastics:* Forms of chemotherapy used intraperitoneally.
- *Tumescents:* Fluid mixed with anesthetic and epinephrine, placed under the skin with a special cannula and pressurized delivery system to make the skin firm for liposuction.
- *Expansion media:* Sterile water, glycine, or saline to create a working space for endoscopy. Care is taken to measure how much goes in and how much comes out. The patient can be at risk for fluid overload.
- *Biologic adhesives:* To adhere delicate tissues together.
- *Perfusion:* For cardioplegia (cardiac cell nutrient and preservation during heart stoppage for heart surgery).
- *Preservatives and fixatives:* For tissues and specimens.
- *Medications:* For injection in a sterile field.

- *Caustics:* Phenols to remove cell layers.
- *Skin cleansers and degreasers:* For skin prep. Detergent forms can denude mucous membranes, causing inflammation and irritation. Some have inherent toxicity.
- *Visualization agents:* Diagnostic chemicals can be used in the form of stains, dyes, or radiopaque contrast media. These chemicals permit observation of body structures by adding colorization of the tissues or by using x-ray.

Solids

Many preoperative and postoperative oral medications are in pill or tablet form. Patients are instructed in their use and about how much water they are permitted to have to swallow them. Small children can be given a medicated pacifier or lollipop that contains preoperative medication, such as a sedative.

Hemostasis can be obtained using woven sheets of hemostatic material. Other sheets of specialized material can be used for adhesion prevention when placed around internal organs.

Suppositories are sometimes used as an adjunct to pediatric or rectal surgery. Some surgeons place a belladonna suppository in the rectum to slow peristalsis and allow healing after hemorrhoidectomy. Timed-release medications such as antibiotics can be implanted in bead form in orthopedic cement during prosthetic joint procedures. Orthopedic surgeons commonly use bone cement impregnated with antibiotic pellets or beads when placing implants into bone. Some of these antibiotic beads are time-released. Gynecologic procedures can include placement of timed-release rings of contraception medication in the uterine cervix.

Powders

Pharmacologic materials in powder form are commonly used in the OR in both dry and diluted forms. Dry powders and fibers used for hemostasis, such as bovine collagen, are applied dry and resorbed by the body in that form. Antibiotic powders are diluted in saline before being used as irrigants in the surgical site or before IV administration.

Sterile talc and tetracycline powder can be placed in solution for a sclerosant action in poudrage of the pleural cavity for the treatment of pleural effusion. These powders are documented in the patient's record. Prepackaged talc has a lot number that should be recorded in the lot log.

Semisolids

Creams, gels, ointments, and lotions are commonly used during surgical procedures. Ideally the product should be double-wrapped and the inner sterile packaging should be placed directly on the sterile field. Many semisolids are supplied in multidose packages and are dispensed to the field carefully without contaminating the rest of the material in the package or tube. Drugs supplied in multidose tubes should have the first half-inch of the product squeezed out into the trash before dispensing a portion to the field for use.

Lubricants are used for many procedures intraoperatively. Most are water-soluble, but those with a petroleum, lanolin, or oil base are not. Postoperatively, petroleum- or oil-based nonadherent dressings are placed on some surgical sites.

Gases

Few substances are used in the OR as gaseous forms. If the gas is used in tank form, the tanks are color-coded. Nitrous oxide (blue), nitrogen (black), helium (brown), carbon dioxide (gray), medical air (yellow), and oxygen (green) are the main gases found in the OR. Of these five gases, nitrous oxide, medical air, and oxygen are administered to the patient in drug-related form through the respiratory tree as an inhalant. Nitrogen is used to power drills and saws, and carbon dioxide is used to create a working space (insufflation) during an endoscopic procedure, but they are not used as drug forms.

In pneumatic retinopexy the ophthalmologic surgeon can use either sulfur hexafluoride (SF_6) or perfluoropropane (C_3F_8) gas injection within the eye to help reposition a torn retina using sterile technique.[2] Medical air can be used if drawn into a 3-mL syringe with a 0.22-μm micropore filter. Between 0.3 mL and 1.2 mL of gas is used to reposition the arc of the retina 45 to 90 degrees in a stable position for healing. The patient is instructed to lie in a certain position to maintain the position of the gas bubble.[2] These gases resorb after a period of time.

Compressed gas cylinders have a valve opening that turns to the left to open (turn on) and to the right to close (turn off). A simple mnemonic to help remember which direction to turn for each function is: Be sure to turn it RIGHT OFF after use and check to see it's not LEFT ON. Another mnemonic is "righty tighty and lefty loosey."

Volatile liquid substances are passed through special vaporizers and warmers to become gaseous inhalant drugs used during general anesthetic delivery.

Medical Gas Terminology

- *Cylinder:* Metal container designed to hold compressed medical gases at a high pressure.
- *Cryogenic vessel:* Metal container designed to hold liquefied compressed medical gases at extremely low temperatures.
- *Compressed medical gas:* Any liquefied or vaporized gas alone or in combination with other gases.
- *Concentrator:* Stand-alone unit that extracts oxygen from room air and delivers concentrated oxygen at a continuous flow rate.
- *Regulator:* Mechanism that controls the flow of a medical gas.

Potential Complications Caused by Pharmaceuticals and Herbal Medicine

Many patients come to the perioperative environment with co-morbidity and polypharmacy. Add to this the use of home remedies and folk medicine, and many complications can arise (Box 23.5).

Some surgical drugs and chemicals increase the effect of home remedies. This action is known as potentiation. Other medicinal substances act as antagonists and interrupt the actions of pre-scribed drugs. The pharmacokinetics of all chemical substances in the body can be altered by drugs given during a surgical procedure. Prolonged use of many physiologic chemicals or drugs can cause the body to develop a tolerance, rendering subsequent doses ineffective.

Many ancient herbs and folk remedies are still used today. Although many are useful, many can cause harm when combined with modern drugs. Most people who use herbal remedies do not have knowledge of how much or how often to use them. Serious complications such as anaphylaxis (allergy) can mask the actual cause of disease. The psychologic effects of some self-administered medications have a placebo effect that causes the patient to believe that symptoms are relieved or diseases are cured. Medical professionals use the placebo effect as a control to test the efficacy of new drugs before they are introduced to the pharmaceutical marketplace.

BOX 23.5 Examples of Medications and Herbal Substances That May Promote Postoperative Complications

Products That Contain Aspirin and Cause Bleeding
- Aleve
- Aspergum
- Bufferin
- Congespirin
- Ecotrin
- Empirin
- Excedrin

Analgesics That Have an Aspirin-Like Effect on Bleeding
- Dolobid
- Norgesic
- Oxycodone
- Pepto-Bismol
- Percodan
- Soma
- Talwin
- Voltaren

Medications That Contain Ibuprofen
- Advil
- Midol
- Naprosyn
- Nuprin
- Ponstel
- Sine-Aid
- Toradol

Anticoagulants
- Coumadin
- Dicumarol
- Heparin
- Panwarfin
- Periactin

Herbal Substances That May Have an Anticoagulant Effect
- Aloe vera
- Chamomile
- Cinnamon
- Clove
- Feverfew
- Garlic
- Ginger
- Ginkgo biloba
- Ginseng
- Licorice
- Some fish oils
- Vitamin E
- Green tea
- Grape seed extract
- Cayenne pepper
- Turmeric

Herbal Substances That Can Increase Blood Pressure
- Ephedra
- Ginseng
- Licorice
- Green tea

Herbs That Can Alter or Prolong Anesthesia
- Kava-kava
- St. John's wort
- Valerian
- Black cohosh

The FDA regulates drugs and pharmaceuticals but not dietary supplements made from herbs.[3] The manufacturers may include a disclaimer that the substance is not approved by the FDA, yet the makers promote their products as treatments for everything from baldness to weight loss. Many of these products have significant effects on the user's physiology, particularly blood pressure and blood function. If a product has been proved to cause serious problems, the FDA intervenes and removes it from the marketplace. One example, ephedra (ma huang), caused serious problems with blood pressure and the cardiovascular system.

Other natural substances such as tea tree oil and aloe vera are used in astringents and makeup formulas. The National Library of Medicine has a database of more than 3000 herbal dietary supplements. Visit www.nlm.nih.gov for additional information.

EVOLVE WEBSITE

http://evolve.elsevier.com/Hornacky/BerryKohn/
- Historical Perspective
- Student Interactive Questions
- Glossary

References

1. U.S. Food and Drug Administration: *Accelerated approval program.* www.fda.gov. Accessed June 20, 2023.
2. Wong I, Wong D: Special adjuncts to treatment. In Schachat AP, editor: *Ryan's retina*, ed 6, Philadelphia, 2018, Elsevier, pp 1957–2006.
3. Hudson I, MacDonald K, Raine J: Regulation of medicines. In *Clinical pharmacology*, ed 12, St. Louis, 2019, Elsevier, pp 63–70.

Bibliography

Bange E, Timlin C, Kabel C, et al.: Evidence for and against green tea and turmeric in the management of chronic lymphocytic leukemia, *Clin Lymphoma Myeloma Leuk* 18(10):e421–e426, 2018.
Pesce M, Esposito G, Sarnelli G: Endocannabinoids in the treatment of gastrointestinal inflammation and symptoms, *Curr Opin Pharmacol* 43:81–86, 2018.
Vallerand A, Sanoski C: *Davis's drug guide for nurses*, ed 16, Philadelphia, 2023, F.A. Davis Company.

24

Anesthesia: Techniques and Agents

CHAPTER OUTLINE

The Art and Science of Anesthesia, 433

Choice of Anesthesia, 433

Anesthesia State, 433

Knowledge of Anesthetics, 434

Types of Anesthesia, 434

Alternatives to Conventional Anesthesia, 464

CHAPTER OBJECTIVES

After studying this chapter, the learner will be able to:

- Identify three methods of general anesthesia.
- Describe the physiologic effects of general anesthesia.
- Discuss the purpose for cricoid pressure.

- Differentiate between general and regional anesthesia.
- List key points in providing safety for the anesthetized patient.

KEY TERMS AND DEFINITIONS

Amnesia Loss of memory.

Analgesia Relief of pain by altering perception of painful stimuli; acts on specific receptors in the nervous system. Does not alter consciousness.

Anesthesia Loss of feeling or sensation, especially loss of the sensation of pain with loss of protective reflexes.

Anoxia Absence of oxygen.

Anticholinergic Antagonist to action of parasympathetic and other cholinergic nerve fibers.

Apnea Suspension or cessation of breathing.

Conduction anesthesia Loss of sensation in a region of the body produced by injecting an anesthetic drug along the course of a nerve or a group of nerves to inhibit conduction of impulses to and from the area supplied by that nerve or nerves (block anesthesia, nerve block anesthesia).

Depolarization Neutralization of polarity; reduction of differentials of ion distribution across polarized semipermeable membranes, as in nerve or muscle cells in the conduction of impulses; to make electrically negative.

Dysrhythmia Ineffective rhythm, as of heart rate or brain waves; term used interchangeably with arrhythmia.

Emergence Return of consciousness, sensation, and reflexes after general anesthesia.

Endotracheal Within the trachea. An endotracheal tube may be placed in the trachea to maintain a patent airway during loss of consciousness.

Epidural anesthesia Loss of sensation below the level of peridural injection of an anesthetic drug into the epidural space in the spinal canal for relief of pain in the lower extremities, abdomen, and pelvis without loss of consciousness.

Extubation Removal of an endotracheal tube.

Fasciculation Abnormal skeletal muscle contraction in which groups of muscle fibers innervated by the same neuron contract together.

Hypercapnia Excessive amount of carbon dioxide in the blood; may also be termed hypercarbia.

Hypnotic Drug or verbal suggestion that induces sleep.

Hypothermia State in which body temperature is lower than the physiologic normal (i.e., below 95° F [35° C]).

Hypoxia, hypoxemia Oxygen deficiency; state in which an inadequate amount of oxygen is available to or used by tissue; inadequate tissue oxygenation.

Induction Period from the beginning of administration of an anesthetic until the patient loses consciousness and is stabilized in the desired plane of anesthesia.

Intrathecal injection Instillation of solution, such as an anesthetic drug, into the subarachnoid space for diffusion in spinal fluid, as for spinal anesthesia.

Intubation Insertion of an endotracheal tube.

Laryngospasm Involuntary spasmodic reflex action that partially or completely closes the vocal cords of the larynx.

Local anesthesia Loss of sensation along specific nerve pathways produced by blocking transmissions of impulses to receptor fibers. The anesthetic drug injected depresses sensory nerves and blocks conduction of pain impulses from their site of origin. The patient remains conscious, with or without intravenous sedation.

Moderate sedation (formerly known as intravenous conscious sedation [IVCS]). Depressed level of consciousness produced by IV administration of pharmacologic agents. The patient retains the ability to continuously maintain a patent airway independently and respond to physical or verbal stimulation. Sedation may relieve anxiety and produce amnesia.

Narcosis State of arrested consciousness, sensation, motor activity, and reflex action produced by drugs.

Narcotic, opioid Drug derived from opium or opium-like compounds, with potent analgesic effects associated with significant alteration of mood and behavior.

Nerve block Loss of sensation produced by injecting an anesthetic drug around a specific nerve or nerve plexus to interrupt sensory, motor, or sympathetic transmission of impulses.

$Paco_2$ Arterial carbon dioxide tension (partial pressure of carbon dioxide in arterial blood). Normal 35 to 45 torr.

Pao_2 Arterial oxygen tension (partial pressure of oxygen in the arterial blood); degree of oxygen transported in the circulating blood. Normal 80 to 100 torr.

pH Expression for hydrogen ion concentration or acidity. In blood, alkalemia values above 7.45; acidemia: values below 7.35; normal 7.4.

Regional anesthesia Loss of sensation in a specific body part or region produced by blocking conductivity of sensory nerves supplying that area. The anesthetic drug is injected around a specific nerve or group of nerves to interrupt pain impulses. The patient remains conscious, with or without intravenous sedation. Regional anesthetic techniques include nerve, intrathecal, peridural, and epidural blocks.

Sedative Pharmacologic agent (drug) that suppresses nervous excitement, allays anxiety, and produces a calming effect. Benzodiazepines, barbiturates, and opioids (narcotics) are the most commonly used drugs for conscious sedation.

Spinal anesthesia Loss of sensation below the level of the diaphragm produced by intrathecal injection of an anesthetic drug into the subarachnoid space without loss of consciousness.

Tachycardia Excessively rapid rate of heart action, heartbeat. The pulse rate is higher than 100 beats/min.

Tachypnea Abnormally rapid rate of breathing.

Topical anesthesia Depression of sensation in superficial peripheral nerves by application of an anesthetic agent directly to the mucous membrane, skin, or cornea.

The Art and Science of Anesthesia

Anesthesiology is the branch of medicine and nursing that is concerned with the administration of medication or anesthetic agents to relieve pain and support physiologic functions during a surgical procedure. It is a specialty that requires knowledge of biochemistry, clinical pharmacology, cardiology, and respiratory physiology. The American Society of Anesthesiologists (ASA), founded in 1905 and incorporated in 1936, has defined anesthesiology as the practice of medicine dealing with the management of procedures for rendering a patient insensible to pain during surgical procedures and with the support of life functions under the stress of anesthetic and surgical manipulations.

The purpose of this chapter is to acquaint the surgical team with several processes associated with the delivery and maintenance of anesthesia and how the team works together to provide a safe surgical procedure for the patient. All perioperative team members should be readily available to assist the anesthesia provider as needed. Continuing education is advised for the entire team.

Choice of Anesthesia

Selection of anesthesia is made by the anesthesia provider in consultation with the surgeon and the patient. The primary consideration with any anesthetic is that it should be associated with low morbidity and mortality. Choosing the safest agent and technique is a decision predicated on thorough knowledge, sound judgment, and evaluation of each individual situation.

The anesthesia provider uses the lowest concentration of anesthetic agents compatible with patient analgesia, relaxation, and facilitation of the surgical procedure. An ideal anesthetic agent or technique suitable for all patients does not exist, but the one selected should include the following characteristics:
- Provide maximum safety for the patient
- Provide optimal operating conditions for the surgeon
- Provide patient comfort
- Have a low index of toxicity
- Provide potent, predictable analgesia extending into the postoperative period

- Produce adequate muscle relaxation
- Provide amnesia
- Have a rapid onset and easy reversibility
- Produce minimum side effects

The patient's ability to tolerate stress and adverse effects of anesthesia and the surgical procedure depends on respiration; circulation; and function of the liver, kidneys, endocrine system, and central nervous system (CNS). The following factors are important:
- Age, size, and weight of the patient
- Physical, mental, and emotional status of the patient
- Presence of complicating systemic disease or concurrent drug therapy
- Presence of infection at the site of the surgical procedure
- Previous anesthesia experience
- Anticipated procedure
- Position required for the procedure
- Type and expected length of the procedure
- Local or systemic toxicity of the agent
- Expertise of the anesthesia provider
- Preference of the surgeon and patient

Anesthesia State

Both the central and the autonomic nervous systems play essential roles in clinical anesthesia. The CNS exerts powerful control throughout the body. The effect of anesthetic drugs is one of progressive depression of the CNS, beginning with the higher centers of the cerebral cortex and ending with the vital centers in the medulla. The cerebral cortex is not inactive during deep anesthesia. Afferent impulses continue to flow into the cortex along primary pathways and excite cells in appropriate sensory areas. Also, the cerebral cortex is integrated with the reticular system.

The brain represents approximately 2% of body weight but receives about 15% of cardiac output. Various factors cause alterations in cerebral blood flow and are of considerable importance in anesthesia. These factors are oxygen, carbon dioxide, temperature, arterial blood pressure, drugs, the age of the patient, anesthetic techniques, and neurogenic factors.

The autonomic nervous system is equally important because of its role in the physiology of the cardiovascular system, the anesthesia provider's ability to block certain autonomic pathways with local analgesic agents, specific blocking effects of certain drugs, and the sympathomimetic and parasympathomimetic effects of many anesthetic agents.

The anesthesia state involves control of motor, sensory, mental, and reflex functions. The anesthesia provider constantly assesses the patient's response to stimuli to evaluate specific anesthetic requirements. Specific drugs are used to achieve the desired results: amnesia, analgesia, and muscle relaxation. The ASA and American Association of Nurse Anesthetists (AANA) have established guidelines and standards for safely administering and monitoring anesthesia care. The ASA also developed the taxonomy for classifying patients by physical status from ASA I, the lowest risk, to ASA VI, the highest risk (Box 24.1). More information about the ASA classification system can be found at http://www.asahq.org/.

Knowledge of Anesthetics

Anesthesia involves the administration of potentially lethal drugs and gases. Interactions of these with human physiology can be profound. Using discerning observation, astute deduction, and meticulous attention to the minutiae, the anesthesia provider delivers skilled induction, careful maintenance of anesthesia, and prophylaxis to avoid postoperative complications.

Being responsible for vital functions of the patient, the anesthesia provider must know physical and chemical properties of all gases and liquids used in anesthesia and their effect on medical conditions. These properties determine how agents are supplied, their stability, systems used for their administration, and their uptake and distribution in the body. Important factors are diffusion, solubility in body fluids, and relationships of pressure, volume, and temperature. The synthesized general anesthetic agents are nonflammable, in contrast with the older agents.

Perioperative and postanesthesia care unit (PACU) nurses need to be cognizant of the pharmacologic characteristics of the most commonly used anesthetics and techniques. Anesthesia and surgical trauma produce multiple systemic effects, which are continually monitored throughout the perioperative care period. The type and level of anesthesia will vary according to the type of surgery being performed. These types are described as follows:

1. *Minimal or light sedation (anxiolysis):* A drug-induced state during which patients respond normally to verbal command. Although cognitive function and coordination may be impaired, ventilatory and cardiovascular functions are unaffected.
2. *Moderate sedation/analgesia (formerly known as conscious sedation):* A drug-induced depression of consciousness during which patients can respond purposefully to verbal commands, either alone or accompanied by light tactile stimulation. No interventions are required to maintain a patent airway, and spontaneous ventilation is adequate.
3. *Deep sedation/analgesia:* A drug-induced depression of consciousness during which patients cannot be easily aroused but respond purposefully after repeated or painful stimulation. The ability to independently maintain ventilatory function may be impaired. Patients may require assistance to maintain a patent airway, and spontaneous ventilation may be inadequate.
4. *Full anesthesia:* General anesthesia and regional anesthesia. General anesthesia is a drug-induced loss of consciousness during which patients cannot be roused, even by painful stimulation. The ability to independently maintain ventilatory function is often impaired. Patients often require assistance to maintain a patent airway, and positive pressure ventilation may be required because of depressed spontaneous ventilation or drug-induced depression of neuromuscular function. Cardiovascular function may be impaired.

Types of Anesthesia

Anesthesia may be produced in the following ways:
- *General anesthesia:* Pain is controlled by general insensibility. Basic elements include loss of consciousness, analgesia, interference with undesirable reflexes, and muscle relaxation.
- *Balanced anesthesia:* The properties of general anesthesia (i.e., hypnosis, analgesia, and muscle relaxation) are produced, in varying degrees, by a combination of agents. Each agent has a specific purpose. This often is referred to as *neuroleptanesthesia.*
- *Local or regional block anesthesia:* Pain is controlled without loss of consciousness. The sensory nerves in one area or region of the body are anesthetized. This is sometimes called conduction anesthesia. Acupuncture is sometimes used.
- *Spinal or epidural anesthesia:* Sensation of pain is blocked at a level below the diaphragm without loss of consciousness. The agent is injected in the spinal canal.

General Anesthesia

Anesthesia is produced as the CNS is affected. Association pathways are broken in the cerebral cortex to produce more or less complete lack of sensory perception and motor discharge. Unconsciousness is produced when blood circulating to the brain contains an adequate amount of the anesthetic agent. General anesthesia results in an unconscious, immobile, quiet patient who does not recall the surgical procedure.

Most anesthetic agents are potentially lethal. The anesthesia provider must constantly observe the body's reflex responses to

• BOX 24.1 ASA Classifications

- ASA I theoretically includes relatively healthy patients with localized pathologic processes. An emergency surgical procedure, designated E, signifies additional risk. For example, a hernia that becomes incarcerated changes the patient's status to ASA I-E.
- ASA II includes patients with mild systemic disease (e.g., diabetes mellitus controlled by oral hypoglycemic agents or diet).
- ASA III includes patients with severe systemic disease that limits activity but is not totally incapacitating (e.g., chronic obstructive pulmonary disease or severe hypertension).
- ASA IV includes patients with an incapacitating disease that is a constant threat to life (e.g., cardiovascular or renal disease).
- ASA V includes moribund patients who are not expected to survive 24 hours with or without the surgical procedure. They are operated on in an attempt to save their lives; the surgical procedure is a resuscitative measure, as in a massive pulmonary embolus. The patient may or may not survive the surgical procedure.
- ASA VI includes patients who have been declared brain dead but whose organs will be removed for donor purposes. Mechanical ventilation and life support systems are maintained until the organs are procured.

TABLE 24.1   Depth of General Anesthesia

From	To	Patient's Responses	Patient Care Considerations
Induction of general anesthesia by IV or inhalant gas	Begins to lose consciousness; will have recall Bispectral state 100	Drowsy, dizzy, amnesic	Close OR doors. Keep room quiet. Stand by to assist. Initiate cricoid pressure if requested.
Loss of consciousness: excitement phase	Relaxation, light hypnosis; low probability of recall Bispectral state 70–50	May be excited, with irregular breathing and movements of extremities; susceptible to external stimuli (e.g., noise, touch)	Restrain patient. Remain at patient's side, quietly, but ready to assist anesthesia provider as needed.
Surgical anesthesia stage of relaxation	Loss of reflexes: depression of vital functions Bispectral state 40: maintenance range	Regular respiration; contracted pupils; reflexes disappear; muscles relax; auditory sensation lost	Position patient and prepare skin only when anesthesia provider indicates this stage is reached and under control.
Danger stage: vital functions too depressed	Respiratory failure; possible cardiac arrest Bispectral state 0	Not breathing; little or no pulse or heartbeat	Prepare for cardiopulmonary resuscitation.

IV, Intravenous; *OR,* operating room.

stimuli and other guides to determine the degree of CNS, respiratory, and circulatory depression during induction and the surgical procedure. No one clinical sign can be used as a reliable indication of anesthesia depth. Continuous watching and appraisal of all clinical signs, in addition to other available objective measurements, are necessary. In this way the anesthesia provider judges the level of anesthesia, referred to as light, moderate, or deep, and provides the patient with optimal care (Table 24.1).

The three methods of administering general anesthetic are inhalation, intravenous (IV) injection, and rectal instillation. The latter method is not commonly used, except occasionally in pediatric patients, because retention and absorption in the colon are unpredictable. Control of each method varies.

Induction of General Anesthesia

Induction involves putting the patient safely into a state of unconsciousness. Fig. 24.1 depicts the levels of unconsciousness associated with general anesthesia. A patent airway and adequate ventilation must be ensured. If one is not already running, an IV infusion is started. The anesthesia provider should wear gloves for venipuncture. A nasogastric tube may be inserted to decompress the gastrointestinal tract and evacuate stomach contents.

Preoxygenation

The anesthesia provider may have the patient breathe pure (100%) oxygen by facemask for a few minutes. This provides a margin of safety in the event of airway obstruction or apnea during induction, with resultant hypoxia.

Loss of Consciousness

Unconsciousness is induced by IV administration of a drug or by inhalation of an agent mixed with oxygen. Because the technique is rapid and simple, an IV drug usually is preferred by anesthesia providers and often requested by patients.

Intubation

A patent airway must be established to provide adequate oxygenation and control breathing of the unconscious patient.

• **Fig. 24.1** Levels of unconsciousness associated with general anesthesia.

The patient's tongue and secretions can obstruct respiration in the absence of protective reflexes.

The anesthesia provider evaluates the airway for the risk for difficult intubation using the Mallampati classification chart (Fig. 24.2). Other measurements include thyromental distance (the distance between the chin and thyroid cartilage), neck flexion/extension range, and the ability to protrude the mandible (prognathism). An oropharyngeal airway, nasopharyngeal airway, laryngeal mask, endotracheal tube, or endobronchial tube (for lung procedures) may be inserted.

Physiologic indicators of a difficult airway include the following:

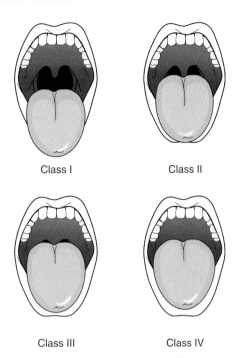

• **Fig. 24.2** Mallampati classification for difficult intubation.

Class I

Class II

Class III

Class IV

• **Fig. 24.3** Short neck or extreme obesity. **A,** Supine position. **B,** Sniffing position.

Trachea

• **Fig. 24.4** Nasotracheal intubation with a Magill forceps.

- Inability to open the mouth less than 4 cm. Patients with previous jaw surgery may have jaw wires in place. Wire cutters should be immediately available in the event of a return to surgery.
- Immobility of the cervical spine. Patients with vertebral disease or injury may not have full range of motion necessary for intubation.
- Chin or jaw deformities. Patients with small jaws or chin may have a difficult airway. Edentulous patients commonly have some bone loss that alters facial contours.
- Dentition can be an issue if the patient has loose teeth or periodontal disease. A tooth can be aspirated during the airway maintenance process. Children between the ages of 6 and 8 commonly have loose baby teeth.
- Short neck or extreme obesity (Fig. 24.3).
- Pathology of the head and neck such as tumors or deformity. An enlarged tongue can be an obstruction to a full view of the glottis.
- Previous tracheostomy scar, which can cause a stricture.
- Trauma.

Intubation is insertion of an endotracheal tube between vocal cords, usually with an oral tube by direct laryngoscopy. A nasotracheal tube may be inserted by blind intubation or with a direct approach using Magill forceps to guide the tube through the pharynx (Fig. 24.4). Epistaxis can be a complication of nasal airway use. This method is contraindicated in anticoagulated patients. Tubes may be made of metal, plastic, silicone, or rubber. Most styles for adult sizes have a built-in cuff that is inflated with a measured amount of air, water, or saline after insertion, to completely occlude the trachea.

The anesthesia provider is informed if a laser will be used in the mouth or throat so that a laser-resistant endotracheal tube can be inserted. The endotracheal tube must be securely fixed in place to prevent irritation of the trachea and maintain ventilation. The anesthesia provider should wear a mask and protective eyewear to prevent secretions splashing in the eyes during intubation. An oropharyngeal suction tip and tubing should be kept close at hand.

Neuromuscular blocking agents are given before intubation to relax the jaw and larynx. Pediatric patients and patients susceptible to malignant hyperthermia may experience jaw tightness, which is referred to as masseter muscle rigidity (MMR) or trismus. Intubation during induction and extubation during emergence from anesthesia are precarious times for the patient. The patient may cough, jerk, or experience laryngospasm from tracheal stimulation. Cardiac dysrhythmias may occur. Hypoxia is a potential complication. Hypoxia commonly precedes dysrhythmia.

Aspiration is also a hazard, particularly in a patient with a full stomach or with increased intraabdominal or intracranial pressure. Any patient who arrives in the operating room (OR) unconscious or who is a victim of trauma should be treated as though they have a full stomach. Pregnant and obese patients should also be considered in this category because of increased intraabdominal pressure in the supine position and possible decreased gastric motility.

Cricoid Pressure

The circulating nurse may be asked to apply pressure to the cricoid cartilage to occlude the esophagus and immobilize the trachea. Referred to as *Sellick maneuver,* this action prevents regurgitation and aspiration of stomach contents. The cricoid cartilage forms a complete ring around the inferior wall of the larynx below the thyroid cartilage prominence. Exerting pressure with one or two fingers to compress the cricoid cartilage against the body of the sixth cervical vertebra obstructs the esophagus (Fig. 24.5).

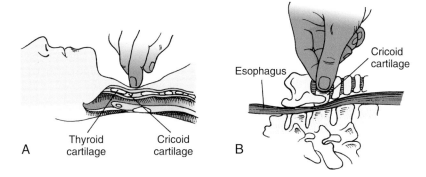

• **Fig. 24.5** Cricoid pressure. **A,** Index finger displaces cricoid cartilage posteriorly, thus obstructing esophagus. **B,** Two-finger technique obstructs esophagus between body of sixth cervical vertebra and cricoid cartilage.

Compression must begin with the patient awake before induction drugs are injected. It must continue until the endotracheal tube cuff is inflated and the anesthesia provider states that it is safe to release pressure. This is the narrowest portion of the pediatric airway. If the patient is younger than 8 years, an uncuffed tube is used to prevent damage to the airway.[1]

Awake Intubation

Based on preoperative physical assessment, the anesthesia provider may determine that intubation must be performed before the induction of general anesthesia (i.e., "awake intubation"). Acromegaly, an anterior larynx, an enlarged tongue, a limited oral cavity, jaw fixation, a short neck, and limited cervical range of motion are the most common indications for awake intubation. These conditions may inhibit visualization of the vocal cords by direct laryngoscopy and thus increase the potential risk for airway obstruction in the absence of protective reflexes, such as after the induction of anesthesia.

Awake intubation can be performed with a fiberoptic or rigid laryngoscope for direct visualization of vocal cords after the administration of IV sedation and application of a topical spray anesthetic to the posterior pharynx. The anesthesia provider may inject a local anesthetic around the laryngeal nerve to suppress the patient's gag and cough reflex. Usually two anesthesia providers work together during awake intubation.

After the patient is sedated and the topical anesthetic agent is applied, one anesthesia provider inserts the endotracheal or nasotracheal tube as the second anesthesia provider gives a rapid-acting barbiturate to induce general anesthesia.

Key Points During Induction

Induction of general anesthesia is a crucial period requiring maximum attention from the OR team. The following key points are critical to the patient's welfare:

1. The circulating nurse should remain at the patient's side during induction to provide physical protection and emotional support, assist the anesthesia provider as needed, and closely observe the monitors.
2. Although induction is quiet and uneventful for most patients, untoward occurrences are possible. Excitement, coughing, breath-holding, retching, vomiting, irregular respiratory patterns, or laryngospasm can lead to hypoxia. Secretions in air passages from irritation by the anesthetic can cause obstruction and dysrhythmias. Induction is gentle and not so rapid as to cause physiologic insult. To prevent these events, the patient must not be stimulated by loud noises, clattering instruments, or opening paper wrappers. Do not move or begin prepping the patient until the anesthesia provider says it is safe to do so.
3. Precautions to be taken during induction include continuous electrocardiogram (ECG) monitoring, use of a precordial chest stethoscope, and having resuscitative equipment, including a defibrillator, readily available.
4. Induction is individualized. For example, an obese or pregnant patient may be induced with the head raised slightly to avoid pressure of the abdominal viscera against the diaphragm. The patient is placed flat, however, if the blood pressure begins to drop. The enlarged pregnant uterus can cause pressure on the vena cava, decreasing venous return. One quick method of relieving pressure is to physically push the uterus toward the patient's left side. Another method for displacing the pregnant uterus is to elevate the patient's right hip by tilting the OR bed toward the left or placing a wedge under the right hip.
5. Small children need gentle handling. The circulating nurse can help the anesthesia provider make the induction period less frightening by staying close to the child. Sometimes a drop of artificial flavoring (e.g., orange, peppermint) put inside the facemask facilitates the child's acceptance of it. Parents are often allowed in for induction according to the institution's policy. After induction, the parent is escorted back to the waiting area by transport personnel.
6. The speed of induction depends on the potency of the agent, administration technique, partial pressure administered, and rate at which the anesthetic is taken up by blood and tissues.

Maintenance of General Anesthesia

The anesthesia provider attempts to maintain the lightest level of anesthesia in the brain compatible with operating conditions. The following are five objectives of general anesthesia:

1. *Oxygenation:* Tissues, especially the brain, must be continuously perfused with oxygenated blood. The color of the blood, amount and kind of bleeding, and pulse oximetry are indicators of the adequacy of oxygenation. Controls on the anesthesia machine and monitors of vital functions keep the anesthesia provider aware of the patient's condition.
2. *Unconsciousness:* The patient remains asleep and unaware of the environment during the surgical procedure.
3. *Analgesia:* The patient must be free of pain during the surgical procedure.

4. *Muscle relaxation:* Muscle relaxation must be constantly assessed to provide necessary amounts of drugs that cause skeletal muscles to relax. Less tissue manipulation is required when muscles are relaxed.
5. *Control of autonomic reflexes:* Anesthetic agents affect cardiovascular and respiratory systems. Tissue manipulations and systemic reactions to them may be altered by drugs that control the autonomic nervous system.

Anesthesia Machine

General anesthesia is maintained by inhalation of gases and IV injection of drugs. An anesthesia machine is always used to deliver oxygen-anesthetic mixtures to the patient through a breathing system.

The anesthesia machine includes sources of oxygen and gases with flowmeters for measuring and controlling their delivery; devices to volatilize and deliver liquid anesthetics; a gas-driven mechanical ventilator; devices for monitoring the ECG, blood pressure, inspired oxygen, and end-tidal carbon dioxide; and alarm systems to signal apnea or disconnection of the breathing circuit.

Breathing tubes of corrugated rubber or plastic carry gases from the machine to the facemask and breathing system. The reservoir (breathing) bag compensates for variations in respiratory demand and permits assisted or controlled ventilation by manual or mechanical compression of the bag. Sterile disposable sets containing tubing, a mask, a Y-connector, and a reservoir bag are commercially available in conductive and nonconductive materials.

Machine design includes fail-safe alarm systems to prevent delivery of a hypoxic gas mixture and to reduce the possibility of human error or mechanical failure. Reference to a daily machine performance checklist by the anesthesia provider before induction should be routine, as recommended by the U.S. Food and Drug Administration (FDA). Studies have shown that many complications associated with the administration of anesthetic could have been avoided if the equipment had been checked before use.

All anesthesia machines have the following features (Fig. 24.6):
1. Sources of oxygen and compressed gases (Fig. 24.7). These may come from piped-in systems, but mounted oxygen tanks are necessary in the event of failure of systems.
2. Means for measuring (flowmeters) and controlling (reservoir bag) delivery of gases.
3. Means to volatilize liquid (vaporizer) and deliver (breathing tubes) anesthetic vapor or gas.
4. Device for disposal of carbon dioxide (carbon dioxide absorption canister).
5. Safety devices:
   a. Oxygen analyzers
   b. Oxygen pressure interlock system or equivalent to automatically shut off the flow of gases in the absence of oxygen pressure
   c. End-tidal carbon dioxide monitors
   d. Pressure and disconnect alarms to notify the anesthesia provider if the flow of oxygen and gases becomes disproportional
   e. Gas scavenger system to collect exhaled gases

Waste Gases. The elimination of waste gas, vented through an exhaust valve into a waste gas scavenger system, controls pollution of the room air. Most waste anesthetic gas removal hoses are purple and are seen exiting the gas machine at the back of the machine. Nitrous oxide (N_2O) and halogenated agents can escape into room air if they are not directed through the scavenger system. Substantial amounts may be an occupational health hazard to OR team members. Prolonged exposure to high concentrations of waste gases (1000 ppm) can cause reproductive abnormalities. Halogenated waste gases should be lower than 2 ppm and N_2O waste gas should be lower than 25 ppm according to safety regulations set by the National Institute for Occupational Safety and Health (NIOSH) and Centers for Disease Control and Prevention (CDC). Additional information can be found at http://www.cdc.gov/.

• **Fig. 24.6** Anesthesia machine for maintenance of general anesthesia. *1,* Anesthetic and respiratory gas monitor; *2,* physiologic monitor (channels include electrocardiograph [ECG], blood pressure, temperature, heart rate, and pulse oximeter); *3,* flow-through vaporizers; *4,* facemask; *5,* reservoir "breathing" bag; *6,* carbon dioxide absorber canister; *7,* patient breathing circuit; *8,* ventilator; *9,* flowmeters for gases; *10,* sphygmomanometer for manual blood pressure.

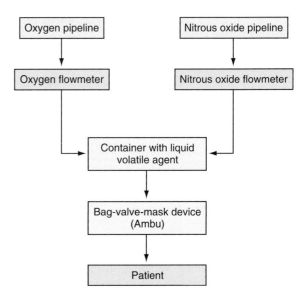

• **Fig. 24.7** Minimum number of components needed for an anesthesia gas machine.

Valves on the machine and tubing connections should be checked daily and must be secure for the system to work properly. Room air should be monitored. This may be done by an infrared spectrophotometer, for example, to monitor the escape of gases from the patient's exhalations and from the anesthetic delivery system. Patients continue to exhale retained gases when they arrive in the PACU. Passive dosimeters may be used to monitor air in team members' personal breathing spaces.

Inhalation Systems. The method for administration of inhalation anesthetics through the anesthesia machine can be classified as semiclosed, closed, semiopen, or open (Fig. 24.8):

- *Semiclosed system:* The most widely used system, a semiclosed system permits exhaled gases to pass into the atmosphere so that they will not mix with fresh gases and be rebreathed. A chemical absorber for carbon dioxide is placed in the breathing circuit. This reduces carbon dioxide accumulation in blood. Induction is slower but with less loss of heat and water vapor than with open methods.
- *Closed system:* A closed system allows complete rebreathing of expired gases. Exhaled carbon dioxide is absorbed by soda lime or a mixture of barium and calcium hydroxide (Baralyme) in the absorber on the machine. The body's metabolic demand for oxygen is met by adding oxygen to the inspired mixture of gases or vapors. This system provides maximal conservation of heat and moisture. It reduces the amount and therefore the cost of agents and reduces environmental contamination.
- *Semiopen system:* With the semiopen system some exhaled gas can pass into surrounding air but some returns to the inspiratory part of the circuit for rebreathing. The degree of rebreathing is determined by the volume of flow of fresh gas. Expired carbon dioxide is not chemically absorbed.
- *Open system:* In an open system, valves direct expired gases into the lower portion of the canister, where they are removed by vacuum. The patient inhales only the anesthetic mixture delivered by the anesthesia machine. The composition of the inspired mixture can be accurately determined. However, anesthetic gases are not confined to the breathing system. High flows of gases are necessary because resistance to breathing varies. Water vapor and heat are lost. Inspired gases should be humidified for respiratory mucosa to function properly, especially for children and during long surgical procedures.

Administration Techniques. Inhalation gases and vapors can be delivered from an anesthesia machine via a facemask, laryngeal mask, or endotracheal tube. Respirations must be assisted or controlled.

Mask Inhalation. Anesthetic gas or vapor of a volatile liquid is inhaled through a facemask attached to the anesthesia machine by breathing tubes. The mask must fit the face tightly to minimize escape of gases into room air. Significant leakage occurs around an ill-fitting mask, particularly in the area above the nose. Several sizes should be available.

Laryngeal Mask. An airway can be maintained by inserting a laryngeal mask airway (LMA) into the larynx. This flexible tube has an inflatable silicone ring and cuff. When the cuff is inflated, the mask fills the space around and behind the larynx to form a seal between the tube and the trachea. All types do not protect against regurgitation and aspiration. OxyMask and ProSeal have a passage for gastric tube placement that provides better protection against regurgitation. Adult and pediatric styles are available and can be useful when intubation and mask ventilation are complex.

Reusable and disposable styles are commercially available (Fig. 24.9). The mask is selected for use by size of the patient, as follows:

- Size 1: 0 to 6.5 kg
- Size 2: 6.5 to 20 kg
- Size 2.5: 20 to 30 kg
- Size 3: 30 to 70 kg
- Size 4: 70 to 80 kg
- Size 5: 80 kg or greater

Endotracheal Administration. Anesthetic vapor or gas is inhaled directly into the trachea through a nasal or oral tube inserted between the vocal cords by direct laryngoscopy. The tube is securely fixed in place to minimize tissue trauma. The patient is given oxygen before and after suctioning of a tracheal tube. Advantages of endotracheal administration are the following:

- It ensures a patent airway and control of respiration. Secretions are easily removed from the trachea by suctioning. Positive pressure can be given immediately by pressing the reservoir bag on the machine without danger of dilating the stomach.
- It protects the lungs from aspiration of blood, vomitus of gastric contents, or foreign material.
- It preserves the airway regardless of the patient's position during the surgical procedure.
- It interferes minimally with the surgical field during head and neck procedures.
- It helps minimize the escape of vapors or gases into the room atmosphere.

Intubation and extubation can cause tracheal stimulation. The patient may cough, jerk, or develop spasms of the larynx (laryngospasm). Other potential complications of endotracheal administration include the following:

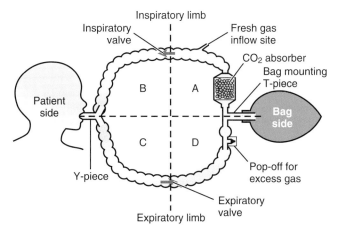

• **Fig. 24.8** Complete anesthesia breathing circuit.

• **Fig. 24.9** Laryngeal mask airway.

- *Trauma to the teeth, pharynx, vocal cords, or trachea:* Postoperatively the patient may experience sore throat, hoarseness, laryngitis, and/or tracheitis. Laryngeal edema is more common in children than in adults. Ulceration of the tracheal mucosa or vocal cords may cause granuloma.
- *Cardiac dysrhythmias:* Cardiac dysrhythmias may occur in light anesthesia or be caused by suctioning through the endotracheal tube.
- *Hypoxia and hypoxemia:* Hypoxia is a common complication during intubation and extubation. Endotracheal tube suctioning can cause hypoxemia.
- *Accidental esophageal or endobronchial intubation:* The latter results in ventilation of only one lung.
- *Aspiration of gastrointestinal contents:* This is a hazard in a patient with a full stomach or a patient who has increased intra-abdominal or intracranial pressure. It can also occur in a patient with intestinal obstruction who is extubated before protective reflexes return.

Controlled Respiration. Respirations may be assisted or controlled. Assistance, to improve ventilation, may easily be given by manual pressure on the reservoir (breathing) bag of the anesthesia machine. Assisted respiration implies that the patient's own respiratory effort initiates the cycle. Controlled respiration may be defined as the completely controlled rate and volume of respirations. The latter is best accomplished by means of a mechanical device that automatically and rhythmically inflates the lungs with intermittent positive pressure, requiring no effort by the patient. Gas moves in and out of the lungs.

The combination of a volume preset ventilator with an assist mechanism maintains the integrity of the respiratory center. Controlled respiration is initiated after the anesthesia provider has produced apnea by hyperventilation or administration of respiratory depressant drugs or a neuromuscular blocker.

Controlled ventilation is used in all types of surgical procedures, especially in lengthy ones. The anesthesia provider's artificial control of respiration or the patient's respiratory efforts influence the minute-to-minute level of anesthesia. Advantages of controlled respiration are the following:

- It provides for optimal ventilation.
- It allows for selective lung deflation for thoracic procedures.
- It provides access to deep regions of the thorax and upper abdomen.
- It permits deliberate production of apnea to facilitate surgical manipulation below the diaphragm, ligation of deep vessels, or obtaining radiographic films.

The patient is taken off the respirator gradually near the end of the surgical procedure, and spontaneous respiration resumes. Assisted ventilation may be continued postoperatively after lengthy procedures until reflexes and spontaneous respirations return.

Inhalation Anesthetic Agents

Inhalation is a controllable method of administration because uptake and elimination of anesthetic agents are accomplished mainly by pulmonary ventilation and selective organ metabolism. The anesthetic vapor of a volatile liquid or an anesthetic gas is inhaled and carried into the bloodstream by passing across the alveolar membrane into the general circulation and on to the tissues.

Ventilation and pulmonary circulation are two critical factors involved in the process. Each can be affected by components of the anesthetic experience, such as a change in body position, preanesthetic medication, alteration in body temperature, or respiratory gas tensions.

In inhalation anesthesia, the aim is to establish balance between the content of the anesthetic vapor or gas inhaled and that of body tissues. The blood and lungs function as the transport system. Anesthesia is produced by the development of an anesthetizing concentration of anesthetic in the brain. The depth of anesthesia is related to concentration and biotransformation (Table 24.1).

Pulmonary blood-gas exchange is important to tissue perfusion. Defective gas exchange can cause hypoxemia and respiratory failure. It also interferes with delivery of the anesthetic. Potent inhalation agents, such as myocardial depressants, affect oxygenation. Most of them induce a dose-related hypoventilation. The deeper the anesthesia, the more depressed ventilation becomes. Surgical stimulation partially corrects depression, but respiration must be controlled to keep oxygen and carbon dioxide exchange constant to prevent hypoventilation and cardiac depression.

Although the respiratory system is used for distribution of the anesthetic, it also must carry on its normal function of ventilation (i.e., meeting tissue demands for adequate oxygenation and elimination of carbon dioxide and helping maintain normal acid-base balance). The amount of anesthetic vapor inspired is influenced by the volume and rate of respirations. Gas or vapor concentration and the rate of delivery are also significant.

Pulmonary circulation is the vehicle for oxygen and anesthetic transport to the general circulation. The large absorptive surface of the lungs and their extensive microcirculation provide a large gas-exchanging surface. In optimal gas exchange, all alveoli share inspired gas and cardiac output equally (ventilation-perfusion match). Because respiratory and anesthetic gases interact with pulmonary circulation, alveolar anesthetic concentrations are rapidly reflected in circulating blood.

Alveolar concentration results from a balance between two forces: ventilation that delivers the anesthetic to the alveoli and uptake that removes the anesthetic from the alveoli. Certain factors influence uptake of the anesthetic and thus induction and recovery. Uptake has two phases:

1. *Transfer of anesthetic from alveoli to blood:* The rate of transfer is determined by the solubility of the agent in the blood, the rate of pulmonary blood flow (related to cardiac output), and the partial pressure of the anesthetic in arterial and mixed venous blood.
2. *Transfer of anesthetic from blood to tissues:* Factors influencing uptake by individual tissues are similar to those for uptake by blood. They are the solubility of the gas in tissues, the tissue volume relative to the blood flow (flow rate), and the partial pressure of the anesthetic in arterial blood and tissues. Tissues differ; thus uptake of the anesthetic differs. Highly perfused tissues (heart) equilibrate more rapidly with arterial tension than does poorly perfused tissue (fat), which has a slow rise to equilibrium and retains anesthetic longer.

Elimination of the anesthetic is affected by the same factors that affected uptake. As an anesthetic is eliminated, its partial pressure in arterial blood drops first, followed by that in tissues.

The most important factors influencing safe administration of any anesthetic are the knowledge and skill of the anesthesia provider. A perfect agent has not been found, and no agent is entirely safe. Commonly used agents are listed in Table 24.2. Advantages and disadvantages are relative.

TABLE 24.2 Most Commonly Used General Anesthetic Agents

Generic Name	Trade Name	Administration	Characteristics	Uses
Inhalation Agents				
Nitrous oxide	None	Inhalation	Inorganic nonvolatile gas; slight potency; pleasant, fruitlike odor; nonirritating; nonflammable but supports combustion; poor muscle relaxation	Rapid induction and recovery; short procedures when muscle relaxation unimportant; adjunct to potent agents. Should be mixed with 30% oxygen to prevent hypoxia.
Desflurane	Suprane	Inhalation	Halogenated liquid with low solubility, desflurane has faster uptake by inhalation and elimination	Not used for induction with children. Can be used for maintenance in adults and children.
Sevoflurane	Ultane	Inhalation	Volatile liquid form, nonflammable and nonexplosive; noted for its rapid induction and rapid emergence qualities	Used for adults and children. Rapid elimination
Isoflurane	Forane	Inhalation	Halogenated methyl ether; potent; muscle relaxant; profound respiratory depressant; metabolized in liver	Rapid induction and recovery with minimal aftereffects; wide spectrum for maintenance
Intravenous Agents				
Thiopental sodium	Pentothal sodium	Intravenous	Barbiturate; potent; short acting with cumulative effect; rapid uptake by circulatory system; no muscle relaxation; respiratory depressant	Rapid induction and recovery; short procedures when muscle relaxation not needed; basal anesthetic
Methohexital	Brevital	Intravenous	Barbiturate; potent; circulatory and respiratory depressant	Rapid induction; brief anesthesia
Propofol	Diprivan	Intravenous	Alkyl phenol; potent short-acting sedative-hypnotic; cardiovascular depressant	Rapid induction and recovery; short procedures alone; prolonged anesthesia in combination with inhalation agents or opioids
Ketamine	Ketaject, Ketalar	Intravenous, intramuscular	Dissociative drug; profound amnesia and analgesia; may cause psychologic problems during emergence	Rapid induction; short procedures when muscle relaxation not needed; children and young adults
Fentanyl	Sublimaze	Intravenous	Opioid; potent narcotic; metabolizes slowly; respiratory depressant	High-dose narcotic anesthesia in combination with oxygen
Sufentanil	Sufenta	Intravenous	Opioid; potent narcotic, respiratory depressant	Premedication; high-dose narcotic anesthesia in combination with oxygen
Fentanyl and droperidol	Innovar	Intravenous	Combination narcotic and tranquilizer; potent; long acting	Neuroleptanalgesia
Diazepam	Valium	Intravenous, intramuscular	Benzodiazepine; tranquilizer; produces amnesia, sedation, and muscle relaxation	Premedication; awake intubation; induction
Midazolam	Versed	Intravenous, intramuscular	Benzodiazepine; sedative; short-acting amnesic; central nervous system and respiratory depressant	Premedication; conscious sedation; induction in children

Synthesis of potent, nonflammable, halogenated, volatile liquids has replaced cyclopropane and ether, which are highly flammable agents. All inhalation agents are administered with oxygen. Volatile liquids are vaporized for inhalation by oxygen, which acts as a carrier, flowing over or bubbling through liquid in the vaporizer on the anesthesia machine. The oxygen picks up 0.25% to 5% concentration of the halogenated agent as adjusted by the anesthesia provider. Known sensitivity to halogenated agents or a history significant for the risk for malignant hyperthermia is a contraindication for their use.

Nitrous Oxide (N₂O)

Generally used as a nonvolatile adjunct to an IV drug, N$_2$O can be inhaled for a comfortable, rapid induction. It has a pleasant, fruitlike odor and is administered by facemask. Relaxation is poor. Excitement and laryngospasm may occur. It is the only true gas in use for anesthesia. The other inhalants used are liquid volatile drugs administered through a vaporizer.

Because it lacks potency, N$_2$O is rarely used alone but rather as an adjunct to barbiturates, narcotics, opioids, and other IV drugs. In combination, the concentration of potent drug is reduced, thereby lessening circulatory and respiratory depression. Because exposure can be an occupational hazard for personnel, measures are taken to minimize levels of N$_2$O in room air.

Advantages. When N$_2$O is used in combination with other forms of inhalants and IV drugs, excessive depth of anesthesia is avoided. N$_2$O is rapidly cleared from the circulation. The incidence of nausea and vomiting is minimal. The gas has a rapid uptake and elimination and few aftereffects except headache, vertigo, and drowsiness. It causes minimal physiologic change, and adverse effects can be quickly reversed. It is an excellent analgesic for procedures not producing severe pain. It does not cause myocardial depression.

Disadvantages. N_2O can cause bowel distention and increased volume in other air pockets. The use of N_2O can cause displacement of tympanoplasty grafts or increased intracranial pressure. It is a potent cerebral vasodilator. It should not be used in pregnant patients because of teratogenic effects.

It should not be used during laparoscopy. N_2O is combustible. There is no muscle relaxation. There is possible excitement or laryngospasm. Hypoxia is a hazard. There is a depressant effect on myocardial contractility.

Halothane (Fluothane)

A rarely used halogenated hydrocarbon, halothane reduces myocardial oxygen consumption more than it depresses cardiac function. Halothane was previously used in a wide spectrum of all types of surgical procedures for adults and children except routine obstetrics, when uterine relaxation is not desired. It is a profound uterine relaxant.

Because its metabolites have a possible effect as a hepatotoxin, some anesthesia providers avoid repeated administration within an arbitrary time (e.g., 3 months) in adults. Recent jaundice and known or suspected liver disease (past or present) are usually contraindications to its use.[2] It is a trigger and contraindicated in patients who are susceptible to malignant hyperthermia. Malignant hyperthermia is covered in depth in Chapter 31.

Advantages. Halothane is nonflammable, potent, versatile, chemically stable, and rapid, and it has a smooth induction.

Disadvantages. Halothane is potentially toxic to the liver and has a profound effect on body temperature control; it may cause hypothermia.[2] Complete elimination of halothane takes some time.

Enflurane (Ethrane)

A nonflammable, stable, halogenated ether, enflurane is similar in potency and versatility to halothane. It is not in common use today. Enflurane was used in a wide spectrum of procedures.

Advantages. Enflurane has a rapid induction and recovery with minimal aftereffects. Pharyngeal and laryngeal reflexes are obtunded easily, salivation is not stimulated, and bronchomotor tone is not affected. The cardiac rate and rhythm remain relatively stable, although caution is advised when it is used with epinephrine. Muscle relaxation is produced, but small supplementary doses of muscle relaxants may be required; nondepolarizing relaxants are potentiated by enflurane.

Disadvantages. Enflurane has a pungent odor. Respiration and blood pressure are progressively depressed with deepening anesthesia. Although biotransformation (metabolism) of enflurane is less than what occurs with other halogenated agents, small amounts of fluoride ion are released. Severe renal disease is a contraindication to use. At deeper levels, an electroencephalographic (EEG) pattern resembling seizures may occur. The agent is absorbed by rubber.

Isoflurane (Forane)

Isoflurane comes closer to ideal than other inhalation agents and is most commonly used. Isoflurane is a nonflammable, fluorinated, halogenated methyl ether similar to halothane and enflurane, yet different. It is a more potent muscle relaxant, but unlike the others, it protects the heart against catecholamine-induced dysrhythmias. Heart rhythm is remarkably stable, with a slightly elevated rate. The blood pressure drops with induction but returns to normal with intraoperative stimulation. A dose-related lowering

of the blood pressure occurs, but cardiac output is unaltered, mainly as a result of an increased heart rate. Isoflurane potentiates all commonly used muscle relaxants, the most profound effect occurring with the nondepolarizing type.

Isoflurane is used for induction and maintenance in a wide spectrum of procedures except routine obstetrics. Isoflurane produces uterine relaxation. Safety to the mother and fetus has not been established. Because the drug is metabolized in the liver, it may be given to patients with minimal renal disease.

Advantages. There is less cardiac depression; there is increased cardiac output with a wide margin of cardiovascular safety. Isoflurane does not sensitize the myocardium to the effects of epinephrine. There are no CNS excitatory effects. There is rapid induction and, especially, rapid emergence with minimal aftereffects (less postoperative nausea and confusion).

Isoflurane is innocuous to organs; it has low organ toxicity because of its low blood solubility and minimal susceptibility to biodegradation and metabolism. It provides superb muscle relaxation. Pharyngeal and laryngeal reflexes are easily obtunded. Isoflurane depresses bronchoconstriction; it may be used in patients with asthma and patients with chronic obstructive pulmonary disease.

Disadvantages. Isoflurane is expensive. It is a profound respiratory depressant and reduces respiratory minute volume. Respirations must be closely monitored and supported. Assisted or controlled ventilation is used to prevent respiratory acidosis. In the absence of intraoperative stimulation, the blood pressure may drop as a result of peripheral vasodilation. Cerebral vascular resistance decreases, cerebral blood flow increases, and intracranial pressure rises but is reversible with hyperventilation. Secretions are weakly stimulated. It also causes coronary vasodilation.

Desflurane (Suprane)

A nonflammable, volatile liquid with low solubility, desflurane has faster uptake by inhalation and elimination than do halothane and isoflurane. Desflurane is used in induction and maintenance of anesthesia in adults. It may be used for maintenance in infants and children, but it is not used for induction because of its potential for causing coughing and laryngospasm. Because it has a high vapor pressure, desflurane is delivered only through a vaporizer specifically designed for this agent. Desflurane vaporizers require electrical power to heat the liquid. It works well for ambulatory surgery patients because of the rapid emergence at the end of the case.

Advantages. There is rapid emergence and recovery from anesthesia. Desflurane resists biotransformation (metabolism) and degradation; it produces few urinary metabolites. The dosage of nondepolarizing muscle relaxants to maintain neuromuscular blockade may be reduced. It can be the inhalant of choice for bariatric procedures.

Disadvantages. Desflurane has a pungent odor that may be irritating during induction. Increasing alveolar concentration may lower the blood pressure, which may be corrected by reducing the inspired concentration. Hemodynamic effects, including an elevated heart rate, preclude use of desflurane by itself in a patient with cardiovascular disease; it may be combined with IV opioids or benzodiazepines.

Sevoflurane (Ultane)

Sevoflurane is a volatile liquid used for inhalation anesthesia. It is nonflammable and nonexplosive. Noted for its rapid induction and rapid emergence qualities, it is commonly used for induction and maintenance of general anesthesia.

Advantages. Sevoflurane is used as an inhalant anesthetic for adults and pediatric patients. It is rapidly eliminated by the lungs. It causes less cerebral vasodilation and can be the inhalant of choice for neurosurgery when the patient has increased intracranial pressure.

Disadvantages. Sevoflurane may cause glycosuria and proteinuria when used for long procedures at low flow rates.

Intravenous Anesthetic Agents

IV anesthesia became popular with the introduction in the 1930s of ultrashort-acting barbiturates. A drug that produces hypnosis, sedation, amnesia, and/or analgesia is injected directly into the circulation, usually via a peripheral vein in the arm. Diluted by blood in the heart and the lungs, the drug passes in high concentration to the brain, heart, liver, and kidneys—the organs of highest blood flow. Concentration in the brain is rapid. With recirculation, redistribution occurs in the body, decreasing cerebral concentration.

Dissipation of effects depends on redistribution and biotransformation. Because removal of a drug from the circulation is impossible, safety in use is related to metabolism. It is advisable for the anesthesia provider to give a small test dose at induction.

Oxygen is always given during IV and inhalation anesthesia. A barbiturate, dissociative agent, or narcotic may be given (see Table 24.2). Each has advantages, disadvantages, and contraindications. They may be supplemented with other drugs.

Thiopental

Thiopental sodium is a sedative-hypnotic used as an IV induction agent and a supplement to regional anesthesia. This drug can be used as a safe adjunct for intubation in patients with head injuries. Cerebral perfusion pressure is maintained while decreasing elevated intracranial pressure. Thiopental is also used as a cerebral protectant in barbiturate narcosis.

Repeated doses are cumulative because of high lipid solubility. Systemic vascular resistance is decreased, causing lowered arterial pressure and lower cardiac output. It decreases uterine blood flow in pregnant patients.

Advantages. Its onset of action is within 30 seconds and short-acting duration is 5 to 30 minutes depending on body mass. It can be used as an anticonvulsant.

Disadvantages. Thiopental is contraindicated in patients with status asthmaticus, chronic renal disease, or hepatic disease. Lower doses are required in the elderly and high-risk surgical patients. Thiopental should not be used in patients who are sensitive to the drug.

Propofol (Diprivan)

An ultrashort-acting alkyl phenol, propofol is a sedative-hypnotic that produces anesthesia. It is used for rapid induction and maintenance of anesthesia for short procedures. It can be used in combination with inhalation agents or opioids for prolonged anesthesia. Propofol is supplied in a sterile, milky soybean, egg lecithin, oil-in-water emulsion. Studies have shown that it is safe to use in egg-sensitive patients because it is not based in egg albumin, which is the primary trigger of egg allergy or sensitivity reactions.

In low doses it produces sedation (i.e., drowsiness, decreased responsiveness). Continued IV administration leads to hypnosis and unconsciousness. Propofol is twice as potent as thiopental sodium.

Propofol is used for general anesthesia for ambulatory surgery patients and for maintenance of moderate sedation during local and regional anesthesia. It is acceptable for patients who are allergic to barbiturates or who have porphyria.

Advantages. Propofol is rapidly distributed, metabolized, and eliminated. Emergence is very rapid, with few postoperative side effects. It can be used for postoperative nausea and vomiting (PONV) and is useful when timed wake-sleep neurologic procedures are performed.

Disadvantages. Propofol produces dose-related cardiorespiratory depression. Cardiovascular depressant action will decrease the blood pressure. Its hypotensive effect is potentiated by narcotics. The solution supports rapid growth of microorganisms if the infusion pump or syringes become contaminated. The vial should be discarded 6 hours after opening.

Propofol is used with caution in geriatric, debilitated, and hypovolemic patients. It is not recommended for pediatrics, obstetrics, and some neurosurgical procedures. Patients with egg albumin or soybean sensitivities may experience an allergic or sensitivity reaction.

Ketamine (Ketalar, Ketaject)

General anesthesia may be produced by a phencyclidine derivative to produce a state referred to as *dissociative anesthesia*. The drug acts by selectively interrupting associative pathways of the brain before producing sensory blockage. This permits a surgical procedure on a patient who appears to be awake (i.e., eyes are open, may move) but who is anesthetized (i.e., unaware, amnesic).

Ketamine may be given IV or intramuscularly (IM) to yield profound analgesia. Ketamine is available in a nasal spray (esketamine) for the treatment of depression in adults. It is swiftly metabolized. Individual response varies, depending on the dose, route of administration, and age. Because of a dose-response relationship, careful patient selection and dose selection are important. Ketamine is used alone or with nitrous oxide. Anticholinergics may be given to decrease hypersalivation.

Ketamine is used mainly in children between the ages of 2 and 10 years and in adults younger than 30 years for short procedures not requiring skeletal muscle relaxation, for plastic and eye procedures when combined with local agents, for diagnostic procedures, as an induction agent before other general agents are used, and to supplement nitrous oxide when adequate respiratory exchange is maintained.[3] For longer procedures, repeated doses are given that may prolong recovery time. If relaxation is needed, muscle relaxants and controlled ventilation are indicated.

Advantages. Ketamine has a rapid induction. Respirations are not depressed unless the drug is administered too rapidly or in too large a dose. A mild stimulant action on the cardiovascular system may elevate the blood pressure. The effects of ketamine are potentiated by narcotics and barbiturates.

Low-dose ketamine (1 mg/kg) has been used as an induction agent for obstetric procedures because of rapid onset, intense analgesia and amnesia, and minimal fetal effects. With its cardiovascular-stimulating properties, it is useful in hypovolemic and hypotensive patients, allowing the use of high oxygen concentration, both in obstetric and trauma procedures.

Disadvantages. Psychologic manifestations (e.g., delirium, vivid imagery, hallucinations, unpleasant dreams) may occur during emergence. These can be reduced by giving preanesthetic diazepam and allowing the patient to lie quietly and undisturbed during recovery except for essential procedures. Reactions are more common in adults than children. A short-acting barbiturate or benzodiazepine such as diazepam may be given to treat emergence delirium.

Ketamine is contraindicated in procedures involving tracheobronchial stimulation because pharyngeal and laryngeal reflexes are usually active. If the drug is used alone, mechanical stimulation of the pharynx should be avoided. Other contraindications include pregnancy, hypertension, increased intracranial pressure, intraocular procedures, and previous cerebrovascular accident because this agent increases cerebrospinal fluid (CSF) and intraocular pressure.

Adjunctive Drugs Used in Anesthesia

Many drugs are used to supplement nitrous oxide, halogenated inhalation agents, and IV drugs to maintain amnesia and analgesia, control hypertension, attenuate the extent of postoperative respiratory depression, or maintain or control other effects of general anesthesia. These drugs must be carefully controlled to avoid adverse drug interactions. For example, morphine sulfate and nitrous oxide have a synergistic action with thiopental sodium (i.e., when they are given together, each potentiates the action of the other). Therefore they are given concomitantly with caution because of their combined respiratory depressant effect.

Some drugs are given preoperatively, during induction, and/or intraoperatively. Adjunctive drugs are used primarily for analgesia and amnesia or to counteract side effects of anesthesia. Some are particularly useful for ambulatory surgery patients because they are short acting.

Narcotics

Historically, natural opiates and synthetic opioids have been given to produce analgesia and sedation preoperatively and postoperatively. In addition, they are used intraoperatively as supplemental agents and/or in combination with oxygen for complete anesthesia for short procedures and in patients with little cardiovascular reserve. Cardiovascular depression must be avoided in these patients. Halogenated agents are contraindicated in patients with liver and renal disease and malignant hyperthermia risk.

Narcotics are popular for general anesthesia, such as the opioids fentanyl (Sublimaze), sufentanil (Sufenta), alfentanil (Alfenta), and the opiate morphine sulfate. Although they are analgesics, to reliably achieve anesthesia, markedly larger doses of narcotics are needed (e.g., 10–30 times as much morphine [3–8 or more mg/kg body weight]). High doses of fentanyl range from 50 to 100 mcg/kg body weight.

The drugs may be given in bolus doses or continuously via IV infusion in combination with inhalant anesthesia. Surprisingly, side effects seem to occur less frequently as the potency of narcotics increases. Some drugs work as agonists to each other. An agonist is a drug or a combination of drugs given to augment each other. In some circumstances, lower doses of each can be given to achieve the desired effect. They reduce adverse physiologic responses to the stress of the surgical procedure, such as increased work of the heart, potential dysrhythmias, sodium and water retention, and increased blood glucose levels. Narcotics produce a dose-related respiratory depression. The respiratory effects of narcotics are as follows:

- Reduction of responsiveness of the CNS respiratory centers to carbon dioxide (less stimulation)

- Impairment of respiratory reflexes and alteration of rhythm (prolonged inspiration, delayed expiration)
- Reduction in the respiratory rate before reduction in the tidal volume
- Production of bronchoconstriction (morphine, meperidine) or rigidity of the chest wall (fentanyl)
- Impairment of ciliary motion

Factors that influence narcotic respiratory actions include age, pain, sleep, urinary output, other drugs, intestinal resorption, and disease.

The neurophysical state obtained by use of large doses of narcotics is not the same as "the general anesthesia state" resulting from use of volatile inhalation agents. Narcotics are more selective in action. Narcotics do not produce muscle relaxation. Conversely, they cause an increase in muscle tone. Neuromuscular blocking agents can block or treat this action or rigidity.

After high-dose narcotic anesthesia, patients are awake and pain-free, with adequate, although not good, ventilation. These patients need careful monitoring by a well-trained PACU staff because narcotization after large doses of narcotics can occur rapidly in an apparently awake and responsive patient. The patient can hypoventilate, become hypoxic, and stop breathing when intraoperative stimuli cease. The vital signs, pupils, and skin color must be monitored.

Clinical signs of narcotic toxicity are pinpoint pupils, depressed respiration, and reduced consciousness. A narcotic antagonist is given to reverse narcotic-induced hypoventilation. Antagonists are used to block cellular receptor sites that bind to a drug. The potential for delayed toxicity after IM injection of narcotics, as opposed to IV administration, exists because absorption from muscle mass may be irregular.

Narcotic Reversal (Narcotic Antagonist). A narcotic antagonist neutralizes or impedes the action of another drug (i.e., reverses its effects). For example, narcotics produce a dose-related respiratory depression that can be reversed by opiate antagonists. These drugs are given IV, IM, subcutaneously (SQ), and nasally.

Naloxone (Narcan). A specific narcotic antagonist, naloxone reverses respiratory depression caused by narcotics. It has no respiratory or circulatory action of its own in the presence or absence of a narcotic or other agonist-antagonist. Complications can include hypertension and tachycardia if naloxone is combined with opioids.

Naloxone has a shorter duration of action than the narcotic being reversed. Respiratory depression can occur. Initial dose is 0.4 to 2 mg diluted in 10 mL of normal saline titrated IV in 1-mL increments every 2 to 3 minutes as needed until adequate reversal is attained. Narcan can be administered SQ, IM, and by nasal spray. The nasal spray is 4 mg and can be repeated every 2 to 3 minutes.

Flumazenil (Romazicon). Flumazenil is a benzodiazepine antagonist used for complete or partial reversal after general anesthesia or conscious sedation. The duration of action is shorter than the action of the drugs being reversed, and resedation can occur. The initial dose is 0.2 mg IV over 15 seconds. This may be repeated in 1-minute intervals up to a total dose of 1 mg. If resedation occurs, the dose may be repeated but is not to exceed 3 mg in 1 hour.

Muscle Relaxants

Skeletal muscle relaxant drugs, referred to as *neuromuscular blockers,* facilitate muscle relaxation for smoother endotracheal intubation and working conditions during the surgical procedure. Their use has eliminated the need for deep inhalation anesthesia to produce relaxation. Administered IV in small amounts at intervals, they interfere with the passage of impulses from motor nerves to skeletal muscles. They act primarily at autonomic receptor sites, the neuromuscular junction, and prejunctional and postjunctional acetylcholine-binding sites, causing paralysis of variable durations. They also can affect transmission of impulses at preganglionic and postganglionic endings in the autonomic nervous system.

Neuromuscular blockers paralyze all skeletal muscles, including the diaphragm and accessory muscles of respiration. Therefore the chief danger in their use is that they decrease pulmonary ventilation, causing respiratory depression. They also may cause circulatory disturbance. Special attention to anesthesia depth, ventilation, and electrolyte balance is required.

The anesthesia provider must constantly verify the degree of paralysis present by noting the amount of relaxation of the abdominal wall or the limpness of extremities or by using a nerve stimulator connected to the patient through needle electrodes. The use of neuromuscular blockers requires surgeon–anesthesia provider teamwork and communication. Use of these drugs always presents the hazard of overdosage, a danger alleviated by the anesthesia provider's familiarity with the surgeon's technique and the requirements of the surgical procedure; thus the anesthesia provider can regulate the dosage of anesthetic and relaxant necessary to produce the conditions required at the appropriate time. For example, a major use of neuromuscular blockers is in intraabdominal procedures.

At different times during the surgical procedure, blockade may be essential. Although tightness of tissues and inadequate exposure may be a result of factors other than relaxation, it is helpful to the anesthesia provider to be told before pertinent action, such as closure of the peritoneum, is taken. Inadequate muscle relaxation makes closure difficult. Controlled respiration during upper abdominal manipulation can prevent descent of the diaphragm into the surgical field.

Neuromuscular blockers are classified as nondepolarizing or depolarizing. Although theoretically they are antagonistic, combinations are used. They may widen the scope of less potent anesthetics, such as nitrous oxide, or lessen the overall amount of anesthetic needed. Depolarizing and nondepolarizing drugs behave differently; depolarizers stimulate whereas nondepolarizers inhibit autonomic receptors. Duration of action should be balanced against duration of effect on ventilation.

Nondepolarizing Neuromuscular Blockers. Nondepolarizing neuromuscular blockers act on enzymes to prevent muscle contraction. They produce tetanic electrical impulses that gradually fade, but they do not cause muscular fasciculation on IV injection. Their effects are decreased by anticholinesterase drugs, acetylcholine, epinephrine, and depolarizing neuromuscular blockers. Action is potentiated by halogenated inhalation agents and some aminoglycoside antibiotics.

Interactions with other drugs can result in delayed recovery. For example, antibiotics may act synergistically to produce prolonged paralysis, such as occurs when the peritoneal cavity is irrigated with an antibiotic solution or antibiotic is injected IV. Box 24.2 lists some antibiotics that can potentiate neuromuscular blockers.

Synergism also occurs with local and inhalation anesthetic agents. They are useful for patients on mechanical ventilators.

> **• BOX 24.2 Antibiotics That Can Potentiate Neuromuscular Blocking Agents**
>
> **Aminoglycosides**
> - Streptomycin
> - Gentamicin
> - Tobramycin
> - Kanamycin
> - Amikacin
> - Netilmicin
>
> **Beta-Lactams**
> - Penicillin G
>
> - Penicillin V
> - Piperacillin
>
> **Miscellaneous Antibiotics**
> - Polymyxin A
> - Polymyxin B
> - Colistin
> - Lincomycin
> - Clindamycin
> - Tetracycline

Nondepolarizing blockers may be referred to as *competitive antagonists*. A peripheral nerve stimulator is useful for assessing neuromuscular transmission as a guide to the dosage, degree, and nature of the blockade, and evidence of muscle-response recovery during and after the use of nondepolarizing agents. The anesthesia provider can choose from several drugs.

Short-Acting Neuromuscular Blocking Agents.
- *Mivacurium (Mivacron):* Blockade lasts 15 to 20 minutes. It has minimal cardiovascular effect but can cause skin flushing.

Intermediate-Acting Neuromuscular Blocking Agents.
- *Atracurium (Tracrium):* With a duration of action of about 30 minutes, atracurium metabolizes more quickly than the other blockers, which may be an advantage in patients with liver or renal disease. Repeated doses are not cumulative. Atracurium causes histamine release, vasodilation, and hypotension.
- *Cisatracurium (Nimbex):* Cisatracurium can cause bradycardia, hypotension, and skin flushing.
- *Vecuronium (Norcuron):* Similar to pancuronium, vecuronium has a shorter duration of action and is more potent. It does not noticeably increase the heart rate or blood pressure unless it is combined with opioids.
- *Rocuronium (Zemuron):* With a rapid onset of action, rocuronium facilitates intubation. The duration of action is about 30 minutes, with minimal overall effect on cardiovascular stability. It can be reversed with neostigmine. Tachycardia is possible. Rocuronium interacts with some antibiotics, including gentamicin, neomycin, and polymyxin B. It must be refrigerated.
- *Other:* Sugammadex (Bridion) is a selective neuromuscular reversal agent specifically for rocuronium, pancuronium, and vecuronium. It is a synthetic cyclodextrin that works by encapsulating the muscle relaxant to reverse paralytic effects.

Long-Acting Neuromuscular Blocking Agents.
- *Tubocurarine (Curare):* Obtained from plants, tubocurarine was used centuries ago by indigenous South Americans for poison arrows. The poison caused death by suffocation from respiratory paralysis. The effects of tubocurarine on the neuromuscular junction were first described in 1856.

Blocking transmission of nerve impulses to muscle fibers results in paralysis, predominantly of voluntary muscles. Tubocurarine releases histamine. Autonomic blockade can cause vasodilation, hypotension, and histamine release. Tubocurarine is used as pretreatment if succinylcholine is used, to decrease the possibility of fasciculation. It is rarely used and has been replaced by other long-acting agents.

- *Gallamine (Flaxedil):* Similar in action and duration to d-tubocurarine, gallamine does not cause hypotension or bronchospasm. It may increase arterial pressure and cause tachycardia. It is contraindicated in patients with iodide and sulfide allergies.
- *Metocurine (Metubine):* Metocurine iodide produces less hypotension and releases less histamine than d-tubocurarine. It is contraindicated in patients with known iodine allergy.
- *Pancuronium (Pavulon):* Pancuronium is similar in action to d-tubocurarine but about five times more potent. It has a vagolytic action that may raise the blood pressure, pulse rate, and heart rate. It can cause dysrhythmia if used with digoxin.
- *Pipecuronium (Arduan):* Pipecuronium can cause decreased arterial pressure with moderate histamine release.

Depolarizing Neuromuscular Blockers. Depolarizing neuromuscular blockers have the opposite effect of the nondepolarizing drugs. They stimulate autonomic receptors. For example, they cause muscular fasciculation (i.e., involuntary muscle contractions). These contractions, the result of depolarization of the nerve-muscle end plate, are seen after injection. They are followed by fatigue. Drugs may be given IM, but IV use is more common.

- *Succinylcholine (Anectine, Quelicin, Sucostrin):* An ultrashort-acting synthetic drug with an onset of action in seconds, succinylcholine produces paralysis for up to 20 minutes. It is used primarily for endotracheal intubation. A dilute solution may be used to provide continuing muscle relaxation.

Repeated IV administration may effect changes in the heart rate and rhythm (i.e., bradycardia and ventricular dysrhythmias) until the drug is metabolized by enzymes. Muscle pain may occur after use unless fasciculation is prevented by a small preliminary dose of a nondepolarizing agent. Succinylcholine is contraindicated in patients with a known or suspected history of malignant hyperthermia. It can cause increased intracranial and intraocular pressures.

- *Decamethonium (Syncurine):* A very potent synthetic with a rapid onset and short duration of action, decamethonium is not cumulative and has little effect on vital systems. It is used for deep relaxation of a short duration, such as for endoscopy, treatment of laryngeal spasm, abdominal closure, and endotracheal intubation. It is excreted through the kidneys. Prolonged blockade may result if decamethonium is given to a patient with renal failure.

Muscle Relaxant Reversal Agents (Cholinergics).
- *Neostigmine (Prostigmin):* Neostigmine inhibits the destruction of acetylcholine released from parasympathetic nerves. It is used to reverse nondepolarizing neuromuscular blocking agents. Use with care in patients with bronchial asthma, bradycardia, seizure disorders, coronary artery disease, and hyperthyroidism. Monitor vital signs, particularly respirations, carefully, and have atropine close at hand. Neostigmine is not for use in patients with peritonitis or bowel or urinary obstruction.
- *Edrophonium (Enlon):* Edrophonium works as a curare antagonist to reverse the nondepolarizing neuromuscular blocking action. It has a rapid onset but short duration. It is contraindicated in patients with bowel or urinary tract obstruction. Monitor vital signs, and have atropine immediately available. It is also used for the Tensilon test in the diagnosis of myasthenia gravis.

Monitoring the Depth of General Anesthesia

The anesthesia provider monitors the level of anesthesia, balancing doses of medications, throughout the surgical procedure. The bispectral index (BIS) is a compact system for monitoring the effects of anesthesia on the brain. The BIS monitor allows the anesthesia provider to accurately track the patient's level of consciousness by using an electrode applied to the patient's forehead that sends EEG-like signals to a small monitor. The digital readout is a single number ranging from 100 (wide awake) to 0 (absence of brain activity).

The device can be used as a stand-alone unit or be integrated into other monitoring devices. The result of its use is decreased amounts of anesthetic administration and a faster postoperative return to alertness. The BIS monitor is not a substitute for clinical judgment and does not detect cerebral ischemia or blood pressure.

Emergence From General Anesthesia

The anesthesia provider attempts to have the patient as nearly awake as possible at the end of a surgical procedure. Pharyngeal and laryngeal reflexes must be recovered to prevent aspiration and respiratory obstruction. The degree of residual neuromuscular blockade must be determined and treated if necessary for respiratory adequacy. The action of nondepolarizing muscle relaxants may be reversed with antagonists, such as long-acting neostigmine (Prostigmin) or pyridostigmine (Regonol) or short-acting edrophonium (Enlon). These anticholinesterase drugs are accompanied or preceded by atropine to minimize side effects, such as excessive secretions and bradycardia.

Extubation is delayed until spontaneous respiration is ensured. The endotracheal tube is carefully removed when this maneuver is deemed safe. A patent airway and adequate manual or mechanical ventilation are maintained until full recovery. In the absence of a means of respiratory control, such as when a maxillofacial procedure endangers the airway, the endotracheal tube may be left in place.

Vomiting and restlessness may accompany emergence. Slight cyanosis, stertorous respiration, rigidity, and shivering are not uncommon as a result of a temporary disturbance of body temperature—regulating mechanisms, thus altering circulation to the skin and muscles. Administering oxygen and pain medication and applying warm blankets help relieve these aftereffects. The anesthesia provider should flush the patient's lungs with oxygen to minimize exhalation of gases in the PACU.

Balanced Anesthesia

Balanced anesthesia has become a widely used technique to achieve physiologic homeostasis, analgesia, amnesia, and muscle relaxation. A combination of agents is used with many possible variations, depending on the condition of the patient and requirements of the procedure. The technique is especially useful for preventing CNS depression in older and high-risk patients.

Induction

Induction can be accomplished with a combination of drugs specific to the patient's needs, such as propofol, inhalation agents, methohexital (Brevital), diazepam (Valium), midazolam (Versed), or other induction agent. Oxygen is administered in physiologic quantities. Neuromuscular blockers permit control of ventilation while providing muscle relaxation during intubation.

Maintenance

Different combinations of narcotics and neuroleptic drugs (tranquilizers) are administered IV, whether they are used alone or in combination with inhalation agents. Neuroleptics reduce motor activity and anxiety; produce a detached, apathetic state; and potentiate hypnotic and analgesic narcotic effects. The dosage can be regulated to produce the desired state.

Emergence

Residual effects of narcotics or muscle relaxants may require reversal by antagonists during and/or at the conclusion of the surgical procedure. Other precautions are taken as for any patient emerging from general anesthesia.

Controlled Homeostasis

Functions controlled by homeostatic mechanisms include body temperature, heartbeat, blood pressure, electrolyte balance, and respiration. These parameters may be altered by anesthetic and other pharmacologic agents and by physiologic stresses during surgical manipulations. In the hands of a skilled anesthesia provider, adjunctive methods of control may be used concurrently with the administration of general anesthesia, but only when the expected outcomes will outweigh the inherent risks.

Induced Hypothermia

Hypothermia is an artificial, deliberate lowering of body temperature below the normal limits (Box 24.3). It reduces the metabolic rate and oxygen needs of the tissues in conditions causing hypoxia or during a decrease or interruption of circulation. Bleeding is also decreased, and less anesthetic is needed. The patient can therefore better tolerate the surgical procedure.

Hypothermia may be used as follows:

- For direct-vision intracardiac repair of complex congenital defects in infants and in other cardiac procedures (most common usage)
- After cardiac resuscitation, to decrease oxygen requirements of vital tissues and limit further damage to the brain after anoxia
- In treatment of hyperpyrexia and some other nonsurgical conditions, such as hypertensive crisis
- To increase tolerance in septic shock
- In neurosurgery, to decrease cerebral blood flow, CSF volume, and venous and intracranial pressures
- To aid in transplantation of organs

Attaining Hypothermia. To achieve hypothermia, heat must be lost more rapidly than it is produced. The following methods may be used:

- *Surface-induced hypothermia:* External cooling of infants and small children weighing less than 20 lbs (10 kg) may be attained by immersion in ice water, packing the body in ice, or alcohol sponging. A hypothermia/hyperthermia machine with a cooling blanket or mattress is used for adults and larger children.
- *Internal cooling:* A decreased or interruption of blood flow can be achieved by placing sterile iced saline slush packs around a

specific internal organ or irrigation of cold fluids within a body cavity, such as intraperitoneal lavage. The cold cardioplegia technique combines cold from saline slush with drugs injected into coronary arteries for myocardial protection during heart surgery. Drugs may be used to lower metabolism and increase resistance to shivering during cooling.

- *Systemic hypothermia:* The bloodstream is cooled by diverting blood through heat-exchanging devices of extracorporeal circulation and returning it to the body by a continuous flowing circuit (e.g., core cooling by cardiopulmonary bypass or IV administration of cold fluids). Systemic hypothermia is used in adults and larger children to 78.8° F (26° C). Oxygen consumption and metabolism of different organs vary, making uniform hypothermia impossible.

The temperature is not deliberately lowered below about 84.5° F (29° C) unless arrest of the heart is desired by means of deep hypothermia (below 78.8° F [26° C]). This is accompanied by perfusion of the rest of the body with the extracorporeal circulation method, permitting an open, motionless dry field while the blood flow is interrupted. A noncontracting heart requires very little oxygen.

The patient is progressively rewarmed at the close of the surgical procedure until the temperature is 95° F (35° C) or until consciousness returns. Sometimes a degree of hypothermia is maintained for a day or two postoperatively to allow the patient to adapt more readily. Oxygen therapy and intubation, if advised, are part of postoperative care.

Complications in the Use of Hypothermia. Hypothermia carries many inherent risks. Primarily it affects the myocardium, decreasing its resistance to ventricular fibrillation and predisposing the patient to cardiac arrest. This is more likely to happen with deep hypothermia or during manipulation of the heart itself. Other dangers are heart block, effects on the vascular system, atrial fibrillation, embolism, microcirculation stasis, undesired downward drift of temperature, tissue damage, metabolic acidosis, and numerous effects on other organs and systems.

Time is required for cooling and rewarming. Shivering and vasoconstriction, normal defenses of the body against cooling, can be problems during the use of hypothermia. This muscle activity greatly increases oxygen needs. Shivering can be overcome by the administration of a muscle relaxant drug or an analgesic such as meperidine.

Rewarming can be accomplished by circulating warmed blood by means of extracorporeal circulation or by using a heating mattress with circulating fluid and warm blankets. If external heat is applied, care should be taken not to burn the patient. Rewarming carries potential problems such as reactive bleeding or circulatory collapse. If the patient is rewarmed too rapidly, vasodilation causes the blood pressure to drop. Organ ischemia can occur from severe shivering. These superficial and systemic events impair perfusion (oxygenation) of tissues. "Rewarming shock" may be prevented by slow warming, adequate oxygenation, and prevention of massive sudden vasodilation or vasoconstriction associated with shivering.

Induced Hypotension

Induced, deliberate hypotension is the controlled lowering of arterial blood pressure during anesthesia as an adjunct to the surgical procedure. Hypotensive anesthesia is used to shorten the operating time, reduce blood loss and the need for transfusion, and facilitate dissection and visibility, especially of tumor margins

---

• BOX 24.3   Hypothermia

- Normal core temperature: 98.2° F to 99.9° F (36.8–37.7° C)
- Systemic hypothermia may be:
  - Light: 98.6° F to 89.6° F (37–32° C)
  - Moderate: 89.6° F to 78.8° F (32–26° C)
  - Deep: 78.8° F to 68° F (26–20° C)
  - Profound: 68° F (20° C) or below
  - Sensorium fades at 91° F to 93° F (32.8–33.9° C)

in radical procedures. Visible vessels are ligated, even in the absence of active bleeding.

Adequate oxygenation of blood and tissue perfusion in vital organs (heart, liver, kidneys, lungs) and in the cerebrum must be maintained to prevent damage. The degree and duration of hypotension must be carefully controlled so the state can be rapidly terminated at any time.

Naturally, controlled hypotension is not indicated as a routine procedure. It is used only when the expected gain for a particular patient requiring a specific surgical procedure outweighs the risks. Hypotension may be specifically induced for the following:

- Surgical procedures in which excessive blood loss is anticipated, such as spinal surgery, to decrease gross hemorrhage or venous oozing.
- Surgical procedures on the head, face, neck, and upper thorax, especially radical dissection, in which the position of the patient allows blood to pool in dependent areas and reduces venous return to the heart and cardiac output.
- Neurosurgical procedures when control of intracranial vessel hemorrhage may be difficult. It reduces leakage, makes an aneurysm less turgid and prone to rupture, decreases blood loss in the case of rupture, and facilitates placement of ligating clips.
- Surgical procedures in which blood transfusions should be avoided, such as when compatible blood is unavailable or transfusion is against the patient's religious belief.
- Surgical procedures on the spine or posterior torso. Blood loss is decreased in the prone position.
- Total hip replacement.

Attaining Hypotension. Several techniques will produce hypotension. The blood pressure may be lowered chemically by direct arterial or venous dilators or by ganglionic blocking drugs. Perfusion pressure drops in proportion to a decrease in vascular flow resistance, but adequate tissue blood flow exists.

Fine adjustment of the desired level of hypotension can be achieved by mechanical maneuvers—namely, alterations in body position or changes in airway pressure, control of the heart rate or blood volume, or addition of other vasoactive drugs in conjunction with hypotensive drugs.[4] Properly used, these maneuvers can reduce the total dose of potentially toxic drugs needed for maintenance of hypotension.

Methods to produce hypotension include:

1. Deep general anesthesia with isoflurane, followed by a vasodilator, produces the desired minute-to-minute effect. With increased concentration, halogenated agents produce hypotension as a result of myocardial and peripheral vascular depression.
2. Sodium nitroprusside is a potent, fast-acting vasodilator that reduces virtually all resistance in vascular smooth muscle (resistance vessels). It also reduces preload and afterload of the heart and pulmonary vascular resistance. To achieve safe arterial pressure control, administration is via a calibrated drug pump. The acid-base status and blood cyanide level are determined frequently to guard against metabolic acidosis and nitroprusside-induced cyanide and thiocyanate toxicity.
3. Nitroglycerin, primarily a vasodilator, directly dilates capacitance vessels. It reduces preload and improves myocardial perfusion during diastole—a protection against potential ischemia. Nitroglycerin for IV infusion (Nitrostat), after dilution in 5% dextrose or physiologic saline, dilates both venous and arterial beds. Arterial pressures are reduced. Nitroglycerin migrates into plastic. To avoid its absorption into plastic

parenteral solution containers, dilution and storage are done in glass parenteral solution bottles. A special nonabsorbing infusion set prevents loss of nitroglycerin.
4. Fentanyl may be used as a basal anesthetic for hypotension. The blood pressure can be maintained at the desired level by the addition of a small amount of a volatile agent. Fentanyl lowers arterial pressure; volatile agents reduce cardiac output.
5. Other drugs such as calcium channel blockers, β-blockers, or angiotensin-converting enzyme (ACE) inhibitors may be used.

Safe lower limits of arterial pressure may vary. Mean systolic value is 50 mm Hg, and values range between 65 and 70 mm Hg, with lower values for short periods only.[4]

Precautions in the Use of Hypotension. Potential complications of hypotensive anesthesia include cerebral or coronary ischemia or thrombosis, reactionary hemorrhage, anuria in acute renal failure, delayed awakening, and dermal ischemic lesions. Primary contraindications are vascular compromise to any vital organ system or the brain. Precautions include the following:

- Careful selection of the patient
- Preoperative cardiac, renal, and hepatic evaluation of the patient to avoid circulatory insufficiency in vital organs
- Selection of an appropriate but not arbitrary level of blood pressure
- Administration and evaluation by expert anesthesia providers
- Use for only a short time and lowering of blood pressure only enough to obtain the desired result
- Maintenance of blood volume at an optimal level by continuous infusion
- Controlled ventilation with adequate oxygenation via an endotracheal tube because hypotension increases susceptibility to hypoxia
- Extensive monitoring: ECG, core temperature, esophageal stethoscopy, urinary output, central venous pressure and arterial catheters, and electrophysiologic brain monitoring or EEG via BIS monitoring

Normovolemic Hemodilution Technique

Intraoperative normovolemic hemodilution has been used in cardiac surgery for several decades but more recently as an adjunct technique in major surgery when large blood loss is anticipated. It is especially useful in infants and children and in patients who, for religious or personal reasons, do not accept administration of blood products.

At the beginning of the surgical procedure, whole blood is withdrawn from the patient to a hematocrit of 14% to 15% and replaced with three times the volume of a balanced electrolyte solution to maintain intravascular volume. This diluted blood is transparent, giving the surgeon a clearer, almost bloodless field. This may decrease operating time. The patient is maintained under controlled hypotension with an inhalation agent and a supplemental narcotic. The body temperature may be lowered to 89.6° F (32° C) or below for moderate hypothermia to help protect vital organs against hypoxia and hypotension.

After significant blood loss has ceased, the patient's own blood is reinfused. Diuresis is stimulated to remove electrolyte solution. Normovolemic hemodilution can make a difficult surgical procedure easier and in some patients makes an otherwise impossible resection possible.

Care of the Anesthetized Patient

Anesthetic agents and drugs vary in potency. Therefore they differ in the amount of analgesia, amnesia, or muscle relaxation produced.

Each patient's ability to detoxify anesthetic agents and to tolerate physiologic stress differs. Impairment of pulmonary function accompanies general anesthesia to some degree. General anesthesia is usually more complicated than local or regional anesthesia.

Considerations

The anesthesia provider keeps the surgeon informed of significant physiologic changes detected by monitoring vital functions. The following should be considered:

1. A deficit in pulmonary and/or cardiac functions is detrimental to the patient's physiologic status. Abnormalities of pulmonary ventilation and diffusion influence the course of anesthesia and diminish tolerance to stress or the insults from the anesthetic and the procedure.
   a. Respiratory patterns vary from breath-holding and apnea to deep breathing and tachypnea.
   b. Drug action affecting respiratory stimulation or depression is related to changes in oxygen tension (Pao_2) or arterial carbon dioxide tension ($Paco_2$).
   c. Hypoxia, anemia, and decreased cardiac output may produce inadequate tissue oxygenation. Subnormal cardiac reserve or oxygen-transporting ability, combined with anemia or hypoxia in an arteriosclerotic patient, for example, can be lethal.
2. Circulation is affected both centrally and peripherally. Individual agents are associated with characteristic hemodynamic patterns. Generally, the agents are circulatory depressants that reduce arterial pressure, myocardial contractility, and cardiac output.
3. The liver is affected by general agents (e.g., the rate of visceral blood flow). Alterations in liver function tests may follow anesthesia. Halogenated hydrocarbons have been associated with hepatotoxicity. The liver metabolizes many anesthetic agents and other medications.
4. Kidney function is affected by disturbances in systemic circulation because kidneys normally receive 20% to 25% of the cardiac output. A reduced renal plasma flow and glomerular filtration rate depress renal functions related to hemodynamics and to water and electrolyte excretion.

Oliguria, with reduced sodium and potassium excretion, accompanies induction. Postoperative fluid retention may result from a reduction in urine volume from anesthesia, intraoperative trauma, and the use of narcotics. In the absence of renal disease, changes in renal function are usually transitory and reversible. Endocrine effects on renal function during anesthesia are important. Many drugs and agents are excreted by the kidneys.

5. Biotransformation of agents varies with metabolites excreted by the kidneys. Urinary excretion of IV agents may be slow and unpredictable. Studies indicate that nitrous oxide may be exhaled as long as 56 hours after anesthesia, and metabolites of halothane have been recovered from patients' urine as long as 20 days after anesthesia.
6. Agents may cause nausea, emesis, or systemic complications. General anesthesia may be contraindicated for the following:
- Elective procedures on patients who are medically at high risk or severely debilitated.
- Elective procedures during the first 5 months of pregnancy. Some anesthesia providers avoid general anesthesia because of unknown teratogenic effects of inhalation anesthetics.
- Emergency surgical procedures on patients who have recently ingested food or fluids. Gastric suction and awake intubation are indicated if the surgical procedure cannot be delayed.

Intraoperative Awareness

Although seemingly anesthetized, the patient may be aware of conversations, noises, and even pain. Is it possible to imagine anything more terrifying than to feel intraoperative maneuvers but be unable to communicate this discomfort? Intraoperative awareness varies, depending on the type of procedure and depth of anesthesia. Monitoring techniques, such as BIS monitoring, may decrease the incidence of intraoperative awareness.

The common use of narcotics and muscle relaxants as adjuncts has consequently decreased the amount of anesthetic used to induce and maintain unconsciousness. This is particularly true in balanced anesthesia. As a result, studies have shown evidence of intraoperative awareness (i.e., recall), consciously or unconsciously, of events and sounds during a state of anesthesia. Even though the patient may not consciously recall or remember the experience, unconsciously it may affect behavior and attitudes postoperatively. Subconscious memory may cause anger, generalized irritability, anxiety, repetitive nightmares, preoccupation with death, or physiologic complications.

Patient awareness of pain is rare in the hands of skilled anesthesia providers. However, hearing is the last sensation to surrender to anesthesia. Therefore perioperative caregivers should be constantly aware of the patient's vulnerability to auditory stimuli, including conversations and room noise. Even potent amnesic drugs may not totally block recall of stimuli, especially disturbing stimuli.

Safety Factors

Team members, especially the anesthesia provider and the circulating nurse, must be constantly aware of potential trauma to the patient because they are unable to produce a normal response to painful or injurious stimuli. The circulating nurse assists the anesthesia provider during the extubation of the patient at the conclusion of the surgical procedure. Although safety factors are stressed throughout the text, important factors in the care of the anesthetized patient are reiterated here for emphasis:

1. The patient's position is changed slowly and gently to allow circulation to readjust (i.e., to compensate for physiologic changes caused by motion or position).
2. Proper positioning and padding are important to avoid pressure points, stretching of nerves, or interference with circulation to an extremity.
3. The patient's chest must be free for adequate respiratory excursion during the surgical procedure. The airway must be patent. Leaning on the patient during the procedure can cause permanent injury.
4. The lungs must be adequately ventilated intraoperatively and postoperatively by either voluntary or mechanical means. Anesthetic agents are basically depressants that affect the vasomotor and respiratory centers, predisposing the patient to postoperative respiratory complications.
5. The anesthesia provider assesses the patient and assists in transferring the patient to a stretcher or bed, safeguarding the head and neck, when it is safe to move the patient. The anesthesia provider calls the count and initiates the move from operating bed to transport cart. The transfer is made carefully and gently to avoid strain on ligaments or muscles

of the patient and the caregivers. The relaxed, unconscious patient is adequately supported.

6. The anesthesia provider gives the PACU nurse a verbal report, including specific problems in regard to this patient, and completes records before the transfer of responsibility. The circulating nurse gives a report of preoperative baselines and intraoperative care to the PACU nurse. The PACU handover exchange report is described in detail in Chapter 30.

Care of General Anesthesia Equipment

The anesthesia equipment is a potential vector in the spread of infection. The anesthesia provider may become the victim of an acquired infection from contact with a patient's body fluids or blood. Studies have found that nearly 20% of anesthesia providers have had hepatitis B infections. The AANA provides guidelines for infection prevention. (More information can be found at http://www.aana.com/.)

Standard Precautions

The need for anesthesia staff to strictly adhere to standard precautions while caring for patients and equipment should be emphasized. Gloves should be worn to prevent skin contact with the patient's blood and body fluids, such as when starting the IV infusion, when intubating and/or extubating, or when suctioning the patient. Soiled gloves should not be worn to open cabinets or press buttons on the monitor.

Protective eyewear should be worn. Hands should be washed when removing gloves and the mask should be changed between patient contacts. Needles must be handled carefully without recapping to avoid accidental needlesticks. All anesthesia equipment that has come in contact with mucous membranes, blood, or body fluids is cleaned, disinfected, or sterilized after use to render it safe for handling and for subsequent patient use. Disposable items are discarded in the appropriate receptacles.

Hazards of Equipment

Anesthesia techniques encompass the use of drugs for parenteral administration and gases and volatile liquids for inhalation administration by means of anesthesia machines. These machines and their component parts (reservoir bags, canisters, connecting pieces, ventilators) accumulate large numbers of microorganisms during use. Consequently, the parts that come in contact with the patient's skin or respiratory tract are sources of cross-contamination.

Inhalation, exhalation, and the forcible expulsion of secretions create moist conditions favorable to the survival and growth of a multitude of organisms (streptococci, staphylococci, coliform bacteria, fungi, yeasts). Therefore the anesthesia circuit can become a veritable reservoir for microorganisms and a pathway for transmission of disease. When the apparatus is used on a patient with a known respiratory disease, such as tuberculosis, the risk for contamination increases.

All used accessories must be terminally cleaned and undergo either high-level disinfection or sterilization before reuse because clinical respiratory cross-infection has been traced to contaminated apparatus. Valves of the breathing circuit become contaminated from essentially healthy patients at an average rate of 35 organisms per minute. *Pseudomonas aeruginosa* has been cultured from carbon dioxide absorption devices. Many microorganisms accumulate in valves and air passages and in soda lime canisters. Although the alkalinity of soda lime inhibits many organisms, it is

neither a dependable germicide nor an effective mechanical filter, nor is it meant to be one. Respiratory therapy equipment, mechanical ventilators, resuscitators, and suction machines and bottles present the same problems.

Resistant strains of organisms, as well as opportunists, have caused health care—associated infections. Patient-to-patient infection must be eliminated. The following are points to remember:

- The patient's respiratory tract is a portal of entry for pathogenic organisms and a source of delivering pathogens into the environment.
- The respiratory tract loses some of its inherent defense mechanisms during anesthesia.
- Aseptic precautions are necessary to prevent needless exposure of air passages to foreign, potentially pathogenic organisms from equipment and hands of anesthesia personnel.
- Anesthesia machines and equipment, unless properly treated, increase the danger of airborne contamination and contact transmission of pathogenic microorganisms capable of causing postoperative wound infections and systemic infections.

In the presence of tuberculosis or a virulent respiratory infection, the anesthesia provider should wear a gown and strictly adhere to standard precautions. Some contacts require donning a mask with high-efficiency particulate air (HEPA) filters. The patient should wear a mask during transportation and until induction of anesthesia.

Disposable Equipment

Disposable equipment warrants use for reasons of safety, efficiency, and convenience. Presterilized disposable airways, endotracheal tubes, tracheotomy tubes, breathing circuits, masks and canisters (with soda lime sealed in the plastic), and spinal trays reduce the hazard of cross-infection. They are especially recommended for the compromised host and the bacteriologically contaminated patient. Single-use components of the anesthesia system are discarded after use. Needles are disposed of in puncture-resistant containers. Needleless syringes that attach into infusion sets should be used when possible to reduce the risk for needlesticks.

Care of Reusable Equipment

All parts of patient-exposed, reusable equipment must be thoroughly cleaned after every use to prevent pulmonary complications. Thorough cleaning to remove organic debris and drying must precede any high-level disinfection or sterilization process. All items that can be sterilized should be sterilized. Manufacturers strive to make the machines that cannot be sterilized more amenable to adequate terminal cleaning and freedom from microorganisms. The following points also should be considered:

1. The anesthesia machine should be disinfected immediately whenever it is soiled by blood and secretions.
2. The surfaces of anesthesia machines, carts, or cabinets should be disinfected after each patient use. The specific work area used for airways, endotracheal tubes, and other items should also be cleaned. The top of a cart or tray should be draped with a disposable impervious material that is changed between patients. All equipment for maintenance of the airway should be set up on and returned to this drape.

Disposable items should be discarded in suitable containers after use. Reusable equipment must be set aside after use for terminal cleaning and testing, thereby diminishing the risk for contaminating clean equipment needed for subsequent patients. A biohazard disposal container should be placed by the anesthesia machine.

3. Monitoring equipment, including ECG and other electrodes and blood pressure cuffs, should be cleaned with a detergent-disinfectant when contaminated and preferably after each use.

4. All equipment that comes in contact with mucous membranes of the patient and the inside of the breathing circuit must be terminally cleaned and sterilized, preferably, or undergo high-level disinfection:

   a. Endotracheal tubes, stylets, airways, laryngoscope blades, facemasks, and suction equipment should be sterile for each patient. Suction catheters and tubing should be sterile, single-use disposable items.

   b. Disposable breathing circuits are preferred to reusable equipment because of the complexities of cleaning and maintaining cleanliness. The interior of reusable breathing circuits remains sterile if they stand unused in their normal position on the machine, but contamination rapidly occurs when the circuits are used on patients. The parts of the circuit nearest the patient are the most heavily contaminated. Therefore reusable corrugated hoses, breathing tubes, and reservoir bags are sterilized or undergo high-level disinfection between each patient use.

   c. Items located farther away, such as circle systems and ventilators, are cleaned and sterilized according to a regular schedule—at least once or twice a month.

5. For cleaning, an automated process is available for decontamination. Machines wash equipment in mild detergent and hot water, and rinse and dry it. Some machines incorporate a chemical disinfection cycle. If automatic equipment is not used, anesthesia and respiratory therapy equipment must be disconnected and manually cleaned before sterilization. Prompt immersion in a detergent-disinfectant solution prevents crusting of secretions. Tubing takes a long time to dry. Commercial dryers are available.

6. Sterilization methods:

   a. Steam is the preferred method for all heat-stable materials.

   b. Ethylene oxide is used for materials that are deteriorated by heat, such as rubber, plastics, mechanical ventilators, and electronic equipment. Thorough aeration, according to the manufacturer's recommendations, is necessary before use to remove all residual gas from the material sterilized. Otherwise, facial burns, laryngotracheal inflammation, and obstruction or bilateral vocal cord paralysis may be caused by use of the equipment.

   c. Buffered glutaraldehyde solution does not impair conductivity of antistatic rubber. Although its use is the least convenient method, it is preferred if ethylene oxide is not available for heat-sensitive items.

   The manufacturer's recommendations should be followed for a 100% kill of *Mycobacterium tuberculosis* by immersion methods. When glutaraldehyde is used, the items must be thoroughly rinsed with sterile water because tap water contains microorganisms.

7. Sterile packaged equipment should be stored in a closed, clean, and dry area. Anesthesia and respiratory therapy equipment should be kept sterile until used.

8. Policies and procedures regarding processing of equipment should be written, available, and reviewed annually.

Checking Anesthesia Equipment

Inhalation systems are tested biologically at regular intervals and checked daily for proper functioning. Preventive maintenance is essential to avoid mechanical failures, which could be fatal. Goals for quality control are to ensure that equipment is available and that it performs reliably when needed. The anesthesia machine and its components should be checked and serviced only by qualified personnel.

Local and Regional Anesthesia

Local and regional anesthetic techniques are used to decrease intraoperative stimuli, thereby diminishing stress response to surgical trauma. Injected at or near the nerves of the surgical site, the anesthetic drug temporarily interrupts sensory nerve impulses during manipulation of sensitive tissues.

When a local anesthetic drug is used, the patient usually remains conscious. Local infiltration anesthesia is particularly advantageous for procedures performed in ambulatory surgery settings from which the patient is discharged to home soon after completion of the procedure. Oral, IM, or IV sedation may be given to relieve anxiety and produce amnesia. IV sedation is commonly used and is referred to as *moderate sedation*.

Anesthetic may be administered locally during general anesthesia for postoperative pain control. When injected before the incision is made, the patient's nervous system is preempted from sensory stimulation associated with the initial trauma of incision. Some surgeons elect to inject local anesthesia drugs before the skin is closed for additional delay of sensory stimulation associated with postoperative pain.

Regional blocks are useful for more extensive procedures. Regional anesthesia may be used, with or without moderate sedation, when general anesthesia is contraindicated or undesired. Nerve blocks, intrathecal blocks, peridural blocks, and epidural blocks are examples of regional anesthesia techniques. These techniques block conduction of pain impulses from a specific area or region. The anesthetic drug is injected around a specific nerve or group of nerves to prevent pain of the surgical procedure.

Local anesthetics and regional blocks, with or without supplementary sedation, are administered as the anesthetic of choice for many diagnostic and therapeutic surgical procedures.

Preparation of the Patient

Preparation of the patient who will receive a local or regional anesthetic depends on the extent of the procedure to be performed and on the anticipated technique of administration. Although it is anticipated that the patient will remain conscious, it is sometimes desirable or necessary to supplement the local or regional anesthesia with moderate sedation. Careful preoperative assessment, history taking, and a clear explanation of what to expect are part of the preparatory process.

Preoperative assessment of the patient who is scheduled for a procedure provides baseline data and identifies risk factors.[5] Data that should be documented include the following:

- Baseline vital signs, blood pressure, laboratory values, and results of ECG monitoring and any other tests that were performed.

- Weight, height, and age; dosage of some drugs is calculated on the basis of body weight in kilograms (milligrams per kilograms of body weight). Some drugs are contraindicated for age extremes (i.e., pediatric or geriatric patients).

- Current medical problem(s) and history of medical events, including a history of substance abuse.
- Current medications or drug therapy, such as insulin for diabetes or hypertensive drugs.
- Allergy or hypersensitivity reactions to previous anesthetics or other drugs.
- Mental status, including emotional state and level of consciousness.
- Communication ability; a patient with hearing impairment or language barrier may be unable to understand verbal instructions during the procedure or respond appropriately.

Preoperative orders regarding the time when the patient should cease taking anything by mouth vary with the circumstances; 6 to 8 hours before the surgical procedure is the usual minimum for adults and children older than 1 year. If possible, the adult patient is instructed to remain on nothing-by-mouth (nil per os [NPO]) status after midnight. Some patients are permitted a few sips of water to take oral medications, such as hypoglycemic or antihypertensive drugs. Other individualized plans for NPO time are considered based on the time of the surgical procedure, patient status, and nutritional and medication needs.

Children younger than 1 year should be NPO for at least 2 hours if they have been on clear fluid. Breastfeeding infants should be NPO for 4 hours. Formula-fed babies should be NPO for 6 hours.

Many ambulatory surgical patients scheduled for same-day procedures have no premedication and are permitted to walk to the OR. Some facilities require the use of a cart or wheelchair for transport. The patient should be transported via cart if sedated.

Intraoperative Patient Care

The patient must be able to respond cooperatively and maintain respiration unassisted. The patient needs careful observation throughout the surgical procedure and for a period afterward for signs and symptoms of delayed reaction or complications. The care the patient will need depends on the type and length of the procedure, the amount of sedation given, and the type and amount of local anesthetic used. Psychologic support and reassurance are given before and during the surgical procedure. The patient should be told what to expect and what is expected of them. The patient should be monitored by qualified personnel and observed for adverse effects of the medication or the procedure.

Local Anesthesia

The surgeon injects the anesthetic drug or applies it topically. The anesthesia provider is not in attendance for this method. Supplemental agents should be available for analgesia or anesthesia, if necessary, or for adverse reactions (Table 24.3). Resuscitative equipment, suction, and oxygen must be at hand before administration of any anesthetic. Qualified personnel should be immediately available to assist in the event of an emergency.

Administration of Local Anesthesia

In the absence of an anesthesia provider, a qualified registered nurse (RN) is responsible for monitoring the patient's physiologic status and safety during local anesthesia. This should be the only activity assigned to this perioperative nurse for the duration of the procedure. Circulating duties should not be done simultaneously.

The perioperative nurse who assumes the responsibility for patient monitoring should have the knowledge, skill, and ability

to use and interpret data from monitoring equipment. The nurse also should be able to recognize signs and symptoms of abnormal reactions to local anesthetic drugs and provide interventions to prevent further complications.

The patient who is under local anesthesia requires observation of physiologic changes in pulse, blood pressure, oxygenation, and respiration. Baseline data obtained during preoperative assessment are compared with intraoperative and postoperative findings. The vital signs, including blood pressure, pulse, and respirations, are continuously monitored. Monitoring devices may include an electrocardiograph and pulse oximeter. Monitoring equipment is used to assess the patient's physiologic status in combination with direct observation.

Data from monitoring and direct observation are documented at frequent intervals (preferably every 5 minutes) and with any significant event, such as the injection of medication or the removal of a specimen. The patient is monitored for reaction to drugs and for behavioral and physiologic changes. It is important for the perioperative nurse to be aware of the maximum dosages of local anesthetics in milligrams per kilogram of body weight.

The total amount of anesthetic and supplementary drugs administered is also recorded in the patient's record. AORN (Association of periOperative Registered Nurses) has established recommended practices for the care of patients receiving local anesthesia. Policies and procedures should be in place to delineate patient care, monitoring activities, and documentation during the use of local anesthetics.

Moderate Sedation

During procedures performed with the patient under local anesthesia, mild sedation may be given by IV infusion. Moderate sedation refers to a mild to moderate depressed level of consciousness that allows the patient to maintain a patent airway independently and respond appropriately to verbal instructions or physical stimulation. A benzodiazepine, such as midazolam (Versed) or diazepam (Valium), is most commonly given either alone or in combination with a narcotic and atropine or scopolamine. Benzodiazepines provide amnesia with sedation, but they also may cause respiratory depression and fluctuations in blood pressure and heart rate and rhythm.

All team members need to understand the objectives and desired effects of moderate sedation. If the primary objective is to allay the patient's anxiety and fear, the therapeutic effects of the drugs given should produce relaxation and some degree of amnesia. Because consciousness is maintained, the patient has intact protective reflexes to respond to physical stimuli. The patient also can be easily aroused with verbal commands as necessary. In this state, vital signs may fluctuate to a minimal extent. Documentation in the patient's record should reflect evidence of continuous assessment and identification of any untoward or significant reactions during administration of local anesthesia with moderate sedation.

The Perioperative Nurse's Role During Local Anesthesia and Moderate Sedation

The patient under moderate sedation should be monitored continuously for cardiac status, blood pressure, pulse, respiration, and oxygen saturation. Monitoring devices may include, but are not limited to, an ECG and pulse oximeter. In the absence of an anesthesia provider, a qualified RN should be assigned to monitor the patient's physiologic state. This nurse should not be assigned

TABLE 24.3   Comparison of Toxicity and Allergy Caused by Local Anesthetic Drugs

Toxic Reaction	Allergic Reaction[a]
Symptoms vary depending on the drug	Immediate localized reaction followed by generalized body reaction
Subjective	
Dizziness, somnolence, paresthesia, nausea, visual/speech problems	Sense of uneasiness, pruritus, agitation, paresthesia
Objective	
Decreased breathing rate and depth, muscle twitches, tremors, slurred speech, seizures, vomiting, unconsciousness, coma	Erythema, urticaria, wheals
Vasovagal	
Dysrhythmias, bradycardia, vasodilation, hypotension, myocardial depression, cardiac arrest	Coughing, wheezing, bronchospasm, hypotension, hypovolemia, vasodilation, cardiovascular collapse, cardiac arrest
Treatment	
Supportive airway management; need intravenous (IV) line; Trendelenburg position; muscular contractions are treated with diazepam (Valium)	Especially with amino ester type: airway management, IV fluids, epinephrine, diphenhydramine, and steroids as needed

[a]Not common with amino amide.

to simultaneously circulate and should be competent in the use and interpretation of monitoring devices.

An anesthesia provider should be in attendance to monitor those patients whose physiologic status is unstable. Policies and procedures should be in place that address the RN's competency in patient monitoring and the nurse's role during the use of moderate sedation.

Monitored Anesthesia Care

When an anesthesia provider's presence is necessary, the surgical procedure is scheduled as monitored anesthesia care (MAC), attended local, or anesthesia standby. Terminology may vary at different institutions. Patients with particular medical problems or age-extreme patients (pediatric or geriatric) may require supervision by anesthesia personnel.

Patients receiving a local anesthetic because they are too ill to undergo general anesthesia should have an anesthesia provider in attendance. The type and length of procedure also may be factors that influence the surgeon's request for an anesthesia provider to be available to give and monitor moderate sedation. The anesthesia provider may initiate and maintain a regional nerve block, such as an axillary brachial plexus block for hand surgery. Moderate sedation and regional blocks with MAC have gained popularity for ambulatory surgery.

Monitoring the Patient Receiving a Local Anesthetic

The extent of monitoring, determined in consultation with physicians in the department of surgery and anesthesiology as applicable, depends on the seriousness of the procedure, sedation required, and/or the patient's condition. The perioperative nurse assigned to monitor the patient receiving a local anesthetic, with or without moderate sedation, continuously attends the patient. This nurse does not have other responsibilities during the surgical procedure. *AORN Guidelines for Perioperative Practice* provides guidance for the perioperative nurse in monitoring the patient receiving a local anesthetic and the patient receiving moderate sedation. The guidelines may be summarized briefly as follows:

1. The patient is monitored for reaction to drugs and for behavioral and physiologic changes. The circulating nurse should recognize and report to the physician significant changes in the patient's status and be prepared to initiate appropriate interventions.
2. The nurse attending the patient should have basic knowledge of the function and use of monitoring equipment, ability to interpret information, and working knowledge of resuscitation equipment. The nurse should have appropriate training and knowledge in pharmacology and the application of the drugs used in the patient's care.
3. Accurate reflection of perioperative care should be documented on the patient's record.
4. Institutional policies and procedures in regard to patient care, including monitoring, should be written, reviewed annually, and readily available. This information should be included in orientation and in-service programs. It should include policies regarding permissible drug administration and emergency interventions by the nurse.

In addition to preoperative assessment and postoperative evaluation for a continuum of care, intraoperative activities include determining and documenting the patient's baseline physiologic status before administration of sedatives, analgesics, and anesthetic drugs and monitoring the patient throughout the procedure. Parameters include, but are not limited to, the following[6]:

- Blood pressure
- Heart rate and rhythm
- Respiratory rate
- Oxygen saturation by pulse oximetry
- Body temperature
- Skin condition and color
- Mental status and level of consciousness

Baseline vital signs are taken when the patient arrives in the OR. These are compared with admission vital signs. Vital signs are taken continually before injection of a drug and at 5- to 15-minute intervals after injection. Changes in the patient's condition are reported to the surgeon immediately. If an adverse reaction occurs, emergency measures should be instituted on request as per policy. These may include maintaining a patent airway, starting oxygen therapy when clinically indicated, and administering IV therapy per the physician's order.

Considerations in the Selection of Local Anesthetics

A local anesthetic depresses superficial peripheral nerves and blocks conduction of pain impulses from their site of origin. Regional nerve blocks interrupt conduction of pain impulses from a specific area or region. These techniques may be used, with or without moderate sedation, when general anesthesia is contraindicated. As with any anesthetic agent, local anesthetics offer advantages in some circumstances but have disadvantages and are contraindicated in others.

Advantages.
- Use of local anesthetic agents can minimize the recovery period. The patient can ambulate, eat, void, and resume normal activity.
- Use of local anesthetic requires minimal equipment and is economical.
- Loss of consciousness does not occur unless anesthesia is supplemented with additional drugs.
- Local anesthesia avoids the undesirable effects of general anesthesia.
- Local anesthesia is suitable for patients who recently ingested food or fluids (e.g., before an emergency procedure).
- Local anesthesia is useful for ambulatory patients having minor procedures.
- Local anesthesia is ideal for procedures in which it is desirable to have the patient awake and cooperative.

Disadvantages.
- Local anesthesia is not practical for all types of procedures. For example, too much drug would be needed for some major surgical procedures; the duration of anesthesia is insufficient for others.
- There are individual variations in response to local anesthetic drugs.
- Rapid absorption of the drug into the bloodstream can cause severe, potentially fatal reactions.
- Apprehension may be increased by the patient's ability to see and hear. Some patients prefer to be unconscious and unaware.
- Local anesthesia is generally contraindicated in patients with the following:
  - Allergic sensitivity to the local anesthetic drug.
  - Local infection or malignancy at the site of injection, which may be carried to and spread in adjacent tissues by injection. A bacteriologically safe injection site should be selected.
  - Septicemia. In a proximal nerve block, a needle may open new lymph channels that drain through a region, thereby causing new foci and local abscess formation from the perforation of small vessels and escape of bacteria.
  - Extreme nervousness, apprehension, excitability, or inability to cooperate because of mental state or age.

Spinal and Epidural Anesthesia

Intraspinal injection of an anesthetic drug is a technique of regional anesthesia performed by a person who has been properly trained and has acquired the necessary skill. Regional anesthesia is delivered to select areas, referred to as *dermatomes*, to affect motor and sensory nerves as desired (Fig. 24.10). The patient's dermatome levels can be tested by touch and by asking the patient to

move specific extremities. Dermatome level T12 is near the iliac crest, T10 is near the umbilicus, and T6 is near the xyphoid.

Assessment of the patient's level of consciousness, pulse, respirations, and blood pressure is essential for early detection of hypotension associated with high spinal anesthesia. If regional anesthesia extends above the level of T4, a full sympathetic block may follow, causing cardiorespiratory arrest. Ventilatory support equipment and naloxone should be immediately available.

Choices in Regional Drugs

The choice of drug depends on factors such as the duration, intensity, and level of anesthesia desired; the anticipated surgical position of the patient; and the surgical procedure (Fig. 24.11).

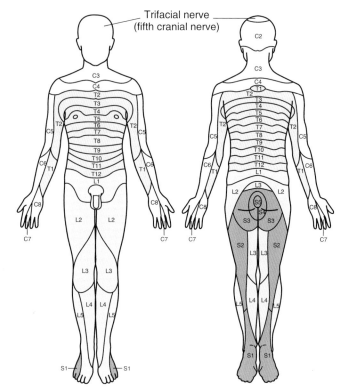

• **Fig. 24.10** Dermatomes of the body.

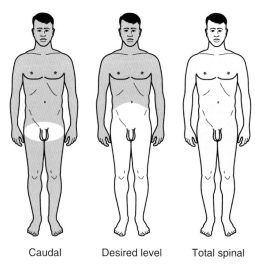

Caudal   Desired level   Total spinal

• **Fig. 24.11** Levels of spinal and epidural anesthesia.

TABLE 24.4 Local and Regional Anesthetic Agents

Generic Name	Trade Name(s)	Uses	Concentration	Duration of Effect (Hours)	Maximum Dosage
Amino Amides					
Bupivacaine	Marcaine Sensorcaine	Local infiltration[a] Regional block[a] Surgical epidural	0.25—0.75%	2—3	400 mg
Dibucaine	Nupercaine Cinchocaine	Local infiltration Peripheral nerves	0.05—0.1%	3—3.5	30 mg
Etidocaine		Peripheral nerves Epidural	0.5—1%	2—3	500 mg
Lidocaine	Xylocaine Lignocaine	Topical Infiltration[a] Peripheral nerves[a] Nerve block[a] Spinal Epidural	2—4% 0.5% 1—2%	0.5—2	200 mg or 4 mg/kg; 500 mg or 7 mg/kg when mixed with vasoconstrictor
Mepivacaine	Carbocaine Polocaine	Infiltration Peripheral nerves Epidural	0.5—1% 1—2%	0.5—2	400 mg
Prilocaine	Citanest	Infiltration Peripheral nerves Regional block Epidural	1—2% 2—3%	0.5—2.5	500 mg
Ropivacaine	Naropin	Infiltration Field block Nerve block Epidural Postoperative pain management Not used for Bier block	0.2% 0.5% 0.75% 1%	2.5 for surgical analgesia; 6—10 for surgical nerve block	200 mg for analgesia; 300 mg for nerve block
Amino Esters					
Chloroprocaine	Nesacaine	Infiltration[a]	0.5%	0.25—0.5	1000 mg
		Peripheral nerves[a] Nerve block[a] Epidural	2% 2% 2—3%		
		Topical	4—10%	0.5	200 mg or 4 mg/kg body weight
Cocaine		Topical anesthesia and vasoconstrictor in ENT surgery	4%	2	1 mg/kg
Procaine	Novocain	Infiltration Peripheral nerves Spinal	0.5% 1—2%	0.25—0.5	1000 mg or 7—10 mg/kg body weight
Tetracaine	Cetacaine Pontocaine	Topical Spinal	2% 1%	2—4	20 mg

ENT, Ear, nose, and throat.
[a]Epinephrine may be used.

Patient factors include the anesthetic history, physical condition, and preference of the patient and surgeon. The duration of action depends on physiologic and metabolic factors. The addition of a vasoconstrictor, usually epinephrine 1:200,000, prolongs the duration.

Diffusion of the drug into the CSF is affected by solubility, molecular weight, and volume. Glucose may be added to make the drug heavier than CSF (hyperbaric). Anesthesia diminishes as the drug is absorbed into the systemic circulation. The most commonly used anesthetic drugs for spinal and epidural anesthesia are listed in Table 24.4.

The anesthesia provider determines the placement site of the injection needle according to the bony landmarks of the spine (Fig. 24.12). The spinal and epidural drugs are injected using

• **Fig. 24.12** Landmarks used for epidural or spinal anesthesia.

specially designed needles with angles and lumens that are specific to the type of anesthesia being delivered (Fig. 24.13).

Spinal Anesthesia

Spinal anesthesia, also referred to as an *intrathecal block,* causes desensitization of spinal ganglia and motor roots. The agent is injected into the CSF in the subarachnoid space of the meninges (the three-layered covering of the spinal cord) using a lumbar interspace in the vertebral column (Fig. 24.14). The subarachnoid space is located between the pia mater (the innermost membranous layer covering the spinal cord) and the arachnoid (the thin, vascular, weblike layer immediately beneath the dura mater, which is the outermost sheath covering the spinal cord). Spinal ganglia, motor nerve roots, and blood vessels pass through the meninges. The drug diffuses into the CSF around ganglia and nerves before it is absorbed into the bloodstream. Absorption into nerve fibers is rapid.

Spinal anesthesia is often used for abdominal (mainly lower) or pelvic procedures requiring relaxation, inguinal or lower extremity procedures, surgical obstetrics (cesarean section without effect on the fetus), and urologic procedures. It is preferred for patients with alcoholism, substance abusers, obese or muscular patients (who would need large doses of general anesthetic and muscle relaxant), and for emergency surgical procedures on patients who have eaten recently. It is also used in the presence of hepatic, renal, or metabolic disease because it causes minimal upset of body chemistry.

The level of anesthesia attained depends on various factors, such as the patient's position during and immediately after injection; CSF pressure; site and rate of injection; volume, dosage, and specific gravity (baricity) of the solution; inclusion of a vasoconstrictor, such as epinephrine; spinal curvature; interspace chosen; uterine contractions with labor; and coughing or straining, which can inadvertently raise the level. Spread of the anesthetic is controlled mainly by solution baricity and patient position.

The period immediately after injection is decisive; the anesthetic is becoming "fixed" (i.e., absorbed by the tissues and unable to travel). Further control of the anesthetic level is attained by tilting the operating bed at that time. The direction of tilting depends on whether the drug is hyperbaric (specific gravity greater than that of spinal fluid) or hypobaric (lighter than spinal fluid). Isobaric anesthetics (same weight as spinal fluid) are made hyperbaric by the addition of 5% or 10% dextrose to the anesthetic before injection.

Immediately after the anesthetic is injected, the anesthesia provider carefully tests the level of anesthesia by pinprick, touch, or nerve stimulation, tilting the bed as necessary to achieve the desired level for the surgical procedure. After anesthetic fixation and with the anesthesia provider's permission, the patient is placed in the surgical position. The patient is asked to relax and let the team turn or position them. Straining or holding the breath can

• **Fig. 24.13** Physical characteristics of four different spinal and epidural needles (not to scale).

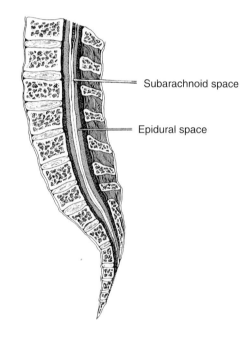

Subarachnoid space

Epidural space

• **Fig. 24.14** Agent is injected into subarachnoid space for spinal anesthesia or into epidural space for epidural anesthesia.

alter the position of the dural sac and precipitate hypotension or an inadvertent rise in the level of anesthesia. The incision is not made until it is certain that anesthesia is adequate. Supplementation of spinal anesthesia is necessary if anesthesia or muscular relaxation is insufficient or the patient is unduly apprehensive. Sometimes the patient is given moderate sedation but can still be roused.

Choice of Agent

The drug used depends on various factors such as the duration, intensity, and level of anesthesia desired, the anticipated surgical position of the patient, and the surgical procedure.

Duration of Agent

The variable duration of anesthesia depends on physiologic and metabolic factors. It is prolonged by the addition of a vasoconstrictor. Anesthesia diminishes as the agent is absorbed into the systemic circulation.

Spinal Anesthesia Procedure

For injection, the patient is placed in the position desired by the anesthesia provider, depending on patient condition, solution baricity, and level of anesthesia to be produced:

- *Lateral position:* The patient lies on the side with the back at the edge of the OR bed or cart. The knees are flexed onto the abdomen, and the head is flexed to the chest. The hips and shoulders are vertical to the OR bed to prevent rotation of the spine (Fig. 24.15).
- *Sitting position:* The patient sits on the side of the OR bed with the feet resting on a stool. The spine is flexed, with the chin lowered to the sternum; the arms are crossed and supported on a pillow on an adjustable table or Mayo stand (Fig. 24.16).

The circulating nurse or an anesthesia technician supports and reassures the patient in an aligned position and assists the anesthesia provider as possible. Attention to asepsis is extremely important. The anesthesia provider dons sterile gloves before handling sterile items. Sterile disposable spinal trays eliminate the need for cleaning and sterilizing of reusable equipment. They also avoid the hazards of sterilizing ampules. The dates on the drugs supplied by the manufacturer should be checked.

A spinal tray usually contains the following:

- Fenestrated drape.
- Ampules of local anesthetic, spinal anesthetic, vasoconstrictor drug, and dextrose.
- Gauze squares, forceps, and antiseptic solution. Some kits include disposable skin prep sponges on plastic applicator sticks.
- Needles: 25-gauge hypodermic needle for infiltration of local anesthetic into the skin; 22-gauge × 2-inch (5-cm) needle for IM injection; blunt 18-gauge needles for mixing drugs; and 22 or 26-gauge × 3½-inch (9-cm) spinal needle with stylets for intrathecal injection.
- Syringes: 5-mL syringes for spinal anesthetic; 10-mL syringes for hypobaric solutions; and 2-mL syringes for superficial anesthesia.

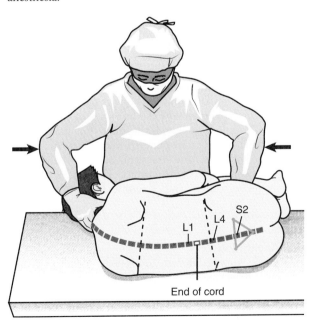

• **Fig. 24.15** Spinal block—lateral position.

• **Fig. 24.16** Spinal block—sitting position.

The puncture site is cleansed with an antiseptic solution and draped with a fenestrated drape. Advise the patient that the prep solution will feel cold and wet. Before the skin is penetrated, the patient should be told that the skin will be numbed with local anesthetic and the spinal needle will be inserted. This prevents the startle effect of the needlestick in the patient. The blood pressure is checked before, during, and after spinal anesthesia because hypotension is common.

Advantages. The patient is conscious if desired. The procedure can be performed with moderate sedation as necessary. Throat reflexes are maintained; breathing is quiet without airway problems because the respiratory system is not irritated. The bowel is contracted. Muscle relaxation and anesthesia are excellent if the procedure is properly executed.

Disadvantages. Spinal anesthesia produces a circulatory depressant effect: hypotension and stasis of blood as a result of interference with venous return from motor paralysis and arteriolar dilation in the lower extremities. A change in body position may be followed by a sudden drop in blood pressure; after fixation of the anesthetic, a slight elevation of the feet and legs may increase venous return to the heart. The agent cannot be removed after injection. Nausea and emesis may accompany cerebral ischemia, traction on viscera and peritoneum, or premedication. There is possible sensitivity to the agent and danger of trauma or infection. The patient has all senses present, such as hearing, sight, and smell, and is able to speak.

Transient or permanent neurologic sequelae from cord trauma, irritation by the agent, lack of asepsis, and loss of spinal fluid with decreased intracranial pressure syndrome are potential complications. Examples include spinal headache; auditory and ocular disturbances, such as tinnitus and diplopia; arachnoiditis; meningitis; transverse myelitis; cauda equina syndrome (failure to regain use of the legs or control of urinary and bowel functions); temporary paresthesias, such as numbness and tingling; cranial nerve palsies; and urinary retention. Late complications include nerve root lesions, spinal cord lesions, and ruptured nucleus pulposus.

True spinal headache caused by a persistent CSF leak through the needle hole in the dura usually responds to supine bed rest, copious oral or IV fluids, and systemic analgesia. Refractory post–spinal headache may be treated by an epidural blood patch: 5 to 10 mL of the patient's own blood is administered at the puncture site. This usually affords prompt relief.

If a high level of anesthesia is reached, extreme caution is essential to prevent respiratory paralysis ("total spinal"), which is an emergency situation requiring mechanical ventilation until the level of anesthesia has receded. Respiratory arrest, although rare, is thought to be a result of medullary hypoperfusion caused by a sympathetic block. Apnea also can be produced by respiratory center ischemia resulting from precipitous hypotension.

The anesthesia machine, oxygen, and IV line must be in readiness before injection. Constant vigilance of respiration and circulation is critical. The blood pressure and heart rate are monitored and maintained at normal levels.

Epidural Anesthesia

The terms *epidural, peridural,* and *extradural* are used synonymously. The epidural space lies between the dura mater, the outermost sheath covering the spinal cord, and the walls of the vertebral column. It contains a network of blood vessels, lymphatics, fat, loose connective tissue, and spinal nerve roots. Injection is made into this space surrounding the dura mater (see Fig. 24.14). The drug diffuses slowly through the dura mater into CSF. Anesthesia is prolonged while the drug is absorbed from CSF into the bloodstream.

The spread of anesthetic and duration of action are influenced by the concentration and volume of solution injected (total drug mass) and the rate of injection. The anesthetic diffuses toward the head (cephalad) and toward the coccyx (caudad). In contrast to spinal anesthesia, patient position, baricity, and gravity have little influence on anesthetic distribution. The high incidence of systemic reactions is attributed to absorption of the agent from the highly vascular peridural area and the relatively large mass of anesthetic injected. Epinephrine 1:200,000 is usually added to retard absorption.

Approaches used for epidural anesthesia and analgesia include thoracic, lumbar, and caudal approaches. Skin and ligaments are infiltrated with a local anesthetic agent before the epidural catheter is placed.

The management and sequelae of epidural anesthesia are similar to those of spinal anesthesia. An epidural approach may be used for lower extremity, abdominal, urologic, anorectal, vaginal, or perineal procedures. It is used commonly for postoperative pain management and in obstetrics during labor and delivery or during and after cesarean section.

A qualified RN attends the patient constantly once the block is initiated for analgesia. Vital signs should be monitored at regular intervals, and any deviation of level of consciousness, pulse, respirations, or blood pressure should be reported immediately to the anesthesiologist. Use of an apnea monitor may be indicated. In an obstetric patient, the fetal heart rate should be electronically monitored continuously because the patient is insensitive to uterine contractions.

Epidural narcotic analgesia may provide sustained postoperative relief or control of pain in patients with intractable or prolonged pain. This may be administered by a percutaneous indwelling epidural catheter, an implanted epidural catheter with infusion port or reservoir and pump, or an implantable infusion device. A patient may come to the OR for placement of an epidural catheter or pump device for ongoing pain management.

An epidural catheter for administration of a narcotic for prolonged postoperative pain relief, usually for 2 or 3 days, may be inserted before induction of general anesthesia, for postoperative use. Morphine, fentanyl, and sufentanil are the drugs most commonly used for prolonged pain relief. Although probability of respiratory depression is less when the epidural route is used compared with spinal narcotics, use of an apnea monitor is advisable.

Side effects include nausea and vomiting, urinary retention, and pruritus. Epidural narcotics block pain at the level of opiate receptors in the dorsal horn of the spinal cord, not in the brain, so the patient is mentally alert and able to ambulate with caution.

Thoracic and Lumbar Approaches

The thoracic and lumbar approaches are peridural blocks. Equipment is similar to that for a spinal block with the addition of a 19-gauge × 3½-inch (9-cm), thin-walled needle with a stylet with a rigid shaft and a short, beveled tip to minimize the danger of inadvertent dural puncture. Insertion of a catheter allows repeated injections for continuous intraoperative and postoperative epidural anesthesia, requiring additional needles, stopcocks, and a plastic catheter in the setup.

Caudal Approach

The caudal approach is an epidural sacral block. Epidural injection is through the caudal canal, desensitizing nerves emerging from the dural sac. The patient position for injection is prone with the hips flexed, sacrum horizontal, and heels turned outward to expose the injection site. The sacral area is prepared and draped, with care taken to protect the genitalia from irritating solution. The left lateral position is used in the pregnant patient. The spread of agents in epidural anesthesia is enhanced in pregnancy, atherosclerosis, and advanced age.

The tray includes the addition of a 20 to 24-gauge × 1½-inch (4-cm) spinal needle with a stylet. Commercial sets are available.

Advantages. Compared with spinal anesthesia, epidural anesthesia has a decreased incidence of hypotension, headache, and potential for neurologic complications, although a higher failure rate is reported.

Disadvantages. There is less controllable height of anesthesia; it is a more difficult technique; there is a greater area of potential infection from anaerobic organisms with the caudal approach; it is unpredictable; it is time-consuming (i.e., a longer time is required for complete anesthesia); a larger amount of agent is injected; and continuous technique may slow the first stage of labor.

Intravascular injection, accidental dural puncture and total spinal anesthesia, blood vessel puncture and hematoma, profound hypotension, backache, and transient or permanent paralysis (paraplegia) are possible complications. The patient may suffer hypoxia, respiratory arrest, and/or cardiac arrest.

Techniques of Administration of Local or Regional Anesthesia

Topical Application

The anesthetic is applied directly to a mucous membrane, a serous surface, or an open wound. A topical agent is often applied to the respiratory passages to eliminate laryngeal reflexes and cough, for insertion of airways before induction or during light general anesthesia, or for therapeutic and diagnostic procedures such as laryngoscopy or bronchoscopy. It is also used in the urethral meatus for cystoscopy.

Mucous membranes readily absorb topical agents because of their vascularity. The onset of anesthesia occurs within minutes. The blood level of a topical agent may equal the same level obtained by IV injection. The duration of anesthesia is 20 to 30 minutes. If a spray or atomizer is used, it should contain a visible reservoir so the quantity of drug administered is clearly observed because droplets vary in size, causing variations in dosages.

Preanesthetic anticholinergics are important before topical application within the respiratory tract. Saliva can dilute the topical anesthetic and prevent adequate duration of contact with mucous membranes. In addition, a dry throat is necessary to prevent aspiration until the anesthetic effect has disappeared and throat reflexes have returned. Adverse reactions to topical anesthetic agents are uncommon when dosage is carefully controlled. Sudden cardiovascular collapse can occur, more commonly after topical anesthesia of the respiratory tract.

Topical local anesthetic ointment may be used on the skin surface before establishing IV access. The ointment should be applied and allowed to remain in contact with the skin for several minutes to an hour for optimal effect. A transparent cover dressing may be placed over the application point to prevent accidental smearing of the medication. Care is taken to prevent contact with the eyes and other mucous membranes.

Cryoanesthesia
Cryoanesthesia involves blocking local nerve conduction of painful impulses by means of marked surface cooling (i.e., freezing) of a localized area. It is used in such brief procedures as the removal of warts or noninvasive papular surface lesions. Cryotherapy units are commercially available.

Simple Local Infiltration
The agent is injected intracutaneously and subcutaneously into tissues at and around the incisional site to block peripheral sensory nerve stimuli at their origin. It is used before suturing superficial lacerations or excising minor lesions.

Regional Injection
The agent is injected into or around a specific nerve or group of nerves to depress the entire sensory nervous system of a limited, localized area of the body. The injection is at a distance from the surgical site. A wider, deeper area is anesthetized than with simple infiltration. There are several types of regional blocks.

Nerve Block. A selected nerve is anesthetized at a given point. Nerve blocks are performed to interrupt sensory, motor, and/or sympathetic transmission. Blocks may be used preoperatively, intraoperatively, and postoperatively to prevent pain of the procedure; diagnostically to ascertain the cause of pain; or therapeutically to relieve chronic pain. Blocks are useful in various circulatory and neurosurgical syndromes, such as reflex sympathetic dystrophy (RSD). For prolonged pain relief (e.g., during a long procedure or to treat chronic pain associated with disease or trauma), a continuous infusion or incremental injections through a catheter may sustain regional anesthesia. Some examples of blocks are as follows:
1. Surgical blocks
   a. Paravertebral block of the cervical plexus for procedures in the area between the jaw and the clavicle
   b. Intercostal block for relatively superficial intraabdominal procedures, such as drain placement
   c. Brachial plexus or axillary block for arm procedures
   d. Median, radial, or ulnar nerve block for the elbow or wrist
   e. Hand and digital block for fingers (an additive vasoconstrictor, such as epinephrine, is not added to the local agent because necrosis can result from inadequate circulation to the digit)
   f. Blocks in other specific areas, such as a penile block for circumcision in adults or femoral block for procedures of the upper leg, knee, and below
2. Diagnostic or therapeutic blocks
   a. Sympathetic nerve ganglion block to produce desired vasodilation by paralysis of the sympathetic nerve supply to the constricting smooth muscle in the artery wall
   b. Stellate ganglion block to increase circulation in peripheral vascular disease in the head, neck, arm, or hand
   c. Paravertebral lumbar block to increase circulation in the lower extremities
   d. Celiac block for relief of abdominal pain of pancreatic origin

Bier Block. A Bier block is a regional IV injection of a local anesthetic to an extremity below the level of a double-cuffed tourniquet. A Bier block is used for upper extremity procedures and for those that last an hour or less.
- A double tourniquet cuff is applied, but not inflated. An IV catheter is inserted in the dorsum of the hand (Fig. 24.17).
- A plastic drape is wrapped around the cuff to seal it off from prep solutions.
- The arm is elevated, prepped, and wrapped with a sterile Esmarch or Ace bandage from the hand to the tourniquet cuff (distal to proximal) to exsanguinate the limb (Fig. 24.18).
- The proximal cuff is inflated, and the wrap is removed. The Esmarch wrap should be rerolled and set aside on the sterile field.
- Local anesthetic is injected into the IV catheter (Fig. 24.19).
- When the anesthetic takes effect over the limb, the lower (distal) cuff of the tourniquet is inflated.
- The upper (proximal) cuff is released.

The patient feels less discomfort related to the tourniquet because the lower cuff is over an anesthetized region.

On release of the tourniquet at the conclusion of the surgical procedure, entry of a bolus of the remaining drug and metabolic waste (lactic acid from ischemia) into systemic circulation may

• **Fig. 24.17** Bier block equipment with double tourniquet in place.

• **Fig. 24.18** Bier block: Exsanguination of limb by elevation and elastic wrap before inflating the proximal cuff and injecting anesthetic.

• **Fig. 24.19** Bier block: Anesthetic is injected and distal cuff inflated. Wrap is removed and proximal cuff deflated.

cause cardiovascular or CNS symptoms of toxicity, such as blindness.

Field Block. The surgical site is blocked off with a wall of anesthetic drug. A series of injections into proximal and surrounding tissues will provide a wide area of anesthesia, as in an abdominal wall block for herniorrhaphy.

Complications of Blocks. Each type of block carries unique complication potential. Examples of complications include the following:

• *Intercostal blocks:* Pneumothorax, atelectasis, total spinal anesthesia, air embolism, transverse myelitis
• *Brachial plexus blocks:* Pneumothorax, hemothorax, recurrent laryngeal nerve paralysis, phrenic paralysis, subarachnoid injection, Horner syndrome (axillary approach may be preferred to interscalene approach)
• *Stellate ganglion blocks:* Pneumothorax

• *Celiac blocks:* Large vessel perforation, pancreatic injury, total spinal anesthesia

Actions of Local and Regional Anesthetics

Local and regional anesthetics interfere with the initiation and transmission of nerve impulses by interacting with the membranous sheath that covers nerve fibers. By physical and biochemical mechanisms, drugs retard and stop the propagation of nerve impulses, eventually blocking conduction.

Drug Pharmacodynamics

The duration of action depends not only on pharmacologic properties of drugs but also on the volume and concentration of the solution and its systemic interactions. Drugs vary in potency, penetration, rapidity of hydrolysis or destruction, and toxicity.

Conduction Velocity. Nerve fibers vary in their susceptibility to drugs. The larger the fiber, the greater the concentration required. The least amount and lowest concentration to achieve the desired effect should be administered. Conduction of a peripheral stimulus is blocked at its origin by topical application or local infiltration of the drug. Transmission of stimuli along afferent nerves from the surgical site is blocked in regional anesthesia. Conductive pathways in and around the spinal cord are blocked for spinal and epidural anesthesia.

Blocking Quality. Drugs of high potency, minimal systemic activity, and prompt metabolism and those that lack local irritation are most effective. Blocking qualities include the following:

• Latency time between administration and maximum effect
• Duration of action
• Regression time between beginning and end of pain perception

Sensory nerves are blocked initially. Motor nerves also are affected, with resultant paralysis of both voluntary and involuntary muscles. Some degree of vasodilation occurs with all local and regional use of anesthetic drugs except cocaine.

Absorption Rate and Additives. Local blood flow, vasodilation, and vascularity of tissues can markedly influence local anesthetic action and systemic absorption of drugs. Fibrous tissue and fat in some injection sites act as diffusion barriers and nonspecific binding sites. Additives to slow uptake include the following:

• *Epinephrine (Adrenalin):* A catecholamine, epinephrine is a potent stimulant. When combined with an anesthetic drug, it causes vasoconstriction to slow circulatory uptake and absorption, thus prolonging anesthesia. It is used to counteract cardiovascular depressant effects of large doses of local anesthetic. It also decreases bleeding, which is a desired effect in many surgical procedures. A concentration of epinephrine that is 1:1000 (1000 mg/1000 mL × 1 mg/mL) to 1:200,000 (0.005 mg/mL) may be optimal for absorptive and hemostatic purposes.

Epinephrine is premixed in commercially prepared solutions. If it is added to an anesthetic drug, it is best to do so with a calibrated syringe to avoid over dosage. Epinephrine can produce an acute adrenergic response: nervousness, pallor, diaphoresis, tremor, palpitation, tachycardia, and hypertension. The patient receiving epinephrine should be well oxygenated.

• *Sodium bicarbonate:* A small amount of carbonation can be added to local anesthetic agents. The carbonation lowers the pH of the solution, causing it to cross the cell membrane more readily. Alkalization results in decreased pain on injection. One potential problem with the addition of bicarbonate is that it may precipitate in the local anesthetic solution.

- *Dextran:* Anesthetic solutions with a pH higher than 8 can be mixed with dextran for prolongation of the localized anesthetic effect.

Toxicity. Allergic reactions to anesthetic drugs can occur but are rare. Toxic reactions occur when the concentration of drug in the blood affects the CNS. Slurred speech, numbness of the tongue, blurred vision, and tinnitus are symptoms of toxicity that can progress to drowsiness and confusion.

The maximum recommended dosage for each drug should not be exceeded. Severe toxic reaction can quickly lead to cardio-vascular collapse. In topical anesthesia, extremely rapid systemic absorption from the mucous membranes explains the relatively high frequency of toxic reactions. In local or regional anesthesia, inadvertent intravascular injection and use of fairly large quantities in highly vascular areas will contribute to local anesthetic toxicity.

Pharmacologic Agent Overview

Many local or regional anesthetic drugs are in use. All are direct myocardial depressants, but the CNS effects precede this depression. Detoxification occurs in the liver. They differ in structure and therefore in action. These drugs are hydrochloride salts of weak bases in solution. They are categorized by chemical structure as amino amides and amino esters (see Table 24.4).

Amino Amides. Amino amides are metabolized in the liver by enzymes and are excreted by the kidneys. Patients with hepatic disease may become toxic with normal dosages because of inef-fective metabolism. The amides include the following:

- *Ropivacaine (Naropin):* Ropivacaine is used for field blocks, nerve blocks, epidurals, and postoperative pain control epidural applications. Four strengths are available: 0.2% (2 mg/mL), 0.5% (5 mg/mL), 0.75% (7.5 mg/mL), and 1% (10 mg/mL). Epidural administration may result in hypotension and bradycardia. The maximum dose for children is 3 mg/kg.
- *Lidocaine (Xylocaine):* Probably the most widely used agent, this potent anesthetic slowly hydrolyzes in circulating plasma. It undergoes hepatic degradation. The dosage should be reduced if hepatic function or blood flow is impaired. Its major advantages are a rapid onset of anesthesia and lack of local irri-tant effect. Allergic reactions are rare.

Used extensively for surgical procedures and dentistry, it has moderate potency and a moderate duration of action. For adult infiltration: 0.5%; for peripheral nerves: 1% to 2% with vasoconstrictor additive; maximum dose is 500 mg or 7 mg/kg body weight. Without a vasoconstrictor, the recommended dose is 4.5 mg/kg, not to exceed 300 mg. It is a good topical anesthetic. For topical use in the respiratory tract: 2% to 4%; maximum dose is 200 mg without vasoconstrictor additive. It is commonly used topically before awake intubation. The maximum dose for pediatric patients is 5 mg/kg.

Clinical indications of lidocaine toxicity usually are related to the CNS, such as complaints of circumoral and tongue numbness. Excessive doses can produce myocardial and circulatory depression. Toxic IV dose is over 300 mg.

- *Mepivacaine (Polocaine, Carbocaine):* Similar to lidocaine, mepivacaine takes effect rapidly but produces a 20% longer duration of anesthesia. It has moderate potency and a moder-ate duration of action. It is commonly used for infiltration and nerve block. It produces minimal tissue irritation and few adverse reactions. Epinephrine may not be added to it

because of its duration of action. For infiltration: 0.5% to 1%; for peripheral nerves: 1% to 2%; maximum dose is 400 mg.

- *Bupivacaine (Marcaine, Sensorcaine):* Four times more potent than lidocaine, bupivacaine has high potency of long duration. The onset of anesthesia is slow, but the duration is two to three times longer than that of lidocaine or mepivacaine.

Cumulation occurs with repeated injection. The drug affords prolonged pain relief after caudal block for rectal procedures. It is contraindicated for obstetric paracervical block and epidural anesthesia and for a Bier block. For local infiltration or a regional block, with or without epinephrine: 0.25% to 0.50%; maximum dose is 175 mg per dose without epinephrine or 225 mg with epinephrine 1:200,000 to a total dose of 400 mg. Pediatric maximum dose is 3 mg/kg.

- *Prilocaine (Citanest):* With prilocaine the onset of anesthesia is slower than with lidocaine, but the duration of action is longer. It is particularly useful for patients with diabetes or cardiovas-cular disease. It is used without epinephrine. For infiltration: 1% or 2%; for regional blocks and peripheral nerves: 2% or 3%; maximum dose is 500 mg. Pediatric maximum dose is 6 mg/kg.
- *Etidocaine (Duranest):* The onset of anesthesia is slower than that of lidocaine, but the block is of greater potency and toxicity, with a longer duration of action. For peripheral nerves: 0.5% to 1%; maximum dose is 400 mg.
- *Dibucaine (Nupercaine, Cinchocaine):* Dibucaine is a very potent drug with a high rate of systemic toxicity. The onset is slow, and the duration of action is long. For infiltration and peripheral nerves: 0.05% to 0.1%; maximum dose is 30 mg.

Amino Esters. Amino esters are hydrolyzed in plasma by pseudocholinesterase enzymes produced by the liver. Para-aminobenzoic acid (PABA), a factor in the vitamin B complex, is a product of this metabolism. Some patients are allergic to PABA. The esters include the following:

- *Cocaine:* The first known local anesthetic, introduced in 1884, cocaine is seldom used. It is a crystalline powder with a bitter taste in solution. It is the most toxic of the local drugs and, in contrast to all but lidocaine, is a vasoconstrictor and a CNS stimulant. Cocaine reduces bleeding and shrinks congested mucous membranes. It causes temporary paralysis of sensory nerve fibers, produces exhilaration, lessens hunger and fatigue, and stimulates pulse and respiratory rates.

Administration is by topical application only because of its high toxicity; the solution rapidly penetrates mucous membranes and spreads into highly vascular tissue. Absorption is self-limiting because of vasoconstrictive properties associated with the drug. Epinephrine should not be added. When applied to the throat, cocaine abolishes throat reflexes. The patient is awake and can cooperate, but its limited use and possible addiction are disadvantages.

Cocaine is used topically in 4% concentration for anesthesia of the upper respiratory tract (nose, pharynx, tracheobronchial tree) in 1 to 2-mL amounts on a cottonoid (pattie). Untoward reactions may occur rapidly in response to even a very small amount of the drug.

Maximum dose is 200 mg or 1.5 mg/kg body weight. Cocaine is metabolized by the liver and excreted by the kidneys. It should be used with caution in patients with impaired liver or kidney function. It is contraindicated in pregnancy because it decreases uterine blood flow.

- *Procaine (Novocain):* Procaine is similar to cocaine but less toxic. Concentrations used: 0.5% for infiltration; 1% to 2% for peripheral nerves. It is injected SQ, IM, or intrathecally. It has low potency, is of short duration, and is ineffective topically. Its advantages include minimal toxicity, easy sterilization, low cost, and lack of local irritation. Newer agents are used more frequently. Maximum dose is 1000 mg (1 g) or 7 to 10 mg/kg body weight.

- *Chloroprocaine (Nesacaine):* Chloroprocaine is possibly the safest local anesthetic from the standpoint of systemic toxicity because of its fast metabolism. It has moderate potency of short duration. It is rapidly hydrolyzed in the plasma. Its action is fast, but it is not active topically. When used in obstetrics, it does not alter neurobehavioral responses of newborn infants in any detectable way. For infiltration: 0.5%; for peripheral nerves: 2%; maximum dose is 1000 mg (1 g). Pediatric dose is calculated by age and weight, should not exceed 11 mg/kg.

- *Tetracaine (Cetacaine):* With tetracaine, the onset of analgesia is slow, but the duration of its effect is longer than that of many other drugs. It has high potency of long duration. It is also more toxic systemically because of the slow rate of destruction in the body, but low total dosage tends to reduce the chances of reaction. It is not used for local tissue infiltration or nerve block. Tetracaine in 2% solution is used only for topical anesthesia on accessible mucous membranes such as the oropharynx. Maximum adult dose is 20 mg. Tetracaine is used primarily for spinal anesthesia. Maximum pediatric dose is 2 mg/kg.

Complications of Local and Regional Anesthesia

Minor or transient complications of local and regional anesthesia are common. Serious complications, although rare, are usually permanent. Complications may be caused by the mechanical effect of needles or pharmacologic effect of the drug administered. As with general anesthesia, the prevention of complications requires patient assessment and preparation, knowledge of anatomy and physiology, and attention to detail.

Proper choice of drug and equipment and constant monitoring are as necessary in local and regional anesthesia as in general anesthesia. Complications of local and regional anesthesia may be summarized briefly as local effects, systemic effects, and effects unrelated to the anesthetic drug.

Local Effects

Tissue trauma, hematoma, ischemia, drug sensitivity, and infection can be minimized by the use of proper drugs and equipment, sterile technique, avoidance of local anesthetics with vasoconstrictors in sites with smaller vascular structures (e.g., digits, penis, pinna), and avoidance of repetitive injection that promotes trauma, edema, tissue necrosis, and infection.

Systemic Effects

Systemic effects are primarily cardiovascular, neurologic, or respiratory (e.g., hypotension, seizure, respiratory depression). Drug interactions also are systemic.

After high blood levels, toxicity that affects more than one system may occur. Blood levels depend on the amount of drug used, its physical characteristics, the presence or absence of

vasoconstrictors, and the injection site. For example, because of vascularity of surrounding tissue, intercostal blocks produce higher anesthetic blood levels in a shorter time than do axillary or epidural blocks. Absorption and the blood level of drugs are related to their uptake and rate of removal from the circulation. A linear relationship exists between the amount of drug administered via a given route and the resultant peak anesthetic blood level.

Predisposing Factors for Hypersensitivity. True hypersensitivity that produces an allergic response can occur, but it is less frequent than reactions from overdosage of pharmacologic agents. The following may predispose a patient to hypersensitivity:

- *Immunologic sensitization:* Allergies are thought to be more common with the amino esters than with the amide group of compounds. An allergic reaction to the preservative in some solutions, such as methylparaben, also is possible. Some local anesthetics release histamine, which is the basis of an allergic response.

True allergy, mediated by antigen-antibody reaction, can cause anaphylaxis, urticaria (skin wheals), dermatitis, itching, laryngeal edema, and possibly cardiovascular collapse.

- *Overdosage:* An excessive amount of drug may enter the bloodstream if the injection exceeds maximum dose or is absorbed too rapidly. The IV method is the most dangerous route of injection because histamine is released into the systemic circulation. The injection site is also pertinent. Hazardous sites involve vascular areas of tracheobronchial mucosa, and tissues of the head, neck, and paravertebral region. The least hazardous areas are subcutaneous tissue of the extremities and trunk (abdominal wall and buttocks).

Precautions. Extraordinary precautions must be taken for a patient with a history of any allergies, hypersensitivities, or reactions to previous anesthetics or other drugs. Atopic individuals, those with a hereditary tendency or multiple allergies, may be more prone to adverse reactions to anesthetics or other drugs. Prediction of allergic reactions is unreliable. If testing for sensitivity to specific drugs is done, it is executed cautiously under well-controlled conditions.

Precautions for preventing adverse drug reactions in all patients include the following:

1. Assessing the patient's preoperative physiologic and psychologic condition to determine potential problems and abnormal stress responses:
   a. Identify all medications the patient has recently received or is currently taking, including any history of substance abuse. If local anesthesia is planned, ask the patient about ever having local anesthesia at the dentist's office and if there were any adverse effects.
   b. Question the patient about known or suspected previous drug reactions. Any chemically related drug is not given.
   c. Help the patient cope with anxiety and fears by giving preoperative instructions and answering questions.
2. Handling drugs with care. Before administering or placing drugs on the sterile table:
   a. Read the label carefully. Check the expiration date.
   b. Discard the ampule or vial if the label is not completely legible or has been disturbed.
   c. Open, unlabeled, undated, multiple-use vials should be discarded and not used.
   d. Observe the solution for clarity, and discard any suspicious ampule or vial.

3. Administering drugs selected by a physician in appropriate concentrations and dosages for anesthesia and moderate sedation:
   a. Give the minimum effective concentration and smallest volume needed. Adjust the precise amount to the weight of the patient in kilograms as appropriate.
   b. Limit the total amount of drug injected or applied to prescribed safe limits. Sterile single-dose ampules and prefilled syringes are recommended.
   c. Inject slowly to retard absorption and avoid overdosage. Use incremental titration of drug.
   d. Pull back on the syringe plunger frequently while injecting tissues to be sure the solution is not entering a blood vessel inadvertently. Intravascular injection of an anesthetic drug can release histamine into the systemic circulation, causing an anaphylactoid (nonimmunologic) reaction.
   e. Exercise caution with drugs that depress respiratory or cardiovascular functions, such as sedatives, when the upper dose limit of the anesthetic drug is used.
   f. Provide continuous IV access for administering drugs for moderate sedation or adverse reactions. An IV line should be established in case of adverse reaction or inadvertent intravascular injection or bolus of anesthetic. A heparin lock device or infusion of IV fluids may be used to maintain continuous access.
   g. Cease administration of the drug immediately at the sign of any sensitivity.
   h. Record the drug name, dosage, route, time, and effects of all drugs or pharmacologic agents used.
4. Monitoring patient continuously:
   a. Observe the patient, including facial expressions, and note responses to conversation and the patient's state of alertness.
   b. Assess the patient's physical signs and symptoms, such as skin color and temperature. Use assessment knowledge and skill, and avoid total reliance on monitoring equipment.
   c. Monitor the patient's vital signs as appropriate (ECG, blood pressure, pulse, oxygen saturation, and respiration).
   d. Know resuscitation measures and be able to assist or initiate them as necessary, as per institutional policies and procedures. Basic cardiac life support certification (BCLS) is required of all RNs who monitor patients. Advanced cardiac life support certification (ACLS) is preferred.

Signs and Symptoms of Systemic Reactions. Signs and symptoms of systemic reaction may be CNS stimulation or depression. Conversely, stimulation may be followed by depression and cardiovascular collapse (see Table 24.3). The cardiovascular system seems more resistant than the CNS to toxic effects of local anesthetics. The seizure threshold may differ enormously in individual patients, as may the relationship of the dose to signs and symptoms of CNS effect. For example, lidocaine usually produces drowsiness before a convulsion whereas bupivacaine may cause sudden seizure, disorientation, decreased hearing ability, paresthesias, muscle twitching, or agitation in a wide-awake patient without premonitory signs. Hypercapnia or hypoxemia from hypoventilation lowers the seizure threshold.

Toxicity of local anesthetics is manifested primarily by CNS effects resulting from high blood levels. Signs and symptoms of systemic reaction include, but are not limited to, the following:
- *Stimulation:* Talkativeness, restlessness, incoherence, excitation, tachycardia, bounding pulse, flushed face, hyperpyrexia, tremors, hyperactive reflexes, muscular twitching, focal or grand mal convulsions
- *Depression:* Drowsiness; disorientation; decreased hearing ability; stupor; syncope; rapid, thready pulse or bradycardia; apprehension; hypotension; pale or cyanotic moist skin; coma
- *Other signs and symptoms:* Nausea, vomiting, dizziness, blurred vision, sudden severe headache, precordial pain, extreme pulse rate or blood pressure change, angioneurotic edema (wheeze, laryngeal edema, bronchospasm), rashes, urticaria, severe local tissue reaction

Systemic reactions or undesired effects of moderate sedation used in combination with local anesthetics may include slurred speech, agitation, combativeness, unarousable sleep, hypotension, hypoventilation, airway obstruction, and apnea.

Other signs and symptoms may be related to specific drugs. Benzodiazepines and sedatives used in moderate sedation may cause somnolence, confusion, diminished reflexes, depressed respiratory and cardiovascular function, and coma. Nystagmus (involuntary eye movements), which may be normal with large doses of diazepam (Valium), may be an abnormal reaction with other drugs. Opioids (narcotics) may cause nausea and vomiting, hypotension, and respiratory depression.

Treatment of Adverse Reactions
Treatment of an adverse reaction is aimed at preventing respiratory and cardiac arrest. Treatment must be prompt. ACLS protocol may be needed.

Administration of the agent thought to produce the reaction is stopped immediately at the first indication of reaction. Therapy is generally supportive, the specifics dictated by clinical manifestations. Treatment consists of the following:
1. Maintaining oxygenation of vital organs and tissues with ventilation by manual or mechanical assistance to give 100% oxygen with positive pressure. Tracheal intubation may be indicated.
2. Reversing myocardial depression and peripheral vasodilation before cardiac arrest occurs. The patient is supine with the legs elevated. IV fluid therapy is begun, and a vasoconstrictor drug may be given IV or IM for hypotension or a weak pulse, which are signs of progressive circulatory depression. The choice of vasopressor is suggested by the signs and symptoms, and the drug is used with caution. Drugs that may be used include the following:
   a. Epinephrine (IV) counteracts hypotension, bronchoconstriction, and laryngeal edema. It also stimulates β- and α-adrenergic receptors and inhibits further release of mediators. It increases arteriolar constriction and force of the heartbeat. When appropriate, application of a tourniquet or subcutaneous injection of epinephrine in an area of drug injection may delay absorption of toxic drug.
   b. Ephedrine and other vasoconstrictors such as phenylephrine (Neo-Synephrine) or mephentermine (Wyamine) cause peripheral vasoconstriction, increased myocardial contraction, and bronchodilation.
   c. Antihistamines block histamine release but generally are not advocated.
   d. Steroids enhance the effect of epinephrine and inhibit further release of histamine. The effect is not immediate, and use is directed toward late manifestations of allergic response.
   e. Isoproterenol (Isuprel) is used predominantly in asthma and heart attacks; it is a bronchodilator.
   f. An antagonist drug may be given in situations in which the causative agent is identified.

3. Stopping muscle tremors or convulsions if they are present because they constitute a hazard for further hypoxia, aspiration, or bodily injury. Diazepam in 5-mg doses or a short-acting barbiturate is given IV to inhibit cortical irritation.

For patients in whom the adverse response is caused by hypersensitivity, the previous measures are applicable. However, aminophylline may be administered to help alleviate bronchospasm, hydrocortisone (IV) to combat shock, and sodium or potassium iodide (IV) to reduce mucosal edema.

The perioperative nurse who is monitoring the patient must know resuscitation measures and be able to assist in or initiate them when necessary. An emergency cart with emergency resuscitative drugs and a defibrillator should be immediately available to the room where local or regional anesthetic with or without moderate sedation is administered. The following equipment should be in the room and ready for use:

- Oxygen and positive pressure breathing device (e.g., Ambu bag and mask)
- Oral and nasopharyngeal airways and endotracheal tubes in an assortment of sizes
- Cardiac and oxygen saturation monitoring equipment
- Suction

Unrelated Effects

A nerve deficit, such as pain or neuritis that occurs in the postoperative period, may be related to a preexisting condition such as multiple sclerosis. Alternatively, it may be from a cause unrelated to the anesthetic drug, such as faulty positioning; trauma from retractors; a tourniquet inflated for an inordinately long period, resulting in ischemia or pressure on peripheral nerves; or an improperly applied cast. Less common causes involve bleeding around the nerve or reaction to epinephrine.

Alternatives to Conventional Anesthesia

When local or regional anesthesia may be contraindicated but consciousness is desirable, acupuncture or hypnoanesthesia may offer alternative methods to control pain. An altered state of awareness of painful stimuli may be advantageous in selected patients.

Hypnosis

Hypnoanesthesia refers to hypnosis used as a method of anesthesia. Hypnosis produces a state of altered consciousness characterized by heightened suggestibility, selective wakefulness, reduced awareness, and restricted attentiveness. Although hypnosis has a long history of misuse, modern application by highly trained medical specialists is appropriate.

Hypnoanesthesia, although seldom used, has been successfully used in adult and pediatric patients. Motivation and concentration on the part of the patient are important factors. The method may be combined with the use of a small dose of a chemical anesthetic or muscle-relaxing drug. Hypnosis should not be used indiscriminately in place of standard treatment and is used as a therapeutic aid in selected patients in the following situations:

- When chemical agents are contraindicated (patient may be kept pain-free, asleep, or awake, without toxic side effects)
- As an adjunct to chemical anesthesia to decrease the amount of anesthesia needed
- When it is desirable to free the patient from certain neurophysical effects of an anesthetic
- When anxiety and fear of anesthesia are so great as to contribute to serious anesthetic risk
- When posthypnotic suggestion may be valuable in the postoperative period
- When it is desirable to raise the pain threshold
- When it is desirable to have the patient respond to questions or commands

Hypnoanesthesia is advantageous for changing burn dressings and debridement of wounds and for patients with severe respiratory or cardiovascular disease or multiple drug allergies. The anesthesia provider must establish rapport with the patient preoperatively so that the patient will listen to and obey hypnotic commands. Hypnosis is a time-consuming method and is unreliable compared with chemical anesthesia.

Acupuncture

The ancient Chinese art of acupuncture has been practiced for more than 5000 years. Its acceptance by Western medical practitioners is fairly recent. Acupuncture is a technique of providing intense stimulation at meridian points, or planes of energy referred to as *Chi* (Fig. 24.20). This stimulation prompts the brain to release endorphins and other chemicals that can relieve or block pain. Some meridians are associated with prevention of nausea and vomiting postoperatively. An example of Chi points in a meridian line for the lung is depicted in Fig. 24.21.

Stimulation is effected by manually rotating or applying electric current to very fine-gauge needles inserted into meridian points. When acupuncture is used for anesthesia, a minute electric

• **Fig. 24.20** Meridians for acupuncture.

• **Fig. 24.21** Example of Chi points in meridian line used in acupuncture for treatment of the left lung.

current is used to speed and enhance analgesia or anesthesia in the desired body region.

The meridian points generally correspond to the area where the somatic nerve supply is located. It is a time-consuming technique. It may be used immediately after premedication is given to reduce postoperative nausea and vomiting after short procedures with the patient under general anesthesia.

Acupuncture is gaining popularity in surgical and dental procedures and for postoperative or intractable pain. The patient remains conscious. Procedures are limited to use by physicians or qualified certified personnel under their direct supervision in keeping with acceptable standards of medical practice.

EVOLVE WEBSITE

http://evolve.elsevier.com/Hornacky/BerryKohn/
- Historical Perspectives
- Student Interactive Questions
- Glossary

References

1. Brockel M, Polaner D, Vemulakouda V: Anesthesia in the pediatric patient, *Urol Clin North Am* 45(4):551−560, 2018.
2. Gyorfi M, Kim P: Halothane toxicity. www.ncbi.nlm.nih.gov. Accessed July 18, 2023.
3. Malamed S. In *Sedation: a guide to patient management*, ed 6, St. Louis, MO, 2018, Elsevier, pp 605−620.
4. Tegegne S, Gebregzi A, Arefayne N: Deliberate hypotension as a mechanism to decrease intraoperative surgical site blood loss in resource limited setting: a systemic review and guideline, *Int J Surg Open* 29:55−65, 2021.
5. Solovitz A, Ivry S, Roner O: Man against the machine: differences in surgical risk evaluation. A cohort prospective study, *Int J Surg* 60:252−256, 2018.
6. Guideline Quick View: Local anesthesia, *AORN J* 109(1):138−140, 2019.

Bibliography

AORN: *Guidelines for perioperative practice*, Denver, CO, 2024, The Association.
Roberts J, Custalow C, Thompsen T: *Roberts and Hedges' clinical procedures in emergency medicine and acute care*, St. Louis, MO, 2019, Elsevier.
Sass E, Heiner J, Nagelhout J: *Nurse anesthesia*, ed 7, St. Louis, MO, 2023, Elsevier.

25

Coordinated Roles of the Scrub Person and the Circulating Nurse

CHAPTER OUTLINE

Division of Duties, 466

Efficiency of the Operating Room Team, 495

CHAPTER OBJECTIVES

After studying this chapter, the learner will be able to:

- Describe the activities of the scrub person.
- Describe the activities of the circulating nurse.
- Discuss the preliminary care of the patient by the circulating nurse.

- Differentiate between counting and being accountable for items used in patient care.

Division of Duties

The circulating nurse and the scrub person should plan their duties so that through coordination of efforts, the sterile and unsterile parts of the surgical procedure move along simultaneously. From the time the scrub person starts the surgical scrub until the surgical procedure is completed and dressings are applied, an invisible line separates the duties of the scrub person (Box 25.1) and the circulating nurse (Box 25.2), which neither person may cross. In this chapter, the duties of the two positions are listed separately, but a spirit of mutual cooperation is essential to move the schedule of surgical procedures efficiently and serve the best interests of the patient.

As a coordinated, systematic effort, the scrub person and the circulating nurse should complete the preparation of the environment as described in Chapter 12, whether it is for the first case of the day or for a subsequent case performed during the course of the day. Establishing a system for performance of roles and adhering to facility policy helps minimize the risk for human error.[1]

Both caregivers should double-check the needs for the procedure before the patient arrives at the room. Table 25.1 contains a systematic checklist of the case flow and case-related activities for the scrub person. Table 25.2 contains a systematic checklist of the case flow and patient care activities for the circulating nurse.

Setting Up the Room

Both the circulating nurse and the scrub person set up the room and position equipment. One suggested room arrangement is illustrated in Fig. 25.1. The case cart and the room furniture are checked by both people as a team. The duties and activities

change when the patient arrives at the room. The circulating nurse begins caring for the patient, and the scrub person continues readying the room. The following activities are performed together before the patient arrives:

1. Place a clean sheet, lift sheet, armboard covers, and safety straps on the operating room (OR) bed. Put a pressure-reducing mattress or gel pads on the OR bed if needed to relieve pressure during a long procedure. A warming or cooling blanket or air conduction system may be needed to heat or cool the patient during a long procedure. Obtain special equipment, such as OR bed attachments, pillows, or padding, needed to position and protect the patient.
2. Obtain appropriate patient monitoring equipment. Sequential compression devices may be indicated.
3. Obtain any specialized equipment that will be needed, such as an electrosurgical unit (ESU), smoke evacuator, sponge counting device (if available), suction apparatus, pneumatic tourniquet, laser, or operating microscope, and check/test each for proper function. Have the appropriate attachments and adjunctive supplies in the room.
4. Gather protective devices such as x-ray–protective gowns and/or lead screens and laser eyewear of the correct optical density as needed. If the C-arm will be used, place gonadal shielding under the bedsheet in the area of the patient's pelvis. The x-ray tube will be positioned under the OR bed and emanate upward.
5. Position the OR bed under the overhead spotlight fixture. Orient the head of the bed for anesthetic access according to the type of procedure to be performed. Patient positioning for some procedures requires the anesthesia provider to be located at the patient's side instead of at the head of the bed. Anesthesia personnel should be responsible for moving

• BOX 25.1   Role of the Scrub Person as Part of the Sterile Team

Prepares
- Sterile instruments and supplies
- Works in concert with the circulating nurse to set up the OR
- Surgeon's specific procedural needs
- Procedure-specific needs
- Hemostatic techniques
- Suture and closure materials

Sterile Technique
- Scrubs, gowns, and gloves using the closed gloving method
- Establishes the sterile field
- Facilitates the surgical procedure
- Anticipates the needs of the sterile team
- Gowns other team members using the open-assisted gowning and gloving technique

Adaptability
- Participates in preincision time out
- Remedies any breach of sterile technique
- Requests and prepares material needed by surgeon
- Keeps the sterile field neat and functional
- Act quickly in an emergency

Accountability
- Establishes baseline counts with circulating nurse
- Informs the circulating nurse of items placed inside patient
- Double-checks items dispensed to the sterile field
- Labels all medication containers and delivery devices
- Reports volume of drug administered to patient for documentation by circulating nurse

Safety
- Manages sharps
- Prevents retained foreign objects in the patient
- Reconciles counts and is accountable for items used in the surgical procedure

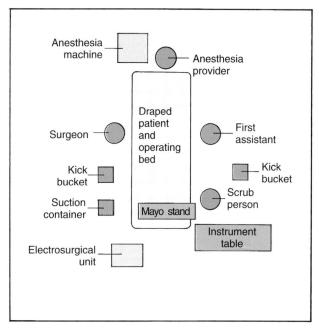

• **Fig. 25.1** Arrangement of the operating room showing sterile field, team members, and unsterile equipment.

the location of the surgeon at the OR bed and to that part of the patient's anatomy that will be encountered during the surgical procedure. The circulating nurse should know how to change the light bulb in case a bulb burns out during a procedure. Newer lights have replacement bulbs in place that activate if one bulb burns out.

7. Connect and check the suction between the receptacle canisters and the wall outlet to be certain suction functions at maximum vacuum. Some facilities use inline filters for specialized equipment. The filters are changed between cases. Gloves and personal protective equipment (PPE) are worn to prevent contact with harmful microorganisms when changing these filters.

8. Place a waterproof laundry bag or antistatic plastic bag in the laundry hamper frame for disposal of reusable woven fabric items.

9. Place appropriately marked receptacles in the room for safe disposal of biohazardous items, such as sharps, disposable drapes, or other biologically contaminated materials. Clean trash containers should be available for noncontaminated trash. Many hospitals do not have in-house incinerators and pay per the pound to have biohazard trash hauled away. Mixed clean and biohazard trash disposal is an unnecessary expense.

10. Line each kick bucket and wastebasket with an impervious plastic liner with a cuff turned over the edge.

11. Arrange furniture with those pieces that will be draped to become part of the sterile field at least 18 inches (45 cm) away from walls or cabinets. They should be kept side by side, away from the laundry hamper, trash container, anesthesia equipment, doors, and paths of traffic. Take emergencies into consideration. A clear path for the crash cart should be maintained at all times. If the patient will be positioned prone, a clear pathway for the transport cart will be needed. A transport cart should be immediately available outside the room to reposition the patient supine if an emergency arises.

the anesthesia equipment to the proper position. The hoses and connections should be checked each time the anesthesia machine is moved. The circulating nurse and scrub person are not trained in this checking procedure.

6. Test the overhead spotlights to check focus and intensity, and pre-position as much as possible. Do not leave the light turned on. The light should be positioned in relationship to

Indirect Patient Care
- Assists with OR preparation
- Opens sterile supplies
- Prepares medication for use in OR
- Maintains patient confidentiality
- Communicates with surgical services personnel
- Pretests equipment
- Plans postoperative care
- Initiates discharge planning

Direct Patient Care
- Patient identification
- Patient assessment
- Identifies correct surgical site
- Transfers patient between cart and bed
- Participates in preoperative time out procedure
- Assists the anesthesia provider
- Provides skin antisepsis
- Provides thermoregulation
- Prevents electrosurgical injury
- Collaborates with patient fluid intake and output
- Monitors vital signs as needed
- Provides dressings and drains

Coordinates
- Plans for each member of the sterile team to enter the sterile field
- Positioning, prepping, and draping
- Connection of surgical machinery
- Laboratory tests
- Multidisciplinary teams
- Diagnostic activities
- Emergency response to patient crisis
- Communication with patient's significant others

Anticipates
- Sequence of the procedure
- Needs of the sterile team
- Breaches of sterile technique
- Hemostatic needs

- Radiation (ionizing and nonionizing) protection for sterile team
- Potential for patient's physiologic changes
- Wound class at conclusion of the procedure
- Patient responses to care
- Significant other's response to patient's condition

Accountability
- Participates in time out
- Validates implants
- Documents patient care
- Specimen care and reporting
- Promotes a culture of safety
- Accountability for instruments, sponges, and sharps
- Patient's advocate
- Evaluates patient outcomes
- Provide handover report to perianesthesia nurse

12. If a case cart system is used, all or most of the needed supplies should be on the cart. Check the case cart sheet/inventory list to ascertain that everything is there and that the wrappings are intact. Position the case cart near the instrument table. Collect additional instruments and supplies according to the preference card or case cart sheet and from cabinets in the room or from another supply area within the OR suite.
13. Obtain an appropriate set of sterile, wrapped instruments from one of the cart shelves and place on top of the case cart. Some facilities use ring stands for opening instrument trays.
14. Place the sterile, wrapped drape pack (or custom pack) on the instrument table so that when opened, the wrapper will adequately drape the table and the drapes will be in their proper place. Open the drape pack first to establish a sterile place to open other sterile items. A splash basin can be opened onto the field near the working end as a catch basin for opening small packages. If a metal basin is used, do not open metal items or blades into the basin. The metal-on-metal strikes can cause damage to honed surfaces and cause free fragments that could end up in patient tissues.
15. Select the correct size gloves and gowns for each member of the sterile team. A prep table can be opened as a sterile gown table. The extra gloves for double-gloving can be opened onto the sterile table.
16. Select the initial sutures to have ready for the surgeon. Open only those needed to begin the case, such as free ties or stick ties. These can be opened into the sterile basin on the main field near the working end of the table. Place unopened but probably needed sutures on top of the case cart for opening as the case progresses.
17. Open the instrument set. If it is a wrapped set, open the wrapper on top of the case cart or ring stand. If the instrument set is in a closed container, open the container by lifting the lid straight up and tilted back toward your body. Do not open any supplies into a rigid instrument container because the edges are not considered sterile.

TABLE 25.1   Systematic Activities for the Scrub Person

Baseline Systematic Activity	Systematic Critical Thinking Activity
Room Setup	
• Plan for patient to enter the room without contaminating the setup. • Plan for position of patient, surgeon, and anesthesia provider.	Determine the position of the surgeon and preference for positioning of the scrub person before setting up table.
Case Cart Contents	
• Instrument set(s) • Custom pack • Gowns • Sterile towels • Prep supplies • Additional soft goods	Check cart contents. Inspect package integrity. Additional instruments may be needed (long instruments). Check for each item listed on case cart sheet. Record preference changes on case cart sheet for computer update.
Items to Have Available	
• Suture • Sponges • Pack of towels • Gloves • Staplers • Dressing	Have extra preferred suture in the room. Extra sponges may be needed.
Table Setup	
• Open the main custom drape pack. The outer wrapper is the sterile table drape. • Determine which part of the table will be closest to the draped patient and establish this area as the working end of the table. Sharps and sutures should be opened onto this location. • Open remaining items into a position of function. Inspect package integrity. • Do not open items into closed container system. Edges are unsterile. • Don eyewear. • Open gown and gloves for self before performing hand and arm cleansing. • Don gown and gloves using closed glove procedure. Remember to tie in. • Set up the working end of the table according to position of patient. • Plan to pass off cords in one direction. • Sterile marker and labels are placed on the sterile instrument table near the working end. • Place items once. Do not leave trash on the field.	The surgical site on the patient establishes the level of the sterile field. Stack drapes in order of use and place away from main instrument setup area of sterile table. Create towel roll(s) for instrument stringers. Align stringer on the roll with shortest instruments closest to the working end of the table. Instrument ratchets are open on the table and closed on the Mayo stand. Establish baseline: Count instruments, sharps, and sponges with circulating nurse. Plan for exchange of scalpel by no touch technique.
Mayo Stand Setup	
• Drape the Mayo stand. Cover surface with one unfolded towel to protect from perforation by sharps. A towel roll can be used to organize instruments on the Mayo stand.	Mayo setup: 2 scalpels, 3 scissors (1 curved and 1 straight Mayo and 1 Metzenbaum), 4 curved Crile hemostats, 2 medium pickups, 4 Allis forceps, and 2 small skin retractors (Army Navy). 2 Light handles, suction tubing and suction tip (Yankauer), electrosurgical unit (ESU) pencil and holder, tip cleaner, and sponges.
Medication and/or Chemicals on the Sterile Instrument Table	
• Place medication cups near edge of field. • Validate all medications and solutions with circulating nurse and then apply labels.	Label syringes and administration devices after the solution or medication has been dispensed to the field. Do not label ahead of time because the wrong drug or solution could be poured. Label states name of product and percent.
Irrigation and Fluids on the Sterile Instrument Table	
• Place basins near edge of sterile field. Label is applied after the solution is poured. • Label all delivery devices.	Normal saline or other solution for irrigation. Sterile water for instrumentation.
Patient Positioning	
• Stand clear and remain sterile because positioning is a nonsterile activity.	Note the presence of safety restraints and padding as the second set of eyes. Drapes and blankets can obscure safety straps.
Team Gowning	
• Assist team to gown and glove using the open-assisted or closed-assisted method. • Contaminated gloves are changed using the open method. Circulating nurse will remove contaminated gloves. Scrub person will reglove the individual.	Do not pass any towels or gowns from the sterile field during the procedure. Biologic contamination is present.

Continued

Systematic Activities for the Circulating Nurse—cont'd

TABLE 25.1

Baseline Systematic Activity	Systematic Critical Thinking Activity
Patient Draping	
• Prep solution must be completely dry. • Patient is draped to establish the level of the sterile surgical field before instrument tables are positioned for use.	Some surgeons use towel clips to secure drapes. Nonperforating styles are preferred. Some surgeons suture or staple specialty drapes in place.
Procedure Start and Flow	
• Position Mayo stand. • Position sterile instrument table. • Hand off ESU cords, tubing, and cables to circulating nurse. • Apply light handles.	Initiate time out before skin scalpel is provided. • Correct patient • Correct site • Correct procedure • Correct supplies/implants
• Two sponges on field adjacent to incision. • Provide scalpel for skin (place skin knife aside on working end immediately after use; disarm and reload as time permits). • Provide ESU for hemostasis (keep in holder when not in use). • Clean the ESU pencil tip. • Keep instrumentation free of debris with moist sponge. • Trade one-for-one sponges and needles. • Open soiled sponges completely before discarding into sponge bucket.	Inform circulating nurse if any uncounted item has been brought into the surgical field. Reconcile all counts by starting at the patient and working toward Mayo stand and then to instrument table. Count sponges and sharps at each cavity within cavity closure. Do closing counts of sponges, sharps, and instruments during surgical site closure. Contain pathology specimen in closed container as possible before passing to gloved circulating nurse.
Dressings and Drains	
• Double-check type of dressing material before circulating nurse dispenses to field. • Dressing is placed over surgical site after incision is cleaned. • Disconnect tubing and cords from field. • Drapes are removed by rolling them off and away from the patient after placement of the surgical site dressing.	Wet sponge followed by dry sponge to clean closed incision. Wound closure strips may be placed over subcuticular closure. Dressing is positioned over cleaned incision before removal of drapes. Skin surrounding the dressing area is cleaned with wet and dry sponges before tape is applied.
Procedure Completion	
• All reusable instruments are opened or disassembled and placed in bins for decontamination in the processing area. Enzyme solution or foam may be applied before transit.	Remove the Bovie tip and place in sharps container. Disarm scalpels. Open all instrument ratchets and box locks and place in mesh tray.
Room Breakdown	**Trash Disposal**
• When patient leaves the room, the table can be broken down completely. • Dispose of sharps in sharps container. • Remove light handles. • Case cart is reloaded with used instrument trays and reusable equipment. • Don examination gloves after removing gown and gloves and washing hands. • Transport the case cart to the processing area.	Dispose of biologic trash in biohazard containers. Dispose of clean trash in regular garbage receptacle. Dispose of linens in hampers. Remove contaminated gown first followed by gloves using peel-off glove-to-glove—skin-to-skin method. Wash hands with soap and water after removing gloves. Clean all case-specific equipment with antiseptic and return to storage.

Systematic Activities for the Circulating Nurse

TABLE 25.2

Baseline Systematic Activity for All Cases	Systematic Patient Care
Patient Assessment and Safety	
• Assess for patient identity and correct site information concerning the planned procedure. Note the presence of correct site markings. • Assess physiologic and psychologic status. • Laboratory work • Current medications and herbals • Allergies and sensitivities • Last intake by mouth • Location of family or significant other	Talk to the patient and determine understanding of the procedure. Observe surgeon's initials on surgical site. Follow facility policy concerning hard-to-mark sites. Check the paperwork/chart/computer for consents, tests, and family/significant other contact information. Check for radiographs, digital information, or scans for use during the procedure. Consult with anesthesia provider and surgeon for information exchange.
Room Setup	
• Ensure a clear path for emergency equipment. • Plan for adequate positioning of the anesthesia provider. • Check the OR bed for correct position. • Make sure lights are in working order.	All necessary positioning aids are available. Plan for entrance of patient without impeding the process of setup or contamination. Plan setup for position of instrument table in relation to surgical field.

TABLE 25.2 Systematic Activities for the Circulating Nurse—cont'd

Baseline Systematic Activity for All Cases	Systematic Patient Care
Standard Room Equipment	
• Appropriate OR bed with armboards • Patient transfer device • Sequential compression device • Two IV poles • Patient-warming device	Check equipment (suction and ESU) for proper function. Place equipment in a position of function. Plan for cords and tubing to be passed off in one direction. Avoid having cords and cables as "trip hazards" if lights are lowered for endoscopy or other procedure in which the lighting is changed. Some facilities use green room lighting for endoscopic cases.
• Mayo stand • Instrument table • Prep stand • Monopolar ESU and dispersive electrode • Suction collection apparatus • Platform steps for team	
Case Cart Contents	
• Instrument set(s) • Custom pack • Gowns • Sterile towels • Prep supplies • Additional soft goods	Check cart contents. Inspect package integrity. Check for each item listed on case cart sheet. Record preference changes on case cart sheet for computer update.
Items to have Available	
• Suture • Sponges • Sterile towels • Gloves • Staplers • Dressings • Speciality items and implants	Have a few sizes available. Only open if necessary. Charge only for items used.
Table Setup	
• Place packs to be opened on clean dry table surface. • Do not open items into closed container system. Edges are unsterile. • Open adequate gowns and gloves for surgeon and first assistant. • Tie gowns of team. • If blades are opened separately, inform scrub person of location on the field.	Open sterile packs in a position of function. Establish and document baseline: Count instruments, sharps, and sponges with scrub person. Provide additional sterile supplies as needed by scrub person.
Medication and/or Chemicals on the Sterile Field	
• Obtain medications and/or chemicals for sterile field using patient identification number. • Dispense medications without aerosolization. • Draw up with needle and syringe. Remove needle before delivering drug to field.	Validate medication type, expiration date, and dose with the scrub person. Validate total amount given and administered. Charge only for drugs used on sterile field.
Irrigation on the Sterile Field	
• Obtain solutions of appropriate temperature for sterile field. • Dispense solutions without aerosolization. Pour in one continuous motion.	Dispense normal saline or other isotonic solution to the field after verifying the date, name, and seal integrity. Do not recap bottles unless saved for nonsterile use. Remaining solution can be used to clean the patient after the dressing is applied and drapes are removed.
Assisting the Anesthesia Provider	
• Assist with positioning during regional anesthesia. • Stand at patient's side during induction of general anesthesia, provide emotional support.	Help anesthesia personnel with IV or intubation if needed. Prepare to apply cricoid pressure as needed during intubation.
Patient Positioning	
• Don nonsterile gloves. • Provide positioning devices as appropriate. • Adequate exposure of surgical site • Appropriate safety restraints • Apply dispersive electrode after patient is positioned. Do not cut or reapply.	The anesthesia provider will indicate when it is safe to start positioning and prepping. The anesthesia provider and surgeon will determine the appropriate safe position for the surgical procedure.

Continued

TABLE 25.2	Systematic Activities for the Circulating Nurse—cont'd	
Baseline Systematic Activity for All Cases	**Systematic Patient Care**
Skin Prep: Determine Patient Potential for Skin Sensitivity	
• One-step • Two-step	Open and set up appropriate skin prep materials. Alcohol-based preps can be a fire hazard if fumes accumulate under drapes. Expose the surgical site without undue exposure. Protect nontarget areas from pooling. Drapes should not be applied until prep has dried completely.
Procedural Positioning of Equipment and Team	
• Assist scrub person to move sterile table adjacent to surgical field. • Attach cords, cables, and tubing to appropriate devices. • Place suction canister in direct view of anesthesia provider. • Provide standing platforms/steps as needed.	Scrub person will hand off cords and cables in one direction. Determine machine settings per surgeon. Scrub person will place sterile Mayo stand over sterile field.
Procedure Start and Flow	**Documentation**
• Initiate the time out, verifying the patient name, procedure, and correct site. • Prepare specimens for pathology. • Communicate with family or significant other within acceptable parameters for patient privacy.	• Procedural times and time out • Additional items not in the baseline count added to field or placed in patient • Ensure that all implants, scans, and procedure-specific items are present before the procedure is started. Validate these items during the time out process and document on the surgical checklist. • Handle specimen containers wearing examination gloves. • Family/significant other updates as appropriate.
Dressings and Drains	
• Dispense dressing materials to sterile field at end of procedure. • Don nonsterile gloves to clean skin edges after patient is undraped. • Tape dressings. Avoid affixing to hairy surface.	One-step prep should not be removed.
Procedure Completion	
• Reconcile closing count with scrub person. Begin count from surgical field on patient to Mayo stand to instrument table. Sponges in sponge bucket are counted in increments of size and initial packaging amounts. • Prepare handover report for postprocedural area nursing staff. • Transport patient to postprocedural area with anesthesia provider.	Give handover report to RN in postprocedural area. • Patient name and age • Allergies or sensitivities • Current procedure and type of anesthesia • Location of incisions, dressings, and drains • Special needs (language, vision, hearing) • Location of family or significant other • Any procedure-specific information • Pertinent comorbidity

Opening Sterile Supplies

The doors to the room should be shut to maintain positive pressure, and each team member present should be wearing appropriate OR attire for the restricted area. Before any sterile supplies are opened, the integrity of each package must be checked for tears and watermarks. If either is present, the package is unsafe to use. The external chemical process monitor should be checked to validate that the package has been through a completed sterilization process. Open packages as follows:

1. Remove tape from packages wrapped in woven fabric wrappers. Laundry machinery can be damaged by wads of tape becoming lodged in the mechanisms. The tape should be opened by breaking the seal on paper or nonwoven material. Removing tape strips from paper-wrapped items increases the risk for tearing the wrapper and exposing the contents to contamination. Check the external chemical indicator tape to be certain the item has been exposed to a sterilization process.

PROS/CONS

Reliance on Scanners and Machines to Validate Sponge and Instrument Counts

Pros

• Computer-assisted handheld counting devices using barcodes tagged with radiofrequency identification (RFID) aid in verifying the manual sponge count. Some facilities also use this technology for instruments. Sponges are the most commonly retained surgical item.
• The scanners are easy to use with proper training and standard operating protocols. Staff members are held accountable by live demonstration and competency on how to use the new technology.

• Every sponge or instrument has an individual barcode/RFID and number making it easy to detect if an item is missing. Scanning sponges and instruments takes place before the start of a case and before wound closure. Instrument trays may have RFID tags that identify the tray location. Individual instruments may have their own individual tag. RFID systems can scan multiple instruments on a sterile field at one time
• In the case of a missing item, the staff at the field has the opportunity to look for it before wound closure; the circulating nurse can check the

Continued

Reliance on Scanners and Machines to Validate Sponge and Instrument Counts

floor, trash cans, or any other unsterile area around the sterile field. Any missing item must be accounted for before the closure of the surgical wound.
- Some scanning systems provide a wand device that can be passed over the patient's body to validate the absence of a retained item before the patient leaves the room.
- Some scanning systems provide permanent documentation of the counting process.
- Assistive technology has the potential to reduce hospital litigation expenses, unreimbursed surgery, surgical delays, and radiation exposure.
- The technology lowers the risk for retained items with the computerized system.

Cons
- During a manual sponge count the paper band should be broken; the sponges should be individually separated from the packed set, counted, and placed on the back table. Scanning the band and fanning the sponges is not an acceptable form of counting.
- Plain radiography is used to locate a retained sponge or instrument. It has a false-negative rate despite the radiopaque marker.
- Counting is not foolproof. Human errors in arithmetic are a cause for inaccurate counts.
- Risk factors for discrepancies in sponge or instrument counts include open procedures, trauma, failure to follow the counting policy, distractions, multitasking, shift change, additional items opened during a case, and poor communication.

- The scanning system can be labor intensive and expensive. The purchase of the equipment, radiopaque sponges, and staff education and training can be costly.
- Reliance on scanning systems should not replace human intervention and common sense. Using counted sponges after the final scanned count can result in a retained sponge.
- Individual variation in counting, timing of counts, poor documentation, communication breakdown, and interpretation of policy can result in counting errors.
- Standardized count policies must be specific to when counts are done, explain the method of counting, and define where to start the count. The policy should contain information for shift changes, emergencies, broken equipment, and what to do if there is a sponge or instrument count discrepancy.
- Reeducation of current standards ensures better patient outcomes.

References
1. Surgical tool tracking with RFID. www.solution.murata.com. Accessed April 26, 2023.
2. U.S. Food and Drug Administration: *Unique device identification system (UDI system)*. www.fda.gov. Accessed April 26, 2023.
3. Aboelmaged M, Hashem G: RFID application in patient and medical asset operations management: a technology, organizational and environmental (TOE) perspective into key enablers and impediments, *Int J Med Inform* 118:58–64, 2018.
4. AORN: *Guidelines for perioperative practice*, Denver, CO, 2024, The Association.

2. Open the drape pack, instrument set, and gown pack on their own individual surfaces so that the inside of each inner wrapper becomes a sterile table cover.

For an envelope-folded wrapper, open the first flap of the wrapper away from yourself. The area touched falls below table level, and the inside of the wrapper remains sterile. Each flap will look triangular. Do not reach over the inside of the sterile table cover or contents of the pack. Pull open each side by pulling the side flaps open, one at a time. Lift the final edge of the wrapper toward you to complete the opening of the sterile field.

For a square side-folded wrapper, open one side, followed by the other side, in a sideways motion so both sides are over the edge of the table. The front and back flaps can be difficult. Both team members should do this step together—one person stands on one side of the table, and the second person stands on the opposite side. Each (simultaneously) grasps a lower edge of both the front and back flaps and opens both flaps together to complete the opening of the pack.

For a square front-back–folded wrapper, the steps for the envelope fold are followed in the same sequences. Each flap will look square. The final square flap will be brought toward your body to create the field (Fig. 25.2).

a. If packs or sets have sequential double wrappers, both layers are opened by the person opening supplies by following the same sequences twice. The outer wrapper is considered the dust cover and the inner wrapper the sterile barrier. The person opening the inner wrapper need not be sterile.

b. Open other packages, such as sponges, gloves, and sutures, maintaining a sterile transfer to the appropriate sterile table. Touch only the outside of the outer wrapper. Avoid reaching over sterile contents and the sterile table. Enclose your hand in the wrapper to the extent possible. Do not slide the inner package over the edge of the peel-pack pouch. Sutures and blades should be opened onto the working edge of the table. Always open blades to the same spot for safety and consistency.

c. If small peel packages are sequentially double-wrapped (i.e., a peel package inside a peel package), only the outer wrapper is removed. Usually the inner wrapper contains several smaller parts that may accidentally fall off the table when dispensed.

d. Instruments processed in rigid, closed container systems are opened by breaking the seal on the sides of the lid and raising it up and away from the tray. The inner basket of instruments is considered sterile, but the container itself is not. Sterile soft goods, sutures, and other individually wrapped items should not be opened into this pan because the edges are not considered sterile.

e. If a sterile package is dropped, the item may be considered safe for immediate use only if it is double-wrapped in an impervious material and the integrity of the package is maintained. Both wrappers should be removed to dispense the item to the sterile field.

f. Mechanical items such as staplers and endoscopic trocars should not be flipped onto the field. The mechanisms can be damaged and may malfunction when used in patient care. Do not open these items until a sterile team member can take them directly from the inner aspect of the package immediately before use. These items should be opened last and extracted from the packaging by the scrub person.

g. Blades should be opened on the working end of the sterile field. The scrub person should be aware of exactly where these are opened. Do not open other items near the blades.

• **Fig. 25.2** Opening square-fold sterile pack. Wrapper is lifted back while keeping hands on the outside. Hands are in folded cuff to avoid contaminating contents of pack. Area touched falls below unsterile table level; sterile inside of wrapper (now table cover) remains sterile.

Do not open blades into metal basins. This dulls the cutting surface. This location should be standardized for systematic safety for the scrub person.

3. The gown and gloves for the scrub person are opened on the Mayo stand or small table separate from the main sterile field. The person establishing the sterile field should not gown and glove from the main field because the risk for contamination is higher than gowning and gloving from a separate surface. The scrub person should glove using the closed gloving method for the first glove layer in double gloving. The outer glove can be applied from the separate table or the main field.
4. The circulating nurse assists the anesthesia provider with patient care preparations if needed as the scrub person sets up the sterile field after scrubbing, gowning, and gloving. If the patient has arrived at the room, the circulating nurse can do the initial assessment and patient check-in.

Scrub Person Duties

When all supplies have been obtained and opened and the room is ready for the patient's arrival, the scrub person prepares for the surgeon's arrival. At all times, the integrity of the sterile field is closely monitored. The principles of aseptic and sterile techniques are followed.

Preparation of the Sterile Field

The gown and gloves are open and ready on a surface separate from the sterile field before the scrub person performs surgical hand hygiene. The scrub person, wearing a mask, dons protective eyewear with side shields and performs a complete surgical hand cleansing according to the facility procedure.

Gown and Glove Using the Closed Gloving Method

If double-gloving, wear gloves one size larger as the first layer and the usual size gloves as the second pair. The larger size underneath provides an air pocket and helps prevent a sensation of tightness around the hands. If hypoallergenic gloves are worn, these should be donned as the first pair, with generic sterile gloves worn as the outside pair. Most facilities no longer use powdered gloves; however, if powdered gloves are used, wipe any powder from gloves with a moist sponge before handling drapes, instruments, and other sterile items. This sponge should be completely opened and dropped into the sponge bucket as part of the count.

When establishing the main sterile field, drape unsterile tables according to the standard departmental setup procedure with drapes from the drape pack. Most facilities will consider the outer wrap of the custom pack as the main sterile table cover. The scrub person may need to drape and set a small table for the patient's skin prep, but more commonly the circulating nurse opens and prepares a disposable or prepackaged prep tray for each surgical site if more than one incision is planned. A second instrument table may be needed for extensive surgical procedures or special types of instrumentation (e.g., tables for preparation of an implant or organ for transplant).

When draping an unsterile table with a separate sterile table drape, unfold it toward yourself to cover the front edge of the unsterile table first; this minimizes the possibility of self-contamination from the edge of the table. Unfold the remainder of the sterile table drape over the surface of the table and away from yourself. The edges are allowed to fall over the ends of the table and are considered contaminated below the tabletop. Avoid leaning over the table.

Place the remaining contents of the drape pack on a corner of the instrument table. Place them once—do not keep moving things from one side to another. Custom packs usually contain disposable supplies that are nested within each other and require minimal handling when setting up the field. Reusable woven fabric drapes may be arranged within the drape pack according to the size or direction of the folds. A standard number of each item is contained within a drape pack. A list of items and their numbers is usually affixed to the outer surface of the pack. The basic drape pack usually contains, at a minimum, the following items:

- One Mayo stand cover
- Four to eight towels
- Two to four medium drape sheets (optional)
- One fenestrated sheet

Draping the Mayo Stand

When draping the Mayo stand, drape both the frame and the tray. The Mayo stand cover is like a long plastic pillowcase with a single sheet of nonwoven fabric that will lie on the flat surface that will hold instruments. It is fan-folded with a wide cuff to protect gloved hands. With hands in the cuff, support the folds of the drape on the arms, in the bend of the elbows, to prevent it from falling below waist level (Fig. 25.3). While sliding the cover on the Mayo stand, place a foot on the base of the stand to stabilize it

• **Fig. 25.3** Starting to drape Mayo stand. Scrub person's hands are protected in cuff of drape. Folds of drape are supported on arms, in bend of elbows, to prevent their falling below waist level. Foot is placed on base of stand to stabilize it.

• **Fig. 25.4** Completing draping of Mayo stand. Hands are protected in cuffs.

(Fig. 25.4). Some sterile custom packs contain an impervious plastic disposable Mayo tray as the bottom layer of the pack. At some facilities, a stainless steel Mayo tray is wrapped snugly and sterilized separately. The tray can be set into the draped Mayo stand or placed on the working end of a Mayfield overbed table.

Basin Setup

If reusable basin sets are used, leave the large solution basin in the ring stand and take the remainder of the basins to the instrument table. The wrapper on the basin set serves as the cover for the ring stand with the large basin. Fabric or paper towels separate the basins. The fabric towels can be folded and placed on the stack of towels on the sterile field. They can be used for wiping instruments or cleaning the patient at the end of the procedure. Many facilities consider all towels as counted items.

Many facilities have discontinued the use of ring stands because they are usually lower than the established sterile field (i.e., the instrument table and the draped OR bed). The use of basins as splash basins is discouraged, but a few surgeons still prefer to use them to wash their gloved hands at the start of the case or during the case as blood and debris accumulate on glove surfaces.

If powdered gloves are used, the splash basin is not highly effective for powder removal because the powder redeposits on the gloves as the hand is withdrawn from the water. If basins are used for this purpose, the circulating nurse should fill them with sterile normal saline or sterile water and remove them from use when the water is grossly dirty. Each time someone rinses their gloves in the basin, debris can be transferred back to the patient, causing foreign body granulomas. Standing water can collect microorganisms from the air and encourage an infection.

The preferred methods for removing powder or blood from gloves is either to use a sterile towel or sponge moistened with sterile saline or to pour sterile saline or sterile water directly over the gloved hands. The basin should not be permitted to sit after being used to rinse glove powder; it should be emptied into the dirty sink in the utility room by the circulating nurse. Any counted sponge should be unfolded and dropped into the sponge bucket for counting.

Some facilities use the large solution basin directly on the sterile field to collect and rinse used instruments. Only distilled sterile water should be used for this purpose because saline is corrosive. Disposable custom packs usually contain plastic basins that can remain on the sterile instrument table.

Separate 1 or 2-liter–sized basins are arranged close to the working edge of the instrument table for holding sterile warm irrigation solution (usually Ringer's lactate or normal saline), for securing the specimen after it is procured, and for moistening sponges.

All basins, containers, and delivery devices should be clearly labeled to identify their contents. The practice of dipping sponges into the irrigation solution should be discouraged because this releases lint into the solution, which in turn can be introduced into the patient during irrigation. Lint can contribute to foreign body reactions and granulomas in the tissues of the patient. An Asepto syringe can be used to moisten sponges with warm saline in their own basin. The runoff should not be used as irrigation.

The basin set also may contain solution cups for the skin prep table and/or a basin specifically intended for trash (waste suture packaging) disposal. Attaching a trash bag to the side of the table compromises the sterility of the field because the bag hangs lower than the sterile table surface. If these bags are used, the inside is not considered sterile because it is below the level of the sterile field. These bags can be hazardous if a needle becomes ensnared in the suture debris and perforates the thin exterior surface of the bag. It could puncture the scrub person during handling. Do not reach into the bag at any time. The use of empty suture packets from the trash is not an appropriate method of accounting for needles during the count.

Arranging the Instrument Table

Arrange other instruments and items on the instrument table (Fig. 25.5). Table 25.3 describes the "Eight Ps" of table and room organization, which can help the scrub person and circulating nurse improve the efficiency of the setup procedure and the case flow.

The instruments for each surgical procedure are selected and placed according to standard basic sets and the preferences of the surgeon. Instruments of suitable size, shape, strength, and function are needed for each step of the surgical procedure. The styles and numbers of instruments are dictated by the type of surgical procedure. Standardization of instrument sets is cost-effective and supports the use of a system for counting and accounting for instruments during the procedure.

Arranging the Mayo Stand

Arrange the instruments and accessory items needed to create the primary incision and control initial bleeders on the Mayo stand. A

• **Fig. 25.5** Example of basic instrument table setup. Contents will vary according to the type of surgical procedure.

TABLE 25.3	The "Eight Ps" of Operating Room and Sterile Field Setup and Management		
The Eight "Ps" to Consider When Preparing for a Surgical Procedure[a]	Environment Considerations for the Circulating Nurse	Sterile Field Considerations for the Scrub Person	
Proper Placement			
Items should be placed so they will not need to be moved during the procedure.	Suction canisters, tourniquet, and the electrosurgical unit (ESU) need to be stationary. The OR lights should be directed toward the field.	The Mayo stand and instrument table should not be moved during the procedure. Drapes may not be moved on the patient's skin.	
Proper Function			
Items should be tested for safety and usefulness before they are needed, to prevent delay in the case.	Test the ESU, tourniquet, laser, and other equipment before the patient enters the room.	Test the efficiency of instruments (e.g., scissors, needle holders, clamps) as they are needed.	
Place it Once			
Items should not be manipulated during the procedure. Energy and attention should not be diverted to resetting the field.	The OR bed should be in the right place for the procedure. The dispersive electrode should not be moved or displaced.	When setting up the field, each item (e.g., a basin) should be placed where it will be used during the procedure with minimal handling.	
Point of Contact			
Items used within the field could cause harm or be rendered useless if they do not reach the intended point of contact.	The circulating nurse should evaluate the delivery of items to the sterile field. Some items (e.g., staplers) should be handed; others can be transferred in other ways.	The scrub person should be aware of the passing of instruments and how they are securely placed in the waiting hand of the surgeon or first assistant.	
Position of Function			
Items should be positioned so they will be usable during the procedure.	The use of a C-arm, laser with articulating arm, or microscope should be preplanned so they may be positioned while the procedure is in progress.	When passing instruments, they should be placed in the surgeon's hand in a usable way. For example, the curve of the instrument should match the curve of the hand.	
Point of Use			
Items should be as close to the area of use as possible.	Pour solutions directly into the basins; open and hand sponges or sutures directly to the scrub person as they are needed.	Basins should be placed close to the edge of the table so the circulating nurse can pour without requiring the basin to be repositioned. The ESU pencil holder should be close to the field for safe containment of the tip.	

TABLE 25.3   Systematic Activities for the Circulating Nurse—cont'd

The Eight "Ps" to Consider When Preparing for a Surgical Procedure[a]	Environment Considerations for the Circulating Nurse	Sterile Field Considerations for the Scrub Person
Protected Parts		
Items and surfaces should be rendered safe for the patient and the team.	Cords, cables, and tubing should be secured and appropriately directed away from the field. Pad the OR bed and patient as appropriate. Use safety belts.	Apply jaw liners to instruments during setup. Hand instruments with care to avoid causing injury with the tip or sharp surface. Do not lay items on or against the patient's body.
Perfect Picture		
Items within and around the field should not be at risk for causing harm or becoming damaged. The environment should not be cluttered.	The entire room should appear neat and tidy. The door should be closed, and the temperature and humidity should be appropriate. Forethought to having a clear path for the crash cart or setup emergency equipment is essential.	The sterile field should remain neat and orderly, with instruments and supplies within easy sight and reach. Consistency fosters a sense of comfort and confidence in the scrub role.

[a]The examples used for each "P" will vary according to the type of procedure and equipment, the position of the patient, and the surgeon's preference. The Eight Ps apply to both the scrub person and the circulating nurse.

• **Fig. 25.6** Example of setup for Mayo stand.

few of each classification of instruments and sponges may be put on the Mayo stand initially. If a local anesthetic will be used, one or two labeled syringes with appropriate size hypodermic needles also are needed.

One possible setup of the Mayo stand is illustrated in Fig. 25.6. As the surgical procedure progresses, additional instruments and supplies can be added or deleted as necessary. Long-handled forceps and clamps and deep retractors can be substituted for those used on superficial structures.

The Mayo stand should be kept neat throughout the surgical procedure. Do not overload it with sponges and sharps. The needle counting magnet or box should not be kept on the Mayo stand because it is easily bumped during the procedure and could

discharge needles into the surgical field. No one should reach over and take things off the Mayo stand. This can cause instruments to fall.

Establishing Baselines

The scrub person should count sponges, surgical needles, other sharps, and instruments with the circulating nurse according to established facility policy and procedure. After completing the initial baseline count with the circulating nurse, a few appropriate size sponges for the initial incision are placed on the Mayo stand. Many different types of precounted sponges and special towels are available (Box 25.3). The gauze sponges may be opened to their full length or left folded. Fix two or three sponges on sponge

Sponges are packaged in increments of 5 or 10 and are embedded with a radiopaque strip. The incremental complement is bound with a paper band or wound onto a cardboard holder or Styrofoam holder. Towels can be specially packed in counted increments for use within the body as retractor padding or as a visceral retainer.

1. Raytec or Raytex with embedded radiopaque string 10 per pack (aka: 4 × 4s, 4 × 8s, pusher, gauze sponge).
2. Laparotomy sponge (with radiopaque loop or strip) 5 per pack (aka: lap tape, lap sponge, lap pad) available in sizes 4 × 8, 12 × 12, 8 × 36, 18 × 18, 8 × 108.
3. Tonsil sponges with long radiopaque string: 5 per pack (aka: tampon) available in small, medium, and large. Available without the string. Radiopaque element is embedded within the fabric of the sponge.
4. Cottonoids with radiopaque strings: 10 per pack (aka: patties or neuro sponges). Some facilities refer to cottonoids by their size in length in inches (i.e., ¼, ½, 1, 2, or 3).
5. Peanuts with embedded radiopaque element: 5 per pack (aka: pusher, cherry, or dissector).
6. Kittner tightly wound dental tape with embedded radiopaque element: 5 per pack (aka: dissector).
7. Surgical towels with radiopaque element in blue or white. Commercially packaged in counted increments of 3 or 5. Not used as drapes.

forceps (if these will be used), but leave the forceps on the instrument table. Sponges and counting procedures/technology are discussed later in this chapter.

Managing Sharps
After completing the baseline counts with the circulating nurse, the scrub person should secure surgical needles and all other sharps, including knife blades. Blades should be opened onto a consistent spot on the field that is agreed upon by everyone who scrubs and circulates. This will help avoid inadvertent cuts to the fingers of the scrub person, who may be unaware of where blades have been opened onto the field.

Surgical needles and sharps should never be loose on the Mayo stand. If eyed reusable needles are used, each needle must be inspected for cleanliness, burrs, and integrity of the eye before threading. Disposable needles are preferred.

Loading Scalpels
Put blades on knife handles. To avoid injury, always use a heavy instrument, such as a Kelly or Pean clamp, to attach the blade; never use the fingers. Avoid using a needle holder because this can weaken the jaws and damage the needle-holding surface. Holding the cutting edge down and away from the eyes and other personnel in the room, grasp the widest and strongest part of the blade above the notch with the heavy clamp, and slip the blade into the groove on the knife handle. A click indicates the blade is in place. To prevent damage to the blade, the instrument should not touch the cutting edge of the blade (Fig. 25.7).

Scalpels should be loaded early in the setup procedure. This is a good habit to acquire because in emergency surgery the surgeon could be opening the patient while the setup ensues. Time can mean a patient's life. The counting process is handled differently during emergency life-and-death procedures and is sometimes aborted in favor of an x-ray.

• **Fig. 25.7** Putting scalpel blade on knife handle. To avoid injury, always use an instrument; never use fingers. The blade is attached with a heavy instrument. Grasp blade at its widest, strongest part, and slip it into groove on handle. The handle and blade are pointed down and away from eyes and other personnel.

Preparing Sutures and Ties for Use
Prepare sutures in the sequence in which the surgeon will use them. The surgeon may ligate (tie off) large blood vessels with a suture ligature shortly after the incision is made, unless electrosurgery is preferred to seal vessels. Prepare ligatures (free ties) first if they will be used. Remove suture material from the packet unless the packet is designed for single-strand dispensing. When trimming the ties to size, work over the instrument table and hold onto the ends of the suture material to prevent strands from dropping over the edge of the table and thus becoming contaminated.

Dispensing reels, relay packets, or strands of ligating material can be placed in a fan-folded towel, with the ends extended far enough for rapid extraction. Place the largest size in the bottom layer along the fold that is farthest away when placed on the Mayo stand or the working end of the instrument table. The next smaller size is placed in the next layer so that the ends are not overriding those below; if three sizes are prepared, the medium size can be placed midway between the other two. The smallest size will be along the closest fold. To prevent possible contamination, strands are pulled out toward the surgical field, never away from it.

A few packets of suture may be opened and prepared for suturing. Seldom is it necessary to prepare large amounts of suture material in advance. Surgical gut suture should not be opened before use if possible. It will dry out and lose tensile strength. If it must be opened for the surgical count, tear the corner of the packet enough to visibly count the needle and close the packet without spilling the liquid contents because it is flammable. Gut suture should not be rinsed before use. Suture materials, preparation, and handling are discussed in detail in Chapter 28.

Handling Medications and Solutions on the Sterile Field
Make labels for the sterile container and the syringe. Sterile labels and marking pens are commercially available for labeling containers for medications, contrast media, dyes, and other solutions used in the sterile field. Labeling is done immediately after the drug is dispensed and should include the name and strength of the solution. An appropriate label should be placed on delivery devices, such as syringes, basins, and medicine cups to prevent inadvertent use of the wrong solution in the wrong manner.

Medications and solutions are dispensed to the sterile field by the circulating nurse after confirming drug identification and expiration with the scrub person. The solution basins and medicine cups should be placed near the edge of the sterile field. If a local anesthetic is to be used, the circulating nurse will dispense the drug to the field after drawing it into a syringe. The drug is not dispensed to the field through the needle because it becomes aerosolized and could expose susceptible people. It is not wise to point a needle for any reason in the interest of safety. Do not spear a bottle held by another person. This is risky and equates with the dangers of recapping needles by hand.

Handling Syringes

Fill the syringe, affix the label, attach an appropriate size needle, and put it on the Mayo stand. This will be the first thing the surgeon will use after the patient is prepped and draped. State the type and percentage of the solution when handing the syringe to the surgeon. Some facilities use a "no touch" technique. This means that the filled syringe is placed in a basin or tray for the surgeon to retrieve. Do not recap any needle by hand. Recapping the needle can be done by laying the cap on the instrument table and sliding the needle inside. Place near the working end of the table with the needle pointing away from you.

Syringes with needles are used for injection and aspiration, and syringes without needles (e.g., Asepto, Toomey) are used for irrigation. Care is taken to determine whether the patient is at risk for latex sensitivity because some syringe plungers or squeeze bulbs might contain latex. Nonlatex injection and irrigation syringes are commercially available. Glass syringes in the same models and sizes are occasionally used. These will be wrapped separately with the barrel and plunger apart. When using a sterile syringe, be very careful not to touch the plunger. Contamination of the plunger contaminates the inner wall of the barrel and thus the solution that is drawn into it. Glove powder and other debris can act as a contaminant and cause a foreign body reaction.

The following types of syringes are commonly used for injection or aspiration:

- *Luer-Lok tip:* This type of syringe has a tip that locks over the needle hub. It is used whenever pressure is exerted to inject or aspirate fluid. Sizes range from 2 to 100 mL.
- *Ring control:* This type of syringe has a Luer-Lok tip. The barrel has a thumbhold and two fingerholds, which give the surgeon a secure grip when injecting with only one hand. Sizes range from 3 to 10 mL.
- *Luer slip tip:* This type of syringe has a plain, tapered tip that may not give a secure connection on a needle hub. It is necessary when using some catheter adapters or a rubber connection for aspiration. Sizes range from 1 to 100 mL.

The size of hypodermic needles is designated by length and gauge. Gauge is the outside diameter of a needle, which gets smaller as the number gets larger (e.g., a 30-gauge needle is smaller than a 20-gauge needle). The length will depend on the intended injection site. Longer needles are used for thicker tissue areas. Although numerous sizes of needles are available, only a few representative sizes and their uses are mentioned here:

- ½ inch (12.7 mm) × 30 gauge, for intradermal local anesthetic
- ¾ inch (19 mm) × 24 or 25 gauge, the usual needle for any subcutaneous injection
- 1½ inches (3.8 cm) × 22 gauge, for subcutaneous or intramuscular injection
- 2 inches (5 cm) × 18 or 20 gauge, for aspiration

- 4 inches (10 cm) × 20 or 22 gauge, for deep injections into joints or for intracardiac injections

The following types of syringes are used for irrigation:

- *Bulb with tapered barrel:* With this type of syringe (commonly referred to by the trade name Asepto syringe), a plastic or rubber bulb is attached to the neck of the barrel. The barrel has a tapered or blunt end (like a turkey baster) and can be made of plastic or glass. It is used for one-hand control of irrigation during many types of surgical procedures. This type of syringe has a solution capacity of 0.25 to 4 ounces (7.6–118 mL).
- *Tapered bulb without barrel:* This type of syringe is a one-piece bulb that tapers to a blunt end. It is used to irrigate small structures, and it may be used for suctioning nasal and oral fluids from neonates during deliveries by cesarean section or used for neurosurgery. This variety is usually disposable because it is not possible to clean the interior of the bulb after use.

To fill an irrigation Asepto syringe, depress the center of the bulb, submerge the tip in solution, and release the bulb. The bulb will reinflate, thus drawing solution into the syringe. Take care not to let the bulb express its contents into the air while withdrawing it from the solution. The liquid can hit unsterile surfaces such as the lights and drip onto the sterile field.

Warm, not hot, solution generally is used for irrigation; check the temperature before giving the syringe to the surgeon. Irrigating solution may be stored in a warmer maintained at a temperature that ranges from 98.6° F to 110° F (37–43.3° C). For use, the solution usually should not exceed the temperature of bath water.

After the Surgeon and Assistant(s) Scrub

Gown and glove the surgeon and assistant(s) as soon as possible after they enter the room, if this is a routine procedure. This procedure should take precedence over other setup activities, but do not interrupt a sharps, instrument, or sponge count to do so; such interruptions lead to incorrect counts. The surgeon and assistant(s) may take their gowns from a separate table that has been set up for this purpose. The scrub person should always glove the remainder of the team by the assisted open-glove method. The team should never take towels, gowns, or gloves from the primary sterile field.

Draping the Patient

After the patient is positioned and prepped, assist in draping according to the type of procedure and the surgeon's preference. Some surgeons use towels secured with towel clips to square off the incision. To prevent reaching over the unsterile OR bed, go to the same side of the table as the surgeon to hand towels and towel clips. For hard-to-drape areas, skin towels may be held in place with sutures or staples rather than clips.

Some surgeons use self-adhering plastic incise sheeting directly over the squared-off incision site; the adherent sheeting may be plain (clear) or impregnated with iodophor. To apply this adherent drape, stand on the opposite side of the OR bed to assist as the surgeon positions the adherent surface over the patient's prepped skin. A large sheet of paper will be pulled from the sticky surface as the sheet adheres to the patient. The circulating nurse should take the paper from the sterile team member and discard it. Take care not to rub the front of the gown on the undraped parts of the OR bed.

The fenestrated drape sheet is placed over this. During the draping process, care is taken not to allow sterile gloves to touch unsterile surfaces such as IV lines or equipment. Drapes are cuffed over the hands as they are positioned. Drapes are not to be moved or repositioned once they are placed. Consider the "place it once" principle.

Once a perforating towel clip has been fastened through a drape, do not remove it because the points are contaminated and the drape now has holes. If it is necessary to remove a perforating towel clip, discard it from the field and cover the punctured area with another sterile drape or towel. A transparent wound dressing (e.g., Opsite) can be stuck over a pinhole from a towel clip in an urgent situation. Nonperforating ball-tip towel clips are preferred for securing drapes.

After patient and OR bed draping is completed, bring the Mayo stand into position over the patient, making sure it does not rest on the patient. Position the instrument table at a right angle to the OR bed. Assist the surgeon in securing sterile light handles for adjustment of the OR light. The beam of light should pass the surgeon's right ear and center at the tip of the index finger of their right hand (or left hand for a left-handed surgeon).

Lay a towel or magnetic pad for instruments below the fenestration (opening) in the drape, and lay two dry sponges on the pad. Some drapes have loopholes or Velcro strips for threading suction tubing and ESU cords through. Allow ample length to reach both the incision area and the equipment. Drop the ends off the side of the OR bed nearest the unit to which the circulating nurse will attach them. It is helpful to have the cables and tubing directed over the same side of the field.

Starting the Surgical Procedure

Initiate a "time out" to validate correct site and correct patient. Place two sponges on the field near the incision site. Pass the skin knife to the surgeon (Fig. 25.8), and prepare to pass a hemostat and suction to the assistant. When passing the knife, take care to direct the blade away from yourself and all other personnel. Hold the hand pronated, with thumb opposed against the tip of the index finger, and flex the wrist. Eye contact is recommended when passing the scalpel.

Some surgeons do not want the knife handed to them but prefer to use a no-passing technique for sharps. When using the no-passing technique, lay the knife on an instrument tray or no-touch pad area for the surgeon to pick up. The surgeon will replace the knife onto this surface or tray after the incision is made.

• **Fig. 25.8** Passing the knife with the blade down and protected. The scrub person's hand is pronated.

The scrub person should not allow the scalpel to remain on the field after its use. It is placed on the instrument table near the working end. Skin is never sterile; therefore the initial skin scalpel is considered contaminated, whether or not the surgeon has cut through a plastic incise skin drape. The skin incision exposes deep skin flora of the hair follicles and sebaceous gland ducts. The blade is removed from the handle with an instrument and a fresh blade applied in readiness as time allows. If an existing scar is excised, it may be sent to the pathology department as a specimen for gross identification (accession). Some surgeons discard this tissue. Determine the surgeon's preferences and the facility policies.

Providing Sponges. Hand up moist sterile sponges if requested for covering skin at the edges of the incision. Open and drop soiled sponges into the appropriate sponge receptacle for counting, and add clean sponges to the field as necessary. If sponges or tapes are added by the circulating nurse during the surgical procedure, break the paper bands and count all of them aloud before use. If an RFID counter is used, pass each pack of sponges through the sensor as part of the count. Do not mix types of sponges and tapes on the table. Keep them separated for ease of identification and tracking. Breaking the paper band signifies that the pack of sponges has been counted, a visible cue for the circulating nurse.

Providing the ESU. The tip of the ESU pencil becomes hot and could burn the patient or a team member. Accidental activation can occur if pressure is exerted on the handpiece; this can cause ignition of the draping material or dry sponges. Therefore attach a container (holder/holster) to the drape with a non-perforating clip for containment of the ESU pencil. When not in use, the tip of the ESU pencil is cleaned on a tip polisher/scraper and placed into the holder. Teflon-coated blades are wiped clean with a damp sponge. The ESU tip should not be cleaned with a scalpel blade. The char should not be permitted to fall into the patient.

Towels and the Sterile Field

If the instrument towel on the sterile field becomes bloody, do not remove it but cover it with a fresh, sterile towel. Stick with the "place it once" principle. Remember that drapes should not be repositioned once they have been placed. Take care not to lay the clean towel over a sponge or instrument.

If the surgeon uses a sterile towel as packing within the wound as a retractor pad or visceral retainer, this is relayed to the circulating nurse immediately and the number of towels is tracked with all other counted items. Surgical towels may have an RFID chip embedded to enable the towel count. The circulating nurse is informed when the packing towel is removed, and it is accounted for at the conclusion of the procedure.

The practice of using towels for intraoperative packing is discouraged unless a mechanism is in place for accounting for their removal from the patient at the end of the procedure. Commercially precounted and packed disposable towels with radiopaque and RFID technology are available from several manufacturers. Reusable towels are processed in-house and do not have x-ray–detectable markers.

Maintaining the Case Flow. Watch the field and try to anticipate the needs of the surgeon and assistant. Keep one step ahead of them in passing instruments, sutures, and sponges and in handing up the specimen basin. Notify the circulating nurse if additional supplies are needed or if the surgeon asks for something not on the table. Ask quietly or signal to the circulating nurse for

PROS/CONS

Surgical Towels on the Sterile Field

Pros

- Radiopaque towels may be used as a retractor or visceral retainer.
- Towel manufacturers have designed towels specifically for visceral packing. They are usually blue or white towels that contain a radiopaque strip. Some towels have the same kind of RFID tag as the radiopaque sponges. Other surgical towels for packing have a microchip that acts as a transducer to pick up radio signals.
- Some packing towels are supplied with metal or plastic radiopaque rings on a twill tape tag designed to remain outside the body when used as packing.
- A handheld scanning device can be used along with a wand that can be scanned over the patient's body to detect any missing RFID packing towels.
- Packing towels are absorbent, low-linting, and prelaundered. The material is a tight weave with a radiopaque marker. White dye-free towels are available. These towels are labeled for single use only.
- Packing towels should be moistened with sterile saline to avoid drying of tissues by osmosis.
- If a packing towel is used, it must be part of the original beginning count. The circulating nurse must immediately be notified if a towel is placed and document the number of towels packed in the body. When a towel is removed, it must be reported to the circulating nurse and documented.

Cons

- Green, blue, or other colored towels are manufactured to be used as part of the draping procedure or to dry hands. Draping towels usually come in custom packs, packed with gowns, or can be opened as a separate pack.
- Towels for draping are not always included as part of the beginning count at all facilities.
- Draping towels are usually made from a different grade of cotton and may be coarser than packing towels. They also contain dye that could cause an allergic or sensitivity reaction if used inside the patient.
- Draping towels do not have the radiopaque marker and are not intended to be used inside of patients.

- Surgeons often use draping towels as packing because they are present on the sterile table and convenient.
- If draping towels get soiled or wet, do not remove them. Cover them with clean towels or a clean drape. Be sure that instruments and sponges are not left under the new drapes because this could cause a miscount.
- Single-use draping towels should never be laundered for reuse. They are designed for use on one patient only. Reprocessing of any medical item, including towels, is governed by the U.S. Food and Drug Administration. Reusable towels should be laundered, delinted, and inspected for holes, stains, and breaks in fabric. Then proper sterilization policies must be followed.
- Towels without a radiopaque strip cannot be easily detected by x-ray. They have been mistaken for masses and hidden by organs and can cause abscesses. Adhesions and encapsulation eventually can lead to the development of a foreign body granuloma. A gossypiboma is a mass formed by a foreign body reaction made up of a cotton matrix. Retained foreign bodies made from fabric are also referred to as textilomas.
- Scanning systems are not 100% foolproof. Failure in scanning systems is not common; however, organs, bone, or extremities of body habitus can obscure the reading. RFID scanners should not be a substitute for the manual count.
- A policy should be in place about counting radiopaque and nonradiopaque towels and the use of nonradiopaque towels on the sterile field.

References

1. Kovacina B, Shepard J, Digumarthy S: The postoperative chest. In Shepard J, editor: *Thoracic imaging: the requisites*, ed 3, St. Louis, 2019, Elsevier, pp 259–278.
2. Tholcke L, Fang W, Gornick B, et al.: Investigating particulate production in the operating suite following the use of waterless alcohol based dry scrub versus traditional hand washing and drying with commonly used surgical towels: an experimental study, *Am J Infect Control* 51(5):551–556, 2023.
3. AORN: *Guidelines for perioperative practice*, Denver, CO, 2024, The Association.

supplies to avoid distracting the surgeon. Consideration is given to the patient, who has received a local or regional anesthetic and may be awake. The patient may hear words like "needle" or "blade" and can become frightened.

When bleeding is obvious, the surgeon needs a hemostatic forceps and/or the ESU pencil. If the bleeding is in a deep wound, the extended ESU pencil tip may need to be attached quickly. After making a deep stitch, the surgeon may want to tag the ends of the suture with a hemostat. Scissors are needed for cutting the suture. Some surgeons use hand signals to indicate the type of instrument needed (Fig. 25.9). These universal signals eliminate the need for talking, but such signs should be clearly understood. An understanding of what is taking place at the surgical site makes these signals meaningful.

Pass instruments in a decisive and positive manner. When instruments are passed properly, surgeons know they have them; their eyes do not need to leave the surgical site. When the surgeon extends their hand, the instrument should be placed firmly into the palm in the proper position for use (Fig. 25.10). Return instruments to the Mayo stand or instrument table promptly after use. Their weight or a sharp tip could injure the patient.

Keep instruments as clean as possible. Wipe blood and organic debris from them with a moist sponge. Remove debris from the

ESU tip. To keep the suction tip and tubing patent, periodically flush the suction tip with a few milliliters of saline or sterile water. Keep track of the amount of solution used to clear the line, and inform the circulating nurse. The volume of fluid in the suction canister may be confused with blood loss.

Suture and Tie Management. Place a ligature (tie) in the surgeon's hand. The surgeon keeps both eyes on the field and does not reach for a ligature except to hold out a hand to receive it. Draw a strand out of the packet and direct it toward the sterile field, grasp both ends, and place the strand securely with an upward sweep in the surgeon's outstretched hand.

The end of a ligature may be placed in a long, curved forceps, such as Adson tonsil forceps or a right-angled clamp, in a maneuver referred to as a *tie on a passer* (Fig. 25.11). This method is used when the structure will be circumferentially tied off instead of being sutured, such as a vessel in the mesentery. When handing a tie on a passer, place the forceps in the surgeon's hand in the same manner used to pass any hemostat. Trail the end of the ligature until it is taken by the surgeon or the assistant during the tying procedure. Be ready with the suture scissors as appropriate.

At all times during the surgical procedure have several sutures armed on needle holders ready. Load the needle into the needle holder in a left- or right-hand manner according to the hand

• **Fig. 25.9** Hand signals. **A,** Clamp. **B,** Scalpel. **C,** Scissors. **D,** Retractor. **E,** Pickups. **F,** Free tie. **G,** Pusher-dissector.

• **Fig. 25.10** Passing a ringed instrument. The scrub person holds the instrument by the hinge and avoids entangling fingers in the rings. Tip is visible, and handle is free. Handle is placed firmly and directly into waiting hand. A soft snap may be heard as the instrument contacts the waiting gloved hand.

• **Fig. 25.11** Tie on a passer.

• **Fig. 25.12** A, Loading a needle holder for right-handed suturing. **B,** Right-handed needle in needle holder. **C,** Hand signal for suture on a needle. **D,** Passing right-handed needle.

dominance of the surgeon or the direction of the suturing motion (Fig. 25.12). As the suture is passed to the surgeon, be sure the surgeon has forceps (pickups) to hold the tissue as it is sutured.

After handing a suture to the surgeon, hand the suture scissors to the assistant and immediately prepare another suture just like it. Account for each needle in its entirety as the surgeon finishes with it because a suture or needle can break. All suture needles should be returned in the needle holder for safety and one-for-one accountability. Check the integrity of the needle as it is returned in the needle holder. Tell the surgeon immediately if a needle is broken so all pieces can be retrieved.

Repeat the size of a suture or ligature when handing it to the surgeon only as appropriate. Obviously, this repetition is not necessary if the surgeon is using a long series of interrupted sutures or many ligatures in rapid succession. Use good judgment.

Be logical in selecting the instruments used for suturing. Give the surgeon long needle holders to work deep in a cavity; short ones may be used for surface work. Give the assistant a needle holder to pull the needle through tissue for the surgeon if the angle of suturing is complex. Have scissors ready when the knot is tied. Hemostats are sometimes used to secure or tag the ends of multiple interrupted sutures placed in rapid succession. Often the knot tying and cutting take place after interrupted (individual) sutures are in position, especially during closure.

Remove the waste ends of suture material from the field, Mayo stand, and instrument table, and place them in the trash disposal container. Put used needles on a magnet, in a numbered needle foam box, or a needle rack (or other container for this purpose) until the needle count is complete. Follow established institutional policy and procedure for securing sharps during the surgical procedure.

Specimen Management on the Sterile Field. Save and care for all tissue specimens according to facility policy and procedure. Some facilities require that all tissue removed from a patient, including exudates, be sent for pathologic examination. Therefore it is advisable to send all tissue to the laboratory even though it may appear to be of no value for examination or diagnostic purposes unless instructed to do otherwise. Any other unusual item such as a retained foreign object should be sent to pathology for accession. Forensic evidence is handled according to facility policy.

Specimens are put in a specimen basin or another container. Never put a large clamp on a small specimen; this may crush cells and make tissue identification difficult. Some specimens have borders or margins that the surgeon will mark with specific colored sutures as tags for the pathologist's identification of and attention to certain areas. Photographs may be taken for the record. In some cases the pathologist may be called to the room for close inspection of the site.

Keep the specimen basin on the field until all tissue has been removed or all contaminated items have been placed in it (e.g., instruments used for appendectomy). Specimens designated as right or left should be kept separate in clearly marked containers (e.g., tonsils, testes, ovaries). Keeping bilateral specimens separated helps prevent confusion if part of the tissue sample is found to be positive for cancer. The skin marking pen can be used to mark on the side of the cup to indicate right or left if labels are unavailable.

When handing a specimen from the field to the circulating nurse, hand it in a basin or appropriate container; never place it on a surgical sponge. Tell the circulating nurse exactly what the specimen is, if there are any identifying notations for the pathologist, or if the specimen is to have special testing (e.g., frozen section). If there are any doubts about the specimen's identification, markers, or processing, ask the surgeon for clarification.

Irrigation of the Surgical Site. Before closure, the surgeon may request several liters of fresh, warm sterile saline irrigation solution to rinse the abdomen (or smaller amounts to irrigate other surgical wounds). Some surgeons may pour the irrigation directly from the basin, and others may request an Asepto syringe. If a Poole suction is used to evacuate the solution, be sure the guard is slipped over the tip to protect the tissues from suction lesions. Keep track of the amount of irrigation used and report it to the circulating nurse for the permanent record.

During Closure. Alert the circulating nurse that closure is about to begin, and hand up the wound closure suture materials. In accordance with established procedures, count sponges, sharps, and instruments with the circulating nurse as the surgeon begins closure of the wound. Verify with the surgeon and circulating nurse that intraabdominal or other cavity-packing materials and towels have been removed.

As time permits, clear unnecessary instrumentation from the Mayo stand, leaving two pairs of tissue forceps (usually Adson pickups with teeth), suture scissors, and four hemostats. Place unneeded instruments and supplies on the instrument table in the original setup position. This makes the instrument count easier than trying to dig through a pile of jumbled instruments. It is also safer by not concealing a sharp tip that could cause a puncture injury.

The instrumentation setup and the Mayo stand should remain sterile until the patient has left the room. Cardiac arrest, laryngospasm, hemorrhage, premature drain extraction, or other emergencies can occur in the immediate postoperative-postanesthesia period. Even though sterile instrument sets are nearby, valuable time can be lost in reopening sterile supplies and every second counts in an emergency situation. Regardless of their previous use, instruments on the Mayo stand can be used for an emergency intervention. These instruments can be lifesaving until other ones become available.

Application of the Dressing. Have a clean, warm, saline-moistened sponge ready to wash blood from the incisional area as soon as skin closure is completed and a separate dry sponge to remove excess solution from the site. Leftover laparotomy tapes and Raytec sponges are useful for cleaning the incision after the count has been completed. Have the sterile dressings ready. Radiopaque sponges are never to be used as dressings. The dressing is held in place by a sterile team member as the patient's drapes are removed. Place the soiled drapes in the appropriate receptacle—not on the instrument table or Mayo stand. The circulating nurse will clean the surrounding skin before applying tape to the dressing.

Circulating Nurse Duties

Before entering the OR at the beginning of the day, circulating nurses should wash their hands and arms as required by institutional policy and procedure, but they do not don sterile gowns and gloves. The circulating nurse is an unsterile team member. Personnel who wear sterile attire touch only sterile items; those who are not sterile touch only unsterile items. The circulating nurse should assist the sterile scrub person by providing and opening sterile supplies needed using aseptic technique to prepare for arrival of the patient and the surgeon. The circulating nurse should test all equipment before bringing the patient into the room.

After the Scrub Person Scrubs

Fasten the back of the scrub person's gown and assist with the wraparound tie. Check with the scrub person to see if additional supplies or instruments are needed. Open any remaining packages of sterile supplies (e.g., syringes, sutures, sponges, gloves) as needed. Use an appropriate method of aseptic transfer to the sterile field. Methods of transfer include, but are not limited to, the following:

1. Place the item on the sterile instrument table with the inside of the wrapper everted over your hand. Never reach over the sterile field and shake an item from its package.
2. Expose the contents so the scrub person can remove the item from the wrapper or package by using a forceps or by grasping the item (Fig. 25.13). The scrub person avoids touching the unsterile outside. Remember that the sterile boundary of a peel-open package is the inner aspect, never the edges.
3. Flip only small, rigid items (e.g., suture), and do so with caution (Fig. 25.14). Flipping an item from a package may result in the item missing the intended sterile surface and landing on the floor. Flipping creates air turbulence and thus is the least preferred method of sterile transfer. Larger items, such as staplers or implants, can become contaminated or damaged and therefore are never flipped.

Check the list of suture materials and sizes on the surgeon's preference card, but verify with the surgeon before opening excess packets. Avoid opening suture packets in advance that may not be used. The surgical procedure might be canceled at the last minute or the patient's condition may warrant something different, and then the sutures would be wasted. If the surgeon's need for sutures cannot be anticipated and further instructions have not been given, dispense only one or two packets ahead of actual need during the surgical procedure.

The scrub person counts the needles with the circulating nurse. Some suture packets incorporate barcode technology. Each packet

• **Fig. 25.13** Scrub person taking contents from suture packet opened and held by circulating nurse. Scrub person avoids touching unsterile outer wrapper.

• **Fig. 25.14** Flipping a packet of suture to the sterile field.

is scanned into the computer system to begin a running tally of which suture and needle has been dispensed to the field. This also generates charges to the patient. Once the surgical procedure is started, additional sutures can be dispensed to the field as needed, preventing waste or overcharging the patient. A manual needle count is done at the end of the procedure by the scrub person and circulating nurse.

Pour warmed solution (usually normal saline) into the round solution basin on the instrument table for irrigation and moistening sponges. Pour sterile water into the instrument basin if one is used. The scrub person will label the basins after the solution is poured. For skin preparation using a two-step prep, pour a small amount of antiseptic agent into the solution cups or prep set on the prep table and obtain sterile gloves for the person doing the prep.

To establish a baseline of table contents for the record, count sponges, sharps, and instruments with the scrub person in the manner described in facility policy and procedure.[2] RFID technology may be used for sponges and instrumentation. An RFID counting device can be mounted on an intravenous (IV) pole near the field or incorporated into a collection unit. The pack of sponges or towels can be passed in front of the scanner on either type of RFID counter to register the number of items within the pack before dispensing to the sterile field. Some commercial RFID collection devices incorporate a collection bin that scans each sponge back into the system. The readout screen indicates if the total number of each item has been returned after use. If all dispensed sponges or towels are not accounted for by the collection bin at the end of the procedure, the readout will indicate exactly what is missing. Some RFID units have a sensor wand that can be covered with a sterile drape and passed over the field to detect the location of the missing item.

If RFID is not used, record the baseline number of sponges and towels immediately on the tally sheet or wipe-off board to begin the ongoing tally. Leave a sufficient space for the listing of items that may be added during the procedure. The baseline instrument counts will be recorded on the instrument tray sheet packed with the set.

Patient Check-in

The circulating nurse attends to the patient while the scrub person continues to prepare the instrument table for the arrival of the surgeon. Although time is limited during the check-in process, the circulating nurse should perform a brief assessment of the patient

and go over the surgical checklist. Assessment data about the patient's health status that can be gathered without using equipment or taking an extraordinary amount of time are listed in Box 25.4.

Greet and identify the patient, introduce yourself, and identify your title and role. Offer the patient a blanket from the warming cabinet. Check the wristband for identification by name and number. Ask the patient to verbally identify themselves by name (can have patient spell name) and birth date and (in their own words) describe an understanding of the surgical procedure. Many patients have similar-sounding names, and a spelling by the patient may be indicated.[3]

If the surgical site is designated left or right, validate the area by having the patient point to the spot. Double-check this spot against the permanent record and the scheduled procedure. The correct surgical site should be marked by the surgeon's initials with an ink marker. If the patient is a minor or is unable to respond, this process is performed in the presence of a parent or legal guardian. Check the plan of care and the patient's chart for pertinent information, including consent and laboratory work. Immediately report any discrepancies or questions to the surgeon and anesthesia provider.

Verify any allergies or environmental and/or chemical sensitivities the patient may have. These may be identified by an additional wristband and by a special notation on the patient's chart. Ask the patient to describe their reaction to the drug or substance.

Entering the OR With the Patient

Be sure the patient's hair is covered with a cap; this prevents dissemination of microorganisms and protects the hair from being soiled. Loosen the neck and back ties on the patient's gown, and untuck the blanket from the foot of the transport stretcher. Align the transport cart with the locked OR bed and lock the wheels. Ask the anesthesia provider or other personnel to stand on the opposite side of the bed as the patient moves over.

Assist the patient as needed, taking care that the patient's gown, blanket, IV infusion tubing, and catheter drainage tubing are not caught between the transport cart and the OR bed. Protect the patient's modesty, and use good body mechanics. Additional personnel should be summoned to help if the patient is unable to move over to the OR bed. If the patient requires the use of a patient roller device, ensure that adequate personnel are available to assist with the move from one surface to the other (see Fig. 13.2).

After the patient has transferred to the OR bed, apply the safety belt over the thighs 2 to 3 inches above the patient's knees, and place their arms on armboards. The safety belt should be placed over the blanket so it is visible at all times, and it should not impair circulation to the extremities. Avoid placing additional blankets over the belt because there is no way to be sure the belt is secure if it is not visible. Other considerations include the following:

1. The patient's legs should not be crossed. A small pillow may be placed under the patient's knees to decrease strain on the lower back. Patients at risk for pressure injury should have gel sacral and heel protectors applied.
2. Remove the patient's arm from the sleeve of the gown (if snaps are not available) before securing it to the armboard. The angle of abduction of the arm on the armboard should not exceed 90 degrees—a right angle with the body. The brachial nerve plexus can be damaged by lengthy, severe abduction of the arm.

• BOX 25.4 Brief Physical Assessment That Can Be Performed by the Circulating Nurse During the Check-in Period Before Entering the Operating Room[a]

Review of Body Systems (Brief History)

- Is the patient a reliable historian, or is a family/significant other translating or communicating on their behalf?
- Is the patient taking any medication on a regular basis (e.g., heart or blood pressure medications)? This should include vitamins, hormones, or herbal preparations.
- Does the patient have any allergies? What are the patient's reactions when exposed to the offending substance? Is the reaction localized or systemic?
- When was the patient's last meal and oral intake? If this is an emergency, what were the foods in this meal? Red foods may falsely imply gastrointestinal bleeding if the patient vomits.
- Has the patient ever had any surgery before? This may reveal a condition that requires special positioning or other modification to the standard plan of care.
- Has the patient experienced any complications during previous surgeries?
- Does the patient wear contact lenses, removable eye lashes, or prosthetic parts?
- Does the patient have any trouble moving limbs?
- Is the patient extremely large or small? This may indicate the need for additional instruments or a weight-appropriate OR bed.
- Is the patient aware of the procedure being performed?
- Are laboratory studies and bloodwork reports included with the chart? Are they current?

Head-to-Toe Assessment (Brief Physical)

- Is the patient here for a scheduled procedure, urgent or emergent care, or possibly a redo from an earlier surgery? This may alter the needed supplies for the case.
- Is the patient a child or adult? Is a parent/guardian present?
- Observe the color of the patient's skin and body tissues.
- Listen to the sound of the patient's voice as they speak. Is it raspy or breathless? Is the patient coughing? Note any odors on breath or body.
- Touch the patient's skin as the dialog progresses. Is it cool, hot, damp, dry, or in any other condition? This assessment can be performed as part of shaking hands. Does the patient have a weak or strong handshake or grasp? Is the patient shaky?
- Is there eye contact, and do the eyes move appropriately?
- Is one or the other eyelid drooping? Is the patient crying?
- Does the patient have enough physical coordination to point to the surgical site? Has the correct site been marked per facility policy and procedure?
- Does the patient appear to understand what is being said? Can the patient speak and respond appropriately?
- Does the patient have a Foley catheter or an ostomy? Is the patient continent?
- Are intravenous fluids running? Is the line infusing? Are additives in the container?
- Is the correct surgical site marked with the surgeon's initials?

[a]Most of these assessment activities can be performed simultaneously in just a few minutes and may lead to additional nursing diagnoses that require a modification of the plan of care.

Help the anesthesia provider as needed. Apply and connect monitoring devices, and assist with IV infusion, induction, and intubation as necessary. Some facilities have anesthesia technicians to assist the anesthesia provider. Before the patient arrives, the anesthesia technician will obtain the following equipment:

- Unsterile gloves for the person who will do a percutaneous venipuncture. Sterile gloves are required for a venous cutdown or insertion of arterial monitoring lines.
- A tourniquet to help expose the vein for percutaneous insertion. An unsterile Penrose drain is sometimes used for this purpose.
- Sponges saturated with antiseptic solution for skin preparation. Thorough skin antisepsis is imperative.
- A sterile IV administration tubing set and Angiocaths of assorted sizes.
- 1½-inch (3.8-cm) × 20 or 21-gauge Angiocaths, which generally are used for IV fluids when blood transfusion is not anticipated; 1½-inch (3.8-cm) × 18-gauge or 2-inch (5-cm) × 20-gauge needles are used when blood transfusion is anticipated.
- Tape strips to firmly secure the needle or catheter and tubing to the patient's skin, which prevents motion that may traumatize the vein. If the patient is sensitive to adhesives, paper tape may be used.
- A stopcock to regulate or stop the flow of solution through the tubing into the vein. Ports should remain covered until needed to prevent microbial migration into the system. Many facilities use nonpuncture IV additive attachments for the anesthesia provider to administer drugs during the procedure.
- IV crystalloid solutions, which include normal saline; dextrose 5% or 10% in water (D5W); dextrose in 0.25% saline; lactated Ringer's solution; and dextrose in lactated Ringer's solution. Dates should be verified. If additives are used, a label is applied stating the drug and dose.

- Fluid warming systems are commonly used to maintain normothermia during the procedure.

When prolonged postoperative fluid therapy or hyperalimentation is anticipated, a radiopaque, plastic, single-, double-, or triple-lumen catheter is inserted through either a venipuncture through the skin (percutaneous insertion) of the neck or subclavian area or a cutdown through a skin incision to expose the vein.

A venous cutdown is performed in other selected situations or during emergencies: for central venous pressure monitoring or if superficial veins are thrombosed or if they are superficially collapsed as a result of shock or prolonged preoperative IV therapy.

A venous cutdown is a sterile procedure that creates an open wound. Sterile gloves, drapes, and a tray of sterile instruments and sutures are needed. Assorted sizes of IV catheters should be available so the anesthesia provider can choose the size best suited to the vein. A soft, pliant catheter takes the contour of the anatomy and is not easily dislodged by movement of the patient. The long-term IV access port will be sutured to the skin.

Check the expiration date, and gently squeeze the plastic IV bag to detect leaks. Check the solution for clarity or discoloration; a cloudy solution is contaminated. A registered nurse (RN) or physician must check the label on the container before the solution is administered. All solutions given are charted and monitored to see that they are infusing at the proper speed. Usually this is the responsibility of the anesthesia provider.

Some vascular or radiologic imaging procedures require the use of IV solutions on the sterile field for use in IV injection. A plastic bag decanter is used to pour the solution into a basin on the field. The solution should be labeled as IV saline or IV Ringer's solution. Sometimes heparin or contrast medium is added. The dosage should be indicated on the labeled container.

During the Induction of General Anesthesia

The circulating nurse remains at the patient's side during the induction of anesthesia. The circulating nurse assists the anesthesia provider during induction and intubation. Maintain a quiet environment. Tactile or auditory stimulation may produce excitement in the patient during induction. Hearing is the last sense lost. A strong startle reaction to sound can provoke life-threatening cardiac dysrhythmias or laryngospasms in any patient. Undue stimulation while the patient is under light anesthesia should be avoided. A quiet, undisturbed induction makes for a much safer and easier maintenance of and recovery from anesthesia. The patient should not be positioned or prepped until the anesthesia provider indicates that it is okay to do so.

After the Patient Is Anesthetized

Attach the anesthesia screen and other table attachments as needed. Reposition the patient only after the anesthesia provider says the patient is anesthetized to the extent that they will not be disturbed by being moved or touched. If the patient is to be placed in the prone position, the induction process is performed on the transport cart before placing the patient prone. Be sure a transport cart remains outside the door for the duration of the procedure in case of an emergency. In the event of cardiac arrest or other emergency, the patient will need to be rapidly turned to a supine position for treatment.

If an ESU is to be used, place the dispersive electrode pad in contact with the patient's skin after the patient is in the final surgical position (Fig. 25.15). Avoid scar tissue and hairy or bony areas. If an excessively hairy area is to be used for the electrode, a small area of hair may be removed with clippers to ensure the electrode adheres to the skin.

Turn on the overhead spotlight and aim the light over the site of the incision. Preoperative medication affects the protective pupillary reflex, and therefore bright light should not be focused on the patient before induction or their eyes are covered.

Expose the appropriate area for skin preparation and/or Foley catheter insertion. Turn the blanket downward and the gown upward neatly to make a smooth area around the surgical site. Other areas are exposed only as necessary. Before prepping and draping begins, note the patient's position to be certain all safety measures have been observed. Double-check the safety belt for security. The circulating nurse or first assistant then prepares the patient's skin with antiseptic solution using the one-step or two-step method. All prep solutions should be completely dry before the patient is draped. Drapes can sequester alcohol fumes and create a fire hazard if not completely dry.

Bag and discard the sponges from a reusable prep tray immediately after use. Prep sponges are not radiopaque. Because they are not included in the sponge count, they are not discarded in the sponge bucket. A totally disposable prep tray may be bagged for disposal with trash at the completion of the surgical procedure. This is not considered a biohazard, but eyewear should be worn to prevent splashes or aerosolization.

After the Surgeon and Assistant(s) Scrub

Assist with gowning the team. Reach inside the gown to the shoulder seam. If a closed gloving technique is used, pull the gown sleeves only so far that the hands remain covered by the knitted cuffs. If an open technique is used, pull each sleeve over the hands so the gown cuffs are at the wrists. Fasten the waist tie first, followed by the neck closure. Securing the back of the gown in this order allows the upper body more freedom of motion for gloving. The scrub person will assist with open-assisted or closed-assisted gloving of the team (Fig. 25.16).

The circulating nurse, as a nonsterile person, should stand by to help with the wrap back tie-in of the gown. The gowned person holds the short tie in the left hand and the long tie attached to a cardboard tab in the right hand. The cardboard tab attached to the long tie is handed to the nonsterile person. The nonsterile person does not actually touch the long tie—only the cardboard tab. The sterile person still holding the short tie slowly turns away from the nonsterile person, causing the long tie to cross over the back of the gown at the waist. The sterile person carefully takes the long tie from the cardboard tab the nonsterile person is holding and ties the two ends together at the waist along the left side of the body. The circulating nurse discards the cardboard tab.

If gloving with powdered gloves, the surgeon and assistant(s) should wipe their gloves with a sterile damp towel or sponge provided by the scrub person to remove glove powder.

Starting the Procedure

Observe for any breaks in sterile technique during draping. Stand near the head of the OR bed to assist the anesthesia provider in fastening the drape over the anesthesia screen or around an IV pole next to the armboard. The drainage bag of the Foley catheter should be placed in view of the anesthesia provider and the circulating nurse.

The scrub person will move the sterile Mayo stand into position over the table. The circulating nurse will move the instrument table into position, being careful not to touch the sterile

Upper arm

Thigh

• **Fig. 25.15** Dispersive return electrode placement.

• **Fig. 25.16** The circulating nurse secures the surgeon's gown as the scrub person performs open-assisted gowning and gloving.

surface of the drapes. Place steps or platforms for team members who need them, or place sitting stools in position for the team that needs to operate while seated. If one person sits, the entire team should be seated to protect the level of the sterile field.

Position kick buckets (sponge buckets) on each side of the OR bed. If an RFID system is used, the scanner and collection bin should remain close to the sterile field. Connect suction, the ESU cord, the dispersive electrode cable, or any other powered equipment to be used. If possible, these cords should be directed off the same side of the OR bed to avoid creating a stumbling hazard. Place foot pedals within easy reach of the surgeon's right foot. Tell the surgeon which foot pedal is placed by which foot (if more than one is used), and confirm and document the desired settings on all machines.

The Time Out Before the Incision

When the entire team is in place, the sterile and nonsterile teams concur that this is the correct patient for the correct procedure on the correct part of the body. Allergies and other pertinent information are validated. All necessary supplies, implants, and equipment are confirmed present. The incision should not be made until all members of the team are in agreement. If the patient is awake, they should be part of the process.

During the Surgical Procedure

Some surgeons want the circulating nurse to communicate updates with family or significant others throughout the procedure. Document the time and the calls in the perioperative nurses' notes.

Be alert to anticipate the needs of the sterile team, such as adjusting the OR light, removing perspiration from brows, and keeping the scrub person supplied with sponges, sutures, warm saline, and other necessary items. Ideally, the circulating nurse watches the surgical procedure closely enough to see when routine supplies are needed and gives them to the scrub person without being asked. The circulating nurse should know how to use and care for all supplies, instruments, and equipment and be able to get them quickly. This is particularly important in emergency situations, such as cardiac arrest or hemorrhage.

Stay in the room. Send a runner for supplies if at all possible. Inform the scrub person if you must leave to get something. Be available to answer questions, obtain supplies, and assist team members.

Sponge Management by the Circulating Nurse

If RFID is not used, keep discarded sponges carefully collected, separated by sizes, and counted according to the increment wherein they are packaged. Examination gloves are used to handle and count sponges. Soiled sponges can be placed in untied clear plastic bags in full view of the scrub person and anesthesia provider. The bags are not tied, in the event a recount must be done. Other collection methods may include a hanging pocket display with an individual pouch for each counted increment of sponges.

Weigh sponges if requested to do so. Gram scales can be brought into the OR for this purpose. Each gram of weight equals 1 mL of blood. The procedure for weighing sponges is described in detail in Chapter 31, Box 31.1.

Monitoring Blood Loss

Assist the surgeon and the anesthesia provider to monitor blood loss. Estimate the blood volume in the suction container by subtracting irrigation and body fluids from the total volume in the container. Determinations of total blood volume may be used for estimation of the surgical blood loss. Obtain blood products for transfusion from the refrigerator as necessary, or send a patient care assistant to the blood bank. If the patient's own blood will be recovered for intraoperative autotransfusion, obtain the necessary equipment.

Know the condition of the patient at all times. Inform the OR manager of any marked changes, unanticipated additional procedure, or delays. In a busy department it may be necessary to rearrange the schedule.

Specimen Management by the Circulating Nurse

Prepare and label specimens for transport to the laboratory. An error in labeling a tissue specimen or culture could cause an inaccurate diagnosis or improper therapy or necessitate another operation. Each container is labeled with the patient's name, identification number, date, surgeon, and type and site of specimen. Avoid labeling the lid because lids could be accidently switched during processing.

Accompanying the specimen is a requisition that specifies the laboratory test requested by the surgeon. The requisition includes the patient identification, date, name of the surgeon, preoperative and postoperative diagnoses, surgical procedure, desired test, and tissue to be examined, including its source. In some cases, previous medications such as antibiotics or hormonal therapy are included for the pathologist. Specimens taken from bilateral aspects of the body, such as tonsils, should be separated and labeled as left and right. This is important if there is a potential for the diagnosis of cancer. More information concerning specific specimens is located in Chapter 22.

Documentation

Complete the documentation in the patient's medical record, permanent OR records, and requisitions for laboratory tests or chargeable items. Information to be included in the documentation of direct intraoperative care is shown in Box 25.5.

During Closure

Count sponges, towels, sharps, and instruments with the scrub person. Hospital policies may require additional items to be included in the final counts. Report counts as correct or incorrect to the surgeon. Complete the count records. Collect used sponges for disposal in the appropriately marked biohazard receptacles.

If another patient is scheduled to follow (TF), the following procedures should be observed:

1. Phone or ask the clerk-receptionist to call the unit where the next patient is waiting and request that preoperative medication or antibiotics be given if ordered; this should be done at least 1 hour to 45 minutes before the scheduled time of the surgical procedure. This process usually is not necessary for the first scheduled patient of the day but is important for subsequent patients when the exact time of the surgical procedure is uncertain. For these patients the anesthesia provider usually orders medication or antibiotics "on call."

2. Send a nursing assistant or transporter for the patient, or notify the unit to transport the patient. The patient should be in the OR designated area 30 minutes before the anticipated time of incision. If a holding area is included in the OR suite, the patient may arrive earlier to receive the preoperative medication there.

- Initial assessment of the patient on arrival to the OR. The identity of the patient and verification of the procedure should be validated. Document the time out. Correct surgical site should be marked by surgeon's initials.
- Significant times, such as arrival, time out, start, completion, and room exit times
- Disposition of sensory aids or prosthetic devices accompanying the patient on arrival in the OR
- Position, surgical safety devices, and/or restraints used during the surgical procedure, and by whom
- Placement of monitoring and electrosurgical unit (ESU) electrodes, tourniquets, and other special equipment and identification of units or machines used, as applicable. The settings and duration of use should be recorded.
- The names and times of all personnel in the room for the procedure
- The type of anesthetic administered, and by whom
- The surgical site preparation, the antiseptic agent administered, and by whom
- Medications, solutions, and doses administered, and by whom
- Time out validation of site, patient, and procedure for the surgical checklist
- A description of the actual surgical procedure performed
- Contact with the patient's family or significant others
- Type, size, and manufacturer's identifying information (lot numbers) of prosthetic implants, or the type, source, and location of tissue transplants or inserted radioactive materials
- Use of x-rays or imaging
- Disposition of tissue specimens and cultures
- Correctness or incorrectness of surgical counts (if incorrect, the remedial measures to locate the lost item)
- Placement of drains, catheters, dressings, and packing. Output is recorded if receptacle is emptied in the OR.
- Wound classification is designated at the end of the procedure
- Charges to patient for supplies, according to hospital routine
- Piece of equipment sent from OR with patient to unit (e.g., tracheotomy set that accompanies patient after thyroidectomy, wire scissors if patient has had teeth wired together). These items are to be returned.
- Disposition of the patient after leaving the OR
- Any unusual event or complication

Check the surgeon's preference card or case cart sheet for the next procedure. Collect supplies that will be needed, and get them organized to the extent possible. These supplies can be assembled and placed on the case cart. They cannot be put on furniture in the room until it is cleaned after completion of the current surgical procedure. Advance preparation for the following case may vary if a case cart system is used. Prepare for room cleanup so that minimal time is expended between surgical procedures:

1. Remove radiographs and scans from the view box, place them in the patient's envelope, and take them to the designated area to be returned to the radiology department. Digital displays should be cleared.
2. Obtain items necessary for the cleanup procedure. Place them on top of the case cart for the scrub person to break down when the current patient leaves the room.

Send for a postanesthesia care unit (PACU) transport cart or an intensive care unit (ICU) bed as appropriate; follow whatever is the institutional procedure. Obtain a transfer monitor and oxygen tank with tubing if needed. Also alert patient care assistants and housekeeping personnel that the surgical procedure is nearing completion so they can be ready to assist in room turnover as needed. This helps shorten the downtime between surgical procedures. Be as systematic as possible so steps are not omitted.

After the Surgical Procedure Is Complete

The scrub person will apply the dressing after the incision is cleaned and dried.

The drapes will be rolled off the patient as a sterile team member holds the dressing in place. Clean the surrounding area of the patient's body before securing the dressing(s) over the surgical wound and the surgical drainage systems. Put a clean, warm gown and blanket on the patient. Place the safety belt over top of the blanket. It needs to be seen at all times.

Open the neck and back closures of the surgeon's and assistants' gowns so they can remove them without contaminating themselves.

Have a patient care assistant bring in the clean transport cart or bed. Check the patient's name on the stretcher or bed if it is the procedure to return the patient to the same one used for transport to the OR suite. Align the cart with the OR bed, and lock the wheels. Remove the leg safety belt.

A lifting frame or patient roller is a great help in moving unconscious and obese patients. The Davis patient roller consists of a series of rollers mounted in a frame long enough to accommodate the trunk of an adult patient. The edge of the roller is placed under the lift sheet and the patient's side. With the patient's head and feet supported by separate team members, the lift sheet is pulled and the patient is rolled onto the stretcher or bed (see Fig. 13.2).

A minimum of four people is required to safely move the patient with this device: one to lift the head and manage the airway (usually the anesthesia provider), one to lift the feet and control the Foley catheter, one beside the stretcher or bed to pull, and one beside the patient to lift them from the OR bed. The action of all four people should be synchronized, and the count of three is called by the person controlling the head, usually the anesthesia provider. The following precautions should be taken in lifting or rolling an unconscious patient:

1. Protect the IV, lines, drains, and urinary drainage bag. Secure IV solution bags on an IV pole. It is preferable to attach the IV pole near the head of the stretcher or bed, where there is less danger of injury to the patient if the bag or IV pole should fall or break.
2. Use the lift sheet to support the arms at the sides so the arms do not dangle.
3. The anesthesia provider guards the head and neck from injury and calls the count for the move.
4. Lift or roll the patient gently and slowly to avoid circulatory depression.

After the patient is safely on the transport cart, remove the lift sheet by logrolling the patient gently from side to side. Brush burns result if the fabric is pulled from under the patient. Place the patient in a comfortable position that is most conducive to the maintenance of respiration and circulation. The appropriate position may vary with the type of surgical procedure; usually the patient should:

- Be supine after a laparotomy, with the head of the stretcher elevated 15 degrees, especially if the patient is still intubated
- Be semiprone after a tonsillectomy, for drainage, if extubated
- Be lateral, on the affected side, after transthoracic surgical procedures, thus splinting the side, usually extubated
- Have the affected extremity supported on a pillow

Raise the side rails before the patient is transported out of the OR. Be sure the completed chart and proper records accompany the patient, and send other supplies as indicated (e.g., tracheostomy obturator). Help transport the patient to the PACU or patient care unit.

Patient Transfer From the Operating Room

During transport, the patient should be constantly observed by someone familiar with their condition. If the patient has had local anesthesia, the circulating nurse and transporter may accompany the patient during the return to an ambulatory unit.

Handover Report to PACU Nurse

Calling to give a handover report before leaving the OR is necessary when special monitoring equipment is needed, such as a ventilator. If the patient has had general anesthesia, the anesthesia provider and circulating nurse should accompany them during transport to the PACU, where they give an updated verbal handover report to the PACU nurse. This postoperative report is important for the continuity of care. A concise verbal handover report from the anesthesia provider and/or circulating nurse includes the following:

- Name and age of the patient
- Type of surgical procedure and name of the surgeon
- Type of anesthesia and name of the anesthesia provider
- Vital signs (baseline, preoperative, and intraoperative), including current body temperature. Body weight should be available in kilograms.
- Types and locations of drains, packing, and dressings. Closure medium should be included.
- Preoperative level of consciousness and current status
- Medications given preoperatively and intraoperatively, as well as those regularly taken by prescription or self-medication
- Medical and surgical history
- Allergies and responses to allergens, substance sensitivity
- Positioning on the OR bed and devices attached to the skin
- Complications during the surgical procedure
- Intake and output, including IV fluids, blood, and urinary output
- Location of the waiting family or significant others
- Special considerations:
  - Sensory and/or physical impairments; eyewear, hearing aids, dentures, or other personal property brought to the OR is returned to the patient when the level of consciousness is appropriate
  - Language barrier and level of understanding
  - Use of tobacco, alcohol, and/or addictive drugs
  - Orders such as "no code," "do not resuscitate (DNR)," "allow natural death (AND)," "or "do not attempt resuscitation"

Sponge, Sharps, and Instrument Counts

The counting of sponges, needles and other sharps, and instruments has been mentioned throughout this chapter. These supplies are crucial to the surgical procedure and must be accounted for throughout every procedure, regardless of size or function. Items are counted before and after use. The types and numbers of sponges, needles and other sharps, and instruments vary for each surgical procedure. The process of counting gives the circulating nurse and the scrub person the opportunity to look at all the supplies and the entire instrument set before the procedure

begins. Missing or defective items can be obtained or replaced without interrupting the continuity of the surgery.

Accountability for counts is a professional responsibility that rests primarily on the scrub person and the circulating nurse. The surgeon and patient rely on the accuracy of this accountability by the team. There are several reasons why it is important for the scrub person and circulating nurse to count and be accountable for all items used during the procedure (Box 25.6). Counts are performed for patient and personnel safety, infection control, and inventory purposes. A retained surgical item in the surgical site after closure is a possible cause for a lawsuit after a surgical procedure.

A retained foreign object made of woven textile is referred to as a *gossypiboma* or a *textiloma*.[4] A foreign body unintentionally left in a patient can be the source of wound infection or disruption. The longer the object remains in the body, the more it incorporates ingrowth of tissue. An abscess can form, and fistulas may develop between organs. The foreign body reaction may be immediate or may be delayed for years. Diagnosis is sometimes difficult and costly, and removal of the object usually requires surgery.

A contaminated sponge or needle that is unaccounted for at the close of the procedure could also inadvertently come into contact with the personnel who clean the room, process instruments, launder the linens, or transport the trash. Blood or body fluids are sources of pathogens such as human immunodeficiency virus (HIV) or hepatitis B virus (HBV). A surgical pattie (cottonoid) that has become saturated with clear cerebrospinal fluid during a neurologic case may be contaminated with Creutzfeldt-Jakob disease (CJD).

Inventory control is monitored by accounting for the instrument set in its entirety. Counting ensures that expensive instruments such as towel clips and scissors are not accidentally thrown away or discarded with the drapes. Injury to laundry and housekeeping/environmental services personnel by the contaminated sharp edges of surgical instruments, blades, and needles is a risk. Surgical instruments also can cause major damage to equipment in the laundry services. Unfortunately, some facilities have felt a need to install metal detectors in the trash and soiled linen areas to monitor for missing instruments.

Counting Procedures

A counting procedure is a method of accounting for items put on the sterile table for use during the surgical procedure. Sponges, sharps, and instruments should be counted and/or accounted for on all surgical procedures. This includes any materials introduced into the patient during the procedure, such as rectal or vaginal packs or sterile towels used to pack off or retain viscera. Inadvertent items such as injection needle caps, cautery tip cleaners, clip cartridges, or suture reels could become retained objects and should be accounted for in their entirety.

Items used during organ procurement procedures should be accounted for in their entirety in the same manner as for any surgical procedure. Respect for the donor should be as important to the surgical team as respect for any patient.

Initial Count When the Instrument Tray Is Assembled

The person who assembles and wraps items for sterilization will count them in standardized multiple units and initial the baseline set contents. Most facilities enclose a copy of this tray inventory count sheet in the instrument set or attach a copy to the outer wrapper.

The effects of enclosing a tray inventory sheet inside the set raises questions of potential exposure of toner and foreign body reaction in the patient. Methods for attaching the tray sheet to the outside of the set should be explored if this is a concern. In commercially prepackaged sterile items (e.g., sponges, disposable towels), this count is performed by the manufacturer and affixed to the outside of the package.

Baseline Count During Setup for the Surgical Procedure

The scrub person and the circulating nurse together count all items before the surgical procedure begins and during the surgical procedure as each additional package is opened and added to the sterile field. These initial counts provide the baseline for subsequent counts. Any item intentionally placed in the wound, such as towels, is recorded. A useful method for counting is as follows:

1. As the scrub person touches each item, they and the circulating nurse number each item aloud until all items are counted.[5]

   There is no need to be disruptive when performing this task. Each pack of sponges will be bound with a paper band that is broken only as each bundle is counted. If RFID devices are used, each item is passed over a scanner. The presence of an intact paper band indicates that the bundle has not been counted yet. Count them one bundle at a time.

2. The circulating nurse immediately records the count for each type of item on the count record or wipe-off board. Preprinted forms are helpful for this purpose.
3. Additional packages should be counted away from counted items already on the table in case it is necessary to repeat the count or to discard an item.
4. Counting should not be interrupted. The count should be repeated if there is uncertainty because of interruption, fumbling, or any other reason.
5. If either the scrub person or the circulating nurse is permanently relieved by another person during the surgical procedure, the incoming person should verify all counts before the person being relieved leaves the room. Personnel who perform the final counts are held accountable for the entire count.

Closing Counts (First Closing Count)

Counts are taken in three areas before the surgeon starts the closure of a body cavity or a deep or large incision. The first count is usually all items except instruments. The instrument count starts as soon as the first count is complete.

1. *Field count:* Either the surgeon or the assistant assists the scrub person with the surgical field count. Additional items (e.g., vaginal or rectal packing, sterile towels used as intraabdominal packing) are accounted for at this time. This area should be counted first. Counting this area last could delay closure of the patient's wound and prolong anesthesia.

2. *Table count:* The scrub person and the circulating nurse together count all items on the Mayo stand and instrument table. The surgeon and assistant may be suturing the wound while this count is in process.
3. *Floor count:* The circulating nurse counts sponges and any other items that have been recovered from the floor or passed off the sterile field to the kick buckets. These counts are verified by the scrub person.

Final Count (Second Closing Count)

The final count is performed to verify any counts and/or if institutional policy and procedure stipulates additional counts before any part of a cavity or a cavity within a cavity is closed. The instrument count is completed once before the second sponge and sharp count begins.

The final count (second count) of sponges and sharps may be taken during subcuticular or skin closure. The circulating nurse totals the field, table, and floor counts. If the final counts match the totals on the tally sheet, the circulating nurse tells the surgeon the counts are correct. In ORs where RFID is used, the circulator can pass a sterile draped circular wand over the patient to verify there are no sponges in the patient.

The scrub person must be alert to the use of a counted instrument such as a malleable retractor for visceral protection. Instruments in use during closure usually are a needle holder, scissors, and pickups unless a stapler is used. Towel clips should not be excluded from accountability.

A count should be reported to the surgeon as correct only after a physical count by number has been completed. Intentionally exposing the patient to x-rays is not a replacement for the physical count.

The circulating nurse documents on the patient's record what was counted, how many counts were performed and by whom, and if the counts were correct or incorrect. There is no need to write all the tallies on the permanent record. An RN should participate to verify that all counts are correct, but the personnel performing the counts are responsible for the accuracy of the counts. The counting procedure, the outcome, and participating personnel should be documented according to institutional policy and procedure. Signatures of all counting personnel may be required according to facility policy.

Omitted counts because of an extreme patient emergency should be recorded on the patient's record, and the event should be documented according to institutional policy and procedure. If a sponge or sponges are intentionally retained for packing or if an instrument intentionally remains with the patient, the number and type should be documented exactly by type and number on the patient's record. Patients in extremis may be brought back to surgery for repeated procedures, and it is important to know what was intentionally left in during the first operation. Any time a count is omitted, refused by a surgeon, or aborted, the reason should be fully documented.

Records can be subpoenaed and admitted as evidence in court. The accountability for all items used during the surgical procedure is placed on the scrub person and the circulating nurse, who jointly perform the counting procedures as defined by institutional policy and procedure. The surgeon and the first assistant facilitate the counting process. It is not the job of the surgeon or the first assistant to actively perform the counts or sign the count reconciliation record.

Incorrect Count

A specific policy and procedure for any count that is incorrect should be defined by each institution and should include, but not be limited to, the following:

1. The surgeon is informed immediately. If RFID technology is used, the surgical site should be scanned by the detection wand. The RFID process can alleviate the need for repeated counts and room searches if the missing item is found during the scan process.

   If RFID technology is not available, the following steps should be followed:

2. The entire count is repeated.
3. The circulating nurse searches the trash receptacles, under the furniture, on the floor, in the laundry hamper, and throughout the room.
4. The scrub person searches the drapes and under items on the sterile field and Mayo stand.
5. The surgeon searches the surgical field and wound.
6. The circulating nurse should call the immediate supervisor to check the count and assist with the search.
7. After all search options have been exhausted, policy should stipulate that an x-ray be taken before the patient leaves the OR. The surgeon may request the x-ray at once, with a portable machine, to determine whether the item is in the wound. Alternatively, the surgeon may prefer to complete the closure first because of the patient's condition or because there is reasonable assurance, based on wound exploration, that the item is not in the patient. Unfortunately, patients' incisions have been reopened after complete closure to retrieve retained objects, such as sponges.
8. The circulating nurse should write an incident report and document on the OR record all efforts and actions to locate the missing item, even if the item is located on the x-ray. This report has legal significance for verification that an appropriate attempt was made to find the missing item. If the item is not found on the x-ray, the report brings to the attention of personnel the need for more careful counting and the control of sponges, sharps, and instruments. A policy and procedure change or update may be advisable.

Sponges

Sponges are used for absorbing blood and fluids, protecting tissues, applying pressure or traction, and blunt dissection. Many types of sponges are available. All sponges on the sterile table and field should be radiopaque. A radiopaque thread or marker made of a barium substance is incorporated into commercially manufactured sponges. RFID-tagged sponges and towels also have a small, encoded tag attached.

Types of Sponges

The following list is representative of the types of radiopaque sponges used:

1. Gauze sponges (which are called swabs in some countries) are supplied sterile, precounted, and folded. When opened out to a single ply during blunt dissection, fibers along the raw edges could become foreign bodies in the wound. These are also called *Raytec* or *Raytex* sponges. All are packed in groups of 10 and bound with a paper band.
2. Laparotomy tapes, also called lap pads, tapes, or packs, are used for retaining the viscera and keeping them moist and warm. Tapes are either square or oblong and have a loop of blue twill tape sewn on one corner. A small radiopaque marker is sewn into one corner of the tape. A metal or plastic radiopaque ring, approximately 1½ inches (3.8 cm) in diameter, may be attached on this twill tape. If rings are used, they remain outside the edges of the incision while the tape is inside. Normal saline solution is commonly used to moisten tapes. Tapes are packaged and paper-banded in groups of five.
3. Dissecting sponges have a self-contained, x-ray–detectable element incorporated into the weave.
   a. Peanut sponges are very small, ovoid soft gauze sponges used for blunt dissection or absorption of fluid in delicate procedures. Cherry sponges are firm ball-shaped dissectors. Both types are clamped into the tip of an Adson, Kelly, or right-angle clamp during use. Both are packaged in groups of five nested in a cardboard or foam holder.
   b. Kittner dissectors are small firm cylindrical rolls of heavy, tightly wound cotton dental tape that are held in a Kelly or Kocher (Ochsner) clamp for use during blunt dissection. They are packaged in groups of five.
   c. Tonsil sponges are soft, ball-shaped, cotton-filled gauze sponges with an attached cotton thread. These come in several sizes and are held in the tip of a forceps for use. They are packaged in groups of five. These sponges are available in larger styles without the thread and are referred to as *tampons*. These can be used in place of a Raytec on a sponge forceps.
4. Compressed absorbent cottonoids (also known as *patties*) are small squares or rectangles made of compressed rayon or cotton; they are very absorbent and resemble a strip of felt. They are moistened with solution or a topical hemostatic agent, such as thrombin, for use on delicate structures such as the nerves, brain, and spinal cord.

   They are pressed out flat after moistening and before handing them to the surgeon. The surgeon will pick up the cottonoid with a forceps (commonly bayonet forceps) and apply it to the area of intended use. Some surgeons will use cottonoids to apply intranasal anesthetic. Cottonoids have a radiopaque element and a thread attached so they can be located in the wound. These range in size from ¼ × ¼ inch to 1 × 3 inches.

5. Towels are occasionally but not universally used for protecting the viscera. The scrub person and circulating nurse are responsible for accounting for the tracking and retrieval of towels or anything placed in the patient. The scrub person informs the circulating nurse that a towel has been used for packing or protecting viscera, and the circulating nurse documents the event. Towels placed inside the patient become part of the count.

   During the first closing count at the conclusion of the case, the circulating nurse checks with the scrub person to verify that the towel has been removed before closure. Disposable varieties of sterile, precounted, packaged towels with x-ray–detectable elements are commercially available. Towels can be white, blue, or green. Some have twill-tape tags with rings like those on lap tapes.

   Retained surgical towels have been the subject of several liability suits. Case law demonstrates that the hospital, on behalf of the scrub person and the circulating nurse, has been successfully sued in cases, whereas the surgeon has been exonerated. The premise for these findings is based on the fact that the scrub person and circulating nurse are responsible for the counts and the fact that the surgeon relies on their accurate performance in this role. Everything temporarily placed inside the patient must be accounted for at the conclusion of the case.

Counting Sponges

Radiopaque, x-ray–detectable gauze sponges, tapes, towels, dissecting sponges, and cottonoid patties are counted in multiples of 5 or 10 per package. The types of sponges and number of different sizes should be kept to a minimum. RFID scanners have helped simplify the sponge-counting process. Conventional counting methods incorporate the following procedure by the scrub person:

1. Hold the entire pack of sponges of whatever type, including tapes, in one hand. The thumb should be over the edges of the folded sponges.
2. Break the paper band. Breaking the band is a good way to designate which stacks have been counted and which ones have not.
3. Shake the pack gently to separate the sponges and loosen the twill-tape tails on tapes.
4. Pick each sponge separately from the pack with the other hand, and number it aloud while placing it in a pile on the sterile instrument table.

If a pack contains an incorrect number of sponges, the scrub person should hand the entire pack to the circulating nurse for removal from the room. There should be no attempt to correct errors or to compensate for discrepancies. The pack should be removed from the room and not used.

Methods of Accounting for Sponges

Regardless of the types and numbers of sponges counted, various methods may be used to help ensure one is not misplaced or left in the patient.

By the Scrub Person

1. Keep sponges, tapes, peanuts, and other such materials separated on the instrument table and far away from each other and from any draping material, especially towels. Dissectors should remain in their holders until needed.
2. Keep sponges far away from small items (e.g., needles, hemostatic clips) that might be dragged into the wound by a sponge or tape.
3. If a moist sponge or towel is given to the surgeon or assistant to wipe their gloves, be sure it is completely opened and dropped into the sponge bucket or RFID scan bin after use.
4. Do not cut sponges or tapes. It may be hard to account for the item in its entirety.
5. Do not remove the radiopaque thread or marker. Either the marker or the sponge could be lost.
6. Never mix sponges and tapes in a solution basin at the same time; this prevents the danger of dragging a small sponge unknowingly into the wound along with a tape. Avoid dipping sponges in the basin to prevent lint dispersal. Moisten with the Asepto syringe.
7. Do not give the pathologist a specimen on a sponge to take from the room; instead, put the specimen on a Telfa pad, in a basin, or on a towel.
8. Discard all soiled sponges into the kick bucket or RFID scan bin after completely opening them and leave no more than two clean sponges on the sterile field at a time. Put up clean ones before removing soiled ones on an exchange basis as part of a systems approach to error prevention.

9. Do not be wasteful of sponges. Besides the economy factor, the more sponges used, the more there are to count and the greater the chance for error.
10. Once the peritoneum is opened or the incision is made and extends deep into a body cavity (where a sponge could be lost), four alternative precautions can be taken:
    a. Remove all Raytec sponges from the field, and use only tapes. Rings, if used, hang outside, over the edges of the wound.
    b. Use folded Raytec sponges on sponge forceps only. Completely unfold and open each one before dropping into the sponge bucket or RFID scan bin.
    c. Give laparotomy sponges to the surgeon one at a time on an exchange basis.
    d. Dissectors are given one at a time clamped inside the tip of an instrument on an exchange basis. Bloody dissector sponges are replaced into the original Styrofoam holder after use. These may not be RFID tagged.
    e. Tonsil sponges (5) and patties/cottonoids (10) should be collected in their packaging increment and rewound on the cardboard supplied in the package. These may not be RFID tagged.
11. With the circulating nurse, count or scan sponges and tapes added during the surgical procedure before moistening or using them. Break the paper band to signify they have been counted. Always start the counts at the field and end at the sponge bucket.
12. Do not add or remove sponges from the surgical field during a sponge count until the count is verified as complete and correct. Before beginning the final count, place one or two tapes or sponges on the field for use while the count is being taken.

By the Circulating Nurse

1. To prevent the possibility of confusion in the count, nonradiopaque gauze sponges used on different trays (e.g., spinal or prep trays) should be bagged and moved away from the field before the incision is made.
2. Each discarded sponge should be examined briefly to be sure no saturated sponges are tangled with them. To avoid the transmission of bloodborne pathogenic organisms, wear gloves and protective eyewear to separate sponges for counting, stacking, and bagging.
3. Count and bag sponges in the same increment in which they are supplied, such as groups of 5 or 10 of like sponges. These numbers should be recorded on the sponge count record and counted. The bagged units are not tied shut or discarded into the trash. The bags are placed aside in full view of the scrub person and the anesthesia provider until the end of the case and all the numbers are reconciled. The anesthesia provider will be observing for blood loss on the sponges.
4. Give additional sponges or tapes to the scrub person when it is convenient for them to count. The scrub person breaks the paper band as the bundle is counted. Broken paper bands are a signal that that particular pack has been counted. The scrub person separates each sponge bundle and counts them, and the circulating nurse records the numbers immediately.
5. Give dressings to the scrub person after the final sponge count. Radiopaque sponges are not used for dressings because they could distort a postoperative x-ray of the site.

6. Do not discard or remove counted sponges from the room for any reason until the patient is out of the room.

Sharps

Sharps include surgical needles, hypodermic needles, knife blades, electrosurgical needles and blades, and instrument tips. Each item must be accounted for. Surgical needles are the most difficult to track and are used in the largest quantity. All surgical needles and other sharps are counted as they are added to the sterile table and/or separated from other instruments in the instrument tray.

Surgical Needle Counts

Surgical needles are used for suturing. The type will determine the method of transfer to the sterile table:

1. Reusable eyed needles put in a needle rack or a suture book are uniformly counted into sets in multiples of two or three of each type and size the surgeon will need. These needles are usually packaged and sterilized separately from the instrument sets. Most facilities have converted to disposable needles and no longer reuse needles.
2. Disposable suturing needles are precounted, packaged, and sterilized by the manufacturer. The label will specify whether the sterile pack contains single or multiple needles. Closure materials are discussed in detail in Chapter 28.

Counting Needles and Other Sharps

Each needle or packet containing needles is separated for individual counting. Suture packets containing swaged needles can remain unopened. The count is taken according to the label on each packet. Some packets contain multiple needles. The scrub person verifies the count when the packet is opened. Counting empty suture packets at the end of the case is not an appropriate method of reconciling a count.

Methods of Accounting for Sharps

If a needle or blade has broken, both the scrub person and the circulating nurse must make sure all pieces are recovered or accounted for. Sometimes the risk of retrieving a piece of a sharp or needle is more hazardous than letting it encapsulate in tissue. The surgeon makes this determination. This must be documented.

Many smaller gauge needles do not appear easily on x-ray unless the technician uses special density calculations or the needles are radiopaque. Needles, knife blades, instrument tips, and other small sharps should never be left loose on the Mayo stand because they could be pulled into the incision or knocked onto the floor. Smallness of the needle is not a valid reason to fail to account for each one.

By the Scrub Person

1. Leave needles swaged to suture material in their inner folder or dispenser packet until the surgeon is ready to use them. These folders or packets can be placed in the edge of a folded towel on the working end of the table.
2. Give needles to the surgeon on an exchange basis; that is, one is returned before another is passed. Account for each needle as the surgeon finishes with it. Needles should only exchange hands within a needle holder.
3. Use needles and needle holders as a unit. The following is a good rule: No needle on the Mayo stand without a needle holder, and no needle holder without a needle.
4. Secure used needles and sharps in a needle-counting box or magnet holder until after the final count. Many methods for efficient handling are available, as follows:

a. Sterile adhesive pads with or without magnets facilitate counting and safe disposal. When a large number of swaged needles will be used, the scrub person and circulating nurse may determine the number of needles a pad will hold and work out a unit system. Disposable plastic boxes of various sizes for the containment of sharps are commercially available.
b. Used eyed needles can be returned to the needle pack. The use of reusable suture needles is not encouraged because they become dulled with use and could harbor microorganisms if not properly cleaned.

By the Circulating Nurse

1. Open only the necessary number of packets of sutures with swaged needles. Overstocking the instrument table not only is wasteful but also complicates the needle count.
2. Counted sharps should not be taken from the OR during the surgical procedure. If a scalpel with a counted knife blade is given to a pathologist to open a specimen, the scalpel must remain in the room after gross examination of the specimen; it is not to be taken to the laboratory with the specimen.
3. A sharp is passed off the sterile field if it punctures, cuts, or tears the glove of a sterile team member. These sharps are retained and added to the table and field counts to reconcile the final sharp count. An empty specimen cup is a good container for a loose sharp.
4. A magnetic roller may be used to locate a surgical needle or blade that has dropped on the floor. A piece of tape is used to retrieve a sharp from the floor. Close the tape over the sharp and place in a specimen cup. Picking up a sharp even with gloved fingers can cause a puncture injury.

Instruments

Surgical tools and devices are designed to perform specific functions that include cutting or dissecting, grasping and holding, clamping and occluding, exposing, or suturing. For each basic maneuver, an instrument of suitable size, shape, strength, and function is needed. Variation in the style and number of instruments will be dictated by the type of surgical procedure and, to some extent, by the personal preferences of the surgeon.

Counting Instruments

Instrument counts are recommended for all surgical procedures. Specific written policies and procedures are followed without deviation. To count instruments, the scrub person should do the following:

1. Remove the top rack of instruments from the instrument tray or container and place it on a rolled towel. Instruments are counted as they are assembled in standardized sets in the processing area. Groups of even numbers of each of the basic clamps facilitate handling and counting.

Some facilities permit "cluster counting," which is a method of counting all scissors, pickups, needle holders, retractors, and other like groups together without having to name each item with its formal name. For example, the tray may contain two pairs each of three different types of scissors. This cluster would be counted as "six scissors" instead of two Mayo, two Metzenbaum, and two suture scissors. This can speed up the count. If an item is not accounted for in the cluster, an itemized individual count ensues. The same can be done for retractors and pickups.

2. Expose all instruments left in the tray for counting. Remove knife handles, towel clips, tissue forceps, and other small instruments from the tray, and place them on the instrument table. Do not put instruments on the Mayo stand until they are counted; they can be put on the stand as they are being counted.

3. Account for all detachable and disassembled parts, such as screws or ratchets. These must be counted or accounted for during assembly and once again during disassembly at the end of the case.

4. Recover and retain all pieces of an instrument that breaks during use. A replacement instrument is added to the count sheet by the circulating nurse.

5. After the initial count is taken, count any instruments added to the table, with one exception. If the circulating nurse decontaminates and sterilizes an instrument for immediate use that has dropped to the floor or has been passed off the table, an adjustment in the count is unnecessary. Instruments that are recovered from the floor or passed off the table and not sterilized are retained by the circulating nurse and reconciled at the closing count. Sterilization for immediate use is not a recommended practice. It is only used when no other alternative is available.

Simplifying Instrument Counts

Counting is easier if the numbers and types of instruments are reduced and if standardized sets are streamlined. Inform the OR manager if unused, unnecessary instruments are routinely included in basic sets. Keep the surgeons' preference cards up to date. Instruments peculiar to specific surgical procedures or surgeons can be wrapped separately and added to the basic foundation set only when needed.

Standard count sheets for each basic instrument set will facilitate the counting process. The sheet accompanies the set. The person who prepares the set verifies the initial count as listed. The circulating nurse can check the items as they are counted with the scrub person.

Efficiency of the Operating Room Team

A discussion of the duties of the scrub person and the circulating nurse would not be complete without consideration of efficiency, productivity, and work habits. Therefore efficiency depends primarily on individual effort and the working relationship among team members.

Productivity

Productivity and efficiency go hand in hand. Productivity is directly related to what a person does and how they do it. Productivity is also the quantity and quality of work (output) in relation to the costs in terms of labor and time (input). To be productive, perioperative nurses and surgical technologists should develop their psychomotor skills, competencies, and mental capacities. This requires an accurate perception of the factors and conditions that affect the patient, surgeon, and other team members. The concept of situational awareness means staying in touch with the environment and thinking ahead in preparing for and participating in the surgical procedure. Productivity is enhanced by a person's ability to do the following:

1. Organize work efficiently and effectively. Efficiency is important to minimize the length of time during which a patient is anesthetized and the anxious family or significant others are waiting.

2. Work rapidly with precision and dexterity. Learn to follow directions quickly and accurately, and give attention to the smallest detail. Carelessness creates waste and unnecessary hazards for the patient and team.

3. Adapt to changes or unexpected situations quickly, calmly, and efficiently. A change in diagnosis during the surgical procedure may require an altogether different setup and a different surgical approach from the one anticipated. Emergencies will arise. Knowing what to do and why to do it in a particular way decreases the anxiety of rapid performance. Exercise good judgment, and learn to prioritize actions and function competently under pressure.

4. Anticipate the needs of the surgeon and the team, and keep one step ahead. The surgeon becomes distracted if handed the wrong instrument or made to wait for supplies. Be alert and try to anticipate procedural needs logically.

5. Maintain physical and emotional stamina. Situational awareness can be compromised by fatigue, poor physical health, and emotional distress. Be sensitive to the health and well-being of other team members.

Time and Motion Economy

Time is money; do not waste it. Know the policies and procedures, and follow them efficiently. Learn to do things right the first time and continue to do them that way; time is wasted in correcting errors. Motions should be productive.

Time Is Costly

Time is an important element in the OR. If time is wasted between surgical procedures, the day's schedule is slowed down and later procedures are delayed. The surgeons' time is wasted, and they then tend to come late because they anticipate delays. The patients and families or significant others become anxious during these delays.

Workers with poor time-management skills tend to become less efficient and drift into poor work habits. Common sense is a great ally. Take time to stop and think. Is there a quicker, easier, or more efficient way of doing the job without compromising technique? Most work habits can be improved. Analyze them in a methodic manner.

Recognizing that a problem exists is the first step toward solving that problem. Gather the facts needed to support the desirability of adopting alternatives. Seek to develop more efficient and more economical work methods.

Associations

Each patient, surgeon, and surgical procedure is unique, but all have commonalities. A logical thought process will simplify the necessary OR preparations for the patient and the surgeon. Supplies and equipment must be ready before the procedure can begin.

Association is a great aid to memory and organization of work. With association, the mention of one article brings to mind the others used with it. For instance, the scrub person knows a suture calls for a tissue forceps to the surgeon, a needle holder to the assistant, and then scissors. Watch for and try to establish associations to increase efficiency. Think of the order in which instruments and supplies are going to be needed, and do first things first (e.g., prepare sutures for closing deep tissue layers before preparing sutures for the skin).

To be proficient, know the organization of work and the relative importance of the factors in accomplishing it. If, as the patient is being prepped, the surgeon requests stainless steel retention sutures for closure instead of the usual sutures, the circulating nurse should realize there is plenty of time to get these sutures after the other duties have been completed. Before getting these closing sutures, the circulating nurse must perform the duties necessary to start the surgical procedure; for example, tie the gowns, supervise the draping, position the instrument table, and connect the ESU and suction. When getting these steel sutures, association tells the circulating nurse to also get wire scissors.

Motion Economy

Wasted motion not only is time consuming but also adds to physical fatigue. Fatigue is the result of body movement. Ten principles of motion economy can reduce fatigue from physical activity and improve personal levels of efficiency:

1. Motion should be productive. Once the steps in a procedure are learned, work to increase speed and the psychomotor skill needed to perform them. Make each movement purposeful; avoid rushed or disorganized motions. Work quietly and quickly. Work as fast as possible without sacrificing accuracy, safety, and technique for speed.

The corollary to this principle is a place for everything and everything in its place. Keep an orderly work area to avoid fumbling and rehandling items. If everything has a place and is in its place, supplies are easily obtained by instinct when needed. A neat and orderly work area is one of the first requirements for productive motions. Consider the workflow so that minimal motions can be made to accomplish productive work.

2. Motions should be simple. Body movements should be confined to the lowest classification with which it is possible to perform work properly.[6] Movements of the upper extremity are classified into five levels:
   a. Class 1 involves the fingers. The knuckle provides the pivot for motion for such tasks as fingering through a card file, turning a setscrew on an instrument, and using a pair of scissors.
   b. Class 2 involves both the hand and the fingers. The wrist is the pivot for motion for tasks such as passing instruments, counting sponges, and picking up or writing on an intraoperative record.
   c. Class 3 includes the forearm. The elbow is used as a pivot to open a peel-open package, unfold drapes, and unwrap small supplies. More effort and time are expended in the third and succeeding classifications because the movements of any one class involve the movements of all classes preceding it. It takes longer and requires more effort to turn the pages of a procedure book or a patient's chart than to thumb through a file of surgeons' preference cards.
   d. Class 4 includes the upper arm. The shoulder pivot is used when opening a door, setting up the Mayo stand, and prepping a patient.
   e. Class 5 adds the torso. The trunk bends or stretches to lift a patient, take supplies from a low shelf or drawer, hang an IV bag, or count the sponges in a kick bucket.

Upper extremity work should be arranged to reduce work to the lowest possible classification. Finger motion is the least fatiguing, and shoulder motion is the most fatiguing. The scrub person should be positioned at the OR bed so that elbow, wrist, and finger motions can be used. To prevent prolonged shoulder motion for both of them, the scrub person should be positioned opposite the surgeon so that both can work with their elbows at their sides. The OR bed should be adjusted for height according to the tallest team member. Steps should be supplied for shorter members.

It is quicker for the circulating nurse to stretch to hang an IV bag than to take time to use finger action to loosen the set screw on an IV pole, lower it with shoulder movement, hang the bag with elbow action, and repeat the sequence in reverse. However, stretching is more fatiguing. Increasing fatigue causes slower motion as the day progresses. Maybe 30 seconds was saved with the first patient of the day, but what happens to the last patient of the day? Time is lost because energy wanes.

3. Motions should be curved. Motions should follow curved rather than straight paths whenever possible. A circular motion to clean the flat surfaces of furniture is less fatiguing than straight push-and-pull strokes.

4. Motions should be symmetric. Motions should be rhythmic and flow smoothly; when possible, both hands should be used symmetrically.

5. Work should be within grasp range. To avoid changes in body position, all work materials should be arranged so they are within grasp range. Grasp range is within the radius from the pivot point of the elbow or shoulder, either horizontally or vertically. The minimum grasp range is within the radius of the arcs formed with only the forearms extended, using the elbows as pivot points on the horizontal plane. The optimum grasp range is within the area where the left-hand and right-hand arcs overlap. This is the area in which two-handed work, such as putting a needle in a needle holder, can be performed most conveniently. The maximum grasp range is within the arcs formed from the shoulder pivots. The overlapping of these arcs is the maximum extent at which two-handed work can be performed within reach without changing body position.

The Mayo stand should be placed over the OR bed at a height and in a position within the minimum and optimum grasp range of the scrub person. It must not rest on the patient, but it can be lowered to an inch or two above the patient. The support pillar of the Mayo stand should be directly in front of the scrub person. The scrub person should be able to adjust the height by using the foot lever.

The instrument table should be positioned as close as possible to the horizontal plane within maximum grasp range. Instruments or supplies that require two-handed work should be placed on the Mayo stand and instrument table as close as possible to the optimum grasp range.

6. Hands should be relieved of work. Hands should be relieved of any work that can be performed more advantageously by other parts of the body. Many electrical instruments have foot pedals to facilitate operation.

7. Work materials should be pre-positioned. Supplies can be arranged for convenient use and minimal handling. Drapes are packaged in order of use so they do not need to be handled by the scrub person, except to move the stack to a corner of the instrument table, until ready to use. Instruments can be arranged in containers so that all of them do not need to be removed until needed.

Economize time and effort by placing items on the instrument table and Mayo stand in the order in which they will be used, and put them in their proper places without rearranging them. Arrange instruments on the Mayo stand in position to hand to the surgeon or assistant.

In passing an instrument, place it in the surgeon's hand in the position in which it will be used so that readjustments will not be necessary. Hold the instrument with the thumb and the first two fingers, far enough away from the handle so the surgeon can grasp it. Hand a needle in a needle holder in the same way, supporting the suture so it does not drag; hand it with the needle pointing in the direction in which the surgeon will start to use it. Hand thumb forceps so the surgeon can grasp the handle; do the same with retractors.

8. Gravity should be used. Dispensers for scrub sponges and brushes operate on the principle that gravity should be used whenever possible. Cabinets for smaller packages in the sterile supply room can be vertical and divided into appropriate size slots. These cabinets can be filled from the top and dispensed from the bottom of each slot. This method is convenient, saves space, and ensures that older items are used first. Shelves for large, heavy packs can be slanted slightly to facilitate handling. Gravity-feed and drop-delivery installations eliminate or reduce motions. The quickest way to dispose of an object is to drop it. Because this also may be the quickest way to break or contaminate the object, the application of this principle requires good judgment.

9. Supplies should be combined. Items should serve two or more purposes whenever possible. For example, sterilizer chemical indicator tape serves a dual purpose: to hold the package closed and to show if it has been exposed to a sterilization process. And only inches, not a yard, of tape accomplish the job. Disposable kits and trays are purchased, or sets are made up of reusable items so that all the supplies and materials needed for a procedure are combined into a single unit. This eliminates opening many separate packages.

10. The worker should be at ease. Tiring body motions or awkward or strained body postures should be avoided. A pleasant, quiet environment is less fatiguing, has fewer psychologic and physiologic adverse effects on team members, and enhances greater efficiency.

Economical Use of Supplies and Equipment

As the cost of supplies increases, circulating nurses and scrub persons should be conscious of ways in which to eliminate wasteful practices. For example, throw away disposable items only. Avoid throwing away reusable items.

The OR suite is one of the most expensive departments of a hospital. Adequate instruments and supplies are necessary for patient care, and cost is not always the primary consideration.

Economy becomes a hazard when exercised beyond the point of safety. Nevertheless, supplies do not need to be used lavishly just because they are available. Remember the principles mentioned in the following sections.

"Just Enough Is Enough"

The varieties and numbers of instruments and supplies needed for each surgical procedure can be kept to a minimum. If the procedure list and surgeons' preferences are kept up to date, articles no longer used can be eliminated. Items to "have available" are not opened unnecessarily. The following procedures should be observed:

1. Pour just enough antiseptic solution for the two-step skin preparation according to the manufacturer's recommendation; it takes only a small amount. Do not open a bottle unnecessarily for a small amount if you know the remainder will not be used.
2. Follow the procedures for draping to provide an adequate sterile field without wasting disposable draping material.
3. Do not open another packet of sutures for the last stitch unless absolutely necessary. A few leftover pieces of the same product may be long enough to complete the closure.
4. Suction tubing, syringes, hypodermic needles, drains, catheters, extra drapes, and other such materials are kept sterile and available. Supplies should be opened only as needed—not routinely "just in case" they may be needed.
5. Do not soak too much plaster or fiberglass casting material when helping with cast applications. Keep just ahead of the surgeon. Ask if more is needed before soaking an extra roll.
6. Turn off lights when they are not needed.
7. Separate trash into contaminated and noncontaminated waste. Contaminated waste is processed at a cost per pound.
8. Recycle all eligible items. This can be cost-effective.

Use Supplies and Equipment for Intended Use

1. Use OR bed appliances according to the manufacturer's instructions for positioning and stabilizing patients.
2. Use unsterile gloves for unsterile procedures in which the use of gloves is for hand protection. Open sterile gloves for sterile procedures only.
3. Do not use hemostats to clamp drapes or tubing; doing so ruins both the hemostat and the tubing. Use a stopcock or a special tubing clamp for tubes, and use a nonpiercing towel clip to secure drapes. Custom drapes come with hook and loop tabs, hook and loop strips, or flaps with holes to secure cords and tubing.
4. Give the assistant a needle holder for pulling needles through tissue for the surgeon. A hemostat can be ruined by using it for this purpose, and the needle can be damaged.
5. Use wire scissors for cutting wire, tissue scissors for cutting tissue, dressing scissors for cutting drains and dressings, and suture scissors for cutting sutures.

Avoid Damage

Handle all supplies and equipment carefully to avoid damage and breakage:
1. Slip off the patient's gown sleeve (if there are no snaps) before the preoperative IV infusion is started. This prevents having to cut off a wet, soiled gown at the completion of the surgical procedure.
2. Rotate sterile and older supplies to prevent items from deteriorating or the integrity of packaging from being compromised.

3. Take special care to preserve the edges of sharp instruments.

4. Follow established procedures for the proper sterilization and care of instruments, electrical equipment, and other materials. If uncertain how to sterilize or care for any equipment, find out; do not ruin items by guessing. Items for gas sterilization should be tagged "for gas" or "heat sensitive" to help prevent the possibility of inadvertent steam sterilization. Moisture-sensitive items such as surgical cameras should be placed back into original case or labeled accordingly.

5. Check drapes to be certain that instruments are not discarded in disposable drapes or sent to the laundry. At the end of the surgical procedure, the scrub person should look for instruments, needles, and equipment before discarding drapes. This is part of the inventory control reason for counting instruments.

6. If an instrument or piece of equipment is defective, immediately remove it from use. Tag the device with a description of the problem, and report the malfunction promptly for corrective action. In addition, report a surgeon's complaints about the function or quality of an instrument or equipment.

7. Adhere to the routine preventive maintenance schedule for equipment.

ⓔ EVOLVE WEBSITE

http://evolve.elsevier.com/Hornacky/BerryKohn/

- Student Interactive Questions
- Glossary

References

1. Bubric K, Biesbroek S, Laberge J, et al.: Prevalence and characteristics of interruptions and distractions during surgical counts, *Jt Comm J Qual Patient Saf* 47(9):556–562, 2021.
2. Kyle E: Preventing unintentionally retained surgical items, *AORN J* 117(3):192–199, 2023.
3. Association of Surgical Technologists: Standards of practice for patient identification, correct surgery site and procedure. www.ast.org. Accessed April 28, 2023.
4. Haidari M, Malakzai H, Haidary A, et al.: Gossypiboma of thigh mimicking soft tissue sarcoma: a case report and review of the literature, *Int J Surg Case Rep* 106:108106, 2023.
5. Carmack A, Valleru J, Randall K, et al.: A multicenter collaborative effort to reduce preventable patient harm due to retained surgical items, *J Qual Saf* 49(1), 2022.
6. Guideline implementation: safe patient handling and movement, *AORN J* 108(6):663–674, 2018.

Bibliography

AORN: *Guidelines for perioperative practice*, Denver, CO, 2024, The Association.

Association of Surgical Technologists: *Surgical technology for the surgical technologists*, ed 5, Boston, MA, 2018, Cengage Learning.

26

Positioning, Prepping, and Draping the Patient

CHAPTER OUTLINE

Preliminary Considerations, 499

Anatomic and Physiologic Considerations, 504

Equipment for Positioning, 506

Surgical Positions, 512

Physical Preparation and Draping of the Surgical Site, 519

CHAPTER OBJECTIVES

After studying this chapter, the learner will be able to:

- Identify the safety hazards associated with moving a patient from one surface to another.
- List the anatomic considerations for positioning.
- Describe the effects of positioning on the patient's body systems.
- Identify key elements of preoperative skin preparation of patients.
- Discuss the implications of chemical and mechanical actions of prepping the patient.
- Describe how a patient is draped using sterile technique.

KEY TERMS AND DEFINITIONS

Abduct Move away from the body.

Adduct Move toward the body.

Anterior In front of.

Antiseptic solution Topical cleansing chemical used to decrease the microbial count on the skin surface.

Body habitus Generalized physiologic configuration of the patient's size, weight, and shape.

Caudad Toward the foot of the patient.

Cephalad Toward the head of the patient.

Circumduct Rotate a joint in a circumferential axis (usually a ball joint).

Circumferential The surface area of the patient's skin that encompasses a limb or other rounded tissue area.

Deep Below the surface layers.

Distal Away from the core.

Dorsal Back of a part.

Extend Flatten a joint (zero-degree flexion).

Flexion Bend at a normal joint, close the angle of the joint.

Hyperabduction Move away from the body in a line more than a safe 90-degree angle.

Hyperadduction Move toward the body, crossing over the neutral plane of the body.

Hyperextend Move beyond the normal flattening of a joint axis.

Inferior Below or beneath.

Lateral Toward the side of the patient.

Medial Toward the midline.

Posterior Behind.

Prone Face down.

Proximal Closer to the core.

Reverse Trendelenburg position Head-elevated position.

Superficial On the surface.

Superior Above.

Supine Face up.

Trendelenburg position Head-down position.

Ventral Front surface.

Preliminary Considerations

Positioning for a surgical procedure is important to the patient's outcome. Proper positioning facilitates preoperative skin preparation and appropriate draping with sterile drapes. Positioning requires a detailed knowledge of anatomy and physiologic principles and familiarity with the necessary equipment. Safety is a prime consideration.

Patient position and skin preparation are determined by the procedure to be performed, with consideration given to the surgeon's choice of surgical approach and the technique of anesthetic administration. Factors such as age, height, weight, cardiopulmonary status, and preexisting disease condition (e.g., arthritis, allergies) also should be incorporated into the plan of care.[1] Preoperatively, the patient should be assessed for alterations in skin integrity, for joint mobility, and for the presence of joint or vascular prostheses.[2] The expected outcome is that the patient will not be harmed by positioning, prepping, or draping for the surgical procedure.

Efficiency of the patient preparation process can be attained by organizing activities in a logical sequence. Table 26.1 illustrates how to coordinate and organize patient preparation activities.

The main objectives for any surgical or procedural positioning are as follows:

- Optimize surgical site exposure for the surgeon.
- Minimize the risk for adverse physiologic effects.
- Facilitate physiologic monitoring by the anesthesia provider.
- Promote safety and security for the patient.

Responsibility for Patient Positioning

The selection of the surgical position is made by the surgeon in consultation with the anesthesia provider. Adjustments are made as necessary for the administration and monitoring of the anesthetic and for maintenance of the patient's physiologic status. The circulating nurse or first assistant may be responsible for placing the patient in a surgical position, with guidance from the anesthesia provider and the surgeon. In essence, patient positioning is a shared responsibility among all team members. The anesthesia provider has the final word on positioning when the patient's physiologic status and monitoring are in question.

In cases of complex positioning or positioning patients who are obese, the plan of care includes the need for additional help in lifting or positioning. Special devices or positioning aids may be necessary. The weight tolerance of the mechanism and balance of the operating room (OR) bed is critical. Manufacturer recommendations should be consulted for guidance in selecting the appropriate bed. To avoid questions or confusion, the weight tolerance should be clearly labeled on every OR bed. Standard OR beds accommodate 350 lbs. Specialty OR beds are available for patients weighing up to 1000 lbs.

Timing of Patient Positioning and Anesthetic Administration

Moving the patient from the transport cart to the OR bed or vice versa requires that both surfaces are securely locked and stable. Someone should be stationed on the far side of the receiving surface to prevent the patient from tumbling off the edge. For any patient under the influence of an anesthetic agent or narcotic medication, personnel should be at the head, foot, and both sides of the patient to prevent dependent parts from sliding off the table. The neck of the patient's gown should be untied to prevent entanglement and choking as the patient moves or is moved from one surface to another.

After transfer from the transport cart to the OR bed, the patient is usually supine (face up on the back; a few exceptions apply and are explained subsequently in this chapter). Privacy is maintained with a warm cotton blanket, and the safety (thigh) strap is positioned in clear sight of the entire team. The patient may be anesthetized in a supine position and then repositioned for the surgical procedure.

Some patients are positioned and then anesthetized if their physiologic status requires special care. If patients undergo a procedure in a prone position and with general anesthesia, they are anesthetized and intubated on the transport cart. A minimum of four people is required to place the patient safely in the prone position on the OR bed. Commonly, more personnel are needed

for a safe transfer between surfaces when the patient is fully under anesthesia and intubated.

Several factors influence the time at which the patient is positioned: the site of the surgical procedure, the age and size of the patient, the technique of anesthetic administration, and whether the patient is conscious and in pain while moving. The patient is not moved, positioned, or prepped until the anesthesia provider indicates it is safe to do so.

Preparations for Positioning

Before the patient is brought into the OR, the circulating nurse should do the following:

1. Review the proposed position by referring to the positioning instructions on the surgeon's preference card or sheet in comparison with the scheduled procedure.
2. Ask the surgeon for assistance if unsure how to position the patient.
3. Assess for any patient-specific positioning and padding needs.
4. Check the working parts of the OR bed before bringing the patient into the room.
5. Assemble and test all table attachments and protective pads anticipated for the surgical procedure and have them immediately available for use. Box 26.1 lists areas that may need specific attention during padding.
6. Review the plan of care for unique needs of the patient.

Safety Measures

Safety measures, including the following, are observed while transferring, moving, and positioning patients:

1. The patient is properly identified before being transferred to the OR bed, and the surgical site is confirmed according to facility policy. The surgeon is required to initial the correct site.
2. The patient is assessed for mobility status, which includes determination of the patient's ability to transfer between the transport cart and the OR bed. Do not plan to have patients move themselves toward an affected limb or toward the blinded eye.
3. The OR bed and transport vehicle are securely locked in position, with the mattress stabilized during transfer to and from the OR bed. Untie the ties of the patient's gown, and take care not to allow the patient's gown or blanket to become lodged between the two surfaces or under the bottom of a moving patient. Velcro strips or other means should be used to maintain the stability of the mattresses of the two surfaces.
4. Two people should assist an awake patient with the transfer by positioning themselves on each side of the patient's transfer path. The person on the side of the transport cart assists the patient in moving toward the OR bed. The person on the opposite side prevents the patient from falling over the edge of the OR bed.
5. Adequate assistance in lifting unconscious, anesthetized, obese, pregnant, or weak patients is necessary to prevent injury. A minimum of four people is recommended, and transfer devices and lifters may be used. The patient is moved on the count of three, with the anesthesia provider giving the signal count. Sliding or pulling the patient may cause dermal abrasion or injury to soft tissues. Dependent limbs can create a counterbalance and cause the patient to fall to the floor. Examination gloves should be worn if the patient is

TABLE 26.1 Planning the Organization of Patient Positioning, Prepping, and Draping

Type of Procedure	Positioning	Catheterization	Preparation Sequence	Drape Tips
Abdominal				
Anterior chest, epigastrium, umbilicus, pelvis Laparoscopy	Supine with arms tucked at sides or secured on armboards. Thigh strap is secured. Legs remain flat. Small pillow under knees to take pressure off lower back, pad heels. Trendelenburg position can increase intraocular and intracranial pressure. Blood pressure and cardiac output decrease. Reverse Trendelenburg position decreases intracranial pressure. Place padded footboard on lower bed segment to support feet. Lateral tilt can be used to elevate the surgical site.	Catheter is placed before the abdomen is cleansed. The urinary drainage bag is placed in view of the anesthesia provider. Female patient is frog-legged for the catheterization procedure. Support legs to prevent extreme external rotation. Complex patients may need ureteral catheters placed preoperatively. This catheter uses cystoscopy setup and two ureteral catheter drainage bags.	Hair is removed during the prep process as desired by the surgeon. Umbilicus is cleansed in sequence as preferred by the surgeon. Urinary meatus is prepped as part of the catheterization process. Abdominal cleansing begins at surgical site and proceeds to the periphery in a circular motion. Avoid pooling of prep solutions under the patient. Safety (thigh) strap is secured after the prep. Before draping, be sure that the safety strap is placed over a blanket so it is visible to entire team.	The dispersive electrode for the monopolar ESU is placed when patient is in the final resting position for the procedure. Do not cut or reposition the electrode. Some surgeons like the surgical site squared off with towels. Some surgeons prefer medium sheets placed above and below the abdominal incision before placing a fenestrated sheet. Some surgeons prefer a clear or impregnated incise sheet. Fenestrated laparotomy sheet is positioned over the surgical site. Additional drapes may be needed to cover the armboards if the laparotomy sheet does not have arm flaps.
Combined abdominal and perineal Abdominal, epigastrium, pelvis Laparoscopy Genitourinary	Patient is anesthetized in the supine position unless epidural or spinal anesthesia is used. Thigh strap is secured during induction. Lithotomy with arms tucked at sides or secured on armboards. Take care not to crush digits in table break. No strap on abdomen. Stirrups should be padded, and the legs should be elevated and lowered simultaneously. Legs are secured in stirrups with straps. Stirrups should be weight appropriate. Pulses should be checked after placement in the stirrups (e.g., popliteal, posterior tibial, dorsalis pedis). Sequential compression devices should remain functional, and tubing unobstructed. Lithotomy position increases autotransfusion from legs. Lowering the legs decreases blood pressure.	Foley catheter is placed before the abdomen is cleansed. The drain bag is placed in view of the anesthesia provider. Rectal irrigation for colon procedures (if necessary) is performed after the catheterization and before the perineal cleansing prep. An impervious, nonsterile, under-buttocks drape should be used to deflect runoff prep solution into a kick bucket. Complex patients may need ureteral catheters placed preoperatively. This catheter uses cystoscopy setup, two ureteral catheters, and a ureteral catheter drainage bag.	Urinary meatus is prepped as part of the catheterization process. Hair is removed during the prep process as desired by the surgeon. Perineum is prepped first, including the vagina, followed by the anus. Abdominal cleansing begins at surgical site and proceeds to the periphery in a circular motion. Thigh strap is secured after the prep. Before draping, be sure that safety strap is placed over a blanket so it is visible to entire team.	The dispersive electrode for the monopolar ESU is placed when patient is in the final resting position for the procedure. Do not cut or reposition the electrode. Under-buttocks, sterile drape is placed first, followed by leggings. Some surgeons like the surgical site squared off with towels. Some surgeons prefer a clear or impregnated incise sheet. Fenestrated laparotomy sheet is positioned over the surgical site. Additional drapes may be needed to cover the armboards if the laparotomy sheet does not have arm flaps. Some surgeons request a sterile drape over the exposed perineum until that portion of the procedure is started. Laparoscopic procedures may require perineal access during the abdominal phase of surgery.

Continued

TABLE 26.1 Planning the Organization of Patient Positioning, Prepping, and Draping—cont'd

Type of Procedure	Positioning	Catheterization	Preparation Sequence	Drape Tips
Lateral				
Thorax, kidney, hip	Patient is anesthetized in the supine position unless epidural or spinal anesthesia is used. Thigh strap is secured during induction. Patient is positioned on the side after the catheter is placed. Padded beanbag vacuum positioning devices may be used. Legs are slightly flexed with pillow between knees. Lower leg is flexed more for stability. Axillary roll is placed under lower axilla. Arms are supported on armboards perpendicular to body. Use wide body strap over the hip and narrow belt loosely over lower leg. Some surgeons prefer to use wide adhesive tape secured to the bed. Table may be flexed to elevate the surgical site.	Catheterization is performed in the supine position. Catheter is placed before the patient is positioned and before the surgical site is cleansed. The drain bag is placed in view of the anesthesia provider. Female patient is frog-legged for the catheterization procedure. Complex patients may need ureteral catheters placed preoperatively. This catheter uses a cystoscopy setup, two ureteral catheters, and a ureteral catheter drainage bag.	Hair is removed during the prep process as desired by the surgeon. Cleansing begins at surgical site and proceeds to the periphery in a circular motion.	The dispersive electrode for the monopolar ESU is placed in the final resting position for the procedure. Do not cut or reposition the electrode. Some surgeons like the surgical site squared off with towels. Some surgeons prefer a clear or impregnated incise sheet. Fenestrated laparotomy sheet is positioned over the surgical site.
Extremity				
Shoulder, arm, wrist, leg, foot, anterior hip	UPPER: Elbow and distal to elbow may require a hand table attachment as a work surface. Sterile or nonsterile tourniquet may be placed. Shoulder procedures may require the patient to be in a supine posture. LOWER: *Supine:* Special orthopedic table may be used with support for unaffected limb and traction for affected limb. *Lateral:* Standard OR bed can be used.	Some patients with lower extremity fractures or joint replacements may need a Foley catheter. Placement of the Foley catheter may require additional help in holding the female patient's legs in position. Frog-legging is not advised with lower extremity fractures. Procedures lasting longer than 2 hours may require a urinary catheter to monitor intake and output.	Extremity is suspended above the surface of the OR bed. Hair is removed as desired by physician. Prep is circumferential. Prevent backflow of prep solution from clean to dirty. Prep from incision to periphery.	The dispersive electrode for the monopolar ESU is placed when patient is in the final resting position for the procedure. Do not cut or reposition the electrode. Do not place electrode on affected leg. Some surgeons like a sterile stockinette placed over the freshly prepped extremity. When a nonsterile tourniquet is used, a plastic impervious drape is placed around the distal aspect of the cuff to protect from prep solution. U-drapes and split sheets are commonly used to isolate the surgical site from the nonaffected areas.

Sitting

Position / Procedure	Positioning	Catheterization / Drainage	Prep	Draping
Sitting Cranial, neck, ear, face, anterior throat, posterior cervical area Abdominoplasty	Patient is anesthetized in the supine position unless epidural or spinal anesthesia is used. Thigh strap is secured during induction. *Many seated variations:* OR bed is in semi-Fowler or high-Fowler position, with the back of the bed elevated between 10 and 45 degrees. Leg break is slightly 5–10 degrees flexed to prevent the patient from sliding down. Sequential compression devices should remain functional and tubing unobstructed to decrease venous pooling in legs. A pillow is placed over the patient's midsection (or overbed table); the arms are placed over the top. Safety strap is placed lightly but securely over the thighs. Padded footboard may be used to maintain position of feet at right angles to legs, protect heels. Intracranial pressure is decreased in the seated position. Abdominal closure for abdominoplasty is facilitated by the flexed body position.	Foley catheter is placed with the patient supine before placement into a seated position. Take care not to kink when repositioning the patient. Drainage bag should be placed in clear view of anesthesia provider.	Hair is removed during the prep process as desired by the surgeon. Patient may want long head hair saved in a plastic bag for personal reasons. Always do this for pediatric patients and their parents. Cleansing begins at surgical site and proceeds to the periphery in a circular motion. Take extreme care not to get prep solution into eyes, nose, mouth, or ears. Clear plastic dressing materials can be placed over the facial orifices of the patient under general anesthesia to prevent exposure. Some surgeons prefer cotton balls or gauze placed in the patient's ears.	The dispersive electrode for the monopolar ESU is placed when patient is in the final resting position for the procedure. Do not cut or reposition the electrode. Cranial procedures use a fenestrated sheet with round aperture. Disposable sheets commonly have an incise sheet built in. Most have an inferior drainage pouch to catch runoff irrigation. Facial and anterior neck procedures require wrapping the head in a towel drape to isolate scalp hair from the field. Full sheets or split sheets can be used to cover the body.

Prone

Position / Procedure	Positioning	Catheterization / Drainage	Prep	Draping
Prone Rectal, spinal, posterior thorax, cervical Modified spinal procedure prone/kneeling	Patient is anesthetized in the supine position on the transport cart unless epidural or spinal anesthesia is used. Safety strap is secured on posterior aspect of calves to prevent leg flexion. Chest rolls or frame prevent constriction of chest and abdomen. Protect genitalia and breasts from compression and shearing force. Gel pads under knees and dorsum of foot to protect the toes. Some special kneeling spinal tables have fabric boots that are fastened around the patient's feet. The boots are attached to the frame to secure the feet. Kneeling tables have padded positioner boards that rest against the patient's buttocks for stabilization.	Foley catheter is placed with the patient supine before placement into the prone position. Drainage bag is placed in the view of the anesthesia provider.	Hair is removed during the prep process as desired by the surgeon. Cleansing begins at surgical site and proceeds to the periphery in a circular motion.	The dispersive electrode for the monopolar ESU is placed when the patient is in the final resting position for the procedure. Some surgeons like the surgical site squared off with towels. Some surgeons prefer a clear or impregnated incise sheet. Fenestrated laparotomy sheet is positioned over the surgical site. Additional drapes may be needed to cover the armboards if the laparotomy sheet does not have arm flaps.

ESU, Electrosurgical unit.

Supine Position
- Occiput
- Heels
- Elbows
- Sacrum
- Scapulae

Prone or Other Face-Down Position
- Anterior knees of kneeling patient
- Face (particularly the forehead) and ears
- Dorsum of foot to protect toes
- Genitalia and breasts

Lateral Position
- Face and ears
- Medial knees
- Axilla
- Ankles and feet
- Arms

incontinent or offers other risk for exposure to blood and body substances.

6. The anesthesia provider guards the head of the anesthetized patient at all times and supports it during movement. The head should be kept in a neutral axis and turned as little as possible to maintain the airway and cerebral circulation.

7. The physician assumes responsibility for protecting an unsplinted fracture during movement.

8. The anesthetized patient is not moved without permission of the anesthesia provider.

9. The anesthetized patient is moved slowly and gently to allow the circulatory system to adjust and to control the body during movement.

10. No body part should extend beyond the edges of the OR bed or contact metal parts or unpadded surfaces.

11. Body exposure should be minimal to prevent hypothermia and preserve dignity.

12. Movement and positioning should not obstruct or dislodge catheters, intravenous (IV) infusion tubing, oxygen cannulas, and monitors.

13. The armboard is protected to avoid hyperextending the arm greater than 90 degrees or dislodging the IV cannula. The surface of the armboard pad and the mattress of the OR bed should be of equal height. Hyperabduction is avoided to prevent brachial plexus stretch.

14. When the patient is supine (on the back), the ankles and legs must not be crossed. Crossing of the ankles and legs creates occlusive pressure on blood vessels and nerves, and pressure necrosis may occur. The patient is then at risk for deep vein thrombosis (DVT).

15. When the patient is prone (on the abdomen), the thorax is relieved of pressure by using chest rolls (subclavicle to iliac crest) to facilitate chest expansion with respiration. The chest rolls should be adequately secured to the table to prevent shifting. The anterior of the pubis should be sufficiently padded to protect the genitalia from pressure.

The abdomen should remain dependent to decrease abdominal venous pressure and facilitate respiratory excursion. Padding

should be placed at the dorsum of the feet to prevent pressure on the toes. In the event of cardiac arrest, a transport cart should be available for immediate emergency repositioning into the supine position and for subsequent resuscitation.

16. When the patient is positioned lateral (on the side), a pillow is placed lengthwise between the legs to prevent pressure on bony prominences, blood vessels, and nerves. This positioning also relieves pressure on the superior hip. The legs are slightly adducted, but not in hyperadduction. Pressure reduction padding is placed beneath the axilla on the unaffected side to protect the arm from body weight. Care is taken to ensure that the padding is not creating undue pressure directly into the axilla.

17. During articulation of the OR bed, the patient is protected from crush injury at the flex points of the OR bed.

18. When the OR bed is elevated, the patient's feet and protuberant parts are protected from compression by overbed tables, Mayo stands, and retractor frames. An adequate clearance of 2 to 3 inches is maintained.

19. Surfaces should not create pressure on any body part. Alternating or pressure-relieving surfaces should be used. Rolled blankets and towels can create pressure because they do not allow for relief of compression at the contact surface. A gel pad or other alternating pressure pad should be used. Fig. 26.1 depicts the tissue layers as they are compressed against a bony prominence.

Anatomic and Physiologic Considerations

A patient's tolerance of the stresses of the surgical procedure depends greatly on normal functioning of the vital systems. The patient's physical condition is considered, and proper body alignment is important. Criteria are met for physiologic positioning to prevent injury from pressure, crushing, pinching, obstruction, and stretching. Each body system is considered when planning the patient's position for the surgical procedure. Complications of positioning are listed in Box 26.2.

Respiratory Considerations

Unhindered diaphragmatic movement and a patent airway are essential for maintaining respiratory function, preventing hypoxia, and facilitating induction by inhalation anesthesia. Chest excursion is a concern because inspiration expands the chest anteriorly. Some positions limit the amount of mechanical excursion of the chest. Some hypoxia is always present in a horizontal position because the anteroposterior diameter of the ribcage and abdomen decreases.

The tidal volume, the functional residual capacity of air moved by a single breath, is reduced by as much as one-third when a patient lies down because the diaphragm shifts cephalad. Therefore there should be no constriction around the chest or neck.

The patient's arms should be at their side, on armboards, or otherwise supported—not crossed on the chest, unless absolutely necessary for the procedure. Patients have additional respiratory compromise if they are obese, smoke, or have pulmonary disease.

Circulatory Considerations

Adequate arterial circulation is necessary for maintaining blood pressure, perfusing tissues with oxygen, facilitating venous return,

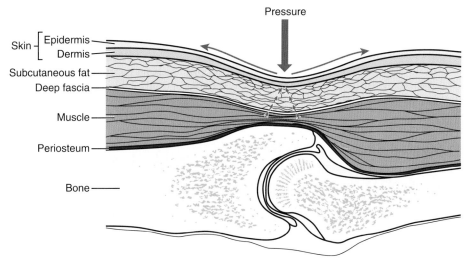

• **Fig. 26.1** Tissues are affected by pressure, which causes deep tissue damage and necrosis.

• BOX 26.2   Complications Caused by Positioning

- Hemodynamic instability from orthostatic position
- Poor ventilation from thoracic compression
- Peripheral nerve injury from compression or stretch
- Tissue damage from crush or shearing force
- Ischemia of hair-bearing scalp, which causes bald spots
- Compartment syndrome
- Pressure necrosis
- Digit amputation in table bends
- Blindness from optic nerve ischemia
- Corneal abrasion
- Ischemic limbs from arterial occlusion
- Venous emboli
- Vertebral injury
- Panic attacks and feelings of claustrophobia in awake patient

---

and preventing thrombus formation. Occlusion and pressure on the peripheral blood vessels are avoided. Body support and restraining straps must not be fastened too tightly. Anesthetic agents alter normal body circulatory mechanisms, such as blood pressure. Some drugs cause constriction or dilation of the blood vessels, which is further complicated by positioning.

Peripheral Nerve Considerations

Prolonged pressure on or stretching of the peripheral nerves can result in injuries that range from sensory and motor loss to paralysis and muscle wasting. The extremities and the body should be well supported at all times. The most common sites of injury in the upper body are the divisions of the brachial plexus and the ulnar, radial, peroneal, and facial nerves; the axons may be stretched or disrupted. Extreme positions of the head and arm greater than 90 degrees can easily injure the brachial plexus and other superficial nerves.

Peripheral nerve injury of the lower body can involve the sciatic, ilioinguinal, and peroneal nerves. If the patient is improperly positioned, the ulnar, radial, and peroneal nerves may be compressed against bone, stirrups, upright retractor posts, or the OR bed.

Arthroscopy leg holders and tourniquets can cause crushed or transected nerve injury. Femoral nerve injury can be caused by retractors during pelvic procedures. Sciatic nerve injury may be caused by tissue retraction or manipulation during hip surgery or extremes of lithotomy position. Facial nerve injury may result from a head strap that is too tight or from manually elevating the mandible too vigorously to maintain the airway.

Musculoskeletal Considerations

A strain on muscle groups results in injury or needless postoperative discomfort. A patient who is anesthetized lacks protective muscle tone. If the head is extended for a prolonged time, the patient may have more pain from the resulting stiff neck than from the surgical wound. Care is taken not to hyperextend a joint, which not only causes postoperative pain but also may contribute to permanent injury to an extremity. Elderly or debilitated patients with osteoporosis or other bone disease may suffer fractures.

When turning a patient, always keep the spine in alignment by grasping the shoulder girdle and hip in a logrolling fashion. Do not turn or elevate a patient by grasping only a hip or shoulder and twisting the spine. Proper body alignment is maintained.

Soft Tissue Considerations

Body weight is distributed unevenly when the patient lies on the OR bed. Weight that is concentrated over bony prominences can cause skin pressure ulcers and deep tissue injury. These areas should be protected from constant external pressure against hard surfaces, particularly in patients who are thin or underweight. In addition, tissue that is subjected to prolonged mechanical pressure (e.g., a fold in the skin under an obese or malnourished patient) is not adequately perfused.

Wrinkled sheets and the edges of a positioning or other device under the patient can cause pressure on the skin. Foam pads are not adequate to relieve pressure because they compress and do not alternate pressure. Towels and sheet rolls do not relieve pressure because they are unyielding to the patient's body weight. Gel pads are preferred. Positioning devices should maintain normal capillary interface pressure of 23 to 32 mm Hg or less to prevent pressure injuries. Blood flow and tissue perfusion are restricted at higher capillary pressures.

Patients should be assessed for risk of pressure injuries. Pressure injuries are more common after surgical procedures that last 1 hour or longer. During lengthy procedures, the head and other body parts should be repositioned if possible. Patients who are debilitated, poorly nourished, or diabetic are at particularly high risk for pressure ulcers and alopecia (permanent bald spots from pressure).[2] Pressure-redistributing padding should be used to prevent pressure injuries.

Accessibility of the Surgical Site

The surgical procedure and patient condition determine the position in which the patient is placed. To minimize trauma and operating time, the surgeon must have adequate exposure of the surgical site.

Accessibility for Anesthetic Administration

The anesthesia provider should be able to attach monitoring electrodes, administer the anesthetic and observe its effects, and maintain IV access. The patient's airway is of prime concern and must be patent and accessible at all times. The anesthesia provider needs to continuously assess urinary output, blood loss, and irrigation use. Consideration for visibility of measuring devices and drainage bags should be incorporated in the plan for positioning.

Individual Positioning Considerations

If patients are extremely obese (e.g., the torso occupies the width of the OR bed), their arms may be placed on armboards. Heavy-duty OR beds are available with side extenders to accommodate wide patients. Patients with arthritis or previous joint surgery may need special individualized care because of limited range of motion in their joints. A patient who has cardiac problems or is obese may experience orthopnea or dyspnea when lying flat.

Pediatric patients, especially infants, need less OR bed length. Some surgeons like the foot portion of the bed lowered or removed to decrease the length of the working surface for accessibility.

Equipment for Positioning

Operating Room Bed

Many different OR beds with suitable attachments are available, and practice is necessary to master the adjustments. OR beds are versatile and adaptable to a number of diversified positions for many surgical specialties; orthopedic, urologic, and fluoroscopic tables are often used for specialized procedures. Fig. 26.2 depicts a typical general-purpose OR bed.

The patient's body habitus may necessitate the use of a specialty OR bed with an increased weight limit. Manufacturer recommendations should be consulted for the operation of each model of OR bed.

Most OR beds consist of a rectangular metal top that measures 79 to 89 inches long by 20 to 24 inches wide (201−225 cm × 51−61 cm) and rests on an electric or hydraulic lift base. Some models have interchangeable radiopaque tops for various specialties.

The surface of the OR bed is divided into three or more hinged sections: the head, the body, and the leg sections. The joints of the OR bed are referred to as *breaks*. Each hinged section can be manipulated, flexed, or extended to the desired position in a procedure called *breaking the OR bed*. Fig. 26.3 shows the range of flexibility of an average general-purpose OR bed.

Some OR beds have a metal body elevator plate between the two upper sections that may be raised up to 5½ inches (14 cm) to elevate an area for a gallbladder or kidney procedure. Care is taken when using this elevator because it can decrease the ability of the chest to expand during ventilation.

The head section is removable, which permits the insertion of special headrests for cranial procedures. An extension may be inserted at the foot of the OR bed to accommodate an exceptionally tall patient. A radiopaque cassette-loading top extends the length of the bed and permits the insertion of an x-ray cassette holder at any area. A self-adhering, sectional, conductive mattress (at least 3 inches [8 cm] thick) covers the surface of the OR bed. Gel-filled alternating surface mattress and pads are commercially available to cover the surface of the OR bed.

• **Fig. 26.2** General-purpose OR bed. *1,* Movable head section; *2,* x-ray cassette tunnel; *3,* kidney elevation bar; *4,* perineal cutout; *5,* lower extremity section; *6,* control box; *7,* pedestal; *8,* base; *9,* casters; *10,* power cord; *11,* side rails; *12,* pads.

• **Fig. 26.3** Flexibility range of general-purpose OR bed. **A,** Lower extremity section lowered. **B,** Range of positions for raised and lowered body and lower extremity sections. **C,** Trendelenburg position and reverse Trendelenburg position. **D,** Lateral tilt.

Standard OR beds have controls for manipulation into desired positions. Some beds are electrically controlled by either remote hand-control or foot-control switches or a lever-operated electro-hydraulic system; older OR beds are controlled with manual hand cranks. Most electric styles have a rechargeable battery that can be used for several weeks without recharging.

The desired sections of the OR bed surface can be articulated by setting the selector control on "back," "side," "foot," or "flex." By activating other selector controls, the surface of the OR bed may be tilted laterally up to 28 degrees from side to side and raised or lowered in its entirety. A tiltometer indicates the degree of tilt between horizontal and vertical for variations in Trendelenburg position. Most styles offer 30 to 40 degrees of Trendelenburg position full-table tilt down or up. All OR beds have a brake or floor lock for stabilization in all positions.

Special Equipment and Bed Attachments

The equipment used in positioning is designed to stabilize the patient in the desired position and thus permit optimal exposure of the surgical site. All devices are clean, free of sharp edges, and padded to prevent trauma or abrasion. Each OR bed has attachments for specific purposes. Many positioning devices to protect pressure points and joints are commercially available. If the devices are reusable, they are washable; some may be terminally sterilized for asepsis between uses.

Safety Belt (Thigh Strap)

For restraint of leg movement during surgical procedures, a sturdy, wide strap of durable material that can be washed or sterilized (e.g., nylon webbing with hook and loop closure, conductive rubber) is placed and fastened over the thighs, above the knees, and around the surface of the OR bed. Some straps are radiolucent. Placement in this location prevents the large muscle groups of the legs from flexing and causing the patient to fall from the OR bed.

Some straps are attached at each side of the bed and fastened together at the center. This belt should be secure but not so tight that it impairs circulation; the circulating nurse should be able to pass two fingers between the strap and the patient. Placement of the belt depends on body position. For prevention of injury to underlying tissue, padding or a blanket should be placed between the skin and the belt. The strap should be placed over, not under, a blanket for easy visualization before prepping and draping.

The safety belt is used during surgical procedures except for certain positions (e.g., lithotomy and seated). Belting across the patient's abdomen during the lithotomy position can cause compression of the abdominal structures. The safety belt is used before and after the procedure, when the patient's legs are in the down position.

Anesthesia Screen

A metal bar attaches to the head of the OR bed and holds the drapes from the patient's face. It is placed after the induction of anesthesia and the positioning of the patient and is used to separate the nonsterile from the sterile area at the head of the bed. The bar is adjustable and allows rotation or angling. Some facilities use two IV poles to secure the drapes at the head of the bed.

Special procedures may require the use of an overbed table that mounts in the same fashion as an anesthesia screen. The socket attachments are secured to the side rail of the bed and are locked onto the frame of this table (Fig. 26.4).

• **Fig. 26.4** Overbed table attachment.

Lift Sheet (Drawsheet)

A double-layer sheet is placed horizontally across the top of a clean sheet on the OR bed. After patients are transferred to the OR bed, their arms are enclosed in the lower flaps of this sheet, with the palms against the sides in a natural position and the fingers extended along the length of the body. The upper flaps are brought down over the arms and tucked under the patient's sides. The sheet should not be tucked under the sides of the mattress because the combined weight of the mattress and the patient's torso may impair circulation or cause nerve torsion.

The full length of each arm is supported at the patient's side, protected from injury, and secured. The hands should not extend into the flex point of the bed or a crush injury may ensue. In addition, a plastic, curved shield, referred to as a sled, can be padded and used to protect and secure the arms from injury (Fig. 26.5).

Tucking of the patient's arms and use of a sled help prevent inadvertent pressure from upright bars of anesthesia screens, table attachments, and stationary retractor poles (Fig. 26.6).

Patients should be told that these methods are used to support the arms when they are anesthetized and relaxed. The word *restraint* is avoided. At the end of the surgical procedure, this sheet, if not soiled or wet, may be used to lift the patient from the OR bed.

Armboard

Armboards are used to support the arms if IV fluids are being infused, if the arm or hand is the site of the surgical procedure, if the arm at the side would interfere with access to the surgical area, if space is inadequate on the OR bed for the arm to rest beside the body, and/or if the arm requires support (as in the lateral position).

The armboard is padded to a height that is level with the OR bed mattress. To minimize the risk for ulnar nerve pressure and abnormal shoulder rotation, the patient's arm is placed palm up (supinated), except when the patient is in the prone position.

The armboard has adjustable angles, but the arm is never abducted beyond an angle of 90 degrees from the shoulder or brachial nerve plexus injury may occur from hyperabduction (Fig. 26.7). A self-locking type of armboard is safest to prevent displacement.

Double Armboard

With a double armboard, both arms are supported, with one directly above the other in lateral position. This type of armboard resembles the wings of a biplane and is sometimes called an airplane support or overbed arm support. Both levels of the armboard are padded (Fig. 26.8). An axillary roll is used to prevent pressure from the weight of the thorax.

• **Fig. 26.5** The patient's arms can be placed at the sides with the lift sheet pulled over the length of the arm and tucked under the patient's body. **A,** Correct way to secure arm at patient's side. **B,** Incorrect placement of patient's arm results in ulnar nerve injury.

• **Fig. 26.6** Tucking the arms can prevent accidental compression against an upright post attached to the bed frame.

More than 90 degrees

90 degrees

• **Fig. 26.7** Position of arm on armboard should not exceed 90 degrees or injury to the brachial plexus may result. **A,** Incorrect positioning. **B,** Correct positioning.

Wrist or Arm Strap

Narrow straps at least 1½ inches (3.8 cm) wide are placed around the wrists to secure the arms to the armboards. The straps are secured without pressure or a tourniquet effect to the hands or arms. Tubing and monitoring lead wires should not be kinked or dislodged.

• **Fig. 26.8** Double armboard with elevated arm positioner.

• **Fig. 26.9** Anteroposterior positioning frames for lateral positioning.

Upper Extremity Table

For a surgical procedure on an arm or hand, an adjustable extremity table may be attached to the side of the OR bed and used in lieu of an armboard. This attachment is sometimes referred to as a hand table. Some types of extremity tables slip under the mattress proximal to the surgical site and extend perpendicular to the patient's trunk, with the distal end supported by a metal leg. Some models attach directly to the OR bed and require no additional floor support.

The upper extremity table provides a large, padded firm surface for the surgical procedure. The surgeon and sterile team usually sit for these types of procedures. The level of the patient determines the level of the sterile field. If one team member sits, the entire team should sit to maintain the level of the sterile field.

Shoulder Bridge (Thyroid Elevator)

When a shoulder bridge is used, the head section is temporarily removed and a metal bar is slipped under the mattress between the head and body sections of the OR bed. The bridge can be raised to hyperextend the shoulder or thyroid area for surgical accessibility. This position can be achieved also by placing a positioning roll transversely under the shoulders, which causes the neck to hyperextend. A perpendicular roll can be placed between the shoulders to cause the shoulders to fall back bilaterally, which elevates the sternum.

Shoulder Braces or Supports

Adjustable well-padded concave metal supports are occasionally used to prevent the patient slipping when the head of the OR bed is tilted down, such as in the Trendelenburg position. Braces should be placed equidistant from the head of the OR bed, with a ½-inch (13-mm) space between the shoulders and the braces to eliminate pressure against the shoulders. The braces are placed over the acromion processes, not over the muscles and soft tissues near the neck. Care is taken to ensure that the patient's total body weight is not borne by the shoulder braces. The leg section can be lowered slightly to minimize shifting of body weight.

To avoid nerve compression, a shoulder brace is not used when the arm is extended on an armboard; in such cases, ankle straps may be used to stabilize the patient. Many surgeons have modified positioning routines to avoid the use of shoulder braces because of inadvertent nerve injury. AORN (Association of periOperative Registered Nurses) does not recommend the use of shoulder braces.[3] Positioning devices such as vacuum-packed, wedge, foam, or gel overlays should be used to prevent movement and nerve injury.

Body Rests and Braces

Body rests and braces are made of metal and have a foam-rubber or gel pad covered with conductive waterproof fabric. These devices are placed in metal clamps on the side of the OR bed and are slipped in from the edge of the OR bed against the body at various points to stabilize it in a lateral position.

Lateral Positioner (Kidney Rests)

Kidney rests are concave metal pieces with grooved notches at the base; they are placed on the body elevator flexion of the OR bed. They are placed snugly against the body for lateral stability in the side-lying kidney position.

Although the kidney rest is padded, care should be taken so that the upper edge of the rest does not press too tightly against the body. Some OR beds have built-in kidney rests that are raised and lowered electrically or with a hand crank.

Anteroposterior positioning frames attach to the bed in the socket attachments for use during spinal endoscopy. All other aspects of positioning should be considered, such as arms, legs, neck, and head (Fig. 26.9).

Body (Hip) Restraint Strap

With a body restraint strap, a wide belt with a padded center portion (to protect the skin) is placed over the patient's hips and secured to the sides of the OR bed. This strap helps hold the patient securely in the lateral position. Some surgeons prefer to use 2 to 3-inch-wide bands of adhesive tape to secure the shoulders and hips of patients in the lateral position. A towel can be placed over the patient's skin before the tape is applied. The ends of the long strips of tape are secured to the underside of the OR bed. Care is taken not to cause compression, stretching, or folding of the skin under the tape.

Positioning for Anal Procedures With Adhesive Tape

For anal procedures, the patient is placed in a prone position (Kraske position). To separate and retract the buttocks, a piece of 3-inch (7.5-cm) adhesive tape is placed on each buttock, 4 inches (10 cm) lateral to the surgical site. For greater security of tape adhesion, benzoin or adhesive liquid is applied to each buttock before the tape strips are applied. Each end of the tape is fastened to the frame of the OR bed.

Adjustable Arched Spinal Frame

An adjustable arched spinal frame consists of two padded arches mounted on a frame that is attached to the OR bed. The patient is placed in the prone position with the ventral surface of the abdomen over this device (referred to as a Wilson frame). The pads extend from the shoulders to the thighs, with the abdomen hanging dependently between the arches. The desired degree of

• **Fig. 26.10** Frames for spinal surgery. **A,** Andrews. **B,** Wilson. **C,** Four-poster Relton frame.

flexion for spinal procedures is achieved by adjusting the height of the arch by means of a crank. Other types of prone positioning frames are available (Fig. 26.10).

Stirrups

Metal stirrup posts are placed in holders, one on each side rail of the OR bed, to support the legs and feet in the lithotomy position. The feet are supported with canvas or fabric loops that suspend the legs at a right angle to the feet. These stirrups are sometimes called "candy cane" or "sling" stirrups (Fig. 26.11).

During extensive surgery, special leg holders may be used to support the lower legs and feet (e.g., Allen or Yellofin [Yellowfin] stirrups). Leg holders are made in different sizes and are weight-specific to support the legs safely. Also available are metal or high-impact plastic knee crutch stirrups that can be adjusted for knee flexion and extension. Even if well padded, these stirrups may create some pressure on the back of the knees and lower extremities and may jeopardize the popliteal vessels and nerves. Gel and foam pads are available for patient protection when stirrups are used (Fig. 26.12).

Metal Footboard

The footboard can be used flat as a horizontal extension of the OR bed or raised perpendicular to the OR bed to support the feet, with the soles resting securely against it. It is padded when the patient is placed in reverse Trendelenburg position. The patient's full body weight should not rest on the soles of the feet.

Headrests

Padded headrests are used with supine, prone, sitting, and lateral positions. They attach to the OR bed to support and expose the

• **Fig. 26.11** **A,** Correct use of candy cane stirrups with feet suspended in cloth slings. **B,** Legs should not rest on stirrup posts or lower leg nerve injury could result. **C,** Hands should be positioned away from bed flex points. **D,** Correct flexion of legs in stirrups.

• **Fig. 26.12** Additional types of stirrups. **A,** Urologic stirrups. **B,** Stirrups used for abdominoperineal and obstetric procedures. **C,** Allen-style stirrups.

• **Fig. 26.13** **A,** Prone position with face in foam or gel-filled donut head positioner ring. **B,** Horseshoe head holder used for prone or supine procedures. **C,** Mayfield headrest with sterile metal pins inserted into patient's scalp for stability. **D,** Prone position with head placed on pillow. Patient can experience ear compression using this method. Donut should be used in place of pillow to allow for zero pressure on ear.

occiput and cervical vertebrae. The head is held securely but without the pressure that could cause pressure injury to the ears or optic nerve ischemic blindness.

Headrests can be shaped like a donut or horseshoe for head and neck procedures; other styles are flat or concave to stabilize the head and neck in alignment. Nonpadded Mayfield metal headrests have sterile skull pins that are inserted into the patient's head for neurologic procedures (Fig. 26.13).

Accessories
Various sizes and shapes of pads, pillows, and beanbags that fit various anatomic structures are used to protect, support, and immobilize body parts. Foam rubber, polymer pads, silicone gel pads, vacuum-shaped bags, and other accessories are covered with washable materials unless they are designed for single-patient use or can be disinfected.

A donut (a ring-shaped foam rubber or silicone gel pad) may be used during procedures on the head or face to keep the surgical area in a horizontal plane. Donuts are used also to protect pressure points such as the ear, knee, heel, and elbow. Protectors made of foam rubber, polymers, silicone gel, or other material also may be used to protect the joints from pressure. Many other types of protectors are available. Some foam padding may be flammable. Some foam pads can create a fire hazard if alcohol prep solution soaks into the surface and remains damp.

Bolsters are used to elevate a specific part of the body (e.g., Kraske pillow to elevate the buttocks for anal procedures). Solid positioning rolls or firm foam under each side of a patient's chest, referred to as chest rolls, raise the chest off the OR bed to facilitate respiration and decrease intraabdominal pressure. Chest rolls extend from the clavicle to the iliac crest bilaterally. Large gel rolls also can be used for this purpose and for axillary elevation during lateral positioning. Commercially available bolsters and elevating pads are commonly used. Because patients may have a latex sensitivity, the manufacturer's literature should be checked for latex content (Fig. 26.14).

• **Fig. 26.14** Common positioning pads.

• **Fig. 26.15** Supine position. Patient lies straight on back, face upward, with arms at sides, legs extended parallel and uncrossed, and feet slightly separated. Strap is placed above knees. Head is in line with spine. Note small pillow under ankles to protect heels from pressure. Arms are secured with lift sheet or placed on armboards.

Pressure-Minimizing Mattress

To minimize pressure on bony prominences, peripheral blood vessels, and nerves during prolonged surgical procedures (more than 2 hours for the average patient, less for a debilitated patient), an alternating pressure mattress is put over the mattress on the OR bed before the patient arrives. This mattress may be a positive-pressure air mattress, a circulating-water thermal mattress, a foam rubber mattress (with indentations similar to an egg crate), a gel pad, or a dry polymer pad.

Unless designed to be placed next to a patient's skin, pressure reduction mattresses and thermal blankets used to induce hypothermia or hyperthermia should be covered with an absorbent sheet or thin pad. Folds and creases in the covering should be avoided to prevent pressure indentations in the skin. Manufacturer instructions should be followed when using these devices.

Surgical Vacuum Positioning System

With the surgical vacuum positioning system, soft pads filled with tiny plastic beads (i.e., beanbags) are placed under or around the body part to be supported. Suction is attached to the vacuum port on the beanbag pad; as air is withdrawn, the pad becomes firm and molds to the patient's body. The suction is then disconnected. A vacuum is created inside the pad, which causes the beads to press together. Friction between the beads prevents them from moving and creates a solid mass that keeps its molded shape. Adequate pressure reduction padding should be placed between the patient's skin and the beanbag. The firm edges of the beanbag should not rest against the patient's skinfolds such as the axilla or groin.

Various sizes and shapes of pads provide firm support while relieving pressure points. To change the patient's position during the surgical procedure, the valve on the pad is squeezed until the pad is slightly soft. The patient is repositioned, and suction is reapplied to remold the pad.

Surgical Positions

Many positions are used for surgical procedures; the most commonly used positions are discussed in the following sections. If IV fluids are infused in the arm during the surgical procedure, the arm is placed on an armboard. This fact is assumed in the following discussion because IV fluids are usually given. If electrosurgery is used, the large reusable electrosurgery smart pad unit is placed on the bed before the patient comes into the OR. The

disposable patient return electrode is placed after the patient is in the final position for the surgical procedure. The electrode may not be moved, shifted, or cut to size. Take care not to kink catheter tubing or dislodge monitoring devices during positioning.

Supine (Dorsal) Position

Fig. 26.15 shows the patient in the supine (**dorsal**) position—the most natural position for the body at rest. The patient lies flat on the back with the arms secured at the sides with the lift sheet; the palms extend along the side of the body in their natural resting position. The elbows may be protected with padded plastic sleds. The legs are straight and parallel and are in line with the head and spine; the hips are parallel with the spine. A safety belt is placed across the thighs 2 inches above the knees.

Small positioning pads may be placed under the head and popliteal area to relieve pressure on the spine as needed. The heels are protected from pressure with a pillow, gel pad, or donut. The feet must not be in prolonged plantar flexion, or nerve stretch injury could result. To prevent footdrop, the soles may be supported by a pillow or padded footboard.

The supine position is used for procedures on the anterior surface of the body, such as abdominal, abdominothoracic, and some lower extremity procedures. Modifications of the supine position are used for the following specific body areas:

- *Procedures on the face or neck:* The neck may be slightly hyperextended by lowering the head section of the OR bed or by placing a shoulder roll. With the patient in the supine position, the head may be supported in a headrest or donut or turned toward the unaffected side.

  The eyes are protected from injury, laser light, and irritating solutions with corneal shields, goggles, or moist eye pads with nonallergenic tape. Before the surgical procedure and prep, contact lenses and removable eyelashes must be removed. The patient's eyes should be lubricated with sterile ophthalmic gel and secured with eye pads taped in place. The eyes should be inspected periodically by the anesthesia provider during the case and at the end of the surgical procedure. No pressure should impair circulation to the optic nerve. If the eyeball becomes ischemic, the patient can be rendered blind.

- *Shoulder or anterolateral procedures:* With the patient in the supine position, a small sandbag, water bag, roll, or pad is placed under the affected side to elevate the shoulder off the OR bed for exposure. The length of the body is stabilized to prevent the spine from rolling or twisting. Hips and shoulders should be kept in a straight plane. The OR bed also can be tilted laterally to elevate the affected part.

- *Dorsal recumbent and modified recumbent position:* For some vaginal or perineal procedures, the patient is in the supine position except that the knees are flexed upward (frog-legged) and the thighs are slightly externally rotated. The soles of the feet rest on the OR bed. Pillows or foam wedges may be placed under the knees for support and prevention of external rotation of the hip (Fig. 26.16). Positioning devices for frog-legging the patient are commercially available. The thighs are widely externally rotated, and the soles of the feet face each other at the medial line of the body. The blanket is placed over the lower legs, and the safety strap is placed over the blanket anterior to the shins to secure the legs from sliding forward.

- *Arm extension:* For surgical procedures of the breast, axilla, upper extremity, and hand, the patient is placed in the supine position; the arm on the affected side is placed on an armboard or upper extremity table extension that locks into position at a 90-degree right angle to the body. The affected side of the body is close to the edge of the OR bed for access to the surgical area.

If the axilla is involved, the arm is placed even with the lower edge of the armboard for accessibility. Hyperextension of the arm is avoided to prevent neural or vascular injury, such as brachial plexus injury or occlusion of the axillary artery. The armboard is well padded.

Trendelenburg Position

With Trendelenburg position, patients lie on their back in the supine position with the knees over the lower break of the OR bed (Fig. 26.17). The knees must bend with the break of the OR bed to prevent pressure on the peroneal nerves and veins in the legs. The safety (thigh) strap is positioned 2 inches above the knees over the blanket. The entire OR bed is tilted approximately 30 to 45 degrees downward at the head, depending on the surgeon's preference. The foot of the OR bed is lowered to the desired angle to help counterbalance the patient's body weight.

Trendelenburg position is used for procedures in the lower abdomen or pelvis when shifting the abdominal viscera cephalad away from the pelvic area for better exposure. Although surgical accessibility is increased, lung volume is decreased and the heart is mechanically compressed by the pressure of the organs against the diaphragm. Intracranial and intraocular pressure is increased. Therefore the patient remains in this position for as short a time as possible. When returning the patient to a horizontal position, the leg section should be raised first and slowly while venous stasis in the legs is reversed. The entire OR bed is then leveled.

A modification of this position may be used for patients in hypovolemic shock. Many anesthesia providers prefer to keep the trunk level and to elevate the legs by raising the lower part of the OR bed at the break under the hips. Others prefer to tilt the entire OR bed downward toward the head. Either position reduces venous stasis in the lower extremities and promotes venous return.

Reverse Trendelenburg Position

With reverse Trendelenburg position, patients lie on their back in the supine position (Fig. 26.18). The entire OR bed is tilted 30 to 40 degrees so the head is higher than the feet; a padded footboard is used to prevent the patient from sliding toward the tilt. The safety (thigh) belt is positioned 2 inches above the knees over the blanket. Small pillows may be placed under the knees. A small pillow or donut is used to stabilize the head.

This position is used for thyroidectomy to facilitate breathing and decrease blood supply to the surgical site (blood pools caudally). It is also used for laparoscopic gallbladder, biliary tract, and stomach procedures to allow the abdominal viscera to fall away from the epigastrium, providing access to the upper abdomen.

• **Fig. 26.16** Modified dorsal recumbent position. Patient lies on back with arms at sides. Knees are slightly flexed, with a pillow under each. Thighs are externally rotated. Referred to as frog-legged.

• **Fig. 26.17** Trendelenburg position. Note knees are over lower break in OR bed, with knee strap above knees. Arms are secured. Shoulder braces are not usually needed with this method of Trendelenburg position.

• **Fig. 26.18** Reverse Trendelenburg position, with soft roll under shoulders for thyroid, neck, and shoulder procedures. (From Rothrock JC: *Alexander's care of the patient in surgery*, ed 14, St. Louis, 2011, Mosby.)

Venous stasis can cause complications, and prevention of deep vein thrombosis (DVT) is an important consideration. The use of sequential compression devices, antiembolic stockings, or foot pumps is suggested to improve venous return.

Semi-Fowler Position

With semi-Fowler position, the patient is supine with the buttocks at the flex in the OR bed and the knees over the lower break. The foot of the OR bed is lowered slightly, flexing the knees. The body section is raised 45 degrees and thereby becomes the backrest. Arms may rest on armboards parallel to the OR bed or on a large soft pillow on the lap. Care is taken that the arms do not fall dependent from the body during the procedure. The safety belt is secured 2 inches above the knees over the blanket. Pressure points such as the coccyx and heels should be padded in seated positions. The entire OR bed is tilted slightly with the head end downward to prevent the patient from slipping toward the foot of the OR bed. Feet should rest on the padded footboard to prevent footdrop. For cranial procedures, the head is supported in a headrest.

In this position, the OR bed looks like a modified armchair. This position may be used for shoulder, nasopharyngeal, facial, and breast reconstruction procedures (Fig. 26.19). Complications of this position include air embolus into the venous system, pelvic pooling or venous stasis, hypotension, positional orthopedic injury, and tissue pressure injury and necrosis.

If an air embolus should enter the patient's right atrium, the patient is immediately repositioned in the left lateral position and the bed is lowered into steep Trendelenburg position. This emergent posture is referred to the Durant position or Durant maneuver. This immediate action causes the air embolus to move from the right ventricular outflow tract. The anesthesia provider places a central venous catheter into the right atrium to aspirate the trapped air bubble and restore cardiac function.

Sitting Position

With the sitting position, the patient is placed in the Fowler position except that the torso is completely in an upright position. The shoulders and torso should be supported with body straps but not so tightly that respiration and circulation are impeded. Pressure points (especially ischial tuberosities) are padded to reduce the risk for sciatic nerve damage.

The flexed arms rest on a large pillow on the lap or on a pillow on an adjustable table in front of the patient (see Fig. 26.4; this table attachment can be secured in the bed sockets in front of the patient as a padded armrest).

The head is seated forward in a cranial headrest for neurosurgical procedures. A padded footboard or large cushioning

• **Fig. 26.19** Modified Fowler position with the shoulder dependent over the edge of the bed for shoulder procedure. Sometimes referred to as the captain's chair.

device under the patient is placed to maintain the patient's feet in an upright position and deter sliding down on the bed.[4]

This position is used on occasion for some otorhinologic and neurosurgical procedures. Air embolism is a potential complication and is treated in the same manner as described for the semi-Fowler position. Antiembolic stockings or sequential compression devices are used to counteract postural hypotension and decrease venous pooling in the extremities and pelvis.

Beach Chair or Modified Sitting Position

With the beach chair or modified sitting position, the patient is supine with the back and legs slightly elevated. The entire spine is somewhat contoured, with the angle of flexion at the hip decreased. Both the head and the feet are elevated 10 to 20 degrees above the level of the heart. The arms are placed across the abdomen, and the safety belt is secured over the thighs. This position is used for several shoulder, nose, neurosurgery, and throat procedures. A large cushioning device should be placed under the patient to prevent injury and movement.

Abdominoplasty and lower abdominal TRAM (transverse rectus abdominis muscle used for breast reconstruction) closure is performed using this position to bring the skin edges closer together after resection of a large abdominal skin flap. The xyphoid-pubic distance is shortened. The arms can be secured with the lift sheet if the hands are not at risk for crush injury at the bed flexion points (Fig. 26.20).

Lithotomy Position

The lithotomy position is used for perineal, vaginal, urologic, and rectal procedures. The patient's buttocks rest along the break between the body and the leg sections of the OR bed. A padded metal footboard is used as an OR bed extension so the patient's legs do not extend over the foot of the OR bed before the legs are placed in the upright position.

Stirrups are secured in sockets on each side of the OR bed rail at the level of the patient's upper thighs. They are adjusted at equal height on both sides and at an appropriate height for the length of the patient's legs to maintain symmetry when the patient is positioned. After the patient is anesthetized, the safety belt is removed and the patient's legs are raised simultaneously by two people (Fig. 26.21). The safety belt should not remain in place

• **Fig. 26.20** Beach chair position. The arms are typically placed across the abdomen, and a safety strap is across the thighs.

• **Fig. 26.21** Lithotomy position. Patient is supine with foot section of OR bed lowered to right angle. Knees are flexed, and legs are elevated to the degree necessary for the type of surgical procedure. Note that buttocks are even with edge of the OR bed and that sometimes a roll is needed under the buttocks to elevate the hips above the level of the bed.

A — Low lithotomy

B — Standard lithotomy

C — Hemi (split) lithotomy

D — High lithotomy

E — Exaggerated lithotomy

F — Tilted low lithotomy

• **Fig. 26.22** Commonly used lithotomy positions.

over the abdomen with the patient in the lithotomy position. It causes increased abdominal venous pressure, which in turn increases the risk for blood loss.

Each person grasps the sole of a foot in one hand and supports the calf at the knee area with the other. The knees are flexed, and the legs and feet are placed inside the stirrups simultaneously. Avoid overflexing the hip toward the abdomen to prevent ilioinguinal nerve compression. For sling or candy cane stirrups, the feet are placed in the fabric slings of the stirrups at a 90-degree angle to the abdomen. One padded loop encircles the sole; the other padded loop goes around the ankle.

Simultaneous movement as the knees are flexed is essential to avoid straining the lower back and causing sudden hemodynamic changes in the venous system. If the patient's legs are properly placed, undue abduction and external rotation are avoided. The leg or ankle must not touch the metal stirrup. Padding is placed as necessary. If the legs are put in stirrups before the induction of anesthesia, the patient can identify discomfort and pressure on the back or legs. The positioning procedure is similar for other types of stirrups. There is no scientific evidence to support raising one

leg at a time. The level of the lithotomy position needed for the surgical procedure is determined by the surgeon (Fig. 26.22).

After the patient's legs are placed in the stirrups, the lower section of mattress is removed and the bottom section of the OR bed is lowered. The buttocks must not extend beyond the edge of the OR bed, which would strain the lumbosacral muscles and ligaments as the weight of the body rests on the sacrum.

The hands should not extend beyond the buttocks if tucked alongside the patient. Hands have been crushed in the break as the leg section of the OR bed was raised at the conclusion of the surgical procedure. Arms may be placed on armboards or loosely cradled over the lower abdomen and secured by the lower end of the blanket. Arms must not rest directly on the chest, which could impede respiration. Lung compliance is decreased by pressure of the thighs on the abdomen, which hinders the descent of the diaphragm.

Venous blood pools in the lumbar region of the torso, especially during prolonged surgical procedures in the lithotomy position. Antiembolic stockings may be worn, or legs may be wrapped in sequential compression devices or foot pumps during the surgical procedure to prevent the formation of thrombi or emboli. The legs should be checked periodically for distal pulses (pedal or posterior tibial), skin color, and evidence of edema. In the lithotomy position, nerve damage or compartment syndrome can occur from direct pressure or ischemia of the muscles, which compromises the viability of tissues. According to AORN, the hemilithotomy position is not recommended and should be used only if necessary because of pressure on the raised leg, which may result in compartment syndrome.

At the conclusion of the surgical procedure, the leg section of the OR bed is raised and the lower section of the mattress is replaced. The patient's legs are removed simultaneously from the stirrups with a minimum of two people. The legs are brought together and lowered slowly to prevent hypotension as blood re-enters the legs and leaves the torso. To prevent external rotation of the hips, the legs are fully extended and brought together as they are lifted from the stirrups. The blanket and safety belt should be reapplied over the thighs during the patient's emergence from anesthesia.

Prone Position

Prone position is used for all procedures with a dorsal or posterior approach (Fig. 26.23). When the prone position is used, the patient is anesthetized and intubated in the supine position on the locked transport cart. The patient's arms are placed along their sides. When the anesthesia provider gives permission, the patient is slowly and cautiously shifted toward the OR bed in the supine position and then turned onto the abdomen onto the OR bed. The patient's body is rotated as if rolling a log; a team of at least four to six people is needed to maintain body alignment during this transfer. The anesthesia provider calls the count. The anesthesia provider controls the patient's head and airway while the rest of the patient's body is moved by the team.

Chest rolls or bolsters under the axillae and along the sides of the chest from the clavicles to the iliac crests raise the weight of the

• **Fig. 26.23** Prone position. Patient is placed on abdomen. Chest rolls are placed under axillae and sides of chest to the level of the iliac crest to facilitate respiration. Knees should be padded, and a pillow is placed under dorsum of feet.

body from the abdomen and thorax. The weight of the abdomen falls away from the diaphragm and keeps pressure off the vena cava and abdominal aorta. This facilitates respiration, although vital capacity and cardiac index are reduced. To ensure cardiac filling and reduce hypotension, venous return from the femoral veins and inferior vena cava is uninterrupted. Female breasts should be moved laterally to reduce pressure on them. Male genitalia should be free from pressure. Pendulous skinfolds should not be crimped under the patient in any manner.

The arms may lie supported along the sides of the body, with the palms up or inward toward the body. An alternative position is to place the arms into a diver's pose by lowering them toward the floor and rotating (circumducting) them upward in a natural range of motion. Care is taken not to dislocate the shoulders. The armboards are reversed on the table, pointing toward the anesthesia provider. The elbows are padded and are slightly flexed no greater than 90 degrees to prevent overextension, and the palms are down. The arms may extend beyond the head, but not so far as to cause brachial plexus compression or stretch.

The head can be turned to one side or positioned face down on a padded headrest to prevent pressure on the ear, eye, and face. Clearance of the airway must be ensured. A serious complication of the prone position is blindness caused by ischemia of the vascular system of the eye.

A pillow or padding under the anterior aspect of the ankles and the dorsa of the feet prevents pressure on the toes and elevates the feet to aid venous return. Do not permit the patient's toes to extend beyond the foot of the bed. Donuts under the knees prevent pressure on the patellae. The safety belt is placed over the calves to prevent flexion of the lower legs. Care is taken not to compress the lower legs. An additional belt can be positioned over the posterior thighs as an added precaution.

Modified Prone Positions

For surgical procedures on the spine, the mattress on the OR bed is adjusted so the hips are over the break between the body and leg sections. A large soft pillow is placed under the abdomen at the lower pelvis. The upper break of the OR bed is flexed, and the OR bed is tilted so the surgical area is horizontal. Some surgeons prefer a special assembly for the orthopedic OR bed, such as an adjustable arch (Wilson frame), a Hastings frame, or an Andrews frame for spinal surgery. In a kneeling Andrews frame, the flexion at the knee with tibial support is between 60 and 90 degrees.

After the administration of anesthesia in the supine position on the transport cart, the patient is carefully lifted and properly positioned on a special table or frame. The patient may be placed in a prone extreme forward sitting or kneeling position with the torso at a right angle to the thighs. The midsection of the abdomen is allowed to hang free. This allows the anesthesia provider to use the hypotensive anesthetic technique for hemostasis.

For neurosurgical procedures, the head rests in a cranial headrest to expose the occiput and cervical vertebrae. The eyes are protected; ophthalmic ointment is applied to protect the corneas and keep the lids closed before turning the patient onto the headrest. The ears are protected with foam support. When the patient is face down on a headrest, the head should be raised periodically to prevent pressure necrosis of the cheeks and forehead. Some anesthesia providers use a small mirror to periodically inspect the face and endotracheal tube position.

Kraske (Jackknife) Position

With the Kraske position, the patient remains supine until anesthetized and is then turned onto the abdomen (prone position) via rotation. The hips are positioned over the center break of the OR bed between the body and leg sections. Chest rolls or bolsters are placed to raise the chest if the patient is under general anesthesia. A Kraske pillow can be placed at the level of the anterior thighs to elevate the buttocks.

The arms are extended on reverse angled armboards with the elbows flexed and the palms down. The head is to the side and is supported on a donut or pillow. The dorsa of the feet and toes rest on a pillow. The safety belt is placed below the knees. The leg section of the OR bed is lowered the desired amount (usually about 90 degrees), and the entire OR bed is tilted head downward to elevate the hips above the rest of the body.

The patient is well balanced on the OR bed (Fig. 26.24). For procedures in the rectal area (e.g., pilonidal sinus, hemorrhoidectomy), the buttocks are retracted with wide tape strips. Because of the dependent position, venous pooling occurs **cephalad** (toward the head) and **caudad** (toward the feet). It is important to slowly return the patient to horizontal from this unnatural position to minimize circulatory complications.

• **Fig. 26.24** Kraske (jackknife) position. (From Rothrock JC: *Alexander's care of the patient in surgery,* ed 14, St. Louis, 2011, Mosby.)

Knee-Chest Position

The knee-chest position is sometimes used for sigmoidoscopy or culdoscopy. For this position, an extension is attached to the foot section. The OR bed is flexed at the center break, and the lower section is broken until it is at a right angle to the OR bed. The patient kneels on the lower section; the knees are thus flexed at a right angle to the body.

The upper portion of the OR bed may be raised slightly to support the head, which is turned to the side. The arms are placed around the head with the elbows flexed in a diver's posture, and a large soft pillow is placed beneath them. The chest rests on the OR bed, and the safety belt is placed above the knees. The entire OR bed is tilted head downward so the hips and pelvis are at the highest point—a modified jackknife position.

Lateral Positions

For lateral positioning, the OR bed remains flat. The patient is anesthetized and intubated in the supine position on the OR bed and then turned to the unaffected side. In the right lateral position, the patient lies on the right side with the left side up (for a left-sided procedure); the left lateral position exposes the right side (Fig. 26.25).

The patient is turned by no fewer than four people to maintain body alignment and achieve stability. The patient's back is drawn to the edge of the OR bed. The knee of the lower leg is flexed, and the upper leg is straight. The knees require padding to prevent pressure and shearing force. In addition, a large soft pillow is placed lengthwise between the legs to take pressure off the upper hip and lower leg to prevent circulatory complications and pressure on the peroneal nerve.

The ankle and foot of the upper leg should be supported to prevent footdrop. Bony prominences are padded. For added stability, a safety belt or a 3-inch-wide (7.5 cm) tape is placed over the hip.

The patient's arms may be placed on a padded double armboard, with the lower arm palm up and the upper arm slightly

• **Fig. 26.25** Left lateral position is when the patient is lying on the left side. Note strap across hip to stabilize body. Pillow between legs relieves pressure on lower legs. Both legs are flexed slightly to alleviate any pressure or stretch. Note that bed is flat, not flexed. Right lateral is directly the opposite position.

flexed with the palm down. Blood pressure should be measured from the lower arm. As an alternative, the upper arm can be positioned on a padded Mayo stand. A pressure reduction pad under the axilla protects neurovascular structures. The shoulders should be in alignment.

The patient's head is in cervical alignment with the spine. The head should be supported on a small pillow between the shoulder and neck to prevent stretching the neck and brachial plexus and maintain a patent airway (Fig. 26.26).

Referred to synonymously as the lateral, lateral decubitus, or lateral recumbent, this position is used for access to the hemithorax, kidney, and retroperitoneal space. This position contributes to physiologic alterations. Respiration is affected by differing gas exchange ratios in the lungs. Because of gravity, the lower lung receives more blood from the right side of the heart; the lower lung therefore has increased perfusion but less residual air because of mediastinal compression and the weight of the abdominal contents on the diaphragm. Positive pressure to both lungs helps control respiratory changes. Circulation is also compromised by pressure on the abdominal vessels. In the right lateral position, compression of the vena cava impairs venous return.

Sims Recumbent Position

With the Sims recumbent position (a modified left lateral position), the patient lies on the left side with the upper leg flexed at the hip and knee; the lower leg is straight. The lower arm is extended along the patient's back, with the weight of the chest on the OR bed. The upper arm rests in a flexed position on the OR bed. This position is preferred for a colonoscopy or sigmoidoscopy. Pregnant nonobstetric patients who are at 16 weeks or more

• **Fig. 26.26** Proper alignment of spinal column in lateral position.

• **Fig. 26.27** Right kidney position for a procedure on the right kidney. Patient is in lateral position with kidney region over OR bed break, or body elevation bar. The table is flexed. Note strap across hip to stabilize body, raised kidney elevator for hyperextending surgical site, and pillow between legs. The lower leg is flexed more than the upper leg. Patient's side is horizontal from shoulder to hip. The arm is supported with a double airplane armboard (not shown).

of gestation should be placed in a left lateral tilt or a wedge should be used under the right hip to prevent hypotension and aortal and inferior vena cava compression.

Kidney Position

With the kidney position, the flank region is positioned over the kidney elevator on the OR bed when the patient is turned onto the unaffected side (Fig. 26.27). The short kidney rest is attached to the body elevator at the patient's back. The longer rest is placed in front at a level beneath the iliac crest to minimize pressure on the abdominal organs. Both rests are well padded. In a large patient, folds of abdominal tissue may extend over the end of the anterior rest and be bruised if caution is not taken. The OR bed is flexed slightly at the level of the iliac crest so the body elevator can be raised as desired to increase space between the lower ribs and iliac crest.

A body strap or wide adhesive tape is placed over the hip to stabilize the patient after the OR bed is flexed and the elevator is raised. The entire OR bed is tilted slightly downward toward the head until the surgical area is horizontal; the upper shoulder and hip should be in a straight line. The upper arm is supported in a double airplane-style armboard. A gel pad is used to support the chest and protect the breasts. An axillary roll is placed to take body weight off the deltoid muscle in the shoulder. Before closure, the OR bed is straightened to allow better approximation of tissues.

The term *kidney position* is used to designate the lateral flexion used to elevate the surgical site. Documentation should clearly state either right or left to indicate which kidney is elevated for the procedure. The kidney position is used for procedures on the kidney and ureter; this position is not well tolerated. Skin and underlying tissue can be damaged by excessive pressure during flexion of the OR bed. OR bed flexion combined with use of the kidney elevator may cause cardiovascular responses. Blood tends to pool in the lower arm and leg. Circulation is further compromised by increased pressure on the abdominal vessels when the kidney elevator is raised. The spine is stressed in a lateral flexed position and can cause strain on the vertebral structures.

Lateral Chest (Thoracotomy) Position

Modifications of the lateral position are used for unilateral transthoracic procedures with a lateral approach. After the patient is turned onto the unaffected side and positioned as described for the lateral position, a second strap may be placed over the shoulder for stability, unless doing so would interfere with skin

preparation. The arms may be extended on a double armboard, or the lower arm is extended on an armboard with the palm up while the upper arm is brought forward and down over a pad to draw the scapula from the surgical area. Position depends on site and length of the chest incision. A gel pad under the axilla elevates the surgical site and relieves pressure on the lower arm.

One lateral body rest is placed at the lumbar area to facilitate respiratory movements and provide support. Another body rest is placed along the chest at the axillary level. This body rest is well padded to avoid bruising the breasts. Vacuum beanbag positioning devices or bolsters may be used instead of body rests. The shoulders and hips should be level. Slight lowering of the head of the OR bed assists postural drainage during the surgical procedure. This position is restrictive to the cardiopulmonary system, especially if used for a prolonged period.

Anterior Chest Position

For thoracoabdominal procedures with an anterior approach, the positioning is more supine than for the lateral chest position. After the patient is anesthetized, a gel pad is placed under the lower axilla; another pillow or wedge is placed behind the buttocks and spine to support the torso. The upper knee is flexed slightly, and a large soft pillow is placed beneath it to relieve strain on the abdominal muscles and upper hip.

The OR bed can be tilted laterally to raise the surgical site. A safety belt is placed across the hip and another above the knees. The lower arm on the unaffected side is supported at the side by an armboard. The upper arm on the affected side is padded well and secured; it can be bandaged loosely to the anesthesia screen above the patient's head with a Kerlix roll. To avoid injury to the brachial plexus, the arm must not be hyperextended or hyperabducted. The head of the OR bed is lowered slightly for postural drainage.

Modifications for Individual Patient Needs

Anomalies and physical defects are accommodated according to each patient's needs. Whether the patient is unconscious or conscious, the avoidance of unnecessary exposure is an essential consideration for all patients. The patient's position should be observed objectively before skin preparation and draping to see that it adheres to physiologic principles.

Protective devices, positioning aids, and padded areas should be reassessed before draping because they could have shifted during the skin preparation procedure or during insertion of an indwelling urinary catheter. Careful observation of patient protection and positioning facilitates the expected outcome.

Documentation

The circulating nurse should document any preoperative limitations in the patient's range of motion, the condition of the skin before and after the surgical procedure, and the position in which the patient was positioned during the surgical procedure, including the use of special equipment. Personnel performing the positioning should be listed by name, role, and title.

Physical Preparation and Draping of the Surgical Site

The type of surgical procedure to be performed, the age and condition of the patient, and the preferences of the surgeon determine specific procedures to be carried out before the incision is made. Consideration must be given to the control of urinary drainage, skin antisepsis, and establishment of a sterile draped field around the surgical site.

Urinary Catheterization

The patient should void to empty the urinary bladder just before transfer to the OR suite unless the procedure requires the bladder to be full, such as for special bladder tone testing procedures. If the patient's bladder is not empty or the surgeon wishes to prevent bladder distention during a long procedure or after the surgical procedure, urinary catheterization may be necessary after the patient is anesthetized.

An indwelling Foley catheter may be inserted by a member of the team. This retention catheter maintains bladder decompression to avoid trauma during a lower abdominal or pelvic procedure, to

permit accurate measurement of output during or after the surgical procedure, and to facilitate output and healing after a surgical procedure on genitourinary tract structures. Catheterization is performed after anesthesia is administered and before the patient is positioned for the surgical procedure, except for a patient who will remain in the lithotomy position.

The Foley catheter should be inserted before the vaginal or abdominal skin preparation to prevent perineal splash to the surgical site. The vagina can be prepped immediately after the Foley catheter is placed. Gloves should be changed and a new prep set used for the abdominal skin prep.

Urinary tract infection can be caused by contamination or trauma to structures during urinary catheterization.[5] Sterile technique must be maintained. A sterile disposable catheterization tray is used unless the patient is being prepared for a surgical procedure in the perineal or genital area. For these latter procedures, a sterile catheter and lubricant may be added to the perineal skin preparation setup. For other surgical procedures, the perineal and meatal areas should be cleansed with an antiseptic agent to reduce microbial flora and remove gross contaminants before the catheterization procedure.[5] Sterile gloves are donned using the open gloving technique (Fig. 26.28).

The catheter should be small enough to minimize trauma to the urethra and prevent necrosis of the meatus; usually a size 14 or 16-Fr catheter is inserted in a woman and a size 16 or 18-Fr catheter is inserted in a man. Silicone Foley catheters are preferred. Some Foley catheters may contain latex, and care is taken not to use these if the patient is latex sensitive. Some manufacturers incorporate silver in the catheter as an antimicrobial agent.

The inflatable balloon size may be 5 or 30 mL (5 mL is used most frequently in adults); 10 mL of sterile water is needed to properly expand a 5-mL balloon, to compensate for volume required by the expansion channel. Foley catheters have a Luer-Lok

• Fig. 26.28 Donning sterile gloves by open glove method for performing patient skin preparation or catheterization. 1, Open sterile glove wrapper. Gloves are in a palm-up position with a short prefolded cuff. 2, To glove the right hand, grasp the inner aspect of the right cuff with the bare left forefinger and thumb. Take care to touch only the inner cuff surface with bare skin. The outer surface of the glove is sterile. 3, Slide right hand into the opening of the glove, taking care not to touch the outer sterile surface. Do not adjust cuff once the glove is on. This is done later. 4, To glove the left hand, use the gloved right hand and slide gloved fingers under the inner sterile aspect of the left cuff. Steady the fingers of the right hand as the bare left hand is slid into the glove. The left cuff is straightened with the right fingers as the final act of donning the glove. 5, Use the sterile fingers of the left hand on the sterile aspect of the right glove to slide the remaining right glove cuff into position. Do not touch the inner aspect (the skin side) of either glove with the outer sterile gloved surface.

valve over the lumen to the expansion channel that is filled using a Luer-Lok syringe. Foley catheter manufacturers do not recommend testing the balloon before insertion. They maintain that doing so causes the balloon to weaken and the small folds of the balloon may cause urethral irritation that could lead to a urinary tract infection. The balloon is tested in the factory at the time of manufacture.

The hand used to spread the labia or stabilize the penis is considered contaminated and should not be used to handle the catheter or prep sponges (Fig. 26.29). To facilitate insertion and minimize trauma, the tip of the catheter is lubricated with a sterile water-soluble lubricant. Urine starts to flow when the catheter has passed into the bladder. The balloon of a Foley catheter is expanded with sterile water only after urine is seen in the tubing, and the bladder is allowed to drain.

If difficulty is encountered during catheter insertion, especially in a geriatric male patient with an enlarged prostate, the catheter should not be forced into the urethra. Stop the catheterization procedure and request help from the surgeon. A flexible catheter stylet of plastic or stainless steel may be needed to pass the catheter through the prostatic segment of the urethra to minimize trauma to the structures.

The catheter is attached to a sterile drainage system, and the drainage bag is positioned in the direct view of the anesthesia provider. The tubing is later attached to the patient's leg, with enough slack in it to prevent tension or pull on the penis or urethra at the conclusion of the case (Fig. 26.30).

Attention is paid to the catheter and tubing during positioning of the patient for the surgical procedure to prevent compression or kinking. Dependent loops of tubing should not be permitted to hang on the floor because this could cause a trip hazard. If the container must be raised above the level of the bladder during positioning, the tubing is clamped or kinked until the container can be lowered and secured under the OR bed to avoid contamination by retrograde or backward flow of urine.

If the catheter is to be removed at the end of the surgical procedure, don examination gloves and use a syringe to withdraw and measure the solution from the Foley balloon expansion port. Cutting off the end with scissors may cause the inflation port to collapse, trapping fluid within the expanded balloon. The urethra can be damaged by withdrawing the expanded balloon.

Principles of Patient Skin Preparation

The purpose of skin preparation is to render the surgical site as free as possible from transient and resident microorganisms, dirt, and skin oil so the incision can be made through the skin with minimal danger of infection from this source.

Many surgeons prefer to have patients bathe with antimicrobial soap the morning of the surgical procedure. The patient should be advised to avoid the use of body emollients, oils, creams, and lotions after washing. Some products decrease the efficacy of antimicrobial soap, and other products prevent adherence of the return electrode and electrocardiographic (ECG) electrodes to the skin.

The perioperative nurse should assess the patient's skin before, during, and after the prepping process. Documentation of the condition of the patient's skin with notation of lesions or other pertinent markings is important. Abnormal skin irritation, infection, or abrasion on or near the surgical site might be a contraindication to the surgical procedure and is reported to the surgeon.

Some patients may have body piercing jewelry that is located on the face, tongue, nose, lip, eyebrow, ears, or other easily identified places. In some cases, the piercing jewelry is located under clothing on the nipples, umbilicus, or genitalia. Body piercing jewelry should be removed for safety reasons before surgery. Certain piercings cannot be removed without a specialized tool. Facilities with patients who commonly have this type of adornment may want to have a removal tool available.

Piercing jewelry could encourage an infection or could cause positioning/pressure injuries. Metals are known to be conductors of electricity and could cause an alternative path burn from a stray current. Oral piercings could become dislodged and enter the patient's airway. Genital jewelry can interfere with urinary catheterization and cause a urinary tract infection. Each facility should have a policy and procedure in place concerning body piercing jewelry. The perioperative nurse should inquire about piercings during the assessment process.

Patients who have been involved in accidents or injured during the commission of a crime may bear physical marks or materials important to the investigation. Objective description of injuries that may include sketches on the record is part of the chain of evidence. Photographs may be taken for the record. Any material on the patient's person could be evidence and should be handled according to facility policy for forensic evidence.

• **Fig. 26.29** Female urinary catheterization. (From Davis JH, Foster RS, Gamelli RL: *Essentials of clinical surgery,* St. Louis, 1991, Mosby.)

• **Fig. 26.30** Secure the urinary catheter. (From Davis JH, Foster RS, Gamelli RL: *Essentials of clinical surgery,* St. Louis, 1991, Mosby.)

Preliminary Preparation of the Patient's Skin

Hair Removal

Hair removal can injure skin, and many surgeons no longer request hair removal. However, hair that surrounds the surgical site may be so thick that removal is necessary. Hair should be removed with clippers. Hair may interfere with exposure, closure, or the surgical site dressing. It may also prevent adequate skin contact with patient return electrodes or ECG leads.

Hair removal is carried out per the surgeon's order as close to the scheduled time for the surgical procedure as possible. Examination gloves are worn. The patient is covered to expose only the area to be clipped. Bath blankets are useful for preventing unnecessary exposure and prevent excess body heat loss during the procedure. The patient may be clipped before the procedure in the holding area or in the OR after the anesthetic has been administered. Care is taken to not let stray hair remain in the surgical field. A wide piece of adhesive tape can be used to collect stray hair.

Clippers

Electric clippers with fine teeth cut hair close to the skin. The short stubble, usually about a millimeter in length, does not interfere with skin antisepsis or exposure of the surgical site. Clipping can be done using short strokes against the direction of hair growth. The blade lies flat against the skin surface. After use, a reusable blade assembly is disassembled, cleaned, and terminally sterilized. The clipper handle is cleaned and disinfected. Cordless handles with rechargeable batteries are available. Disposable clipper heads are preferred over reusable styles for sharpness and optimal function.

Razor

Shaving is not the preferred method of hair removal and should be performed as near the time of incision as possible if this method must be used. Avoid making nicks and cuts in the skin. Gloves should be worn to prevent blood exposure if a nick should occur. Nicks made immediately before the surgical procedure (i.e., up to 30 minutes) are considered clean wounds. However, nicks and abrasions made several hours before the procedure may present as inflamed wounds at the time of surgical incision. The surgeon should be notified if the skin is not intact at the surgical site. This could be cause for cancellation of the surgical procedure. The time lapse between the preoperative shave and the surgical procedure may increase the risk for postoperative infection.

Wet shaving is preferable to dry shaving, which can leave the skin abraded. Soaking hair in lather allows keratin to absorb water, which makes hair softer and easier to remove. A sharp clean razor blade should be used. The skin is held taut and is shaved by stroking in the direction of hair growth. Blades are discarded in the appropriate sharps container.

Skin Degreasing

The skin surface is composed of cornified epithelium with a coating of secretions that include perspiration, oils, and desquamated epithelium. These surface sebaceous lubricants are insoluble in water. Therefore a skin degreaser or fat solvent may be used to enhance adhesion of ECG or other electrodes. It also may be used before skin preparation to improve adhesion of self-adhering drapes or to prevent smudging of skin markings. Isopropyl alcohol and acetone are effective fat solvents. A fat-solvent emollient is incorporated into some antiseptic agents. Some solvents, such as alcohol, are flammable and must be allowed to completely dry before draping. Vapors can become a fire hazard if trapped beneath surgical drapes.

Surgical Skin Cleansing Fundamentals

Before beginning the positioning and prepping sequence, ask the patient to verbally state the location for the procedure and to point to and touch the site if possible. The correct site should have been marked with indelible ink by the surgeon before the patient was brought to the OR, as part of the identification process. Before amputation of an extremity, expose the opposite limb also for comparison. Check with the surgeon, the permit, and the notes in the chart. Confirm that the correct area is identified by the surgery schedule as well. Double-check the radiographs to be sure they have not been hung in the view box backward.

After the patient is anesthetized and positioned on the OR bed, the skin at the surgical site and an extensive area surrounding it is exposed and cleansed with an antiseptic agent immediately before draping. The person performing the prep must wear personal protective equipment (PPE) to prevent a splash to the eyes.

Towels should be tucked in at the patient's sides to catch any runoff. The two-step skin prep using scrub soap and paint is performed wearing sterile gloves. The one-step skin prep is essentially a layer of alcohol-based solution performed while wearing nonsterile examination gloves. The end result of antisepsis of the skin is essentially the same. Keep in mind that skin is never sterile regardless of surgical cleansing method used.

Care is taken when prepping areas of the body that may be delicate or where prepping may be potentially harmful to the patient, such as carotid arteries, occluded vessels, tumor masses, distended abdomen, traumatic wounds, eyes, ears, trachea, and questionably stable tissues. Never rub a tumor or infectious mass. Areas marked by the surgeon preoperatively should be gently cleansed, so as not to wash off the markings. Some surgeons use surgical marking pens or surgical dyes, such as methylene blue, brilliant green, or alcohol-based gentian violet. Others may use heavy-duty black markers to delineate the surgical site.

Setup and Procedure for a Two-Step Skin Prep

Some disposable skin preparation trays include gloves, disposable towels, prep sponges, and cotton-tipped applicators. Some disposable trays have containers of premeasured antiseptic cleansing solution (Fig. 26.31). Disposable trays without antiseptic agents

• **Fig. 26.31** Contents of a two-step skin prep tray depicted with textured sponges.

can be packaged sterile or unsterile. These are referred to as *dry trays* and require the addition of the antiseptic cleansing solution of choice. If prepackaged disposable trays are not used, a sterile table is prepared by the scrub person with the following sterile items:

- Small table drape to create the sterile field.
- Sterile gloves.
- Two absorbent towels used to prevent pooling under body parts along the sides of the area and to define the upper and lower limits of the area to be prepped.
- Two or three small basins for solutions (antiseptic scrub detergent, antiseptic paint solution, and sterile water or alcohol if requested by the surgeon). About 1 or 2 ounces of solution in each basin usually is sufficient.
- Gauze sponges (nonradiopaque). The number varies according to the size of the area intended for the surgical procedure. These are not counted sponges from the instrument table and should be discarded in a trash container separate from the sponge bucket. Textured foam sponges may be preferred.
- Cotton-tipped applicators as necessary.

The antiseptic solutions are poured into each of the basins. Do not preheat the prep solutions because the fluid portion can evaporate and cause concentration of the antiseptic chemical. One-half ounce of warm sterile water is added to the scrub soap basin to allow sudsing action of the agent. Do not pour the remainder of the water into a basin on the sterile field because once the water is poured, the lip is considered contaminated. The water can be recapped and used for cleaning the patient's skin at the end of the surgical procedure before tape is applied.

Sterile gloves are donned by the person doing the prep using the open glove method for the two-step prep. A sterile prep setup is commonly used. Skin is mechanically cleansed and chemically decontaminated to reduce skin flora.

The surgical site is bordered by sterile towels after donning the sterile gloves. The sides of the patient are protected by towels to prevent runoff of excess solution. The cotton-tipped applicators are dipped into the soapy solution and used to cleanse the umbilicus if the umbilicus is part of the surgical site. The soiled applicators are discarded into the trash. Several sponges are placed into the soapy solution, and several are placed into the paint solution. A few sponges are reserved for use at the end of the prep if the surgeon incorporates an alcohol rinse. Each sponge is squeezed into the corresponding basin so as to not soak the patient and the surrounding bed linens.

The soapy antiseptic sponges are used to mechanically and chemically cleanse the skin in a circular or linear motion from the incisional site to the periphery (Fig. 26.32). The soap decreases the surface tension of the skin and permits the sponge to pick up and remove dirt and microbes from the skin. The sponge should not backtrack over the already prepped area. Each sponge is discarded in the trash after use and not placed in the sponge bucket. A towel is used to blot the soap from the site. It is fully opened and placed over the site and carefully lifted off without rubbing or dragging the fabric over the cleansed area.

The paint-style antiseptic solution is applied in the same manner, with a circular motion from the incisional site to the periphery. This solution is not blotted or wiped off. It should be allowed to dry. If the surgeon prefers, an alcohol sponge is sometimes used to complete the skin prep procedure. If alcohol is used, it is allowed to dry completely before drapes are applied, to minimize the risk for fire from trapped vapors.

• **Fig. 26.32** Abdominal antiseptic skin preparation. Patient is in supine position. Area includes breast line to upper third of thighs, from table line right to table line left. *Shaded area* shows anatomic area to be cleansed with antiseptic. *Arrows* within area show direction of motion for skin preparation.

• **Fig. 26.33** One-step skin prep applicator.

Setup and Procedure for a One-Step Skin Prep

A one-step skin prep is a self-contained unit constructed of a sponge applicator tip and a chamber that contains antiseptic solution (Fig. 26.33). The unit is packaged in a blister pack with two cotton-tipped applicators. A pack of sterile towels is opened and used to tuck in at the patient's sides and periphery of the surgical site. When taken from the package, the applicator is not handled under sterile conditions. Users wear nonsterile examination gloves to prevent the solution from getting on their hands. The product should not be permitted to come into contact with reusable equipment such as basins because it does not readily wash off.

To apply the prep solution, the unit is compressed at the working end to break the seal of the inner chamber and allow the solution to saturate the applicator tip. The cotton-tipped applicators are dipped into the saturated sponge and used to clean the umbilicus; these cotton-tipped applicators are then discarded. The sponge end is inverted and allowed to become the applicator end.

The area to be prepped is painted in the same stroke direction as for a two-step skin prep. These one-step prep antiseptics have a thicker texture, dry like shellac, and are not blotted off in any manner after application. Some preps are tinted pink, blue, or orange for easy visibility and verification that all areas of the surgical site have been prepped. The risk for pooling is minimized with these products because of their consistency. They mechanically hold cells in place over the skin surface and chemically kill microorganisms. The alcohol-based skin prep products form a barrier over the skin.

The manufacturer recommends not removing the product after the procedure but rather allowing it to wear off over time to provide a lasting antisepsis for up to 3 days. Alcohol can be used to remove the product if necessary, or remover solution is commercially available. A package insert includes patient take-home instructions about the product and the purpose for its presence on the skin.

The chemical action is the actual antiseptic agent (iodophor or chlorhexidine) in combination with an alcohol base. The alcohol base can pose a fire hazard if not permitted to dry completely before draping. These items should not be heated in any way. They contain an ampule that can pressurize and explode in the presence of heat. Prepackaged antiseptic soapy prep sponges are available without alcohol for sensitive areas such as the face or perineum. These one-step soapy prep sponges are used in urology rooms.

Preparing Areas Considered Contaminated

Umbilicus
Although the umbilicus is considered a contaminated area, prepping this central area of the abdomen after the surgical site can cause contamination of a freshly prepped abdomen. Most surgeons prefer the umbilicus to be cleaned with cotton-tipped swabs before the main abdominal incision is prepped to prevent debris from the contaminated site splashing on the freshly prepped incision. This is a logical conclusion.

Stoma
Intestinal stomas are contaminated with fecal material and intestinal flora. The stoma should be isolated with a sterile clear plastic adhesive dressing and prepped last. If the stoma is to be incorporated with the surgical incision, it is prepped and dried last and covered with a sterile clear plastic adhesive dressing to prevent fecal material from entering the wound. Some surgeons pack the open end of the stoma with a povidone-iodine (Betadine)-soaked radiopaque sponge. This sponge should be accounted for in the count tally at the end of the procedure. A nonradiopaque gauze sponge should not be used as stoma packing in the sterile field because it could become misplaced and be unaccounted for in the procedure.

Other Contaminated Areas
Other areas such as draining sinuses, skin ulcers, the vagina, and the anus are also considered contaminated areas. In all of these areas, the general rule of scrubbing the most contaminated area last with separate sponges applies. Use logic when determining the sequence for surgical skin prep.

Foreign Substances
Adhesive, grease, tar, and similar foreign materials are removed from skin before the area is mechanically cleansed with an antiseptic agent. A nonirritating solvent should be used to cleanse the skin. The solvent should be nonflammable and nontoxic. Do not allow the solution to collect underneath the patient. Take care that the foreign substance in itself is not hazardous or flammable. Some chemicals can ignite when exposed to water or moisture.

Traumatic Wounds
In the preparation of an area in which the skin is not intact because of a traumatic injury, wound irrigation may be part of the skin preparation procedure. The wound may be packed or covered with sterile gauze while the area around it is thoroughly scrubbed and shaved if necessary. The extent and type of injury determine the appropriate procedure. Protective gloves, eyewear, and a mask should be worn during the irrigation.

Solutions that are irritating to a denuded area must not be used. Small areas may be irrigated with warm sterile normal saline solution with a bulb syringe. When a bulb syringe is used, care must be taken not to force debris and microorganisms deeper into the wound. The wound is irrigated gently to dislodge debris and flush it out. Soft nylon brushes are sometimes used. This is useful for industrial injuries and motorcycle accidents.

Copious amounts of warm sterile solution may be needed to flush out a large wound. A container of warm sterile normal saline or Ringer's lactate solution attached to IV tubing can be hung on an IV pole near the area to be copiously irrigated. If the area is on an extremity, a sterile irrigating basin with a plastic drape fitted over the top is placed under the extremity. During irrigation, solution runs from the wound into the basin. Suction tubing placed in the basin removes the irrigating solution into a kick bucket, suction canister, or machine.

Dry towels or sheets may be necessary under the patient if the area has not been protected during irrigation. A moisture-proof pad placed under the wound before irrigation helps channel solutions into a drainage pan.

Debridement of the wound (excision of all devitalized tissue) usually follows irrigation. The surgeon may request to have sterile tissue forceps and scissors on the prep table for removal of nonviable tissue.

Areas Prepared for Grafts
Separate setups are necessary for skin preparation of recipient and donor sites before skin, bone, or vascular grafting procedures. The donor site is usually scrubbed first.

The donor site for a skin graft should be scrubbed with a colorless antiseptic agent so that the surgeon can properly evaluate the vascularity of the graft postoperatively. The recipient site for skin grafts is usually contaminated (e.g., after a burn or other traumatic injury). Items used in preparation of the recipient site must not be permitted to contaminate the donor site. Also, microorganisms on the skin of the donor site must not be transferred to a denuded recipient site.

Antiseptic Solutions
The infection control committee usually determines the chemical antiseptic or antimicrobial agents to be used in the OR for skin preparation. Products selected by the OR committee are commonly the same ones selected for use as hand and skin antisepsis of the sterile team. The maximum concentration of a germicidal agent that can be used on skin and mucous membranes is limited by the agent's toxicity for these tissues. The ideal antiseptic skin-cleansing agent should have the following qualities:
- It has broad-spectrum antimicrobial action and rapidly decreases the microbial count. It should be virucidal and active against protozoa and yeasts.
- It can be quickly applied and remains effective against microorganisms.

- It can be safely used without skin irritation or sensitization. It should be nontoxic.
- It effectively remains active in the presence of alcohol, organic matter, soap, and detergent.
- It should be nonflammable when dried for use with laser, electrosurgical, and other high-energy devices.

Chlorhexidine Gluconate

Chlorhexidine gluconate was discovered in 1950 in England. A solution of 2% to 4% chlorhexidine gluconate is used as an antiseptic skin-cleansing soap preoperatively. A tincture of 0.5% chlorhexidine gluconate in 70% isopropyl alcohol (Hibitane) is sometimes used. A broad-spectrum, rapid-acting antimicrobial agent, it binds to negative charges on microbial cell walls to produce irreversible damage and death. It has minimal activity against yeasts, spores, and tuberculosis. It is effective against most viruses.

Activity is adversely affected by traces of soap and is reduced in the presence of organic matter. If chlorhexidine is used in combination with personal soaps and shampoos for preoperative bathing, it is inactivated. The patient should be instructed to shampoo the hair with personal shampoo and thoroughly rinse before applying chlorhexidine as a body wash. Body lotion should not be applied after bathing because this nullifies the residual bacteriostatic properties of the compound. The patient should be instructed to keep chlorhexidine out of the eyes and ears.

This agent is not absorbed through intact skin but binds with mucous membranes. It significantly reduces and maintains a reduction of microbial flora, such as bacteria and yeasts, for at least 4 hours.[6] The prolonged effect is inhibited if chlorhexidine is combined with iodine preparations. Its activity increases at elevated temperature because it binds with the stratum corneum. It is available either tinted for color demarcation of the skin area being prepped or nontinted if the surgeon needs to observe the skin color. Because it is an irritant to the eyes and ototoxic, it is contraindicated for facial antisepsis. If chlorhexidine gets on clothing, chlorine bleach is avoided because it permanently stains the fabric. Clothing should be rinsed with cold water until all traces of the product have been removed.

Iodine and Iodophors

Discovered in 1812, iodine was first used in wound care in 1839. A solution of 1% or 2% iodine in water or in 70% alcohol is an excellent antiseptic. However, potential hazards of skin irritations and burns led to a decline in its use. If used, iodine should dry and then be rinsed off with 70% alcohol to neutralize the damaging effect.

Iodophors are iodine compounds that may be combined with detergents. Povidone-iodine has a surfactant, a wetting and dispersive agent, in an aqueous solution such as Betadine surgical scrub, a commonly used detergent form of iodophor. The detergent form should be rinsed off. Iodophor solution without detergent can be used for rinsing. Iodophor in 70% alcohol also is available. Iodophors are excellent cleansing agents that remove debris from skin surfaces while slowly releasing iodine. They are broad-spectrum antimicrobial agents that have some virucidal and sporicidal activity. Iodophors are relatively nontoxic and virtually nonirritating to skin or mucous membranes.

The brown film left on the skin after application of the solution clearly defines the area of application. This should not be wiped off because microbial activity is sustained by the release of free iodine as the agent dries and color fades from the skin. The

solution should remain on the skin for at least 2 minutes. To hasten drying of the skin, alcohol may be painted on the area without friction before a self-adhering drape is applied. The alcohol must not be permitted to pool and must be completely dry before draping.

Iodophors are used with caution to prep the skin of patients who are sensitive or allergic to iodine. True iodine allergy is very rare. The association with an actual allergy is more an issue with systemic problems as opposed to topical sensitivity and is exceedingly rare. Studies have shown that seafood allergy is associated with fish protein and not iodine.[7]

The type of preparation, concentration of iodine, and presence of surfactants affect the microbial activity of products. Povidone-iodine complexes are available in solution, spray, and gel forms. Tinctures are in an alcohol-based solution. Manufacturer instructions are strictly followed for the product in use. The concentration of povidone-iodine may be altered by evaporation if the solution is warmed. Skin irritation may be caused by an increase in iodine concentration. Manufacturer recommendations should be followed.

Alcohol

Isopropyl and ethyl alcohols are broad-spectrum agents that denature proteins in cells. A 70% concentration with continuous contact for several minutes is satisfactory for skin antisepsis if the surgeon prefers a colorless solution that permits observation of true skin color. Because alcohol coagulates protein, it is not applied to mucous membranes or used on an open wound. Isopropyl alcohol is a more effective fat solvent than is ethyl alcohol. Both are volatile and flammable. They must not pool around or under the patient, especially if an electrosurgical unit (ESU) or laser will be used. Vapors can accumulate under the drapes and become a fire or explosion hazard.

Parachlorometaxylenol

Originally developed in 1948 in Europe as a hair conditioner, parachlorometaxylenol (PCMX) has bactericidal properties useful for skin antisepsis. It is effective against some fungi, tuberculosis, and viruses. PCMX has residual properties with repeated use. It is nontoxic to the skin, eyes, and ears.

Skin Preparation for Specific Anatomic Areas

Head and Neck

Eye

1. The eyebrows are never shaved or removed unless the surgeon deems this essential. Eyebrows do not grow back completely or evenly.
2. The eyelashes may be trimmed, if ordered by the surgeon, with fine iris scissors coated with sterile water-soluble lubricant to catch the lashes.
3. The eyelids and periorbital areas are cleansed with a nonirritating antiseptic agent and then rinsed with warm sterile water. The prep starts centrally and extends to the periphery (i.e., from the center of the lid to the brow and cheek).
4. The conjunctival sac is flushed with a nontoxic agent, such as sterile normal saline solution, with a bulb syringe. Some surgeons use a dilute iodophor solution (not the detergent or alcohol form). The patient's head is turned slightly to the affected side. The solution is contained with sponges or an absorbent towel. Care must be taken to prevent prep solution from entering the patient's ears.

Chlorhexidine is contraindicated for facial preps. Chlorhexidine gluconate can cause corneal damage if accidentally introduced into the eyes and can cause sensorineural deafness if the agent enters the inner ear (e.g., through a perforated tympanic membrane).

Ears, Face, and Nose

1. Usually, defining the area with towels is not easy. As much of the surrounding area is included as is feasible and consistent with aseptic technique. Skin surfaces should be cleansed at least to the hairline.
2. Cotton applicators are used for cleansing the nostrils and external ear canals.
3. Protect the eyes with a piece of sterile plastic sheeting. If the patient is awake, ask that the eyes be kept closed during the prep. Cotton balls or nonradiopaque gauze should be placed in the ears to prevent runoff. Cotton balls may leave small fibers in residual cerumen in the ear that can cause irritation.

Neck

1. One sterile towel is folded under the edge of the blanket and gown, which are turned down almost to the nipple line.
2. The area includes the neck laterally to the table line and up to the mandible, tops of the shoulders, and chest almost to the nipple line.
3. For combined head and neck surgical procedures, include the face to the eyes; the shaved areas of the head, ears, and posterior neck; and the area over the shoulders.

Chest and Trunk

Lateral Thoracoabdominal Area

1. The gown is removed. The blanket is turned down well below the lower limit of the area to be prepared. A towel is folded under the edge of the blanket.
2. The arm is held up by an assistant during the prep.
3. Beginning at the site of incision, the area may include the axilla, chest, and abdomen from the neck to the iliac crest. For a surgical procedure in the region of the kidney, it extends up to the axilla and down to the pubis. The area also extends beyond midlines, anteriorly and posteriorly, and may include the arm to the elbow (Fig. 26.34).

Chest and Breast

1. The anesthesia provider turns the patient's face toward the unaffected side.
2. One towel is folded under the blanket edge, just above the pubis. Another is placed on the OR bed under the shoulder and side.
3. The arm on the affected side is held up by grasping the hand and raising the shoulder and axilla slightly from the OR bed.
4. The area includes the shoulder, upper arm down to the elbow, axilla, and chest wall to the table line and beyond the sternum to the opposite shoulder (Fig. 26.35). Breast procedures generally require both breasts to be prepped.

Shoulder

1. The anesthesia provider turns the patient's face toward the opposite side.
2. A towel is placed under the shoulder and axilla.
3. The arm is held up by grasping the hand and elevating the shoulder slightly from the OR bed.
4. The area includes the circumference of the upper arm to below the elbow, from the base of the neck over the shoulder, scapula, and chest to the midline.

Rectoperineal Area

1. With the patient in the lithotomy position, a moisture-proof pad is placed under the buttocks and extends to the kick bucket that receives solutions and discarded prep sponges.
2. The area includes the pubis, external genitalia, perineum and anus, and inner aspects of the thighs (Fig. 26.36).
3. Begin the scrub over the pubic area, scrubbing downward over the genitalia and perineum. Discard the sponge.
4. The inner aspects of the upper third of both thighs are scrubbed with separate sponges, working from groin to distal aspect of thigh.

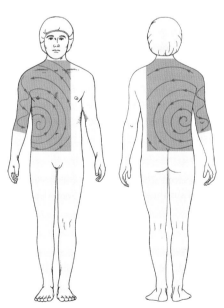

• **Fig. 26.34** Lateral thoracoabdominal antiseptic skin prep. Patient is in lateral position. Area includes axilla, chest, and abdomen from neck to iliac crest. Area extends beyond midline, anteriorly and posteriorly.

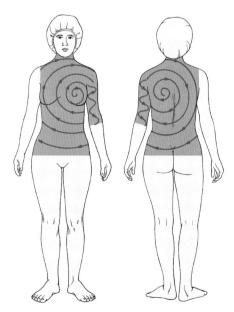

• **Fig. 26.35** Chest and breast antiseptic skin prep. Area includes shoulder, upper arm down to elbow, axilla, and chest wall to table line and beyond sternum to opposite shoulder. If patient is in lateral position, back is prepped also.

• **Fig. 26.36** Rectoperineal and vaginal antiseptic skin prep. Area includes pubis, vulva, labia, perineum, anus, and adjacent area, including inner aspects of upper third of thighs. The inner aspect of the vagina is prepped after the external vulva is prepped. The anus is prepped last.

5. The anus is prepped last.
6. The rectoperineal area is prepped before the abdomen, using a separate prep set and gloves if an abdominal approach is planned.

Vagina

1. Sponge forceps should be included on the preparation table for a vaginal prep because a portion of the prep is done internally. A disposable vaginal prep tray, with sponge sticks included, is available.
2. With the patient in the lithotomy position, a moisture-proof pad is placed under the buttocks and extends to the kick bucket that receives solutions and discarded prep sponges.
3. A towel is folded above the pubis.
4. Urinary catheterization is performed if indicated. Vaginal and anal flora should not be permitted to enter the sterile environment of the urinary bladder.
5. The external area includes the pubis, vulva, labia, perineum, anus, and adjacent area, including inner aspects of the upper third of the thighs (see Fig. 26.36).
6. Begin over the pubic area, scrubbing downward over the vulva and perineum. The inner aspects of the thighs are scrubbed with separate sponges from the labia majora outward.
7. The vagina and cervix are cleansed with sponges on sponge forceps or disposable sponge sticks. The cleansing agent should be applied generously in the vagina because vaginal mucosa has many folds and crevices that are not easily cleansed.
8. After thorough cleansing of the vagina, wipe it out with a dry sponge to prevent the possibility of the fluid entering the peritoneal cavity during the surgical procedure on pelvic organs.
9. The anus is prepped last to prevent intestinal florae from entering the vaginal vault.

Extremities

1. A moisture-proof pad should be placed on the OR bed under an extremity to retain runoff solution. This is removed after the prep so the bed is dry under the surgical site. The extremity is supported by personnel wearing sterile gloves and remains elevated until sterile drapes are applied under and around the prepped area.
2. A full circumferential extremity prep may be done in two stages to provide adequate support to joints and to ensure that all areas are scrubbed. It may include the foot for hip, thigh, knee, and lower leg procedures.
3. Caution must be taken to prevent solution from pooling under a tourniquet. The padding absorbs the solution and could cause tissue maceration. If a nonsterile pneumatic tourniquet

• **Fig. 26.37** Hip antiseptic skin prep. Area includes abdomen on affected side, thigh to knee, buttock to table line, groin, and pubis.

is used, it is positioned before the prep and protected with a sterile clear plastic drape. A towel tucked around the tourniquet cuff absorbs excess solution. This is removed before the tourniquet is inflated.

Upper Arm

1. A towel is placed under the shoulder and axilla.
2. The arm is held up by grasping the hand and elevating the shoulder slightly from the OR bed.
3. The area includes the entire circumference of the arm to the wrist, the axilla, and over the shoulder and scapula.

Elbow and Forearm

1. A towel is placed under the shoulder and axilla.
2. The arm is held up by grasping the hand.
3. The area includes the entire arm from the shoulder and axilla to and including the hand.

Hand

1. Towels may be omitted. The anatomy of the hand furnishes sufficient landmarks to define the area, and towels are apt to slip over the scrubbed area.
2. The arm must be held up by a gloved person supporting it above the elbow so that the entire circumference can be scrubbed.
3. The area includes the hand and arm to 3 inches (7.5 cm) above the elbow.

Hip

1. One towel is placed under the thigh on the OR bed. Another towel is placed on the abdomen and folded under the edge of the gown, just above the umbilicus.
2. The leg on the affected side is held up by supporting it just below the knee.
3. The area includes the abdomen on the affected side, the thigh to the knee, and the buttocks to the table line, the groin, and the pubis (Fig. 26.37).

Thigh

1. One towel is placed under the thigh on the OR bed. Another towel is placed on the abdomen and folded under the edge of the gown, just below the umbilicus.

2. The leg is held up by supporting the foot and ankle.
3. The area includes the entire circumference of the thigh and leg to the ankle, over the hip and buttocks to the table line, the groin, and the pubis. Take care not to allow the solution to pool under the patient's buttocks.

Knee and Lower Leg
1. A towel is placed over the groin.
2. The leg is held up by supporting it at the foot.
3. The area includes the entire circumference of the leg and extends from the foot to the upper part of the thigh (Fig. 26.38).

Ankle and Foot
1. Towels are omitted.
2. The foot is held up by supporting the leg at the knee. A leg-holder device is useful.
3. The area includes the foot and entire circumference of the lower leg to the knee.

Documentation

Details of the preoperative skin condition and preparation should be documented in the patient's intraoperative record. These should include, but are not limited to, the following:
- The condition of the skin around the surgical site and placement sites of the return electrodes
- Hair removal, if done, including the method and location, and areas for attachment of monitors or electrodes
- Antiseptic solutions, fat solvents, irrigating solutions, and any other agents used
- The skin area prepped and skin reaction, if any
- The name of the person who did the prep

Draping

Draping is the procedure of covering the patient and surrounding areas with a sterile barrier to create and maintain an adequate sterile field. An effective barrier eliminates or minimizes passage of microorganisms between nonsterile and sterile areas. Criteria to be met in establishing an effective barrier are that the material must be:

- Blood and fluid resistant to keep drapes dry and prevent migration of microorganisms. Material should be impermeable to moist microbial penetration (i.e., resistant to strike-through) and resistant to tearing, puncture, or abrasion that causes fiber breakdown and thus permits microbial penetration.
- Lint-free to reduce airborne contaminants and shedding into the surgical site. Cellulose and cotton fibers can cause granulomatous peritonitis or embolize arteries.
- Antistatic to eliminate risk for a spark from static electricity. Material must meet standards of the National Fire Protection Association (NFPA).
- Sufficiently porous to eliminate heat buildup so as to maintain an isothermic environment appropriate for the patient's body temperature.
- Drapable to fit around contours of the patient, furniture, and equipment.
- Dull and nonglaring to minimize color distortion from reflected light.
- Free of toxic ingredients, such as laundry residues and nonfast dyes.
- Flame resistant to self-extinguish rapidly on removal of an ignition source. This is a concern with use of lasers, ESUs, and other high-energy devices that provide an ignition source at the sterile field. Drapes become fuel for a fire. Some materials are more flammable than others; some are fire-retardant.

Draping Materials

Self-Adhering Sheeting

Sterile, waterproof, antistatic, and transparent or translucent plastic sheeting may be applied to dry skin.

Incise Drape. The entire clear plastic drape has an adhesive backing that is applied to skin. This may be applied separately, or the sheeting may be incorporated into the drape sheet. The skin incision is made through the plastic.

Antimicrobial incise drapes have an antimicrobial agent impregnated in the adhesive or the polymeric film. A film coated with an iodophor-containing adhesive, for example, slowly releases active iodine during the surgical procedure to effectively inhibit proliferation of organisms from the patient's skin. The antimicrobial may be another agent that does not contain iodine. The skin may be prepped with alcohol and allowed to dry before the drape is applied. Time is a factor in microbial accumulation from resident bacteria. Antimicrobial incise drapes are used to sustain suppression, particularly for procedures that last more than 3 hours.

Towel Drape. A nonwoven towel drape has a band of adhesive along one edge. Used as a draping towel, it remains fixed on skin without towel clips. This is advantageous when clips might obscure the view of a part exposed to x-rays during the surgical procedure. It also is used to wall off a contaminated area, such as a stoma, from the clean skin area to prevent spilling contents and causing infection or chemical irritation.

Aperture Drape. Adhesive surrounds a fenestration (opening) in the plastic sheeting. This secures the drape to the skin around the surgical site, such as an eye or ear. Caution is used in applying this type of drape around the face of a patient who is awake. The patient must have breathing space. If oxygen is used during a local procedure, it can build up under the drape creating a fire hazard if cautery is used. Some patients experience claustrophobia. Fabric towels may not feel as confining.

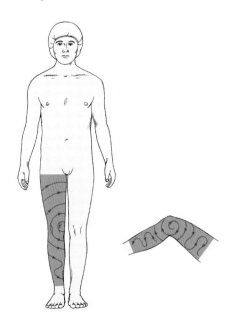

• **Fig. 26.38** Knee and lower leg antiseptic skin prep. Area includes entire circumference of affected leg and extends from foot to upper part of thigh. Upper extremity is prepped in the same manner.

Advantages of Self-Adhering Drape Material

- Resident microbial flora from skin pores, sebaceous glands, and hair follicles cannot migrate laterally to the incision.
- Microorganisms do not penetrate the impermeable material.
- Landmarks and skin tones are visible through the transparent plastic.
- Inert adhesive holds drapes securely, eliminating the need for towel clips and possible puncture of the patient's skin.
- Plastic sheeting conforms to body contours and has elasticity to stretch without breaking its adhesion to skin.

Some self-adhering drapes have sufficient moisture-vapor permeability to reduce excessive moisture buildup that could macerate the skin or loosen adhesive. A nonporous material should not cover more than 10% of the body surface because it may interfere with the patient's thermal regulatory mechanism of perspiration evaporation. The heat-retaining property of plastic causes the patient to perspire excessively, but its nonporous nature prevents evaporation.

This material is used in the following manner:

1. The usual skin prep is done.
2. The scrubbed area must be dry. It may dry by evaporation, or excess solution may be blotted with a towel.
3. Transparent plastic material is applied firmly to the skin, with the initial contact along the proposed line of incision. The drape is smoothed away from the incision area.
4. Regular fabric drapes are applied over the plastic sheeting unless plastic is incorporated into the fenestrated area of the drape.

Nonwoven Disposable Drapes

Most nonwoven disposable materials are compressed layers of synthetic fibers (e.g., rayon, nylon, or polyester) combined with cellulose (wood pulp) and bonded together chemically or mechanically without knitting, tufting, or weaving. This material may be either nonabsorbent or absorbent. Polypropylene and foil also are used in some types. Those fabrics that comply with criteria for establishing an effective barrier have the following advantages as disposable drapes:

- They are moisture-repellant; they retard blood and aqueous fluid moisture strike-through to prevent contamination. Not all nonwoven fabrics have this characteristic; only nonabsorbent materials or those laminated with plastic are impermeable to moisture.
- They are lightweight, yet strong enough to resist tears.
- They are lint-free unless cellulose fibers are torn or cut.
- Contaminants are disposed of along with drapes.
- They are antistatic and flame-retardant for OR use.
- They are prepackaged and sterilized by the manufacturer, which eliminates washing, mending, folding, and sterilizing processes.

Some drapes have a reinforced area of multiple layers that surrounds the fenestration. The outer layer absorbs fluids, but the underneath layer is impermeable to strike-through. An antimicrobial may be incorporated into this reinforced area. Other drapes have an impermeable layer around the fenestration. Drapes that are completely laminated with a plastic layer may be used for an extremity or for instrument table covers. They are not used over the entire body of the patient because of their heat retention property.

Many nonwoven drapes have pouches or troughs incorporated close to the fenestration or along the sides of the drape to collect fluids, such as amniotic or arthroscopy fluid. The pouch may have drainage ports, or fluid may be suctioned out. Some drapes also have pockets, skid-resistant instrument pads, or devices for holding cords incorporated in them (Fig. 26.39).

Laser-Resistant Drape. Nonwoven drapes that contain cellulose ignite and burn easily. Polypropylene drapes do not ignite, but they can melt. An aluminum-coated drape may be safest for use with lasers, especially around the oxygen-enriched environment of the head and neck area.

Thermal Drape. An aluminum-coated plastic body cover reflects radiant body heat back to the patient to reduce intraoperative heat loss. A sterile, nonconductive, radiolucent thermal drape may be used as the final drape. The patient may be wrapped in nonsterile reflective covers (thermal drape) in the preoperative holding area. These may remain in place through the surgical procedure under standard sterile drapes and during postoperative recovery in the postanesthesia care unit (PACU). A reflective blanket or thermal drape is recommended when more than 60% of the body surface can be covered and when the surgical procedure will last more than 2 hours.

Nonwoven, disposable drapes are supplied prepackaged and presterilized by the manufacturer. A sterile package may contain a single drape, or it may have all of the drapes needed for a procedure, including towels, a Mayo stand and instrument table covers, and gowns. Unused disposable drapes and gowns should not be resterilized.

Woven Textile Fabrics

The thread count and finish of woven natural fibers determine the integrity and porosity of reusable fabrics. Tightly woven textile fabrics may inhibit migration of microorganisms. Cotton fibers swell when they become wet. This swelling action closes pores or interstices so that liquid cannot diffuse through tightly woven fibers. The fabric can be treated to further repel fluids (i.e., be impermeable to moisture strike-through).

Reusable drapes may be made of pima cotton of 270 or 280 thread count with a Quarpel finish. This fluorochemical finish combined with phenazopyridine or a melanin hydrophobe produces a durable water-resistant fabric. However, this fabric has essentially the same heat-retaining qualities as plastic lamination, so it cannot be used for complete patient draping. This treated

• **Fig. 26.39** Fenestrated laparotomy drape sheet with reinforcement around fenestration.

material can be used as reinforcement around fenestrations in otherwise untreated drapes.

Tightly woven 100% polyester reusable fabrics are hydrophobic (repel water droplets) but allow vapor permeation. Other reusable fabrics with different construction but similar barrier properties may be used.

The following points about reusable woven textile drapes should be considered:

- Material must be steam-penetrable and must withstand multiple sterilization cycles.
- When packaged for sterilization, drapes must be properly folded and arranged in sequence of use. Drapes may be fanfolded or rolled.
- Material must be free from holes and tears. The person who folds the drape is responsible for inspecting it for holes. Those detected may be covered with heat-seal patches. Tears or punctures (e.g., from towel clips or sharp instruments) compromise the barrier qualities of drapes.
- Drapes should be sufficiently impermeable to prevent moisture from soaking through them. Moisture has a wicking action that can cause migration of microorganisms.
- Reusable fabrics must maintain barrier qualities through multiple launderings. Densely woven, treated cotton becomes moisture permeable after about 75 washings; untreated cotton becomes moisture permeable after as few as 30 washings. Repeated drying, ironing, and steam sterilizing also alter fabric structure. The number of uses, washings, and sterilizing cycles should be recorded, and drapes that are no longer effective as barriers should be taken out of use.

Styles/Types of Drapes

Towels

Disposable or reusable sterile towels may be used to outline, or square off, the surgical site after prepping the skin. The folded edge of each towel is placed toward the line of incision to square it off. Towels are usually packaged in groups of four by the in-house laundry and can be secured with nonperforating towel clips or may be sutured or stapled to skin.

Radiopaque towels in counted packages are commercially available. Some disposable types have adhesive strips to hold them in place.

Surgical towels are traditionally used as draping material; however, in some facilities they are considered counted items. If a surgical draping towel is placed in the surgical incision, it becomes an item that must be accounted for and is listed using the same mechanism that is in place to track any other counted items.

The scrub person reports to the circulating nurse that a towel has been placed in the incision. The circulating nurse writes down the number of towels placed inside the patient on the count tally sheet or wipe-off board. At the conclusion of the surgical procedure, the scrub person reports how many towels have been removed and the number is validated by the circulating nurse during the final count. Counts are documented as correct or incorrect per facility policy.

The literature is replete with horror stories about surgical towels that carelessly become retained foreign objects when the team fails to account for them. Anything that becomes part of the incisional packing is considered a counted item.

Fenestrated Sheets

The drape sheet has an opening (fenestration) that is placed to expose the anatomic area where the incision will be made. Many styles of disposable nonwoven or reusable woven fabrics are available for specific uses. The size, direction, and shape of the fenestration vary to give adequate exposure of the surgical site. The sheet is long enough to cover the anesthesia screen at the head and extend down over the foot of the OR bed. Fenestrated sheets are usually marked to indicate the direction in which they should be unfolded. This may be an arrow or label designating the top or head, bottom or foot. It is wide enough to cover one or two armboards.

Reinforcement around the fenestration (see Fig. 26.39) for both nonwoven and woven fabrics provides an extra thickness to minimize the passage of microorganisms by capillary action to the sterile field. The reinforced area is usually 24 inches (60 cm) wide.

The drapes described are basic styles of fenestrated sheets.

Laparotomy Sheet. The laparotomy sheet is often referred to as a lap sheet; the longitudinal fenestration is placed over the surgical site on the abdomen, back, or comparable area (see Fig. 26.37). The opening is large enough to give adequate exposure in the usual laparotomy. The sheet is at least 108 × 72 inches (274 × 183 cm). Pediatric sizes are available. Lap sheets with a vertical fenestration can be used in some spinal procedures. Specialty lap sheets for cesarean sections may have an oval fenestration.

Thyroid Sheet. The thyroid sheet is the same size as a laparotomy sheet. The fenestration is transverse or diamond shaped and is positioned closer to the top of the patient over the neck area.

Chest Sheet. The chest sheet is similar to a laparotomy sheet except that the fenestration provides for a larger exposure. It is used for chest and breast procedures. Some chest sheets have a horizontal fenestration.

Hip Sheet. The hip sheet is similar to the laparotomy sheet but somewhat longer to completely cover the orthopedic fracture table. The fenestration may be oval and used in conjunction with an impervious stockinette.

Perineal Sheet. The perineal sheet is of adequate size to create a sterile field with the patient in the lithotomy position. Some styles have large leggings incorporated into it to cover the legs in stirrups. It may have one or two openings to accommodate the perineum or rectum.

Laparoscopy Sheet. A laparoscopy sheet is a combination laparotomy and perineal sheet. It is used for gynecologic laparoscopy in lithotomy or combined abdominoperineal resection with the patient in the lithotomy position. The fenestrations are located on the abdominal portion and the perineum. Some styles have built in leggings.

Separate Sheets

Although fenestrated sheets are used for most surgical procedures, they are not always practical. The openings may be much too large for small incisions, such as specimens for biopsies or procedures on the hands or feet. Smaller separate sheets may be used for these purposes to leave exposed only the small surgical area or to provide additional drapes on the surgical field. Many of these are disposable.

Split Sheet. The split sheet is the same size as a laparotomy sheet. Rather than the sheet being fenestrated, one end is cut longitudinally up the middle at least one-third the length of the sheet to form two free ends (tails). The upper end of this split may be in the shape of a U. Adhesive strips on each tail approximately 8 inches (20 cm) from the end of the split adhere together to snug the drape around an extremity or head. Shorter styles have adhesive strips the full length of the inner aspect of the tails for circumferential wrapping.

Minor Sheet. The minor sheet is 36 × 45 inches (91 × 114 cm). It has many uses. Wrapped around an extremity, it permits the extremity to remain on the sterile field for manipulation during the surgical procedure. It is used under an arm to cover an armboard for shoulder, axillary, arm, and hand procedures.

Medium Sheet. The medium sheet is about 36 × 72 inches (91 × 183 cm). It is used to drape under legs, as an added protection above or below the surgical area, and for draping areas in which a fenestrated sheet cannot be used.

Single Sheet. The single sheet is 108 × 72 inches (274 × 183 cm). Folded lengthwise, it is placed above the sterile field to shield off the anesthesia provider and anesthesia machine or other equipment near the patient's head or sterile field. A single sheet also is used to cover the patient and OR bed below the surgical area around the face.

Leggings. Leg drapes are supplied in pairs to cover the legs of a patient in the lithotomy position. A rectangle, approximately 36 × 72 inches (91 × 183 cm), is closed on two sides to form a tentlike pocket. One open edge is folded into a cuff to protect gloves from contamination during application.

Stockinette. Stockinette is a tubular drape used to cover an extremity. This seamless tubing of stretchable woven material contours snugly to the skin. The material is porous and absorbent, so it is not a microbial barrier. Therefore, when used as a drape, it may be covered with a layer of plastic.

A two-ply tubular disposable drape is available that has an inner layer of stockinette and an outer layer of vinyl to make it impervious. An opening is cut through the material over the line of incision. Edges may be secured with a plastic incise drape before the incision is made, or it may be clipped to the wound edges after the incision. Rolled elastic Ace or Coban bandage is sometimes used for this purpose. Care is taken to use nonlatex materials for patients sensitive to latex.

Principles of Draping

The entire team should be familiar with the draping procedure because draping is an important step in the preparation of the patient for a surgical procedure. The scrub person should be knowledgeable and ready to assist with draping. The scrub person is responsible for seeing that necessary articles are arranged in proper sequence on the instrument table. Once a drape is placed it cannot be moved without contamination.

The person responsible for draping the patient may vary, as do materials and styles of drapes used to create a sterile field. The surgeon or assistant usually places the self-adhering incise drape or towels and towel clips to outline the surgical site. The scrub person assists with placing the remainder of the drapes.

During any draping procedure, the circulating nurse should stand by to direct the scrub person as necessary and watch carefully for breaks in technique. A contaminated drape or exposure of a nonsterile area is a potential source of infection for the patient.

Basic principles regarding draping are as follows:

1. Place drapes on a dry area. The area around or under the patient may become damp from solutions used for skin preparation. The circulating nurse removes damp items or covers the area to provide a dry field on which to lay sterile drapes.
2. Allow sufficient time to permit careful application.

3. Allow sufficient space to observe sterile technique. Do not reach across a nonsterile surface.
4. Handle drapes as little as possible.
5. Never reach across the OR bed to drape the opposite side; go around it.
6. Take towels and towel clips, if used, to the side of the OR bed from which the surgeon is going to apply them before handing them up.
7. Carry folded drapes to the OR bed. Watch the front of the sterile gown; it may bulge and touch the nonsterile OR bed or blanket on the patient. Stand well back from the nonsterile OR bed.
   a. Hold drapes high enough to avoid touching nonsterile areas, but avoid touching the overhead operating light.
   b. Hold a drape high until it is directly over the proper area, and then lay it down where it is to remain. Once a sheet is placed, do not adjust it. Be careful not to slide the sheet out of place when opening the folds.
   c. Protect gloved hands by cuffing the end of the sheet over them. Do not let gloved hands touch the skin of the patient or other nearby items, such as the IV.
8. When unfolding a sheet from the prepped area toward the foot or head of the OR bed, protect the gloved hand by enclosing it in a turned-back cuff of sheet provided for this purpose. Keep hands at table level.
9. If a drape becomes contaminated, do not handle it further. Discard it without contaminating gloves or other items.
   a. If the end of a sheet falls below waist level, do not handle it further. Drop it, and use another.
   b. If in doubt as to its sterility, consider a drape contaminated.
   c. If a drape is incorrectly placed, discard it. The circulating nurse peels it from the OR bed without contaminating other drapes or the prepped area.
10. A piercing towel clip that has been fastened through a drape has its points contaminated. Remove it only if absolutely necessary, and then discard it from the sterile setup without touching the points. Cover the area from which it was removed with another piece of sterile draping material.

Unusual Circumstances Considered Potentially Contaminated

1. If a hole is found in a drape after it is laid down, the hole must be covered with another piece of draping material (or Opsite) or the entire drape discarded. Use judgment concerning whether covering or discarding the drape is appropriate. Discarding the drape is the ideal if at all possible.
2. A hair found on a drape during a procedure in process must be removed, and the area covered immediately. Ideally the drape should be discarded and replaced if possible. The source of a hair is usually unknown and would cause a foreign body tissue reaction or infection in a patient if it got into the wound. If the drape cannot be removed, remove the hair with a hemostat, and hand the instrument off the sterile field; cover the area with a towel or another piece of draping material.

Procedures for Draping the Patient

Draping procedures establish the sterile field. Standardized methods of application should be practiced using adequate draping materials. The most common procedures are discussed here merely to elaborate the principles. The following section details procedures that use only absorbent woven draping materials because establishing a microbial barrier with them is more complex. The draping procedure is simplified when single-thickness impermeable materials are used. A procedure book should be consulted for specific draping procedures.

Laparotomy

The term *laparotomy* refers to an incision through the abdominal wall into the abdominal cavity. All flat, smooth areas are draped in the same manner as the abdomen. These areas include the neck, chest, flank, and back. The draping procedure is as follows:

1. Hand up four towels and towel clips (if the surgeon uses them). With practice, these can be held in the hands at the same time and separated one by one as the surgeon takes them. Go to the side of the OR bed on which the surgeon is draping to avoid reaching over the nonsterile table. The surgeon places these towels within the prepped area, leaving only the surgical area exposed.
2. Hand one end of a fan-folded medium sheet across the OR bed to the assistant, supporting the folds, keeping the sheet high, and holding it taut until it is opened; then lay it down. Place this medium sheet below the surgical site with the edge of it at the skin edge, covering the draping towel.

This sheet provides an extra thickness of material under the area from the Mayo stand to the incision, where instruments and sponges are placed, and closes some of the opening in the laparotomy sheet if necessary. This sheet may be eliminated if a self-adhering incise drape or impermeable drapes are used.

3. Place a laparotomy sheet with the opening directly over the prepped area outlined by the towels, in the direction indicated for the foot or head of the OR bed (Fig. 26.40). Drop the folds over the sides of the table. However, if an armboard is in place, hold the folds at table level until the sheet is opened all the way. Open it downward over the patient's feet first and then upward over the anesthesia screen (Fig. 26.41). Sheets with appropriate fenestrations are used to expose the surgical site.
   a. For the neck, use a thyroid sheet.
   b. For the chest, with the patient in either the supine or lateral position, use a breast sheet.
   c. For the flank, with the patient in the kidney position for transverse incision, use a kidney sheet.
   d. For the back, use a laparotomy sheet, the same as for the abdomen.
4. Place a large single sheet crosswise on the OR bed above the fenestrated site. This sheet provides an extra thickness above the area and closes some of the opening in the laparotomy sheet if necessary. It also covers the armboard if one is in use. A single sheet may be needed for this latter purpose even if an impermeable laparotomy sheet is used.

Head

An overhead instrument table may be positioned over the patient for neurologic procedures. The table drape is extended down over the patient's shoulders to create a continuous sterile field between the instrument table and the surgical site. The draping procedure is as follows:

1. The surgeon places four towels around the head and secures them with towel clips or affixes them in place with sutures or skin staples. Towel clips and staples are not used if x-rays will be taken during the surgical procedure.
2. Hand one end of a fan-folded medium sheet to the assistant. Holding it taut, unfold and secure it over the head end of the OR bed below the surgical site at the skin edge of the draping towel.
3. Place a fenestrated sheet with the opening over the exposed skin area of the head. Unfold the sheet across the front edge of the overhead table, and secure it before allowing the remainder of the drape to drop over the head of the OR bed toward the floor. Some disposable fenestrated head sheets have transparent plastic adhesive incise sheeting to cover the incisional site. The incise sheet may be impregnated with iodophor for additional wound protection during the procedure.

Face

Even if the surgical site is unilateral, the surgeon may want the entire face exposed for comparison of skin lines. The draping procedure is as follows:

1. The surgeon places a drape under the head while the circulating nurse or assistant elevates the head. This drape consists of an open towel placed on a medium sheet. The center of the

• **Fig. 26.40** Draping with sterile laparotomy sheet. Scrub person carries folded sheet to table. Standing far back from OR bed, with one hand, scrub person places the fenestration of the sheet on patient so that opening in sheet is directly over prepped skin area. A second sterile team member helps complete the opening of the drape over the body from the opposite side of the table.

• **Fig. 26.41** Unfolding upper end of laparotomy sheet over anesthesia screen. Note that hands approaching unsterile area are protected in cuff of drape and that sheet is stabilized with other hand.

towel edge is 2 inches (5 cm) in from the center of the sheet edge. The towel is drawn up on each side of the face, over the forehead or at the hairline, and fastened with a small nonperforating towel clip. This leaves the desired amount of the face exposed.

2. Hand up three additional towels and four towel clips. These towels frame the surgical site.
3. Place a medium sheet just below the site. This sheet must overlap the one under the head.
4. A fenestrated drape may be placed to complete draping.
5. Cover the remainder of the foot of the OR bed, as necessary, with a single sheet.

If the patient is receiving inhalation anesthesia, use a minor sheet instead of a towel on a medium sheet for the first drape under the head. A minor sheet is large enough to draw up on each side of the face and to enclose the endotracheal tube and oropharyngeal monitoring probes from the anesthesia machine for a considerable distance, thus keeping them from contaminating the sterile field.

If the surgical procedure on the face is unilateral, the anesthesia provider may sit along the unaffected side, near the patient's head, with the anesthesia screen placed on the same side of the OR bed.

Skin staples or sutures may be used to affix towels around the contours of the face and neck of the patient under general anesthesia. Each staple or stitch overlaps the skin and edge of the drape.

Eye

After skin preparation, the unaffected eye is protected by covering it with a sterile eye pad before draping the patient. The draping procedure is as follows:

1. The surgeon places two towels and a medium sheet under the head while the circulating nurse holds the head up, as described for a face drape. One towel is drawn up around the head, exposing only the eyebrow and affected eye, and fastened with a clip without pressure on the eyes.
2. Hand up four towels and towel clips to isolate the affected eye. Some surgeons prefer a self-adhering aperture drape.
3. Cover the patient and remainder of the OR bed below the surgical area with a single sheet.

If local anesthetic will be administered, the drapes are raised off of the patient's nose and mouth to permit free breathing. A Mayo stand or anesthesia screen positioned over the lower face before the draping is one method to elevate the drapes. Oxygen, 6 to 8 L/min, can be supplied under the drapes via tube or nasal cannula. If the patient has chronic obstructive pulmonary disease (COPD), the oxygen level should not exceed 3 L/min. Take extreme caution that oxygen does not build up under the drapes. An ignition source such as a cautery or laser could spark a fire beneath the drapes.

For a microsurgical procedure, a sterile, padded, U-shaped steel wrist rest for the surgeon and assistant is fastened to the head of the OR bed. Towels are put around the patient's head before the rest of the facial and body draping is completed.

If irrigation will be used, a plastic fenestrated drape is placed over the four towels to keep them dry if an aperture drape is not preferred.

Ear

The basic draping procedure is the same as for draping a face or eye, except that only the affected ear is exposed. The head is turned toward the unaffected side. Oxygen can be supplied under the drapes, as previously described. The anesthesia provider is usually positioned at the side of the OR bed near the patient's face.

Chest and Breast

While the arm is still being held up by the assistant after skin preparation:

1. Place a minor sheet on an armboard, under the patient's arm, extending the sheet under the side of the chest and shoulder. The prepped arm is lowered to the sterile draped armboard. The distal portion of the arm may be encased in sterile stockinette so that the arm can be manipulated during the surgical procedure.
2. The patient's body is draped with a sterile medium sheet.
3. Hand up towels and towel clips; five or six are necessary.
4. Apply a breast sheet so that the axilla is exposed for anticipated axillary dissection. Many breast procedures require both breasts to be prepped and exposed for comparison during the procedure.

Shoulder

While the arm is still being held up by the assistant after skin preparation:

1. Place medium sheets over the chest and under the arm.
2. Place a minor sheet under the shoulder and side of the chest.
3. The surgeon outlines the surgical site with towels and secures them with clips.
4. Place a minor sheet over the patient's chest, covering the neck. Keep this sheet even with the edge of the towel that borders the surgical site laterally.
5. Wrap the arm in a minor sheet or encase it in a sterile stockinette, and secure it with a sterile gauze or elastic bandage.[8] At this point, a sterile team member relieves the unsterile person who has been holding the arm.
6. Place a medium sheet above the area, and secure these sheets together with towel clips. Sticky split sheets can be used one above and one below the area.
7. A laparotomy or breast sheet may be used. Pull the arm through the opening. Or a single sheet may be placed above the area, and the foot of the OR bed is covered with a medium sheet.
8. If irrigation will be used, an arthroscopy drape with a large packet for fluid collection and a connection for suction tubing is available.

Elbow

While the arm is still being held up by the unsterile assistant after skin preparation:

1. Place a sterile medium sheet across the chest and under the arm, up to the axilla.
2. The surgeon defines the surgical area on the upper (proximal) arm by placing a towel around the upper arm and securing it with a towel clip.
3. Wrap the hand in a sterile towel. At this point, a sterile team member relieves the unsterile person who has been holding the arm by grasping the wrapped hand, maintaining the arm in an elevated position.[8]
4. The hand is grasped with a sterile stockinette, which is pulled down over the entire arm toward the axilla, over the surgical site.[8] An elastic bandage is wrapped around the arm starting at the distal end (hand) to the proximal area (axilla).

5. Place a medium sheet across the chest, on top of the arm, even with the towel on the upper arm and covering it. Secure this sheet around the arm with a towel clip.
6. An extremity sheet is drawn over the hand and the arm. The extremity sheet is opened in its entirety across the patient's body.

Hand

While the arm and hand are still being held up after skin preparation:
1. Place an impervious minor sheet, folded in half, on the extremity table.
2. The surgeon places a towel around the lower arm, limiting the exposed area to the affected hand, and secures it with a towel clip.
3. Pull a stockinette over the hand and up over the length of the arm. At this stage in draping, the unsterile person is relieved of holding the arm. The draped arm is laid on the draped extremity table.
4. Place a minor sheet across the extremity table just above the surgical site.
5. Place an extremity sheet over the hand. Do not drop folds below the level of the armboard. Open the sheet across the patient's body toward the feet first. Attach the top end to the IV poles at the head of the bed.

Perineum

With the patient in the lithotomy position for a genital, vaginal, or rectal procedure:
1. Place a medium sheet under the buttocks. The circulating nurse can grasp the underside and assist in placement. With the patient's legs elevated in stirrups, this drape hangs below the level of the OR bed and covers the lowered section of the OR bed.
2. Slide leggings over each leg, protecting the gloved hands in the folded cuffs.
3. The anus is covered if it is not part of the surgical site. An adhesive towel drape may be used for this purpose.
4. Place a medium sheet across the abdomen, from the level of the pubis, extending over the anesthesia screen or attached to IV poles at the head of the bed.
5. A fenestrated perineal sheet may be used rather than a medium sheet over the abdomen. To use a perineal sheet with built-in leggings, hand one end of the sheet to the assistant, opening out folds, and draw the leggings over the feet and legs simultaneously. The hands are kept on the outside of the sheet to avoid contaminating the gloves and gown.

Hip

The patient is in a lateral position. If the leg will be manipulated during the surgical procedure, while the leg is still being held up after skin preparation:
1. Place a medium sheet on the OR bed under the leg, up to the buttock.
2. Place another medium sheet on the OR bed, overlapping the first one, to cover the unaffected leg. Some surgeons prefer to use an incise sheet or a lower extremity stockinette.
3. The surgeon wraps the foot and leg with an elastic bandage, covering the stockinette. The leg, held up to this point, is laid on the OR bed.

4. Place a minor sheet lengthwise of the OR bed on each side of the exposed area, even with the skin. The sheets under the leg and above the site do not overlap. Some surgeons prefer to draw the leg through the opening of a hip sheet or place a split sheet under the leg with the tails crossed over it toward the patient's head.
5. Place a medium sheet above the exposed area. Secure these last three sheets with towel clips.
6. Place a single sheet above the surgical area and over the anesthesia screen.

If manipulation of the leg is not necessary during the surgical procedure, drape the same as for a laparotomy, using a hip sheet instead of a laparotomy sheet.

Knee

While the leg is still being held up after skin preparation:
1. Place a medium sheet lengthwise on the OR bed, under the leg, up to the buttock. Take care not to contaminate sterile gloves on the unsterile tourniquet if used.
2. Place another medium sheet on the OR bed, overlapping the first sheet, to cover the unaffected leg.
3. The surgeon limits the sterile field above the knee by placing a towel around the leg and securing it with a towel clip.
4. Lay a minor sheet on the sterile sheets under the leg. The person who has been holding the leg lays it on this minor sheet. The surgeon wraps the leg in the minor sheet and secures it with a sterile bandage. Stockinette may be preferred for this step.
5. Place a medium sheet above the exposed area, at the skin edge, over the draping towel, and fasten it with a towel clip.
6. Place a laparotomy or extremity sheet, with the opening on the foot and the longer part of the sheet toward the head of the OR bed. Open it, and draw the leg through the opening. A split sheet may be used instead. If water will be used for arthroscopy, a drape with a fluid collection pocket should be opened according to the diagram so the pocket is in the correct position.

Lower Leg and Ankle

While the leg is still being held up after skin preparation:
1. Place a medium sheet under the leg and over the unaffected leg to above the knees.
2. The surgeon limits the sterile field by placing a towel around the leg above the area of the intended surgical site and securing it with a towel clip.
3. Put a stockinette over the foot and draw it up over the leg to above the skin edge of the towel. The person who has been holding the leg is relieved, and the leg is held by a sterile team member.
4. Place a medium sheet above the surgical area, and secure it around the leg with a towel clip.
5. Place a laparotomy, extremity, or split sheet with the leg drawn through the opening.
6. Cover the remainder of the OR bed over the anesthesia screen with a single sheet as necessary.

Foot

The general method of draping a foot is the same as that for the hand. While the foot is still being held up after skin preparation:
1. Place a medium sheet on the OR bed under the foot.

2. The surgeon limits the exposed area to the foot by placing a towel around the ankle and securing it with a towel clip.

3. Enclose the foot in a stockinette. A sterile team member relieves the unsterile person who has been holding the leg.

4. Place a medium sheet above the foot, and secure it around the ankle with a towel clip.

5. Place a laparotomy or extremity sheet with the opening over the foot and longer part of the sheet toward the head of the OR bed.

Draping of Equipment

A pneumatic tourniquet frequently is used to control bleeding during surgical procedures on the upper and lower extremities. A nonsterile tourniquet cuff is placed around the extremity before skin preparation and is covered with the draping material. An impervious towel that delineates the upper limit of the surgical area is placed around the extremity below the tourniquet cuff.

Equipment that is brought into the sterile field but cannot be sterilized must be draped before it is handled by sterile team members. The following applies to draping of equipment:

1. Tailored, disposable, clear plastic drapes are available to cover equipment, such as the operating microscope and the C-arm, so that they can be manipulated in the sterile field by the sterile team.

2. If x-rays are to be taken during the surgical procedure and it is not a digital system, a cassette holder may be placed on the OR bed, under the mattress, before the patient is positioned, prepped, and draped. The circulating nurse raises the edge of the sterile drape for the radiology technician to place and remove the x-ray cassette. The cassette may be covered with a sterile Mayo stand cover or specially designed disposable cover and placed on sterile drapes when a lateral view is needed.

3. Cords, cables, attachments, and tubing that are not sterile are inserted into sterile plastic sleeves before they are placed on the sterile field.

Nonsterile equipment that must stand near the sterile field is isolated from the sterile area with a barrier drape. IV poles frequently are used to attach drapes to shield off power-generating sources of mechanical and electrical equipment, such as electrosurgical and cryosurgical units, fiberoptic lighting units, and air-powered or electrical instruments. The drape over the patient or a separate single sheet is extended from the OR bed upward in front of or over the nonsterile equipment. The circulating nurse fastens the drape to IV poles on each side of the equipment that stands above the level of the sterile field or near it.

Heat-generating equipment must have adequate ventilation to dissipate heat. Impermeable, heat-retaining materials cannot completely encase these units. Ends of fiberoptic light cables should not make prolonged contact with drapes, or a fire may result.

Some nonsterile equipment, of necessity, is moved over the sterile field. The sterile field is protected using additional draping material as follows:

1. Sterile disposable drapes are available to cover x-ray equipment and image intensifiers.

2. When ready to move an x-ray tube or image intensifier over the sterile field, cover the field with a sterile minor sheet. The circulating nurse discards this sheet after use because it is considered contaminated.

3. Photographic equipment and video cameras should be draped as much as is feasible when used over the sterile field. Some video cameras fit directly into the headlamp of the surgeon or in the overhead spotlight and require no special draping.

Plastic Isolator

A patient isolation drape may be used in conjunction with a fracture table. The isolation drape literally divides the room in half vertically. It isolates the sterile field from equipment, such as the C-arm image intensifier used for hip procedures. The drape is suspended from a steel frame on one side of the special orthopedic table but does not enclose the patient. The drape may have an incise portion that may be impregnated with a timed-release iodophor. Storage holsters and irrigation pouches are commonly incorporated into the side. Care is taken not to perforate the plastic surface when placing items in the pouches.

ⓔ EVOLVE WEBSITE

http://evolve.elsevier.com/Hornacky/BerryKohn/

- Historical Perspective
- Student Interactive Questions
- Glossary

References

1. Armstrong M, Moore RA: Anatomy, patient positioning. www.ncbi.nlm.nih.gov. Accessed May 12, 2023.

2. Spruce L: Prevention of perioperative pressure injury, *AORN J* 117(5):317−323, 2023.

3. Stanton C: Guideline for positioning the patient, *AORN J* 115(5):5−7, 2022.

4. Roman A, Tufegdzic B, Lamperti M, et al.: Before the knife: a detailed step-by-step description of an optimized semi-sitting position in posterior fossa surgery, *World Neurosurg* 172:e241−e249, 2023.

5. Croke L: Best practices for indwelling urinary catheter use in the surgical population, *AORN J* 109(1):7−9, 2019.

6. Lucero S, Dryden M: Antisepsis, asepsis and skin preparation, *Surgery* 37(1):45−50, 2019.

7. Beaty AD, Lieberman PL, Slavin RG: Seafood allergy and radiocontrast media: are physicians propagating a myth? *Am J Med* 121(2):158.e1−158.e4, 2008.

8. Lee D, Neviaser R: Positioning, shoulder and elbow surgery. In Miller M, Browne J, Cole B, et al., editors: *Operative techniques*, ed 2, St. Louis, 2019, Elsevier.

Bibliography

AORN: *Guidelines for perioperative practice*, Denver, CO, 2024, The Association.

Phillips NM, Hornacky A: *Pass CNOR!*, St. Louis, 2019, Elsevier.

27

Physiologic Maintenance and Monitoring of the Perioperative Patient

CHAPTER OUTLINE

Monitoring Physiologic Functions, 535

CHAPTER OBJECTIVES

After studying this chapter, the learner will be able to:

- Identify pertinent body systems that should be monitored during a surgical procedure.
- Discuss the differences between invasive and noninvasive means of patient monitoring.

- Discuss why personnel monitoring a patient should be knowledgeable about the monitoring devices used.
- Describe how monitoring parameters provide information about interrelated body systems.

KEY TERMS AND DEFINITIONS

Core temperature Temperature inside the body.

Expiration Exit of waste gases from the body through the mouth and nose.

External respiration Exchange of gases between the lungs and blood at the alveolar level.

Hemodynamics Study of blood circulation, blood pressure, peripheral vascular physiology, and cardiac function.

Internal respiration Exchange of gases between the blood and cells at the capillary/tissue level.

Monitoring Observing, evaluating, and reporting physiologic function.

Pulse Palpable sensation of blood passing through an artery.

Respiration Exchange of oxygen (O_2) and carbon dioxide (CO_2) at the molecular level.

Sinus rhythm Electrical impulse in the heart that originates at the sinoatrial node of the right atrium of the heart, passes through the atrioventricular node at the atrial-septal junction, and continues down the length of the Purkinje fibers in the ventricular septum, causing contraction of the ventricles.

Ventilation/inspiration Bringing air into the lungs through the mouth, nose, or tracheal stoma.

The development of successful controllable anesthesia has made modern surgery possible. Because anesthesia is an adjunct to most surgical procedures, familiarity with various anesthetic agents, their interaction with certain drugs, and potential hazards is a necessity. The perioperative nurse responsible for patient monitoring may detect the onset of complications and help avert an undesired outcome.

Working with anesthesia providers in the perioperative environment gives the learner an unparalleled opportunity to master immediate resuscitative measures and their effectiveness, and an understanding of the care of unconscious and critically ill patients. For example, the learner daily observes endotracheal intubation, ventilatory control, insertion of arterial and venous cannulas, fluid replacement, and sophisticated hemodynamic monitoring.

No surgical procedure is minor. Surgery and anesthesia impose certain inescapable risks, even in supposedly ideal circumstances.

Overall, however, the anesthetic-related surgical mortality rate is relatively low. Preexisting patient factors, such as age and medical condition, and those related to the circumstances of the surgical procedure, such as type, duration, and elective versus emergency procedure, are more significant in determining surgical mortality.

The American Society of Anesthesiologists (ASA) has established standards for basic perioperative monitoring. Specialization in monitoring equipment and the use of computers to record monitoring data are facets of contemporary anesthesia practice.

Monitoring Physiologic Functions

Preoperative patient assessment establishes a baseline and provides valuable information with which intraoperative and postoperative patient care is planned and evaluated. Establishing a preoperative baseline enables the caregiver to be alerted to changes in the patient's physiologic condition that may require prompt attention.[1]

Surgical and anesthetic techniques have become increasingly complex, which allows many critically ill patients of all ages to undergo surgical procedures. The anesthesia provider carefully monitors the patient's condition through the entire perioperative process and keeps the surgeon informed of important changes.

Monitoring implies keeping track of vital functions. During extensive surgery with the patient under anesthesia, the body is subjected to physiologic stress. Bleeding, tissue trauma, potent drugs, large extravascular fluid shifts, multiple transfusions, and a surgical position that may inhibit breathing and circulation all contribute to altered physiology. These factors can induce significant cardiopulmonary dysfunction.

Patients under local anesthesia are frequently monitored with electrocardiographs (ECG). If the patient has a known cardiac condition, such as atrial fibrillation (AF), the atrial dysrhythmia is felt by the patient and demonstrated on the ECG machine. If the patient has had atrial ablation treatments, an AF rhythm may be measured by the ECG monitor and not felt by the patient.[2] It is important to use subjective and objective measures to evaluate the patient's condition.[2]

Evaluation of the patient's responses to surgical stressors includes observation, auscultation, and palpation. The assessment is enhanced with the use of electronic or mechanical devices that reveal physiologic trends and subtle changes and indicate responses to therapy. Most of this equipment is expensive and is incorporated into the anesthesia machine. Compact precise devices with miniaturized circuitry, better visibility, and easier maintenance are incorporated into portable models that allow for continued monitoring after the patient leaves the operating room (OR).

Computers improve and expedite analysis of data. They are sophisticated data collection and management tools that assist in physiologic assessment, diagnosis, and therapy. Clinical computers vary from single-function devices to complex, multifunction, real-time systems that acquire, store, and display data; organize information; display trends; and perform calculations.

Personnel who use electronic and computerized monitoring equipment must understand its use and function, be experienced in its interpretation, and be able to determine equipment malfunction easily. Instrumentation should augment, not replace, careful observation of the patient. Monitoring equipment can be inaccurate. Information from monitors should be compared with physical assessment data.

Perioperative nurses involved with patient monitoring should remain current in the knowledge of physical assessment and the use of the equipment. Periodic competency testing should be performed. Written policies, procedures, and guidelines should be available for reference.

The spectrum of monitoring devices is broad. It ranges from noninvasive to invasive. Noninvasive monitors do not penetrate the body or a body orifice. Conversely, invasive monitors penetrate skin or mucosa, or they enter a body cavity. Some parameters can be measured with both noninvasive and invasive methods. Perioperative nursing responsibilities may include assisting with sophisticated hemodynamic monitoring to evaluate the interrelationship of blood pressure (BP), blood flow, vascular volumes, and physical properties of blood, heart rate, and ventricular function.

Detection of early changes in hemodynamics allows prompt action to maintain cardiac function and adequate cardiac output (CO). Monitoring facilitates rapid, accurate determination of decreased perfusion. It reflects immediate response to therapeutic measures and stress.

Invasive Hemodynamic Monitoring

Hemodynamics is the study of the movement of blood. Measurements of CO and intracardiac pressures provide information related to functions of the heart and other major organ systems.

Invasive hemodynamic monitoring uses basic physiologic principles to detect and treat a wide variety of abnormalities. Its purpose is to avoid problems in high-risk patients and accurately diagnose and treat patients with established life-threatening disorders. Hemodynamic monitoring involves direct intravascular measurements and assessments by means of indwelling catheters connected to transducers and monitors.[3]

Pressures and forces within arteries and veins are converted to electrical signals by the transducer, a device that transfers energy from one system to another. These electrical signals are then processed and amplified by the monitor into a continuous waveform displayed on an oscilloscope or monitoring screen that reproduces images received via the transducer, or the monitor may digitally display the values.

These measurements yield specific information that is otherwise not usually attainable or as accurate. Although these measurements may be pertinent in guiding patient care, they present additional risks because obtaining them requires invasion of the great vessels or heart. The benefits of invasive monitoring must be balanced against the risks.

Various types of equipment, monitors, and catheters are in use. Everyone caring for patients with invasive monitors must have knowledge of anatomy and physiology and an understanding of the entire monitoring circuit. Every precaution must be taken to ensure patient safety. Strict adherence to policies and procedures, manufacturer instructions for use, and sterile technique is absolutely essential to minimize complications and misinterpretation of data that could lead to errors in therapy.

Indwelling arterial, venous, and intracardiac catheters permit rapid accurate assessment of physiologic alterations in high-risk patients. Intravascular access is justified because of the high yield of information with minimal discomfort to patients. But hemodynamic monitoring techniques must not be abused.

Cardiac dysrhythmias, thrombosis, embolism, and infection are serious, sometimes fatal, complications of intravascular cannulation. Some facilities require the patient to sign a consent form before insertion of an invasive catheter.

Intravascular Cannulation

Intravascular catheters usually are inserted before induction of anesthesia by the anesthesia provider. They may be inserted percutaneously or by cutdown, depending on the type of catheter, intended purpose, and location of the vessel to be cannulated. Intracardiac catheters may be placed under fluoroscopic control, or their position may be verified on a chest radiograph after insertion. In addition to their use in hemodynamic monitoring, intravenous (IV) catheters can be used to administer blood, drugs, and nutrients. Catheters may be inserted into the right atrium or pulmonary artery via the vena cava through a subclavian, jugular, brachial, or femoral vein.

Intraarterial catheters are inserted for direct pressure measurements and to obtain blood for arterial blood gas (ABG) analyses.

Potential sites for cannulation include the radial, ulnar, axillary, brachial, femoral, and dorsalis pedis arteries. The radial artery is most commonly used if ulnar circulation to the hand is adequate. A Doppler ultrasound device may be used to determine a dominant artery and locate a weakly palpable one. When radial artery dominance exists, the ulnar, brachial, or other artery is used.

As a precaution, adequacy of perfusion to the extremity below the catheter should be established before insertion in case thrombosis or occlusion occurs. A radial artery distal to a brachial artery previously used for cardiac catheterization is avoided because of the possibility of distorted pressures or occlusion. Some physicians cannulate the femoral artery if the catheter is to remain in place for more than 24 hours. The incidence of thrombosis is lower when a large vessel is used.

Thrombosis may result from irritation of the vessel wall or hypercoagulation or inadequate flushing of the catheter and line. The larger the catheter in relation to the arterial lumen, the greater the incidence of thrombosis. Other complications of arterial cannulation include embolic phenomena, blood loss from a dislodged catheter or disconnected line, bruise or hematoma formation, arteriovenous fistula or aneurysm formation, systemic infection, and ischemic fingers from arterial spasm.

Intravascular Catheters

Most catheters are radiopaque and have centimeter calibrations. They are flexible. They may be made of silicone, polyethylene, polyvinyl chloride, polytetrafluoroethylene (Teflon), or polyurethane. Those with soft pliable tips are safer than are stiff catheters. Shearing of a vessel with extravascular migration of the catheter has occurred from stiffness and sharpness of the catheter and movement of the patient. Soft catheters are introduced over a guidewire or with flow-directed balloons. The catheter and related introducer, guidewire, and caps may be supplied as a prepackaged sterile kit.

Many catheters have an outer coating to prevent clot formation. Polyurethane or other uncoated catheters are available for the patient who is allergic to heparin. Some catheters also have an antimicrobial coating such as chlorhexidine-silver sulfadiazine or minocycline- rifampicin to prevent infection.[4] The catheter is kept open with a slow continuous infusion. Routine flushing of the catheter is necessary. Normal saline solution may be used if heparin is unnecessary or contraindicated. Continuous-flush devices with fast-flush valves release small amounts of solution. Limited pressure diminishes the possibility of ejecting a large clot. The catheter usually is fast-flushed both hourly and after blood samples are withdrawn. Air bubbles in the line must be avoided. After flushing, the drip rate in the drip chamber is checked.

A catheter may have a single lumen or two or three lumens. The catheters discussed are used for hemodynamic monitoring of the following:
- ABGs and pressure via a single-lumen intraarterial catheter
- Central venous pressure (CVP) via a central venous, Hickman, or Broviac catheter
- Pulmonary artery pressures (PAPs) via a pulmonary artery or Swan-Ganz catheter

Catheter Insertion

Catheter insertion is a sterile procedure. The necessary sterile supplies should be collected before the patient arrives. Many sterile kits are available that contain the necessary supplies. Although catheters are different, the technique for insertion is basically the same for all types. Insertion is a team effort. The circulating nurse's responsibilities may vary but usually include the following:

1. Explain the procedure and reassure the patient. If the patient will be awake, sedation may be ordered.
2. Document the patient's vital signs and pulse distal to the selected insertion site if the arm is the insertion site. If the pulse weakens after cannulation, circulation may be inadequate in an extremity and the catheter may need to be removed.
3. Position the patient as appropriate.
   a. For radial artery cannulation, affix the forearm to an armboard with the hand supinated and wrist dorsiflexed to an angle of 50 to 60 degrees over a towel. Avoid extreme dorsiflexion; this can obliterate the pulse. Tape the thumb to the armboard to stabilize the artery at the wrist.
   b. For subclavian or jugular vein insertion, place the patient in a 25 to 30-degree Trendelenburg position to reduce the potential for air embolism. Elevate the right scapular area with padding or a rolled towel underneath the shoulders to allow the physician to identify anatomic landmarks and locate the vein more easily. Turn the patient's head away from the insertion site.[5]
4. Prepare the skin per routine procedure. Wearing sterile gloves, the anesthesia provider then drapes the area. Warn patients if their face will be covered.
5. Inform patients, if awake, that they may have a burning sensation for a few seconds when the local anesthetic is injected before the area becomes numb. Explain that pressure, but not pain, may be felt during insertion. The skin and subcutaneous tissues are infiltrated with a local anesthetic because the skin is incised to facilitate entrance of the catheter. A cutdown, or opening of the skin and tissues to access a vein, may be necessary.
6. Assist the anesthesia provider as appropriate. Be familiar with and follow manufacturer directions for the brand of catheter and monitoring equipment used.
7. Make sure the connections between the catheter and infusion line are secure after the catheter has been inserted and properly placed. The catheter is sutured in place with a synthetic monofilament suture to prevent inadvertent advancement or removal and is taped to the skin. Lumens on the three-way stopcock and catheter may be capped to prevent fibrin deposits and retrograde contamination.
8. Connect the catheter line to the transducer or monitor, and take baseline pressure readings.
9. Dress the puncture site. An antibacterial ointment may be put around the site. Tape must not apply pressure directly over the insertion site or catheter. A transparent dressing is preferable. The catheter beneath it must not be bent or curled.
10. Take the patient's vital signs. Use a sphygmomanometer with the BP cuff on the arm opposite from the insertion site, and check the BP to compare with the monitor's pressure reading to verify the monitor's accuracy. The monitor may read higher systolic and lower diastolic pressures than the BP cuff readings.
11. Document the procedure and initial readings. Include the insertion site; type and gauge of catheter; type of infusion solution and amount of heparin, if added; flow rate and pressure; pulse before and after insertion; tolerance of the procedure; color, sensation, and warmth of the area distal to the insertion site; time of insertion; and names of insertion team members.

Frequent checks of circuitry and calibrations are necessary to validate the recorded data. Conscientious attention to every detail is mandatory during catheter insertion and monitoring. An ultrasound can be used to check for the tip placement of the central venous catheter to ensure there has been no perforation or other catheter misplacement.[5] Ultrasound is a quick method that does not expose the patient to unnecessary x-ray exposure.

Drawing Blood Samples

When the arterial or venous catheters are in place, the perioperative nurse may be asked to collect blood samples for analysis or to take measurements, although this is not universal practice. These procedures require special training, skill, and knowledge of equipment and hazards involved.

Samples for ABG measurements are sometimes drawn from an indwelling catheter line kept open with a continuously running infusion. The tubing incorporates a plastic three-way stopcock, usually close to the catheter insertion site. One lumen of the stopcock goes to the infusion solution, one to the cannulated vessel, and one to outside air. The lumen to outside air is normally closed or covered with a sterile cap, or a sterile syringe is kept inserted in the lumen to prevent bacteria and air from entering. With a three-way stopcock, two of the three lumens are always open.

In drawing blood samples from an indwelling catheter, always use strict sterile technique. Blood may be drawn through a stopcock on a single-lumen catheter or from one lumen of a multilumen catheter. A sterile ABG monitoring kit with administration tubing and pressure transducers may be used for intraarterial pressure monitoring. Manufacturer instructions should be followed for turning the stopcock to draw blood samples and to flush lines. Drawing blood from a multilumen catheter is simplified when an injection port can be used. Many styles do not use needles, but use a double Luer-Lok tip to connect. The basic procedure is similar to the following, using a stopcock (always wipe the stopcock or end of the catheter with alcohol before entering the system):

1. Wear sterile gloves. A sterile heparinized or saline syringe is used to prevent the blood samples from clotting. Follow the recommended heparin protocol. To heparinize, draw 1 mL of aqueous heparin 1:1000 into a 10-mL syringe. While rotating the barrel, pull the plunger back beyond the 7-mL calibration. With the syringe in an upright position, slowly eject the heparin and air bubbles while rotating the barrel.
2. Attach a sterile 5-mL syringe to the stopcock lumen going to outside air. Turn off (close) the infusion lumen. This automatically opens the line between the patient and the syringe. Aspirate to clear the line of fluid, and close the lumen to the patient. Discard this diluted sample.
3. Quickly attach the sterile syringe to a lumen to outside air, and open the lumen to the patient. This closes the lumen to the infusion, permitting aspiration of undiluted blood for analysis. Arterial pressure forces blood into the syringe. Withdraw 3 to 5 mL of blood. Hold the barrel and the plunger of the syringe to avoid their separation. Cap the syringe for placement in a properly labeled specimen bag.
4. Close the lumen to the patient, and flush the line and stopcock by letting the infusion solution run through them to prevent clot formation inside the catheter wall or stopcock, which could result in arterial embolization.
5. Close and recap the lumen to outside air (being careful not to contaminate the cap), thereby restarting the infusion to the patient. Regulate the infusion rate with the clamp on the infusion tubing.
6. If air bubbles are in the syringe, remove them. Send the samples immediately to the laboratory. If more than 10 minutes elapses between blood drawing and analysis, the analysis cannot be considered accurate. In the event of delay, the syringe with blood should be immersed in ice immediately and refrigerated at near-freezing temperature. Iced specimen bags may be used.
7. Attach the appropriate laboratory slips that include information such as the patient's name and location, the time and date, and whether the patient is receiving supplemental oxygen or breathing room air.

Physiologic Parameters Monitored

Noninvasive methods can be used to monitor some cardiopulmonary and neural functions and determine body temperature and urinary output (Box 27.1). Both noninvasive and invasive techniques are used for monitoring hemodynamic parameters to show minute-to-minute changes in physiologic variables. Normal ranges of hemodynamic parameters are given in Table 27.1.

• BOX 27.1 Noninvasive Methods of Monitoring Vital Functions

Cardiopulmonary Functions

- *Blood pressure (BP):* Measurement of pressure exerted against arterial vessel walls to force blood through circulation.
- *Capnometry:* Measurement of end-tidal concentration of carbon dioxide, by exposing expired air to infrared light.
- *Cardiac index (CI):* Measurement of cardiac output in relation to body surface, with use of ultrasound.
- *Chest x-ray study:* Determination via radiology of the position of intravascular catheters and endotracheal or chest tubes.
- *Echocardiogram:* Assessment of intraventricular blood volume by observing two-dimensional color images of the beating heart produced by an ultrasonic probe placed in the esophagus.
- *Electrocardiogram (ECG):* Recording of electrical forces produced by the heart to evaluate changes in rhythm, rate, or conduction.
- *Near-infrared reflectance:* Determination of the amount of oxygen in hemoglobin being delivered to the brain, with use of a niroscope (near-infrared reflectance scope [NIRS]).
- *Pulse oximetry:* Determination of arterial hemoglobin oxygen saturation with measurement of the optical density of light passing through tissues.
- *Respiratory tidal volume (V_T):* With use of a respirometer, measurement of the volume of air moved with each respiration.
- *Stethoscopy:* Detection of cardiac rate and rhythm and pulmonary sounds, with auscultation.
- *Total blood volume (TBV):* Measurement of plasma and red blood cell volumes, with use of an electronic device.

Neural Functions

- *Electroencephalogram (EEG):* Recording of electrical activity in the brain.
- *Evoked potentials:* Recording of electrical responses from the cerebral cortex after stimulation of a peripheral sensory organ.

Other Functions

- *Temperature:* Measurement of core body temperature, with use of a thermometer probe.
- *Urinary output:* Measurement of urine to assess renal perfusion, with use of an indwelling catheter attached to a calibrated collection device.

TABLE 27.1 Hemodynamic Monitoring Parameters

Parameter	Abbreviation	Normal Range for Adults
Arterial oxygen content	Ca_{O_2}	17–20 mL/dL blood
Blood pressure	BP	Systolic 90–130 mm Hg Diastolic 60–85 mm Hg
Cardiac index	CI	2.8–4.2 L/min/m^2
Cardiac output	CO	4–8 L/min
Central venous pressure	CVP	2–8 mm Hg, 3–10 cm H_2O
Cerebral perfusion pressure	CPP	80–100 mm Hg
Coronary perfusion pressure	CPP	60–80 mm Hg
Ejection fraction	EF	60–70%
Glomerular filtration rate	GFR	80–120 mL/min
Heart rate	HR	60–100 beats/min
Intracranial pressure	ICP	0–15 mm Hg
Left ventricular end-diastolic pressure	LVEDP	8–12 mm Hg
Mean arterial pressure	MAP	70–105 mm Hg
Mean pulmonary artery pressure	MPAP	9–19 mm Hg
Oxygen saturation in arterial blood	Sa_{O_2}	95–97.5%
Oxygen saturation in mixed venous blood	Sv_{O_2}	75%
Partial pressure of carbon dioxide in arterial blood	Pa_{CO_2}	34–45 mm Hg (torr)
Partial pressure of oxygen in arterial blood	Pa_{O_2}	80–100 mm Hg (torr)
Partial pressure of oxygen in venous blood	Pv_{O_2}	40 mm Hg (torr)
Pulmonary artery pressure	PAP	Systolic: 15–25 mm Hg Diastolic: 8–15 mm Hg
Pulmonary capillary wedge pressure	PCWP	6–12 mm Hg
Right atrial pressure	RAP	3–6 mm Hg
Right ventricular pressure	RVP	Systolic: 15–25 mm Hg Diastolic: 0–5 mm Hg
Stroke volume	SV	60–130 mL/beat
Systemic vascular resistance	SVR	800–1600 dyne/s/cm
Total blood volume	TBV	8.5–9% of body weight in kg
Venous oxygen content	Cv_{O_2}	15 mL/dL blood

Electrocardiogram

Every heartbeat depends on the electrical process of polarization. Muscles in the heart wall are alternately stimulated and relaxed. An ECG is a recording of electrical forces produced by the heart and translated as waveforms (Fig. 27.1). It shows changes in rhythm, rate, and conduction, such as dysrhythmias, appearance of premature beats, and block of impulses. An ECG does not provide an index of CO. Cardiac monitoring has become standard procedure in the OR and postanesthesia care unit (PACU).

Cardiac monitoring systems generally consist of a monitor screen; a cathode ray oscilloscope, on which the ECG is continuously visualized; and a printout system, which transcribes the rhythm strip to paper to permit comparison of tracings and provide a permanent record. The printout may be controlled or automatic. A heart rate meter may be set to print out a rhythm strip and sound an alarm if the rate goes above or below a preset figure. Lights and beeps may provide appropriate visual and audible signals of the heart rate.

Monitor leads or electrodes are attached to the chest or extremities. These electrodes detect electrical impulses that the heart generates. Connecting lead wires and cables transmit them to the cardiac monitor. A complete cardiogram includes 12 different leads, but usually only two or three electrodes are used. Careful placement of leads is important to show waves and complexes on the ECG rhythm strip. Leads to the anterior, lateral, or inferior cardiac surfaces, where ischemia most often occurs, provide myocardial ischemia monitoring. Use of multiple leads allows better definition of dysrhythmia and ischemia—the main reason for cardiac monitoring in the OR.[6] The choice of leads is made by the anesthesia provider or by the surgeon in cases of unattended local anesthesia use.

• **Fig. 27.1** Electrocardiogram complex. P wave before each QRS complex represents atrial depolarization. PR interval of sinus rhythm occurs between each P wave and R wave. PR segment represents conduction of impulse through atrioventricular (AV) node, bundle of His, bundle branches, and Purkinje fibers. QRS complex after each P wave represents ventricular depolarization and occurs at regular intervals, but rate can vary. T wave represents ventricular repolarization.

When placing disc electrodes, the underlying skin must be clean and dry for adequate adherence. The sites are shaved, if necessary, because hair can interfere with adherence. The skin is abraded slightly with a gauze pad or rough material to facilitate conduction. The backing is peeled off the disc with care to not touch the adhesive. The conductive gel within the pad at the center of the disc is checked. If it is not moist, another is used. The electrode is placed on the desired site, adhesive side down, and secured tightly by applying pressure. Begin at the center and move outward to avoid expressing gel from beneath the electrode. Placing gel over a bony area is avoided because bone interferes with conduction.

One ECG tracing is taken as a baseline before induction of anesthesia. An ECG is especially valuable during induction and intubation, when dysrhythmias are prone to occur. Early detection and rapid identification of abnormal rhythms and irregularities of the heart's actions permit treatment to be more specific.[6] Tracings may show changes related to the anesthetic itself or to oxygenation, coronary blood flow, hypercapnia (increased $PaCO_2$), or alterations in electrolyte balance or body temperature.

The ECG tracing becomes a flat line when heart action ceases, but preceding tracings may define the type of cardiac arrest, which is of value in treatment. It is beyond the scope of this text to describe normal and abnormal cardiac rhythms interpreted by the ECG. However, perioperative nurses who monitor patients under local anesthesia should become familiar with them. Box 27.2 shows the characteristics of sinus rhythm, and Fig. 27.2 shows an example of sinus rhythm in each of 12 leads.

The ECG monitors should be insensitive to electrical interference. Occasionally, recordings may be affected by a high-frequency electrosurgical unit. If a tracing problem occurs, lead contacts, the integrity of the leads, and the choice of monitoring axis are checked.

• BOX 27.2 Characteristics of Sinus Rhythm

- P wave is present before each QRS complex.
- Equal space exists between P wave and R wave (PR interval) in each complex.
- QRS complex follows each P wave (ratio 1:1).
- P wave and QRS complex occur at regular intervals (rate can vary).

The ECG monitor may be connected to a computer for analysis and storage of data. From the ECG readings, a device within the computer may be able to measure the amount of blood being pumped by the heart. This gives a continuous assessment of pumping capacity and CO. Impedance cardiography also provides data based on the mechanical activity of the heart. This is also a noninvasive computer-assisted measurement of CO, an alternative to the thermodilution technique.

Echocardiogram

Sound waves from a sonar-like device provide two-dimensional color images of the beating heart. An ultrasonic probe on the end of a small gastroscope is placed in the esophagus during the surgical procedure. Also referred to as transesophageal echocardiography, this form of echocardiogram can help the anesthesia provider immediately assess intraventricular blood volume, which can be useful information for the surgeon during cardiac surgery.

Stethoscopy

Auscultation of the chest (listening to the chest) is used to detect both cardiac rate and rhythm and pulmonary sounds. A stethoscope is taped over the precordium (the region over the heart and

• **Fig. 27.2** Example of normal sinus rhythms as they appear in each of 12 leads. (From Kinney MR, Packa D: *Andreoli's comprehensive cardiac care,* ed 8, St. Louis, 1996, Mosby.)

stomach at the level of the diaphragm), or a pressure-sensitive detector may be placed within the patient's esophagus. With the trachea protected by a cuffed endotracheal tube to prevent aspiration, the thin flexible tube stethoscope is inserted into the esophagus to the level of the heart. Esophageal stethoscopy is especially valuable during thoracic and abdominal procedures, when auscultatory monitoring is ineffective because of tissue manipulation or movements of the members of the operating team. Esophageal stethoscopes are available in disposable models with an added temperature monitor.

Arterial Blood Pressure

BP signifies the pressure exerted against vessel walls to force blood through the circulation. Evaluation of BP during anesthesia requires consideration of blood volume, CO, and the state of the sympathetic tone of the vessels. Tissue perfusion is dependent on these factors. Arterial BP is used to assess hemodynamic and respiratory status during every surgical procedure, with very few exceptions.

The BP measures contraction of the heart (systolic pressure) and relaxation of the heart between contractions (diastolic pressure). Blood is forced through the arteries between contractions. Pressure is higher during systole and lower during diastole. Many factors can cause BP to vary. It is measured in millimeters of mercury (mm Hg). Normal range is 120 mm Hg or less for systolic and 80 mm Hg or less for diastolic.

The arm used for measurements should be opposite the one cannulated for IV fluid therapy or invasive monitoring and should be protected from contact with team members standing beside the OR bed. BP readings can be obtained using indirect or direct methods, either intermittently or continuously.

Sphygmomanometer

A pneumatic cuff is wrapped around the circumference of the upper arm. When the cuff is inflated, measurements are obtained on the sphygmomanometer as the cuff deflates. Through a stethoscope placed over the brachial artery distal to the cuff, the systolic pressure is heard when blood begins to flow through the artery. The diastolic pressure is noted by a change in sound. This is an indirect noninvasive method for intermittent monitoring of BP.

Doppler Ultrasound Flowmeter

With ultrasound, BP can be monitored automatically at preset intervals. The Doppler ultrasound flowmeter monitor automatically inflates the cuff, takes a reading, and deflates the cuff. It can be programmed to sound an alarm if systolic pressure reaches a preset high or low level. The readings are more accurate than with sphygmomanometer pressure cuff monitoring because the ultrasonic transducer amplifies blood flow sounds. Automated noninvasive BP monitors function well in a noisy environment. However, they do not provide continuous BP measurement or detect extremely low pressures. Frequent inflations of the cuff can bruise the skin, especially of geriatric patients.

Infrared Beams

Noninvasive infrared beams (Finapres technique) may be used to indirectly monitor BP. A small cuff fits on a finger. The beams from the cuff shine through tissue. They continuously measure arterial pressure from one heartbeat to the next.

Direct Arterial Pressure

From an invasive modality, beat-to-beat direct pressures are obtained through an artery, usually the radial or femoral, via an indwelling catheter inserted percutaneously. A very slow drip of slightly heparinized sterile saline or plain sterile saline solution keeps the catheter open. The fluid-filled tubing from the catheter is connected to a mechanical electric transducer. The transducer is attached to an amplifier. A waveform of the amplified pulse, which represents force imposed on the transducer, is displayed. The monitor also converts waveforms into numeric measurements of systolic and diastolic rates. An alarm sounds if deviations are significant.

Arterial lines can be used to measure arterial pressure curves that in turn provide information about cardiac output. Studies are in process to determine if an arterial line provides the same information as pulmonary artery catheters.

Mean Arterial Pressure

Mean arterial pressure (MAP), calculated by most monitors and shown on digital display, portrays perfusion pressure of the body. This is significant in the evaluation of myocardial perfusion. Normal MAP is between 70 and 105 mm Hg. Direct intraarterial pressure monitoring is valuable in patients with major multiple trauma or burns, inaccessibility of an extremity, unstable vital signs, or inaudible BP. Other indications are complex extensive procedures, such as a cardiopulmonary bypass with an open chest; major vascular surgery with large potential fluid shifts or blood loss; total hip replacement; and major neurosurgery with the patient in the sitting position. Also included are patients in shock or with preexisting cardiac or pulmonary disease who must undergo major surgery.

Direct pressure monitoring is necessary in deliberate hypotensive anesthesia, and in treatment of hypotensive or hypertensive crisis with continuous infusion of vasopressor or hypertensive drugs.

Blood Gases, Oxygenation, and pH

Monitoring of tissue perfusion is indispensable in the evaluation of pulmonary gas exchange and acid-base balance. Measurements are considered in relation to other parameters, such as vital signs, venous pressure, and left atrial pressure. Oxygen (O_2) and carbon dioxide (CO_2) in blood exert their own partial pressures (P). Measurements are expressed in millimeters of mercury or torr. They may be differentiated as arterial (Pa) or venous (Pv). The gas being measured is identified. The partial pressure of oxygen is expressed as Po_2, or specifically in arterial blood as Pao_2 and in venous blood as Pvo_2. Oxygen saturation (So_2) in arterial blood (Sao_2) is expressed in percentages. The partial pressure of carbon dioxide is specified as $Paco_2$ or $Pvco_2$ (see Table 27.1 for normal ranges). Monitoring techniques can be either noninvasive or invasive.

Pulse Oximetry

A pulse oximeter measures arterial oxyhemoglobin saturation (Sao_2). It provides a reading within seconds by measuring the optical density of light passing through tissues. A sensor probe is clipped on each side of a pulsating vascular bed. Fingers, toes, earlobes, and the bridge of the nose are suitable sites. The patient's skin should be clean and dry. An area with fingernail polish should be avoided or the polish removed. Skin integrity under the sensor must be intact.

The sensor must be maintained flush with the skin surface and positioned so that the light source and photodetector are in direct alignment. The sensor is attached to an oximeter, which is plugged into a power source. Some power sources are battery powered. The oximeter may have an earphone adapter and an alarm system. The alarm is usually set for audible alert within 10 seconds if the oxygen saturation falls below the preset range.

Wavelengths of red (660 nm) and infrared (940 nm) light pass through tissues from the light source side of the probe. Light is picked up by a receptor in the sensor on the opposite side of the tissue. The oximeter continuously calculates the amount of oxygen present in the blood by processing the ratio of red to infrared light absorbed. The presence of oxygen in hemoglobin influences this absorption (oxyhemoglobin).

The oximeter reading should remain above 95%. A reading less than 90% probably signifies developing hypoxia. Some patients have significant respiratory disease and prolonged trends of low readings. Oximeters give no information about the retention of carbon dioxide and are not indicators of respiratory failure caused by carbon dioxide retention. In some circumstances, the readings that indicate gas exchange can be altered with the administration of supplemental oxygen.

Falsely high readings may occur in cigarette smokers because carbon monoxide (CO) (carboxyhemoglobin) can prevent red blood cells from picking up oxygen. Carboxyhemoglobin closely resembles oxyhemoglobin and is perceived by the sensor to be oxygenated. These cells may absorb light from the oximeter, however, so the reading may be higher than the actual Sao_2. Other factors may influence reliability, such as shielding of the sensor, excessive ambient light, patient movement, and intravascular dyes (methylene blue). Patients undergoing a surgical procedure with local anesthesia may exhibit an average consistent with 2% of baseline oxygenation.

Oximeter readings always should be compared with patient assessment. (Information about competency testing for the use of pulse oximetry can be found at the National Institutes of Health [NIH] website: www.ncbi.nlm.nih.gov.)

Capnometry

Changes in exhaled carbon dioxide reflect changes in internal respiration, circulation, and metabolism. Capnometry measures end-tidal concentration of carbon dioxide. Normal concentration is 38 torr (5%). Carbon dioxide production is in direct relationship to cellular metabolism. Monitoring external respiration of carbon dioxide can detect the onset of inadvertent hypothermia or malignant hyperthermia. Capnometry, a noninvasive technique, also can be used to detect anesthesia equipment problems, inadvertent esophageal intubation, inadequate neuromuscular blockage, air embolus, and a ventilation-perfusion problem.

A mainstream or sidestream adapter is placed in the breathing circuit as close to the facemask as possible so that expired carbon dioxide approximates alveolar concentration. The analyzer, attached to the adapter, exposes expired air to infrared light. The amount of light absorbed by carbon dioxide determines the end-tidal concentration. A sidestream analyzer can be used to monitor patients receiving local or regional anesthesia by placing the sampling end of the tubing in the patient's nostril or mouth.

A capnographic waveform printout provides data to evaluate respiratory rate and rhythm. Some gas monitors continuously measure carbon dioxide, oxygen, and nitrous oxide parameters of the patient's airway. Digital values are displayed on the monitor.

Optode

An optode is an optical fiber inserted through an 18 or 20-gauge radial artery cannula. The tip contains chemicals that react to oxygen, carbon dioxide, and acidity of the blood. The optode is connected to a monitor that generates light through the fiber. The chemicals produce luminosities that vary in intensity for oxygen and carbon dioxide. These are measured. Readings are instantaneously and continuously shown on a digital display. Precautions must be taken to maintain sterile technique with this equipment as with other methods of percutaneous radial artery cannulation.

Direct Arterial Blood Gas Analysis

Blood samples may be drawn intermittently from arterial or venous indwelling catheters. ABG determinations of Pao_2, Pco_2, and So_2 are used to monitor adequacy of oxygenation and carbon dioxide elimination. This is especially important in patients who need mechanical ventilation. The tidal volume, respiratory rate, and concentration of oxygen can be appropriately adjusted. ABG monitoring also permits laboratory analyses of pH, base excess, bicarbonate, and electrolytes to evaluate metabolic processes and acid-base status. Differentiation of respiratory or metabolic acidosis or alkalosis is a guide to appropriate treatment. Samples may be taken for other analyses (e.g., glucose or coagulation factors).

Hypoventilation, uneven ventilation in relation to blood flow, impairment of diffusion, and venous-to-arterial shunting lead to anoxemia unless oxygen in inspired air is increased. Hypoventilation of the whole lung or a major portion leads to retention of carbon dioxide and predisposes the patient to cardiac dysrhythmias. Disturbances of acid-base balance have many serious consequences in many organs. They must be corrected to achieve normal physiologic functioning.

Central Venous Pressure

Because it accurately measures right atrial BP, which in turn images right ventricular BP, central venous pressure (CVP) monitoring assesses function of the heart's right side. It measures the pressure under which blood returns to the right atrium and reflects pressure in the venous system as blood returns to the heart. In other words, CVP represents the amount of venous return and filling pressure of the right ventricle. This information helps determine the patient's circulatory status.

CVP monitoring also aids in the evaluation of blood volume and the relationship between circulating blood volume and the pumping action of the heart (i.e., adequacy of volume presented to the heart for pumping). Therefore CVP monitoring is a useful guide in blood or fluid administration to avoid circulatory overload in patients with limited cardiopulmonary reserve. Too great or too rapid replacement can cause pulmonary edema. Generally, a low CVP indicates that additional fluid can be given safely. CVP monitoring may be used during shock or hypotension to judge the adequacy of blood replacement. However, CVP is not a measure of blood volume per se or of CO.

Indications for CVP monitoring include major surgical procedures in patients with preexisting cardiovascular disease, in surgical procedures in which large volume shifts are anticipated (e.g., open heart surgery), in critically ill patients (e.g., massive trauma, malignant hyperthermia), in surgical procedures in which venous air emboli are a risk (e.g., craniotomy in a sitting position), and in rapid administration of blood or fluid.

Although CVP monitoring provides valuable data for assessment of the adequacy of vascular volume, it only indirectly reflects the function of the left side of the heart. There is no direct relationship between right and left ventricular filling pressures. Because of the distensibility (compliancy) of the pulmonary blood vessels, the lungs can accept a marked increase in blood flow before significant congestion appears. Backup of blood caused by impaired function of the left ventricle and a subsequent increase in pulmonary vascular resistance (PVR) may occur before this increased pressure affects the right side of the heart, as exhibited by CVP values. CVP does not correlate with left-sided heart performance in patients with left ventricular dysfunction or pulmonary congestion.

Central Venous Cannulation

CVP may be monitored with a single-lumen or multilumen radiopaque catheter. A double-lumen or triple-lumen Hickman or Broviac catheter is used most commonly. The right atrial lumen of a Swan-Ganz pulmonary artery catheter also can be used to obtain CVP readings. The lumens are labeled and color-coded on multilumen catheters.

The catheter is inserted, preferably percutaneously through a subclavian vein. A brachial, external or internal jugular, or femoral vein may be used or, via cutdown, the antecubital vein. If patients are awake, they are asked to bear down (Valsalva maneuver) as the vein is punctured. This increases intrathoracic pressure and counteracts negative pressure from the vein, thus reducing the possibility of air embolism.

The catheter is threaded through the vein and advanced into the superior vena cava or right atrium. This may be done by fluoroscopy, or a chest radiograph may be taken to verify accurate placement of the catheter tip.

The catheter may be attached to a transducer and monitor. Pressure readings are expressed in millimeters of mercury. The catheter can be attached to a fluid-filled manometer that measures pressure in centimeters of water (cm H_2O).

To set up this line, the IV solution bag is connected to the tubing, the manometer is inserted into the line by attaching it to the stopcock between the IV tubing and the extension tubing, air is expelled from the line, the line is clamped, and the manometer is secured upright to an IV pole. The hub of the catheter lumen is connected to the stopcock. Connections to the three-way stopcock should be taped to prevent inadvertent disconnection and air leaks. Cyclic variations in intracaval venous pressure occur; pressure becomes negative during atrial filling and respiratory inspiration. Sucking of air into the system during negative venous pressure can result in an air embolus.

Baseline measurement is taken as soon as the catheter is in place and attached to the monitor. This is also a presumptive check for proper placement of the cannula tip. Because expansion of the lungs increases intrathoracic pressure and deflation decreases it, fluid in the manometer should fluctuate with each breath.

To obtain a CVP reading on the manometer, adjust the scale to zero level with the patient's right atrium. The lumen of the stopcock to the catheter is shut off, which allows the IV fluid to run into the manometer to the desired level. The infusion is shut off, and the catheter is opened. After the reading is obtained, the infusion lumen to the catheter is opened to keep the line open.

Electronic transducer systems provide continuous monitoring of venous pressure. Continuous monitoring supplies good measurement of the right side of the heart and portrays the trend of heart function that is more valuable than are isolated readings obtained with a manometer. CVP values may vary somewhat, but normal readings range from 2 to 8 mm Hg, or 3 to 10 cm H_2O.

Multilumen central venous catheters provide access for administration of drugs, blood, fluids, and hyperalimentation. Blood can be removed for blood gas analyses or autotransfusion. These catheters also provide access for removal of air emboli.

Pulmonary Artery Pressure Monitoring

Because a pulmonary artery catheter measures function of both the right and the left sides of the heart, it provides faster, more accurate indication of impending left ventricular failure than does CVP alone. Pressures of the left side of the heart are reflected in pulmonary artery and pulmonary capillary wedge pressures, measured with the pulmonary artery catheter. This is more sensitive to rapid changes in the cardiovascular system than is CVP and is more sensitive to the ability of the heart to accommodate fluid loads.

Measurement of pulmonary pressures enables precise rapid assessment of the left ventricle's ability to eject adequate CO. Continuous evaluation of left ventricular function is extremely important in patients whose left-sided heart dysfunction has a greater direct effect on CO, circulating volume, and respiratory function than does impaired right-sided heart function. Data procured include pulmonary artery pressure (PAP), pulmonary capillary wedge pressure (PCWP), right atrial pressure (RAP), and CO computation. These pressures reveal the hemodynamic status of cardiovascular and pulmonary functions. They also serve as guidelines for administration of fluids, diuretics, and cardiotonic drugs to obtain optimal CO.[7]

Indications for pulmonary artery monitoring include preexisting cardiac or pulmonary disease in a patient undergoing a major vascular, intraabdominal, or neurosurgical procedure and a potential risk for development of cardiopulmonary instability from the stress of the surgical procedure. Other conditions may include shock, burns with large fluid shifts, renal failure with low CO, and pulmonary emboli. Pulmonary artery catheters may be used in patients who need long-term monitoring.

Some multipurpose catheters may be used with ventricular and atrial pacing wires in patients with heart block or severe bradycardia. These catheters may be used to measure CO in patients with intracardiac shunts or during titrated drug administration.

Contraindications to invasive pulmonary catheter monitoring are abnormal cardiac anatomy in the patient, inadequate monitors, and lack of personnel trained in the use of the monitors.

Pulmonary Artery Cannulation

Various pulmonary artery catheters are available. The number of lumens varies from two to five, depending on the range of functions desired. These catheters are used with transducers for monitoring. The type of transducer varies according to the balloon flotation device in the catheter.

In setting up the monitoring system, manufacturer instructions must be followed explicitly. All equipment, including the oscilloscope, should be checked. The stopcocks and flush devices in the lines to the transducer heads need to be attached. Preassembled tubing systems and disposable transducer domes are commercially available. If the patient also will have a peripheral arterial line, two transducers and a triple stopcock manifold are needed. Simultaneous monitoring of PAP and RAP is thus possible. The transducer dome is back-flushed. The monitor should be balanced and calibrated according to manufacturer directions. There must be no air bubbles remaining in the lines or system.

Before the catheter is inserted, the physician inspects it for defects. If recommended by the manufacturer, the balloon may be tested for leakage by inflating it, submerging it in sterile saline solution, and watching for air bubbles. The balloon must then be deflated. Moistening the catheter tip with saline solution or lidocaine reduces the possibility of venospasm at insertion.

Vital signs are taken before insertion of the catheter. ECG readings should be monitored for dysrhythmias during insertion. With the introducer set, the catheter is inserted and advanced rapidly to prevent kinking or knotting. It is advanced through the vein into the inferior or superior vena cava and on into the right atrium.

Continued manipulation irritates or damages vessel walls. Watching the increment markings on the side helps determine how far the catheter has advanced. It is possible to keep pushing the catheter while it is not going into the right place. It can coil up and knot in the ventricle.

When the catheter tip reaches the right atrium and a right atrial waveform appears on the oscilloscope screen or readout strip, the balloon is inflated slowly with air with a tuberculin syringe to enable it to float with the flow of blood. The balloon is never inflated without a visible oscilloscope trace. If the patient is awake, a voluntary cough confirms the position of the catheter in the thoracic cavity if the right atrial wave fluctuates. The amount of air is specified by the manufacturer (usually about 1.3–1.5 mL). Overinflation could rupture the balloon.

Carbon dioxide (CO_2) is used for balloon inflation in patients with intracardiac shunts. If the balloon ruptures in arterial circulation, carbon dioxide is more soluble than ambient (room) air in blood. A feeling of resistance should accompany inflation. Absence of resistance is a sign of a ruptured balloon; inflation should be stopped immediately. Fluid is never used for inflation because it prevents proper catheter flotation and complete deflation.

Passing through the tricuspid valve, the catheter enters the right ventricle. A typical right ventricular waveform should appear. If dysrhythmia develops or is persistent, a bolus of lidocaine may be injected. Then, after the catheter floats through the pulmonary semilunar valve into the pulmonary artery, a pulmonary artery tracing should appear on the monitor. This waveform has a steep upstroke at the beginning from right ventricular ejection and opening of the pulmonic valve, followed by a dicrotic notch on the downstroke at the closing of the pulmonic valve.

Pulmonary artery blood flow carries the balloon into one of the artery's smaller branches. When the vessel diameter becomes too narrow for it to pass, the balloon wedges in the vessel and occludes it. A PCWP waveform should appear. After recording of this wedge pressure, the physician permits the balloon to deflate passively; air is not aspirated with the syringe.

The catheter then slips back into the main branch of the pulmonary artery. A PAP waveform should reappear on the monitor. The physician depends on these sequential characteristic pressure waveforms to reveal the catheter tip's location at all times. The circulating nurse records pressure at each location. The catheter remains in the pulmonary artery with the balloon deflated, continuously recording the PAP, except when a PCWP reading is desired. The balloon may be ruptured if a PAP waveform persists and a PCWP reading is unobtainable or if resistance is not felt with an attempt to inflate the balloon.

An x-ray is taken to confirm the catheter position. In the case of rupture, the catheter may be left in place to record the PAP, provided it has not slipped back to the right ventricle. The physician may also elect to remove it. The balloon is always inflated during catheter advancement and deflated during catheter withdrawal.

For prevention of an air embolus after catheter insertion, the catheter must not be attached to the monitoring system until all air has been expelled. All lines and transducers should be checked for secure connections and patency. Each transducer's balancing port must be leveled with the patient's right atrium. RAP, PAP, and PCWP waveforms and the patient's response to the procedure must be documented.

Swan-Ganz Thermodilution Catheter

The no. 7 Swan-Ganz thermodilution catheter has four separate lumens or passages within its outside wall. It is versatile and widely used to measure right-sided heart pressure and CO. Critical conditions such as heart failure, cardiac tamponade, pulmonary hypertension, and other causes of shock can be diagnosed and monitored with a Swan-Ganz catheter.

The catheter is 43¼ inches (110 cm) long, with 10-cm increments marked on the side to permit observation of how far the catheter has advanced during insertion. Like all pulmonary artery catheters, it is a balloon-tipped flotation catheter that is inserted into a major vein and advanced to the inferior or superior vena cava.

When inflated, the thin latex balloon at the tip permits the catheter to float with the flow of blood through the right atrium, tricuspid valve, right ventricle, pulmonary semilunar valve, and pulmonary artery and to wedge in a small pulmonary artery branch (arteriole) for recording of the PCWP during occlusion of the vessel. When the balloon is not inflated, the catheter lies in the pulmonary artery to record the PAP. Proper catheter placement is essential to minimize the risk for vessel damage and complications and to validate pressure readings.

The end of the catheter inserted in the patient is referred to as the distal end; the opposite one is the proximal end. The proximal end has several external ports that provide access to the lumens used in patient monitoring. The pulmonary artery port is used for monitoring PAP and PCWP. A syringe is connected to the balloon port for the desired balloon inflation. The thermistor port is used for CO calculation. The right atrial port is used for measurement of RAP. This port also can be used to administer fluids or can be connected to a flush system for maintenance of catheter patency. For CO measurement, normal saline or dextrose solution is injected into the cardiovascular system via the proximal lumen. The pulmonary artery and right atrial ports should be labeled.

The catheter has four separate lumens or passages. The pulmonary artery lumen, the largest and most distal, terminates in the opening at the catheter's tip. With proper catheter positioning, this opening lies in the pulmonary artery. In this position, with the balloon deflated, pulmonary artery systolic, diastolic, and mean pressures are recorded on the monitor. These are indicative

of pulmonary function. When the balloon is inflated and the catheter migrates to a pulmonary artery branch to wedge, the PCWP is recorded. PCWP is sometimes referred to as pulmonary artery wedge pressure (PAWP) or pulmonary artery occlusion pressure (PAOP).

Occlusion of a pulmonary artery branch creates a no-flow system, thereby blocking blood flow from the right side of the heart to the lungs and permitting pressure equilibration in the pulmonary vascular bed distal to the catheter. Occlusion of an arteriole and low resistance of the pulmonary systems give a pressure measurement equal to the left atrial pressure (LAP), which in turn is equal to the left ventricular end-diastolic pressure (LVEDP).

To prevent pulmonary infarction, ischemia, and hemorrhage from prolonged wedging, the balloon is always deflated immediately after a reading is taken. The catheter floats back into the main pulmonary artery. The pulmonary artery lumen can provide blood samples for blood gas measurements and mixed venous blood, which is also of value in evaluating cardiac function.

The balloon lumen opening, which permits inflation and deflation, is about 1 cm from the catheter tip. When inflated, the balloon surrounds, but does not cover, the opening in this tip.

The thermistor lumen opening is about 4 cm from the catheter tip. This lumen contains temperature-sensitive wires that run its length and transmit the temperature of blood flowing over them from the thermistor to the computer for determination of CO using the thermodilution technique.

The proximal right atrial lumen opening is about 30 cm from the catheter's tip. This opening lies in the right atrium to monitor RAP when the catheter is in place.

Interpretation of Pressures

The range of normal pressure values may vary slightly from one authority to another. Characteristic waveforms appear on the oscilloscope or screen, depending on the location of the catheter tip during insertion and continuous monitoring. These waveforms must be watched carefully to ascertain that the catheter is in the desired position. The catheter enters the right atrium via the vena cava.

Right Atrial Pressure. Normal RAP is 3 to 6 mm Hg. RAP reflects right atrial filling diastolic pressure, equivalent to CVP, and right ventricular end-diastolic pressure (RVEDP), pressure at the end of filling just before contraction. A rise in RAP may indicate right or left ventricular failure, volume overload (hypovolemia), or air embolism. A fall in RAP may indicate vasodilation, hypovolemia, or peripheral blood pooling.

Right Ventricular Pressure. Normal right ventricular pressure (RVP) is 15 to 25 mm Hg systolic and 0 to 5 mm Hg diastolic. A rise in RVP may indicate mitral insufficiency, congestive heart failure, hypoxemia, or left ventricular failure.

Pulmonary Artery Pressure. Normal PAP is 15 to 25 mm Hg systolic and 8 to 15 mm Hg diastolic; the mean is 9 to 19 mm Hg. These pressures estimate venous pressure in the lungs, and mean filling pressure of the left atrium and left ventricle. They reflect right ventricular function, unless the patient has pulmonary stenosis, because the pulmonary artery systolic pressure commonly approximates the right ventricular systolic pressure. Changes in pulmonary artery systolic and mean pressures indicate changes in PVR.

Alterations in PVR occur in hypoxemia, respiratory insufficiency, pulmonary edema, pulmonary emboli, shock, and sepsis.

Thus these pressures are indices of pulmonary function. A rise in PAP may indicate left ventricular failure; increased pulmonary arteriolar resistance, as in pulmonary hypertension and hypoxia; or fluid overload.

Pulmonary Capillary Wedge Pressure. Normal pressure is 6 to 12 mm Hg. Pulmonary artery diastolic pressure and PCWP are prime determinants of function of the left side of the heart because they reflect LVEDP just before the left ventricle contracts, except in patients with mitral valve impairment.

Normally, when the mitral valve between the right atrium and right ventricle is open (ventricular diastole), flow of blood from the pulmonary artery to the pulmonary veins and left side of the heart is unimpeded. Then, pressures throughout the pulmonary circulation and left side of the heart are comparable. Because PCWP usually approximates LAP, an indicator of left heart function, it is an important determinant of left ventricular preload.

Intraoperative monitoring of PCWP usually can give early disclosure of left ventricular dysfunction. A rise in PCWP may indicate left ventricular failure, mitral insufficiency, pulmonary hypertension, fluid overload, or pulmonary congestion. A rise also may occur during anesthesia induction. A fall in PCWP may indicate a reduction in LVEDP and CO, or hypovolemia.

Complications of Pulmonary Artery Catheter Monitoring

Invasion of the great vessels and heart carries many inherent perils. Probably the most common during insertion is cardiac dysrhythmia, especially premature contractions. Other problems include local or systemic infection (septicemia, endocarditis), thrombus formation, pulmonary emboli, pulmonary infarction, pneumothorax, hemothorax, major vessel or heart chamber perforation, kinking or knotting of the catheter, balloon rupture, postoperative bleeding, and erroneous diagnosis from misinterpretation of data.

Although rare, pulmonary artery perforation is very serious. Predisposing factors are pulmonary hypertension, anticoagulation therapy, hyperthermia, or an overinflated balloon or catheter. Hemoptysis and sudden hypotension are signs and symptoms of pulmonary artery rupture. Equipment for endobronchial intubation, chest tube insertion, and surgical intervention must be available.

Complications that are potentially life-threatening increase markedly after 48 to 72 hours of indwelling catheterization. The physician must be notified of any change in patient status. Catheter withdrawal is performed by and at the discretion of a physician. For prevention of injury to the heart valves, the balloon is slightly inflated until the catheter is withdrawn to the right atrium. Then the balloon is completely deflated for withdrawal. Dysrhythmias may occur.

Pressure is applied to the percutaneous insertion site to prevent bleeding. The pulse and BP are checked before and after withdrawal. A postwithdrawal dressing is applied. The patient is monitored for at least 24 hours.

In addition to patient problems, monitoring problems may arise. Each requires a specific intervention. A major problem is a damped pressure or PAP waveform, which means decreased amplitude in pressure tracings or loss of sharpness in the image that suggests a defect in the circuit.

Common causes are air in the system or blood in the transducer; loose connections; a kinked, overwedged, or malpositioned catheter; falling systolic pressure in the patient; or a clot in the

monitor system. If the last-mentioned cause is suspected, gently try to aspirate blood. If no blood can be aspirated, the catheter should not be flushed. Flushing could dislodge a clot. The physician should be notified and may withdraw the catheter.

Another problem involves a sudden change in configuration of a pressure tracing. Potential causes include the following:
- The transducer is not at the right atrial level.
- The transducer needs calibration.
- The transducer connection to the catheter is not secure.
- The catheter is no longer in the proper position.
- A loss of pressure in the pressure bag has occurred.

If a PCWP waveform persists after a reading, the balloon may not be completely deflated or the distal catheter tip may be caught in the wedge position, which requires immediate attention. Circulating nurses should be familiar with the appropriate interventions in both patient problems and monitoring problems, in addition to being knowledgeable about the causes and preventive measures. Only in this way can patient safety be maximized in invasive monitoring.

Cardiac Output

Cardiac output (CO) is measured using the thermodilution technique to determine liters of blood pumped per minute by the left ventricle into the aorta. Normal resting value is 4 to 8 L/min. A known amount of fluid at a known temperature is injected into a lumen of an arterial catheter, and a temperature gradient at a point downstream is measured via a second lumen. Iced-cold or room-temperature physiologic saline solution or 5% dextrose in water (10 mL) generally is used.

Blood flow supplies the thermal dilution; for example, saline solution mixes with blood in the superior vena cava or right atrium, depending on the catheter location, which reduces the temperature of blood in the heart. The cooled blood flows past a transistorized intravascular thermistor in the thermodilution catheter that detects changes in blood temperatures that are then used to compute CO. When the solution is injected via the proximal right atrial lumen of a pulmonary artery Swan-Ganz catheter, a digital display of CO is seen within 4 to 5 seconds.

CO reflects the mechanical activity of the heart and represents total blood flow to all tissues and vascular shunts. It depends on the heart rate, the contractile strength of the heart muscle (myocardial contractility), the peripheral resistance of vessels, and venous return. Inotropic agents such as digitalis or epinephrine increase contractility and CO, except in patients with loss of functioning ventricular muscle (e.g., after myocardial infarction or an aneurysm of the left ventricle). Agents such as β-blockers decrease the work of the heart by reducing contractility and CO. Calculation of the left ventricular stroke work index reflects pumping ability.

During systole, the ventricle does not totally eject the blood received during diastole. The amount of blood ejected with each contraction is referred to as the stroke volume (SV). Normal resting SV is 60 to 130 mL/beat. Determinants of the SV are the LAP, afterload, contractile state of the myocardium, and LVEDP. The ejection fraction (EF), a commonly used indicator of ventricular function, is the percentage value of the SV. Normal EF is 60% to 70%. Major SV determinants of CO are preload, contractility, and afterload. Only in limited circumstances does adjustment of the heart rate therapeutically enhance CO.

Preload, the amount of blood in the ventricle at the end of diastole, may be referred to as left ventricular end-diastolic volume (LVEDV) or filling pressure (LVEDP). Assessment of changes in volume and measurement of changes in filling pressure help describe cardiac function. The Starling principle concerns the relationship between volume, stretch, and contractility. It relates myocardial fiber length to the force of the contraction. The greater the preload and stretch of myocardial fibers, the greater the subsequent contraction, which thereby increases the SV until at some point ventricular failure commences. Fiber overstretch weakens contractions.

As the pumping ability decreases, the left ventricle is unable to empty completely. Residual blood, combined during diastole with incoming oxygenated blood from the pulmonary veins and left atrium, increases workload and elevates the left ventricular volume and pressure. As ventricular efficiency declines, CO falls. Retained blood in the left ventricle backs up into the left atrium and pulmonary circulation, increasing these pressures. Pulmonary edema and respiratory insufficiency result as fluid is impelled into the alveoli. The CVP catheter measures the right-sided heart preload; the pulmonary artery catheter measures left atrial and left ventricular end-diastolic pressures.

Cardiac function may be classified as normal, compromised, or failing. In healthy hearts, maximum ventricular performance seems to be achieved at filling pressure of 8 to 12 mm Hg. In compromised hearts, this pressure is higher.

A reduced CO results in decreased perfusion of the capillary circulation. During hemorrhage, when circulating blood volume is reduced, the resulting diminished venous return and preload lead to a lowered CO. Atrial fibrillation also can modify the filling of the ventricles. Venous dilation contributes to pooling of blood, with subsequent decreased venous return to the heart. Low CO states result from reduced preload, as in hypovolemia, venous dilation, or cardiac tamponade; reduced contractility, as from anesthetic drugs, ischemia, infarction, or cardiac decompensation; dysrhythmias; or increased afterload, as in hypertension, pulmonary emboli, or an elevated or diminished heart rate.

Body position can influence circulation, as can age, body surface area, oxygen consumption, body temperature, basal metabolic rate, and activity. Thus many factors can affect CO.

Afterload indicates the resistance the heart must overcome to eject blood into the systemic circulation. This impedance to flow is called systemic vascular resistance (SVR). Left ventricular pressure must exceed pressure in the aorta to open the aortic valve and force blood from the heart into the circulation. Afterload, not a direct measure, is deduced by calculating the SVR. An elevated afterload can produce increased left ventricular wall tension in an attempt to generate adequate intracavitary ventricular pressure to overcome resistance and permit systolic ejection. The subsequent increase in myocardial oxygen demand must be met, or ventricular function deteriorates.

Diminution of afterload reduces wall tension, thereby improving ventricular contraction. Improving cardiac function involves cost in myocardial oxygen consumption. Augmenting CO by increasing the heart rate and contractility increases myocardial oxygen consumption. Improving CO by augmenting preload or by reducing afterload results in relatively little oxygen cost to the myocardium.

A comprehensive view of cardiac function can be obtained with measurements of filling pressure, CO, and calculation of peripheral resistance. Repeated measurements offer evaluation of treatment.

Cardiac Index
The cardiac index (CI) is used to assess the heart's ability to meet the body's need for oxygen and other nutrients. With noninvasive

ultrasound, the CI measures CO in relation to body surface. A CI less than 2 L of blood/min/m² of body surface identifies high risk for untoward cardiovascular events during or after anesthesia. The BP may drop; irregular heartbeats may develop. If these adverse events are anticipated, they can be prevented or treated.

Total Blood Volume
Blood volume is useful in determining the total amount of blood replacement necessary. An accurate method of total blood volume (TBV) measurement involves measuring plasma and red blood cell volumes separately and then adding the results together. For measurement of red blood cell volume, cells are tagged with detectable, nontoxic, radioactive chromium, subsequently injected IV, and counted after an appropriate mixing time. Or radioactive iodinated human serum albumin, in standard-dose packages, can be injected, mixed, and counted. Counting may be done rapidly using an electronic device. This technique may be used in place of estimation of blood loss.

Respiratory Tidal Volume
The respiratory tidal volume (V_T), the volume of air moved with each respiration and expiration, may be measured with a respirometer placed on the expiratory limb of the anesthesia machine or mechanical ventilator. Alarms may be incorporated to signal disconnection, failure to cycle, and excessive pressure.

Body Temperature
The body continuously produces heat through metabolic activities and loses heat through convection, evaporation, conduction, and radiation. The production of heat causes increased oxygen consumption by the body's cells. When the rate of heat production is equal to the rate of loss, a heat balance of constant core body temperature is maintained. Core temperature is that of the interior of the body as opposed to the body surface temperature. Normal core temperature ranges from 98° F to 100° F (36.8–37.7° C).

Under anesthesia, the average adult loses 0.9° F to 2.7° F (0.5–1.5° C) of body temperature; the greatest loss occurs during the first hour, through convection from exposure to the environment, through evaporation via respiration, through conduction from contact with cool surfaces, and through radiation from tissues. Intraoperative hypothermia, or core temperature less than 96° F (36° C), is a common complication of surgery under general anesthesia, especially in pediatric and geriatric patients.

Some anesthetic agents inhibit heat production: halogenated agents cause vasodilation that contributes to surface cooling, and muscle relaxants prevent shivering, which is a thermoregulatory protective reflex.

Other factors can change core temperature. Hyperthermia (retention of heat) may be caused by premedication, drapes, a closed anesthesia breathing circuit, hypermetabolic crisis, or fever from sepsis. Physical reactions are not seen in the anesthetized patient; therefore the body temperature should be continuously monitored for metabolic changes.

Electronic thermometers with digital readouts measure body and surface temperatures with thermistor or thermocouple probes. A core temperature probe can be inserted into a body orifice (e.g., nasopharynx, esophagus, bladder, rectum). An esophageal probe measures body temperature at the level of the right side of the heart and is responsive to changes in body heat. A rectal probe responds slowly to changes in body temperature and can be inaccurate because of the presence of stool. These probes are available in various sizes and have flexible tips; some are disposable. The sensor of a bladder probe is in the tip of a sterile Foley catheter. A Foley temperature probe can be misread if the bladder is irrigated during the surgical procedure.

A sterile catheter probe may also be inserted into the pulmonary artery. A probe can be placed on the tympanic membrane via the external auditory canal of the ear to measure temperature closest to the hypothalamus, which is the thermoregulatory center in the brain.

Skin surface probes have either small tips or discs that are attached to the skin, often on an extremity, with an adhesive-backed foam pad. Cutaneous liquid crystal thermography, with temperature-sensitive chemicals laminated within an adhesive plastic strip, may be used for surface monitoring. The strip is usually applied to the forehead; its chemicals visibly change color with a temperature variation. Proximity to major arteries, insulation from the external environment, and the location of an inflammatory process and the surgical site are considerations in the choice of the temperature monitoring site.

Urinary Output

Urinary output can be measured with an indwelling Foley catheter attached to a calibrated collection bag. The sterile disposable collection system must be below the level of the bladder to prevent distention and allow flow without reflux. Output is valuable in assessing effective blood volume and fluid administration, except when a diuretic is given. Volume, electrolytes, osmolarity, and pH are important.

Any change in urine color can signal a change in the patient's condition. Brown urine can mean the presence of hemoglobin or myoglobin caused by rhabdomyolysis in a hypermetabolic crisis, such as malignant hyperthermia. Frank blood or clots may indicate an injury to the kidney, ureter, or bladder from iatrogenic cause or other trauma. IV dye, such as methylene blue, turns the urine green as it perfuses through the renal system. The blue dye is sometimes used during a surgical procedure to demonstrate renal function, but it can be used for chromopertubation of the fallopian tubes and be resorbed into the systemic circulation. Pulse oximeter readings can be altered by the dye.

A reduction in urinary volume may indicate reduced renal perfusion. Oliguria can result from stress of the surgical procedure, antidiuresis from the anesthetic agent, impending renal failure, or reduced volume of circulating blood. Urinary output greater than 30 to 60 mL/h usually shows adequate intravascular volume and BP.

The collecting system should be able to accurately measure a half-hour output between 1 and 200 mL and provide observation of the urine. Hemoglobinuria can be a manifestation of transfusion of incompatible blood.

An electronic monitoring system is available with digital display of data that can be fed into a computer. The system records output in milliliters for both the present and the immediately past hours. It also shows the number of minutes elapsed in the current hour. Early warning of possible cardiovascular or renal problems is facilitated by visual alert signals if urine flow falls below 15 mL/h or ceases.

Chest Radiograph

A chest radiograph is essential for checking the position of the pulmonary artery (Swan-Ganz) catheter, CVP line, endotracheal tube, and chest tube and for observing changes in the lungs and heart during the perioperative care period.

Electroencephalogram

Electrical activity of the nervous system reflects neurologic function; therefore electrophysiologic monitoring provides information about the functional integrity of the central nervous system during anesthesia and is especially valuable in patients undergoing high-risk neurosurgical, cardiac, vascular, and orthopedic procedures.

Electrodes placed on the scalp transmit the electrical signals, or alpha rhythms, from brain activity. Alpha rhythms normally occur at a rate of 8 to 13 waves/second. On the electroencephalogram (EEG), these wave patterns vary among individuals in response to anesthetics, drugs, and pathologic and physiologic changes. They reveal the presence of organic brain damage, abnormal physiologic alterations, and actions of drugs.

Regional cerebral blood flow correlates well with EEG activity. Computer analysis offers visual recognition of cerebral hypoperfusion or ischemia. The EEG is used particularly in surgical procedures that involve expected localized brain ischemia caused by intentional surgical occlusion. An EEG also is a means of determining cessation of circulation, an index of expected prognosis, and brain vitality.

Scalp electrodes (cups or discs of silver/silver chloride, gold, or tin) are fixed in place with conductive gel. Subdermal platinum electrodes can be used. Electrodes are placed over areas of cerebral cortex according to a system that uses measurements of head circumference, distance between the ears, and distance from the nasion (point where the sagittal plane intersects the frontonasal suture) to the inion (external protuberance of the occipital bone). The small neurophysiologic signals recorded are amplified for analysis and display. Multiple channels are necessary to detect regional versus global alterations in function. As many as 8 to 32 channels may be recorded simultaneously.

Paper records or strip-charting provides comparisons of EEG activity during crucial periods, with the activity seen before anesthesia induction or surgical manipulation. Methods of EEG analysis that permit automated pattern recognition and alarm generation enhance monitoring in the OR and intensive care unit (ICU). Devices are available that process EEG signals to simplify and facilitate the complex EEG analysis.

Cerebral Function Monitor

The cerebral function monitor provides trend recording of amplitude and amplitude variability for a single channel of the EEG and is useful mainly for detection of marked global alterations in EEG activity during cardiopulmonary bypass, induced hypotension, or metabolic coma. During carotid endarterectomy, paired monitors can detect EEG asymmetries. Although they simplify monitoring, they may be less sensitive to ischemia than the 16-channel strip-chart recording.

Compressed Spectral Array

Compressed spectral array (CSA) programs may give a time-compressed mountain-and-valley representation of brain activity. The mountains move to the left with slower brain activity and to the right with faster activity. CSA helps determine whether the brain is ischemic because of a lack of contralateral circulation during vascular surgery, such as carotid endarterectomy. This type of computerized EEG can be run on general-purpose mini-computers or microcomputers.

Neurometrics Monitor

A neurometrics monitor is a single-channel device for displaying processed EEG signals. From 4 to 32 minutes of EEG can be seen at one time, but trends are less easily seen.

Bispectral Index Monitoring

Bispectral index (BIS) monitoring is a noninvasive method of monitoring the anesthesia level through processed EEG parameters. Electrodes are placed on the patient's forehead, and the brain signals are relayed to a monitor. Readings are displayed as a single number (100 [wide awake] to 0 [absence of brain electrical activity]) and indicate the level of anesthesia.

The BIS electrodes are placed after the induction of general anesthesia while the patient is in a neutral supine position. The baseline reading is recorded by the anesthesia provider. BIS readings change with positional adjustments, such as Trendelenburg and reverse Trendelenburg positions. The reading increases in Trendelenburg position and decreases in reverse Trendelenburg position. The change is generally attributed to increased or decreased intracranial and intraocular pressure caused by position shift.

The results are reduced drug use, faster wake-up time, and decreased risk for patient awareness during the surgical procedure. This potentially translates into faster discharge for ambulatory surgery patients.

Evoked Potentials

Sensory information (sight, sound, smell, taste, touch) evokes an electrical response when it reaches the brain. Evoked potentials are those electrical responses recorded from the cerebral cortex after stimulation of a peripheral sensory organ. A computer is programmed to average the brain's repetitive responses to the stimuli. The computer displays these as waves on a video screen or prints them on a plotter.

Auditory Evoked Potentials

A clicking sound is delivered in the ear to stimulate the auditory nerve. Brain waves are recorded using the evoked potential computer. The evoked potentials can be used to assess function of the auditory nerve (e.g., during removal of acoustic neuroma). Because the auditory nerve enters the brainstem, evoked responses provide an indirect assessment of brainstem activity.

Somatosensory Evoked Potentials

Intraoperative monitoring of somatosensory evoked potentials is used to continuously assess spinal cord function and protect the cord from injury during orthopedic or neurosurgical procedures on the spine or spinal cord. Because hypotension increases the insult of direct pressure on the cord and heightens damage to cord function, the spinal cord is monitored when induced hypotension is used for spinal surgery.

Impulses generated below the site of the surgical procedure travel over lateral afferent neural pathways and through the operative spinal area and are recorded using electrodes at the brain level. Abnormal brain responses are marked by changes in the arrival time of electrical impulses or amplitude of the waves on a graph. Change in latency and amplitude of the recorded signal, which normally averages 30 to 50 evoked responses, alerts the team to the danger of spinal cord compression or ischemia. Corrective measures taken immediately can prevent serious sequelae. Evoked responses then return to normal.

Intracranial Pressure Monitoring

Intracranial pressure (ICP) is the result of cerebrospinal fluid (CSF) production-absorption or arterial blood flow–venous drainage in the cranium. Average ICP in adults is 8 to 15 mm Hg/cm H_2O. ICP is lower when the head is elevated and higher when the head is lowered. Increased pressure within the thoracic cavity causes pressure in the skull to rise. The patient is maintained in 30 to 45-degree semi-Fowler position. The zero reference point of the calibrated fluid tube is mounted level with the outer canthus of the patient's eye, which falls relatively even with the foramen of Monroe.

ICP is measured with a fluid-filled monitoring system and an intraventricular catheter. Placement of and care for the catheter are sterile procedures. Cap, mask, eyewear, and sterile gloves are worn. Only sterile 0.9% preservative-free saline solution is used. Heparinized solution is contraindicated. The tubing has a stopcock to drain CSF and take samples for testing. Only 2 mL is drained at a time to prevent cerebral decompression. Never flush the ICP catheter. The fluid should be clear, with no traces of blood.

Contraindications to ICP monitoring include coagulopathies, anticoagulation therapy, cerebral edema with ventricular collapse or shift, and known scalp infection.

The normal flow of CSF is slow because it is secreted and absorbed at the same constant rate. The average adult has 75 mL of CSF present at any given time. Approximately 500 to 700 mL flows through the dural sheath. The blood flow through the intracranial circulation is influenced by systemic BP in normal circumstances. Pressure in the cranium rises in response to several factors: a rise in CSF production, a decrease in CSF resorption, increased blood flow, and decreased venous drainage. The fluid volume-pressure relationship can fluctuate with cardiac dysrhythmia (bradycardia vs. tachycardia) by increasing and decreasing.

Signs of decompensation include change in the patient's level of consciousness, sudden confusion, seizures, altered breathing, vomiting, and coma. Immediate treatment includes hyperventilating with 100% oxygen and evaluation of the pressure. Complications include infection, hemorrhage, air leak into the ventricle, CSF leak around the catheter, occluded catheter, ventricular collapse, and brain herniation.

A prolonged pressure of 18 to 20 mm Hg is considered elevated. The cerebral perfusion pressure (CPP) is calculated by subtracting the ICP measurement from the MAP. When the CPP falls below 50 mm Hg, the brain is at significant risk for deterioration.

Extremes of pressure cause herniation of the brain into the foramen magnum, which creates an ischemic environment for the brainstem and brain death. Cerebral blood flow is restricted when the pressure rises above normal.

(e) EVOLVE WEBSITE

http://evolve.elsevier.com/Hornacky/BerryKohn/

- Historical Perspective
- Student Interactive Questions
- Glossary

References

1. Thanavaro JL: Cardiac risk assessment: decreasing postoperative complications, *AORN J* 101(2):201–212, 2015.
2. Dorian P: Whom do you believe? The patient or the ECG? *Heart Rhythm* 12(4):666–667, 2015.
3. Simmons B: Hemodynamic monitoring. In Parsons PP, Wiener-Kronish JP, Stapleton RD, et al., editors: *Critical care secrets*, ed 6, St. Louis, 2019, Elsevier, pp 83–90.
4. Casimero C, Ruddock T, Hegarty C, et al.: Minimizing blood stream infection; developing new materials for intravascular catheters, *Medicines* 7(9):49, 2020.
5. Eiting E, Kim H: Arterial puncture and cannulation. In Roberts JR, Custalow CB, Tomsen TW, editors: *Roberts and Hedges' clinical procedures in emergency medicine and acute care*, ed 7, St. Louis, 2019, Elsevier, pp 377–393.
6. Callans DJ, Epstein AE: Reflections on the lowly PVC, *Heart Rhythm* 12(4):714–715, 2015.
7. American Cancer Society: *Intravenous IV lines, catheters, and ports for cancer treatment*. www.cancer.org. Accessed March 22, 2023.

Bibliography

Wells A, Hutchinson P: The management of traumatic brain injury, *Surgery* 36(1):613–620, 2018.

28

Surgical Incisions, Implants, and Wound Closure

CHAPTER OUTLINE

The Surgical Incision, 551

Surgical Landmarks, 556

Wound Closure, 559

CHAPTER OBJECTIVES

After studying this chapter the learner will be able to:

- Describe the anatomy of the skin and underlying tissues.
- Discuss the rationale for placement of the surgical incision.
- Identify several surgical incisions and their associated surgical procedure.

- Identify several absorbable sutures and their application.
- Identify several nonabsorbable sutures and their application.
- List several different types of needles and their application.

KEY TERMS AND DEFINITIONS

Allogeneic graft Tissue taken from the same species for implantation into a different individual of the same species.

Approximation Bringing the edges of an incision together.

Autologous graft Tissue taken from one area of a person's body for implantation into another area of the same person's body.

Evert edges Turning the edges of the skin outward with pickups for approximation.

Figure of 8 Suturing method used to provide hemostasis of a large vessel.

Free tie Strand of suture without a needle.

Fusiform (elliptical) Oval-shaped incision that follows the natural lines of tension in the integument.

Implantation Process of placing material or tissue into a surgical site.

Ligature Strand of suture material used to tie or bind. Suture ligature is a free tie. Tie on a passer is a tie held in the tip of a clamp.

Prosthesis Artificial part worn on the outside or implanted inside the body.

Purse string Circular suturing method for closure of a round opening.

Stick tie Suture on a needle in a needle holder.

Suture Strand of material used for sewing tissue together or ligating a structure.

Undermine Method of releasing the skin edges by sharp dissection to approximate skin. Care is taken not to interrupt circulation to the tissue.

Xenograft Tissue taken from one species for implantation into another species.

The Surgical Incision

Anatomy and Physiology of the Integument

Tissue structure and function vary according to location in the body. Basic tissue types are described in Table 28.1.

The skin contributes to the health and well-being of the patient. Intact skin is an effective barrier to most harmful elements. Wounded, nonintact skin is an open avenue for microbial entry. Wounds occur intentionally or unintentionally. When treated properly, most wounds heal without incident. Unfavorable outcomes occur when wound healing is disrupted by poor circulation, infection, or immune dysfunction.

Skin is a multifunction body cover, and skin assessment is an important measurement of generalized wellness. Skin color, texture, and condition can be the best predictors of how well a surgical site will heal. The most intricate procedure can be done in deep tissue layers, but the superficial layers are what the patient sees and measures the outcome against. Durability and viability of the skin of the perioperative patient are influenced by many factors. Within reasonable limits, in the absence of hemorrhage and sepsis, wound healing is predictable. Disregard for the principles of tissue handling and wound management can lead to complications. The intent of this chapter is to provide an overview of body tissues, surgical incisions, and surgical site closure.

TABLE 28.1	Four Basic Histologic Tissue Types	
Histologic Tissue Type	**Description**	**Implications to Surgical Team**
Epithelial Tissue		
A. Types		
1. Simple	Single layer of cells (endothelium) that lines the blood vessels, heart, and lymphatics	Delicate tissue that is easily damaged by rough handling
2. Stratified	Several layers of cells that form the skin, gastrointestinal tract, genitourinary (GU) tract, reproductive tract, and oropharynx; lines area that serves as a passage; reduces friction with mucus; can convert into keratin	Superficial layer of body cover; surface modifications are performed here; forms hair and nails
3. Transitional	Combination of simple and stratified layers found in ureters and bladder	Encountered during GU reconstruction and neoconstruction
B. Cellular surface structure		
1. Squamous	Flat	
2. Columnar	Tall, cylindric	
3. Cuboidal	Square	
Connective Tissue		
A. Fluid	Blood, lymph, chyle, cerebrospinal fluid, synovium vitreous and aqueous, and mucinous material	Care with body substance isolation and provision of hemostasis
B. Fibrous		
1. Areolar	Loose network forming the frame for subcuticular tissue	Reorganized during liposuction and fat transplantation procedures
2. Adipose	Fat that fills the loose network; visible in fetus at 14 weeks' gestation; not found in eyelid, penis, scrotum, labia minora, cranium, and lung tissue	
3. Reticular	Forms firmer framework for organs and vessels	
C. Supportive		
1. Cartilage	Avascular, no lymphatics or nerves	Structural integrity is altered during rhinoplasty and otoplasty; cartilage may be used as graft material; radical neck reconstruction may involve tracheal rings or laryngectomy for multidisciplinary treatment
a. Hyaline	Translucent, articular, and rubs against other articular surface; forms the epiphyseal line in long bone, portions of the nose, and tracheal rings	
b. Costal elastic	Becomes fibrous with age; found in ribs, nose, trachea, and larynx	
c. White fibrocartilage	Forms circular menisci in joints and between vertebrae	
d. Yellow elastic	Found in auricle of ear, eustachian tubes, and epiglottis	
2. Erectile	Found in corpus cavernosa, clitoris, and nose	
D. Hard	Bony surfaces covered with periosteum except at articulations and cartilaginous areas of insertion points	Reconstruction requires framework of underlying bone or graft material; autologous bone may be harvested from graft site for neoconstruction; donor bone may be used as transplant material
1. Cancellous bone	Spaces are filled with red marrow; erythroblasts and smaller vessels	
2. Compact bone	Hollow center filled with yellow marrow (higher fat content) and larger vessels	

TABLE 28.1	Four Basic Histologic Tissue Types—cont'd	
Histologic Tissue Type	**Description**	**Implications to Surgical Team**
Muscle Tissue		
A. Visceral	Smooth, involuntary muscle; hollow organs, vessels, glands, areola, scrotum, iris of eye	Skeletal muscle may be used to replace bulk lost to debridement; vascularized flaps replace radical tissue excisions
B. Skeletal	Cylindric, striated, voluntary cells	
C. Cardiac	Branching cells, nonnucleated, less fibrous connective tissue	
Nerve Tissue		
A. Types		
1. Neuron	Cells generate and conduct nerve impulses; has multiple cytoplasmic fibers on one side (dendrites) and a single myelinated extension from the other side (axon)	Nerves may be injured during any procedure
2. Neuroglia	Insulate and support neurons in central nervous system	
B. Classification by activity type		
1. Afferent	Sensory	
2. Efferent	Motor	

From Fortunato NM, McCullough SM: *Plastic and reconstructive surgery,* St. Louis, 1998, Mosby.

The skin is the largest and heaviest organ of the body. The two main layers that compose the integument are the *epidermis* and the *dermis*. The thickness of the skin and its layers is determined by its location. The combined thickness of the epidermis and dermis ranges from 4 mm on the back to 1.5 mm on the scalp. Fig. 28.1 shows a cross-section of the integument (skin) and its layers. Areas involving bone will incorporate vascularized periosteum over the bone.

There are two basic skin types: glabrous and hairy. Glabrous, smooth skin is very thick and is found on the palms and soles. The surface is marked by ridges and sulci arranged in unique configurations referred to as *dermatographics*, or fingerprints. These ridges first appear in the fingertips during the 13th week of fetal life. A marked absence of hair follicles and oil glands is characteristic of this tissue. Hairy, thin skin has hair follicles, sweat glands, and oil glands.

Langer Lines

Natural lines of tension are formed by the relationship of the skin to the underlying musculature (Fig. 28.2). Austrian anatomist Karl Langer (1819–1887) described how incisions could be more cosmetic if natural cleavage lines were followed when planning the surgical incision. The collagen fibers in the epidermis and dermis form an elliptical shape when the skin is incised in fusiform fashion along the natural lines. The angle of the incision should be no more than 30 degrees at each margin. The surgeon may undermine the tissue to minimize the distance between the skin edges. Closure is better when the edges meet during approximation. As the incision heals, tension of the skin is relaxed, causing minimal pulling and widening of the bridge of scar tissue.

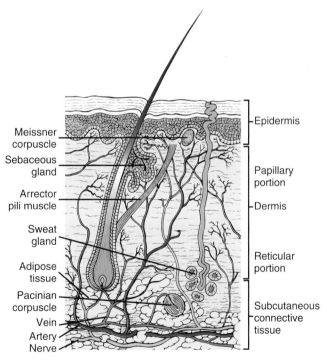

• **Fig. 28.1** Anatomy of the skin.

Epidermis

The epidermis is the outermost layer of skin. It is organized into five levels of stratified squamous epithelium and contains no organs, glands, nerve endings, or blood vessels. This layer renews

• **Fig. 28.2** Langer lines. **A,** Anterior view. **B,** Posterior view. **C,** Forearm. **D,** Relaxed skin tension lines of face. From Fortunato NM, McCullough SM: *Plastic and reconstructive surgery,* St. Louis, 1998, Mosby.)

itself every 15 to 30 days, depending on the body surface area, the age of the individual, and the individual's generalized condition. The basic anatomy and physiology of epidermal layers are as follows:

- *Stratum corneum:* Keratinized cells make up 75% of the epidermal thickness. Cells are shed from this level, which is referred to as the *horny layer.* It is thinner in hairy, thin-skinned areas.
- *Stratum lucidum:* Cells are flattened. Organelles and nuclei are absent.
- *Stratum granulosum:* This level is arranged in three to five layers. Mitotic activity creates cells for renewal of epidermal layers.
- *Stratum spinosum:* This layer creates cells for renewal of epidermal layers.
- *Stratum basale:* A single cell layer that lies between the junction of the epidermis and the dermis. Intense mitosis in this layer in combination with the basal layer and the spinosum causes epidermal regeneration. As cells are generated they migrate upward, toward the surface. Melanocytes, located between basal cells and in hair follicles, create melanin, which causes skin pigmentation. Melanin enters and accumulates in keratocytes, causing superficial skin tone and providing ultraviolet protection. Exposure to sunlight causes

darkening of existing melanin and accelerated generation of new melanin.

Each epithelial layer consists of keratin-producing cells (keratinocytes). Keratin is modified into functional components such as hair and fingernails on select body surfaces. Overactivity of the spinosum and basal levels can increase epidermal thickness in normally thin areas, causing psoriasis.

Dermis

The dermis is composed of papillary and reticular layers of flexible connective tissue. Superficially, the dermis has an irregular surface of papilla-like fingers that project into the strata basale of the epidermal layers. The dermis, regardless of location, is a loose, areolar connective tissue that contains pain and touch receptors, glands, blood vessels, and lymphatics. It is the key layer in wound repair and tissue healing.

Glandular Structures and Ducts in the Integument

Oil Glands (Sebaceous Glands)

Sebaceous and sudoriferous glands are found within the dermal layers of the skin. Sebaceous glands are referred to as *holocrine glands* because the oily secretion sebum also carries cellular debris. The sebaceous duct empties into a hair follicle or, on nonhairy areas, directly onto the surface of the skin. Sebum is a lubricant with minor antibacterial and antifungal properties. The palms and soles lack sebaceous glands, but these glands are numerous on the scalp and face and around natural body orifices. Oily skin types sometimes have increased scar formation because the oil forms a mechanical barrier to healing.

Sweat Glands (Sudoriferous Glands)

Sudoriferous glands are found on every area of the body except the lips, nipples, and glans penis. Eccrine and apocrine glands are two types of sudoriferous glands. Eccrine glands are widely distributed over the entire surface of the body and are responsible for producing 700 to 900 g of sweat per 24 hours. These simple structures are embedded in the dermis and have a funnel-shaped exit path (pore) leading directly to the skin's surface. Secretions are produced in response to physical activity and cool the body by evaporation. These glands are most numerous on the palms, soles, and forehead.

Apocrine glands are located only in the axillary, perineal, and areolar areas in combination with eccrine glands. Apocrine glands are larger than eccrine glands and are embedded in subcutaneous tissue. These glands secrete a viscous fluid and have ducts that open into hair follicles. Initially the secretion is odorless, but it quickly develops an odor caused by bacterial decomposition. These glands secrete in response to stress or excitement. In animals, apocrine and sebaceous glands are thought to release pheromones, which are hormones thought to cause sexual attraction. Modified apocrine glands are found in the ear canals and secrete cerumen (earwax).

Blood Supply and Innervation

The dermis contains a rich supply of blood and lymph. In some areas, arterial and venous communication is by direct shunting, without using a capillary mechanism. Arteriovenous shunts allow for thermoregulation and blood pressure control. Capillary networks are located in the papillary layer to nourish the epidermis. *Effector innervation* of the dermis is derived from postganglionic fibers of the sympathetic ganglia. *Affector innervation* is a superficial dermal network of free nerve endings, hair follicles, and encapsulated sensory organs.

Tissue Layers Under the Integument

Subcutaneous Adipose Layer

Underneath the dermis is a loose, fatty layer that is referred to as the *subcutaneous layer*. Beneath the subcutaneous tissue is a layer of striated muscle. The looseness of this structure allows for movement of the skin over supporting musculature. In males the distribution is through the nape of the neck, deltoids, triceps, abdomen, lumbosacral region, and buttocks. In females the fatty layer extends through the breasts, abdomen, buttocks, epitrochanteric area, and anterior thighs.

Fascia

The fascia is a fibrous areolar tissue that supports the superficial skin layers and encases the muscle. Fascia throughout the body covers the muscles anteriorly and posteriorly. The superficial fascia is located directly underneath the integument and is the point to which injection of a local anesthetic agent should extend for the best effect. Sensory nerve fibers run through this area, and an anesthetic agent is easily absorbed. Adipose cells occupy areolar spaces, rendering the fascia soft and pliable and permitting vessels, nerves, and lymphatics to pass through the layers.

The deep fascia is tough and less pliable. It runs the length of the muscle bundle and terminates in fibrous tendons that attach to bones beneath the periosteum. The anterior fascia of the abdomen is arranged in three layers that merge around the rectus abdominis muscles. The internal and external oblique muscles cover and surround the rectus muscles to the level of the linea circularis, or the landmark known as the *arcuate line*, sometimes called the *semicircular line of Douglas* (Fig. 28.3). The arcuate line

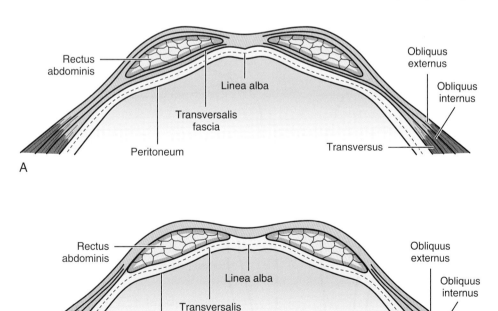

• **Fig. 28.3** Abdominal tissue layer at the arcuate line. **A,** Above the arcuate line. **B,** Below the arcuate line.

is formed by three fascial merges one-third the distance between the umbilicus and the pubis. Below the level of the arcuate line the fascial layers are fully anterior with no posterior fascial component. The rectus abdominis is behind the layered fascia.

Peritoneum

Lying beneath the posterior fascia of the abdomen is the peritoneum—the thin, two-layer serous membrane that lines the interior of the abdominal cavity (parietal peritoneum) and surrounds the organs (visceral peritoneum). The inferior aspect of the peritoneum overlies or is superior to the dome of the urinary bladder. In other words, the bladder is infraperitoneal, or below the peritoneal cavity. The stomach is superior to the peritoneal sac with the fundus situated supraperitoneally. The kidneys and the aorta are behind the peritoneum (retroperitoneal).

Accessory Appendages to the Integument

Modifications in the epidermal layer cause varied degrees of keratin deposition. Thickness and durability are functionally related to the location of keratinization. Hair and fingernails are modified keratin.

Other skin appendages include glands, blood vessels, and sensory organs. Glands arise in the dermis, and some exit the body through ducts that penetrate the epidermis. Other glands empty into the superior segment of hair follicles.

Hair Follicles

Hair follicles are keratinized epidermal epithelium that terminates in the dermal layers. The follicle is nourished by a capillary bed. Loss of this blood supply results in death of the follicle. Small bundles of smooth muscle cells, referred to as *arrector pili,* form attachments to the surrounding connective tissue in a diagonal fashion. As arrector pili contract, the shaft of the hair is straightened to an upright position. This contraction causes the superficial skin to dimple and pucker, creating "goose bumps."

Nails (Ungues)

The dorsal tip of each phalanx is tipped with a plate of specialized keratinized cells. Proximally, the nail root is covered by stratum corneum, which is referred to as the *eponychium,* or cuticle. The nail plate rests on a bed of epidermis (nailbed). Nails are chemically similar to the surface epidermis. Peripheral blood supply may be assessed through the translucent nail plate but should not be the sole determinant of oxygenation and well-being of the patient.

Surgical Landmarks

The primary reference point for abdominal incisions is the umbilicus. Secondary surface landmarks include the xyphoid, the pubis, and the iliac crests. Incisions may be vertical, horizontal, or oblique and may occur in various areas of the torso (Fig. 28.4). Specialty incisions, such as those involving the head, limbs, breast, reconstructive procedures, and other organ systems, are described in their respective chapters.

The direction of the incisional line is determined by the anatomic plane in the body (Fig. 28.5). Some specialty instruments are constructed to dissect, debulk, or separate layers in a specific pattern according to the angle of the natural tissue arrangement. One example is a sagittal saw that is designed to cut bone along the sagittal plane.

Placement of the Surgical Incision

Before the procedure begins the surgeon chooses the most suitable incision for the procedure being performed. All incisions incorporate, with varying degrees of success, certain characteristics that include the following:
- Condition of the patient
  - Knowledge of previous surgery in the same region and the presence of adhesions
  - Ease and speed of entry into tissues

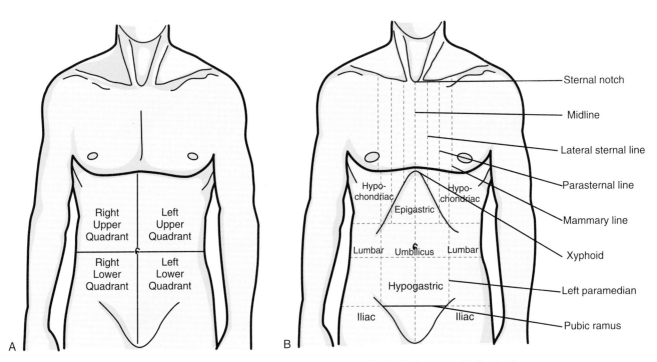

• **Fig. 28.4** Surgical landmarks. **A,** Surgical quadrants. **B,** Surgical topographic landmarks.

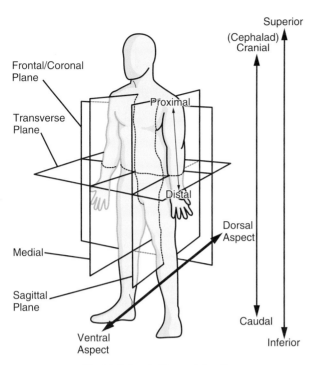

• **Fig. 28.5** Surgical lines of direction.

• Size of the body habitus and the natural lines of tissue tension (Langer lines)
• Maximum exposure of intended surgical site and adjacent structures (i.e., muscles, nerves, vessels, lymphatics)
  • Ability to extend the incision if necessary
  • Least amount of disfiguration as possible
• Minimum trauma and scar formation
• Least postoperative discomfort
• Maximum postoperative wound strength

Abdominal Surgery

A laparotomy involves surgically opening the abdominal wall and entering the peritoneal cavity (Fig. 28.6). The skin and subcutaneous tissue are incised, and the blood vessels are ligated or electrocoagulated. Both the posterior fascia and the peritoneum may be cut at the same time, thus exposing the contents of the abdominal cavity. Various types of incisions are used in a laparotomy, but each follows essentially the same technique.

Types of Abdominal Incisions

The incisions discussed in the following sections are applicable to open abdominal or pelvic procedures for specific organs or organ systems. The usual anterior surface incisions are depicted in Fig. 28.7.

Laparoscopy is performed through either one puncture or multiple (usually one to five) incisions that are smaller (usually 5–10 mm), separate, and distinct. Endoscopy and laparoscopy are discussed in detail in Chapter 32.

Midline Incision

A midline incision can be upper abdominal, lower abdominal, or a combination of both going around the umbilicus. The patient may have thicker deposits of adipose tissue under the planned incision line. Depending on the intended procedure, a full

midline incision can begin in the epigastrium at the level of the xyphoid process and may extend inferiorly to the suprapubic region. The surgeon is careful to avoid cutting bowel that may be close to the surface in the peritoneal cavity. Most surgeons curve the incision around the periphery of the umbilicus to avoid cutting through the structure.

An upper midline incision above the umbilicus offers excellent exposure of and rapid entry into the epigastric region. The upper midline incision is made carefully to accommodate the position of the falciform ligament of the liver. A lower midline incision can begin inferior to the umbilicus and extend to the pubis for lower bowel, gynecologic, or obstetric pelvic procedures. Care is taken at the lower margin to avoid perforating the urinary bladder. An indwelling urinary catheter can help keep the bladder decompressed.

The midline incision enters the body through fascial planes that are relatively avascular. Many vessels and nerve endings are spared. The muscles are easily separated and retracted for visualization, and when the procedure is complete it is easy to close. If the incision must be lengthened, the extension is easier to make. When closing, the surgeon may request a visceral retainer to protect the underlying organs and prevent an inadvertent suture from passing through the bowel.

Paramedian Incision

The paramedian incision is a vertical incision made approximately 4 cm (approximately 2 inches) lateral to the midline on either side in the upper or lower abdomen. After the skin and subcutaneous tissue are incised, the rectus sheath is split vertically and the muscle is retracted laterally. This incision allows quick entry into and excellent exposure of the abdominal cavity. It limits trauma, avoids nerve injury, is easily extended, and gives a firm closure. Examples of use include access to the biliary tract or pancreas in the right upper quadrant and access to the left lower quadrant for resection of the sigmoid colon.

Subcostal Upper Quadrant Oblique Incision

A right or left oblique incision begins in the epigastrium and extends laterally and obliquely just below the lower costal margin. One example is the Kocher incision in the right subcostal region, which was developed by Swiss surgeon and Nobel laureate Emil Theodor Kocher (1841–1917). It continues through the rectus muscle, which is either retracted or transversely divided. Although this type of incision affords limited exposure except for upper abdominal viscera, it provides good cosmetic results because it follows skin lines and produces limited nerve damage. Despite being painful, it is a strong incision postoperatively. Examples of use include biliary procedures.

Bilateral subcostal incisions that join in the midline may be preferred for procedures that involve the stomach and/or pancreas. A modified bilateral subcostal incision (chevron incision or rooftop incision) is made for increased visibility during a liver transplantation or resection. The chevron incision can be extended superiorly toward the xyphoid to create the Mercedes incision for greater access to the inferior aspect of the diaphragm.

McBurney Incision

Charles McBurney (1845–1913) described a method of diagnosing appendicitis in 1889 by pressing on the right lower quadrant, just below the umbilicus and 4 cm (2 inches) medial from the anterior superior iliac spine. This area of the abdomen is referred to as *McBurney point*.

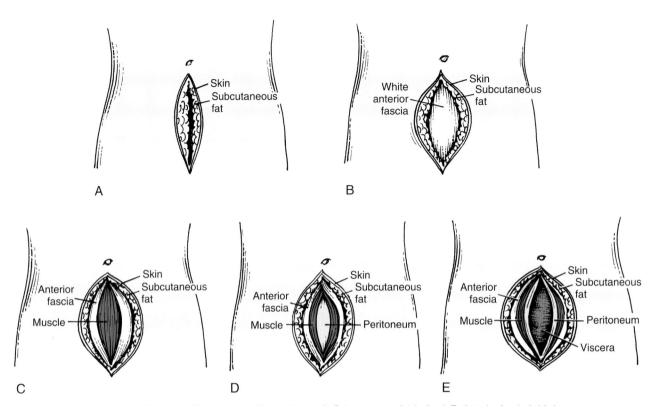

• **Fig. 28.6** Dissecting tissue layers of the abdomen. **A,** Subcutaneous fat *(yellow)*. **B,** Anterior fascia *(white)*. **C,** Muscle *(red)*. **D,** Skin through muscle dissected. This white peritoneum is shown for dissection. **E,** Open peritoneum with viscera beneath.

Anterior Surface Incisions

A. Sternotomy
B. Kocher (Subcostal)
C. Supraumbilical
D. Infraumbilical
E. McBurney appendectomy
F. Transverse
G. Maylard transverse muscle-cutting
H. Pfannenstiel

I. Thyroidectomy
J. Tracheotomy
K. Infraareolar
L. Inframammary
M. Midline
N. Paramedian
O. Rockey-Davis

P. Mercedes
Q. Chevron
R. Epigastric (upper midline)
S. Lower midline
T. Pararectus
U. Gibson (hand-assisted laparoscopy)
V. Inguinal
W. Femoral
X. Clamshell
Y. Subclavicular
Z. Carotid

• **Fig. 28.7** Anterior surface incisions.

McBurney incision involves a muscle-splitting incision that extends through the fibers of the external oblique muscle. The incision is deepened, the internal oblique and transversalis muscles are split and retracted, and the peritoneum is entered. This is a fast and easy incision, but exposure is limited. Its primary use is for appendectomy. Some surgeons modify this incision in a transverse plane referred to as the *Rockey-Davis* or *Lanz* incision to conceal the scar in a natural skinfold.

Thoracoabdominal Incision

For a thoracoabdominal incision the patient is placed in a lateral position. Either a right or a left incision begins at a point midway between the xyphoid process and umbilicus and extends across the abdomen to the seventh or eighth costal interspace and along the interspace into the thorax. The rectus, oblique, serratus, and intercostal muscles are divided in the line of incision down to the peritoneum and pleura. This converts the pleural and peritoneal cavities into one main cavity, thus allowing excellent exposure for the upper end of the stomach and lower end of the esophagus. Examples of use include esophageal varices and the repair of a hiatal hernia.

Midabdominal Transverse Incision

The midabdominal transverse incision starts on either the right or left side and slightly above or below the umbilicus. It may be carried laterally to the lumbar region between the ribs and crest of the ilium. The intercostal nerves are protected by cutting the posterior rectus sheath and peritoneum in the direction of the divided muscle fibers.

Transverse abdominal incisions are sometimes used for infants because the abdomen is wider than it is long. Better exposure to the intraabdominal cavity is attained. In some cases the same is true for extremely short, stout adults with large abdominal girth.

The advantages are rapid incision, easy extension, a provision for retroperitoneal approach, and a secure postoperative wound. Examples of use include choledochojejunostomy and transverse colostomy.

Pfannenstiel Incision

German gynecologist Herman Johannes Pfannenstiel (1862–1909) developed the Pfannenstiel incision, a curvilinear transverse incision across the lower abdomen and within or superior to the hairline of the pubis. The incision follows the Langer lines of the natural skinfolds. The rectus fascia is incised transversely below the arcuate line, and the muscles are separated. The peritoneum is incised vertically in the midline. This lower curved incision provides good exposure and strong closure for pelvic procedures. Its primary use is for urologic and gynecologic procedures and cesarean section. One disadvantage is that exposure may be limited. The scar is obscured by the patient's pubic hair.

One modification is the Maylard transverse incision. This incision is not curved but straight. It is made above the level of the curvilinear Pfannenstiel incision for greater access to the pelvic and urologic organs.

Inguinal Incision (Lower Oblique)

An oblique incision of the right or left inguinal region extends from the pubic tubercle to the anterior iliac crest, slightly above and parallel to the inguinal crease. Incision of the external oblique fascia provides access to the cremaster muscle, inguinal canal, and spermatic cord structures. Great care is taken not to entrap ilioinguinal nerves or the spermatic cord. Its primary use is for inguinal herniorrhaphy.

Wound Closure

Closure of a surgical site or other wound is performed after necessary hemostasis has been achieved. Wounds include deep and superficial structures. Methods of wound closure include sutures, staples, clips, tapes, and glues.[1]

Suture Basics

The noun form of suture is used for any strand of material used for ligating or approximating tissue; it is also synonymous with stitch. The verb *to suture* denotes the act of sewing by bringing tissues together and holding them in approximation until healing has taken place.

If the material is tied around a blood vessel to occlude the lumen, it is called a ligature or *tie*. A suture attached to a needle for a single stitch for hemostasis is referred to as a stick tie or *suture ligature*. A free tie is a single strand of material handed to the surgeon or first assistant to ligate a vessel. A tie handed to the surgeon in the tip of a forceps or clamp is referred to as a *tie on a passer*.

Suturing Techniques

Halsted Suture Technique

The education a physician receives during postgraduate surgical training exerts a lasting influence on their surgical techniques. The classic example of the influence of a professor on his students is that of Dr. William Stewart Halsted (1852–1922).

Halsted, a professor of surgery at Johns Hopkins Hospital in Baltimore from 1893 to 1922, perfected and brought into use the fine-pointed hemostat for occluding vessels, the Penrose drain, and rubber gloves. He is best known for his principles of gentle tissue handling. The silk suture technique he initiated in 1883, or a modification of it, is in use today. Its features are as follows:

1. Interrupted individual sutures are used for greater strength along the wound. Each stitch is taken and tied separately in a figure of 8 pattern for deeper tissues. If one knot slips, all the others hold. Halsted also believed that interrupted sutures were a barrier to infection; he thought that if one area of a wound became infected, the microorganisms traveled along a continuous suture to infect the entire wound.
2. Sutures are as fine as is consistent with security. A suture stronger than the tissue it holds is not necessary.
3. Sutures are cut close to the knots. Long ends cause irritation and increase inflammation. Only external stitches have tails for ease of removal after healing.
4. A separate needle is used for each skin stitch.
5. Dead space in the wound is eliminated. Dead space is that space caused by separation of wound edges that have not been closely approximated by sutures. Serum or blood clots may collect in a dead space and prevent healing by keeping the cut edges of tissue separated.
6. Two fine sutures are used in situations usually requiring one large one.
7. Silk is not used in the presence of infection. The interstices (braid pattern) can harbor microorganisms.
8. Tension is not placed on tissue. Approximation versus strangulation preserves the blood supply.

Halsted's principles were based on use of the only suture materials available to him: silk and surgical gut. With the advent of less reactive synthetic materials, wound closure may be safely and more quickly performed with different techniques without complications.

Principles of Suturing

The strength of the wound is related to the condition of the tissue and the number of stitches in the edges. Care is taken not to place more sutures than necessary to approximate the edges. The amount of tissue incorporated into each stitch directly influences the rate of healing.[2] The adequacy of the blood supply to the tissue needs to be preserved for healing to take place.

Methods of Suturing

The edges of the wound are intentionally directed by the placement of sutures during closure. Suturing techniques are depicted in Fig. 28.8. Examples of suturing techniques that direct the wound edges for specific healing mechanisms include, but are not limited to, the following:

1. *Everting sutures:* These interrupted (individual stitches) or continuous (running stitch) sutures are used to evert edges.
   a. *Simple continuous (running):* This suture can be used to close multiple layers with one suture. The suture is not cut until the full length is incorporated into the tissue (see Fig. 28.8, *A*).
   b. *Continuous running/locking (blanket stitch):* A single suture is passed in and out of the tissue layers and looped through the free end before the needle is passed through the tissue for another stitch. Each new stitch locks the previous stitch in place (see Fig. 28.8, *B*).

   c. *Simple interrupted:* Each individual stitch is placed, tied, and cut in succession from one suture (see Fig. 28.8, *C*).
   d. *Horizontal mattress:* Stitches are placed parallel to wound edges. Each single bite takes the place of two interrupted stitches (see Fig. 28.8, *D*).
   e. *Vertical mattress:* This suture uses deep and superficial bites, with each stitch crossing the wound at right angles. It works well for deep wounds. Edges approximate well (see Fig. 28.8, *E*).
2. *Inverting sutures:* These sutures are commonly used for two-layer anastomosis of hollow internal organs, such as the bowel and stomach. Placing two layers prevents passing suture through the lumen of the organ and creating a path for infection. A single layer is placed for other structures, such as the trachea, bronchus, and ureter. The edges are turned in toward the lumen to prevent serosal and mucosal adhesions. The number of layers is proportional to the quality of the blood supply. Stitches can be interrupted or continuous.
   a. *Halsted suture:* A two-layer modification of the horizontal mattress suture used for friable tissue.
   b. *Connell suture:* A continuous single-layer suture of gut used for hemostasis in the inner layer of bowel with a separate outer inverting layer of alternating horizontal and vertical mattress sutures.
   c. *Cushing suture:* A continuous vertical mattress suture that unites half of the lumen, followed by a second continuous vertical mattress suture that completes the second half of the circumference.
   d. *Grey-Turner sutures:* A series of inverted interrupted horizontal or vertical mattress stitches.
   e. *Purse string suture:* A continuous stitch that encircles and closes a lumen while inverting the edges.

Knot Placement

Each suture placed in tissue usually requires the placement of a knot to secure the ends. Interrupted stitches require individual knots, and therefore placement of each knot can influence how well the wound heals and the cosmetic result. The following list of principles concerns knots and knot tying:
1. The knot should be tied away from:
   a. Vital structures, such as the eye
   b. Sources of contamination, such as the mouth
   c. Potential irritants, such as the nares
   d. Potential sources of increased inflammation, such as the incision line
2. The knot should be tied toward:
   a. The better blood supply
   b. The area that provides the best security of the knot
   c. Where the mark would be less noticeable, if possible

Cutting Sutures

Care is taken to prevent excess suture from remaining in the wound. Suture tails are trimmed close to the knot inside the body, but a short tail may be left for external stitches to facilitate removal. Considerations for cutting suture include the following:
1. Scissors are stabilized by the index finger on the screw (tripod stance), the blades are angled slightly and slide down to the area just above the knot, and the suture is cut with the tips of the scissors.
2. The tips of the scissors must be visible to ensure that other structures are not injured by the cutting motion.

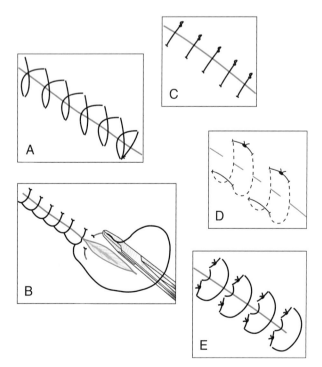

• **Fig. 28.8** Examples of suturing techniques. **A,** Simple continuous. **B,** Continuous locking. **C,** Simple interrupted. **D,** Horizontal mattress. **E,** Vertical mattress.

3. A hemostat and/or a second suture should be available in the event the knot is inadvertently cut, releasing the sutured tissue.
4. A hemostat may be placed on one of the suture ends to stabilize the suture to be cut.
5. If removing a suture, a forceps is used to grasp the suture at the knot. Cut the suture between the knot and the skin. Extract the cut suture with the forceps.

Retention Sutures

Interrupted nonabsorbable sutures are placed through tissue on each side of the primary suture line, a short distance from it, to relieve tension on it. Heavy strands are used in sizes ranging from 0 through 5. The tissue through which retention sutures are passed includes skin, subcutaneous tissue, and fascia and may include rectus muscle and peritoneum of an abdominal incision.

After abdominal surgical procedures, retention sutures are used frequently in patients in whom slow healing is expected because of malnutrition, obesity, carcinoma, or infection; in geriatric patients; in patients receiving cortisone; and in patients with respiratory problems.[3]

Retention sutures may be used as a precautionary measure to prevent wound disruption when postoperative stress on the primary suture line from distention, vomiting, or coughing is anticipated. Retention sutures should be removed as soon as the danger of sudden increases in intraabdominal pressure is over, usually on the fourth or fifth postoperative day. Retention sutures are also used to support wounds for healing by second intention and for secondary closure after wound disruption for healing by third intention.

Retention Bridges, Bolsters, and Bumpers

To prevent heavy retention suture from cutting into skin, several different types of bridges, bolsters, or bumpers are used:
- Bridges are devices placed on the skin to span the incision. The retention suture is brought through the skin on both sides of the incision and through holes on each side of the bridge and is fastened over the bridge. Foam plates are available to prevent suture pull-through and to protect skin. One type allows adjustment of tension on the edges of the incision during the postoperative healing period.
- Bumpers are segments of materials such as foam, plastic, or rubber tubing. One end of the suture is threaded through the tubing before the suture is tied. It covers the entire retention suture strand that is on the skin surface to prevent irritation (Fig. 28.9). Compression bolsters are made from material such as polyethylene foam held in place with buttons to secure and distribute tension of retention sutures.
- Buttons, discs, beads, and plates are used as bolsters and bumpers to prevent the suture from retracting or cutting into skin or friable tissue. The suture is pulled through holes and tied over a foam-padded plate, sterile button, or other device (e.g., with pull-out tendon sutures). Beads may be placed on the ends of pull-out subcuticular skin sutures. The devices are used most frequently in abdominal, plastic, and orthopedic surgery.

Traction Suture

A traction suture may be used to retract tissue to the side or out of the way, such as the tongue in a surgical procedure in the mouth. Usually a nonabsorbable suture is placed through the part. Other materials that may be used to retract or ligate vessels include the following:

- *Umbilical tape:* Aside from its original use for tying the umbilical cord on a newborn, cotton umbilical tape may be used as a heavy tie or as a traction suture. It may be placed around a portion of bowel or a great vessel to retract it. These should be counted and accounted for at the end of the procedure. Cotton should be moistened with sterile saline before use. Umbilical tapes should not be cut into pieces.
- *Vessel loop:* A length of thin flat silicone can be placed around a vessel, nerve, or other tubular structure for retraction. It can be tightened around a blood vessel for temporary vascular occlusion. These should be counted and accounted for at the end of the procedure. Vessel loops should not be cut into pieces.
- *Aneurysm needle:* An aneurysm needle is an instrument with a blunt needle on the end for passing suture. The eye is on the distal end of the needle. The needle forms a right or oblique angle to the handle, which is one continuous unit with the needle. The needles are made in symmetric pairs, right and left. The surgeon uses them to place a ligature around a deep, large vessel, such as in a thyroidectomy or in thoracic surgery. They can be used to pass a suture tape around an incompetent cervix to perform cerclage. These should be counted and accounted for at the end of the procedure (refer to Chapter 34, Fig. 34.19).

Endoscopic Suturing

Endoscopic sutures are available as ligatures and preknotted loops or with curved or straight, permanently swaged needles for use through an endoscope. The ligatures are fashioned into loosely knotted loops before being passed through the endoscope to tie off vessels and tissue pedicles. After the loop is placed around the target site, the knot is slid into position and tightened. The ends are cut with endoscopic scissors and removed through the endoscope. Suture with a permanently swaged needle is placed through either a 3-mm suture introducer for a straight needle or an 8-mm suture introducer for a curved needle. Used to suture vessels, reconstruct organs, approximate opposing tissue surfaces, and anastomose tubular structures, the technique varies according to the method used for knot tying.[4] The methods of endoscopic knot tying are as follows:
- *Extracorporeal method:* The swaged needle and both ends of the suture are brought outside the body through the trocar. The needle is cut off, and the knot is loosely fashioned. The knot is reintroduced into the body through the trocar by means of a knot-sliding cannula. It is snugged into position and tightened against the tissue. The ends of the suture are cut close to the knot with endoscopic scissors. Excess suture ends are removed through the endoscope.
- *Intracorporeal method:* The needle and suture are passed through the tissue with an endoscopic needle holder. Endoscopic instruments are used to tie the knot and cut the suture inside the body.

Specifications for Suture Material

- It must be sterile when placed in tissue. Sterile techniques must be rigidly followed in handling suture material. For example, if the end of a strand drops over the side of any sterile surface, discard the strand. Almost all postoperative wound infections are initiated along or adjacent to suture lines. Affinity for bacterial contamination varies with the physical characteristics of the material.

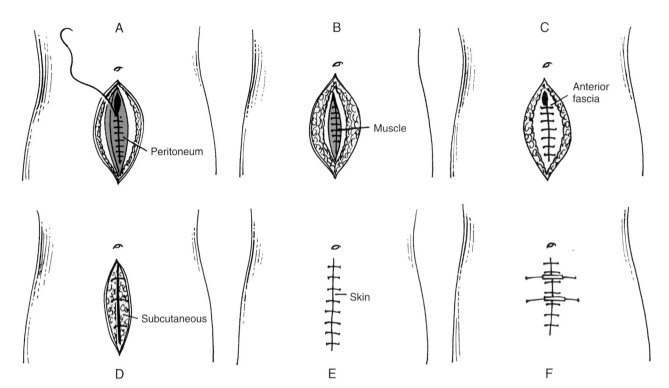

• **Fig. 28.9** Suturing incised abdominal tissue layers. **A,** Peritoneum (continuous stitch, taper-point needle). **B,** Muscle (interrupted stitch). **C,** Anterior fascia (interrupted stitch, cutting needle). **D,** Subcutaneous (not always sutured, taper-point needle). **E,** Skin (interrupted stitch, cutting needle). **F,** Retention sutures. Note bumpers to protect skin.

• It must be predictably uniform in tensile strength by size and material. Tensile strength is the measured pounds of tension or pull that a strand will withstand before it breaks when knotted. Minimum knot-pull strengths are specified for each basic raw material and for each size of that material by the U.S. Pharmacopeia (USP). Tensile strength decreases as the diameter of the strand decreases.

• It must be as small in diameter as is safe to use on each type of tissue. The strength of the suture usually needs to be no greater than the strength of the tissue on which it is used. Smaller sizes are less traumatic during placement in tissue and leave less suture mass to cause tissue reaction. The surgeon ties small-diameter sutures more gently and thus they are less apt to strangulate tissue. A small-diameter suture is flexible, easy to manipulate, and leaves minimal scar on skin.

• USP-determined sizes range from heavy 10 (largest) to very fine 12-0 (smallest); ranges vary with materials. Taking size 1 as a starting point, sizes increase with each number above 1 and decrease with each 0 (zero) added. The more zeroes in the number, the smaller the size of the strand. As the number of zeroes increases, the size of the strand decreases. In addition to this system of size designation, the manufacturer's labels on boxes and packets may include metric measures for suture diameters. These metric equivalents vary slightly by types of materials. Box 28.1 shows how suture gauge is measured on a scale in numeric descriptions from smallest to largest.

• It must have knot security, remain tied, and give support to tissue during the healing process. However, sutures in the skin are always removed 3 to 10 days postoperatively, depending on the site of incision and cosmetic result desired. Because they are exposed to the external environment, skin sutures can be a source of microbial contamination of the wound that inhibits healing by first intention.

• It must cause as little foreign body tissue reaction as possible. All suture materials are foreign bodies, but some are more inert (less reactive) than others.

Choice of Suture Material

The surgeon selects the type of suture material best suited to maintain tensile strength and promote healing. Fig. 28.10 shows the labeling of a generic suture packet. When selecting a suture, specific notations about the characteristics of each suture are listed on the box and the packet. Surgical sutures are classified as either absorbable or nonabsorbable:

1. *Absorbable sutures:* Sterile strands prepared from collagen derived from healthy mammals or from a synthetic polymer. They are capable of being absorbed by living mammalian tissue but may be treated or coated to modify resistance to absorption. Some synthetic sutures are coated with a Triclosan or chlorhexidine antimicrobial chemical.[5] They may be colored by a dye approved by the U.S. Food and Drug Administration (FDA).

2. *Nonabsorbable sutures:* Strands of natural or synthetic material that effectively resist enzymatic digestion or absorption in living tissue. During the healing process, suture mass becomes encapsulated and may remain for years in tissues without producing any ill effects.

Sutures may be dyed with a color additive approved by the FDA. They may be modified with respect to body, texture, or capillarity. Capillarity refers to a characteristic of nonabsorbable

• BOX 28.1   Suture Gauge Diagram

SMALLER GAUGE	ZERO	LARGER GAUGE
12-0 11-0 10-0 9-0 8-0	7-0 6-0 5-0 4-0 3-0 2-0 0 1 2 3 4 5 6	7 8 9 10

Each packet is color-coded by type of suture composition for ease of identification when selectiong for a procedure. The package colors are similar between manufacturers for type and chemical makeup of suture.

METHOD TO SELECT A SUTURE FOR A SURGICAL PROCEDURE
1. Identify by color (Trade name)
2. Gauge of suture (more zeros indicate smaller gauge)
3. Size and configuration of needle/tip (actual needle and tip image)
   Double needle image indicates a needle on each end
4. Number of strands/needles per pack (Most packs have one needle/suture combination) (some packs have 3 or 8 swaged-on needles) (Ties can be single, very long, or 12 precut strands)

GAUGE OF SUTURE (size USP)   Order number/Letter suffix # per box
Length of suture strand   RFID scan box
# of strands/needles per pack

TRADE NAME OF SUTURE™
Generic composition name of suture
Color and texture of suture
Special attributes (*coated or antimicrobial*)
Sterility statement
Absorbable/Nonabsorbable data
No reprocessing disclaimer
MANUFACTURER'S COMPANY NAME

SHADOW IMAGE OF ACTUAL NEEDLE SIZE
NOMENCLATURE NAME OF NEEDLE
Icon image configuration of needle tip
Numeric size of needle curve (fraction)
Needle composition   Bar code and Expiration date
                                                              Lot #

• **Fig. 28.10** Suture packet generic information.

sutures that allows the passage of tissue fluids along the strand, permitting infection, if present, to be drawn along the suture line. Suture materials may be untreated or may be treated to reduce capillarity. Noncapillarity is the characteristic of some nonabsorbable sutures in which the nature of the raw material or specific processing meets USP tests that establish them as resistant to wicking transfer of body fluids.

The two classifications of suture materials are subdivided into monofilament and multifilament strands:

1. *Monofilament suture:* A strand consisting of a single threadlike structure that is noncapillary. Monofilament suture is generally less traumatic when pulled through tissue. The smooth surface glides easily without catching on tissue. Some monofilament suture retains its curved shape when removed from the packet. This is referred to as *memory.* Manufacturers recommend that the suture not be tugged on to straighten the strand. It can weaken the integrity.
2. *Multifilament suture:* A strand made of more than one threadlike structure held together by braiding or twisting. This suture strand is capillary unless it is treated to resist capillarity

or is absorbable. Multifilament suture has a rougher surface and can be somewhat traumatic as it is pulled through tissue layers. Gut suture has memory and will weaken if stretched for straightening.

The following factors influence suture choice:
- Biologic characteristics of the material in tissue (e.g., absorbable vs. nonabsorbable, capillary vs. noncapillary, or inertness).
- Healing characteristics of tissue. Tissues that normally heal slowly, such as skin, fascia, and tendons, usually are closed with nonabsorbable sutures. Absorbable suture placed through the skin may cause a stitch abscess to develop because it is inclined to act as a culture medium for microorganisms in the pores of the skin. Tissues that heal rapidly, such as stomach, colon, and bladder, may be closed with absorbable sutures. Braided suture can be the nidus for stone formation if placed in moisture reservoirs, such as the urinary bladder.
- Location and length of the incision. Cosmetic results desired may be an influencing factor. The choice of suture is made by determining the best method of closure for minimizing scar formation.

- Presence or absence of infection, contamination, and/or drainage. If infection is present, sutures may be the origin of granuloma formation with subsequent discharge of suture and sinus formation. Foreign bodies in potentially contaminated tissues may convert contamination to infection. Foreign bodies in the presence of some body fluids may cause stone formation, as in the urinary or biliary tract. Braided suture is not used in the presence of infection.
- Patient problems such as obesity, debility, advanced age, and diseases, which influence the rate of healing and time desired for wound support.
- Physical characteristics of the material such as ease of passage through tissue, knot tying, and other personal preferences of the surgeon.

Absorbable Sutures (Table 28.2)

Surgical Gut. Surgical gut is collagen derived from the submucosa of sheep intestine or serosa of beef intestine. Many elaborate mechanical and chemical cleaning processes occur before intestinal ribbons of collagen are spun into strands of various sizes, ranging from the heaviest (size 3) to the finest (size 6-0). Gut is packed in an alcohol solution that is potentially flammable. The manufacturer recommends that gut suture not be rinsed before use. Although the larger sizes are made from two or more ribbons (multifilament), the behavior of surgical gut is that of a monofilament suture. Surgical gut is digested by body enzymes and absorbed by tissue so that no permanent foreign body remains.

Gut is available in plain (untreated) or chromic (treated with chromium salts). Plain surgical gut loses tensile strength relatively quickly. It is used to ligate small vessels and to suture subcutaneous fat. It is not used to suture any layers of tissue likely to be subjected to tension during healing. Fast-absorbing plain surgical gut is specially treated to speed absorption and tensile strength loss. It may be used for epidermal suturing where sutures are needed for no more than a week.

Chromic surgical gut is treated in a chromium salt solution to resist absorption by tissues for varying lengths of time, depending on the strength of the solution and duration and method of the process. Chromic surgical gut is used for ligation of larger vessels and for suture of tissues in which nonabsorbable materials are not usually recommended because they may act as a nidus for stone formation, as in the urinary or biliary tracts.

TABLE 28.2 Absorbable Suture

Suture Name	Strand Formation	Sizes Available	Colors	Tensile Strength	Notes
Plain gut	Twisted multifilament	6-0 to 3	Yellow Blue Black	5—10 days	Natural; duration 70 days; packed in alcohol solution; not used in presence of infection
Chromic gut	Twisted multifilament	7-0 to 3	Brown Blue Black	14—21 days	Natural; duration 90 days; packed in alcohol solution; not used in presence of infection
Collagen	Twisted multifilament	4-0 to 8-0	Blue		Natural; available as plain or chromic; used in eye surgery; not used in presence of infection
Maxon[a]	Monofilament	7-0 to 2	Green Clear	60 days	Synthetic; duration 6 months; nonantigenic, nonpyogenic; prolonged approximation without stress; hydrolytic absorption by tissues; can be used in presence of infection
PDS, PDSII[a]	Monofilament	9-0 to 2 10-0 to 7-0	Violet Blue Clear	90 days	Synthetic; duration 6 months; nonantigenic, nonpyogenic; prolonged approximation without stress; hydrolytic absorption by tissues; can be used in presence of infection; antibacterial Irgacare (a form of triclosan)
Monocryl[a]	Monofilament	6-0 to 2	Golden Clear Undyed Violet	21 days	Synthetic; duration 91—119 days; antibacterial Irgacare (a form of triclosan)
Vicryl[a]	Braided	Coated 9-0 to 2 Undyed 8-0 to 1	Violet Undyed	40 days	Synthetic; duration 90 days; coating is a lubricant; available as 42-day fast absorbing Vicryl Rapide; antibacterial Irgacare (a form of triclosan); not used in presence of infection
Velosorb[a]	Braided	6-0 to 1	Violet Undyed	5—10 days	Synthetic; duration 40—50 days; not used in presence of infection
Polysorb[a]	Braided	8-0 to 2	Violet Undyed	21 days	Synthetic; duration 56—70 days; not used in presence of infection
Biosyn[a] Caprosyn[a]	Monofilament	6-0 to 1	Violet Undyed	10 days to 3 weeks	Synthetic; duration 90—110 days (Biosyn) duration 56 days (Caprosyn)

[a]Trade name.

Collagen Sutures. Collagen sutures are extruded from a homogeneous dispersion of pure collagen fibrils from the flexor tendons of beef. Both plain and chromic types are similar in appearance to surgical gut and may be dyed blue. Sizes range from 4-0 through 8-0. These sutures are used primarily in ophthalmic surgery.

Handling Characteristics of Surgical Gut and Collagen.

1. Most surgical gut and collagen sutures are sealed in packets that contain an alcohol solution to keep the material pliable. This solution is mostly alcohol and water but may be irritating to ophthalmic tissues. Hold the packet over a basin and open carefully to avoid spilling fluid on the sterile field or splashing it into your own eyes. Rinsing is necessary only for surgical gut or collagen sutures to be implanted into the eye. Do not soak or the suture will weaken.

2. Surgical gut and collagen sutures should be used immediately after removal from their packets. When the material is removed and not used at once, the alcohol evaporates and the strand loses pliability. Excessive exposure to water or saline will reduce the tensile strength. Before unwinding, the strand can be dipped momentarily in water or saline solution at room temperature; heat will coagulate the protein.

3. Unwind the strand carefully. The suture is stiff and has folded memory. Handle it as little as possible. Never pull or stretch surgical gut; this weakens it. Do not straighten suture by running fingers down the length of the strand; excessive handling with gloves can cause fraying that causes the strand to weaken.

Synthetic Absorbable Polymers. Polymers, either dyed (colored) or undyed (white or clear), are extruded into absorbable suture strands. These synthetic sutures are absorbed by a slow hydrolysis process in the presence of tissue fluids. They are used for ligating or suturing except when extended approximation of tissues under stress is required. They are inert, nonantigenic, and nonpyrogenic and produce only a mild tissue reaction during absorption. They may be monofilament or multifilament, coated or uncoated.

Handling Characteristics of Synthetic Absorbable Polymers.

- Synthetic absorbable sutures have an expiration date on the package. Therefore rotate stock. "First in, first out" is a good rule to follow.

- Synthetic absorbable sutures are packaged and used dry. Do not soak or dip in water or normal saline solution. The material hydrolyzes in water, so excessive exposure to moisture will reduce the tensile strength. It is smooth and soft and will retain its pliability.

Nonabsorbable Sutures (Table 28.3)

Surgical Silk. Surgical silk is a natural animal product made from the fiber spun by silkworm larvae in making their cocoons. From the raw state, each fiber is processed to remove natural waxes and gums. Fibers are braided or twisted together to form a multifilament suture strand. Braided silk is used more frequently because surgeons prefer its high tensile strength and better handling qualities. Surgical silk is treated to render it noncapillary. The fibers lose tensile strength if wet. Therefore silk sutures should not be moistened before use.

Silk is not a truly nonabsorbable material. It disappears within 2 years. It causes less tissue reaction than does surgical gut, but it is not as inert as most of the other nonabsorbable materials. It is used frequently in the serosa of the gastrointestinal tract and to close fascia in the absence of infection.

Surgical Cotton. Cotton is a natural cellulose fiber. Suture is made from individual, long-staple cotton fibers. Single-strand cotton suture is rarely used because it causes an inflammatory reaction. Cotton umbilical tapes are used to tie umbilical cords or retract tissue structures during a surgical procedure. It should be moistened before it is handed to the surgeon. Moisture prevents clinging to the surgeon's gloves.

Surgical Stainless Steel. Stainless steel sutures are drawn from 316L-SS (L for low carbon) iron alloy wire. This is the same metal formula used in the manufacture of surgical stainless steel implants and prostheses. Two different kinds of metal alloy should not be embedded in the tissues simultaneously. This combination creates an unfavorable electrolytic reaction. Some implants and prostheses are made of Vitallium, titanium, or tantalum. Suture material in the wound must be compatible with these metals.

Before the availability of surgical stainless steel from suture manufacturers, commercial steel was purchased by weight, using the Brown and Sharpe (B&S) scale for diameter variations. Many surgeons still refer to surgical stainless steel size by the B&S gauge, from 18 (the largest diameter) to 40 (the smallest). One manufacturer labels surgical stainless steel with both B&S gauge and equivalent USP diameter classifications. Both monofilament and twisted multifilament stainless steel strands are available.

Surgical stainless steel is inert in tissue and has high tensile strength. It gives the greatest strength of any suture material to a wound before healing begins and supports a wound indefinitely. Some surgeons use stainless steel for abdominal wall or sternal closure or for retention sutures to reduce the danger of wound disruption in the presence of contributing factors. It may be used in the presence of infection or in patients in whom slow healing is expected. It is used for secondary repair or resuturing after wound disruption.

Unlike most other suture materials, steel lacks elasticity. A suture secured too tightly may act as a knife and cut through tissue. Stainless steel sutures are harder to handle than any other suture material. A painstaking knot-tying and twisting technique with a nonserrated instrument is required. The serrations of the instrument will create weak areas along the suture. Wire suture is cut only with wire scissors.

Handling Characteristics of Surgical Stainless Steel Suture.

1. Surgical stainless steel strands are malleable and kink rather easily. Kinks in the strand can make it practically useless. Therefore use care in handling to keep the strand straight.

2. Barbs on the end of a strand can tear gloves, puncture the skin, or traumatize tissue. Sternal wire suture has been known to extrude through the skin if the cut end is not buried deep into the tissue.

3. If surgical stainless steel must be threaded through a needle, some surgeons prefer one or two twists of the end around the strand just below the eye of the needle to prevent unthreading during suturing.

Synthetic Nonabsorbable Polymers. Synthetic nonabsorbable sutures have higher tensile strength and elicit less tissue reaction than does silk. They retain their strength in tissue. Knot tying with most of these materials is more difficult than with silk. Additional throws are required to secure the knot. The surgeon may sacrifice some handling characteristics and ease of knot tying for strength, durability, and nonreactivity of the synthetics. These advantages may outweigh the disadvantages. Synthetic nonabsorbable sutures are available as monofilament or braided strands.

| | | TABLE 28.3 **Nonabsorbable Suture** | | | |

Suture Name	Strand Formation	Sizes Available	Colors	Tissue Effects	Notes
Silk Sofsilk[a] Perma-hand[a]	Braided	9-0 to 5	Black White	Acute tissue inflammation	Natural fiber coated with silicon or wax; encapsulates; not used in presence of infection; not detectable after 2 years
Cotton[a]	Twisted strands	Umbilical tape	White	Minimal tissue inflammation	Natural fiber; moisten before use; single-strand suture rarely used
Ethilon[a]	Monofilament	11-0 to 2	Black Green Clear	Minimal tissue inflammation	Synthetic nylon
Nurolon[a]	Braided	6-0 to 1	Black	Minimal tissue inflammation	Synthetic nylon; not used in presence of infection
Dermalona Monosof[a]	Monofilament	11-0 to 2	Blue Black Clear	Minimal tissue inflammation	Synthetic nylon; uncoated
Surgilon[a]	Braided	6-0 to 1	Black White	Minimal tissue inflammation	Synthetic nylon; silicone coated; not used in presence of infection
Prolene[a]	Monofilament	10-0 to 2	Blue Clear	Minimal tissue inflammation	Synthetic; can be used in a contaminated wound; available with attached Teflon pledgets
Pronova[a]	Monofilament	8-0 to 5-0	Blue	Minimal tissue inflammation	Synthetic; can be used in a contaminated wound
Surgipro II[a]	Monofilament	8-0 to 2	Blue	Minimal tissue inflammation	Synthetic; can be used in a contaminated wound
Vascufil[a]	Monofilament	7-0 to 2-0	Blue	Minimal tissue inflammation	Synthetic; less memory; can be used in a contaminated wound
Novafil[a]	Monofilament	7-0 to 2	Blue Clear	Minimal tissue inflammation	Synthetic; can be used in a contaminated wound
Ti-Cron[a]	Braided	7-0 to 5	Blue White	Minimal tissue inflammation	Synthetic; coated with silicone; available uncoated; available with precut pledgets; not used in presence of infection
Surgidac[a]	Braided	6-0 to 4-0	White	Minimal tissue inflammation	Synthetic; not used in presence of infection
Mersilene[a]	Braided Monofilament	10-0 to 5	Green White	Minimal tissue inflammation	Synthetic; braided form not used in presence of infection
Ethibond[a]	Braided	7-0 to 5	Green White	Minimal tissue inflammation	Synthetic; coated with polybutilate; encapsulates; available with attached Teflon pledgets; not used in presence of infection
Steel	Monofilament Multifilament	6-0 to 7	Silver	Minimal tissue inflammation	Low carbon alloy; do not handle with serrated instrument; only use wire scissors to cut; do not use with metal implant of different alloy

[a]Trade name.

Surgical Nylon. Nylon is a polyamide polymer derived by chemical synthesis from coal, air, and water. It produces minimal tissue reaction. Nylon has high tensile strength, but it degrades by hydrolysis in tissue at a rate of about 15% to 20% per year. It may be used in all tissues where a nonabsorbable suture is acceptable, except when long-term support is critical. It is available in three forms: monofilament, uncoated multifilament, and coated multifilament.

Polyester Fiber. A polymer of terephthalic acid and polyethylene, Dacron polyester fiber is braided into a multifilament suture strand that is available in two forms: uncoated fiber and coated fiber.

1. Uncoated polyester fiber suture is closely braided to provide a flexible, pliable strand that is relatively easy to handle. However, uncoated braided polyester fiber suture tends to drag and exert a sawing or tearing effect when passed through tissue. It may be used in all tissues in which a multifilament nonabsorbable suture is indicated.
2. Coated polyester fiber suture has a lubricated surface for smooth passage through tissue. Sutures are available with different coating materials:
   a. Polybutilate is the only coating developed specifically as a surgical lubricant. This polyester material adheres strongly to the braided polyester fiber. Polyester fiber coated with

polybutilate provides a strand superior to any other braided material, coated or uncoated, in decreasing drag through tissue.

b. Polytetrafluoroethylene (PTFE), a commercial product known by the name Teflon and manufactured by DuPont, is used as a coating bonded to the surface or impregnated into spaces (interstices) in the braid of the polyester fiber strand. Minute particles of this coating can flake off the strand. Because these particles are insoluble and resistant to enzymes, foreign body granulomas may be produced.

c. Silicone, a commercial lubricant, provides a slippery coating but does not bond well to polyester fiber. It can become dislodged in tissues as the strand is tied.

Polypropylene Suture. A polymerized propylene is extruded into a monofilament strand. It is the most inert of the synthetic materials and almost as inert as stainless steel. Polypropylene is an acceptable substitute for stainless steel in situations in which strength and nonreactivity are required, and it is easier to handle. The suture may be left in place for prolonged healing. It can be used in the presence of infection.

Handling Characteristics of Synthetic Nonabsorbable Polymers.

1. Physical damage to suture materials can occur from the time the suture is removed from a packet if the strand is mishandled. Handle all sutures and needles as little as possible. Avoid pulling or stretching. Sutures should be handled without using instruments except when grasping the free end during an instrument tie. Clamping instruments—especially needle holders and forceps with serrations—on strands can crush, cut, and weaken them.

2. All synthetic materials require a specific knot-tying technique. Knot security requires additional flat and square ties. Multifilament materials are generally easier to tie than are monofilament sutures.

Barbed Suture (Table 28.4)

Barbed Suture. This synthetic self-anchoring suture is used for low-tension suturing without the need of knotted ends. Barbed synthetic suture is available in absorbable and nonabsorbable material. Handling barbed suture is done with care. The barbs are tiny but still can snag on sponges or drapes. Use of barbed suture has many applications in several specialties. Barbed suture has two different configurations: unidirectional barbs and bidirectional barbs.

Unidirectional barbed suture has a needle on one end and a loop on the other end. The loop can be used to anchor the suture in place of a knot. The barbs are designed to pull through the tissue in one direction and maintain placement without moving. At the completion of closure the needle can be cut off without losing stability of the wound.

Bidirectional barbed suture is double-armed and has raised barbs that are angled from the center to the ends in both directions. During closure the suture is placed with a slight reverse torque to anchor the barbs into the dermis from the center in one direction, and then the reverse is performed in the opposite direction. The result is a well-approximated incision line.

TABLE 28.4 Barbed Suture

Barbed Suture	Corza Medical	V-Loc Medtronic/Covidien	Stratafix Ethicon
Unidirectional Knotless Loop end	Polypropylene: Clear or blue Nonabsorbable Size 3-0 to 2	V-Loc PBT: Polybutester: Blue Nonabsorbable Size 3-0 to 1 Endo 3-0 to 0	Polypropylene: Undyed Nonabsorbable, spiral Size 4-0 to 1
	Monoderm: Violet or clear Absorbable Size 4-0 to 0 90—120 days	V-Loc 180: Green or clear Absorbable Size 4-0 to 0 Endo 3-0 to 0 180 days	PGA-PCL: Clear Absorbable, spiral Size 4-0 to 0 90—120 days
	PDO: Violet Absorbable Size 4-0 to 2 180 days	V-Loc 90: Violet or undyed Absorbable Size 4-0 to 2-0 90—110 days	PDO: Violet Absorbable, spiral Size 4-0 to 1 210 days
Bidirectional Double-armed Knotless	Polypropylene: Clear Nonabsorbable Size 2-0 to 2		Polypropylene: Clear Nonabsorbable, spiral Size 4-0 to 1
	Nylon: Blue Nonabsorbable Size 1 to 2		
	Monoderm: Violet or clear Absorbable Size 5-0 to 0 90—120 days		PGA-PCL: Violet or clear Absorbable, spiral Size 4-0 to 1
	PDO: Violet Absorbable Size 4-0 to 2 180 days		PDO: Violet Absorbable, spiral Size 5-0 to 1 210 days

Surgical Needles

Except for simple ligating with free ties, surgical needles are needed to safely carry suture material through tissue with the least amount of trauma. Each packet is opened and counted during the initial sharps count. The best surgical needles are made of high-quality tempered steel that is:

- Strong enough that it does not break or fracture easily
- Rigid enough to prevent excessive bending, yet flexible enough to prevent breaking if bent
- Sharp enough to penetrate tissue with minimal resistance (yet it need not be stronger than the tissue it penetrates)
- Approximately the same diameter as the suture material it carries to minimize trauma in passage through tissue
- Appropriate in shape and size for the type, condition, and accessibility of the tissue to be sutured
- Free from corrosion and burrs to prevent infection and tissue trauma

Because needles are made of steel, theoretically they are detectable by x-ray if inadvertently lost in tissue. The location in tissue may preclude the needle from appearing on a radiograph. For example, the angle of the needle or its position behind bone may obstruct detection. The smaller the size of the needle, the more likely the image is to be obstructed. All needles should be accounted for in their entirety so that they do not become foreign bodies in tissue. Lost needles can become embedded in linen or trash, causing harm to unsuspecting support personnel.

Many shapes and sizes of surgical needles are available. Names vary from one manufacturer to another; general classification only, not nomenclature, is standardized. They may be straight like a sewing needle or curved. All surgical needles have three basic components: the point, the body (or shaft), and the eye. They are classified according to these three components.

Point of the Needle

Points of surgical needles are honed to the configuration and sharpness desired for specific types of tissues. The basic shapes are cutting, tapered, and blunt (Fig. 28.11).

Cutting Point

A razor-sharp, honed cutting point may be preferred when tissue is difficult to penetrate, such as skin, tendon, and tough tissues in the eye. These make a slight cut in tissue as they penetrate. The location and degree of sharpness of cutting edges vary. Cutting needles are less traumatic as they pass through tissues.

Conventional Cutting Needles. Two opposing cutting edges form a triangular configuration with a third edge on the body of the needle. Cutting edges are on the inside curvature of a curved needle. Cutting edges may be honed to precision sharpness to ensure smooth passage through tissue and a minute needle path that heals quickly.

Reverse-Cutting Needles. A triangular configuration extends along the body of the needle. The edges near the point are sharpened or honed to precision points. The two opposing cutting edges are on the outer curvature of a curved needle.

Side-Cutting Needles. Relatively flat on the top and bottom, angulated cutting edges are on the sides. Used primarily in ophthalmic surgery, they will not penetrate underlying tissues. They split through layers of tissue.

• **Fig. 28.11** Configurations of needle points. **A,** Conventional cutting and reverse cutting. **B,** Side cutting. **C,** Cutting edge at end of tapered body with **D,** trocar point, **E,** taper, and **F,** blunt.

Trocar Point

Sharp cutting tips are at the points of tapered needles. All three edges of the tip are sharpened to provide cutting action with the smallest possible hole in tissue as it penetrates.

Taper Point

These needles are used in soft tissues, such as intestine and peritoneum, which offer a small amount of resistance to the needle as it passes through. The needle points tend to push the tissue aside as they go through, rather than cut it. The body tapers to a sharp point at the tip.

Blunt Point

These tapered needles are designed with a rounded blunt point at the tip. They are used primarily for suturing friable tissue, such as liver and kidney. Because the blunt point will not cut through tissue, it is less apt to puncture a vessel in these organs than is a sharp-pointed needle. Blunt needles also may be used in some tissues to reduce the potential for needlesticks, especially in general and gynecologic surgery.

Body of the Needle

The body, or shaft, varies in wire gauge, length, shape, and finish. The nature and location of tissue to be sutured influence the selection of needles with these variable features. Most manufacturers have designated a specific alphanumeric code to describe each needle they produce. Examples of alphanumeric codes for taper-point needles can be found in Table 28.5.

Considerations relating to the body of the needle are as follows:
1. Tough or fibrosed tissue requires a heavier gauge needle than the fine-gauge diameter needed in microsurgery.
2. The depth of the bite (placement) through tissue determines the appropriate needle length.

3. The body of the needle may be round, oval, flat, or triangular. The point determines the shape: round or oval bodies have trocar, taper, or blunt points; flat or triangular bodies have cutting edges. The shape also may be straight or curved (Fig. 28.12).

   a. Straight needles are used in readily accessible tissue. They have cutting points for use in skin, which is their most frequent use, or tapered points for use in intestinal tissue held by a purse string device. They are not used with a needle holder.

   b. Curved needles are used to approximate most tissues because quick needle turnout is an advantage. The curvature may be ¼, ⅜, ½, or ⅝ circle; half-curved with only the tip curved; or compound curved. Curved needles always are armed in a needle holder before being handed to the surgeon.

   c. J-shaped needles range from 15.5 cm to 17.5 cm in length. The width of the J bend at the tip is available in 7 to 9-mm curvature. They are used for 10 to 14-mm fascial incisions created for trocar use during laparoscopy. They are multiuse needles that can be threaded with the suture of the surgeon's choice at the point of use. Their unique shape enables the surgeon to close the deep layers of the wound without perforation of underlying organs while visualizing closure of the accessory ports with the laparoscopic camera.

4. Curved needles that have longitudinal ribbed depressions or grooves along the body on the inside and outside curvature can be cross-locked in the needle holder. This feature virtually eliminates twisting or turning of the needle in any position in the needle holder.

5. In all needles the body must have a smooth finish. Many needles have a surface coating of microthin plastic or silicone to enhance smooth passage through tissue. Others have a black surface finish to enhance visibility at the surgical site.

Eye of the Needle

The eye is the segment of the needle where the suture strand is attached. Surgical needles are classified as eyed, French eye, or swaged or atraumatic. Swaged-on suture is inserted directly into the end of the needle by the manufacturer (Fig. 28.13, *C*).

Eyed Free Needle

The closed eye of an eyed surgical needle is like that of any household sewing needle. Needles that are threaded by the scrub person are referred to as *free needles*. The shape of the enclosed eye may be round, oblong, or square. The end of the suture strand is pulled 2 to 4 inches (5—10 cm) through the eye so the short end is about one-sixth the length of the long end. Unlike regular sewing thread, there is no knot placed in the end of the suture.

Disposable varieties are preferred. Some specialty needles will be packed in-house on a needle rack. Care is taken when handling these needles. Careful counting and accountability are required. In

Purpose	Ethicon	Medtronic/ Covidien	Configuration
General closure	CT	GS 24	½ circle taper 40 mm
General closure	CT 1	GS 21	37 mm
Cardiovascular	RB	EV 23	17 mm
Gastrointestinal	SH	EV 20	25 mm
Multilayer closure	CTX	GS 25	48 mm
Cardiovascular	BB	CV 15	⅜ circle taper 17 mm
Urologic	UR 6	GU 46	⅜ circle taper 27 mm

TABLE 28.5 Select Examples of Common Taper-Point Needles (Alphanumeric Codes) and Representative Manufacturers

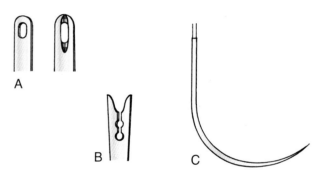

• **Fig. 28.13** Eyes of free needles and swaged-on needles. **A,** Oblong eyes. **B,** French eye. **C,** Swaged.

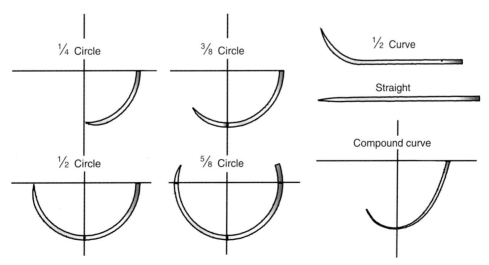

• **Fig. 28.12** Shapes of needle bodies.

some cases, if a swaged suture breaks during a procedure, the surgeon may request a free needle to complete the suturing process.

French Eye Needle

Sometimes referred to as *spring eye* or *split eye*, a French eye needle has a slit from the inside of the eye to the end of the needle through which the suture strand is drawn. To thread a French eye after arming the needle in a needle holder, 2 to 3 inches (5–7.5 cm) of the strand is secured between the fingers holding the needle holder. The strand is pulled taut across the center of the V-shaped area above the eye and drawn down through the slit into the eye (Fig. 28.13, *B*, and Fig. 28.14).

French eye needles, as a general rule, are used with pliable braided materials, primarily silk and cotton, of medium or fine size. These needles are not practical for surgical gut; the strand may fray, or the eye may break because the diameter is usually too large for the slit.

Handling of Free Needles. Eyed and French eye needles have the following disadvantages for the scrub person, surgeon, and patient:

- Each needle must be carefully inspected by the scrub person before and after use for dull or burred points and defects in the eye.
- Care must be taken to avoid puncturing gloves with the needle point when threading.
- If the scrub person must choose an appropriate needle to thread, the needle should be the same approximate diameter as the suture size requested by the surgeon.
- Needles can unthread prematurely. This is an annoyance to the surgeon and prolongs operating time for the patient. To avoid this, the surgeon may prefer the suture strand threaded double with both ends pulled the same length through the eye. The scrub person may lock the suture strand by threading the short end through the eye twice in the same direction.
- Two strands of suture material are pulled through tissue when threaded needles are used. The bulk of the double strand through the eye creates a larger hole than the size of the needle or suture material, causing additional trauma to tissue.

Swaged-on Needle

A swaged-on needle is a continuous unit with the suture strand. The needle is swaged onto the end of the strand in the manufacturing process. This eliminates threading at the operating

room (OR) bed and minimizes tissue trauma because a single strand of material is drawn through tissue (Fig. 28.15). The diameter of the needle matches the size of the strand. The surgeon uses a new sharp needle with every suture strand. Usually referred to as *swaged needles,* three types of swaged-on needle-suture attachments are available.

1. *Single-armed attachment:* One needle is swaged to a suture strand. Some larger closure needles can have the end looped back into the needle. This suture is much longer and can be used to form looped-locking closure.
2. *Double-armed attachment:* A needle is swaged to each end of the suture strand. The two needles are not necessarily the same size and shape. These are used when the surgeon wishes to place a suture and then continue to approximate surrounding tissue on both sides from a midpoint in the strand. Barbed suture is packed this way, for example.
3. *Controlled-release needle attachment:* This attachment is secure, so the suture strand will not separate from the needle inadvertently, but it will release rapidly when pulled off intentionally. It is usually only single-armed. The surgeon grasps the suture strand just below the needle, pulling the strand taut, and releases the needle with a straight tug of the needle holder on the needle. This facilitates fast separation of the needle from the suture when desired. This type of needle is referred to as a *pop-off needle.*

Placement of the Needle in the Needle Holder

Needle holders have specially designed jaws to securely grasp surgical needles without damage if they are used correctly. Care is taken not to use needle holders for anything other than holding needles. The jaw can weaken or spring, causing the needle to twist and turn when suturing. The scrub person should observe the following principles in handling needles and needle holders:

1. Select a needle holder with appropriate-size jaws for the size of the needle to be used. An extremely small needle requires a needle holder with very fine tipped jaws. As the wire gauge

• **Fig. 28.14** To thread French eye needle, pull strand taut across center of V-shaped area and draw down through slit into eye.

• **Fig. 28.15** Tissue effects of needle penetration. **A,** Threaded. **B,** Swaged atraumatic.

• **Fig. 28.16** Correct position of curved needle in needle holder for right-handed surgeon, about one-third down from swage or eye.

of the needle increases, the jaws of the needle holder selected should be proportionately wider and heavier. Curved jaws or angulated handles may be needed for placement of the needle in tissues.

2. Select an appropriate-length needle holder for the area of tissue to be sutured. When the surgeon works deep inside the abdomen, chest, or pelvic cavity, a longer needle holder will be needed than is needed in superficial areas.

3. Clamp the body of the needle in an area one-fourth to half the distance from the eye to the point (Fig. 28.16). Never clamp the needle holder over the swaged area. This is the weakest area of a swaged-on needle because it is hollow before the suture strand is attached. Pressure on or near the needle-suture juncture may break the needle.

4. Place the needle securely in the tip of the needle holder jaws, and close the needle holder in the first or second ratchet. If the needle is held too tightly in the jaws or the needle holder is defective, the needle may be damaged or notched in such a manner that it will tend to bend or break on successive passes through tissue.

If the needle breaks, it must be accounted for in its entirety. All pieces and fragments must be retrieved from the patient's body and the surrounding environment for personnel safety.

5. Pass the needle holder with the needle point up and directed toward the surgeon's thumb when grasped so it is ready for use without readjustment. If a hands-free technique is preferred, place the needle holder on a tray or magnetic mat with the needle point facing down.

6. Hand the needle holder to the surgeon so the suture strand is free and not entangled with the needle holder. Hold the free end of the suture in one hand while passing the loaded needle holder with the other hand. Protect the end of the suture material from dragging across the sterile field. The assistant may take hold of the free end to keep the strand straight for the surgeon and to keep it from falling over the side of the sterile field. This is referred to as *trailing the suture.*

7. Hand the needle holder to an assistant to pull the needle out through tissue. A hemostat or other tissue forceps is not used for this purpose because the instrument may be damaged or may damage the needle. The needle should be grasped as far back as possible to avoid damage to the point or cutting edges.

Considerations in the Choice of Sutures and Needles

The surgeon chooses from available types and sizes of sutures and needles, the ones that best suit each purpose. In general, fine sizes are used for plastic, ophthalmic, pediatric, and vascular surgery; medium sizes are used for all other kinds of surgery; heavy sizes are used for retention and for anchoring bone. In general, cutting needles are used in tough tissue such as skin, fascia, tendon, and

mucous membranes, including the cervix, palate, tongue, and nose. Medium tissue calls for round taper-point or cutting needles. Round taper-point needles generally are used for nerve, peritoneum, muscle, and other soft tissue, such as lung and intestine, subcutaneous tissue, and dura.

It is almost impossible to learn the needle–tissue–suture–surgeon combinations by memory alone because of the unlimited number of combinations. Learning the general classification of needles, sutures, and tissues is the first step; practical experience is necessary to remember the combinations. Try to learn the suture and needle combinations most commonly used.

The preference card usually lists the surgeon's usual suture-needle routine by tissue layer. Some cards list swaged-on sutures by order number, but this can be confusing. Some of the order numbers include alphanumeric labels that refer to how many sutures are packed in a box. This has nothing to do with the suture itself. Others list sutures by size and materials and needles by size and shape, which is easier to follow. Suture and needle sizes are as variable as patient sizes. Therefore the surgeon may unexpectedly request a smaller or larger size out of routine for a particular patient's situation.

Each manufacturer produces different needle styles. Most types have a comparable counterpart in another brand name. Table 28.5 describes cross-referencing of needle types by alphanumeric codes among different manufacturers.

Packaging and Preparation of Sutures and Needles

Suture material is individually packaged and supplied sterile by the manufacturer. It is sterilized by cobalt-60 irradiation or ethylene oxide gas. Reprocessing of suture material is not recommended. It can be damaged and is not guaranteed to be sterile.

Swaged needles come in sterile packets attached to the suture material. The suture needles are counted as the packet is dispensed to the field and confirmed as they are opened. When the swaged-on suture is opened in the field the contents are verified. Discard the outer sterile packet as soon as the suture is opened. Saving the empty packet on the field is not a reliable way to keep track of the number of suture needles used.

Disposable eyed and French eye needles are individually packaged and sterilized by the manufacturer. Needles are counted when dispensed to the sterile field one at a time and only as needed. Single-use needles ensure a sharper point with less tissue trauma.

Preparation of Reusable Needles

Standard sets of reusable eyed and French eye needles may be prepared for each surgical procedure where they are used. This necessitates preparing more needles in a package than will actually be used. The margin for error in counting increases when too many needles are present on the field. Choose needles for each procedure according to each surgeon's preferences as listed on the preference card.

Packaging of Suture Materials

A strand of sterile suture material is supplied with as many as four coverings.

Box

Each box is sealed in cellophane and contains one, two, or three dozen packets of sterile suture material. The label on the box may be color-coded by suture material (e.g., light blue for silk, tan for chromic gut, yellow for plain surgical gut). Competing manufacturers frequently select similar colors for box labels and suture material identification. Most boxes fit into a suture cabinet rack. Many synthetic sutures have expiration dates because the material degrades with time. Each box is provided with a lot number that corresponds to the lot number on the individual suture packets.

Overwrap

Each individual suture packet has a sealed outer overwrap. The overwrap is peeled back to expose the inner primary sterile packet for aseptic transfer to the sterile table. The circulating nurse must not contaminate the sterile inner primary packet as the overwrap is peeled apart and the packet is transferred onto the sterile table or presented to the scrub person.

Primary Sterile Packet

Suture material, with or without swaged needles, is sealed in a sterile primary inner packet that is to be opened by the scrub person. The primary packet may be made of foil, paper, or plastic, or combinations of these. Labels may be color-coded by material, the same as the box. If a swaged needle is enclosed, a silhouette of the needle is included on the label, along with the size and type of suture material.

A single strand of material or multiple strands may be in the primary packet. The packet may be designed for dispensing individual strands from a multiple suture packet. Packaging configurations and considerations include the following:

1. Suture packets should be opened only as needed, to minimize waste.
2. Custom kits with multiple suture packets within a single package facilitate dispensing sutures to and organizing them on the sterile table. The kit may have appropriate sutures, with or without swaged needles, to meet the requirements of a particular surgeon or procedure. The packets are organized in order of use. The contents are listed on the cover of the package to facilitate counts. Expiration date will be printed on the outer label if synthetic suture is inside.
3. Sterile suture packets are labeled "Do Not Resterilize." Component layers of the packaging materials cannot withstand exposure to the heat of steam sterilization without potential physical damage to the contents and packets. The manufacturer will not guarantee product stability or sterility for packets resterilized in the hospital or in secondary processors, or for strands removed from packets and sterilized.
4. Some suture materials have an expiration date stamped on the box and primary packet to indicate the stability of the material. Oldest sutures should be used first. Sutures should not be used past this expiration date because the chemical composition may have started to degrade, and the safety and stability of the suture is in question.

Inner Dispenser Matrix

Suture material is contained within the primary sterile packet in a manner that facilitates removing or dispensing it. This may be a paper folder, reel, or plastic tray that may or may not be removed with the suture strands. The inner matrix keeps the suture from tangling as it is pulled out for use.

Preparation of Suture Material

The length of each strand of suture material within the primary packet varies; the shortest is 5 inches (approximately 13 cm), and the longest is 60 inches (152 cm). The most commonly used lengths range from 18 to 30 inches (46–76 cm). The length the surgeon prefers should be noted on the preference card. The scrub person may have to cut the strands to the desired length, depending on the lengths available.

Standard Length

The term *standard length* refers to a 60-inch (152-cm) strand of nonabsorbable material or a 54-inch (137-cm) strand of absorbable material without a swaged needle referred to as a *free tie*. It is not handed to the surgeon in this length. The scrub person may cut it into a half-length or third-length for use as a free tie (suture ligature), or thread it for a stick tie or suture, as shown in Figs. 28.17 and 28.18.

Ligating Reels

Twelve-foot (approximately 4-m) lengths of nonabsorbable or 54-inch (137-cm) lengths of absorbable suture are wound on disposable plastic reels. These reels are color-coded by material and have size identification. The surgeon keeps the reel in the palm of the hand for a series of free ties. The reel is radiopaque in case it is inadvertently dropped in a body cavity. These are counted items.

Precut Lengths

Most suture materials are supplied in precut lengths of 12 to 18 inches and are ready for use as free ties or for threading. These facilitate handling for the scrub person. They are dispensed individually from some primary packets or may be removed and placed in a fold of a towel near the sterile field. Packets contain from 3 to 17 strands, depending on the material.

Swaged Needle-Suture

The manufacturer predetermines lengths of sutures; however, the surgeon has a wide variety of choices to meet all suturing needs. The scrub person must remember that a strand can be shortened but not extended. An appropriate length for location of tissue must be handed to the surgeon. A packet may contain one suture strand armed with a single or double needle(s) or multiple strands with swaged needles.

The sterile package will depict the needle image of a single-armed suture or two needles in a double-armed suture. The package will also indicate how many sutures are enclosed. The

• **Fig. 28.17** Scrub person preparing one-third–length sutures. One free end of full-length strand is passed from right to left hand. At the same time, loop is caught around third finger of right hand. Other loop is caught around third finger of left hand while each end is held and suture is adjusted to equal lengths (thirds). Then each loop is cut with scissors.

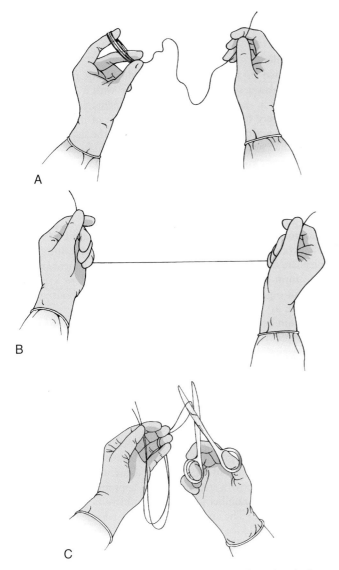

Fig. 28.18 Sequence of scrub person preparing half-lengths. **A,** Suture loops are separated by fingers of left hand while unwinding. **B,** Full length is gently unwound and straightened before cutting. Scrub person does not pull hard or test strand, but keeps firm grasp on both ends to prevent suture from snapping away and possibly becoming contaminated. **C,** Suture is bent in half, and loop is cut.

number of suture needles recorded on the pack is reported to the circulating nurse during the count.

Surgical Staples

Surgeons can join many tissues with staples. This involves inserting stainless steel or titanium staples through tissues with a stapler—a device specifically designed for this purpose. Some surgical procedures have become simplified or feasible since the advent of surgical stapling techniques. Titanium internal staples are preferred.

As Hümer Hültl recognized in 1908, for internal stapling to be successful, fine wire as the basic material must form a B shape when stapled into tissue. This shape allows blood to flow through tissues, preventing necrosis secondary to devascularization beyond

the staple line. Sufficient pressure must be exerted, however, to provide hemostasis of cut tissues.

Skin staples form a D shape when placed with the stapler. The box shape of the staple allows for adequate blood flow through the dermal layers. The length and width of the staples must accommodate tissue being approximated or transected. The number of staples varies with the length of the staple line.

Individual titanium ligation clips used for hemostasis form a completely occlusive, flat closure. Unlike the protection of blood flow in the shape of internal staples and skin staples, complete closure of the clipped structure is critical to prevent blood loss.

Advantages of Using Staples

Staples can be used safely in many types of tissues and have a wide range of applications.

- Stapling is a rapid method of ligating, anastomosing, and approximating tissues. The time saved, compared with suturing techniques, reduces blood loss and total operating and anesthesia time for the patient.
- Wound healing may be accelerated because of minimal trauma and the nonreactive nature of metallic staples.
- Staples produce an even surface and an airtight, leakproof closure.
- Staples can be placed through an endoscopic trocar.

Stapling Instruments

Each stapler is designed for stapling specific tissues (e.g., skin, fascia, bronchus, gastrointestinal tract, vessels). The surgeon selects the correct instrument for the desired application. The consequences of an erroneous staple application, however, are much more difficult to correct than those of manually placed sutures. The surgeon must learn when and how to use each instrument. Whether the stapler is reusable or a single-use disposable, the basic technical mechanics of stapling are the same.

Staplers either fire a single staple or simultaneously fire straight or circular rows of staples. The rows can be double- or triple-staggered staple lines. A different instrument must be used for each type of staple cartridge.

Skin Stapler

To approximate skin edges, the stapler fires a single staple with each squeeze of the trigger. Edges of both cuticular and subcuticular layers are aligned, with the edges slightly raised in an everted direction with Adson pickups (forceps) with teeth, as close to their original configuration on the horizontal plane as possible. Care is taken not to perforate the skin with the tips of the pickups. The stapler is positioned over the line of incision so that the staple will be placed evenly on each side. The staple forms a rectangular D shape over the incision. As many staples as needed are placed to close the incision.

Skin staplers are supplied preloaded with different quantities of staples in varying widths (i.e., crown span). The most appropriate stapler should be chosen for the selected use. For example, an average range of 28 to 35 staples is needed to close most abdominal incisions. More may be needed to close the chest; fewer may be needed for an inguinal herniorrhaphy.

Skin staples are removed 5 to 7 days postoperatively. Extractors are used for this purpose. As it heals, the skin flattens out to form an even surface with excellent cosmetic results if the staples have been properly placed lightly over the skin. Embedded staples are difficult to remove, and results may be less than desired.

Internal Staplers

Internal staplers are used to separate, anastomose, or occlude vessels and internal organs. They are manufactured as reusable stainless steel instruments with cartridges, single-use instruments with cartridges, or single-use single-fire disposable instruments.

Several internal staplers used for separation and anastomosis have self-contained knives. Some occlusion models do not have knives. They create only a reinforced staple line. The surgeon can trim away excess tissue along the staple line with a scalpel.

Staplers with cartridges and knives can be used on the same patient throughout the entire procedure. As the staples are fired and the knife used, the scrub person carefully changes the cartridge without disturbing the next load of staples. Fig. 28.19 shows the three most common styles of internal staplers that can be reloaded or purchased as single-fire instruments.

To avoid unnecessary contamination of a sterile instrument, the package should not be opened until the surgeon determines the correct size for the intended use of the stapler. Staplers should never be flipped or dumped onto the field. The impact can cause misalignment of the staples or internal knife and result in misfire. This could cause problems during the procedure and possibly cause an anastomotic leak postoperatively. The circulating nurse should open the package aseptically, and the scrub person should lift the instrument out of the sterile pack. A misfired stapler and its packaging should be given to the supervisor in charge for inspection by the manufacturer.

The numbers and sizes of staples in cartridges vary; the length of the linear jaws or the diameter of the circular head varies for internal use. Internal staplers are available with either stainless steel or titanium staples. The surgeon may prefer titanium because it creates less distortion when computed tomography (CT) scans are used. Titanium staples are safer for use in magnetic resonance imaging (MRI) because they are nonmagnetic. Care is taken to discard any used staple device in the designated container at the end of the surgical procedure for the safety of the surgical services personnel.

Linear Stapler

Two staggered or side-by-side straight double or triple rows of staples are placed simultaneously in tissue with a linear stapler. This stapler is used throughout the alimentary tract and in thoracic surgery for transection and resection of internal tissues. The tissue is positioned in the straight jaws of the stapler. The gap between the jaws must be adequate for the thickness of tissues. Terminal anastomosis (thoracoabdominal [TA]) staplers have no built-in knife. Excess tissue is trimmed away after firing with a scalpel before the instrument is removed. TA is commonly used to close a side or end of a structure such as a segment of bowel or the lobe of a lung.

Gastrointestinal anastomosis (GIA) staplers have a knife that is run between the two staple lines to separate tissue after firing. GIA staplers are commonly used to join two tubular segments side by side to form a pouch. They also can be used to close a terminal end of an organ. GIA is commercially available without a knife, referred to as *SGIA*.

The number of staples that will be fired depends on the length of the stapler jaws. The TA and GIA instruments can be reloaded with a second staple cartridge for use on the same patient. The instrument is discarded at the end of the surgical procedure. Single-use disposable models are available.

Intraluminal Circular Stapler

With the circular stapler a double row of staggered staples is placed in a circle for intraluminal end-to-end anastomosis (EEA) of tubular hollow organs in the gastrointestinal tract. Because the diameter of the lumen of organs in the alimentary tract varies, the surgeon must choose a stapler with an appropriate head circumference size. The number of staples the instrument fires depends on its head size. The instrument can be reloaded with a new staple-cutting head for second use on the same patient. Single-fire models are available. The EEA stapler is available curved or straight.

A circular knife within the head of the EEA stapler trims tissue to produce a round lumen as the stapler is fired. The result is a circular anastomosis and two distinct tissue rings, intact circles of tissue from the anastomosed region referred to as *doughnuts*. These are sent as two separate specimens to be examined for intactness. Care is taken to keep the distal and proximal tissue circles separate, so if cancerous margins are present, they will be correctly identified if a second resection is required.

Ligating and Dividing Stapler

A double row of two staples each ligates tissue and vessels that are then divided simultaneously between the staple lines with a cutting knife incorporated into the stapler. The staple configuration after firing is flat like a ligating clip. Hemostasis is attained. This disposable stapler is used primarily to ligate and divide omental vessels or other small, soft tubular structures. The working end is curved to encircle the vessel as it is ligated and cut. Some types have built-in carbon dioxide (CO_2) cartridges referred to as *powered LDS* (ligate–divide–staple).

Endoscopic Stapler

Endoscopic staplers are available for ligating and dividing and for linear stapling. The stapling device is passed through an 11 or a

• **Fig. 28.19** Internal staplers. **A,** Terminal end stapler. **B,** Internal anastomosis stapler with linear knife. **C,** End-to-end stapler with circular knife.

12-gauge laparoscopic trocar. It may be reloaded several times with staple cartridges for multiple firings. The stapler is discarded in the sharps container after single-patient use.

Clips

Multiload or single-load ligating clips are used to completely occlude vessels as needed. Titanium is the usual composition. Clips are applied to individual vessels with a clip application instrument and are designed to close flat. They do not cut tissue. The purpose is to permanently occlude the vessel. The instrument can be a reusable ring-handled stainless instrument or a disposable preloaded plastic applicator. Care is taken not to prematurely squeeze the handles as the instrument is passed to the surgeon. Squeezing will cause the clip to fall from the jaws of the instrument before it can be applied to the vessels.

Tissue Adhesives

Conventional suturing and stapling materials hold tissues in apposition during the healing process. Sutures and staples will not fuse or bond tissues. Ancient Egyptians used resins and gums to hold tissue surfaces together. Research is ongoing for an ideal tissue adhesive that will bond tissue, effect hemostasis, promote regeneration of cells, and serve as a barrier to microbes, fluid, and air. Biologic and synthetic tissue adhesives have extensive potential applications for wound closure and reconstruction.

Biologic Adhesives

Fibrin sealants, most commonly called *fibrin glue,* act as biologic adhesives and hemostatic agents. The components are fibrinogen, cryoprecipitate from human plasma; calcium chloride; and reconstituted thrombin of bovine origin. When applied directly to tissues, thrombin converts fibrinogen to fibrin to produce a clot. Fibrin sealants can be applied to deeper tissues as a liquid, gel, or aerosol spray to control bleeding and approximate tissues technically difficult to approximate by suturing, especially after resections or traumatic injuries of friable or highly vascular tissues, such as liver, spleen, and lung. Each component is applied simultaneously with separate syringes to prevent congealing before application to the tissue site. It is not mixed ahead of use or it will congeal and be useless. A sample formula and supplies for fibrin glue compound are found in Box 28.2.

• BOX 28.2   Sample Fibrin Glue Compound and Supplies

Sterile specimen cup
Two 2-mL disposable syringes
Two 14-gauge intravenous (IV) catheters
6 units thawed cryoprecipitate
1 ampule calcium chloride (CaCl) (10%, 1 g)
50,000 units thrombin

Instructions

Mix CaCl and thrombin in the specimen cup. Draw into the 20-mL syringe, and attach a 14-gauge IV catheter. Draw cryoprecipitate into the second syringe with a 14-gauge IV catheter on the end. Both syringes are discharged over the wound at the same time. The fibrin glue will form a clot over the wound. This method can be used if commercial fibrin glue is unavailable.

Fibrin glue may be used for microsurgical anastomoses of blood vessels, nerves, and other structures such as fallopian tubes; for reconstruction of the middle ear; to fix ocular implants; to close superficial lacerations and fistula tracts; and to secure some skin grafts. It may be used as a carrier for demineralized bone powder to promote osteoregeneration.

Tisseel is a topical fibrin sealant produced by Baxter Healthcare Corporation that can be applied by a duo syringe or a spray. Tisseel is derived from the human blood proteins fibrin and thrombin and is applied in the same manner as earlier forms of fibrin sealant. No bovine components are used. Aprotinin is an antifibrinolytic protein ingredient that may cause an allergic reaction in some patients. The risk for transmissible viral or prion disease is low, but it still must be considered. Tisseel is used alone and cannot be used with any other hemostatic material—an embolic event can occur. Tisseel is commercially available in freeze-dried or prefilled syringe kits. Frozen kits need to thaw for at least 30 minutes before use. Quick-thaw instructions are written in the packaging material. Care is taken to follow the exact steps so the product works effectively. More information is available at http://www.tisseel.com/ and http://www.fda.gov/.

Autologous or Homologous Plasma

Plasma collected from the patient (autologous) or a single donor (homologous) is processed into a cryoprecipitate containing clotting factor XIII to produce fibrinogen. Autologous plasma is obtained preoperatively and prepared either in the blood bank or in the OR. A single donor must be tested and found to be negative for human immunodeficiency virus (HIV) and hepatitis before plasma is processed.

Autologous or homologous fibrinogen is warmed to 98.6° F (37° C) immediately before use. Thrombin is reconstituted to 1000 units/mL. Equal volumes of fibrinogen and thrombin are applied simultaneously.

Pooled-Donor Plasma

Fibrin glue commercially prepared from pooled-donor plasma (i.e., blended from multiple donors) has significantly greater bonding strength than does autologous or single-donor plasma. The fibrinogen must undergo purification and viral inactivation to prevent transmission of bloodborne pathogens. VISTASEAL is a human fibrin and human thrombin combination sealant used to control mild to moderate bleeding. It is available in different amounts, comes frozen, is quick to thaw, and comes in dual applicator kits.[6]

Synthetic Adhesives

Synthetic glue-like adhesive substances that polymerize in contact with body tissues effect hemostasis and hold tissues together.

Cyanoacrylate

Butyl cyanoacrylate and octyl cyanoacrylate derivatives may be used for topical skin closure (skin glue). Both types of synthetic adhesives are applied to clean, dry, easily approximated wounds and require no additional dressing material. The glue is introduced over the edges of the approximated wound. The adhesive forms a closure over the incision and secures the closure over the skin. The incision remains visible for inspection and the adhesive forms a protective, occlusive antimicrobial barrier. Conversely, if the wound is contaminated, an infectious process can be sequestered.

Skin glue is available from several manufacturers and comes in blue, violet, and clear varieties. Before using skin glue, check the expiration date. The glue dries after 2.5 minutes and remains on the wound for 5 to 10 days. The glue is applied with an applicator along approximated, clean wound edges that are not under tension. The product can be applied in a long strand or in a series of closely aligned dots. Thick layers can produce an exothermic effect, and the patient can experience a burning sensation. This can be minimized by applying thin layers over top of each other. Adherence is compromised by a hairy or greasy surface. A protective dressing or splint can be applied after the glue is completely dry. The patient should be instructed to keep the area dry for 48 hours and not to apply any ointments, which could cause the glue to peel off prematurely. If the glue must be removed from tissue sooner, acetone can be used.

Methyl Methacrylate

Methyl methacrylate is used to augment fixation of pathologic fractures and to stabilize prosthetic devices in bone. It is an acrylic, cement-like substance commonly referred to as *bone cement*. It is a drug supplied in two sterile components that must be mixed together immediately before use. One component is a colorless, highly volatile, flammable, liquid methyl methacrylate monomer in an ampule. The powder component may contain antibiotic gentamycin or tobramycin.

This powerful liquid solvent must be handled carefully. The other component is a white powder mixture of polymethyl methacrylate, methyl methacrylate–styrene copolymer, and barium sulfate in a packet. The barium sulfate provides radiopacity to the substance. When the powder and liquid are mixed, an exothermic polymeric reaction forms a soft, pliable, dough-like mass. This reaction liberates heat as high as 230° F (110° C). As the reaction progresses, the substance becomes hard in a few minutes. The mixing and kneading of the entire contents of the liquid ampule and powder packet must be thorough and should continue for at least 2 to 4 minutes. Time may vary by the amount of powder and additives. The substance must be adequately soft and pliable for application to bone. The completion of polymerization occurs in the patient. After it hardens, it holds a prosthesis firmly in a fixed position.

A hazard to OR personnel has been reported in regard to the use of methyl methacrylate in the OR. Some personnel have experienced dizzy spells, difficulty breathing, and/or nausea and vomiting after mixing of methyl methacrylate. The fumes can cause severe eye irritation in people wearing gas-permeable contact lenses during the use of this chemical compound. The monomer and several of its ingredients are potent allergenic sensitizers when vapor is inhaled. Disposable mixing bowls with covers and vapor suction ports should be used. Closed containment models are available.

Patients can experience physiologic symptoms when the bone cement is used. Most common problems include hypoxia, hypotension, cardiac dysrhythmia, pulmonary vascular resistance, and cardiac arrest. The anesthesia provider must monitor the patient closely and should be alerted to the placement of the cement. The chemicals in the cement can cause many of these symptoms, but other causes, including fat embolism, have been cited.

Implantable Materials

Tissue deficiencies may require additional reinforcement or bridging material to obtain adequate wound healing. Sometimes edges of fascia, for example, cannot be brought together without excessive tension. In large or older patients the fascia cannot withstand this tension because of weakness caused by the infiltration of fat. Other implantable materials are used to produce subsurface modifications, such as breast enlargement.

Biologic or synthetic mesh materials are used to fill congenital, traumatic, or acquired defects in fascia or a body wall and to reinforce fascia, as in hernia repair.

Implants must be sterile and compatible with the recipient's tissues. The surgeon should note any allergies or sensitivities to metallic substances if any are to be used. Care is taken to ensure the correct size and handling regardless of the type of implantable used. Powderless gloves are recommended to prevent particulate distribution in the wound.

Administrative controls concerning implantable materials include documentation of the source material, the lot number in case of a recall, and special preparatory handling. The circulating nurse dispenses the implant to the sterile field and the scrub person readies the material for use. Implants should not be handled excessively to prevent damage to the surface or contamination with particulate or lint from the field.

Examples of implant uses and characteristics include, but are not limited to, the following:

- Dimensional subsurface space-holding devices, as in tissue expanders
- Load bearing as in orthopedic implants
- Passage creation as in a stent
- Bone integration for increased density
- Flexion with low friction, as in hernia mesh
- Subsurface modification such as testicular implants to replace missing parts
- Mechanical-electrical regulation of a body system such as pacemakers
- Drug delivery devices

Implants can be permanent or temporary and composed of many materials. Any implant that is removed (explanted) is usually sent to the pathology laboratory for accession (gross identification). Refer to Fig. 28.20 for a collective comparison of implants for tissue repair and replacement.

Biologic Materials

Fascia Lata

Strips of fascia lata are obtained from the fibrous connective tissue that covers thigh muscles of beef cattle. In lieu of commercial fascia lata (allogeneic graft), the surgeon may strip a piece of fascia from the patient's thigh (an **autologous graft**). Fascia lata also is obtained from cadavers and freeze-dried (an **allogeneic graft**). Fascia lata contains collagen. It increases the amount of tissue already present and becomes a living part of the tissue it supports. It is used to strengthen weakened fascial layers or to fill in defects in fascia.

Synthetic Materials

Synthetic Meshes

Synthetic meshes offer several advantages for reinforcing or bridging fascial or other tissue deficiencies:

1. They are easily cut to desired size for the defect.
2. They are easily sutured underneath the edges of tissue to create a smooth surface.
3. They are pliable to preclude erosion into major structures.

NATURAL (BIOLOGIC)				SYNTHETIC			
Autologous	**Allogeneic**	**Xenograft**	**Biomaterials**	**Chemical**	**Metallic**	**Polymer**	**Mechanical**
Skin	Bone	Porcine dermal collagen	Biodegradable fixation S-1 (CO_2 and H_2O)	Glial antibiotic disc	Plates/screws	Solid	Pacer
Cartilage	Tendon and ligament	Tricalcium phosphate	Hydroxyapatite ceramic	Bone cement	Rods	Expandable	Penile hydraulics
Bone	Cornea	Porcine heart valve	Bioengineered stent endothelial	Drug-eluting stent	Stent	Shunts	Medication pump
Muscle	Alloderm	Bovine xenograft screws	Bovine collagen polyester graft	Conduit graft	Joint	Stents	Cochlear components
Gut	Tissue matrix: Periosteal Chondrium	Calcium alginate gel	Bioengineered vessels	Mesh graft	Grid	Thermoplastic polymer	Heart assist device
Hair follicles	Fascia	Coral		Drug-eluting birth control device: IUD	Clips and staples	Liquid	Internal cardiovertor defibrillator
Vessels	Saphenous veins	Bovine collagen dressing			Metallic oxide, ceramic	Polyethylene	Nerve stimulator
Adipose	Heart valve	Bovine collagen matrix			Zirconium oxide	Polyurethane	
Stem cells	Ossicles	Porcine collagen matrix			Chromium oxide	Nonabsorbable ligating clip	
Mesenchyme	Bone marrow				Aluminum oxide	3D printed polymer reconstruction forms	
					Dental ceramic		

• **Fig. 28.20** Implants: tissue repair and replacement materials. *3D*, Three-dimensional; *IUD*, intrauterine device.

4. They are inert to avoid inflammatory response and minimize foreign body tissue reaction.
5. They are porous to allow free drainage of exudate.
6. Fibrous tissue easily grows through openings to incorporate mesh into tissue to maximize tensile strength.

The manufacturer's instructions must be followed for each type of mesh product. Unused mesh should be discarded and not reprocessed.

Polyester Fiber Mesh (Mersilene Mesh). Mesh remains soft and pliable in tissue but has limited elasticity. It is the least inert of the synthetic meshes. It is not preferred in the presence of infection or in contaminated wounds because of its multifilament construction. Polyester fibers are knitted by a process that interlocks each fiber juncture to prevent unraveling when cut. However, a minimum of 1 × 4 inch (6.5 mm) of mesh should extend beyond the suture line.

Polyglactin 910 Mesh (Vicryl Mesh). Mesh is knitted fibers of undyed and uncoated polyglactin 910. Because it is absorbed by hydrolysis, this mesh is intended for use as a buttress to provide temporary support during healing. The mesh acts as a scaffold for ingrowth of connective tissue. It may be used to support a traumatized spleen, kidney, or abdominal wall and to support facial fascia. Absorption is essentially complete in 60 to 90 days.

Polypropylene Mesh (Prolene Mesh, Marlex Mesh). Knitted mesh of polypropylene has high tensile strength and good elasticity. However, Marlex mesh is stiffer and exhibits greater fiber fatigue than does Prolene mesh. Because polypropylene is inert, it may be used in the presence of infection or during healing by second intention. Mesh is used to span and reinforce traumatic abdominal wall defects, incisional ventral hernias, large inguinal hernias, and other fascial deficiencies. It stimulates rapid tissue ingrowth through interstices of mesh. Mesh remains soft and pliable in tissues. It will not unravel when cut.

Polytetrafluoroethylene (Gore-Tex Soft Tissue Patch). A sheet of expanded PTFE may be used to repair hernias and tissue deficiencies that require prosthetic material. This material is flexible, soft, and porous to allow tissue ingrowth. It is not used in the presence of infection. It must be handled only with clean gloves or rubber-shod forceps.

Tissue Replacement Materials

For centuries surgeons have sought materials to replace parts of anatomy. Tissue may be absent or distorted because of congenital deformity, traumatic injury, degenerative disease, or surgical resection. Replacement or substitution of tissue may be possible with biologic dressings or implanted materials, or with synthetic prosthetic materials implanted in the body. An overview of the types of biologic and synthetic tissue replacement materials is given here. Their uses are referenced in other chapters by surgical specialty or procedure.

Tissue replacement materials may require reconstitution with sterile saline before use. The circulating nurse should record the lot number of the replacement material and the lot number of the saline used for preparation. Avoid the use of saline with preservative when preparing tissue replacement material. Small vials of saline diluent may contain a bacteriostatic preservative and may alter the tissue. IV saline is suitable for this process because it has no preservative.

Biologic Wound Cover

A biologic dressing temporarily covers an open surface defect in skin and underlying soft tissues. Although defects are usually the result of trauma such as burns, vascular or pressure necrosis can cause skin ulcers. Open wounds quickly become contaminated. The dressing arrests loss of fluid, reduces or eliminates microbial growth, and minimizes scarring. It promotes production of granulation tissue and epithelialization before healing by second or third intention. A fibrin-elastin biologic bonding adheres the dressing to exposed surfaces. Biologic dressings are dermal replacements. The source determines the type of dressing. Dermal substitutes are a matrix of different components such as human collagen, fibroblasts, and growth factors to regenerate skin cells.

Autograft

Skin is grafted from one part of the patient's body to another part. Skin grafts are described in Chapter 40 of this text.

Allograft

Human tissue obtained from one genetically dissimilar person (i.e., unmatched donor) is grafted to another person. This is referred to as an *allograft*. Negative HIV and hepatitis B virus (HBV) status of donor and recipient should be determined and documented before use. Any natural body tissue transferred from one human to another must be free of infection.

Cryopreserved Skin. Allograft skin provides a protective covering that initially acquires, and then eventually loses, vascular connection with underlying tissue. A cadaver usually is the source of skin for a dermal allograft. Cryopreservation maintains viability of skin during prolonged storage. Skin is frozen by cooling at a rate of 1.8° F to 9° F (−16.8° C to −12.8° C) to −94° F (−70° C) until frozen and then stored in a liquid nitrogen freezer.

Immediately before use, skin is warmed by immersion in sterile water at 107.6° F (42° C), the maximum compatible with cellular viability.

Skin should be warmed at a rate of 90° F to 126° F (32−52° C) per minute. (The patient's own skin can be cryopreserved for prolonged storage for later use as an autograft.) Allografts may be obtained from a skin bank.

For storage of allografts or autografts up to 14 days, skin may be placed in isotonic saline solution or tissue nutrient medium and refrigerated at 33.8° F to 50° F (1−10° C).

Amniotic Membrane. Prepared from human placenta, amniotic membranes can be used as biologic dressings to promote the healing of burns, skin ulcers, and infected wounds and cover defects such as spina bifida. The placenta has two loosely connected membranes: amnion is used for partial-thickness wounds, and chorion is used for full-thickness defects.[7] Membranes are prepared by cleaning blood and clots from the placenta immediately after delivery, placing the placenta in an iodophor solution, and refrigerating it at 39° F (4° C). Membranes should be stripped from the placenta within 36 hours after delivery. Amnion can be used fresh, preserved, frozen, or dried. It may be obtained from a tissue bank that prepares and stores amniotic membranes.

Xenograft

With xenograft, skin obtained from a dissimilar species may be placed on human tissue as a temporary dressing.

Porcine Dermis. Porcine (pig) skin is used to cover body surfaces denuded of full-thickness skin until permanent skin grafting can be accomplished. Vascularization does not occur, but the xenograft adheres tightly while reepithelialization proceeds underneath it. It may remain in place for as long as 2 weeks before it dries up and peels off spontaneously. Porcine biologic dressings are available in rolls or strips. They may be prepared fresh for refrigeration, fresh frozen, irradiated and then frozen, or dried. Some dressings are soaked in an iodophor and should not be placed on a patient allergic to iodine. Dressings must be prepared and used according to the manufacturer's instructions.

Artificial Skin. A skin substitute may be prepared from a layer of collagen obtained from the dermis of a calf or pig and coated with autologous epithelium obtained from the recipient. Another type is synthesized from a bilayered polymeric membrane. The top layer is silicone elastomer. The bottom layer is a porous, cross-linked network of collagen and glycosaminoglycan. This artificial skin is biodegradable, but it can be used as a temporary covering that is similar to porcine xenografts.

Biologic Materials

Autologous tissues may be grafted or transferred from one part of the patient's body to another. Allograft tissues or organs may be transplanted from another human. Xenograft biomaterials may be used to supplement tissues.

Standards are set by the American Association of Tissue Banks for screening donors and retrieving, processing, and preserving allogeneic tissues, including skin, cartilage, bone, and blood vessels. Potential donors of allografts are tested for HIV and HBV. Excluded from donating are people who are HIV-positive or who have a history of hepatitis, an active infection, an immune disorder, or a suspected prion disease.

Bone Grafts

A bone graft affords structural support and a pattern for regrowth of bone within a skeletal defect. Cancellous bone is porous. Its porosity permits tissue fluid to reach deeper into it than into cortical bone, and thus most of the bone cells live. Cortical bone is used for bridging large skeletal defects because it gives greater strength. It may be fixed in the recipient site by means of metallic sutures or screws. Bone obtained from the crest of the ilium or a rib is cancellous and cortical bone; cortical bone is obtained from the tibia. The main purpose of a bone graft is to stimulate new bone growth.

Autologous bone, which is obtained from the patient, usually is taken from the ilium, tibia, or ribcage at the time of the surgical procedure. Calvarial bone from the frontal, parietal, or occipital cranial bones may be harvested for maxillofacial bone grafts. A free bone graft with its vascular pedicle, such as a free fibular graft, may be obtained for revascularization by microvascular anastomosis after removal of dead (avascular) bone. A separate, small sterile table may be prepared for the instrumentation required for the donor site. If the recipient area is potentially contaminated, the donor site must not be cross-contaminated from the recipient site.

Allogeneic bone, which is obtained from a cadaver, is dead bone. This bone is weaker than autologous bone, thus requiring a longer time of immobilization. Union occurs from bone regeneration in the recipient with this type of bone graft. It may be desirable, however, to spare the patient the added operating time and trauma of removing an autologous graft.

Composite bone grafts are freeze-dried allografts combined with autologous particulate cancellous bone and marrow. A crib formed from a cadaver bone (e.g., rib) is packed with the patient's bone particles and marrow. When implanted to reconstruct bony defects, the composite graft induces bone regeneration in the recipient site. The freeze-dried allograft is biodegradable by slow resorption. Eventually it is replaced by mature, functional bone.

Decalcified bone and demineralized bone chips or powder, prepared from homogeneous bone, also are used to stimulate bone regeneration or to fill defects in bone. This material is sterilized and stored at room temperature. For use, it is soaked in lactated Ringer solution. The powder then becomes a paste that can be used to fill a depressed area or to caulk an irregularity (e.g., in craniofacial reconstruction).

Bone Bank. Bone may be preserved and stored in a bone bank until needed. Autologous bone may be preserved after the surgical procedure by storage in a bone bank for subsequent grafting into the same patient. Bone such as a rib or femoral head may be salvaged from patients (i.e., living donors) who are free of malignancy or infection for an allogeneic graft into another person. Bone also may be obtained from cadavers (i.e., nonliving donors).

Bone used for allografts must be clean and sterile. Immediately after removal, bone marrow, fat, and blood are rinsed out with sterile distilled water or normal saline solution. The bone may be put in sterile nested glass jars or double plastic or metal containers. If it is to be used for an allogeneic graft, a small piece of bone is put into a sterile Petri dish and sent to the laboratory for culture tests. Bone should never be used until negative results of culture and serology are received. Several methods are used to preserve bone:

- Freezing is the most common method of preserving bone. Bone is quick-frozen in a freezer at $-94°$ F ($-70°$ C) or in liquid nitrogen. If bone will be used within 6 months, it can be stored in a refrigerator freezer at $-4°$ F to $-5°$ F ($-20°$ C to $-20.6°$ C). For prolonged storage of more than 6 months, the freezer temperature must be maintained below $-4°$ F ($-20°$ C) to avoid damage from a buildup of ice crystals.

Bone frozen by liquid nitrogen is stored in vapor at about $-238°$ F ($-150°$ C). The container initially is placed on a shelf labeled "Not Ready for Use." It is labeled "Sterile" and moved to the freezer compartment labeled "Ready for Use" when negative results of culture and serology tests are recorded on the identification card. Bone is thawed rapidly immediately before grafting.

- Freeze-drying requires specialized equipment that removes moisture as the freezing process takes place in a condenser with a vacuum cycle.

- Ethylene oxide sterilization ensures safety of bone. It must be aerated for 72 hours before storage at room temperature or in a refrigerator. When protected from air and contamination, sterilized bone can be stored indefinitely, although a 1-year expiration date is recommended if bone is placed in a heat-sealed, peel-apart package.

- Packaged bone may be shipped in dry ice to a center equipped to sterilize it by gamma irradiation.

- Formaldehyde solution, 0.25% to 1% concentration, may have a bacteriostatic effect around the graft site in infected or contaminated wounds, such as in osteomyelitis. During storage, temperature is maintained at 35.6° F to 39° F (2–3.8° C) in a refrigerator.

The container must be labeled with donor information and not used until laboratory reports are available. The donor must be seronegative for hepatitis B surface antigen and HIV. Bone from a living donor is quarantined for 90 days, awaiting results of a repeat test for HIV.

Xenograft Bone Implant

Coralline hydroxyapatite, which is composed of skeletons of sea coral, and collagen may be used to replace facial or cranial bone. This material has hardness, mineral content, and porosity similar to that of human bone. These implants stimulate bone growth into the porous architecture of the coral.

Organ Transplants

Some whole body organs can be transplanted from one human to another. This is done in an effort to sustain life by compensating for physiologic deficits or inadequate function of vital organs. Organ transplants are discussed in Chapter 45 of this text.

Tissue Transplants

Skin and blood vessels are frequently transplanted from one part of the body to another. These are referred to as *autografts* because the patient is both donor and recipient. The transplanted tissue becomes a part of the living tissue in the recipient site.

Some tissues can be transplanted from one person to another to restore function, such as the cornea, or to provide support in structures, such as cartilage in nasal reconstruction. These are referred to as *allografts*. Some allografts are commercially prepared, such as lyophilized human dura mater and human umbilical cord vein graft.

Human Dura Mater. A trimmed and measured piece of cadaver dura mater is freeze-dried, sterilized by exposure to ethylene oxide, and stored in a vacuum container. It may be stored at room temperature indefinitely, provided the vacuum is maintained. The graft is reconstituted by the addition of normal saline solution to the container for a minimum of 30 minutes. Most of these grafts are used for closure of dural defects, but they also may be used to repair abdominal and thoracic wall and diaphragmatic defects.

Neurologic tissue for transplant may harbor the prion responsible for the development of Creutzfeldt-Jakob disease (CJD). Routine sterilization does not render this material safe for use in the presence of CJD. Routine testing does not reveal CJD contamination.

Human Umbilical Cord Vein Graft

A cryopreservation process converts an umbilical vein into an inert, antithrombogenic graft. A polyester mesh covering over the outer surface allows tissue ingrowth and provides added strength. Commercially supplied, an allograft-modified human umbilical vein graft is an acceptable graft material for arterial reconstruction when an autologous saphenous vein is not available.

The graft is thoroughly rinsed with sterile saline, heparinized saline, or lactated Ringer's solution before implantation. A series of three basins filled with sterile solution of choice are used for the rinse process. The basins should be set up on a separate sterile surface, away from the main sterile field, and discarded after use.

After rinsing, the graft should remain moist until implanted. Only noncrushing clamps should be used to avoid damage to the graft during handling.

Xenograft Biomaterials

In addition to porcine skin used as biologic dressings, artificial skin derived from the collagen of a calf or pig, allogeneic bone, and other materials derived from animals are commercially prepared for tissue replacement. Some are supplied in glutaraldehyde solution and require rinsing before use. Follow the recommended rinsing instructions.

Arteriovenous Shunts. Enzymatically treated bovine carotid artery xenografts are used for blood access in patients on hemodialysis therapy who have poor blood vessels or in whom it is difficult to create either fistulas or shunts. Femoral arteriovenous bovine shunts can be punctured innumerable times with a low incidence of thrombus formation.

Collagen. Collagen is used in its natural form, such as a processed bovine graft and microfibrillar hemostatic powder, and restructured into membranes or films. It can be injected into middle to deep dermis to fill and smooth nasolabial furrows and facial creases. It is implanted to correct soft tissue defects and contours. The duration of effect is 4 to 6 months. Collagen can be altered by a variety of techniques to change its physical properties and duration of action in tissue.

Corium. Corium implants are prepared from porcine dermis to replace tissue loss or to support tissues. They can be used as a fascia lata substitute or dural replacement or to repair tympanic membrane, hernia, or bladder sling. Corium will form a collagen matrix to close a defect in soft tissues around teeth.

Human Skin Equivalent. Bioengineered skin product, referred to as Apligraf, is derived from bovine collagen and human tissue taken from discarded foreskins of circumcised newborns. The mixture takes 5 days to generate and grow under sterile conditions in the laboratory. It is specially ordered for each patient and cannot be stored for additional uses. The cell culture mixture is applied to nonhealing wounds, such as venous stasis ulcers after debridement. More information can be found at http://www.apligraf.com/.

Synthetic Materials

A prosthesis is a permanent or temporary replacement for a missing or malfunctioning structure. Some synthetic implants replace vital structures, such as diseased heart valves and blood vessels. Devices such as pacemakers assist the function of vital organs. Other materials are used to repair or replace defects.

Care is taken to determine whether the patient has an allergy to any metals.[8] Some metallic devices can have a nickel component, and patients who are sensitive to nickel can have an augmented inflammatory response to the metal. Prosthetic materials implanted into the body must:

- Be compatible with physiologic processes
- Produce no or minimal tissue reaction
- Be sterile so they will not cause infection or become a culture medium
- Be noncarcinogenic or other disease causative
- Have viable and adequate tissue coverage, unless used as a biologic dressing over denuded skin surfaces
- Have adequate blood supply through or around them
- Be stable so that they will not degenerate or change shape if used for permanent function
- Contour or conform to normal tissue configuration as desired

Permanently implanted devices can provide support, restore function, and augment or restore body contour. Inorganic substances cannot unite with tissue, however. Their physiologic responses may be predictable. All synthetic materials implanted in contact with blood will activate coagulation and promote the process of thrombosis. The surface of some materials is less thrombogenic (i.e., less likely to form clots) than those of others.

The magnitude of the inflammatory response they stimulate varies in patients. An immune response may cause chronic inflammation from bacterial adhesion, such as biofilm. Infection that develops around a prosthesis usually necessitates its removal. Most infections arise from microorganisms inoculated into the wound at the time of implantation. Therefore meticulous sterile technique is mandatory.

Prosthetic implants must not be flash sterilized. They must be sterilized in a standard cycle for the agent used (see Chapter 17). The cycle should be monitored with a biologic indicator, and a negative biologic test result should be confirmed before the implant is used. Implants sterilized by the manufacturer are preferred because the sterilization controls are closely monitored. Biologic testing is imperative for any implant.

Carbon Fiber

Pure carbon fibers braided into a strip are used for ligament replacement and articular resurfacing. Inert in tissue, carbon fiber stimulates regrowth of connective tissue and cartilage. The fibers may be braided with polypropylene or coated with a resorbable gelatin or lyophilized dura. The prosthesis should be soaked in normal saline solution before implantation to facilitate handling.

Metal

Stainless steel, a cobalt alloy (with the trade name Vitallium), and titanium are manufactured into prosthetic implants. Used primarily for stabilization of bone, metal implants must be strong enough to withstand the stress of weight bearing or muscular action and must not corrode in body tissues. They are never reused because of the weakening that can occur with use.

Special care must be taken in handling metal implants to protect the surfaces. A simple scratch on a metal implant can lead to its corrosion in the body. The implant will be bathed continuously by weakly chloride body fluids. If corrosion begins, the implant may fail and have to be removed. It is very important therefore that all metal implants be protected from scratches. This can be accomplished by:

1. Wrapping each implant individually, or wrapping sets with each size implant (i.e., screws and plates) in a separate compartment, for both storage and sterilization. Most prostheses come from the manufacturer in protective coverings or cases. Some of these are suitable for adequate sterilization, with subsequent placement in the sterile field to minimize handling before implantation.
2. Preventing implants from coming into contact with other hard surfaces of metal or glass, both during storage and sterilization and on the instrument table.
3. Not handling or transferring an unprotected implant with any type of forceps. Implants of one metal should not come into contact with those of another metal because an electrochemical reaction occurs between metals. Two different metals are not implanted in the same patient for this reason. Instruments used for insertion also should be of the same metal as the implant (e.g., a stainless steel screwdriver and screw).

Methyl Methacrylate

A highly refined methyl methacrylate mixture can be molded and shaped to fit a defect in bone. When it hardens, this material looks and feels very much like bone. It is used to repair a skull. In some patients the chemicals in the cement can cause neurotoxic effects.

Polyester Fiber

Polyester fibers (Dacron) woven or knitted into seamless cylinders are used to replace major arteries.

Polyethylene

Polyethylene tubing may be inserted into structures such as fallopian tubes or ureters to give support during healing or to bridge a defect in tissue continuity. Polyethylene may be combined with silicon to produce a thromboresistant coating for vascular grafts and artificial hearts.

Implants of porous polyethylene are used for anatomic reconstruction, such as of the external ear. The porosity of the implant encourages both soft tissue and vascular ingrowth. Collagen deposited along the framework adds strength. Porous polyethylene is a strong, flexible material that can be molded or shaped to the desired configuration. When dipped into boiling normal saline solution, the material becomes pliable for molding by hand. An implant can be shaped by cutting with a scalpel blade. Glove powder, lint, and dust particles must not adhere to the implant because they can cause a foreign body reaction around the implant.

Polytetrafluoroethylene (Teflon)

Some prostheses or parts of prosthetic devices are made of the polymer PTFE. It may be woven into a fabric for arterial grafts, extruded into tubing for struts, or molded into a solid configuration for valves or joints. Its flexibility makes it a useful replacement for tissues when motion is desirable.

Silicone

Silicone is one of the most inert of the synthetic polymers used for implantation. It has a durable and nonthrombogenic surface. It is used in many forms: gel, sponge, film, tubing, liquid, and preformed molded anatomic structures. It may be coated with polyurethane or polyester or used as an elastomer to coat

polyester. A medical-grade silicone elastomer (Silastic) in one form or another is used in virtually every surgical specialty for tissue reconstruction or replacement. Silicone may migrate from a ruptured or leaking gel or liquid-filled implant and cause systemic illness.

Complete instructions for cleaning and sterilizing silicone implants before use are supplied by the manufacturer with each type of prosthesis. These instructions must be followed meticulously. Implants are not handled with bare hands, and care must be taken to ensure they do not pick up lint and dust. Gloves worn during handling must be entirely free of powder. Skin oil, lint, dust, powder, and other surface contaminants can evoke foreign body reactions around the implant in tissue.

Skin Closure

In addition to sutures, staples, and skin glue, other materials may be used to hold skin edges in approximation.

Wound Silo

A sterile, clear plastic, round or tubular cover can be placed over areas of evisceration or dehiscence until the abdomen can be primarily closed. The silo is sometimes referred to as a *Bogotá bag* after the Colombian surgeons who described its use after performing open fasciotomies of the abdomen in compartment syndrome. This device is useful in covering congenital gastroschisis of the abdomen in newborns until a repair can be made.

The silo creates a see-through barrier over the abdomen and viscera as a temporary closure device. It can be used with a wound vacuum dressing. Some facilities use empty sterilized 3-L intravenous (IV) bags sutured or clipped to the skin. Commercial silos are available in adult and pediatric sizes.

Skin Closure Strips

Adhesive-backed strips of microporous nylon (Proxi-Strip) or polypropylene (Steri-Strip) or rayon acetate are placed at intervals across the line of incision. They may be used to approximate skin edges of superficial lacerations, as the primary closure of skin in conjunction with subcuticular suture, or in conjunction with interrupted skin sutures or staples. Often they are used after early suture or staple removal to support the wound during healing. A skin tackifier, such as tincture of benzoin, may be recommended by the manufacturer for ensuring adhesion to skin.

Sterile strips are available in various widths and lengths. They are ethylene oxide gas—sterilized in peel packets by the manufacturer. Skin closure strips have the following advantages:

- They may be used in the emergency department on superficial lacerations to eliminate the need for sutures that would require local anesthesia for placement and subsequent return of the patient for suture removal.
- They eliminate foreign body tissue reaction of suture material in skin.
- They have enough porosity to permit adequate ventilation of clean or contaminated wounds.
- They permit removal of sutures within 32 to 48 hours postoperatively. Crosshatch scarring (referred to as *railroad tracks*) and the possibility of infection are reduced when sutures are removed early. Skin closure strips provide long-term wound reinforcement and support.
- They permit visibility of the healing wound so that the surgeon can see how well the wound edges have coated. Some strips are

translucent; others have a color tone or opacity that does not afford this advantage.

- They minimize skin irritation because they are hyporeactive.
- They can be applied and removed rapidly.
- They can be easily cut to meet exact length requirements.

The team should keep in mind that the external part of the closure is what the patient sees and on which an opinion of the entire surgical experience is based. The shape of the repaired site and scar formation can lead the patient to believe that surgery was unsuccessful. Proper closure and wound care can help minimize scarring and preserve the patient's self-esteem.

Ⓔ EVOLVE WEBSITE

http://evolve.elsevier.com/Hornacky/BerryKohn/

- Historical Perspective
- Student Interactive Questions
- Glossary

References

1. Robinson K: Materials for wound closure. www.emedicine.medscape.com. Accessed May 17, 2023.
2. Lista F, Austin R, Ahmad J: Reduction mammoplasty with short scar techniques. In, Nelican PC, editor: *Plastic surgery*, vol. 5. St. Louis, MO, 2018, Elsevier, pp 160−173.
3. Lammers R, Scrimshaw L: Methods of wound closure. In Roberts JR, Custalow CB, Thomsen TW, editors: *Roberts and Hedges' clinical procedures in emergency medicine and acute care*, ed 7, St. Louis, MO, 2019, Elsevier, pp 655−707.
4. Lee S, Garrett K, Milsom J: Combined endoscopic and laparoscopic surgery (CELS), *Semin Colon Rectal Surg* 29(4):237−243, 2018.
5. Miyoshi N, Shiki F, Junichi N: Effectiveness of triclosan-coated sutures compared with uncoated sutures in preventing surgical site infection abdominal wall closure in open/laparoscopic colorectal surgery, *J Am Coll Surg* 234(6):1147−1159, 2022.
6. Danker W, DeAnglis A, Ferko N, et al.: Comparison of fibrin sealants in peripheral vascular surgery: a systemic review and network meta-analysis, *Ann Med Surg* 61, 2021.
7. Anitua E, Nurden P, Prado R, et al.: Autologous fibrin scaffolds: when platelet and plasma derived biomolecules meet fibrin, *Biomaterials* 192:440−460, 2018.
8. Christensen T, Samant S, Shin A: Making sense of metal allergy and hypersensitivity to metallic implants in relation to hand surgery, *J Hand Surg Am* 42(9):737−746, 2017.

Bibliography

AORN: *Guidelines for perioperative practice*, Denver, CO, 2024, The Association.

29

Wound Healing and Hemostasis

CHAPTER OUTLINE

Mechanism of Wound Healing, 584

Types of Wounds, 585

Factors Influencing Wound Healing, 586

Hemostasis, 589

Wound Management, 598

Complications of Wound Healing, 604

Postoperative Wound Infections, 606

Wound Assessment, 607

Basic Wound Care, 607

CHAPTER OBJECTIVES

After studying this chapter, the learner will be able to:

- Identify tissue layers specific to the anatomic site of a wound.
- List several factors that affect wound healing.
- Describe the three mechanisms of wound healing.

- List three complications of wound healing.
- Describe three dressing materials and their application.

KEY TERMS AND DEFINITIONS

Adhesion Band of scar tissue that holds together or unites surfaces or structures that are normally separated.

Chronic wound Tissue with an injury in a patient with an underlying condition that takes longer than average to heal.

Cicatrix Firm avascular scar tissue.

Contracture Formation of extensive scar tissue over a joint.

Dead space Space caused by separation of wound edges or by air trapped between layers of tissue.

Debridement Removal of damaged tissue and cellular or other debris from a wound to promote healing and prevent infection.

Decubitus ulcer A chronic wound caused by prolonged pressure.

Dehiscence Partial or total splitting open or separation of the layers of a wound.

Devitalized Tissue that is nonviable, necrotic.

Edema Abnormal accumulation of fluid in interstitial spaces of tissues.

Epithelialization Epithelial cells regenerate over a wound.

Eschar Granular tissue around the edges of a chronic wound. It can be firm and dark or soft and beige.

Evisceration Protrusion of viscera through an abdominal incision.

Exsanguination Tissue is drained of blood.

Extravasation Passage of blood, serum, or lymph into tissues.

Exudate Fluid, cells, or other substances that have been discharged from vessels or tissues. It contains white blood cells, lymphokines, and growth factors that stimulate healing.

Friable tissue Tissue is fragile and bleeds easily.

Granulation tissue Formation of fibrous collagen to fill the gap between the edges of a wound healing with contraction (i.e., second intention).

Granuloma Inflammatory lesion that forms around a foreign substance, such as glove powder or a suture knot.

Hematoma Collection of extravasated blood in tissue.

Hemostasis Arrest of blood flow or hemorrhage; the mechanism is via coagulation (formation of a blood clot).

Hypertrophic scar Excessive raised dense scarring that does not exceed the border of the wound.

Iatrogenic Condition caused by treatment or procedure performed by medical personnel.

Incision Intentional cut through intact tissue (synonymsurgical incision).

Inflammation Increased blood flow to injured tissue as part of the healing process.

Ischemia Decrease of blood supply to tissues.

Keloid Overgrowth of firm rounded scar that extends beyond the border of the wound. Can be painful and may bleed if injured.

Necrosis Death of tissue cells; devitalized tissue.

Occlusive dressing A dressing that permits air, but prevents the passage of fluids in or out of the covering. Sealed over all edges.

Scar Deposition of fibrous connective tissue to bridge separated wound edges and restore continuity of tissues.

Seroma Collection of extravasated serum from interstitial tissue or a resolving hematoma in tissue.

Tensile strength Ability of tissues to resist rupture.

Tissue reaction Immune response of the body to tissue injury or foreign substances.

Ulcer Skin layers are lost as a result of decreased arterial circulation or obstructed venous drainage.

Wound disruption Separation of wound edges.

Mechanism of Wound Healing

Interruption of tissue integrity, either intentional or unintentional, requires understanding of the mechanism and factors that cause wounding and influence wound healing. When tissue is cut, the body's inherent defense mechanisms respond immediately to begin repair. Three mechanisms of wound healing are recognized: first intention/primary union, second intention, and third intention/delayed primary closure (Fig. 29.1). Each mechanism has practical applications in the making and closing of incisions or traumatic wounds. The degree of contamination and the amount of viable tissue are factors in the determination of which method of healing is used.

First Intention/Primary Union

Healing by first intention is desired after primary union of an incised, aseptic, accurately approximated wound. Well-approximated wounds form a fibrin bridge that aids healing. A closed system drain may be used. Key elements of first-intention closure include the following[1]:

- No tissue loss
- Well-approximated edges with suture, wound sealant, or wound-closure strips

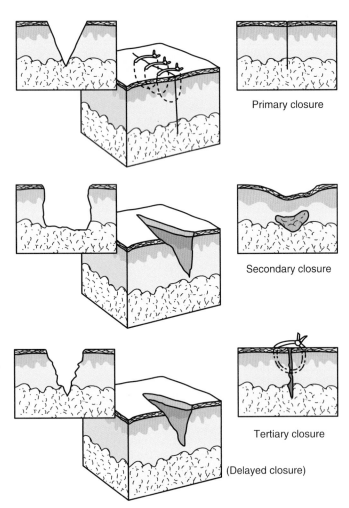

Primary closure

Secondary closure

Tertiary closure

(Delayed closure)

• **Fig. 29.1** Mechanisms of wound healing. (From Trott AT: *Wounds and lacerations: emergency care and closure,* ed 3, St. Louis, 2005, Mosby.)

- Minimal or no postoperative swelling
- No serous discharge or local infection
- No separation of wound edges
- Minimal scar formation

The rates and patterns of wound healing differ in various tissues. In general, first-intention wound healing consists of three distinct phases:

1. *Lag phase of acute inflammatory response:* Tissue fluids containing plasma, proteins, blood cells, fibrin, and antibodies exude from the tissues into the wound, depositing fibrin, which weakly holds the wound edges together for the first 5 days.

   Fibrin and serum protein dry out and form a scab that seals the wound from further fluid loss and microbial invasion. At the same time, fibroblasts, fibrous tissue germ cells, and epithelial cells migrate from the general circulation. Subsequent adhesion of these cells, a process known as fibroplasia, holds the wound edges together. Leukocytes and other white blood cells produce proteolytic enzymes to dissolve and remove damaged tissue debris. Macrophages and neutrophils ingest foreign material, cellular debris, and bacteria.

2. *Healing or proliferative phase of fibroplasia:* After the fifth postoperative day, fibroblasts multiply rapidly, bridging wound edges and restoring the continuity of body structures. Collagen, a protein substance that is the chief constituent of connective tissue, is secreted from the fibroblasts and formed into fibers.

   Reepithelialization causes the rapid gain in tensile strength and pliability of the healing wound. Tensile strength is the ability of the tissues to resist rupture. The healing phase begins rapidly, diminishes progressively, and terminates on about the 14th day. It may continue for up to 20 days.

3. *Maturation or differentiation phase:* From the 14th postoperative day until the wound is fully healed, scar formation occurs by deposition of fibrous connective tissue. The collagen content remains constant, but the fiber pattern reforms and cross-links to increase the tensile strength. Wound complete closure occurs over a period of weeks up to 6 months. As collagen density increases, vascularity decreases and the scar grows pale. The scar tissue is only 80% as strong as the original tissue.

Second Intention

The mechanism of second-intention healing is by granulation, eventual reepithelialization, and wound contraction rather than with suturing closed by first intention. The wound heals from the bottom up; it heals spontaneously if the dermal base is preserved. The following are considerations with this type of healing:

1. Infection, excessive trauma, loss of tissue, and poorly approximated tissue are common. Inflammatory response is exaggerated.

2. The wound is left open and allowed to heal from the inner toward the outer surface. Eschar forms around the edges and can be softened and removed with chemical treatment. Devitalized tissue is debrided.

   a. In some wounds, the use of maggot therapy is useful for debridement.

   b. Debridement of devitalized tissue can be performed with scissors or a knife.

c. The wound can be packed with dressing material that attaches to the necrotic tissue. When the packing is removed, the dead tissue separates from the wound bed, leaving a red beefy surface.
3. Healing is delayed. The wound may need grafting.
4. Healing may produce a weak union, which may be conducive to incisional herniation later.
5. The risk for secondary infection is proportional to the amount of necrotic tissue present in the wound and to compromised immune response in the patient. Repeated debridement may be necessary.
6. Scar formation is excessive.
7. Contracture of skin is pronounced. After healing is complete, the scar may need revision or release.

Third Intention/Delayed Primary Closure

Approximation and suturing are delayed or secondary for the purpose of walling off an area of gross infection or an area where extensive tissue was removed (e.g., in a debridement or from a traumatic injury). The edges are closed 4 to 6 days postoperatively after meticulous debridement.[2] The following are considerations in healing by third intention:
1. The wound is cleaned and debrided.
2. The defect is packed with moist gauze to promote drainage and granulation.
3. Antibiotic therapy is implemented.
4. The wound may be an old traumatic or septic wound.
5. The area should not be devascularized, and deep sutures should be avoided. Granulomas can form.
6. Two clean surfaces of granulation tissue are brought together for later closure.
7. A deeper and wider scar usually results.

Types of Wounds

A wound is an injury, either intentional or unintentional, that disrupts the continuity of body tissues with or without tissue loss. Wounds may be surgical (intentional), traumatic, incidental, or chronic.

Intentional Wounds
Surgical-Site Incision or Excision

An incision is a cut or an opening into intact tissue. An excision is removal of tissue. A sterile sharp scalpel, scissors, curette, or other cutting instrument may be used to separate skin and underlying tissues. Thermal instruments that both cut or vaporize tissue and coagulate surrounding blood vessels are used for incision and excision. The location, length, and depth of an incision must be planned.

The surgeon spreads the skin taut between the thumb and index finger in preparation for the skin incision. With one stroke of evenly applied perpendicular pressure on the scalpel, a clean incision is made through the epidermis and dermis into the subcutaneous layers. The following factors influence the ease with which a primary skin incision is made:
• Sharpness, shape, and size of the knife blade
• Resistance of self-adhering plastic drapes
• Toughness of skin or scar tissue
• Thickness of subcutaneous tissue
A clean stroke with a sterile surgical scalpel, followed by attention to all of the principles of sterile technique and tissue

handling, is the best insurance for healing by first intention. The line of direction of the incision in relation to the natural lines of direction of the skin may be a factor in wound healing. Excess tension on the healing wound can delay wound healing. Wounds heal side to side, not end to end.

Other Types of Intentional Wounds
Occlusion Banding
Hemorrhoid ligation results in ischemia and degeneration of a hemorrhoid. A Silastic band is placed around the hemorrhoid using a special spring-loaded applicator. Other types of occlusion banding are performed on fallopian tubes with ligatures, Silastic bands, or plastic clips through a laparoscope. Portions of tissue distal to the occlusion point separate from perfused tissues, interrupting the continuity of the lumen of the part in the banding process.

Chemical Wounds
Chemicals can be intentionally applied to skin or other tissue surfaces to denude or coagulate the area. These chemicals cause inflammation and reepithelialization of the surface. This procedure is common in facial peels used in plastic and dermatologic surgery.

Traumatic Wounds

After traumatic injury, preservation of life is the first critical concern. The patient's general condition is of prime consideration, and the plan of care is individualized to meet the patient's needs. Injuries are evaluated, and those that pose the greatest hazards to life or to return to normal function are cared for first.

The primary objective after life support is wound closure with minimal deformity and functional loss.[3] Minor injuries are cared for in the emergency department (ED). Patients with major injuries undergo treatment in the ED before going to the operating room (OR) as quickly as the condition warrants. Traumatic wounds can be considered closed or open, simple or complicated, clean or contaminated. Wound closure is predicated on the type, location, severity, and extent of injury.

Closed Wounds
Skin is intact in a closed wound, but underlying tissues and/or organs are injured. A blister filled with serum or a hematoma of blood and serum may form under the epidermis. Torn ligaments and simple fractures are closed wounds.

Open Wounds
In open wounds, the skin is broken by abrasion, laceration, or penetration.

Simple Wounds
Continuity of skin is interrupted in simple wounds but without loss or destruction of tissue and without implantation of a foreign body. These lacerations are usually caused by a sharp-edged object cutting or penetrating at a low velocity. These wounds can be closed by first intention unless underlying structures or organs have been injured.

Complicated Wounds
In complicated wounds, tissue is lost or destroyed by crush or burn or a foreign body is implanted by high-velocity penetration. If a penetrating wound was made by an object, such as a knife or

bullet, this object is not removed until the surgeon explores the wound in the OR. The device should be stabilized to prevent additional injury. Movement of a foreign object may cause further trauma. The depth of a penetrating wound is irrigated and may be excised.

The complicated wound may be closed by second or third intention. Skin grafting may be necessary if the dermis has been destroyed. Any object removed from the patient's wound may be forensic evidence. The hospital's policy and procedure manual should be consulted for guidance on handling potential police evidence.

Clean Wounds

Clean wounds heal by first intention after closure of all tissue layers and wound edges. The cosmetic care of lacerated areas is important, as is treatment to provide normal function and satisfactory appearance of a part.

Contaminated Wounds

When dirty objects penetrate skin, microorganisms multiply rapidly. Within 6 hours, contamination can become infection. Debridement is performed to remove devitalized tissue, and the wound is irrigated. Devitalized tissue is removed because it acts as a culture medium. The wound may be left open to heal by second or third intention. Closure may be delayed for several days.

The patient's history should be assessed for tetanus bacillus immunization. Tetanus is most likely to occur in deep wounds contaminated by soil or animal feces. Adsorbed tetanus toxoid (0.5 mL) may be given as an initial immunizing dose or as a booster if the patient has been immunized within the previous 5 years. Tetanus immune globulin (human, 250–500 units) also should be given to any patient who has a severe wound or who has had the wound for more than 24 hours and has not been immunized within the previous 10 years.

Delayed Full-Thickness Injury

Industrial accidents commonly include crush injury or deep injection of substances, such as paint or printer's ink, beyond the level of the dermis. The full extent of the tissue damage may not be apparent for several days after the event because the effects of the injury cause increasing tissue loss. The patient may have occlusive dressings or casting for the initial apparent injuries but should be continually assessed for signs of increasing tissue necrosis or full-thickness tissue loss. Electrocution or lightning strikes act similarly by causing deep tissue necrosis several days after the initial wounding.

Incidental and Chronic Wounds

Pressure sores and decubitus ulcers may result from compromised circulation over bony prominences or other pressure points for extended periods. Positioning and padding considerations in the plan of care can help prevent incidental pressure-related injuries in the perioperative environment.

Ulcers

Venous stasis or arterial insufficiency in the legs may cause chronic skin ulcers. Arterial ulcers are pale, dry, and circumscribed. Venous ulcers are wet and irregular in shape. Tissue necrosis may occur after radiation therapy. These chronic wounds have tissue loss and usually have heavy bacterial contamination. Topical application of fibronectin (a platelet-derived wound-healing

formula) or some other preparation of growth factors from the patient's own blood may help control infection and promote healing. Growth factors stimulate the growth of tissue, capillaries, and skin. If a wound fails to heal by second intention with formation of granulation tissue, debridement and skin grafting may be necessary.

Iatrogenic Wounds

Iatrogenic wounds can happen as the result of therapy or treatment such as radiation burns. Accidental injuries such as trocar wounds on unintended organs caused during a surgical procedure can be classified as iatrogenic. The treatment and healing vary according to the mechanism of injury.

Factors Influencing Wound Healing

Each patient has internal and external forces that influence healing. Most wounds progress to healing unless the closure is poor, an infection ensues, or the tissue is devitalized by other forces. Hemostatic and inflammatory responses must be intact for healing to take place.

The degree of wound contamination is evaluated, and the potential risk for postoperative wound infection is considered. At the conclusion of the surgical procedure, the wound is assigned a classification.

Surgical Wound Classification

The surgical site may be clean or contaminated when the surgeon makes the initial incision. A clean site may become contaminated depending on the type of wound, the pathologic findings or circumstances that create the need for the surgical procedure, the anatomic location, and the techniques of the OR team. After completion of wound closure, the circulating nurse should verify the wound classification with the surgeon.

The wound class should not be assigned until the dressing is applied. This is documented in the patient's intraoperative records. Surgical sites are classified by the degree of microbial contamination or exposure that may predispose a patient to a postoperative wound infection.[4]

According to the Centers for Disease Control and Prevention (CDC), risk for infection increases in proportion to contamination of the incision and surrounding tissues exposed during the course of the surgical procedure. The true extent of risk cannot be evaluated until the procedure is completed. The wound is classified at the end of the surgical procedure as one of the following four types (Box 29.1):
1. Clean
2. Clean-contaminated
3. Contaminated
4. Dirty and infected

Generalized Health Condition of the Patient

Chronic diseases alter normal physiology. Diseases such as diabetes, uremia, fibrocystic disease, cirrhosis, active alcoholism, and leukemia can delay wound healing.

Circulatory Status

Cardiovascular and respiratory insufficiency inhibits tissue perfusion. Oxygenation is essential to wound healing and to inhibition

Classification of Surgical Wounds From the CDC

Clean Wound (Infection Rate: 1–5%)
- Elective procedure with wound made in ideal operating room conditions
- Primary closure; wound not drained
- No break in sterile technique during surgical procedure
- No inflammation present
- Alimentary, respiratory, and genitourinary tracts or oropharyngeal cavity not entered

Clean-Contaminated Wound (Infection Rate: 3–11%)
- Primary closure; wound drained
- Minor break in technique occurred
- No inflammation or infection present
- Alimentary, respiratory, and genitourinary tracts or oropharyngeal cavity entered in controlled conditions without significant spillage or unusual contamination

Contaminated Wound (Infection Rate: 10–17%)
- Open fresh traumatic wound of less than 4 hours' duration
- Major break in technique occurred
- Acute nonpurulent inflammation present
- Gross spillage/contamination from gastrointestinal tract
- Entrance into genitourinary or biliary tracts with infected urine or bile present

Dirty and Infected Wound (Infection Rate: 27–40%)
- Old traumatic wound of more than 4 hours' duration from dirty source or with retained necrotic tissue, foreign body, or fecal contamination
- Organisms present in surgical field before procedure
- Existing clinical infection: acute bacterial inflammation encountered, with or without purulence; incision to drain abscess
- Perforated viscus

of growth of anaerobic microorganisms. If oxygen does not circulate, the wound does not heal.

Smoking

Vasoconstriction caused by smoking decreases blood supply and oxygenation to the wound. Carbon monoxide in smoke binds with hemoglobin (forming carboxyhemoglobin) and further diminishes oxygenation. Smoking contributes to respiratory complications. This can cause forceful coughing that can raise intraabdominal pressure and create increased strain on an abdominal wound and impair healing.

Age

Loss of skin turgor and muscle tone and elasticity is a natural characteristic of the aging process. Thickened connective tissue, decreased subcutaneous fat, diminished capillary blood flow, and reduced vascularity are age-related factors that may delay wound healing. The tension of sutures on aged skin can further inhibit tissue perfusion. Sutures and skin staples should be reinforced with wound-closure strips. Newborn infants, especially those who are preterm, and geriatric patients are especially prone to infection.

Nutritional Status

Wound healing is impaired by deficiencies in proteins, carbohydrates, zinc, and vitamins A, B, C, and K. Protein provides essential amino acids for new tissue construction. Carbohydrates are necessary energy sources for cells and prevent excessive

metabolism of amino acids to meet caloric requirements. Vitamin B complex is necessary for carbohydrate, protein, and fat metabolism. Vitamin C permits collagen formation. Although vitamin A and zinc are known to be important in collagen synthesis, their mechanism in wound healing is not well understood. Vitamin K is involved in the synthesis of prothrombin and other clotting factors. Copper and iron assist in collagen synthesis. Calcium and magnesium are important in protein synthesis. Manganese serves as an enzyme activator.

Malnutrition, whether primary or secondary to disease, can be a major factor in wound healing and infection. Impairment of physiologic functions associated with a body weight loss that is greater than 10% and protein energy malnutrition increase the risk for postoperative complications. Liver function, skeletal and respiratory muscle function, overall physical and mental activity, and inflammatory response to wound healing are altered in the patient who is malnourished.

Protein and fat deficiency is especially significant in patients with extensive burns or multiple injuries who have greatly increased caloric requirements. Malnutrition caused by anorexia or cachexia has a deleterious effect on wound healing. Hyperalimentation with vitamin, trace element, and mineral supplements preoperatively and postoperatively usually is indicated for patients who are malnourished.

In overweight patients, the bulk and weight of adipose tissue cause difficulty in confining excess fat and securing good wound closure. To minimize dead space, the surgeon may place drains and sutures in subcutaneous fat; both may actually potentiate infection. Of all tissues, fat is the most vulnerable to trauma and infection because of its poor vascularity. Many patients who are extremely obese, more than 100 lb (45.4 kg) over ideal body weight, have cardiac decompensation and respiratory insufficiency.

Fluid and Electrolyte Balance

The body's system for balancing fluids and electrolytes is extremely complex. As a result of illness, injury, or infection, the patient may not be able to maintain normal fluid and electrolyte balance. Fever associated with infection, for example, can raise fluid requirements as much as 15% for each 1.5° F (or 1° C) rise in body temperature.

Body fluid is intracellular (ICF [within cells]) and extracellular (ECF [outside cells as intravascular plasma and interstitial fluid between cells]). The electrolyte content differs. ECF contains more sodium than ICF; ICF has more potassium than ECF. Changes in this balance can affect kidney function, cellular metabolism, oxygen concentration in the circulation, and hormonal function. Adequate ECF volume is necessary for circulation of blood to tissues.

Hematology

The presence of an abnormal or pathologic condition that affects the blood should be carefully evaluated preoperatively. A low hemoglobin level (low red blood cell count) associated with anemia can result in tissue hypoxia, which alters synthesis of collagen and epithelialization. A hematocrit value below 20% lowers oxygen tension in tissues, which disrupts cell regeneration. An elevated leukocyte level (white blood cell count) indicates the presence of infection in the body.

Inflammatory and Immune Responses

The body repairs tissues at the cellular level in response to injury or exposure to foreign substances. It triggers an inflammatory response to mobilize cellular components associated with healing. Some foreign materials cause more inflammatory reaction than do others.

Extremes of inflammation may result in response to allergy, infection, or chronic irritation and may delay wound healing. Inflammation should not be confused with infection, which has a pathogenic microbe that causes the complications. Patients with an impaired immune response have an altered inflammatory response and do not heal appropriately.

Allergic Response

Hypersensitivity to substances inhaled, ingested, injected, or in contact with skin causes an acute allergic reaction. The type of allergic response displayed by the patient should be considered. A localized sensitivity response may appear as a rash or hives. A systemic allergic response may be more severe and include signs of airway obstruction and cardiac dysrhythmias.

Immunosuppression

The patient's immunologic response may be deficient because of a congenital or acquired immunologic disease, drugs, or radiation therapy. Patients with immunosuppression are easily infected with potentially pathogenic flora within their own bodies. They may not have the usual signs and symptoms of infection, such as initial inflammatory response. Lack of integrity of the immune system, such as leukopenia or defective immunoglobulin synthesis, can be life-threatening.

Drug Therapy

Wound healing occurs basically through collagen synthesis. Agents that interfere with cellular metabolism have a potentially deleterious effect on the healing process. Prolonged high dosage of steroids, such as cortisone preoperatively, inhibits fibroplasia and collagen formation.

Some antineoplastic agents used as chemotherapeutic adjuvants to surgery also may delay systemic wound healing or cause localized tissue necrosis from extravasation at the site of injection. Immunosuppressants are given to transplant patients to prevent organ or tissue rejection. Leukopenia and susceptibility to infection are common sequelae to administration of these drugs. Other drugs that interfere with wound healing include anticoagulants, antiinflammatory agents, and colchicine.

Radiation Therapy

Healing is delayed if the patient has had radiation in large doses preoperatively. The blood supply in irradiated tissue is decreased, and rapidly growing cells, including healthy cells, are destroyed. However, little change from the normal healing pattern occurs if radiation has been given in low doses and the surgical procedure is performed within 4 to 6 weeks of radiation.

Surgical Technique

Devitalized tissue caused by laser or electrosurgery cannot regenerate. Interruption of blood supply and innervation decreases circulation and prevents epithelialization. Excess tension on the suture line that inhibits tissue perfusion prolongs healing time.

Aseptic Technique

Healthy tissues can combat a certain amount of contamination. Microorganisms are normally present in skin and air. Devitalized tissues have little power of resistance. Infection may occur from any one of a variety of causes that result in a breakdown of the wound postoperatively. The surgeon gives meticulous attention to sterile technique throughout the surgical procedure to minimize contamination of the surgical site.

The entire OR team carefully carries out aseptic and sterile techniques. In addition, many precautions are taken by all OR personnel. Strict adherence to housekeeping techniques, air engineering, sterilization procedures, and all of the principles of aseptic technique is necessary. Infection may be caused by a break in the chain of asepsis.

Method of Hemostasis

Complete hemostasis must be achieved to prevent loss of blood and hematoma (blood clot) formation. Blood loss is caused by tissue trauma. The method of dissection and coagulation of bleeders can cause devitalization of tissue. Devitalized tissue cannot heal; it only necroses. Delivery of oxygen to healing tissues is affected. Any condition that lowers circulating blood flow and the delivery of oxygen to the tissues impairs healing.

Tissue Handling

All tissues should be handled gently and as little as possible throughout the surgical procedure. The surgeon makes an incision that is just long enough to afford sufficient operating space. Careful consideration is given to underlying blood vessels and nerves to preserve as many as possible. Retractors are placed to provide exposure without causing undue pressure on tissues and organs or tension on muscles. Trauma to tissue in dissecting, handling with instruments, ligating, or suturing may cause edema and necrosis with resultant slow healing. The body must rid itself of necrotic cells before the healing phase of fibroplasia takes place.

Tissue Approximation

Tissue edges are brought together with precision, avoiding strangulation and eliminating dead space, to promote wound healing. A closure that is too tight or closure under tension causes ischemia, a decrease of blood supply to tissues. Approximation is critical to the healing of flaps and grafts. Constricted or interrupted blood supply can cause flap failure or loss of a vascularized graft.

Dead space is caused by separation of wound edges that have not been closely approximated or by air trapped between layers of tissue. Serum or blood may collect in a dead space and prevent healing by keeping cut edges separated. Wound edges not in close contact cannot heal. A drain may be inserted to aid in removal of fluid or air from the surgical site postoperatively, or a pressure dressing may be applied over a closed wound to help obliterate dead space.

The choice of wound-closure materials and the techniques of the surgeon are prime factors in the restoration of tensile strength to the wound during the healing process.

Wound Security

The quality of approximated tissue and the type of closure material are two factors that determine the strength of the wound. Tensile strength of the tissues themselves varies; some tissues are more friable than others. Drains or catheters may be placed in the wound to evacuate serum or fluid and prevent it from accumulating in the dead space postoperatively. Drainage tubes may cause a weak spot in the incision, and underlying tissue may protrude. Also, drains may provide an inlet for microorganisms, as well as an outlet for drainage. When possible, drains are placed through a stab wound in the skin rather than through the surgical incision.

When sutures are used, the suture material provides all of the strength of the wound immediately after closure. Closely spaced sutures give a stronger suture line. The strength of a suture should not be greater than the strength of the tissue in which it is placed. To minimize tissue reaction to sutures, the fewest and the smallest sutures consistent with the holding power of the tissues should be used. Inert surgical staples are used to approximate some tissues.

Immediately after closure, tissue along the incision is at about 40% of its original strength. It reaches its greatest strength in 7 to 15 days. The wound is about one-third healed on the sixth postoperative day and two-thirds healed on the eighth day. The condition of the patient, the type of surgical procedure, and many other factors may cause variance from the average patient response. As tensile strength of the wound increases, reliance on other support for wound security gradually lessens.

Postoperative Complications

Edema, vomiting, or coughing can place stress on the healing wound before fibroplasia takes place. Complications in other parts of the body, far from the surgical site, such as pneumonia, thrombus, or embolus, can inhibit oxygen supply to the wound site.[5] Collagen synthesis is partly a function of the oxygenation of tissues; therefore oxygen perfusion to tissues contributes to the rate of healing, tensile strength of the wound, and resistance to infection. This is particularly important in arterialized and microvascular tissue grafts and flaps used to cover soft tissue defects and in organ transplantation. Ischemic tissue is more susceptible to infection than is well-vascularized tissue.

Physical Activity

Early ambulation postoperatively is one of the most important factors in recovery for the surgical patient. Ambulation may be started immediately after recovery from anesthesia if the patient's condition does not contraindicate it. Some surgeons exempt only the patient whose blood pressure (BP) is not stable, the patient who has a cardiac problem, or the patient whose general condition is poor. If the patient's physical condition does not safely permit ambulation, the surgeon orders otherwise.

Ambulation is started gradually, with the patient first turning onto one side. The patient sits up with the feet over the side of the bed and then stands on the floor for a minute before returning to bed. After repeating this several times, the patient takes a few steps and finally increases the distance walked. Sitting in a chair for prolonged periods is discouraged because this contributes to stasis of blood in dependent parts. The patient must understand the value of early ambulation, which includes the following:

- Early ambulation improves circulation, which aids in the healing process and eliminates stasis of blood, which may result in thrombus and embolus formation.
- The patient is better able to cooperate in deep-breathing exercises to raise bronchial secretions; thus pulmonary complications are reduced.
- Early ambulation decreases gas pain, distention, and the tendency toward nausea and vomiting. It helps prevent constipation. Bodily functions return to normal more readily.
- Increased exercise aids digestion. Thus the patient's oral intake progresses sooner after the surgical procedure, so that less

supplementary intravenous (IV) fluid is necessary for hydration and nutrition.
- Early ambulation eliminates the general muscle weakness that follows bed rest.
- Fewer pain-relieving drugs are necessary.
- Early ambulation boosts patients' morale with the knowledge that they will be out of bed early after the surgical procedure, able to care for themselves, and soon ready to go home. This helps the mental outlook and, through it, the physical recovery.
- Early ambulation shortens hospitalization.

Hemostasis

Hemostasis, the arrest of a flow of blood or hemorrhage, is essential to successful wound management. The mechanism is coagulation, or the formation of a blood clot. The clotting of blood takes place in several stages by enzyme reaction.

Hemostatic Process

When severed by incision or traumatic injury, a blood vessel constricts and the ends may contract. Platelets rapidly clump and adhere to connective tissue at the cut end of a constricted vessel. Interaction with collagen fibers causes platelets to liberate adenosine diphosphate (ADP), epinephrine, and serotonin from their secretory granules. In turn, ADP causes other platelets to clump to the initial layer and to each other, forming a platelet plug. This may be sufficient in small vessels to provide primary hemostasis.

The reaction of plasma from vessels with connective tissue cells at the site of injury activates clotting factors and causes a series of other reactions. Prothrombin, normally present in blood, reacts with thromboplastin, which is released when tissues are injured. Prothrombin and thromboplastin, along with calcium ions in the blood, form thrombin. This requires several minutes. Thrombin unites with fibrinogen, a blood protein, to form fibrin, which is the basic structural material of blood clots. This last reaction is very rapid.

The fibrin strands reinforce the platelet plug to form a resilient hemostatic plug capable of withstanding arterial pressure when the constricted vessel relaxes. Massive thrombosis within the vessels would occur once coagulation was initiated, if it continued. However, fibrin is digested during the process. The products of this digestion, and antithrombins normally present in blood, act as anticoagulants. The coagulation mechanism rapidly and efficiently inhibits excessive blood loss so that excessive coagulation does not occur (Fig. 29.2).

Bleeding During a Surgical Procedure

Two types of bleeding occur during surgical procedures: pulsating arterial bleeding and venous oozing from denuded or cut surfaces. Although the need to control gross bleeding is obvious, insidious but continuous loss of blood from small veins and capillaries can become significant if oozing is uncontrolled. Complete hemostasis, gentle tissue handling, elimination of dead space, precise wound closure, and a protective wound dressing are essential to minimize trauma to tissue and enhance healing.

Incomplete hemostasis may cause the formation of a hematoma. A hematoma is a collection of extravasated blood in a body cavity, space, or tissue caused by uncontrolled bleeding or oozing. It may be painful and firm to the touch. Some hematomas require evacuation to prevent infection; others reabsorb with time.

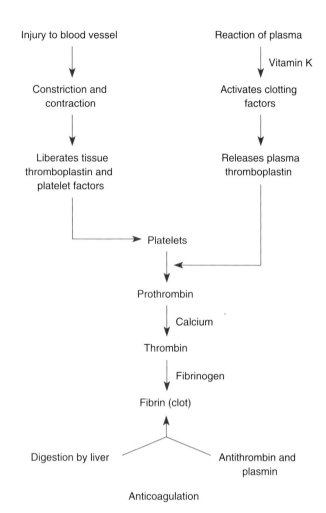

• **Fig. 29.2** Mechanism of hemostasis.

Methods of Hemostasis

Numerous agents, devices, and sophisticated pieces of equipment are used to achieve hemostasis and wound closure. These various methods can be classified as chemical, mechanical, or thermal.

Chemical Methods of Hemostasis

Chemical forms of topical hemostasis interact with blood to form a clot. Some materials reabsorb during the healing process. Hemostatic materials should not be packed into closed spaces, as in the spinal canal, where they might swell and cause pressure on nerves or other tissues. The material can be applied in confined areas until hemostasis is achieved but removed before closure.

Absorbable Gelatin

Available in either powder or compressed pad form, gelatin (Gelfoam) is an absorbable hemostatic agent made from purified porcine gelatin solution that has been beaten to a foamy consistency, dried, and sterilized by dry heat. As a pad, it is available in an assortment of sizes that can be cut as desired without crumbling. When it is placed on an area of capillary bleeding, fibrin is deposited in the interstices and the sponge swells, forming a substantial clot.

The gelatin sponge is not soluble; it absorbs 45 times its own weight in blood. It is denatured to retard absorption, which takes

place in 20 to 40 days. It is frequently soaked in thrombin or epinephrine solution, although it may be used dry after compression.

Before a gelatin sponge is handed to the surgeon, it is dipped into warm saline solution, if used without thrombin or epinephrine, and pressed between the fingers or against the sides of the basin to remove air from it. The same procedure is used with thrombin (human or bovine) or epinephrine solution.

In powder form, gelatin is mixed with sterile saline solution to make a paste (slurry) for application to cancellous bone to control bleeding or to denuded areas of skin or muscles to stimulate growth of granulation tissue.[6] Gelatin film can be used in neurologic, ophthalmic, and otorhinologic procedures.[7] Gelatin hemostatic products should not be used in infected areas.

Absorbable Collagen

Hemostatic sponges (Collastat, Superstat, Helistat), felt (Lyostypt), or membranes and plugs of bovine collagen origin are applied dry to oozing or bleeding sites. The collagen activates the coagulation mechanism, especially the aggregation of platelets, to accelerate clot formation. The material dissolves as hemostasis occurs.

Any residual material absorbs in the wound. Because of an affinity for wet surfaces, the material must be kept dry and should be applied with dry gloves or instruments. Absorbable collagen is contraindicated in the presence of infection or in areas where blood or other fluids have pooled. It is applied directly to the bleeding surface as supplied from the sterile package. Collagen hemostatics absorb within 8 to 10 weeks. Do not let this material accumulate in the skin incision because it creates a mechanical barrier to healing and causes scars.

Microfibrillar Collagen

Available in compacted nonwoven web form or in loose fibrous form, microfibrillar collagen (Avitene, Instat, Surgiflo) is an absorbable topical hemostatic agent. It is produced from a hydrochloric acid salt of purified bovine corium collagen. It is applied dry. When it is placed in contact with a bleeding surface, hemostasis is achieved by adhesion of platelets and prompt fibrin deposition within the interstices of the collagen. The collagen can swell to 20% of its volume within 10 minutes. Bovine products should not be used in patients with known allergy to bovine proteins.

Tissue cohesion is an inherent property of the collagen itself. It functions as a hemostatic agent only when it is applied directly to the source of bleeding from raw oozing surfaces, including bone and friable tissues, or directly to active bleeding from irregular contours, from crevices, and around suture lines. Firm pressure is applied quickly with a dry gauze sponge, which is held either by the fingers in accessible areas or by using forceps in less accessible areas.

The material must be compressed firmly against the bleeding surface before excessive wetting with blood can occur. Effective application is evidenced by a firm adherent coagulum with no breakthrough bleeding from either the surface or edges. Excess material should be removed from around the site without recreating bleeding. The remaining coagulum absorbs during wound healing.

Oxidized Cellulose

Absorbable oxidation products of cotton cellulose or oxidized regenerated cellulose (rayon) are available in the form of a pad or in a knitted fabric strip that is of low density (Surgicel) or high density (Surgicel Nu-Knit). These products are applied dry and may be sutured to, wrapped around, or held firmly against a bleeding site or laid dry on an oozing surface until hemostasis is obtained.

When oxidized cellulose comes into contact with whole blood, a clot forms rapidly. As it reacts with blood, it increases in size to form a gel and stops bleeding in areas in which bleeding is difficult to control by other means of hemostasis.

Except in situations in which packing is required as a lifesaving measure, only the minimal amount necessary to control capillary or venous bleeding is used. If left on oozing surfaces, it absorbs 10 times its own weight with minimal tissue reaction. It is not recommended for use on bone unless it is removed after hemostasis because it may interfere with bone regeneration. Oxidized regenerated cellulose has some bactericidal properties, but it is not a substitute for antimicrobial agents and is absorbed in 1 to 2 weeks. Thrombin is inactivated in the presence of oxidized cellulose. During the absorption period, the cellulose can look like an abscess on x-ray.

Zeolite Beads

Trauma patients may arrive in the OR with wounds packed with bags of zeolite beads used for emergency hemostasis by emergency squads in the field. The intact sterile gauze bag is radiopaque and can be placed directly into the wound. Pressure is applied. It is packaged in 3.5-ounce gauze bags wrapped in foil. The large volume is necessary to have enough to fill a traumatic wound.

The beads are derived from a form of volcanic pumice that has an exothermic reaction in the presence of moisture. The beads absorb the water from blood and reach temperatures around 140° F to 155° F (60−68.3° C). Later generations of zeolite hemostatic material have been impregnated into dressing material and have minimal exothermic action. Zeolite dressings are available with silver granules embedded for antimicrobial properties.

The OR team removes the bead pack or emergency zeolite dressing as part of the trauma surgery because the beads are not biodegradable and could cause a foreign body reaction.

Kaolin-Based Product

Kaolin (QuikClot) has been incorporated into products for hemostasis and is used in the same manner as the dressing materials impregnated with zeolite beads. It is available in various size gauze pads and rolls with radiopaque markers. No exothermic reaction occurs with kaolin. Kaolin is a natural mineral form of hydrated aluminum silicate that is insoluble in water. QuikClot contains no animal, human, botanical, or shellfish protein.

Used in treatment of hemorrhage, the kaolin dressings provide excellent hemostasis by activating factor XII, part of the coagulation cascade. In its powder form, it can be used as a sclerosing agent for pleurodesis in pneumothorax. Care is taken to avoid inhaling the powder because it can cause respiratory complications.

QuikClot is approved by the U.S. Food and Drug Administration (FDA) for uncontrolled emergency bleeding and is used for eviscerating wounds. The foil-wrapped packet can be stored in warm or cool temperatures and has a shelf life of 3 years. Prolonged exposure to the air diminishes the effectiveness of the product once opened. American troops have used this product for combat and trauma since 2005. It is also used by emergency personnel for trauma. More information about this kaolin-based product can be found at www.quikclot.com.

Oxytocin

Oxytocin is a hormone produced by the pituitary gland. It can be prepared synthetically for therapeutic injection (Pitocin, Syntocinon). During cesarean section, oxytocin (10 units) may be directly injected into the uterine muscle to cause contraction after delivery of the baby and placenta. It is a systemic agent used to control hemorrhage from the uterus, rather than a local hemostatic agent per se. Oxytocin is sometimes used to induce labor. It also causes contraction of the uterus after delivery of the placenta.

Ergonovine, another oxytocic drug commonly referred to as ergotrate maleate, can be used to treat uterine bleeding after childbirth or abortion after the delivery of the placenta. It causes sustained uterine contractions over a period of 3 hours. The drug is derived from ergot, a form of rye. Ergotrate should be stored in a cool, dry area and protected from light.

Monsel Solution

Persistent intrauterine bleeding at the placental attachment site can be treated IV with additional oxytocin and topically during a cesarean section with Monsel solution (20% aqueous ferric subsulfate). A surgical laparotomy tape saturated with approximately 16 mL of Monsel solution can be used to tamponade the bleeding internal endometrial surface. Monsel solution is acidic and is used with care to prevent contact with perineal surfaces; it can cause denaturation of the tissues. It can also cause dermal tattooing. Additional hemostatic material such as Surgicel can be applied to the area when the pack is withdrawn after several minutes.

Monsel solution can be used to create hemostasis over denuded areas caused by shave biopsies of the skin or anorectal or uterine cervix punch biopsies. Ferric subsulfate is applied using a cotton swab and causes the vessels to occlude by denaturing protein. Monsel solution was developed by Leon Monsel (1816−1878), a French pharmacist, and is recorded in use during 1852 in the Crimean war, in which Florence Nightingale served with her nurses.

Styptics

A styptic is an agent that checks hemorrhage by causing vasoconstriction. Styptics have the disadvantage of being rapidly carried away by the bloodstream.

Epinephrine

A hormone of the adrenal gland, epinephrine (Adrenalin) is prepared synthetically for use as a vasoconstrictor to prolong the action of local anesthetic agents or to decrease bleeding. Used in some local anesthetic agents to constrict the vessels locally, epinephrine keeps the anesthetic concentrated within the area injected and reduces the amount of bleeding when the incision is made. It is rapidly dispersed, leaving little local effect. Within the incision, gelatin sponges soaked in 1:1000 epinephrine may be applied to bleeding surfaces. These are especially useful in ear and microsurgical procedures in which localized hemostasis of capillaries is critical. Excess epinephrine can be absorbed systemically and cause cardiac stimulation.

Silver Nitrate

Crystals of silver nitrate in 20% to 50% solution or mixed with silver chloride and molded into applicator sticks are applied topically for vasoconstriction. Both an astringent and an antimicrobial, silver nitrate is commonly used in the treatment of burns or other moist wounds. Silver nitrate can be used to seal areas of previous surgical incisions that are left open to heal by secondary intention. Silver nitrate should not be used on the face because it may cause discoloration of the skin. The staining darkens to black in the presence of light.

Aluminum Chloride (25–35%)

Aluminum chloride is applied with a cotton swab to cause the formation of coagulum over a denuded area. It is not as effective as Monsel solution and does not cause skin discoloration. The area should be covered with an occlusive dressing to prevent drying of the wound.

Zinc Chloride

Zinc chloride causes coagulation over a denuded area. Zinc chloride paste or solution is sometimes used after Mohs micrographic surgery.[8]

Tannic Acid

A powder made from an astringent plant, tannic acid is used occasionally on mucous membranes of the nose and throat to help stop capillary bleeding.

Thrombin

An enzyme extracted from human or bovine blood is used as a topical hemostatic agent in 5000 to 20,000-unit solutions. Thrombin accelerates coagulation of blood and controls capillary bleeding. It unites rapidly with fibrinogen to form a clot. Topically, it may be used as a dry powder to sprinkle on an oozing surface or as a solution, alone or to saturate a gelatin sponge. Topical thrombin may be sprayed on areas of capillary bleeding that do not lend themselves to other means of hemostasis, such as sealing a skin graft onto a denuded area. It should not be allowed to enter large vessels. Systemic absorption can cause intravascular thrombosis.

Thrombin is used for topical application only. It is never injected. Recommendations are that thrombin be mixed just before use because it loses potency after 3 hours. Thrombin solution should be labeled with the name of the drug and the concentration and kept separate from any other solutions on the instrument table. Manufacturer instructions should be followed for mixing solution. Bovine thrombin is contraindicated if the patient is allergic to bovine products. Human thrombin may carry the risk for viral or prion contamination.

Sclerotherapy

A caustic sclerosing solution may be injected into veins, as in the mucosal lining of the esophagus or anus, to stop or prevent venous bleeding. The solution may be a mixture of equal parts of dehydrated alcohol, bacteriostatic saline, and sodium tetradecyl in a contrast medium base. Other sclerosants are mixtures of absolute ethanol or ethanolamine.

Bentonite Powder

In 2018 the FDA approved an inorganic aluminum phyllosilicate clay powder (Hemospray) for topical use in the upper and lower gastrointestinal tract.[9] The powder is administered from a handheld spray device powered by a carbon dioxide cartridge. The single-use endoscopic device sprays the powder through a catheter to the bleeding site. The powder forms a gel layer and stops bleeding within 5 minutes. More information can be found at www.fda.gov.

Embolization

A hemostatic agent can intentionally be placed inside a vessel to occlude the blood supply to a tumor. Several substances are used as embolic agents to intentionally thrombose a vessel. The embolization depends on the amount of thrombus formed within the substance of the hemostatic agent. Patients on anticoagulant therapy may not form an adequate clot to embolize the desired area. In some circumstances, the embolized area can recannulate in 4 to 6 weeks and become patent. In ischemic tissues, distal embolization may take place.

The hemostatic agent is delivered under fluoroscopy to the site via injection mixed as a suspension or slurry in contrast medium and sterile saline solution for intravascular use. Albumin or dextran can be used to create a more viscous suspension. A commonly used agent is polyvinyl alcohol foam fibers.

Other "off label" materials used in embolization include the following:

- Gelfoam powder can be used as a slurry. The occlusion can last several weeks or months, depending on the physiology of the area to be embolized.
- Avitene provides quick embolization that lasts 2 to 3 months.
- Dehydrated alcohol can be used to embolize low-pressure venous lesions. It is mixed with contrast medium to perform the injection under fluoroscopic guidance.
- Ethiodol (oil-based) can be mixed with chemotherapeutic agents for hepatic chemoembolization. Ethiodol has contrast medium properties.

Other embolization devices, such as coils in various shapes, can be placed via the endovascular route to an area of aneurysm by catheter technique. Coils can be soaked in thrombin. Some lesions can develop collateral circulation, and repeating the coil procedure may not be possible if the blood supply is persistent distal to the coil placement. Several coils can be placed at one time and may take varying amounts of time to be effective.

Silicone balloons can be deployed into a vessel that develops a distal and proximal thrombus at each end of its structure. The balloon deflates over time because it is somewhat permeable, but the lasting thrombus maintains the desired occlusion. Latex balloons are less permeable but pose a risk to patients with latex sensitivity or allergy.

Mechanical Methods of Hemostasis

External Mechanical Methods

Mechanical hemostasis is achieved by occluding severed vessels until normal forces of blood have time to form a clot. During the surgical procedure, the surgeon uses many mechanical devices to apply pressure or create a mechanical barrier to the flow of blood. Pressure also is used prophylactically preoperatively and postoperatively to control the tone of blood vessels and aid venous return.

Mechanical external pressure devices may be applied before the patient arrives in the OR or after the patient is transferred to the OR bed. The intended purpose may be prophylactic to prevent venous stasis, deep vein thrombosis (DVT), or pulmonary embolus (PE) intraoperatively and postoperatively. Or the function may be therapeutic to control internal hemorrhage preoperatively or hematoma postoperatively. A bloodless surgical field also can be created by external pressure devices.

Antiembolic Stockings. Elastic stockings may be applied to the lower extremities to prevent thromboembolic phenomena. Static compression on the legs helps prevent venous stasis. Stockings are available in knee-length and groin-length sizes. To apply the stockings, the circulating nurse rolls the stocking from top to toe. After placement over the patient's toes, the stocking is gently unrolled over the leg from foot to ankle to calf.

Sequential Compression Device. Inflatable double-walled vinyl or woven fabric leg wraps use alternating compression and relaxation to reduce the risk for DVT in the legs of patients at high risk who are undergoing general anesthesia or experiencing extremes of intraoperative positioning. The leg wraps may be used over antiembolic stockings on each leg, although the compression device alone is sufficient in the prevention of DVT. The patient's foot is not encased within the wrap. The circulating nurse should measure the patient's thigh or calf for the correct size selection (i.e., small, medium, large, or extra-large) for either full-leg (thigh-high) or knee-high leg wraps. Proper selection and application are essential for effective compression. Disposable leg wraps are commercially available.

A motorized pump, attached by tubing to each wrap, sequentially inflates leg wraps at the ankles, then at the calves, and then at the thighs for full-leg compression. The pressure of this wavelike action is greatest at the ankles. The leg wraps are divided into chambers so that pressure can be regulated by preset or adjustable gauges. Pressure between 40 and 50 mm Hg applied for 12 seconds and then released for 48 seconds empties blood from deep leg venous sinuses. The action prevents venous stasis and accumulation of clotting factors in deep veins. The pumping action is started before induction of anesthesia because general anesthesia reduces venous return and causes vasodilation.

The circulating nurse should regularly check operation of the pump and periodically inspect the leg wraps and tubing. Care is taken to ensure that the patient is not lying on the tubing. The type of device, time started, pressure and cycle settings, and time discontinued must be documented on the intraoperative record. If the surgeon wants leg wraps to remain on the patient postoperatively, the device is transported to the postanesthesia care unit (PACU) or intensive care unit (ICU) with the patient. Frequently, sequential compression is continued for 24 hours postoperatively or until the patient is fully ambulatory after an abdominal, hip, or neurosurgical procedure.

MAST Pneumatic Counterpressure Device. Although the concept dates back to 1903, external counterpressure was not a popular medical device until the Vietnam War. There it was used to control hemorrhagic shock until definitive hemostasis became available to casualties. Circumferential pneumatic compression counteracts postural hypotension, maintains venous pressure, and controls hemorrhage. Several types of pneumatic antishock garments (PASGs) are used, primarily to treat hypovolemic shock.

The acronym MAST can refer to medical antishock trousers, military antishock trousers, or a military antigravity suit. An inflatable waterproof garment is fastened around the patient from ankles to ribcage. The trouser chambers are inflated first, to prevent venous stasis in the legs. The entire suit or only specific chambers of it can be inflated from the feet up. Each chamber is inflated separately with a foot pump. By increasing pressure on vessel walls of the legs and abdomen, systemic vascular resistance of peripheral vessels increases blood flow to the heart, lungs, and brain. Compression of torn vessel walls reduces the size of the laceration and diminishes blood loss.

The MAST device may be in place when the trauma patient arrives in the OR. Deflation begins after induction of anesthesia,

beginning with the abdominal chamber. Leg chambers may remain inflated for counterpressure if BP remains unstable. Deflation must be slow and gradual. The MAST suit is never cut off the patient. Rapid deflation reduces cerebral and cardiopulmonary circulation, with resultant shock. BP is monitored; it should not drop more than 5 mm Hg.

Pneumatic counterpressure devices may be used to prevent air embolism during some head and neck procedures performed with the patient in a sitting position. The increased venous filling produced decreases the possibility of an air embolism. Also, these devices may be used postoperatively to reduce bleeding or stabilize the patient's condition after massive blood loss during the surgical procedure.

Tourniquets. A tourniquet is a device used to provide hemostasis by constricting the flow of blood in an extremity. It is frequently used on the proximal aspect of an extremity to keep the distal surgical site free of blood. A bloodless field makes dissection easier and less traumatic to tissues and reduces surgical time. Bleeding must be controlled before pressure is released.

Precautions for tourniquet application and use are observed. A tourniquet should not be used when circulation in an extremity is impaired or when an arteriovenous access fistula for dialysis is present. A tourniquet can cause tissue, nerve, and vascular injury.[9] Paralysis may result from excessive pressure on nerves. Prolonged ischemia can cause loss of innervation and circulation in the extremity. Tourniquet time should be kept to a minimum. Metabolic changes may be irreversible after 1 to 1.5 hours of tourniquet ischemia. Consideration for latex sensitivity may be an issue for some devices used as tourniquets. Rubber materials should be latex-free if the patient is sensitive to latex products.

A tourniquet is dangerous to apply, to leave on, and to remove. A tourniquet may be applied by the surgeon, first assistant, or circulating nurse on the surgeon's orders.

Pneumatic Tourniquet. Similar to a blood pressure cuff, although heavier and more secure, the pneumatic cuff consists of a rubber bladder shielded by a plastic insert inside a fabric cover with a Velcro closure. Many different types of cuffs are available. Some are straight and cylindric; others are contoured. A cuff of appropriate length and width must be used, and various sizes are available. Cuffs are inflated automatically with compressed gas (air or oxygen) by means of tubing interconnected between the cuff and a pressure cartridge, piped-in system, or battery-powered unit.

The desired pressure is uniformly maintained by a pressure valve and registered on a pressure gauge. The tourniquet console, a pressure regulator with a gauge, may be contained in a unit mounted on a portable stand or hung on an IV pole. An automated tourniquet with a computerized microprocessor control signals both audible alarms and visual indicators for deviations from preset pressure and for elapsed time of inflation.

Correct pressure is the minimum amount necessary to produce a bloodless field. The calculation of tourniquet cuff pressure is according to the systolic blood pressure. An exact pressure to which the cuff should be inflated has not been determined. In a healthy adult, upper extremity pressure 30 to 70 mm Hg higher than the systolic value of the blood pressure may be sufficient to suppress arterial circulation.

Tourniquet pressure on an average adult arm usually ranges from 200 to 250 mm Hg (up to 6 lbs). In the lower extremity, cuff pressure should be higher than the systolic pressure by one-half the value. This may require 250 to 300 mm Hg on the thigh.

Thin adults and children need less pressure; muscular and obese extremities may need more. Inflation time also should be kept to a minimum. If needed for more than 1 hour on an arm or 1.5 hours on a leg, the tourniquet may be deflated at intervals periodically at the discretion of the surgeon. The limb should be exsanguinated before reinflation of the tourniquet.

A pneumatic tourniquet should be used and maintained according to the manufacturer's written instructions. These and institutional policies and procedures should be available to users of this complex equipment. The cuff, tubing, connectors, gauges, and pressure source should be maintained in working order. Precautions to be taken when using a pneumatic tourniquet include the following:

1. Inspect and test the pneumatic tourniquet equipment before each use.
   a. Inspect the inflatable cuff, connectors, and tubing for cleanliness, integrity, and function.
   b. Ensure that the cuff and tubing are intact and that the connectors are securely fastened to the tourniquet pressure source.
   c. Check the pressure gauge for accuracy. An aneroid pressure gauge can be checked by comparing it with a mercury manometer. Pressure drifts can be detected by wrapping the cuff around a rigid cylinder, inflating it to 300 mm Hg, and observing for pressure variations.
2. Protect the patient's skin under the tourniquet cuff.
   a. Place a single layer of wrinkle-free padding around the extremity. A length of stockinette or lint-free cotton sheet wadding may be used (Webril). Disposable padded covers are commercially available.
   b. Keep the padding and cuff dry. Antiseptic solutions and other fluids should not contact or accumulate under the cuff. Skin maceration or burns could result. Placement of an impervious drape around the cuff prevents the pooling of fluids.
3. Position the cuff at the point of maximum circumference of the extremity.
   a. Avoid vulnerable neurovascular structures. Nerves and blood vessels may be compressed against bone when the cuff is inflated. Soft tissue provides padding for underlying structures. The cuff should be placed on the upper arm or proximal third of the thigh.
   b. Select a cuff of appropriate width for the size and shape of the extremity. A wide cuff occludes blood flow at a lower pressure than does a narrow cuff.
   c. Select a cuff with adequate length to overlap at least 3 inches (7.5 cm) but not more than 6 inches (15 cm).
   d. Apply the cuff smoothly and snugly over padding before prepping the extremity.
   e. Apply a sterile cuff, if used, after prepping and draping. A sterile cuff may be used for an immunocompromised patient.
4. Preset pressure gauges. The surgeon determines the pressure setting according to the patient's age, limb size, and systolic blood pressure and the width of the cuff to be used.
5. Exsanguination of the elevated extremity after prepping and draping, but before cuff inflation, prolongs the tourniquet time and provides a bloodless field. An Esmarch bandage can be latex or nonlatex. Check for patient's allergies before the case begins.
   a. Elevate the limb during the preparation and keep elevated for 2 minutes after the skin prep to encourage venous

drainage. Inflation of the cuff over blood-filled vessels may cause intravascular thrombosis and lead to embolus.
   b. A sterile team member spiral-wraps an Esmarch bandage around the extremity to compress the blood vessels. The wrap begins distally at the digit tips and progressively spirals proximally up to the tourniquet cuff. After the limb is completely wrapped, the cuff is inflated and the Esmarch is removed.
   c. The scrub person rerolls the Esmarch bandage and keeps it sterile on the back table for potential reuse during the case.
6. Inflate the cuff rapidly to occlude arteries and veins simultaneously to predetermined minimum pressure.
7. Monitor safety parameters during use of the pneumatic tourniquet.
   a. Monitor the pressure gauge to detect pressure fluctuations within the bladder of the cuff.
   b. Monitor the duration of inflation. Inform the surgeon when the cuff has been inflated for 1 hour and every 15 minutes thereafter. In some ORs the circulating nurse posts the tourniquet time on a tally board in view of the surgeon and anesthesia provider.
8. Document the use of a tourniquet on the intraoperative record.
   a. Record the times the tourniquet is applied, inflated, deflated, and removed. The anesthesia provider also records the inflation time on the anesthesia sheet when a tourniquet is used with a Bier block for regional anesthesia.
   b. Record the location of the cuff, who placed it, and the pressure setting.
   c. Record the model and serial number of the tourniquet used.
   d. Document assessment of the skin condition of the extremity preoperatively and evaluation of skin and tissue integrity after removal of the cuff.
9. Clean and inspect the pneumatic tourniquet after each patient use.
   a. Wash the reusable cuff and bladder according to manufacturer instructions. An enzymatic detergent should be used if blood or body fluid came in contact with the cuff. A disposable cuff cover facilitates cleaning.
   b. Rinse and dry the cuff and bladder. Water droplets inside the bladder can damage the pressure mechanism if forced backward during subsequent deflation. Care should be taken to prevent water from getting into the bladder during washing.
   c. Wipe the connecting tubing with a disinfectant.
   d. Test the cuff, tubing, connectors, and gauges before storage between uses. A malfunctioning device must be removed from service until repaired and tested by appropriate personnel.

A pneumatic tourniquet is used most frequently to produce a bloodless surgical field. Tourniquets without pressure measurement gauges can cause damage to tissues. Other types of tourniquets used occasionally include the following:

- *Blood pressure cuff:* The cuff is inflated with ambient air. The surgeon determines the amount of pressure to be sustained. The regulator valve is tightened. The pressure gauge or sphygmomanometer must be monitored for pressure deviations.
- *Rubber band:* This may be used as a tourniquet for a finger or toe. The surgeon puts a sterile rubber band on the digit after draping. This method is not used for patients with latex sensitivity.

- *Rubber tubing:* When an IV infusion is started, a small length of rubber tubing is tied around the extremity, usually an arm, while the needle is inserted. This stops venous return and makes the vein more visible for venipuncture. A Penrose drain is commonly used as a tourniquet.
- *Rubber bandage (Esmarch bandage):* Friedrich von Esmarch (1823–1908), a German military surgeon, introduced an elastic bandage for the control of hemorrhage on the battlefield in 1869. Known today as the Esmarch bandage, a 3-inch (7.5-cm) roller bandage is used to compress superficial vessels as an emergency tourniquet.

Contraindications for Tourniquet Use. Tourniquets are not used in the presence of infection or venous stasis in the limb. A bolus of infectious material or a clot could become dislodged. Other situations in which a tourniquet is not used include, but are not limited to, the following:

1. Malignant disease in the limb (may cause spread)
2. Vascular access ports or shunts (can destroy the patency of the structure)
3. Known peripheral vascular disease or history of DVT
4. Extremes of age: neonate or elderly
5. Rheumatoid arthritis
6. Skin grafts

Pressure Dressings. Pressure on the wound in the immediate postoperative period can minimize the accumulation of intercellular fluid and decrease bleeding by eliminating dead space. Pressure dressings are used on some extensive wounds to decrease edema and potential hematoma or seroma formation. They may be used as an adjunct to wound drainage to distribute pressure evenly over the wound.

Packing. Packing is used with or without pressure to achieve hemostasis and eliminate dead space in an area where mucosal tissues need support, such as the vagina, rectum, or nose. Packing impregnated with an antibiotic ointment or antiseptic agent, such as iodoform gauze, may be used to ensure closure of an incision from the wound base toward the outside (i.e., healing by second intention), as in a large abscess cavity. The surgeon inserts sterile packing as the final stage of the surgical procedure. It is usually removed in 24 to 48 hours. The intraoperative record and patient's chart should reflect the type, amount, and location of packing.

Internal Mechanical Methods

Meticulous hemostasis during the surgical procedure is essential to control bleeding and minimize blood loss. The surgeon uses many mechanical tools to achieve hemostasis.

Hemostatic Clamps. Clamps for occluding vessels are used to compress blood vessels and to grasp or hold a small amount of tissue. The hemostat is the most frequently used surgical instrument and the most commonly used method of hemostasis. This instrument has either straight or curved jaws that narrow to a fine point. Often the pressure of clamping an instrument is sufficient to constrict and seal a vessel with minimal trauma or adjacent tissue necrosis. A wide variety of hemostatic clamps are used for vessel occlusion, including noncrushing vascular clamps that do not damage large vessels.

Ligating Clips. When placed on a blood vessel and pinched shut, clips occlude the lumen and stop the bleeding from the vessel. Metallic clips, such as stainless steel or titanium clips, are small pieces of thin serrated wire that are bent in the center to an oblique angle. Absorbable polymer clips are similar in configuration. Clips are most frequently used on large vessels or those in anatomic locations difficult to ligate by other means. Many surgeons use clips for ligating vessels, nerves, and other small structures. A specific forceps is required for the application of each type available.

Single clips may be mounted in a sterile plastic cartridge that can be secured in a heavy stainless steel base to facilitate loading the applier forceps. Disposable manual and powered appliers preloaded with multiple clips also are available. Some disposable clip appliers ligate as they apply the clip to a vessel.

Ligating clips were devised in 1917 by Dr. Harvey Cushing for use in brain surgery. Cushing clips are made of silver. Titanium clips are more common today because they cause less interference with computed tomography (CT) and magnetic resonance imaging (MRI) examinations. The serrations across the wire prevent slipping off the vessels. Polymeric clips have a locking device to secure them on vessels.

Metallic clips also may be used to mark a biopsy site or other anatomic areas to permit radiographic visualization and thus detect postoperative complications. For example, migration of a marker clip could indicate the presence of a hematoma in the wound. The artifacts (i.e., distortion) caused by stainless steel clips may be a disadvantage in future radiologic studies or MRI scans. Titanium and absorbable polymeric clips are preferred to eliminate or decrease image distortion of CT and MRI scans.

Ligatures. A ligature, commonly called a tie, is a strand of material that is tied around a blood vessel to manually occlude the lumen and prevent bleeding. Frequently the ligature is tied around a hemostat and slipped off the point onto the vessel and pulled taut to effect hemostasis. Vessels are ligated with the smallest size strand possible and include the smallest amount of surrounding tissue possible. Ends are cut as near the knot as possible.

Large and pulsating vessels may require a transfixion suture. A ligature on a needle (stick tie) is placed through a "bite" of tissue and brought around the end of the vessel. This eliminates any possibility of its slipping off the vessel. All bleeding points should be ligated before the next layer of tissue is incised.

Pledgets. Small pieces of Teflon felt are used as a buttress under sutures when bleeding might occur through the needle hole in a major vessel or when friable tissue might tear, such as cardiac muscle during cardiomyotomy. Placed over an arteriotomy site, they exert pressure to seal off bleeding. Pledgets are used most frequently in cardiovascular surgery and remain in place as part of the suture. Commercially prepared sutures with pledgets attached are available.

Packs. Packs are used to sustain pressure on raw wound surfaces and keep viscera from becoming injured during a procedure. The application of sponges or laparotomy tapes effectively controls capillary ooze by occluding the capillaries. The surgeon usually wants these packs moistened, often with room-temperature but sometimes with warm normal saline solution. Warm packs promote hemostasis by accelerating the coagulation mechanism. Warm saline does promote vasodilation and could augment venous oozing. Do not soak sponges or packs in the irrigation basin. Lint could be transferred to the patient, causing adhesions.

PROS/CONS

Irrigation, Solution Basins, and Dispersing Lint

Pros

- Irrigation is a major part of the intraoperative and postoperative processes of surgery. The purpose of irrigation is to keep tissues moist, flush out debris, keep the surgical field visible, wipe instruments clean, and decrease surgical site infections.
- Sponges and towels are two of the most frequently used items in surgery. Moist sponges are used to soak up blood, clean instruments, and retract or pack body cavities. Moist towels are also used as visceral retainers.
- Irrigation should be applied to sponges and towels by an Asepto syringe to avoid dispersing particulate in the solution basin. If necessary, a separate basin of solution can be used for this purpose.
- Surgeons may request several liters of fresh warm irrigation during the surgical procedure. They may ask for the solution in an Asepto syringe or pour directly from the basin into the patient.
- Warm fresh irrigation may be requested to irrigate the surgical site before closure. A clean Poole suction tip with the guard in place should be used to suction large amounts of irrigation fluid.
- Products used in the OR should be powder free and low linting.
- Solutions used on the sterile field as irrigation should be accounted for in their volume entirety to prevent confusion with estimated blood loss.
- Education regarding irrigation and sponges should include moistening all towels and sponges with an Asepto syringe in a separate basin or impervious area of the sterile field. If a towel or sponge is dipped into an irrigation basin, that irrigation is not safe for use inside the patient.

Cons

- During a procedure, a surgeon may request a wet sponge or towel. The scrub person commonly dips the sponge or towel and rings it out back into the basin before handing it to the surgeon. Dipping sponges and towels in the irrigation basin disperses fibers and lint into the solution. Floating particulate can be seen on the surface of the solution.

- Sponges and towels lose lint during routine use. This can lead to complications such as inflammation, granuloma or textiloma formation, adhesions, infection, thrombus formation, and tissue necrosis.
- High-lint cotton sponges and towels should be avoided. Cotton balls and cotton gauze should not be used in open body cavities because they shed the most fibers.
- Cases of coronary embolization from fiber fragments during the flushing of catheters with irrigation have been documented. Fibers were found in the solution where sponges were dipped. The catheter-flushing syringe was filled from the same irrigation basin and introduced the particulate and fibers into the patient's vascular system.
- Fibers and particulate have been found on guidewires and instrumentation that came into contact with the sponges, towels, and irrigation on the sterile field.
- Lack of standardization and understanding in perioperative practice puts patients at risk for foreign body reaction from fiber particles.
- Dipping sponges and towels in irrigation without measuring the amount used does not support accurate measurement of irrigation used during the procedure.

References

1. Barnes S, Spencer M, Graham D, et al.: Surgical wound irrigation: a call for evidence-based standardization of practice, *Am J Infect Control* 42(5):525–529, 2014.
2. Haidari M, Malakzai H, Haidary A, et al.: Gossypiboma of thigh mimicking soft tissue sarcoma: a case report and review of the literature, *Int J Surg Case Rep*, 106, 2023.
3. Laird JR: Reducing the risk of foreign body embolization during interventional procedures: keeping the room out of the patient, *Endovasc Today* 13(10): 96–99, 2014.

Compressed Absorbent Patties. Compressed absorbent radiopaque patties (cottonoids) are used for hemostasis when placed on the surface of brain tissue and to absorb blood and fluids around the spinal cord or nerves. These patties are available in an assortment of sizes. Before use, the scrub person counts and moistens them with normal saline solution, presses out excess solution, and keeps them flat. Some surgeons prefer an antibiotic, thrombin, or epinephrine solution to moisten the patties for hemostasis.

Bone Wax. Composed of a sterile nonabsorbable mixture of beeswax, isopropyl palmitate, and a softening agent, bone wax provides a mechanical tamponade barrier to stop oozing from cut bone surfaces. Each foil packet contains 2.5 g of wax and is opened just before use to minimize drying. The scrub person can warm wax to the desired consistency by manipulating it with the fingers or by immersing the unopened packet in warm solution. Small pieces can be rolled into 1-cm balls and placed around the rim of a medicine cup or bowl. When needed, the cup can be presented to the surgeon. Some surgeons prefer to use a freer elevator to apply the wax to the bleeding bone edge.

Bone wax is used in some orthopedic and neurosurgical procedures and when the sternum is split (sternotomy) for cardiothoracic procedures. Bone wax should be used sparingly and is contraindicated when rapid bone regeneration is desired. The wax is not soluble and is a mechanical barrier that can persist for years; it may impede ossification sund bone union. It is contraindicated

in the presence of infection. Some patients may be sensitive and can develop a foreign body reaction or osteomyelitis.

The product is cobalt sterilized, and the expiration date should be checked before use. It should not be stored in areas that exceed 77° F (25° C).

Bone Wax Alternatives. Biodegradable water-soluble material that looks and feels like bone wax is a physical mechanical barrier on cut bone edges and is intended to be used sparingly. One type, Ostene, is an inert alkylene oxide copolymer, derived from ethylene oxide and propylene oxide. Ostene contains no beeswax and does not cause an inflammatory response like beeswax. It is supplied in 1- to 3-g foil packets for sterile use. More information can be found at www.ostene.com.

Bone wax alternative is sterilized by irradiation and cannot be reprocessed. It should be warmed to body temperature and worked into soft 1-cm balls just like bone wax. It has no biophysical cellular action, and its presence in the wound does not impair osteogenesis. It is contraindicated in the presence of infection.

Digital Compression. When digital pressure is applied to an artery proximal to the area of bleeding, such as in traumatic injury, hemorrhage is controlled. The main disadvantage of digital pressure is that it cannot be applied permanently. Firm pressure is applied on the skin on both sides as the skin incision is made to help control subcutaneous bleeding until vessels can be clamped, ligated, or cauterized. Pressure is applied while the surgical area is sponged to locate a bleeding vessel.

Suction-Irrigation. Suction is the application of negative pressure, either continuously or intermittently. It is used during surgical procedures for removal of blood and tissue fluids from the surgical field, primarily to enhance visibility. An appropriate diameter and style of tip for evacuation of blood is attached to sterile disposable suction tubing. The scrub person hands the end of the tubing to the circulating nurse, who attaches it to a suction collection container.

A powered suction-irrigation system may be used to simultaneously irrigate the wound and evacuate solution. The irrigation may be pulsed (i.e., intermittent to remove debris and clots) or continuous with gravity flow. The surgeon adjusts the flow of irrigation and suction with controls on the disposable tip assembly. Spatter screens that fit around the tip of the irrigator like a cone to minimize splashes and aerosolization are commercially available.

Drains. Postoperatively, drains aid in removal of blood, fluid, and air from the surgical site to obliterate dead spaces and enhance approximation of tissues, thus preventing hematoma and seroma formation. Drains usually are placed through a stab wound in the skin adjacent to the primary incision.

Thermal Methods of Hemostasis

Hemostasis may be achieved or enhanced by application of either cold or heat to body tissues.

Cold Methods of Hemostasis

Cryosurgery. Cryosurgery is performed with the aid of special instruments for local freezing of diseased tissue without harm to normal adjacent structures. Extreme cold causes intracapillary thrombosis and tissue necrosis in the frozen area. Frozen tissue may be removed without significant bleeding during or after the surgical procedure. Cryosurgery is also used to alter cell function without removal of tissue. It tends to be hemostatic and lymphostatic, particularly in highly vascular areas.

Extreme cold is delivered to extract heat from a small volume of tissue in a rapid manner. Liquid nitrogen is the most commonly used refrigerant; however, carbon dioxide gas may be used. The liquid or gas is in a vacuum container and comes through an insulated vacuum tube to a probe. All but the tip of the probe is insulated. Freezing of tissue at this tip is a result of the liquid nitrogen at the lowest temperature of $-320°$ F $(-196°$ C$)$ becoming gaseous. In the process, heat is removed from the tissue. A ball of frozen tissue gradually forms around the uninsulated tip. The extent of tissue destruction is controlled by raising or lowering the temperature of cells surrounding the lesion from $-4°$ F to $> -6°$ F $(-20°$ C to $> -21°$ C$)$.

The machines vary in range of temperatures obtained according to their design and type of refrigerant used. Some are nonelectric with foot switch–operated probes. Special miniature, presterilized, disposable models for single-patient use are particularly suitable for ophthalmic applications.

Because the process is rapid, involves less trauma to destroy or remove tissue, controls bleeding, and minimizes local pain, cryosurgery is used to alter the function of nerve cells and destroy otherwise unapproachable brain tumors. Other techniques for which it is used include removal of superficial tumors in the nasopharynx and the skin, destruction of the prostate gland, removal of highly vascular tumors and some otherwise non-resectable liver tumors, removal of lesions from the cervix and anus, cataract extraction, and retinal detachment. The amount of tissue destroyed is influenced by the size of the tip of the probe, temperature used, duration of use, kind of tissue and its vascularity, and skill of the surgeon.

Hypothermia. Cooling of body tissues to a temperature as low as $78.8°$ F $(26°$ C$)$ in adults and large children and $68°$ F $(20°$ C$)$ in infants and small children, well below normal limits, decreases cellular metabolism and thereby decreases the need for oxygen by tissues. The decreased requirement for oxygen decreases bleeding. Hypothermia lowers blood pressure to slow the circulation and increases the viscosity of blood. This process results in hemoconcentration, which contributes to capillary occlusion and microcirculatory stasis to provide an essentially dry field for the surgeon. Hypothermia may be localized or generalized (systemic). Hypothermia is used as an adjunct to anesthesia, particularly during heart, brain, and liver procedures.

Hot Methods of Hemostasis

Diathermy. Oscillating high-frequency electric current generates enough heat to coagulate and destroy body tissues. Heat is generated by resistance of tissues to passage of alternating electric current. A short-wave diathermy machine produces a high frequency of 10 million to 100 million cycles per second. The machine should not be activated until the surgeon is ready to deliver this current. Diathermy is useful in stopping bleeding from small blood vessels. It is used primarily to repair a detached retina and to cauterize small warts, polyps, and other small superficial lesions.

Electrocautery. A small battery-operated pencil with a tiny thin wire loop heated by a steady direct electric current to red heat coagulates or destroys tissue on contact. Heat is transferred to tissue from the preheated wire. Electrocautery pencils are commonly used for plastic surgery, eye procedures, and vasectomies.

The hot point of the cautery should be at least 24 inches (61 cm) from the anesthesia machine and the patient's oxygen source (facemask or endotracheal tube), which is an oxygen-rich environment. Cautery should not be used in the mouth, around the head, or in the pleural cavity. Cautery should not be used when any flammable agent is present. To prevent fire, only moist sponges should be permitted on the field while any cautery is in use.

Electrosurgery. High-frequency electric current provided from an electrosurgical unit (ESU) frequently is used to cut tissue and coagulate bleeding points. The concentration and flow of current generate heat as it meets resistance in passage through tissue. Because air has low electrical conductivity, an active electrode tip delivering radiofrequency energy must be in direct contact with tissue. Both cutting and coagulating currents are used in many open and minimally invasive surgical procedures. Some surgeons prefer electrosurgery to other methods of cutting and ligating vessels. ESU is not used on the skin.

Coagulated tissue is devitalized and causes a foreign body reaction that must be resorbed by the body during healing. If a large amount of coagulated tissue is present, sloughing and necrosis may result.

Because the high-frequency electric current goes through the patient's body during monopolar use, a return electrode is applied to the patient and plugged into the grounded generator. When a bipolar ESU is used, the current does not pass through the patient's body and a return electrode is not needed. Smoke, or plume, from use of the ESU should be removed from the air with a smoke evacuator. Combined ESU and smoke evacuator units are commercially available. ESUs are described in detail in Chapter 20.

Fulguration. Sparks of high-voltage electric current char the surface of tissue, producing a thin coagulated crust (eschar) without damaging underlying tissues. Fulguration uses a spark-gap monopolar generator that emits a higher-frequency current than does electrocoagulation from an ESU. This high-voltage arcing, described as spray coagulation, is used primarily for transurethral bladder and prostate procedures. A return electrode pad is used on the patient.

Argon Beam Coagulator. Argon gas in combination with an ESU pencil effectively delivers radiofrequency energy to tissue in a coaxial, noncontact, white-light beam for the purpose of rapid hemostasis monopolar coagulation. The argon beam coagulator directs a gentle flow of ionized argon gas from a generator to a pencil-shaped handpiece. The nonflammable gas flow over tissues clears blood and fluid from the target site and allows creation of a superficial eschar directly on tissue by the ESU pencil.

Less necrotic tissue is produced than with the high-current density of electrocoagulation because the temperature never exceeds 230° F (110° C) and penetration is approximately half the depth, which minimizes tissue destruction.

The depth of penetration depends on the power, duration of application, and electrical characteristics of the tissue. Coagulation occurs through the arcing effect of electrical energy, not through the action of the argon gas. The coaxial flow of gas delivers monopolar current that coagulates the surface with practically no smoke or odor. A return electrode is applied to the patient to complete the electrical circuit.

The argon beam coagulator is used to control hemorrhage from vascular structures, surface bleeding of an organ such as the liver, and diffuse oozing and to achieve hemostasis of bone marrow. Handpieces and electrodes are available for use through endoscopes, but they are not used in fluid environments, such as joints.

Hemostatic Scalpel. The sharp steel blade of the hemostatic scalpel seals blood vessels as it cuts through tissue. The disposable blade, size No. 10, 11, or 15, has a heating and sensing microcircuitry between the steel and a layer of copper coated with electrical insulation and a nonstick surface. The blade fits into a reusable handle that contains control switches.

The scrub person hands the end of the electrical cord attached to the handle to the circulating nurse, who plugs it into the controller unit. When the surgeon activates the handpiece, the blade transfers thermal energy to tissues as the sharp edge cuts through them. An audible sound is emitted to signal the activation of the device. The temperature can be adjusted between 230° F and 518° F (110−270° C). The surgeon can raise or lower the temperature in increments of 50° F (10° C). After use, it remains hot to the touch for 30 to 40 seconds. The blade also can be used cold, like any other scalpel.

The hemostatic scalpel can be used to incise skin, soft tissues, and muscle in a long smooth stroke. This is particularly advantageous in vascular areas, such as the scalp, head and neck, and breast. The blade is kept clean by wiping with a damp surgical sponge. Scraping the surface of the blade on a tip polisher decreases its efficiency. Care is taken not to touch the hemostatic scalpel blade to an active ESU tip so that the circuitry is not damaged.

This scalpel may be used to debride burns. Blood flow into the incised area is minimal, which provides the surgeon with a clear dry field, thus shortening surgical time. The rapid hemostasis with minimal tissue damage promotes wound healing and may eliminate a need for blood replacement. It is not effective in a bloody field or for vessels larger than 1.5 mm. Because electric current from the microcircuitry does not pass through the patient's body, a return electrode is not required. This also prevents muscle contractions.

Plasma Scalpel. The plasma scalpel vaporizes tissues and stops bleeding as it simultaneously cuts and coagulates tissue. Within the instrument, which looks like a large ballpoint pen, argon or helium gas passes through an electric arc that ionizes it into a high thermal state. These gases are inert and noncombustible. As the instrument moves over tissue, the gas that flows from the tip is visible, which allows the surgeon to see the depth and extent of the incision.

Tissue damage, with resultant inflammatory response during wound healing, is greater than that caused by a steel knife blade but less than that caused by other electrosurgical instruments and lasers. Because it coagulates blood vessels up to 3 mm in diameter, the plasma scalpel is useful in highly vascular areas.

Ultrasonic-Harmonic Scalpel. The titanium blade of the scalpel moves with a rapid ultrasonic motion that cuts and coagulates tissue simultaneously. The portable generator, a microprocessor with piezoelectric discs, converts electrical energy into mechanical energy. This energy is transmitted through a handpiece to a single-use blade. All three parts of the system lock into a frequency of 55,500 movements per second. When this happens, the system is said to be in harmony: thus the name harmonic scalpel.

The scalpel can be used for sharp or blunt dissection without damage to adjacent tissues. Vibrations from the blade denature protein molecules as it cuts through tissue, producing a coagulum that seals bleeding vessels. The continuous vibration of the denatured protein generates heat within the tissue to cause deeper coagulation. This action does not raise tissue temperature above 176° F (80° C), so that char or smoke is not produced. A fatty particulate mist may be generated. The vibrating blade also produces a cavitation effect (as it cuts through tissue with high water content) that disrupts cell walls and separates tissue, which aids in dissection.

The ultrasonic scalpel is used primarily for laparoscopic and thoracoscopic procedures. Blades and accessories for open procedures make this technology available to all surgical specialties. Because electricity is not required for effects on tissue, a return electrode is not necessary.

Laser. Laser light is used for control of bleeding or for ablation and excision of tissues in organs that can be exposed or are accessible endoscopically. The laser furnishes an intense and concentrated light beam of a single wavelength from a monochromatic source of nonionizing radiation. Thermal energy of this beam may simultaneously cut, coagulate, and vaporize tissue.

The laser wound is characterized by minimal bleeding and no visible postoperative edema. The amount of tissue destruction is predictable by adjusting the width and focus of the beam. Different lasers have selective uses. Lasers are described in detail in Chapter 20.

Photocoagulation. The photocoagulator uses an intense multiwavelength light furnished by a xenon tube to coagulate tissue. Its use is limited to ophthalmology.

Wound Management

Providing appropriate conditions for wound healing has been a quest through the ages. In ancient mythology, the Greek god Hermes carried a staff entwined with two snakes. This signified the snake's ability to repeatedly shed and regenerate its skin. Although humans do not shed their skin, they can regenerate tissue cells if the wound is protected from accumulations of blood and serum, mechanical injury, impaired circulation, and infection.

Drains

The use of devices to drain fluids and pus from the body dates back to the writings of Hippocrates. He wrote of insertion of a hollow tin or silver tube with flushings of wine and tepid oil to treat empyema. This was the first wound drainage system. In the 19th century, glass tubes, to be replaced by rubber catheters, were commonly used for gravity drainage.

In 1897, Dr. Charles B. Penrose (1862–1925), an American gynecologist, described a passive tubular drain made of gutta-percha, the coagulated latex from rubber trees, with a gauze wick inserted through the length of the lumen. This latex drain, which still bears his name, is in use today to maintain a vent for the escape of fluid or air or to wall off an area of exudate in the wound. Sump drains, commercially introduced in 1932, offered advantages, such as use with suction apparatus. Suction drainage has been used since 1947. Closed-wound drainage systems, first introduced in 1952, are used to enhance wound healing.

The use of gravity drainage through various types of tubes versus capillary drainage through wicking devices historically has been a controversial issue. Even today, surgeons do not universally agree on the use of systems currently available. The location and purpose of the drain determine the surgeon's selection from the many types available. Drains may be used prophylactically or therapeutically during the surgical procedure or postoperatively.[10] Drains and drainage reservoirs are disposable.

Intraoperative Drainage

Used prophylactically to evacuate gastric contents, intestinal fluids, or urine, intraoperative drainage and decompression help prevent tissue trauma and restore organs to normal function.

Gastrointestinal Decompression

A plastic or rubber nasogastric tube inserted through a nostril down into the stomach or small intestine removes flatus, fluids, and other contents. The tube has holes in several locations near the tip to permit withdrawal of the contents. Several types of nasogastric tubes are used; the most common are the Levin tube into the stomach and the Dobhoff tube into the small intestine. A vented tube, such as the Salem sump tube, is preferable for use with nasogastric suction. Tubes can be single lumen or double lumen.

To prevent aspiration of stomach contents, the anesthesia provider may insert a nasogastric tube preoperatively to empty the stomach before an emergency surgical procedure. The surgeon may ask the anesthesia provider to insert a tube during an intra-abdominal procedure for one of the following purposes:
- Decompression of the gastrointestinal tract
- Relief of distention that obstructs the view of the surgical site
- Measurement of blood loss from gastric hemorrhage
- Evacuation of gastric secretions during intestinal anastomosis

The nasogastric tube may remain in place postoperatively to prevent vomiting and distention caused by decreased peristalsis after anesthesia, manipulation of the viscera during the surgical procedure, or obstruction from edema of tissues at the surgical site. For this purpose, the tube is connected to a suction apparatus. The tube also may be used for nasogastric feeding during the healing process after a surgical procedure on the upper alimentary canal.

Urinary Drainage

Urethral or ureteral catheters inserted preoperatively provide constant drainage from the bladder or kidneys during the surgical procedure. The purpose may be to keep the bladder decompressed or to prevent extravasation of urine into the tissues around the surgical site during and after genitourinary procedures.

Postoperatively, the inflated balloon of an indwelling Foley catheter maintains an even pressure on the bladder neck, which may help control bleeding after prostatectomy, for example. An indwelling Foley catheter may be connected to a bladder irrigation or gravity drainage system until the bladder resumes normal function postoperatively. A suprapubic urinary catheter may be inserted percutaneously to assist with urinary drainage after pelvic surgery.

Postoperative Drainage

Drains are used therapeutically in the presence of purulent or necrotic material. Prophylactically, they may be inserted to evacuate fluids, including blood, or air from a wound or body cavity postoperatively.[10] Drains are usually placed in a separate small stab wound adjacent to the surgical incision and secured with a nonabsorbable monofilament suture. Drains can stimulate a walling-off process around a surgical site in which subsequent drainage may accumulate. This enhances wound healing by the following:
- Eliminating fluid accumulation
- Obliterating dead space
- Allowing apposition of tissues
- Preventing formation of hematomas or seromas
- Preventing tissue devitalization or wound margin necrosis
- Minimizing a potential source of wound contamination
- Decreasing postoperative pain
- Minimizing scarring

The action of drains may be either passive or active.

Passive Drains

Passive drains provide the path of least resistance to the outside. They function by overflow and capillary action through the drain to the absorbent dressing. They are influenced by pressure differentials and may be assisted by gravity.

Penrose Drain. A Penrose drain is a thin-walled cylinder of radiopaque latex. Nonlatex Penrose drains are commercially available. The diameter may be ¼ to 2 inches (6 mm to 5 cm), depending on the surgeon's preference. The drain is usually supplied to the sterile field in a 6 to 12 inch (15–30 cm) length for the surgeon to cut as desired. Penrose drains are commercially available prepackaged and sterilized. However, if they are prepared for onsite steam sterilization, a gauze wick is inserted to permit steam penetration of the lumen.

Although Penrose drains generally are used without a wick, the surgeon may prefer that the wick of gauze packing be left in the lumen to absorb drainage from the wound. This is referred to as a "cigarette" drain. For use without a wick, the drain is moistened in normal saline solution before it is handed to the surgeon. After it is placed into the surgical area and brought out through a stab wound in the skin, the drain is secured with a skin suture, or a sterile safety pin is attached on the outside close to the skin to keep the drain from retracting into the wound. The head of the safety pin should be crimped closed with a large forceps to prevent it from opening and piercing the patient.

Constant Gravity Drainage

A drain may be inserted for drainage by gravity flow from the gallbladder, bladder, or kidney. Each OR suite has a supply of sterile rubber or silicone tubes and catheters. Those used for drains, such as a T-tube, should be radiopaque. Some have inflatable balloons (e.g., Foley catheters) or enlarged bulbous ends (e.g., mushroom, Malecot, Pezzer catheters) to help hold them in place. A monofilament nonabsorbable suture may be used to circumferentially secure the drain in place.

A closed or semiclosed system is used to collect drainage. The scrub person keeps the end of the tube or catheter sterile until it is connected to the sterile end of the constant drainage tubing. Tubing should be connected or clamped as soon as the drain is brought through a stab wound in the skin or a tube or catheter is inserted into an organ. The circulating nurse connects tubing to a drainage bag. Constant drainage bags are marked in gradations from 500 to 2000 mL. The bag must be in a dependent position, lower than the site of the drain, to avoid retrograde reflux.

Active Drains

Active drains are attached to an external source of vacuum to create suction in the wound. A constant gentle negative-pressure vacuum evacuates tissue fluid, blood, and air through a silicone, polyvinyl chloride, or polyurethane drain. Suction levels vary, depending on the system, to create the negative pressure (less than atmospheric).

Closed Wound Suction Systems. These systems are used when suction must be applied to an uninfected closed-wound site in the chest wall (e.g., after mastectomy), in the upper part of the abdomen, and in areas of joint replacement. They also are placed under large tissue flaps or in subcutaneous spaces in obese patients to eliminate dead space and hold tissues in apposition.

The sterile plastic drain has round or flat perforated and nonperforated tubing connected to a sharp stainless steel trocar. The trocar makes a small stab wound through the underlying tissues adjacent to the surgical incision and is brought up through the skin. The trocar is cut off and the nonperforated part of the drain tubing is pulled through the stab wound to the outside of the body. The perforated segment remains within the body. The nonperforated part of the tubing is attached to the disposable drainage collection reservoir. A monofilament nylon suture is used to stitch the tubing in place on the skin to minimize the risk for pulling out.

Several different units are available with reservoirs of different capacities and sizes of drainage tubing. Calibrations on the side of the container measure the drainage, and a line designates when it should be emptied or changed. These units are made entirely or partially of clear plastic so the surgeon can inspect drainage. The drain is radiopaque or has radiopaque markings to aid in checking its location on a radiograph, if desired.

The drainage reservoir can be attached immediately after placement of the tubing or after wound closure; then the vacuum is activated. Directions printed on each unit must be followed to activate the vacuum. The amount of suction in these systems varies depending on the method of creating the vacuum. Manually activated, spring-loaded devices (Hemovac) and grenade-type or bulb evacuators (Reliavac, Jackson-Pratt) have variable preset suction levels between 30 and 125 mm Hg (Fig. 29.3).

A portable, battery-powered device (VariDyne) can provide a constant and continuous vacuum at any setting between 10 and 350 mm Hg. With this system, the surgeon can determine the suction level on the basis of the material and area to be evacuated. With closed-wound suction systems, the drainage container does not need to be in a dependent position. An antireflux valve guards against backflow of fluids. Great care is taken not to dislodge the drainage tube when moving the patient from the OR bed to the transport cart after surgery.

Sump Drains. Sump drains may be used for aspiration, irrigation, or introduction of medication. Either flat or round, a sump drain has a double or triple lumen. Usually made of radiopaque silicone, it has large lateral openings to minimize clogging. The drain is brought out through a separate stab wound near the surgical site. Sump drains create equalized negative pressure at the site to be drained, usually in the abdomen.

Sump drains are connected to a constant drainage system, with or without suction. Irrigation of the surgical site and connection to suction as soon as possible enhance function. Levels of suction between 80 and 120 mm Hg are desirable. The tubing may be attached to a piped-in (wall) or portable vacuum system. The drain must be clamped when not attached to suction or connected to a closed container. It functions as a passive drain if peripheral suction is not used and must be in a dependent position.

Chest Drainage. Drainage of the pleural cavity ensures complete expansion of the lungs after surgery. Air and fluid must be evacuated from the pleural space after surgical procedures within the chest cavity. One or more chest tubes are inserted. If the surgeon inserts two, the upper tube evacuates air and the lower tube drains fluid. After the chest tube is inserted during closure, the end is covered with sterile gauze until it can be connected to a sterile closed water-seal drainage system. The drainage system must prevent outside air from being drawn into the pleural space during expiration. Water in the collection unit seals off outside air to maintain a negative pressure within the pleural cavity (Fig. 29.4).

Two tubes vent the leakproof top of the collection unit. A short air-outlet tube extends 1 inch (2.5 cm) or more above the stopper to about 3 inches (7.5 cm) below it into the collection unit. The long inlet tube extends from above the stopper, through it, to about 1 inch (2.5 cm) from the bottom of the collection unit. Sterile water is poured into the collection unit to a level 1 to 2 inches (2.5–5 cm) above the end of the long inlet tube. Clear sterile tubing connects the inlet tube to the tube placed into the pleural space. On the patient's initial expiration, water rises a short distance up into the inlet tube. With each subsequent inspiration-expiration, the water level in the tube fluctuates. If the water level in the tube remains stationary, the chest tube or connecting tubing may be clogged or kinked. The collection unit must be kept well below chest level to prevent water from entering the chest and to keep the tubing free of kinks.

Fluid drains by gravity from the chest into the water. The collection unit should be calibrated so drainage can be measured. Air bubbles through the water and escapes through the outlet tube.

If gravity drainage is not adequate for reexpansion of the lungs, suction may be applied at 15 to 20-cm water pressure to ensure evacuation of air and fluid. This requires the addition of one or two collection units to the system to act as a pressure regulator and the addition of a suction machine to maintain negative pressure. Disposable chest drainage units are available as a single unit or in a series of two or three. Some units have modifications based on the principle described for a closed water-seal system. Manufacturer directions should be followed for use. The unit must be properly connected before the patient leaves the OR.

With some units, the chest tube may be clamped during transportation as a safety measure. The surgeon should be

• **Fig. 29.3** Closed system active drainage. **A,** Hemovac drain reservoir. **B,** Bulb vacuum reservoir. **C,** Balloon pump hard canister reservoir. **D,** Activation of a Hemovac drain reservoir.

• **Fig. 29.4** Chest drainage. **A,** Placement of drains. **B,** Scrub person pours sterile water into the unit to create a water seal. **C,** Tubing attachment to three-chamber collection unit.

consulted as to whether clamping is contraindicated. Indiscriminate clamping can create a mediastinal shift of the thoracic organs. Only tube clamps are used to occlude the tubing, not crushing clamps such as a Kocher clamp.

Digital chest drainage systems (Thopaz$^+$) are available that have smart technology for alerts for malfunction.[11,12] More information can be found at www.medelahealthcare.com.

Patient Care Considerations

Drains, tubes, catheters, drainage tubing, and adapters are used for one patient only; they are never reused for another patient. If not properly handled by the scrub person and circulating nurse, a drain can be a source of wound contamination or irritation. When the surgeon inserts a drain, the following considerations should be kept in mind:

1. Drains, tubes, and catheters are kept sterile, ready for the circulating nurse to open if needed. They are available in many styles and sizes. They are patient charge items. Do not open until the surgeon specifies the style and size. A monofilament nonabsorbable suture on a small cutting needle is used to secure the drain to the skin. A Penrose drain may need a sterile safety pin. Remember to crush the head of the pin with a large clamp to prevent injury to the patient.

2. If the patient has a sensitivity to latex, do not use a drain, tube, or catheter with any latex components. Most drains are available in silicone.

3. The scrub person keeps the end of the drain sterile until it is connected to the sterile end of the drainage tubing.

4. Tubing connections must be physically tight and secured. Do not completely obscure connections by wrapping tape around them.

5. The drain site is dressed separately from the incision site. A nonadherent dressing can be used as the contact layer around the drain. Gauze dressings can be slit in a Y shape to fit around the base of the drain.

6. Avoid tension on the drain and kinks in the drain and tubing. A gentle loop can be made and secured with tape at the time of dressing application.

7. Collection bags or containers connected to passive drains, including chest tubes, must be kept well below the level of the body cavity where the drain is inserted and below the level of the drainage tubing to prevent retrograde flow. The amount of drainage should be recorded.

8. The circulating nurse must check the suction level to be certain it is consistent with the surgeon's orders or should activate the suction as appropriate for the system being used.

9. An x-ray may be taken for verification of placement of the drain or tube.

10. The type of drain, size, and its location are documented on the intraoperative record and reported to the PACU nurse.

Dressings

Most skin incisions and surgical wounds are covered with a sterile dressing for at least 24 to 48 hours to provide an optimal physiologic environment for wound healing. The dressing serves several functions:

- To keep the incision free of microorganisms, both exogenous and endogenous
- To protect the incision from outside injury, especially in children
- To absorb the drainage of exudates and secretions from the wound
- To maintain a moist environment that supports healing
- To give some support to the incision and surrounding skin, or to immobilize surrounding tissue
- To provide pressure to reduce edema or prevent hematoma
- To conceal the wound aesthetically

The function of a dressing is determined by its structure. The overall dressing should be:

- Large enough to cover and protect the wound site and tissue around it
- Permeable to gas and vapor, allowing circulation of air to the skin
- Secure to prevent slippage
- Comfortable for the patient

Types of Dressings

In considering the components to assemble for the dressing, the needs of the particular wound should be kept in mind. One wound may require a dressing that provides a function different from that needed for another type of wound. The dressing materials should be tailored to the location and condition of the wound site (Fig. 29.5).

One-Layer Dressing

A clean incision that is primarily closed with sutures, staples, or skin-closure tapes in which no or slight drainage is expected may be covered with an adhering occlusive dressing (e.g., Bioclusive, Opsite). These sterile, transparent, polyurethane film dressings are available in various sizes. The patient can bathe or shower with these in place. They usually are removed in 24 to 48 hours. Liquid collodion or other waterproof material may be used.

Skin-Closure Dressing

A transparent plastic film with an adhesive backing (Opsite) can be placed over the entire length of the incision to hold the skin edges in apposition. The film is vented to allow the escape of exudate. An additional wound dressing may be overlaid to further splint and reinforce approximation of the skin edges. These dressings are available in various sizes.

Dry Sterile Dressing

A single-layered or multilayered dressing is applied dry over a clean incision from which no or slight drainage is expected. Dry gauze is not used on a denuded area because it adheres and acts as a foreign body. Granulation tissue grows into it; bleeding can be reactivated when it is removed. A dry sterile dressing can be applied over a dry wound. It is secured with adhesive tape. A circumferential wrap may be preferred on an extremity, but it must not compromise circulation.

Three-Layer Dressing

When moderate to heavy drainage is expected, a complete dressing consists of at least three layers.

Contact Layer. The contact layer acts as a passageway for the secretion and exudates that emanate from a draining wound. It has a wicking action to help reduce the risk for infection and skin maceration. It must conform to body contours regardless of the site and extent of the wound and must stay in intimate contact with the wound surface for at least 48 hours yet be nonadherent for painless removal. Some dressings contain silver nanoparticles for antimicrobial properties with antibiotic intervention.[12] The contact layer may be:

Overlapping tape ⎫
                  ⎬ Outer wrap
Cushioning layer ⎭

Absorbent layer

Lubricant (contact) layer

• **Fig. 29.5** Anatomy of a dressing.

- *Nonocclusive:* Nonadherent materials, such as gauze sponges or compressed material on a thin plastic or aluminum film, draw secretions from the wound but remain air-permeable. The looser the weave of the material, the more nonocclusive it is.
- *Semiocclusive:* Hydroactive materials, such as foams, hydrogels, collagen, and hydrocolloids, provide a mechanical surface with permeability properties. Some of these agents help debride the wound or promote healing.
- *Occlusive:* An airtight seal prevents drying of the wound. The dressing is impermeable to air and water but allows passage of exudates. This is usually a fine mesh gauze dressing impregnated with an oil emulsion, such as petrolatum, Xeroform, iodophor, antibiotic ointment, or scarlet red. It is nonadherent to the skin or wound.

Intermediate Layer. This layer absorbs secretions passing through the contact layer. To provide adequate capacity, it should be layered (e.g., with gauze sponges) to the thickness required by the particular wound. It should not be excessively bulky. It must not unnecessarily apply pressure that could compromise circulation.

Outer Layer. This layer holds the contact and intermediate layers in proper position. It should be conforming, stretchable to avoid constriction if edema develops, and capable of clinging to itself so that it stays in position without telescoping if mobility is desired. The following materials are used for this purpose:

1. Nonallergenic tape is used most frequently. Other types of tape in various widths from ½ to 4 inches include foam tape, silk, paper, and linen cloth adhesive.
2. An elastic bandage provides gentle, even pressure to hold bulky dressings in place or to bind a splint onto an extremity. It stretches to conform to body contours, does not constrict, and yet gives firm support. The types available include the following:
   a. Four-ply crinkled-gauze bandage
   b. Cotton elastic bandage
   c. Cotton elastic bandage with adhesive on one side, which is especially useful in holding dressings on the chest because it is firm yet permits chest expansion
3. Montgomery straps are used to hold bulky dressings that require frequent changes or wound inspections. These are pairs of adhesive straps in assorted widths with gauze strings attached to one folded end of each strap. The other end of each strap is secured to the skin on each side of the dressing. The strings are tied across the dressing to hold it in place, usually on the abdomen.
4. Stockinette is put over the dressing on an extremity before application of a rigid cast used for immobilization. Available in several widths, stockinette is a seamless tubing of stretchable knitted cotton.
5. Mesh undergarments can be used to secure perineal dressings on male and female patients. The mesh is a loosely woven elastic fabric that is not compressive, but supports dressings in areas that are not easily taped in place.

Pressure Dressing

Bulky dressings are added to the intermediate layer of a three-layer dressing after many extensive surgical procedures, especially in plastic surgery and surgical procedures on the knee or breast. Pressure dressings are used for the following purposes:

- To eliminate dead space and prevent edema or hematoma
- To distribute pressure evenly
- To absorb extensive drainage
- To encourage wound healing and minimize scarring by influencing wound tension
- To immobilize a body area or support soft tissues when muscles are moved
- To help provide comfort to the patient after surgery
  Materials used for pressure dressings include the following:
- Fluffed gauze
- Combine pads, which are gauze-covered absorbent cellulose
- Single-piece bulk dressings, which are available for use on the trunk and extremities and save time in application
- Cotton rolls, which are used, for example, to apply pressure on each side of a knee after a surgical procedure on that joint
- Foam rubber

Stent Dressing

Stent fixation is a method of applying pressure and stabilizing tissues when it is impossible to dress an area, such as the face or neck. A form-fitting mold may be taped over the nose. Long suture ends can be crisscrossed over a small dressing and tied.

Bolster/Tie-Over Dressing

Dressing materials may be sutured in place to exert an even pressure over autografted wounds to prevent hematoma or seroma formation. Sterile gauze may be rolled into a tubular shape and tied with the ends of the wound closure suture (Fig. 29.6).

Wet-to-Dry Dressing

Dressing materials soaked in sterile normal saline solution are applied to the wound and allowed to dry thoroughly. The dried dressing is then removed, taking adhering tissue layers with it. This process is used to facilitate new tissue growth and is commonly used on burn wounds. Because this method of debridement is extremely painful, it is frequently performed in the OR with the patient under general anesthesia.

Wet-to-Wet Dressing

Dressing materials are soaked in sterile normal saline solution or other medicated solution and applied wet. This method provides little mechanical debridement and is less painful for the patient. The dressing material may be changed in the OR or under sterile conditions on the patient care unit.

Silicone Dressing

Silicone dressings are used as a measure of scar reduction and prevention. The sheet of silicone can be cut to fit and is snugly adherent to the wound to prevent overgrowth of the cicatrix. Conventional dressing tape can be used but is not usually necessary. The dressing can be rinsed off and reapplied by the patient during the healing period. The sheets should be worn a minimum of 6 hours per day and are replaced once per week.

The natural tackiness of the silicone sometimes causes difficulty when gloves are worn for placement of the sheet. Plastic surgeons use this material frequently.

Dialkylcarbamoyl Chloride–Coated Dressing

Dressings coated with dialkylcarbamoyl chloride attract bacteria to coated fibers.[13] The bacteria are inactivated and remain attached to the coating. The bacteria are removed with dressing changes.

Negative Pressure Dressing

The negative pressure dressing is an active dressing providing a barrier while augmenting even pressure over the site. These are sometimes called wound vacuum dressings (wound vac). Negative pressure dressings are multilayer wound covers attached to a suction unit for even pressure maintenance. The dressing consists of a fenestrated nonadherent piece of plastic with encapsulated foam, which is placed over the wound and then covered with a

sheet of foam material. This multilayer wound cover is sealed with a plastic adherent sheet that is connected to negative pressure.

Application of Dressings

Application of sterile dressings is regarded as part of the surgical procedure. The scrub person and circulating nurse assist the surgeon or first assistant in dressing the surgical site post-operatively. The procedure is as follows:

1. The circulating nurse opens sterile dressings after the final sponge count is completed. Radiopaque sponges are not used because they could distort a postoperative x-ray or cause an incorrect count if the patient's incision must be reopened.
2. Skin surrounding the incision is cleaned of blood with a sponge moistened with sterile saline solution and dried by a sterile team member.
3. The incision and wound drainage sites are dressed separately unless the drain comes out through the incision. The scrub person cuts a Y-shaped slit in dressings to go around the drain.
4. Sterile dressings are applied and held in place by a sterile team member as the drapes are removed. When the drapes are off, the circulating nurse, wearing examination gloves, helps clean and dry the surrounding skin.
5. Benzoin or some other tackifier adhesive substance may be applied on the skin around the intermediate layer before tape is applied, to increase its adhesion.
6. The circulating nurse applies tape or Montgomery straps (as appropriate) firmly but not tightly to avoid wrinkling and traction on skin. Traction and wrinkling can cause skin irritation. If a patient has a known sensitivity to regular adhesive tape, hypoallergenic tape should be used. It is lightweight, yet strong; sticks well; is porous; and allows skin to breathe.
7. The surgeon or first assistant applies elastic wrap bandages, pressure dressings, stockinette and casts, and splints. The circulating nurse provides the necessary supplies and assists as appropriate. A patient care assistant may help hold the patient's torso or extremity during application of an elastic wrap bandage or cast. Cast application is discussed in Chapter 36.

Complications of Wound Healing

The surgeon gives meticulous attention to sterile technique, hemostasis, tissue handling and approximation, and selection of wound-closure materials, including drains and dressings. The entire OR team carries out strict aseptic and sterile techniques to prevent infection and other possible complications of wound healing.

Hematoma/Seroma

Collections of blood or serum in a wound can act as a mechanical barrier to margination of the wound. Circulation can be interrupted, and neovascularization cannot take place. Studies have shown that biochemical action of the collection causes tissue destruction and promotes bacterial growth. Hematomas in deep tissue can lead to abscess formation.

Scar/Surgical Cicatrix

After the natural process of wound healing, a scar (cicatrix) remains on the skin surface. To achieve a cosmetically acceptable scar, the surgeon attempts to make the surgical incision along natural creases or within natural skinfolds or hairlines. The location and

• **Fig. 29.6** Bolster/tie-over dressing.

direction of the incision affect scarring. Tension needed for approximation of wound edges during closure and subsequent movement of underlying tissues can affect wound healing and scar formation. Wounds in mobile skin contract, resulting in a smaller scar.

Hypertrophic scars, which are a result of excessive fibrin formation within the borders of the scar, can develop from too much tension on the wound, poor approximation of wound edges, or infection. Some suture materials may contribute to hypertrophy. Burn wounds are also conducive to excessive scarring. The patient may wish to have an unsightly scar revised at a future time.

Keloids develop when the inflammatory response and fibroblast proliferation are overactive during wound healing (Fig. 29.7). This is an inherited trait, most common among Africans, Asians, and people with dark skin tones or those who freckle. Keloids extend beyond the borders of the scar and can continue to grow and become very large and painful over a prolonged period after the surgical procedure.

A keloid may be painful, itchy, and prone to bleeding. They can be excised, leaving a small border of scar tissue. The edges are approximated using skin staples or fine monofilament nonabsorbable suture. If a patient is known to have keloids form, an antiinflammatory agent may be injected into tissue before closure. A pressure dressing is useful in minimizing keloid formation. Application of silicone gel sheeting placed over healed bulky tissue scars for 24 hours over a period of 2 weeks can reduce the size of the scar. Use of the neodymium:yttrium-aluminum-garnet (Nd:YAG) laser can decrease the size of the scar.

Nodules and granulomas may form in the scar if excess suture material is used. Scar tissue hypertrophies around the suture, particularly the knot. Some patients extrude suture pieces through the incision line for several months or years postoperatively. This may represent a sensitivity to the suture material.

Adhesions

An **adhesion** is a fibrous scar band that binds together two surfaces or structures that normally are separate. Fibrous bands that develop in the peritoneal cavity can hold viscera together, sometimes causing bowel obstruction or female infertility.

The most common cause is previous abdominal or pelvic surgery, but acute appendicitis or peritonitis can cause adhesion

• **Fig. 29.7** Keloid scars can form over chest and neck of susceptible patients as a complication of wound healing.

formation. Serosal injury caused by abrasion from sponges or gloves, tissue handling, infection, and tissue ischemia may be a precipitating factor. Other substances, such as blood and biologic debris, can contribute to adhesion formation. Granulomas that form from powder on gloves, lint on sponges, or other foreign material left in the wound also predispose the patient to adhesion formation.

Techniques to prevent peritoneal adhesions include gentle tissue handling, careful irrigation with sterile saline or lactated Ringer solution, and prevention of foreign body introduction, such as glove powder and lint. Placement of a flap of omentum over the affected organ before closure is another acceptable method.

A single-layer, knitted, absorbable adhesion barrier sheet, such as Interceed (TC7), can be placed over abdominal organs after attaining hemostasis and before closure. It is composed of oxidized regenerated cellulose and absorbs in about 4 weeks. This product is contraindicated in the presence of known infection.

One type of barrier sheet, composed of sodium hyaluronate and carboxymethylcellulose (HA/CMC), can be used over organs at risk for adhesion formation. Once moistened, it adheres to the surface of the organ. No suturing is necessary. It converts to a gel form and is absorbed by the body in 7 days. Bioabsorbable translucent spray barriers such as SprayShield are available.

Postoperative Wound Disruption

Failure of a wound to heal or closure material to secure it during the healing process leads to **wound disruption**—a separation of wound edges. Disruption usually occurs between the 5th and 10th postoperative days. This is the lag period in healing, the time when the wound is not yet strong. Wound disruption is caused not by a single factor but by a combination of predisposing factors that influence healing.

Although it may occur in any body area, acute wound disruption most frequently follows abdominal laparotomy, surgical incision into the peritoneal cavity. It starts with a small opening in the peritoneum, which allows a wedge of omentum to slip through it. This omentum becomes edematous and extends the opening along the line of incision and upward through other layers of the abdominal wall. Disruption is usually precipitated by distention or a sudden strain, such as vomiting, coughing, or sneezing. Terms used to describe abdominal wound disruption include the following:

- *Dehiscence:* Partial or total separation of the superficial layers of the wound. The strength of the tissues and extent of separation determine whether the wound must be reclosed. Strangulated sutures can cause devitalized wound edges that may fail to heal. Wound infection can cause dehiscence.
- *Evisceration:* Protrusion of viscera through the full thickness of the abdominal incision. Although wound disruption of any degree calls for emergency care, an evisceration requires immediate replacement of viscera and reclosure of the incision.
- *Herniation:* The surface layers remain intact, but the deep layers separate, permitting the underlying muscles or organs to bulge.
- *Fistula:* Draining tunnels may form between two organs, such as between loops of bowel and the bladder.
- *Sinus tract:* An abscess may form in deeper tissues and form a tunnel to the outside of the body.

Symptoms

Patients who subsequently experience wound disruption often do not have a smooth course immediately after surgery. They may have undue pain, discomfort, nausea, drainage, slight fever, vomiting, or hiccups. Acute symptoms of wound disruption include the following:

- Tachycardia
- Vomiting
- Abnormal serosanguineous discharge
- Change in contour of the wound
- Sudden pulling pain during straining (the patient feels something "give")

Any seepage of serosanguineous fluid is suspicious and should be sent for culture and sensitivity before the skin prep is started. A swab culture for both aerobic and anaerobic microorganisms should be obtained. If the patient has had antibiotic therapy, this should be noted on the laboratory request. The patient's wound, rather than the eschar, should be swabbed. Gloves should be worn when culturing a patient's wound or handling dressing material.

Any of these symptoms should be investigated at once. Examination of the wound may show it gaping somewhat, or viscera may appear at the skin surface.

Treatment at the Bedside

1. Place an emergency call for the surgeon. Have a nasogastric tube ready for insertion to relieve distention (if appropriate).
2. Reassure the patient.
3. Apply sterile towels over the wound and saturate them with saline solution to keep the area moist.
4. Give drugs according to the surgeon's order.
5. Do not give the patient anything by mouth.
6. Prepare the patient for return to the OR. Treatment in the OR consists of secondary wound closure. Grossly infected wounds may require delayed primary closure.

Compartment Syndrome

Extreme inflammation can cause swelling between the fascial layers in any plane of the body. Compartment syndrome is frequently seen in limbs, although it can happen in any area of the body where skeletal muscle is encapsulated with fascia. Fluids, exudates, and transudates build up between the tissue layers and cause tissue ischemia and destruction of cells.

Compartment syndrome is a surgical emergency that requires linear fascial incisions (fasciotomy) to release the pressure within the capsule. Fasciotomy is performed to save the tissue from necrosis. The fascial incisions are left open to drain for weeks or months. Primary closure is complex after repeated debridement, and the wound may remain open at various degrees for several months. Scarring is deep and disfiguring because much vital tissue is lost. Skin grafts may be necessary.

Postoperative Wound Infections

Wound healing can be interrupted by infection at almost any phase. Infection results from introduction of virulent microorganisms into the receptive wound of a susceptible host. Moisture and warmth in the wound create an environment conducive to bacterial growth. Wound infections warrant special attention because many occur in clean wounds as a result of microorganisms introduced at the time of the surgical procedure. Secondary contamination is uncommon because fibrin seals the wound within hours after the surgical procedure.

A postoperative wound infection may occur in the incision or in deep structures that were entered or exposed. Its nature and severity vary because of local, systemic, technical, and environmental factors. Each factor is important; all are interrelated in clinical infection. Usually a postoperative infection is localized, but severe systemic reaction is possible. The specific pathogen and site of infection determine its gravity. Postoperative wound infections are classified as follows:

- *Incisional infection:* An infection occurs at the site of the incision within 30 postoperative days. It involves skin, subcutaneous tissue, or muscle. The incisional area is usually inflamed and sore. Purulent drainage or an organism identified by culture is present. The surgeon usually must open and drain the wound.
- *Deep wound infection:* An infection occurs at the surgical site within 30 postoperative days if a prosthesis was not implanted or within 1 year around the site of an implant. The infection involves tissues or spaces at or beneath the fascia. Pus may be present. The wound may spontaneously dehisce. The surgeon may need to open and drain the wound or remove an implant. Infection that involves an implant or gross necrotic tissue is prone to serious sequelae.

Compromised patients and geriatric patients are highly likely to develop an endogenous infection. Procedures on potentially contaminated areas, such as the gastrointestinal tract, are more apt to result in postoperative infections. Wound infections can progress to septicemia and multisystem organ failure.

Necrotizing Fasciitis

Necrotizing fasciitis is also known as flesh-eating bacteria. Signs of the acutely rapidly spreading infectious condition are swelling, bright red surface, pain, and fever. Mortality is high because the toxic effects of the necrosis become system-wide rapid destruction of organ systems. Surgical treatment requires wide debridement of muscle and fascia. The three types of necrotizing fasciitis are:

1. *Type I:* Aerobic (gram-negative) and anaerobic (gram-positive) microorganisms
   a. Streptococci other than group A
   b. *Escherichia, Enterobacter, Klebsiella,* and *Proteus*
   c. *Corynebacterium*
2. *Type II:* Most common type
   a. Beta-hemolytic *Streptococcus*
   b. *Staphylococcus aureus* (less common)
3. *Type III:* Water-borne microorganisms from fish or insects
   a. *Vibrio*

Prevention of Wound Infections

Prevention of wound infection and a successful outcome of surgical intervention are goals of the team administering perioperative care to surgical patients. In summary, preventive measures should focus on the following:

- Adherence to aseptic and sterile techniques and standard precautions with all patients
- Control of endogenous infection
- Meticulous surgical technique and wound closure

- Reduction of exogenous or environmental sources of contamination, such as airborne microorganisms
- Thorough prompt cleansing and debridement of traumatic wounds
- Prevention of intraoperative contamination of a wound
- Appropriate use of prophylactic antibiotics
- Frequent handwashing
- Sterile technique for dressing changes

Serious sequelae, such as wound disruption or septicemia, may follow wound infection. Therefore they must be assiduously prevented so that wound healing can occur naturally.

Wound Assessment

The stages of wound healing vary among individuals according to generalized health and age. Other factors influence the mechanism and should be considered when assessing the progress of healing postoperatively.

Objective Inspection of the Postoperative Wound

The perioperative nurse should inspect the patient's wound and document its condition. The nurse should have a basic understanding of the mechanism of the injury or the source of the wound, such as a surgical incision, and should be able to assess the wound for complications. All complaints of pain should be investigated and referred to the physician. Gloves should be worn during wound assessment. Sterility should be maintained as appropriate. Assessment of the wound should include the following:

1. Location of single or multiple sites.
   a. Laparoscopy can yield multiple puncture sites. If a uterine manipulator was used, some vaginal tenderness may occur.
   b. Trauma can cause multiple wounds that vary in type.
   c. Some injuries are not immediately visible, such as organ trauma.
   d. Incidental wounds, such as pressure sores, may not be obvious for several days postoperatively.
   e. Iatrogenic injury may manifest as a change in vital signs, indicating bleeding or severe inflammatory response. Sepsis from bowel perforation may not be evident for several days postoperatively.
2. Color of the wound and surrounding tissue. It may be a combination of one or many colors. Estimate the volume of each color in percentages of the total wound.
   a. A red, beefy wound bed indicates healing granulating tissue. Pink indicates epithelialization. The edges may have tan or beige eschar.
   b. Yellow to yellow-white color indicates exudate caused by microorganisms. The color can range from greenish to beige, depending on which organism is present and whether antibiotic therapy is in place.
   c. Black indicates necrotic tissue that can interfere with healing and supports the growth of microorganisms.
   d. Redness combined with swelling surrounding the edges of the wound may indicate infection.
   e. Macerated tissue around a wound may indicate the need for thicker dressing material or a pouch to collect drainage.

3. Perfusion of the patient's tissues.
   a. Capillary refill should be assessed.
   b. Blanching of surrounding tissues may indicate lack of blood flow.
4. Size in length, width, and depth.
   a. The wound should be measured in centimeters.
   b. The depth can be measured with a sterile cotton-tipped swab.
   c. Tunneling should be noted for direction and depth.
   d. Anatomic description pertaining to lines of direction should be described like the face of a clock. The direction of the patient's head should be considered as 12 o'clock.
5. Temperature of the site and the patient.
   a. Hot to warm tissue surrounding the wound may indicate infection.
   b. Elevated body temperature may indicate systemic sepsis.
6. Dressing type and condition.
   a. Is the dressing wet or dry?
   b. Is the dressing constrictive?
   c. Is the dressing effective for its intended purpose?
7. Drainage or drainage device.
   a. Odors usually indicate drainage and infection.
   b. The presence of embedded material may become obvious as the wound bed sloughs. Traumatic or industrial wounds may entrap foreign material that could be extruded in exudate.
   c. Drainage of more than 50 mL/day should be pouched for collection.
   d. Gastrointestinal contents, such as bile, stool, or pancreatic enzymes, should not be permitted to contact surrounding skin. An ostomy appliance should be used.

Basic Wound Care

Gloves are worn for all dressing change procedures. Eye protection or full face shields should be worn if syringes are used for irrigation. The wound should be cleansed before the dressing is replaced. Rinsing with sterile normal saline solution provides a moist environment for healing and promotes granulation formation. Some antiseptics, such as povidone-iodine, hydrogen peroxide, and acetic acid, can cause tissue injury and delay wound healing. The wound should be cleaned before the surrounding area is cleaned to prevent contamination of the open site. Gauze used for cleansing surrounding tissue should not drag across the open wound.

Debridement may be necessary. Nonsurgical methods of debridement include chemical autolysis and mechanical packing materials. Autolysis involves placement of proteolytic enzymes in the wound to break down necrotic tissue. The viable tissue is unaffected. Mechanical debridement is accomplished using wet-to-dry dressings. The results of debridement are fresh granulation tissue and a clean wound bed. Surgical debridement may be performed with dissection instruments, such as scissors or a scalpel. A laser is sometimes used, although it can cause devitalization of tissue by charring.

Dressing material and wound care products are determined by physician orders. Types, advantages, and disadvantages of various wound care materials can be found in Table 29.1.

TABLE 29.1	Wound Care Materials				
Dressing Material	**Composition and Properties**	**Indications for Use**	**Advantages**	**Disadvantages**	**Notes**
Alginate	Originates from brown seaweed; highly absorbent; becomes a gel when exposed to exudate, creating a moist environment	Used for infected and noninfected wounds with moderate to heavy drainage; some are used for tunneling wounds	Can absorb 20 times its own weight in fluid; rehydrates wound and facilitates debridement; requires secondary dressing cover	Contraindicated for use with light exudate or dry eschar; can promote bacterial growth if used with occlusive dressing cover; not used with third-degree burns	Packaged as ropelike fibers or pad; do not use with alkaline solutions; packaged sterile; remains in place 2–4 days
Composite	Composed of 2 or more moisture-enhancing materials in combination with absorbent material	Used for partial-thickness or full-thickness wounds with moderate to heavy exudate; can also be used over fresh granulation or necrotic tissue	Facilitates debridement and allows for moisture/vapor exchange; safe for use over healthy or infected tissue; easy to apply and remove	Should be placed in area with border of healthy intact tissue for anchoring; should not be used for light exudate; may cause excess moisture loss; can become very adherent	Check manufacturer recommendations about use with adjunct topical medications
Exudate absorber	Added to wound surface to eliminate dead space and absorb exudate; minimizes odors	Used for full-thickness wounds with moderate to heavy exudate; can be used with necrotic wounds; some can be used as lining material before packing and surface dressing	Can absorb 5 times its own weight in fluid; rehydrates wound and facilitates debridement; requires secondary dressing cover	Contraindicated for use with light exudate or dry eschar	Supplied in bottles or packets; clean wound and irrigate before use; fill the wound cavity to eliminate dead space and line the defect
Foam	Semipermeable, either hydrophilic or hydrophobic	Creates a moist environment and affords thermal insulation	Nonadherent; repels contaminants and is easy to apply and remove; absorbs light to moderate exudate; can be used with compression dressings; requires secondary dressing cover	Not used for dry wounds; can cause maceration of adjacent skin	Some erythema or itching may occur during the first 24 hours; not used with occlusive dressings; change more frequently if exudate is heavy
Gauze	Composed of woven or nonwoven materials; can be impregnated; used as primary or secondary dressing; can be natural or synthetic material; nonocclusive	Used for wound protection, wicking, and absorption; can be used wet or dry; packaged in rolls, pads, or strips	Moderately absorbent; less expensive to use and can be used in combination with other material; can be used as packing	Needs to be changed frequently; can leak or strike-through; can dry out, causing injury to healing tissue	If applied wet and allowed to dry, gauze can be debridement agent; may be saturated with oils, iodophor, bismuth, petroleum jelly, scarlet red
Hydrocolloid	Occlusive, adhesive wafer; the contact layer may differ in composition; creates a moist environment; supplied in packets, tubes (paste), oral discs, and wafers; can be cut to fit	Clean wounds granulate, and necrotic wounds debride autolytically	Impermeable to contaminants; self-adhesive and can remain in place for 3–5 days without tissue damage; slight to moderate absorption	Not used with heavy exudate, sinus tracts, or infection; not intended for full-thickness wounds exposing bone; visualization of the wound not possible; occlusive properties inhibit air exchange; can injure fragile tissue at wound edges	Safe to use under compression devices and wraps; can be used at ostomy sites or areas affected by incontinence
Hydrogel	Water- or glycerin-based gel, gauze, or sheet dressing that has high moisture content; supplied in tubes, packets, spray, liquid	Used for partial- and full-thickness wounds; good for burns, necrosis, and irradiated tissue	Very soothing; can rehydrate dried tissues; used to fill dead space and facilitate debridement	Not used for absorption of exudate because of inherent moisture content; can dry out easily; not a bacterial barrier; may be difficult to secure to wound	Keep covered after application to prevent evaporation of the gel
Transparent film	Adhesive, semipermeable membrane; bacterial and water barrier permeable to oxygen	Waterproof, but permeable to air and moisture vapors; bacterial barrier	Promotes a moist environment for new granulation and autolysis of necrotic tissue	Not used for infected wounds; periphery of wound needs to be intact to apply the film; may be hard to apply	Used for superficial and partial-thickness wounds with minimal exudate
Skin sealant	Barrier film applied in liquid form that dries to form a plastic-like barrier coating; supplied in liquid form and individual wipes	Used on intact skin surrounding a wound or ostomy site or over a surgical incision closed by primary intention	Waterproof barrier	Can sting raw skin when applied; has alcohol base to cause drying by evaporation	Some have vapors that may be harmful to inhale as product evaporates

EVOLVE WEBSITE

http://evolve.elsevier.com/Hornacky/BerryKohn/
- Historical Perspective
- Student Interactive Questions
- Glossary

References

1. Moore A, Marshall C, Nauta A, et al.: Scarless wound healing: from experimental target to clinical reality. In Atala A, Lanza R, Mikos T, et al., editors: *Principles of regenerative medicine*, ed 3, St. Louis, MO, 2019, Elsevier, pp 65–92.
2. Staruch R, Hettiaratchy S: Warzone trauma and surgical infections, *Surgery* 37(1):58–63, 2019.
3. Acker A, Leonard J, Seamon M, et al.: Leaving contaminated trauma laparotomy wounds open reduces wound infections but does not add value, *J Surg Res* 232:450–455, 2018.
4. Butler M, Zarosinski S, Rockstroh D: Improvement of surgical wound classification following a targeted training program at a children's hospital, *J Pediatr Surg* 53(12):2378–2382, 2018.
5. Veith J, Collier W, Kim J, et al.: A national analysis of readmissions for wound healing complications following the repair of lower back, hip, and buttock pressure ulcers using the nationwide readmissions database, *Am J Surg* 217(4):658–663, 2018.
6. Serrato-Avilla JL, , Navarao-Fernández JO, Hernández-Reséndiz R: Gelatin paste as an alternative cost effective hemostatic agent in cranial surgery: doing more with less, *World Neurosurg* 122:224–228, 2018.
7. Paulo D, Semonche A, Choudhry O, et al.: History of hemostatics in neurosurgery, *World Neurosurg* 124:237–250, 2018.
8. Brooks N: Treatment of melanoma excision wound with 50% zinc chloride solution astringent—Mohs melanoma surgery without the paste, *J Clin Aesthet Dermatol* 13(3):15–16, 2020.
9. Jensen J, Hicks R, Labovite J: Understanding and optimizing tourniquet use during extremity surgery, *AORN J* 109(2):171–182, 2019.
10. Mujagic E, Zeindler J, Coslovsky M, et al.: The association of surgical drains with surgical site infection: a prospective observational study, *Am J Surg* 217(1):17–23, 2018.
11. Barazzi L, Biagio L, Meneguzzi M, et al.: Novel, digital, chest drainage system in cardiac surgery, *J Card Surg* 35(7):1492–1497, 2020.
12. Rybka M, Mazurek L, Konop M: Beneficial effect of wound dressings containing silver and silver nanoparticles in wound healing—from experimental studies to clinical practice, *Life (Basel)* 13(1):69, 2022.
13. Totty JP, Bua N, Smith GE: Dialkylcarbamoyl chloride (DACC) coated dressings in the management and prevention of wound infection: a systematic review, *J Wound Care* 26(3):107–114, 2017.

Bibliography

AORN: *Guidelines for perioperative practice*, Denver, CO, 2024, The Association.
Phillips NM, Hornacky A: *Pass CNOR!*, St. Louis, MO, 2019, Elsevier.

30

Postoperative Patient Care

CHAPTER OUTLINE

Postanesthesia Care, 610

Admission to the Postanesthesia Care Unit, 612

Discharge From the Postanesthesia Care Unit, 614

CHAPTER OBJECTIVES

After studying this chapter the learner will be able to:

- List several functions of a postanesthesia recovery unit.
- Discuss the role of the perianesthesia nurse.

- Define the differences in postanesthesia phases as compared with patient condition.

KEY TERMS AND DEFINITIONS

Dermatome Segment of skin and subcutaneous tissue innervated by a single dorsal afferent sensory nerve root. Level is named for the area of the spine from which the afferent nerve originates.

Dermatome map Topographic outline of bilateral sensory nerve root distribution, beginning with the cervical spinal nerves and ending at the sacral spinal nerves.

Myotome Group of muscle fibers innervated by a single anterior efferent motor nerve root. Level is named for the area of the spine from which the efferent nerve originates.

Perianesthesia nursing Providing patient care before and after the administration of anesthesia for a surgical procedure.

Postanesthesia Care

Surgical procedures are performed in many diverse settings, including surgeons' offices, ambulatory surgery centers, and hospital-based surgical suites and specialty units. In general, the selection of the surgical setting is influenced by the anticipated complexity of the procedure, the patient's health status, available technology, and financial resources.

Regardless of the surgical setting or procedure, the patient should be observed and monitored postoperatively for physiologic and psychologic condition in a controlled postsurgical or postanesthesia environment before transfer to a patient care unit or discharge from the facility.

The postoperative phase of the surgical patient's perioperative experience begins after the surgical or interventional procedure is completed and the patient is admitted to a postprocedure area (usually a postanesthesia care unit [PACU] or an intensive care unit [ICU]) or discharged to home.

Ideally, an area is designated for the postoperative or postprocedure care of patients. It may vary in name or location according to its specific function within the health care facility. In some settings in which only local anesthetics are used, the patient has a brief postoperative observation period in the room where the procedure was performed. When the patient's condition is determined to be physiologically stable using criteria set by the surgeon, the patient is discharged from the facility. Dental, podiatric, and dermatologic offices often function in this capacity.

Immediate postoperative patient care is usually provided in a designated area of the hospital or ambulatory care facility. This area may be called the recovery room (RR) or postanesthesia recovery (PAR) unit. In this text the term *postanesthesia care unit (PACU)* is used to describe a specialized area for patient care during recovery from anesthesia. Institutional policies and procedures guide patient care activities in the PACU according to protocol established by the anesthesia and surgical services departments. The American Society of Anesthesiologists (ASA) has devised a scale of physical assessment ratings in which patients are categorized by perioperative or perianesthesia risk and outcome (Table 30.1). The ASA score is assessed and documented at admission and discharge from the PACU.

Organized in 1980, the American Society of PeriAnesthesia Nurses (ASPAN), formerly known as the American Society of Post Anesthesia Nurses, has established standards of practice for the postoperative care of diverse populations, such as pediatric, adult, and geriatric patients. ASPAN has identified specific phases of care, as follows:

- *Preanesthesia phase:* Focuses on the emotional and physical preparation of the patient before a surgical procedure. The patient is assessed to establish the nursing diagnoses for the perianesthesia period. Baselines are established for the patient's preoperative physiologic and psychologic condition.

American Society of Anesthesiologists Physical (P) Status Classification

Status[a]	Definition
ASA1	A healthy patient
ASA2	Mild systemic disease without functional limitations
ASA3	Severe systemic disease associated with definite functional limitations
ASA4	Severe systemic disease that is an ongoing threat to life
ASA5	Patient is unlikely to survive 24 hours without the surgical procedure
ASA6	Patient is brain dead and being prepared as an organ donor

With ASA2, ASA3, and ASA4, the systemic disease may or may not be related to the cause for surgery. If a patient (ASA1–ASA5) needs emergency surgery, an E is added to the physical status (e.g., ASA1E, ASA2E).
From *American Society of Anesthesiology classification* (https://www.ncbi.nlm.nih.gov/books/NBK441940/).

- *Postanesthesia phase I:* Focuses on providing immediate postoperative care from an anesthetized state to a condition that requires less acute intervention. The patient's condition may be ASA III or IV. The patient's condition is compared to the baseline set in the preanesthesia phase. The patient transitions from phase I to phase II.
- *Postanesthesia phase II:* Focuses on preparing the patient for self-care or care in an extended-care setting.
- *Extended care level:* Focuses on the patient who is preparing for discharge to home or other care facility.

The goal of postanesthesia or postprocedure care is to assist the patient in returning to a safe physiologic level after receiving an anesthetic agent or undergoing a surgical procedure.[1] In some settings, perianesthesia nurses follow up with the patient through a phone call to the patient's home within 24 to 48 hours of discharge. (More information about ASPAN position statements concerning patient care is available at http://www.aspan.org/.)

Postanesthesia Care Unit

Located in proximity to the operating room (OR), the basic PACU design consists of a large room divided into a series of individual cubicles (approximately 80 ft²) separated by privacy curtains. The beds should be a minimum of 4 ft apart, and equivalent spacing should be between the bedside tables and walls. Each cubicle has a cardiac monitor, pulse oximeter, blood pressure measurement device, suction apparatus, and oxygen administration equipment.

Additional supplies that are available include warming devices, airway management equipment, intravenous (IV) fluids and administration sets, dressing reinforcement materials, medications, indwelling Foley catheters and drainage systems, emesis basins, and bedpans. Lead screens and lead shielding should be available for surrounding patients and staff when x-ray scans are performed.

Other equipment, including crash carts with defibrillators, should be positioned strategically throughout the room for easy accessibility. More than one emergency setup should be immediately available in case the other is in use. Foot-controlled or elbow-controlled handwashing stations should be in proximity to patient care areas. Hand sanitizer should be readily available. Trashcans should have foot-controlled lids.

Some facilities include isolation rooms for patients who are highly contagious or highly susceptible to infection. If the PACU does not have a partitioned isolation area, these patients may be placed at one end of the room and separated from other patients with screens or curtains. Isolation procedures should be used in handling bedding and equipment per institutional policy. All patients have the right to receive the same level of care regardless of extenuating circumstances.

Ideally, the amount of cubicle space is allotted according to the number of ORs in the OR suite. This allotment may vary between one and a half to two cubicles per OR and is based on the caseload, duration of surgical procedures, and room turnover time in the OR. A rapid succession of short procedures could easily fill the PACU and leave no vacancy for additional patients. This scenario is more common in facilities in which the PACU doubles as a special procedure care unit for ambulatory patients who are receiving nerve blocks for pain therapy.

Some institutions allow an uncomplicated endoscopy to be performed in the PACU. The rationale behind this practice is that patients undergoing special procedures need to be monitored by experienced personnel for a short time after a treatment or test. For some procedures the PACU nurse monitors a patient receiving IV sedation and may assist the physician, thus depleting the staff available for postoperative care.

In larger institutions where prolonged and complex surgical procedures are performed (e.g., transplantation, multiple trauma), patients may remain in the PACU for more than 24 hours because of the potential need to return to the OR for an additional surgical procedure. In such cases the PACU doubles as a surgical ICU.

Increased patient load and acuity increase the need for adequate staffing, space allocation, education of personnel, and management of resources. The consolidation of facilities and personnel should not jeopardize the delivery of safe postoperative patient care. Use of the PACU as an overflow ICU depletes the resources intended for the adequate care of postsurgical patients.[2]

Postoperative Observation of the Patient

The duration and type of postoperative observation and care vary according to the following factors:
- Patient's condition (e.g., alert and oriented vs. unresponsive)
- Need for physiologic support (e.g., ventilator-dependent vs. awake and extubated)
- Complexity of the surgical procedure (e.g., open laparotomy vs. laparoscopy)
- Type of anesthetic agent administered (e.g., a general inhalation agent vs. local infiltration)
- Need for pain therapy (e.g., intermittent analgesic administration vs. continuous epidural infusion)
- Prescribed period for monitoring parameters for evaluation of physiologic status (e.g., stable vs. unstable vital signs)

Perianesthesia Patient Care Personnel

Adequate numbers of personnel should be available to monitor patients and provide appropriate care as needed.[3] The education and training of PACU nurses should include knowledge and skill in the following areas:

- Airway management techniques, including positioning, chin lift, jaw thrust, suctioning, bagging, and placement of an airway
- Circulatory assessment, including hemodynamics, neurovascular condition, and renal function
- Neurologic condition, such as level of consciousness or dermatome level associated with epidural infusion (Box 30.1 and Fig. 30.1)
- Neuromuscular activity in myotome groups after neuromuscular blockade anesthetic
- Anesthetic agents and their actions (e.g., physiologic depression associated with general anesthesia; anesthetic techniques are discussed in detail in Chapter 24)
- Medications and their actions (e.g., narcotics, opioids, and tranquilizers)
- Most invasive and minimally invasive surgical procedures (e.g., open laparotomy, laparoscopy)

• BOX 30.1 Dermatome Sensory Somatic Landmarks

C2	Occiput
C5	Shoulder
T1	Little finger
T4	Nipple line
T6	Xyphoid process
T12	Iliac crest
L1–L5	Groin to dorsum of foot
S1	Dorsum of foot
S3	Heel, lateral foot to sole of foot
S5	Genitalia and perineal area

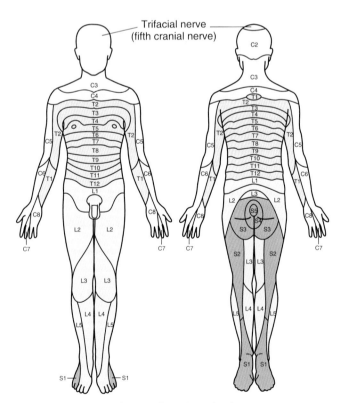

• Fig. 30.1 Dermatome levels.

PACU nurses should demonstrate competency in the following:
- Physical assessment (e.g., heart, lung sounds)
- Recognition of physiologic complications (e.g., airway obstruction, hypothermia, malignant hyperthermia, pain, hydration, nausea or vomiting, and oropharyngeal aspiration)
- Management of physiologic emergencies (e.g., airway obstruction, hemorrhage, cardiac arrest, and malignant hyperthermia). Postoperative complications are discussed in detail in Chapter 31
- Interpretation of monitoring data from electrocardiogram (ECG) and oximetry devices (patient monitoring is discussed in Chapter 27)

Additional competencies should include current certification in CPR, both basic cardiac life support (BCLS) and advanced cardiac life support (ACLS). If pediatric patients are involved, credentials should include pediatric advanced life support (PALS). Reviews and drills should be planned and implemented by the perianesthesia nurse manager.

Professional Activities

In 1986, ASPAN developed specialty certification for perianesthesia nurses. Eligible nurses must have a current active nursing license in the state of practice and 1200 hours of PACU patient care within 2 years of the examination. A baccalaureate degree is not required. Eligibility includes 1200 hours of perianesthesia direct care nursing experience as a caregiver, manager, educator, or researcher. A nurse who specializes in the care of phase I postanesthesia patients in hospital-based or extended-recovery care facilities may attain certification as a certified postanesthesia care nurse (CPAN) by taking and passing an examination offered by the American Board of Perianesthesia Nursing Certification (ABPANC).

In ambulatory surgery settings, nurses who specialize in the postanesthesia care of patients who move rapidly from phase I to phase II can attain board certification from ABPANC in ambulatory postanesthesia care (CAPA).

The certification for both CAPA and CPAN is valid for 3 years and can be renewed by passing a written examination or by obtaining 90 contact hours of continuing education credits. A perianesthesia nurse may hold both credentials simultaneously. Current active licensure and a minimum of 900 hours in perianesthesia nursing are required during the 3-year term of certification. ASPAN has produced a core curriculum as an additional reference for perianesthesia nurses who plan to take the certification examination. Additional information about PACU certification can be found at http://www.cpancapa.org/.

Other personnel in the PACU may include licensed practical nurses or licensed vocational nurses (LPNs/LVNs) and other unlicensed patient care personnel. These caregivers are supervised by a registered nurse (RN), who is responsible for their training and assignments within the PACU. Their duties vary according to the needs of the department and their level of knowledge and skill.

Admission to the Postanesthesia Care Unit

Before the phase I or phase II patient leaves the OR, the circulating nurse should call the PACU nurse to give the estimated time of arrival in the PACU and advise of a need to have special life support equipment on standby for immediate use.

As the patient enters the PACU, the immediate physiologic and psychologic status is reported to the PACU nurse by the accompanying personnel (usually the circulating nurse, first assistant, anesthesia provider, or resident). This reporting is referred to as the *handover report*. Any necessary life support equipment, such as a ventilator, is connected. The PACU nurse connects the ECG electrodes, attaches a pulse oximeter lead, and places a blood pressure cuff on the patient.

Many PACUs are supplied with automatic or computerized equipment that provides an immediate display of vital signs and physiologic data from monitors that are attached to the patient in the OR and remain on the patient during transport. The phase I PACU nurse simultaneously assesses the patient and assimilates the data. The flow of activity is fast paced but directed toward the immediate physiologic needs and support of the patient.[3]

Postoperative Handover Report

The postoperative handover report provides information from the anesthesia provider (if one was in attendance), the surgeon (or appropriate designee, such as the first assistant), and the circulating nurse. Much of the report is delivered verbally, but postoperative orders and pertinent information regarding the patient's condition and intraoperative care are documented in writing. If the surgeon gives a verbal order, they should cosign the chart within 24 hours. The content of the postoperative report to the PACU nurse should include, but is not limited to, the information discussed in the following sections.

Anesthesia Provider's Report

- Patient's name, sex, age, preoperative and postoperative diagnosis, surgical procedure, and surgeon
- Type of anesthesia and the patient's response
- Baseline preoperative vital signs and summary of vital sign flow during the surgical procedure up to the point of discharge from the OR
- Sensitivities and allergies, including reaction to allergen
- Any physiologic changes or existing conditions and interventions to counteract them (e.g., diabetes, chronic obstructive pulmonary disease, previous myocardial infarction, hypertension)
- Medications administered preoperatively, intraoperatively, and postoperatively (e.g., preoperative sedation, intraoperative antibiotic, continuous infusion of medication)
- IV fluid administration and body fluid output (e.g., blood products and estimated blood loss, urine, ascites, gastric contents)
- Specific patient care orders to be performed in the PACU or in the immediate postoperative period (e.g., aerosol or mist mask)

Surgeon's Report

- Postoperative orders that pertain to immediate treatments or therapies to be performed in the PACU or in the immediate postoperative period (e.g., passive range-of-motion device, radiographic study to check placement of central line catheter)
- Serial diagnostic tests that are to be initiated in the PACU and continued through the immediate postoperative period (e.g., blood counts at specified intervals)
- Specific interventions that pertain to care of the surgical site (e.g., dressing change, reinforcement)

Circulating Nurse's Handover Report

- Baseline physiologic and psychologic assessment data

- Positioning and skin preparation, including the condition of the skin preoperatively and postoperatively
- Condition of patient return electrode site
- Use of specialized surgical equipment (e.g., laser, endoscope)
- Intraoperative irrigation fluids
- Administration of medication, hemostatics, contrast media, or dyes in the surgical field
- Any implants, transplants, or explants
- Type of dressings and the presence of drains or stents
- Intraoperative urinary catheterization and output
- Patient's indication of pain (verbal score of 0 to 10 or nonverbal grimace, crying, restlessness)
- Any pertinent information not reported by the anesthesia provider or surgeon
- Location of family member or significant other who may be waiting

Postoperative reports vary according to the type of anesthesia and the surgical procedure, the preferences of the anesthesia provider and surgeon, and institutional policy and procedure. The main emphasis is the patient's needs in the immediate postoperative period. This continues until the patient transitions to phase II and is discharged from the PACU.

Patient Care Activities

The application of physiologic and psychosocial knowledge, principles of asepsis, and technical knowledge and skills is necessary to promote, restore, and maintain the patient's physiologic processes in a safe, comfortable, and effective environment.[2] Particular attention is given to monitoring of oxygenation, ventilation, and circulation. PACU care includes maintaining adequate ventilation, alleviating postoperative nausea and vomiting (PONV), preventing shock, and alleviating pain.[2]

Patient Assessment for Pain

Patients are assessed for vital signs and level of discomfort. Pain is referred to as the fifth vital sign. Pain has been described as both physiologic and psychologic. The adult patient is offered an opportunity to describe pain according to a numbered scale of 0 to 10. The patient's ethnicity and sex can influence the expression of pain. Some groups consider showing pain to be a form of weakness.

The perianesthesia nurse should be aware that the patient's demeanor may not adequately relate to the patient's comfort level.[4] Pediatric patients may better describe pain according to the Wong-Baker pain-rating FACES scale (see Fig. 8.2). Before administration of medication for pain, the patient's communication level should be determined regardless of age. Assessing for vision, speech, language, and hearing can give the perianesthesia nurse significant clues about patient understanding of the pain scales in use.[4]

Some patients have alternative methods for managing pain, such as imaging, breathing exercises, meditation, reiki, and acupressure. Other nonpharmacologic methods of pain management include electronic nerve stimulators applied to the skin, such as TENS, or implanted within the neural pathway. Alternative therapies should not be considered replacements for medications when providing comfort for the patient.

Postoperative Care Orders

Postoperative medical orders are coordinated by the anesthesia provider and the surgeon and include monitoring requirements, oxygen and fluid therapies, pain medications, and other special considerations. Patients are evaluated continually using appropriate monitoring methods and frequent observations by the perianesthesia nurses. Clinical evaluation of each patient's status through listening, watching, and feeling is augmented by electronic monitoring devices. Machines should not be the only method of determining the patient's condition.

As in all other patient care areas, standard precautions are carried out for the disposal of needles and the handling of any item contaminated by blood and body fluids. Handwashing is essential after each patient contact to prevent cross-contamination.

Family members or significant others are notified when a patient is admitted to the PACU to let them know the surgical procedure is complete, which helps relieve the anxiety experienced during the hours of waiting. Depending on institutional policy, some facilities allow parents or other visitors in the PACU.[5] No special attire is required unless the patient is in an isolation setting.

Postsurgical Overflow Considerations

PACU nurses are very knowledgeable and skilled in the care of critically ill patients. This measure of versatility sometimes places the PACU nurse in the position of keeping and monitoring patients who should be housed in the ICU. Sometimes the ICU does not have readily available bed space for the critical postoperative patient, and therefore the PACU nurse provides this care. In some circumstances the general postoperative patient population is maintained in the PACU when space is not immediately available on the patient care floors. Some facilities have developed a specialty float pool to work in combination with the PACU team to manage the patient load.

Patients who are normally discharged to the patient care unit from the PACU can be consolidated with float pool nurses to relieve the PACU nurses for more postprocedure or postoperative patient care. Consideration must always be given to the availability of appropriate qualified staff and bed space for care of immediate postanesthesia patients, despite the extra load of patients who should be housed elsewhere.

The perianesthesia nurse manager should collaborate with the OR scheduling personnel and OR manager to preview pending schedules a day or two before the schedule commences to plan for staffing needs. Patient overflow conditions cannot always be predetermined, but the managers of both areas should be apprised of extremely full OR schedules so they can plan for the event of emergent admissions over the usual caseload.

Documentation

Most facilities have implemented electronic medical records. The charting may be done on a computer and can be reviewed in real time by physicians and staff as the patient progresses through the perianesthesia phases of care. Institutional policies and procedures should be followed in documenting PACU care.

Observations of respiratory and circulatory functions and level of consciousness are recorded at frequent intervals. Postoperative physiologic and psychologic status are documented at the time of any significant event (e.g., the administration of medication) and routinely at 5 to 7-minute intervals for the first hour and at 15 to 30-minute intervals for the second hour and thereafter. Pertinent observations are recorded as appropriate or necessary.

Discharge From the Postanesthesia Care Unit

Most patients remain in the PACU at least 1 hour or until they have sufficiently recovered from anesthesia so their vital signs have stabilized and they are capable of reasonable self-care. The patient's condition is scored using a postanesthesia scoring system according to vital signs, activity level, and consciousness; several standardized formats are available for this purpose. The anesthesia provider assesses the patient as necessary and may determine when the patient's condition is stable enough for discharge from the PACU. After discharge from the PACU, the patient is transported to a patient care unit or an ICU or is released from the ambulatory care facility.

A physician is responsible for the patient's discharge from the PACU. The anesthesia department staff and medical staff may approve discharge criteria for the PACU nurse to use in determining readiness for discharge. These criteria should be consistent with the standards of the ASA and the accreditation standards of The Joint Commission (TJC) or the Accreditation Association for Ambulatory Health Care (AAAHC).

The continuity of care is maintained when the PACU nurse provides a handover report to the RN at the receiving patient care division. The handover report should include the following information:

1. Patient name, age, and sex
2. Physiologic condition and assessment, allergies, vital signs, preoperative medical and surgical history. May include information about physiologic ability (e.g., paralysis)
3. Surgeon and the procedure performed
4. Anesthetic used and patient's response
5. Any unusual circumstances during the procedure. May include known infectious findings
6. Blood loss and fluid replacement (includes intake and output)
7. All medications given in PACU for pain, PONV, IV. Medication report should include any special circumstances, such as addiction or recreational drug use/alcohol abuse
8. Dressings and drains, including Foley catheter
9. Tests and treatments performed in PACU and any postoperative orders
10. Valuables and their disposition (e.g., prosthetics, eyeglasses, hearing aid)
11. Location and contact information for significant other or caregiver. May include social information such as communication barriers (language or cognition)

Postoperative Evaluation of Expected Outcomes

Ideally, the perioperative nurse who preoperatively assessed the patient and intraoperatively developed and implemented the plan of care can assess or interview the patient postoperatively and evaluate patient care outcomes.[3] An assessment is performed in person if possible, or the patient may be interviewed with a follow-up telephone call within 24 to 48 hours of discharge.

The plan of care should be evaluated in terms of the attainment of expected outcomes. The identification of influencing factors provides a foundation for ongoing improvement of perioperative patient care services. Considerations for the design of the postoperative evaluation include, but are not limited to, the following:

1. Was a preoperative visit made, and was it helpful to the patient?
2. Were the patient and family adequately prepared for the surgical procedure physically, psychologically, emotionally, and spiritually? Did the patient receive written preoperative instructions?
3. What could have been improved?
4. Were all pertinent patient needs, problems, and health status considerations identified in the nursing diagnoses?
5. Did the plan of care address the nursing diagnoses?
6. Did the patient experience any complications?
7. Was preoperative teaching used? Was it adequate and helpful?
8. What were the patient's perceptions of the surgical experience?
9. Were the expected outcomes achieved to the patient's satisfaction?
10. To what degree do the patient's observable physiologic and psychosocial responses indicate the attainment of expected outcomes?
11. Was the patient given a follow-up survey of satisfaction to complete and return to the department?

The evaluation of patient outcomes helps identify environmental influences and procedural activities that may need to be modified by the OR staff. For example, if the patient has had a reddened pressure area develop over a bony prominence, was the positioning equipment at fault or was the area unpadded? A reevaluation of products currently being used may be indicated. Injury to skin may be caused by the pooling of skin prep solutions under the patient, inadequate padding of bony prominences, or faulty electrical equipment.

The subjective data received from the patient help evaluate how much discomfort the patient is experiencing, especially paresthesia (a numb, tingling sensation). Neurovascular injuries may be related to positioning on the OR bed. Each level of the dermatome map should be evaluated. The perioperative nurse may suggest comfort measures to help this patient, but an adverse outcome indicates a need to improve positioning procedures for subsequent patients.

The postoperative assessment or follow-up telephone call terminates the direct perioperative nurse–patient relationship. The evaluation of the degree of attainment of expected outcomes completes the perioperative nursing process.

To be successful, a postoperative evaluation program requires the cooperative effort of and input from all personnel involved with patient care, including RNs, technicians, and physicians.[1]

Administrative personnel may seek specific information and should be consulted for input. They should participate in structuring the program at its inception to avoid duplication of action and to promote a collegial effort. Postoperative evaluation data may be collected through the following measures:

- Interview and assessment of the patient
- Conferences with physicians, nurses, and other caregivers
- Review of responses on the patient evaluation form

The postoperative evaluation program should be reviewed periodically and revised as necessary. An interdisciplinary conference is an effective medium for the accomplishment of these objectives. An effective perioperative evaluation program and positive patient experiences promote good public relations and demonstrate a caring image to the public it serves.[1]

EVOLVE WEBSITE

http://evolve.elsevier.com/Hornacky/BerryKohn/

- Historical Perspective
- Student Interactive Questions
- Glossary

References

1. Ead H: How tuned in are you to the patient experience? *J Perianesth Nurs* 30(3):236–238, 2015.
2. Byrne MD: Virtually sensing the future of perianesthesia nursing, *J Perianesth Nurs* 30(1):64–67, 2015.
3. McVay S: Finding joy, gratitude, and meaning in routine PACU tasks, *J Perianesth Nurs* 30(2):160–163, 2015.
4. Lovich-Sapola J, Smith CE, Brandt CP: Postoperative pain control, *Surg Clin North Am* 95(2):301–318, 2015.
5. Marshak C: The evidence supports visitation in the PACU: let's do it, *J Perianesth Nurs* 29(5):18–19, 2014.

Bibliography

American Society of PeriAnesthesia Nurses (ASPAN): *2019–2020 Standards of perianesthesia nursing practice*, Cherry Hill, NJ, 2019, The Association.

AORN: *Guidelines for perioperative practice*, Denver, CO, 2024, The Association.

Doyle DJ, Hendrix JM, Garmon EH: *American Society of Anesthesiology classification*, Treasure Island, FL, 2023, StatPearls. www.ncbi.nlm.nih.gov.

31

Potential Perioperative Complications

CHAPTER OUTLINE

Potential for Complications During and After Surgery, 616

Respiratory Complications, 617

Cardiovascular Complications, 620

Fluid and Electrolyte Imbalances, 632

Blood Volume Complications, 634

Shock, 641

Metabolic Crises, 642

Iatrogenic Injury, 646

CHAPTER OBJECTIVES

After studying this chapter the learner will be able to:

- Describe several respiratory complications that are possible in the perioperative period.
- Identify three potential dysrhythmias that may complicate the patient's perioperative course.
- Demonstrate the procedure for weighing surgical sponges in the operating room.
- List the primary drugs used in the management of an acute malignant hyperthermic crisis.
- Identify three methods for preventing hypothermia in the perioperative patient.

KEY TERMS AND DEFINITIONS

Anabolism Buildup of tissues or properties.

Anaphylaxis Life-threatening form of allergy.

Anemia Reduction of the number of functioning red blood cells capable of containing enough hemoglobin to transport oxygen.

Anoxia Absence of oxygen; not synonymous with hypoxia.

Aspiration Entry of gastric, oropharyngeal, or other substance into the lungs.

Atelectasis Collapsed or airless lung.

Cardiotonic Drug that increases the tone of the heart, such as digitalis.

Catabolism Breakdown of tissues or properties.

Coagulopathy Disorder that causes problems with blood clotting.

Dysrhythmia Abnormal, disordered, disturbed rhythm.

Embolus Blood clot or other substance, such as air, plaque, amniotic fluid, or fat, that occludes a segment of the cardiovascular system.

Hemoglobinopathy Any one of a group of blood diseases that are characterized by abnormal forms of hemoglobin in the blood.

Hemorrhage Abnormal internal or external loss of blood from an arterial, venous, or capillary source.

Hypertension Elevated blood pressure. If on several occasions the systolic pressure is greater than 140 mm Hg or the diastolic pressure is greater than 90 mm Hg, the patient is considered hypertensive.

Hypotension Low blood pressure. If on several occasions the systolic pressure is lower than 100 mm Hg, the patient is considered hypotensive. This should be compared with other assessment parameters.

Hypoventilation Reduced rate and depth of breathing that causes an increase in circulating carbon dioxide.

Hypoxia Decreased concentration of circulating oxygen.

Metabolic crisis Physical and chemical changes that cause catabolic or anabolic activity that may be life-threatening.

Thrombus Blood clot within a blood vessel.

Vasoconstrictor Drug that causes narrowing of a blood vessel.

Vasodilator Drug that causes relaxation of a blood vessel or causes opening (dilation).

Potential for Complications During and After Surgery

Many facilities use scoring systems as guidelines to predict the potential for complications during the perioperative care period. The patient receives care from a multidisciplinary team that plans for their safety by assessing risks and benefits of the surgical procedure. Preoperatively the patient is assessed by the anesthesia provider using the American Society of Anesthesiologists (ASA) scoring system. Intraoperatively the patient's risk for infection is assessed using the Centers for Disease Control and Prevention (CDC) wound classification scheme. In the postanesthesia care area the patient's readiness for discharge is scored according to one of several predictive indicator grids based on their physiology. All of the scoring systems add up to a number that is used in decision-making concerning the plan of care and progression toward wellness.

The purpose of this chapter is to acquaint the caregiver with the potential complications that patients experience during and after surgery. A satisfactory score in one care period is not always a predictor of how the patient will do in subsequent phases of care after the physical changes associated with surgery.

Each organ system interacts with other organ systems to produce homeostasis in the patient. An alteration in one organ system will affect all of the others, causing the potential for a poor outcome. Morbidity and mortality can be minimized with prompt detection and precise intervention.

Respiratory Complications

One of the primary areas of postoperative complications is the respiratory system. The patient's potential for developing pulmonary problems depends on several factors. Any preexisting lung disease, such as emphysema, infection, or asthma, predisposes the patient.[1,2] Smokers have the highest risk for succumbing to postoperative pulmonary problems because of chronic irritation of the respiratory tract with consequent production of excess mucus. Chest wall deformities, obesity, and extremes of age are other pertinent preoperative influences.[2] Intraoperative factors include the following:

- Types of preoperative medications
- Type and duration of anesthesia
- Type and duration of assisted ventilation
- Position of the patient during the surgical procedure
- Extent of the surgical procedure

Postoperatively one of the most critical factors is the patient's ability to mobilize secretions by deep breathing, coughing, and ambulation.[2] Patients undergoing chest and abdominal surgery are likely to breathe shallowly because of pain and therefore may not adequately raise accumulated secretions. Development of one pulmonary complication often predisposes the patient to development of another. Acute respiratory distress syndrome (ARDS), also known as *progressive pulmonary insufficiency* or *shock lung,* may develop in the first 24 to 48 hours after a traumatic injury.[1]

Aspiration

Aspiration of gastric contents into the lungs may occur because of decreased throat reflexes when the patient is unconscious or is conscious with the throat anesthetized, as for bronchoscopy. Residual effects impede lung function and blood-gas exchange.

A chemical pneumonitis results from aspiration of highly acidic gastric juices. Edema forms, alveoli collapse, ventilation-perfusion mismatch occurs, and hypoxemia results. Aspiration of solids in emesis results in edema, severe hypoxia, and respiratory obstruction. Bronchospasm and atelectasis may be followed by pneumonitis or bronchopneumonia. Most aspirate is irritating, but it can be infectious if nasopharyngeal or gastric flora are aspirated. Pneumonia or lung abscess may result with necrosis of the pulmonary parenchyma.

Etiology

Every patient who has food in the stomach is a poor risk for anesthesia. Increased intragastric pressure is an aspiration hazard and may result from conditions such as diaphragmatic hernia, gastrointestinal bleeding, intestinal obstruction, or gas forced into the stomach by application of positive pressure ventilation without use of a cuffed endotracheal tube.

Symptoms

Symptoms include central cyanosis, dyspnea, gasping, and tachycardia, followed by cardiac hemodynamic embarrassment, lung collapse, and consolidation.

Treatment

Most effective treatment occurs during the first minutes after aspiration. The strategy is to remove as much aspirate as possible and limit the spread of what is left in the lung. The head of the operating room (OR) bed is lowered with a right lateral tilt for postural drainage; the right mainstem bronchus bifurcates slightly higher than the left mainstem bronchus. The oropharynx and tracheobronchial tree are suctioned. If the patient has aspirated particulate matter that causes obstruction of the airways, bronchoscopy must be performed to remove the aspirate. Suctioning must be interrupted every 10 to 15 seconds to administer oxygen. Oxygenation and carbon dioxide removal are high priorities.

Aspiration of acid gastric content injures the alveolar capillary interface, resulting in intrapulmonary shunting and pulmonary edema. Intensive pulmonary care is aimed at improving ventilation-perfusion ratios and decreasing abnormal gas exchange.[2] This may require endotracheal intubation for mechanical ventilation with continuous positive pressure. Most cases of severe hypoxemia occur rapidly within the first 30 to 60 minutes after aspiration. Careful cardiovascular monitoring and frequent blood-gas and acid-base determinations guide therapeutic measures to maintain intravascular volume. Prophylactic antibiotics may be given for aspiration of bowel-contaminated fluid to prevent infection, and a bronchodilator may be used to treat spasm. Most cases of permanent injury or death result from the initial hypoxemia.

Prevention

Prevention involves adequate preoperative preparation (withholding oral intake 8–10 hours before induction) and careful administration of anesthetic agents. The anesthetic is decreased near the end of the surgical procedure, hastening the return of throat reflexes. All trauma and obstetric patients receiving general anesthesia should be treated as if they have a full stomach and therefore should be intubated using cricoid pressure (Sellick maneuver). The cricoid pressure should be released after verification of endotracheal tube placement. Gastric evacuation is delayed during labor and by analgesic medications. A nasogastric tube may be inserted preoperatively or intraoperatively.

Laryngospasm and Bronchospasm

Laryngospasm is a partial or complete closure of the vocal cords as an involuntary reflex action. Bronchospasm is contraction of smooth muscle in the walls of the bronchi and bronchioles, causing narrowing of the lumen. Spasms or abnormal narrowing is produced by a marked increase in smooth muscle tone of the airway walls. Marked elevation of airway resistance profoundly alters gas flow into and out of the lungs. Accompanying changes result in a decreased ventilation-perfusion ratio with a subsequent reduction in Pao_2 and rise in $Paco_2$. Many factors can precipitate spasm.

Etiology

Etiologic factors for laryngospasm and bronchospasm include mechanical airway obstruction, use of certain anesthetics and drugs, allergic conditions such as asthma, vagal reflex, stimulation of the pharynx and larynx with the patient under light anesthesia, traction on the peritoneum, foreign material in the tracheobronchial tree, movement of the head or neck or traction on the carotid sinus, and painful peripheral stimuli. The degree of spasm varies from mild to severe.

Symptoms

Symptoms include wheezing respirations or stridor, reduced compliance, central cyanosis, and respiratory obstruction.

Treatment

Treatment depends on the precipitating factor. Methods generally used include positive pressure ventilation, oxygen, tracheal intubation, and neuromuscular blockers for relaxation. Bronchodilator drugs such as aminophylline, isoetharine, and metaproterenol are given with caution because they act as cardiac stimulators and, in the presence of hypoxia, may contribute to cardiac dysrhythmia and cardiac arrest.

Patients may be refractory (unresponsive) to bronchodilators because of acid-base abnormalities. Correction can reduce the side effects and augment the beneficial effects of bronchodilators. If the etiologic factor is an allergy, steroids and antihistamines may be given. Vagal reflexes are inhibited by atropine. If reflex is the cause, anesthesia is deepened. Drying agents are given for excessive secretions. Immediate effective treatment is mandatory to counteract hypoxia and prevent cardiac arrest.

Prevention

Prevention involves maintenance of a patent airway, appropriate premedication such as glycopyrrolate, avoidance of factors stimulating the vagal reflex, and treatment of the predisposing pulmonary condition.

Airway and Respiratory Obstruction

An airway is maintained with an oral airway or endotracheal tube. Airway obstruction is the most frequent cause of respiratory difficulty in the immediate postoperative period. The patient may exhibit paradoxic respiration (i.e., downward movement of the diaphragm occurring with contraction rather than expansion of the chest), resulting in hypoxia and carbon dioxide retention. As the condition worsens the patient becomes restless, diaphoretic, cyanotic, and, finally, unconscious. If not relieved within seconds, this serious complication may lead to cardiac arrest.

Etiology

Etiologic factors include blocking of the airway by the tongue, soft tissue, excessive secretions, or a foreign body; laryngospasm or bronchospasm; or positioning of the head with the chin down.

Symptoms

Symptoms of respiratory obstruction include increased respiratory effort with inadequate ventilatory exchange, visible use of accessory muscles, and respiratory motion of the chest and abdomen without audible air movement at the airway. If the airway is totally obstructed, breath sounds will be absent; if it is partially obstructed, a snoring sound will be elicited. The pulse is rapid and thready.

Assessment of oxygenation is essential if the patient's airway patency is in question. Visual inspection of the patient may reveal peripheral cyanosis (i.e., pallor, duskiness, or bluish color of the nail beds and extremities). This is caused by a decrease in capillary oxygen levels. Peripheral cyanosis is not always indicative of impending danger to the patient. It can be caused by hypothermia, stress, medications, or other physiologic factors that cause peripheral vasoconstriction.

If the patient is in an arterial hypoxemic state, they will exhibit central cyanosis—pallor, duskiness, or bluish color of the lips, face, and generalized body surface. Central cyanosis is a serious sign that requires immediate airway and ventilatory assessment followed by emergent treatment.[3] Central cyanosis may develop more slowly if the patient has been breathing a high concentration of oxygen.[2]

Treatment

Suctioning blood, mucus, or emesis, gently hyperextending the neck, and elevating the chin may eliminate the cause of obstruction. Oxygen is administered by positive pressure; a nasal airway or endotracheal intubation may be necessary. If the anesthesia provider has been unable to manually ventilate or intubate the patient in two or three attempts, it may be necessary to establish an indirect airway by opening the patient's anterior neck; a needle is inserted through the cricoid cartilage for a cricothyrotomy or, if time permits, a tracheotomy.[3]

Hypoventilation

Hypoventilation, the ability to oxygenate, depends on the condition of the lungs, hemoglobin concentration, cardiac output (CO), and oxygen saturation. Inadequate or reduced alveolar ventilation can cause a deficit in oxygenation. This can lead to hypoxia (a decreased level of oxygen in arterial blood and tissues), hypoxemia (a decreased level of oxygen in arterial blood), and hypercapnia, also known as *hypercarbia* (an elevated level of carbon dioxide in arterial blood).

The body compensates for mild hypoxia with increased heart and respiratory rates, bringing oxygen to the blood and tissues at a faster rate. If hypoxia progresses, this compensation is inadequate. If hypoxia is prolonged, cardiac dysrhythmias or irreversible brain, liver, kidney, and heart damage result. Retention of carbon dioxide also leads to acidosis.

Etiology

Contributing factors to hypoventilation include alveolar impairment, pain, faulty positioning, a full bladder, or a short, thick neck. Inadequate pulmonary ventilation from depression of the medullary center in the brain by narcotics or anesthetics, neurologic effects of spinal or epidural drug administration, reduced CO, severe blood loss, obstruction to the respiratory passages, or abnormality of the ventilation-perfusion ratio also can contribute to hypoxia and hypercapnia.

Symptoms

Symptoms of hypoventilation and hypoxia include an increased pulse rate, pallor or central cyanosis from hypoxia or a flushed or reddened appearance from hypercapnia, decreased volume of respirations, stertorous or labored respirations, and dark blood in the surgical field. The acid-base balance can be affected.

Treatment

The immediate administration of oxygen in the proper dosage is the treatment of choice for hypoventilation and hypoxia.[4] Oxygen is a medication requiring proper dosage for safe, effective administration. In the healthy patient, changes in the concentration of carbon dioxide in the blood stimulate the primary central chemoreceptor (respiratory center) in the medulla of the brain. In response to this stimulation the patient takes a breath to increase oxygenation.[2]

Patients with chronic obstructive pulmonary disease (COPD) have higher than normal levels of circulating carbon dioxide and exhibit a decreased primary chemoreceptor response. They rely on secondary chemoreceptors in the carotid and aortic bodies to sense the changes in carbon dioxide levels in the blood. High concentrations of oxygen decrease the sensitivity of the secondary chemoreceptors in patients with COPD, causing respiratory depression known as *carbon dioxide narcosis*.

To minimize the risk for respiratory arrest in patients at risk for carbon dioxide narcosis, a 2 to 3-liter per minute (L/min) flow of oxygen per nasal cannula is recommended postoperatively.[4] An endotracheal tube may be left in place postoperatively to support assisted ventilation in select patients.

Patients are encouraged to cough and breathe deeply postoperatively. If a patient received naloxone hydrochloride (Narcan) to reverse the respiratory depressant effect of a narcotic, the patient may awaken rapidly and cough, inadvertently causing extubation. The patient must be watched closely during recovery.

Prevention

A patent airway, appropriate oxygenation, and proper positioning help prevent hypoventilation. Intraoperative measurements of arterial pH, P_{CO_2}, and P_{O_2} enable the anesthesia provider to evaluate oxygenation and carbon dioxide gas exchange. To prevent hypoventilation and hypoxia, patients may be given oxygen and assisted ventilation during transport to the recovery area.

Emboli

Pulmonary embolus (PE) is a major cause of death during a surgical procedure and in the immediate postoperative period. Some intraoperative problems may extend into postoperative recovery.

PE is an obstruction of the pulmonary artery or one of its branches by an embolus, most often a blood clot, but can be fat or other material. The most common cause of PE is stasis of blood, particularly in the low-pressure regions such as deep veins of the legs and pelvis, where the majority of thrombi arise. These clots become detached and are carried to the lungs.

Injury to the intima of vessel walls and coagulative changes in blood also are important factors. A prolonged period on the OR bed may decrease blood flow to the lower extremities by more than 50%. Blood flow is impaired further if the knees are raised on a hard, rolled towel, putting occlusive pressure on the deep veins of the legs.

Venous stasis also is correlated with obesity, dehydration, congestive heart failure, and atrial fibrillation. Local trauma to a vein or venous disease enhances the chance of thrombus formation. Hypercoagulability may coexist with conditions such as pregnancy, fever, myocardial infarction, and some malignancies

and after abrupt cessation of anticoagulant therapy. Prevention consists of a regimen of prophylactic anticoagulants or antiplatelets for high-risk patients and routine measures to prevent venous stasis, such as intermittent compression or antiembolic stockings.

Because of the origin of thrombi in deep veins, it is important to observe the patient postoperatively for thrombophlebitis, evidenced by heat, edema, redness, pain in the calf, or a positive Homans sign, which is pain in the calf on forceful dorsiflexion of the foot.

Nonspecific symptoms depend on whether the embolism is mild or massive. The patient may have dyspnea, pleural pain, hemoptysis, tachypnea, crackles, tachycardia, mild fever, or persistent cough. Patients with massive emboli have air hunger, hypotension, shock, and central cyanosis. Treatment of pulmonary emboli consists of bed rest, oxygen therapy, anticoagulant therapy, thrombolytic agents, and sometimes a surgical procedure to remove the emboli or place a vena cava filter to prevent additional clots reaching the lungs.

Fat embolism occurs primarily after fracture of a long bone, the pelvis, or ribs. However, it sometimes occurs after a blood transfusion, cardiopulmonary bypass, or renal transplant. Fat globules enter a venous sinus and become bloodborne. Symptoms develop when globules block pulmonary capillaries, causing interstitial edema and hemorrhage.

Frequently, ARDS ensues 24 to 48 hours after injury, with hypoxia and decreased surfactant production, resulting in collapse of the alveolar membrane and microatelectasis. The syndrome develops most often in patients older than 10 years, especially those who have traveled long distances with an immobilized fracture. Symptoms include disorientation, increased pulse rate, elevated temperature, tachypnea, dyspnea, crackles, and pleuritic chest pain.[4] Other significant signs are fat in the sputum and urine and a petechial rash on the anterior chest. Treatment is supportive. Mortality is high.

Air embolism may occur intraoperatively with the patient in a sitting position for a craniotomy or posterior cervical operation. Cerebral diploic veins are noncollapsible; venous sinuses in the skull remain open. The pull of gravity on the venous drainage exerts a significant negative pressure that sucks air into the veins and into the right atrium of the heart. The air embolus blocks the tricuspid valve. This can be a complication in handling central venous catheters and using syringes to obtain blood for gas analysis.

Cardiac dysrhythmias and unexplained hypotension are prime signs and symptoms. A characteristic heart murmur may be audible with a precordial stethoscope or Doppler. Immediate treatment of air embolus is to place the patient into Trendelenburg position with the right side slightly elevated (Durant procedure). The anesthesia provider can place a central venous catheter into the patient's jugular vein and pass it into the right atrium to evacuate the air with a large syringe.

Intrauterine fetal death, abruptio placenta, or placenta previa may precipitate an embolism of amniotic fluid. Also, tumors may cause emboli from primary or metastatic sites. Other material such as plaque or hemostatic material can embolize, causing injury or death to the patient.

Pneumothorax

Although it is rare, insertion of a needle into the thoracic cage can occur during a nerve block or subclavian catheter insertion.

Excision of a breast mass close to the chest wall can precipitate pneumothorax. The primary symptoms are pain and shortness of breath. Confirmation is made by x-ray. If the pneumothorax is extensive and the lung fails to reexpand, a chest tube with an underwater seal is required.

Patients with pleural effusion may require thoracentesis, which involves draining the chest for relief of symptoms. Careful placement of the needle can prevent pneumothorax.

Intercostal Muscle Spasm

A "rigid chest" may occur after large doses of IV fentanyl or on emergence from general anesthesia. It may reverse itself, or neuromuscular blockers may be needed.

Atelectasis (Pulmonary Collapse)

Partial collapse of a lung, atelectasis, is one of the most common postoperative problems. If mucus obstructs a bronchus, air in the alveoli distal to the obstruction is resorbed. That segment of lung then collapses and consolidates. Retained mucus becomes contaminated by inhaled bacteria; the patient may develop bronchopneumonia.

Etiology

Factors that promote increased production of mucus (e.g., certain irritating anesthetics) and decreased mobilization of mucus (e.g., from a tight abdominal dressing) predispose the patient to pulmonary collapse. Furthermore, normal respiration includes a deep sigh several times an hour to help keep the lungs expanded. This natural sigh is inhibited by anesthetics, narcotics, and sedatives. Oxygen and carbon dioxide are absorbed into the pulmonary blood flow, and the alveoli collapse. Low tidal volume intensifies the problem. High concentrations of oxygen remove nitrogen from the lungs, leaving oxygen, carbon dioxide, and water in the alveoli.

Symptoms

Atelectasis increases the temperature, pulse, and respiratory rate. The patient may appear cyanotic and uncomfortable, with shallow respirations and pain on coughing. Breath sounds are diminished, with fine crackles. Chest x-ray reveals collapsed areas of the lungs as patch opacities, generally involving the lung bases.

Treatment and Prevention

Measures to help prevent or treat atelectasis are abstention from smoking, a regimen of coughing and deep breathing, and early ambulation. An upright position allows for better lung expansion. Medication for pain, when appropriate, before breathing exercises or ambulation improves the ability to breathe deeply and cough effectively. Splinting the thoracic or abdominal incision with a pillow also helps decrease the pain of coughing. Repeated vigorous coughing is contraindicated in some patients (e.g., after cataract extraction, craniotomy, herniorrhaphy).

Pulmonary Edema

Pulmonary edema may be defined as an abnormal accumulation of water in extravascular portions of the lungs, including both alveolar and interstitial spaces. In surgical patients the most probable cause is increased microvascular pulmonary capillary permeability or capillary endothelial injury. Blood stagnates in the pulmonary circulation. Fluid exudes from capillaries into the alveoli and interstitial spaces. Reduction of capillary membrane perfusion leads to hypoxia. Symptoms, usually seen postoperatively in the postanesthesia care unit (PACU) or intensive care unit (ICU), may include a bounding, rapid pulse; crackles; dyspnea; and engorged peripheral veins.

Cardiovascular Complications

The emotional and physical stresses to which a surgical patient is subjected may lead to cardiovascular complications. The patient who fears dying while under anesthesia runs a greater risk for cardiac arrest on the operating bed than do patients with known cardiac disease. Psychologic stress can have physiologic manifestations. Extreme preoperative anxiety predisposes the patient to a difficult induction and intraoperative period and postoperative discomfort.

Patients with a history of cardiovascular problems are prone to develop complications. These may include dysrhythmias, hypotension, thromboembolism and/or thrombophlebitis, myocardial infarction, or congestive heart failure. Cerebral thrombosis or embolism may result in prolonged coma. Patients must be closely monitored for symptoms of cardiovascular complications. Anoxia, the complete or almost total absence of oxygen from inspired gases, arterial blood, or tissues, is a precursor to cardiovascular collapse. Cardiac arrest can result in death in the OR.

Hypotension

Reduced blood pressure (BP), with resultant inadequate circulation, may accompany depression of the myocardium, depression of the vasomotor center in the brain, a decline in CO, or dilation of the peripheral vessels. Hypotension also may occur when positive pressure is applied to the airway. Progressive deepening of general anesthesia usually produces peripheral vasodilation and diminished myocardial contractility. Adequate blood flow to the brain and heart, the two most vulnerable vascular beds because of their high metabolic demand, must be maintained. If arterial hypotension is uncontrolled, it may cause a cerebrovascular accident, myocardial infarction, or death.

Etiology

Overdosage of general anesthetic agents or rapid vascular absorption of local agents may result from the patient receiving an amount of the agent that exceeds their tolerance. Tendency for overdosage occurs during prolonged anesthesia with large amounts of drugs absorbed, in age-extreme patients, or with unrecognized hypothermia during lengthy abdominal or thoracic procedures. Circulatory effects of spinal or epidural anesthesia, such as diminished CO or reduced peripheral resistance, also produce hypotension.

Other causes of hypotension include the following:
- Volume depletion and/or hemorrhage
- Circulatory abnormalities (e.g., cardiac tamponade, heart failure)
- Cerebral or pulmonary embolism (fat embolism from fracture sites, amniotic fluid emboli during delivery, or air emboli from introduction of air into the circulation during an infusion or procedure)
- Myocardial ischemia or infarction
- Changes in position, especially if executed rapidly or roughly

- Excessive preanesthetic medication (postural hypotension may follow narcotic administration)
- Epidural or spinal anesthesia above the level of T6 (sympathetic block)
- Potent therapeutic drugs (e.g., tranquilizers, adrenal steroids, antihypertensives) given before the anesthetic
- Hypoxia

Surgical manipulation may mechanically induce hypotension by obstructing venous return to the heart with packs, retractors, or body rests, or hypotension and bradycardia may result from a vagal-induced reflex precipitated by intraperitoneal traction, manipulation in the chest or neck area, rapid release of either increased intraabdominal pressure or overdistention of the bladder, anorectal stimulation, or stimulation of the periosteum or joint cavities. Other causes are transfusion reaction (suggested by accompanying cyanosis and oozing at the surgical site), septic shock, severe hyperthermia, and anaphylactic reaction.

Symptoms

Early reversible shock is accompanied by unstable BP, vasoconstriction, and elevated serum pH and catecholamine levels. Late manifestations are pallor or central cyanosis, clammy skin, dilated pupils, decreased urinary output, tachycardia, decreased bleeding in the surgical field, or pallor of organs caused by compensatory vasoconstriction, nausea, vomiting, sighing respirations, or air hunger in conscious patients.

Diagnosis

Determination of arterial BP and pulse rate and estimation of pulse volume are indicative of the volume of cardiac ejection. Arbitrary figures of measured BP are not as important as individual circulatory status. A specific measurement in a healthy adult may be relatively insignificant, whereas the same figure in a geriatric patient could be hazardous. In critically ill patients, direct arterial pressure, central venous pressure (CVP), and urinary output are monitored.

Treatment

Treatment must be prompt to avoid circulatory collapse. The aim is to increase perfusion of the vital organs and treat any specific cause while giving general supportive therapy. Supportive measures include oxygen by mask with assisted respiration; elevation of the legs to increase BP by draining pooled blood, especially after sympathetic blockade; and rapid IV fluid therapy to increase blood volume.

Because the volume of fluid is more vital than its composition, various solutions are applicable for early treatment in an emergency. If whole blood is not available, crystalloid solutions (e.g., lactated Ringer's solution), 5% dextrose in water (D_5W), physiologic saline solution (0.9% saline), plasma or serum albumin, or 6% dextran (plasma expander) may be given. Rapid infusion under pressure may be necessary. Vasoactive drugs are given as necessary; these are usually vasopressors to constrict arterioles and veins while increasing the myocardial contractile force. Blood gases should be monitored.

Prevention

The causes must be reversed or avoided. Therefore the patient should be observed constantly throughout anesthesia. In individuals suspected of having hypotension the cardiovascular response to the desired surgical position should be tested before induction. Overdosage of premedication and anesthetic drugs is avoided. The patient's position is changed slowly, tissue is manipulated gently, and blood and fluid loss are replaced promptly. The anesthesia provider administers a minimal amount of the anesthetic and takes adequate time to induce and deepen anesthesia so as not to raise the blood level of the anesthetic too rapidly. Positive pressure is applied to the airway prudently.

Some narcotics and anesthetic agents, surgical trauma, anoxia, and blood loss can lead to postoperative hypotension. When combined, these factors interfere with the complex physiologic mechanisms that support BP. Peripheral vessels dilate. A degree of cardiovascular collapse ensues. Vasoconstriction reduces renal blood flow, causing decrease or failure of kidney function. Patients must be monitored postoperatively for sudden drops in BP or other signs of shock. Vasoactive drugs and oxygen may be administered. To avoid hypotension, fluid management is critical to renal function after restoration of systemic BP.

Hypertension

Abnormal elevation of the BP, hypertension, may occur, especially in a hypertensive or arteriosclerotic patient. Even mildly hypertensive patients are prone to myocardial ischemia (inadequate blood flow to the heart) during induction of and emergence from anesthesia. Intubation stimulates the sympathetic nervous system. Other predisposing factors include pain, shivering, hypoxia, hypercapnia, effects of vasopressor drugs, or hypervolemia from excessive replacement of fluid losses. Treatment consists of administration of oxygen, diuretics, and antihypertensive β-blocker drugs as indicated. If not controlled, hypertension may precipitate a cerebrovascular accident or myocardial infarction. It may cause bleeding from the surgical site or may threaten the integrity of a vascular bypass.

Venospasm

If caused by cold IV fluid infusion, venospasm may manifest as very slow flow. It may result from pressure infusion or extravasation. IV procaine relieves spasm. Thrombophlebitis may follow venospasm.

Coronary Thrombosis

Coronary thrombosis can occur from severe hypoxia and lack of oxygen to coronary vessels. Sometimes its occurrence is the reason for a patient not to regain consciousness after a surgical procedure.

Venous Stasis

Venous return of blood from the lower extremities can be slowed by the effects of general or spinal anesthesia and by the position of the legs during prolonged surgical procedures. The venous stasis that develops in most patients during a surgical procedure can be effectively counteracted. To prevent thrombophlebitis and thrombosis in patients with thromboembolic disease, anticoagulants may be administered. Antiembolic stockings, with or without a sequential pneumatic compression device, augment venous flow from the legs. Elevation of the legs as little as 15% above horizontal can assist in venous return.

Postoperatively the patient may be placed in Trendelenburg position with the legs elevated. Flexion and extension of the legs and feet, frequent turning, and early ambulation, unless contraindicated, aid circulation.

Deep Vein Thrombosis

Venous stasis, changes in clotting factors in the blood, and damage to vessel walls are the primary causes of deep vein thrombosis (DVT) in the lower extremities. Age, obesity, immobility, and a history of thromboembolic or other cardiovascular disease are predisposing factors. The type, location, and extent of the surgical procedure can contribute also. Preoperative prophylactic interventions, including anticoagulants, sequential compression devices, or antiembolic stockings, can reduce the risk for postoperative pulmonary embolism, which is a life-threatening complication of DVT.

Disseminated Intravascular Coagulation

Although it occurs rarely, disseminated intravascular coagulation (DIC) is a life-threatening syndrome. It is a complex derangement of clotting factors. The hemostatic process involves vasoconstriction with platelet aggregation and clotting. In DIC the normal clotting mechanisms do not function. Instead, a repetitive, overactive cycle of clot formation (coagulopathy) and simultaneous clot breakdown (fibrinolysis) occur. This leads to consumption of platelets and coagulation factors and release of fibrin degradation products that act as potent anticoagulants.

DIC can follow hemorrhage, thrombi, emboli, infection, or allergic reaction to an incompatible blood transfusion. It may be precipitated by septic shock, abruptio placenta during pregnancy, or massive soft tissue damage of extensive trauma or burns. As blood becomes depleted of platelets and major clotting factors, coagulation is initiated throughout the bloodstream, especially in microcirculation.

Prolonged bleeding may be noted; hematomas and cutaneous petechiae may appear. Massive hemorrhage and ischemia of vital organs may ensue. Bleeding may be noted from various sites, such as through the nasogastric tube or IV site.

The patient may have hypotension and oliguria. Postoperatively the patient may have nausea and vomiting, severe muscular pain, and convulsions and may lapse into a coma. Diagnosis is based on laboratory blood studies. Treatment begins with control of the primary condition. Blood, plasma, and dextran can be administered IV. Heparin and clotting factors, if given early, may prevent hemorrhage.

Cardiac Dysrhythmias

An alteration of normal cardiac rhythm may decrease CO, exhaust the myocardium, and lead to ventricular fibrillation or cardiac arrest. Bradycardia is the slowing of the heart or pulse rate. Tachycardia is an excessive rapidity of the heart's action. Ventricular tachycardia and ventricular fibrillation are the dysrhythmias of most serious consequence and thus most feared.

Etiology

Etiologic factors include hypoxia; hypercapnia; acidosis; electrolyte imbalance; coronary disease; myocardial infarction; vagal reflexes; anesthetic agents; toxic doses of digitalis, epinephrine, or other drugs; and laryngospasm and coughing initiated by the presence of secretions in the airway after induction. Other causes may be hypotension, hemorrhage, hypovolemia, pneumothorax, and mechanical injuries.

Ventricular Dysrhythmias

An impulse originating in the ventricles must travel to the rest of the myocardium from one ventricle, then proceeding to the other. Because the impulse does not travel via the rapid, specialized conduction system, depolarization of both ventricles takes longer and is not simultaneous. The complexes of dysrhythmias have an abnormal appearance on an electrocardiogram (ECG) compared with normally initiated and conducted impulses.

Premature Ventricular Contraction

An ectopic focus in the ventricles stimulates the heart to contract or beat prematurely before the regularly scheduled sinoatrial impulse arrives (Fig. 31.1). Primary precipitating factors are electrolyte or acid-base imbalance, myocardial infarction, digitalis toxicity, and caffeine. The premature ventricular contraction (PVC) must be distinguished from a premature atrial contraction (PAC). Isolated PVCs may not require treatment, but those occurring in clusters of two or more, or more than five or six per minute, require therapy. The aim is to quiet the irritable myocardium and restore adequate CO.

Treatment consists of a lidocaine bolus followed by a continuous drip by infusion, correction of the cause (e.g., hypoxia), and other antidysrhythmic drugs if indicated . Temporary pacing may be used for severe bradycardia. Paired PVCs pose an increased danger of ventricular tachycardia.

Ventricular Tachycardia

A rapid heart rate (100–220 beats/min) may be caused by ventricular ischemia or irritability, anoxia, or digitalis intoxication. The heart rate does not allow time for ventricular filling (Fig. 31.2). The resultant reduced CO predisposes the patient to

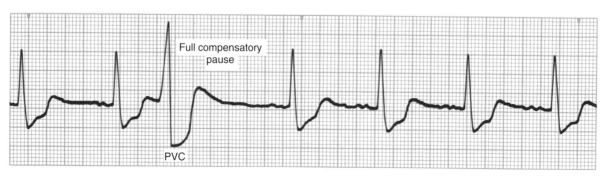

• **Fig. 31.1** Premature ventricular contractions.

• **Fig. 31.2** Ventricular tachycardia.

• **Fig. 31.3** Ventricular fibrillation.

ventricular fibrillation or cardiac failure. Ventricular tachycardia is treated by prompt IV administration of lidocaine or other medication.

Synchronized cardioversion of 10 to 200 joules may be used if the BP is palpable. This is the application of a high-intensity, short-duration electric shock to the chest wall over the heart to produce total cardiac depolarization. This countershock is timed to interrupt an abnormal rhythm in the cardiac cycle, thereby permitting resumption of a normal one. Cardioversion is usually applied in instances of nonarrest for a dangerous ventricular tachycardia. It may be an elective or emergency treatment. Asynchronous cardioversion is used if the patient is pulseless. Treatment includes correction of the underlying cause.

Ventricular Flutter

Often called fine ventricular fibrillation, the flutter appears as a transient state between ventricular tachycardia and ventricular fibrillation. The patient will show signs of poor CO.

Ventricular Fibrillation

The most serious of all dysrhythmias, fibrillation is characterized by total disorganization of ventricular activity (Fig. 31.3). There are rapid and irregular, uncoordinated, random contractions of small myocardial groups without effective ventricular contraction or CO. Circulation ceases. The patient in fibrillation is unconscious and possibly convulsing from cerebral hypoxia.

Treatment

Because respiratory and cardiac arrest quickly follow, ventricular fibrillation is rapidly fatal unless successful defibrillation is effected as follows:

1. *Precordial thump:* In a monitored patient a fast, sharp, single blow to the midportion of the sternum (using the nipple line as a landmark) may be delivered with the bottom fleshy part of a closed fist struck from 8 to 12 inches (20 to 30 cm) above the chest. The blow generates a small electrical stimulus in a heart that is reactive. It may be effective in restoring a beat in cases of asystole or recent onset of dysrhythmia. A precordial thump can be used in a witnessed, monitored cardiac arrest.

2. *Asynchronous cardioversion:* Prompt defibrillation by short-duration electric shock to the heart produces simultaneous depolarization of all muscle fiber bundles, after which spontaneous beating (conversion to spontaneous normal sinus rhythm) may resume if the myocardium is oxygenated and not acidotic. Defibrillation of an anoxic myocardium is difficult. The start time of the fibrillation should be noted. The electric shock is coordinated with controlled ventilation and cardiac compression. Cardiopulmonary resuscitation (CPR) begins as soon as fibrillation is identified. Many variables may affect defibrillation, such as body weight, paddle position, electrical waveform, and resistance to electric current flow. Procedures follow an established protocol.

3. *Adjunct drug therapy:* Drugs are given as necessary: vasopressor, cardiotonic, and myocardial stimulant drugs to maintain a useful heartbeat; vasodilator or antidysrhythmic drugs to prevent recurrence; and sodium bicarbonate to combat acidosis. Continuous monitoring of the heart and laboratory analysis of arterial blood gases are essential.

Defibrillation: Equipment and Technique. Necessary equipment for defibrillation includes a defibrillator machine and two paddle electrodes. Defibrillators use direct electric current. Most have integrated monitors; monitor and defibrillator switches may be separate or combined. An operational monitor does not always indicate that the fibrillation power is on.

Many monitor-defibrillator units can monitor the ECG from the paddle electrodes, as well as from separate patient leads. These paddles and patient leads cannot operate simultaneously, however. Depending on the type of defibrillator, the electrical cord must be plugged in or batteries charged. All defibrillators should be checked regularly with suitable test equipment. Paddles must be cleaned immediately and prepared for reuse. This is emergency equipment and must be available at all times.

External Defibrillation. External defibrillation of the heart is used unless the chest is already open, as for intrathoracic surgery. Standard electrode paste or jelly or saline-soaked 4 × 4-inch gauze pads reduce the resistance of the skin to passage of the electric current. If paste is used on paddles, it should not extend beyond the electrodes or onto any part of the handles.

Gel pads between the paddles and the patient's skin provide the advantage that if external cardiac compression is resumed after defibrillation, hands will not slip on the chest. The large diameter of the paddles increases the area of skin contact, thus reducing the possibility of skin burns by spreading of the current. The paddles must be held flat against the skin and more than 2 inches (5 cm) apart to prevent electrical arcing. They must be kept scrupulously clean because foreign material reduces the uniformity of the shock. The electrodes must be pressed firmly against the chest wall for good contact. One of two external paddle positions may be used:

1. *Standard position:* One electrode is placed just to the right of the upper sternum below the clavicle. The other is positioned to the left of the cardiac apex (i.e., left of the nipple at the fifth intercostal space along the left midaxillary line). The delivered current flows through the long axis of the heart.
2. *Anterior-posterior position:* One electrode is placed anteriorly over the precordium between the left nipple and the sternum. The other is positioned posteriorly behind the heart immediately below the left scapula, avoiding the spinal column. This allows for more energy passage through the heart, but placement is more difficult.

Internal Defibrillation. For internal defibrillation, sterile electrodes are placed on the myocardium—one over the right atrium and the other over the left ventricle. If these electrodes are gauze covered, they are dipped in sterile saline solution before use. Minimal current is needed when paddles are placed directly on the heart.

Perioperative team members must understand the functioning of the defibrillator for the patient's safety as well as their own. The person holding the electrode paddles delivers the electric charge by pressing a switch on the handle or a foot switch. The safest method is to activate both paddles simultaneously for discharge of electrical energy. The operator should have dry hands and stand on a dry floor.

To avoid possible self-electrocution when using a defibrillator, neither the person holding the electrodes nor anyone else should touch the metal frame of the OR bed or the patient while the current is being applied. No part of the operator's body should touch the paste or the uninsulated electrodes. Loud verbal warning is given before discharge. Countershock is repeated at intervals if fibrillation persists. Transthoracic impedance falls with repetitive, closely spaced electrical discharges. After each countershock, the ECG and pulse should be reassessed.

Myocardial damage resulting from defibrillation efforts is in direct proportion to the energy used; therefore maximal settings, when not required, may increasingly impair an already damaged myocardium. The energy level delivered through a specific ohm load should be indicated on the front panel of the defibrillator. Delivery output ranges vary among machines.

The strength of the countershock is expressed in energy as joules or watt-seconds—the product of power and duration. If the patient's chest muscles do not contract, no current has reached the patient. The defibrillator's connection to the electrical source and the "off" button to the synchronizer circuit should be checked. If the machine is battery operated, the battery must be charged enough to energize the capacitor. Personnel must be familiar with and follow operating instructions for the defibrillator in use.

Appropriate preoperative sedation and skillfully administered anesthetic help prevent hazardous cardiovascular reflexes. Because PVCs are precursors to ventricular fibrillation, in itself a precursor

to cardiac arrest, any cardiopulmonary emergency in a prearrest phase requires the following procedures:

1. *Monitoring of the heart rhythm and rate:* The ability to recognize the rhythms that precede arrest permits intervention that may prevent arrest. If the cardiac status is not under constant monitoring, hypoxia and acidosis may be present and require correction before other therapeutic modalities can be used effectively.
2. *Establishment of an IV lifeline:* Venous cannulation provides access to peripheral and central venous circulation for administering drugs and fluids, obtaining venous blood specimens for laboratory analysis, and inserting catheters into the right side of the heart and pulmonary arteries for physiologic monitoring and electrical pacing. If cardiac arrest appears imminent or has occurred, cannulation of a peripheral or femoral vein should be attempted first so as not to interrupt CPR. To keep the infusion open, the rate should be kept slow. The usual complications to all IV techniques should be guarded against.

Cardiac Arrest

In cases of cardiac arrest there is cessation of circulatory action; the pumping mechanism of the heart ceases. Cardiac standstill represents total absence of electrical cardiac activity (asystole), reflected as a straight line on an ECG rhythm strip.[5] It may occur as primary cardiac failure or secondary to failure of pulmonary ventilation. The types of circulatory arrest are profound cardiovascular collapse, electromechanical dissociation, ventricular fibrillation, and ventricular asystole or standstill.[6] Cardiac arrest may precede or follow failure of the respiratory system because the systems are interrelated.

CPR should be started immediately, either manually or mechanically, if the person is to survive. Emergency medical personnel have a mechanical device that provides continuous chest compressions for an extended period while transporting a patient to a health care facility. The device can accommodate a sternum height up to 14.5 inches and a chest width up to 22 inches. The device eliminates provider fatigue and allows medical personnel to do other patient care tasks.

Incidence

Arrest may occur during induction of anesthesia, intraoperatively, or postoperatively. Occurrence during cardiac surgery or after massive hemorrhage is not uncommon. Patients prone to arrest include those at age extremes and those with previously diagnosed paroxysmal dysrhythmias, primary cardiovascular abnormalities, myocarditis, heart block, or digitalis toxicity. An unexpected arrest is one that happens in a patient of general good health who is undergoing a low-risk or relatively routine procedure. These arrests are associated with major morbidity and mortality.

Etiology

A single factor or combination of factors may precipitate cardiac arrest, but the general cause is inadequate coronary arterial blood flow. Defective respiratory function produces systemic hypoxemia, causing myocardial hypoxia and depression. It also increases myocardial irritability and the heart's susceptibility to vagal reflexes.

Some of the specific precipitating factors are dysrhythmias, emboli, extreme hypotension or hypovolemia, respiratory obstruction, aspiration, effects of drugs, anesthetic overdosage, excessively rapid or unsmooth induction, sepsis, pharyngeal stimulation, metabolic abnormalities (acidosis, toxemia, electrolyte imbalance), poor cardiac filling caused by positioning, manipulation of the heart, central nervous system trauma, anaphylaxis, and electric shock from ungrounded or faulty electrical equipment.

Symptoms

Symptoms include loss of heartbeat and BP; sudden fixed, dilated pupils; sudden pallor or cyanosis; cold, clammy skin; absence of reflexes; unconsciousness or convulsions in a previously conscious patient; respiratory standstill; and dark blood or absence of bleeding in the surgical field.[5,6]

Diagnosis

The ECG monitor readily detects arrest during anesthesia, with absence of BP and precordial heart sounds and the lack of a palpable carotid pulse. The onset of pupillary dilation is within 45 seconds after cerebral anoxia; full dilation is reached about 90 to 110 seconds after cessation of cerebral circulation.

Treatment

CPR is initiated immediately to restore oxygenation to vital organs.[5] Defibrillation may be needed for ventricular fibrillation. IV drugs generally are used to improve cardiopulmonary status.

Prevention

Optimal psychologic preoperative assessment to identify the level of anxiety and testing for abnormalities and sensitivities is an important preoperative preparation. Intraoperative precautions include the following:
- ECG and temperature monitoring
- No stimulation during induction
- Maintenance of an adequate airway
- Oxygen and carbon dioxide monitoring
- Arterial BP monitoring
- Medications
- Appropriate positioning and slow position changes with the patient under anesthesia; no weight on the patient
- Gentle handling of tissues with minimal traction and manipulation
- Skillful anesthetic administration

Intravenous Cardiovascular Drugs

An important factor in optimal anesthesia management is prompt recognition of the causes of hypotension, shock, and other complications that could lead to cardiac arrest. Prompt correction of reversible precipitants is critical. Many intravenous (IV) drugs are used to correct hypoxia and metabolic acidosis, manipulate cardiovascular variables, or treat pulmonary edema.

Pharmacodynamics

Uptake, movement, binding, and interactions of drugs vary at the tissue site of their biochemical and physiologic actions. Drug action is determined by how the drug interacts in the body. Some drugs alter body fluids; others, such as anesthetics, interact with cell membranes; most act through receptor mechanisms.

Receptor Mechanisms
Most drugs mimic naturally occurring compounds and interact with specific biologic molecules to produce biologic responses. For example, some cardiovascular drugs are sympathomimetics. They evoke physiologic responses comparable to those produced by the sympathetic nervous system. A receptor is a structural protein molecule on a cell surface or within cytoplasm that binds with a drug to produce a biologic response. Three types of receptors are noteworthy in understanding the drugs used to counteract complications that may occur during anesthesia.

Adrenergic Receptors. Adrenergic receptors are innervated by sympathetic nerve fibers and activated by epinephrine or norepinephrine secreted at the postganglionic nerve endings. These receptors are classified as alpha or beta, depending on their sensitivity to specific adrenergic activating and blocking drugs. The α_1 and α_2 receptors are located primarily in peripheral and renal arteriolar muscles; β_1 receptors predominate in the heart; β_2 receptors are primarily in smooth muscle of the lungs and blood vessels.

Cholinergic Receptors. Cholinergic receptors are sites where acetylcholine exerts action to transmit nerve impulses through the parasympathetic nervous system to regulate the heart rate and respirations.

Opiate Receptors. Opiate receptors are regions in the brain capable of binding morphine in areas related to pain.

Drug Interactions
No drug has a single action. Each modifies existing functions within the body by interactions to stimulate or inhibit responses. The desired action may be accompanied by side effects or an exaggerated response. An allergic reaction may occur immediately after exposure or may be delayed.

Anaphylaxis is a life-threatening, acute allergic reaction in which cells release histamine or a histamine-like substance.[7] Anaphylaxis, a form of vasogenic shock, causes vasodilation, hypotension, and bronchial constriction. Within seconds of receiving a drug that induces an allergic reaction, the patient will exhibit edema, wheezing, cyanosis, and dyspnea. Treatment includes epinephrine and antihistamines to control bronchospasm. Isoproterenol, vasopressors, corticosteroids, and aminophylline also may be administered.[6,7]

In combination with local, regional, or general anesthetics, drugs must be carefully administered and monitored. The action of one drug may counteract the action of another drug. Patients who do not respond to one drug (e.g., a catecholamine) may respond to another. Physicians do not always agree on the use of potent drugs. For example, a vasoconstrictor used to treat hypotension may possibly cause ischemic damage to organs. The physician's orders should be followed for all drugs.

Intravenous Administration
The speed of administration and dosage will depend on the drug and its intended action. Dosages given in this text vary according to individual patient circumstances. The technique of IV administration also varies.

Continuous Intravenous Drip. The drug is diluted in a volume of dextrose or normal saline solution. The rate of administration is regulated by adjusting the number of drops per minute from the solution container into the IV tubing. A drug that might be absorbed by plastic should not be added to solution in a plastic infusion bag.

Bolus. A bolus is a single rapid injection of the full dosage of a drug that cannot be diluted. It is usually given through an existing IV line, and it may be injected directly into a vein or an intrathecal catheter. Some drugs can be given via an endotracheal tube for absorption through the alveoli or mucous membranes. The drug quickly reaches peak level in the bloodstream.

Intravenous Push. A drug may be injected slowly into an IV line or through an intermittent infusion pump over a period of minutes. The total dose may be diluted and given in repeated doses over a period of hours. An infusion pump may be used to control the rate of delivery precisely.

Titration. Dosage is calculated on the basis of body surface area (BSA) and hemodynamic parameters. CO is evaluated in terms of BSA. This may be determined by the ratio of the patient's height and weight on the BSA scale or by thermodilution. The patient's physiologic responses also will determine total dosage.

Considerations for Drug Administration

Some drugs are inactivated by others. The IV tubing should be flushed or changed to avoid precipitation, such as can occur with sodium bicarbonate. Many potent drugs should be infused through an IV catheter, which is safer than a needle to prevent extravasation. If a drug extravasates at the site of injection, the area must be promptly infiltrated with an appropriate drug (e.g., phentolamine, Regitine) or saline flush to prevent the necrosis that can result from some vasoactive drugs.[8]

Drugs by Classification

Pharmacokinetics includes the mechanisms of absorption, distribution, and metabolism of drugs in the body and elimination from the body. Nurses must have knowledge of drug actions and of how to prepare and administer drugs. The following drugs are classified by their pharmacodynamics to counteract adverse cardiovascular and pulmonary status.

Sympathomimetics are used most often for the following purposes:

- To increase force (inotropic effect), maintain contractility (noninotropic effect), or decrease the stroke volume of myocardial contractions
- To increase the pulse rate
- To increase or decrease arterial BP
- To correct dysrhythmias
- To increase renal blood flow
- To stimulate the central nervous system
- To treat bronchospasm
- To prolong the effect of local anesthetics
- To manage life-threatening emergencies

Patients receiving any of the following drugs must be carefully monitored.

Antidysrhythmics

Antidysrhythmics control the heart rate and rhythm. They may induce a decreased rate and CO. They may reduce cardiac conduction and increase dilation of peripheral vessels.

Lidocaine (Xylocaine). Lidocaine increases the threshold for ventricular irritability by exerting a focal anesthetic effect on the myocardial cell membrane. It is used for ventricular tachycardia and fibrillation, especially if resistance to defibrillation effort occurs. It can be given IV, intrathecally, or by endotracheal tube. Dosage is 1 mg/kg or 75 to 100 mg by IV push over 30 to 60 seconds, followed by half the initial dose every 5 to 10 minutes to a total of 3 mg/kg if ectopic heartbeats continue. After conversion, a maintenance dose of 1 to 4 mg/min can be given by IV

drip. Half these dosages are used to treat shock or pulmonary edema.

Amiodarone. Amiodarone is the first line of treatment in shockable rhythms such as ventricular fibrillation, supraventricular tachycardia, or pulseless ventricular tachycardia. Dosage is 15 mg/kg IV over 10 minutes, followed by 1 mg/kg/min over 3 hours. Total should not exceed 100 mg over 24 hours. Amiodarone is not used in second- or third-degree atrioventricular (AV) block unless a pacemaker is present or in electrolyte imbalance of potassium or magnesium. Complications include the potential for thyroid, liver, or lung tissue damage. Amiodarone can interact with oral anticoagulants, digoxin, and other class I antidysrhythmics.

Bretylium (Bretylol). Bretylium lowers the defibrillation threshold, permitting otherwise refractory rhythms to be electrically converted. It is indicated in cases of ventricular tachycardia and fibrillation unresponsive to other therapy. Dosage is 5 mg/kg by rapid IV bolus, followed by defibrillation. If fibrillation continues, the dose can be doubled and repeated as necessary. For ventricular fibrillation, 300 to 600 mg may be required. The drug may be diluted for continuous IV drip at a dosage of 1 to 2 mg/min for ventricular tachycardia and to prevent fibrillation. Some degree of hypotension may occur.

Procainamide (Pronestyl). Procainamide suppresses PVCs and recurrent tachycardia. This drug may be used if lidocaine is contraindicated or has not controlled ventricular tachycardia. Dosage is 100 mg by IV push every 5 minutes until dysrhythmia ceases, or to a total of 1 g. Maintenance IV drip is 1 to 4 mg/min. Marked hypotension may occur if infusion is too rapid.

Adenosine (Adenocard). Adenosine slows AV node conduction. This action converts supraventricular tachycardia to normal sinus rhythm. Dosage is 6 to 12 mg by IV bolus followed immediately by a saline bolus. Incremental doses of 0.05 mg/kg can be given as necessary. This drug is contraindicated for patients with asthma.

Verapamil (Isoptin). A calcium channel blocker, verapamil inhibits calcium ions to slow myocardial contractility, the heart rate, and the demand for oxygen. It is used as an antidysrhythmic to treat paroxysmal supraventricular tachycardia, acute atrial flutter, and atrial fibrillation. Dosage is 5 to 10 mg (0.075–0.15 mg/kg adult body weight) by slow IV push over 2 minutes; may be repeated after 30 minutes. This drug is not given to patients with severe hypotension, malignant hyperthermia (MH), or cardiogenic shock, nor is it given concurrently with an IV β-adrenergic blocker, such as propranolol.

Propranolol (Inderal). A β-adrenergic receptor blocking agent, propranolol is used to control supraventricular dysrhythmias and treat hypertension. It reduces myocardial oxygen consumption by blocking catecholamine-induced increases in the heart rate, BP, and cardiac contractions. It may be used if control of ventricular fibrillation is not achieved with lidocaine or other drugs. Dosage is 1 to 3 mg by IV push, not to exceed 1 mg/min, titrated for heart rate and rhythm. This drug is contraindicated for patients with asthma, bronchospasm, or cardiac depression.

Isoproterenol (Isuprel). A β-adrenergic receptor stimulant, isoproterenol stimulates the sympathetic tone, rate, and strength of myocardial contractions and CO. It increases the myocardial demand for oxygen. It may be used for ventricular dysrhythmias, but it may produce tachycardia or dysrhythmia. It is indicated to control hemodynamically significant bradycardia in a patient who has a pulse but is unresponsive to atropine. It is a vasodilator and bronchodilator. Dosage is IV drip of 1 mg to 500 mL of dextrose or saline solution at the rate of 1.25 mL/min, titrated according to the heart rate and rhythm.

Antimuscarinics/Anticholinergics

Antimuscarinics/anticholinergics block passage of impulses through the parasympathetic nerves to the heart and smooth muscles. When both the sympathetic and parasympathetic components of the autonomic nervous system are stimulated, the parasympathetic dominates to slow the heartbeat and respirations. An anticholinergic allows the desired sympathetic action.

Atropine. Atropine reduces cardiac vagal tone, enhances AV conduction, and increases CO. It accelerates the cardiac rate in sinus bradycardia with severe hypotension or in bradycardia associated with hypoxia and reduced CO. It may restore cardiac rhythm in AV block or ventricular asystole. It is a primary drug used in cardiopulmonary arrest. Atropine may be given IV, intrathecally, or via an endotracheal tube. Dosage is 1 mg by IV bolus for asystole, 0.5 mg for bradycardia, at 5-minute intervals until the desired rate is achieved or to a total dose of 3 mg. Full vagal blockage could result from overdosage.

Vasodilators

Vasodilators are noninotropic drugs that relax smooth muscle in the capillaries and cause peripheral dilation. They dilate arteries and veins almost equally without increasing myocardial contractility. This reduces venous return to heart. They are used to alter blood flow and lower BP in patients who have severely reduced CO or are in hypertensive crisis.

Sodium Nitroprusside (Nipride, Nitropress). Sodium nitroprusside acts rapidly as a direct peripheral vasodilator to increase CO and redistribute cardiac work in patients with pump failure. It increases tissue perfusion without reflex tachycardia. Dosage is IV drip, not to exceed 10 mcg/kg/min, of 50 mg dissolved in 2 to 3 mL of dextrose added to 250 to 1000 mL of 5% dextrose in water for infusion. An infusion pump or microdrip-regulating system ensures a precise flow rate. The solution deteriorates in light, so it must be protected by opaque material such as a dark bottle or aluminum foil. No other drug should be injected into the IV line while sodium nitroprusside is infusing.

Nitroglycerin (Nitrostat IV, Nitrol IV, Tridil). Nitroglycerin decreases venous return to the heart and reduces preload and afterload, thus lowering myocardial oxygen demands. It is used for control of BP in hypertension associated with cardiovascular procedures or endotracheal intubation or in the immediate postoperative period. Dosage is up to 50 mcg/min by IV push. The drug should be titrated to increase the dose, and the time intervals between infusions should be adjusted, depending on lowering of the BP. This potent drug must be diluted in dextrose or saline solution. It is absorbed by polyvinyl chloride plastic, so glass solution bottles and tubing that is not made of polyvinyl chloride should be used. The drug is also light sensitive.

Cardiotonics

Cardiotonics combine inotropic effect on the contractility of muscle with vasodilation of blood vessels. They stimulate myocardial function. Vasodilation reduces cardiac afterload, thereby improving cardiac performance and correcting peripheral vascular compensations.

Inamrinone (Inocor). Inamrinone possesses significant vasodilator activity to improve tissue perfusion, especially to the kidneys, and improve CO. It is used for short-term effect in patients with ischemic heart disease and severe heart failure. The BP and heart rate remain unchanged, whereas peripheral arteriolar resistance falls. Dosage is 0.5 to 2.5 mg/kg by IV bolus followed by IV drip of 5 to 10 mcg/kg/min. Titrated to hemodynamic response, a second bolus can be given after 30 minutes.

Dobutamine (Dobutrex). A synthetic derivative of dopamine, dobutamine increases myocardial contractility while producing little systemic arterial constriction. It is used for short-term treatment of refractory heart failure, cardiogenic shock, and hemodynamically significant hypotension. Dosage is 2.5 to 10 mcg/kg/min IV drip. Tachycardia or dysrhythmia may result from a larger dose. It is incompatible with alkaline solutions and drugs such as sodium bicarbonate.

Catecholamines

Catecholamines are vasoconstrictors that improve tissue perfusion by maintaining perfusion pressure, preventing or diminishing blood loss, decreasing tissue vascularity, and improving coronary blood flow. Among indications for their use are anesthetic overdose, hypotension associated with blood loss, and adrenergic insufficiency. They raise the BP. They are antispasmodic.

Epinephrine (Adrenalin). An endogenous catecholamine and α-adrenergic receptor stimulant, epinephrine plays an essential role in restoration of spontaneous circulation in asystole; therefore the drug epinephrine is the first drug administered in instances of cardiac arrest. By increasing systemic vascular resistance, it improves coronary perfusion pressure and CO produced by cardiac compression during CPR. It improves myocardial contractility and tone and causes vasoconstriction of arteries.

Epinephrine may be given IV, intrathecally, by endotracheal tube, or by intracardiac injection. Dosage is 0.5 to 1 mg by IV bolus, repeated every 5 minutes as necessary. It is available in preloaded syringes of 1:10,000 dilution (1 mg/10 mL). It may be added to an IV infusion of 250 mL of 5% dextrose in water. It is inactivated by alkaline solutions. Continuous infusion may increase the heart rate, BP, and CO. Side effects include elevated myocardial oxygen demand and possible PVCs or ventricular fibrillation.

Norepinephrine (Levophed). An endogenous catecholamine, norepinephrine restores and maintains BP. It may be given after peripheral vascular collapse as a result of severe hypotension or cardiogenic shock. It constricts renal and mesenteric vessels and may cause severe peripheral vasoconstriction. Dosage is 16 mg/L administered at the rate of 0.5 to 1 mcg/min and titrated up to 30 mcg/min IV drip in 5% dextrose in water, titrated to the desired BP; average dose range is 2 to 4 mcg/min. The drug is toxic if extravasation occurs. Hypotension from hypovolemia is a contraindication.

Diuretics

Diuretics increase the amount of urine excreted. Potent diuretics are used to treat pulmonary edema and postarrest cerebral edema. They inhibit resorption of sodium. They are used with caution because they may have a direct vasodilating effect or may lead to fluid and electrolyte depletion. The following two drugs are the most commonly used:

- *Furosemide (Lasix):* 0.5 to 2 mg/kg injected slowly over 1 to 2 minutes by IV push; the dose can be repeated in 2 hours
- *Ethacrynate sodium (Sodium Edecrin):* 40 to 50 mg or 0.5 to 1 mg/kg injected slowly by IV push

Vasopressors

Vasopressors exert an inotropic vasoconstriction action on arterioles and veins through stimulation of α-adrenergic receptors, and they increase the heart rate, BP, and myocardial contractility by activation of β-adrenergic receptors. These drugs cause vasomotor depression of the peripheral circulation but increase coronary flow. They may increase ventricular contractile force, alter sinoatrial nodal activity, constrict smooth muscles, and dilate renal and mesenteric blood vessels. They may produce ventricular dysrhythmia, which can be intensified by hypoxia or hypercapnia. Drug effectiveness is reduced in the presence of respiratory or metabolic acidosis.

Dopamine (Intropin). In high dosages (greater than 10 mcg/kg/min IV drip), dopamine causes peripheral vasoconstriction to increase CO and BP. It may be used during cardiogenic shock, severe hypotension, and asystole and then be titrated to the desired BP. Discontinuance should be gradual. A low dose, 1 to 5 mcg/kg/min IV drip, dilates renal and mesenteric blood vessels to maintain urinary output but may not increase the heart rate or BP. The drip rate may be increased until organ perfusion is evidenced by the BP and urinary output. Tachydysrhythmias are an indication for reduction in dose or discontinuation. Dopamine is inactivated in alkaline solution and by sodium bicarbonate. It is caustic if it extravasates. It should be diluted immediately before use.

Metaraminol (Aramine). Metaraminol produces marked vasoconstriction and increases CO and BP, which may be useful to treat severe hypotension. It may be given IV or via endotracheal tube. Dosage is 0.4 mg/min IV drip in 5% dextrose in water.

Other Vasopressors. These drugs have various actions. Selection will depend on the action needed. Drugs that may be used include the following:
- Isoproterenol (Isuprel)
- Methoxamine (Vasoxyl)
- Mephentermine (Wyamine)
- Norepinephrine (Levophed)
- Phenylephrine (Neo-Synephrine)
- Vasopressin (antidiuretic hormone)
- Dobutamine (Dobutrex, catecholamine)

Other Drugs
Multiple drugs are used for specific problems. Life-threatening acid-base or electrolyte imbalances associated with cardiovascular or pulmonary complications may need to be corrected (e.g., after CPR). All drugs must be used with caution and given at the appropriate time for the correct reason.

Sodium Bicarbonate. Metabolic acidosis secondary to accumulation of lactic acid produced by respiratory metabolism may need to be corrected. Bicarbonate binds with hydrogen ion from lactic acid to produce carbonic acid that breaks down into carbon dioxide and water. Sodium bicarbonate may be given after other resuscitation measures to reverse acidosis. Dosage is 1 mEq/kg by IV bolus initially, titrated according to blood gas analyses for subsequent doses, usually no more than 0.5 mEq/kg at 10 to 15-minute intervals. An excessive dose can produce metabolic alkalosis. Sodium bicarbonate should not be mixed in an IV line with any other drug; it will precipitate calcium salts and inactivate catecholamines.

Cardiopulmonary Resuscitation
CPR is aimed at rapidly restoring oxygen delivery to vital organs to reverse the processes that lead to death. To prevent irreversible

brain damage, resuscitative measures must be instituted immediately, within 3 to 5 minutes after the arrest. The combination of anoxia and acidosis can make restoration of normal function impossible.[5]

Resuscitation in the OR is not a one-person job. The team must be completely familiar with the preplanned routine before the necessity for its use arises. Success depends on prompt diagnosis and immediate effective treatment.[5] Outcome is directly related to the rapidity with which a functional, spontaneous heart rhythm can be restored. Patients who experience arrest in an OR may be on monitors with an IV line already in place and resuscitation equipment on hand. These arrests are referred to as *witnessed arrests*. The time of onset of arrest should be noted and the time-elapsed clock started. Basic life support is instituted at once to reestablish oxygenation and restore the heartbeat.

Basic Cardiac Life Support
Basic cardiac life support (BCLS) is that particular phase of emergency cardiac care that prevents circulatory or respiratory arrest or insufficiency through prompt recognition and intervention. BCLS can and should be initiated by any person present when cardiac arrest occurs. The process begins with chest compressions to maintain circulation of the oxygen present in the circulatory system.[5] This is referred to as *hands-only CPR*. In adults the compression depth should be at least 2 inches, followed by allowing the chest to fully recoil. In infants or children the compression depth should not exceed one-third the anteriorposterior diameter of the chest.

When the arrested patient is in the OR, anesthesia providers and other team members are present. In a witnessed arrest the carotid pulse is palpated. The carotid artery is located in the groove between the trachea and muscles of the side of the neck. Palpation of the femoral artery is an acceptable option. If pulse and breathing are not immediately restored, CPR is begun.

If ventricular fibrillation or tachycardia without a pulse is evident, countershock is delivered as soon as possible (DC 200–300 joules delivered energy in an adult; 2 joules/kg or 1 joule/lb in an infant or child). If this is unsuccessful, additional countershocks and medications are given as ordered or per protocol. In open heart defibrillation, between 5 and 40 joules is delivered, beginning with lower energy levels.

In infants and small children a hand is placed over the precordium to feel the apical beat or the brachial pulse is checked in lieu of a carotid pulse. The brachial pulse is on the inside of the upper arm midway between the elbow and the shoulder. The index and middle fingers are used to implement chest compressions. A precordial thump is not given to an infant or child. In infants and children, bradydysrhythmias and heart block lead to cardiac arrest more commonly than does ventricular fibrillation.

Ventilation
During general anesthesia either an oropharyngeal or nasopharyngeal airway or endotracheal tube may be in place to maintain a patent air passage. Oxygen (100%) can be delivered at once under positive pressure by manual ventilation.

A cuffed endotracheal tube permits continuous delivery of high oxygen concentration without the hazard of stomach distention or aspiration. It facilitates adequate ventilation because with its use interposed breaths are not necessary, thereby permitting a faster, uninterrupted cardiac compression rate of 100 beats/min. When ventilation is combined with cardiac compression, tissues receive oxygen. In the OR the anesthesia provider manages ventilation. The following principles apply:

1. If attempts to ventilate the patient are unsuccessful despite proper opening of the airway, further attempts to remove the obstruction should be made. Laryngoscopy, cricothyrotomy, or tracheotomy may be indicated.
2. Tracheal suctioning should last no longer than 5 seconds at a time without ventilation, to prevent hypoxia.
3. If spinal injury is suspected or present, extension of the neck is avoided and a modified jaw-thrust technique is used. The head, neck, and chest are kept aligned.
4. Ventilation is assessed by seeing the chest rise and fall and hearing and feeling air escape during the patient's exhalation.

Circulation

This may be accomplished by external closed-chest cardiac compression: the rhythmic application of pressure over the lower half of the sternum above the xyphoid process (Figs. 31.4 and 31.5). Cardiac compression must be performed with knowledge

• **Fig. 31.4** Cross indicates correct spot to place hands for performing closed-chest cardiac compression: over lower half of sternum and above xyphoid process.

• **Fig. 31.5 Closed-Chest Cardiac Compression.** Patient is supine on hard, flat surface. Resuscitator places heel of one hand over lower half of sternum with heel of other hand on top. Fingers are arched upward to avoid exerting force on ribs. Elbows are straight and locked, with shoulders straight over hands.

and care. All physicians and patient care personnel must be trained and certified in CPR at least to the minimal BCLS level.

Because the heart occupies most of the space between the sternum and the thoracic spine, intermittent sternal compression of 2 inches raises intrathoracic pressure and produces CO. Blood is forced from the heart into the pulmonary artery and aorta. During relaxation of pressure, negative intrathoracic pressure causes venous blood to flow back into the heart from the pulmonary and systemic circulatory systems.

Basic principles are the same for infants and children.

CPR should not be interrupted for more than 5 seconds at a time except for endotracheal intubation. If intubation is difficult, the patient must be ventilated between short attempts. CPR is never suspended for more than 10 seconds, except during defibrillation (Fig. 31.6). Manual external cardiac compression causes fatigue, leading to variation in CO; therefore it is advisable to have additional relief personnel available.

Elevation of an adult's legs to a 60-degree angle aids venous return and augments circulation. Cardiac compression is successful only if the heart fills with blood between compressions and the resuscitator can move an adequate volume of oxygenated blood. The carotid or femoral pulse is checked every few minutes to indicate compression effectiveness or return of a spontaneous, effective heartbeat.

Complications of external compression are minimized by careful attention to detail. Compression must be performed with extreme caution to prevent injuries such as rib or sternal fracture, costochondral separation, fat embolism, laceration of the liver, lung contusion, pneumothorax, and hemothorax. To prevent fractures, the xyphoid process at the tip of the sternum is never compressed and pressure is never exerted on the ribs.

Internal Cardiac Compression. Internal cardiac compression is instituted if the patient's chest is already open, such as during a cardiothoracic procedure. Thoracotomy may be performed and internal compression administered in instances in which external compression may be ineffective (e.g., internal thoracic injuries, such as penetrating wounds of the heart, flail chest, pericardial tamponade caused by hemorrhage, chest or spinal deformities). The advantages of internal compression are (1) more complete ventricular emptying with greater outflow of blood into the circulation and (2) rapid diastolic filling for a faster stroke rate than with external compression. Less blood flows in a retrograde manner. The disadvantages are (1) delay in compression, (2) potential trauma to the lungs and myocardium, and (3) possible infection.

Checking the Effectiveness of Cardiopulmonary Resuscitation

Signs suggestive of effective compression are constricted, reactive pupils; a palpable peripheral pulse; an audible heartbeat; and improvement in color of the mucous membranes, skin, and blood. Additional signs indicative of potential recovery are prompt return of spontaneous respiration and consciousness. Continuous compression is stopped when arterial BP remains above 70 to 90 mm Hg and a strong spontaneous pulse is resumed. CPR may be performed intermittently as necessary to assist the restored heart.

Persistent dilation of the pupils and lack of reaction to light are ominous signs usually indicative of brain damage. Cell destruction is also manifested by convulsions, hyperpyrexia, and persistent coma. Survival in relation to these symptoms is usually accompanied by tragic consequences such as decerebration or paralysis.

• **Fig. 31.6** The team in action during cardiac resuscitation.

Advanced Cardiac Life Support

Advanced cardiac life support (ACLS) consists of definitive therapy intended to reinstitute spontaneous oxygenation. It includes BCLS, use of adjunctive equipment and special techniques for establishing and maintaining effective ventilation and circulation, cardiac and supplemental monitoring, recognition and control of dysrhythmias, defibrillation, establishing and maintaining an IV infusion route, drug administration, and postresuscitation care. It requires the supervision and direction of a physician. It should be initiated immediately to improve long-term functional survival. Subsequent insertion of an arterial line supplies access for direct pressure monitoring and arterial blood gases. Capnography is used to measure the quality of cardiac compression and may be an indicator of returned circulation.

Intravenous Drugs

Compression is usually accompanied or followed by judicious use of drugs, administered IV, to manipulate cardiovascular variables, such as hypoxia and acidosis. These drugs may improve the patient's cardiopulmonary status by increasing the perfusion pressure during cardiac compression, stimulating spontaneous or more forceful myocardial contractions, accelerating the cardiac rate, and suppressing abnormal ventricular activity.

Oxygen, epinephrine, and atropine are the mainstays of pharmacologic management in CPR. Used in combination with basic life support, lidocaine, and defibrillation, they correct most CPR oxygen-delivery problems. Each additional drug serves as a vital adjunct in definitive therapy and postresuscitation care.

Crash Cart

An emergency arrest cart should be available at all times in all critical care areas (i.e., OR, emergency department [ED], PACU, and ICU). Specific drugs and equipment vary, depending on how well equipped the anesthesia provider is for emergencies. Equipment on a portable cart usually includes the following list:
• Oxygen and resuscitation equipment, including oxygen cylinder, tubing, mask, Ambu bag, or bag-valve-mask
• Capnography monitor
• Laryngoscope tray, blades, endotracheal equipment and tubes, assorted airways (oral and nasal), stylet, padded tongue blades

- Tracheotomy tray
- Sterile gloves, sterile gauze sponges, prep swabs, adhesive tape, tourniquets, sutures, armboard, drapes
- Suction machine, catheters, suction tips
- IV infusion solutions and sets, IV needles and catheters (14 and 16 gauge), tubing stopcocks, infusion pump, medication additive labels
- Equipment for intraosseous access
- Cutdown tray, venous cannulas, wire-guided catheters
- Assorted sterile syringes: 3, 5, 10, 20, and 50 mL
- Assorted sterile needles: 25 gauge × $^5/_8$ inch; 20 gauge × $1^1/_2$ inches; 18 gauge × $1^1/_2$ inches; 20 gauge × 3 inches (intracardiac); spinal needles
- Arterial blood sampling kit with needles, saline or heparinized syringes; arterial line tray
- Disposable scalpels, hemostats
- Emergency thoracotomy set, including scalpel with No. 20 blade, rib retractor, self-retaining retractor
- ECG monitor, leads, recording sheets
- Cardiac arrest board to provide a firm surface under the patient for compressions
- Defibrillator with paddles (adult, pediatric, external, internal), electrode jelly or paste, saline pads
- Cardiac arrest record for treatment documentation/flow sheets
- Cardiac pacemaker
- Drugs—mainly vasoconstrictors, cardiotonics, vasopressors, cardiac depressants, anticholinergics, cerebral dehydrating agents, pulmonary dehydrating agents (many frequently used emergency drugs are available in sterile, commercially prefilled syringes to avoid delay in preparation; they are routinely checked for expiration dates)
- CVP manometer
- Nasogastric tube and bulb syringe
- Flashlight and batteries for checking pupils

Personnel Responsibilities

During CPR, team members must remain calm but react quickly and act efficiently. Cardiac arrest in the OR during business hours may be more easily managed because more personnel may be on the premises. Codes after business hours are more complex and may involve minimal personnel who are required to perform multiple functions. The following outline is a suggestion of expected behaviors of team members during a code situation:

1. *Director of the code:* One person, the most knowledgeable in resuscitation efforts and patient physiology, usually the anesthesia provider, commands resuscitation efforts. The director is assisted by surgeons, nurses, surgical technologists, and other available personnel. A cardiologist is usually summoned (if available). Resuscitation teams are multidisciplinary.

   The person in charge directs lifesaving interventions that entail minute-to-minute decisions such as medications and defibrillation. To avoid confusion the director of the code issues orders for others to follow. Every circulating nurse should be qualified and prepared to organize and assign tasks to members of the support staff in the event of cardiac arrest during off-shift times.

2. *Circulating nurse:* Initiate the code and summon help.
   a. Start the time-elapsed clock (if available), and record the time of arrest.
      (1) Remain calm and support calmness in the team.

(2) Documentation is performed according to facility policy. Most have preprinted code sheets.
   b. Activate the emergency alarm to alert the OR manager and summon assistance.
      (1) Several physicians and registered nurses should respond to form the code team.
      (2) Support staff should respond to become runners.
   c. Help reposition the patient as necessary into the supine position for CPR. Lower the OR bed and provide the resuscitator with a standing platform to facilitate cardiac compression. The circulating nurse must be able to perform chest compressions if an additional resuscitator is not immediately available.
      (1) Prone patient's transport cart should be immediately available.
      (2) A firm surface should be placed under patient's back.
      (3) If patient is on an irregular surface (e.g., fracture table), compressions may be difficult.
   d. Send a runner for the crash cart. Prepare necessary equipment from the crash cart, such as medications, the defibrillator, and the ECG if it is not already in use.
      (1) During off-shift times, the scrub person may have to break scrub and become the runner.
      (2) The circulating nurse remains in the room to assist the director of the code.
      (3) Record drugs, times, routes if a recorder has not been assigned.
   e. Control traffic. Exclude unauthorized personnel from the room. Students should either be instructed to stand back or enlisted to obtain supplies as able. Provide an optimal environment for successful resuscitation.
   f. Help with and observe IV and monitoring lines, such as an arterial line. Assist in collection of blood samples.
   g. Maintain accuracy of sponge, needle, and instrument counts and sterility to best of ability if wound closure progresses (but sterility is secondary to resuscitation efforts).
      (1) Counts may be aborted, but accountability remains important.
      (2) X-rays may be taken as patient condition permits.
   h. Document all medications given, the time and amount, and the sequence of procedures performed. Documentation is important in guiding therapy and providing legal protection.
   i. Supervise termination of the procedure as necessary.
      (1) Arrange for crash cart replacement.
      (2) Place restocked crash cart in the designated location for future use.
   j. In unsuccessful resuscitation, follow protocol regarding notification of family or significant others, care of the deceased, specimens to be saved, and forms to be filled out after a death in the OR.
      (1) Observe respect for the patient's dignity as possible.
      (2) The family or significant others may request to see the patient's body. A designated place should be available for this purpose.

3. *Scrub person:*
   a. Remain sterile and keep the tables sterile if possible. If arrest occurs during a noncardiac surgical procedure, when the chest is not open, the surgical site is packed with saline-soaked sponges and covered with sterile drape, and the patient is repositioned as necessary for CPR. If the

surgical site is in an area that can be closed rapidly during resuscitation, this may be done.

(1) During regular business hours support staff should be the runners.

(2) During off-shift times the support staff is minimal; it is necessary to break scrub and be the runner.

(3) Obtain the crash cart.

b. Keep track of sponges, needles, and instruments. Counts are completed as possible, and the surgical site is closed as soon as possible despite the outcome. In a life-threatening emergency the surgeon may order that counts be aborted. Follow the written institutional policy and procedure for counts during emergency situations.

(1) Keep all unnecessary instruments and supplies off the field.

(2) Push back table off to the side of the room. Move the Mayo stand away from the patient.

c. Give attention to the field and the surgeon's needs. If the patient is hemorrhaging, keep suction tubing clear and tapes available.

d. If the circulating nurse is performing chest compressions and no other support personnel are available, assist as required.

4. *OR manager (on duty during business hours):*

a. Assign professional and assistive support personnel to augment the team (e.g., an extra circulating nurse, medication nurse, runners [personnel to obtain supplies or handle laboratory samples]).

b. Notify the attending physician, if not present, and appropriate administrative personnel.

c. Alert the ICU of a potential patient admission.

d. Reassign subsequent patients' scheduling.

e. Keep track of resuscitation progress.

f. Evaluate the arrest procedure and emergency equipment; verify the documentation.

g. Support the team as necessary. Keep the surgical suite running smoothly during the emergency. Order another fully stocked crash cart.

Duration of Cardiopulmonary Resuscitation

CPR may be done as long as necessary to restore circulatory function if adequate ventilation and a good peripheral pulse have been restored. It is not uncommon for a second arrest to occur after successful resuscitation. The time frame for survival is shortened drastically if the arrest is unwitnessed. When the patient's condition is adequately stabilized and the surgical site is closed, the patient is transferred to the ICU.

The decision to discontinue resuscitative efforts in the OR is made by a physician. The decision is based on assessment of cerebral and cardiovascular status. The end point of cardiovascular unresponsiveness is suggested as the most reliable basis for this decision.

Appropriate administrative personnel and services, such as the nursing unit, ICU, and clergy, as well as the patient's family, are notified of the cardiac arrest as required. In case of death, the surgeon notifies the family.

Postresuscitation Care

Postarrest supportive therapy depends on the cause and duration of arrest. Care centers on cardiac and cerebral preservation, maintaining circulation and ventilation, and minimizing sequelae such as cerebral edema. The patient must be carefully monitored and closely observed for 48 to 72 hours postarrest. In select patients, hypothermia may be used to reduce oxygen needs.

Vital signs, acid-base and electrolyte balances, and urinary output are closely watched. Seizures should be controlled to prevent further anoxia. The patient is observed for signs of embolism, pulmonary edema, fractured ribs caused by chest compressions, and hemopericardium. A chest x-ray is taken as soon as feasible after the arrest. An IV fluid lifeline must be left in place. If cerebral damage is evident, the prognosis is guarded.

Staff Education

Practice sessions of a cardiac arrest emergency and CPR with subsequent evaluation and revision are valuable to review the protocol and prepare the OR staff before need for implementation. Current CPR/BCLS certification for health care providers is required of all OR personnel. Many ORs require yearly BCLS review, with recertification every 2 years. ICU personnel are required to be ACLS-certified.

Fluid and Electrolyte Imbalances

Fluid and electrolyte imbalances may be caused by many different factors and may be manifested by numerous symptoms. Maintenance of correct balance, which greatly influences the outcome of surgical intervention, is a very relevant aspect of intraoperative and postoperative care.

Fluid loss is replaced by IV infusion. Usually normal saline or dextrose (5% or 10% in water or saline) solution is started initially. Electrolytes may be added to the solution as needed. Two other IV solutions are commonly used to maintain balance:

1. *Mannitol:* An osmotic diuretic agent; has an effect on renal vascular resistance. Depending on the percentage of drug in solution, it can either increase or decrease renal blood flow. It may be given prophylactically to prevent renal failure. It is used also to decrease intracranial and intraocular pressure. It is rapidly excreted by the kidneys.

2. *Ringer's lactate solution:* A physiologic salt solution; may be infused when the body's supply of sodium, calcium, and potassium has been depleted or for improvement of circulation and stimulation of renal activity. Its electrolyte content is similar to that of plasma.

Changes in fluid and electrolyte balances affect renal function, cellular metabolism, and oxygen concentration in the circulation.[8]

Acid-Base Balance

For enzyme systems to function, a normal balance must be maintained between acidity and alkalinity of body fluids located within intracellular and extracellular compartments. The symbol pH represents the hydrogen ion concentration that determines acidity or alkalinity of a solution; neutral pH is 7, below 7 is acid, and above 7 is alkaline. Urine is usually acid, with a pH range between 4.6 and 8. Normal serum pH is 7.40, within a range of 7.35 to 7.45.

Hydrogen ions do not exist as separate electrolytes in body fluids but are maintained in balance with other electrolytes to ensure neutrality. Because most metabolic processes produce acids, chemical buffers interact with hydrogen ions. Carbonic acid and a hydrogen ion form bicarbonate (HCO_3)—the most important buffer. The kidneys and lungs regulate this system by excreting or retaining needed ions in body fluids. Abnormal acid-base balance results from the following factors:

1. Respiratory malfunction in handling carbon dioxide produced from carbonic acid
   a. *Acidosis:* pH less than 7.35 with carbon dioxide above 45 torr
   b. *Alkalosis:* pH more than 7.45 with carbon dioxide below 35 torr
2. Metabolic abnormality in balance between hydrogen and serum HCO_3
   a. *Acidosis:* pH less than 7.35 with HCO_3 less than 22 mEq/L
   b. *Alkalosis:* pH more than 7.45 with HCO_3 more than 26 mEq/L

Electrolytes

Compounds that separate into ions, which are charged particles capable of conducting electrical impulses, are essential in maintaining fluid and acid-base balance and regulating cell functions. The primary electrolytes in the body (Table 31.1) are as follows:

1. *Sodium:* A key regulator in water balance, sodium is necessary to the normal function of muscles and nerves. Large amounts are in extracellular fluid in concentrations of 136 to 145 mEq/L; intracellular concentration is 10 mEq/L. This balance is necessary for normal metabolism.
   a. Hyponatremia (insufficient serum sodium) usually accompanies excessive fluid loss or adrenal insufficiency. Muscle twitching, hypovolemia, hypotension, and tachycardia may be symptoms.
   b. Hypernatremia (elevated serum sodium) may be caused by hyperglycemia or administration of mannitol. Diaphoresis (sweating) may be the only obvious symptom. Convulsions can occur.

TABLE 31.1 Normal Blood Chemistry Laboratory Values

Parameter	Normal Values for Adults
Alanine aminotransferase (ALT)	10–35 international units/L
Aspartate aminotransferase (AST)	4–36 international units/L
Base excess of blood	0 ± 2 mmol/L
Bicarbonate (HCO_3)	22–26 mEq/L
Bilirubin (total)	0.1–1 mg/dL
Blood urea nitrogen (BUN)	5–20 mg/dL
Calcium (Ca)	9–10.5 mg/dL
Carbon dioxide (CO_2) in serum	23–30 mEq/L
Chloride (Cl)	90–110 mEq/L
Creatinine	0.7–1.5 mg/dL
Creatine phosphokinase (CPK)	12–80 units/L
Glucose	70–115 mg/dL
Magnesium (Mg)	1.6–3 mEq/L
pH of serum	7.35–7.45
Phosphate (P)	2.5–4.5 mg/dL
Potassium (K)	3.5–5 mEq/L
Sodium (Na)	136–145 mEq/L

2. *Chloride:* Essential to electrochemical reactions for acid-base regulation, chloride is in extracellular fluids in large amounts. Chlorides are retained or excreted by the kidneys to offset HCO_3 excretion. Sodium tends to carry chloride with it.
   a. Hypochloremia (loss of chloride) may occur from vomiting, suctioning, sweating, and diuresis. It produces symptoms of metabolic alkalosis: slow, shallow respirations and muscle tightening.
   b. Hyperchloremia (excessive chloride) can result in renal failure. Acidosis develops, and breathing becomes labored.
3. *Potassium:* One of the main constituents of cell protoplasm, potassium is primarily (98%) in intracellular fluid. It is essential for electrochemical reactions for cellular functions.
   a. Hypokalemia (shift of potassium from the blood to the cells or depletion of potassium from the body) can be associated with metabolic alkalosis. Cardiac dysrhythmias can occur when the serum potassium level falls.
   b. Hyperkalemia (increase in serum potassium) may be caused by renal failure and may lead to respiratory and/or cardiac arrest. Metabolic or respiratory acidosis can occur.
4. *Calcium:* Essential to normal muscle physiology, calcium also is an integral part of the blood-clotting mechanism.
   a. Hypocalcemia (decreased calcium intake or absorption) may be a result of increased excretion. This can cause cardiac dysrhythmias.
   b. Hypercalcemia (increased serum calcium) may be a result of a shift of calcium from the bones to plasma, decreased excretion, or increased uptake and absorption. It causes neuromuscular depression and cardiac dysrhythmias.
5. *Magnesium:* Essential to electrochemical reactions for normal body functions, magnesium is primarily in intracellular fluid. An imbalance may be accompanied by calcium and/or potassium imbalances.
   a. Hypomagnesemia (low magnesium level) usually is associated with hypokalemia. This may be the most undiagnosed electrolyte deficiency in geriatric patients or those who have illnesses associated with malabsorption in the intestine or kidneys. It may cause cardiac dysrhythmias and nervous system and muscular irritability, and it may exaggerate drug toxicities.
   b. Hypermagnesemia (elevated serum magnesium) can inhibit nerve and muscle responses. It may lead to respiratory depression and cardiac arrest.
6. *Phosphate:* Normally in intracellular fluid, phosphate allows electrochemical reactions for metabolic functions. Phosphate and calcium vary inversely; thus phosphate will buffer acidosis from a rising calcium level.
   a. Hypophosphatemia (low serum phosphate level) may produce tissue hypoxia.
   b. Hyperphosphatemia (increase in phosphate) usually occurs in renal failure. It is associated with hypocalcemia.

Disturbances in fluid and electrolyte balance can result from:
- *Acid-base imbalances associated with chronic disease or organ dysfunction:* Acidosis increases serum chloride, potassium, and calcium; alkalosis decreases chloride, potassium, calcium, and phosphate.
- *Cell destruction leading to hyperkalemia:* Cellular potassium is depleted, with serum potassium increase.
- *Shift of potassium from blood into cells, causing hypokalemia:* This may be caused by the effects of epinephrine, insulin, bicarbonate, hypothermia, or cardiopulmonary bypass.

- *Changes in blood lipids:* Calcium and magnesium are depleted by poor absorption.
- *Fever:* Metabolic rate is increased; water and electrolytes are lost.
- *Stress:* Glucose tolerance is diminished, and blood glucose and serum potassium levels are increased.
- *Gastric drainage:* Sodium and chlorides are lost.
- *Fluid loss from drainage tubes, diaphoresis, vomiting, or diarrhea:* Sodium, chloride, and potassium are lost.
- *Maxillofacial injury:* Oral intake is inhibited.
- *Radiation enteritis:* Magnesium and potassium are diminished.
- *Disease of the bowel, liver, or biliary tract; intestinal tract obstruction; or gastrointestinal fistula:* Calcium and phosphate are poorly absorbed.
- *Loss of muscle mass as a result of preoperative malnutrition:* Nitrogen loss is increased.
- *Drugs:* Metabolic balance can be adversely affected; losses of potassium, magnesium, and chloride from diuretics are examples.
- *Inadequate oxygen/carbon dioxide exchange:* Acid-base balance is disrupted.

Hypovolemia

Hypovolemia is a decreased circulating blood volume from loss of blood and plasma or a deficit of extracellular fluid volume commonly referred to as *dehydration*. When excessive fluid loss is greater than absorption of interstitial fluid into the circulation, the patient may go into hypovolemic shock.

Etiology

Etiologic factors include reduced fluid intake, hemorrhage, plasma loss (e.g., through extensive burns, wound drainage), and dehydration from loss of gastrointestinal fluids (e.g., by vomiting), or diaphoresis (caused by fever, from diuresis). Impaired renal function and metabolic acidosis are predisposing factors. Prolonged cardiopulmonary bypass can cause hypovolemic shock.

Signs and Symptoms

Signs and symptoms include dry skin and mucous membranes; depressed BP; elevated pulse; oliguria; decreasing CVP and blood volume determinations; and deep, rapid respirations.

Treatment

Hypovolemic shock resulting from hemorrhage or underestimated blood loss is most often seen in the OR. This is usually reversed by prompt restoration of circulating blood volume. The extent of hypovolemia will determine treatment, which may include the following:

1. *Fluid volume replacement:* Whole blood, plasma expander, or infusion of lactated Ringer solution or other IV fluid is indicated to increase blood volume. Hypervolemia must be avoided in replacement.
2. *Position:* Elevation of the legs may aid venous return and CO except in severe oligemia (low total blood volume [TBV]).
3. *Temperature:* The patient is kept warm but not overheated. Perspiration increases fluid loss. Shivering can cause hypothermia.
4. *Oxygen:* Oxygen is administered when PO_2 is low because the circulation is not delivering enough oxygen to tissues.
5. *Drugs:* Drugs are administered as needed to maintain BP, correct acidosis, or protect the kidneys from failure.

Prevention

Decreased blood volume, if present preoperatively, increases surgical risk and morbidity. It should be treated, and the electrolyte imbalance should be corrected. Fluids, blood gases, and blood loss must be monitored intraoperatively.

Hypervolemia

Hypervolemia is an excess of extracellular fluid in the blood, commonly referred to as *fluid overload* and *edema*. IV infusions given too rapidly or in excessive amounts, especially isotonic saline solution, can cause hypervolemia. Prolonged administration of adrenocorticosteroids is also a predisposing factor. Hypervolemia may progress to pulmonary edema.

Dyspnea, coarse crackles, an elevated pulse and respiratory rate, and diminished urinary output are symptomatic of hypervolemia. Increasing CVP may indicate fluid overload with venous distention. Diuretics and fluid restriction ameliorate hypervolemia and prevent pulmonary edema.

Blood Volume Complications

Blood Loss Considerations

Some blood loss is inevitable whenever tissues are severed by intent or traumatic injury. Blood loss is computed as a percentage of total blood volume (TBV). TBV averages from 6% to 8% of total body weight. This equals about 75 mL/kg in the average healthy adult man and 60 to 70 mL/kg in the average woman. Calculation of TBV depends on the venous hematocrit value. Normal hematocrit, the volume of red blood cells expressed as a percentage of the volume of whole blood, is 42% to 52% in men and 37% to 47% in women. An infant reaches these blood volume levels at approximately 3 months of age.

An increase in hematocrit indicates a decrease in plasma volume, normally by dehydration and loss of sodium. A decrease in hematocrit indicates a decrease in the number of red blood cells, but this does not necessarily reflect blood loss; it may be caused by overhydration. Fluid and electrolyte balance are important for maintenance of blood volume. Inadequate fluid replacement can lead to a decrease in CO and cardiovascular collapse.

A decrease in red blood cells (erythrocytes) and in hemoglobin, the chief oxygen-carrying component of these cells, causes hypoxia if values fall below normal (Table 31.2). Therefore determination of intraoperative blood loss may be critical to physiologic functions.[9] The extent of blood loss will depend on the location and magnitude of the surgical procedure. Blood loss can be categorized as follows:

- *Minor:* Loss of 500 to 700 mL is about 15% of TBV.
- *Moderate:* Loss of 750 to 1500 mL is about 15% to 30% of TBV. A resultant decrease in pulse pressure and slight tachycardia (rapid heart rate) may progress to tachycardia, tachypnea (rapid breathing), and postural hypotension (reduced BP on position change).
- *Major:* Loss of 1500 to 2250 mL is about 30% to 45% of TBV. The BP drops, the skin becomes cold and clammy, and urinary output decreases.
- *Catastrophic:* Loss of more than 2250 mL is greater than 45% of TBV. Hypoxia (decrease in oxygen level) develops from loss of hemoglobin (red blood cells). Prolonged hypoxia leads to irreversible heart, brain, liver, and kidney damage.

TABLE 31.2	Normal Values of Blood[a]		
	Males	Females	Children
Red blood cells (RBCs)	4.7—6.1 million/mm^3	4.2—5.4 million/mm^3	3.8—5.5 million/mm^3
Hemoglobin (Hgb)	14—18 g/dL	12—16 g/dL	11—16 g/dL
Hematocrit (Hct)	42—52%	37—47%	31—43%
Prothrombin time (PT)	11.0—12.5 seconds	Same	Same
Platelets	150,000—400,000/mm^3	Same	Same after 1 week of age
Partial thromboplastin time (PTT)	30—40 seconds	Same	25—35 seconds

[a]Values vary depending on calibration of testing equipment in the laboratory that services the health care facility.

Hemorrhage

Severe bleeding into or from a wound is a major contributing factor to intraoperative and postoperative morbidity and mortality. If bleeding is uncontrolled, exsanguination can occur. Massive hemorrhage may cause hypovolemic shock, ventricular fibrillation, or death as a result of marked decrease in CO. Common symptoms are arterial hypotension, pale or cyanotic moist skin, oliguria, bradycardia from hypoxia or tachycardia after moderate to marked blood loss, restlessness, and thirst in the conscious patient.[9]

In the OR, hemorrhage is readily visible. Meticulous hemostasis during every step of the surgical procedure and good nutritional status of the patient preoperatively are crucial to prevention. Preoperative evaluation of the patient's clotting time and history of bleeding (personal and familial), type and crossmatch of blood, and insertion of an IV line before incision are necessary precautions. In treating hemorrhage the surgeon locates the source of bleeding and applies digital compression to severed or traumatized blood vessels until noncrushing vascular clamps can be placed to occlude the vessel proximal and distal to the site of bleeding. The vessel is then ligated, clipped, electrocoagulated, or sutured. Circulating blood volume must be restored promptly.

If allogeneic blood is transfused, it must be fresh and warmed to limit electrolytic changes. Sodium bicarbonate may be given IV to reduce acidosis. Multiple IV infusion routes can be used, by cutdown if necessary, to infuse blood under pressure.[9] Lactated Ringer's solution or other plasma expanders are used when blood is contraindicated (e.g., for religious reasons). Oxygen is administered to combat hypoxia. Accurate measurement of blood and fluid losses intraoperatively, followed by adequate replacement, will help prevent hypovolemic shock. Autotransfusion may be feasible.

Hemorrhage can be detected postoperatively by observation of blood-soaked dressings. The patient must be checked frequently for both observable and nonobservable symptoms of hemorrhage. Slipping or sloughing of a ligature or the passage of clots from ligated or coagulated vessels can cause internal bleeding.

Estimation of Blood Loss

An accurate determination of TBV involves measuring plasma and red blood cell volumes separately and then adding these values together. This may be done rapidly by an electronic counting device. In lieu of this, blood loss is estimated in all surgical procedures in which a major loss is anticipated. This can be done by the following steps:

- Visual inspection of blood on drapes and the floor by the anesthesia provider.
- Estimation of blood in the suction container. Allowance must be made for the presence of other body fluids and irrigating solution, if used. The scrub person must estimate the amount of solution suctioned into the container through irrigation of the wound and/or tubing. This can be done by knowing the capacity of the irrigation syringe in use and keeping track of the number of times it is used. The circulating nurse subtracts these amounts to estimate the volume of blood in the container.
- Visual inspection of blood in sponges by the anesthesia provider.
- Measurement of blood in sponges by weighing them. Sponges are weighed after use as they are discarded from the surgical field.

Weighing Sponges

Some anesthesia providers and surgeons prefer to have sponges weighed to determine blood loss rather than visually estimating the loss (Box 31.1). A scale calibrated in grams is used. The dry and wet weights of each type of sponge must be known. Wet weight is that of a sponge soaked in normal saline solution and wrung out until almost dry. A chart of these weights should be available; often it is attached to the scale. The number of sponges being weighed is multiplied by the appropriate dry or wet weight.

Each type must be weighed separately, with the dry sponges separated from the wet ones. To allow for (i.e., by subtracting) dry or wet weights and the weight of a moisture-proof cover on the scale platform or a container, the scale is adjusted to register at zero. When blood-soaked sponges are weighed, the reading on the scale equals the blood loss; 1 g equals 1 mL. The scale is checked at each use for readjustment to zero. Some scales are controlled by a microprocessor that automatically makes calculations.

The circulating nurse must weigh sponges before they dry out. Blood loss is recorded each time sponges are weighed, adding new weight to previous ones to keep a current total. A tally board for this purpose may be mounted on the wall where the anesthesia provider and surgeon can read it. The estimated blood in the suction container can be recorded here also. Irrigation solutions used for moistening sponges should be carefully measured and documented.

Use a scale that measures in grams. Always wear personal protective equipment (PPE). This method helps subtract the weight of the actual sponges and the container they are weighed in. One gram of weight equals one millimeter of blood (1 g = 1 mL).

Weighing Dry Sponges

1. Obtain a small plastic sponge basin and one pack of each type of sponge used for the procedure.
2. Weigh a complete unwrapped complement of each type of sponge in the plastic sponge basin (e.g., 10 unwrapped Raytec, 5 unwrapped laparotomy sponges of the correct size).
   - *Raytec:* Place the open pack of dry Raytec in the plastic sponge basin on the scale and set the dial to zero. This will account for the weight of the sponges and the basin without the blood.
   - Remove the dry sponges from the plastic basin and set aside.
   - Place the counted bloody sponges into basin.
   - Take the weight reading. The number of grams of weight is recorded.
   - *Laparotomy sponges:* Place the open pack of dry laparotomy sponges in the plastic sponge basin on the scale and set the dial to zero. This will account for the weight of the sponges and the basin without the blood.
   - Remove the dry sponges from the plastic basin and set aside.
   - Place the counted bloody sponges into the basin.
   - Take the weight reading. The number of grams of weight is recorded.

Weighing Sponges Premoistened With Saline

Repeat the previous steps with the following changes:
1. Dip the complete set of dry Raytec or laparotomy sponges into water and wring out all excess liquid. This will simulate the dampening of the sponges with the sterile saline.
2. Place the damp set into the plastic basin and set the dial on the scale to zero. This accounts for the weight of the damp sponges and the container.
3. Remove the moist sponges and replace them with the same number and type of bloody sponges.

Reduction of Blood Loss

When significant bleeding can be anticipated, several techniques are used to reduce red blood cell loss during the surgical procedure or eliminate blood transfusion requirements.

Hemodilution

Acute normovolemic or isovolemic hemodilution reduces red blood cells but maintains normal or equal blood volume. After induction of anesthesia, a physician, usually the anesthesia provider, withdraws blood through an arterial or venous catheter. The blood is drawn into bags containing anticoagulant, usually citrate. Citrate metabolizes rapidly, thus minimizing the risk for systemic anticoagulation when blood is reinfused. The amount withdrawn depends on the anticipated blood loss and the patient's estimated TBV and hematocrit.

A plasma volume expander is given by IV infusion while blood is removed, to restore blood volume. This hemodilution technique reduces red blood cell loss during the surgical procedure because the hematocrit has been lowered. The surgical procedure begins when the hematocrit is between 27% and 30%. Adequate intravascular volume and oxygenation are maintained. Urinary output must be measured.

Each bag of blood must be labeled with the patient's name and identifying number and the time of withdrawal. Blood may be stored at room temperature for 6 hours or in a refrigerator for 24 hours. At the conclusion of the surgical procedure, or sooner if

indicated, the blood is reinfused IV to raise the hematocrit back to the preoperative level. Units are reinfused in reverse order of withdrawal (i.e., last one first) so that the unit with the highest concentration of red blood cells and coagulation factors is infused last. (More information is available at the website of the American Association of Blood Banks, www.aabb.org.)

Blood Volume Expanders

Crystalloid or colloid solutions are administered IV for fluid replacement and plasma volume expansion. They are not the sole replacements for blood loss. They must be used with caution. The following list comprises the most commonly used plasma volume expanders.

- *Dextran:* This crystalloid polymer of glucose acts by drawing fluid from tissues to decrease blood viscosity. It remains in circulation for several hours. It interferes with the crossmatching of blood; thus a blood sample for this purpose must be drawn before dextran is infused. It may be used until blood or blood products are available or for hemodilution. As a 6% or 10% solution, it may be mixed in water with glucose or sodium chloride.
- *Lactated Ringer's solution:* This crystalloid physiologic salt solution is infused for the improvement of circulation and stimulation of renal activity and in patients in whom the body's supply of sodium, calcium, and potassium has been depleted.
- *Hetastarch (Hespan):* This colloid polymer expands plasma volume slightly in excess of the volume infused. It approximates the action of serum albumin. Large volumes may alter coagulation factors. It can be used for hemodilution.

Pharmacologic Agents

The action of specific pharmacologic agents either stimulates or retards the coagulation mechanism. This action may reduce blood loss and help provide hemostasis in patients with hematologic disorders. Some of these disorders are associated with cardiovascular disease or end-stage renal disease. Others are congenital or acquired coagulopathies. Three types of agents affect bleeding.

Desmopressin Acetate

Desmopressin promotes hemostasis in patients with von Willebrand disease and shortens the bleeding time in patients with uremia. When given prophylactically, this synthetic vasopressin analog can decrease surgical blood loss in patients undergoing spinal surgery and reduce blood loss after cardiac surgery.

Vasodilators

Vasodilators lower systemic BP, thus decreasing bleeding. Sodium nitroprusside, nitroglycerin, and other drugs are used.

Anticoagulants

Anticoagulants minimize the tendency of blood to clot, yet do not lead to excessive bleeding during or after the surgical procedure. These agents provide adequate anticoagulation with a minimum of hemorrhagic complications. They help prevent venous stasis to reduce the incidence of DVT and PE. They may be given orally (PO), subcutaneously (SQ), or IV, beginning preoperatively, especially in patients who have a history of thromboembolic disease. The action of each anticoagulant is different and is described as follows:

- Heparin acts to inhibit conversion of prothrombin to thrombin. This prolongs clotting time. It may be administered

SQ to keep activated partial thromboplastin time in the high-normal range between 30 and 40 seconds. Given IV, heparin is effective immediately. It may be used as a flush to keep IV lines open or to flush the lumen of a blood vessel (1 mL of heparin in 100 mL of normal saline solution). Heparin does not dissolve a thrombus, but it will prevent a clot from becoming larger.

- Coumarin derivatives depress blood prothrombin and decrease the tendency of blood platelets to cling together, thus decreasing the normal tendency of blood to clot. They also interfere with action of vitamin K to prevent the synthesis of prothrombin and fibrinogen. Warfarin sodium is the most commonly used coumarin derivative.
- Low-molecular-weight dextran reduces platelet adhesiveness and aggregation to prevent sludge from forming in the bloodstream. It coats blood platelets to keep them from massing together.
- Aspirin diminishes clumping of platelets by inhibiting the release reaction of platelet factors and action of vitamin K.

Vitamin K enables the liver to produce clotting factors in blood, including prothrombin. To reduce the possibility of intraoperative hemorrhage, patients who have been receiving anticoagulant therapy and those who have faulty metabolism or absorption of vitamin K are given it preoperatively. It also is given to geriatric or debilitated patients before intraocular surgery, to newborns preoperatively, and to mothers just before delivery. The latter helps prevent postdelivery hemorrhage and ensures that the baby has an adequate prothrombin level until a sufficient amount is produced by the liver.

Hypotensive Anesthesia

In selected situations in which excessive blood loss is anticipated or encountered, arterial BP may be deliberately lowered to produce an essentially bloodless field. When induced, hypotension is carefully controlled by the anesthesia provider.

Hematologic Disorders

Some hemolytic and hemorrhagic disorders require special consideration during perioperative care to minimize risks of surgical intervention. Concern is for the maintenance of adequate tissue perfusion and oxygenation and for hemostasis and coagulation in patients at risk. Patients at risk for intraoperative bleeding or who have a known hematologic disorder should have a complete blood count, complete blood chemistry panel, and urinalysis done preoperatively. Hemoglobin, hematocrit, and red blood cell counts are critical determinants for blood replacement requirements preoperatively and intraoperatively.[9] Precautions can be taken to minimize the risks of surgical intervention with adequate blood replacement.

Anemia

Anemia is a symptom of a deficiency in either the quantity or quality of red blood cells (erythrocytes). Hemoglobin, the chief component of these cells, delivers oxygen to tissues. Normal hemoglobin values are 14 to 18 g/dL of blood in males, 12 to 16 g/dL in females, and 11 to 16 g/dL in children. These values are lower in anemic patients. Thus anemia may result in tissue hypoxia. The various types of this disorder may be caused by the following factors:

- Blood loss from massive bleeding (e.g., from a traumatic injury) or chronic blood loss (e.g., from a gastric or intestinal

ulcer): This blood loss can be replaced by transfusion of blood products.
- Dietary deficiency of sufficient iron, protein, vitamins, and minerals to form red blood cells or produce hemoglobin: Dietary supplements are given to correct the deficiency.
- Diseases or drugs that inhibit the bone marrow from producing blood cells, such as tumors or chronic renal disease: The cause must be diagnosed and treated.
- Destruction of red blood cells (hemoglobinopathy) by an overactive reticuloendothelial system in the spleen or liver: A splenectomy may be indicated for hypersplenism or hereditary spherocytosis, for example.
- Destruction of red blood cells by foreign substances entering the circulatory system (e.g., through an incompatible blood transfusion): Neonatal anemia may necessitate an exchange transfusion.
- Abnormal blood cells produced by the bone marrow: These are usually caused by genetic or hereditary factors.
- Myelodysplastic syndromes in which the bone marrow fails to produce blood cells in sufficient numbers: Bone marrow suppression can be the result of disease or treatment of disease. Some patients have the genetic disposition for bone marrow failure known as trisomy 8 that develops in the older adult. It is manifest by low hemoglobin concentration, marked decrease in red cells, and significantly low platelet formation.

The average normal life span of red blood cells is 120 days. In patients with any one of the many forms of hemolytic anemia, red blood cells have a shortened life span. Hemolytic anemias may be acquired or inherited. All must be adequately assessed preoperatively.

Sickle Cell Hemoglobinopathies

A severe, chronic, inherited hemolytic disorder, sickle cell anemia is most prevalent among blacks of African descent. It may be found in other ethnic groups, particularly people of Mediterranean descent. Pairing of identical abnormal recessive genes causes substitution of a single amino acid for glutamic acid in the polypeptide chain, which alters the hemoglobin. These abnormal cells, known as hemoglobin S, become distorted in shape when exposed to low oxygen tension in the venous circulation. Dehydration, cold, infection, and physical or emotional stress may precipitate crisis periods that vary in duration and intensity when sickling occurs.

A crisis may also occur spontaneously without apparent cause. The resultant sickle-shaped red blood cells occlude the microcirculation through the capillaries, arterioles, and venules. Occlusion results in blood stasis, hypoxia, vasospasm, ischemia, and necrosis, which cause pain and ultimately permanent damage to tissues and organs. Stasis ulcers and biliary tract disease are common complications that may require surgical intervention. Elective surgical procedures are performed when the patient is not in crisis, but these patients are always at risk for crisis.

Sickle cell trait is present when one abnormal gene is inherited. The red blood cells have both hemoglobin A (normal) and hemoglobin S (sickle cell). People with this trait usually are asymptomatic and tolerate routine anesthesia and surgical intervention well. However, when they are stressed by hypothermia, acidosis, or hypoxemia, local or regional sickling can occur during the surgical procedure. Sickle cells have a life span of 15 to 30 days.

The severity of the hemolytic process is proportional to the amount of hemoglobin S in the blood. Hemoglobin in patients with sickle cell anemia usually ranges from 6 to 9 g/dL, with a hematocrit of 25% to 30%. Patients of African descent and other susceptible people should be tested preoperatively. Electrophoresis is the standard laboratory test for hemoglobin S. Consideration must then be given to the following in the perioperative management of patients with sickle cell anemia or sickle cell trait:

1. Transfusion of whole blood, packed cells, or low-molecular-weight dextran may be administered preoperatively, especially if the patient's hemoglobin is 5 g or less.
2. Urea may be given PO or IV prophylactically to prevent a sickle cell crisis. It also may be used to reverse a crisis.
3. Systemic antibiotics are initiated preoperatively because these patients are susceptible to postoperative infection.
4. Normal body temperature must be maintained. Any lowering increases the requirement for oxygen. The patient must be kept warm to avoid hypothermia.
   a. Add extra blankets during transport to the OR suite.
   b. Avoid drafts from the air-conditioning system in the holding area, OR, and PACU.
   c. Cover the patient's head for warmth.
   d. Raise the temperature in the OR to 80° F to 85° F (27–29° C).
   e. Place the patient on a hyperthermia blanket on the OR bed.
   f. Monitor the patient's temperature intraoperatively with an electronic probe.
   g. Place warm blankets over the patient before transfer to the PACU.
5. Oxygen is administered during induction of anesthesia, intraoperatively, and after extubation to prevent deoxygenation of the sickle cells and subsequent ischemic infarction in tissues.
6. Blood gases are monitored to avoid hypoxia, acidosis, hypotension, and hypovolemia. Fluid and blood replacement intraoperatively reduces the risk for crisis from dehydration.
7. Scheduling an elective surgical procedure early in the morning minimizes dehydration after a period of nothing by mouth (NPO).

Hemorrhagic Disorders

Patients with a disorder in the mechanism of blood coagulation have abnormal bleeding tendencies. These may be related to the following:

- Hemorrhagic diseases, such as a type of purpura in which spontaneous bleeding occurs under the skin, through mucous membranes, or in the gastrointestinal tract, that is idiopathic (cause unknown) or secondary to a systemic or an infectious disease or to exposure to chemical agents
- Platelet deficiency in the blood, such as thrombocytopenia as a result of decreased production of platelets by bone marrow or excessive destruction of platelets in the peripheral circulation
- Abnormal clotting factors, such as in hemophilia and von Willebrand disease, which are inherited genetic disorders

A baseline of blood values should be established preoperatively. The baseline consists of a complete blood count, including platelets, plasma clotting time, bleeding time, prothrombin time, and partial thromboplastin time. Adequate blood replacement of the deficient factors must be available during the surgical procedure and postoperatively.

Hemophilia

The term *hemophilia* refers to a group of genetic bleeding disorders characterized by abnormal clotting factors.

Hemophilia A, the classic disorder, is caused by a deficiency of functional factor VIII, the antihemophilic globulin in plasma. Hemophilia B, also known as Christmas disease, is caused by a lack of functional factor IX—the plasma thromboplastic cofactor. A carrier mother transmits to her son this sex-linked recessive trait of the specific clotting factor. Hemophilia occurs most commonly in males of Russian-Jewish descent.

The severity of the disorder depends on the percentage of functional versus nonfunctional factor in the blood. Partial thromboplastin times or thromboplastin generation times are the standard tests for this determination. These patients have normal vasculature and platelets ($150,000-400,000/mm^3$ of blood); thus bleeding time (1–3 minutes by the Duke method) and prothrombin time (11–12.5 seconds) test results are normal.

Severely affected hemophiliacs have spontaneous bleeding episodes into the skin, muscles, and joints, most commonly the ankles, knees, wrists, and elbows. If untreated, joint deformities can result. Bleeding will be excessive from even a minor wound such as a bruise or cut.

For hemostasis during a severe bleeding episode, replacement therapy must be initiated to raise the clotting factor to between 60% and 100% (normal individuals have clotting factor levels of 60–120%). In hemophiliacs, fibrin clots do not form and bleeding continues. The missing clotting factor must be raised temporarily to control hemorrhage. This is started preoperatively for elective surgery. Concentrates available for replacement therapy include the following:

1. Factor VIII for hemophilia A
   a. Lyophilized concentrate products, such as Hemofil M and Koate or HS reconstituted with diluent provided by the manufacturer
   b. Cryoprecipitate
   c. Fresh-frozen plasma or concentrate
2. Factor IX for hemophilia B
   a. Lyophilized concentrate products, such as Konyne and Profilnine reconstituted with diluent provided by the manufacturer
   b. Fresh-frozen plasma
3. Lyophilized concentrate with inhibitors to neutralize the antibody that prevents clotting

Lyophilized concentrates are made from pooled normal human plasma obtained by plasmapheresis, a process of separating red blood cells by centrifugation. The circulating nurse should obtain factor concentrate from the blood bank and must be familiar with how to prepare it. The dosage for factor deficiency is calculated on the basis of the plasma volume, half-life of the factor, and percentage of the deficit. It is given by IV infusion intraoperatively and postoperatively.

Blood Loss Replacement

Despite meticulous hemostasis and methods to reduce blood loss, blood replacement is necessary during many extensive surgical procedures, particularly cardiovascular, orthopedic, organ transplantation, and trauma surgery. Surgeons limit the use of transfused blood whenever possible. However, to compensate for blood loss of more than 1200 mL or a hematocrit value below 30% and to prevent shock, transfusions of whole blood, fresh-frozen plasma, packed red blood cells, platelets, serum albumin, or blood substitutes must be carried out according to policy. Transfusions may be allogeneic, autologous, or a blood substitute.

Informed consent should be obtained before blood loss replacement methods are selected.

Allogeneic Blood

Allogeneic blood is that drawn from one individual for transfusion into another. It must be compatible (i.e., not cause a reaction). Therefore blood typing and crossmatching are essential to determine compatibility between donor and recipient. The four main blood types are A, B, O, and AB. In addition, many subgroups of antigens exist in red blood cells. Also, agglutinogens, known as Rh factor, may be present (i.e., Rh positive or negative). If these are not present in red blood cells, the blood is Rh negative.

A recipient must receive donor blood of the same type and Rh factor. In extreme emergency situations, O-negative blood, referred to as universal donor blood, may be given until the patient's blood can be typed and crossmatched or until compatible blood can be obtained. Conversely, type AB is considered to be the universal recipient, being compatible with A, B, O, and AB.

A transfusion of the wrong blood type can be fatal. Transmission of hepatitis B or C, human immunodeficiency virus (HIV), and other viruses and infections is a potential danger, even with current testing of all donor blood. Other diseases that require deferral of blood donation include the following:

- Syphilis
- Hepatitis B, C
- HIV
- Human T-lymphotropic virus (HTLV) 1 and 2
- Cytomegalovirus (CMV)
- Malaria
- Babesiosis
- Toxoplasmosis
- Chagas disease
- Lyme disease
- Creutzfeldt-Jakob disease (and patients who have had injections of human pituitary hormone or human dura mater tissue implants)

Consequently, because of many transmissible disease subjects, many patients prefer "directed donors." When blood replacement is anticipated before a surgical procedure, a family member or friend with a compatible blood type can be asked to donate blood to be held in the blood bank for the patient. Directed donations are not necessarily safer than nondirected voluntary donations supplied from the blood bank, however.

When multiple units of blood must be transfused, packed cells, fresh-frozen plasma, and platelets usually are given to supplement units of whole blood. These components are not part of whole blood replacement.

All established measures must be strictly observed for the patient's safety. The following basic rules apply to the transfusion of all allogeneic blood products:

1. Blood products are obtained from the blood bank by a person responsible for signing them out to a specific patient.
2. To have blood nearby, a refrigerator with controlled temperature may be installed in the OR suite. Blood products for transfusion are kept at a constant temperature between 34° F and 43° F (1−6° C), verified by a recording thermometer on the outside and a standard one inside. Both audible and visible alarms are activated if a dangerous temperature is reached. Fluctuations in temperature cause red blood cells to deteriorate. Microorganisms can multiply in unrefrigerated blood. If blood is brought into the OR and then not needed, it should be

TABLE 31.3	Shelf Life of Blood Products According to the American Association of Blood Banks	
Blood Products	**Shelf Life**
Red blood cells	42 days refrigerated
Frozen red blood cells	10 years
Platelets	5 days at room temperature
Fresh-frozen plasma	1 year
Cryoprecipitated antihemophilic factor	Frozen 1 year
Granulocytes	Transfuse within 24 hours of collection

returned immediately to the refrigerator in the suite or blood bank. Do not allow whole blood or its derivatives to stand unrefrigerated in the OR. Before use, each blood product should be checked for the expiration date. Each product has a specific shelf life (Table 31.3).

3. Blood products are administered by a physician or nurse after a careful comparison of the label on the bag with the identity of the patient. A second professional person confirms the data. The label stays on the container while the blood product is being transfused.
4. Cold, refrigerated blood may induce hypothermia. Blood should be warmed as it is transfused by immersion of administration tubing in a controlled water bath or through coils in a temperature-modifying device. The temperature must be maintained between 89° F and 105° F (32−41° C). Hemolysis may occur if the temperature exceeds 110° F (43° C).
5. Another solution may be infused immediately before a blood product is administered. In changing to the blood product, avoid the possibility of air entering the tubing. A blood filter must be used for transfusion. The filter should be changed after the second or third unit of whole blood to avoid the filter becoming clogged with microaggregates.
6. The anesthesia provider records on the anesthesia record the following information for each unit transfused:
   a. The name of the person who started the transfusion.
   b. The type and amount of product transfused (i.e., whole blood, plasma, packed cells, platelets, albumin).
   c. The time started and drops per minute.
   d. Information on the label, including the blood group, Rh factor, and number.
7. The patient is observed closely for any type of reaction. This probability increases in direct proportion to the number of units transfused. The most common type of reaction is allergic; febrile is almost as common, and hemolytic reactions are possible. Transfusion reactions with the patient under anesthesia may be accompanied by profound hypotension, temperature change, blood in urine, and/or skin rash. The common physical reactions and chills are not seen in an anesthetized patient. If any suspicious reactions occur:
   a. Stop the transfusion. Keep the IV line patent with IV solution as directed by the physician.
   b. Return unused blood to the blood bank along with a sample of the patient's blood.
   c. Send a urine sample to the laboratory as soon as possible.
   d. Take vital signs (temperature, pulse, respirations, BP) every 5 to 10 minutes until the patient is stable.

e. Have emergency medications and resuscitation equipment available.

f. Document on the patient's chart the type of reaction, action taken, patient's response, and other documentation as required by the institution.

Autologous Blood

Autologous blood is blood recovered from the patient and reinfused. Referred to as autotransfusion, this process is the preferred method of replacement for either elective or emergency procedures. The patient's own blood is the safest form of transfusion; it eliminates concerns about compatibility/reactions and transmission of exogenous organisms. Autologous blood is equal or superior in quality to allogeneic blood. It may be obtained preoperatively from patients and returned to them intraoperatively or postoperatively as needed.

Some patients who, because of religious beliefs, will not accept allogeneic blood may accept autotransfusion in the form of cell salvage, red cell fractions, plasma fractions, white cell fractions, or platelet fractions. Jehovah's Witnesses, for example, believe that receiving blood or blood products violates a biblical prohibition against consumption of blood.[10] They have the right to refuse transfusion, and that should not be interpreted as a death wish. Some will accept blood fractions as a personal decision. Informed consent should be obtained from all patients for whom autotransfusion or administration of blood fractions is contemplated.

Preoperative Blood Donation

One or more units of whole blood or blood components can be obtained by phlebotomy from the patient preoperatively and stored in the blood bank. Blood may be donated as often as every seventh day for a period of 6 weeks if the hemoglobin remains at least 11 g/dL or the hematocrit is 33%, with the final unit donated no less than 72 hours before the scheduled surgical procedure. If two or more units are donated, a PO or IM iron supplement may be prescribed because as much as 10% of iron stores are lost with each donation. Epoetin alfa, a glycoprotein, can be administered SQ or IV for up to 6 weeks preoperatively to stimulate red blood cell production. Red blood cell stimulation can be continued postoperatively and is effective if iron stores are adequate. The patient's body replenishes the fluid lost in donation within 24 hours.

Autologous blood is usually stored in a liquid state as whole blood or packed red blood cells. Whole blood with anticoagulant can be stored for 35 days, and red blood cells with preservative for 42 days. Red blood cells and plasma can be frozen for prolonged storage. The same protocol is used in the OR for reinfusing autologous blood as described for allogeneic transfusions. If the patient does not need reinfusion, the blood is discarded. The blood is not given to another patient.

Intraoperative Autotransfusion

Recovery of blood as it is lost requires sterile equipment that suctions blood from the surgical site, filters and anticoagulates it, and contains it for IV reinfusion to the patient with minimal damage to cells. Intraoperative blood salvage is widely used when potential blood loss may exceed 20% of the patient's blood volume. Blood can be suctioned directly from a body cavity or the wound. Any plastic devices, including suction tubing and pouches, used for blood recovery must be approved by the U.S. Food and Drug Administration (FDA).

Blood is not salvaged if microfibrillar collagen (Avitene) has been used for hemostasis. This may not wash out when red blood cells are processed and can predispose the patient to DIC or ARDS. In addition, blood contaminated with enteric organisms or amniotic fluid is not salvaged. If a malignant tumor can be resected intact, autotransfusion may benefit the patient with cancer. Most cancer cells will filter out of processed blood. Autologous blood is not collected from patients with known systemic infections or from open traumatic wounds. Other patients, of all ages, are candidates for autotransfusion.

The autotransfusion unit must be easily and quickly assembled because it may be lifesaving for a trauma patient in an emergency situation. All fluid paths should be disposable and must be sterile. Three basic systems are used for intraoperative autotransfusion, as follows:

1. *Automated cell salvage processor:* Blood is suctioned through double-lumen tubing. An anticoagulant solution of heparinized saline or citrated dextrose mixes with blood at the tip end of the tubing. The aspirate passes through a 140-mm filter before entering the collection reservoir. This filter removes fat and debris.

When a sufficient quantity to be processed has accumulated, the blood is pumped into a centrifuge bowl. The centrifugal force separates red blood cells from plasma, platelets, white blood cells, and other debris, including anticoagulant. These red blood cells are washed with normal saline solution. A suspension of red blood cells in saline solution is pumped into a reinfusion bag. Each bag contains about 250 mL of washed packed red blood cells with a hematocrit of 50% to 55%, ready for IV reinfusion. The entire cycle takes 3 to 7 minutes.

Some autotransfusion units have automatic, programmed cycles, including process air and foam detectors; others operate manually. Platelet-rich plasma suitable for autotransfusion can be sequestered from some units.

2. *Canister collection method:* Blood is suctioned and anticoagulated as described for the cell processor. From the tubing, the blood collects in a reservoir with a disposable liner. When the reservoir becomes full, or at the end of the surgical procedure, the liner is removed. The contents are washed in a standard red blood cell washer before being reinfused.

This equipment may be located in the blood bank. The liner must be labeled with the patient's name and identifying number if it leaves the OR for washing. Autologous blood obtained using this technique has a high hematocrit level and is nearly free of protein, anticoagulant, and debris.

3. *Salvage collection bag:* An anticoagulant, usually citrate, is added to blood collected directly into a single-use, self-contained transfusion bag. The blood is not washed but reinfused through a blood filter. This simple method is most appropriate when profuse bleeding occurs in areas that form pools that can be easily suctioned, such as the abdominal or chest cavities.

All three methods are safe when used according to the manufacturer's instructions. The automated cell salvage devices are the most sophisticated and complex. Only properly trained personnel should operate them. OR personnel may be trained to set up the sterile suction and containers.

Postoperative Autotransfusion

Autologous blood may be collected, processed, and bagged during a surgical procedure for reinfusion postoperatively. Bags must be labeled with the name and identifying number of the patient and the time of processing. Autologous blood also can be salvaged postoperatively from a drainage tube placed into the surgical wound, most commonly a chest tube. The tube may be connected to a cell washer in a portable unit that attaches to wall suction in the PACU or ICU.

Another method collects wound drainage by suctioning it directly into a filtered collection bag. With both of these methods, blood is anticoagulated. It may be collected for a maximum of 6 hours. The concentrated red blood cells, either washed or unwashed, are reinfused IV. Whether obtained intraoperatively or postoperatively, unwashed blood can be kept at room temperature for 4 hours and washed blood can be kept for 6 hours at room temperature or refrigerated for 24 hours at 39.2° F (4° C).

Blood Substitutes

Oxygen-carrying blood substitutes offer another alternative for transporting oxygen. Since the 1970s, researchers have sought to develop hemoglobin-based oxygen carriers to serve as blood substitutes for emergency use. The ideal blood substitute has not been developed that satisfies clinical testing and safety for patient use. Chemically modified hemoglobin from outdated human blood or bovine blood has been used in the research effort.

Oxygenation of body tissues is a serious subject when the patient's blood volume or hemoglobin level is decreased because of blood loss. These substitutes might be used in anemic patients, in people who refuse blood or blood products for religious reasons, or when compatible allogeneic blood is not available. A number of blood substitutes are being studied and tested in animals and humans.[11]

- *Fluorovent:* Oxygen-carrying perfluorocarbon (PFC) can be used for preterm infants with underdeveloped lungs and in both adults and children with ARDS. It is a liquid instilled directly into the lungs to act as a surfactant. It encourages the exchange of oxygen and carbon dioxide. Patients with COPD may benefit from its use as well. Clinical trials were postponed for safety reasons.
- *Oxycyte:* This IV form of PFC carries five times the amount of oxygen carried in hemoglobin. The oxygen-hemoglobin exchange ratio is extremely efficient because the molecules are 1/70 the size of a red blood cell and can reach tiny capillary surfaces. It can be stored at room temperature and requires no crossmatching. It was rejected for FDA approval; more studies are ongoing.
- *Hemopure:* This bovine hemoglobin–based polymer solution has been used in clinical trials in the United States and Europe.[11] It is stable for 3 years at room temperature and requires no crossmatching. It is given by IV infusion and is compatible with all blood types. The FDA allows the product to be used only if no options are available for survival, although it is not approved by the FDA.
- *PolyHeme:* Human polymerized hemoglobin is processed from outdated human red blood cells. The product is screened for infectious disease, pasteurized, and polymerized. It is safe for use with any blood type. The shelf life is 12 months. It was rejected for FDA approval.
- *Oxyglobin:* This red blood cell alternative for veterinary services is compatible with all blood types. It was approved by the FDA for use in animals.

Complications of Blood Loss or Replacement

The patient is constantly monitored to detect any complications that might be developing as a result of blood loss or replacement

or as a compromise of the cardiovascular system. Hemorrhage can cause shock and DIC. Earlier PFC emulsions caused pulmonary complications, such as hyperinflated, noncollapsible lungs. Traces of older PFC emulsions can persist systemically and cause the threat of accumulation in fatty tissue. Accumulation could compromise developing neonatal nervous tissue, which has a high fatty content.

Early blood substitute products have been associated with gastrointestinal problems, myocardial infarction, stroke, coagulopathies, kidney and liver dysfunction, fever, and vasoconstriction.

Research is being done on growing red blood cells in a laboratory from adult donor cells. Small amounts of red blood cells have been successfully bioengineered and could be a safer alternative to treat blood loss in the future.

Shock

Shock is a state of inadequate blood perfusion to parts of the body. If untreated, it will become irreversible and result in death. George W. Crile (1864–1943), one of the founders of the Cleveland Clinic, was the first surgeon to systematically study physiologic shock and its relationship to hypotension in the surgical patient.

Hemorrhagic shock results from a decrease in circulating blood volume caused by loss of blood, plasma, or extracellular fluid. Fluid loss is excessive when it is greater than compensatory absorption of interstitial fluid into the circulation. Shock resulting from hemorrhage or inadequate blood volume replacement, as seen in the OR and PACU, usually is reversed by prompt restoration of circulating blood volume.

Shock is a complex phenomenon, a life-threatening condition in which circulation fails for one or several reasons. Loss of circulating blood volume, loss of the pumping power of the heart, or loss of peripheral resistance can result in insufficient flow of blood for adequate tissue perfusion or oxygenation. If it is prolonged, inadequate organ blood flow with deficient microcirculation profoundly depresses vital processes. Because the objective of circulation is achieved in the capillaries, defective cellular metabolism derived from shock interferes further with the body's inherent defenses, and metabolic acidosis occurs.

Normal defense mechanisms are reflex vasoconstriction and increased pulse rate, which tend to redistribute the flow of blood to the heart and brain at the expense of the other vital organs. If shock is promptly recognized, treated, and reversed, permanent damage is avoided. If it progresses to irreversibility, death ensues from cellular dysfunction and organ hypoperfusion.

Multiple types and causes of shock present problems in relationships among the heart, circulatory system, and blood volume. Circulatory inadequacy may originate from a marked decrease in CO, venous return to the heart, or peripheral vascular resistance. All forms of shock carry high mortality rates. The best treatment is prevention. Shock is classified according to the cause of inadequate tissue perfusion.

Hypovolemic and Traumatic Shock

Fluid loss is greater than compensatory absorption of interstitial fluid into the circulation. The vascular capacity is low, causing a decrease in diastolic filling pressure. Damage to the capillaries caused by soft tissue trauma increases capillary permeability, with loss of blood volume into the tissues and decreased urine production. This state is aggravated by pain, which inhibits the vasomotor center, leading to vasodilation and hypovolemia. Toxic factors associated with intravascular coagulation lead to pulmonary, renal, and/or multiple organ failure.

Hemorrhagic Shock

Shock results from hemorrhage or inadequate blood volume replacement. This is characterized by significant blood loss, more than can be replaced for physiologic equilibrium. The loss of blood causes the BP to decrease to levels too low to perfuse vital organs.

Cardiogenic Shock

The pumping action of the left ventricle is insufficient to pump enough blood to vital organs. Cardiogenic shock may be precipitated by congestive heart failure, myocardial contusion or infarction, coronary air embolism, mechanical venous obstruction, or hypothermia. In addition to drugs, various mechanical devices may be used, such as an auxiliary ventricle or counterpulsation with an intraaortic balloon pump (IABP), to temporarily increase left ventricular function.

Neurogenic Shock

Loss of vasomotor tone in peripheral blood vessels leads to sudden vasodilation and pooling of blood. Vasodilation produces hypotension. Peripheral resistance is too great for compensation by increased CO, increasing the risk for congestive heart failure and PE. Causes may be brain damage, deep anesthesia, emotional trauma, vagal reflex from pain or surgical manipulation, or spinal cord injury.

Vasogenic Shock

Anaphylaxis and septic shock (toxic shock) from infection are the most common types of vasogenic shock. CO decreases as the heart muscle weakens and the CVP is unstable.

Metabolic Crises

Convulsions

Convulsions occur most often in patients with a hyperactive metabolic rate, especially in dehydrated or febrile children. Anoxia and death can occur.

Etiology

Etiologic factors include severe hypoxia and carbon dioxide retention, hypernatremia, hyperthermia, overdose of regional anesthetic drugs, air embolism, and epilepsy.

Symptoms

Symptoms include muscular twitching, dilated pupils, rapid snorting respirations, rapid pulse, grimacing, and cyanosis.

Treatment

Oxygen is administered to maintain respiration, and diazepam (a rapid-acting barbiturate) or a neuromuscular blocker is given to stop muscular activity. Mechanical ventilation may be needed for apnea or to support circulation.

Prevention

Metabolic crises are prevented by maintaining normal body temperature and fluid and electrolyte balance.

Inadvertent Hypothermia

A decrease in the patient's core body temperature to below 96° F (35° C) can affect vasoconstriction and vasodilation, CO, and renal function. Depending on the degree of body heat loss, hypothermia is categorized as follows:
- Mild (down to 90° F [32° C])
- Moderate (down to 85° F [29° C])
- Deep (down to 80° F [27° C])

If core temperature falls below 68° F (20° C), brain activity ceases. Patients can emerge from anesthesia with a body temperature below normal. Inadvertent hypothermia occurs spontaneously intraoperatively; it is not to be confused with induced hypothermia. Age-extreme, thin, and debilitated patients are most susceptible, as are patients undergoing neurosurgical, cardiovascular, thoracic, and abdominal procedures.

Etiology

Anesthesia inhibits the protective reflexes that generate body heat (i.e., shivering). It also depresses the thermoregulatory center in the hypothalamus, decreases the basal metabolic rate, and increases vasodilation for heat loss by radiation and conduction. Core body heat is lost by exposure to a cool external environment (e.g., during skin preparation) and through the surgical incision.

Other factors include preoperative sedation, use of general versus regional anesthesia, adjunctive drugs, the length of the surgical procedure, blood and fluid loss and replacement, the room temperature, and evaporative loss through the skin and respiratory tract.

General anesthesia commonly causes a 1° F to 1.5° F decrease in core temperature during the first hour, extending the action of propofol by 30%. The greatest risk for hypothermia is in the patient who has had combined general and epidural anesthesia. Protective central inhibition of the thermoregulatory center in the hypothalamus and peripheral nervous system is delayed.

Symptoms

Hypothermia can cause adverse cardiovascular, hematologic, immunologic, metabolic, and neurologic effects.[12] Cardiac dysrhythmias, hypoxia, metabolic acidosis, hyperglycemia, and dilated pupils may be a result. A depressed central nervous system, which can lead to coma, may not be evident until the postoperative period.

Shivering, impaired speech, muscle rigidity, peripheral or central cyanosis, a weak pulse, falling BP, and dysrhythmias seen in the PACU may be symptoms of hypothermia. The incidence of ventricular tachycardia is doubled, causing an increased incidence of postoperative myocardial infarction.

Treatment

The hypothermic patient must be rewarmed as soon as possible. However, postanesthesia shivering during the rewarming process can be hazardous. Shivering is an involuntary rhythmic contraction of muscle groups with irregular and intermittent relaxation. This physiologic response to cold is activated when the hypothalamus senses that the core temperature has dropped. Some postanesthesia shivering is caused by anesthetic agents. Untreated shivering leads to increased oxygen consumption as a result of muscular activity and to increased cardiac stress as a result of hypoxia.

In the PACU a forced-air skin surface warmer or an ultraviolet or infrared heat lamp directed at the lightly covered patient is an effective means for raising the body temperature. A temperature-regulating hypothermia/hyperthermia machine, set at 104° F to 107° F (40–42° C), may be used with a heated blanket beneath the patient. Any warming device placed under the patient should be closely monitored to prevent burns and used according to the manufacturer's instructions. If mechanical warmers are not available, heated blankets placed over and underneath the patient should be changed at 15-minute intervals. Blankets can be heated to 105° F (40.5° C) for an adult or 100° F (38° C) for a small child or infant. The patient should wear a cap. Warmed, humidified oxygen and warm IV fluid should be administered. Coniine (an α₂-adrenergic agonist) or analgesics such as meperidine or morphine derivative may suppress shivering.

Prevention

Prevention of hypothermia is the best treatment. Prevention begins before the patient arrives in the OR and continues during the procedure:
1. Place a hypothermia/hyperthermia mattress or reflective blanket on the OR bed. A radiant heat source can be placed over an infant.
2. Check the room temperature and humidity.
3. Apply warmed blankets as soon as the patient arrives in the OR and immediately after drapes are removed.
4. Limit skin exposure during positioning and skin preparation (i.e., keep the patient covered as much as possible).
5. Minimize the time of exposure between skin antisepsis and draping.
6. Keep the sheet under and the drapes over the patient and around the surgical site dry to provide insulation, prevent heat loss, and maintain asepsis. Dry the area after skin preparation.
7. Warm antiseptic, irrigating, and IV solutions, including blood, before administration. Anesthetic gases, including oxygen, can be warmed also.
8. Monitor body temperature.
9. Leave a cap on the patient; a plastic head covering retains more heat than do other materials.

Malignant Hyperthermia

Malignant hyperthermia (MH) is a hypermetabolic crisis in susceptible people. It is triggered by potent halogenated anesthetic agents and depolarizing skeletal muscle relaxants. MH, a potentially fatal complication of inhalant anesthesia, is characterized by uncontrolled acceleration of muscle metabolism accompanied by tremendous oxygen consumption and production of heat and carbon dioxide.

Elevated body temperature is a later sign of an MH crisis. The body temperature can rapidly rise at a rate of 1.8° F (1° C) every 5 minutes if MH is untreated. A temperature as high as 117° F (47° C) has been recorded, but 111.2° F (44° C) is probably the highest with survival. The survival rate with appropriate treatment is between 80% and 90%. The mortality rate without appropriate treatment is around 90%; thus MH is of significant concern.

Etiology

The exact cause of MH is unknown. It is understood that certain patients are susceptible and some anesthetic agents may trigger this metabolic crisis.

Susceptible Patients

A familial genetic transmission exists as an autosomal dominant trait with variable multifactor inheritance patterns. The genetic defect manifests by increasing calcium levels in skeletal muscles. The crisis results from a hereditary inability of the sarcoplasmic reticulum, a skeletal muscle cell membrane, to control intramyoplasmic levels of calcium.

Skeletal muscle undergoes contraction as a result of release of calcium ions in response to drugs or stress. A rapid increase of calcium in muscle fiber leads to generalized catabolism of the cells, an interruption of normal anabolism. As biochemical reactions occur, the body produces heat and carbon dioxide.

Susceptible patients also include those with any type of myopathy or acquired muscle disease, such as ptosis, strabismus, hernia, muscle weakness or hypertrophy, or muscular dystrophy. The incidence of MH is higher in children than in adults. Patients, especially children, with rheumatoid arthritis are particularly susceptible to MH. MH may occur in a patient's first exposure to anesthesia or in a later one; one-third of reported cases of MH have occurred in a second or subsequent anesthesia.

Triggers

Succinylcholine, halothane, enflurane, desflurane, and isoflurane are the main triggers of MH in susceptible individuals.

Symptoms

Clinical signs and symptoms occur according to the swiftness of onset. The onset may be rapid, occurring immediately after induction, or may occur after several hours of general anesthesia or even in the postoperative recovery period.

Spasm of the jaw muscles with rigidity of the masseter muscles (trismus) or severe fasciculation after succinylcholine administration may suggest MH development to the anesthesia provider, although this activity is not uncommon in pediatric patients.

The most common presenting sign of MH is unexplained ventricular dysrhythmia, primarily tachycardia or PVCs. This is associated with an unexplained increase in end-tidal carbon dioxide, tachypnea, cyanosis, skin mottling, and unstable BP. Blood in the surgical field may appear dark as a result of central venous desaturation.

When a sudden, generalized hypermetabolic state is produced, the temperature rises rapidly as more heat is produced than the body can eliminate. This is not a first sign. Elevated temperature may be a late sign or may be absent in MH syndrome. Fever, hot skin or tissues, and diaphoresis are symptoms of heat buildup. A favorable prognosis decreases when excessive heat in the tissues is noted through the surgeon's gloves or when the anesthesia provider senses heat in the reservoir bag or soda lime canister on the anesthesia machine. The body tries to adjust by vasodilation and increased CO.

If rapidly increasing tissue demands are not met, hypoxia, central venous hypercapnia, and severe respiratory and metabolic acidosis occur, progressing to cardiovascular collapse. Blood tests will reveal increased serum levels of potassium, magnesium, creatine phosphokinase (CPK), and myoglobin. Excessive myoglobin release caused by rapid muscle destruction (rhabdomyolysis) can cause renal failure and lead to anuria.

Late clinical findings include hyperkalemia; acute renal failure; left-sided heart failure; DIC; skeletal muscle swelling or necrosis from hypoxia and acidosis; pulmonary edema; neurologic sequelae, including paraplegia and decerebration; and coma from ischemia secondary to hypoxia. Recurrence of MH crisis can occur 24 to 72 hours postoperatively.

Monitoring

Parameters and studies to be monitored routinely in patients at risk for MH who undergo general anesthesia are heart rate and rhythm, BP, core temperature by esophageal probe, pulse oximetry, capnometry, nerve stimulation to measure the level of muscle relaxation, and precordial stethoscopy. A rise in temperature greater than 0.5° F per hour should raise suspicion for MH.

Treatment

Success is contingent on complete preparedness (preplanned action, written protocol, immediate equipment supply), early diagnosis, and vigorous therapy. The following treatment outline is the suggested protocol established by the Malignant Hyperthermia Association of the United States (MHAUS). (Emergency therapy wall charts can be ordered online at www.mhaus.org.) Institutional policies and procedures should be in place as follows to guide the perioperative team in caring for a patient in MH crisis:

1. Discontinue inhalant anesthesia and stop the surgical procedure immediately. The anesthesia provider immediately institutes hyperventilation with 100% oxygen at a high flow rate of at least 10 L/min. Research has shown that the breathing circuit and anesthesia delivery machine need not be changed because the high concentration of oxygen delivery clears the machine of anesthetic gases very rapidly. If the surgical procedure cannot be interrupted, safe agents may be used to maintain anesthesia during the stabilization period.

2. Immediately start drug therapy. Administer:
   a. Dantrolene sodium (Dantrium, Revonto, Ryanodex), 2 to 3 mg/kg in an initial IV bolus and repeat every 5 to 10 minutes until the maximum dose of 10 mg/kg is given or the MH episode is controlled. Large volumes are needed; therefore a central line is necessary.

   Patients generally respond to the drug quickly. The onset of action is usually 2 to 3 minutes. Occasionally doses higher than 10 to 20 mg/kg are needed.

   Dantrolene is a specific drug for treatment of MH. It directly blocks accumulation of calcium within the muscles by preventing its release from the sarcoplasmic reticulum and by uncoupling excitation-contraction, thus relaxing skeletal muscle. It has no effect on cardiovascular or respiratory functions. Calcium channel blockers may not be given with dantrolene because they may cause hyperkalemia, myocardial depression, and cardiovascular collapse. Verapamil is contraindicated.

   Given IV, Dantrium and Revonto are supplied in 65-mL vials as a sterile, lyophilized powder that contains 20 mg of dantrolene and 3 g of mannitol. Each vial must be reconstituted before use with 60 mL of sterile water for injection without a preservative agent. The large quantities of sterile water that are needed would contain the preservative agent in toxic amounts. A semiautomatic fluid-dispensing syringe expedites mixing. If this is not available, additional personnel should help with the reconstitution process because large quantities of the diluted drug will be needed and each vial will require

vigorous shaking to mix. A central line is the best route for administration of large quantities of the drug. Peripheral vessel constriction can make IV administration difficult. In extreme circumstances the drug may be given through a filter to remove particulate from the solution.

   Ryanodex is a rapidly prepared formulation of dantrolene sodium supplied in 250-mg vials with 125 mg of mannitol. This form of the drug requires 5 mL of nonbacteriostatic sterile water to reconstitute the solution in 20 seconds. This allows rapid administration to stabilize the patient with minimal risk for fluid overload. A central line may not be needed if the peripheral veins are patent. Reconstituted Ryanodex and other forms of dantrolene must be used within 6 hours of mixing and must be protected from direct sunlight. Dantrolene sodium solution will be yellow-orange when mixed. More information can be found at www.ryanodex.com/.

   If other IV solutions have been running, the line should be flushed with sterile water before dantrolene is injected; this will prevent precipitation. Do not use lactated Ringer's solution because it will increase the level of acidosis. An additional IV site should be established to infuse iced normal saline solution at the rate of 15 mL/kg every 15 minutes for at least 45 minutes.

   Dantrolene is continued postoperatively at a minimum of 1 mg/kg every 6 hours for 24 to 72 hours postepisode. After the initial 48 hours, 1 mg/kg every 6 hours may be given orally for 24 hours. No serious side effects have been reported with short-term use, but muscle weakness may be evident for 24 to 48 hours after administration. A few isolated reports of nausea, vomiting, and fatigue have been documented. Prolonged administration may lead to hepatotoxicity.
   b. Procainamide (Pronestyl), 15 mg/kg diluted in 500 mL of physiologic saline solution IV over 60 minutes. Procainamide treats cardiac dysrhythmia if required.
   c. Sodium bicarbonate, 1 to 2 mEq/kg IV stat and repeat as guided by blood gas analysis. An alkali, sodium bicarbonate raises pH temporarily. It combats acidosis and antagonizes hyperkalemia by lowering the plasma potassium level. It can cause rebound acidosis. Monitoring of arterial pH and P_{CO_2} is necessary to determine subsequent doses.
   d. Regular insulin, 10 units in 50 mL of 50% dextrose in water IV. Insulin offsets the high glucose metabolic demands and improves glucose uptake. It shifts potassium back into the cells to help treat hyperkalemia. Blood glucose and potassium levels must be monitored.
   e. Calcium chloride, 2.5 mg/kg, to treat severe cardiac toxicity caused by hyperkalemia.
   f. Mannitol, 0.25 g/kg IV, and furosemide (Lasix), 1 mg/kg IV, up to four doses each. These drugs dislodge myoglobin from the renal tubules and sustain urinary flow. Urinary output greater than 2 mL/kg/h must be maintained to prevent renal failure. The dose is calculated in consideration of the mannitol contained in the dantrolene sodium solution.

3. Begin active cooling. Administer refrigerated or iced normal saline IV. Lavage the stomach and rectum. Avoid irrigating the bladder if at all possible because accurate measurement of urinary output and urinalysis are important. If the

peritoneal or thoracic cavity is open, cool sterile saline may be poured into the opening.

Cool the body surface by placing the patient on a plastic sheet and applying ice bags and ice water, or use a hypothermia blanket. If readily available, use extracorporeal perfusion apparatus for partial (femoral-to-femoral) cardiopulmonary bypass to cool the viscera. Body temperature must be carefully monitored to avoid accidental cooling to dysrhythmic levels. Medication may be given to limit shivering, normally a heat-retaining mechanism that also increases oxygen consumption. Surface cooling is considered more effective in children because of their high ratio of surface area to body volume. Cooling that is too vigorous can result in inadvertent hypothermia and cardiac arrest. To avoid hypothermia, cooling should be discontinued when the core temperature reaches 100° F (38° C).

4. Correct the electrolyte imbalance on the basis of blood sampling of electrolytes, pH, and blood gases. After the presumed onset of MH, an arterial line must be established if one is not already in place. Blood samples are taken at 10-minute intervals for pH, P_{CO_2}, P_{O_2}, sodium, potassium, chlorides, calcium, magnesium, and phosphate. Hypocalcemia and hyperkalemia followed by hypokalemia may be expected.

Also measured are CPK, aspartate aminotransferase (AST, formerly serum glutamic-oxaloacetic transaminase [SGOT]), alkaline phosphatase, and lactate dehydrogenase for indication of muscle destruction. Blood urea nitrogen (BUN) for kidney function, bilirubin for liver function, coagulation studies, blood lactate and pyruvate, and serum thyroxine levels may be ordered.

5. CVP should be monitored. A CVP line may need to be inserted if one is not already in place.

6. Urinary output is monitored via an indwelling Foley catheter. In addition to the measurement of volume, urine is sampled for hemoglobin and myoglobin. The urine may be brown as the amount of hemoglobin and myoglobin increases.

Supplies for Malignant Hyperthermia

Supplies should be kept in a specific location and must be immediately available for both adult and pediatric patients. A cart marked for use in MH is convenient. Supplies that may be needed include the following:

1. Monitors, including ECG, electronic temperature probes, recorder
2. IV equipment, including blood administration sets and pumps; CVP line setup; IV solutions—12 bags, 1000 mL each, of physiologic saline kept in a refrigerator
3. Arterial line setup
4. Intubation equipment
5. Ice chips and plastic bags, hypothermia blankets
6. Gastric lavage set, three-way indwelling catheter for insertion into the rectum, 50-mL syringes
7. Blood sampling and arterial blood gas equipment
8. Indwelling Foley catheter, urometer bag
9. Drugs:
   a. Thirty-six 20-mg vials of dantrolene sodium (the quantity needed to treat and stabilize a 70-kg adult)
   b. Thirty-six 60-mL vials of sterile water without a preservative agent to reconstitute dantrolene (the quantity needed for a 70-kg adult is 2100 mL)

c. Five 100-mL prefilled syringes of sodium bicarbonate 5%
d. Six 1-g ampules of procainamide
e. Ten 50-mL vials of 20% mannitol
f. Four 2-mL (20-mg) prefilled syringes of furosemide
g. One 100-unit vial of regular insulin
h. Two 50-mL vials of 50% dextrose in water
i. Three 1000-unit vials of heparin
j. Ten 250-mg vials of hydrocortisone sodium succinate (Solu-Cortef)

10. Associated needles and syringes
11. Extracorporeal perfusion apparatus if available
12. Defibrillator machine and electrodes

Prevention

Identification of susceptible patients is the best prevention. The preoperative history should routinely include questions about the patient's previous anesthesia experiences, unexplained incidents or death of family members who underwent anesthesia, and known muscular abnormalities or episodes of heatstroke in the patient or relatives. Hereditary predisposition has been detected in three generations; however, the patient's family history frequently is not known.

The most prominent clue to identification of a patient susceptible to MH is a family history of unexplained death while under general anesthesia. Genetic counseling of the patient and family is advised. Although the crisis usually occurs when the patient is under general anesthesia, it can occur during periods of emotional or physical stress. Susceptible people should wear a Medic-Alert bracelet or tag.

Diagnosis of susceptibility to MH can be accomplished by preoperative muscle biopsy. A 1-g specimen of skeletal muscle is excised from the thigh with the patient under local anesthesia. The specimen is removed from the muscle as a strip and outstretched between the prongs of a double-tipped clamp. Evaluation of the muscle response to caffeine-induced contracture during exposure to halothane reveals sensitivity. Although a local anesthetic is used to obtain the muscle biopsy, dantrolene should be readily available in the unlikely event of an episode of MH.

The blood CPK level may be elevated in susceptible patients, but it also can be influenced by alcohol consumption or strenuous exercise. A normal CPK level does not ensure absence of the MH trait. Nuclear magnetic resonance imaging using phosphorus also may detect susceptibility, but it is not always a reliable indicator.

Prophylaxis

Dantrolene may be given preoperatively to susceptible patients. The suggested dose is 1-mg/kg increments every 4 to 6 hours PO up to a total dose of 4 mg/kg, followed by 2.5 mg/kg IV 30 minutes before induction of general anesthesia. Intraoperative monitoring is mandatory. When nontriggering anesthetic agents are used, prophylactic dantrolene therapy may be unnecessary. Each patient should be evaluated individually. Some indications for dantrolene prophylaxis may include:

- Previous history of suspected MH episode
- Family history of MH (actual or suspected)
- Known MH susceptibility
- Prolonged procedure anticipated in an MH-susceptible patient
- Underlying disease or physiology causing suspicion of MH susceptibility

Nontriggering anesthetic agents should be administered to MH-susceptible individuals. Barbiturates, benzodiazepines, narcotics, and opioids are considered safe. Nitrous oxide by inhalation or IV propofol or ketamine hydrochloride can be administered for general anesthesia. Most of the synthetic nondepolarizing neuromuscular blockers are safe muscle relaxants. Amino amide and ester agents can be used safely for local anesthesia.

Postoperatively the patient should be continuously monitored in the ICU for 24 to 48 hours. If the vital signs remain stable during this time, the patient may be discharged. (More information is available from MHAUS at www.mhaus.org.)

Iatrogenic Injury

Physiologic injuries are many and varied. The anesthesia provider may inadvertently loosen teeth or damage dental work during endotracheal intubation. Nerves can be injured from faulty positioning, such as hyperabduction or extension of the arm. Pressure sores may develop on poorly padded areas. Fingers and body parts can be pinched in OR bed flexures. Careless handling of an anesthetized patient can result in paralysis, fractures, or postoperative pain.

Eyes can be injured from irritating anesthetics or facemasks or from drying or scratching of the cornea if the eyelids are not closed. Patients with protruding eyes, faces covered by drapes, or those in prone positions are at high risk for eye injury. Use of an ocular lubricant protects the cornea from drying, and taped eyelids prevent corneal abrasions.

Extravasation, thrombophlebitis, and air emboli are associated with IV infusions. IV cannulas should be visible and not entirely hidden beneath drapes; infusions should be checked frequently. Precaution is the best prevention of injuries.

ⓔ EVOLVE WEBSITE

http://evolve.elsevier.com/Hornacky/BerryKohn/

- Historical Perspective
- Student Interactive Questions
- Glossary

References

1. Taylor A, DeBoard Z, Gauvin JM: Prevention of pulmonary complications, *Surg Clin North Am* 95(2):237−254, 2015.
2. Randles D, Dabner S: Applied respiratory physiology, *Anaesth Intensive Care Med* 16(2):63−67, 2015.
3. Baker P: Preparedness and education in airway management, *Anesthesiol Clin* 33(2):381−395, 2015.
4. Bauchmuller K, Faulds MC: Care of the critically ill patient, *Surgery* 33(4):165−171, 2015.
5. Wyckoff M, Greif R, Morley P, et al.: 2022 International consensus on cardiopulmonary resuscitation and emergency cardiovascular care science with treatment recommendations: summary from the basic life support; advanced life support; pediatric life support; neonatal life support; education, implementation, and teams; and first aid task forces, *Circulation* 146:483−557, 2022.
6. Stefanescu A: Arrhythmias and cardiogenic shock as a presentation of hyperthermia, *J Am Coll Cardiol* 65(10):616, 2015.
7. Moore LE, Kemp AM, Kemp SF: Recognition, treatment, and prevention of anaphylaxis, *Immunol Allergy Clin North Am* 35(2):363−374, 2015.
8. Yen C, Johar S, Lim W: Case series of neonatal extravasation injury: importance of early identification and management, *Cureus* 14(1):e21179, 2022.
9. Douglas WG, Uffort E, Denning D: Transfusion and management of surgical patients with hematologic disorders, *Surg Clin North Am* 95(2):367−377, 2015.
10. Khan F, Singh K, Friedman M: Artificial blood: the history and current perspectives of blood substitutes, *Discoveries (Craiova)* 8(1):e104, 2020.
11. Doshi HH, Giudici MC: The EKG in hypothermia and hyperthermia, *J Electrocardiol* 48(2):203−209, 2015.

Bibliography

American Society of PeriAnesthesia Nurses (ASPAN): *2019−2020 Standards of perianesthesia nursing practice*, Cherry Hill, NJ, 2019, The Association.
AORN: *Guidelines for perioperative practice*, Denver, CO, 2024, The Association.

32

Endoscopy and Robotic-Assisted Surgery

CHAPTER OUTLINE

Eight Essential Elements of Endoscopy, 647
Knowledge and Skill for a Safe Endoscopic Environment, 655
Types of Endoscopic Procedures, 655
Care of Endoscopes, 658

Considerations for Patient Safety, 659
Duties of the Assistant for Flexible Endoscopy, 660
Robotic-Assisted Endoscopy, 660

CHAPTER OBJECTIVES

After studying this chapter, the learner will be able to:

- Describe the difference between rigid and flexible endoscopy.
- List the eight essential elements necessary for all endoscopy.

- Identify three potential hazards of puncture endoscopy.
- List three considerations for patient safety during endoscopy.

KEY TERMS AND DEFINITIONS

Endoscopy Examination of a body part or cavity with an optical system in a tubular structure.
Insufflation Act of filling with gas. Laparoscopy is performed with carbon dioxide gas (CO_2).
Laparoscopy Endoscopic examination of the peritoneal body cavity through a percutaneous access portal, placement of expansion medium to create a working space, and manipulation of intraabdominal organs.
Percutaneous Puncture through the skin.

Pneumoperitoneum The peritoneal cavity is filled with CO_2.
Trocar Surgical instrument that consists of a sheath with a sharp pyramidal or blunt conical obturator used to puncture or penetrate multiple layers of tissue. The sheath remains in place as the obturator is removed. Additional instrumentation is passed through the sheath.
Veress needle Spring-loaded needle that delivers CO_2 for the creation of a pneumoperitoneum.

Eight Essential Elements of Endoscopy

Endoscopic technology, regardless of whether it is performed with a rigid scope or a flexible scope, has the following eight elements in common (Box 32.1):

1. Access portal
2. Working space
3. Illumination
4. Vision
5. Manipulation
6. Capture
7. Evacuation
8. Closure

These essentials of endoscopy are described in more detail in the following sections.

Access Portal Into the Body

1. Natural orifice or functional stoma
   a. Oral, nasal, aural, vaginal, anal, urethral. Some rigid scopes have an obturator (a blunt-tipped rod placed through the lumen) to permit smooth insertion of the instrument, such as into the anus.
   b. Natural orifice transluminal endoscopic surgery (NOTES).[1] This is a form of incisionless surgery.

   The surgical procedure is performed by entering the mouth, vagina, or anus. The endoscope is passed into the passage and traversed to a point where an incision can be made into an organ wall to access a structure within the peritoneum. Target structures include the stomach (weight loss procedures and fundoplication), adjacent structures, hernia, gallbladder, and

• **Fig. 32.1** Single-site laparoscopic port.

appendix. Research is underway for diaphragmatic pacing wires, pancreatic biopsy, and percutaneous endoscopic gastrostomy (PEG) tube revision.

Advantages of NOTES procedures include no scar, less pain, fewer complications, shorter hospital stays, and faster recovery.

The surgeon can enter the mouth and pass the endoscope into the stomach, where an incision is made through the gastric wall. The working instruments are used to excise the gallbladder and remove it from the body through the mouth. One point of concern is the closure of the gastrotomy and the potential for bleeding and leakage.

For gynecologic procedures (using vaginal natural orifice transluminal endoscopic surgery [vNOTES]), the endoscope is inserted through the vaginal wall to perform a hysterectomy or tubal and ovarian procedures.[2] A supportive retractor may be used to maintain the working space. Women with previous hysterectomies may have adhesions and may not be candidates for a transvaginal approach to the peritoneal cavity. Previous surgery of any kind may be problematic for vNOTES procedures.

Other procedures can be performed transrectally, but there are concerns for bowel contents entering the peritoneal cavity. Research is being done on the feasibility of transesophageal NOTES to enter the thoracic cavity for node staging without an external incision.

   c. Ear canal: Small specula are used to perform procedures within the ear.

2. Puncture or incision: Placement of the initial devices to introduce the expansion medium for creation of the working space requires interruption of the body's intact surface. Some surgeons use preemptive analgesia with a local anesthetic injection at the port sites at the start of the laparoscopic surgical procedure. Some surgeons inject local anesthetics at the end of the case.

   a. Multiple sites based on the type of cavity or space and the location of landmarks and blood supply.

  (1) *Open method:* An incision is made into the skin, and a 5 to 10-mm blunt Hasson trocar and sheath are placed into the cavity or space. No Veress needle is used. Expansion medium (carbon dioxide [CO_2]) can be placed through a port into the cavity or space. This procedure may be used for the patient who has many adhesions or has had multiple previous surgeries.

Single-port **laparoscopy** (single-incision laparoscopy [SIL], single-port access [SPA], one-port umbilical surgery [OPUS], and laparoendoscopic single site [LESS])[3]: One periumbilical incision is created, and a semiflexible port platform with three or four lumens is inserted. **Insufflation** is performed through accessory tubing attached to the device. The laparoscope and instrumentation are used through the lumens in the multilumen platform (Fig. 32.1).

The single-site multilumen platform can be used in robotic applications.[4] The instrumentation styles are curved or articulated and permit triangulation of placement and two-handed manipulation of internal structures. Robotic procedures can incorporate single-port incisions.

  (2) *Closed method:* A tiny nick is incised into the skin, and a Veress spring-loaded insufflation needle is placed through the skin into the peritoneal cavity for the delivery of an expansion medium such as CO_2 gas.

The surgeon can test placement of the **Veress needle** in three ways. The first way is the *manometer* test. The surgeon inserts the Veress needle and begins insufflation. If the needle is not completely in the peritoneal cavity, the manometer reading on the gas machine reads high. The gas is turned off, and the needle is advanced until the flow of the gas is unobstructed. The second method of Veress needle placement testing is by the *hanging drop* method. A small drop of sterile saline is placed at the opening of the Veress needle and is "sucked" in by the negative pressure of the peritoneal cavity. The third method of Veress needle placement is the *aspiration* test. The Veress needle is inserted with a syringe attached at the end. The surgeon attempts to aspirate through the needle. If the syringe does not permit aspiration, the placement is correct. If any fluid, blood, or other material enters the syringe, the needle has entered a viscus or vessel.

   b. Access devices for insufflation and creation of a working space.

  (1) *Veress needle:* A tiny 1 to 2-mm nick is made with the scalpel at the inferior edge of the umbilicus. The Veress needle is inserted by blind puncture **percutaneously**

(through the skin) into the abdominal cavity. This needle has an exterior sharp bevel and an interior spring-loaded ball-tip obturator that retracts as it passes through tissue.

The valve key on the top should be closed for insertion. As the sharp bevel passes through the tissue layers, the rounded obturator snaps forward to guard against inadvertent punctures of nontarget tissue.

Slight popping noises are made by the needle and spring mechanism as the needle passes through each layer. The last sound is the peritoneal perforation.

The CO_2 tubing is connected for insufflation of a working space when the surgeon is reasonably assured that the Veress needle tip is in the correct space. The gas flow is started at 1 L/min and increased to 2 L/min. The intra-peritoneal pressure should remain at 15 mm Hg for the average adult patient. Methods of placing the Veress needle into the peritoneal cavity include:

(a) *One-hand placement:* The surgeon grasps and lifts the lower abdominal (hypogastric) segment midway between the umbilicus and the superior margin of the pubis. As the abdomen is raised, the surgeon directs the Veress needle through the tissue layers until the peritoneal cavity is entered. A towel clip may be used at the infraumbilical midline to grasp and raise the abdominal wall.

(b) *Two-hand placement:* The surgeon and the first assistant grasp the abdominal tissue on either side of the umbilicus and lift. Some surgeons use Allis forceps or perforating towel clips to grasp the sides of the umbilicus. The surgeon introduces the Veress needle through the abdominal wall into the peritoneal cavity. In the average patient the needle is inserted at a 45-degree angle. In overweight patients a 90-degree angle can be used.

(2) *Trocar and sheath (sleeve):* A trocar consists of a sharp or blunt obturator and a sheath or sleeve. The primary sheaths have ports with key valves for instillation of fluids or gases. The trocars are inserted with the key valve closed to prevent evacuation of the expansion medium used to create the working space. In arthroscopy the medium is fluid. In laparoscopy the expansion medium is CO_2. The primary access portal will be the appropriate size in millimeters to accommodate the laparoscope.

(a) Sharp trocar

(i) *Pyramidal or conical tip:* Describes the configuration of the tip.

(ii) *Shielded:* A spring-loaded shield drops down and protects the sharp tip of the trocar when it is not actively cutting through tissue. Studies have shown that this mechanism does not necessarily reduce the incidence of iatrogenic trocar-induced punctures.

(b) *Blunt trocar:* The trocar tip is rounded. The blunt trocar and sheath (Hasson) are introduced through a small infraumbilical incision in the open technique. The tissue layers are retracted with S-shaped retractors. Traction sutures are placed at the level of the fascia and brought out through the skin incision. The sheath has graduated threads that permit the device to create a seal when placed through the abdominal layers. The traction sutures are tied to the sheath to stabilize and seal the pneumoperitoneum. Insufflation with CO_2 for creation of a working space is

performed through the key valve. A Veress needle is not used.

Another style of blunt trocar has a distal balloon that is inflated to anchor the trocar in place. It is placed using the open technique. A small foam collar seals the external portion of the incision.

(c) *Dilating sleeve:* The initial trocar/obturator and primary sleeve are small diameter (between 1.9 and 2.1 mm) and are introduced through a small nick in the inferior aspect of the umbilicus. The trocar is rigid, and the sheath is a flexible plastic meshwork with a stopcock for insufflation of the pneumoperitoneum.

As the initial trocar is removed, larger diameter instrumentation can be introduced through the radially dilating sleeve, causing it to dilate or "step up." The texture of the sleeve expands to accommodate a variety of diameters, such as 5, 7, 10, 11, and 12-mm instrumentation.

The skin puncture stretches and forms a seal around the access portal, anchoring it in position. The fascial puncture can be stretched to accommodate 12-mm instrumentation. The wounds measure around 4 mm when the sleeve is withdrawn and rarely need closure with suture.

c. Secondary insertion of accessory trocars for manipulation within the working space can be inserted under direct vision after the laparoscope is inserted into the primary port. Additional trocars and sleeves may be used in a triangular position around the umbilicus or primary trocar. Instrumentation for manipulation and capture is placed though these ports.

Working Space Within the Body

1. Structural working space
   a. Abdominal lift device for creation of a gasless, tent-shaped working space. No expansion media used. The working space is somewhat smaller than that created from gas insufflation. The bowel is not compressed and may be distended. Visualization is affected by the small working space. Care is taken when placing the abdominal lift hooks so as not to snare the omentum or bowel.

   The lift devices are sometimes difficult to remove without ensnaring abdominal contents. Trocar insertion is sometimes difficult because there is no back pressure or resistance to the force of placement. Blind puncture is not commonly used.

   An expandable balloon can be used to bluntly dissect and separate the abdominal wall from the abdominal contents for instrumentation placement. It takes some of the pressure off the actual lift device as it pulls upward on the abdominal wall.

   (1) Linear lift requires a frame such as an arc above the patient that attaches to a cable system placed through the patient's abdominal wall. The shape of the working space may be irregular.

   (2) Planar lift uses a corkscrew-like hook or a fanlike retractor that is placed through the abdominal wall and suspended

from an articulating arm attached to a frame on the OR bed. The shape of the working space is more trapezoid than domed like a pneumoperitoneum.
  b. Physiologic muscularity or structural framework, such as cartilage in the trachea and bronchus for upper aerodigestive flexible or rigid endoscopy.
  c. Speculum support between muscular layers such as the vaginal speculum or anoscope.
2. Expansion media
  a. *Fluid:* The bladder, uterus, and joint spaces can be expanded with fluid to create a working space.
  b. *Gas:* The peritoneal cavity is filled with CO_2 gas, creating a gas lake called a pneumoperitoneum, before a laparoscope is inserted into the primary trocar through the abdominal wall. The pneumoperitoneum expands the abdomen and provides a working space (Fig. 32.2).

With the tip of a No. 11 or 15 scalpel blade, a small incision (1–2 mm) is made into the abdominal wall at the infraumbilical margin. The spring-loaded 14-gauge Veress needle measuring 70 to 120 cm (average) to 150 cm is inserted through the tiny incision at the thinnest portion of the abdominal wall. Great care is taken when a Veress needle is used for blind puncture. The major vessels of the abdomen are at risk for injury.

Some surgeons will check for entrance into the peritoneal cavity with a syringe. Some surgeons will aspirate to check for blood or bowel contents, and others may use a saline-filled syringe to introduce a few milliliters into the opening of the Veress needle to check for any obstruction.

The CO_2 tubing is attached to the Veress needle and the gas is delivered by an insufflator, which is a specially designed machine that allows a metered flow of gas at a controlled pressure of between 12 and 18 mm Hg depending on the patient's body size and health condition. Pressure gauges on the machine will indicate if the flow is commencing appropriately.

The gas passes through sterile disposable tubing with an inline, single-use hydrophobic filter that prevents particulate matter and condensation from the gas tank from entering the abdominal cavity.

The insufflation tubing filters particulate as small as 0.2 μm. The insufflator should be positioned higher than the patient's abdomen for maximum performance. If the cylinder is placed below the level of the patient, the pressure gradient on the patient's side increases, causing a backflow of biologic contaminants into the insufflator. As a result, the internal aspect of the insufflation machine can become biologically contaminated. This can be the source of cross-contamination between patients.

The CO_2 gas itself is not sterile and is delivered to the body cold, around 73.4° F (23° C), when not passed through a heating and humidifying element. Studies have shown less hypothermia in patients when the gas is delivered at temperatures between 86° F and 95° F (30–35° C). The patient is at risk for hypothermia if core body temperature is less than 36° C. Studies have shown a decrease of 32° F (0° C) body temperature for each 50 L of CO_2 cycled through the patient.

Once the pneumoperitoneum is established, a 10 or 12-mm trocar is inserted and the insufflation tubing is attached to a port on the side of the trocar sleeve. The average adult can accommodate 5 to 6 L of CO_2 in the peritoneal cavity to create the working space. A secondary 5 or 7-mm trocar with a gas port will be inserted.

  c. *Air:* Ambient room air can be delivered into a natural body orifice by a hand pump bulb or machine to expand the lumen of the bowel for sigmoidoscopy or colonoscopy.
  d. *Balloon expansion between tissue planes:* A balloon device can be inserted between tissue layers and expanded with saline to separate and bluntly open the preperitoneal plane of dissection. After blunt dissection and expansion, the

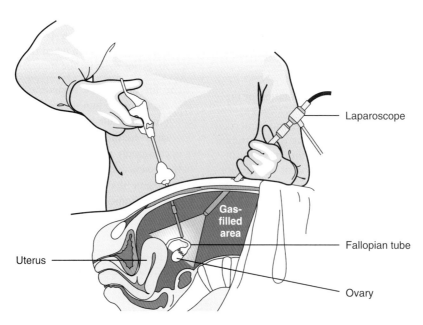

Uterus

Laparoscope

Gas-filled area

Fallopian tube

Ovary

• **Fig. 32.2** Surgeon working with laparoscopic instruments within a CO_2-filled pneumoperitoneum.

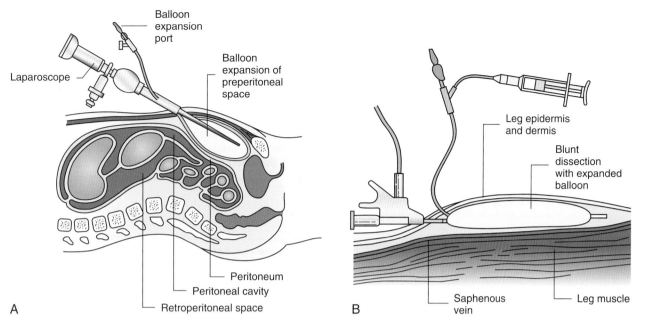

• **Fig. 32.3** Balloon expansion of surgical planes. **A,** Preperitoneal expansion. **B,** Saphenous vein harvest using balloon dissection technique.

balloon is deflated and withdrawn. The space is then insufflated. This is useful for extraperitoneal laparoscopic hernia repair procedures. Saphenous vein harvests and spinal surgery can be performed using this method (Fig. 32.3).

Illumination of the Working Space

Illumination within the body cavity is essential for visual acuity. The light source may be through a fiber-optic bundle or, rarely, from an incandescent lightbulb. The light carrier may be an integral part of the viewing sheath, as in flexible scopes and rigid telescopes, or it may be a separate light carrier accessory to a hollow rigid scope. The power source is usually electricity, but some handheld rigid scopes can use batteries.

1. *Fiber-optic light:* With fiber-optic lighting, an intense cool light illuminates body cavities, including those that cannot be seen with other light sources. Light is conducted through a bundle of thousands of coated glass fibers encased in a plastic sheath attached to a light source generator. Each fiber is drawn from optical glass into a strand 10 to 70 mm in diameter that is coated to minimize loss of light by reflection. Light entering one end of the fiber is transmitted by refraction through its entire length.

   The light produced through the bundle of fibers is nonglaring and evenly distributed on the area to be visualized. Although it is of high intensity, the light is cool. A minimal rise of temperature in the tissues exposed to it may occur. Although the light inside the patient is cool, the cable should not be allowed to lie on the drapes because it is a potential source of ignition and fire.

   Both ends of the fiber-optic cable must have the correct fittings to attach to the lamp and to the endoscope or removable light carrier. The diameter of the cable varies from 2 to 5.5 mm to be compatible with the aperture for the light source. Cable lengths also vary from 6 feet (183 cm) to 9 feet (274 cm), so the projection lamp can be positioned at a distance from a sterile field.

   Before use, the fiber-optic cable should be checked for damage. One end of the cable is held toward a low-power light, such as the overhead operating room (OR) light. Broken fibers in the cable will appear as dark spots like pepper, even to the naked eye. The cable should be replaced if more than 20% of the area appears dark. Newer light cables have a clear sheath for easier visualization of broken fibers.

   A xenon, quartz-halogen, mercury, or halide lightbulb provides an intense light source for transmission of light through a fiber-optic bundle to the distal end of the scope. Usually a portable, compact, self-contained unit, the light has an intensity that may be regulated from 400 foot-candles to as much as 5200 foot-candles, and up to 5500 Kelvin daylight in some illuminators.

2. *Other*
   a. Incandescent bulbs screw into the fitting at the end of a removable light carrier or at the end of a built-in lens system. Electric current is conducted through a single-filament wire to illuminate the tiny incandescent lightbulb. Very few instruments use this lighting system. Older-model rigid laryngoscopes are an example.
   b. Indirect lighting is used with specula, such as vaginal, nasal, or anal.

Vision Within the Working Space

1. *Scope:* The length of the scope varies but is appropriate to reach the desired structure. The surgeon views anatomic structures through a telescopic lens. The diameter of the scope

varies from the 1.7-mm needle fetoscope to the 5 mm or less of the arthroscope to the 10 to 12 mm of a laparoscope.

a. *Rigid:* A rigid scope is a telescopic rod-lens system that permits viewing in a variety of directions, such as a cystoscope. The direction of a telescope lens can be straightforward (0°) or angled (30°, 45°, 90°). Laparoscopes are made in two styles—diagnostic and operative. The diagnostic laparoscope is a single telescopic rod-lens with no accessory ports (Fig. 32.4, *A*). The operating laparoscope has the rod-lens system with one working channel (see Fig. 32.4, *B*). Operating laparoscopes have been in use since the 1970s and were the first scope to use an umbilical single-incision approach. Gynecologic surgeons used the operating laparoscope for tubal ligation and exploratory procedures.

Rigid telescopes are metal and use fiber-optic illumination. Disposable models are available. The rigid telescope used in laparoscopy is placed into the body through the primary trocar sheath.

b. *Rigid hollow:* Disposable plastic sigmoidoscopes, anoscopes, and otoscopes are available. Illumination is from a separate light carrier rod. Rigid bronchoscopes have additional side ports for administration of oxygen or anesthetics. These scopes are used through a natural body orifice.

c. *Flexible:* Flexible scopes have a directional adjuster dial that contours the lensed tip into and around anatomic curvatures to permit visualization of all surfaces of the wall of a hollow structure, such as the upper and lower gastrointestinal tract (Fig. 32.5).

The user can look directly into the eyepiece, or an attachment can be placed over the eyepiece to project the image onto a video screen. Flexible endoscopes have working channels that permit the manipulation of flexible biopsy forceps and laser fibers. A separate suction channel is on the opposite side. Two trumpet valves located near the eyepiece control suction and insufflation with air to create a viewing and working space. The covering of flexible endoscopes is made of silicone-plastic material and is usually latex-free.

2. *Camera:* A camera can be mounted to the eyepiece of the endoscope. Some cameras are used sterile, and others are high-level disinfected and covered with a sterile camera drape. The camera consists of a coupler that attaches to the eyepiece of the endoscope, a camera head, a connecting cable, and a connector to attach the camera to the camera controller box. Hi-tech cameras and monitors provide clear images (Fig. 32.6).

a. *Video:* Endoscopes may be attached to a still or video camera so that organs or lesions can be photographed during a procedure. Video cameras with recorder/player/printer equipment require high-powered light sources for photographic applications and video documentation.

By viewing high-resolution monitor(s), the endoscopist can manipulate instruments for diagnostic examination or to perform a therapeutic procedure. Video documentation can be obtained by recording the examination or procedure on a flash drive or to a CD. Microcomputer imaging systems with a printer can reproduce these images into still photographs. This equipment is either kept on a mobile cart or permanently placed in ceiling-mounted articulated booms (Fig. 32.7).

b. *Monitor:* More than one video monitor is recommended for ease of viewing the image transmitted by the endoscope by the entire team. Placement of the monitors in the direct line of vision of the surgeon and the first assistant eliminates the need to turn the head away from the field and prevents stiff neck and fatigue.

Flat-panel monitors can be suspended from the ceiling on articulated arms that permit the user to place the viewing plane in a position of function.

Other Visual Devices

1. *Wireless capsule endoscopy:* An endoscopic camera can be ingested to visualize the small bowel. The camera weighs around 4 g and measures 11 mm—about the size of a jellybean.

The endoscopic capsule contains four light-emitting diodes (LED) and a color camera. It travels by peristalsis through the small bowel, taking up to 50,000 images over an 8-hour period. The patient wears adhesive reception pads

• **Fig. 32.4** Basic rigid endoscopes. **A,** Standard rigid endoscope. **B,** Single-puncture laparoscope with working channel.

• **Fig. 32.5** Flexible endoscope.

• **Fig. 32.6** Camera and video setup for endoscopy.

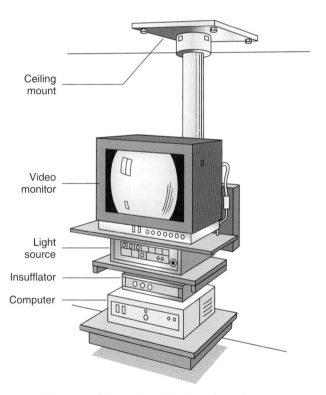

• **Fig. 32.7** Ceiling-mounted endoscopic equipment.

that transmit to a small receiver worn on a belt. No food may be consumed for 4 hours; however, liquids can be taken 2 hours after swallowing the capsule. The capsule endoscope is excreted naturally in the feces after a few days. If the capsule is not expelled, an x-ray should be taken to rule out a stricture causing entrapment of the device.

The diagnostic capabilities have proven effective even when a negative finding was noted by other means. This method of video endoscopy is useful for patients who weigh more than 20 kg and children older than 10 years.

2. *Microscopic attachments:* The optical system of some endoscopes can be attached to a specially designed operating

microscope such as the colpomicroscope (colposcope). The illumination of the endoscope and binocular magnification of the microscope permit study of abnormal tissues and/or therapeutic procedures in areas otherwise inaccessible without an open surgical procedure. Many microscopes have manipulators or "joysticks" that permit the use of laser during the procedure.

3. *Ultrasonic imaging:* A high-frequency ultrasound transducer at the end of a fiber-optic endoscope provides visualization of the heart, liver, pancreas, spleen, and kidneys. Interventional use during diagnosis of mediastinal, retroperitoneal, and gastrointestinal disease is enhanced by the use of endoscopic ultrasound scopes.

    a. *Radial echoendoscope:* Provides rotational ultrasonic imaging between 270 and 360 degrees of circumference at the tip of the endoscope. The radial scope has no access port for fine-needle aspiration.

    b. *Linear array endoscope:* Provides straightforward imaging. It has a working channel for fine-needle aspiration and a Doppler for sensing vascular structures.

    c. *Single ultrasound probes:* Provides vision similar to the radial ultrasound endoscope, but is introduced through a regular fiber-optic endoscope.

4. *Radiographic assisted:* Fluoroscopy may be preferred to video images for visualization of certain procedures such as radioactive implantation.

    a. *Contrast media:* Radiopaque contrast can be injected into the lumen of the biliary system or other structure to observe for patency or obstruction.

    b. *Radioisotopes:* Radioisotopes can be injected and traced with sensitive detector probes.

Manipulation and Maneuverability Within the Working Space

For puncture endoscopy, one or more 5 to 12-mm secondary trocars are inserted through the abdominal wall under direct video visualization at strategic points. This is to create working access portals for graspers, cutters, dissectors, staplers, and suturing devices for tissue manipulation. These accessory instruments can be passed through channels in the endoscope to, for example, remove fluid or tissue; coagulate or ligate bleeding vessels; or inject fluid, contrast

• **Fig. 32.8** Examples of instrumentation used in endoscopes.

media, or dye to distend cavities. The accessories will be determined by the type of endoscope and purpose of the procedure.

1. *Instrumentation:* Dissectors, graspers, hooks, spatulas, snares, clamps, needle holders, specimen catch bags, and probes are available for tissue manipulation through the endoscope (Fig. 32.8). The length and diameter are appropriate to the type of endoscope in use. The handle and shaft of the instrument can be rigid or flexible for procedure-specific maneuverability.

   Laparoscopic tip designs include duckbill (flat straight), dolphin (pointed straight), Babcock (tubular grasper), and Maryland (curved). Most have ring handles. Some handles lock and others simply grasp. The surface of the jaws can be smooth, serrated, or toothed and can be articulated, single action, or double action. Some of the jaws rotate. Special dissectors such as a peanut or Kittner are available on long probes for use in blunt dissection.

2. *Suturing, stapling, and clipping instrumentation:* Laparoscopic suturing instruments have one fixed and one mobile jaw. The handles lock to securely hold the needle for complex intracorporeal stitches. Knot pushers slide the knot into place. A special suturing device that shuttles the needle back and forth through tissues can be operated with one hand. To reverse the direction of the needle the surgeon presses a lever. LAPRA-TY clips can be used to secure sutures without tying a knot.

   Endoscopic gastrointestinal anastomosis (GIA) linear stapling and cutting instruments require a 12-mm port. The jaws have markings to help the surgeon line up the tissue for manipulation and stapling. Linear staplers are available to create three- to four-row staple lines without cutting. These can be used to close an enterotomy. Care is taken not to staple across a second staple line or incorporate Ligaclips in the dissection plane.

   Laparoscopic clip appliers require a 10 or 12-mm access port. Most disposable styles have a rotating jaw and a self-loading mechanism. Clips range in size from 6 to 11 mm.

3. *Functional energy-driven devices (laser, ultrasonics, suction, irrigation, electrosurgery):* A laser beam can be focused through some endoscopes. Argon, potassium titanyl phosphate (KTP), holmium:yttrium aluminum garnet (Ho:YAG), and neodymium:yttrium aluminum garnet (Nd:YAG) lasers will

pass light through a fiber. The CO_2 laser can be directed through a rigid endoscope or the interior mirror system of a multiarticulated arm of the operating microscope. The beam is then focused through the endoscope, which is held in a self-retaining device.

- A distal smoke-evacuation suction device clears plume to maintain visibility through the scope and at the site of lasing. The endoscopes are specifically designed for adaptation to the articulated arm of the CO_2 laser (e.g., the CO_2 laser laparoscope and CO_2 laser bronchoscope).
- Ultrasonic waves can be used through an endoscope to disassociate tissue or materials such as stones for removal from the body via suction or retrieval devices. Other forms of ultrasonic dissection are found in the harmonic scalpel, which moves at more than 50,000 vibrations per second to denature protein without heat. It seals small vessels by coagulation as it incises.
- An active electrode connected to a monopolar electrosurgical unit (ESU) may be used through an endoscope for surgical procedures or a resectoscope for transurethral surgery in urology. A variety of electrodes, both disposable and reusable, are available in many lengths and configurations. They must have adequate insulation and be inspected for defect before use. Care is taken not to activate the ESU tip when it is touching any of the metal staples or hemostatic clips because they may conduct the energy, causing tissue injury.
- Electrical energy transfers by capacitance from the activated electrode through intact insulation into other nearby conductive materials. Unless a safe path is provided for current to return to ground, the current induced by capacitance might cause an unintentional burn on nontargeted tissue.
- Direct coupling occurs when the activated electrode touches other metal instruments, particularly the laparoscope. An all-metal trocar/cannula system allows accidental contact to dissipate through the abdominal wall. The surgeon should avoid activating the electrode unless it is in direct contact with the tissue.
- A shielding and monitoring system is commercially available for monopolar endoscopic electrosurgical electrodes. Bipolar instruments, including dissectors, scissors, and graspers, eliminate the potential hazard of stray currents with monopolar electrodes.

4. *Adjunct organ displacement:* A uterine manipulator such as a tenaculum can be placed through the vagina to the inside of the uterus or attached to the cervix. This manipulator can be reusable or disposable and may have a channel for the instillation of colored dye for chromopertubation or radiopaque contrast medium to observe for uterine configuration and tubal patency by x-ray. The uterus can be displaced into the desired position by moving the exterior portion of the device cephalad, laterally, anteverted, or retroverted to view the pelvic structures. Some devices have a disposable patient intrauterine cannula with a reusable handgrip (e.g., RUMI or HUMI [Harris-Kronner uterine manipulator-injector]).

   Retractors can be placed through the laparoscope to provide additional exposure or displacement of organs in the endoscopic field. The expanding styles (fan-type) have hinged joints so they can be passed through the trocar sheath into the peritoneal sac and then opened widely to retract organs.

5. *Robotics:* A voice-actuated articulated arm can be used as a steady camera-holding device. The surgeon uses a programmed voice card to instruct the arm where to position and reposition the camera. Adjunct robotic manipulators can be used by a surgeon seated at a control panel manipulating joysticks to activate instrumentation inside the patient.

6. *Hand-assisted access sleeves:* Larger organs may require a tactile sense for diagnosis or excision that cannot be attained by endoscopic instruments alone. The surgeon can make a small 3-inch incision and insert a sterile inflatable or gel sleeve through which they can insert a hand into the incision without losing the pressurized field.

After sleeve assembly is placed in the incision, pneumoperitoneum can be established. Organs can be palpated or grasped by hand and removed. This method is particularly good for laparoscopic abdominal, bowel, kidney, splenectomy, and any specimen greater than 5 to 8 cm. Darker gloves are suggested for less light reflection on the video monitor.

Capture of Specimens Within the Working Space

1. Graspers and snares can be used through an endoscope to remove tissue specimens through the same access portals as the trocars. Some specimens are too large to pass through the trocar sheath, so the sheath is removed and the specimen is withdrawn through an enlarged incisional puncture or hand-assist portal site.

Instrumentation used in tissue capture can be used through all forms of endoscopes. Some instruments of this type have electrosurgical capabilities to provide hemostasis in the process.

2. Pouches with drawstrings can be introduced through the trocar sheath to capture an entire specimen for delivery to the surface via the access portals created for the trocars. Pouches are available in many sizes, including capacity for a 2-kg specimen.

Evacuation of Gases, Fluids, and Solids From the Body

1. Gases, fluids, and solids can be evacuated through an endoscope. Suction irrigators are commonly used. Ultrasonic dissectors use this principle for the evacuation of tissue through the suction port on the endoscopic instrument. The substances are biohazardous because they contain blood and body fluids.

2. Containment is used when evacuating CO_2 after the procedure is completed. The gas should not be evacuated into the room air because it contains biologic particles.

Closure or Minimizing of the Access Portal(s)

1. Closure of target internal organs with suture or other media such as staples and clips can be performed through the

endoscope. Intraabdominal ligation is achieved with loops of chromic or plain surgical gut (Endoloop ligatures). After the applicator is passed through the scope, the loop is placed around the tissue and pulled taut. An endoscopic swaged needle-suture is passed in a needle holder for suturing. Intracorporeal (inside body) and extracorporeal (outside body) knotting techniques are used to secure sutures. Endoscopic ligating clips and staples also are used for ligation and tissue approximation.

2. External punctures and incisions are closed. In adults, incisions of 5 mm are closed at the subcutaneous level; however, 10-mm incisions are closed at the fascial level to prevent herniation. In pediatric patients, 5-mm incisions are closed at the fascial level proportionate to body size.

3. Natural closure by physiologic structures such as muscular sphincters requires no intervention by the surgeon. Rigid tubular anatomy, such as bronchi, is unaffected and requires no specific closure.

Knowledge and Skill for a Safe Endoscopic Environment

Attributes of the Endoscopic Team

Each member of the endoscopic team has an important role in the performance of the surgical procedure. The intricacies of the instrumentation and the limits of the visual field require strict attention to detail and awareness of each step in the endoscopic process. The attributes of the team members complement each other within their own scope of practice. Together, they provide the knowledge and skill necessary for the safe and effective performance of an endoscopic procedure. Each member anticipates the needs of the other and is prepared to convert to an open procedure at a moment's notice.

Attributes of the Surgeon

The surgeon must have an expert knowledge of anatomy and physiology. Landmarks can look distorted and unusual through an endoscope. An inexperienced person would not be able to recognize physiologic structures in this visual context. Manual dexterity is critical for all phases of the procedure. During a puncture laparoscopy, major vascular and digestive structures are in significant jeopardy if an insufflation needle is blindly placed or if a trocar is aimed in the wrong trajectory.

Eye-hand coordination is essential for specimen capture and tissue suturing. The inability to directly view target structures with the naked eye may present some distortion of the field. Working from a monitor screen instead of using direct vision can be awkward because the eyes are not directed to the area of manipulation.

Surgeons go through extensive training and assessment before performing live surgery. Many facilities require laparoscopic certification as a requirement to practice.

Types of Endoscopic Procedures

Not all endoscopic procedures are performed as sterile procedures; some are aseptic (high-level disinfection). An endoscope is introduced into the gastrointestinal tract through the mouth or anus. It touches only intact mucous membranes. The gastrointestinal tract normally harbors resident and transient microorganisms.

Although the procedure is not considered sterile, patients and personnel are protected from cross-contamination.

Endoscopes are thoroughly cleaned and terminally sterilized or undergo high-level disinfection after use. The Spaulding classification recommends sterilization for semicritical items, including endoscopes. Accessories or instrumentation such as biopsy forceps that come into contact with nonintact tissue should be sterile. High-level disinfected flexible endoscopes should be hung from a rack after terminal processing. Instruments should be stored according to the manufacturer's recommendations. Many endoscopic procedures are performed in an endoscopy unit rather than in the OR.

Endoscopy is performed as a sterile procedure if body tissue will be incised or excised or if a normally sterile organ or body cavity is entered, such as the bladder or uterus. Ideally, the endoscope and all accessories should be sterile regardless of the point of entry. Consider the entry of the vascular system when taking biopsies and the possibility of microbial contamination.

Control of scheduling endoscopic procedures and adequate instrumentation will help provide sterile endoscopes for every patient. Written policies and procedures must specify accepted practices for patient care and infection control. AORN (Association of periOperative Registered Nurses) has developed recommended practices for the use and care of endoscopes to be used as a guide in establishing processing procedures.

Only sterile endoscopes and accessories should be used on patients with suppressed immune systems, such as from chemotherapy or steroid therapy or human immunodeficiency virus (HIV)-related diseases. Disposable endoscopes are available.

Routine practices should be established to reduce the risk for potential patient injuries and complications. These practices include, but are not limited to, the following:

- Training for and demonstrating competence in the use and care of endoscopic equipment by surgeons and perioperative personnel
- Providing complete sets of properly prepared, functional instruments
- Monitoring the patient for changes in physiologic status (e.g., development of hypercapnia and/or hypothermia can be caused by CO_2 insufflation)

All patients should be prepped and draped for conversion to an open procedure when warranted because of recognized or potential complications. Instrumentation and supplies for an open procedure should be readily available. The surgeon should inform the patient preoperatively of this possibility and should obtain an informed consent.

Laparoscopic Procedure

After the patient has been anesthetized, intubated, prepped, catheterized, and draped, the OR bed may remain flat or be tilted approximately 5 to 10 degrees into a slight Trendelenburg position. A Veress needle, blunt Hasson trocar, or single-port access device is inserted into the peritoneal cavity through a small infraumbilical incision to create the primary access portal. The anterior abdominal wall is thinnest and less vascular at the lower edge of the umbilicus, along the linea alba, which makes this area easiest for penetration of a single layer of fascia and peritoneum with minimal interruption of skin and dermal blood vessels.

The average adult peritoneal cavity is insufflated with CO_2 to an intraoperative pressure of 12 to 15 mm Hg to create the working space. Overweight patients may need higher insufflation pressures to counteract the weight of the abdominal wall. The circulating nurse monitors this pressure during insufflation; it should not fall below 8 mm Hg or rise above 18 mm Hg.

After sufficient pneumoperitoneum is established, the patient is placed in a slight reverse Trendelenburg position to shift abdominal contents caudad for upper gastrointestinal procedures. A padded footboard should be in place to prevent the patient from sliding downward on the OR bed. Moderate Trendelenburg position is used for lower pelvic procedures to shift abdominal contents cephalad.

If a Veress needle is used to create the working space with CO_2 gas, it is replaced by a trocar and sheath, which is inserted into the peritoneal cavity. The insufflation tubing is disconnected from the Veress needle and attached to the inlet port of the trocar sleeve. The sharp obturator is then removed from the trocar sheath. A rigid 7 or 10-mm, 0° laparoscope with a light cable is introduced into the abdomen through the trocar sheath. The sheath matches the size of the laparoscope.

If the Hasson blunt trocar is used, the trocar is placed percutaneously through the abdominal wall. The surgeon will make an incision and enter the peritoneal cavity. The edges of the deeper tissue will be held with traction sutures or S-retractors as the trocar is introduced. Once in position, the Hasson will be attached to the insufflation tubing and used to insufflate, creating the working space without the blind puncture technique. Once the working space is established, the blunt obturator will be removed and the laparoscope is inserted. The use of a Hasson trocar is referred to as *open laparoscopy.*

The cold CO_2 gas flowing through the primary access portal sleeve may cause the lens to fog as the scope enters the warm peritoneal cavity. Some surgeons use a sterile antifog solution on the laparoscope lens. Commercial scope warmers that look like a thermos canister may be used. The container should contain only warm sterile water. Saline use can be corrosive to instrumentation. Disposable active charcoal scope warming sleeves are available. They are easy to use and convenient.

If a single-port device is not used, one or two secondary 5, 7, or 10-mm trocars are inserted through the abdominal wall under direct vision through the laparoscope. Placement of multiple secondary trocars will form a triangular pattern on the abdomen for insertion of multiple instruments. The CO_2 insufflation tubing can be connected to a secondary port inlet to minimize the effect of the cold gas against the laparoscope lens that could cause fogging inside the warm body of the patient.

If a 10, 12, or 15-mm trocar is used, sizing caps or lumen reducers can be used to reduce the opening of the sheath for the use of smaller endoscopic instruments and probes. The use of size-reducing caps prevents the escape of pneumoperitoneum.

A sterile camera attached to the laparoscope transmits images on video monitor(s). Two monitors, one on each side of the OR bed, generally are used. Without straining their necks, the surgeon and the team can view the manipulation of instruments inserted through secondary ports in the direct line of vision.

At the conclusion of the procedure, the CO_2 should be evacuated through the suction port on the trocar into the vacuum system and not expelled directly into the room air. The expelled gas contains plume, blood, and body fluids that cause airborne contamination. Personal protective equipment, such as masks and eyewear, should be worn by all personnel in the room.

Some surgeons prefer to use a gasless method for displacing and expanding the abdomen during laparoscopy. A device referred to as an *abdominal lift* can be used to elevate the abdominal wall for minimal access procedures without the use of CO_2. Shorter instrumentation can be used because the internal organs are closer to the surface.

Pediatric Endoscopy

Pediatric endoscopy is a common method of diagnosis and treatment. Procedures such as appendectomy, pyloromyotomy, fundoplication, orchiopexy, nephrectomy, ureteral procedures, and cancer staging are examples of endoscopic surgery performed successfully in children. Robotic approaches are generally successful; however, the procedural time may be increased. One advantage is the robotic instrument tips are much smaller than the surgeon's hands and can accomplish delicate maneuvers relatively easier.

Procedural Considerations for Laparoscopy in Children

Anatomic differences between children and adults are most pronounced between the ages of birth to 8 years. Infants have large umbilical vessels that are easily damaged and may even be permeable to CO_2. The processus vaginalis at the inguinal ring may be weak and easily opened inadvertently by a pneumoperitoneum. The aortoiliac axis is nearer the surface and may be punctured by the trocars or instrumentation. The left epigastrium or the right hypochondrium is a good site for initial insufflation. A 1-year-old child may accommodate a 1-L working space. Smaller, shorter instruments and scopes should be used.

The visual field is limited by the small size of the child, sometimes as small as 4 to 5 mm. Hasson trocars and sheaths may be preferred to other methods if CO_2 insufflation must be used. In some circumstances, abdominal wall lift devices are more appropriate for a safe and effective procedure.

General anesthesia is used, and the child should have an empty bladder. The bladder is higher in the abdomen than it is in adults. A Foley catheter and a nasogastric tube are useful for decompression of internal structures before a laparoscopy. After the skin prep and sterile draping, the infraumbilical incision is made. A mosquito hemostat is inserted into the incision and opened to stretch the wound slightly.

Some surgeons prefer to use an open laparoscopic method as opposed to a blind puncture. A radial dilating trocar can be placed in the tiny incision and can be sequentially enlarged with instrumentation to the desired size. It can be secured with suture to prevent dislodgment. Pneumoperitoneum is established with CO_2 insufflation at 8 mm Hg to the desired level. Pressure should not exceed 8 mm Hg for infants and 12 mm Hg in children to 8 years of age. Smaller telescopes are usually adequate with a 0° to 30° viewing angle. Secondary trocars are inserted sharply under direct vision of the laparoscope.

Endoscopy and the Pregnant Patient

Endoscopy can be performed on pregnant patients. The usual risks for laparoscopy are present with addition of the risk to the fetus and the potential for preterm birth. The team must keep in mind that two patients are involved with the procedure. The risk for spontaneous abortion is ever present. If the fetus is viable, the team must be prepared for a surgical preterm delivery.

The most common laparoscopic applications include appendectomy, cholecystectomy, and ovarian procedures. Other procedures include laparoscopic cerclage of the uterine cervix for patients with cervical insufficiency (formerly known as cervical incompetency). The isthmus of the cervix can be banded with Mersilene tape before the 13th week of gestation.

Laparoscopy during the first trimester potentially increases the risk to the developing fetus as a result of the anesthetic. The severity of the mother's disease such as infection or preeclampsia plays a role. Second-trimester laparoscopy increases the risk for nontarget organ or vessel damage because the typical landmarks are distorted. Visceral displacement by the enlarging uterus changes the landscape of the internal structures.

Recommended techniques include using the open laparoscopic method using the Hasson trocar and minimizing operative times. The patient should have her right side slightly elevated to displace the uterus from the inferior vena cava and a Foley catheter to keep the urinary bladder empty.[5] Antiembolic hose should be applied to decrease the risk for deep vein thrombosis (DVT). If x-ray will be used, the fetus should be completely shielded. Uterine manipulators are not used.

Placement of the primary trocar depends on the height of the fundus. The open technique using a Hasson trocar is a safe method. A Veress needle can be used under ultrasound guidance. A subxyphoid approach between 2 and 6 cm above the umbilicus is a common location. An alternative site is Palmer point in the left upper quadrant, 2 cm below the costal margin at the midclavicular line. The secondary trocars can be placed under direct visualization. Single-incision ports have been used with some success.

End-tidal CO_2 should be monitored closely and maintained between 25 and 30 mm Hg to prevent fetal acidosis. The intraperitoneal pressure should be between 12 and 15 mm Hg. If the fetus is of viable age (around 24 weeks), a transvaginal ultrasound should be used. Any sign of fetal distress indicates the need to release the pneumoperitoneum immediately. If the fetus is not of viable gestational age, a Doppler should be used to document heart tones preoperatively and postoperatively. More information about pregnant patients and endoscopy can be found at www.sages.org.

Hazards of Endoscopy

Endoscopy is not without its hazards. Minimally invasive surgery requires appropriate credentialing. Surgeons who wish to perform laparoscopy and other endoscopic techniques should be credentialed through the medical staff department. Personnel who are responsible for scheduling endoscopic procedures should confirm the surgeon's practice privileges. Serious complications of endoscopy include the following:

1. *Perforation:* Perforation of a major organ or vessel is a constant cause for concern when sharp trocars and rigid scopes are used. Flexible fiber-optic endoscopes have decreased this danger, but it remains a potential complication. Patient positioning from supine to Trendelenburg position shifts the intraabdominal anatomy, causing elevation of the major vessels of the lower abdominal cavity. Care is taken to prevent inadvertent injury to these structures while holding cameras or other devices situated in intraabdominal trocar sleeves during repositioning of the OR bed.

   The sharp obturator should be examined briefly after it is withdrawn from the trocar sleeve. The presence of gross blood, stool, bile, or other unidentified substance may indicate perforation of an intraabdominal organ.

2. *Bleeding:* Bleeding can occur from a biopsy site, pedicle of a polyp, or other area where tissue has been cut. Endoscopic sutures or clips can become dislodged. Care is taken to observe for pooling of blood in the body cavity that may indicate venous oozing or other vessel disruption.

3. *Hypothermia:* CO_2 is colder than body temperature. The patient may experience moderate to severe hypothermia if other warming measures, such as forced-air warming or heating blankets, are not used. Hypothermia can alter the effects of propofol and increase the incidence of hypothermic coagulopathy.

4. *Preperitoneal insufflation:* If the Veress needle was not inserted completely into the peritoneal cavity, the CO_2 can be insufflated into the preperitoneal tissues. The trocar can be inserted and the gas evacuated through the inlet side port. The gas is a biocontaminant and should be evacuated via the suction.

5. *Gas embolism:* Gas in the vascular system can cause a cardiovascular collapse. Signs include dysrhythmias, tachycardia, cyanosis, and pulmonary edema. Treatment includes stopping the CO_2 flow, placing the patient in a left lateral position, elevating the right side slightly, hyperventilating with 100% O_2, and the anesthesiologist can pass a right CVP catheter to aspirate blood from the right atrium (Durant procedure).

6. *Incidental iatrogenic injury:* Robotic attachments or frames attached to the OR bed can cause pressure against the patient's body. Brachial plexus injury can occur after laparoscopic or robotic procedures caused by placement of the equipment. Stirrups and other table-positioning devices can cause iatrogenic injury if not used safely.

Electrical systems used with endoscopy must conform to the standards and be subjected to the routine maintenance procedures prescribed by the National Fire Protection Association code for electrical safety. Two major electrical hazards associated with endoscopy are as follows:

1. *Improperly grounded electrical equipment:* If the surgeon will be using a monopolar ESU, place the return electrode on the patient with adequate skin contact to allow return of electric current. Only solid-state generators, and preferably bipolar active electrodes, should be used to avoid variances in voltage. A new return electrode should be placed if the patient is repositioned from a lithotomy to supine position for an open abdominal procedure. The return electrode may gape and lose sufficient contact with the skin when the legs are moved. Pads should not be removed and repositioned. The adhesive may have weakened after the first application. If the large Megadyne bed pad is used, the patient should be positioned correctly on the pad.

2. *Unsuspected current leaks:* Corrosion or accumulation of organic material can inhibit flow of current across the screw fitting between the light carrier and the bulb. Current can leak through the instrument to the patient. Ideally, endoscopes should not contain electrically conductive elements or metals that can corrode. Corrosion can be caused by repeated exposure to body fluids, hard water, or chemical agents.

Microorganisms, such as *Mycobacterium tuberculosis,* can be transmitted from one patient to another via a bronchoscope. Disposable bronchoscopes are available. *Streptococcus pneumoniae, Pseudomonas aeruginosa, Clostridium* organisms, and bloodborne pathogens also present potential hazards of cross-contamination. Personnel are exposed to potentially infectious body fluids and blood from aerosols, splashes, and contact with contaminated instrumentation. Gloves, masks, protective eyewear, gowns, and/or aprons are worn during endoscopic procedures and cleaning of equipment. Personnel should use standard precautions during endoscopic procedures and when handling and processing contaminated endoscopes and accessories.

Care of Endoscopes

Endoscopes are delicate and expensive instruments. Rough handling, jarring, or bending of parts should be avoided. They should never be piled on top of each other or mixed with other instruments. Endoscopes should be cleaned and flushed at the point of use with the manufacturer's recommended cleaning solution. Contaminated endoscopes should be transported to the processing area in a biohazard container. Facility policies should be in place for handling contaminated endoscopes for personnel safety.

All parts of endoscopes and accessories are thoroughly disassembled, mechanically cleaned, and terminally sterilized or subjected to high-level disinfection after use. The primary causes of infection, such as herpes, hepatitis, or condylomata transmitted endoscopically, are inadequate cleaning and disinfection or sterilization of endoscopic equipment.

Cleaning

All parts of the endoscope should be cleaned as soon as possible after use while organic debris is still moist. Mucus, blood, feces, and protein-type residue can become trapped in the channels of the scope. This material is difficult to remove if it dries and may render the scope useless.

Endoscopes should be washed in warm, never hot, water and a neutral, nonresidue liquid-detergent solution. A pipe cleaner or small brush may be used to clean inside the lumens of all channels. The stopcocks on some scopes should be thoroughly disassembled for cleaning, too, because dirty valves will stick. Stopcocks are opened for cleaning; they should never be forced but can be loosened with a drop of solvent or lubricant.

Particular attention should be paid to lens cleanliness, or viewing will be obstructed. Debris can be carefully removed from around the lens with a fine toothpick. Special lens paper is used on the lens itself. Lensed instruments should not be cleaned with any substance that could dissolve cement around the lens. Consult the manufacturer's recommendations.

The endoscope is rinsed thoroughly and dried well. If scopes are to be sterilized in ethylene oxide gas, they must be thoroughly dry. Ethylene oxide combines with water on items that are damp to form ethylene glycol. Alcohol on cotton can be used on a stylet or a pipe cleaner to dry insertion tubes. Air can be forced through channels to dry inside them. Because organisms will multiply in a moist environment, all parts should be dry during the interval before further processing or storage.

An endoscope processor is available to clean long, flexible fiberoptic scopes, such as a colonoscope. It has two modes of operation to process the scope and its channels: a wash-and-dry cycle and a cycle of wash, disinfectant soak with activated recommended cleaning solution, rinse, and dry. Some endoscopes are cleaned with a solution of hydrogen peroxide and peroxyacetic acid.[6] This equipment is an automated washer/disinfector.

Accessories are scrupulously cleaned. All debris is removed to ensure adequate steam sterilization. Disposable, single-use biopsy forceps and cytology brushes are recommended because the configurations of these accessories are particularly difficult to clean. Some trocars, scissors, and forceps have disposable or replaceable points or tips on reusable shafts or handles. These combination instruments facilitate cleaning and ensure a sharp cutting edge with each use.

Scopes and accessories should be inspected for damage after cleaning. Preferably, all endoscopic equipment should be terminally sterilized; otherwise it should be high-level disinfected after thorough mechanical cleaning.

Sterilization

After cleaning and drying, each endoscope with all of its parts disassembled is placed in a well-padded perforated tray of convenient size. Some endoscopes, such as an arthroscope, are supplied in a perforated case lined with foam cut to fit each disassembled part. The tray or fitted case is wrapped for sterilization. Instruments should be wrapped and sterilized by the method recommended by the manufacturer.

Some parts of endoscopes can be safely steam sterilized and therefore should be. Hollow, rigid metal sheaths, such as a sigmoidoscope, can be terminally steam sterilized after use but then may be stored to keep clean rather than sterile for a surgically aseptic procedure. Some fiber-optic cables also can be steam sterilized. Reusable biopsy forceps should be steam sterilized.

Parts with lenses and some fiber-optic carriers, such as a colonoscope, cannot be steam sterilized. High temperature and moisture will soften the cement holding lenses or fiber-optic fibers in place. The flexible shafts of some accessory instruments may erode when steam sterilized. These parts should be sterilized in ethylene oxide gas, hydrogen peroxide plasma, or soaked in a chemical sterilant solution if ethylene oxide or hydrogen peroxide is not available.[6] The lumens must be completely dry before sterilization.

The manufacturer may recommend that the pressure not exceed 5 lbs during ethylene oxide sterilization of a fiber-optic lighting system. The manufacturer's instructions for handling, using, cleaning, and sterilizing these items should be followed. Aeration is necessary after ethylene oxide sterilization. Ethylene oxide is a vesicant if it comes into contact with skin. It also can cause eye irritation.

If endoscopes and accessories are immersed in activated glutaraldehyde or acetic acid, a plastic tray should be used without a towel in the bottom. Prolonged use of a stainless steel tray may create an electrolytic action between the metals and can cause metallic deposits on instruments. Scopes and all accessories should be well rinsed in sterile distilled water before they are used, to prevent tissue irritation from solution.

Peracetic acid, another chemical sterilant in solution, is commercially available for sterilizing endoscopes for immediate patient use. The STERIS system has specialized tray assemblies for endoscope processing. These tray assemblies are not intended for long-term storage of sterilized instruments, but for immediate patient use.

Storage

If endoscopes are not wrapped for sterilization and storage, they are terminally sterilized by chemical means or at least undergo high-level disinfection before being returned to their respective storage cabinets. Clean, dry, unwrapped rigid instruments should be stored on a soft material such as plastic sheeting or foam. Towels hold a residue of laundry detergent that can tarnish metal. Flexible endoscopes with detachable parts should be stored disassembled, hung in a vertical position with the distal end pointed downward. Accessories also may be hung. The lumens should be flushed with alcohol to facilitate fluid evaporation.

The scope should be subjected to high-level disinfection or peracetic acid sterilization before use in patient care.

Considerations for Patient Safety

Endoscopy through a natural body orifice is usually performed on a patient who is not under general anesthesia. The following considerations should be included in the plan of care:
1. The patient should be monitored for signs and symptoms of reaction to drugs. Endoscopy is frequently performed with the use of sedatives and a topical or local anesthetic agent or with no anesthetic at all. The patient is awake during these procedures. Drugs such as midazolam (Versed), diazepam (Valium), propofol (Diprivan), opioids, and narcotics may be administered intravenously as an adjunct to other preoperative sedation to produce relaxation and cooperation during the procedure and amnesia afterward. Respiratory depression and transient hypotension can occur. Antagonistic drugs should be available to reverse narcotic depression. Emergency resuscitation equipment should be available.
2. A topical agent is frequently applied to nasal or oral and pharyngeal mucosa before introduction of an endoscope into the tracheobronchial tree or gastrointestinal tract. A topical agent may be instilled into the urethra before introduction of a cystoscope.
3. The teeth, gums, and lips are protected if the endoscope is introduced through the mouth. Dentures are removed. A mouthpiece is inserted.
4. Hydrogen and methane gases are normally present in the colon. These gases are flushed out with carbon dioxide (CO_2) before laser surgery or electrosurgery through the colonoscope to avoid the possibility of explosion within the colon.
5. Power sources and lights should be tested before each use and after cleaning. They should be kept in working order.
6. The heat generated from the projection lamp of a fiber-optic illuminator is dissipated. It should not be enclosed in drapes because the heat could set them on fire. If the unit contains a fan for heat regulation, the direction of airflow should be away from the patient and the sterile field to minimize airborne contamination.
7. Endoscopes should be smooth, with no nicks on the surface. A scratch on the sheath could injure tissue or the mucous membrane lining of an orifice. Metal endoscopes should be individually wrapped and sterilized to prevent surface scratches from contact with other metallic instruments. Metallic endoscopes should be handled only with gloved hands.
8. Extreme care should be taken to observe patients after endoscopic procedures for effects of respiratory or circulatory system distress caused by gas absorption, trauma, or medication.

Many flexible endoscopic procedures are performed on ambulatory outpatients. The patients must not leave the facility until vital signs are stable and side effects have passed. Follow-up phone calls are suggested within 24 to 48 hours to monitor patient progress and answer questions. Any patient concerns should be directed to the surgeon. Additional follow-up phone calls may be necessary.

Duties of the Assistant for Flexible Endoscopy

Often only a circulating nurse assists the surgeon with a minimally invasive procedure. The assistant's duties are as follows:

1. Set up the supplies and equipment as much as possible before the patient and surgeon arrive. Consult the procedure book. Remember that sterility must be maintained for a sterile procedure.
2. Explain the steps of the procedure to the patient as appropriate. It is important that the patient know the reasons for any discomfort that may be experienced so that symptoms of discomfort will be recognized as normal.
3. Explain the position and need for it before positioning the patient. The position the patient must assume during the procedure is often uncomfortable.
4. Drape the patient properly to prevent unnecessary exposure.
5. Adjust room lighting. The surgeon may want the room in semidarkness. A dimmer on the room light is helpful, but if one is unavailable, the radiograph view boxes may be illuminated to provide indirect lighting.
6. Divert the patient's attention as much as possible during the procedure. The patient may complain of pain more than is justified as a way of expressing displeasure at the invasion of the endoscope or the position required during the procedure. The circulating nurse should stay with the patient to offer reassurance and emotional support. Suggest that slow, deep breaths may help relaxation and lessen the discomfort. Soft music may help the patient relax. The surgeon may allow the patient to watch the procedure through a viewing attachment on the endoscope or on a video monitor.
7. Evaluate the patient's level of discomfort, and inform the surgeon of unusual reactions. The circulating nurse also monitors the patient's respiratory status, blood pressure, and pulse. Pulse oximeter and automated blood pressure devices may be used routinely. Vital signs should be documented before the procedure begins, every 15 minutes during the procedure, and again at the conclusion. Additional vital signs should be recorded when medication is given or tissue samples are excised.
8. Know how to assemble the different scopes and their accessories and how to operate them. When passing the suction tube or biopsy forceps, place the tip directly at the lumen of the scope so the surgeon can grasp the shaft and insert it without moving their eyes from the scope.
9. Care for surgical specimens as appropriate.
10. Take care not to drop endoscopic instruments; they are delicate and expensive. Fiber-optic bundles are glass; do not kink or bend them.

Endoscopic procedures are considered minimally invasive except for ophthalmoscopy because the scope is placed into a body orifice or cavity. Many require one or more small skin incisions for insertion of the scope and accessories. Endoscopy is used for many diagnostic and surgical procedures.

AORN has developed recommended practices for endoscopic minimally invasive surgery.

Robotic-Assisted Endoscopy

The first robotic-type system available in the United States, AESOP (Automated Endoscopic System for Optimal Positioning), provided a stable laparoscopic telescope/camera holder with a bed-mounted articulated arm controlled by a voice-actuated computer.[7] The device is voice actuated by the surgeon who wears a microphone headset during the procedure to verbally direct the aim and direction of the laparoscope. The robot discerns verbal commands because a voice card trained with the surgeon's spoken word is inserted into a microprocessor housed in the base of the unit. Each command causes the sterile-draped articulated arm to respond by assuming the exact position requested by the surgeon.

Intuitive Surgical later developed Navigator to hold the laparoscope/camera assembly steady and to change the visual field from micro to macro without causing the sensation of "seasickness" in the team as they visualize the surgical site on the monitor. The Navigator regulates the temperature of the laparoscope to prevent fogging. In 2000, the da Vinci robotic system was approved by the U.S. Food and Drug Administration (FDA). It has continued to update its technology to meet the needs of patients and surgeons.

In 2019, the Versius system was introduced to the OR. It is a portable robot that can be transported to any room. It is easy to set up and does not take up much space. In 2021, the FDA approved the first robotically assisted surgical device for transvaginal hysterectomy called the Hominis. Other robotic systems are also in use.

Robotic technology has revolutionized the endoscopic approach to surgery. The devices currently found in operating rooms around the world range from simple camera holders to full room control at the command of the surgeon. Examples of contemporary robotic-integrated components include the following:
- Environmental control computer platform
- Functional peripheral equipment
- Instrument manipulating robot
- Master control console

Environmental Control by Robotics

Environmental control robotic systems are built into a computer-directed platform in which the surgeon verbally controls other computer-generated activities such as lights, bed motion, and other devices during the surgical procedure.

Environmental control systems have been developed by which peripheral equipment such as the ESU, lights, OR bed, insufflator, light source, and other mechanized devices in the OR are voice controlled by the surgeon. The surgeon can address the system through a headset and request a preloaded computed tomography (CT) scan to appear on a computer monitor.

Real-time verbal and video documentation is recorded for the permanent record. The surgical report is generated by electronic media, and a hard copy is printed simultaneously. Many companies such as STERIS, Skytron, Stryker, Storz, Olympus, Medtronic, Ethicon Endosurgery, and CONMED have coordinated with more than 16 robotic companies to develop compatible devices.

Functional Peripheral Equipment

Machines used during the surgical procedure can be controlled by the environmental control computer platform. All the endoscopic equipment such as light source, insufflator, electrosurgery unit, irrigator, aspirator, image recorder, and video monitor can be activated, adjusted, and directed by the surgeon's touch on a foot pedal or command into a headset. Other devices in the room such as the spotlights and OR bed respond in kind to the direction given by the surgeon. Casual conversation is ignored by the computer.

Instrument-Manipulating Robot and the Master Console

Surgical robots are hands-free systems wherein the surgeon sits or stands at a master console several feet away from the field (Fig. 32.9). The surgeon remotely manipulates three to four articulated arms with joysticks while observing each precision action with a three-dimensional (3D) binocular laparoscope and a 3D digital camera on a 3D high-definition video touch screen with

full depth of field (Fig. 32.10). The camera system can work with low levels of light.

Early robotic features included a double console with a communication intercom that permits two surgeons to collaborate and work simultaneously. The system offered the surgeons more control over the video, audio, and customized ergonomic settings. Surgeons in training find this technology engaging and efficient for learning robotic technology. The foot pedals permit the primary surgeon to switch between energy modalities. Other features include a multi-image viewer that can tile the images for comparative views. The one-piece drape for the robot streamlines the setup procedure.

Most robots offer magnified 3D high definition with true depth perception. The design allows for freedom of robotic cart positioning over all four quadrants of the patient. The da Vinci Xi does not require focusing, white balancing, or other calibration before use.

• **Fig. 32.9** Layout of a robotic system. *3D,* Three-dimensional; *OR,* operating room.

4-arm robot   Surgeon console

• **Fig. 32.10** Robotic components.

• **Fig. 32.11** Surgeon at robotic console.

The surgeon has 1 cubic foot of comfortable space wherein to work the controls and switch views in real-time action. The da Vinci robot will not operate if the surgeon's forehead is not seated inside the face port viewer. The unit will lock and remain immobile until the surgeon's head is again placed in the correct position (Fig. 32.11).

The backup battery will run for 20 minutes in the event of a power failure. The robot runs on a dedicated circuit and requires 24 hours to recharge the battery. Each robot has an emergency stop button in the event of malfunction. There is an override switch to continue the surgery if the fault is a false alarm.

Each instrument is specially designed with a microchip that communicates with the computer to log each use. The computer tracks the function of the instrument and reports when it needs to be changed or repaired. Only instruments made by Intuitive Surgical or created by agreement with specific permissions work with the da Vinci robot (e.g., harmonic scalpel, dissectors). Reposable instruments are available and should be cleaned with sterile water, never saline because of the corrosion potential. Most reposable instruments are good for 12 to 18 uses and may be

marked with a permanent marker to document each use. Sterile wrenches are included in the instrument set in case of emergency conversion to an open procedure. The articulating arms can be disengaged at the field without contamination.

The system is voice actuated and may be controlled by a surgeon who is many miles away by telecollaboration, although this is not the intent of current technology. Many cardiac, prostatic, gynecologic, and general surgery procedures have been successfully performed by the surgeon using robotic technology. The articulated arms perform the procedure using a three- or four-arm laparoscopic system that offers a circumferential 360-degree wrist-like movement for precision grasping, manipulation, dissection, clamping, and suturing of tissues. Hand tremor is eliminated, and ambidextrous movement is facilitated with natural hand-wrist motion.

Motions are described in geometric terms aligned with seven degrees of freedom in human wrist and arm-articulated motion. These motions are described as follows:
• Roll—rotation or circumduction
• Pitch—up and down
• Yaw—side to side
• Grip—open and close
• Insertion—back and forth
• Clockwise
• Counterclockwise

Most specialty services (cardiac, vascular, urology, gynecology, spine, orthopedic) use robotics. Orthopedics and neurosurgery use robotic systems such as ROBODOC, ORTHODOC, and Neuromate by Intuitive Surgical. ROBODOC is a computer-controlled robot that drills bones for prosthetic implants and can remove old bone cement. ORTHODOC displays CT images for preoperative planning for arthroplasty. Neuromate is a surgical robot to assist with stereotactic brain surgery.

The Mako robotic arm system by Stryker uses CT preoperative scans for planning, intraoperative cutting technology, and joint balancing for total knee, partial knee, and total hip arthroplasty.

PROBOT assists with urologic surgery for prostatectomy. Instrumentation used through the access portals includes monopolar and bipolar electrodes, ultrasonics, sharp and blunt dissectors, graspers, clip appliers, and needle holders. Numerous robotic companies have designed robots with technology for use in specific surgeries such as ENT, spine, vascular, hysterectomy, and cardiovascular surgery. The Magellan robotic system is designed for vascular catheterization. Emerging robotic systems can reach challenging areas with clear visualization and precise movement.

Virtual Reality

Virtual reality is the computer science of simulating real-life motion, time, and space. Computer-generated images mimic real-life situations. Some facilities have initiated virtual reality training programs for surgeons and operators of complex technologic equipment. The surgeon-in-training practices a procedure without touching a real patient. The surgeon dons a specialized headset/visor and sensor gloves and selects the training scenario to be practiced. The computer displays a 3D video of human anatomy in the headset/visor. The sensor gloves signal motion, direction, and pressure to a computer and in turn create a sensation of touch for the surgeon. The entire activity looks, feels, and responds as if the surgeon were performing surgery on an actual patient. This investigative technology can allow for "practice surgery" while evaluating the skill and dexterity of the surgeon.

The possibilities for integrating advanced technologies to simplify surgery and make it less painful and safer for patients seem endless as surgeons develop and refine innovative techniques. The challenges for all members of the OR team are to learn about technologic advances and monitor the quality of patient care in their application. Engineering performance (i.e., clinical application of biotechnology) is measured by reliability, safety, maintenance, and effectiveness of equipment. Clinical performance is measured by the skills of users to achieve desired results—a successful outcome for the patient.

Human Intervention During Robotic-Assisted Procedures

A sterile team is at the sterile field to guide tiny 1- to 2-cm incisions through the skin, place the Veress needle or trocars, and perform typical activities, such as draping, sponging, and dressing the surgical site.

The FDA requires the manufacturers to provide training for surgeons. Facilities using robotics require credentialing before the surgeon can schedule procedures. The surgeon should be mentored for 15 or more procedures before operating solo.

Although referred to as *robotic,* the procedures performed using machines require the surgeon's hands to manipulate the joysticks so the articulated arms and tips can mimic motions on a microscopic level. None of these devices have the power of decision-making and cannot run without human intervention.

Advantages and Disadvantages of Robotic-Assisted Surgery

Advantages of robotic-assisted techniques include greater precision than the human hand can provide alone and greater freedom of motion, without the tremor and fatigue associated with maintaining a position for a long period.

Disadvantages of the computerized systems include start-up costs, the learning curve, and time in training. Long-term studies need to be done to establish the full range of uses and efficacy. Many standardized procedures will need revision to be suited to new technology. Additional consideration should be given to the size and positioning of the robotic arms, draping, and console units. Computerized technology requires adequate space for the additional machinery and team members. Ceiling-mounted booms may provide consolidation of essential endoscopic machinery, thereby reducing the floor space used by the large pieces of equipment. The use of the room is limited for other surgical procedures when the mounted equipment cannot be easily rotated out of the field.

Some surgeons state that the "haptic sense" is lacking, meaning that the tactile sense, or touch, of tissues is not as sensitive as working inside an open patient for some procedures.

ⓔ EVOLVE WEBSITE

http://evolve.elsevier.com/Hornacky/BerryKohn/

- Historical Perspectives
- Tips for the Scrub Person and Circulating Nurse
- Student Interactive Questions
- Glossary

References

1. Simek C, Kaan H, Aihara H: Future directions for robotic endoscopy—artificial intelligence (AI), three-dimensional (3D) imaging, and natural orifice transluminal endoscopic surgery (NOTES), *Techn Innov Gastrointest Endosc* 25(1):95−101, 2022.
2. Baekelandt J, Kapurubandara S: A novel approach using vaginal natural orifice endoscopic surgery to repair a symptomatic uterine isthmocele, *Fertil Steril* 119(2):328−330, 2023.
3. Carrara A, Lauro E, Fabris L, et al.: Endo-laparoscopic reconstruction of the abdominal wall midline with linear stapler, the THT technique: early results of the first case series, *Ann Med Surg* 38(1−7), 2019.
4. Bang JY, Amoletti JP, Holt B: An endoscopic transluminal approach, compared with minimally invasive surgery, reduces complications, *Gastroenterology* 156(4):1027−1040, 2019.
5. Das Deepanjana D, Propst K, Wechter ME, et al.: Evaluation of positioning devices for optimization of outcomes in laparoscopic and robotic-assisted gynecology surgery, *J Minim Invasive Gynecol* 26(2):224−252, 2019.
6. Molloy-Simard V, Lemyre JL, Martel K, et al.: Evaluating the standard of endoscope processing: terminal sterilization of duodenoscopes using a hydrogen peroxide-ozone sterilizer, *Am J Infect Control* 4(3):243−250, 2018.
7. Garstka M, Alameer E, Awwad S, et al.: Conventional robotic endoscopic thyroidectomy for thyroid cancer, *Endocrinol Metab Clin North Am* 48(1):153−163, 2018.

Bibliography

AORN: *Guidelines for perioperative practice,* Denver, CO, 2024, The Association.

Bishoff J, Kavoussi L: *Atlas of laparoscopic and robotic urologic surgery,* ed 4, Philadelphia, 2023, Elsevier.

Kamboj A, Hoversten P, Leggett C: Upper gastrointestinal bleeding: etiologies and management, *Mayo Clin Proc* 94(4):697−703, 2019.

Novitsky Y: *Atlas of robotic general surgery,* St. Louis, 2022, Elsevier.

33

General Surgery

CHAPTER OUTLINE

Special Considerations for General Surgery, 664

Breast Procedures, 666

Abdominal Procedures, 670

Liver Procedures, 674

Splenic Procedures, 675

Pancreatic Procedures, 675

Esophageal Procedures, 676

Gastrointestinal Surgery, 677

Intestinal Procedures, 682

Colorectal Procedures, 686

Abdominal Trauma, 688

Anorectal Procedures, 691

Hernia Procedures, 692

Amputation of Extremities, 694

CHAPTER OBJECTIVES

After studying this chapter, the learner will be able to:

- Describe the pertinent surgical anatomy of the breast.
- Describe the surgical procedures used to diagnose breast cancer.
- Identify the pertinent anatomy of the abdominal organs within the peritoneal cavity.
- Discuss the differences between laparoscopic and open cholecystectomy.

- List the types of anastomoses used for intestinal surgery.
- List several surgical diagnostic procedures used to evaluate abdominal trauma.
- Differentiate between direct and indirect inguinal hernia.
- Discuss the psychologic effects of limb amputation on the patient under regional anesthesia.

KEY TERMS AND DEFINITIONS

-itis Inflammation of an organ or part.

-ectomy Removal of an organ or part.

-otomy Opening into an organ.

-ostomy Creation of an opening in an organ or part intended to remain open permanently or for an extended time.

-orrhaphy Repair and fixation of an organ or part.

Anastomosis Surgically joining two lumens to create a patent passage.

Laparotomy Surgically opening the abdomen for an exploratory or definitive surgical procedure.

Resection Removal of a segment of an organ or part.

Stoma A surgically created opening in an organ that forms an exit from the body.

Special Considerations for General Surgery

The discipline of general surgery provides the fundamentals for surgical practice, education, and research. The definition of general surgery agreed on by the American Board of Surgery and the Accreditation Council for Graduate Medical Education (ACGME) serves as the basis of graduate education and certification as a specialist in surgery.[1] The following principles are inherent in general surgery:

- A central core of knowledge and skills common to all surgical specialties (e.g., anatomy, physiology, metabolism, pathology, immunology, wound healing, shock and resuscitation, neoplasia, and nutrition)

- The diagnosis and preoperative, intraoperative, and postoperative care of patients with diseases of the alimentary tract, the abdomen and its contents, breast, head and neck, endocrine system, and vascular system (excluding intracranial vessels, the heart, and vessels intrinsic and immediately adjacent thereto)

- Responsibility for the comprehensive management of trauma and critically ill patients with underlying surgical conditions

In a community hospital, the practice of general surgery usually encompasses many aspects of surgical care. In larger teaching facilities, general surgery services are commonly specialized (e.g., breast, biliary tract, gastrointestinal, or colon and rectal surgery). The introduction of surgical specialties was the outgrowth of increased knowledge of the etiology of disease and specialized treatment of all parts of the body. General surgery, the basis for all specialties, has decreased in breadth as specialization has increased. The anatomic parts not specifically delegated to specialists have remained in the realm of the general surgeon. Other surgical disciplines depend on general surgeons for clinical collaboration in reconstruction involving the gastrointestinal and vascular systems.

The scope of this chapter focuses on procedures commonly categorized as general surgery. Technologic advances characterize many aspects of surgical practice. The general surgery team of today should be familiar with endoscopic techniques for diagnosis and treatment. Electrosurgery, lasers, and surgical staplers are part of the setup for standard general surgery. Patients are best cared for when the entire perioperative team understands the principles of available technologies and has clinical experience in the safe use of these technologies. The following are examples of technologic applications and the associated aspects of patient care:

1. Malignant lesions, especially those of the breast, thyroid, and gastrointestinal tract, account for a large percentage of surgical interventions. The extent of the surgical excision of a lesion is determined only after thorough exploration during a surgical procedure, sometimes scheduled as a diagnostic laparoscopy or biopsy and frozen section.
   a. Although the patient has been informed preoperatively of an anticipated procedure, the unknown factor is cause for apprehension. The circulating nurse should provide comfort while the patient is awake. A biopsy or endoscopic procedure may be performed with the patient under local anesthesia and with or without moderate sedation.
   b. A definitive open or laparoscopic surgical procedure is performed on the basis of results of the biopsy and frozen section or endoscopic examination while the patient is under anesthesia. The scrub person should be prepared with two draping and instrument setups, depending on the diagnosis established and the surgeon's plan for the surgical procedure. Anticipated equipment and supplies should be available without delay.
2. The types of anesthesia administered are as varied as the types of surgical procedures. Blood pressure, pulse, respiration, electrocardiogram (ECG), and pulse oximetry should be monitored for all patients, regardless of the anesthetic used. Personnel responsible for monitoring patients should be qualified to interpret data, assess the patient, and effect corrective action in the event of an untoward reaction.
3. Patients are placed in the supine position for many general surgical procedures. Extra padding and accessory positioning aids should be available for other positions. The average operating room (OR) bed can accommodate 350 lb of body weight. Overweight patients require a suitable bed capable of managing body weight.
4. Draping for abdominal incisions is usually standardized. Modifications are necessary for other sites, such as the breast or neck.
5. Instrumentation is varied and suited to function in a specific anatomic area. For example, gastrointestinal procedures require crushing clamps (e.g., Pean clamps to occlude the intestinal lumen before resection) and atraumatic clamps (e.g., Bainbridge clamps to protect delicate tissues). Included in all procedures are instruments for exposing, dissecting, grasping, clamping, suctioning, and suturing. For atraumatic

retraction, various lengths of umbilical tape, hernia tape, or vessel loops may be placed around vessels or other structures to retract them. These materials should be included in the count.
6. Some procedures require minimal access and are adaptable to ambulatory surgery; others are extremely extensive. More complex procedures, such as colectomy and cholecystectomy, are often performed endoscopically and require less in-house hospitalization.
7. The electrosurgical unit (ESU), argon beam coagulator, laser, endoscope, laparoscope, and/or ultrasound transducer may be used during the procedure.
8. In complex open and laparoscopic abdominal and pelvic procedures, the following should be noted:
   a. Indwelling Foley or ureteral catheters may be inserted preoperatively to decompress the urinary bladder and monitor urinary output. Some surgeons may request the placement of ureteral catheters to stent and outline the ureters for complex dissection of abdominal organs. This will require a sterile cystoscopy setup, stirrups, and a urologist before the general surgery procedure of the abdomen begins.
   b. Nasogastric (NG) tubes may be passed before or during the surgical procedure to decompress the stomach and bowel. The anesthesia provider inserts the NG tube after the induction of anesthesia. The NG tube may be removed at the end of the surgical procedure.
   c. After the abdominal cavity is entered, single free 4×4-inch sponges should be removed from the field. They are used only while folded and secured on a sponge stick. Wet or dry laparotomy sponges are used in the abdominal cavity. A small dissector (peanut, cherry, or Kittner) is always clamped in a forceps before being handed to the surgeon.
   d. Before the peritoneum is incised, suction should be available and ready for immediate use, especially in biliary or intestinal procedures or when fluid or blood may be anticipated in the peritoneal cavity. If a cell saver is used for blood salvage, the suction tip for blood is kept separate from the suction tip for other fluids. Hemostatic agents should not be used with a cell saver.
   e. Drains may be exteriorized through a stab wound in the adjacent abdominal wall before closure. A nonabsorbable monofilament suture on a small cutting needle will be used to secure the drain to the skin. Drains are discussed in Chapter 29.
   f. Contaminated items, such as those used to dissect and/or anastomose intestinal segments, are isolated in a basin on the back table.
   g. Before closure, the wound is irrigated with warm, sterile, normal saline solution to remove blood and debris.
   h. Retention sutures may be used to give additional strength to wound closure. Rubber or silicone bumpers or a wound bridge may be used to protect the skin from tension exerted by the adjunct wound closure sutures. Wound closure is discussed in Chapter 28.
9. Assorted sizes of drains, tubes, drainage bags, and wound suction systems should be available. Care is taken to ensure that the patient is not latex sensitive.
10. Irrigating solutions should be body temperature (not to exceed 110° F [43° C]) when used. All radiopaque contrast

media, anticoagulants, and solutions on the instrument table and their delivery devices are clearly labeled to avoid any error in administration. Hypodermic syringes with needles are not recapped by hand. Care is taken to monitor the volumes of fluid used for irrigation.

11. Blood loss and urinary output are recorded on the perioperative record. Anesthesia personnel document the amount of intravenous (IV) solution and medications administered during the case.

12. Specimens are carefully labeled and sent for processing as appropriate. Care of specimens is discussed in Chapter 22.

Breast Procedures

The mammary glands are bilateral organs (modified sweat glands) lying in the superficial fascia of the pectoral area (Fig. 33.1). They are attached to the underlying muscles by loose areolar tissue and suspended by Cooper ligaments. The breasts extend from the border of the sternum to the anterior axillary line (tail of Spence) and from approximately the first to the seventh ribs.

The breasts are highly vascular. The blood supply is derived laterally from the thoracic branches of the axillary, intercostal, and internal mammary arteries (Fig. 33.2). Venous drainage forms an anastomotic circle around the base of the nipple, with branches draining the circumference of the gland into the axillary and internal mammary veins. Lymphatic drainage follows the same path as the venous system and empties into the thoracoabdominal and lateral thoracic vessels. Innervation arises from the anterior and lateral cutaneous nerves of the thorax.

General surgery on the breast for males and females includes diagnostic procedures and those performed for known pathologic disease, such as cancer. Diagnostic techniques include mammography, ultrasonography, fine-needle aspiration (FNA), computed tomography (CT), magnetic resonance imaging (MRI), and the traditional tissue biopsy.

The desired surgical procedure should be determined on an individual basis after careful diagnostic studies and histologic diagnosis.[2] Size, location, and type of diseased tissue and stage of malignancy are important considerations. No single surgical procedure is suitable for all patients.

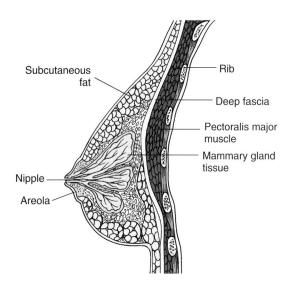

• **Fig. 33.1** Sagittal section of normal breast in relation to chest wall and ribcage.

Incision and Drainage

Surgical opening of an inflamed and suppurative area is most often carried out because of infections in the lactating breast. The cavity is usually irrigated, and the wound is packed and allowed to heal by granulation. The causative organism is often *Staphylococcus*.

Breast Biopsy

The average size of lumps found by women who do and do not practice breast self-examination (BSE) is illustrated in Chapter 22 (see Fig. 22.3). All breast masses are considered malignant until proved benign. To determine the exact nature of a mass in the breast, tissue is removed for pathologic examination. The size and location (Fig. 33.3) of the lesion influence the type of biopsy:

- *Fine-needle aspiration:* A 22 or 25-gauge needle attached to a syringe is inserted into the tumor mass. A few cells are aspirated and sent to the pathology laboratory for cytologic studies. This may be performed in conjunction with a mammogram (mammographic breast biopsy) or as an office procedure. FNA also may be used to evacuate fluid from benign cysts.
- *Core biopsy:* For this type of incisional biopsy, a large-bore trocar needle, such as a Tru-Cut or Vim-Silverman biopsy needle, is inserted into the mass. A core of suspected tissue is withdrawn for histologic examination. Any retrieved fluid is also sent to the pathology laboratory.
- *Stereotactic breast biopsy:* The patient is placed prone on a special x-ray table, and the breast is placed in an opening in the table. A computer-guided system is used to digitally locate and pinpoint nonpalpable breast lesions. The biopsy is obtained with a vacuum-assisted Mammotome device while the patient is under local anesthesia.
- *Incisional biopsy:* The mass is incised, and a portion is removed for histologic examination.
- *Excisional biopsy:* The entire mass is removed for pathologic study.
- *Sentinel node biopsy:* The breast mass is injected with a radioisotope (technetium) in the radiology department several hours before the planned surgical procedure. In the OR, the tumor is injected with a dye containing isosulfan blue that is taken up by the lymph nodes of the breast. The nodes are excised before the primary mass.
  - A sterile Geiger counter probe is used on the field to locate the areas of radioactivity. The specimens are sent to pathology for immunohistochemical staining.
  - Lead containers are used to house the specimens for 24 hours before the pathologist examines them.
- *J-wire or needle localization in radiology department:* The mass is identified on mammography, and the patient undergoes the insertion of a wire into the mass in the radiology department under fluoroscopy (Fig. 33.4). The wire remains taped in place as the patient is taken to the OR. The mass is excised with the wire intact (Fig. 33.5). The specimen is taken back to the radiology department to be x-rayed as a confirmation that the wire is still in the mass. After the confirmatory x-ray, the specimen is taken to pathology.
- *Fiberoptic ductoscopy:* A flexible 0.9-mm scope with a 0.2-mm working channel is used in the ductal lumens of the breast. Studies have shown that 85% of breast cancer originates in the ductal system in the epithelial lining. The image is enlarged to 200 times by magnification. The scopes are approved for 10 uses each by the U.S. Food and Drug Administration (FDA).

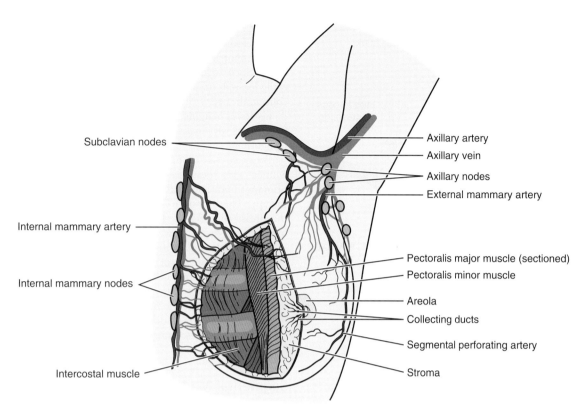

• **Fig. 33.2** Normal anatomy of the breast, including vessels and lymph nodes.

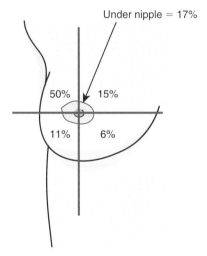

• **Fig. 33.3** Breast cancer location by quadrant.

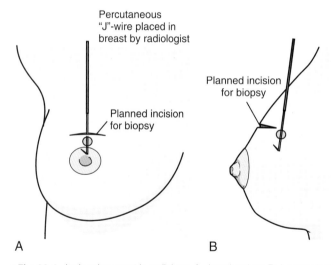

• **Fig. 33.4** J-wire placement in radiology. **A,** Anterior view. **B,** Lateral view.

• Anesthetic cream is applied to the nipple. A fine catheter is introduced, and sterile saline is instilled. Specimens can be obtained by this method, and ductal lavage is performed for cell studies.

• The ducts may need to be dilated with fine lacrimal probes before inserting the catheter. Additional anesthetic can be introduced via the catheter.

Preoperatively, the surgeon discusses with the patient possible findings and treatment options. The patient may agree to an immediate definitive surgical procedure such as mastectomy or lumpectomy if warranted by the biopsy and frozen section results.

Two separate prepping, draping, and instrument sets are necessary to avoid mixing cancerous cells of the breast specimen with the freshly prepared reconstructive site. The team should change gown and gloves.

To minimize disfigurement, many women with early operable breast cancer (a mass smaller than 5 cm) opt for limited resection followed by radiation and chemotherapy (Fig. 33.6). The difference between tumor and deep tumor-free resection margin remains an important consideration in determining the most appropriate type of mastectomy incision (Table 33.1).

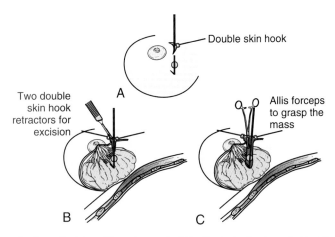

• **Fig. 33.5** Excision of breast mass in OR with J-wire in place. **A,** Visualization of mass. **B,** Increased exposure. **C,** Removal of mass.

• **Fig. 33.6** Common conservative breast incisions followed by radiation therapy.

Lumpectomy

Lumpectomy, a partial mastectomy, consists of removal of the entire tumor mass along with at least 1 to 2 cm of surrounding nondiseased tissue. This procedure is recommended for peripherally located tumors that measure less than 5 cm. Lumpectomy is contraindicated if breast size precludes postoperative radiation or if negative margins around the tumor cannot be obtained. Compared with mastectomy, the lumpectomy incisions are less disfiguring.

Breast conservation, the surgical treatment of choice for many women with breast cancer, includes a lumpectomy to excise a primary tumor and axillary node dissection followed by radiation therapy. This approach maintains the appearance and function of the breast (Fig. 33.7). The surgeon may prefer to perform the lumpectomy first, followed by axillary dissection (Fig. 33.8).

The patient should be reprepped and redraped between procedures. A separate set of instruments is used for each procedure to avoid possible tumor cell implantation in the axilla. A transverse incision for axillary dissection, approximately 1 cm below the axillary hairline, extends from the pectoralis major muscle anteriorly to the latissimus dorsi muscle posteriorly. Lymphoareolar tissue between these muscles is removed—usually at least 10 lymph nodes.

Segmental Mastectomy

In a segmental mastectomy, a wedge or quadrant (quadrantectomy) of breast tissue is removed; this wedge includes the tumor mass and the lobe in which it is growing. Some surgeons explore the axilla and take a few lymph nodes for histologic studies.

Simple Mastectomy

In a simple mastectomy, the entire breast is removed without lymph node dissection. A simple mastectomy may be performed for a malignancy that is confined to breast tissue with negative nodes, as a palliative measure for an advanced ulcerated malignant tumor, or for the removal of extensive benign disease. Skin grafting may be necessary if the primary closure of skin flaps

TABLE 33.1	**Stages of Breast Cancer**			
	Stage I	**Stage II**	**Stage III**	**Stage IV**
Size	<1–2 cm	2–5 cm	>5 cm	Large and fully integrated with surrounding tissue
Location	Confined to breast	Breast mass with or without suspicious axillary lymph nodes	Breast mass with palpable, fixed axillary, and/or subclavicular lymph nodes	Distant metastasis; extension to skin
		May or may not extend to pectoral fascia or muscle	Mass may be adherent to surrounding tissue	Lymphedema above or below the clavicle
		No distant metastasis	No distant metastasis	
Surgical Options	Segmental mastectomy	Total mastectomy	Modified or radical mastectomy	Radical or extended radical mastectomy
	Breast conservation surgery for stages I and II lumpectomy with axillary node dissection and radiation therapy			

• **Fig. 33.7** Common mastectomy incisions. **A,** Bilateral. **B,** Alternative incisions based on tumor location, **C,** Unilateral.

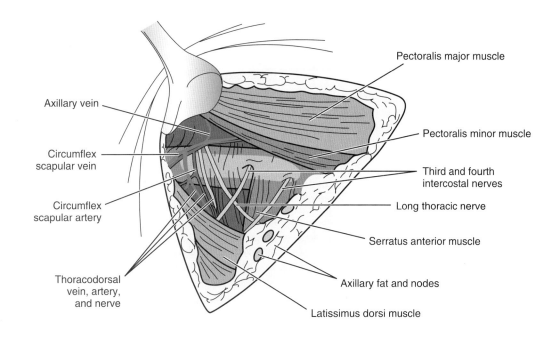

Pectoralis major muscle

Axillary vein

Circumflex scapular vein

Pectoralis minor muscle

Circumflex scapular artery

Third and fourth intercostal nerves

Long thoracic nerve

Serratus anterior muscle

Thoracodorsal vein, artery, and nerve

Axillary fat and nodes

Latissimus dorsi muscle

• **Fig. 33.8** Axillary lymph node dissection for breast cancer.

would create unacceptable tension. Skin flaps are then loosely approximated, and grafts taken from the thigh are applied to the remaining defect. A latissimus dorsi or transverse rectus abdominis myocutaneous (TRAM) flap may be preferred for reconstruction.

A subcutaneous mastectomy may be performed for patients with chronic cystic mastitis who have had multiple previous biopsies, for patients with multiple fibroadenomas or hyperplastic duct changes, and for patients with central tumors that are noninvasive in origin. Some patients with a strong family history of breast cancer may have prophylactic mastectomies as a precaution. All breast tissue is removed, but the overlying skin and nipple remain intact. A prosthesis may be inserted at the time of the surgical procedure, depending on the surgeon's decision and the patient's wishes.

Modified Radical Mastectomy

A modified radical mastectomy is usually performed for infiltrating ductal and localized small malignant lesions. The term *modified* encompasses various techniques, but all include removal of the entire breast (total mastectomy). In addition, all axillary lymph nodes are resected. The underlying pectoralis major muscle is left in place; the pectoralis minor muscle may or may not be removed. In patients with small lesions and no metastases, breast reconstruction may be performed immediately or a few days after the procedure.

Radical Mastectomy

A radical mastectomy is performed to control the spread of malignant disease from large infiltrating cancers. After a positive finding on the tissue biopsy, the entire involved breast is removed along with the axillary lymph nodes, the pectoral muscles, and all adjacent tissues. During the surgical procedure, skin flaps and extensive exposed tissue are covered with moist packs for protection. The chest wall and axilla are irrigated with sterile water before closure. Skin grafts are usually required to cover the defect.

Extended Radical Mastectomy

Cancer is a disease that grows both deeply and laterally. An extended radical mastectomy is indicated when malignant disease is present in the medial quadrant or subareolar tissue because it tends to spread to the internal mammary lymph nodes. The involved breast is removed en bloc along with the underlying pectoral muscles, axillary contents, and upper internal mammary (mediastinal) lymph node chain. This procedure is more difficult than a classic radical mastectomy.

Considerations for Female Breast Procedures

For a breast procedure, the patient is placed in the supine position; the involved side is positioned close to the edge of the OR bed, and the arm on the affected side is extended on an armboard. The affected side is elevated with a small pillow, or the OR bed is tilted. The anterior part of the chest is prepped from the chin to the umbilicus and from the axilla on the affected side to the nipple line of the opposite breast. The entire arm on the affected side is included in this preparation. General anesthesia is usually preferred for a mastectomy because local infiltrate may obscure a tumor.

Because of the vascularity of breast tissue, a laser or ESU is commonly used for hemostasis. Larger vessels may require a tie. Patients undergoing a mastectomy should be watched for excessive bleeding. Some surgeons prefer to irrigate the mastectomy wound with sterile water, instead of sterile normal saline solution, for osmotic cytolysis to crenate (shrivel or shrink) cancerous cells.[3] The circulating nurse should check with the surgeon about the care of the specimen for the pathologist. The specimen is placed in sterile normal saline solution if estrogen or progesterone receptor studies are to be performed. Formalin is used for permanent sections.

A bulky compression dressing and Surgi-Bra may be applied in the OR. Depending on the amount of tissue resected, a closed-wound suction system may be inserted to remove blood and serum and to prevent pressure necrosis of skin flaps.

Lymphedema of the arm on the affected side is a possible complication after mastectomy causing the arm to painfully swell and lose function.[4] The patient is highly susceptible to infection. When axillary dissection is performed, the lymphatic structure of the arm is compromised, causing primary lymphedema. Secondary causes include radiation, extreme inflammation, or infection. Although lymphedema can be an immediate problem, it most frequently builds up over time during the postoperative period. The severity is classified by the degree of pitting and loss of arm mobility. Patients experience neck and back pain as the arm becomes heavier with accumulated lymph. Obesity significantly increases the risk for lymphedema development. The enlarged arm causes self-perception issues and is a constant reminder of cancer treatment.

Management of lymphedema involves one or more of the following: (1) manual drainage, (2) compression garment/sleeve, (3) physical exercise, and (4) meticulous skin care. Some patients are candidates for a liposuction procedure to reduce the size of the arm. The patient must wear a compression sleeve at all times after a reduction procedure for life to keep the arm in a reduced state. Lymphatic grafts to the axilla from the medial thigh have been used with some success; however, the risk for lymphedema of the donor leg is possible.

Patients who have undergone a mastectomy are often referred to The American Cancer Society's Reach to Recovery rehabilitative program. In this program, volunteers who have had mastectomies visit patients, share information with them, and give them encouragement. Information can be found at www.cancer.org.

Abdominal Procedures

Biliary Tract Procedures

The gallbladder is located in the right upper quadrant in a fossa under and immediately adjacent to the right lobe of the liver (Fig. 33.9). The gallbladder is a thin-walled sac and has a normal capacity of 50 to 75 mL of bile. Bile secreted by the hepatic cells enters the intrahepatic bile ducts and progresses to the common bile duct. When not needed for digestion, bile is diverted through the cystic duct into the gallbladder, where it is stored. When bile is needed, the gallbladder contracts and empties bile into the cystic duct; the bile flows into and through the common duct into the duodenum.

Gallstones are concretions of elements of bile, particularly cholesterol (about 50%), and may be found in the gallbladder or in any portion of the extrahepatic biliary duct system. Brown stones are usually fatty acids, and black stones are composed of inorganic salts. The incidence of stones, referred to as cholelithiasis, increases with age and is more prevalent in women and in people who are overweight.

Acute or chronic inflammation of the gallbladder, common duct stones (choledocholithiasis), carcinoma, and the congenital absence of bile ducts (biliary atresia) are the most common indications for a surgical procedure. Obstructive jaundice, which is potentially fatal, may be a sign of ductal cholelithiasis or the presence of a neoplasm. The cause of jaundice should be determined and the condition relieved to spare the patient irreversible progressive liver damage. Biliary stones are sent as dry specimens if removed separately.

The greatest hazards of biliary tract surgery are associated with the anatomic relationships of the ducts and the cystic artery and with pathologic changes in the gallbladder. Complications include hemorrhage and injury to the extrahepatic biliary duct system. Spilled bile can cause peritonitis postoperatively.

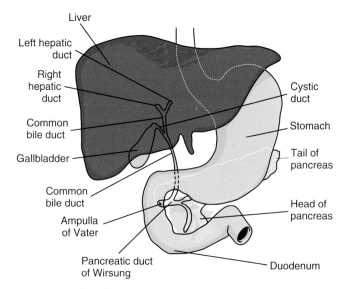

• **Fig. 33.9** Normal anatomy of the biliary system and portal system.

Ultrasonography, nuclear imaging such as hepatic intraductal assay (HIDA) scan, and CT scanning are used for the diagnosis of gallbladder disease. Oral (PO) and IV cholecystography may be used for visualization of the gallbladder in the initial evaluation of patients with biliary symptoms.

Endoscopic retrograde cholangiopancreatography also may be performed, usually by a gastroenterologist, to identify stones, tumors, inflammatory lesions, or an obstruction. A flexible fiberoptic duodenoscope is introduced with the patient under IV sedation and with the use of a topical anesthetic to control the gag reflex.

Contrast media is injected to opacify the entire biliary tract and pancreatic duct under fluoroscopy. Care is taken when preparing the contrast in the syringe without air bubbles. Air bubbles will appear like stones on radiographs. Some definitive therapy is possible during this procedure, such as stone retrieval (endoscopic papillotomy), stent insertion, and sphincterotomy. A percutaneous transhepatic puncture is used to resect tumors for biopsy, dilate strictures, place stents in the bile duct, and establish temporary drainage through ducts. A contrast medium can be injected for a cholangiogram.

Cholecystectomy

Gallbladder disease is cured by removal of the gallbladder in a procedure referred to as a *cholecystectomy*—the most common surgical procedure performed on the biliary tract. A cholecystectomy is performed to relieve the gastrointestinal distress common in patients with acute or chronic cholecystitis (with or without gallstones); it also removes a source of recurrent sepsis. Persistent infection in the biliary tract may cause recurrent stones.

For an open cholecystectomy, the patient is placed in the supine position. As requested by the surgeon, the right upper quadrant may be slightly elevated on a gallbladder rest or pillow after the induction of general anesthesia. The OR bed may be tilted slightly into a reverse Trendelenburg position so the abdominal viscera gravitate downward, away from the surgical area.

Open Abdominal Cholecystectomy

With an open abdominal cholecystectomy, the gallbladder is usually exposed through a right subcostal incision (Kocher incision) that may be extended over to the midline at the level of the xyphoid. The incision should be adequate for good exposure of the gallbladder and bile ducts. After exploration of the abdominal cavity, laparotomy packs are used to wall off the surrounding organs for exposure.

The bilious contents of the gallbladder may be aspirated to prevent bile from spilling into the peritoneal cavity—a potential source of peritonitis, especially if the gallbladder is inflamed and tightly distended. The cystic duct, cystic artery, hepatic ducts, and common bile duct are accurately identified.

After palpation of the ducts for stones, the cystic duct and artery are ligated with hemostatic clips and divided. Using blunt dissection, the gallbladder is freed and removed from the liver and its fossa (Fig. 33.10). Some surgeons use ESU and/or neodymium:yttrium aluminum garnet (Nd:YAG) or holmium:yttrium aluminum garnet (Ho:YAG) laser for sharp dissection and coagulation. Stones removed as part of the specimen should be sent to pathology for analysis and documentation. If bile leakage or hemorrhage has been excessive, a sump drain or closed-wound suction drain may be placed in the subhepatic space and brought out through a stab wound after copious intraabdominal irrigation.

Laparoscopic Cholecystectomy

With a laparoscopic cholecystectomy the patient is supine in a slight to moderate reverse Trendelenburg position. A rigid fiberoptic laparoscope is inserted through a sheath into the peritoneal cavity. In conventional laparoscopy, multiple trocars are inserted through triangulated puncture wounds in the right upper quadrant: one or two just right of midline, with the uppermost trocar slightly below the xyphoid and costal margin and the other midway to the umbilicus; one laterally in an anterior axillary line above the iliac crest at the costal margin; and another in a midclavicular line slightly above the level of the umbilicus and 2 cm below the rib. The location of puncture sites will vary according to patient size and surgeon preference (Fig. 33.11).

Single-port access technology uses an open laparoscopic method in which a single incision is made at the umbilicus and a flexible multilumen port is inserted through which insufflation and additional instruments are placed. A Veress needle is not used. Single-incision laparoscopy is discussed in Chapter 32.

A camera attached to the laparoscope allows the surgeon to view the manipulation of instruments through the sheaths of these trocars. Viewing monitors are positioned on each side of the head of the OR bed (Fig. 33.12). With this procedure, the fundus of the gallbladder is grasped through one or more lateral ports and held by the assistant. After careful dissection, the surgeon ligates and divides the cystic duct and artery with suture loops or clips. A laser, an ESU, or microscissors may be used to transect these structures.

The gallbladder is freed, most often by using an ESU or by using argon, potassium titanyl phosphate (KTP), or a contact Nd:YAG or Ho:YAG laser. The gallbladder is usually lowered into an Endo Catch pouch and aspirated to remove bile and collapse the sac. It then may be removed in one piece or cut into sections and withdrawn through the periumbilical incision.

The perioperative team must be ready to convert from laparoscopic to an open procedure in the event of bleeding or other difficulty during the procedure. Supplies and instrumentation should be immediately available. It is advantageous to have precounted sets in the room during these procedures.

Common Bile Duct Exploration

Concomitant exploration of the common duct is often but not routinely performed during cholecystectomy. Curved stone

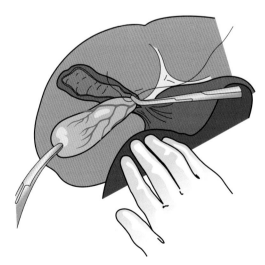

• **Fig. 33.10** The gallbladder is dissected from the liver bed.

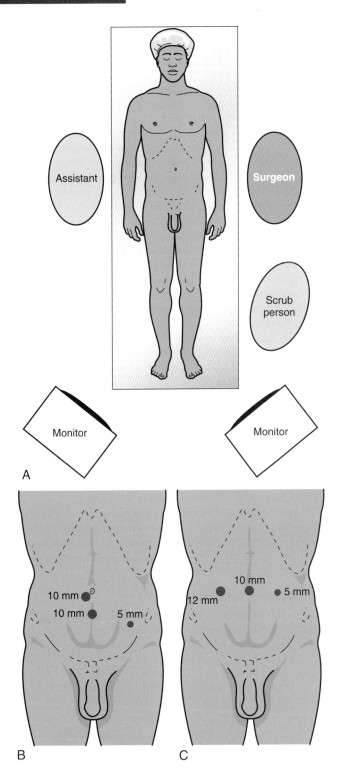

• **Fig. 33.11** Laparoscopic setup. **A,** Position of personnel for a basic laparoscopy. **B,** Trocar placement is determined by the target organ position. **C,** Trocars used vary in size according to position of function for dissection and hemostasis.

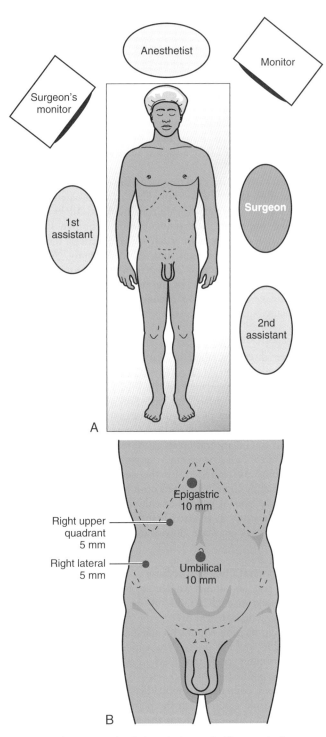

• **Fig. 33.12** Laparoscopic cholecystectomy. **A,** Placement of personnel and monitors for gallbladder removal. **B,** Trocar placement for gallbladder removal.

forceps, small malleable scoops, dilators of various sizes, balloon catheters, stone baskets, and nylon brushes are useful in clearing the hepatic and biliary ducts of stones to prevent them lodging in the duct and causing subsequent obstructive jaundice.

Palpable stones, jaundice with cholangitis, and dilation of the common bile duct are indications for exploration. A T-tube drain may be inserted to stent the duct and provide postoperative drainage. The surgeon may choose other intraoperative techniques to identify unsuspected stones, pathologic conditions, or anatomic variations in the hepatic duct system.

Intraoperative Cholangiograms

X-rays are obtained during either open abdominal or laparoscopic procedures. The radiology department is notified in advance if a cholangiogram is anticipated. To check for patient position, scout films may be obtained when the patient is initially positioned on the OR bed, before the procedure is started. The circulating nurse should assess the patient for allergies or sensitivities to contrast media and should ensure that the OR bed has an x-ray top or can be equipped for x-ray or fluoroscopy. Most facilities use digital x-rays.

The radiology technician returns to the OR when the surgeon is ready for films. Cholangiograms may be obtained after the gallbladder is removed or before the cystic duct and artery are ligated. A radiopaque contrast medium, usually diatrizoate sodium (Hypaque or Renografin), is injected into the cystic duct or common bile duct with a 30 to 60-mL syringe.

Unless fluoroscopy is used, a series of three or four radiographs are obtained and displayed in digital format. Before each exposure, the surgeon injects contrast media through a Cholangiocath (a plastic catheter inserted into the cystic or common duct), cannula, or direct needle puncture in the common duct (Fig. 33.13). Instruments are removed from the field to the extent possible to minimize the obstruction of structures on the radiographs. The field is covered with a sterile barrier before the x-ray machine or C-arm is positioned over the patient. Sterile x-ray tube and C-arm covers are commercially available. All other radiologic precautions for patient and personnel safety and shielding should be observed.

Ultrasonography

Ultrasonography, a noninvasive technique, takes less time and does not have the radiation hazards of intraoperative cholangiograms. A sterile ultrasound probe is manipulated along the common bile duct from the liver to the duodenum. The probe transmits high-frequency sound waves back to the ultrasound unit in the form of echoes, which are displayed on a screen as black-and-white real-time images. To enhance the transmission of ultrasound waves, the abdominal cavity is irrigated with warm normal saline solution. Density in tissue causes sound waves to

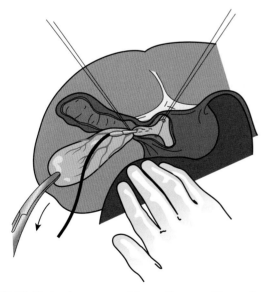

• **Fig. 33.13** Cholangiograms are taken with x-ray. The cystic duct is ligated.

echo in altered patterns and directions. Gallstones appear as bright echoes, often with an acoustic shadow. Photographs or video can be obtained to document the findings of ultrasonography.

Choledochoscopy

Intraoperative biliary endoscopy provides image transmission and illumination, thus allowing the surgeon visual guidance in exploring the biliary system. Intrahepatic and extrahepatic bile ducts can be visualized with a flexible fiberoptic choledochoscope introduced into the common duct. To provide distention of the biliary tract, normal saline solution must continuously flow through the irrigation channel.

Stones are easily seen and are usually free-floating under the pressure of the irrigating solution. A flexible stone forceps, a basket, or a balloon-tipped biliary catheter may be inserted through the instrument channel of either a rigid or flexible scope to allow manipulation of a stone under direct vision. A biopsy forceps may be inserted to obtain a tissue sample. An Nd:YAG laser fiber may be used through the choledochoscope to crush bilirubin stones in the distal common hepatic duct; this allows easy removal of the stones.

Cholelithotripsy

Cholelithotripsy is a noninvasive procedure in which high-energy shock waves are used to fragment cholesterol gallstones. The procedure is performed under IV sedation or general anesthesia. The patient is usually placed in the prone position but may also be in the supine or lateral position, on a lithotripter table, or submerged in a water bath. Spark-gap shock waves generated from an electrode pass through a fluid medium into the body until they reach the stone, which is focused with an ultrasound probe and computer.

The shock waves are synchronized with the R waves of the patient's cardiac rhythm, which is monitored by ECG to avoid dysrhythmias. Each shock pulverizes the stones into small fragments, which then pass through the bile duct. This passage may be aided by oral administration of deoxycholic acid (ursodiol) taken daily after lithotripsy to dissolve the fragments.

Choledochostomy and Choledochotomy

With choledochostomy, a T-tube is used to drain the common bile duct through the abdominal wall. A choledochotomy is the incision of the common bile duct for the exploration and removal of stones. Intraoperative cholangiography may be performed before and after exploration and/or stone removal. The duct is irrigated after calculi are removed. Patency of the duct and of the ampulla of Vater is investigated, often through a choledochoscope. If a neoplasm is found during exploration, resectability is determined; many tumors of the liver or pancreas are inoperable.

Cholecystoduodenostomy and Cholecystojejunostomy

Either a cholecystoduodenostomy or cholecystojejunostomy is performed to relieve an obstruction in the distal end of the common duct. Through anastomosis, these procedures establish continuity between the gallbladder and either the duodenum or jejunum. Careful evaluation precedes the surgical procedure.

Cholecystoduodenostomy and cholecystojejunostomy are bypass procedures to avoid further obstructive jaundice, but they do not solve the problem. Common causes of the obstruction are calculi, stricture of the duct, or neoplasms of the duct, ampulla of Vater, or pancreas.

Choledochoduodenostomy and choledochojejunostomy are side-to-side anastomoses between the duodenum or jejunum and the common duct. These procedures are carried out for difficult or recurrent biliary or pancreatic obstruction as a result of benign or malignant disease.

Liver Procedures

The liver, the largest gland in the body, is divided into left and right segments (or lobes) and is located in the upper right abdominal cavity beneath the diaphragm (Fig. 33.14). Part of the stomach and duodenum and the hepatic flexure of the colon lie directly beneath the liver. A tough fibrous sheath, the Glisson capsule, completely covers the organ; the tissue within this capsule is very friable and vascular. The hepatic artery, a branch of the celiac axis, maintains the arterial supply. Blood from the stomach, intestine, spleen, and pancreas is carried to the liver by the portal vein and its branches.

The many functions of the liver include forming and secreting bile, which aids digestion; transforming glucose into glycogen, which it stores; and helping regulate blood volume. The liver is vital for the metabolic functioning of the body. It metabolizes fats, proteins, and carbohydrates; synthesizes cholesterol; excretes bilirubin; and secretes hormones. The liver has remarkable regenerative capacity, and up to 80% of it may be resected with little or no alteration in hepatic function.

Liver function tests are used to assess the degree of functional impairment and to evaluate liver activity and reserve. Most of these tests involve taking a series of blood samples from the patient for specific studies. Ascites may result from impaired liver function.

Liver Needle Biopsy

A percutaneous needle biopsy may help establish a diagnosis of liver disease. Because the procedure is performed with the patient

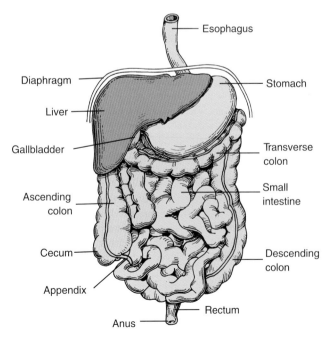

• **Fig. 33.14** Abdominal organs within peritoneal cavity.

under local anesthesia, moderate sedation, or monitored anesthesia care (MAC), the patient should be instructed to take several deep breaths and then hold the breath and remain absolutely still while the needle is inserted. Failure of the patient to cooperate can cause needle penetration of the diaphragm or hepatic injury and result in hemorrhage, a serious complication. Leakage of bile into the abdominal cavity may produce chemical peritonitis, an additional hazard.[5]

After skin preparation and the induction of local anesthesia (with the patient in the supine position), a Franklin-Silverman, Tru-Cut, or EchoTip ProCore biopsy needle is introduced into the liver via a transthoracic intercostal or transabdominal subcostal route. The needle is rotated to separate a small core of tissue, and it is then withdrawn to remove the specimen. As soon as the needle is removed, the patient is told to resume normal breathing and is assisted to turn onto their right side to compress the chest wall at the penetration site and prevent the seepage of bile or blood.

Slight bleeding may follow a liver biopsy; the patient's prothrombin time is checked. This method of biopsy is not used if the patient has a coagulopathy.

In select patients under local anesthesia, a laparoscopic-assisted approach may be used to enhance visualization of the biopsy site. The anterior abdominal wall is elevated with a low volume of carbon dioxide insufflation or a planar lift device without insufflation. The biopsy needle is inserted through the abdominal wall as described previously. A topical hemostatic gelatin sponge or other topical chemical hemostatic agent is laparoscopically applied to the biopsy site on the liver. The patient remains supine after this procedure.

Drainage of Subphrenic and Subhepatic Abscesses

Abscesses in and around the liver may be caused by a variety of microorganisms or as a result of secondary infections from abdominal organs. In general, these abscesses are treated by incision and drainage. A catheter may be introduced into the abscess cavity, which has been localized on a CT scan. The location of the abscess determines the percutaneous approach (i.e., transpleural, subpleural, transperitoneal, or retroperitoneal). Care must be taken to avoid contamination of the pleural or peritoneal cavity.

Intraoperative Hepatic Ultrasound

Intraoperative ultrasound can be used to identify anatomic structures or liver densities associated with a primary tumor or metastasis. Before rotating the liver forward and excising diseased or injured lobes or segments, it is necessary to divide the appropriate ligamentous attachments and to ligate the veins and arteries. Lesions not accessible for resection may be treated with cryosurgery or a Cavitron ultrasonic surgical aspirator (CUSA). These techniques may be used in conjunction with resection. An ultrasonic aspirator permits the precise removal of tissue and controls bleeding during resection.

Hepatic Resection

The standard anatomic resections of the liver are right or left lobectomy, right or left trisegmentectomy, and left lateral segmentectomy. Because it is a vital organ, the entire liver cannot be removed without liver transplantation. Lobectomy or segmental resection is indicated for cysts, benign or malignant tumors, or severe penetrating or blunt trauma. Depending on the location of the lesion to be resected, a right or bilateral subcostal incision or an upper midline incision is made and can be extended as needed for exposure and exploration. The liver is the most commonly injured abdominal organ. Hepatic parenchymal injuries usually cause intraperitoneal hemorrhage and shock.

Liver tissue is very friable. The prevention or arrest of hemorrhage is a prime concern. Omental flaps, falciform ligament, or a Gerota fascia flap may be used for coverage and tamponade of bleeding surfaces in conjunction with local hemostatic substances. Microfibrillar collagen, oxidized cellulose, or spray hemostatic agents are often used to control bleeding. Large, blunt, noncutting needles are used to suture the liver. Drains are usually placed in the wound and brought out through stab wounds. Equipment for blood replacement, portal pressure measurement, and chest drainage should be available.

Portosystemic Shunts

Portal hypertension, bleeding esophageal varices, or massive gastrointestinal hemorrhage may necessitate an emergency surgical procedure for decompression of the portal venous system. Often the patient has an alcohol dependence disorder, with cirrhosis, poor nutrition, and unstable blood volume, or generally is a poor surgical risk. A portosystemic shunt is a vascular anastomosis between the portal and systemic venous systems. The surgeon may select one of several techniques for a portacaval or mesocaval shunt. In patients with portal hypertension and hypersplenism, a splenorenal shunt may be performed in conjunction with a splenectomy for portal decompression.

Splenic Procedures

The highly vascular spleen is located in the upper left abdominal cavity and lies beneath the dome of the diaphragm; it is protected by the lower portion of the ribcage. The capsule of the spleen is covered with peritoneum and is held in place by numerous suspensory ligaments. The splenic artery furnishes the arterial blood supply, and the splenic vein drains into the portal system.

As the largest lymphatic organ of the body, the spleen has an intimate role in the immunologic defenses of the body and acts as a blood reservoir. The main functions of the spleen involve the formation of blood elements. Radionuclide scanning and other radiographic studies provide information for analysis.

Splenectomy

The most common reason for removal of the spleen is hypersplenism—overactivity that causes a reduction in the circulating quantity of red cells, white cells, platelets, or a combination of them. Splenectomies are often scheduled at specific times because patients often require the administration of whole blood immediately before a surgical procedure. Often these patients are also receiving steroid treatment, and provisions are made to maintain therapy during the surgical procedure and postoperatively.

Hematologic disorders, tumors, or accessory spleens may also necessitate surgical intervention. A splenic rupture requires an immediate surgical procedure to prevent fatal hemorrhage and may require a splenectomy. In certain patients with benign

disease, a laparoscopic approach has been successfully used for splenectomy.

In performing a splenectomy, a left rectus paramedian, midline, or subcostal incision is used to enter the peritoneal cavity, and the spleen is displaced medially by careful manual manipulation. The splenorenal, splenocolic, and gastrosplenic ligaments are ligated and divided. Great care should be exercised in ligating the splenic artery and vein because these vessels are often friable. Hemorrhage is the principal intraoperative hazard. After removal of the spleen and before closure, careful inspection for bleeding from the splenic pedicle and retroperitoneal space is essential.

Splenorrhaphy

After a splenectomy, patients—especially children—are immunologically impaired (i.e., more susceptible to infection), which sometimes can produce catastrophic results. To protect the patient's immune competence, surgeons attempt to salvage splenic tissue after splenic trauma. Splenorrhaphy, or splenic repair, can be accomplished in several ways. Once the spleen is mobilized, actively bleeding vessels are ligated and devitalized tissues are debrided. The spleen then can be sutured or stapled along the edge of a partial splenectomy. Microfibrillar collagen or absorbable gelatin sponges can be placed over a small laceration or capsular tear to effect hemostasis. The splenic artery may be ligated.

The spleen may be wrapped in omentum or synthetic mesh. Segments can be reimplanted into an omental pouch in the intraperitoneal space to preserve splenic function. In patients with extensive trauma, a drain that is exteriorized through a stab wound may be inserted into the left subdiaphragmatic space.

Pancreatic Procedures

The pancreas is both an endocrine gland and an exocrine gland. The islets of Langerhans form the endocrine division and secrete the hormones insulin and glucagon, both of which are essential to the metabolism of carbohydrates and the storage of calories. Acini and the ducts leading from them constitute the exocrine portion, which secretes pancreatic juice into the duodenum. Pancreatic juice neutralizes stomach acid; the loss of pancreatic juice results in severe impairment in the digestion and absorption of food.

The pancreas lies transversely across the posterior wall of the upper abdomen behind the stomach. The head, or right extremity of the pancreas, is attached to the duodenum; the tail, or left extremity of the pancreas, is in proximity to the spleen.

Disorders of the pancreas generally include acute and chronic inflammation, cysts, and tumors. The head of the pancreas is the most common site of a malignant pancreatic tumor. Cancer in the body or tail of the pancreas is often asymptomatic until advanced and beyond surgical resection. Malignancies are more common in males than females. It is rare before the age of 45 years and is most common after the age of 60. Accuracy in the diagnosis of pancreatic problems is difficult, but evaluation by ultrasonography, endoscopic retrograde cholangiopancreatography (ERCP), and scanning has led to significant improvements in planning surgical treatment.[6]

An exploratory laparotomy is the most reliable means of diagnosing and evaluating pancreatic trauma. Pancreatitis is associated most often with pancreatic duct stones, gallstones, or alcoholism. Corrective biliary tract procedures usually alleviate gallstone pancreatitis.

Pancreaticojejunostomy

Pancreaticojejunostomy may be performed for relief of pain associated with chronic alcoholic pancreatitis and pseudocysts of the pancreas. There are several types of procedures for the drainage of obstructed ducts or pseudocysts. These methods involve anastomosing a loop of the jejunum (Roux-en-Y loop) to the pancreatic duct. Hemorrhage and leakage of bile are complications to be avoided.

Pancreaticoduodenectomy (Whipple Procedure)

Pancreaticoduodenectomy is an extensive procedure performed on patients with carcinoma of the head of the pancreas or the ampulla of Vater. A gastrointestinal setup is used for this procedure. The abdominal cavity is exposed through one of several possible anterior incisions, but a long right paramedian incision is usually made. The abdominal and pelvic cavities are explored for distant metastases. Because many vital structures and organs are involved in resecting the diseased proximal portion of the pancreas, careful dissection of vessels is necessary to prevent hemorrhage, which complicates the procedure. Resection includes the distal stomach, the duodenum distal to the pylorus, the distal end of the common bile duct, and all but the tail of the pancreas.

Several methods of reconstructing the digestive tract are possible, but all include anastomosis of the pancreatic duct, common bile duct, stomach, and jejunum. Most surgeons reestablish biliary-intestinal continuity by end-to-side choledochojejunostomy (Fig. 33.15). The stomach and pylorus may be preserved in patients with benign disease or localized, small tumors. After pancreatic and biliary reconstruction, the divided end of the duodenum is anastomosed to the side of the jejunal limb used for the reconstruction. A watertight seal of all anastomoses is essential to prevent peritonitis or pancreatitis. Drains are inserted.

Improvements in preoperative and postoperative care and the refinement of technical details have increased the survival rate of patients who undergo this potentially hazardous radical surgical procedure. The most common postoperative complications of pancreaticoduodenectomy are shock, hemorrhage, renal failure, and pancreatic or biliary fistula. If a fistula should occur, wound suction is continued until the fistula closes. In general, the fistula will close spontaneously if adequate nutrition and electrolyte balance are maintained.

Pancreatectomy

Subtotal distal pancreatectomy is usually performed to resect a benign tumor or for chronic pancreatitis. The distal tail is resected to the head of the pancreas. A splenectomy is usually performed with this procedure because the blood supply to the tail of the pancreas comes from splenic vessels that are sacrificed. A total pancreatectomy allows a wide resection of a primary malignant tumor and its multifocal sites in the pancreas. A patient who has undergone a total pancreatectomy will have endocrine and pancreatic insufficiency.

Pancreaticoduodenal Trauma

Combined injuries of the pancreas and duodenum from penetrating wounds or blunt trauma are among the most complicated to treat. A midline incision is used to explore the abdomen. Suturing to control bleeding, debridement of devitalized tissue, and draining are the initial therapies. Pancreatic fistulas and abscesses are potential complications. Extensive injury of the head of the pancreas and duodenum may require pancreaticoduodenal resection with gastrojejunostomy.

Esophageal Procedures

The esophagus is the 25 to 30-cm-long musculomembranous tube between the pharynx in the throat and the stomach in the abdomen. It is composed distally of striated skeletal muscle and proximally of smooth muscle. It passes through the thoracic cavity and enters the abdominal cavity through the esophageal hiatus (opening) in the right crus of the diaphragm; it joins the right medial surface of the stomach. The esophagus propels food by peristalsis. Within the abdominal cavity, the esophagus is bordered by the liver anteriorly and the aorta posteriorly and slightly to the left (with the spleen on the left) and between the right and left branches of the vagus nerve. The blood supply is derived from the inferior thyroid arteries and the bronchial, gastric, and phrenic branches directly off the aorta.

Patients with long-standing (more than 5 years) gastroesophageal reflux with erosive esophagitis can develop Barrett esophagus.[7] This can happen when the cellular structure at the gastroesophageal junction has changed from squamous cells to columnar cells. It is more common in males than females and starts between the ages of 40 and 60 years.

Although there is no cure, further damage can be prevented with appropriate medical treatment. If strictures form, frequent

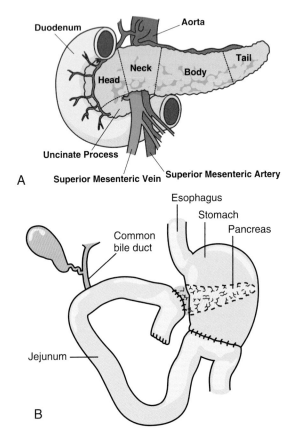

• **Fig. 33.15** **A,** Surgical anatomy of the pancreas. **B,** Whipple procedure.

dilation with bougie (pronounced boogee) instrumentation may be necessary. The bougies range in size from 16 to 60 French. The risk for developing cancer is between 5% and 10%, and patients with Barrett esophagus are frequently assessed and screened by esophagoscopy and biopsy.

Surgical options include antireflux surgery (hiatal hernia repair), endoscopic ablation (with laser, radiofrequency, or cryosurgery), endoscopic mucosal resection, or esophagectomy.

Diverticula (pouches or pockets) can be present at the distal end of the esophagus near the dorsal aspect of the throat at the level of C5-C6. These pockets can herniate and collect food and can progressively become larger. These pockets are referred to as Zenker diverticula, which account for 65% of all diverticula in the esophagus. They can become infected and necrotic or engorged to the point of rupture, which then becomes a surgical emergency. Some texts refer to a herniated diverticula as Killian dehiscence.

Esophageal Hiatal Herniorrhaphy

When intraabdominal pressure exceeds pressure in the chest, the abdominal esophagus and a portion of the stomach may slide through the esophageal hiatus and into the thoracic cavity. Although this condition (referred to as hiatal or diaphragmatic hernia) is common, a surgical procedure is indicated when the resultant esophagitis causes ulceration, bleeding, stenosis, or chest and back symptoms. Reflux esophagitis and sphincter incompetence also may have other causes that necessitate a surgical procedure.

The abdominal approach to correct the problem involves a midline or left subcostal incision. Because visualization of the hiatal area may be difficult, the incision may be extended over the lower ribcage. The patient may be placed in a slight reverse Trendelenburg position. Organs and vital structures should be protected with moist sponges and gently retracted to expose the hiatus. Long-handled clamps are needed. After mobilization, the hiatus is narrowed with heavy sutures, and the fundus of the stomach is anchored against the diaphragm to prevent recurrent herniation and gastroesophageal reflux.

Prevention of reflux is one of the prime objectives of fundoplication because it was the cause of the patient's previous esophagitis. Lengthening the intraabdominal esophagus and increasing pressure on the lower esophageal sphincter also help control reflux. The esophagus is secured by wrapping the proximal stomach (fundus) around the gastroesophageal junction in one of two ways: either by a total 360-degree wrap (Nissen fundoplication) or by a 180 to 200-degree wrap (Toupet partial fundoplication) (Fig. 33.16). The fundus of the stomach acts as a flap valve

to create pressure around the distal esophagus, thus decreasing reflux. As an alternative to fundoplication, some surgeons insert an antireflux collar-like prosthesis around the esophagus just above the gastroesophageal junction.

A laparoscopic fundoplication, which may be performed in select patients, has similar advantages to laparoscopic cholecystectomy. The procedure involves mobilizing the esophagogastric junction and repairing the hiatal defect with a continuous suture technique. This is followed by a total fundoplication to fix the anterior margin of the diaphragmatic hiatus proximally and the esophagogastric junction distally. The laparoscopic approach has been successful in treating gastroesophageal reflux as a minimally invasive procedure.

Esophagogastrectomy

Removal of the lower portion of the esophagus and proximal stomach may be indicated to resect malignant tumors, benign strictures, or perforations at or near the esophagogastric junction. A left thoracoabdominal or upper midline incision is made. After the esophagus and stomach are mobilized and divided, an end-to-end esophagogastric anastomosis may be completed with staples and/or sutures. An end-to-side anastomosis with plication of the stomach around the distal part of the esophagus may be preferred. Depending on the extent of esophageal resection, other options for restoring continuity of the alimentary tract may be necessary.

Surgical Procedures for Esophageal Varices

Esophageal varices are tortuous, dilated veins in the submucosa of the lower esophagus that may extend up into the esophagus or down into the stomach. This condition is caused by portal hypertension and is usually associated with obstruction within a cirrhotic liver. The rupture of esophageal varices can cause massive hemorrhage. The patient may come to the OR with a Sengstaken-Blakemore tube in place to control bleeding by the use of pressure from the inflated balloon in the tube. An NG tube may be inserted through the central lumen to drain stomach contents and blood.

During the surgical procedure, varices may be sclerosed through an esophagoscope. A sclerosant is injected via a needle puncture into each varix. Several injections may be necessary to achieve complete hemostasis.

Sclerotherapy is usually attempted before more radical procedures are performed. The lower esophagus may be transected and the distal segment anastomosed with a circular stapler just proximal to the stomach. A portosystemic shunt procedure may be performed for portal decompression.

Gastrointestinal Surgery

Advances in the surgical management of patients with gastrointestinal problems have lessened the mortality rate. Interference with the gastrointestinal tract affects its functioning; specific deficiencies may result from gastrointestinal surgery depending on the site and extent of the surgical procedure.

Massive resection of the small intestine can produce long-term nutritional problems such as weight loss and malabsorption of most nutrients. Metabolic bone disease may follow gastric surgery because of poor absorption of calcium and vitamin D. Patients who have undergone extensive gastrointestinal procedures should

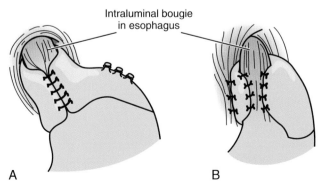

Intraluminal bougie
in esophagus

A   B

• **Fig. 33.16** Hiatal hernia repair. **A,** Nissen. **B,** Toupet.

have a periodic nutritional evaluation. Biochemical tests monitor nutritional status and include serum proteins, albumin-globulin ratio, and blood urea nitrogen (BUN). Body weight is also significant. If caloric intake is inadequate, protein is converted to carbohydrates for energy and as a result protein synthesis suffers.

Considerations for Gastrointestinal Surgery

The separation of instruments used for resection and anastomosis and for abdominal closure is a matter of preference of the surgeon and institution. Two distinct setups may be used, but the single setup is most commonly used. The single setup consists of identifying and using only selected instruments and supplies for resection, anastomosis, and abdominal closure and discarding contaminated instruments and equipment from the field after use. Acid secretions from the gastric resection site are very irritating and may cause peritonitis. In addition, the intestinal tract harbors many microorganisms. Leakage into the peritoneal cavity can be a source of generalized peritoneal sepsis. Gloves should be changed after anastomosis is completed; gowns also may be changed.

An NG tube is often inserted for the aspiration of gastric contents or for decompression of the intestinal tract. A variety of gastrointestinal tubes should be available for aspiration and irrigation.

Normal saline solution is used in abdominal procedures to moisten laparotomy sponges. Normal saline is an isotonic solution and has the same osmotic quality as blood serum and interstitial fluid. It will not alter sodium, chloride, or fluid balance because it does not cross cell membranes. (Hypotonic solutions cause cells to swell; hypertonic solutions cause them to shrink.) Normal saline is used for intraperitoneal irrigation unless the surgeon prefers to use a solution such as lactated Ringer's solution. Antibiotic solutions also may be needed for irrigation.

ESUs are used routinely by many surgeons for electrocoagulation of bleeding vessels in the abdominal wall, omentum, and mesentery. Ligating clips or suture ligatures are used for large vessels. To reduce tissue trauma, the jaws of intestinal forceps are protected with soft covers made of silicone.

Stapling devices are preferred by most surgeons for mechanical organ anastomosis. An intraluminal circular stapler can be used for end-to-end, end-to-side, or side-to-side anastomoses from the esophagus to the rectum. A straight linear stapler may be preferred for some gastrointestinal anastomoses and resections. Because the size of the lumen varies in different organs of the gastrointestinal tract, the circulating nurse should not open a sterile disposable stapler until the surgeon determines the appropriate head size or cartridge length for the instrument to be used.

The technical principles that guide the surgeon for all gastrointestinal anastomoses include the following:
- Good blood supply
- No tension
- Adequate lumen
- Watertight and leakproof
- No distal obstruction

A hand-sutured anastomosis produces an inverted suture line with serosa-to-serosa approximation. Many surgeons prefer anastomosing the inner seromuscular layer with absorbable interrupted or continuous sutures and the outer layers with either absorbable or nonabsorbable interrupted stitches.

A stapled anastomosis results in anastomosed mucosa-to-mucosa apposition.

Gastric Procedures

The stomach, a hollow muscular organ, is situated in the upper left abdomen between the esophagus and duodenum (see Fig. 33.20). Anatomically, it is divided into the fundus, body, and pyloric antrum. The two borders of the stomach, the lesser and greater curvatures, are important surgically because of their relation to the major vascular and lymphatic systems that supply the stomach.

The blood supply is derived from the celiac axis. The gastroduodenal artery and the right and left gastric arteries are the main tributaries. The splenic artery gives rise to the gastroepiploic arteries that are located at the greater curvature. The venous drainage follows the arterial supply but empties into the portal circulation of the liver.

The lymphatics empty into the pancreaticosplenic nodes and into the cisterna chyli via the celiac group. Omentum, a double fold of peritoneum attached to the lesser and greater curvatures, loosely covers the stomach and small intestine.

The innervation is both sympathetic and parasympathetic. The vagus nerve controls the reflex activities of movement and the secretions of the alimentary canal and is significant in rhythmic relaxation of the pyloric sphincter.

Food entering the stomach is reduced to chyme, a semiliquid, and then passes through the duodenum and small intestine. The chyme is absorbed through the lacteals of the intestine into the lymphatics, where it is converted to a milky white chyle. The chyle flows into the cisterna chyli and into the thoracic duct.

The main functions of the stomach are motor, secretory, and endocrine. The motor aspect moves the food along. The secretory actions cause the food to break down. The endocrine component is responsible for the release of gastrin and somatostatin. Gastrin causes the release of acid, and somatostatin inhibits the release of gastrin.

The interference of gastric motor activity or muscular contractions results in gastrointestinal complaints of abdominal pain, nausea, vomiting, hemorrhage, and dyspepsia. Some diseases, such as cancer, may not produce symptoms until the condition is far advanced. A surgical procedure is indicated when the presence of disease is established after laboratory tests such as gastric analysis, gastroscopy, and/or x-ray studies.

After gastric surgery, dumping syndrome may be experienced by patients shortly after eating. This complication occurs when food and fluids empty rapidly into the jejunum. It is characterized by nausea, vomiting, weakness, dizziness, pallor, sweating, palpitations, and diarrhea. Dumping syndrome after eating may persist for 6 months to 1 year postoperatively.

Gastroscopy

Gastroscopy involves the passage of a flexible fiberoptic gastroscope. This procedure is usually performed while the patient is sedated, with a topical anesthetic applied in the oropharynx to control the gag reflex. The operator visually inspects the mucosal walls of the stomach, and tissue specimens are sometimes obtained. Bleeding points may be coagulated with a laser, ESU, or sclerosing agent.

Gastrostomy

Establishment of a temporary or permanent opening in the stomach may be indicated for gastrointestinal decompression or to provide alimentation for a prolonged period when nutrition cannot be maintained by other means. A gastrostomy tube eliminates the incidence of aspiration that may occur around an NG tube. Often the patient is too debilitated to tolerate a major surgical procedure or may have an inoperable esophageal tumor or oropharyngeal trauma. A Foley, Malecot, Pezzer, or mushroom catheter may be inserted percutaneously into the stomach.

Simple Gastrostomy

With the patient under general anesthesia, the stomach is exposed through a small upper left abdominal or midline incision. The catheter is inserted into the anterior gastric wall and is held in place with purse-string sutures; it is brought out through a separate stab wound in the left upper quadrant. The stomach is sutured to the abdominal wall at the exit site of the catheter. After an abdominal procedure on a critically ill patient, the surgeon may prefer to place a small-bore catheter into the jejunum rather than the stomach for enteral hyperalimentation.

Percutaneous Endoscopic Gastrostomy

With percutaneous endoscopic gastrostomy, the patient is placed under IV sedation and an endoscopist introduces a fiberoptic gastroscope and insufflates the stomach with air to create a working space and a turgid surface to the stomach.[8] Light from the scope is directed anteriorly for transillumination through the abdominal wall. The surgeon infiltrates the skin with a local anesthetic at a selected gastrostomy site, usually approximately one-third of the distance along the left costal margin at the midclavicular line. The gastrostomy tube is introduced through a percutaneous puncture and secured with sutures.

Gastric Resections

The stomach may be totally or partially resected for removal of a malignant tumor or for benign chronic ulcer disease. Although surgical resection is the only cure, gastric carcinomas are often inoperable because of metastases to the liver or extension into surrounding tissues. In such cases, palliative procedures may be performed. The appropriate procedure is determined after thorough exploration of the abdominal cavity by the surgeon. Circular staplers are commonly used for anastomosis after resection. Leakage at the site of anastomosis leads to peritonitis. Some surgeons oversew the staple line.

Total Gastrectomy

With a total gastrectomy, the entire stomach is excised for malignant lesions through a bilateral subcostal, long transrectus, or thoracoabdominal incision. A total gastrectomy necessitates reconstruction of esophagointestinal continuity by establishing an anastomosis between a loop of jejunum and the esophagus. This anastomosis may be end-to-side with a lateral jejunojejunostomy or end-to-end with a Roux-en-Y jejunojejunostomy. The purpose of the jejunojejunostomy is to prevent the reflux of bile and pancreatic fluids into the esophagus. Some surgeons create a jejunal pouch for this purpose.

Subtotal Gastrectomy

Partial resections of the stomach, originally described by Theodor Billroth (1829–1894), are often referred to as Billroth procedures. A benign lesion (usually an ulcer) or a malignant lesion located in the pyloric half of the stomach requires removal of the lower half to two-thirds of the stomach. In a patient with a gastric or duodenal ulcer, a partial resection limits gastric acidity and relieves pain, bleeding, vomiting, and weight loss.

In this procedure, the peritoneal cavity is entered through a right paramedian or upper midline abdominal incision. A variety of surgical procedures may be used to reestablish gastrointestinal continuity. Anastomosis of the remaining portion of the stomach to the duodenum (gastroduodenostomy, antrectomy, or Billroth I, Fig. 33.17) or to a loop of the jejunum (gastrojejunostomy or Billroth II, Fig. 33.18) is often performed. A truncal vagotomy, which is discussed in the following section, is performed to eliminate the possibility of postoperative peptic ulceration.

Common modifications of the Billroth I procedure are the Schoemaker and von Haberer-Finney techniques. The Schoemaker procedure involves end-to-end anastomosis of the stomach and duodenum after the lesser curvature of the stomach is sutured

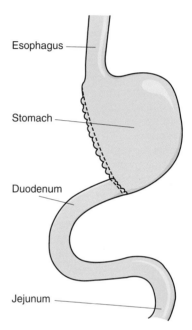

• **Fig. 33.17** Billroth I gastrectomy with anastomosis to duodenum.

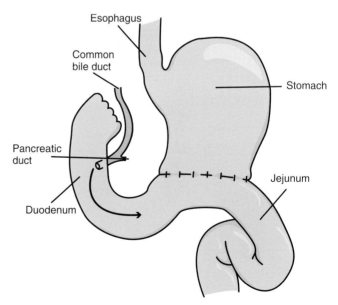

• **Fig. 33.18** Billroth II subtotal gastrectomy with anastomosis to jejunum.

to make the anastomosis site the same size as the duodenum. With the von Haberer-Finney method, the lateral wall of the duodenum is brought up to the stomach so that the entire end of the stomach is open for direct anastomosis.

Popular modifications of the Billroth II procedure include the Polya and Hofmeister techniques, both of which involve variations of end-to-side gastrojejunostomy.

Vagotomy

Chronic gastric, pyloric, and duodenal ulcers that do not respond to medical treatment cause patients severe pain and difficulty in eating and sleeping. Vagotomy, the division of the vagus nerves, may be recommended to interrupt vagal nerve impulses, thus lowering the production of gastric hydrochloric acid and hastening gastric emptying. Vagotomy can be performed at several different locations along the course of the vagus nerve (Fig. 33.19).

Proximal gastric vagotomy, also known as parietal cell vagotomy, divides the vagal nerve fibers to the proximal stomach but maintains the entire stomach and vagal nerves to the antrum. These sections of the vagal nerve inhibit the release of gastrin, a stimulant of gastric secretion.

Truncal vagotomy and selective vagotomy require a concomitant drainage procedure because these procedures denervate the stomach. A gastroenterostomy is performed with a truncal vagotomy, which divides the vagal trunks at the distal esophagus. An antrectomy is performed with a selective vagotomy, which transects the gastric branches. Vagotomy with drainage is a compromise procedure and is restricted to high-risk patients or those with severe duodenal deformity.

Pyloroplasty, enlarging the pyloric opening between the stomach and duodenum, may be performed in patients with an obstructing pyloric ulcer or in conjunction with vagotomy to treat bleeding duodenal ulcers. Duodenal dilation or duodenoplasty may be indicated.

Vagotomy procedures, which are conservative surgical therapies compared with gastrectomy, decrease the surgical risk for select patients with chronic ulcers. It is now known that ulcers caused by the *Helicobacter pylori* organism can be cured with antibiotics.

Gastrojejunostomy (Roux-en-Y Gastroenterostomy)

A procedure may be necessary to reestablish continuity between the stomach and intestinal tract, such as after a partial gastrectomy or when the lower end of the stomach is obstructed by an ulcer or

a nonresectable tumor. A gastrojejunostomy may be performed to treat alkaline reflux gastritis, postgastrectomy syndromes such as postvagotomy diarrhea, and dumping syndrome. Except in geriatric patients, a concomitant vagotomy is necessary to prevent a postoperative gastrojejunal ulcer when the acid-forming portion of the stomach is not resected.

In this procedure, a loop of jejunum may be anastomosed to either the anterior or the posterior wall of the stomach; both approaches have advantages and disadvantages. In a Roux-en-Y gastrojejunostomy, the jejunum is divided. The distal end is anastomosed to the side of the stomach, and the proximal end is anastomosed to the side of the jejunum at a lower level. The result is a Y-shaped double anastomosis that diverts the flow of bile and pancreatic enzymes directly into the jejunum, bypassing the created gastric stoma.

An adaptation of a Roux-en-Y anastomosis is also used to drain the biliary tract or other organs, such as the pancreas or esophagus, directly into the jejunum to bypass the stomach and prevent the reflux of intestinal contents.

Bariatric Surgery

The study of morbid obesity, or bariatrics, has led to the development of a subspecialization in general surgery: bariatric surgery.

Bariatric surgery can be performed as an open abdominal surgery or as a laparoscopic procedure. The surgical landmarks are altered in overweight patients because the body habitus is large and extends beyond the borders of the average-sized patient. Insufflation via Veress needle may not be performed at the umbilicus. An alternative site is Palmer point because the risk for injury is less (Fig. 33.20). The umbilicus, for example, lies several inches lower on a pendulous abdomen. Using the infraumbilical or supraumbilical area of the patient as an inflation or primary trocar site could cause injury to nontarget organs (Fig. 33.21).

Bariatric procedures produce three types of results:
1. Restricted intake caused by an inflatable silastic band (Fig. 33.22)
2. Bypass the food and decrease absorption (Fig. 33.23)
3. Bypass absorption and restrict intake

People who have a body mass index (BMI) of 40 or more, weigh 100 lbs (45.4 kg) more than their ideal weight, and have failed to lose weight despite years of medical treatment are potential candidates for bariatric surgery. Patients with a BMI of 35 to 40 and have serious comorbid disease, such as obstructive sleep apnea, cardiomyopathy, and type 2 diabetes, may be candidates

Celiac axis

Truncal

Selective
or
gastric

Highly selective
or
parietal cell vagotomy

• **Fig. 33.19** Vagotomy.

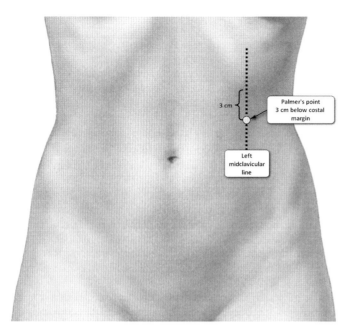

• **Fig. 33.20** Palmer point for alternative insufflation when the umbilical area is not safe. (From Granata M: Are we underutilizing Palmer's point entry in gynecologic laparoscopy? *Fertil Steril* 94(7):2716–2719, 2010.)

• **Fig. 33.22** Gastric banding. **A,** Gastric band with port. **B,** Gastric band in place.

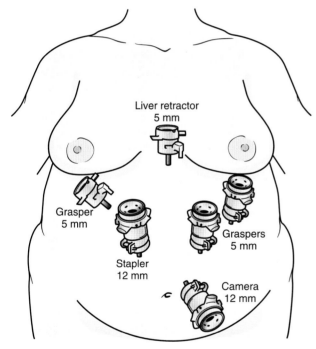

• **Fig. 33.21** Laparoscopic ports for a bariatric procedure. Note the displacement of the umbilical landmark.

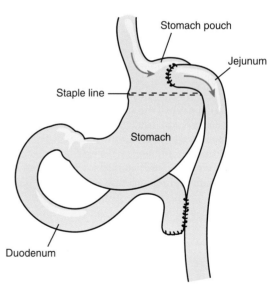

• **Fig. 33.23** Gastric bypass for a bariatric procedure.

after careful screening. The plan of care requires the patient to have psychologic and physiologic support during the process, or the procedure could be a failure. Some facilities have extended the procedure to overweight adolescents aged 11 years and older, with varying degrees of success. The average age for adolescent bariatric surgery is 15 to 19 years old.[9]

The physical size of a patient who is overweight presents special needs with respect to transporting and positioning, selecting instrumentation, and providing psychologic and physiologic support. The OR bed must support the patient's weight and fit the length and width of the patient's body habitus. The standard OR bed cannot do these things safely, so a special OR bed must be used.

Many extremely overweight patients have medical complications such as hypertension, peripheral vascular disease, cardiac disease, degenerative arthritis, gallbladder disease, or diabetes mellitus.[10] Consideration is given to pressure-reducing surfaces, such as gel pads and positioning devices designed to hold large limbs.

The plan of care for overweight patients usually includes the application of antiembolic stockings and the insertion of an NG tube, a Foley catheter, IV and arterial lines, and central venous pressure (CVP). Because respiratory distress is a potential complication during the induction of anesthesia, intubation while the patient is awake may be the technique of choice. Many overweight patients have short, wide necks, so positioning head support in a "sniffing posture" may be necessary to establish a secure airway.

The types of surgical procedures performed for bariatric surgery can be done via open or endoscopic methods. Natural orifice transluminal endoscopic surgery (NOTES) is feasible, but not widely developed for the gastric alterations necessary to restrict absorption or reduce volume in weight-loss surgery. The procedures and instrumentation for any approach are modified to suit the patient's size. Single-incision laparoscopy has been adapted to accommodate longer instrumentation and a deeper port matched to the thickness of an overweight patient's abdominal wall. The average surgical landmarks are not reliable because of adipose layers and redundant skin. This in combination with adhesions from previous abdominal surgery can disqualify the patient from a single-incision approach.

Bariatric procedures for gastric restriction are not without risks. Nutritional deficiencies, anemia, wound infection, and a failure of staple lines have occurred postoperatively. The capacity of the stomach is reduced to approximately 30 mL to restrict food absorption or intake. Patients lose at least 25% to 60% of their excess body fat.

Gastroplasty

In gastroplasty, which is usually referred to as a vertical banded gastroplasty, four linear staple lines are placed vertically on the lesser curvature side of the stomach just left of the gastroesophageal junction in addition to a gastric band to cause restriction of intake. This creates a small channel for the passage of gastric contents from the proximal to the distal segments. The total intake at any given time is about 1 ounce. The stomach is divided between staple lines and oversewn with sutures.

To prevent dilation, the outlet at the end of the staple line is usually reinforced with a silastic band. This method does not have the same restricted absorption as gastric bypass. Some patients do not lose satisfactory amounts of weight because they take in excess high-calorie liquids and sugary foods.

Gastric Bypass

In a gastric bypass procedure, the capacity of the stomach is restricted by creating a small pouch in the fundus (the proximal segment of the stomach) and bypassing portions of the small intestines to decrease the absorptive qualities of the gastrointestinal tract (see Fig. 33.23). The stomach is transected horizontally with a linear stapler, and the proximal jejunum is divided. A Roux-en-Y gastrojejunostomy is constructed between the 1-ounce-sized pouch, vertically oriented stomach pouch, and the jejunum, bypassing the remainder of stomach to establish intestinal continuity for the passage of gastric contents. The proximal jejunal segment is anastomosed end to side to the distal segment for drainage of gastric, biliary, and pancreatic fluids.

Patients are advised not to eat concentrated sugars because doing so stimulates dumping syndrome. Nutrient supplements, such as vitamins, iron, and calcium, are necessary to prevent anemia and osteoporosis.

Intestinal Procedures

Anatomically, the intestines are divided into the small (upper) and large (lower) intestines, and there are subdivisions of each.

The small intestine extends from the pylorus to the ileocecal valve. The three sections include the duodenum (proximal portion), the jejunum (middle section), and the ileum (distal portion that joins the large intestine). The ileocecal valve, a sphincter muscle, lessens the backflow of material that has been discharged to the large intestine. The blood supply to the small bowel is divided into arcades with several subdivisions (Fig. 33.24).

The large intestine, or colon, extends from the ileum to the rectum and is generally divided into the ascending, transverse, descending, and sigmoid colon. The cecum is the pouch formed where the large intestine joins the small intestine. The blood supply to the large bowel is united on the mesenteric border by the marginal artery of Drummond with widely dispersed arcades of vessels (Fig. 33.25).

The mesentery, a peritoneal fold, attaches the small and large intestines to the posterior abdominal wall and contains the arteries, veins, and lymph nodes that supply the intestines.

Inflammation, intestinal obstruction, and disruption in absorption and motility are disorders that may lead to surgical intervention. Etiologic factors determine the surgical procedure. Segments of bowel can be removed, and the continuity can be reestablished by anastomosis (Fig. 33.26).

Resection of the Small Intestine

Tumors, as well as strangulation from adhesions, volvulus, obstruction, and regional ileitis, usually are treated by resection of the involved segment. An abdominal incision is made over the suspected or known site of disease. After exposure, clamps are placed above and below the diseased segment of the bowel and mesentery to avoid spillage. The involved area is resected, and an end-to-end, end-to-side, or side-to-side anastomosis is performed to restore continuity.

Variations of this technique are used for other related problems of the small intestine, such as extensive perforation. Bowel strangulation and obstruction necessitate an immediate surgical procedure to prevent necrosis, peritonitis, and death.

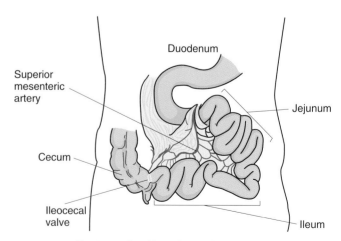

• **Fig. 33.24** Small bowel arterial blood supply.

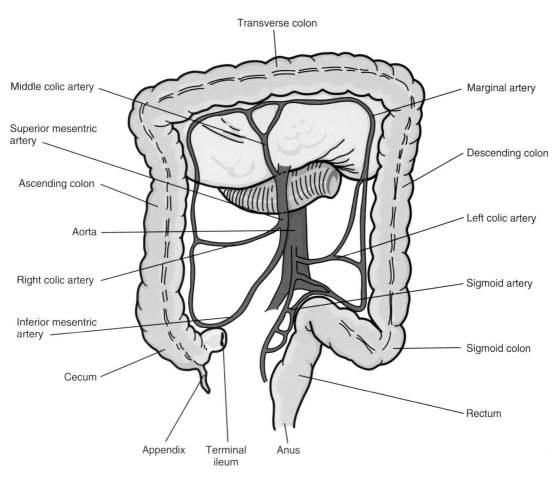

• **Fig. 33.25** Large bowel arterial blood supply.

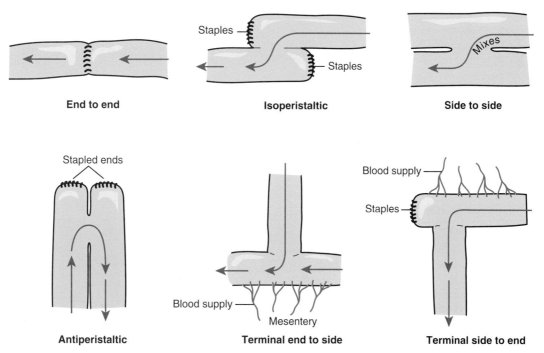

• **Fig. 33.26** Intestinal anastomoses. Intestinal anastomoses can be performed with sutured anastomoses or with circular or linear staplers, as shown here. Same principles apply to other anastomoses, such as vascular structures.

Hemicolectomy, Transverse Colectomy, Anterior Resection, and Total Colectomy

Colitis, diverticulitis (or diverticulosis), obstruction, and neoplasms are the most common reasons for surgical intervention to remove a diseased segment of the colon. Most surgical procedures involve opening the abdomen, walling off the peritoneal cavity, incising and clamping at the points where resection is to be carried out, and, finally, reestablishing continuity by anastomosis.[11] In select patients, a laparoscopic approach may be used to mobilize the segment of the large or small bowel to be resected. The resected bowel is removed through a small minimal-access incision in the abdominal wall. Stomas also can be created with the laparoscopic technique.

The perioperative plan of care includes preoperative administration of intestinal antibiotics, bowel-cleansing methods, and diet restrictions (e.g., a clear liquid diet). Bowel cleansing can cause depletion of electrolytes and is performed only as necessary.

Intraoperatively, contaminated instrument technique should be used during the procedure. Instruments used on the interior aspect of the bowel should not be used on other tissues and should be isolated after use.

An NG tube may be inserted before the surgical procedure begins and may remain in place until partial healing of the anastomosis occurs and effective peristalsis returns. Fluid and electrolyte balance is maintained.

Intestinal Stomas

An intestinal ostomy is a surgically created opening, or *stoma*, that extends from a portion of the bowel to the exterior via the abdominal wall. This procedure may be performed to divert intestinal contents so inflamed bowel can heal, to decompress pressure caused by an obstructive lesion, or to bypass an obstruction such as a benign or malignant tumor. A stoma can be created from the large or small bowel. Some intestinal stomas are temporary; others are permanent.

The type and level of the lesion determine whether an ileostomy, a cecostomy, or a colostomy is indicated. Preoperatively, the patient's abdomen will be assessed for stoma placement based on the type of stoma, body size, and belt line. The stoma site is marked so the patient's clothing will not interfere with the collection appliance. Most facilities have stoma nurses available to assist with stoma planning and teaching. An ileostomy will be positioned on the right side of the lower abdomen. The output will be more frequent and liquid. A colostomy is usually positioned on the left side of the abdomen. The output will be more formed.

In patients with a temporary stoma, intestinal continuity is reestablished after healing, through closure of the opening in the bowel and anastomosis of the previously separated ends. If the stoma will be permanent, the patient will wear a collection appliance at all times.

The patient's acceptance of these procedures is as varied as an individual's emotional reactions. Each patient requires a rehabilitation plan based on personal needs. These plans should include care of the collection appliance, maintenance of skin integrity, proper diet, odor control, and comfortable clothing. Patient participation is an integral part of the preparation for self-care and enhances self-confidence.

Ileostomy

An ileostomy is performed for conditions such as chronic ulcerative colitis or after removal of the colon (colectomy). In this procedure the proximal end of the transected ileum is exteriorized

through the abdominal wall (Fig. 33.27). The usual stoma site is the midportion of the right rectus sheath, approximately 3 cm below the level of the umbilicus. First, a disk of epithelium the size of the planned stoma is excised. The anterior and posterior sheaths are then incised, and the rectus sheath is divided with a muscle-splitting incision. The proximal end of the ileum is brought out through the peritoneum and muscle to the skin; here the edges are everted and sutured to the skin (Fig. 33.28). Liquid

• **Fig. 33.27** Ileostomy. Proximal end of transected ileum is brought out through peritoneum and muscle. The end is everted and sutured to skin. Stoma site is in midportion of right rectus sheath below level of umbilicus.

A

B

• **Fig. 33.28** Ileostomy stoma is brought through an opening in the skin and sutured into place. **A,** The edges of the intestinal mucosa are aligned with subcuticular tissues by sutures. **B,** The stoma is formed by everting the mucosa and tying the sutures.

or semisolid discharge is collected in an ileostomy bag placed over the stoma. The surrounding skin requires special care to prevent excoriation and irritation.

The entire cecum and colon, as well as the rectal mucosa (mucosal proctectomy), are resected in an endorectal-ileoanal pull-through procedure. The ileum is anastomosed to the anus with a circular stapler. The rectal and anal muscles are preserved for anal continence.

In a multistage procedure, a pouch can be constructed for use as a fecal reservoir using loops of the terminal ileum. This procedure can be performed as an open surgery or laparoscopically. Pouch configurations can resemble a J, W, or S. Studies have shown that the J pouch is the preferred method overall. A 20-cm J pouch is fashioned of the ileum with a linear stapler. The lower curve of the J is anastomosed to the rectal stump with a circular stapler side to end (Fig. 33.29). During the healing period, a temporary ileostomy may be in place. Fecal material will pass through the ileostomy, pouch, and the rectum. The anal anastomosis is closely monitored during this time for integrity. Once it is confirmed that the pouch is healed and the anastomosis is secure, the ileostomy will be closed as a final step in the process.

Although not without complications, these procedures offer acceptable alternatives to a permanent ileostomy stoma, especially in children and young adults.

• Fig. 33.29 Ileorectal anastomosis of a J pouch created from a loop of ileum. Anastomosis is 1.5 cm superior to dentate line performed with a circular stapler (end-to-end anastomosis [EEA]). (From Khatri VP: *Atlas of advanced operative surgery*, Philadelphia, 2013, Saunders.)

Cecostomy

With a cecostomy, an opening is created in the cecum, and a tube is inserted for decompression of the massive distention caused by colonic obstruction. The tube is placed into the cecum through the lower right side of the abdomen. Less severe distention may be relieved by suction and irrigation through a colonoscope and the insertion of an intestinal tube through the anus to the cecum. Cecostomy or colonoscopic decompression may precede subsequent colon resection.

Colostomy

An opening anywhere along the length of the colon to the exterior skin surface creates an artificial anus (Fig. 33.30). The section of colon to be exteriorized depends on the location of the lesion to be resected or treated. For example, a low anterior bowel resection necessitates a sigmoid colostomy. A permanent colostomy in the sigmoid colon forms an artificial anus after a combined abdominoperineal resection for rectal carcinoma (see Fig. 33.30, *A*). The rectum is removed. A collection device for fecal material is not needed after a patient's bowel evacuation becomes regulated. Most patients wear a stoma cap even when they are in the process of regulation.

Either a double-barreled or a loop colostomy may be performed as a temporary measure. In a double-barreled colostomy (see Fig. 33.30, *B*), the transverse colon is divided and both ends are brought out to the margins of the skin incision. The proximal stoma serves as an outlet for feces, and the distal opening leads to the nonfunctioning bowel. In a loop colostomy (see Fig. 33.30, *C*), a loop of colon is brought out onto the abdominal wall. A plastic rod or ostomy bridge is placed under the loop to hold it out on the exterior abdominal wall. The peritoneum is closed, and the wound around the colostomy is sutured.

Appendectomy

Appendicitis can occur at any age but is seen most often in adolescents and young adults. It may imitate other conditions such as a ruptured ovarian cyst or ureteral calculus. Some appendices are retrocecal, which makes diagnosis and excision more difficult (Fig. 33.31). Classic symptoms of early appendicitis include pain in the right lower quadrant at McBurney point, rebound tenderness, nausea, and moderate elevations in temperature and white blood cell count.

An emergency appendectomy is necessary to prevent a progression to gangrene and the perforation of friable tissue, with subsequent peritonitis. Most appendectomies can be performed via laparoscopy. The open abdominal approach involves a muscle-splitting incision in the right lower quadrant, over McBurney point. The blood supply to the appendix is ligated and severed. A crushing clamp is applied to the appendiceal base, which is then ligated and severed from the cecum. After amputation, the surgeon may elect to cauterize the stump or wipe it with a sponge soaked with an iodophor (povidone-iodine [Betadine]) to reduce contamination. The stump is then inverted into the cecum as a purse-string suture is tightened around the stump (Fig. 33.32). Instruments used in the appendectomy are isolated as contaminated and not used on other tissues.

Drainage is indicated in the presence of an abscess, appendix rupture, or any gross contamination of the wound. An appendectomy is usually an uncomplicated procedure with rapid convalescence unless life-threatening peritonitis results.

• **Fig. 33.30** Comparison of intestinal stomas. **A,** Colostomy. **B,** Transverse double-barrel colostomy. **C,** Ileostomy. **D,** Continent ileostomy.

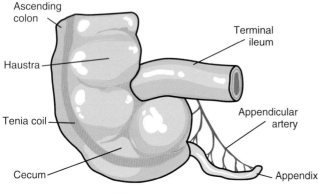

• **Fig. 33.31** Cecum and appendix.

Laparoscopic Appendectomy

After creation of a peritoneal working space with carbon dioxide, trocars are placed, the laparoscope is inserted through the infraumbilical incision, and the patient is placed in Trendelenburg position. If a single-lumen approach is not used, secondary trocars are inserted in the suprapubic area and left lower quadrant for placement of graspers and dissectors. The appendix is located and hemostatically dissected from the mesoappendix with endoscopic clips or staples. Endoloop ligatures are placed at the base of the appendix, and endoscopic scissors are used to transect it. Grasping forceps are used to place the appendix into an Endopouch collection reservoir to prevent the extrusion of contents during evacuation through the infraumbilical trocar.

Colorectal Procedures

Colorectal carcinoma is one of the most common abdominal malignancies, with the highest incidence in people older than 60 years. Resection of the carcinoma is the surgical procedure of choice; radiation and chemotherapy are adjuvant therapies or palliative therapies for advanced disease. Early diagnosis and prompt treatment of asymptomatic carcinoma improve the survival rates.

Diagnostic procedures are routinely performed in patients with bowel or rectal bleeding, chronic diarrhea, or a history of intestinal polyps and/or carcinoma of the colon. Serial guaiac stool tests may detect the presence of occult blood. A barium enema provides a complete radiographic study of the colon. Colonoscopy is commonly done in place of a barium enema. An endoscopic examination is routine. Some therapeutic procedures may be accomplished with laser or ESU through an endoscope.

Sigmoidoscopy

Sigmoidoscopy is direct visual inspection of the sigmoid and rectal lumens by means of a flexible fiberoptic or rigid lighted sigmoidoscope. The flexible scope is more comfortable for the patient and gives the surgeon better visualization of the mucosal surface to evaluate the left colon and rectosigmoid. It may be used intraoperatively to check an anastomosis or for preoperative diagnosis. Water-soluble lubricant is used to help ease insertion of the scope.

The patient is prepared preoperatively with enemas and colon cleansing. Placing the patient in the left lateral position allows for

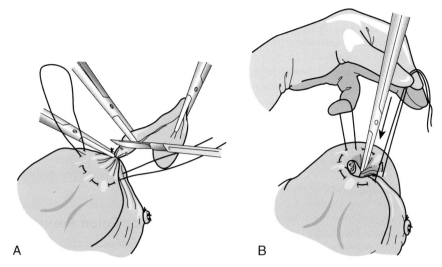

• **Fig. 33.32** Ligation of the appendiceal stump. **A,** A purse-string suture is placed around the base of the appendix. It is double-clamped and dissected with a scalpel. **B,** The appendiceal stump is inverted into the circumference of the purse-string suture. The suture is tightened as the stump is buried within.

anatomic positioning of the sigmoid colon. The knee-chest or Kraske position allows the sigmoid colon to fall forward into the abdomen. The Sims or lithotomy position may be used for an extremely overweight or extremely ill patient.

The surgeon may inflate room air into the colon with a hand-pumped bulb to create a working space during insertion of the well-lubricated scope to better visualize the mucosal walls and folds. This insufflation stimulates the stretch receptors of the bowel, causing a feeling of desire to defecate, which necessitates reassurance of the patient. Have the suction handy for evacuation of air from the colon at the conclusion of the procedure.

Colonoscopy

Colonoscopy provides visual inspection of the lining of the entire colon. This is facilitated by placing the patient in left lateral position so that the folds of the large intestine will be in anatomic alignment (Fig. 33.33). The colonoscope is flexible and consists of two channels: one for suctioning and irrigating and one for operating. Its greatest uses are to examine the lumen of the colon, to perform a biopsy of tissues, and to search for and excise or ablate polyps. Other indications are for the study of inflammatory bowel or diverticular disease, the passage of blood in the feces (hematochezia), or a change in bowel habits; as a preoperative screen before colostomy closure; for confirmation of radiographic findings; and as a follow-up for patients who have undergone intestinal procedures. Argon and Nd:YAG lasers or ESU is used through a colonoscope to ablate some tumors and to treat polyps, arteriovenous malformations, and bleeding disorders.

Because the presence of stool in the rectum prevents adequate examination with the scope, the patient should have a preoperative bowel evacuation prep. Colonoscopy without moderate sedation is contraindicated if the patient is uncooperative. Relative contraindications may include acute, severe, or radiation-caused inflammatory disease or complete obstruction. Perforation can occur. Vital signs should be monitored during the procedure.

Complications of colonoscopy include electrical burn during polypectomy, tearing or perforation of the colon by tip pressure, tearing of the liver or spleen by air pressure, and tearing of diverticula resulting from the introduction of air into them.

• **Fig. 33.33** Correct anatomic left lateral position for colonoscopy.

Polypectomy

Most surgeons and pathologists agree that adenomatous mucosal polyps in the colon are potentially malignant and should be removed. A polypectomy is usually performed through a fiberoptic colonoscope. Polyps, which are often familial, may be single or multiple and are easily excised at the base. The colonoscope may be used intraoperatively to locate polyps.

If the polyps are pedunculated, they are cauterized at the stalk and retrieved by a snare for microscopic examination. Electrocoagulation or lasing of the base provides hemostasis. Some polyps or the involved segment of colon is removed by laparotomy or laparoscopy. After a polypectomy, patients should have annual colonoscopic examinations.

Abdominoperineal Resection

Abdominoperineal resection (also known as the Miles procedure) is a radical type of colectomy and excision of the rectum and anus performed for colon cancer or extreme inflammatory disease. This procedure may include not only the lower sigmoidal segment but also any portion up to the entire colon. The distal resection is too deep to permit anastomosis of the colon or ileum to the anal region. The patient will have a permanent colostomy or, if the entire colon is removed, a permanent ileostomy.

Preoperative preparations include presurgical bowel prep to evacuate the bowel contents. The patient will be positioned supine in low lithotomy using boot-style stirrups after the administration of general anesthesia. Sequential compression devices should be used on the legs. The anesthesia provider will insert an NG tube to decompress the gastrointestinal tract. The circulating nurse will open two prep sets: one for the perineum and a separate one for the abdomen.

Some surgeons prefer to use ureteral stents to make ureteral identification and preservation easier. This requires a cystoscopy setup and two ureteral catheters prepared for the urologist. The perineum is prepped, and the urologist inserts the ureteral catheters that will be connected to ureteral drainage collection. A Foley catheter is inserted at this time because the ureteral catheters will be removed postoperatively and the indwelling catheter will remain in place. The cystoscopy table should be kept sterile at the side of the room in case the urologist needs the instrumentation to remove the stents at the conclusion of the procedure.

If ureteral stents are not used, two prep sets are necessary. The perineum is prepped first, and a Foley catheter is inserted. Using the second prep set, the abdominal skin is prepped from the xyphoid to the pubis.

The instrumentation is set up on two separate tables and requires two separate teams (abdominal and perineal) to work simultaneously. The perineal team will drape the patient using a lithotomy drape pack with leggings. The abdominal team will then drape the abdomen. Great care is taken to keep the instrumentation and counted items separated. Usually one circulating nurse can manage the separation of the materials. Both teams work at the same time.

The abdominal team will open the abdomen with a full midline incision from subxyphoid to the pubis. Some surgeons use a left paramedian incision. The surgeon will "take down" the colon from its mesenteric attachments. When the colon is mobilized, the distal rectum is divided with a linear stapler (GIA). The remaining proximal end of the resected colon will be clamped and transected from the segment being removed. Some surgeons tie off the remaining bowel segment with saline-moistened cotton umbilical tapes. The bowel specimen is removed and handed off in a basin to the circulating nurse. The abdominal surgeon mobilizes the remaining rectal stump remnant in preparation for its removal by the perineal team. The pelvic floor is reperitonealized, and the anorectal stump is removed by the perineal team. The abdomen is irrigated with sterile normal saline and suctioned using a Poole tip to protect the organs. The terminal portion of bowel will be exteriorized to form a stoma.

The abdominal tissue layers are closed with suture, and the skin is usually closed with staples. One or more drains may be used. Dry sterile dressings are applied. A stoma appliance will be positioned to collect intestinal contents.

The perineal team will close the anus with a heavy silk purse-string suture or staples and simultaneously direct the elliptical dissection from distal to proximal, separating the perianal tissues from the tip of the coccyx to midperineal floor and circumferentially from the anus toward the rectal margins. The lower blood supply arises laterally from the middle hemorrhoidal artery at the point where the abdominal resection and the perineal dissection meet. The anorectal stump is removed from the perineum. The levator ani muscles are approximated if possible, and the skin layers closed with suture. Some surgeons use a Penrose drain in the perineal incision for 24 to 48 hours. Fluff gauze and mesh pants are commonly used as dressings.

Postoperatively, the NG tube may remain in place for 24 hours and the Foley catheter may stay in for several days. If ureteral stents were used, they will be removed before the patient leaves the OR. The patient will be taken to the PACU and remain there until stable enough to be discharged to the patient care division. Sequential compression devices should be used on the legs until the patient is ambulatory to minimize the risk for deep vein thrombosis.

Low Anterior Colon Resection

The sigmoid colon and rectum lie within the bony pelvis, which makes the resection of tumors in the lower sigmoid colon, rectosigmoid, and rectum technically difficult. The objective is to achieve wide local excision with en bloc resection of the lymphatics and perirectal mesentery (Fig. 33.34). Intraluminal and linear staplers facilitate colorectal anastomosis in a low anterior colon resection. The distal colon is transected after closure with a linear stapler. The intraluminal stapler, with the anvil removed, is introduced through the anus and rectal stump either through or adjacent to the linear staple line. After the anvil is replaced, an intraluminal end-to-end or end-to-side anastomosis with the proximal segment of colon is completed.

Total excision of the mesorectum is necessary to prevent recurrence of the tumor in the pelvis or at the staple line; a distal tumor clearance of at least 2 cm is necessary. With this technique for low anterior colorectal anastomosis, colorectal continuity is restored and anal sphincter control is maintained without necessitating a permanent colostomy; with an abdominoperineal resection, a permanent colostomy is necessary.

The surgeon may check the colorectal anastomosis with a sigmoidoscope at the completion of the surgery before closing the abdomen. The sigmoidoscope will be placed in the rectum, and room air will be used to insufflate and expand the anastomosed segment. The abdomen will be simultaneously filled with warm saline irrigation. The anastomotic line will be observed for air leak. If a leak is present, air bubbles will rise to the surface of the irrigation solution. If no leak is present, the irrigation is suctioned out of the abdomen using a Poole tip with a guard. The sigmoidoscope is withdrawn, and the air is permitted to escape.

Abdominal Trauma

Trauma is the major cause of death in people younger than 40 years. Bleeding from the disruption of solid organs or major vessels in the abdomen (including the pelvis) and infection from perforation of a hollow viscus are life-threatening injuries.

Abdominal trauma is usually caused by one of the following:
- Blunt trauma caused by direct impact, rapid deceleration, shearing forces, and/or increased intraluminal pressure can rupture or sever multiple structures, including those that are retroperitoneal.
- Penetrating injuries involve structures within the path of the weapon; gunshot wounds may also injure adjacent structures through the blast effect or cavitation. A stab or gunshot wound of the abdomen can penetrate across the diaphragm into the chest or vice versa.

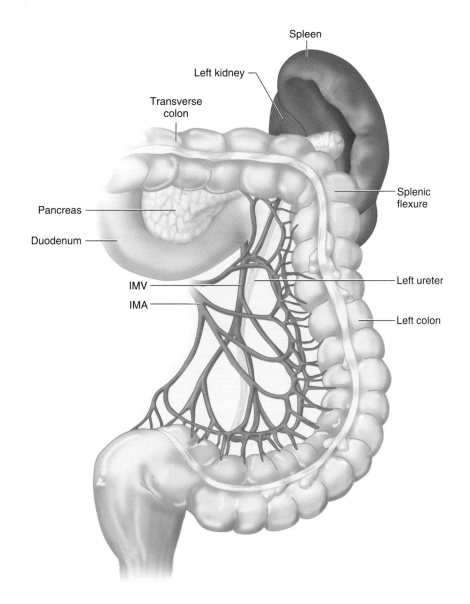

Spleen

Left kidney

Transverse
colon

Pancreas

Duodenum

IMV

IMA

Splenic
flexure

Left ureter

Left colon

• **Fig. 33.34** Left colon resection. *IMA*, Inferior mesenteric artery; *IMV*, inferior mesenteric vein. (From Fleshman JW, Birnbaum E, Hunt S et al: *Atlas of surgical techniques for colon, rectum, and anus*, Philadelphia, 2013, Saunders.)

Planning Perioperative Care for Abdominal Trauma Patients

Many patients have multiple injuries that affect more than one body system. These patients require a comprehensive approach to diagnosis and treatment by a multidisciplinary team. The philosophy of trauma management has changed from that of an individual surgeon treating an injured patient in the emergency department and OR to a system that begins at the site of the accident with stabilization by trained personnel and continues with definitive care, including rapid surgical intervention and rehabilitation. This section will concentrate on abdominal trauma and its surgical evaluation and treatment.

Systematic Approach to Evaluation

When dealing with abdominal trauma patients, the first thought is hemorrhage or fecal spill. Other injuries such as biliary or pancreatic spillage are less common. Severe penetrating trauma can be complicated by evisceration.

Ultrasonography, x-ray, and CT scan are useful presurgical diagnostic tests to assess the extent of abdominal injuries and determine indications for surgical intervention. Free air in the abdomen generally indicates a ruptured organ, such as the bowel. This necessitates immediate laparotomy to locate the torn organ and control seepage of bowel contents. CT scan and ultrasonography provide additional assessment data.

Peritoneal Lavage

The patient who is hypotensive with left upper quadrant pain requires a peritoneal lavage to determine active intraabdominal bleeding. Before the procedure, the patient is positioned supine and an NG tube placed to decompress the stomach and observe contents (if not contraindicated by upper body or facial injury). A

Foley catheter should be inserted to decompress the bladder and observe the urine.

The peritoneal lavage procedure is done under local anesthesia by creating a 2-cm midline incision in one of two planes: infraumbilical or supraumbilical (if the patient is pregnant or has a fractured pelvis). The incision extends to the peritoneal membrane, which is anesthetized and grasped with hemostats. The peritoneum is incised only under direct vision. If blood is seen immediately rushing from the peritoneal incision, a rapid-sequence induction is performed by the anesthesia provider, and an immediate exploratory laparotomy is performed.

If no immediate hemorrhage is seen, proceed by instilling body-temperature lactated Ringer's solution or sterile normal saline, 10 mL/kg. The circulating nurse and anesthesia provider document all fluids into or out of the patient's abdomen. Allow the solution to sit in the abdomen for a few moments. The organs can be slightly agitated by hand and the solution drained into a basin or container with a lid. The circulating nurse labels the irrigant and sends it to the laboratory for a rush cell count. The laboratory personnel look for blood cells, stool, vegetable matter, or any other indicator of intraabdominal injury. Negative findings mean that the patient needs no further intraabdominal surgery at that time but will be monitored closely for any change in condition.

Keep in mind that retroperitoneal bleeding may not be diagnosed with peritoneal lavage. Many major structures such as the great vessels and kidneys are retroperitoneal. Injuries to the great vessels require an immediate surgical procedure to control bleeding and restore vascular continuity. Major organ injuries mandate an open laparotomy for repair or reconstruction or to resect severely damaged tissues.

Emergency Exploratory Laparotomy

The patient is positioned supine and prepped from chin to groin. An NG tube is placed and a Foley catheter inserted. The surgeon makes a midline incision from xyphoid to pubis in some cases. The surgeon carefully displaces the abdominal contents laterally to examine each angle of the individual organs (Fig. 33.35). After careful inspection of the viscera, the surgeon manually palpates the entire length of the bowel, starting at the duodenum and ending at the sigmoid flexure. This process is referred to as "running the bowel" (Fig. 33.36).

After the exploration, any injuries to the organs caused by the trauma are repaired, and the abdomen is closed. If the exploratory procedure was extensive, the patient's tissue may be extremely edematous and might not approximate without undue tension. The patient's abdomen may have to remain open for several days and the patient brought back to the OR for a delayed primary closure.

Each surgeon has a routine for protecting the patient's open incision until the edges can be approximated. Commercial sterile wound packs are available. Some surgeons use sterile silastic sheeting circumferentially stapled to the wound edges to form a temporary cover. If silastic sheeting is not available, some surgeons have cut sterile 3000-mL IV bags to fit like a patch (referred to as a Bogota or silo bag). A bulky dressing is placed over the area, and the patient is transferred to intensive care for stabilization and monitoring.

Great care is taken to count and be accountable for instruments, sharps, and items used in the emergency procedure. The organized team works in concert to perform counts as possible based on the patient's condition. Some surgeons order a routine x-ray of the patient's abdomen before transfer to the unit. If laparotomy sponges or towels must be left inside the patient as visceral retainers, the circulating nurse documents the exact number placed inside the patient and communicates the same information to the surgeon and the intensive care nurse in the handover report. This information could be valuable if the patient crashes in the unit and some of the sponges must be removed outside the OR.

Non-OR personnel may accidentally discard the sponges by not realizing that they are counted items. When the patient is brought back to the OR for closure, the sponges are to be accounted for in their entirety and documented as being retrieved. Care again is taken not to mix the removed sponges with the sponges used for the closure procedure.

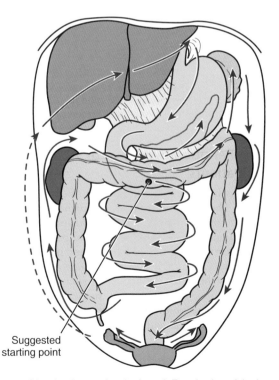

• **Fig. 33.36** Direction for running the bowel. Examination of the bowel for injury after trauma.

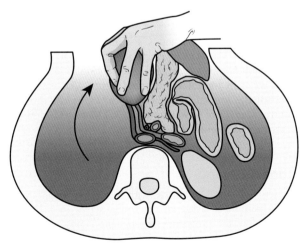

• **Fig. 33.35** Displacing organs during exploratory laparotomy.

Complications of Abdominal Surgery

Patients are particularly prone to pulmonary complications after abdominal surgery. They are also subject to a variety of fluid and electrolyte imbalances because they generally have nothing-by-mouth (NPO) status postoperatively. They may also lose sodium, potassium, chloride, and water through NG suction. If great quantities of alkalotic pancreatic secretions are lost through decompression of the small bowel, metabolic acidosis may result. The loss of acidic stomach secretions may lead to metabolic alkalosis.

Peritonitis and wound infection may result after gastrointestinal surgery because of spillage of contaminants from the lumen of the gastrointestinal tract. *Escherichia coli* and *Bacteroides fragilis* are the most common organisms; *Clostridium perfringens* (endospore-forming bacteria), the chief cause of gas gangrene, can be found in the intestinal tract. Blood supply can be compromised, causing ischemic bowel. Wound infection can cause wound disruption and/or the formation of scar tissue; the latter is enhanced by peritonitis or postoperative radiation therapy. Even years after an abdominal procedure, increased intraabdominal pressure may induce an incisional hernia through an old scar that has weakened.

Adhesions are the most common cause of postoperative intestinal obstruction. They are caused by an outpouring of fibrin from traumatized tissue, which causes intestinal surfaces to stick together and thus limits mobility.

Foreign bodies in the peritoneal cavity can produce granulomas that stimulate fibrin. Glove powder, lint from sponges, and some powerful antibiotics also can produce granulomas. Some patients must return to the OR for lysis of adhesions. Adhesions may present a contraindication for future laparoscopic surgery.

Anorectal Procedures

Hemorrhoids, abscesses, fissures, and fistulas are often indications for surgical intervention. The anal region is well supplied with nerves, and these procedures often cause much discomfort. Patients are also sensitive and embarrassed because of the surgical site. After rectal surgery, patients may have an initial difficulty voiding and usually experience considerable pain, which requires medication and sitz baths.

Anoscopy, Proctoscopy, and Sigmoidoscopy

Endoscopic diagnostic procedures such as anoscopy, proctoscopy, and sigmoidoscopy are used for visual examination of the mucosa of the anus, rectum, and sigmoid. Sigmoidoscopy is routinely performed before rectal surgery. Some surgeons prefer a sigmoidoscope setup to be available for all colorectal procedures for periodic anastomosis checks. Fiberoptic equipment has aided in the early detection and treatment of tumors, polyps, and ulcerations.

Hemorrhoidectomy

Hemorrhoidectomy is the surgical removal of varicosities of veins or prolapsed mucosa of the anus and rectum that do not respond to conservative treatment. Hemorrhoids are classified as internal (occurring above the internal sphincter and covered with columnar mucosa) or external (appearing outside the external sphincter and covered with skin). Often both types are present in the patient. External hemorrhoids cause pruritus and pain, whereas the internal type often bleed and may become thrombosed and edematous. Rectal bleeding cannot be assumed to be a result of hemorrhoids; a thorough investigation is required to rule out gastrointestinal disease.

The usual procedure for a hemorrhoidectomy consists of dilating the sphincter, ligating the hemorrhoidal pedicle with suture ligatures, staples (circular stapler), or silastic bands, and excising each hemorrhoidal mass with a sharp dissection, laser, ESU, or cryosurgical unit. Sclerotherapy can be done by injecting a hypertonic solution to shrink the hemorrhoidal veins, this is usually done on smaller hemorrhoids. The Kraske position generally is used, with the patient's buttocks retracted by wide adhesive strips that are fastened to the edges of the OR bed (Fig. 33.37).

Some surgeons prefer to position female patients in the lithotomy position to avoid contamination of the vagina with bloody anal fluid. When lithotomy is used for males, the scrotum gets in the way and may need to be retracted with temporary stay sutures or superficial skin staples. Petrolatum gauze packing may be inserted in the anal canal, or a fluff gauze dressing with antibiotic ointment and mesh pants are applied at completion of the surgical procedure. Some surgeons insert a belladonna suppository to suppress peristalsis during the healing period.

As an alternative to a surgical procedure, McGivney rubber band ligation of internal hemorrhoids is a common office procedure. After infiltration of a local anesthetic, the hemorrhoid is visualized with an anoscope and grasped with the McGivney ligating instruments (Fig. 33.38). Two bands are placed around the base of each hemorrhoid. Sloughing of the avascular hemorrhoid occurs in 7 to 10 days.

Incision and Drainage of an Anal Abscess

Localized infection in tissues around the anus results in abscess formation. Early incision and drainage are essential to prevent spreading of the infection.

Fistulotomy and Fistulectomy

An anal fistula often develops after incision and drainage or the spontaneous drainage of an anorectal abscess. A fistulous tract may be opened (fistulotomy) to allow drainage and healing by

• **Fig. 33.37** Patient positioning for hemorrhoidectomy.

• **Fig. 33.38** Hemorrhoid banding instrument.

granulation, or the tract may be excised (fistulectomy). Injection of a dye or the use of a probe and grooved director aids in identifying the tract.

Fistulas tend to follow a predictable path along the ischiorectal or supralevator planes. The prediction of the path (origin and exit) is referred to as the Goodsall rule of anal fistulas (Fig. 33.39). A Seton drain can be placed to assist drainage and healing of abscess collections. Surgical excision is staged to prevent injury to the anal sphincter.

Fissurectomy

When a benign ulcerative lesion occurs in the lining of the anal canal, the anus is dilated, and the infected tissue is excised. Some fissures can be vaporized with a laser. Fecal incontinence caused by damage to the anal sphincter is a potential complication that the surgeon tries to avoid.

Treatment of Rectal Tumors

Surgeons prefer to resect a small rectal cancer instead of performing a radical surgical procedure. Many cancers within 20 cm of the anal verge are amenable to local treatment with endoscopic, laser, or cryosurgical techniques. Electrosurgical cutting and coagulating can be combined to remove superficial anorectal and pararectal lesions. For electrosection, the lesion should be small, mobile, and polypoid, with no palpable lymph nodes. The procedure may be performed for palliation to relieve bleeding, painful sphincter spasms (tenesmus), or severe constipation. Interstitial radiation therapy is sometimes used for small anorectal squamous cell carcinomas. The protocol may include external radiation, but bleeding lesions do not respond well to radiation.

In a procedure called transanal endoscopic microsurgery (TEM), tumors in the upper half of the rectum may be excised through an operating rectoscope. This long, tubular instrument improves the surgeon's visual image by incorporating a binocular stereoscope. With TEM, carbon dioxide (CO_2) is insufflated to hold open the walls of the rectum. Tissue graspers, a high-frequency knife, suction, needle holders, and other instruments can be inserted through ports in the airtight eyepiece on the rectoscope. TEM may be used to remove benign lesions and some malignant tumors.

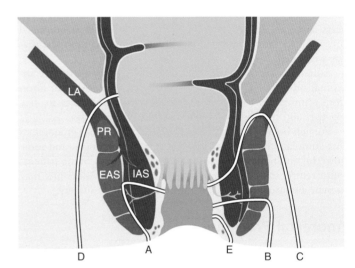

• **Fig. 33.39** Pathways of perianal fistulae. Park Classification: **A,** intersphincteric, **B,** transsphincteric, **C,** suprasphincteric, **D,** extrasphincteric, **E,** superficial. *EAS,* External anal sphincter; *IAS,* internal anal sphincter; *LA,* levator ani; *PR,* puborectalis. (From Yassin NA, Day N, Phillips R: Imaging of anal fistulas, *Semin Colon Rectal Surg* 25(4):176–182, 2014.)

Excision of Pilonidal Cysts and Sinuses

A painful draining cyst with fistulous tracts may occur in the soft tissues of the sacrococcygeal region. When the cyst becomes infected, drainage is necessary to relieve pain, swelling, and suppuration. The cyst and sinus tracts are excised or marsupialized to prevent recurrence. Marsupialization is the suturing of cyst walls to the edges of the wound after evacuation; this permits the packed cavity to close by granulation. A Z-plasty may be preferred for primary closure to produce a strong transverse scar, or the wound may be closed with a rotational pedicle flap. Surgical judgment determines whether primary closure or healing by granulation is chosen.

Hernia Procedures

A hernia is the protrusion of an organ or part of an organ through a defect in the supporting structures that normally contain it.

A hernia may be congenital, acquired, or traumatic. Most occur in the inguinal or femoral region, but umbilical, ventral, and hiatal hernias also occur (Fig. 33.40). A hernia is usually composed of a sac (covering), hernial contents, and an aperture (opening), but in some locations the sac is absent. Some surgeons send the excised hernia sac to pathology, but minimal pathology is ever found and the processing is an unnecessary cost to the patient.

A hernia is called *reducible* when the hernial contents can be returned to the normal cavity by manipulation. If this cannot be done, the hernia is called *irreducible* or *incarcerated*. Bowel present in an incarcerated hernia not only may lack adequate blood supply but also may become obstructed. This is referred to as a *strangulated hernia*, and an immediate surgical procedure is necessary to prevent necrosis and gangrene of the strangulated bowel.

Inguinal Herniorrhaphy

An inguinal hernia is often repaired with the patient under local anesthesia. An oblique inguinal incision on the affected side is extended through external oblique aponeurosis. The hernia sac is emptied of its contents, ligated, and excised, and the floor of the inguinal canal is reconstructed. Prosthetic mesh is sometimes needed to reinforce a large or recurrent defect.

Repair depends on whether the inguinal hernia is direct or indirect. In both types of inguinal herniorrhaphies in male patients, the spermatic cord and blood supply to the testes are protected from injury. The spermatic cord is retracted with a Penrose drain moistened with saline. Infarction of a testis can occur if the blood supply is compromised. The female round ligament, the homolog of the spermatic cord, passes through the inguinal ring.

Direct Hernia

A direct hernia protrudes through a weakness in the abdominal wall in the region between the rectus abdominis muscle and

inguinal ligament and medial to the inferior epigastric artery. This area is a surgical landmark referred to as the Hesselbach triangle. This hernia is the most difficult type to repair and is more common in men.

An acquired weakness of the lower abdominal wall, a direct inguinal hernia often results from straining, such as heavy lifting, chronic coughing, or straining to urinate or defecate. Prompt surgical repair prevents possible discomfort and the threat of later complications.

Indirect Hernia

With an indirect hernia, the peritoneal sac containing intestine protrudes through the internal inguinal ring and passes down the inguinal canal outside Hesselbach triangle. It directs laterally to the inferior epigastric vessels. It may descend all the way into the scrotum. An indirect inguinal hernia is more common in male patients but can be present in females and originates from a congenital defect in the fascial floor of the inguinal canal. Most inguinal hernias are indirect.

Laparoscopic Repair

A laparoscopic procedure may be used to repair either an indirect or a direct reducible inguinal hernia using mesh behind the hernial defect. This procedure is particularly advantageous for repairing bilateral or recurrent hernias. A transabdominal preperitoneal (TAPP) or intraperitoneal approach may be used, or a transextraperitoneal procedure (TEPP) can be performed. Polypropylene mesh is inserted to reinforce the wall of the inguinal canal; this is sutured, stapled, or tacked in place.

Femoral Herniorrhaphy

Femoral herniorrhaphy involves repairing the defect in the transversalis fascia below the inguinal ligament and removing the peritoneal sac protruding through the femoral ring. The transversalis fascia is normally attached to Cooper ligament, which prevents the peritoneum from reaching the femoral ring. To repair this defect, it is necessary to reconstruct the posterior wall and close the femoral ring. These hernias are more common in women.

Umbilical Herniorrhaphy

Repair of an umbilical hernia consists of closing the peritoneal opening and uniting the fasciae above and below the defect to reconstruct the abdominal wall surrounding the umbilicus. This type of hernia is seen most often in children and represents a congenital defect of protrusion of the peritoneum through the umbilical ring. It also may be acquired by women after childbirth.

Ventral (Incisional) Herniorrhaphy

Impaired healing of a previous surgical incision, usually a vertical abdominal incision, may cause an incisional hernia. Often the result of a weakening of abdominal fasciae, projections of peritoneum carrying segments of bowel protrude through fascial perforations. It is necessary to reunite the tissue layers to close the defect. After excising the old scar, the peritoneal sac is opened, the hernia is reduced, and the layers are firmly closed. If existing tissue is not sufficient for repair, synthetic mesh may be used to reinforce the repair. Incisional hernias are sometimes the aftermath of postoperative hematoma, infection, or undue strain.

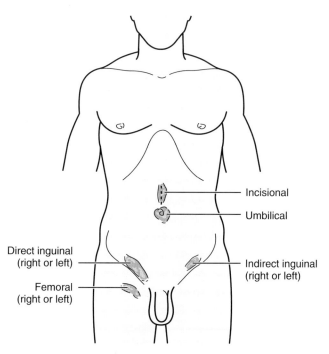

Incisional

Umbilical

Direct inguinal (right or left)

Femoral (right or left)

Indirect inguinal (right or left)

• **Fig. 33.40** Hernia locations.

Ventral hernias have a high recurrence rate when mesh is placed on the outside of a large repair. Through an intra-abdominal laparoscopic approach, omentum can be placed over the mesh or the peritoneum can be put back over the mesh.

Hiatal (Diaphragmatic) Herniorrhaphy

A hiatal hernia results when a portion of the stomach protrudes through the hiatus of the diaphragm. Ten percent of the population has this condition, but not all cases are symptomatic. The hiatus is the opening for the esophagus through the diaphragm, the chief muscle of respiration. A weakening in the hiatus permits violation of the muscular partition between the abdomen and the chest.

Symptoms are caused mainly by inflammation and ulceration of the adjacent esophagus, which result from the reflux of gastric juices from the herniated stomach. Symptoms include pain, blood loss, and difficulty in swallowing (dysphagia). Diagnosis is made by radiologic and endoscopic studies. This is not the cause of gastroesophageal reflux.

Surgical treatment is appropriate when medical therapy fails to alleviate the problem. The surgical approach may be thoracoabdominal or via the abdomen or chest; each approach offers certain advantages. The abdominal approach is generally preferred, but opening the chest may provide a better view of the hiatal region and thus may be preferred.

Amputation of Extremities

Amputation is the total or partial removal of any extremity. The need for amputation is associated most often with massive trauma, a malignant tumor, extensive infection, and vascular insufficiency. Orthopedic or vascular surgeons may perform these procedures.

In preparing the patient for a lower extremity amputation, the patient's chart is checked, and both legs are exposed for comparison before skin preparation. It must be made absolutely certain that the correct leg is prepared. The surgeon must initial the correct surgical site. During the "time out" phase of incision, the limb is confirmed again for correctness.

Many lower extremity amputations are performed with the patient under spinal anesthesia. It must be ensured that the specimen is never within the patient's sight. Policy is followed in regard to the patient's permission for disposal of an extremity.

In general, two types of amputations are performed: open (guillotine) and closed. The guillotine procedure is regarded as an emergency procedure and is rarely performed. Patients who are severely ill or toxic or who experience severe trauma (e.g., an extremity caught under an immovable object) are candidates for this procedure. In the guillotine procedure, tissues are cut circularly with the bone transected higher to allow soft tissues to cover the bone end. Blood vessels and nerve endings are ligated, but the wound is left open. The surgical procedure is often followed by prolonged drainage and healing, muscle and skin retraction, and excessive granulation tissue. A second procedure is often required for final repair.

The conventional flap or closed type of amputation is more desirable. Fashioning curved skin and fascial flaps before amputation of the bone allows deep and superficial fasciae to be approximated over the bone end before closure of the loose skin. Drainage by catheter or suction apparatus may be required. The wound usually heals in approximately 2 weeks.

Amputations of the Lower Extremity

Amputations of the lower extremity are classified as above-knee (AK), below-knee (BK), toe, transphalangeal, transmetatarsal, or the Syme amputation. The level of amputation is determined by the patient's general health, vascular status, and potential for rehabilitation.

Above-Knee Amputation

Amputation at the lower third of the thigh is selected when gangrene or arterial insufficiency extends above the level of the malleoli. A midthigh amputation involves making a circular incision over the distal femur, creating large anterior and posterior skin flaps, and transecting fasciae and muscles. Vessels and nerves such as the femoral and sciatic nerves, respectively, are ligated and severed. Sharp bone edges of the stump are smoothed and debulked with a rasp. The wound is irrigated with sterile normal saline solution before closure of tissue layers.

Hemostasis is important to prevent massive hemorrhage or painful hematoma. Drains may be used depending on the surgeon's preference. A noncompressive dressing is applied. AK amputation is a more extensive procedure than BK amputation, and thus a longer time is required for rehabilitation. In general, a prosthesis is fitted 4 to 6 weeks after amputation.

Below-Knee Amputation

Amputation at the middle third of the leg provides for more functional prosthesis fitting and the reduction of phantom limb pain; it also permits a more natural gait (Fig. 33.41). An immediate postoperative prosthesis (IPOP) can be applied in the OR. The IPOP dressing requires a stump sock, padding, and a rigid plaster dressing. The dressing not only protects the stump but also aids in controlling the weight placed on it. The prosthesis is metal and provides a pull on the stump. The pylon (foot) may be attached before the patient returns to the unit. If the patient is overweight or debilitated, weight-bearing may be delayed for several days.

Toe and Transmetatarsal Amputations

Toe and partial foot amputations are generally performed for gangrene and osteomyelitis.

• **Fig. 33.41** Below-knee (BK) amputation.

• Fig. 33.42 Syme amputation of the foot.

Syme Amputation

A Syme amputation is usually performed for trauma and involves the distal part of the foot. The amputation is above the ankle joint. The skin of the heel is used for the flap (Fig. 33.42).

Hip Disarticulation and Hemipelvectomy

Hip disarticulation and hemipelvectomy involve total removal of the right or left pelvis, including the innominate hipbone, along the ipsilateral lower extremity. A multidisciplinary team of orthopedists and general surgeons perform the procedure because it involves massive soft tissue resection and bony excision.

The division of bone may be carried through the sacroiliac joint, or a portion of iliac bone and crest may be preserved. An internal hemipelvectomy includes the removal of innominate bone with adjacent muscles. The large defect created may be covered by a myocutaneous flap of the quadriceps femoris muscle and the overlying skin and subcutaneous tissue. The neck of the femur rests against the soft tissues. These radical procedures are indicated for malignant bone or soft tissue tumors and extensive traumatic injuries. Specialized prosthetic devices are available to permit ambulation.

Amputations of the Upper Extremity
Amputations of the Hand

Hand amputations usually result from trauma and include part or all of the distal phalanges of the digits. Attention is directed to keeping the hand as a working unit when one or more fingers are removed. Every effort should be made to save the thumb; the smallest stump is better than a prosthesis.

Forearm and Forequarter Amputation

Wrist, elbow, and humerus disarticulations are radical procedures performed for malignant tumors or extensive trauma.

Rehabilitation

Postoperative considerations for any amputation include control of bleeding and phantom limb sensations, stump care, immediate fitting of a functional terminal prosthesis, exercises to prevent flexion contractures, and ambulation or use of a hand or arm.

The loss of an extremity involves major psychologic and physical adjustments. The rehabilitative process is very important and is often affected by the emotional reactions of the patient. Patients with an early postoperative prosthesis have a more positive outlook about their loss. Morale is boosted by being able to walk the first postoperative day or soon thereafter (which, in the case of a leg amputation, depends on the surgeon's orders for the weight-bearing program). This in turn aids in ambulation.

Phantom limb pain is particularly distressing to many patients. The nerves have been severed, but the patient has the sensation that the amputated part is still present. This sensation is often associated with painful paresthesia (i.e., tingling, prickling, tickling, burning). The pain is real. It usually responds to aspirin, acetaminophen (Tylenol), or a similar agent, but narcotics may be necessary to control pain. The combined efforts of the patient, family, significant others, and interdisciplinary professional personnel are needed for successful rehabilitation.

ⓔ EVOLVE WEBSITE

http://evolve.elsevier.com/Hornacky/BerryKohn/

- Historical Perspective
- Tips for the Scrub Person and Circulating Nurse
- Student Interactive Questions
- Glossary

References

1. Steiman J, Sullivan S, Scarborough J, et al.: Measuring competence in surgical training through assessment of surgical entrustable professional activities, *J Surg Educ* 75(6):1452–1462, 2018.
2. Sibbering M, Courtney CA: Management of breast cancer: basic principles, *Surgery* 37(3):157–163, 2019.
3. Nandurkar R, Sluka P, Davis I, et al.: Lytic effects of water on cancer cells: implications for post-operative irrigation, *ANZ J Surg* 92(1–2):157–161, 2022.
4. McDuff S, Mina A, Brunelle C, et al.: Timing of lymphedema after treatment for breast cancer: when are patients most at risk? *Int J Radiat Oncol Biol Phys* 103(1):62–70, 2018.
5. Barbier L, Calmels M, Gauss L, et al.: Can we refine the management of blunt liver trauma? *J Visc Surg* 156(1):23–29, 2018.
6. Barresi L, Tacelli M, Ligresti D, et al.: Tissue acquisition in pancreatic cystic lesions, *Dig Liver Dis* 51(2):286–292, 2018.
7. Homatsu Y, Newhams K, Jobe B: Enhancing the detection of Barrett esophagus, *Thorac Surg Clin* 28(4):453–464, 2018.
8. Bream P, Krohmer S, Pillai A, et al.: Percutaneous gastrostomy: how to recognize, avoid, or get out of trouble, *Tech Vasc Interv Radiol* 21(4):255–260, 2018.
9. Karasko D: Weight loss in adolescents after bariatric surgery: a systematic review, *J Pediatr Health Care* 33(1):26–34, 2018.
10. Nudel J, Sanchez V: Surgical management of obesity, *Metabolism* 92:206–216, 2018.
11. Zivanovic O, Sonoda Y: Small bowel and large bowel resection and anastomosis. *Principles of gynecologic oncology surgery*, (vol 17), St. Louis, MO, 2019, Elsevier, pp 227–244.

Bibliography

AORN: *Guidelines for perioperative practice*, Denver, CO, 2024, The Association.
Han MG, Cho E, Park CH, et al.: Self-expandable metal stents for choledocholithiasis in Billroth II gastrectomy patients, *Hepatobiliary Pancreat Dis Int* 17(6):546–552, 2018.
Iezzoni J: Diagnostic histochemistry in hepatic pathology, *Semin Diagn Pathol* 35(6):381–389, 2018.
Leopold B: Saks E: hemorrhoids. In Ferri FF, editor: *Ferri's clinical advisor*, St. Louis, MO, 2019, Elsevier.

CHAPTER OUTLINE

Anatomy and Physiology of the Female Reproductive System, 697

Gynecology: General Considerations, 700

Diagnostic Techniques, 701

Robotic Procedures, 706

Vulvar Procedures, 706

Vaginal Procedures, 707

Abdominal Procedures, 710

Perioperative Obstetrics, 714

Complicated Birth, 718

Assisted Reproduction, 722

Nonobstetric Surgical Procedures and the Pregnant Patient, 725

CHAPTER OBJECTIVES

After studying this chapter the learner will be able to:

- Identify the anatomy of the female genitourinary system.
- Describe the physiology of the female reproductive system.
- Differentiate between adolescent and adult gynecologic health.

- Describe the pertinent considerations when caring for a pregnant patient.

KEY TERMS AND DEFINITIONS

Abortion Termination of pregnancy. Several descriptions include elective voluntary surgical ending of pregnancy, incomplete natural termination of pregnancy before the age of viability, missed abortion, spontaneous abortion, and threatened abortion.

Amenorrhea Absence of menstrual periods.

Cesarean birth Surgical delivery of a fetus through an abdominal incision. Also known as cesarean section or C-section.

Chromopertubation Instillation of dye through the fallopian tubes as a test of patency.

Dilation and curettage (D&C) Progressive enlargement of the opening of the uterine cervix is to permit instrumentation for debulking the endometrium and other surgical procedures.

Elective voluntary surgical ending of pregnancy First trimester: pregnancy is terminated during first 3 months of gestation. Second trimester: pregnancy is terminated during second 3 months of gestation. Late: pregnancy is terminated after the second trimester has ended.

Endometrium Lining of the uterus that is normally shed during menstruation.

Fundus The round top or dome of uterus.

Leiomyofibroma Term for fibroid tumors. Also known as myoma (e.g., uterine muscle tumor).

Graafian follicle Mature ovum.

Gravid Pregnant.

Incomplete natural termination of pregnancy before the age of viability Products of conception are partially retained and may need surgical removal to prevent sepsis in the mother.

Menarche Beginning of menstruation.

Menometrorrhagia Bleeding between menstrual periods in a premenopausal woman that is surgically treated by dilation and curettage, endometrial ablation, or hysterectomy.

Menorrhagia Excessive bleeding at menstruation that is surgically treated by dilation and curettage, endometrial ablation, or hysterectomy.

Menstruation The shedding of the endometrium during periodic hormonal cycles.

Missed abortion Natural termination of gestation before the age of viability. Products of conception must be surgically removed to prevent sepsis in the mother.

Neoplasia New tissue overgrowth. Potentially cancerous.

Retained products of conception (RPOC)/retained secundus - Products of conception retained either at delivery of a viable fetus or at the time of incomplete abortion. Placental remnants.

Spontaneous abortion Natural termination of pregnancy before age of viability. Products of conception are expelled without surgical intervention.

Tanner stages Incremental measurement of sexual development from first signs of puberty to maturity in both sexes.

Thelarche The beginning of breast development that is measured in stages.

Threatened abortion Pregnancy is diagnosed at risk for natural termination before the age of viability. Medical and/or surgical management may be attempted to prevent full natural termination.

Anatomy and Physiology of the Female Reproductive System

The female genitourinary system comprises the organs, glands, secretions, and other elements of reproduction referred to as the *pudendum*. Components of the female reproductive system are both external and internal organs.

External Female Genitalia

The term *vulva* is used collectively for the female external genitalia (Fig. 34.1). This sensitive, delicate area is highly vascular, with an extensive superficial and deep lymph supply and rich cutaneous sensory innervation. It includes the labia majora, labia minora, clitoris, vestibule, Bartholin glands, hymen, and perineum.

Labia Majora

The labia majora are two large folds, or lips, containing sebaceous and sweat glands embedded in fatty tissue and covered by hair-bearing skin. They join anteriorly in a fatty pad, the mons veneris, which overlies the pubic bone (symphysis pubis). In the adult female this area is covered with a triangular pattern of hair. Sebaceous secretions of the labia lubricate the proximal area. The labia majora atrophy and hair follicles decrease in number after menopause, making the labia minora more prominent.

Labia Minora

The labia minora, or small lips, lying within the labia majora, are flat folds of connective tissue containing sebaceous glands. Anteriorly these labia split into two parts. One part passes anteriorly over the clitoris to form a protective prepuce, or foreskin. The other passes behind the clitoris to shape a frenulum, a fold of mucous membrane. Posteriorly they join across the midline behind the vagina to form the fourchette, or fold of skin, just inside the posterior vulvar commissure.

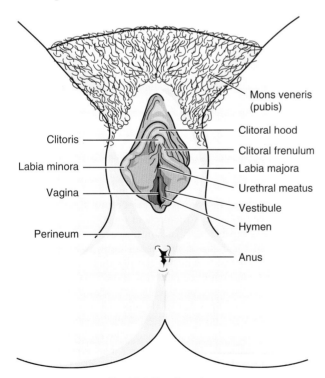

• **Fig. 34.1** Female perineum.

Clitoris

The clitoris is the female erectile organ, the homolog of the penis. It is composed of bilateral cavernosa and a glans. The clitoris is attached by ischiocavernosus musculature to the pubic rami by a suspensory ligament. It is located at the apex of the labia minora, which join to form a prepuce, or hoodlike covering. The clitoris measures about 4 inches in length, but less than 1 inch is visible at the prepuce.

The mucous membrane covering the glans contains many nerve endings and is a source of sexual stimulation for the female. The blood supply is derived from a terminal branch of the pudendal artery, which is a terminal division of the internal iliac artery. The venous drainage is continuous with the labial plexus. Innervation is from the sacral plexus.

Vestibule

The vestibule is the space, or shallow elliptic depression posterior to the clitoris, enclosed by the labia minora. The urethral opening is located in this region posterior to the clitoris and anterior to the vagina. The fourchette forms the posterior boundary where the labia meet anterior to the perineum.

Bartholin Glands

Small, bilateral Bartholin glands lie deep in the posterior third of the labia majora, within the bulbocavernosus muscle. The mucous secretion is a vaginal lubricant. These glands can become inflamed and infected, causing pain and discomfort.

Hymen

The hymen is a thin, vascularized connective tissue membrane that surrounds and may partially or completely occlude the vaginal orifice. It varies in thickness and elasticity among individuals. The central aperture permits passage of menstrual flow and vaginal secretions. This structure will vary according to individual anatomy and physical activity. In some patients the aperture may be imperforate or divided by a septum, requiring surgical intervention. The presence or absence of a hymenal ring is not an indicator of sexual activity.

Perineum

The perineum is a diamond-shaped wedge of fibromuscular tissue between the vagina and the anus. It is divided by a transverse septum into an anterior urogenital triangle and a posterior anal triangle. It consists of the perineal body and perineal musculature. With fibers of six muscles converging at its central point, the perineum forms the base of the pelvic floor and helps support the posterior vaginal wall.

These muscles are the bulbocavernosus (vaginal sphincter), the two superficial transverse perineal muscles, the two levator ani muscles, and the external anal sphincter. The levator ani muscles are the largest muscles and, in contrast to the other superficial muscles, are deep. The most important muscles in the pelvis, the levator ani muscles form a hammock-type suspension (pelvic diaphragm) from the anterior to the posterior pelvic wall, beneath the pelvic viscera. These muscles retain the organs within the pelvis by offering resistance to repeated increases in intraabdominal pressure, such as coughing, bearing down in labor, and straining at stool.

Internal Female Reproductive Organs

The internal female reproductive organs (Fig. 34.2) lie within the pelvic cavity, protected by the bony pelvis. Bones and ligaments

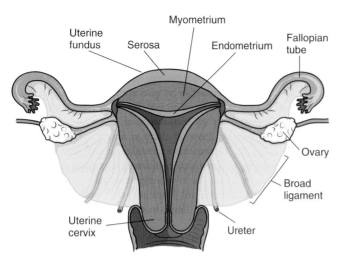

• **Fig. 34.2** Female reproductive system.

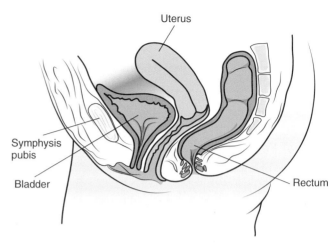

• **Fig. 34.3** Female reproductive anatomy in sagittal view.

form the pelvic outlet. The dilated cervix of the uterus and the vagina constitute the birth canal.

Vagina

The vagina is a thin-walled, 8-cm fibromuscular tube extending from the vestibule obliquely backward and upward to the uterus, where the cervix projects into the top of the anterior wall. The vagina is elastic and capable of distention during intercourse and parturition. The bladder lies anteriorly; the rectum lies posteriorly. It is lined with mucous membrane and contains glands that produce a cleansing acid secretion.

The anterior vaginal wall is shorter than the posterior wall. The upper third of the posterior wall is covered by peritoneum reflected onto the rectum. Normally the anterior and posterior walls relax and are in contact. However, the lateral walls remain rigid because of the pull of the muscles and therefore are in close contact with pelvic tissues.

A rich venous plexus in the muscular walls makes the vagina highly vascular. Uterine and vaginal arteries supplying the area are branches of the internal iliac artery. Branches of the vaginal artery extend to the external genitalia and the adjacent bladder and rectum. Lymphatic drainage is extensive. The upper two-thirds of the vagina drain into the external and internal iliac nodes; the lower third drains into the superficial inguinal nodes.

The vault (upper part of the vagina) is divided into four fornices, or arches (Fig. 34.3). During digital pelvic examination, pelvic organs can be palpated through the thin walls of the vault. The anterior fornix, in front of the cervix, is adjacent to the base of the bladder and distal ends of the ureters.

The pouch of Douglas (retrouterine cul-de-sac) directly behind the larger posterior fornix lies behind the cervix. This pouch separates the back of the uterus from the rectum anteriorly by the uterine peritoneal covering, which continues down to cap the posterior vaginal fornix, and posteriorly by the anterior wall of the rectum. Lateral uterosacral ligaments embrace the lower third of the rectum. The floor of the pouch, about 7 cm above the anus, is formed by reflection of the peritoneum from the rectum to the upper vagina and uterus.

The posterior cul-de-sac is the route of entry for a number of diagnostic or surgical procedures because the pouch of Douglas (the lowest part of the peritoneal cavity) is separated from the vagina only by the thin vaginal wall and peritoneum.

The lateral fornices lie on either side of the cervix, in contact with anterior and posterior sheets of the broad ligaments surrounding the uterus. Proximal structures are the uterine artery, ureters, fallopian tubes, ovaries, and sigmoid colon.

Uterus

The uterus is the female organ of gestation. It receives and holds the fertilized ovum during development of the fetus and expels it during childbirth. Resembling an inverted pear in shape, this hollow, muscular retroperitoneal organ is situated in the bony pelvis. It lies between the bladder anteriorly and the sigmoid colon posteriorly. The uterus is divided transversely by a slight constriction into a wider upper part (the body or corpus uteri) and a narrower lower part (the 2–3-cm cervix uteri or ectocervix that protrudes into the vagina).

The corpus meets the cervix at the internal os. Peritoneum covers the corpus externally; the endometrium, ranging in thickness from 2 to 10 mm, lines it internally. This mucous membrane is uniquely adapted to receive and sustain the fertilized ovum. The fundus, or rounded top portion of the uterus, lies above the uterine cavity.

The shape of the uterine cavity (endometrial cavity), flattened from front to back, is roughly triangular in the nonpregnant female. The upper lateral angles extend out toward openings of the fallopian tubes, which enter bilaterally through the uterine walls at the cornua. The apex of the triangle is directed downward to the cervix. The cavity within the cervix, the endocervical canal, narrows to a slit at the distal orifice, where the cervix communicates with the vagina via the external os. The endocervix is the glandular mucous membrane of the cervix. The corpus of the uterus and the cervix are considered individually in relation to disease and therapy because they differ in structure and function.

The uterus is capable of expansion to accommodate a growing fetus. Much of the bulk of the corpus consists of involuntary muscle, the myometrium, which is composed of three layers. The inner layer prevents reflux of menstrual flow into the tubes and peritoneal cavity, which could result in endometriosis. It also contributes to the competency of the internal os to prevent premature expulsion of the fetus. The middle layer encloses large blood vessels. These muscle fibers act as living ligatures for hemostasis after delivery. The outer layer has expulsive action, ejecting menstrual flow and clots, an aborted embryo, or the fetus at term.

Usually the uterus lies forward at a right angle to the vagina and rests on the bladder. Although the cervix is anchored laterally by ligaments, the fundus may pivot about the cardinal ligaments widely in an anteroposterior plane. Mobility rather than position is the criterion for normality.

Fallopian Tubes (Salpinges)

The fallopian tubes (small, hollow musculomembranous tubes, sometimes called *oviducts* or *uterine tubes*) run bilaterally like arms from each side of the upper part of the uterus to the ovaries. Near each ovary, the open end of each tube expands into the infundibulum, which divides into fimbriae, or fingerlike projections, that sweep up the ovum (the female reproductive cell) as it is expelled from the ovary. Ciliated cells move the ovum toward the uterus.

The lumen of the tube becomes very narrow where it penetrates the uterine wall to reach the uterine cavity. Contractions in the muscular walls change the shape and position of the tubes. At ovulation, they move the fimbriated ends into close apposition with ovarian surfaces. The fallopian tubes serve as a continuous passage from the external environment into the abdominal cavity via the vagina, cervix, and uterine body. Infectious diseases and other substances can enter the peritoneal cavity through this route.

Ovaries

The ovaries are oval glandular gonads located in shallow peritoneal fossae on the lateral pelvic walls, from which they are suspended by the infundibulopelvic ligaments. They are attached to the posterior layer of the broad ligament by the mesovarium (a peritoneal fold) and to the uterus by the ovarian ligament (a fibromuscular cord).

The ovaries, the counterpart of the male testes, contain ova. Each ovary measures 2×3 cm and consists of a center of cells and vessels surrounded by the cortex. This main portion contains the stroma or fibrous framework in which the ovarian follicles are embedded. Of the approximately 200,000 primordial follicles present at birth, fewer than 400 are likely to produce a mature ovum (graafian follicle) during the reproductive years. A serous covering derived from peritoneum surrounds the ovaries. In addition to protecting maturing ova, the ovaries, which atrophy after menopause, produce female sex hormones.

The ureters course along the retroperitoneum bilaterally and lie close to the ovarian blood supply just anterior to the common iliac arteries. The ovaries, when diseased, may be adherent to the ureters. Some surgeons will have a urologist place ureteral catheters to make the structural identification easier during dissection.

Muscles and Ligaments

Muscles and ligaments support and suspend the uterus and fallopian tubes in the normal position in the center of the pelvic cavity.

Broad Ligaments

Bilateral broad ligaments are composed of a broad double sheet of peritoneum extending from each lateral surface of the uterus outward to the pelvic wall. Between these two layers of peritoneum, the fallopian tubes are enclosed in the free upper borders (mesosalpinx), with the tubal ostia opening directly into the peritoneal cavity.

Round Ligaments

The round ligaments are fibromuscular bands that extend from the anterior surface of the lateral borders of the fundus to the labia majora. They run beneath the peritoneum and anterior sheet of the broad ligament down, outward, and forward through the inguinal canal to the labia.

Cardinal Ligaments

The lower portion of the broad ligaments, the cardinal ligaments, are attached to the lateral vaginal fornices and supravaginal portion of the cervix. They act as a supportive pivot.

Uterosacral Ligaments

The uterosacral ligaments are peritoneal folds containing connective tissue and involuntary muscle. They arise on each side from the posterior wall of the uterus at the level of the internal os, pass backward around the rectum, and insert on the sacrum at the level of the second sacral vertebra. They pull on the cervix to keep the uterus anteverted and, through the cervix, the vagina in position as well.

Physiology

The function of the female reproductive organs is to conceive, nurture, and produce offspring. The development and function of these organs are influenced by the hormonal secretions of the ovaries and adrenal, thyroid, and pituitary glands. These hormonal relationships also affect primary and secondary sex characteristics.

The physiologic hormonal cycle prepares the uterus for the fertilized ovum. Hormone production stimulates the endometrium and breasts, resulting in thickening of tissue and increased blood supply.

Each month during the years from puberty to menopause, one (or both) of the ovaries matures a follicle from within. When the matured graafian follicle ruptures, it discharges the enclosed ovum, which enters the fallopian tube at the fimbriated end. The process of maturation and discharge of the egg is called *ovulation,* resulting in a fertile period that lasts several days. Changes in cervical mucus and vaginal epithelium also accompany ovulation.

Union of the ovum with a viable mature male germ cell (spermatozoon), which has ascended to the fallopian tube from the vagina, results in fertilization within 12 hours of ovulation. The union takes place in the outer third of the tube and travels toward the uterus over a period of 3 days. The fertilized ovum normally proceeds to the cornu of the uterus, where it enters to implant in the endometrium within 14 days of fertilization. By day 17 the blood supply of the fetal and maternal blood vessels is functional. The placental circulation is established. The ensuing pregnancy will last approximately 266 days, or 9 calendar months, if carried to full term.

The ovarian hormone estrogen, together with progesterone, causes a sequence of changes in the endometrial lining of the uterus to prepare for implantation of the fertilized ovum. Estrogen also produces the development of secondary sexual characteristics. Progesterone is responsible for maintaining pregnancy until hormones from the placenta assume this role.

Menstruation is the periodic discharge of blood, mucus, disintegrated ovum, and uterine mucosa formed during the hormonal cycle if pregnancy does not take place. The duration of the menstrual period varies but averages 3 to 5 days. The amount of blood lost varies greatly. The menstrual cycle, the time between the onset of each period, is approximately 28 days.

Regularity of menstruation can be disturbed by disease conditions and emotions, in addition to the onset of pregnancy. This physiologic cycle continually recurs throughout the reproductive life of the woman. Assessment of the female patient should include documentation of the age of menarche (first menses), the date of the last menstrual period (LMP), use of contraception, and sexual history. The possibility of pregnancy should be considered if the female patient is within childbearing age, regardless of age, social status, or vocation. A surgical procedure and/or the administration of anesthetic agents could be hazardous to a developing embryo.

Gynecology: General Considerations

The emotional preparation of gynecologic patients presents a special challenge to the operating room (OR) team. Anticipation of physical exposure, potential loss of sexual function, infertility problems, or termination of pregnancy can create severe anxiety. Some surgical procedures terminate reproductive capability and produce menopause. Patients must be able to express concerns, ask questions, and receive reassurance and support.

Examination With the Patient Under Anesthesia

Bimanual examination of the pelvis with the patient in the lithotomy position and relaxed from anesthesia usually precedes vaginal and abdominal gynecologic surgical procedures. This allows the surgeon to thoroughly assess the size, outline, consistency, position, and mobility of the uterus, fallopian tubes, and ovaries. This examination also helps the surgeon determine or confirm the approach for the procedure and whether a lesion is resectable. This is helpful in evaluating women experiencing pain or nervous tension and those who are overweight. The vaginal vault and perineum are prepped, and the examination is performed before prepping the abdomen for a diagnostic laparoscopy or exploratory laparotomy.

Special Features of Gynecologic Surgery

Diagnostic and surgical procedures may be carried out through a vaginal or an abdominal approach or the two approaches may be combined. The procedure can be done with an open, laparoscopic, or robotic approach. Each requires a different position and different preparation, drapes, and setup. Surgical techniques for general abdominal procedures apply to gynecologic surgery. Diagnostic and definitive surgical procedures are often combined and done in one surgical procedure.

The following procedures apply to both vaginal and abdominopelvic procedures:

1. Spinal, epidural, or (more commonly) general anesthesia is used. An epidural catheter may be inserted preoperatively for postoperative pain control.
2. A Foley catheter may be inserted after the administration of the anesthetic agent to prevent the bladder becoming distended during the procedure and to record urinary output. The circulating nurse and the anesthesia provider should check the urinary drainage bag frequently and report urine volume or evidence of blood. This could indicate injury to the bladder or ureters. Percutaneous insertion of a cannula directly into the bladder through the abdominal wall (suprapubic cystostomy) provides an alternative indwelling urinary drainage system in select patients.

3. An electrosurgical unit (ESU), with either monopolar or bipolar electrodes, is frequently used.
4. Argon, carbon dioxide (CO_2), and neodymium:yttrium aluminum garnet (Nd:YAG) lasers are used, generally in conjunction with a colposcope or laparoscope and the operating microscope for some procedures.
5. Closed-wound suction drainage, or another type of drain, may be used to prevent hematoma or serum accumulation in the pelvis and/or the wound.
6. Prophylactic preoperative anticoagulation with subcutaneous heparin, antiembolic stockings, sequential compression devices, and early ambulation are especially important in pelvic surgery because of the potential for deep vein thrombosis (DVT) and subsequent pulmonary emboli (PE).

Vaginal Approach

1. The patient is in the lithotomy position. Care is taken not to lean on the patient's legs during the procedure.
2. Instrumentation must be of sufficient length for use within the vaginal canal and uterine cavity. In addition to retracting, cutting, holding, clamping, and suturing instruments, vaginal setups include dilation and curettage (D&C) instruments for intrauterine procedures (Table 34.1).
3. A laser, an ESU, or a cryosurgical unit may be used to remove hypertrophied tissue or certain benign neoplasms.
4. A suction system, including a Poole suction tip with guard, tubing, and collection canister, is part of the setup.
5. Raytec sponges are rolled and secured on sponge forceps in deep areas (also referred to as *sponge sticks*). Long, narrow, 4 × 18-inch sponges (tapes) with radiopaque markers on the end are used for packing off abdominal viscera in vaginal procedures. All counts are very important in these procedures.
6. Vaginal packing is inserted after certain procedures for hemostasis and/or therapeutic purposes. Antibiotic or hormone cream may be applied to the packing during insertion.

TABLE 34.1	Instruments for Dilation and Curettage
Purpose	**Instruments**
To expose	Vaginal speculum Posterior retractor Weighted posterior retractor Narrow lateral Heaney retractors
To grasp and hold	Single- and double-toothed tenacula
To measure uterine cavity	Uterine sound (graduated probe)
To dilate cervix	Graduated dilators Goodell dilator
To scrape tissue	Sharp and blunt, large and small uterine curettes
To obtain specimen	Endometrial biopsy suction curette
To carry sponges	Sponge forceps
To remove polyps and biopsy tissue	Polyp and biopsy forceps
To insert packing	Uterine dressing forceps
To promote hemostasis	Electrosurgical unit

Impregnated vaginal packing is commercially available. The packing should be recorded on the patient's chart and removed at the surgeon's order.

7. At the completion of the surgical procedure a sanitary pad is placed against the perineum between the patient's legs. Mesh underwear can be applied to hold the pad in place. Care is taken not to disturb drains or the Foley catheter.

Abdominal Approach

1. The supine or Trendelenburg position is used for abdomino-pelvic procedures to displace pelvic organs cephalad. Preparation and drapes are the same as for abdominal laparotomy. Abdominal incisions commonly used in gynecologic open procedures are shown in Fig. 34.4.
2. When a large abdominal mass is present or the pelvic organs are pushed from their normal relationships, ureteral catheters may be inserted via cystoscopy, before the surgical procedure, to facilitate identification of the ureters to prevent inadvertent dissection. Severing of the ureters during the procedure greatly increases postoperative morbidity and mortality if the injury is not immediately detected and corrected.
3. Instrumentation includes the basic laparotomy setup with the addition of long instruments for deep manipulations within the pelvis and uterine graspers, such as a Somer uterine elevator or a tenaculum.
4. At the completion of the surgical procedure a sanitary pad is placed against the perineum between the patient's legs. Mesh underwear can be applied to hold the pad in place. Care is taken not to disturb drains or the Foley catheter.

Abdominal Complications

Injuries to ureters, which can lead to loss of renal function if unrecognized, can occur during the surgical procedure because of their relationship to pelvic structures. The surgeon must identify and isolate the ureter on the affected side to prevent accidental crushing or kinking.

Adhesions after pelvic surgery can cause infertility, intestinal obstruction, and/or chronic abdominal pain. The surgeon may place a biodegradable fabric (e.g., Interceed Absorbable Adhesion Barrier) over tissues and pelvic organs before closing the peritoneal

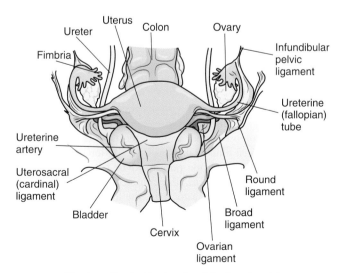

Uterus
Ureter Colon Ovary
Fimbria
Infundibular pelvic ligament
Ureterine (fallopian) tube
Ureterine artery
Uterosacral (cardinal) ligament
Round ligament
Bladder Broad ligament
Cervix
Ovarian ligament

• **Fig. 34.4** Surgical landmarks of the female pelvis.

cavity. This satin-like knitted fabric acts as a physical barrier to prevent adhesion formation during the healing process. Within 8 hours the fabric becomes a gelatinous protective coating, which is completely absorbed within 28 days.

Combined Vaginal-Abdominal Approach

If vaginal and abdominal surgery is indicated, a combined procedure is planned. For example, the patient may be scheduled for a total abdominal hysterectomy with anterior vaginal colporrhaphy. In such instances the vaginal procedure is performed first. The patient is then removed from the lithotomy position and repositioned in the supine position, and the abdominal preparation and surgical procedure are performed. Care is taken to ensure the dispersive electrode has not been displaced, and a new one should be applied when the patient is repositioned.

The following considerations apply:

1. Because of the possibility of infection, separate sterile setups are used for vaginal and abdominal procedures performed concurrently.
2. Vaginal preparation precedes exploratory pelvic laparotomy in readiness for the unexpected or for a D&C scheduled to precede an abdominal procedure. A separate sterile prep table is used for the external genitalia and vagina. Another sterile setup is used for the abdominal preparation. The vaginal area is prepped first to prevent splashing up to a freshly prepped abdomen.

Diagnostic Techniques

The gynecologist uses both noninvasive and invasive diagnostic techniques. Some are performed as office or ambulatory procedures, especially those using the vaginal approach.

A pelvic examination includes inspection and palpation of the external genitalia; bimanual abdominovaginal and abdominorectal palpation of the uterus, fallopian tubes, and ovaries; and speculum examination of the vagina and cervix. This inspection is augmented by a cytologic study of smears of cervical and endocervical tissue obtained by scrapings.

The Papanicolaou (Pap) smear has significantly facilitated diagnosis of cervical cancer and premalignant lesions. Characteristic cellular changes in cervical epithelial cells are identified. Cytologic aspiration from within the endocervical canal may reveal unsuspected carcinoma of the endometrium, fallopian tubes, or ovaries and occult cervical cancer.

The Schiller test involves staining the vaginal vault and cervical squamous epithelium with Lugol solution. Glycogen in normal epithelium takes up the iodine. Abnormal tissues, with little or no glycogen, do not stain brown and thereby pinpoint sites for biopsy. Abnormal cytologic findings are an indication for further evaluation by histologic tissue study. Patients susceptible to iodism should not be exposed to Lugol solution.

Uterine cancer consists of two entities: cervical cancer and endometrial cancer. These differ by age-groups, types, and consequences. Cancer of the cervix appears most often in association with coitus at an early age, multiple partners, nonbarrier contraceptives, poor sexual hygiene, a chronically infected cervix, or a history of sexually transmitted infections (STIs). These include infection with herpes simplex virus (HSV), human papillomavirus (HPV), cytomegalovirus (CMV), *Chlamydia trachomatis,* and *Trichomonas vaginalis.* A higher frequency of abnormal Pap smear findings is associated with these infections.

HPV produces condylomata (venereal or genital warts), which have been identified as a possible cause of cervical carcinoma.[1] HPV screening is part of the routine gynecologic examination. HPV vaccination, a series of two injections given over a 6-month period, may be administered. The Centers for Disease Control and Prevention (CDC) speculate that 90% of sexually active men and 80% women will experience HPV infection (genital warts) during their lifetime.[1] HPV-related cancers have decreased 40% among vaccinated individuals.[1]

Cancer of the endometrium occurs primarily in postmenopausal women and is more common than cervical cancer. It is often associated with obesity, low parity, late menopause, hypertension, and diabetes mellitus.

Biopsy of the Cervix

Cervical cancer may not present symptoms in the early stage and may progress to invasion before discovery. Spotting, postmenopausal bleeding, or chronic cervicitis may be the first visible sign. The condition may be suspected by results of cytologic examination or visual inspection, but diagnosis is made by biopsy.

Excisional Biopsy

In excisional biopsy an attempt is made to excise the entire cervical lesion by sharp dissection. Sutures or an ESU is used for hemostasis. Packing may be needed.

Incisional Biopsy

Incisional biopsy involves the use of a scalpel, punch biopsy, or other instrument to obtain tissue for diagnosis but not to remove the lesion. If a malignancy is diagnosed, additional evaluation and further treatment are carried out by additional surgery and/or radiation therapy.

Cone Biopsy

Patients diagnosed by Pap smear as having severe cervical dysplasia or intraepithelial carcinoma of the cervix require conization to remove the lesion and rule out invasive carcinoma. The biopsy, obtained with a laser, scalpel, or cervitome (cold knife conization), includes the squamocolumnar junctions of the ectocervix (transformation zone) and is tapered to include the endocervical canal to the level of the internal os (Fig. 34.5). Most of the lesions categorized as cervical intraepithelial neoplasia (CIN), dysplasia, or carcinoma in situ are found in this area. Conization of the cervix provides the most comprehensive specimen to diagnose a premalignant or malignant lesion. Multiple blocks and sections are examined by the pathologist to determine the extent of invasive disease.

Complications include hemorrhage, infection, cervical stenosis, an incompetent cervix, and infertility. The CO_2 laser used for conization minimizes these risks. Hemostasis is secured with sutures or ESU as needed.

Cervical dysplasia can occur in sexually active females ages 12 years and older; the peak incidence is between the ages of 25 and 35 years. Used therapeutically for chronic inflammation and for premalignant lesions in women of childbearing age, conization may be performed by scalpel, electrosurgery, or laser. Laser conization is used to treat severe dysplasia and carcinoma in situ.

Loop electrosurgical excision procedures (LEEPs) use a stainless steel or tungsten loop electrode to excise a central core of tissue from the transformation zone of the endocervical canal. Large loop excision of the transformation zone (LLETZ) is

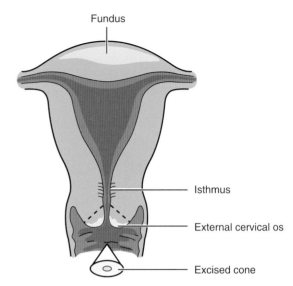

• **Fig. 34.5** Cone biopsy for cervical cancer.

performed with minimal bleeding and few complications. These procedures may be performed in the OR or office setting with local anesthesia. Future childbearing is unaffected. Although the specimen is comparable in size to that obtained with cold knife conization, the specimen has superficial desiccation and may be inferior in quality. Wide conization may result in scarring and obstruction of the os.

Fractional Curettage

Tissue is obtained for histologic examination by scraping the uterine cavity. Fractional curettage differentiates specimens between the endocervix and the endometrium in a series of two steps. A biopsy specimen may be taken from the cervix, if indicated by the Schiller test, in association with endocervical curettage. A small curette is introduced into the endocervical canal, which is scraped from the internal to the external os. The specimen is placed on a Telfa pad, and both are put into a container. This scraping precedes cervical dilation to avoid dislodging tissue from above the internal os.

After cervical dilation a different curette is inserted into the uterine cavity for curettage of the endometrium. The endometrial specimen is placed in a container separate from the one used for the specimens obtained by endocervical curettage.

Colposcopy

Illumination and binocular magnification afforded by the colpomicroscope permit identification of abnormal epithelium to target for biopsy. The colposcope has a cool, intense white light that can be fitted with a green filter to improve visualization of the vascular pattern. With the colposcope positioned in front of the vulva, without touching the patient, the colposcopist can focus light through a speculum on the ectocervix, the lower part of the cervical canal, and the vaginal wall.

The cervix is swabbed with 3% acetic acid to eradicate mucus and facilitate viewing the surface and vasculature. Biopsies are performed for histologic confirmation of the diagnosis. Endocervical curettage also may be performed. A video camera or still camera can be attached to a colposcope to photograph lesions.

Vaginal condylomata from HPV and adenoses, preinvasive lesions of the cervix, cervical dysplasia, CIN, and other vaginal and cervical lesions can be treated by laser with the colpomicroscope. Visualization, unobstructed by instruments, is excellent. Condylomata can incubate for 3 weeks to 6 months and will appear as white, raised areas when exposed to 3% acetic acid. Full-strength acetic acid solutions will burn the patient's tissues.

The CO_2 laser permits selective destruction of large areas of vaginal epithelium without vaginal or cervical stenosis. It cuts, coagulates, seals, and sterilizes simultaneously. This results in less blood loss, a shorter period of vaginal discharge after treatment of the cervix, and a lower incidence of infection than in other surgical treatment modalities.

Electrosurgery and cryosurgery are other options to ablate lesions. Care is taken to avoid contact with the plume from viral lesion ablation.

Culdocentesis and Colpotomy

Culdocentesis

In culdocentesis, blood, fluid, or pus in the cul-de-sac is aspirated by needle via the posterior vaginal fornix for suspected intraperitoneal bleeding, ectopic pregnancy, or tuboovarian abscess. Clear, straw-colored peritoneal fluid is a negative finding. Blood can indicate an ectopic pregnancy, trauma, or tumor. Bloody fluid should be sent to the laboratory in a heparinized specimen tube. A flat plate of the kidneys, ureters, and bladder (KUB) (x-ray examination without contrast medium) may reveal air under the diaphragm, which is indicative of a ruptured organ. Air under the diaphragm appears as dark patches on x-ray.

Posterior Colpotomy

In posterior colpotomy a transverse incision is made through the posterior vaginal fornix into the posterior cul-de-sac to facilitate diagnosis by intraperitoneal palpation, inspection of the pelvic organs, or determination of free fluid, blood, or pus in the pouch of Douglas. Pus from a pelvic abscess or blood, possibly a sign of ectopic pregnancy or a ruptured ovarian cyst, is evacuated. Tubes and ovaries are inspected. If they are normal, the incision is closed. A drain may be inserted.

Some surgical procedures, such as aspiration of an ovarian cyst or reproductive sterilization by tubal ligation, can be performed through the incision, although exposure and visualization are limited. A tube or ovary is sometimes removed through the vagina.

Fallopian Tube Diagnostic Procedures

Tubal Perfusion

To test tubal patency, chromopertubation is performed. Methylene blue or indigo carmine dye in a solution of sterile normal saline is introduced into the uterine cavity via a 50-mL syringe or intravenous (IV) tubing attached to a cervical cannula. The surgeon views the ends of the fallopian tubes through a laparoscope. Dye seen coming from one or both tubes indicates patency.

Tubal Insufflation

Uterotubal insufflation may be used to test the patency of the fallopian tubes. It usually is done as an office procedure to study infertility. The test may be therapeutic in relieving minor obstructions. Contraindications include genital tract infection, possible pregnancy, and uterine bleeding.

A cannula with a seal (e.g., RUMI, HUMI, Kahn, Kronner, or Jarcho) is inserted into the cervicouterine canal and connected to an insufflation apparatus. CO_2 is introduced slowly under controlled flow. A relationship exists between tubal patency and the pressure required to force gas through the fallopian tubes into the peritoneal cavity.

Resistance to flow (i.e., backpressure) is measured on a mercury manometer. To prevent gas embolism, the Rubin test is done before—never after—curettage. Open vessels could introduce an air embolus. Intraabdominal irritation before total absorption of CO_2 from the peritoneal cavity causes referred pain in the shoulders. The patient may refer to the feeling as "gas pains."

Hysterosalpingography

X-ray study of the uterus and tubes may afford further evaluation of infertility after repeated negative Rubin test findings. The patient is placed in the lithotomy position, and the vagina is prepped. The cervix is grasped with a single-toothed tenaculum. A cannula is inserted into the cervical canal, and 10 mL of a water-soluble radiopaque contrast medium is instilled with a syringe through the cannula (Fig. 34.6). This contrast medium ascends into the corpus uteri and fallopian tubes to yield information about structure and function. Serial x-rays may be taken to assess postprocedure tubal spillage. In some patients, tubal spasms prevent immediate passage of the contrast medium through the tubes.

Pediatric and Adolescent Gynecology

Pelvic examination of an infant or child is rarely performed unless there is disease or trauma. Any indication of physical or sexual abuse must be reported to legal authorities. The facility should have a procedure in place for reporting child abuse.

The preadolescent has no hormonal stimulation and has not developed sexual characteristics such as rounded labia or pubic hair. In infants the uterus regresses in size until the age of 6 years, when it regains the size it was at birth. The cervix is not palpable, and the uterine body is difficult to differentiate from surrounding tissues.

From the age of 7 years, the body begins to respond to estrogen stimulation. The mons thickens, and the vagina begins to elongate. The uterus has a growth spurt at age 9 to 10 years and begins to have the pear shape of the adult uterus. The endometrium

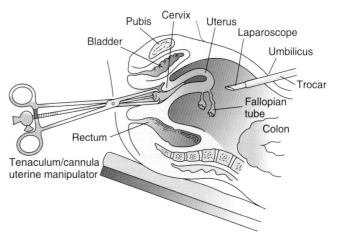

• **Fig. 34.6** Uterine cannula and tenaculum.

develops and proliferates. The vagina extends to its full length of 10 to 12 cm, and the external genitalia resemble those of an adult. Thelarche (first breast development) begins as nipple buds at about 10 years of age.

Menarche (first menstruation) is common between the ages of 10 and 15 years (12 years is common), and averages 3 years from the onset of breast development and within 6 months of the appearance of axillary hair. The first routine gynecologic examination is recommended at between ages 13 and 15 years for an external exam and to answer questions about reproductive health. An internal examination should be done if necessary.

Routine examinations will be individualized according to the needs and sexual activity of the girl. Sexually transmitted disease (STD) testing is performed. Incidences of STD must be reported to the health department.[2] The presence of an STD may indicate an abusive situation.

Females who have not developed secondary sex characteristics and menstruated by age 15 years should seek a gynecology consult. Sexual maturation is measured on a scale of Tanner stages. Each physical secondary sex characteristic happens between specific ages. Breast development and body hair precede menstruation. Menarche can be delayed by anorexia nervosa or other dietary practices that diminish body fat stores below 17%. Menstruation can be obstructed by an imperforate hymen.

Adolescent Pregnancy

According to the CDC the adolescent pregnancy rate is the lowest it has been in 30 years. The decline in the 10 to 14-year-old group has remained steady, while the birth rates for 15 to 19-year-olds has declined. Births to young mothers place them at high risk for problems, resulting in preterm birth and cesarean delivery. Many of these young girls have had no prenatal care and are subject to preeclampsia (pregnancy-associated hypertension). Often the babies are of low birthweight and are small for gestational age (SGA).

Gynecologic Pathology in Infants

The female infant should be thoroughly examined from a gynecologic standpoint at birth. Clitoral anomalies may be related to androgenic sexual hormones or a true genetic anomaly. If a vagina cannot be visualized, the hymen may be imperforate, or there may be vaginal agenesis. Digital rectal examination is performed, and a slight central mass representing the rudimentary uterine cervix may be palpated. Ovaries are not large enough to be palpable unless a pathologic condition is present. Ultrasonography may need to be performed to differentiate anatomic structures.

Pelvic Endoscopy

Pelvic endoscopy is an established part of the gynecologist's diagnostic and therapeutic regimen. It permits detailed intraperitoneal inspection of the pelvic organs without laparotomy. These procedures are not without danger, however. Inadvertent perforation of vessels or a hollow viscus and/or infection are major potential hazards. Operator expertise, careful patient selection, adequate anesthesia, and safe equipment are essential. Pelvic endoscopy is a sterile procedure. Vaginal and abdominal approaches are used for direct visualization of pelvic organs and adjacent structures.

Culdoscopy

A culdoscope is introduced into the peritoneal cavity via the posterior vaginal fornix and pouch of Douglas. Some gynecologists prefer culdoscopy to investigate ovaries or posterior surfaces in the lower pelvis. Local or caudal anesthesia is used. The patient is placed in the knee-chest or lithotomy position. With the posterior lip of the cervix held by a tenaculum and retracted anteriorly, the uterus is elevated while counterpressure is applied to the posterior vaginal wall by the speculum.

This maneuver stretches the posterior vaginal fornix while a trocar and cannula or sheath penetrate the thin wall and enter the pelvis between the uterosacral ligaments. When the trocar is removed with the cannula in place, air enters the cul-de-sac because of the negative intraabdominal pressure produced by the knee-chest position. Air displaces the bowel to create a working space, and the scope may be inserted through the cannula.

At the completion of the procedure the culdoscope is removed. Before the cannula is removed, the OR bed is straightened and the patient is laid flat while as much air as possible is evacuated by hand pressure on the abdomen into low suction. Care is taken not to aerosolize body substances. Some surgeons place a suture in the puncture site.

Hysteroscopy

A rigid fiberoptic hysteroscope, introduced vaginally through the uterine cervix, provides direct inspection of the interior of the uterus to diagnose disease or treat conditions such as menorrhagia and uterine fibroids. The hysteroscope may also be used to identify and remove polyps, lost intrauterine devices (IUDs), or intrauterine adhesions. Adequate expansion of the uterine cavity is a prerequisite for viewing endometrial surfaces and tubal orifices. Fluid is instilled to expand the uterine cavity to create a working space.

Hysteroscopy systems have been developed that use sterile normal saline as an expansion medium to create the working space. The fluid should be delivered through a pressure-controlled infusion pump that tracks volume instilled. Intrauterine pressures should be maintained at or below the mean arterial pressure. Use of a continuous-flow pump makes it difficult to monitor intrauterine pressures.

The circulating nurse monitors inflow and outflow of the uterine expansion fluid medium and informs the surgeon and the anesthesia provider of any discrepancy in excess of 1500 mL. Visibility is further enhanced with a video camera and monitor screen. The procedure may be videotaped.

Hysteroscopy is used to perform endometrial ablation using a laser (Nd:YAG, argon, or potassium titanyl phosphate [KTP]) or ESU to stop or decrease uterine bleeding.

The Nd:YAG laser is the best choice for deep photocoagulation, causing endometrial destruction and scarring the uterine lining. The entire endometrial lining is treated from the fundus to about 4 cm above the external cervical os. The tip of the laser fiber can be held away from tissue (i.e., blanching technique) or in contact with endometrium (i.e., dragging technique). A specialized electrosurgical rollerball electrode is an alternative method to using a laser. This can provide relief from menorrhagia (i.e., excessively heavy menses). The destruction of the endometrium causes the woman to have amenorrhea, thereby causing sterility. Hormonal activity is unchanged.

Air or gas is not used for uterine insufflation or laser fiber cooling during hysteroscopy because of the risk for air or gas embolism. In addition, 32% dextran 70 in dextrose (Hyskon) is not used as an irrigant or uterine expansion medium for endometrial laser ablation because of the systemic effects of fluid absorption through open capillaries. Precise measurements of intake and output are critical to patient safety and prevention of fluid overload. Symptoms of fluid overload include hyponatremia, hypotension, bradycardia, nausea and vomiting, confusion, and congestive heart failure. Hysteroscopy can be performed as an ambulatory surgery or office procedure.

Laparoscopy

Procedures using a 10 or 12-mm fiberoptic laparoscope with a 0° or 30° angle lens inserted into the peritoneal cavity permit direct observation of pelvic and abdominal organs and peritoneal surfaces. Single-port or multiple-port laparoscopic methods can be used. Endoscopic techniques may be used to diagnose and treat ectopic pregnancy; inspect the ovaries for evidence of follicular activity and retrieve ova for in vitro fertilization; visualize and reduce pelvic masses; and determine the cause of infertility, endocrinopathies, or amenorrhea. Many pelvic diseases, such as endometriosis, adhesions, and ovarian cysts, may be identified and treated through the laparoscope and its accessory instrumentation.

The gynecologist can perform myomectomy, salpingectomy, oophorectomy, hysterectomy, and other procedures such as tuboplasty and incidental appendectomy without the need for a large abdominal incision. Surgical procedures such as tubal sterilization by electrocoagulation with or without partial resection, placement of a clip or silicone ring on the tube, or biopsy can be performed.

A general anesthetic agent is administered. The patient is placed in a modified lithotomy position with the stirrups adjusted so the legs are at a 45-degree angle to the axis of the OR bed. Improper positioning can result in lower leg neuropathy.

The vaginal area is prepped, followed by the abdominal prep. The patient is straight-catheterized, or an indwelling Foley catheter is inserted to monitor output and keep the bladder decompressed. The patient is draped for a combined abdominovaginal procedure. The sterile drapes must provide two exposures (i.e., an abdominal opening and a perineal opening) and cover the legs.

A tenaculum is placed on the anterior lip of the cervix. A cannula is inserted into the uterine cervix for instillation of dye and for manipulation of the uterus during the procedure to provide greater visibility (Fig. 34.7). A D&C may be performed as part of the procedure after the injection of dye or contrast media.

Insertion of the scope is preceded by a pneumoperitoneum of CO_2 to create a working space in the abdomen and pelvis. The infraumbilical midline area is most commonly used if no scars, with possible adherent viscera beneath, are present. This area is preferred because it has no abdominal wall vessels that might be injured. The firm attachment of the fascia to the peritoneum facilitates entry. Great care is taken to avoid injury to the great vessels or intraabdominal organs. Insufflation can be performed with a Veress needle or a blunt trocar, such as a Hasson (open laparoscopy).

The patient is placed in a 10-degree Trendelenburg position to shift the abdominal organs cephalad. A small, infraumbilical skin incision is made in the anterior abdominal wall. Through it a sharp trocar and sheath are introduced into the peritoneal cavity via blind puncture, if a blunt Hasson is not used. Some sharp

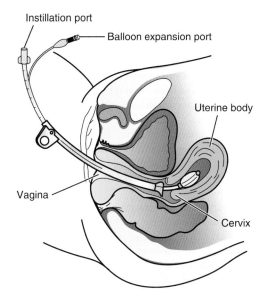

• **Fig. 34.7** Kronner uterine manipulator for laparoscopy.

trocars and sheaths have spring-loaded end guards that cover the sharp tip and protect the underlying structures after penetration of abdominal tissue layers. The trocar is removed, and a telescope of the same caliber is inserted through the trocar sheath, which remains in the cavity. Some sheaths have threads that are used to anchor it into position.

Additional secondary trocars and sheaths can be placed in the suprapubic hairline (see Fig. 34.12, later in this chapter). These trocars may be inserted into the peritoneal cavity under direct vision through the endoscope, which offers good transillumination for the puncture when the room lights are dimmed, or visualization on the video monitor. A secondary trocar should have a gas port to which the CO_2 tubing can be attached to prevent the cold gas from causing the scope to fog. The suction-irrigation tubing is attached to a side port on the secondary sheath.

Before use, warming the tip of the telescope in a warm moist towel or normal saline solution can prevent fogging of the distal lens of the endoscope caused by the intraperitoneal temperature and moisture. (Sterile antifog solution and devices are commercially available.) The telescope is connected to the light source by a fiberoptic cable. Because of the potential fire hazard to drapes, the light source is not activated until the cable is attached to the telescope. The video camera is draped and connected to the telescope. The camera may not be sterile and must be draped to prevent contamination.

At completion of the surgical procedure, the CO_2, video monitor, and light source are turned off, accessory instruments and sheaths are removed, and the patient is leveled into a flat, supine position. Hemostasis is surveyed before the telescope is removed from the primary trocar site.

The valve of its sheath closes as the telescope is withdrawn to prevent escape of CO_2 gas into the room air. The pneumoperitoneum contains aerosolized blood and body fluids and should be evacuated through the suction tubing into the suction canister. Electrosurgical plume also should be suctioned from the peritoneal cavity because it binds with hemoglobin and causes the arterial oxygenation to decrease. The patient can become hypoxic.

The large fascial incisions are sutured, and the skin can be closed with wound glue. Small dressings or adhesive bandages (Band-Aids or Steri-Strips) are applied.

The patient requires close monitoring by the anesthesia provider because increased intraabdominal pressure may lead to cardiovascular disturbances from vagal reflex. This reflex is caused by stretching of the peritoneum, retention of CO_2, or compression of the inferior vena cava.

Postoperative shoulder pain may follow the use of a pneumoperitoneum. This is referred pain caused by pressure on the diaphragm, which is somewhat displaced by CO_2 during the procedure. Slight elevation of the head after recovery from anesthesia relieves this pain.

Although numerous complications have been reported, the most common are perforation of the intestine or major blood vessel, hemorrhage from a biopsy site, gas embolism from intravascular injection, and burns of the abdominal wall and bowel. Some injuries, such as viscus puncture or thermal damage, may not be immediately apparent. Symptoms may not be present until 48 to 72 hours postoperatively, when tissue necrosis or sloughing occurs.

Robotic Procedures

Many gynecologic procedures can be done with the robotic-assisted approach. Patient positioning is dependent on the target area. The surgeon and assistant must have extensive training to manage and manipulate instrumentation. Some surgeons use a disposable single-site trocar with multiple valves, such as the SILS or TriPort+. Single-site trocars may have up to five valves. They may have three 5-mm valves and a 10 to 15-mm valve. Some devices have a built-in air seal pressure system. Multiple instruments can be used at one time. Patients may have only an umbilical incision.

Vulvar Procedures

Benign growths on the vulva, although rare, consist mainly of fatty and fibrous tumors. These growths are excised if large. Suspicious lesions should be removed for pathologic examination. Cancerous lesions may be multicentric, with the majority found on the labia majora and a lesser percentage on the labia minora, vestibule, clitoris, and posterior commissure. Vaginal smears should be taken to determine the presence of metastatic growth to the vaginal wall. Treatment depends on the size of the primary lesion, involvement of nodes, and extent of metastasis. Mutilative procedures require emotional adjustment to permanent change.

Diseases of the Vulva

Wide local excision of a single well-localized area with no premalignant changes elsewhere may be performed. Punch biopsies may be obtained. Leukoplakia and preinvasive lesions of the vulva may be treated with a laser or ultrasonic aspirator.

Simple Vulvectomy Without Node Dissection

The labia majora and minora, part of the mons veneris, and the hymenal ring, including the clitoris, may be removed for premalignant lesions and early microinvasive cancer of limited penetration. The clitoris and perianal region are spared if the lesion is small. The incision must be wide to avoid local recurrence.

Total Vulvectomy

Basal cell carcinoma usually does not metastasize but is often locally extensive and prone to recur. Treatment consists of wide total vulvectomy, also without node dissection.

Radical Vulvectomy With Bilateral Inguinal-Femoral Lymphadenectomy

Radical vulvectomy is performed for invasive vulvar cancers or melanoma and is usually done in one stage. Resection lines may vary depending on the location and size of the lesion (Fig. 34.8). The procedure involves abdominal and perineal dissection, and both areas, including the thighs to the knees, are prepped. Structures generally removed include all of those from the anterior surface of the pubis to the perianal region posteriorly, with wide lateral excision beyond the vulva, to fascial depth. More specifically, large areas of abdominal and groin skin, the labia majora and minora, the mons, clitoris, Bartholin, and periurethral glands, and bilateral inguinal lymph nodes are removed en bloc. Inguinal skin flaps are retained for closure. Deep pelvic node dissection is carried out if examination of frozen sections determines these nodes are cancerous. If the vagina, urethra, and/or anus are involved, they are removed also. Anal involvement may require a colostomy.

Lymphadenectomy is carried out with the patient in the supine position. Two teams may perform bilateral dissection. The patient is then placed in the lithotomy position for vulvectomy. Reconstruction of the pelvic floor and vaginal walls may be necessary. The legs are abducted for easier approximation of subcutaneous tissue during primary closure with sutures or staples. Closed-wound suction drainage is used postoperatively to avoid fluid collection beneath skin flaps. A pressure dressing is applied.

Bartholin Glands

Obstruction of the secretory duct of the Bartholin gland may be caused by inflammation. A cyst may be prone to secondary infection or abscess formation.

Marsupialization of Bartholin Gland Cyst

A cyst enlarges as mucous secretions accumulate. Marsupialization establishes drainage from within the vagina by creation of a new, enlarged ductal opening. The cyst is incised linearly in the region of the normal opening and evacuated. The edges of the vaginal mucosa and cyst wall are sutured together to produce epithelialization so that the cyst cannot recur. An abscess may be drained.

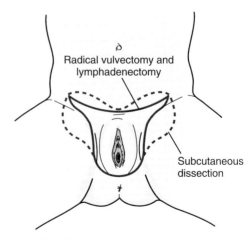

• **Fig. 34.8** Incisions for radical vulvectomy.

Vaginal Procedures

The vaginal wall, cervix, and uterus may be approached with the patient in the lithotomy position. Tumors, benign or malignant, may be confined to any one of these structures or may involve adjacent tissues. Herniation or fistula formation may require repair of the vaginal wall and adjacent structures. Excision or repair may require a combined vaginal-abdominal procedure.

Vaginal Wall

Excision of a Vaginal Lesion

A biopsy taken from an epithelial tumor should be studied histologically to rule out adenocarcinoma. Vaginal adenosis and gross cervical abnormalities, as well as clear cell adenocarcinoma of the vagina, have occurred in female offspring of women who received diethylstilbestrol (DES) or similar synthetic estrogen during the first trimester of pregnancy to avoid spontaneous abortion. Adenosis may be treated with a laser.

Vaginectomy

Vaginectomy (partial or complete) is performed for carcinoma in situ or carcinoma of the vagina. Vaginoplasty is necessary for reconstruction. External radiation and radium implants, with possible eventual pelvic exenteration, is the treatment for advanced invasive malignancy. The proximity of the bladder and rectum makes therapy difficult.

Radical vaginal or abdominal hysterectomy and vaginectomy with extraperitoneal lymphadenectomy sometimes are combined for carcinoma of the upper and middle thirds of the vagina if the bladder or rectum is not involved.

Vaginoplasty

A vagina may be constructed in patients with congenital absence of the vagina (Rokitansky syndrome) or, more commonly, in those with stenosis after radiation therapy or after surgical removal of the vagina. Care must be taken to avoid damage to the urethra, bladder, and rectum.

The vaginal space is created by blunt and sharp dissection. If a large part of the surface of the space is denuded, a skin or amnion graft is shaped around a vaginal mold. The mold is placed in such a way that the graft will take. With the use of dilators to prevent stenosis and with the use of estrogen cream to assist in epithelialization of the cavity, an adequate functional vagina can be created in many patients. A pseudovagina is created for transsexual surgery.

Procedures for Repair of the Pelvic Outlet

Injury to muscles and fascial layers of the perineum and/or genital tract, usually during childbirth, may result in extensive vaginal relaxation (Fig. 34.9). Manifestation of perineal hernias may be delayed until later years, when generalized loss of elastic tissue develops. Downward pressure is exerted on other structures, such as the bladder. Moderate to severe degrees of herniation of viscera require surgical intervention to restore pelvic floor integrity and sphincter competency.

Vaginal plastic procedures for genital prolapse consist of narrowing and reconstructing the damaged pelvic floor. Vaginal repairs are referred to as vaginal plastic procedures.

Anterior Colporrhaphy

Anterior colporrhaphy, known as the Kelly procedure, is performed for prolapse of the anterior vaginal wall to repair a

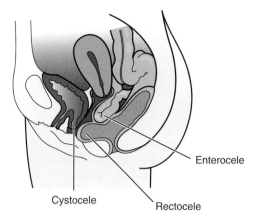

• **Fig. 34.9** Cystocele, rectocele, and enterocele.

urethrocystocele (herniation of the bladder into the vaginal canal). The wall is incised, and a strip of redundant vaginal mucosa is excised, the extent of which depends on the severity of the prolapse. The bladder is dissected free from the vaginal septum and returned to normal position by suturing the pubocervical ligaments beneath it. Approximation of the pubococcygeus muscles provides further suburethral support. The vaginal wall is closed with sutures.

By improving support to the bladder neck region, restoring the posterior urethrovesical angle, and narrowing the urethral opening, stress incontinence (urine leakage with coughing, sneezing, or laughter) is relieved. The surgical procedure also prevents voiding difficulty and the recurrent cystitis that accompanies retention of urine caused by a cystocele bulging below the bladder neck.

Posterior Colpoperineorrhaphy

Repair of the posterior vaginal wall for rectocele, a herniation of the rectum into the vagina, consists of a triangular excision of redundant vaginal mucosa and separation of the vagina from the rectum. Support is reestablished by suturing together rectovaginal fascia, as well as the levator ani, as high as possible. Perineal muscles are reconstructed to restore continuity of support. A lacerated perineum also may be sutured. The surgical procedure relieves fecal incontinence and/or constipation.

Repair of an Enterocele

An abnormally deep hernial sac may contain a segment of intestine, referred to as an enterocele or cul-de-sac hernia. Repair consists of opening the sac, reducing its contents, excising the sac, closing the aperture or weakness that allowed the sac to descend into the rectovaginal septum, and strengthening the normal anatomic coverings. Approximation of the uterosacral ligaments and levator ani in the midline removes the cul-de-sac defect.

Repair of a Prolapsed Uterus

Various surgical procedures correct and restore support of the prolapsed uterus (procidentia; Fig. 34.10). *Correction* of prolapse anteverts the uterus and shortens an elongated cervix and cardinal ligaments. In a Manchester colpoperineorrhaphy, for example, the cervix is amputated and the cardinal ligaments are united in front of it. The anterior vaginal wall is plicated, and the posterior pelvic floor is reconstructed.

Often, cystocele and rectocele are present and are simultaneously repaired. In complete prolapse both the cervix and the

• **Fig. 34.10** Prolapse of the uterus, in varying degrees.

uterine body protrude through the vaginal aperture, and the vaginal canal is inverted. Bleeding ulceration of exposed tissues may ensue. Vaginal hysterectomy is done for severe prolapse or prolapse accompanied by stress incontinence when childbearing is no longer desired. A vaginal pessary to support a retrodisplaced or prolapsing uterus may be inserted in a woman who presents a poor surgical risk.

Repair of Vaginal Eversion

Outward protrusion of the vagina can occur after obstetric or surgical trauma or from inherent weakness in vaginal muscle tone, particularly in a woman's postmenopausal years. The fascia of the vagina is attached to the sacrospinous ligament, located within the coccygeus muscle. The resultant scarring and fibrosis fixate the vagina in a normal anatomic position.

Colpocleisis

Colpocleisis, or the Le Fort procedure, is an obliteration of the vagina by denuding and approximating the anterior and posterior walls. The procedure is generally reserved for geriatric patients and those who present a poor surgical risk.

Procedures for Repair of Genital Fistulas

A genital fistula is an abnormal communication between a part of the genital canal and either the urinary or the intestinal tract. Various dye tests, cystoscopy, and pyelography help pinpoint a urinary tract fistula. Injury during parturition, surgical trauma (especially radical procedures for cancer), penetrating extension of cervical carcinoma, and radiation necrosis are common etiologic factors.

Repair of a Vesicovaginal Fistula

A vesicovaginal fistula, which develops between the bladder and vagina, is the most common type of genital fistula. A small opening permits seepage of urine, although the patient may void normally. Total incontinence may result from a large fistulous aperture and cause irritation of the vagina, vulva, and thighs. Through a vaginal approach, the anterior vaginal wall is dissected free. The fistula to the bladder is closed, and the attachment of the bladder to the vagina is reestablished. The repair should be made with at least three layers of tissue. The bladder should be decompressed by an indwelling Foley catheter postoperatively. Antibiotics may be administered judiciously to prevent infection in the healing site.

If the vesicovaginal fistula is high in the vagina, a better result will be obtained by entering the bladder via suprapubic incision

for direct repair rather than by using a vaginal approach. Care must be taken not to occlude ureteral orifices. This is accomplished by insertion of ureteral catheters, which can be removed after the procedure. Attention is given to excision of any infected tissue, closure with multiple layers, and bladder decompression by the Foley catheter.

Repair of a Rectovaginal Fistula

A fistula between the rectum and vagina may occur after episiotomy or obstetric perineal lacerations, vaginal or rectal surgery, radiation therapy, trauma, or infection. Fecal incontinence and fecal material in the vagina are characteristic, although the anal sphincter is intact. Preoperative bowel preparation, including prophylactic antibiotic therapy, is important because of the contaminated surgical area. A temporary colostomy may be advisable before the surgical procedure to divert the fecal stream from the repair site. With a vaginal approach a plastic repair of the perineum is done. Scar tissue and the fistulous tract are excised, and the edges of the perineal muscles and fascia are approximated.

Cervix

Surgical treatment of an abnormal cervix should be preceded by tests such as a Pap smear to rule out early malignant change.

Cauterization

The cervix may be cauterized by electrocautery to treat chronic inflammation and/or leukorrhea (i.e., vaginal discharge).

Trachelorrhaphy

Lacerations of the cervix may result from childbirth. Repair (i.e., trachelorrhaphy) involves reconstruction of the cervical canal as necessary. A vaginal plastic setup is used.

Trachelectomy

The cervix may be amputated to remove an intraepithelial cancer. Most surgeons prefer total hysterectomy to cervical amputation because the remaining uterine component may become cancerous.

Removal of the uterine cervix in early-stage cancer with lymphadenectomy is a fertility-sparing option for some women. Studies demonstrated that 52% live births resulted from known pregnancies after trachelectomy.[3] Cesarean birth was required for most of these deliveries, and most of these infants were born preterm. Complications noted in the studies included preterm labor and spontaneous abortion.

Uterus

Dilation and Curettage

The most frequently performed gynecologic procedure, dilation and curettage (D&C) is done for diagnostic and/or therapeutic purposes. The main purpose of a D&C is to establish the cause of abnormal uterine bleeding so the gynecologist can plan definitive treatment.

The procedure is performed for women with postmenopausal bleeding or symptoms suggestive of endometrial cancer, even when cytologic smear findings are negative. It may be performed in infertility studies or to confirm preoperative diagnosis before amputation of the cervix or hysterectomy. D&C is performed therapeutically to relieve dysmenorrhea by cervical dilation only, to remove polyps or benign endometrial pathologic conditions, to remove residual tissue and arrest bleeding after incomplete abortion, or to perform voluntary abortion before the 13th week of pregnancy. A regional paracervical block or general anesthesia is required.

With the anterior lip of the cervix held in a tenaculum and the posterior vaginal wall retracted, a uterine sound is introduced into the uterus to determine the depth and direction of the intrauterine cavity. It is important that the surgeon know the shape and position of the uterus to avoid perforation. The cervical os is sequentially dilated with graduated metal probes. A small curette is introduced into the endocervical canal, which is scraped from the internal to the external os. Submucosal fibroids are usually discernible as the curette passes over them. Exploration of the fundus with a polyp or placental forceps usually extracts any polyps present in the endometrium.

Intrauterine Thermal Balloon Ablation

Three types of intrauterine ablation devices are available: microwave, radiofrequency, and thermal.[4] A specialized electrically heated latex balloon probe can be introduced into the uterine cavity through the cervical os to treat menorrhagia (Fig. 34.11). The intrauterine probe is attached to a cable system controlled by a microprocessing unit that measures temperature, pressure, and time. The thermal balloon is expanded by the computer to fill the capacity of the uterine cavity and heated to 188.6° F (87° C). A depth of approximately 3 to 5 mm of endometrium is ablated within 8 minutes of contact. This procedure is suitable for patients who have regularly shaped uterine cavities with a capacity of less than 30 mL or 10 cm in depth. A larger or irregularly shaped uterine cavity would not evenly accommodate the expansion of the balloon.

Intrauterine thermal balloon therapy is contraindicated for women who wish to have future pregnancies. The thermal process destroys the endometrial lining that supports the placental attachment during pregnancy. As per all latex devices, use of a latex balloon is contraindicated for patients sensitive to latex products.

Vaginal Hysterectomy

Vaginal hysterectomy is performed for severe uterine prolapse or prolapse accompanied by stress incontinence and for patients with pelvic relaxation or a history of myomas, irregular uterine bleeding, or a treated premalignant lesion. The procedure can be done totally through the vagina or by laparoscopic-assisted methods. In laparoscopy the abdominal attachments are taken down via the laparoscopic instruments and the uterus is removed through the vagina.

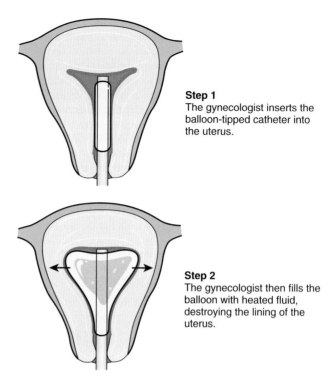

Step 1
The gynecologist inserts the balloon-tipped catheter into the uterus.

Step 2
The gynecologist then fills the balloon with heated fluid, destroying the lining of the uterus.

• **Fig. 34.11** Endometrial thermal ablation with balloon.

The uterus is removed through the vagina with incision of the vaginal wall and the pelvic cavity. Urinary incontinence caused by an enterocele and/or a rectocele may be simultaneously repaired by anterior and posterior colporrhaphies and with reconstruction of the pelvic floor. Advantages of the procedure include restoration of a normal anatomic relationship and preservation of vaginal function. The ovaries are not always removed. Contraindications are immobility of pelvic organs, a large uterus, a pathologic condition such as an ovarian mass, or pelvic cancer.

The vaginal wall is incised anteriorly, and the bladder is separated from the cervix. The incision is continued around the cervix. The peritoneal cavity is entered through the posterior cul-de-sac and the anterior uterovesical pouch. Ligaments supporting the uterus and uterine vessels are ligated and cut. The fundus is delivered, the upper pedicles are sutured, the uterus is removed, and the peritoneum is closed. Suturing the cardinal and uterosacral ligaments together and to the vaginal vault supports the vault and prevents prolapse of the vagina.

Potential complications include injury to the ureters, bowel, or bladder and massive hemorrhage from the uterine vessels. An unopened laparotomy setup should be available in case it is necessary to open the abdomen.

Radical Vaginal Hysterectomy

A surgical approach to early carcinoma of the cervix, radical vaginal hysterectomy (i.e., the Schauta procedure) does not permit pelvic lymph node dissection but is useful in select patients (e.g., obese patients). It includes vaginal removal of the uterus, upper third of vagina, fallopian tubes, and ovaries. Damage to the ureters or bladder is a potential complication.

Laparoscopic-Assisted Vaginal Hysterectomy

In laparoscopic-assisted vaginal hysterectomy (LAVH) an abdominal endoscopic approach is used to dissect the uterus from its supporting ligaments and vasculature. Trocar placement is depicted in Fig. 34.12. Endoscopic clips, linear staplers, sutures, electrosurgery, or a laser may be used to enhance hemostasis. Once the intraperitoneal attachments of the uterus are ligated and divided, a vaginal approach is used to separate the bladder from the anterior aspect of the uterus as in a standard vaginal hysterectomy. Direct visualization of the bladder flap dissection through the endoscope from above enables the surgeon to avoid damage to adjacent structures (Fig. 34.13). The uterine vascular pedicles are ligated vaginally. In the Heaney technique the uterus is inverted and removed fundus-first through a posterior colpotomy. The uterosacral ligaments are sutured to the posterior aspect of the vaginal cuff, and the colpotomy is closed.

This method is used in moderate prolapse of the uterus. In the Döderlein technique a nonprolapsed uterus is inverted and

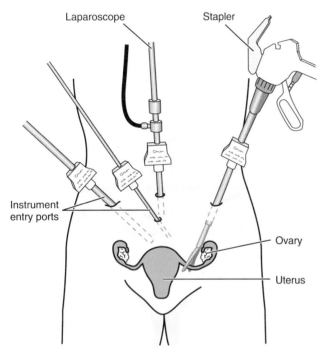

• **Fig. 34.12** Access portals for laparoscopically assisted vaginal hysterectomy.

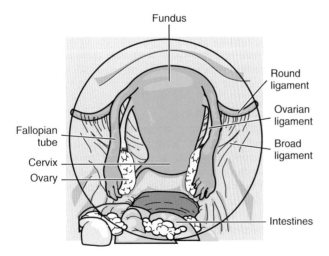

• **Fig. 34.13** Laparoscopic view of the uterus.

removed fundus-first through an anterior colpotomy. This technique provides greater visibility of the uterine vessels and a more effective vaginal suspension. LAVH is the procedure of choice when a minimally invasive procedure is desired, when salpingo-oophorectomy may be necessary, and when the uterus is only moderately enlarged.

Abdominal Procedures

The open abdominal approach may be used for a fixed or enlarged uterus; exploration; inflammatory disease; and most malignant lesions of the uterus, fallopian tubes, and ovaries. This approach permits inspection of pelvic and abdominal organs and lymph glands for biopsy or treatment. Open laparotomy or minimally invasive endoscopic procedures are performed as appropriate to achieve desired outcomes.

Congenital Abnormal Uterine Development

The uterus can assume abnormal configurations during fetal development (Fig. 34.14). Abnormal uterine formation can include single cornu, double fundi, absent cornu or vagina, full or partial septum, or a complete duplication of the female reproductive tract. Ovaries may or may not be affected. Select patients may be candidates for uterine repair, or hysteroplasty. A uterine septum or bicornate uterus is sometimes repaired surgically. The uterine scar from hysteroplasty alters the integrity of the uterine wall and may necessitate cesarean delivery if the woman becomes pregnant (Fig. 34.15).

Myomectomy

The most frequent indication for abdominal hysterectomy is leiomyofibroma, commonly known as benign fibroids or myomas. Fibroids are composed of coiled muscle and fibrous connective tissue. They may be single or multiple and most often are present in the wall of the uterus (intramural) (Fig. 34.16). Some may be attached by a pedicle (pedunculated) or protrude into and distort the uterine cavity (submucous).

In myomectomy, single or multiple fibroid tumors are removed from the uterine wall in premenopausal women who may still desire pregnancy. The procedure is especially adaptable to pedunculated tumors, which may become necrotic from interference with the blood supply. Removal of large submucous fibroids may require opening the uterus, which poses the significant risk for blood loss and potential for rupture during pregnancy (depending on location on the uterine body).

Fibroids, which are usually slow growing, are treated conservatively if they are small and present no problems. If symptoms such as menometrorrhagia, bladder or bowel pressure, pelvic discomfort, or rapid tumor growth develop, surgical treatment is essential. The tumor has no active growth during pregnancy and after menopause because of hormonal changes.

Fibroid Embolization Through the Uterine Artery

Symptomatic uterine fibroids are sometimes treated with occlusion of the arterial blood supply, causing the substance of the fibroid to diminish. An intravascular placement of guidewires and catheters in an interventional radiology suite facilitates delivery of embolization materials, such as hemostatic gelatin particles or sclerosing solution. The location of the target fibroid and its direct

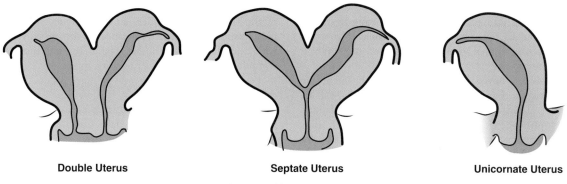

Double Uterus   **Septate Uterus**   **Unicornate Uterus**

• **Fig. 34.14** Uterine anomalies.

• **Fig. 34.15** Hysteroplasty.

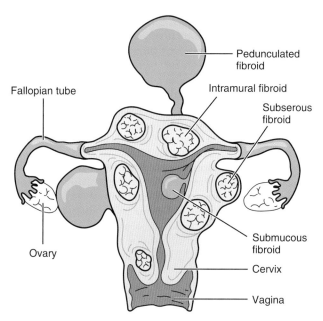

Pedunculated fibroid

Intramural fibroid

Subserous fibroid

Fallopian tube

Submucous fibroid

Cervix

Ovary

Vagina

• **Fig. 34.16** Uterine fibroids.

blood supply are carefully determined by x-ray during the procedure.

Decreasing the uterine blood supply can impair future childbearing, and other fibroid management options should be explored before uterine artery embolization is performed. Embolizing submucous fibroids can cause endometrial sloughing, infection, fever, and sepsis. Pedunculated submucous fibroids should be removed hysteroscopically.

Abdominal Hysterectomy

Medical, psychosocial, and sexual ramifications must be considered when contemplating hysterectomy (removal of the uterus). Medically, the procedure may be lifesaving in patients with a malignant lesion or severe hemorrhage. However, the gynecologist has an obligation to consider the individual patient's attitudes when another mode of therapy is available as an alternative to hysterectomy.

Because it signals the end of the patient's reproductive potential, a hysterectomy may cause psychologic stress and a sense of incompleteness, even though sexual responsiveness is not dependent on the uterus. Patients whose families are complete, however, may welcome reproductive sterilization.

The uterus is removed through an abdominal incision and opening of the peritoneal cavity.

Differential diagnoses include dysfunctional uterine bleeding caused by disturbed endocrine function, tubal or ovarian masses, and pelvic cancer. In addition to these indications, hysterectomy is performed for uterine prolapse, extensive endometriosis, and cervical or uterine cancer. Various types of hysterectomies are performed.

Total Abdominal Hysterectomy

The entire uterus, including the cervix, is resected. Normal ovaries are preserved for hormone production whenever possible in women younger than 45 years. Studies have shown that after hysterectomy, women have an increased risk for ovarian cysts within 5 years of the surgical procedure. Bilateral oophorectomy followed by hormone replacement therapy has eliminated the need for subsequent surgery for ovarian pathologic conditions.

The abdominal peritoneal cavity is entered through a vertical midline or a transverse Pfannenstiel incision. Vertical incision facilitates exploration. The patient is placed in a deep Trendelenburg position. Incision through the uterine peritoneum is carried out laterally.

The abdominal organs are retracted and protected with laparotomy packs moistened with warm sterile normal saline solution. The fallopian tubes and round and broad ligaments are clamped, cut, and ligated. The ovaries, when not removed, are suspended to avoid adherence to the vaginal vault. With the uterus forward, posterior sheets of the broad ligaments are incised, the ureters are identified, and the uterine vessels and uterosacral ligaments are clamped, divided, and sutured. All uterine-supporting ligaments must be divided and ligated. The bladder is mobilized from the cervix and vagina, the vaginal vault is incised, and the cervix is dissected from the vagina.

After the uterus is removed, the connective tissue ligaments are anchored to the vagina. The vaginal mucosa and muscular wall are approximated by absorbable sutures or staples, and the bladder, vault, and rectum (i.e., pelvic floor) are reperitonealized (i.e., covered with peritoneum). Abdominal layers are closed as for laparotomy. The following considerations apply:

1. When the surgeon is closing the vaginal vault after removal of the uterus, the needle, suture, needle holder, or stapler and all instruments used on the cervix and vagina are considered contaminated and isolated from the main instrumentation. Separate instruments are used for abdominal closure.
2. Complications of hysterectomy include injury to the ureters with possible fistula formation or renal failure, injury to the bladder or bowel with fistula formation, and massive hemorrhage from damage to major vessels.
3. Some surgeons have a urologist place ureteral catheters before the hysterectomy begins so that they are easily identified during the procedure. This is referred to as ureteral stenting and requires the use of a separate cystoscopy setup. The cystoscopy setup should remain sterile in the room after the stenting procedure in case an adjustment is necessary during the case. This saves creating another setup midprocedure.

Radical Hysterectomy With Pelvic Lymph Node Dissection

A radical Wertheim procedure, essentially a hysterectomy with pelvic lymph node dissection, may be performed for early stages of invasive cervical cancer and sometimes for endometrial cancer. It involves wide en bloc removal of paracervical and uterosacral tissues (uterus, tubes, ovaries, ligaments) and at least the upper third of the vaginal canal. Bilateral pelvic lymph nodes and channels surrounding the external iliac artery and vein, the hypogastric artery and vein, and the obturator fossae are also dissected and removed. Some surgeons perform a modified Wertheim procedure for microinvasive carcinoma. This is somewhat less extensive than the radical procedure and may omit lymphadenectomy.

Because radical hysterectomy involves excision of paracervical and paravaginal tissue, bladder innervation is disrupted. This results in bladder dysfunction postoperatively, sometimes for as long as 6 months. Bladder complications are related to the extent of dissection.

Salpingo-oophorectomy

Fallopian tubes and ovaries are removed along with the uterus. This procedure may be done for endometrial, tubal, or ovarian cancer; excessive vaginal bleeding; or large fibroids. In postmenopausal women for whom total hysterectomy is indicated, bilateral salpingo-oophorectomy is often performed to avoid future ovarian pathologic conditions.

Pelvic Exenteration

An ultraradical procedure for invasive, persistent carcinoma, exenteration is not performed for palliation but rather only when a possibility of cure exists. The extent of the disease determines the amount of exenteration.

In anterior exenteration the reproductive organs, the distal part of the ureters, the bladder, and the vagina are removed. This modification is performed for cancer of the cervix, vagina, or vulva with extension to the bladder. The ureters are diverted to an ileal conduit, whereas the bowel remains intact.

Posterior exenteration removes the reproductive organs, sigmoid colon, and rectum. It is done for cervical carcinoma involving the rectum or advanced rectal carcinoma involving the uterus and posterior vaginal wall. The urinary system remains intact; fecal diversion is by colostomy.

Total or complete exenteration, rarely performed, involves en bloc dissection of the bladder, reproductive organs, perineum, rectum, and pelvic lymph nodes. Two setups are needed: abdominal and perineal. These procedures affect structure, function, body image, and sex life and should be preceded by intensive physical and psychologic preoperative preparation.

Numerous complications may occur involving any major system. Anesthesia and procedure times are long. Blood replacement and extensive monitoring are essential. Multiple stomas and gross pelvic defect with much dead space predispose the woman to infection; therefore several wound drains are used. Vascularized omental and myocutaneous flaps are used to fill pelvic defects.

Fallopian Tube Procedures

The fallopian tubes are also referred to as the uterine tubes, oviducts, and salpinges.

Tubal Ligation for Reproductive Sterilization

Tubal ligation should be considered a permanent method of reproductive sterilization because reversal cannot be guaranteed. Thorough preoperative counseling of the patient and her husband or partner should preface this procedure.

Various open surgical techniques can be used for tubal ligation. They are essentially similar, involving (1) removal of a portion of the middle part of the fallopian tube on each side for pathologic confirmation and (2) ligation of both the distal and proximal ends to prevent the cut ends from growing together. Frequently performed by laparoscopy, tubal ligation by open abdominal approach may be done alone, in conjunction with other abdominal surgery, immediately postpartum, or for patients in whom laparoscopic technique is contraindicated.

Ligation may be performed through a small transverse incision in the pubic hairline area. An infraumbilical incision is used for postpartum patients. This is referred to as minilaparotomy. Tubal ligations are often performed immediately after cesarean delivery and closure of the uterine wall. No additional instruments are required other than those used for the cesarean section.

The Pomeroy technique of ligation is the most reliable, provides a surgical specimen of each tube, and causes minimal tubal destruction. The tube is tied with suture material, and a section is removed. The tube eventually pulls apart, destroying the passage between the ovary and uterus.

Sterilization also may be performed after vaginal delivery, on the first to third postpartum day, through an infraumbilical incision. In the cauterization technique the bipolar electrosurgical electrode transects and seals the ends of the fallopian tube or excises a section of the tube and seals the ends.

Laparoscopic application of a stretchable silastic band (Falope ring) or spring-loaded ligating clips (Hulka or Filshie) also produces occlusion. In some patients, however, the Pomeroy and other occlusion techniques may be reversible by a subsequent reparative procedure. An estimated 1% of sterilized women will seek reversal because of sterilization at an early age, remarriage, or death of a child.

Tuboplasty

Removal of an obstruction may restore tubal patency to reverse infertility caused by diseased, damaged, or occluded tubes. Microsurgical techniques with fine suture materials and lasers have vastly improved results of tubal reconstructive procedures. Success depends on the extent of abnormal tissue or tubal destruction and/or the site of obstruction. The location of the previous ligation and normality of tissues at the severed ends of the tubes will influence the reversibility of a tubal ligation.

Although tubal patency may be restored, abnormal function may persist in tubes scarred by previous surgery or ectopic pregnancy or damaged by pelvic inflammatory disease (PID). The chance of successful uterine pregnancy may remain limited. The risk for a tubal pregnancy can increase after tuboplasty.

Preoperative assessment may include a hysterosalpingogram to determine the length and patency of tubal segments and/or laparoscopy with tubal dye perfusion or ultrasound imaging with instillation of sterile normal saline solution to demonstrate patency. Contraindications for tuboplasty include active infection or disease and a tube that is less than 3 cm long.

Tuboplasties are microsurgical procedures performed through an abdominal incision. They include the options described in the following sections.

Salpingolysis

Adhesions caused by an inflammatory process, such as a ruptured appendix or ovarian cyst, may surround the fallopian tubes. The tubes may function normally after lysis of adhesions.

Salpingostomy

Tubal mucosa and/or fimbriae may become occluded secondary to PID or other infectious process. A salpingostomy creates an opening in a distally obstructed tube. A CO_2 laser may be used through the microscope to open fimbriated ends and to divide adhesions in blocked tubes. An incision in a tube also may be performed to evacuate an early small tubal pregnancy (ectopic pregnancy).

Tubal Anastomosis

A proximal obstruction in the tube is resected. The remaining patent segment is then reimplanted into the uterus and anastomosed at the cornu. Salpingitis usually occludes the tube near the cornu, which may need to be shaved to reach healthy tissue. A previous sterilization procedure usually occludes the midisthmus. This anastomosis will be midtubal in the ampulla.

Salpingectomy and Salpingo-oophorectomy

Salpingectomy (removal of a fallopian tube) is often performed in association with salpingo-oophorectomy (partial or total removal of the corresponding ovary). Procedures may be unilateral or bilateral. Indications are extensive damage from PID or endometriosis, cysts, primary adenocarcinoma of the tube, and ectopic pregnancy.

Total abdominal hysterectomy and bilateral salpingo-oophorectomy may be performed for bilateral disease. Removal of a large tuboovarian abscess is essential to prevent rupture and dissemination of pus in the abdominal cavity.

Ovaries

Ovarian pain usually is referred to the lower abdomen just above either groin, making differential diagnosis from abdominal disease pertinent. Pelvic endoscopy, ultrasonography, and computed tomographic (CT) scans assist diagnosis. An ovarian mass requires exploration for evaluation. The mass may be a cyst or a tumor. Ovarian tumors may be benign or malignant, cystic or solid. Epithelial ovarian cancer begins as a cystic intraovarian growth. It usually is asymptomatic until malignant cells have spread into the peritoneal cavity.

Ovarian cancer is usually confined to the peritoneal cavity and retroperitoneal lymph nodes, but advanced ovarian carcinoma can obstruct the urinary and intestinal tracts. Ovarian cancer is the leading cause of gynecologic cancer deaths in the United States.

Screening for Ovarian Cancer

This disease is particularly deadly because 80% of symptomatic women present to their physician with advanced disease. Screening modalities include ultrasound, CT, pelvic ultrasound, serum CA125, and physical examination. Unfortunately, early diagnosis does not ensure a decrease in mortality.

Benign cysts, more common than tumors, may arise from the graafian follicle, corpus luteum, or epithelium (dermoid). As they grow, ovarian cysts can cause menstrual disturbances, pain, and abnormal uterine bleeding. They may leak contents into the peritoneal cavity, causing irritation, or they may rupture, causing massive bleeding that necessitates immediate laparotomy.

Cysts or solid tumors, even if asymptomatic, should be removed as a precaution because they may degenerate into a malignant lesion, increase in size, or lead to twisting of the pedicle. The type of procedure depends on the type of cyst or tumor, the age of the patient, and the importance of childbearing potential.

Excision or Biopsy

The surgeon examines the ovaries. If a cyst or tumor is found in one ovary, the surgeon inspects the other ovary to rule out a neoplasm. Pelvic washings may be obtained and tested for cancer cells. If ovarian cancer is highly suspected, the entire ovary is removed for tissue sampling to avoid dissemination of cancerous cells throughout the pelvis. Biopsy specimens also may be taken from paraaortic and pelvic lymph nodes.

Ovarian Cystectomy

A procedure to remove an ovarian cyst may be scheduled as an oophorocystectomy, cysto-oophorectomy, or ovarian cystectomy. Many benign ovarian cysts and tumors are treated by local excision with preservation of the ovary. A large cyst may be aspirated before removal. Immediately after removal, the surgeon incises the cyst for examination to determine its character because gross appearance and frozen section are both important. If there is reasonable assurance that the lesion is benign, removal of only the cyst or resection of a diseased portion (e.g., endometrioma) is justified, with preservation of normal tissue.

Oophorectomy

The most frequent indications for oophorectomy (removal of an ovary) are benign ovarian tumors. Many gynecologists believe that cystadenomas and all solid benign ovarian tumors should be treated by unilateral salpingo-oophorectomy because of the difficulty of clean dissection and the questionable assurance of their benign nature. In postmenopausal women, both ovaries, both tubes, and the uterus are removed to avoid future cancer.

If there is a strong probability or proof of malignancy in any ovarian cyst or mass, total hysterectomy and bilateral salpingo-oophorectomy are usually performed, regardless of age. Partial or complete omentectomy may be included because the rich blood supply of omentum contributes to rapid metastases. The extent of the surgical procedure is determined by the lesion. In malignant tumors a differentiation is made between primary and metastatic ovarian cancer, which influences treatment.

As much tumor as possible is removed—a procedure referred to as *debulking*—for management of advanced ovarian cancer. An ultrasonic aspirator may be used for debulking. The procedure may require resecting parts of small and large intestines and the urinary tract.

After debulking, most patients receive chemotherapy. This often is followed by a "second-look laparotomy" to reassess the peritoneal cavity for further palliative or therapeutic therapy.

Intraoperative Intraperitoneal Chemotherapy

Ovarian cancer is primarily a peritoneal disease that is sensitive to chemotherapy. The goal of intraperitoneal instillation is to expose the greatest number of ovarian cancer cells with the least amount of systemic toxicity. Earliest used agents include 5-fluorouracil and methotrexate in large quantities of irrigant to cover the greatest surface of the peritoneal cavity; however, a cisplatin and paclitaxel infusion may be used. The best results have been seen with minimal extensions of the disease, but it does seem to prolong life in advanced disease. Great care is taken when handling chemotherapeutic agents.

Muscles and Ligaments of the Pelvic Floor
Urinary Stress Incontinence Procedures

Urinary stress incontinence is the sudden, involuntary, and intermittent release of urine as a result of muscular changes around the proximal urethra, bladder neck, and bladder base. Differential diagnosis from fistulas, bladder neuropathies, and primary lesions is established by urethroscopy, a cystometrogram, and urodynamics. Surgical correction attempts to restore support. Three basic approaches are used. Anterior colporrhaphy with plication (i.e., reducing the size of the bladder neck) often is satisfactory. In a urethral sling procedure a musculofascial sling is placed beneath the bladder neck and urethra; usually this is a combined vaginal and abdominal procedure.

Urethral suspension procedures reposition the urethra and bladder neck retropubically by suspending the urethra in a plane with the symphysis pubis through a transverse abdominal incision. Sometimes a combined abdominoperineal approach is necessary for urethral suspension. Variations of these procedures have been devised, including an endoscopic suspension of the bladder neck.

Marshall-Marchetti-Krantz Vesicourethral Suspension

After mobilization through an extraperitoneal abdominal approach into the prevesical space, the urethra and bladder neck are suspended to the posterior border of the symphysis pubis. Sutures are placed through the anterior vaginal wall on each side of the urethra and brought through the periosteum on the posterior surface of the symphysis pubis. Sutures also may be placed adjacent to the bladder neck and through the rectus muscle fascia to suspend the bladder neck.

This procedure may be performed in conjunction with other pelvic surgery. It is 85% effective in the treatment of stress incontinence in women. A suprapubic catheter may be used for bladder drainage for 48 to 72 hours postoperatively. Urinary retention is a common complication for up to 7 days.

Perioperative Obstetrics

Diagnostic techniques such as ultrasonography, specialization in fertility problems, and techniques of fetal monitoring and management have brought significant changes in the field of reproductive biology. Perioperative personnel become involved in the care of obstetric patients, in both elective and emergency procedures, for both obstetric and nonobstetric procedures. The pregnant woman experiencing trauma or an acute surgical disease, such as appendicitis, presents challenges to the perioperative team. The well-being of the fetus depends on maternal physiologic factors. Anesthesia and positioning are especially critical concerns. The anatomic changes of pregnancy alter the appearance and location of commonly identified surgical landmarks. Laboratory values are altered as a result of the growing fetus within the mother's uterus (Table 34.2).

Planning care for the surgical obstetric patient includes determination of the expected date of confinement (EDC). The size of the uterus, competency of the placenta, and condition of the growing fetus are prime considerations.

Considerations for the Care of the Pregnant Patient

Oxygen consumption increases about 20% during pregnancy and as much as 100% above normal during labor in response to the increased metabolic demand. Hypoxia and hypercapnia develop rapidly. Fetal oxygenation varies in direct relation to that of the mother in normal and abnormal situations. In treating fetal distress, continuous 100% oxygen is administered to the mother until delivery or relief of the distress. Hypoventilation and hyperventilation are potentially harmful because they induce hypoxemia and hypercapnia in both the mother and the fetus.

Maternal hypotension and hypovolemia diminish uterine blood flow and fetal perfusion. Hypoxia and acidosis threaten fetal well-being. The mother is safeguarded by appropriate anesthetic technique and selection of drugs. The fetus is protected by adequate uteroplacental perfusion and fetal monitoring by trained personnel. The patient should not be left alone in the holding area or OR. The fetal heart rate and uterine contractions are monitored continually. The procedure involves the care of two patients.

Positioning the Pregnant Patient

Uterine displacement to the left during transport and until after delivery is necessary to shift the uterus away from the large abdominal vessels. The positional effect on cardiac output is of major importance in avoiding maternal hypotension and maintaining fetal well-being. In the supine position the enlarged uterus compresses the inferior vena cava and aorta, resulting in diminished venous return to the heart, stroke volume, and cardiac output. This is further complicated if the patient is obese with a large central body habitus.

The patient is positioned supine with the right side slightly elevated by a wedge or small roll to tilt the uterus to the left

		Change in	
Test	**Nonpregnant Females**	**Pregnant Females**	**Gestational Timing**
Hemoglobin (Hgb)	12–16 g/dL	↓ 1.5–2 g/dL	Drops to lowest point between 30th and 34th weeks, then stable
Hematocrit (Hct)	37–47%	↓ 4–7%	Drops to lowest point between 30th and 34th weeks, then stable
White blood cells (WBCs)	5000–10,000/cm³	↑ 3.5 × 103	Gradual increase throughout pregnancy
Platelets	150,000–400,000/mm³	↓ Slightly	Gradual decrease throughout pregnancy
Fibrinogen	200–400 mg/dL	↑ 50%	Gradual increase throughout pregnancy
Calcium (Ca)	9–10.5 mg/dL	↓ 10%	Gradual decrease throughout pregnancy
Sodium (Na)	136–145 mEq/L	↓ 2–4 mEq/L	Decreases before 20th week, then stable
Chloride (Cl)	90–110 mEq/L	↑ Slightly	Gradual rise, almost negligible
Potassium (K)	3.5–5 mEq/L	↓ 0.2–0.3 mEq/L	Decreases before 20th week, then stable
Creatinine clearance	95–125 mL/min	↑ 40%	Rises through 20th week, then stable
Blood urea nitrogen (BUN)	5–20 mg/dL	↓ 50%	Drops during first trimester, then stable
Glucose (fasting)	70–115 mg/dL	↓ 10%	Gradual decrease throughout pregnancy
Uric acid	2–6.6 mg/dL	↓ 33%	Decreases during first trimester, then stable
Albumin	3.2–4.5 g/dL	↓ 1 g/dL	Rapid drop before 20th week, then stable

TABLE 34.2   Altered Laboratory Values of Pregnancy

(Fig. 34.17). The OR bed may be tilted 30 degrees to the left. A slight Trendelenburg position assists venous return in the patient.

Anesthesia

Anesthesia is selected on an individual basis. Regional anesthesia, such as spinal or epidural, is preferred because it has a lesser effect on the physiology of the mother and her fetus. It is advantageous in patients with diabetes because of reduced metabolic expenditure, low incidence of vomiting, and earlier return to oral intake. General anesthetic is administered when the mother or fetus is in jeopardy and delivery is crucial, as in the presence of hemorrhage or severe fetal distress. The choice also depends on the reason for the surgical procedure, degree of urgency, and the patient's condition and preference. A cesarean section can be done with local anesthesia in an extreme emergency when an anesthesia provider is not immediately available.

The anesthesia provider chooses the method safest for the mother and fetus. Gastric motility and emptying are inhibited by fear, pain, labor, and narcotic administration. Patients requiring emergency surgery may have eaten recently. A pregnant patient should always be regarded as having a full stomach.

Spinal or epidural anesthesia allows the mother to see her newborn in the OR. It also reduces neonatal depression and risk for maternal aspiration. Hypotension is treated with IV fluid infusion and/or IV ephedrine given to increase blood pressure. Ephedrine, mephentermine (Wyamine), and metaraminol (Aramine) do not cause undesired uterine vasoconstriction. Other vasopressors can cause fetal hypoxia.

Placentally transmitted drugs depressant to the fetus are avoided. A single injection of morphine may be given through the epidural catheter at the conclusion of the surgical procedure. With injection into the pain path, the drug significantly reduces postoperative pain for 24 to 36 hours with minimal side effects. General anesthesia provides more rapid induction, less

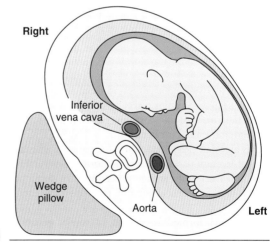

• **Fig. 34.17 A,** Pressure on aorta and vena cava caused by gravid uterus. **B,** Pressure is relieved by placing a wedge under right hip.

hypotension, greater cardiovascular stability, and better control of the airway and ventilation.

Preoxygenation Precedes Induction

Rapid-sequence induction and intubation are used if general anesthesia must be administered. Cricoid pressure during intubation occludes the esophagus to prevent regurgitation. Induction-to-delivery time is directly related to fetal hypoxia. Intervals greater than 3 minutes may lead to a lower pH of blood (metabolic acidosis) and respiratory depression of the infant from altered uteroplacental perfusion.

All efforts are made to deliver the newborn as rapidly as possible, consistent with safety, to minimize anesthesia and surgical time and to protect the fetus. With general anesthesia, all preparations, such as patient skin preparation, insertion of an indwelling Foley catheter, draping, gowning, and gloving, are done before induction of anesthesia.

Threatened Abortion

Cerclage

Patients with painless dilation and effacement of the cervix during the second trimester may be at risk for preterm delivery caused by cervical incompetence. The pregnant patient at risk should be assessed for a history of previous preterm rupture of membranes or spontaneous abortion. The initial primipara cervical incompetence is rarely evident before 16 weeks' gestation.

Diagnosis of threatened abortion for cervical incompetence is commonly made between 18 and 26 weeks' gestation. Gestational ages appropriate for elective treatment of known cervical incompetence range between 12 and 16 weeks' gestation, before the cervix has dilated beyond 2 to 3 cm. Some patients may be suitable for this procedure up to 20 weeks' gestation.

Cerclage is not usually performed after 26 weeks' gestation because the cervix is often too short to support suturing. Most cerclage is performed as an ambulatory procedure.

Occasionally, cerclage may be performed as an emergency procedure when the cervix is dilating and membranes are bulging, as long as the membranes have not ruptured or premature labor has not begun. The patient is placed in a deep Trendelenburg position to take the uterine pressure off the cervix. No vaginal prep is performed, to prevent accidental rupture of the membranes. It may be necessary to simultaneously perform transabdominal amniocentesis to decompress the membranes for the cerclage procedure. A sterile amniocentesis setup will be required.

General anesthesia is commonly used to provide relaxation of the uterine muscle. Cerclage is contraindicated in active infection, ruptured membranes, bleeding, or active labor. Cerclage is performed with ligature tape and a suture passer (Fig. 34.18).

Rarely, transabdominal cervicoisthmic cerclage (TCIC) may be performed as an open pelvic procedure for patients who have had severe cervical lacerations, congenital malformations of the cervix, or multiple failed cervical cerclage procedures. In some patients, laparoscopy is used for cervical banding to support the uterus for a pregnancy.

TCIC can be performed as early as 11 weeks' gestation after ultrasonographic documentation of a viable pregnancy. A 5-mm Mersilene tape is sutured around the cervical isthmus in an avascular plane. This procedure has been successful in preventing pregnancy loss characterized by painless cervical dilation and pregnancy loss during the third trimester.

• **Fig. 34.18** Suture passer.

Shirodkar Procedure

A small incision is made in the anterior vaginal mucosa at the level of the bladder reflection and at the posterior cervix—cul-de-sac junction (Fig. 34.19). A tunnel under the cervical mucosa is then made to join the anterior and posterior incisions. A polyester (Mersilene) tape is drawn around the internal os and tied. The knot is secured posteriorly to prevent erosion into the bladder. The suture tail is cut long so it can be located and released at 37 to 38 weeks' gestation or if active labor begins (before delivery). Mucosal incisions are closed. A cesarean section may be necessary at term.

McDonald Procedure

The polyester suture tape is placed around the cervix with a circumferential running stitch without mucosal dissection. Cervical scarring is less, and the procedure is quicker to perform. The tape can be removed at term for vaginal delivery.

Aborted Pregnancy

Termination of pregnancy may be spontaneous or induced. The procedure will depend on the gestational age of the fetus. Ultrasonography may be used to determine the stage of intrauterine pregnancy and the implantation site of the placenta.

Some patients are psychologically repulsed by the word abortion. They may associate the word with elective termination (elective voluntary abortion) regardless of natural causes or therapeutic need. Religious or personal beliefs may influence decision-making about a pregnancy that cannot continue to full term. In some circumstances the patient may accept and understand the word *miscarriage* and feel freer to select appropriate treatment options without fear of reprisal or rejection.

Consideration for the support of psychologic coping mechanisms of the patient in crisis is more important than using absolute words such as *abortion*. Females with Rh-negative blood types are candidates for immune globulin (RhoGAM) injections to prevent sensitization from the potentially Rh-positive fetus and complications with other pregnancies.

Suction Curettage

Intrauterine contents can be aspirated for elective abortion or for incomplete abortion (spontaneous abortion) within the first 20 weeks of pregnancy.

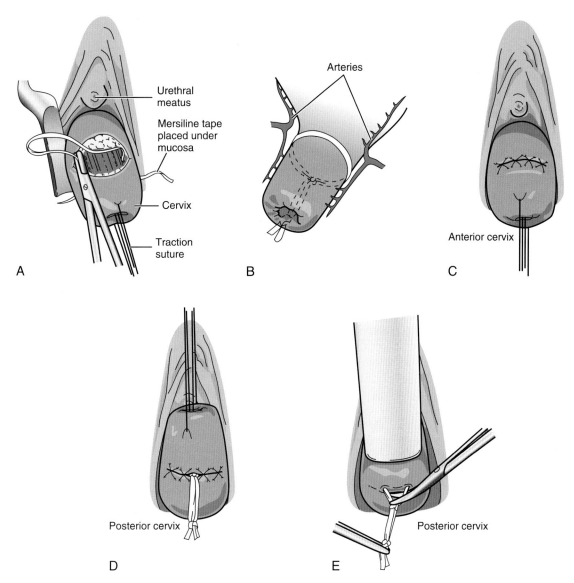

• **Fig. 34.19** Steps in the Shirodkar Procedure for Closure of an Incompetent Cervix. **A,** A ligature is placed below the mucosa circumferentially around the neck of the cervix. **B,** The uterine arteries are preserved and the ligature is tied on the posterior aspect of the cervix. **C,** The mucosal tissue is approximated with absorbable suture. **D,** A short length of ligature tape is left in place as a grasping tail. **E,** At term, the ligature tape is clipped to permit the cervix to open for the delivery of the fetus.

Uterine Evacuation

A small, flexible plastic tip or cannula is inserted into the uterus in the first 8 weeks of pregnancy. Suction created by drawing back on the plunger of a large syringe attached to the cannula is sufficient to evacuate the contents of the uterus. Disposable equipment for suction curettage not requiring dilation or anesthesia is commercially available.

Dilation and Evacuation

For pregnancies of 8 to 16 weeks' duration, dilation and evacuation (D&E) must be performed. Cervical dilation is adjusted to the stage of pregnancy and the necessary cannula. A laminaria tent (i.e., a cone-shaped expansion plug) may be inserted preoperatively to gradually dilate the cervix, usually for 4 to 24 hours. Dilation with the laminaria, which is removed before the procedure, is gentler than instrument dilation, which can cause cervical tearing. Some instrument dilation may be necessary.

A vacuum aspirator—cannula is inserted into the uterine cavity and connected by tubing to an adjustable electric vacuum pump. With gentle suction, the uterine contents are collected in a vacuum canister. Additional curettage with uterine curettes may be necessary to completely remove the remaining uterine contents (**retained products of conception (RPOC)**/retained secundus). The curetted contents are sent to the pathology department for gross examination. After an incomplete spontaneous or **missed abortion**, it is vital to remove all retained products of conception to prevent infection, especially from anaerobic bacteria, which may progress to septic shock.

A D&C setup and suction curettage are used. The tissue is sent for culture and pathologic examination. Some patients may

• **Fig. 34.20** Ectopic pregnancy.

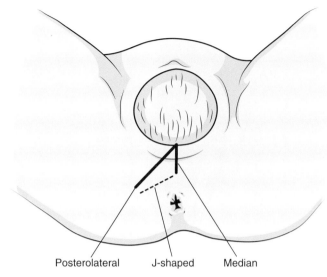

• **Fig. 34.21** Episiotomy.

request baptism of an aborted fetus for religious reasons. Perioperative personnel may perform this function or request hospital clergy to assist. This has deep meaning for many patients.

Ectopic Pregnancy

A fertilized ovum may become implanted outside the uterine cavity. Referred to as an ectopic pregnancy, rarely does this fetus develop to full term. This type of pregnancy usually involves the fallopian tube (95%) but can develop in the uterine cervix, on the ovary, or intraabdominally (Fig. 34.20).[5]

Symptoms of ectopic pregnancy are irregular growth patterns of the uterus, abdominal pain, and vaginal bleeding. Diagnosis is made by ultrasonography, laparoscopy, or detection of blood in the cul-de-sac by aspiration. Hemorrhage results from extensive trauma to the tube and mesosalpinx. The patient often goes into severe shock. Immediate surgical intervention is necessary.

Ruptured ectopic pregnancy is a true obstetric-gynecologic emergency. The affected tube is opened, and the products of conception are removed; hemostasis is attained; and the pelvic cavity is irrigated. The surgeon may attempt to repair the affected tube. Removal of the associated tube and possibly the ovary depends on the extent of damage from the rupture.

If an ectopic pregnancy is diagnosed by ultrasound or laparoscopy before rupture, conservative surgery may be able to restore fertility. Tubal pregnancy can be removed through a linear salpingostomy or by segmental resection, followed by tuboplasty. Laparoscopic techniques may be used. Some ectopic pregnancies can be managed through a vaginal colpotomy incision or abdominal minilaparotomy.

Complicated Birth

Difficult Vaginal Delivery

Routine episiotomy allows for vaginal delivery in some parturient mothers (Fig. 34.21). The obstetrician uses scissors to cut the vaginal outlet to make room for the presenting part of the fetus. An episiotomy helps prevent lacerations into the rectum or urethra that could later develop into a fistula. Perineal tears can still happen, and the team needs to know how to assist with repairs. Complicated deliveries can include a torn cervix that later requires

surgical reconstruction. If the obstetrician suspects a potential complication, the surgical team will be set up and on standby.

Placental Problems

Placental implantation problems can complicate birth. The placenta normally implants into the inner third of the myometrial layer and separates at the decidual layer during birth. Predisposition for implantation problems increases in patients with a history of previous placental problems, uterine deformity, or previous uterine surgery.[6,7] Improper placental implantation can be diagnosed with ultrasound.

When the placenta implants improperly and the chorionic villi invade beyond the normal implantation depth, the placenta cannot separate during delivery. This is known as *placenta accreta*. Extremely deep implantation is known as *placenta increta*.[6,7] As the placenta tries to separate during delivery, there is uncontrolled maternal hemorrhage. Further complications arise if the placenta invades through the myometrium to the level of the serosa, which is known as *placenta percreta* (Fig 34.22)

The depth of placental implantation is negatively affected by uterine contractions. The blood supply to the placenta is impeded by myometrial compression during labor contractions, depriving the fetus of oxygen. Other organs, such as the bladder, can be affected by an invasive placenta. Placenta percreta can invade the bladder wall as it grows through the serosal layer of the uterus.

In severe cases the mother may present with intractable hemorrhage necessitating a cesarean hysterectomy to stop the bleeding. The team should have a cystoscopy setup available for the placement of ureteral catheters and inspect for bladder damage. The hysterectomy should be performed with the patient in the low lithotomy position for rapid access to the bladder with the cystoscope.

Difficulties arise when the uterus unexpectedly ruptures along a previous cesarean section (C-section) scar. The fetus is delivered as quickly as possible. If the bleeding cannot be controlled, the uterus can be removed totally or supracervically if the placenta has not invaded the cervical tissue.

Perimortem C-section (at the death of the mother after longer than 5 minutes) is not usually successful before 24 weeks' gestation. The surgeon may elect to try to save the fetus by immediately

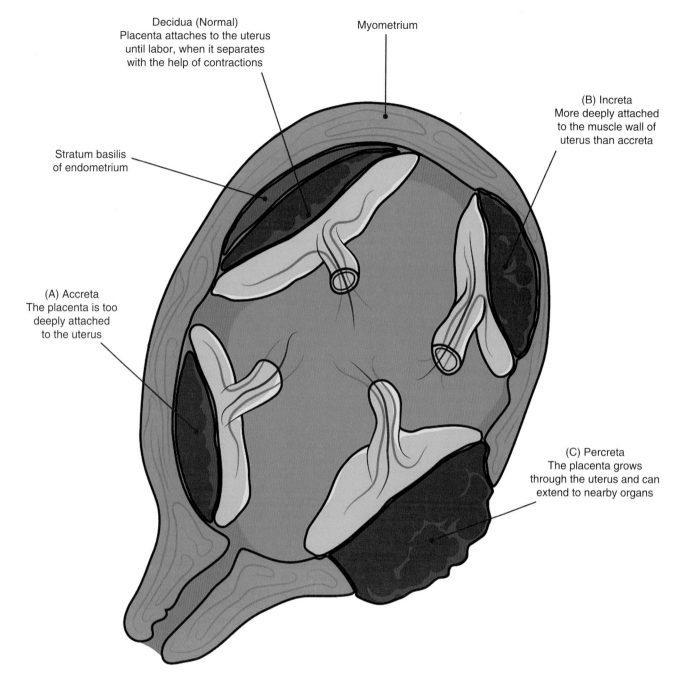

Decidua (Normal)
Placenta attaches to the uterus
until labor, when it separates
with the help of contractions

Myometrium

(B) Increta
More deeply attached
to the muscle wall of
uterus than accreta

Stratum basilis
of endometrium

(A) Accreta
The placenta is too
deeply attached
to the uterus

(C) Percreta
The placenta grows
through the uterus and can
extend to nearby organs

• **Fig. 34.22** Abnormal placental implantation that can cause serious hemorrhage during delivery and necessitate hysterectomy.

cross-clamping the aorta (to conserve placental blood) and quickly performing a hysterotomy for delivery.

Cesarean Birth

A cesarean section is a method of delivery by abdominal and uterine incisions. Cesarean delivery may take place in the labor and delivery department or in the OR. Pregnancy and labor produce many physiologic alterations. Both the mother and the newborn have specific needs requiring comprehensive care. To promote a positive experience, the perioperative team should be cognizant of these physiologic and psychologic needs and of the reasons for transabdominal delivery.

A C-section is a significant family event. Partners or support persons may be permitted in the OR, and mothers are given regional anesthesia and are usually awake.

The frequency of cesarean delivery is attributed mainly to diagnosis and management of uterine dystocia (ineffective labor), failure to progress, and fetal distress detected by fetal monitoring. A C-section is performed when safe vaginal delivery is questionable or immediate delivery is crucial because the well-being of the mother or fetus is threatened.

Indications for C-section include hemorrhage, placenta previa (low implantation), abruptio placenta (premature separation), invasive placenta (accreta, increta, or percreta), toxemia, fetal malpresentation, cephalopelvic disproportion (CPD), chorioamnionitis, genital herpes in the mother within 6 weeks of delivery, fetal distress, or prolapsed umbilical cord.[7] The multiparous pregnant patient who has had previous cesarean delivery may attempt vaginal delivery or may elect to schedule a planned cesarean birth.

Severe, unanticipated complications, such as bleeding or fetal distress during late pregnancy or labor, adversely affect the mother and/or fetus, creating an emergency. For these patients, preparations for immediate delivery are rapid. The patient easily senses a loss of control, especially if she participated in a childbirth education program for vaginal delivery. She needs special support. Most mothers fear more for the survival of the fetus than for themselves.

An elective patient is admitted the morning of surgery. The patient is taken to the delivery suite. An emergency patient will go directly to the delivery room from the labor area. The pediatrician and neonatal personnel from the nursery are notified before the procedure so they will be available to resuscitate and care for the infant in the delivery room. Sterile pediatric resuscitation equipment and supplies are made available.

Setup

Routine abdominal skin prep, draping, and setup are used for C-sections. Instruments are essentially those for a major gynecologic laparotomy with the addition of delivery forceps, a cord clamp, and a mucus aspiration bulb for infant suctioning on the field. A Foley catheter is inserted to decompress the bladder and monitor urinary output. The patient is placed supine with the right side of the OR bed elevated or a small pillow under the right hip to displace the uterus from the inferior vena cava.

All preparations are made for the setup before the anesthetic is administered to the patient. If regional anesthesia is planned, the setup, counts, and preliminary routines can be performed simultaneously with the anesthesia procedures. The patient is prepped, catheterized, and draped after the anesthetic has taken effect. If general anesthesia is to be used, the setup, prep, catheterization, and draping are performed before the anesthetic is administered to prevent prolonged depression of the fetus.

Incision and Delivery

A low transverse Pfannenstiel, or low midline vertical, incision is made in the skin and underlying tissue layers. The skin incision and uterine incision may be made in different anatomic planes. The length varies with the size of the fetus. Dissection is expeditious. As the uterus is incised, the amniotic sac will be opened. The amniotic fluid will escape rapidly, requiring suction. Retractors are removed, and the fetal head or the presenting part is delivered as gentle fundal pressure is applied (Fig. 34.23).

The uterine incision is made by one of the following methods (Fig. 34.24):

- *Low transverse (Kerr incision).* The bladder is dissected off the uterus and retracted gently downward. The lower uterine segment is entered through a low horizontal curvilinear incision. This approach causes less intraoperative blood loss and a decreased chance of rupture with subsequent pregnancies. Some patients will be able to have vaginal deliveries in future pregnancies.
- *Low vertical midline (Kronig incision).* An 8-cm vertical incision is made in the lower uterine segment after the bladder is separated and retracted away. This incision is used when the fetus is small, preterm, and in the breech position. It is also used when cesarean hysterectomy may be performed after delivery.

• **Fig. 34.23** Fundal pressure.

- *Classic uterine incision.* The uterus is incised vertically above the attachment of the bladder. The bladder is not dissected off the lower uterine segment. This approach is rarely used but may be necessary for a fetus in transverse presentation or for multiple fetuses. It may be indicated for a low anterior placenta, varicosities of the lower uterine segment, or cervical cancer. A major disadvantage is the high incidence of rupture with subsequent pregnancy.

Immediately on emergence of the head, the nares and mouth are aspirated with a bulb syringe to clear them of amniotic fluid (Fig. 34.25). Newborns delivered by C-section have respiratory secretions. Delivery is completed, and the umbilical cord is double-clamped and cut between the clamps with sterile scissors. The newborn is transferred via a sterile sheet to the neonatal resuscitation team.

The circulating nurse or neonatal team member who receives the newborn should wear protective eyewear, a gown, and gloves until all blood and amniotic fluid are wiped off the infant. The risk for exposure to blood and amniotic fluid warrants the same adherence to standard precautions as with any other contact with blood and body fluids. The neonate is placed under a radiant warmer for resuscitation.

Oxytocin, 10 to 20 units, is administered IV to the mother to promote uterine contraction, minimize blood loss, and facilitate expulsion of the placenta and membranes. The placenta is delivered, visually inspected, and placed in a specimen basin. The uterine fundus is palpated for firmness and massaged as necessary to prevent hemorrhage from relaxation. Intrauterine injection of 10 units of oxytocin may be necessary to firm up an atonic uterus.

The patient is returned to a horizontal supine position. The uterine incision is closed in layers with absorbable sutures, and hemostasis is ensured.[8] Clots and excess intraperitoneal fluid are evacuated. After inspection of the pelvic organs and possible tubal ligation, the peritoneum and abdominal incision are closed.

Intraoperative assessment is the same as for any surgical patient. Sponges, tapes, and needles are counted before closure of the uterus and again before closure of the peritoneum, fascia, and skin.

Postpartum surveillance of the patient is essential. Lochia is observed. Abnormal bleeding, such as rapid saturation of the perineal pad, is immediately reported to the physician and recorded. Nurses' notes should include the mother's contact with the infant, the mother's emotional reaction to the surgical

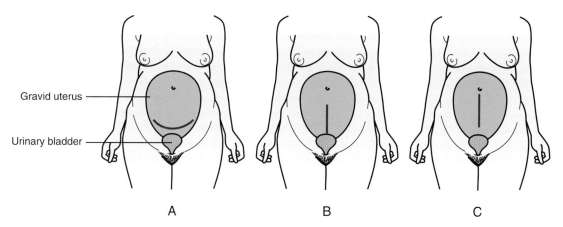

Gravid uterus

Urinary bladder

A   B   C

• **Fig. 34.24** Uterine Incisions for Cesarean Birth. **A,** Low transverse Kerr incision is the most commonly used. **B,** Low midline Kronig incision may be used for smaller or preterm fetus. **C,** Higher midline incision is referred to as a classic C-section and is used only in extreme circumstances. This method has a higher incidence of rupture in subsequent pregnancies.

Low incision in uterus

• **Fig. 34.25** Cesarean delivery after incising uterus and fetal membranes. As head is lifted through low uterine incision, pressure usually is applied to fundus of uterus through abdominal wall to help expel fetus.

procedure, and personnel in attendance, in addition to physical assessment data.

Neonate

Immediate postdelivery care is given in the OR by the neonatal team. The infant is taken to the nursery after careful examination by a pediatrician. The neonate traditionally has been evaluated by the Apgar score, acid-base status, and neurobehavioral examination. The Apgar score, first published by American anesthesiologist Virginia Apgar (1902–1974) in 1953, is an excellent screening tool for vital functions immediately (at 1- and 5-minute intervals) after birth, but the subtle effect of drugs may be overlooked. The Neurologic and Adaptive Capacity Score does not use noxious stimuli but emphasizes neonatal tone. Drugs that will produce significant neurobehavioral changes in the newborn must be avoided during labor and delivery.

In the newborn the apical pulse is the most accurate. Oxygenation is extremely important. Hypoxia (too little oxygen) can lead to intracranial hemorrhage, brain damage, or necrotizing enterocolitis. Hyperoxia (too much oxygen), administered at a rate in excess of 40% concentration, can cause bronchopulmonary dysplasia or retrolental fibroplasia.

Father or Support Person in the Delivery Room

Paternal or support-person participation in the birthing process is well established for vaginal delivery to provide support to the mother, a family-centered birth, and immediate bonding with the infant. However, the presence of the father/partner or support person in the OR during cesarean delivery is not universal and requires the surgeon's consent. Hospitals adopting this policy report favorable experiences. This person is informed of the conditions permitting and excluding their presence. Those who have attended a structured childbirth education course have more understanding of pregnancy and birth. In compliance with hospital policy, donning of OR attire and supervised handwashing with an antimicrobial soap before entrance to the OR are stressed.

The father/partner or support person sits by the mother's head. They may accompany the infant to the newborn examining area after delivery. If the newborn and the mother's conditions permit, the father/partner or support person may rejoin the mother in the OR for bonding.

Prenatal Testing

Potentially useful for management of some congenital developmental disorders or genetic defects, prenatal diagnostic studies are performed during pregnancy in select patients. Fetal anomalies are found in 2% of all women tested. Disorders in the fetus may be cause for induced abortion, elective cesarean delivery, or intrauterine fetal surgery.

Ultrasonography

Ultrasound is the standard tool for fetal imaging in utero. Ultrasonography, a noninvasive technique, permits accurate location of the placenta, determination of the gestational size of the fetus, assessment of fetal heart activity, and reliable diagnosis of structural defects (e.g., hydrocephalus, spina bifida). Other defects, such as missing limbs or conjoined twins, may be diagnosed.

Blood and Chorionic Villus Sampling

Ultrasound is also used for catheter or cannula guidance to obtain percutaneous umbilical blood samples or transcervical chorionic villus samples. Through direct fetal blood samples, anemia and some metabolic and chromosomal abnormalities can be diagnosed and treated in utero. Intravascular blood transfusions can be given to correct fetal anemia. Chorionic villi are a source of fetal genetic information. When obtained between the 8th and 12th weeks of gestation, chorionic villi can aid in accurately diagnosing some enzymatic defects and in detecting the sex of the fetus.

Amniocentesis

Amniotic fluid is aspirated from the amniotic sac under ultrasound direction at 16 to 20 weeks' gestation for chromosomal analysis. This highly accurate test is indicated for known or suspected risk for chromosomal abnormality because of advanced maternal age, known parental translocation carrier, or a history of previous pregnancy with chromosomal defect in the fetus or infant. Maternal serum α-fetoprotein (AFP) measurement can predict neural tube disorders (e.g., myelomeningocele) or other defects in the fetus.

Fetoscopy

Fetoscopy permits direct visualization of the fetus. A fiberoptic needle scope (fetoscope) is inserted into the amniotic cavity to view fetal parts, to obtain a biopsy of skin, or to sample fetal blood. The fetoscope is 1.7 mm in diameter with a visual field of 70°. To ensure an adequate volume of amniotic fluid, fetoscopy is done after 16 weeks of pregnancy. Because of the intent to view specific structures, the position of the fetus must first be determined and the procedure performed under sonographic-assisted visualization.

Placental localization is important, especially in the area of umbilical cord insertion. Hemoglobinopathies and coagulation problems (e.g., hemophilia) may be rapidly diagnosed by aspiration of fetal blood from the placenta or umbilical cord. Congenital skin disorders and albinism may be detected through biopsy. Direct viewing of the fetus may reveal characteristic abnormalities of various congenital syndromes. The procedure is not without complications and should be performed only by trained physicians when genetic information is critical.

Intrauterine Fetal Surgery

Improvement and expansion in prenatal diagnosis have led to rapidly developing antenatal surgical intervention—intrauterine fetal surgery. Diagnostic screening by ultrasound, AFP, or some other method during gestation reveals abnormalities heretofore diagnosed after delivery. Some disorders can be treated in utero. Other conditions fall within the province of the surgeon. Prerequisites for fetal therapy include accurate diagnosis, known pathophysiology, workable treatment, and technical capability. Fetal surgery teams are composed of radiologists, perinatologists, pediatric surgeons, anesthesia providers, obstetric nurses, perioperative nurses, and surgical technologists.

Most correctable malformations may be detected in utero but are best remedied by a surgical procedure after delivery at term. A full-term infant is a better surgical risk than is the fetus. Surgical treatment in utero is reserved for fetuses in whom continuing organ development could be normal if surgically treated (e.g., diaphragmatic hernia, spina bifida, tracheal stenosis, hydronephrosis caused by urinary tract obstruction).

Minimally invasive procedures facilitate the placement of shunts and catheters. Highly invasive procedures require hysterotomy (opening of the uterine wall) (Fig. 34.26). Preoperative preparation includes the administration of tocolytic drugs (indomethacin suppository) to prevent the onset of labor caused by

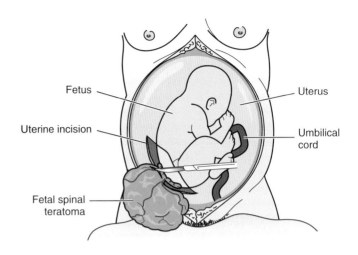

• **Fig. 34.26** Intrauterine fetal surgery.

uterine manipulation. An irritable uterus requires cancellation of the procedure.

The procedure is performed in the late second trimester with the patient under general anesthesia, using isoflurane because it is considered less hazardous to the fetus.

The uterus is exposed through an abdominal incision, and a cannula is inserted through the uterine wall to decompress some of the amniotic fluid. The uterine anterior fundal incision is carefully extended down to the amnion. The sac is opened, and the edges are secured to the uterine edges with Raney clips. Meticulous hemostasis is necessary. ESU use is avoided. Small doses of fentanyl and pancuronium are administered to the fetus for anesthesia. A sterile pulse oximeter and electrocardiographic (ECG) leads are sutured to the fetus to monitor oxygenation and cardiac activity.

Great care is taken to avoid manipulation of the placenta or cord. Warmed sterile saline irrigation is continuously perfused through the amniotic cavity during the procedure. After the repairs are complete, a small, wireless transducer is placed in the fetal chest for continued postoperative monitoring of the fetus in utero. This transducer is removed after birth. If fetal repairs require thoracotomy and diaphragmatic patching, the pleural space is maintained with warmed lactated Ringer solution to allow for continued lung growth.

On completion of the procedure the amnion is sutured closed and fibrin glue is applied. The uterus is sutured, and the abdominal incision is stapled. The fetal wound healing is nearly scarless because of decreased inflammatory response and neotissue generation associated with continued fetal development. The pregnancy continues as long as possible after the open procedure, preferably to a minimum of 32 to 36 weeks' gestation. Lung maturity is the key issue for success.

Preterm labor usually precipitates cesarean birth. Vaginal delivery is contraindicated because a classic uterine incision of the fundus is used for open intrauterine fetal surgery and may predispose the uterus to rupture during contractions.

Assisted Reproduction

Infertility, the inability to conceive a child after a year or more of repeated attempts, can be emotionally devastating. Both partners undergo extensive testing to determine possible organic or functional causes. These may include a structural defect in either partner, past or present infections, genetic and/or immunologic abnormalities, or an endocrine imbalance or deficit. In the woman a hostile cervix, antibodies to sperm, endometriosis, or exposure to DES in utero may prevent conception.

Tubal occlusion is the most frequent cause of infertility. A male partner may have an inadequate number, quality, or mobility of sperm or an absence of live spermatozoa in semen. When conventional infertility therapy has failed to produce a pregnancy, other options are available to assist in achieving pregnancy and birth of a mature, live infant.

In Vitro Fertilization

The term *in vitro* means "in glass." Fertilization literally takes place in a culture dish or test tube. In vitro fertilization (IVF) refers to removal of ova from the prospective mother via endoscopy, fertilization with the husband's or a donor's sperm, and incubation in the laboratory with subsequent embryo transfer to the uterus. Ovulation may be stimulated by administration of hormones. Multiple follicles may mature, and several ova are procured. The first documented birth from IVF and embryo transfer, performed by Dr. Robert Edwards and Dr. Patrick Steptoe, took place in England in 1978 by cesarean section. The first "test tube" baby has since grown and had a child of her own. The first IVF clinic in the United States using the Edwards-Steptoe method was established in Virginia in 1980.

IVF is most successful in women younger than 30 years. In women younger than 34 years, the success rate is 45% to 55% for delivery per ovum retrieval. The success of this technology for pregnancy in women older than 42 years is less than 10%. However, reports of a live birth by this method to a woman 60 years of age are found in the literature.

Patient Selection

IVF is accepted therapy for women with severely damaged or nonfunctioning fallopian tubes, for men with scarce or absent sperm, or for infertility of unknown cause. Contraindications include a uterine myoma, single uterine cornu, or bicornate or septate uterus. The woman is evaluated preoperatively for a normal uterine cavity, an accessible ovary, and evidence of ovulation. These parameters are measured by pelvic ultrasonography and serum estrogen levels. A laparoscopy, endometrial biopsy, and hysterosalpingogram may be part of preoperative testing. Semen analysis is done to check the sperm condition and count of the male partner.

Some patients may be unable to provide an ovum, conceive, or carry a fetus to full term. In select situations a surrogate mother will carry the developing fetus to term, surrendering the neonate at birth to the adoptive mother. Family members, such as a sister or other, may participate. Ethics and legal issues surround this event. Patient confidentiality is protected.

Induction of Ovulation

IVF is coordinated with timing of the ovulatory cycle. The medical protocol is prescribed for the individual couple. From day 2 or 3 of the menstrual cycle through day 6 or 7, the woman takes fertility drugs to stimulate growth and maturation of ovarian follicles. These drugs are a combination of clomiphene citrate (a synthetic hormone) and human luteinizing and follicle-stimulating hormones. Follicular growth is monitored daily,

beginning about the eighth day, by ultrasonography and serum estrogen levels. The fluid-filled follicles on the surface of the ovaries contain ova (oocytes). When follicles reach a diameter of 15 to 20 mm, the woman is given human chorionic gonadotropin (hCG) intramuscularly to stimulate maturation of the ova.

Ovum Retrieval

The patient is scheduled for retrieval of mature ova about 35 hours after hCG injection. Ovum retrieval may be accomplished through ultrasound-assisted transvaginal, transvesical, or transabdominal approaches. The procedure is performed with the patient under general anesthesia or IV sedation. Transvaginal ovum retrieval is the procedure of choice, but the approach depends on accessibility of the ovary.

With the patient in the lithotomy position, the ultrasound probe with an aspiration needle guide attached is advanced through the cervix, uterus, and fallopian tube to the ovary. The needle guide is directed toward the follicle, as seen on a monitoring screen. The follicle is punctured with a 14-inch × 17-gauge needle. Follicular fluid is aspirated into a 5-mL syringe. Ova procured from the graafian follicle are placed in sterile solution designated by the treating gynecologist.

Extensive scarring in tubes may make ovaries inaccessible via the transvaginal approach. For a transvesical approach the ultrasound probe is inserted through the urethra and posterior bladder wall to the ovary. With the patient positioned supine, a retrieval probe can be inserted percutaneously through the abdominal wall to reach the ovary in the pelvic cavity.

Ova can be retrieved by laparoscopy. The surgeon visualizes the ovaries. The follicle is punctured with an 8-inch × 14-gauge needle and aspirated directly into a test tube through a catheter attached to the needle. All instruments and solutions used for retrieval are kept at a normal physiologic temperature of 98.6° F (37° C). After completion of aspiration, the syringe or test tube is carefully handed to the circulating nurse using aseptic technique.

To avoid contamination, fluid should not be exposed to the environment, including light. Dimmed room light also enhances the surgeon's view on the video monitor. The circulating nurse labels the specimen and sends it immediately to the laboratory for confirmation of ovum retrieval while instrumentation is still in place. If the report is negative, the search for another ovum continues until the laboratory gives a positive response of retrieval. The procedure may be repeated on the contralateral ovary. Many surgeons prefer to retrieve at least three to five ova for fertilization. Other women can be suitable volunteer donors of ova for women who have been unable to provide a suitable ovum.

Fertilization

The aspirated ova are placed in a culture dish containing a nutrient mixture similar to tubal secretions at midcycle, which prepares the ova for fertilization. Fresh semen obtained an hour or so before the woman undergoes ovum retrieval, or previously collected frozen sperm from a partner or donor, is added. Care is taken to confirm identification of the ovum and sperm to prevent error.

The culture dish is incubated for 40 to 48 hours for fertilization to take place. Cell division is detected by microscopic examination. When the embryo reaches the 4 to 8-cell stage of development, it is ready for transfer to the uterus.

Multiple oocytes can be fertilized, and embryos can be stored frozen for a period of up to 3 years for later implantation if desired. Embryos frozen at the 2, 4, 8, or 16-cell stage, after thawing, have a viability rate of 60% to 80%. The embryo is transferred during a natural ovulatory cycle for the best results.

Embryo Transfer

Approximately 48 hours after retrieval, the woman returns for embryo transfer. She is placed in the knee-chest position. Anesthesia is unnecessary. A catheter prepared in the laboratory, containing the embryo in culture medium, is inserted into the uterus. The patient remains in the knee-chest position for at least an hour to allow the embryo to gravitate to the upper uterine fundus. Immediately after embryo transfer, an injection of progesterone is given. Necessary for implantation, injections are given daily for the next 12 to 15 days. Implantation is necessary for progression of the cell mass to an embryo. The woman's own ovarian function sustains early gestation, as confirmed by ultrasonography.

Failure to implant may result from escape of the embryo from the uterus with removal of the catheter, excess uterine contractility, inadequate luteal phase affecting the endometrium, mechanical disturbance of the endometrium, or encapsulation of the embryo in blood or mucus.

Gamete Intrafallopian Transfer

The procedure for gamete intrafallopian transfer (GIFT), developed in 1984, is similar to IVF but is always done laparoscopically. The woman must have at least one patent, functional fallopian tube. Ovulation is induced as described for IVF. Laparoscopy is scheduled 34 or 35 hours after injection of hCG. Fresh semen is obtained from the partner at least an hour before this procedure and is centrifuged and incubated at body temperature until use.

Ovum retrieval via laparoscope is accomplished as described for IVF. The follicular fluid is sent immediately to the laboratory, where an embryologist selects two or three ova. These and the sperm, along with the culture medium, are loaded into a catheter and sent back to the OR. The surgeon passes the catheter through the laparoscope and injects fluid into the ampulla of the fallopian tube. One or both tubes may receive an injection.

Other procedures, such as laser vaporization of endometriosis or lysis of adhesions, may be performed while the surgeon waits for the catheter. Additional ova may be inseminated and cryopreserved for IVF if GIFT is unsuccessful. Many implants may precede conception; it may never be successful.

Artificial Insemination

In vivo fertilization by artificial insemination of sperm may provide a reproductive option for a fertile woman. Homologous insemination deposits the partner's sperm into the upper vagina, cervical canal, or uterine cavity. Whole ejaculate is used when the man is unable to deposit sperm into the partner's vagina because of psychologic or physiologic factors. Washed sperm are used for intrauterine injection. Semen or sperm may be frozen and stored in a sperm bank for future use if reproductive capacity is threatened, such as by illness. Artificial insemination is coordinated with the recipient's ovulation for conception to occur.

Donor insemination involves the same techniques, but sperm are obtained from a donor. Donors are screened for STIs, including infection with human immunodeficiency virus (HIV) and hepatitis B virus (HBV). Genetic screening also may be required. Donor sperm may be sought when the partner has a genetically transmitted disease or defect. The couple may have concerns about donor selection.

Uterus Transplants

The first successful uterine transplants were performed in 2014 at the Sahlgrenska University Hospital in Gothenburg, Sweden by Dr. Mats Brännström. Uterine transplants in humans became possible after 10 years of research using animals. The early studies concluded that living donors were preferred because cadaver organs would possibly have a prolonged ischemic time. With the living donor the ischemic time was approximately 2.5 hours. With a cadaver uterus the ischemic time would be greater. The procurement and the transplant were performed simultaneously to minimize the time element.

Of the 33 women who received donor uterine transplants, 21 of the recipients were from living donors. As of 2022, 21 babies have been born after uterine transplants.[9] One of the women has successfully carried two pregnancies.

The original recipient women were O-positive blood type and ranged from 30 to 36 years in age. They were categorized as "absolute uterine factor infertility" because they did not have a uterus. Most of the women were born with vaginal-uterine dysgenesis, and one had a hysterectomy for cancer in her 20s. The condition is known as Mayer-Rokitansky-Küster-Hauser syndrome (MRKH) and presents as a congenital absence of a uterus and in some cases the upper segment of vagina. Functional ovaries are present, but not located in the pelvis. They are located higher in the abdomen, having failed to descend during fetal development. Mature ova are retrieved transabdominally, fertilized in vitro, grown to a 4-cell stage, and frozen in preparation for transfer to the transplanted uterus.

The donor organs were procured from family members in all but one case; the donor uterus used in the first birth was from a friend aged 61 years. The postmenopausal donor was given hormones to stimulate the endometrial lining in preparation for donation. Criteria for uterine donation include good general health, previous childbearing, nonsmoking, and appropriate tissue matching. The donation surgery can take 8 to 10 hours in some cases. The donated organs were taken complete with long pedicles of round ligament, sacrouterine ligament, paravaginal tissue, uterine arteries, and veins. There is no innervation of the transplanted uterus.

The implanted uterine vasculature was attached end to side with the internal iliac arteries and veins with 7-0 and 8-0 nonabsorbable monofilament suture. Perfusion was quickly evident. The ligamental tissue was secured for support. A tiny Doppler probe was attached to the uterine artery for postoperative monitoring of the blood supply. The end of the thin probe cable was exteriorized through the abdomen and was extracted by the third postoperative day. The recipient uterus transplant procedure took around 5 hours.

The recipients were given immunosuppressant drugs and 23 of the 33 uteri were still viable at 1 year after implantation. Menstruation began within 43 days in the first patient and began to regularly cycle within 3 months. The other recipients also began to have regular menstrual cycles. Periodic cervical biopsies were done to monitor the viability of the tissue. The first embryo was transferred 1 year after the transplant. Pregnancy tests returned positive 3 weeks after the first embryo transfer. Fetal heartbeat was present 2 weeks later.

Criteria for the uterus recipient patients include the informed consent that only one fertilized embryo will be implanted, only two pregnancies would be permitted per patient, the births would be by cesarean section 1 month preterm, and the uterus will be removed to prevent the need for long-term immunosuppression. Transplanted uteri are not considered a "life-long" organ, but rather a temporary means to have a baby when absolute uterine factor infertility is the diagnosis.

Nonobstetric Surgical Procedures and the Pregnant Patient

The pregnant surgical patient who is brought to the OR for reasons other than childbirth presents a unique challenge to the perioperative team. The plan of care includes consideration for two patients: the mother and her developing fetus. The effects of surgical intervention can be disastrous to a pregnancy, but it is necessary in some situations to save the mother and/or the fetus. A developing fetus is intolerant of hypovolemia and hypoxemia. These considerations apply to all pregnant patients.

The average gestation, or duration of pregnancy, is 38 to 40 weeks, or 9 calendar months. This gestation period is divided into trimesters (3-month segments). Each trimester represents a specific developmental and viability concern (Box 34.1). Maternal anatomic and physiologic changes occur during each trimester of pregnancy (Table 34.3). Modifications to the plan of care vary according to these changes.

Risks associated with surgical intervention may be specific to the fetus. During the first trimester, spontaneous abortion of the developing embryo (until the end of the eighth week) or fetus (from the eighth week) can occur. Preterm labor and/or delivery may be precipitated during the second and third trimesters. The surgeon and anesthesia provider should discuss the risks, benefits, and potential outcome with the patient and her family.

Nonobstetric surgical procedures on pregnant patients are usually performed for an urgent or emergent reason, such as cholecystitis, appendicitis, or trauma. Urgent surgical procedures are delayed until the second or third trimester, if possible. Emergency procedures are performed immediately, regardless of gestational stage. If the maternal condition is critical, the primary concern is to save the mother. Elective surgical procedures should be deferred until after delivery of the neonate and when the anatomic and physiologic changes of pregnancy have returned to normal.

Anesthesia Considerations in Pregnancy

The surgeon and anesthesia provider collaborate closely because the risks of anesthesia and surgical procedures are high for both the mother and the fetus. Perinatal morbidity and mortality are affected by maternal health, fetal viability, the type of anesthetic, and the surgical procedure. The incidence of preterm labor, low birthweight, and fetal death increases if a general anesthetic agent must be administered. The objectives of anesthesia management in the pregnant surgical patient include, but are not limited to:

1. *Maternal safety:* The pregnant patient always should be treated as if she has a full stomach. Nausea and vomiting are common and place the patient at risk for aspiration of regurgitated stomach contents during induction of anesthesia, intubation, and extubation. The condition of the mother directly affects the outcome of the pregnancy.

• BOX 34.1   Stages of Fetal Development and Viability Concerns

First Trimester (1–3 months, 1–12 weeks)
- Zygote implants in uterine wall by 14 days.
- Communication of venous sinus and arterial supply of maternal circulation is completed at 17 days.
- Teratogens can impair organogenesis until 14th week.
- Primitive placental system with umbilical cord is established by 7th week.
- Heart rate is detectable on ultrasound at 10–12 weeks.
- Facial features and external genitalia are present by 12th week.
- Crown-to-rump length is 6–7 cm by 12th week.

Second Trimester (4–7 months, 13–27 weeks)
- Arms and trunk grow rapidly.
- Little muscle tone.
- Scalp hair, tiny nipples, and external ears develop by 20th week.
- Meconium is present in intestine.
- Body weight is 300 g.
- Skeletal calcification is seen on x-ray.
- Sucks thumb and moves freely at will.
- Fetal heart rate is audible with fetoscope at 120–160 beats/min at 20th week.
- Fingertip pressure causes ballottement (fetal rebound) in amniotic sac during 16th–32nd weeks.
- Teratogens may cause minor structural and functional abnormalities, especially endocrine, brain, and special senses, from 10th week to term.
- Body is covered with vernix (gray-white cheeselike substance) and lanugo (soft, downy hair).
- Eyebrows and eyelashes are present.
- Body weight is 454–630 g (1–1.4 lb) by 24th week. May be viable.

Third Trimester (7–9 months, 28–38 to 40 weeks)
- Subcutaneous fat begins to develop.
- Crown-to-rump length is 25 cm.
- Testes are descended in males.
- Body weight is 1100 g (2.5 lb).
- Surfactant is present in alveoli of lungs by 28th week.
- Increased chance of survival.
- Body weight is 1361–1814 g (3–4 lb) by 32nd week.
- Body is fuller and rounded.
- Muscle tone is good.
- Less vernix and absence of lanugo by 36th week.
- Body weight is 3402–3629 g (7.5–8 lb) by 38–40 weeks.
- Crown-to-rump length is 36 cm.

---

2. *Avoidance of teratogenic drugs:* Many anesthetic drugs cross the placenta and enter the fetus through the uteroplacental circulation. Some drugs that adversely affect the fetus during the first trimester are nitrous oxide, halogenated agents, sedatives, tranquilizers, antidepressants, and amphetamines.
   - Halogenated agents and nitrous oxide have been given without teratogenicity in emergency situations during the second and third trimesters. Only short-acting drugs should be used. The fetal liver is immature and metabolizes tranquilizers and other narcotics slowly. Neonatal respiratory depression is common if these drugs have been used.
   - Agents used in local and regional anesthesia have not shown teratogenicity in animal studies and may provide a safer anesthetic alternative than those agents used for general anesthesia when a surgical procedure must be performed.

TABLE 34.3 Maternal Anatomic and Physiologic Changes of Pregnancy

System	First Trimester (1–3 Months, 1–12 Weeks)	Second Trimester (4–7 Months, 13–27 Weeks)	Third Trimester (7–9 Months, 28–38 to 40 Weeks)
Cardiovascular	Cardiac output begins to increase at 6th week.	Cardiac output increases 30–50% by 16th week.	Cardiac output decreases slightly by 30th week.
	Plasma volume begins to increase.	Plasma volume continues to increase. Hypervolemic and hemodiluted.	Plasma volume increase peaks 50% at 32–36 weeks.
		Red blood cell (RBC) production increases 20%. White blood cell (WBC) production increases 30–40%.	RBC increases, peaks at 33%.
	Breast veins dilate.	Capillary engorgement can cause epistaxis (nosebleeds) and epulis (bleeding gums).	May develop hemorrhoids, varicosities in leg veins. Increased risk for venous thrombosis.
	Vasculature increases to vulva and vagina.	Heart rate increases 15–20 beats/min.	Factors VII, IX, X increase, causing hypercoagulative state. Plasma fibrinogen increases 40–50%.
		Slight hypotension caused by decreased peripheral vascular resistance.	Normotensive by 26th week.
		Uterus presses on vena cava when supine.	Uterine circulation is 1 L/min by 38th–40th weeks.
		Physiologic anemia: hemoglobin, hematocrit, and platelets decrease.	
Pulmonary	Lung compliance and pulmonary diffusion remain constant throughout pregnancy.	Diaphragm is displaced upward by rising fundus; thoracic circumference increases by 6 cm.	Diaphragm is displaced 4 cm by rising fundus; thoracic breathing replaces abdominal breathing.
	Vital capacity and partial pressure of oxygen (Po_2) are unchanged.	Tidal volume increases 30–40%.	Venous stasis increases risk for thrombus formation and pulmonary emboli.
		Respiratory rate increases 15% to accommodate increasing metabolism.	
		Mild dyspnea. Chronic state of compensated respiratory alkalosis.	
		Nasal congestion caused by estrogen-induced edema.	
Gastrointestinal	Nausea and vomiting.	Nausea and vomiting diminish.	Gastric emptying time is decreased.
	Constipation.	Incidence of cholecystitis is increased.	
	Salivation increases.	Progesterone causes decreased gastrointestinal motility. Esophageal sphincter tone is decreased; at risk for gastric reflux.	Gallbladder sluggish, gallstones frequently develop.
Neurologic	May feel some slight Braxton Hicks contractions starting at 8th week.	Intraocular pressure decreases. Some temporary visual changes develop; vision returns to prepregnant state after delivery.	Braxton Hicks contractions increase and become regular.
Endocrine	Human chorionic gonadotropin hormone secreted by corpus luteum of ovary is present in serum 9 days after conception.	Protein binding causes increase in circulating hormones. Thyroid and adrenal hormone levels are elevated. Insulin production increases.	Prolactin increases and peaks at delivery.
	Progesterone production increases.	Erythropoietin increases by 20th week.	
	Basal metabolic rate decreases. Blood glucose level decreases.	Metabolism increases.	

TABLE 34.3	Maternal Anatomic and Physiologic Changes of Pregnancy—cont'd		
System	**First Trimester (1–3 Months, 1–12 Weeks)**	**Second Trimester (4–7 Months, 13–27 Weeks)**	**Third Trimester (7–9 Months, 28–38 to 40 Weeks)**
Genitourinary			
Ureters and renal pelves and calyces dilate, increasing risk for urinary tract infection. Dilation is present throughout pregnancy.	Urinary frequency is caused by uterine pressure on bladder.	Bladder pressure decreases as fundus elevates. Bladder is displaced superior to pelvis.	Lateral position facilitates renal blood flow and increases urinary output.
		Glomerular filtration rate increases 30–50%. Drugs are excreted faster.	Frequency is increased as presenting part enters pelvis.
Integumentary	No appreciable change.	Striae gravidarum (stretch marks) appear on breasts and abdomen.	Dark line (linea nigra) appears between umbilicus and pubis.
			Increased pigmentation of face (chloasma).
Musculoskeletal	Feels fatigue.	Feels energetic.	Energy declines.
	Weight loss first few weeks caused by nausea and vomiting. Average weight gain 2.2 lb (1 kg) by 10–12 weeks.	Weight gain 1 lb (0.45 kg) per week; desirable weight gain between 12th and 20th weeks is 8 lb (3.62 kg). Gains 0.5–1 lb (0.24 kg–2.2 kg) per week between 20th and 38th weeks.	Ideal weight gain 25–30 lb (11–13.6 kg) total for entire pregnancy.
		Progressive lordosis to compensate for shifting center of gravity causes backache.	Increased lordosis as uterus expands and protrudes forward.
	Leg cramps.	Leg cramps increase by 24th week.	Pelvic joints relax, and slight separation of symphysis pubis can be seen on x-ray.
Reproductive	Menstruation ceases.	Uterine fundus elevates halfway between symphysis pubis and umbilicus by 12th–16th weeks but rises above umbilicus by 24 weeks.	Uterine fundus elevates halfway between umbilicus and xyphoid process by 28th week and reaches xyphoid by 32nd week. Fundus decreases in height (caused by uterine weight) by 38th week. Uterine weight at term is 1100 g.
	Progesterone causes uterine lining to thicken.	Fetal movement is felt by 18th–20th weeks.	
	Estrogen causes uterine body to hypertrophy, anteflex, and become globular; by 3rd month, fundus reaches pelvic brim.		
	Cervix softens, and vulva and vagina appear blue (caused by increasing vascularity). Vaginal discharge increases.	Lower uterine segment elevates in pelvis.	
	Breast tissue enlarges and becomes sensitive.	Areolae darken.	Breasts feel full and tender. May secrete colostrum (precursor to milk).

3. *Prevention of fetal asphyxia:* Maternal hypoxia rapidly affects the oxygenation of the fetus. The oxygenation capability depends on the hemoglobin content and arterial oxygen tension of maternal blood and uteroplacental perfusion. Maternal hypotension and decreased uterine blood flow cause fetal hypoxia.

4. *Prevention of preterm labor:* Studies have shown no association of any single anesthetic agent with an increase or decrease in preterm labor. Manipulation of the gravid uterus can cause preterm labor. The use of halogenated agents in advanced pregnancy decreases uterine tone and prevents uterine contractions. Vasopressors and drugs used to reverse muscle relaxants may stimulate the uterus to contract and initiate preterm labor.

Special Considerations
Intraoperative Care of the Pregnant Patient

Both the mother and the fetus should be monitored during the surgical procedure. The mother's physiologic and psychologic condition rapidly affects the well-being of her fetus. Changes in the fetal condition may be the first indicators of a physiologic change in the mother. Intraoperative care and monitoring of the pregnant surgical patient include special considerations regarding the following objectives:

1. *Minimize the patient's time under anesthesia:* Skin preparation and draping should be done before induction of general anesthesia. Devices for electronic fetal and uterine monitoring should be in position and in proper working order.

2. *Monitor maternal oxygenation:* Pulse oximetry is useful for noninvasive measurement of oxygenation in hemoglobin. Readings should remain above 94% to prevent fetal hypoxia. Continuous oxygen is usually administered.

3. *Monitor the fetal heart rate:* An electronic fetal heart monitor (EFM) should be used by appropriately trained personnel for continuous monitoring. Fetal tachycardia may be the first indicator of maternal hypoxia. EFM is most effective after 16 weeks' gestation. Personnel qualified in EFM should be assigned this role.

4. *Monitor the uterine tone:* The uterus should be palpated frequently during the surgical procedure to detect contractions. Uterine manipulation, bladder stimulation, and several anesthetic drugs may cause preterm labor.

5. *Prevent aspiration:* Assist the anesthesia provider during intubation by providing cricoid pressure (Sellick maneuver) as directed.

6. *Prevent maternal hypotension:* If the uterus is enlarged to the level of the umbilicus or above (17−20 weeks' gestation), place a small pad or folded sheet under the right hip to laterally displace the uterus to the left. This redistributes the weight of the gravid uterus off the vena cava and abdominal aorta and facilitates a normotensive state. Renal perfusion is also improved.

7. *Monitor urinary output:* Minimum urinary output should be 25 mL/h. Palpate the bladder every 30 minutes. Bladder distention can cause uterine irritability and preterm labor. The bladder is displaced above the pelvis during the second and third trimesters and is easily injured. An indwelling Foley catheter should be inserted if the surgical procedure is anticipated to exceed 1 hour.

8. *Maintain a normothermic environment:* Warm the room to 75° F (24° C) and maintain a consistent temperature during the surgical procedure. Maternal hypothermia causes decreased uteroplacental perfusion and can cause fetal bradycardia. Use prewarmed blankets and irrigating solutions. Keep the mother's head covered.

9. *Prepare for emergency cesarean birth or preterm delivery:* In the event of untimely rupture of the membranes, preterm labor, or fetal distress, it may be necessary to perform a cesarean section or precipitous delivery in an effort to save a viable fetus. A preterm fetus requiring immediate delivery after 24 weeks' gestation or 1 lb (500 g) weight may be considered viable. Fetal viability is individualized by measurement of lung maturity, body weight, and ability to sustain life after removal from the uterus.

10. *Protect the fetus from hazards in the environment:* The pregnant uterus at any stage of gestation should be shielded from ionizing radiation. During the first trimester, radiation may cause teratogenic damage. This may be unavoidable in trauma surgery.

11. *Reassure the mother:* Explain that she and her fetus will be monitored closely and that they will be carefully protected.

Intraoperative Risks

The enlarging uterus displaces abdominal organs and distorts anatomic landmarks, making diagnoses of trauma or a pathologic condition complex. A motor vehicle accident (MVA) is a common cause of abdominal trauma. A seat belt (lap belt) without a shoulder restraint can cause compression injury to the enlarged uterus. Spontaneous laceration and/or rupture can occur. Peritoneal lavage, if used to assess for intraabdominal bleeding, should be done through an incision above the umbilicus to avoid injuring the uterus.

Surgical procedures for reasons other than trauma, such as pathologic causes, require careful differential diagnosis. Anatomic and physiologic changes of pregnancy must be considered. For example, the appendix is displaced to the upper right quadrant and may mimic cholecystitis. In advanced pregnancy, chest drainage tubes should be inserted one or two intercostal spaces higher, if needed. Diagnosis is complicated because laboratory tests are altered by the progressing pregnancy and results vary according to the gestational stage.

Assessment of the patient's condition is difficult because compensatory mechanisms of pregnancy cause alterations in vital signs. The arterial blood pressure is lower than prepregnant values, and the pulse is elevated to accommodate an increase in circulatory volume. Decreased peripheral vascular resistance prevents overt physiologic signs of shock, such as cool, clammy skin.

Circulating blood volume can be reduced 30% to 35% before the patient shows any signs of hypovolemic shock, such as lowered blood pressure and increased pulse rate. In hypovolemic shock, blood is shunted away from the uteroplacental circulation at the expense of the fetus. The fetus becomes hypoxic. Fetal demise rate is 80% in maternal hypovolemic shock.

An EFM can detect early signs of fetal hypoxia and uteroplacental insufficiency. Use of a fetal monitor is recommended during surgical procedures after 16 weeks' gestation. Personnel appropriately trained in fetal monitoring should perform this assessment throughout the perioperative period, including during the surgical procedure and postanesthesia recovery.

In the immediate postoperative period the pregnant patient must be assessed for uterine irritability, vaginal bleeding, and/or ruptured membranes. Any combination of these signs may signal impending labor and possible preterm delivery and must be reported to the physician immediately. Bladder distention can cause uterine irritability and stimulate preterm labor. The bladder should be palpated frequently. A distended bladder is felt as a bulge above the symphysis pubis that is slightly cooler than the surrounding skin.

Psychologic Considerations

For most patients and their families, pregnancy is a time of joy and excitement. Their happiness is shattered when they are faced with the prospect of a surgical procedure and its inherent risks. In urgent and emergency situations the family has little time to adjust to the pending procedure.

The outcome is uncertain, and the risks to the mother and her fetus are great. The patient and family are also facing the possibility of a preterm delivery.

The perioperative team should consider the special needs of the pregnant patient and her family and provide as much reassurance as possible. Preterm emergent C-section after 25 weeks' gestation has a 45% fetal survival rate.

EVOLVE WEBSITE

http://evolve.elsevier.com/Hornacky/BerryKohn/

- Historical Perspective
- Tips for the Scrub Person and Circulating Nurse
- Student Interactive Questions
- Glossary

References

1. Centers for Disease Control and Prevention: HPV vaccine. www.cdc.gov. Accessed June 5, 2023.
2. Hertweck SP, Rothstein DH: Challenges and opportunities in adolescent gynecology patients with surgically-treated congenital and acquired anomalies: transition of care from pediatric to adult surgery, *J Pediatr Adolesc Gynecol* 32(2):103–109, 2019.
3. Chen T, Li J, Zhu Y, et al.: The oncological and obstetric results of radical trachelectomy as a fertility-sparing therapy in early stages cervical cancer patients, *BMC Womens Health* 22:424, 2022.
4. Boles T, Salcedo M, Lorenzoni C, et al.: Overview of thermal ablation devices for treating precancerous cervical lesions in low resource settings, *J Glob Health* 12:03089, 2022.
5. Brincat M, Bryant-Smith A, Holland TK: The diagnosis and management of interstitial ectopic pregnancies: a review, *Gynecol Surg* 16(1):1–15, 2019.
6. Chen L, Wang X, Wang H, et al.: Clinical evaluation of prophylactic abdominal aortic balloon occlusion in patients with placenta accreta: a systematic review and meta-analysis, *BMC Pregnancy Childbirth* 19(1):1–8, 2019.
7. Fadl SA, Linnau KF, Dighe MK: Placental abruption and hemorrhage: review of imaging appearance, *Emerg Radiol* 26(1):87–97, 2019.
8. Stegwee SI, Jordans IPM, van der Voet LF, et al.: Single- versus double-layer closure of the caesarean (uterine) scar in the prevention of gynaecological symptoms in relation to niche development—the 2Close study: a multicentre randomised controlled trial, *BMC Pregnancy Childbirth* 19(1):1–11, 2019.
9. Johnannesson L, Richards E, Reddy V: The first 5 years of uterus transplant in the US: a report from the United States Uterus Transplant Consortium, *JAMA Surg* 157(9):790–797, 2022.

35

Urologic Surgery

CHAPTER OUTLINE

Anatomy and Physiology of the Urinary System, 730

Special Features of Urologic Surgery, 733

Surgical Procedures of the Genitourinary System, 738

Bladder Flap Urethroplasty, 748

Male Reproductive Organs, 749

Endocrine Glands, 758

Transsexual Surgery (Sex Reassignment), 758

Postoperative Complications of Urologic Surgery, 759

CHAPTER OBJECTIVES

After studying this chapter, the learner will be able to:

- Identify the organs of the male genitourinary system.
- Compare the differences between male and female urinary systems.

- Describe the procedures performed for urinary incontinence.
- Describe the procedures performed for prostate cancer.

KEY TERMS AND DEFINITIONS

Diversion Redirection of urine flow into a neobladder or stoma.

Extraperitoneal Outside the peritoneal cavity.

Hemolyze Blood cells dissolve, releasing hemoglobin.

Hyponatremia Low salt concentration of the blood.

Impotence Inability to have an erection.

Incontinence Inability to control bladder or bowels.

Isosmotic Solution having the same osmotic pressure as blood.

Litho- Stone; calculi.

Meatotomy Incising the meatus (distal opening) of the urethra.

Neobladder A urine collection reservoir fashioned from a segment of bowel.

Neurogenic Caused by the nerves within the area. Loss of bladder control caused by nerve injury or malfunction.

Orthotopic Autologous tissue used to create a structure or a replacement structure within the body. Used here to describe the creation of a bladder reservoir from bowel tissue that communicates with the urethra.

Retroperitoneal Behind the peritoneal cavity.

Transurethral Through the urethral canal.

Anatomy and Physiology of the Urinary System

The urinary system provides the vital life-sustaining functions of extracting waste products from the bloodstream and excreting them from the body. Organs of this system include bilateral kidneys and ureters, the bladder, and the urethra (Fig. 35.1). An obstruction to blood flow in the renal arteries or any part of the urinary system can cause renal damage, which ultimately results in uremia (a biochemical imbalance) or renal failure if left undiagnosed and untreated. Vascular hypertension, hypotension, obstruction, tumors, infection, trauma, and other systemic or neurogenic disorders are of major concern to a urologist.

Kidneys

The kidneys are large, bean-shaped, glandular organs located bilaterally in the retroperitoneal space of the thoracolumbar region behind the abdominal cavity. The arterial blood supply (renal artery) of the kidney originates from the aorta and enters the hilum on the medial aspect. Venous drainage flows through the renal vein and into the inferior vena cava. The lymphatics drain into the lumbar nodes. Innervation is from the autonomic nervous system originating in the lumbar sympathetic trunk and vagus nerve.

Each kidney is enclosed in a thin, fibrous capsule referred to as Gerota fascia. The renal parenchyma, the substance of the kidney within the capsule, is composed of an external cortex and internal medulla. The medulla consists of conical segments called renal pyramids. Each pyramid and its surrounding cortex form a lobe. Within these pyramids are the essential components of renal function: the nephrons (Fig. 35.2). As the urine forms, it drips from the papillae at the tips of the pyramidal structures.

Ren is the Latin word for kidney—hence the adjective *renal* and combining forms of *ren-* and *reno-* in terms pertaining to the

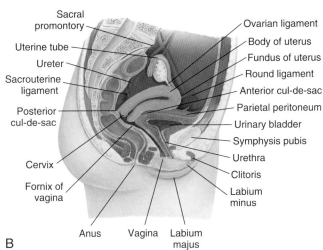

• **Fig. 35.1** Anatomy of the urinary tract. **A,** Male urinary tract. **B,** Female reproductive organs and urinary system. (*B,* From Thibodeau GA, Patton KT: *Anatomy and physiology,* ed 5, St. Louis, 2007, Mosby.)

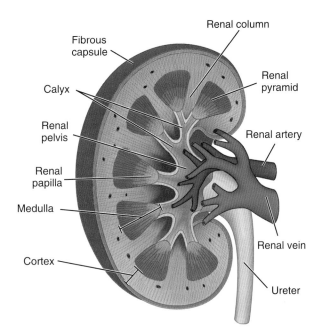

• **Fig. 35.2** Cross-section of the kidney. (From Thibodeau GA, Patton KT: *Anatomy and physiology,* ed 5, St. Louis, 2007, Mosby.)

kidney as part of the renal system. The purposes of the kidney are as follows:

• To remove metabolic waste, excess substances, and toxic substances from the blood
• To regulate and maintain body fluid and pH balance
• To help regulate and respond to blood pressure by producing the hormone renin
• To produce the hormone erythropoietin to control the rate red blood cells are produced by the bone marrow
• To assist in the production of water-soluble vitamin D, which is important for the metabolism of calcium

Each nephron consists of a glomerulus, glomerular capsule, and tubules. A glomerulus is an aggregation of capillaries formed by an afferent branch of the renal artery. These capillaries unite to form an efferent vessel. This capillary network is enclosed in a glomerular capsule (capsule of Bowman), which is the dilated beginning of the renal tubule. From the capsule, the tubule becomes tortuous and forms the proximal convoluted tubule. The

distal portion forms the descending and ascending limbs of the medullary loop (loop of Henle) (Fig. 35.3).

Nitrogenous wastes, salts, toxins, and water filtered from the capillary network form urine, which flows through the medullary loop and into the collecting tubule. The collecting tubules converge at the papilla (apex) of each renal pyramid. Urine flows continuously from each papilla into a calyx. Each kidney has between 4 and 13 minor calyces that lead into 2 or 3 (rarely 4) major calyces that form the renal pelvis. The renal pelvis forms the dilated proximal end of the ureter.

Urine forms at the glomerulus by filtration. Hydrostatic pressure forces the plasma minus the blood cells and large molecules through the system. The amount of blood filtered is approximately 1700 quarts, from which is derived 200 quarts of filtrate. As this filtrate passes through the tubules, 99% of the water is resorbed and approximately 1 to 2 quarts of urine are produced. Cardiac function is closely related to the perfusion of the kidneys. Every time the heart beats a small drop of urine is formed. Cardiac failure leads to renal failure. Failure of both kidneys to function is followed by death within a few weeks.

Ureters

The ureters are connecting tubes between the kidneys and bladder; they are 4 to 5 mm in diameter, have a 0.2 to 1-cm lumen, and are approximately 12 inches (25–30 cm) long. They lie bilaterally beneath the parietal peritoneum and descend along the posterior abdominal wall to the pelvic brim. From there, they pass along the lateral wall of the pelvis and curve downward, forward, and inward along the pelvic floor to the bladder.

The wall of each ureter is continuous with the renal pelvis and is composed of mucous membrane, longitudinal and circular muscles, and an outer layer of fibrous and elastic tissue. Slow, rhythmic, peristaltic contractions carry urine from the kidneys to the bladder in response to filling of the renal pelves.

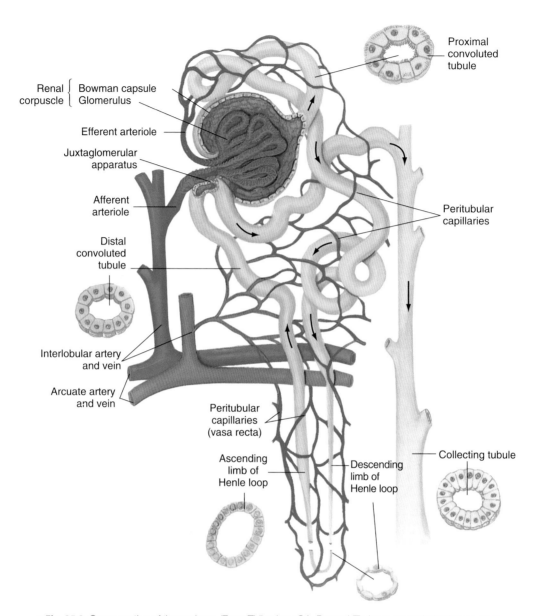

• **Fig. 35.3** Cross-section of the nephron. (From Thibodeau GA, Patton KT: *Anatomy and physiology,* ed 5, St. Louis, 2007, Mosby.)

Urinary Bladder

The bladder is a hollow muscular reservoir lined with mucous membrane; it is located extraperitoneally in the anterior pelvic cavity behind the symphysis pubis. The ureters enter the bladder wall obliquely on each side. The triangular area between the ureteral and urethral orifices is called the *trigone.* Folds of mucous membrane in the bladder wall act as valves to prevent the backflow of urine into the ureters. Urine collects in the bladder until an autonomic nerve stimulus from the sacral reflex centers causes micturition (urination) through the urethra. This stimulus opens the muscle fibers that form an internal sphincter at the bladder neck, the vesicourethral junction.

The arterial supply of the urinary bladder is derived from the hypogastric arteries that branch from the internal iliac arteries. The venous drainage empties into the hypogastric veins. The lymphatics drain into the internal and common iliac nodes.

The autonomic innervation of the bladder controls filling and emptying of the bladder. The parasympathetic fibers from S3 to S5 promote emptying by contraction of the detrusor muscles. The sympathetic nerve fibers that originate from L1 to L2 cause relaxation of the detrusor muscles and closure of the internal urinary sphincter, allowing the bladder to fill. Somatic innervation of the external urinary sphincter responds to somatic fibers arising from S2 to S4 and is voluntarily controlled to contract the musculature. Spinal cord injury at or below the level of L5 can result in inability to empty the bladder.

Urethra

The male urethra is approximately 25 to 30 cm long and has a diameter of 7 to 10 mm. It consists of two segments (proximal and distal) that are further subdivided into three segments referred to as the *prostatic,* the *membranous,* and the *cavernous* urethral segments. The proximal (posterior) prostatic urethra passes from the bladder orifice, through the prostate gland, and to the pelvic floor. The membranous urethra passes from the pelvic floor to the base of the penis. The distal (anterior) segment consists of parts of the membranous, bulbous, and anterior urethral segments that pass through the penis to the external urethral orifice at the meatus. The membranous and anterior urethras also serve as a passageway for secretions from the male reproductive system (see Fig. 35.1, *A*). The urethra is lined with urothelium that is continuous with the lining of the bladder.

The female urethra is approximately 3 to 5 cm long and 6 to 8 mm in diameter. It is firmly embedded posterior to the clitoris and anterior to the vaginal opening. The Skene glands are situated bilaterally near the opening of the urethral meatus. Females are predisposed to urinary tract infections because the urethra is anatomically located near the vagina and the anus, both of which have resident flora that can cause infection if introduced into the urethra. Mechanical injury during coitus and the use of a pessary for vaginal support or diaphragm for contraception may be contributing factors to chronic urinary tract infection (see Fig. 35.1, *B*).

Special Features of Urologic Surgery

Urologic Endoscopy

Cystoscopic diagnostic procedures and some conservative urologic procedures approached through the urethra are performed in a specially designed and equipped area that is often referred to as the "cysto" room or suite. This area may be located within the operating room (OR) suite or in the urology clinic. X-ray control booths, developing units, and digital imaging are located adjacent to or within the area. Because x-ray procedures are often performed, the walls and doors of the room should be lined with lead and personnel remaining in the room with the patient during x-rays or fluoroscopy should wear lead aprons. Patients should be protected with gonadal and thyroid shields whenever feasible.

To protect the welfare of the patients and personnel, all safety regulations apply in the cysto room as they do elsewhere in the OR suite. All lighted instruments and electrical equipment should be checked for proper function before and after each use. Excess fluid should not be permitted to accumulate on the floor.

Proper OR attire is worn by all personnel entering the room. Personal protective equipment such as eyewear and masks should be worn if there is a possibility of splash or aerosolization. Many urologists don a water-repellant apron before scrubbing. It is recommended that the urologist wear a sterile gown and sterile gloves. Procedures performed in the cysto room should be performed as in a sterile field to prevent introducing microorganisms into the patient. Adherence to the principles of aseptic technique should be practiced to prevent urinary tract infection.

Urologic Bed

A urologic bed differs from the standard OR bed in that it provides an x-ray–compatible base, a drainage system, and lithotomy knee supports with safety belts (Fig. 35.4). Some urologic beds incorporate electrosurgical units (ESUs). Urologic radiographic studies use conventional x-rays, fluoroscopy and image intensification, and tomography. The imaging system is an integral part of the urologic bed. Some beds have a built-in automatic x-ray

• **Fig. 35.4** Urologic bed.

• **Fig. 35.5** Knee crutch stirrup commonly used with urologic table.

film–handling system, others have a film cassette holder, and others adapt to a C-arm.

The drainage system may have a drainage pan with tubing to drain port or single-use drainage bags. Under-knee/calf supports with gel pads and Velcro straps provide patient comfort in the lithotomy position (Fig. 35.5). Urologic beds are equipped with hydraulic or electric controls to adjust height and tilt. Some have tray attachments for the light source and auxiliary equipment such as an ESU or laser, as well as hooks for irrigating solution bags.

Patient Preparation for a Cystoscopic Examination

1. Unless the procedure will be performed with the patient under general or regional anesthesia, the patient may be encouraged to drink fluids before coming to the cysto room. Fluids ensure rapid collection of a urine specimen from the kidneys. Some tests require the ability to void for bladder strength studies or while contrast medium passes through the urinary system. Electromyographic (EMG) data may be gathered during the process.
2. Intraurethral procedures are often performed with topical agents or local infiltration anesthetics. The patient should be reassured that the procedure usually can be performed with only mild discomfort. Respect the patient's modesty by providing appropriate drapes and keeping the cysto room door closed.

3. The patient is assisted into the lithotomy position with the knees resting in padded knee supports or stirrups. Gel pads behind the legs and knees help avoid undue pressure in popliteal spaces. Velcro straps are used to secure the patient's legs. Some cystoscopic procedures are performed with the male patient in the supine position.

4. The drainage area is located under the lower break of the urologic bed. The drainage area is visible for draping after the patient's legs have been positioned on knee supports and the foot of the bed has been lowered or removed.

5. The pubic region, external genitalia, and perineum are mechanically and chemically cleansed with an antiseptic agent according to routine skin preparation procedure. Scrub soaps can be diluted with warmed sterile saline or water for the comfort of the patient.

6. Topical anesthetic agents are instilled into the urethra at the end of the prep procedure. A viscous liquid or jelly preparation of lidocaine hydrochloride, 1% or 2%, may be used. This medium remains in the urethra rather than flowing into the bladder.

   a. *For the female:* The female urethra is most sensitive at the meatus. A small, sterile cotton-tipped applicator dipped into the anesthetic gel and placed in the meatus is sufficient anesthesia for local urethral procedures. The applicator is removed when the urologist is ready to introduce an instrument. Cone-shaped syringes are commercially available for intraurethral instillation of local lidocaine 2% jelly.

   b. *For the male:* A disposable cylinder with an acorn tip can be used for intraurethral insertion. The agent is injected into the urethra, and the penis is compressed with a noncrushing spring-loaded penile clamp for a few minutes to retain the drug.

7. A sterile filter screen is placed over the drainage pan. The patient is draped as for other perineal procedures in the lithotomy position. The urologist may need to have access to the rectum. The perineal sheet has two fenestrations: one exposes the genitalia, and the other fits over the screen on the drainage pan. A mesh filter is incorporated into this latter fenestration to capture resected tissue. Tissue specimens are collected as irrigating fluid passes through a collecting basket. The sterile mesh filter collects any specimen that is missed by the collection basket.

8. The urologist may prefer to wear a sterile disposable plastic apron over their gown.

Urologic Endoscopes

Urologic endoscopic instruments and catheters are available in sizes to suit infants, children, and adults. The sizes of these instruments and catheters are measured on the French (Fr) scale: the diameter in millimeters (mm) multiplied by 3. The smallest ureteral catheter is 1 mm in diameter, or 3 Fr; the largest is 14 Fr.

Each type of procedure requires specific endoscopic equipment. All rigid urologic endoscopes have the same basic components, which are discussed in the following sections (Fig. 35.6).

Sheath

The hollow sheath, through which the urologic endoscope passes, may be concave, convex, or straight in configuration at the distal end (the end inserted into the urethra) (Fig. 35.7). The other end has a stopcock attachment for irrigation. Sheath sizes range from

A

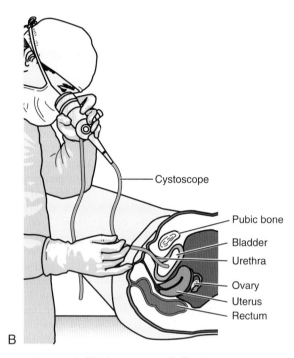

B

• **Fig. 35.6 A,** Rigid cystoscopy. **B,** Flexible cystoscopy.

• **Fig. 35.7** Cystoscope, bridge, and sheath.

11 Fr for infants to 30 Fr for adults. Space is provided within the sheath to accommodate instruments for work in the bladder or urethra. Other instruments and catheters can be inserted through the sheath into the ureters and/or kidneys for diagnostic or therapeutic procedures.

Obturator

The stainless steel obturator, which is inserted into the sheath, occludes the opening of the sheath and facilitates introduction into the urethra without trauma to the mucosal lining.

Telescope

Telescopes are complex precision optical systems; they are costly, delicate instruments that are handled gently at all times. Each telescope contains multiple finely polished optical lenses that relay the image from the distal end inside the bladder or urethra to the ocular (eyepiece) used by the urologist to view internal structures. Additional rod-shaped elements (i.e., field lenses) are located between each pair of relay lenses. Properly spaced throughout the length of the telescope, the lenses provide undistorted and clear vision at the desired angle and with some magnification. All telescopes are stainless steel and have a Bakelite or heat-resistant plastic ocular. Some telescopes have operating or working elements incorporated into them.

The optical systems provide several angles of vision (Fig. 35.8):

- Direct forward or 0° vision is useful for viewing the urethra and for use with the optical urethrotome (an instrument for sharp resection of tissue in the urethra).
- Right-angle or 30° vision is most suitable for viewing the entire bladder and insertion of ureteral catheters.
- Lateral, which deviates 70° but includes an additional visual field at a right angle in the line of vision, is used for wide-angle viewing within the bladder.
- Foroblique, which is a forward vision with an oblique view somewhat in front of a right angle, is used to examine the urethra and for transurethral surgical procedures.
- Retrospective, which provides an approximate 55° angle of retrograde vision, is used to inspect the bladder neck.

Light Source

The light source is a fiber-optic bundle and may be an integral part of the sheath or the telescope. A cable connects the instrument to a fiber-optic light source.

Types of Urologic Endoscopes

Many different types of urologic endoscopes and accessories are used, including nephroscopes introduced into the kidney and

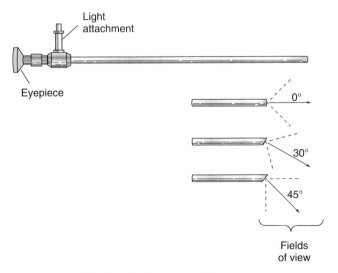

• **Fig. 35.8** Viewing angles of telescopes.

cystoscopes introduced through the urethra into the bladder. Before instrumentation is placed on the sterile instrument table, the preferred type and size of the endoscope for the examination and/or treatment should be verified with the urologist. The endoscopes and accessories most commonly used in the cysto room are described in the following sections.

Brown-Buerger Cystoscope

The stainless steel sheaths of the Brown-Buerger cystoscope range in size from 14 to 26 Fr. Size 21 Fr is the size most often used in adults; it has a right-angle examination telescope for routine inspection of the bladder. Size 24 or 26 Fr is used to accommodate larger instruments and catheters that cannot be used through size 21 Fr. The sheath contains the light carrier.

A Brown-Buerger cystoscope set usually consists of two sheaths—one concave and one convex, each with its own obturator—and two or three right-angle telescopes. Along with the basic examination telescope, the set may have a combination operating and double catheterizing telescope (i.e., a convertible telescope), or the operating and double catheterizing functions may be in separate telescopes. The convertible operating and catheterizing telescopes have a small, deflectable lever on the distal end to aid in directing ureteral catheters or flexible stone baskets into the ureters. All corresponding parts of each set must be the same French size.

Blue Light Video Cystoscope

The blue light cystoscope uses photodynamic diagnostic (PDD) technology. Cystoscopes are available in both rigid and flexible styles. The blue light system is used specifically for the diagnosis of bladder cancer after instillation of a photoactive substance. Hexaminolevulinate (HAL) is instilled into the bladder 1 hour before the procedure. Tumor cells absorb the drug because they have less ferrochelatase enzyme. The blue light (375–440 nm) from the cystoscope is absorbed by the drug and gives the tumor cells a pink or red color. The surgeon can distinguish the normal cells from tumor cells, which could have been missed with white light cystoscopy.[1]

McCarthy Panendoscope

The stainless steel sheaths of the McCarthy panendoscope range in size from 14 to 30 Fr. These are used most often with the Foroblique telescope for viewing the urethra. Other telescopes are available for bladder visualization. The telescopes are interchangeable with all sizes of sheaths. A bridge assembly is required to fit the telescope properly to the sheath. The light is supplied through the telescope.

Wappler Cystourethroscope

The Wappler cystourethroscope combines the functions of the Brown-Buerger cystoscope and the McCarthy panendoscope. The stainless steel sheaths range in size from 17 to 24 Fr. The Foroblique and lateral telescopes, which also supply the light, are interchangeable with all sheaths. A visual obturator may be used to permit visualization and irrigation during the introduction of the sheath into the urethra.

Resectoscope

The resectoscope uses electric current to excise tissue from the bladder, urethra, or prostate (Fig. 35.9). Components of this instrument include the sheath, obturator, telescope, working element, and cutting electrode. The sheath, usually 24 to 28 Fr, is

• **Fig. 35.9** Resectoscope.

made of Bakelite or fiberglass to prevent a short circuit of the electric current. If the short beak post sheath is used with a wide-angle telescope, a Timberlake obturator is used to introduce the sheath into the urethra.

The working element of the resectoscope, which is inserted through the sheath, has a channel for the telescope and cutting electrode. The types of working elements differ by the method in which the cutting electrode moves:

- The Iglesias resectoscope uses a thumb control on a leaf spring—lock mechanism. The working element can be adapted for simultaneous irrigation and suction to control hydraulic pressure in the bladder.
- The Nesbit resectoscope uses a thumb control on a spring.
- The Baumrucker resectoscope uses finger control on a sliding mechanism.
- The Stern-McCarthy resectoscope uses a rack and pinion to move the loop forward and back. This requires two hands.

The cutting electrode is the most critical component of a resectoscope. Because it cuts and coagulates tissue, the electrode must be stabilized in the working element so it retracts properly into the sheath after each cut. The electrode has a cutting loop from which electric current is passed through tissue, an insulated fork, an insulated stem, and a contact that is inserted into the working element. Several loop sizes are available; the stem is usually color-coded by size. Loop size corresponds to the French size of the sheath. The electrode is malleable and therefore is checked before use to be certain the insulation is intact and the loop is not broken. Disposable styles are preferred.

Electric current is applied only when the loop is engaged in tissue, and it is inactivated after a cut is completed. The sheath can be charred if electric current is maintained after the cutting loop has been retracted into it. Conductive lubricants may provide a pathway for electric current and therefore should never be used on the sheath. Cleanliness of the sheath and all other components is essential to proper function.

Endoscopic Accessories

Ureteral catheters, bougies, filiforms and followers, stone baskets, and sounds are commonly used by urologist-endoscopists. Other accessories, such as retractable baskets and graspers, are used to remove tissue or calculi (stones).

Electrodes

In addition to the cutting loops used with the resectoscope, primarily for transurethral resection (TUR), other types of electrodes with tips of various shapes are used in the bladder. One type, referred to as a *Bugbee,* is inserted through the operating telescope

• **Fig. 35.10** Y-tubing for cystoscopy.

of the Brown-Buerger cystoscope or Wappler cystourethroscope. The Bugbee is used mainly for fulguration of bladder tumors, coagulation of bladder vessels to control bleeding after biopsy, and ureteral meatotomy. More electric current is needed when working in solution (as in the bladder) than when working in air.

A spark-gap generator is commonly used for transurethral resection and fulguration. A spark-gap ESU requires high-voltage arcing, which is described as spray coagulation. Spark-gap generator use requires the patient to be grounded with a return electrode. The power control settings on the ESU should be as low as possible. Recommended practices as suggested by AORN (Association of periOperative Registered Nurses) for the use and care of electrosurgical equipment (e.g., return electrodes) apply also to urologic procedures. Additional information about ESUs can be found in Chapter 20.

Lasers

Argon, neodymium:yttrium aluminum garnet (Nd:YAG), and holmium:yttrium aluminum garnet (Ho:YAG) lasers can be adapted for use with urologic endoscopes. These are particularly useful for the ablation of hemangiomas and vascular tumors in the bladder and kidneys. The argon-pumped tunable dye laser is used for photodynamic therapy on solid bladder tumors. A flash lamp—pulsed dye laser will fragment a calculus in a ureter.

Lasers used through endoscopes require most of the same equipment as needed for standard urologic endoscopy. The bladder expansion medium can be either saline or water to create the working space because, unlike with the ESU and electrodes, no ionic charge is emitted from the laser.

Irrigating Equipment

Continuous irrigation of the bladder is necessary during cystoscopy (cysto) to do the following:

- Distend bladder walls to create a working space so the urologist can visualize them.
- Wash out blood, bits of resected tissue, or stone fragments to permit continuous visibility and collection of specimens.

A sterile, disposable, and closed irrigating system is used because it prevents airborne contamination of the solution. The tubing is Y shaped (Fig. 35.10). Two or more liters of sterile irrigating solution may be needed for a single examination.

Disposable tandem sets may be used to connect several containers together. Tandem sets allow for a continuous flow and replacement of containers without interruption of flow.

Sterile disposable irrigating tubing is connected to the irrigating solution container before it is hung on a hook on the urologic bed, in the ceiling, or on a stand placed beside the bed. The solution container should be at a level 2.5 feet (0.75 m) above the bed; a lower level decreases flow, and a higher level increases hydraulic pressure with consequent fluid absorption by the tissues of the patient. Tubing should be filled with solution before being attached to the sheath of the cystoscope or resectoscope. The plastic tubing from the container to the instrument is for individual patient use only and is discarded after use.

Sterile isosmotic irrigating solutions that are nonhemolytic and nonelectrolytic are generally preferred by most urologists. Sterile distilled water may be used for visualization procedures and during resection or fulguration of bladder tumors with an ESU. Water may hemolyze red blood cells if a sufficient amount enters the circulation through open blood vessels. As much as 3 to 6 L of solution may be absorbed during a transurethral prostatectomy.

Saline is contraindicated for use with a monopolar ESU because the electrons in saline act as a conductor and disperse the current when the ESU is used. Newer bipolar resectoscopes use saline irrigation without problems.

Isosmotic solutions of 1.5% glycine (an amino acid) or sorbitol (an inert sugar) premixed in distilled water are commercially available in 1.5 and 3-L containers.

Glycine solution is sometimes used for TUR with an ESU; however, it can cause serious complications in some patients. Overabsorption of glycine can occur during TUR, causing water intoxication with resultant hyponatremia and acid-base imbalance (acidosis). This process has been called transurethral resection syndrome and is hallmarked by dilutional hyponatremia.

During a cysto procedure, the flow of solution into the endoscope is controlled by the stopcock on the sheath where the tubing attaches. Rubber tips or sealing caps are used to seal other openings on the instrument to prevent solution from escaping during a procedure. The openings through which catheters or instruments are to be inserted are closed with rubber sealing caps that have a central hole. The accessory can be inserted through this hole with the seal maintained. Silicone caps should be used instead of rubber caps if the patient or surgeon has a latex sensitivity.

The irrigating solution flows away from the instrument and into the drainage pan through the filter screen when the urologist needs to divert the flow. Solution drains from the pan, through the tubing, and into a collecting container that is emptied after each patient use. Fluid collection receptacles can provide the surgeon with accurate patient fluid output. Some older cysto rooms have floor drains, which are a source of environmental contamination unless cleaned thoroughly. If large quantities of solution are used, the level of drainage into the container should be observed to prevent overflow onto the floor or around the foot pedal of the ESU, which can be an electrocution hazard.

Evacuators

Evacuators may be attached to the endoscope to irrigate the bladder and aspirate stone fragments, blood clots, or resected tissue. Stone or tissue fragments collected in the evacuator are retrieved and sent to the pathology laboratory. The two most commonly used types are the Ellik evacuator and the Toomey evacuator, as follows:

• **Fig. 35.11** Ellik evacuator for flushing prostate tissue from the bladder during transurethral resection of the prostate (TURP).

• **Fig. 35.12** Toomey irrigator.

- *Ellik evacuator:* The Ellik evacuator is a double bowl-shaped glass or firm disposable plastic receptacle (Fig. 35.11). It contains a trap for fragments so they cannot be washed back into the sheath of the endoscope during irrigation with pressure on the compression-bulb attachment.
- *Toomey evacuator:* The Toomey evacuator is a syringe-type evacuator with a wide opening into the barrel (Fig. 35.12). It may be used with any endoscope sheath. A metal adapter permits its use with a catheter.

Care and Preventive Maintenance of Urologic Endoscopes

1. Sterilization is recommended before use. The bladder is considered a sterile space. Endoscopes and reusable accessories must be free of debris and residue for sterilization and/or high-level disinfection techniques to be effective.
   a. Disassemble all parts and open all outlets.
   b. Clean all parts in an appropriate liquid detergent solution. Clean the interior of sheaths and openings with a soft brush.
   c. Rinse in clean water, and dry thoroughly.
   d. Wipe lenses gently with a soft, dry cloth.
2. After cleaning, place endoscopes on a towel to drain. With air, blow-dry the lumens. Moisture in the channels can dilute chemical sterilants and, if ethylene oxide is used, will form ethylene glycol, which is toxic to tissues.
3. Check the function of all moving parts, the clarity of vision through telescopes, and the patency of channels through instruments and catheters.
4. Keep sets of sterile sounds, bougies, and filiforms and followers together so the urologist has a complete range of sizes readily accessible.
5. Wrap items for sterilization after cleaning. Flexible instruments should be protected by a rigid container.
6. Clean and dry stone baskets before sterilizing by low-temperature sterilization methods, such as plasma vapor,

peracetic acid, or ethylene oxide. Retractable stone baskets are sterilized in the open position.

7. The principles and methods of sterilization apply to urologic endoscopy equipment.

8. Endoscopic processors and sterilizers are useful for sterilizing instrumentation between patient uses. The instrumentation is used immediately after processing and is not stored in the processing tray.

9. Because the interior of the bladder is considered sterile, the recommended practice is to use only sterile instrumentation.

Surgical Procedures of the Genitourinary System

Most patients commonly seen by urologists are in the preadolescent or older age-groups. Congenital and common pediatric problems are discussed in Chapter 8. This chapter focuses on adult problems, most of which occur in men older than 50 years who have prostatic disease and women who have urinary incontinence. Female bladder problems are addressed in Chapter 34.

An open surgical procedure is performed only after conservative treatment fails or examination of the genitourinary (GU) tract confirms a condition that does not yield to treatment. Fortunately, most urologic conditions can be diagnosed and treated conservatively through a urologic endoscope and its accessories. Some laparoscopic and robotic procedures are performed to remove a kidney (nephrectomy) or obtain lymph nodes for biopsy. When a congenital or acquired condition does not respond to conservative therapy, the urologist performs open surgical procedures to repair, revise, reconstruct, or remove organs.

Obstructive and neuromuscular disorders are common problems in the urinary tract. Renal calculus disease and tumors in the urinary tract are most commonly diagnosed in middle age. These conditions may cause obstruction and subsequent infection in the kidneys, ureter, or bladder.

Kidney

Definitive renal surgical procedures are justified for the management of renal neoplasms, large cystic lesions that compromise renal function and/or produce obstruction, inflammatory diseases that necessitate drainage, or renal vascular disease. Chronic degenerative disease or severe traumatic injury can produce irreparable damage to renal cells. Computed tomography (CT) and magnetic resonance imaging (MRI) identify the site, size, and extent of tumor involvement.

Ultrasonography and intravenous (IV) urograms and pyelograms differentiate among solid tumors, stones, and cystic disease. A radionuclide scan may indicate renal function; arteriograms and venograms indicate the extent of renal vascular disease.

The kidney is usually approached posteriorly with the patient in a lateral position (Fig. 35.13). The kidney rest may be raised,

• **Fig. 35.13** Surgical position for open kidney procedure.

and the bed flexed until the flank muscles become tense. After the patient is secured in position, the bed is tilted in Trendelenburg position until the flank is horizontal to the floor. A flank incision is made parallel to and just below or over the 11th or 12th rib; the 12th rib may be removed. The retroperitoneum is opened to expose the kidney. The peritoneal cavity is not entered.

The kidney can be approached anteriorly through a transverse, subcostal, or midline incision. A thoracoabdominal incision may be preferred in an obese patient or to reach a lesion in the upper pole of the kidney. These incisions, with the patient in the supine position, are often used for exposure of the aorta and vena cava for renovascular procedures. An anterior approach may be advantageous when prompt control of blood supply is important in renal trauma.

Nephrectomy

Removal of a lobe or the entire kidney is indicated when tumor, disease, or traumatic injury has resulted in the absence of renal function. The entire kidney can be removed during a laparoscopic procedure. Hand-assisted laparoscopy (HALS) can use used.[2] The organ is dissected, fragmented, and aspirated; vascular pedicles are stapled. This alternative technique is used primarily for benign renal disease.

Partial Nephrectomy or Heminephrectomy

Partial excision of the kidney may be sufficient when a lobe has been destroyed by localized disease or injury but the remainder of the kidney remains functional. The vascular supply to the segment to be removed must be identified, ligated, and divided. The parenchyma of the lobe is resected from the capsule by blunt dissection. The renal pelvis and remaining capsule are closed.

Radical Nephrectomy

In a radical nephrectomy, the renal vessels are dissected free, ligated, and divided. Prerenal fat and fascia are dissected to remove the kidney. The ureter is ligated and divided close to the bladder. The renal pedicle is ligated and divided, and the kidney is removed. Massive hemorrhage from the renal artery and veins is a potential complication, as is injury to adjacent structures (i.e., inferior vena cava, aorta, and duodenum on the right side or spleen on the left side).

A nephrectomy is performed in the OR on a living donor (unilateral) or a cadaver donor (bilateral) to procure the kidney(s) for transplantation. Meticulous dissection is necessary to free the kidney, its blood vessels, and the ureter with minimal trauma. The ureter is dissected free and transected while the renal blood supply remains intact to ensure adequate urinary output. A kidney from a living donor may last longer than a kidney from a cadaver because the organ ischemic time is less and transplantation takes place sooner. A living donor kidney can be obtained by HALS.

The left kidney is most commonly used for living donor transplant because it is easier to access. The anatomy is more complex on the right side because of the renal vein structure and requires a longer surgical time, causing a longer scar. Dr. Rizk El-Galley developed a special angled clamp that permits HALS right nephrectomy by excising a cuff of vena cava with the renal vein for added length of the vessel.

Bilateral Nephrectomy

Removal of both kidneys may be indicated before transplantation in a patient maintained on chronic dialysis who has severe

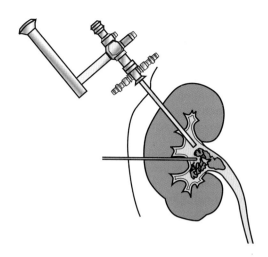

• **Fig. 35.14** Percutaneous nephrostomy.

hypertension. If rejection is uncontrollable after kidney transplantation, the donor kidney may have to be explanted and the patient returned to chronic hemodialysis. This is less likely after transplantation from a live donor than from a cadaver.

Nephrostomy or Pyelostomy

An incision through the renal parenchyma or into the renal pelvis may be necessary to establish temporary or permanent drainage when an obstruction prevents the flow of urine from the kidney (Fig. 35.14). A percutaneous tube is placed in the kidney through the skin. A cutaneous nephrostomy tube may be used to drain a kidney postoperatively during healing after renal reconstruction or revascularization. Silastic tubes placed internally through a cystoscope via the ureter eliminate the need for an open surgical procedure for a temporary urinary diversion.

More commonly, temporary urinary diversion is performed percutaneously under fluoroscopic or ultrasound guidance by a radiologist and/or urologist. A plastic disc is applied to the skin to secure the catheter, which is attached to a drainage bag in a manner to prevent tension. The tubing may be connected to a leg bag to avoid tension on the catheter during ambulation.

Pyeloplasty

Revision or reconstruction of the renal pelvis is performed to relieve an anatomic obstruction in the flow of urine by creating a larger outlet from the renal pelvis into the ureter. This may be performed to repair or excise damaged tissue so kidney function will be restored without a partial or total nephrectomy.

Either a rigid or a flexible fiber-optic nephroscope may be used to visually inspect the renal collecting system. A laser fiber may be used to ablate some tumors.

Renal Revascularization

Stenotic lesions of renal arteries are surgically correctable causes of hypertension. Renovascular reconstructive procedures (renal angioplasty) are designed to either improve blood flow through the stenotic area to the kidney or bypass the stenotic area.

Revascularization procedures may have a dual purpose: to correct hypertension and preserve renal function. The patient is placed in the supine position for these procedures because the renal arteries are approached through an abdominal incision.

In Situ Vascular Reconstructive Techniques

Obstruction of the renal artery most often occurs as a result of atherosclerotic stenosis at the origin of the artery or fibromuscular dysplasia (abnormal development) confined to the main renal artery. The obstruction is most often resected and replaced by an aortorenal saphenous vein bypass graft. A reversed segment of proximal saphenous vein, gently distended and irrigated, is anastomosed first to the aorta and then to the renal artery.

Prosthetic woven Dacron grafts may be used instead of an autologous vein graft for renal artery bypass combined with distal aortic replacement. Segmental resection of diseased arterial segments with primary end-to-end anastomosis may be performed. Thromboendarterectomy is more often performed than is the latter procedure. All of these procedures may be performed bilaterally or as staged bilateral renal artery reconstructions. Percutaneous transluminal angioplasty may be preferred to these open procedures.

Ex Vivo Extracorporeal Kidney Surgery

When stenotic disease or another obstructive lesion extends into the branches of the renal artery, in situ reconstruction may be difficult, hazardous, or impossible. In these patients, a temporary nephrectomy with microvascular repair followed by autotransplantation of the kidney may be performed; this is referred to as *workbench surgery*. The kidney is completely mobilized from the retroperitoneal space. If one kidney is to be reconstructed, the ureter can remain intact and reconstruction is performed on a sterile bench (Mayo tray) placed over the patient's lower abdomen.

For a bilateral reconstruction, one kidney is detached from its ureter to permit complete removal from the abdomen. A second team works on the contralateral kidney in situ while the other kidney is reconstructed at an adjacent dissecting bench (table) ex vivo.

Extracorporeal perfusion is necessary for renal preservation during reconstruction. This may be accomplished either with perfusion of cold lactated Ringer's solution or other hyperosmolar solution by gravity flow or with a continuous hypothermic perfusion through a Belzer pump machine. A simple cold storage in saline slush also may be used for renal preservation. Dry ice is never used.

A kidney may be autotransplanted into the patient's pelvis for revascularization of the kidney, removal of renal tumors or calculi, or repair of ureteral injuries.

Traumatic Injury

Serious hemorrhage may result if a kidney is ruptured or injured by blunt trauma or a bullet or stab wound. This requires an immediate surgical procedure. The surgeon makes every effort to save kidney tissue and the ureter. A Foley catheter is inserted to keep an accurate record of urinary output and check for the presence of hematuria preoperatively and postoperatively. Gross hematuria preoperatively usually indicates injury to the bladder or urethra. Kidney damage is diagnosed by the presence of blood seen microscopically.

Dialysis

End-stage renal disease and acute renal failure are potentially fatal conditions unless they can be controlled or reversed. Uremia and hypertension develop if renal failure is prolonged. Renal dialysis is the procedure of removing waste products and excess intravascular fluid from the body of a patient in acute or chronic renal failure by diffusion through a semipermeable membrane. This may be accomplished by either hemodialysis or peritoneal dialysis. The treatment modality alleviates the acute manifestations of uremia and controls many of the chronic long-term complications of end-stage renal disease.

Grossly undernourished and anemic patients with severe electrolyte imbalances must be adequately stabilized by dialysis before kidney transplantation. Some patients require dialysis for the remainder of their lives. Patients undergoing chronic dialysis must have a means of arterial-venous access established for long-term maintenance.

Patients with chronic renal failure can tolerate extensive surgical procedures with minimal complications. Their management in the OR must include strict attention to maintaining a patent hemodialysis access shunt, fistula, or catheter; careful monitoring of fluid and electrolyte balance; and avoiding postoperative infections. After kidney transplantation, the patient may require postoperative dialysis; thus access must remain patent during and after the surgical procedure.

Hemodialysis

In hemodialysis, waste products are removed from the blood through the semipermeable membrane of a dialyzer (artificial kidney machine). An arteriovenous (AV) shunt or fistula is created subcutaneously in either an arm or a leg to provide access to the patient's circulation (Fig. 35.15).

The Quinton-Scribner double-lumen shunt, developed in 1960, consists of two tips attached to tubing. One tip is placed in the artery and the other in a nearby vein. The tubing from each tip is exteriorized through a subcutaneous tunnel to form a loop. The arterial and venous blood mix in this shunt. Variations and modifications of this basic external shunt are used to create an AV conduit; some have self-sealing devices to minimize the potential problems of clotting and infection.

An anastomosis, usually between the radial artery and the cephalic vein in the forearm, creates an arterialized peripheral vein that permits dialyzer connections to be made by venipuncture. Needles are placed in the venous limb of the AV fistula for blood outflow and return (Fig. 35.16). The Brescia-Cimino radiocephalic AV fistula, first described in 1966, is easiest to construct and has the fewest complications. If creation of an AV fistula by direct anastomosis is not feasible, a biologic or synthetic graft may be interposed between the artery and the vein.

Cryopreserved human vein, saphenous or other autologous vein, bovine carotid artery heterograft, and polytetrafluoroethylene (PTFE) grafts are used.

Peritoneal Dialysis

For acute, intermittent, or continuous peritoneal dialysis, a Tenckhoff silicone catheter is placed into the peritoneal cavity (Fig. 35.17). A paramedian incision generally is used to place a section of the catheter in subcutaneous tissue. The catheter has one or two synthetic fiber cuffs to anchor it in subcutaneous tissue and block bacterial invasion along the catheter into the peritoneal cavity.

Dialysate is instilled over time into the peritoneal cavity to draw solutes from body fluids into the dialyzing solution across the peritoneal membrane. This process selectively removes electrolytes, metabolites, toxins, and water normally excreted by the kidneys.

Dialysate that has been warmed to body temperature is instilled, allowed to remain for a specified number of hours, and then withdrawn by a cycling machine or by gravity drainage. A Y-set disconnect system attached to the catheter allows separation of inflow and outflow. Peritonitis is always a potential complication.

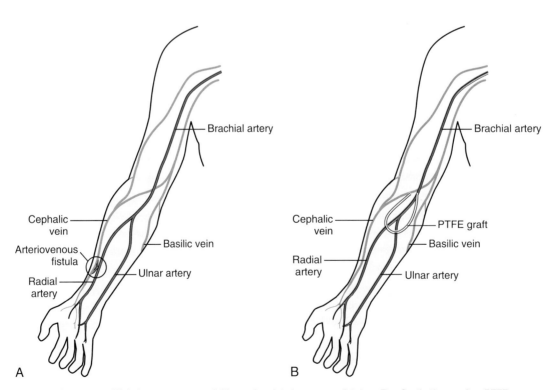

• **Fig. 35.15** Dialysis access modalities. **A,** Arteriovenous fistula. **B,** Synthetic graft. *PTFE,* Polytetrafluoroethylene.

• **Fig. 35.16** Arteriovenous fistula and dialysis machine.

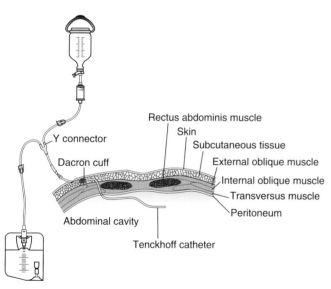

• **Fig. 35.17** Tenckhoff catheter for peritoneal dialysis.

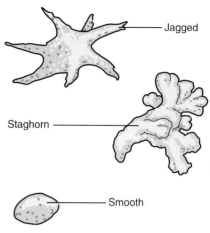

• **Fig. 35.18** Kidney stones.

and the appearance and volume are recorded on the intraoperative record.

Urolithiasis (Urinary Calculus)

A renal calculus (kidney stone) is a solid deposit or deposits of minerals and salts (Fig. 35.18). These deposits are called calculi and accumulate in the renal collecting system. Kidney stones are more common in white males living in warm climates and nearly 30% to 50% experience recurrence 5 to 10 years after initial treatment. Diagnosis in adults is best made with CT scan. Ultrasound is best used to diagnose kidney stones in children. Calculi can be the result of cystinuria (amino acid metabolic disorder), hypercalcemia (immobility or hyperparathyroidism), oxalate (oxalic and glycolic acid in urine), and uric acid (dietary purines).

Renal colic is an intense pain caused when a calculus or fragments of calculi partially or completely obstructs the calyces or renal pelvis. Renal calculi often dislodge and move from the renal pelvis into the ureter. A nidus (e.g., an infection or an exposed suture postoperatively) can be the focal point for the formation of a calculus in the ureter. If calculi are small enough, they pass into the bladder and are voided. Those that remain lodged, causing obstruction to outflow from any part of the urinary tract, must be removed.

Preservation of renal function is the primary objective of surgical procedures for urolithiasis. Lithotomy is removal of a calculus. Lithotripsy is fragmentation of a stone followed by removal. Chemolysis is dissolution with a chemical substance.

After removal from any location in the GU tract, urinary calculi should be placed in a dry container and sent to the pathology laboratory for chemical analysis.

Percutaneous Nephrostolithotomy or Nephrolithotripsy

With percutaneous nephrostolithotomy or nephrolithotripsy, a guidewire inside a transluminal angioplasty needle is introduced, under fluoroscopy, through the flank into the renal pelvis. The access point is carefully closed. This procedure may be performed in the radiology department with the patient under local anesthesia. In the OR, dilators are placed over the guidewire to enlarge a nephrostomy tract for introduction of a nephrostomy tube or nephroscope. The patient is placed in a modified prone position to elevate the surgical side slightly.

Renal calculi may be removed with stone forceps or baskets, or they may be fragmented with a lithotriptor. Lithotripsy is

Infection is often treated by adding antibiotics to the dialysate. Heparin is added to prevent fibrin clots in the catheter. The patient may perform this routine at home several times per week, usually during the evening hours.

A patient being treated with peritoneal dialysis may come to the OR for an unrelated surgical procedure. Respiratory excursion may be impaired by pressure of retained dialysate under the diaphragm. A slight reverse Trendelenburg position may alleviate respiratory discomfort. Additional suction containers should be available if the abdomen must be evacuated while the patient is in the OR. Fluid removed from the peritoneal cavity is measured, necessary for large calculi such as a staghorn calculus, which branches from the renal pelvis into the calyces and may extend into the ureter. Size, density, composition, and location influence the urologist's choice of lithotripsy.

Ultrasonic Lithotripsy. With ultrasonic lithotripsy, ultrasonic waves are used to shatter the calculus into fragments. This procedure is usually performed with the patient under spinal or general anesthesia. Either a rigid or a flexible fiber-optic nephroscope is inserted percutaneously; a hollow, metal ultrasonic probe, which emits high-frequency sound waves, is inserted through the nephroscope. The probe is visually placed in contact with a calculus that is localized in the renal pelvis as identified on x-ray or by fluoroscopy.

As the ultrasonic energy is absorbed, the calculus fragments and shattered particles are aspirated by suction through the probe. A nephrostomy tube may be placed in the renal pelvis for temporary drainage postoperatively; this tube is usually removed after 2 weeks.

Electrohydraulic Lithotripsy. With electrohydraulic lithotripsy, an electrohydraulic lithotriptor is used to create an electrical discharge in fluid; this discharge is transformed into a hydraulic shock wave. The calculus disintegrates when the probe is directed at it. Larger fragments may be removed with Randall stone forceps, and smaller ones are flushed out with irrigation. A tube is left in the nephrostomy tract for continued irrigation for several days after lithotripsy. This procedure may be performed with a local anesthetic with IV sedatives and analgesics.

Nephrolithotomy or Pyelolithotomy

A large staghorn renal calculus that does not dislodge from the calyces or renal pelvis may need to be removed through an open incision. A nephroscope may be used during the surgical procedure for direct visual examination of the nephrons to locate and remove residual calculi. Ultrasound also may be used to identify retained fragments. Localized hypothermia provides the surgeon with a bloodless surgical field and lengthens the time in which the renal artery may be clamped safely without a loss of renal function during the search for and extraction of calculi.

Extracorporeal Shock Wave Lithotripsy

Many patients are scheduled for x-ray immediately before a noninvasive extracorporeal shock wave lithotripsy (ESWL) procedure. A ureteral stent may be inserted to facilitate the passage of stone fragments. The ureteral stone may be manipulated back up into the renal pelvis. An x-ray may be obtained to check the location of the calculus.

The long-term effects of ESWL are under study, but to date the results are inconclusive. Potential long-term effects may be related to the underlying organs adjacent to the location of the stone as it is fragmented. Shock waves delivered directly over the kidney may injure the renal tissue, causing the development of hypertension or chronic renal disease. The proximal location of the pancreas in the retroperitoneum exposes the organ to shock waves. The question is raised as to the potential development of diabetes. Peripheral organ damage is an area for future research.

Water Bag Lithotripsy

With a water bag lithotripsy, the patient first receives a continuous epidural or general anesthetic and then is positioned against a large fluid-filled pad on the OR bed. The calculus is visualized by fluoroscopy and approximately 1500 ultrasonic waves are generated over a period of 60 minutes by rapid high-voltage sparks that are discharged from the bottom of the OR bed and transmitted through the water bag to enter the body. The shock wave energy is generated electromagnetically and focused with an acoustic lens. The impact of the sonic waves against the calculus causes fragmentation.

After each series of 150 to 200 waves, the focus on the calculus is rechecked by fluoroscopy. Each shock wave is synchronized with the patient's respirations and resting phase of the heartbeat; an electrocardiogram (ECG) monitors the patient's R waves to avoid disrupting the cardiac rhythm. A loud report sounds in the room each time a spark is fired, and therefore both the patient and personnel must wear protective earplugs.

Shock waves also may be produced by piezoelectric transducers activated by an electronic generator. These transducers are mounted on a bowl-shaped spherical dish; a soft, fluid membrane over this dish maintains contact with the patient's skin. Ultrasound images produced from an ultrasound localization system are used to position the stone at the focal point of the shock waves.

Ureters

The ureters are the vital anatomic structures for the flow of urine from the kidneys to the bladder. An obstruction to urinary flow must be either corrected or diverted. The ureters may be approached through either an endoscope or an open incision.

Ureteroscopy

Both rigid and flexible, short and long, fiber-optic ureteroscopes allow direct visualization of the ureteral tumors, calculi, and strictures. These scopes are introduced percutaneously or cystoscopically. Biopsies of tumors can be performed, and strictures can be corrected by balloon dilation. Ureteral calculi can be extracted with stone baskets or forceps or fragmented using ultrasound or lasers.

Percutaneous endoscopic techniques can be used in conjunction with x-ray. A complete x-ray implies that the procedure extends beyond the bladder into the ureters. Another term for a single radiograph of the abdomen is *KUB* (kidneys, ureters, and bladder). Some surgeons refer to a KUB as a "flat plate." This procedure may be performed for the following reasons:

- Drainage of the renal pelvis for differential diagnosis or renal function
- Insertion of ureteral catheters to provide constant drainage for one or both kidneys or outline the ureters for a difficult pelvic surgical procedure
- Insertion of a ureteral stent for internal drainage of an obstructed ureter
- Transluminal dilation of a ureteral stricture
- Manipulation and removal of a calculus
- Ureteral meatotomy to enlarge the opening of one or both ureteral orifices into the bladder

Ureteral Catheters

Made of flexible woven nylon or other plastic material, ureteral catheters range in caliber from size 3 to 14 Fr and are approximately 30 inches (76 cm) in length. Sterile, prepackaged disposable catheters are available. Most are radiopaque so they can be visualized on x-ray.

The urologist visualizes the ureteral orifice through the cystoscope. The catheter is inserted through the scope and introduced into the ureter.

• **Fig. 35.19** Ureteral catheter tips. **A,** Whistle. **B,** Olive. **C,** Round. **D,** Flexible filiform. **E,** Blasucci curved. **F,** Braasch bulb. **G,** Acorn/cone. **H,** Garceau tapered.

The catheter has graduated markings in centimeters so the urologist can judge the distance that the catheter has been inserted. The urologist will request a size and style of catheter tip best suited for the intended purpose. The most common tips are shown in Fig. 35.19.

- *Whistle tips:* Used for drainage, as ureteral markers, or for the injection of a radiopaque contrast medium for retrograde pyelography. The largest sizes are used to dilate ureters to facilitate passage of a calculus.
- *Olive tips:* May be used for the same purposes as whistle tips.
- *Round tips:* May be preferred for drainage.
- *Flexible filiform tips:* May be used to bypass an obstruction for drainage.
- *Blasucci curved tips:* May be used to bypass a ureteral stricture more easily than straight tips.
- *Braasch bulb with whistle tips:* Preferred to dilate the ureter or to inject contrast medium for a ureterogram.
- *Acorn or cone tips:* May be preferred for a ureterogram.
- *Garceau tapered tips:* Used to dilate ureters.

Ureteral catheters that are left indwelling to provide drainage must be attached to a sterile, closed urinary drainage system. Because ureteral catheters are smaller in diameter than standard urinary drainage catheters, an adapter is used. This adapter may be a small rubber tip or nipple placed on one end of a straight connector or on both ends of a Y-connector. The catheters are put through the hole in the tip(s).

The distal end of the connector is attached to a constant drainage system with sterile tubing. A separate drainage system for each catheter is usually desired by the urologist. Each drainage container is labeled to identify the right and left ureteral catheters.

Ureteral Stent

An indwelling ureteral stent is inserted for long-term drainage in a wide variety of benign and malignant diseases that cause ureteral obstruction.

• **Fig. 35.20** Ureteral stone removal.

A stent also may be indicated for temporary drainage or marking a ureter for abdominal surgery. Placement of ureteral stents requires a cysto setup separate from the main surgical field. The table should be left intact for the duration of the abdominal procedure in the event a second cysto is necessary.

Several types of stents are used. They can be made of durable and biocompatible silicone, polyurethane, or another copolymer. The stent may have a collar, a double-J configuration, a pigtail, or a coil to minimize migration up into the renal pelvis or down into the bladder. The stent is passed through the cystoscope and over a guidewire into the ureter, and it remains fixed for internal urinary drainage. As described for ureteral catheters, some types of stents are used to identify ureters and provide external drainage intraoperatively.

Percutaneous Ureterolithotomy

As described for percutaneous nephrolithotomy and lithotripsy, a calculus lodged in the renal pelvis or upper tract of the ureter can be extracted or fragmented through a ureteropyeloscope.

Transurethral Ureteroscopic Lithotripsy or Lithotomy

A urologic endoscope can be introduced transurethrally for direct visualization and lithotripsy or for extraction of a calculus that is obstructing a ureter (Fig. 35.20). Ultrasonic and electrohydraulic lithotripsy can be performed through a ureteroscope.[3]

Laser Lithotripsy

The use of laser technology has improved the minimally invasive treatment of calculi. A flash lamp–pulsed dye laser beam is directed through a flexible fiber-optic ureteroscope to a calculus in the lower tract. The fine tip of the laser fiber probe extends beyond the end of the scope and is placed in direct contact with the calculi to produce fragmentation without ureteral injury.

This pulsed laser has a green wavelength and is attracted to the yellow color of a calculus. The energy generated through the intermittent laser pulses fragments the yellow calculus by mechanical action without increasing its temperature to more than 50° F (10° C). This procedure may be performed with the patient under epidural or general anesthesia. Shattered calculi will pass with the patient's urine. An indwelling ureteral stent may be left in place for 48 hours and removed by the urologist in the office postoperatively.

Ureteral Stone Extraction

A flexible-shaft, basket-type stone-capture device (stone basket) is inserted into the ureter through a cystoscope in the bladder for extraction of a ureteral calculus. Several types of stone baskets are available, including the Dormia, Johnson, Levant, Pfister-Schwartz, and Lomac. These instruments have a fine wire or nylon basket that can be expanded through the shaft to ensnare a calculus located in the lower third of the ureter. Specialized stone baskets have a laser fiber port for calculus fragmentation. The basket is used to retrieve the central core after the exterior portion of the calculus is shattered.

Stone baskets must be cleaned promptly after use in a non-residue liquid-detergent solution to remove debris. Removable parts must be disassembled. Debris should be brushed away from the junction of the basket and shaft with a small, soft brush. Inspection of the basket wires is critical during cleaning. If the wires are cracked or broken at the end closest to the shaft, the basket may be passed into the ureter but cannot be withdrawn without trauma.

Ureterolithotomy

If a calculus fails to pass spontaneously through the ureter or cannot be removed with a stone basket, an open surgical procedure may be necessary. If the calculus is high in the ureter near the kidney, the patient is positioned for a lateral flank incision below the 12th rib. An abdominal incision is used to reach a calculus in the lower segment near the bladder. The exposed ureter will be dilated proximal to the calculus and collapsed distal to it. The surgeon makes a small incision directly over the calculus and extracts it from the ureter with a stone forceps.

Litholapaxy and Cystolithotomy

Calculi usually can be removed from the bladder through the urethra. Crushing a urinary calculus in the bladder is referred to as *litholapaxy* or *lithotrity*. If a litholapaxy is unsuccessful or contraindicated, the removal of a calculus by incision into the bladder may be necessary; this surgical procedure is a *cystolithotomy*. For a litholapaxy, a lithotrite (Fig. 35.21) is introduced into the bladder through the urethra and is used to pulverize and remove calculi. The instrument used may be a lithotrite with hinged jaws, an ultrasound lithotriptor, or an electrohydraulic lithotrite. The electrohydraulic lithotrite generates energy shock waves at the tip of a flexible probe inserted through a cystoscope by direct vision. The stone fragments are then irrigated from the bladder.

Ureteroneocystostomy

Implantation of the ureters into the bladder wall can be performed to relocate the ureters into a different site for correction of ureterovesical reflux, reestablish urinary flow after temporary

• **Fig. 35.21** Lithotrite for crushing bladder stones.

diversion or ureteral injury, or establish urinary flow from a kidney transplant after bilateral nephrectomy and ureterectomy.

Ureteroureterostomy

Anastomosis of two segments of one ureter is usually performed to reestablish ureteral continuity after traumatic injury. A ureteral catheter may be inserted as a stent and the ureter sutured over it. This procedure, a transureteroureterostomy anastomosis, may be indicated to bypass a ureteral stricture or to eliminate ureteral reflux that may be the result of trauma. Injury to a ureter can occur as a complication of pelvic or abdominal surgical procedures, as well as from external penetrating wounds.

Ideally, a transureteral anastomosis can be made 2 to 4 cm above the pelvic brim because the ureters are close at this point and the recipient ureter has a straight course into the bladder.

Vesico-psoas Hitch Procedure

The loss of a large segment of a middle or distal ureter can result from trauma or ureteral resection for tumor or stricture. A vesico-psoas hitch may be the procedure of choice when the length of the remaining ureter is insufficient for ureteroneocystostomy or ureteroureterostomy. The bladder is mobilized through an extraperitoneal approach into the retroperitoneal space. It is attached (i.e., hitched) to the psoas muscle to reposition the bladder cephalad. The segment of proximal ureter is brought through and sutured to the bladder wall. The kidney also may be mobilized and attached to the psoas muscle if too much tension will be placed on the ureterovesical anastomosis.

Urinary Bladder

The bladder may be opened through a suprapubic incision when a neoplasm, calculus, obstruction of the bladder neck, or traumatic injury is not amenable to treatment through the cystoscope. Diagnosis is usually established through urodynamics (the study of bladder function) and direct visualization via a cystoscope.

Cystometrogram

A cystometrogram measures voiding pressure within the bladder to determine muscle tone and check nerve supply. A calibrated recording tidal irrigator cystometer is used for this measurement. The patient should feel a desire to void when 350 mL of solution is put into the bladder. Carbon dioxide gas is used with some electronic transducers or radio pressure gauges. The normal maximum capacity of the bladder is 450 to 550 mL. Normal bladder pressure is 40 to 50 mL of water. If the problem is neurogenic, the cystometric findings are not higher than normal. If the problem is a hypertonic bladder, these measurements are higher than normal.

Cystoscopy

Cysto is a visual examination of the interior walls and contents of the bladder. This term is used broadly because various concurrent procedures may be carried out by using specially designed instruments through the cystoscope. Complete cysto and litholapaxy have been described. A plain cysto is a routine examination of the bladder. In conjunction with plain cysto, the following procedures also may be performed within the bladder:
- Biopsy of a tumor with a flexible-shaft biopsy forceps to obtain specimens
- Cystogram for diagnostic x-rays after injection of a contrast medium into the bladder

- Blue light cystoscopy with hexaminolevulinate (Cysview)[1]
- Fulguration of a tumor by use of an electrode to destroy tissue
- Resection of or incision into a bladder neck obstruction with a resectoscope
- Coagulation of a hemangioma with an argon laser, vaporization of a superficial tumor of the bladder wall with an Nd:YAG laser, or photodynamic therapy to a solid tumor with an argon-pumped tunable dye laser
- Removal of a foreign body with a flexible-shaft, foreign-body forceps
- Insertion of interstitial radionuclide seeds

Suprapubic Cystostomy

With a suprapubic cystostomy, urinary drainage from the bladder is established via a catheter inserted through a suprapubic incision or trocar puncture into the bladder (Fig. 35.22). If the bladder or urethra is injured by trauma associated with bony and soft tissue injuries of the pelvis, the bladder may be drained with a catheter placed above the pubic arch. This method of drainage is also preferred after some ureteral, bladder, prostatic, and urethral surgical procedures to decrease tension on sutures, ensure a patent route for urinary drainage, and minimize urinary retention.

A suprapubic catheter also can be used when the surgeon wants the patient to void some urine voluntarily via the urethra to maintain urethral function and tone, such as after bladder or vaginal repairs. Suprapubic catheters are connected to a sterile, closed, constant drainage system before the patient leaves the OR. The following are the most commonly used catheters for cystostomy drainage:
- Foley, 30-mL balloon, sizes 20, 22, or 24 Fr
- Foley, 5-mL balloon, 24 Fr, three-way irrigating catheter (third lumen can be used for continuous irrigation)
- Bonanno suprapubic catheter

Cutaneous Vesicostomy

In a cutaneous vesicostomy, urinary drainage is established directly from the bladder into a collecting device affixed on the abdomen rather than through a suprapubic catheter. The bladder is opened through a transverse suprapubic incision, and a flap is raised at the dome. A skin flap is raised in the midline of the

• **Fig. 35.22** Suprapubic cystostomy for urinary drainage.

abdomen below the umbilicus. The bladder flap is sutured to the defect created in the skin and then covered with the skin flap. A transparent adhering skin dressing and collection device form a seal around the resultant bladder stoma. A cutaneous vesicostomy may preserve renal function and/or improve upper urinary tract structure in patients with a neurogenic or atonic bladder, urinary incontinence, or bladder outlet obstruction.

Cystotomy and Cystoplasty

An incision into the urinary bladder through a suprapubic incision (cystotomy) may be performed to repair (cystoplasty) a bladder laceration or rupture as a result of trauma or a defect in the bladder wall.[4] Various techniques are used to restore the capacity and function of the bladder. Free fascial grafts, seromuscular grafts, myouterine flaps, and segments of stomach, ileum, or sigmoid colon are used to close defects.

To stimulate regeneration of tissue, the defect may be covered with peritoneum, omentum, lyophilized human dura, gelatin sponge, or a biodegradable or synthetic material. The bladder is also incised to perform a Y-V–plasty to relieve a stricture or contracture of the bladder neck by broadening the outlet of the bladder into the urethra.

Cystectomy

In a cystectomy, the bladder is removed for invasive malignant disease. The bladder can be removed by an open procedure or by robot-assisted laparoscopy. A radical total cystectomy with en bloc pelvic lymph node dissection is usually performed. The neurovascular bundle, which is required for penile erection, may be preserved in a male patient as possible, or a penile prosthesis may be implanted during a subsequent surgical procedure.

A salvage or partial cystectomy with intraoperative radiation therapy may be an alternative to a total cystectomy. If a urinary diversion procedure (previously described) has not been performed before removal of the bladder, transplantation of the ureters into the skin or into the intestinal tract for urinary drainage is required at the time of cystectomy. A gastrocystoplasty may be the procedure of choice after a partial cystectomy, especially in a patient with impaired renal function.

Continent Urinary Diversion Procedures

The ureters may be permanently or temporarily transplanted to maintain the patency of urinary excretion from the body. The bladder may be bypassed or absent. Bilateral transplantation for permanent urinary diversion is performed when bladder function is impaired by neoplasm, chronic infection, congenital anomaly, trauma, or other cause.

The procedure follows completion of a total cystectomy (removal of the bladder), a radical cystoprostatectomy in a male patient, or radical hysterectomy with salpingo-oophorectomy and cystectomy in a female patient, with or without pelvic lymphadenectomy. The ureters may be implanted into the intestinal wall, but more commonly they are transplanted to an isolated loop or a detubularized segment of intestine that becomes a reservoir for urine. Ideally, a urinary reservoir collects and stores urine and expels it under voluntary control (i.e., functions as the lower urinary tract).

The upper urinary tract should be protected from urine reflux, which can lead to kidney infection. Normal renal function and electrolyte balance also must be preserved. These objectives are not easily attained. Various procedures are used for urinary diversion.

With a continent reservoir, an intestinal pouch is created with bilateral antirefluxing ureteroenteric anastomoses. This high-capacity (up to 800 mL), low-pressure pouch provides an intraabdominal reservoir (neobladder) for the storage of urine. A one-way outflow valve provides continence (i.e., the ability to control function). A cutaneous stoma also may be created to empty the reservoir (Fig. 35.23, *A*). The procedure is performed through a low midline incision.

Several techniques are used to create the reservoir from a segment of ileum. Anastomoses may be stapled or sutured to reestablish intestinal continuity. Some types use the appendix as the external conduit. For some procedures, the umbilicus can be used as the stoma site. This is done for cosmesis, particularly in children.

Although creating a continent reservoir is a lengthy surgical procedure, the resultant quality of life for the patient makes this procedure, which prevents involuntary urinary leakage, the procedure of choice unless contraindicated by the patient's tolerance or pathologic condition. Two components are important to the creation of a continent reservoir: (1) a urinary collection reservoir is created from segments of bowel and (2) a catheterizable stoma is fashioned on the abdomen or in the umbilicus.

Indiana Pouch. The Indiana pouch, developed in 1987, is constructed by mobilizing a segment (6–8 inches [15–20 cm]) of terminal ileum, cecum, and ascending colon. The ureters are anastomosed to the colonic segment, inferiorly on each side of the pouch, to prevent reflux. The terminal ileum is exteriorized to form a continent stoma for self-catheterization. This is the most common form to date and demonstrates a 93% continence rate during the day.

Kock Pouch. With a Kock pouch, developed in 1982, a U-shaped pouch is created from a segment (28–32 inches [70–80 cm]) of ileum. Nipple valves are created on two sides by intussusception (i.e., a portion of ileum is ensheathed in another portion). The afferent inflow valve prevents reflux. The ureters are anastomosed end to side distally near this inflow valve. The efferent outflow valve provides continence.

Absorbable staples and/or mesh is used to help stabilize the valves. The reservoir will gradually increase in capacity to as much as 750 to 800 mL of urine. The patient does not wear a collection device but must use a catheter every 4 to 6 hours to empty the reservoir through the exteriorized cutaneous stoma. This form can have as high as a 25% failure rate.

Mainz II Pouch. With a Mainz pouch, a reservoir is formed by mobilizing a segment (4–8 inches [10–20 cm]) of cecum and ascending colon and detubularizing two small segments of equal length of terminal ileum. The walls of the pouch are formed by anastomoses of the ascending colon and cecum with the ileal segments. The ureters are implanted into the ascending colon in an antirefluxive manner. To increase capacity, this pouch can be anastomosed to the urinary bladder remnant after partial cystectomy.

Mitrofanoff Technique. Continent diversion can be achieved by inverting the appendix into the cecum and exteriorizing the intussuscepted appendiceal mucosa to form a continent stoma for self-catheterization. In the absence of a healthy appendix, an additional segment of ileum (3–5 inches [8–13 cm]) can be used to create a continent umbilical stoma.

Ureterosigmoidostomy. With a ureterosigmoidostomy, the ureters may be anastomosed to a nonrefluxing segment of sigmoid colon. Urine diverted into the colon may cause physiologic complications, making this alternative for permanent urinary diversion the least desirable therapeutically. The transverse colon is commonly used. However, the patient does retain an intact body image.

Orthotopic Neobladder. Orthotopic neobladder is constructed from a segment of ileum or colon and anastomosed directly to the urethra. Care is taken to preserve the urethral musculature. To empty the bladder, the patient increases the abdominal pressure while relaxing the external sphincter.

Studer Pouch. First introduced in 1989, it is commonly used today as a neobladder that is anastomosed to the urethra. This type of pouch works well with short ureter segments (Fig. 35.23, *B*).

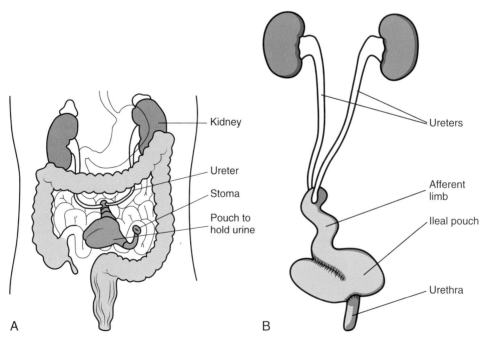

• **Fig. 35.23** Urinary diversion. **A,** Continent ileal reservoir with stoma. **B,** Studer pouch connected to urethra (orthotopic).

Camey Pouch. An orthotopic ileocystoplasty can be performed on a male patient if a U-shaped segment (approximately 16 inches [41 cm]) of ileum reaches the urethra at the pelvic floor without tension. The ureters are anastomosed through small enterostomies to the distal ends of the mobilized and divided ileum.

A urethroileal anastomosis in the midsection of the ileal reservoir allows the patient to void through the urethra. Continence is maintained by spontaneous contraction around the outflow valve at the site of anastomosis. Micturition occurs by relaxation of the perineal muscles and a Valsalva maneuver (i.e., a forced expiratory effort). Urine passes out the urethra.

Augmentation Bladder. Scientists in Germany have performed tests in pigs that demonstrate that bladder cells can be grown in a matrix of bovine collagen to create a new bladder. A segment of ileum is harvested and stripped of its mucosal layer. The epithelium-impregnated matrix acts as a scaffold for the growing cells, and blood vessels begin to form. The scientists believe that this is a step in augmenting a deficient bladder at this time but hope that this work will form the basis of total bladder replacement. Scaffolds can be used for the replacement of surgical mesh and can be adapted to repair other body parts.

Transcutaneous Urinary Diversion

Ileal Conduit. In the creation of an ileal conduit, a procedure popularized by Bricker in the 1950s, both ureters are anastomosed to an isolated segment of the terminal ileum near its proximal end. The distal end is everted and sutured to a predetermined stomal site on the skin, usually on the right side of the abdomen below the waist.

A urinary collection appliance is secured over the stoma before the patient leaves the OR. An ileal conduit with an incontinent external stoma (Fig. 35.24) creates the psychologic stress of an altered body image for the patient, but it may be the procedure of choice for the patient who will receive systemic chemotherapy after radical cystectomy. As a secondary procedure after chemotherapy, an incontinent ileal conduit may be converted to a continent ileal reservoir.

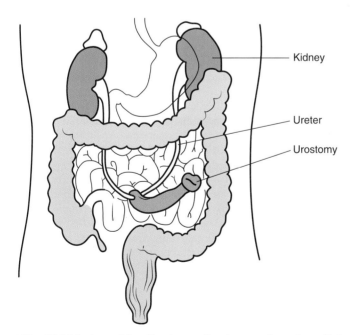

Kidney

Ureter

Urostomy

• **Fig. 35.24** Ileal conduit with stoma. Requires urostomy bag. Not continent.

Cutaneous Ureterostomy. To create a cutaneous ureterostomy, the end of the ureter closest to the bladder is brought through the abdominal wall to the skin. This procedure can be performed unilaterally or bilaterally with a single cutaneous stoma or double-loop stoma. The patient must be fitted postoperatively with an appliance for collecting urine directly from the ureter to the exterior of the body.

This procedure may be performed as a temporary emergency measure after trauma to the bladder, such as a ruptured bladder.

Urinary Incontinence

Involuntary, uncontrollable voiding may accompany congenital or acquired physiologic conditions, such as a loss of bladder control after spinal cord injury or neurogenic disease. Urinary incontinence may develop in males because of loss of sphincter control after prostatectomy and in females after obstetric injury, radiation therapy, or severe pelvic fractures. Surgical intervention is often necessary for stress incontinence—the intermittent leakage of urine as a result of a sudden increase in intraabdominal pressure (e.g., during coughing or sneezing) on weakened urethral sphincter muscles at the bladder neck. Various surgical procedures are performed as determined by urodynamics.

Gynecologists perform some bladder suspension procedures (e.g., Marshall-Marchetti-Krantz suprapubic vesicourethral suspension), and urologists perform other procedures. Laparoscopic approaches have been developed for bladder neck suspension. Surgical procedures that suspend, support, or reposition the bladder can correct urinary incontinence or improve urinary continence.

Transvaginal Bladder Neck Suspension

Pereyra Procedure. In the Pereyra procedure, the bladder neck is elevated with sutures suspended from the anterior rectus fascia. The primary difference between this procedure and the Stamey procedure is that a Pereyra ligature carrier needle is passed blindly down through the retropubic space and out into the vagina.

Both procedures relocate the proximal urethra and bladder neck into the zone of intraabdominal pressure without necessitating open pelvic surgery. The Pereyra procedure is used for uncomplicated recurrent urinary stress incontinence and is 80% effective for long-term resolution of urinary leakage.

Stamey Procedure. In the Stamey procedure, sutures are placed on both sides of the urethrovesical junction from the anterior rectus fascia into the vagina. The patient is positioned in a modified lithotomy position so the legs extend laterally to flatten the lower abdomen. Short suprapubic incisions, right and left of midline, are extended to the anterior rectus fascia. The vagina is incised transversely and dissected from the urethra to expose the trigone of the bladder. The urethrovesical junction is located by palpating the balloon of the Foley catheter inserted into the bladder. A straight or angled Stamey needle is passed through the rectus fascia, along the internal vesicle neck, and out through the vaginal incision.

The cysto equipment should be set up on a separate sterile table because contamination of the eyepiece is unavoidable. A cystoscope is inserted to ascertain correct needle placement without injury to the bladder. A heavy nylon suture threaded onto the needle is drawn from the vagina to the suprapubic incision; the needle is inserted again. The vaginal end of the suture is passed through a 1-cm length of polyester tubular graft before it is threaded onto the needle. When the suture is drawn to the abdominal wall, it establishes a suspending loop on one side of the bladder neck. The suture is tied over the anterior rectus fascia with enough tension to elevate the bladder neck by traction on the adjacent vaginal fascia. This procedure is repeated on the contralateral side.

Artificial Urinary Sphincter

A prosthesis may be implanted to apply pressure to the urethra to maintain continence between periods of voiding. The pressure-regulating mechanism has a reservoir, urethral cuff, and a pump constructed of silicone rubber. A reservoir with a desired pre-determined pressure is positioned intraabdominally beside the bladder.

Depending on the preferred surgical approach, the cuff en-circles either the bladder neck or the bulbous urethra. The pump is placed in the subcutaneous tissue of the scrotum (in males) or labium (in females). A control assembly lies subcutaneously adjacent to the external inguinal ring; tubing connects the com-ponents. A sterile radiopaque isotonic solution is used to fill the prosthesis. When a patient squeezes the pump, solution is trans-ferred from the cuff into the reservoir, thus releasing pressure on the urethra and permitting urine to flow.

Neurostimulation for Bladder Control

The detrusor muscle can be unstable and require electro-stimulation. Electrostimulation simulates the signals from S2 to S4 to mimic the autonomic activity necessary for bladder control. The patient is placed prone, and the leads are placed in the back through an incision. On completion of the lead placement, the patient is placed in a lateral position. A pocket is created in the flank for the small generator. Postoperatively the patient is taught to avoid metal detectors, theft devices in stores, and any large magnets. The patient is given a special magnet to turn the device on or off as needed.

Periurethral Injection of Bulking Agent

Collagen or Teflon may be injected into the tissues surrounding the urethra proximal to the external sphincter. The injection swells the tissue, narrowing the urethra sufficiently for sphincteric control. This procedure is performed in select patients with moderate to severe urinary incontinence, such as in a male after a transurethral resection or a female in whom a suspension pro-cedure has been unsuccessful. The injection is made transur-ethrally with a flexible syringe through a fiber-optic cystourethroscope. A suprapubic catheter is used for 3 to 5 days postoperatively to allow some voluntary passage of urine from the urethra. Postoperative complications include urinary retention, urethral fistulas, and infection.

Bladder Flap Urethroplasty

A bladder flap urethroplasty procedure is advisable when urody-namics show a resistance to urinary flow in a female with a neurogenic bladder. A lesion of the nervous system can cause bladder dysfunction.

Urethra

The urethra functions as the outlet for urine to pass from the bladder. Obstruction or dysfunction of the urethra may cause urinary retention or incontinence. Enlargement of the prostate

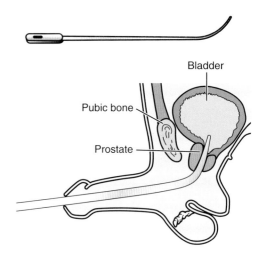

• **Fig. 35.25** Van Buren sound is curved for safe use in male urethral dilation.

may cause obstruction. Gonorrhea, other disease processes, or traumatic injury may cause a stricture.

Perineal Urethrostomy

When indwelling or intermittent urethral catheterization is contraindicated in a male patient with an obstructed or trau-matized urethra, urinary drainage may be established through a perineal incision. An indwelling catheter is inserted into the bladder through an incision into the membranous urethra. Male patients may have a perineal urethrostomy after a total penectomy.

Urethral Dilation

Periodic dilation may be necessary for weeks to years after an infection or a trauma that has caused a urethral stricture. Balloon dilators, woven filiforms and followers, bougies, or metal sounds are used. If the latter are preferred, curved metal Van Buren sounds (Fig. 35.25) are used to dilate a male urethra; straight sounds are used for a female urethra. A short urethral stent may be inserted.

Urethral Stent

To prevent collapse of the lumen caused by stricture, a spring-loaded stainless steel mesh stent can be placed into the male urethra via a cystoscope at a level proximal to the bulbar urethra and distal to the external urinary sphincter. The stricture is measured and dilated or incised by internal urethrotomy. To be effective, the stent selected should measure 1 cm greater than the length of the stricture.

A special deployment applicator is used to place the stent in the urethra. The stent becomes a permanent urethral implant and is useful for males who have benign prostatic hypertrophy. It is contraindicated in bleeding disorders or for males who are receiving anticoagulation therapy. After the procedure, antibiotics are administered as a prophylactic measure.

Urethrotomy

An Otis urethrotome may be used to cut into a urethral stricture. After the instrument is passed into the urethra, the blade is released to cut the stricture. If a specimen of the urethra is taken for biopsy, a rigid biopsy forceps is used through a cystourethroscope. This scope also is used with a laser to open a urethral stricture.

Urethroplasty

Reestablishment of continuity without stricture is the ultimate objective after a traumatic urethral injury and is usually associated with pelvic fractures in males. Scrotal inlay urethroplasty or another method of urethral reconstruction is usually delayed until the extent of injury can be fully evaluated by urethrograms. A suprapubic cystostomy catheter inserted as an emergency measure can maintain urinary drainage for several weeks to months. Insertion of a urethral catheter into a ruptured urethra in the immediate posttraumatic period can produce periurethral infection, stricture, and other irreparable damage.

Perineum and Genital Surface Procedures
Ablation of Condylomata Acuminata

Condylomata are caused by a sexually transmitted human papillomavirus (HPV). Referred to as genital warts, this condition can affect the genitalia, perineum, perianal region, and mucous membranes of males and females. The incubation period is 1 to 2 months after exposure, but longer periods have been reported. HPV has been implicated in cervical cancer.

In an office setting or OR and with the patient under local anesthesia, condylomata are surgically ablated with a carbon dioxide (CO_2) laser. Before the procedure, 3% acetic acid is applied to the area to make the lesions visible by causing them to turn white and raised. As with all other laser procedures, laser precautions (e.g., appropriate eyewear for all persons in the room, proper instrumentation) are followed.

Viral mutation in laser plume has been documented, and personal protective equipment is required. Appropriate laser eyewear and masks should be worn by the staff and the patient to prevent contamination of respiratory and ocular mucosa with virus-laden plume. The eyewear also protects from laser light. Surgical plume is removed and filtered from the surgical field with an evacuation device.

Male Reproductive Organs

The primary functions of the male reproductive organs are procreation, sexual gratification, and hormone secretion. These organs are both internal and external (Fig. 35.26).

Testes

The testes, or testicles, are both endocrine glands and male reproductive organs and are bilaterally suspended in the scrotum, which is divided by a membranous septum referred to as the median raphe. The testes contain a series of tubules, where spermatozoa are formed. As the sperm mature they move to the epididymis, where they are stored until ejaculated. The epididymis secretes seminal fluid to carry the mature sperm through the vas deferens between the lobes of the prostate into the seminal vesicles. The ejaculatory ducts empty sperm and prostatic secretions into the posterior urethra.

The Leydig cells of the testes secrete hormones that influence growth and development, sexual activity, the production of spermatozoa, and the development of secondary sex characteristics. Disorders in or around one testis or both testes that inhibit sexual activity or reproductive capability or cause discomfort in the scrotum may necessitate a surgical procedure. If both testes are

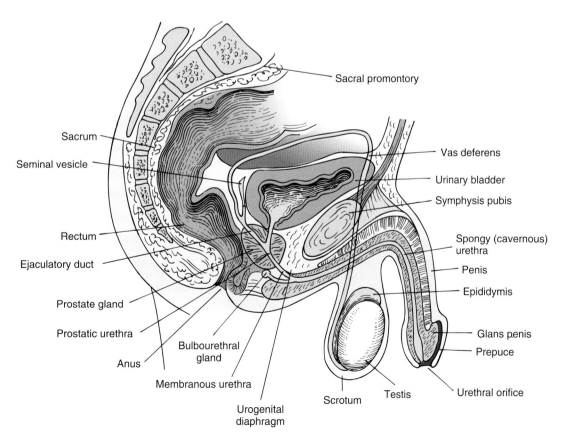

• **Fig. 35.26** Male reproductive organs in sagittal section.

excised (a bilateral orchiectomy), the patient becomes sterile and deficient in male hormones.

Male patients should be instructed to conduct a monthly testicular self-examination (TSE), which should be completed when the scrotum is relaxed (after a warm bath or shower). When performing a TSE, each testis is gently rolled between the thumb and forefingers. The testis should feel smooth and oval, should be without lumps or hardened areas, and should move freely within the scrotal sac. Palpation should be pain free. Testicular cancer affects males in the 15 to 35-year age range.

Orchiectomy

A bilateral orchiectomy may be performed in patients with prostatic cancer to alter the hormonal environment. After this relatively simple procedure, control of the disease is attempted before the urologist considers other endocrine surgery, such as an adrenalectomy. Psychologic preparation is important to help the patient accept the sterilization and the other body changes (e.g., breast enlargement) that may occur as a result of the alteration in the hormonal system.

In this procedure, bilateral oblique incisions in the inguinal canals extend into the upper anterior surface of the scrotum over the testes. The testes are removed from the scrotum after ligation of the spermatic cords at the external or internal inguinal rings. Silicone rubber prostheses may be implanted in the scrotal sac to improve aesthetic appearance, which helps with the psychologic rehabilitation of the patient.

The removal of one testis (unilateral orchiectomy) does not sterilize the patient. This procedure may be indicated after traumatic injury or infection, but it is more commonly performed to remove a tumor. Primary testicular tumors may be right- or left-sided; germ cell tumors may develop bilaterally. Accurate histologic findings and clinical evaluations of the type of tumor and stage of disease are mandatory for determining the appropriate therapy. CT and lymphangiography or lymphoscintigraphy are valuable diagnostic tools.

Unilateral radical orchiectomy via an inguinal incision may be followed by radiation or chemotherapy and retroperitoneal lymph node dissection. The spermatic cord and vas deferens are ligated and divided separately at the internal ring so these structures can be identified if further dissection is needed for metastatic disease.

Retroperitoneal Lymphadenectomy

A transabdominal midline incision is made for exposure of the lymph nodes and sympathetic nerve fibers in the paraaortic plane, usually along the anterolateral aspect of the aorta in the retroperitoneal space. A unilateral lymphadenectomy usually is performed on the ipsilateral (same) side as the tumor unless regional metastases have spread via lymphatic invasion, in which case a bilateral dissection is indicated. If possible, the neurovascular bundles extending from the hypogastric plexus to the corporeal tissues of the penis are preserved. These nerve fibers are identified and placed in vessel loops before lymphadenectomy is carried out, thus preserving ejaculatory function.

Scrotal-Testicular Trauma

An injury may require exploration of the scrotum to ligate bleeding vessels or insert a Penrose drain. Infection is likely to develop after a penetrating wound; therefore extraperitoneal spaces in the scrotum must be drained thoroughly.

Testicular Torsion

The testicle can become twisted on the spermatic cord, causing extreme pain. Immediate correction is necessary or the testicle will become ischemic and tissue death will follow. Manual detorsion may be tried, but surgical intervention is indicated if reduction is not successful within 1 hour of onset.

Hydrocelectomy

A hydrocele is an accumulation of peritoneal fluid in the sac of the tunica vaginalis of the testis. Through an anterior incision into the scrotum, the hydrocele sac is dissected away from the testis and removed from the scrotum. There is a 5% incidence in newborns, most of which will resolve spontaneously. Hydrocele is more common in preterm babies because they may have been born before 32 to 38 weeks' gestation (the average gestational age at which closure vaginalis occurs). Hydrocele is also more common in children who have increased fluid in the peritoneum (i.e., ventriculoperitoneal shunt to drain hydrocephalus or peritoneal dialysis).

Spermatocelectomy

A small mass attached to the epididymis may be palpated in the scrotum superior to the testis. This painless cyst is a collection of testicular fluid and sperm cells. These cysts are repaired if they become annoying to the patient.

Varicocele Ligation

Dilation of the spermatic veins in the pampiniform plexus of the spermatic cord can cause a soft, elastic, often uncomfortable swelling in the scrotum. This condition, known as a varicocele, occurs more often on the left side. It can cause a loss in testicular mass and a decrease of sperm density associated with male infertility caused by increased temperature. Ligation of the spermatic vein can improve sperm count if the testis has not atrophied.

The spermatic vein is ligated above the inguinal canal lateral to the inferior epigastric vessels or in the retroperitoneal space lateral to the iliac artery. In the latter approach, a transverse abdominal incision starts at the anterior superior iliac spine and extends toward the lateral aspect of the rectus abdominis muscle. The hemiscrotum must be manually emptied of all blood before the vein is ligated or the varicocele may persist postoperatively.

Laparoscopic approaches have been developed for spermatic vein ligation. In such a procedure, the internal inguinal ring is located laparoscopically and the spermatic cord and blood vessels are identified. The spermatic vein is dissected free, ligated with two endoscopic clips, and cut between the clips with endoscopic scissors. Most patients are able to return to work within 2 days of the procedure.

Vas Deferens

The vasa deferentia are the small fibromuscular excretory ducts that carry sperm upward through the spermatic cords from the epididymides (which lie along the upper portion of each testis) to the seminal vesicles, the pouch-like glands in front of the urinary bladder near the prostate gland. Interruption of or obstruction to a vas deferens inhibits normal spermatogenesis.

Vasectomy

Elective bilateral vasectomy is an established method of male sterilization and is usually performed as an ambulatory surgical

• **Fig. 35.27** Completed vasectomy.

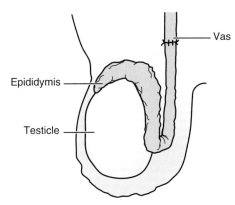

• **Fig. 35.28** Vasovasostomy.

procedure. In a vasectomy, a segment of each vas deferens is removed and sent to the pathology department in individually labeled specimen cups (Fig. 35.27). Depending on the preference of the urologist, the cut ends are either ligated with suture or clips or the endothelium of the lumen is coagulated with the ESU.

Techniques vary, but all patients should be informed that spontaneous regeneration of a severed vas deferens does occur in a small percentage of patients and that sterility is not immediate. Follow-up care includes semen testing for sperm count; repeat testing should continue until no sperm is found in the seminal fluid. Patient teaching includes instructions to use alternative birth control methods until the seminal fluid contains no sperm.

Vasovasostomy

Recannulization of the vas deferens for the restoration of fertility requires an unobstructed anastomosis. The vas deferens has a tough 2-mm outer diameter and an inner diameter of 1 mm or less at the distal end, as well as dilation at the proximal end. This makes precise anastomosis under the operating microscope preferable to nonmicrosurgical techniques, in which it is difficult to see the lumen of the vas deferens on the distal side. One-layer microscopic anastomosis and splinting techniques for a vasectomy reversal often result in a stricture caused by scarring within the lumen of the vas deferens, which inhibits the passage of sperm.

After a scrotal incision is made to expose the vas deferens above and below the site of previous ligation, the two ends are cut to excise scar tissue and open the lumen. Under magnification of the operating microscope, interrupted sutures are placed in the mucosal lining of the lumen to create a fluid-tight anastomosis (Fig. 35.28). Muscularis is approximated separately. A CO_2 milliwatt laser may be used to weld tissue to overcome the scarring and stricture that may be associated with suturing. Sperm counts return to normal soon after the surgical procedure.

Male Infertility

Primary infertility is diagnosed after a failure to conceive during a period of 1 year of unprotected sexual intercourse. Causes of infertility include abnormality in the female and/or male reproductive systems. Male infertility can be the result of deficient sperm production, obstructed sperm passage, a mechanical inability to pass sperm, hormonal imbalance, testicular disease or injury, a low sperm count, and antibodies against sperm.

The history and physical examination should be concurrent with the female partner's gynecologic evaluation. Issues assessed should include sexual history, previous pregnancies, health history, the use of lubricants, drug use, radiation exposure, and timing and frequency of intercourse. Childhood illnesses such as high fevers and viral infections may be factors. A previous sexually transmitted disease can cause scarring that prevents the transport of sperm. Endocrine testing includes follicle-stimulating hormone, luteinizing hormone, testosterone, and prolactin levels. Urinalysis is performed to rule out infection and/or retrograde ejaculation.

The semen analysis includes determining ejaculate volume, sperm count and motility, morphology, and the presence or absence of white blood cells or red blood cells in the seminal fluid. The patient is advised to abstain from sexual intercourse for 2 to 3 days before the testing is performed.

Prostate Gland

The prostate gland, a musculoglandular organ in males, is encased in a fibrous capsule and surrounds the posterior urethra at the bladder neck. It is divided into five lobes. The arterial supply is derived from the pudendal, inferior vesicle, and hemorrhoidal arteries that terminate into two large groups of bilateral prostatic vessels. The venous drainage is through the dorsal vein divided into three bundles bilaterally. The innervation is from parasympathetic fibers arising at S2 to S4 and from the sympathetic nerve fibers at the thoracolumbar nerve from the hypogastric nerve. This forms the pelvic plexus that innervates the bladder, ureters, seminal vesicles, prostate, and cavernous nerves of the corpus cavernosa of the penis. Lymphatics drain into the internal iliac and sacral nodes into the intestinal trunk to the cisterna chyli.

The normal function of the prostate gland is to provide alkaline secretions to the seminal fluid for sperm mobility during ejaculation. The standard of care includes an annual digital prostate examination and prostate-specific antigen (PSA) testing after 55 years of age.[5]

Although the prostate gland normally weighs 20 g, in most men it will enlarge to some degree by 50 years of age. Fifty percent of all men older than 80 years will have prostatic cancer. Enlargement of the prostate gland can obstruct the urethra and interfere with voiding; this difficulty in voiding is what most often brings men with prostatic disease to the urologist. The urologist will examine the prostate and order a PSA blood test. If the tests indicate benign prostatic hypertrophy/hyperplasia (BPH), surgery is not the first treatment method of choice.

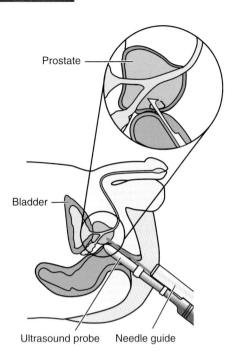

• **Fig. 35.29** Transrectal ultrasound-guided prostatic biopsy.

Conservative treatment for benign enlargement of the prostate includes administration of oral tamsulosin (Flomax). If the prostate does not respond to drug therapy by shrinking, then balloon dilation, stenting, or other surgical procedure may be indicated.

The entire prostate gland or one or more lobes can be resected from its capsule transurethrally (transurethral resection of the prostate [TURP]). Prostatectomy also can be performed robotically or through a suprapubic or retropubic abdominal approach or a perineal incision.

A radical prostatectomy, performed through a retropubic abdominal or perineal incision, includes extirpation of the prostate, periprostatic tissue, seminal vesicles, and vas ampullae en bloc. The approach and procedure depend on the urologist's preference for removing the type of pathologic condition.

Transrectal aspiration, core biopsies, or ultrasonography helps establish the correct diagnosis (Fig. 35.29). Prostatic carcinoma may be treated by surgical removal, interstitial and external beam radiation, chemotherapy, and/or hormonal therapy. Management depends on the stage of the disease and the age and condition of the patient. Carcinoma of the prostate is the second most common cause of cancer-related deaths in men in the United States. BPH is a common indication for prostate intervention in men older than 50 years if the prostate symptoms do not respond to drug therapy. Men younger than 50 years may not qualify for definitive treatment if prostate enlargement is caused by prostatitis. Conservative antibiotic therapy is the treatment of choice.

Balloon Dilation and Stenting of Prostatic Urethra

During a cystoscopy, a balloon dilation probe can be inserted into the urethra and expanded to relieve obstruction caused by prostatic hypertrophy. One or more titanium stents can be deployed to maintain patency of the lumen. The stent remains in the lumen and becomes overgrown with urothelium. This procedure permanently relieves urinary retention (Fig. 35.30).

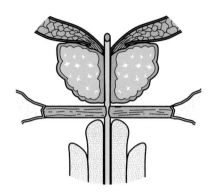

• **Fig. 35.30** Prostatic stent.

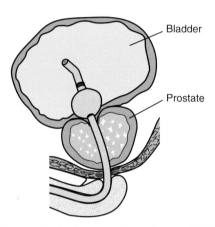

• **Fig. 35.31** Transurethral microwave thermotherapy (TUMT) probe delivers microwaves to the prostate tumor.

Transurethral Microwave Thermotherapy

With transurethral microwave thermotherapy (TUMT), ultrasound guidance is used to insert a microwave probe into the urethra to the level of the prostate blockage (Fig. 35.31). Microwaves are generated by a console and transmitted to the distal aspect of the probe. Heat generated by the microwave probe is absorbed by the urethral portion of the prostate for 1 hour.

The probe is cooled with water circulation at 68° F (20° C) to protect nearby structures. A rectal probe is used to record rectal temperature. The heated tissue sloughs, which causes the urethral stricture to release. Most patients can void with ease, although a few patients require a Foley catheter for several days postoperatively.

Transurethral Needle Ablation

With transurethral needle ablation (TUNA), an ambulatory procedure, cystoscopic guidance is used to insert a probe into the urethra to the level of the prostate stricture. Two small needles are passed from the side of the telescopic probe into the hypertrophied prostatic tissue (Fig. 35.32). Radio waves are transmitted selectively into the tissue via the needles.

Prostatic tissue in contact with the needles is ablated; nearby structures, such as nerves and vessels, are spared. Up to six select areas of stricture can be precisely ablated in the same procedure.

Each application creates a defect in the prostate. The tissue reabsorbs over a period of 3 months, causing the stricture to release. The patient may complain of urinary retention or burning on urination for 24 to 96 hours after the procedure. The main side effect is the potential for retrograde ejaculation.

Transurethral Prostatectomy

Transurethral resection, also referred to as *transurethral resection of the prostate* (TURP), involves the removal of all or part of the glandular tissue within the prostatic capsule by electroresection through the urethra (Fig. 35.33). A resectoscope, via cysto sheath, is introduced into the prostatic urethra. Using alternating currents from the ESU through the cutting loop electrode, the urologist resects tissue and coagulates bleeding vessels. The bladder is distended with solution to create a working space during resection. Irrigation solution (10–12 L) may be needed. Glycine was used with older equipment, but newer bipolar resectoscopes are designed to work with sterile normal saline.

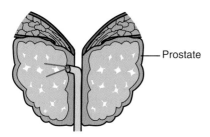

• Fig. 35.32 Transurethral needle ablation (TUNA) probe delivers selective radiofrequencies to prostate via directed needles.

Sterile water as an expansion medium can cause complications related to intravascular hemolysis. Care is taken not to permit the patient to absorb excessive amounts of solution through the prostatic venous sinuses, or TUR syndrome may occur. This can cause dilutional hyponatremia less than 125 mEq/L. Glycine is a neurotransmitter inhibitor that is metabolized into glycolic acid and ammonium. Ammonia has been noted to be elevated during TUR syndrome. Risk factors include the following:

- Height of the solution bags (extremes of height increase the amount of pressure of the fluid as it enters the bladder)
- Deep resection (which allows for increased venous absorption of solution)
- Amount of tissue resected in excess of 45 g
- Duration of the procedure (risk increases when the procedure exceeds 90 minutes)
  Signs of TUR syndrome include the following:
- Mental confusion
- Nausea and vomiting
- Hypertension followed by hypotension
- Symptoms of fluid overload and pulmonary edema
- Bradycardia and dysrhythmia
- Visual disturbances
- Seizures and twitching
- Coma
  Treatment of TUR syndrome includes the following:
- Administration of IV hypertonic saline
- Monitoring of serum sodium levels
- Diuretics

Resected prostatic tissue is collected in an Ellik or other evacuator. After the surgical procedure, tissue fragments must be sent to the pathology department for analysis and weighing. The urologist may insert a three-way 30 or 50-mL Foley catheter for

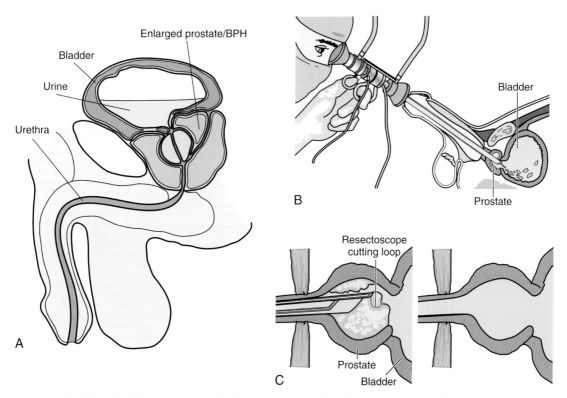

• Fig. 35.33 A, Enlarged prostate. **B,** Transurethral resection of enlarged prostate with resectoscope (TURP). **C,** Obstructive prostate is removed with cutting loop. *BPH,* Benign prostatic hyperplasia.

irrigation and hemostasis. The large, inflated balloon compresses against the bladder neck fossa to form a tamponade to help control bleeding. Some urologists place the Foley catheter under direct tension by taping the catheter to the patient's leg or abdomen to increase the tamponade effect for hemostasis. The third lumen provides a means for continuous postoperative irrigation to prevent the formation of clots in the bladder.

Benign nodular hyperplasia of glands less than 50 g in size is the usual indication for TURP. This approach has the potential complications of impotence and urinary incontinence. The technique is one of the most difficult for a urologist to master. Although electroresection is used most commonly, transurethral incision of small prostate glands (less than 25 g), balloon dilation of the prostate, laser surgery, and cryosurgery are other invasive techniques for treating BPH. TURP may be performed for the diagnosis or treatment of localized cancer.

Suprapubic Prostatectomy

The suprapubic approach for prostatectomy is limited almost exclusively to the removal of a large, benign, hypertrophied gland weighing more than 50 g. Through a midline vertical incision above the symphysis pubis, the superior bladder wall is opened to expose the prostatic urethra (Fig. 35.34, *A*). The prostatic lobes are enucleated with a finger that is inserted through an incision into the mucosa of the urethra. This procedure may be termed *transvesicocapsular prostatectomy* because the prostatic capsule is approached through the bladder.

Hemostatic agents are usually packed into the extremely vascular prostatic fossa to help control bleeding. Pressure from the Foley catheter balloon inserted after closure of the urethra also helps obtain hemostasis. A suprapubic cystostomy tube is inserted to facilitate urinary drainage from the bladder during the healing process.

Retropubic Prostatectomy

In the retropubic approach, the prostate gland is exposed below the bladder neck through a vertical or transverse abdominal incision above the symphysis pubis. The bladder is not opened. The gland is removed through an incision in the prostatic capsule; this procedure is called a transcapsular prostatectomy. The periprostatic tissue, seminal vesicles, and vas ampullae also may be excised. This method is common for prostate glands larger than 50 g.

Radical Retropubic Prostatectomy

A limited pelvic lymph node dissection is performed for carcinoma with no evidence of spread beyond the prostatic capsule. This radical procedure may be carried out as initial curative therapy or after transurethral prostatectomy. After dissection of the lymph nodes, one of two approaches may be used to totally remove the prostate:

1. *Campbell technique:* An incision is made at the bladder neck, and the urethra is transected. The prostate and periprostatic tissue are widely dissected anterograde from the bladder. The bladder neck is reconstructed for the vesicourethral anastomosis. The patient will be impotent because the nerves responsible for erection are transected. A penile prosthesis may be implanted.
2. *Walsh technique:* The prostate is resected retrograde beginning at the urethra, working back to the bladder neck. Dissection is carried out close to the prostatic capsule to preserve the neurovascular bundle and thus maintain potency. The vesicourethral anastomosis is completed.

Nerve-sparing procedures have been developed to preserve sexual potency. A device referred to as CaverMap can be used during the open prostatectomy procedure to locate nerves that control erection (Fig. 35.35). A sensor band is placed around the penis, and a handheld device with a nerve-stimulating probe is used to sense nerve impulses responsible for causing erection. Studies performed by the American Urological Association show that between 40% and 70% of radical prostatectomy patients experienced erectile dysfunction of varying degrees after the surgery. Some patients are unable to achieve erection until after 18 months postoperatively. The CaverMap helps locate the nerves but does not ensure the ability to achieve erection postoperatively. The ProPep nerve monitoring system is used for robotic surgery.

Perineal Prostatectomy

The perineum affords the most direct open surgical approach to the prostate through a relatively avascular field (see Fig. 35.34, *B*).

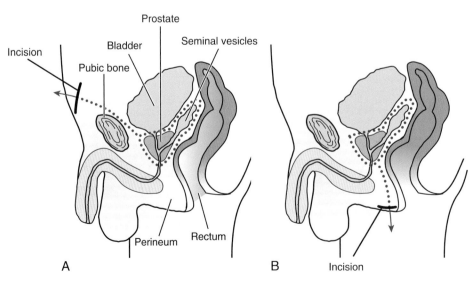

• **Fig. 35.34 A,** Suprapubic prostatectomy. **B,** Perineal prostatectomy.

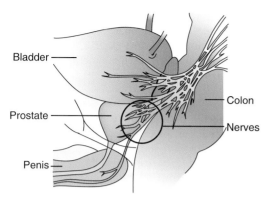

• **Fig. 35.35** Innervation of the male genitourinary organs and the relationship between prostatic and penile nerves.

• **Fig. 35.36** High lithotomy position.

With the patient in an extreme lithotomy position, the perineum is incised between the scrotum and the anal sphincter (Fig. 35.36). The rectum is dissected from the posterior surface of the prostate, or dissection may be carried out between the external anal sphincter and the rectum.

The perineal approach may be used to enucleate the prostate gland from its capsule or for radical cystoprostatectomy. This latter procedure includes removal of the entire prostate gland, its capsule, the seminal vesicles, and a portion of the bladder. The classic radical perineal prostatectomy with pelvic lymph node dissection may be the surgical procedure of choice to reduce the morbidity of prostatic carcinoma. Urinary incontinence and impotence are common outcomes with this procedure. Laparoscopic methods can be used to sample intraabdominal lymph nodes.

Robotic-Assisted Prostatectomy

The robotic-assisted laparoscopic approach used is dependent on the method used to dissect the seminal vesicles and the vas deferens away from the rectum. Enucleation of the prostate is facilitated by traction on the Foley catheter.

Robotic-assisted prostatectomy has become the preferred method of choice. When it was initially started, about 8% of urologists used robotic equipment for prostatectomy. Currently, the use of robots exceeds 85% of all prostatectomies and has been beneficial for the patients. Blood loss is minimal at 100 to 300 mL compared with open prostatectomy at 450 to 800 mL. Patients have demonstrated better urinary continence and preserved sexual function when robotics were used. Refined preservation of two key nerve bundles that innervate the prostate and urinary sphincters has been possible using robotics.[6] Surgeon experience and technique play a large part in the success of the procedure. Robotic surgery is discussed in Chapter 32.

Transperineal Prostatic Cryoablation

Transperineal prostatic cryoablation offers an alternative to radical prostatectomy in select patients with cancer of the prostate. This procedure is performed in the cysto room with the patient under general or spinal anesthesia. The entire prostate and periprostatic tissues are frozen. With the patient in the lithotomy position, an ultrasound probe is placed in the rectum for guidance in positioning five cryoprobes. Each cryoprobe is placed transperineally through a hollow sheath inserted in a small (18-gauge) needle puncture site. Liquid nitrogen is delivered to each probe from the cryosurgical device/console.

Care must be taken to avoid freezing the rectum. Warm water is run through a urethral catheter to keep the urethra warm to prevent tissue sloughing, a potential complication of transurethral cryosurgery. Both the prostate gland and the tumor cells are destroyed. The side effects of this procedure include a high risk for impotence (80–90%) and urinary incontinence (30%).

Pelvic Lymphadenectomy

A pelvic lymphadenectomy involves either a low abdominal incision into the extraperitoneal space or a laparoscopic approach. The lymph nodes are dissected bilaterally from the iliac vessels, obturator spaces, and hypogastric vessels. These nodes may be examined by frozen section to detect early and subtle metastases from prostatic carcinoma. If several nodes are positive for cancer, the patient is unlikely to benefit from a radical prostatectomy.

If the nodes are negative, the urologist may proceed with a radical retropubic prostatectomy. Pelvic lymphadenectomy also may be performed as a staged procedure before radical perineal prostatectomy. If feasible, at least one neurovascular bundle is preserved.

Penis

The penis is the cylindric erectile male organ of copulation. Because it contains the urethra, a deviation or malformation in structure may affect normal urinary flow from the bladder. Circumcision or surgical procedures to repair congenital anomalies of the penis are usually performed during infancy and childhood. Penile anatomy consists of the glans at the distal section, the corpus spongiosum circumferentially the length of the urethra, and the corpus cavernosa bilaterally the length of the shaft (see Fig. 35.26). The distal portion where the urethra exits is referred to as the glans. In its natural state, the glans is covered by redundant skin, which is referred to as foreskin. Some cultures electively remove this skin covering from males in infancy by circumcision. The U.S. Centers for Disease Control and Prevention (CDC) guidelines recommend circumcision as prevention for HIV. Studies have shown that the foreskin is vulnerable to the virus because of its cellular structure.[7]

The arterial supply of the penis arises from the inferior pudendal arteries. Venous drainage is from the venules in the periphery of the corpora and the superior and deep dorsal veins into the cavernosal and pudendal plexuses. Innervation is from both sympathetic and parasympathetic origin combined with autonomic reflexes.

The erection and ejaculatory responses are neurologically mediated by afferent and efferent pathways. Sacral efferent parasympathetic innervation causes both psychogenic and reflex erections. Destruction of these nerves during abdominal-perineal resection and radical prostatectomy results in impotence in 70% to 100% of patients. At the level of the penis, innervation is from adrenergic nerves in the arteriolar smooth muscle.

Complete transection of the spinal cord can result in impotence. Reflex erections may be found in patients with lesions of the upper cord. An exact locus of impulses in the brain has not been identified.

Adult Male Circumcision

Difficulty in the retraction of the foreskin is referred to as phimosis. Paraphimosis occurs when the foreskin retracts to expose the glans and cannot be repositioned back. These conditions may necessitate circumcision or removal of the foreskin to prevent necrosis and gangrene. In some patients, a small cut in the foreskin, a dorsal slit, is sufficient to release the constriction. An erection that cannot be released because of tight foreskin is a medical and possibly a surgical emergency. Attempts to drain the penis are made by injecting vasodilators. Once the penis is flaccid, a determination is made as to surgical intervention.

Adult male circumcision requires more dissection and ligation than does a pediatric procedure (Fig. 35.37). The patient is placed in the supine position. The foreskin is retracted to prep the glans penis. ESU should be available; however, a small battery-operated cautery is usually sufficient to provide hemostasis for pinpoint bleeders. Some surgeons prefer fine absorbable free-ties. The tissue

around the foreskin is dissected, incised, and trimmed away. The remaining edges are circumferentially sutured with fine interrupted absorbable sutures. Vaseline gauze is used as a dressing. A scrotal suspension strap may be used to hold the dressings in place and provide support.

Impotence

The cause of erectile dysfunction (ED), or impotence, can be classified as organic or psychogenic. Patients are thoroughly evaluated by a urologist and properly selected for surgical therapy. Organic causes are confirmed by angiography, neurologic testing, and papaverine injection—induced erection studies. A test dose of sildenafil (Viagra) delineates vasculogenic causes from psychogenic causes. Viagra is ineffective if neurologic damage has occurred. Other ED drugs include tadalafil (Cialis). Tadalafil is also used to treat BPH. Side effects of ED drugs include hypotension and decreased circulation to the blood supply to the eye. Some patients may experience priapism (prolonged erection over 4 hours) and may need emergency treatment to prevent permanent damage to the penile vascular system in the corpus cavernosa.

Studies of penile activities include the measurement of erections during the rapid eye movement (REM) phases of sleep. A small band attached to a pressure-sensitive machine is placed around the penis. Erections, referred to as nocturnal penile tumescence, are recorded during sleep. This helps rule out organic causes of impotence.

Psychogenic causes are suspected after organic causes have been ruled out. Some psychogenic causes may be attributed to a fear of sexual relations after a heart attack or surgical procedure. Antidepressants and psychologic counseling may be helpful.

• **Fig. 35.37** Adult male circumcision.

Most procedures for the diagnosis and treatment of organic impotence are performed with the patient under regional anesthesia.[8] Consideration for the patient's privacy should be included in the plan of care.

Dorsal Vein Ligation

A failed erection can be caused by inadequate filling or inadequate storage of blood in the erectile tissue of the corpus cavernosa of the penis. Some patients can achieve erection but cannot maintain it for more than a few minutes because of a cavernosal leak. The diagnosis is made by the dynamic infusion cavernosometry and cavernosography (DICC) procedure. In select patients with this condition, the urologist may elect to ligate the dorsal vein and several collateral vessels of the penis to delay the venous return from the erectile tissue and help sustain erection. This procedure is not always successful.

Penile Prosthesis

Implantation of a penile prosthesis as treatment for organic impotence can enable some men to achieve a satisfactory return of sexual activity within 4 to 6 weeks postoperatively. Complications include scar tissue formation and erosion of the implant through the penile tissue. Penile prosthetic implants are of three types: semirigid silicone, semiflexible silicone, and an inflatable hydraulic device:

- The semirigid prosthesis consists of two silicone rods that are inserted into the corpus cavernosum on each side of the penis, usually through a vertical incision in the perineum underneath the scrotum. The suitable-size prosthesis is selected from available lengths. This prosthesis maintains a permanent semierection.
- A semiflexible prosthesis is constructed of malleable material and silicone.
- An inflatable hydraulic device is inserted through a midline incision that extends from the base of the penis to a point midway between the symphysis pubis and the umbilicus. Silicone cylinders are implanted into each corpus cavernosum (Fig. 35.38). Tubing connected to these cylinders at the base of the penis is brought into the left inguinal canal, the prevesical space, and the right inguinal canal, where it is connected to tubing from the pump-release mechanism placed in the scrotum.

A reservoir filled with solution is sutured into the abdominal fascia of the prevesical space; the tubing from this reservoir is also connected to the pump-release mechanism. To achieve an erection, the patient squeezes the pump in the scrotum. Multiple manufacturers make implants, and the patient can select the type of prosthesis to suit their needs (Fig. 35.39).

Penectomy

Cancer of the penis is uncommon in the developed world.[9] It accounts for 1.3% of all cancers occurring in men.[3,10] Penile cancer is more commonly found in men between 55 and 70 years of age, although 20% are younger than 40 years.[9] The common factor in the majority of penile cancer cases is an intact foreskin, which has a cancer rate of 25% to 60%. Jewish males, who are circumcised 8 days after birth, rarely develop penile cancer. Any treated lesion of the glans that does not clear in 2 to 3 weeks should be investigated as a cancerous or precancerous lesion, especially in an uncircumcised man.[9] Another common factor is HPV infection in the presence of an intact foreskin; 45% to 48%

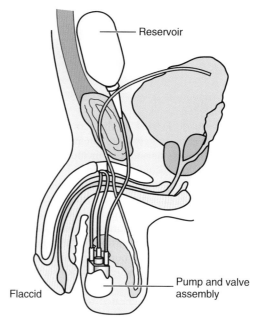

• **Fig. 35.38** Inflatable penile prosthesis in position.

• **Fig. 35.39** Inflatable penile prosthesis components.

of penile cancers are related to HPV.[9] The incidence increases with the number of sexual partners.

Approximately 78% of all penile cancers are located between the coronal sulcus and the distal aspect of the glans.[9] Fewer than 5% are located on the shaft. Nearly 30% to 60% of males presenting with penile cancer have positive palpable inguinal lymphadenopathy on examination. Sentinel node biopsy can be used to guide inguinal node dissection. Diagnosis of superficial lesions can be done with Mohs microscopic mapping. A clear margin of 2 cm is desired. Treatment of penile cancer with chemotherapy has not been very successful.

The penis may be partially or completely resected because of neoplasm or trauma. A partial penectomy may allow the patient enough length for upright voiding. Cosmetic reconstruction may be possible in some patients. Invasive disease may necessitate a complete penectomy, including removal of the scrotum and testes (orchiectomy). Reconstruction after a complete penectomy includes urethral diversion to the perineum. The plan of care should include consideration for psychologic counseling.

Endocrine Glands

Two pairs of glands in the endocrine system are of primary interest to the urologist: the adrenal glands in both sexes and the testes in the male.

Adrenal Glands

The adrenal glands are located in the retroperitoneum on the superior margin of each kidney. The adrenal cortex is the outer covering and produces hormones, including glucocorticoids (cortisol) and mineralocorticoids (aldosterone), which control the body's metabolic processes and help regulate fluid and electrolyte balance. With low levels of cortisol or aldosterone, the body is not able to respond adequately under minimal physical or emotional stress, including change in temperature, exercise, or excitement. The adrenal medulla is the inner portion of the gland and secretes the stimulants epinephrine and norepinephrine and assists the body in coping with stress. The adrenal glands secrete hormones that stimulate the sexual organs.

An adrenalectomy may be indicated to remove a benign, malignant, or metastatic tumor within the adrenal medulla or eliminate adrenal hormonal secretions. Pheochromocytoma, a tumor of the adrenal medulla, causes excessive amounts of these stimulants to be released, resulting in hypertension. Pheochromocytoma is most commonly found in younger patients. Only a small percentage of the lesions are malignant.

The adrenal glands are a rich source of estrogens, and estrogens may stimulate a recurrence or metastasis from prostatic or breast cancer. A bilateral adrenalectomy may be performed as a supplemental treatment of advanced prostatic or breast cancer to reduce the hormonal environment within the body.

For an open unilateral adrenalectomy, the adrenal gland is usually approached posteriorly through a lateral incision into the retroperitoneal space. The 12th rib is usually resected on the right side because the adrenal gland lies above the kidney, behind the liver. The surgeon may also prefer a posterior approach for a bilateral adrenalectomy with the patient placed in a modified prone position for the bilateral incisions. Other surgeons prefer an anterior thoracoabdominal or transabdominal incision into the retroperitoneal space with the patient in the supine position.

The circulating nurse must verify with the surgeon the preferred position before the patient is positioned, prepped, and draped. Depending on the preoperative diagnosis, the thoracoabdominal incision may be preferred to extend the incision across the costal margin into the eighth or ninth intercostal space for exposure and exploration of the extraadrenal paraganglion system. Laparoscopic and robotic methods are commonly used by many surgeons with good results.

Transsexual Surgery (Sex Reassignment)

Transsexual surgery may be the only acceptable alternative for a patient who psychologically desires to become a member of the opposite sex—both physically and emotionally.[10] Before having surgery, the patient is usually required to live in the desired sex role for a period of 1 year. This type of surgery presents challenges to both the urologic and the gynecologic teams.

Sex transformation requires a stable personality, psychiatric counseling for feasibility, and careful preparation and support.[10] The patient changes legal identity and social status. Adolescents who have gender dysphoria may choose to live as the sexual identity in which they feel comfortable, but may experience resistance from parents and friends. They are not necessarily candidates for transsexual surgery, but in some circumstances may be permitted to dress and live in the gender role they choose. Hormonal changes at puberty can be altered by hormone therapy under the guidance of a physician.[10]

The World Professional Association for Transgender Health (WPATH), formerly the Harry Benjamin International Gender Dysphoria Association Standards of Care, safeguards both transsexual people and the men and women who provide professional services for them.[10] This set of standards divides the transition process into a series of discrete steps that enable the patient to progress at a livable pace during transition. These steps maximize the chance that the sex change process will be successful. The first step a transsexual should make is to locate a therapist who is familiar with the standards of care. It is also important to find a good support group.

Male to Female

Surgical techniques have been developed to eliminate the external genitalia of a male by dissecting the penile structures, shortening the urethra, and removing the testes. Preservation of the sensitive erogenous tissues was pioneered and perfected by Dr. Georges Borou in Morocco in the early 1960s. The patient undergoes counseling and feminization with female hormones (estrogen) preoperatively.

The patient is placed in the lithotomy position for the procedure. The process is performed in several steps:

1. The perineum is dissected, and the penile shaft and scrotal skin are preserved for construction of a neovagina and labia.
2. A tissue tube is created from portions of the scrotal skin and sutured to the inverted penile skin for length.
3. A tunnel is created in the perineum between the urethra and the rectum at the space of Douglas and packed with lap tapes.
4. The corpus spongiosum is dissected, and the urethra is cut to length. A Foley catheter is used to stent the urethral placement.
5. The dorsal vessels and nerves are spared as the glans is separated from the corpus cavernosa. The glans and a pedicle stalk are all that remain of the penile shaft. A clitoris is fashioned from the remaining glans and sutured into position. The lower abdomen is tunneled transversely and retracted superiorly so the pedicle of nerves and vessels can be nested into the retropubic space. Some procedures retain a thinly trimmed glans as a neocervix in an inverted penis-to-vagina transition.
6. The vaginal skin tube is placed inside the vaginal tunnel like a graft and sutured into place after removing the lap tapes. The neovagina is packed with vaginal packing to create equal pressure on the walls circumferentially.
7. The edges of the abdominal skin and dorsal penile tissue are pulled up and over the edge of the pubic bone and sutured into place as the anterior perineum. The remaining scrotal skin and perineal tissue are fashioned into the new posterior perineum and labia majora. The urethra is exteriorized and positioned by sutures. The apex at the superior margin is joined to form a clitoral hood and labia minora at a later procedure.
8. Drains are placed in the groins bilaterally, and the neovagina is packed.

CHAPTER 35 Urologic Surgery **759**

9. The lateral edges of the left and right labia majora are approximated with temporary stay sutures to provide compression to the perineum to prevent dependent hematoma and loss of the vulvar flap. These sutures are removed several days postoperatively when the danger of hematoma is passed.

Breast implants are placed at a later date after enlargement with tissue expanders. Some patients prefer to have breast implants before the feminization procedure to make the transition preoperatively. Most patients have lived as a woman for several years before undergoing genitalia surgery. Suppression of beard and body hair, redistribution of adipose tissue, voice change, and removal of pronounced thyroid cartilage (Adam's apple) are gradual processes that are managed surgically or chemically over time.

The prostate and seminal vesicles are retained so that clitoral orgasm with emission from the urethra is possible, although sperm are not produced. The actual success rate for orgasm potential is estimated at 25%. The resultant newly created vulva is realistic in form and function.

Female to Male

Female-to-male transsexual surgery is also possible in satisfactory candidates. Management of this change is complex. A treatment schedule of hormonal substitution (i.e., androgens [male hormones] in the female patient) is begun well in advance of the procedure.

In a one-stage procedure, a bilateral subcutaneous mastectomy or reduction, total abdominal hysterectomy, and bilateral salpingo-oophorectomy are performed. Three to five additional stages are necessary to complete the transformation, as follows:

1. Urethral elongation and reconstruction, to the tip of the enlarged clitoris. Some patients do not opt for urethral lengthening and maintain its natural position in the perineum. Urethral reconstruction can be performed using buccal tissue from inside the mouth.[11]
2. Revision of the labia for penile lengthening and scrotal construction.
3. Flaps or grafts to create a penile shaft.
4. Placement of penile erection implants. Rigid implants are commonly used.
5. Prosthetic testicular implantation.

An understanding, nonjudgmental, unembarrassed attitude on the part of health care personnel can help the patient adjust psychologically, as well as recover physically, after the radical change. Consideration should be given to the patient's family and significant others because they, too, must adjust. The patient may have married and produced children while in the role of their birth sex. In addition to confusion about parental roles, the patient may experience rejection or revulsion from offspring, family members, and others. Referral for family/significant others and individual counseling should be included in the plan of care.

Postoperative Complications of Urologic Surgery

Oliguria, the diminished capacity to form urine, is often seen after urologic surgery. Water and sodium are conserved by antidiuretic hormone, aldosterone, epinephrine, and norepinephrine secreted during stress; this decreases urinary output. Dehydration, shock, cardiac failure, renal failure, or third-space loss (e.g., edema, ascites) may contribute to oliguria. Because prolonged oliguria may result in renal failure, a urinary output of less than 30 mL/h should be reported to the surgeon. Treatment depends on the cause.

Because of the introduction of the catheter and instruments, the patient should be watched for infection after all urinary tract procedures. Cloudy urine, dysuria, frequency, urgency, and pain or burning on urination are symptoms of urinary tract infections. Damage to bladder sphincters from instrumentation or urethral infection may lead to incontinence. Sharp abdominal pain after cysto or the manipulation of a ureter to remove calculi may suggest peritonitis from bladder or ureteral perforation. Susceptibility to infection accompanies urinary diversion.

ⓔ EVOLVE WEBSITE

http://evolve.elsevier.com/Hornacky/BerryKohn/
- Historical Perspective
- Tips for the Scrub Person and Circulating Nurse
- Student Interactive Questions
- Glossary

References

1. Rakarja P, Haruid A, Mochtar C, et al.: Recent advances in optical imaging technologies for the detection of bladder cancer, *Photodiagnosis Photodyn Ther* 24:192–197, 2018.
2. Choi CI, Kim DI, Chung YS, et al.: Initial experience with hand-assisted laparoscopic living donor nephrectomy: training and clinical practice as a general surgeon, *Transplant Proc* 50(10):3113–3120, 2018.
3. Fontenelle L, Sarti T: Kidney stones: treatment and prevention, *Am Fam Physician* 99(8):490–496, 2019.
4. Roth J, Cain M: Neuropathic bladder and augmentation cystoplasty, *Urol Clin North Am* 45(4):571–585, 2018.
5. Ivlev I, Jerbkova S, Mishia M, et al.: Prostate screening patient decision aids: a systematic review and meta-analysis, *Am J Prev Med* 55(6):896–907, 2018.
6. Steineck G, Bjartell A: Degree of preservation of the neurovascular bundles during radical prostatectomy and urinary continence 1 year after surgery, *Eur Urol* 67(3):559–568, 2015.
7. Nelson R: New CDC guidelines recommend circumcision to cut HIV risk, *Lancet Infect Dis* 15(3):269–270, 2015.
8. Eswara J, Ko D: Minimally invasive techniques in urology, *Surg Oncol Clin N Am* 28(2):327–332, 2018.
9. Engelsgjerd J, LaGrange C: *Penile cancer*, Treasure Island, FL, 2023, StatPearls. www.ncbi.nlm.nih.gov. (Accessed 6 June 2023).
10. Coeman E, Radix A, Bouman W, et al.: Standards of care for the health of transgender and gender diverse people, version 8, *Int J Transgend Health* 23(Suppl 1):S1–259, 2022.
11. Scarritt M, Murdock M, Badylak S: Biologic scaffolds composed of excellular matrix for regenerative medicine. In Atala A, Lanza R, Mikos T, et al., editors: *Principles of regenerative medicine*, St. Louis, MO, 2019, Elsevier, pp 613–626.

Bibliography

AORN: *Guidelines for perioperative practice*, Denver, CO, 2024, The Association.

Bishoff J, Kavoussi L. In *Atlas of laparoscopic and robotic urologic surgery*, ed 4, Philadelphia, PA, 2023, Elsevier.

O'Connor E, Greenwell T: Urological complications following gynaecological surgery, *Obstet Gynaecol Reprod Med* 29(1):6–11, 2018.

Shergill A, Wang D, Thipphauong S, et al.: Comprehensive imaging and surgical review of urinary diversions: what the radiologist needs to know, *Curr Probl Diagn Radiol* 48:161–171, 2018.

36

Orthopedic Surgery

CHAPTER OUTLINE

The Art and Science of Orthopedic Surgery, 761

Anatomy and Physiology of the Musculoskeletal System, 762

Special Features of Orthopedic Surgery, 765

Extremity Procedures, 770

Fractures, 771

Joint Procedures, 775

Repair of Tendons and Ligaments, 784

Cast Application, 785

Complications After Orthopedic Surgery, 788

CHAPTER OBJECTIVES

After studying this chapter the learner will be able to:

- Identify the pertinent anatomy and physiology of the musculoskeletal system.
- Discuss several types of fractures and the stabilization of each.

- Describe several common specialty orthopedic instruments.
- Discuss bone healing.
- Discuss the process for applying a cast.
- Describe the care of a patient undergoing orthopedic surgery.

KEY TERMS AND DEFINITIONS

Arthrodesis Fusion of a joint.

Avascular necrosis Disruption of the blood supply to a bone, resulting in death and irreversible decay of the osseous tissue.

Bivalved cast Cast cut into two parts—front and back—for removal and reapplication.

Bone cement implantation syndrome (BCIS) Adverse physiologic response of the patient to placement of bone cement in the medullary canal.

Cast material Used to encase and stabilize a structure. Casts are made of plaster or fiberglass.

Closed reduction Closed reduction (CR) of a fracture without opening the skin.

Compartment syndrome Swelling between layers of fascia that causes damage to tissue. Toxins cause death of tissue.

Exothermic Generating heat.

Exsanguinate Evacuation of blood from a limb before inflating a tourniquet to create a bloodless field.

Fasciotomy Emergency procedure to release pressure on region of compartment syndrome.

Laminar airflow Specialized clean air delivery to the orthopedic operating room. The direction of airflow is carefully calculated to enter and exit the room without generating airborne particulate.

Open reduction and internal fixation (ORIF) of a fracture The fractured limb is opened surgically, and the bone is repaired with plates and screws.

Osteoblasts Basophilic cells that synthesize collagen and glycoprotein to form bone matrix.

Osteoclasts Cells in the bone that influence growth and regeneration by breakdown and resorption of existing cellular material.

Osteomyelitis Bone infection.

Union Healing process of bone. Nonunion is the failure of the bone to align and heal.

The Art and Science of Orthopedic Surgery

The word *orthopedics* is derived from two Greek words: *orthos,* meaning "straight," and *paithee,* meaning "child." As the name implies, orthopedics began with the treatment of crippled children by means of rest, braces, and exercise. Degenerative diseases and disabilities affecting the musculoskeletal system cause loss of function and impair activity of the aged. Consequently, orthopedic surgeons treat a large number of geriatric and pediatric patients compared with other surgical populations.

Orthopedic patient care is individualized. As a branch of medicine and a contemporary surgical specialty, orthopedics is concerned with the diagnosis, care, and treatment of musculoskeletal disorders—that is, injury to or disease of the body's system of bones, joints, ligaments, muscles, and tendons. Conservative, noninvasive medical and physical methods are used, if possible, to restore form and function.

Orthopedics depends on many disciplines to help evaluate and treat patients. Diagnostic imaging, bioengineering, electrobiology, genetics, microbiology, oncology, and transplantation are only a few of these. Professional registered perioperative nurses who specialize in orthopedic patient care are eligible for certification by examination through the Orthopaedic Nurses Certification Board (ONCB).

Eligibility for the certification includes current licensure in the United States or Canada and a minimum of 2 years' experience as a registered nurse with a minimum of 1000 hours of nursing practice in orthopedic patient care in the preceding 3 years. The certification period is 5 years and can be renewed through 75 contact hours (at least 50 orthopedic, 25 general) of continuing education, 1000 hours of practice, or by successful passage of the certification examination. (More information about certification and the National Association of Orthopaedic Nurses [NAON] is available at www.oncb.org/exam-eligibility.)

Anatomy and Physiology of the Musculoskeletal System

Structures that make up the musculoskeletal system provide bone shape, support, and stability; protect vital organs; and enable parts and the body as a whole to move. The musculoskeletal system includes bones, cartilage, joints, ligaments, muscles, and tendons. Orthopedic surgery is concerned primarily with these structures in the upper and lower extremities, including the shoulder and hip joints, and the vertebral column. Neurosurgeons also specialize in vertebral column surgery.

Bones

The human skeleton (Fig. 36.1) has 206 separate bones. The bony framework of the human body is divided into the axial skeleton, which consists of 80 bones that comprise the skull, vertebrae, and ribcage, and the appendicular skeleton, which consists of 126 bones that make up the limbs. Each upper extremity is composed of 32 bones, and each lower extremity is composed of 31 bones. Bones are classified according to shape: long, short, flat, and irregular. The humerus in the upper arm, radius and ulna in the forearm, femur in the thigh, and tibia and fibula in the lower leg are long bones.

The end of a long bone is referred to as the *epiphysis,* and the shaft is referred to as the *diaphysis.* Thin plates of cartilage are found in the ends of long bones. In immature bone this is the area of growth and elongation and accounts for 18% of pediatric

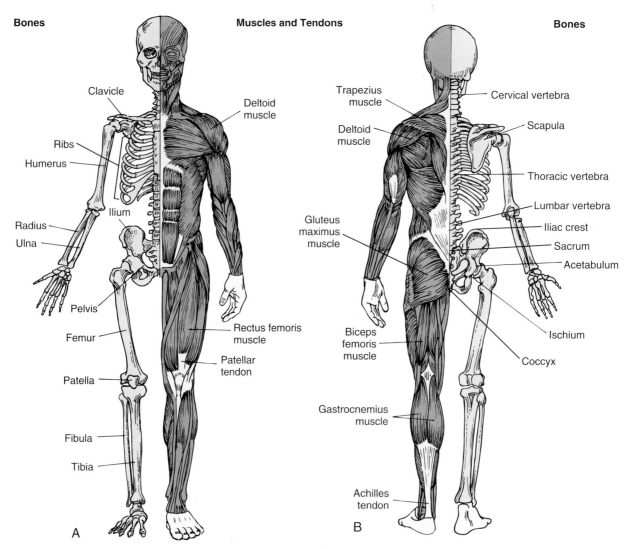

• **Fig. 36.1** Musculoskeletal system. **A,** Anterior view. **B,** Posterior view.

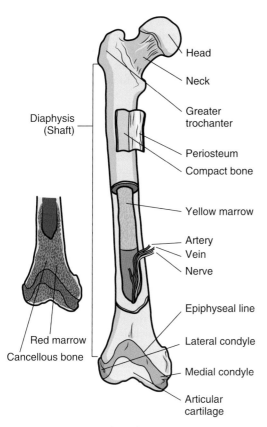

• **Fig. 36.2** Long bone anatomy.

fractures.[1] A child's x-ray may appear normal even when the epiphysis is fractured.[1] In mature bone these plates are ossified and do not grow (Fig. 36.2). The bones in the hand and foot are short bones. The scapula and patella are examples of flat bones. The vertebrae are irregular bones.

The cortex (outer layer) of bone is compact, hard connective tissue. This cortical osseous tissue surrounds porous, spongy, cancellous tissue. The innermost substance is bone marrow and is classified as either red or yellow according to its location and function (see Fig. 36.2).

The red marrow is found in the ends of long bones, porosities of cancellous bone, and flatter bones, such as the skull, sternum, and pelvic bones. This type of marrow is responsible for erythropoiesis, which is the formation of red blood cells and certain white blood cells. Yellow marrow is found in the medullary canals, or shafts of long bones, and has a higher adipose content.

Periosteum, a strong fibrous membrane, covers bone, except at joints. Pediatric periosteum is thicker and more pliable, allowing for less fracture displacement.[1] The blood supply and innervation penetrate periosteum and enter the bone through structures known as Volkmann canals. Lengthwise, lamellar structures, referred to as haversian canals, provide weight-bearing strength and passage for additional blood supply (Fig. 36.3). The inner aspect of bone is lined with endosteum, which is tissue similar to periosteum. In small children this layer contains osteoclasts that destroy bone to enlarge the marrow cavity for circumferential growth.

Bone Healing

Broken bones heal by a process referred to as union. Union of bones takes place in a series of steps (Fig. 36.4):

1. *Hematoma formation:* Blood accumulates in the area of break or injury. The inflammatory process ensues, and extravascular

• **Fig. 36.3** Vascular structure of bone. (From Mourad LA: *Orthopedic disorders,* St. Louis, 1991, Mosby.)

blood converts from liquid to a semisolid clot. Active phagocytosis removes necrotic tissue and debris.

2. *Callus formation:* Fibrin cells form a network around the injured area. The damaged periosteum is stimulated to generate osteoblasts, forming new bony substance referred to as *osteoid.* Minerals begin to accumulate in the network, forming a collagen callus. A callus is visible on radiograph within 1 to 2 weeks of injury.

3. *Calcification process:* Calcification begins and establishes support of the injury. Connective tissue proliferates across the site and is usually completely calcified within 6 weeks.

4. *Remodeling phase:* Excess cellular material is resorbed, and the bone resumes its preinjury strength and configuration. This remodeling phase is enhanced by stress and exercise. Depending on the site and severity of the injury, complete remodeling can take 6 months to 1 year to complete.

Cartilage

Cartilage, a smooth, relatively firm, compressible connective tissue, cushions most articular surfaces at the ends of bones. It does not have a direct blood supply and is devoid of lymphatics and nerves. Cartilage derives its nutrition from synovial fluid and maintains a high water content except in pathologic states.

Joints

Bones give stability, but the body must bend and flex for locomotion. The ends of bones come together at joints. The articular cartilage and construction of the joint prevent bones from scraping against each other. Tough, fibrous connective tissue forms the outside capsule of the joint, and a finer membranous lining secretes synovium, which is similar to egg albumin. The synovial fluid contains macrophages and white blood cells that keep the joint free of debris and bacteria that could interfere with mobility.

Joints are classified by variations in structure that permit movement (Fig. 36.5). The hip and shoulder are ball-and-socket joints; the knee, ankle, elbow, and phalangeal joints of the fingers are hinged; the wrist is a condyloid joint; and the thumb is a saddle joint. The proximal and distal bone ends are held securely in place by the joint capsule attached to both bone shafts and by ligaments.

• **Fig. 36.4** Bone healing stages.

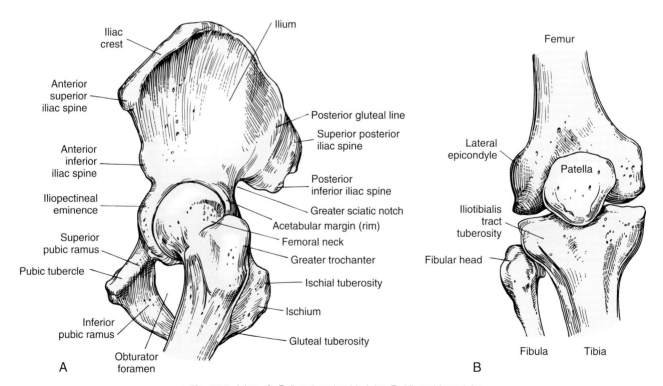

• **Fig. 36.5** Joints. **A,** Ball-and-socket hip joint. **B,** Hinged knee joint.

Ligaments

Ligaments are bands of flexible, tough fibrous tissue that join the articular surfaces of bones and cartilage. They become strong when the parallel configuration of their collagen fiber is oriented against the forces applied to them (e.g., the cruciate ligaments stabilize the knee joint). Ligaments are avascular and heal slowly. They do not readily reattach to bone when torn and are prone to subsequent reinjury.

Muscles

The human body has hundreds of muscles. Muscles are all the contractile tissues of the body and are classified as smooth (involuntary), branching (cardiac), or striated skeletal (voluntary). Muscles have a rich arterial supply because they require oxygen to perform many functions, and they have a multilevel venous drainage system because they perform as the venous pumps for resaturation by the lungs. They contract when an electrochemical impulse from the brain crosses the myoneural junction, causing fibers to shorten. Groups of muscles work together (i.e., contract simultaneously to bring about body movement).

Skeletal muscle is the largest category of muscle tissue. There are more than 600 skeletal muscles in the human body. Skeletal muscle constitutes approximately 23% of small female body weight and 40% of larger male body weight. Each muscle fiber is a single cell that ranges in length from 0.04 to 3 inches (1—80 mm). The fibers are bound together into fascia-covered bundles referred to as fasciculi. Several fascia-bound fasciculi constitute a skeletal muscle and contract in response to signals mediated by the nervous system and neurotransmitters, such as acetylcholine.

The peripheral attachment is referred to as the origin. The distal attachment is referred to as the insertion.

Tendons

Tendons are bands of extremely strong, flexible fibrous tissue that attach muscle bundles to the periosteum of bones (see Fig. 36.1 and Fig. 36.31, later in this chapter). They are encased in the synovial membrane sheath of movable joints.

Special Features of Orthopedic Surgery

The orthopedic surgeon, also referred to as an orthopedist or orthopod, attempts to restore function of the musculoskeletal system lost as a result of injury or disease. Surgical procedures may be performed to repair traumatic injuries, such as fractures, dislocations, torn ligaments, or severed tendons. Other procedures reconstruct joints, eradicate a benign or malignant disease process, or correct postural disabilities.

In addition to conventional x-rays, computed tomography (CT), magnetic resonance imaging (MRI), and bone densitometers allow evaluation of conditions amenable to surgical correction. Arthroscopy enhances diagnosis and treatment of joint disorders, especially those caused by sports injuries. Highly sophisticated implants and instrumentation make many orthopedic procedures possible. A large percentage of orthopedic surgical procedures involve contaminated traumatic wounds or tissues highly susceptible to infection.

The occurrence of osteomyelitis (infection in bone) can happen after a bone is injured in an accident, or a nonhealing ulcer, or after a surgical repair.[2] Acute osteomyelitis may cause nonunion of fractures. Microorganisms may harbor in a hematoma or in soft tissues and spread directly to bone via the circulatory system. The most common microorganisms that cause osteomyelitis are *Staphylococcus aureus, Staphylococcus epidermis,* and *Streptococcus* species.[2] Osteomyelitis spreads via hematogenous seeding from soft tissue or direct contamination during surgical treatment. Soft tissue spread is common in the lower legs, feet, and toes of persons with diabetes. Most ulcers heal, but 20% lead to amputation within 18 months.[2]

The incidence of osteomyelitis is highest among males of all age-groups. The risk increases by 50% with each decade of life.[2] The most prevalent microorganism is *S. aureus* (44%), which has been further complicated by antibiotic resistance. Chronic osteomyelitis is often associated with peripheral vascular disease.

Meticulous attention to sterile technique is critical in all orthopedic procedures to prevent or at least minimize the devastating effects of infection.[3] Sterility of implants and fixation devices is absolutely essential.[3] Medical management of the patient receiving an implant should include a minimum of 6 months between any active infection and the placement of a prosthetic.

Precautions also must ensure protection for the orthopedic surgeon and team, especially when caring for a trauma victim. Manipulation of sharp bony fragments and instrumentation can be hazardous. Transmission of bloodborne pathogens is readily possible because of aerosolization of bone and debris during drilling and sawing, using powered irrigation units, and using heavy instrumentation. In addition to standard precautions recommended by the Centers for Disease Control and Prevention (CDC), the American Academy of Orthopaedic Surgeons (AAOS) recommends:

1. Wearing protective attire.
    a. Wear knee-high, waterproof shoe covers or boots. Blood and body fluids frequently splash to the floor and lower legs. Shoe covers should be removed and changed if they become contaminated.
    b. Wear a fluid-impervious gown and/or a waterproof apron under the gown. Copious irrigation frequently is used.
    c. Double-glove at all times, and/or have additional protection for fingers. Cloth gloves or glove liners of woven Kevlar may be worn between latex gloves in cases of trauma and major reconstructive procedures, when sharp instruments and mechanical devices are used.
    d. Wear protective eyewear at all times. A full-face shield should be considered when splatter is anticipated. Powered bone instruments can produce a fine mist. A hooded suit—type helmet should be considered when powered bone instruments are used. See Fig. 16.7 for orthopedic helmeted attire.
2. Avoiding inadvertent penetration of the skin of personnel during the surgical procedure.
    a. Use instrument ties and other no-touch suturing and sharp instrument techniques whenever possible.
    b. Pass sharp instruments on a tray or magnetic mat, not hand to hand.
    c. Announce when instruments are being passed.
    d. Cover exposed internal wires and pins that extend through the skin with appropriate tubing, cork stoppers, or plastic caps.
3. Wearing clean gowning and gloving (i.e., the scrub person should change contaminated gloves before gowning and gloving another team member during the surgical procedure).

Instrumentation

Each orthopedic procedure must have the correct instrumentation for that particular bone, joint, tendon, or other structures the surgeon will encounter. An instrument used on a hip procedure is not appropriate for a hand procedure. Large bone orthopedic instruments are heavy—often large and bulky, resembling carpentry tools—but also delicate. Each instrument has a specific purpose and requires special care and handling. Orthopedic instruments can be divided into categories by functional design.

Exposing Instruments

To expose a bone or joint, special retractors and elevators are used (Fig. 36.6). Retractors are contoured to fit around the bone or joint without cutting or tearing muscles. Periosteal elevators are semisharp instruments used to strip periosteum from bone without destroying its ability to regenerate new bone. They are used for blunt dissection.

Grasping Instruments

Grasping instruments are required to hold, manipulate, or retract bone. Bone-holding forceps should be selected appropriately for the size of the bone in the surgical field. Bone hooks are used for retraction and leverage (Fig. 36.7). Heavy clamps are needed to hold smaller bones or grasp a joint capsule, such as a meniscus clamp for fibrocartilage in the knee.

Dissecting and Debulking Instruments

Cutting instruments are used to remove soft tissue around bone; to cut into, cut apart, or cut out portions of bone; and to smooth jagged edges of bone. The surgeon's armamentarium includes

osteotomes, gouges, chisels, curettes, rongeurs, reamers, bone-cutting forceps, meniscotomes, rasps, files, drills, and saws (Fig. 36.8). These have sharp edges. Extra care should be taken not to nick or damage cutting edges; they should always be protected on the instrument table and during cleaning, sterilizing, and storing. Fitted sterilizable cases (see Fig. 36.8, *E*), trays, foam towels, metal, or canvas cases are used to keep sets together by sizes (e.g., osteotomes, gouges, chisels, curettes), as well as to protect cutting edges.

Cutting instruments must be sharp. Osteotomes, chisels, gouges, and meniscotomes can be sharpened with handheld hones or a honing machine designed for this purpose. Most manufacturers provide a service for sharpening and repairing instruments. Curettes, rongeurs, and reamers should be returned for sharpening. Small drill bits and saw blades usually are disposable (Fig. 36.9).

Power-Driven Cutting Instruments

Instruments powered by electricity or compressed air or nitrogen offer precision in drilling, cutting, shaping, and beveling bone. The instrument may have rotary, reciprocating, or oscillating action. Rotary movement is used to drill holes or insert screws, wires, or pins. Reciprocating movement, a cutting action from front to back, and oscillating cutting action from side to side are used to cut or remove bone.

Some instruments have a combination of movements and can be changed from one to another with hand controls. In some the change may be made by adjusting the chuck forward or backward and locking it into the desired position. Powered instruments increase speed and decrease the fatigue caused by the use of manually driven drills, saws, and reamers. They also reduce blood loss from bone by packing tiny particles into cut surfaces.

Measuring Devices

Rulers, calipers, depth gauges, and flexible devices are standard use instruments for measuring angles and depth. Technologic devices such as digital angle gauges and computer scanning technology such as CT and robotic systems are important for the appropriate sizing of implants and selective bone cutting. Measurements of bone diameter are performed when selecting a joint prosthesis (Fig. 36.10).

Implant-Related Instruments

Drivers, clamps, and retractors are used for inserting, securing, or removing fixation and prosthetic implants. Each type of implant requires its own instrumentation. Instruments used for insertion

• **Fig. 36.6** Exposing instruments. **A,** Periosteal elevators. **B,** Bennett retractor.

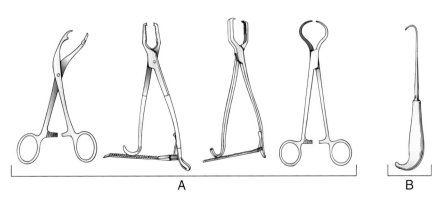

• **Fig. 36.7** Grasping instruments. **A,** Bone-holding forceps. **B,** Bone hook.

• **Fig. 36.8** Cutting instruments. **A,** Osteotome, curved or straight tapered blade. **B,** Gouge, curved, straight, or angled tip. **C,** Chisel, straight blade. **D,** Curette with assortment of sizes of cutting loops. **E,** Sterilizing case for set of osteotomes, gouges, chisels, or curettes. **F,** Rongeur. **G,** Bone cutter, straight or angled blade.

or extraction of metallic implants must be of the same metal as the implant to prevent galvanic reaction.

Materials and Equipment Used Frequently

The items discussed in this section are used frequently in many orthopedic procedures.

Bone Grafts

When necessary to provide structural support, a piece of bone from one part of the skeletal system may be obtained from the patient to reinforce another part of the skeletal system. Autologous cancellous and cortical bone is obtained from the crest of the ilium, and cortical bone is obtained from the fibula.

Free vascularized fibular grafts may be preferred to replace avascular (dead) bone or large segments of long bones after trauma or tumor resection. Autologous bone may not have adequate shape or strength, it may not be available in sufficient quantity, or the surgeon may deem it undesirable to subject the patient to a secondary incision or added operating time.

Allograft bone, coralline hydroxyapatite, or a bone graft substitute of tricalcium may be used. Donors, both living and cadaver, should be tested for human immunodeficiency virus (HIV) antibody before a graft is transplanted. Living donors should be retested 90 days after procurement if possible. People who are HIV positive, have any immune disorder or active infection, or have a history of hepatitis are excluded as donors. The probability of transmission of HIV in frozen or freeze-dried bone is remote. Secondary sterilization by ethylene oxide or ionizing radiation may increase the margin of safety but will reduce the biologic effectiveness of the graft.

Soft Tissue Allografts

Cartilage, ligaments, and tendons obtained from cadavers may be frozen or freeze-dried for use to augment soft tissue repairs.

Fixation Devices

External and internal fixation devices are used to stabilize or immobilize bone, usually after skeletal injury. External devices provide temporary support during healing. Many types of screws, plates, pins, and nails are used for temporary or permanent internal fixation of fractures or bone segments after a reconstructive procedure. Devices are also used to stabilize the vertebral column.

Oscillating saw blades

Reciprocating saw blades

Drill bits

Sagittal saw blades

• **Fig. 36.9** Saw blades and drill bits. (From Gregory B: *Orthopaedic surgery,* St. Louis, 1994, Mosby.)

• **Fig. 36.10** Measuring devices used in orthopedics. (From Gregory B: *Orthopaedic surgery,* St. Louis, 1994, Mosby.)

Prosthetic Implants

Prosthetic implants are used to permanently replace bone, joints, or tendons. They are made of nonmagnetic and electrolytically inert metals such as stainless steel, cobalt, and titanium alloys or polymers such as silicone and polyethylene. Some modular implants are made of several materials. All metals have some corrosion factors and can create a sensitivity reaction that results in a rash or dermatitis over the metallic implant.[4] Others have a polymeric or porous coating for tissue ingrowth over a portion of the implant. The design of the prosthesis is balanced and sized to fit according to body motion and measurements. The principles of biomechanics have revolutionized orthopedic surgery.

Polymethylmethacrylate (bone cement, PMMA) may be used to reinforce fixation or increase the strength of the implant. An orthopedic implant must withstand stresses within the internal environment. Fatigue strength, corrosion resistance, biocompatibility, and biomechanics are critical factors in selecting an implant.

Because of the high cost of prosthetics and fixation implants such as plates and screws, the inventory is kept as low as possible, yet large enough to ensure availability when needed.

Expensive implants are patient-charge items; they cannot be reused even if they are temporary. After measurements are taken, an implant of the correct size, shape, and design is selected from the sets available. Only the implant to be used is handled, without the others being touched. Sterilized sets of screws and plates are packaged in slotted trays according to size. Several graduated sizes are included in each set. Always check that the set includes the appropriate screwdriver for the type of screws in the set.

An infection around a fixation or prosthetic implant may require its removal, often resulting in permanent deformity or disability.[4] Sterility at the time of implantation is imperative. Joint implants are supplied sterile by the manufacturer. They can be stocked by consignment. Some facilities have the vendor bring in the needed sizes the day before surgery. Implant sizes and availability should be checked before the patient is brought to the operating room (OR). Confirmation of the correct implants is part of the "time out" process.

Implants, such as plates and screws, should not be flash-sterilized for any reason. Only standard cycles with appropriate biologic monitoring should be used. Some implants cannot withstand the heat of steam sterilization; ethylene oxide or some other appropriate method is used. Aeration time is necessary after ethylene oxide sterilization. Each sterilization cycle containing an implant(s) should be biologically tested per load and internal biologic monitoring. The implant(s) are not considered safe for use until a negative biologic test result is known. The manufacturer's recommendations should be followed.

A metal implant should not be removed from a package with an instrument. The surface could be scratched. An implant with a scratched or dented surface cannot be used because an electrolytic reaction will occur in the body. Team members who handle prosthetic implants should have clean, sterile gloves.

Specifics about the device or prosthesis and fixation method must be recorded in the patient's intraoperative record. This includes the type, size, and other identifying information, such as the manufacturer's lot number. Lot numbers are recorded in the departmental lot number log as appropriate in case of recall.

Lasers

Although not used as commonly as in other surgical specialties, lasers are used in some orthopedic procedures. They are useful in confined areas (e.g., through an arthroscope) to minimize bleeding.

Carbon Dioxide (CO_2) Laser

PMMA can be vaporized with a carbon dioxide (CO_2) laser to remove a cemented joint implant during a revision arthroplasty. Care is taken to use a smoke evacuator during the procedure. The CO_2 laser cannot penetrate a fluid environment; therefore the joint is insufflated with CO_2 gas to create a working space. The vaporization of cellular water destroys soft tissue. The CO_2 laser is useful in arthroscopic surgery for synovectomy and sculpturing articular cartilage. The joint is irrigated after the laser use to evacuate charred tissue.

Holmium:Yttrium Aluminum Garnet Laser

Used primarily in the knee, ankle, shoulder, and elbow, the holmium:yttrium aluminum garnet (Ho:YAG) laser was approved for spine in 2023.[5] The 2.1-mm wavelength with low penetration depth combined with pulsed high energy is delivered through a fine fiberoptic fiber. The Ho:YAG laser acts on water in cells without charring or damaging tissue extensively. It can ablate dense cartilage, bone, and soft tissue. It is used through an arthroscope to cut, shape, smooth, and sculpt cartilage and tissues in joints.

Neodymium:Yttrium Aluminum Garnet Laser

The neodymium:yttrium aluminum garnet (Nd:YAG) laser is used primarily in arthroscopy of the knee and shoulder joints on articular cartilage. It vaporizes protein and bonds collagen. It can be used for percutaneous disk procedures. Delivered fiberoptically, the Nd:YAG laser may have a reusable sapphire tip or a disposable, single-use ceramic contact tip. The Nd:YAG laser may be passed through a potassium titanyl phosphate (KTP) crystal, which has good cutting properties, to vaporize protein.

Bone Wax

Bone wax is used for hemostasis on cut bone. The surgeon's preference card should be checked before the packet is opened to the sterile field. The inner sterile foil packet can be placed in warm saline irrigation to soften the wax for use. Alternative bone edge hemostasis can be attained with Gelfoam slurry or synthetic non–bee's wax copolymers. Bone wax and other bone edge hemostatics are discussed in Chapter 29.

Nerve Stimulator

A nerve stimulator is used occasionally to identify neural tissue during a partial nerve resection to control spastic muscles such as in cerebral palsy or muscular dystrophy. When the popliteal nerve, for example, is stimulated with the nerve stimulator, the foot jerks. Both direct electric current and sterile disposable battery-operated stimulators are available.

Sutures

Ligaments, tendons, periosteum, and joint capsules are fibrous tissues. They are primarily tough, stringy collagen and contain few cells or blood vessels. As a result, they heal more slowly than do vascular tissues. Nonabsorbable synthetic materials are used to suture ligaments, tendons, and muscles involved in movement of the bony skeleton. Absorbable suture is preferred to suture periosteum. The surgeon's preferences should be checked before the suture packets are opened to the sterile field.

Casts and Braces

A cast, brace, or other rigid support is a means of obtaining external fixation of a fracture or a part after tendon repair, arthrodesis, or other surgical procedures. It is the means of putting a part at rest for healing after surgery or attempting to correct an injury or structural abnormality. (More information about casting is located at the end of this chapter.)

Cast Room

Casts may be applied in a cast room located outside of the OR suite, sometimes referred to as the plaster room. Closed reduction (CR) and other noninvasive structural support procedures are performed in the cast room. It keeps plaster dust from the perioperative environment—an important aspect of aseptic environmental control.

Laminar Air System

Special care must be used to carry out strict asepsis. Infection is the most serious, dreaded, and costly complication of orthopedic surgery. Some surgeons prefer to operate within an ultraclean air system, especially for total joint replacement procedures. Orthopedic surgeons use laminar airflow more frequently than do other surgical specialists.

A surgical patient isolation drape may be used to isolate the sterile field from personnel and equipment. Surgical helmets are available that isolate airborne contaminants shed from each team member. Hoses exhaust exhaled air. Masks are not worn under the helmet. Fig. 16.7 depicts the team wearing the helmet system. This system can be used independently or in conjunction with a laminar airflow system. Laminar airflow design is described and illustrated in detail in Chapter 10.

Isolation suits are fully contained gowns with acrylic plastic face shields and a battery-powered air filtration system. Because the suits retain heat, the OR may be kept at 70° F (21° C) for the comfort of team members. The patient should be maintained in a normothermic state with forced-air warming or protected by some other independent warming method.

Fracture Table

An orthopedic OR bed, often referred to as the fracture table, is used for many surgical procedures requiring traction, x-ray image intensification, and/or cast application. The patient is anesthetized on the transport cart before being positioned on the fracture table. The many available attachments make possible any desired position and traction on any part of the body. The table can be raised, tilted laterally, or put into Trendelenburg or reverse Trendelenburg position.

Attachments are designed not only for stabilizing the patient in the desired position but also for exerting traction to help reduce a fracture and for providing a means of evaluating the diagnosis or surgical site by real-time x-ray imaging. Bakelite or some other radiolucent material that does not interfere with x-ray studies is used for attachments that might otherwise obscure the findings.

Essential standard component attachments on all models of orthopedic tables include narrow, three-section patient body supports, a lateral body brace, a sacral rest, perineal post, and traction apparatus.[5] Optional accessories are available to accommodate the types of procedures performed and the model of the OR bed. When the fracture table is used, the following preparations are considered:

1. Consult the surgeon's preferences and manufacturer's manual for attachments needed for each desired position. The fracture table is used for supine procedures and cannot accommodate lateral positioning.
2. Check the patient's height and weight in kilograms. Each style of OR bed has specific weight limits. The weight limit is printed on the base of the table.
3. Assemble the necessary attachments. Pad all parts of the OR bed and attachments to prevent pressure on joints, the sacrum, and the perineum.
4. Attach the standard components and accessories to the OR bed frame so all is in readiness for positioning the patient after the administration of anesthesia. The patient may have a spinal or general anesthesia. Patients with several comorbidities usually have spinal anesthesia to avoid any complications associated with general anesthesia.[6]

5. Arrange appropriate staff to move the patient from one surface to another. The patient will be a full lift whether general or regional anesthesia is used. Placement on the fracture table is somewhat precarious because the body section is very narrow. It is easy for the patient to fall if not carefully positioned and secured.

6. Secure the patient with recommended safety devices.

X-ray Equipment

Conventional x-ray equipment and fluoroscopy frequently are used during orthopedic procedures. Considerations for patient safety and personnel protection described in Chapter 13 apply to the use of x-ray for all invasive or noninvasive orthopedic procedures performed in the OR suite. Special positioning and draping techniques may be necessary, especially when C-arm fluoroscopy is used.

Often both anteroposterior (AP) and lateral views are necessary to assess the alignment of a bone or determine the position of a fixation device or prosthetic implant. Radiographs or C-arm fluoroscopic images document the work of the surgeon for the permanent record.

Special Considerations in Orthopedic Surgery

1. Unit beds are used to transport patients in traction apparatus. Beds, frames, and transport carts can be decontaminated in the vestibule/exchange area.

2. A cast should be removed preoperatively in the cast room. If the OR suite does not have a cast room, a cast may be bivalved (cut) in the patient's room and then removed in the OR to minimize the dispersal of particulates in the air.

3. Positioning the patient intraoperatively and postoperatively should be directed by the surgeon. Immobilization and good body alignment contribute to patient comfort and prevention of neurovascular injury. Pillows or other supports should not cause pain, impair function of unaffected muscles and joints, or compromise circulation.

4. Transcutaneous electrical nerve stimulation (TENS) may be used for postoperative analgesia. The electrode pads are affixed to the skin along the sides of the incision when a dressing is applied. Before application, the skin should be cleansed with water. (Saline is a conductor, so it cannot be used for cleansing.) The wires are connected to the stimulator in the postanesthesia care unit (PACU) or after recovery from anesthesia. The patient can be taught preoperatively how to use TENS for relief of pain postoperatively.

5. Electrostimulation promotes cellular responses in bone and ligaments. Mechanically stressed bone generates electrical potentials related to patterns of bone regeneration. If stimulated, healing may accelerate.

Both internal direct-current stimulators and external pulsating electromagnetic field or electrical capacitor devices are used to stimulate bone and neural regeneration, revascularization, epiphyseal growth, and ligament maturation.

Extremity Procedures

Although instrumentation varies by procedure and the size of structures involved, basic techniques apply to handling both upper and lower extremities.

General Considerations

1. A sterile irrigating basin or pan is placed under an extremity to catch solution if an open wound is to be cleansed, irrigated, and debrided, as for a compound fracture. If an irrigating basin is not used, the runoff is collected by an absorbent pad under the prepped limb. A staff aide wearing gloves can elevate the limb during the prep procedure.

2. A pneumatic tourniquet is commonly used for a surgical procedure on or below the elbow or knee to provide a blood-free field. The tourniquet cuff is applied before the extremity is prepped. Prevent prep solution from running under the tourniquet cuff by covering the cuffed area with a sticky drape or towel. The tourniquet is not inflated until the limb is elevated and exsanguinated using a sterile Esmarch bandage. It is important to exsanguinate the limb to ensure a bloodless field and prevent blood clots. Do not discard the Esmarch bandage in case it is needed again. Reroll it and place on the back table.

Always check the pressure setting with the surgeon before inflating a tourniquet. Ischemia time is a critical factor in patient safety. Notify the surgeon of the time lapse after the first hour and every 15 minutes thereafter throughout tourniquet inflation. Document the tourniquet location, time, pressure, and unit identifying number.

3. The extremity is elevated for the skin prep. A dry, sterile drape is positioned under the limb by the scrub person before it is lowered to the sterile field.

4. A self-adhering incise drape may be used as the first drape applied over the incision site. If the extremity must be manipulated during the surgical procedure, the entire circumference must be draped free with sterile stockinette.

5. Stockinette may be used over a self-adhering plastic drape or to cover skin and wrapped with Coban or Ace bandage to keep the circumferential drape in place. This wrap is cut with bandage scissors over the line of the incision. An extremity sheet or split sheet may be used over the wrapped stockinette as a body drape. A large sterile glove can be placed over the foot to protect the sterile field during lower limb surgery.

6. A fluid-control drape collects blood and irrigating fluids in a pouch to prevent strike-through of and runoff from drapes. Fluids can be drained or suctioned for disposal. Blood may be suctioned directly from the surgical site for autotransfusion if blood loss is more than 400 mL, as in some procedures.

7. After a surgical procedure on a knee joint, a pressure dressing is usually applied to prevent serum accumulation. This may be a Robert Jones dressing, which includes a soft cotton batting roll, sheet wadding, and cotton elastic bandage. A cotton roll or other bulky material may be placed on each side of the knee and held in place with sheet wadding. A four-ply, crinkled-gauze bandage or cotton elastic bandage over this provides even, gentle pressure. Depending on the surgical procedure, a plaster splint or some other type of knee immobilizer may be preferred.

8. After a surgical procedure on a shoulder, the arm may be bound against the side of the chest for immobilization. An absorbent pad or a large piece of cotton or sheet wadding is placed under the arm to keep skin surfaces from touching because they may macerate. The arm is held in a shoulder immobilizer that supports the humerus and wrist, or it may be bound firmly to the side of the chest with a cotton elastic bandage.

9. Postoperatively the extremity is elevated on a pillow placed lengthwise. This facilitates venous return, decreases swelling, and minimizes pressure on nerves. The hand should be elevated above the level of the heart; the toes must be higher than the nose.

Indications for Orthopedic Surgery

Preoperative assessment of an acute or chronic disability affecting the musculoskeletal system of an extremity includes evaluation of the extent of bony or soft tissue involvement with or without concomitant neurovascular compromise.

Assessment for signs and symptoms of neurovascular impairment in an extremity includes the six Ps: *p*allor, *p*ulses, *p*ain, *p*aresthesia, *p*uffiness, and *p*aralysis. The six Ps are assessed postoperatively and monitored until support devices, such as casts or splints, are removed from the surgical site.

Adult orthopedic surgery is usually necessitated by trauma or by a degenerative disease process. Surgical procedures on the following major anatomic classifications of structures are discussed in this chapter:

- Fracture of bones
- Reconstruction of joints
- Repair of tendons and ligaments

Fractures

Intact bones are essential to the stability and mobility of upper and lower extremities. A comminuted (splintered) or fractured (broken) bone can cause malfunction and pain. Fractures vary by cause, location, type of fracture line, and extent of injury. Typical long bone fracture lines are depicted in Fig. 36.11. They are either traumatic or pathologic.

1. *Traumatic fracture:* The impact, forced twisting, or bending of an accidental injury can break one or more bones in the body. Traumatic fractures can occur when bone has become fatigued from overwork or has inadequate muscle support during exertion; a stress fracture may result (e.g., in the tibia or fibula of an athlete). Traumatic fractures are either closed or open.
    a. *Closed fracture:* Sometimes referred to as *simple fractures,* broken fragments do not protrude through adjacent tissue

to puncture the skin. The fracture is named for the direction of the line of breakage (e.g., spiral, transverse, oblique).
    b. *Open fracture:* Also referred to as a *compound fracture,* the proximal or distal end of bone, or both, protrude from the fracture site through adjacent tissues and skin. Because of the risk for infection developing in the exposed bone, an open fracture is a surgical emergency.

2. *Pathologic fracture:* Demineralization of bone (e.g., from osteoporosis or the aging process) and primary or metastatic malignant bone disease can spontaneously fracture a bone without undue stress. Although they are technically simple fractures, pathologic fractures may require more than simple fixation of bone fragments.

Bone allografts or autografts may be needed. Methylmethacrylate bone cement may be used to increase the strength of a fixation implant or as an adjunct to fill a bone defect (e.g., after removal of a tumor around a pathologic fracture). Bone grafts can be biologic, synthetic, or a combination (bioengineered) of substitutes. The patient's own bone can be ground in a bone mill to autograft the fixation. A compound made from collagen protein mixed with ceramic material may serve to stimulate creation of cartilage and osteoblasts (bone-forming cells).

Mechanical means are used to reduce a fracture and immobilize the parts, maintaining the fragments in proper alignment. Fractures must be handled gently with support above and below the site to prevent further trauma. The surgeon should assume responsibility for supporting the fracture site during transfer of the patient from one bed surface to another. Other personnel must be instructed regarding the special care needed to move a patient. The surgeon removes or directs removal of temporary splints or traction. An adequate number of personnel must be available so the patient can be lifted gently. More lifters should be on the affected side because this helps support the fracture during transfer.

In treating a fracture the surgeon seeks to accomplish a solid union of bone in perfect alignment, return joints and muscles to normal position, prevent or repair vascular trauma, and rehabilitate the patient as early as possible. Treatment of fractures usually includes three distinct phases: reduction, immobilization, and rehabilitation. The methods of treating fractures include the following:

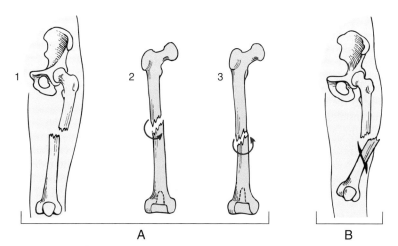

• **Fig. 36.11** Fractures of a long bone. **A,** Simple closed fractures. *1,* Transverse break runs across bone; *2,* oblique break runs in slanting direction across bone; *3,* spiral break coils around bone. **B,** Compound open fracture protrudes through skin.

- Closed reduction (CR) with immobilization
- Skeletal traction
- External fixation
- Open reduction and internal fixation (ORIF)
- Electrostimulation

Closed Reduction

A fracture may be manipulated (set) to replace the bone in its proper alignment without opening the skin. This technique is referred to as a closed reduction (CR). Many fractures of the lower leg or arm can be treated by CR.

Often performed in the emergency department, CR with the patient under anesthesia and application of a device for immobilization may be done in the cast room of the OR suite.

A plaster, fiberglass, or other lightweight synthetic cast, cast-brace, or molded plastic fracture-brace may be used to hold the reduced fracture site in alignment during union.

Skeletal Traction

Traction is the pulling force exerted to maintain proper alignment or position. In skeletal traction the force is applied directly on the bone after insertion of pins, wires, or tongs placed through or into the bone. A small sterile setup is required. Traction is applied by means of pulleys and weights. Weights provide a constant force; pulleys help establish and maintain constant direction until the fractured bone reunites.

Forearm or Lower Leg

A Kirschner wire (K-wire), either plain or threaded, or a Steinmann pin is drilled through the bone (preferably cortical) distal to the fracture site. For forearm fractures the wire or pin must be strong enough to prevent side-to-side, angular, and rotary motion while the fracture is healing. A traction bow is attached to the protruding ends of the wire or pin. The pulleys are fastened to this bow. The ends of the wire or pin are covered with corks or plastic tips to protect the patient and personnel from the sharp ends.

Finger

A fine K-wire may be drilled through the distal phalanx. The ends may be attached to a banjo splint. Or a cast may be applied to the forearm with a loop of heavy wire incorporated in it that fans out beyond the fingers. The K-wire is fastened to this loop by a rubber band.

External Fixation

External fixation devices are used for the treatment of selected types of skeletal injuries, especially to the pelvis and extremities, with marked soft tissue loss and instability. Skeletal pins and connecting bars permit rigid fixation but with access to devitalized skin and soft tissue for wound management, especially for open injuries of the tibia. Fixation devices used for unstable pelvic fractures allow early ambulation.

Femur and Tibia

External fixation applies tension and compression forces to bone. Tension stimulates bone growth. Compression helps control infection and promotes union in fractures without bone loss. External fixators also can be used for correcting bone deformities and for lengthening the femur and tibia after osteotomy for limb length discrepancy. Several types of devices used on the lower extremities allow the patient to ambulate.

Stabilization Bar

Two or more pins or screws aligned parallel to each other are inserted into the cortex of each fragmented section of bone. These may be connected to a metal bar, such as the dynamic axial fixator, that runs parallel to the bone on one side of the leg, or the pins may protrude through the leg and be clamped onto bars on both sides, such as with the Hoffman external fixation system.

Ilizarov Technique

Particularly useful for salvaging infected and nonunion fractures, the Ilizarov external fixator frame consists of a series of stainless steel rings connected by rods, nuts, and bolts. It can be assembled in various configurations and lengths. Wires are inserted percutaneously through the bone and connected under tension on both sides of the rings. Usually two wires are attached to each ring, at the proximal and distal levels, to stabilize bone fragments. The placement of wires is checked under C-arm fluoroscopy. Threaded rods are placed parallel to each other and in line with the longitudinal axis of the bone to connect and stabilize rings.

The system has more than 120 interchangeable components, including wrenches, pliers, and wire cutters. Wire insertion is a sterile procedure. The frame is assembled on the sterile field. It weighs approximately 8 lb (3.6 kg) when fully assembled.

Open Reduction and Internal Fixation

Internal fixation is necessary for fractures that are not amenable to CR and stabilization with cast or brace immobilization, skeletal traction, or external fixation methods. Open reduction exposes the fracture site for realignment under direct visualization; CR sometimes precedes the insertion of an internal fixation device. The fracture is reduced to align fragments. If vascular structures have been traumatized, internal fixation followed by vascular repair may be necessary to restore arterial tissue perfusion and adequate venous drainage.

The procedure may be performed with the patient under regional block anesthesia, especially in patients in poor physical condition, such as a geriatric patient or one who has suffered multiple traumas. Intravenous (IV) moderate sedation may be given to dull the patient's awareness of the sound of drills and mallets.

Excellent results can be obtained with internal fixation of a fracture soon after it occurs. This method provides firm immobilization and close approximation of the fragments so that the gap between the ends is not too great for the callus to bridge. It reduces to a minimum the space between fragments and movement at the fracture site (Fig. 36.12). Healing seems to take place faster. The patient starts non–weight-bearing exercises and progresses to ambulation early, which reduces joint stiffness and muscle atrophy and prevents a long period of rehabilitation.

A Colles fracture of the radial bone in the wrist is sometimes surgically stabilized with plates and screws (Fig. 36.13, *A*) or CR under finger trap distraction (see Fig. 36.13, *B*).

Screws, Plates, and Nails

Many types of rigid fixation implants are available. The surgeon chooses the type best suited to serve its purpose. The implant may remain permanently, or it may be removed after the fracture has healed, especially in a young person. For example, a plate can

• **Fig. 36.12** Open reduction and internal fixation of femur with plates and screws. Note that one screw has been transfixed across the fracture line for stability.

cause a stress fracture from the shielding forces exerted over time along its rigid edges on the less rigid underlying bone. If osteomyelitis develops, an implant must be removed.

Screws, plates, nails, rods, and pins are made of stainless steel 316 L, titanium, or cobalt alloys. These metals are nonmagnetic and electrolytically inert. Only one kind of metal is used in a patient. The instrumentation used to implant it must be of the same metal. Semirigid carbon fiber–reinforced plastic plates also are used in some situations.

Biodegradable screws, plates, and rods provide stability during osteogenesis. A plate may be affixed to cortex of the bone, or an intramedullary rod can be inserted into the bone. The type and size of implant(s) must be documented in the patient's record and logged according to institution policy and procedure.

Screws

Screws alone may be used for fixation of an oblique or spiral fracture of a long bone. Screws must be long enough to penetrate both cortices. Hard cortical bone gives the best fixation, and two cortices generally hold better than one. Screws are available in various lengths and diameters. Not all screws have the same type of head (e.g., heads may be single slot, cross slot, concave cross slot, hexagon, or Phillips) (Fig. 36.14). The correct screwdriver must be used with each type of screw.

Compression Plates and Screws

Many fractures requiring open reduction are rigidly fixed through the compression method. Compression plates are heavy and strong. They are held in place by specially designed cortical lag screws. The threads of these screws are deeper than those on other types of screws and are farther apart, which allows a larger amount of bone between the threads. This construction gives maximum holding power and rigid fixation. Locking compression plates (LCPs) are available, which gives the surgeon two options: placement of a conventional screw in one side or use the threaded hole to place a threaded screw to prevent movement or loosening.

A compression instrument may be used. It is connected to the end of the plate and then fastened to the bone with a short screw. When the nut on the compression instrument is tightened, the bone fragments are brought tightly together. The remaining screws are put into the plate, and the fracture is fixed. Screws alone are used only in selected situations. A cast may or may not be applied.

After ORIF of an acetabular fracture, a compression plate may be bent to conform to the contour of the acetabulum and secured with long cortical and cancellous lag screws.

Eggers Plate and Screws

The plate is slotted, which permits the muscle tone of the extremity to keep the ends of the fragments pressed closely together. The pressure stimulates osteogenesis.

Sherman Plate and Screws

The appropriate-size plate is fitted to the contour of the bone, by bending it slightly if necessary, before the screws are applied. With a drill guide, holes for the screws are drilled with an electric or air-powered drill in the center of the screw hole and perpendicularly to the plate. The drill bit should be slightly smaller than the screws. The screws should pass through both cortices of the bone.

Nails

An intertrochanteric or subtrochanteric fracture of the neck of the femur may be treated by inserting a nail, compression screw, or multiple pins through the neck into the head of the femur (Fig. 36.15). Many different types of nails are used. They are usually inserted over or alongside a guidewire. The nail may form a continuous angulated unit with a plate that fits on the outer lateral cortex of the femur, or the plate may be attached and the nail, screws, or pins inserted separately. Screws secure the plate to the shaft of the femur before or after the nail is inserted, depending on the design of the implant.

The patient is positioned supine on the fracture table. The surgeon and assistants assume responsibility for moving and positioning the patient. Fig. 36.16 shows the position for nailing the left hip. The procedure may be performed with C-arm fluoroscopic image intensification rather than conventional x-ray machines. All sterile tables are positioned on the affected side.

Intramedullary Nailing. An intramedullary nail, rod, or pin is driven into the medullary canal through the site of the fracture (Fig. 36.17). This brings the ends together for union, splints the fracture, and eases pain. It permits early return of function so the patient can be ambulatory. Intramedullary implants also provide a method of holding fragments in alignment in comminuted fractures. Rigid implants generally are used for pathologic fractures or an impending fracture of diseased bone. Flexible intramedullary rods may be preferred for some traumatic fractures, particularly femoral fractures. The length, size, and shape of the nail or pin depend on the bone to be splinted.

The patient with a femoral or tibial fracture is positioned on the fracture table. This permits traction as needed to maintain reduction. Fig. 36.18 shows the position of the patient for intramedullary nailing of the left tibia. C-arm fluoroscopy is used.

The fracture may be repaired by either ORIF or CR procedures. In some situations the medullary canal must be reshaped or enlarged before an implant is inserted. The implant may be removed after union at the fracture site has taken place, especially

A

Ulnar
styloid

C

B

• **Fig. 36.13 A,** Mechanism of Colles fracture of wrist with incision for open reduction. **B,** Common Colles fractures. **C,** Closed reduction of Colles fracture on wrist positioning frame.

if it causes pain. If nonunion occurs, the implant may need to be removed.

Interlocking Nail Fixation. After CR of the fracture, an intramedullary rod or nail is inserted down the length of the shaft of a long bone without exposing the fracture site. This technique is called closed intramedullary nailing and may be used for transverse or short oblique fractures of the midshaft of the femur or tibia. An incision is made to expose the femoral trochanter or tibial tuberosity.

To stabilize more oblique, comminuted fractures and those beyond the midshaft region, transfixion screws are also used with locking nails. These screws pass through the cortices of the bone and holes in the intramedullary nail. This method of closed interlocking nail fixation may be static or dynamic, depending on the location and configuration of the fracture. In the static method, screws are inserted in both the proximal and distal fragments; in the dynamic method they are proximal or distal. Several types of interlocking nail systems are available based on patient's need. All systems prevent gliding and rotation of fragments, as well as shortening of the limb from bone loss.

Joint Procedures

Joint function depends on the quality of its structures. Articular cartilage covers the two ends of bone where they meet to form the joint. Bones are held securely in place at their articulation by ligaments and the joint capsule attached to both bone shafts. The synovial membrane lining the joint capsule secretes synovial fluid to lubricate the joint. When the joint is injured or altered by arthritis or some other degenerative disease, normal joint motion is impaired and/or painful.

Compression plate

Sherman screw hole plate

Eggers slotted plate

Bone screws

Concave cross slot head

Single slot head

Cross slot head

Simulated Phillips head

• **Fig. 36.14** Fixation plates and screws.

• **Fig. 36.16** Position on orthopedic table for nailing left hip. Note arm on affected side suspended from screen to remove it from surgical field. Note traction on affected leg and support under knee. Elevated right leg permits C-arm x-ray to be adjusted below for lateral view.

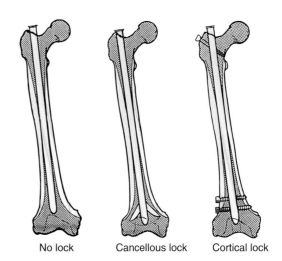

No lock   Cancellous lock   Cortical lock

• **Fig. 36.17** Examples of intramedullary nail and rod devices. (From Gustilo RB, Kyle RF, Templeman DC, editors: *Fractures and dislocations,* St. Louis, 1993, Mosby.)

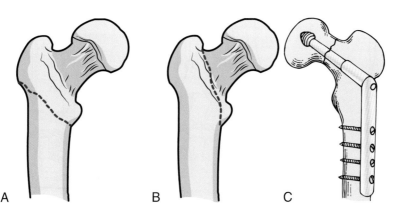

A   B   C

• **Fig. 36.15** Fractured hip. **A,** Type I fracture. **B,** Type II fracture. **C,** Compression hip screw for fixation of fracture of femoral neck.

Dislocations

Dislocation of one or more bones at a joint may occur with or without an associated fracture. Tendons, ligaments, and muscles are deranged. The articular surface of the bone is displaced from the joint capsule. The force of displacement damages the capsule and tears ligaments and surrounding tissues. Blood vessel and nerve damage can occur, impeding circulation and causing changes in sensation and muscle strength.

CR, with or without skeletal traction, may be necessary at the time of an acute injury. If CR fails to stabilize the joint and prevent recurrence, ORIF may be necessary. Surgical procedures to stabilize chronic recurrent dislocations are most frequently performed on the shoulder.

Arthrodesis

Fusion of a joint may be achieved by removing the articular surfaces and securing bony union or by inserting a fixation implant that inhibits motion. Arthrodesis may be performed after resection of a recurrent benign, potentially malignant, or malignant lesion that involves the ends of the bones and joint. After resection of the diseased portion of the bones, the joint may be stabilized with a bone graft or an intramedullary fixation implant.

• **Fig. 36.18** Position on orthopedic table for intramedullary nailing of left tibia. Note left foot anchored to foot holder and knee resting on elevated curved knee rest. Right foot is anchored, and knee rest is adjusted for support of leg. A post is placed between the legs once the patient is positioned for safety.

Arthrodesis is performed most frequently for lesions in the distal femur and proximal tibia around or including the knee joint. It also may be performed to relieve osteoarthritic pain or stabilize a joint that does not respond to other methods of treatment after injury, such as instability of the thumb. Because arthrodesis limits motion, other joint reconstructive procedures are usually attempted first.

Triple arthrodesis of the ankle is performed to correct deformity or muscle imbalance of the foot. The subtalar, calcaneocuboid, and talonavicular tarsal joints are fused. Staples are sometimes used to hold bones together (Fig. 36.19).

Arthroplasty

Arthroplasty (reconstruction of a joint) may be necessary to restore or improve range of motion and stability or relieve pain.[7] This may be done by resurfacing, reshaping, or replacing the articular surfaces of the bones. The incisional approach to the hip joint can vary according to the technique used. Traditional incisions were longer than current methods used (Fig. 36.20). Hip arthroplasty is performed using several methods (Fig. 36.21).

Femoral and Humeral Head Replacement

A metal Austin-Moore prosthetic implant can replace the femoral or humeral head and neck to articulate with the existing acetabulum (Fig. 36.22). Austin-Moore prostheses have a shaft that is driven into the medullary canal of the bone. The head of the natural femur is removed. In some cases the femoral head is ground into bone graft matrix for reimplantation around the prosthesis. The neck is shaped or removed as necessary for accurate placement of the prosthesis. A reamer may be used to enlarge the canal for insertion of the prosthesis. These prostheses are used for the following purposes:

- To mobilize the joint in arthritic patients
- To replace a comminuted fractured head when soft tissue attachments are destroyed
- To replace the head if avascular necrosis or nonunion occurs after reduction of fractures

A free vascularized fibular graft may be preferred to decompress the femoral head, provide structural stability, and vascularize bone in an area of avascular necrosis. This procedure preserves the femoral head rather than replacing it with a prosthesis after removal of dead bone. The peroneal artery and vein are preserved with the graft. Under the operating microscope the vessels are

A   B   C

• **Fig. 36.19** Ankle arthrodesis. **A,** Incision for internal ankle fusion (arthrodesis). **B,** Fusion. **C,** External fixator during fusion.

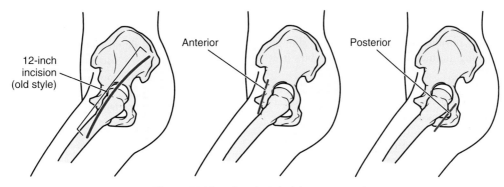

• **Fig. 36.20** Hip arthroplasty incisions compared.

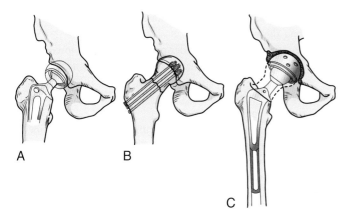

• **Fig. 36.21** Hip arthroplasty methods.

• **Fig. 36.22** Austin-Moore prosthesis to replace femoral head and neck in hemiarthroplasty. Shaft is driven into medullary canal of femur.

anastomosed to branches of the femoral circumflex vessels. Restoration of vascularization prevents progression of necrosis and stimulates osteogenesis (new bone formation).

Femoral Head Surface Replacement

As an alternative to femoral head replacement a concentric metal shell is cemented over the femoral head. A high-density polyethylene shell is cemented into the acetabulum. Surface replacement to relieve severe hip pain and disability is reserved for young adults with good femoral and acetabular bone stock.

Patients with sclerotic, well-vascularized subchondral bone of hypertrophic osteoarthritis, for example, may be candidates for this procedure. Resurfacing induces healing and reduces stress on the hip joint.

Total Joint Replacement

The surgeon's goal in total joint arthroplasty is to alleviate pain and create functional mobility and stability.[7] The prosthesis must maintain normal anatomic relationships and biologic fixation to bone. Correct alignment and fit of component parts are crucial aspects of their function.

Although prosthetic implants for some joints have not been as well developed as those for others, total joint replacement is an accepted therapeutic modality, especially for the hip, knee, ankle, and elbow joints. Usually performed to improve mobility and relieve the pain of severe arthritic joints, total joint replacement may be indicated when other therapeutic measures have failed to correct a congenital defect, traumatic injury, or degenerative disease.

A functional design for the prosthesis must consider a combination of load bearing, strain-stress, and kinetics in association with the pathologic condition. Positioning of the prosthesis influences the distribution of stress and rate of wear.

The bones on both sides of the joints are replaced or resurfaced. Both component parts must be solidly anchored to avoid movement of the prosthesis and wear on surrounding tissue. All movement must be between the smooth articulating surfaces of the prosthesis. Various alloys, ceramics, and high-density polyethylene or silicone are used; component parts of many prostheses are made of more than one material.

Metal-to-plastic joints are self-lubricating. Natural synovial fluids help lubricate other types. The rate of wear on parts must be low so the prosthesis will remain functional over many years (the exact number is undetermined). The major complication of total joint arthroplasty is loosening of the prosthetic components over time, particularly in weight-bearing joints of obese and/or active patients. Configuration, surface features, and the method of fixation of component parts influence the mechanical stability of an "artificial" joint. The orthopedic surgeon must consider the following factors:

1. *Biomechanics:* Ideally a prosthesis provides full range of motion. The support provided by cartilage, ligaments, and the articular capsule surrounding the prosthesis influences its stability. Prostheses may be constrained or nonconstrained.

a. A constrained prosthesis provides a stable joint but restricts motion to a single plane or limits motion in all planes.

b. A nonconstrained prosthesis allows gliding and shifting motions resembling normal range of motion, but it is inherently unstable.

2. *Biophysical components:* A total joint prosthesis has at least two components—one for each side of the articulation. To determine the size and shape of components to fit the patient, measurements of bones that form the joint may be obtained preoperatively by developing templates (i.e., patterns on grids) from the patient's radiographs. If templates have not been obtained, x-rays and measurements are taken at the surgical field. The surgeon also takes trial measurements at the site to verify the correct selection of the implant.

a. Solid components have a predetermined configuration. The surgeon must select the most appropriate size from those available. Bone may need to be reshaped to accommodate the prosthesis.

b. Modular systems have interchangeable components so the surgeon can customize the prosthesis at the OR bed. For example, the width, depth, or length can be adjusted to the patient's anatomy. A quick-setting silastic mold may be formed for precise matching in three dimensions. The mold is sent to a laboratory, where the prosthesis is customized with the use of a laser scanner and a computer-guided milling machine.

c. Computer-assisted arms and robotic surgical techniques use CT technology to preplan the surgical procedure.[8] Exact models of the patient's anatomy are created in three-dimensional format for precise measurements and implant size. The surgeon guides the robot or arm to drill or make precision cuts for improved implant position and better outcomes. This technology can be used for most joint replacements.

3. *Fixation:* The bone into which the component part is implanted and the surface of the prosthesis will determine the method of fixation.

a. Press-fit fixation relies on direct bone-to-prosthesis contact. This can be achieved by a variety of methods, including reshaping the bone to the size and/or configuration of the implant and/or securing threads, pegs, or screws on the prosthesis into bone.

b. Biofixation refers to a surface on the implant that allows tissue ingrowth for stability. Ingrowth is defined as the development of bony tissue in an empty hole. A portion of the implant has a porous or rough surface. Bone grows into pores or interstices. Many types of coatings are used, such as tricalcium phosphate or coralline hydroxyapatite sprayed on the surface.

Others have a porous material, such as polysulfone, bonded to metal. Surfaces that are porous enough for bone ingrowth without greatly expanding the surface area or weakening the implant are most desirable. Cementless prostheses require a precise fit in bones. They are particularly suited for young, active patients.

c. PMMA fixation uses self-curing thermoplastic acrylic cement to provide long-term fixation. It is not a type of glue but rather a space-filling fixation material. Several different preparations of PMMA, commonly referred to as bone cement, are available. Several types contain antibiotics such as gentamicin or tobramycin. Although antibiotics may be a component, these types are not recommended for use in a joint with active infection.

The powder and liquid components are mixed at the instrument table in a vacuum container immediately before insertion into the intramedullary canal of a long bone or socket of a joint. It becomes like dough when mixed. PMMA cures, or hardens, in response to an exothermic reaction that reaches 114° F (46° C) and destroys surrounding cells.

Cement is produced in low, medium, and high viscosity. Low-viscosity cement has a 3-minute sticky phase and cures in 1 to 2 minutes. Medium-viscosity cement has a 3-minute working phase and a 1.5 to 2.5-minute curing time. High-viscosity cement has a short, sticky phase and cures in 1 to 2 minutes. Low environmental temperature can prolong the curing time.

Bone cement is injected under pressure to fill the interstices of bone. When the implant is placed, the cement fills the cancellous spaces around it for a secure fit. Cement can crack or break and cause loosening of the prosthesis over time.

The liquid portion is highly flammable and should not be placed in proximity to the cautery. Use of appropriate venting devices during mixing provides an extra measure of safety for the team. Users should not wear gas-permeable contact lenses because fumes can penetrate and bind with the lens material. A second pair of gloves should be worn when handling bone cement and discarded when handling is complete.

Physiologic responses to bone cement are varied. Some patients experience hypotension and can suffer an embolus or cardiac arrest during the cementing process, a condition known as bone cement implantation syndrome (BCIS). Rarely a tiny fragment of cement can enter the venous system and embolize to the lungs. Causes of BCIS are not exactly known but are attributed to several of the following situations:

- Exothermic effects of the cement
- Gas embolism by the polymerization of PMMA
- Emboli (clots, fat, or cement) from pressurized cementing process in the cancellous bone
- Enhancement of halogenated anesthetic gas by fumes of the cement
- Increased cardiac depression and hypotension

Close collaboration with the anesthesia provider during the use of bone cement affords the patient an additional measure of safety.

d. Hybrid fixation refers to a combination of fixation methods. Some components are cemented; some are press-fitted or held by screws or some other noncemented technique.

e. Bone grafts may be needed to replace bone loss around the joint. Either autologous or fresh-frozen allograft bone may be used.

Total Hip Replacement

Total hip prostheses have greatly reduced the number of arthroplasty procedures previously described, especially in patients older than 50 years who have degenerative hip disease. Several types and sizes of prostheses are available. Each has its own advantages and disadvantages. The surgeon must select the appropriate one for each patient's particular condition.

With the patient lateral on the OR bed, an incision approximately 6—10 inches (15.24—25 cm) long is made along the lateral aspect of the thigh to remove the greater trochanter (Fig. 36.23). Removal of the greater trochanter facilitates exposure to prepare sites for insertion of the prosthesis. However, its removal can cause abductor muscle weakness, instability, and other complications. Therefore some surgeons prefer an anterior approach to the hip joint with the patient supine on a radiolucent table. Anterior incisions are approximately 4 inches (10 cm).

With all approaches the femur is disarticulated from the acetabulum. The femoral head is removed at the neck and replaced with a prosthesis. The prosthesis is a metal head, usually titanium, on a metallic stem that is seated into the medullary canal of the femur. Before the femoral prosthesis is inserted, the acetabulum is reamed to the configuration of the cup-shaped acetabular component (Fig. 36.24). This may be high-density polyethylene or metal with a smooth, rough, or porous outer surface. The inner surface is smooth polyethylene to articulate with the smooth finish on the head of the femoral prosthesis. The acetabular component is fixed in the socket. Then the femoral prosthesis is positioned. This sequence is reversed if a silastic mold is made for a customized femoral component.

Computer-assisted surgical modeling or robotics may be used to help the surgeon plan the surgical procedure, select the most appropriate type and size of prosthesis, and prepare the surface of the bone.[9] A drill in the end of the robotic arm precisely drills the cavity in the femur to hold the implant stem. Robotic systems provide better implant alignment and prevent removal of too much bone.

Three types of robotic systems are available: active, semiactive, and passive systems. Some systems may show images on a computer screen.[9]

Active systems: The robot performs the image-based preplanned procedure with the surgeon monitoring and guiding the robot. The robotic arms do the work.

Semiactive: The system assists the surgeon with feedback for placement accuracy of cutting guides and component placement.

Passive: The system provides positioning coordinates while the surgeon does all manual labor.

Many manufacturers make different robotic systems. A few examples include:

- MAKO: Image-based, semiactive
- ROBODOC: CT image-based, active
- CORI: Imageless, semiactive
- OMNIBotics: Imageless, passive

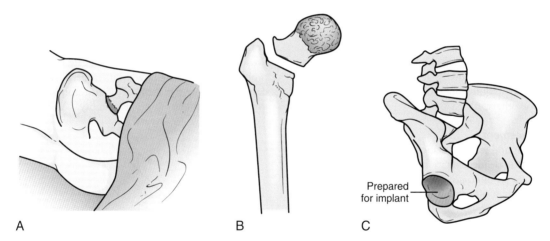

A   B   C

• **Fig. 36.23** **A,** Lateral position of the patient for total hip arthroplasty. **B,** The diseased femoral head is removed. **C,** The diseased acetabulum is reamed to receive the acetabular cup implant.

Plastic liner
Femoral head
Femoral stem
Titanium acetabular cup

• **Fig. 36.24** Components of a total hip joint replacement.

- NAVIO: CT image, handheld system; hand control cutting functions that calibrate to the patient's images

Total Knee Replacement

Insertion of a total knee prosthesis may be indicated to provide for mechanical deficiencies in the function of the knee. The patient, usually older than 60 years, may have significant chronic pain and joint destruction as a result of arthritis, an inflammatory condition, or an autoimmune disorder. One or both knees may be affected. Bilateral total knee replacement can be performed safely in a patient who has the ability to actively participate in postoperative rehabilitation.

Selection of the appropriate prosthesis from among the types available depends on the deformity of the femorotibial articulation, patellofemoral articulation, and structure of the cruciate and collateral ligaments. The prosthesis consists of a multiradius femoral component, a modular tibial component, and a patellar component (Fig. 36.25). The tibial and patellar components of high-density polyethylene articulate with the polished metallic surface of the femoral component.

With the patient supine on the OR bed, the knee is maintained in a flexed position (Fig. 36.26). Numerous commercial devices are available for this purpose. The pneumatic tourniquet cuff is placed on the thigh before prepping. The knee will be draped free.

A vertical midline incision is made over the anterior knee. After the distal femur and the proximal tibia are measured and cut, a trial prosthesis is inserted. The knee is taken through a range of motion to assess alignment, ligament balance, and patellar positioning before the components are fixed in place.

To achieve stability, permanent bone ingrowth into a porous coated or rough-surface implant is desirable. Prostheses of this construction may not require bone cement for fixation. Hybrid fixation is used for others.

Total Ankle Replacement

Rheumatoid arthritis and posttraumatic osteoarthritis are the most common causes of ankle degeneration. Ankle joint replacement may be indicated as an alternative to arthrodesis in selected patients, usually older than 60 years, to relieve pain and secondarily to increase motion and provide stability in the tibiotalar joint.

With the patient positioned supine, an anterior incision may be made from the base of the second metatarsal to the crest of the tibia. A posterior approach, with the patient positioned prone, may be preferred for wider exposure of anatomic structures. Procedures vary depending on the type of prosthesis to be implanted.

The nonconstrained type allows normal dorsiflexion, plantar flexion, and rotation of the foot but is inherently unstable; the constrained type restricts motion to a single plane but is inherently more stable. The tibial components of both types are high-density polyethylene, and the talar components are metal.

Total Metatarsophalangeal Joint Replacement

Hallux rigidus and hallux abductus valgus deformities can lead to pain and altered gait. Through joint replacement the deformity can be realigned with stability and motion. Several types of implants are available. The silastic hinge toe, a double-stemmed silicone prosthesis with a hinge, is a popular choice to restore motion of the great toe and lesser metatarsophalangeal joints.

Total Shoulder Replacement

Shoulder replacement may be indicated for severe destruction by disease or posttraumatic degeneration of the humeral articular surface with resultant loss of motion, instability, and pain. The prosthesis replaces the humeral head and resurfaces the glenoid cavity, the articular surface of the scapula (Fig. 36.27). Preferred if ligamentous or capsular support is sufficient, a nonconstrained prosthesis has a plastic component for the glenoid socket and a metal humeral head. Only the articular surfaces are replaced with these gliding metal-to-plastic components.

A stable fixed-fulcrum, constrained prosthesis with interlocking components may be required to prevent dislocation. The patient is placed in a semi-Fowler position with the affected shoulder slightly off the edge of the OR bed for these surgical procedures.

Total Elbow Replacement

Prosthetic replacement may be indicated to correct intraarticular problems within the elbow joint, especially one with severe surface damage. Surface replacement with a nonarticulating, constrained prosthesis provides internal stability. A hinged or articulated,

• **Fig. 36.26** Positioning device for knee surgery.

• **Fig. 36.25** Components of total knee joint replacement.

• **Fig. 36.27** Components of total shoulder joint replacement.

nonconstrained capitellocondylar prosthesis improves the functional range of motion in the humeroulnar articulation. Both the metallic humerus and ulnar components are cemented in place after shaping the bones. High-density polyethylene bushings facilitate articulation of the hinge assembly connecting the humoral and ulnar components.

Total Wrist Replacement

Silicone rubber implants are used to replace the radiocarpal joint in the wrist, primarily to improve function. A resection arthroplasty is done, usually from an anterior approach. The proximal row of carpal bones (i.e., scaphoid, lunate) and the trapezium are resected. Stems of the flexible, hinged implant are inserted into the intramedullary canals of the radius proximally and capitate carpal bone distally. A silicone cap is placed over the distal end of the ulna. Flexion and extension of the wrist are possible through free sliding of stems within the medullary canals. Some other types of prostheses have fixed stems.

Trapeziometacarpal Joint Replacement

A metal ball–to–plastic socket prosthesis restores function of the thumb. This prosthesis is cemented in place.

Metacarpophalangeal Joint Replacement

Known as implant replacement arthroplasty for small joints in the hands, the head of the affected metacarpal or proximal phalanx is removed in a metacarpophalangeal joint replacement. The silicone rubber implant bridges the excised joint. One stem fits into the medullary canal of the proximal metacarpal, and the other fits into the distal phalanx. The hinged body of the implant keeps the bones separated and mobile.

Patient Care Considerations in Arthroplasty

Patients of all ages may have debilitating and painful arthritis; many are older than 65 years. Attention must be paid to support all joints during moving and positioning of these patients. Other unique aspects of joint replacement should be kept in mind:

1. The prosthesis must be handled carefully.
   a. Use only instruments specifically designed for implantation of the prosthesis.
   b. Avoid causing dents and scratches.
   c. Avoid glove powder and lint. Silicone implants should not be placed on fabrics; place the implant in a metal basin or transfer it directly to the surgeon.
   d. Open sterile packages just before use, after the surgeon determines the size and style.

2. Bone cement, if needed, must be mixed by the scrub person immediately before use.
   a. Follow the manufacturer's instructions for handling this material. The scrub person should know by feel and appearance when the cement is of the correct consistency. A practice session is helpful before mixing for the first time during an actual surgical procedure.
   b. Avoid excessive exposure to vapors. In addition to causing irritation to the eyes, vapors may damage gas-permeable contact lenses if worn. A scavenging system should be used.
   c. Avoid getting lipid solvent on gloves. It can diffuse through the latex to cause allergic dermatitis. Wear a second pair of gloves during the process and then discard them when the task is complete.
   d. Cement is poured into a syringe for injection into the intramedullary canal for joints such as hip or shoulder joints. Cement may be shaped manually for hinged joints.
   e. The temperature of the room can affect the time necessary for cement to set or "cure."
   f. Be aware that some patients have an alteration in vital signs (e.g., hypotension, cardiac dysrhythmias) during placement of the cement in the medullary canal.

3. A silastic mold, if used to customize the prosthesis, must be prepared at the sterile field. The scrub person mixes the catalyst and silicone quickly and thoroughly and then pours the mixture into the injector tube immediately before it is inserted into the bone. The customized prosthesis must be steam-sterilized when it arrives from the laboratory. A standard sterilization cycle with internal and external biologic monitoring, not flash-sterilization, is used.

4. Air-powered drills, saws, and reamers must be properly connected with adequate pressure. Check the pressure in tanks of compressed air or nitrogen before the surgical procedure begins. It must be more than 500 lbs. Turn on the tank by turning the knob to the left. Turn off the tank by turning the knob to the right.

5. Suction tubing must be kept open and collection containers changed as necessary to maintain suction for irrigation during the surgical procedure.

6. Blood loss should be appropriately monitored. It can be extensive during total hip arthroplasty. Blood may be salvaged from the sterile field with a separate suction tube and processed (e.g., through a cell saver) for autotransfusion.

7. Closed-wound suction drainage generally is used, especially after hip, knee, and shoulder arthroplasty.

8. The exhaust system for personnel wearing helmets must be functioning properly if the surgical procedure is performed within a laminar airflow system. Air circulation is affected by ambient airflow, causing misdirection of the clean air.

9. Traffic through the OR should be restricted to minimize air turbulence. Infection is a major potential hazard of all bone and joint surgery. It can be both disabling and expensive.

10. The type of prosthesis used must be documented, including the manufacturer's identifying information. The label of a sterile implant can be affixed to the patient's record.

Arthroscopy

Arthroscopy, the visualization of the interior of a joint through an arthroscope, allows diagnosis and conservative treatment of some cartilaginous, ligamentous, synovial, and bony surface defects. Arthroscopy is used for definitive treatment of meniscal, articular cartilage, and ligamentous defects in the knee. An arthroscope also may be used in the shoulder, ankle, elbow, wrist, and hip. Examples of arthroscopic port placement for the knee and wrist are shown in Fig. 36.28. Fiberoptic arthroscopes have diameters

ranging from 1.7 to 6 mm to accommodate the size of the joint. Angles of the viewing lenses also vary from 0° to 90°.

Sterile irrigating solution, either lactated Ringer's or normal saline solution, at room temperature is necessary to create a working space in the joint. The solution is injected initially via a needle and syringe. Then through a small stab wound, a cannula is inserted into the medial aspect of the knee, for example, for inflow of irrigation. Outflow tubing is connected to the metal sheath of the arthroscope. It can be attached to suction or placed in a drainage bucket and allowed to drain by gravity.

The sheath (sleeve) over a sharp trocar is inserted through a stab wound in the skin at the selected site of entry for the arthroscope. When the trocar penetrates the capsule, the capsule and synovium form a tight seal around the sheath. The sharp trocar is replaced with a blunt obturator to advance the sheath into the joint. The obturator is removed, and the arthroscope is inserted through the sheath. The inflow and outflow irrigating tubes are connected to the stopcocks on the sheath.

An operating arthroscope may have a channel for passage of long, thin, manually operated instruments such as probes, hooks, scissors, knives, punches, and grasping forceps. Or these instruments may be manipulated through separate access portals into the joint under visualization through the scope. Power-driven shavers are also used to smooth rough articular cartilage or bony surfaces.

A pulsed-energy Nd:YAG, Ho:YAG, or CO_2 laser may be adapted to some arthroscopes for use in a confined area and to minimize bleeding. A video camera attached to the eyepiece allows projection of the view to a closed-circuit television monitor so that the surgeon can manipulate instruments with precision. Some cameras attach to the side of a beam splitter on the scope. Discussion of endoscopy and the essential elements is found in Chapter 32 of this text.

Patient Care Considerations in Arthroscopy

1. All metal components of the arthroscope are steam-sterilized. Some optical systems and fiberoptic cords can be steam-sterilized; others require STERIS, STERRAD, or ethylene oxide (EO) gas sterilization. Protective sterilizing cases are recommended to protect the optics when the components are batch processed. Follow the manufacturer's recommendations for sterilization of the arthroscope and its component attachments.

2. The scrub person checks all sterile equipment and instruments while setting up.
   a. Check the arthroscope for clean lenses and unbroken optics.
   b. Check the patency of the inflow and outflow irrigation stopcocks and ports.
   c. All component parts must be the correct size; the optics, trocar, and obturator must fit securely into the sheath. Surgical instruments must pass through the channel. The fiberoptic cord must fit the arthroscope and projection lamp.
   d. Inspect the edges of cutting instruments, such as blades, burrs, knives, and scissors, under magnification. Blades must be sharp, set properly, and glide smoothly.
   e. Assemble power equipment. Rings must fit tightly. Forward and reverse rotating actions must function smoothly. Blades must be locked properly. The power source should be checked.

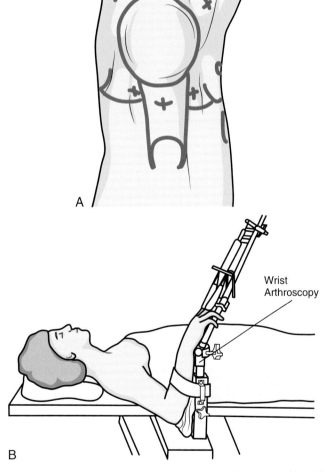

A

B

Wrist Arthroscopy

• **Fig. 36.28** Examples of arthroscopic access port placement. **A,** Knee. **B,** Wrist on frame.

3. The circulating nurse checks all nonsterile equipment (e.g., fiberoptic light source, video equipment, fluid delivery elevation stand, laser).

4. The video camera and cable must be enclosed in a sterile cover unless the camera has been sterilized. The scrub person and circulating nurse coordinate draping.

5. The extremity must be firmly supported in a leg or arm holder that allows flexion of the joint (Fig. 36.29). A tourniquet is applied for arthroscopy of the knee, ankle, elbow, or wrist. Care is taken not to allow prep solution to run under the tourniquet cuff.

6. The patient is prepped and draped as for any sterile procedure on the extremity, with extra precautions to provide a waterproof barrier against contamination by irrigating solutions.

7. The circulating nurse hangs bags of sterile normal saline or lactated Ringer's solution on an IV pole at least 3 feet (1 m) above the joint. This ensures adequate hydrostatic pressure to keep the joint distended to create a working space and maintain the flow of the irrigating solution. Some facilities use irrigation pumps. Two to four 3000-mL bags may be needed.

The solution is maintained at room temperature to avoid hyperemia from warm solution, which may appear as inflammation of synovium, or blanching, which produces an avascular appearance from cold solution. Used solution should be disposed of per biologic waste protocol.

8. Equipment must be appropriately attached after the patient is draped.
   a. The scrub person secures, for example, drainage tubes, fiberoptic cord, suction, and air-power cables to drapes in a location that will not impede movement of the extremity.
   b. The circulating nurse attaches, for example, tubing to irrigating and suction systems and cords to power sources.

Arthrotomy

Arthrotomy (i.e., incision into a joint) may be necessary to remove bone or cartilage fragments or to repair a defect in the synovium or joint capsule. Synovectomy may be the procedure of choice for relief of pain and control of inflammation in a rheumatoid arthritic joint. If a joint is ankylosed (fused), fibrosed, or deranged, open arthrotomy rather than arthroscopy may be necessary. Occasionally during arthroscopy, an injury or disease process that cannot be adequately treated requires arthrotomy while the patient is anesthetized or it may be performed at a later time. In the knee, for example, potential neurovascular complications may preclude arthroscopic repair.

Bunionectomy

Hallux valgus, a lateral deviation in position of the great toe, increases the prominence of the adjoining metatarsal head. Pressure at the base of the first metatarsophalangeal joint causes inflammation that creates formation of an exostosis or bunion beneath the bursa and joint capsule. A bunionectomy is performed to remove a painful exostosis and functionally or cosmetically correct the deformity (Fig. 36.30).

A capsulotomy must be performed to enter the first metatarsophalangeal joint. The procedure may be done with the patient under local infiltration anesthesia and IV sedation. A pneumatic tourniquet around the ankle provides hemostasis, unless contraindicated in a patient with a circulatory problem in the foot. One of several procedures may be selected.

- *Keller arthroplasty:* The proximal third of the proximal phalanx of the great toe is resected. A silicone implant may be placed in the intramedullary canal to stabilize the metatarsophalangeal joint.
- *Metatarsal osteotomy:* The metatarsal alignment is corrected by moving the metatarsal head laterally.
- *McBride operation:* The abductor tendon is fixed to the lateral portion of the metatarsal neck, and the sesamoid bone is excised.
- *Silver bunionectomy:* The medial aspect of the exostosis is removed from the first metatarsal head.

Bunionectomies are only one of many procedures performed by podiatrists, as well as orthopedic surgeons, in the treatment of foot-related disorders, including degenerative diseases and injuries of the foot and ankle.

Hammer Toes

A hammer toe is a deformity of the second, third, and/or fourth toes. The affected toe is bent at the middle joint and therefore resembles a hammer. Hammer toes are flexible at first and can be corrected conservatively, but if they persist, they can become fixed

• **Fig. 36.29** Arthroscopy limb holder.

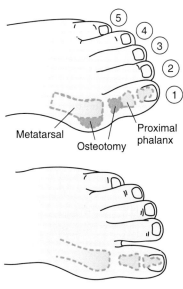

• **Fig. 36.30** Bunionectomy.

and require a surgical procedure, such as osteotomy, to shorten the angle of the toe.

Hammer toe can form in the presence of bunions that cause walking in an unbalanced gait. Improperly fitted shoes cause the toes to bend. The external surface of the affected toes develops painful calluses and makes wearing shoes very painful.

Neurolysis

Neuropathy caused by entrapment of a nerve produces tingling, numbness, and a burning sensation with radiating pain and compromise of function. Known as a tunnel syndrome, this most frequently occurs in the wrist from entrapment of the median nerve (i.e., carpal tunnel syndrome). It may originate from compression of the radial nerve in the lower arm (i.e., radial tunnel syndrome) or from the posterior tibial nerve in the foot (i.e., tarsal tunnel syndrome).

The cause of formation of scar tissue or adhesions around the nerve may be related to repetitive stress, trauma, or inflammatory disease. Neurolysis, freeing of the nerve from the surrounding structures, relieves pain and restores sensation and function. For example, in the wrist the transverse carpal ligament overriding the median nerve is incised. A segment may be excised and a synovectomy may be performed to relieve the symptoms of carpal tunnel syndrome. Release of the median nerve may also be accomplished endoscopically.

Repair of Tendons and Ligaments

Tendons and ligaments may be severed, torn, or ruptured. These injuries are frequently seen in athletes. Total or partial avulsion of the major ligaments and tendons torn from their attachments in or around an extremity joint requires repair to stabilize the joint.

Tendons can be lengthened, shortened, or transferred. When a surgical procedure is indicated, tendon repair is a meticulous but tedious procedure. Tenorrhaphy (close apposition of the cut ends of tendons, particularly extensor tendons) is imperative to successfully restore function. Tendons heal slowly.

Nonabsorbable or slow-absorbing suture is widely used in tendon repair because of its durability and lack of elasticity. A tendon may be wrapped in a silicone membrane to prevent adhesions after repair. Artificial tendons are made of a polyester center covered with silicone rubber. A double-velour polyester prosthesis is used for ligament repair of a shoulder separation.

Hand Surgery

Hand reconstruction has become a subspecialty of both orthopedics and plastic surgery. Tendon surgery is within the realm of orthopedic surgeons; however, many plastic surgeons also perform tendon repair and transfer for hand reconstruction. Restoration of function is the goal of the hand surgeon.

The surgeon often manages surgical correction of fractures and rotational deformities of the fingers. Tenosynovectomy (excision of the tendon sheath) may be performed to release arthritic contractures.

Sports Medicine

Sports medicine deals with the anatomic, biochemical, physiologic, and psychologic effects of motion, strength, and coordination on physical activity. Public awareness of and surgeons' concerns about athletic injuries have led to the development of sports medicine centers that emphasize physical conditioning, injury prevention, and rehabilitation of athletes.

Sports medicine is a rapidly growing area of orthopedics, primarily as a result of interest in exercise among the general population. The intensity of a sports activity places physical demands on the musculoskeletal system that can result in injury. Most injuries involve ligaments, tendons, and muscles rather than broken bones. Most injuries, such as a strained muscle or tendon, do not require surgical intervention. MRI is a reliable method of assessing intraarticular injuries, either acute or chronic.

The knee, shoulder, and ankle are most prone to athletic injuries of ligaments and dislocations of joints. Arthroscopy is useful in the diagnosis and treatment of some injuries. Others require open surgical reconstruction to regain joint stability. For example, a complete ligament tear usually requires surgical repair. Some procedures combine arthroscopy and arthrotomy. Postoperative rehabilitation aims to restore range of motion, minimize muscle atrophy, and reestablish muscle endurance and joint position. The patient should commit to a long-term conditioning program to prevent reinjury.

Knee Injuries

The knee is the joint that is most vulnerable to both contact and noncontact sports injuries. For example, hyperextension can result from a noncontact activity. Contact sports can result in a combination of injuries to the cruciate and collateral ligaments, meniscus, and posterior capsule (Fig. 36.31).

Anterior Cruciate Ligament

Knee stability is influenced by the dynamics of the anterior and posterior cruciate ligaments. Injuries to these ligaments are the most common and most serious types of knee injuries. The anterior cruciate ligament (ACL) can be partially or completely torn, ruptured, or avulsed. The extent of the injury determines the method of reconstruction. Arthroscopically, the ACL may be

• **Fig. 36.31** Normal internal knee anatomy and typical sports injuries treated with surgery.

transferred into the posterior aspect of the lateral femoral condyle and secured with sutures, staples, or screws.

After an autograft is harvested through an open incision, the knee may be reconstructed through the arthroscope. One technique places a bone-patellar tendon-bone autograft and fixes it with cancellous or interference bone screws into tibial and femoral tunnels. In another method a composite of autogenous semitendinosus muscle with a polypropylene ligament augmentation device sutured to it extends from the tibial attachment across the joint and is stapled to the distal femur. In the open Insall procedure, a bone-block graft with an iliotibial band of fascia lata is secured to the tibial tubercle.

Artificial ligamentous substitutes may be preferred for ACL reconstruction. These materials also are used to stabilize torn or ruptured ligaments in the ankle. Expanded polytetrafluoroethylene (PTFE) can be secured with screws. Allograft ligaments also are used. Woven bovine collagen, bovine and carbon fiber material, or a partially absorbable matrix of polylactic acid polymer and filamentous carbon may be used as a scaffold for new collagenous tissue ingrowth for disrupted ligaments. Concomitant partial meniscectomy or meniscal repair may be performed with ACL reconstruction.

Meniscus

Partial meniscectomy or repair of a meniscal tear may be done by open arthrotomy or closed arthroscopy. Neurovascular injury is a potential complication of these procedures. Patients selected for arthroscopy usually have a single vertical longitudinal tear that can be debrided. Localized synovium can be abraded. Sutures must be placed to reduce displacement and stabilize the meniscus.

Ankle Injuries

Ankle sprains are commonly caused by inversion injury. Ankle fractures are usually eversion injuries. Fractures of the malleoli are referred to as Pott fractures. Internal fixation of the inferior margins of the tibia and fibula to the superior surface of the talus may be required.

Rupture of the Achilles tendon can occur spontaneously during a physical activity, such as basketball or racquet sports, usually from indirect trauma. A gap is palpable at the back of the ankle. Severed ends of the tendon may be brought together through an open or percutaneous repair with heavy size 2 nonabsorbable suture.

Ankle arthroscopy may be the procedure of choice for placing internal fixation devices or removing osteophytes (bony outgrowths) in the joint after healing of an ankle fracture.

Shoulder Injuries

Many anterior glenoid labrum and minor rotator cuff tears, the most common acute injuries, can be repaired arthroscopically. Some recurrent dislocations also can be stabilized with sutures, staples, or screws. For a major rotator cuff tear, an open Bankart repair usually is necessary to suture the labrum and reattach the glenohumeral ligament. An open Putti-Platt correction for recurrent dislocation will limit external rotation of the shoulder.

Cast Application

For CR of fractures, traction, and postoperative applications, many orthopedic appliances must be available and at hand when needed. An orthopedic cart can provide the necessary items for these situations (Box 36.1). The items may vary somewhat at different hospitals, but many are universally used. The cart can be taken wherever needed in the OR suite. One higher shelf should be designated for sterile items.

Casting supplies are commonly found on the orthopedic cart. A cast is a rigid form of dressing used to encase and support a part of the body. It supports and immobilizes the part in optimum position until healing takes place. A cast usually includes the joints above and below the affected area. It may suffice as a conservative mode of treatment (e.g., fractures). It can be fitted to any body contour or position and can be worn for months. The following are requirements of a cast:
- It must fulfill its intended function of maintaining position of the desired parts.
- It must not be too tight and must have no pressure areas. Postapplication pain is an important symptom and must be promptly investigated to ensure that circulation is not impaired.
- It must not be too loose. It must be as light as possible, yet strong enough to withstand usage.
- It must be comfortable, with no binding or chafing.

Fiberglass Casts

A woven fiberglass tape impregnated with a water-activated polyurethane resin can be used for casting or bracing. Polypropylene stockinette is applied over the patient's skin. Polypropylene web wrap may be used for extra padding over bony prominences and pressure points. The person applying the cast must wear gloves to facilitate smoothing and blending the layers of the fiberglass tape and to prevent resin pickup on the hands. The resin is activated by lukewarm water. The tape is applied in the same manner as plaster.

The fiberglass cast is lighter and thinner, yet stronger, than a plaster cast and is more porous, providing better ventilation. The outside may get wet without deterioration. X-rays penetrate synthetic materials better than they do plaster to evaluate the healing process. A combination of plaster and synthetic resin on a gauze backing produces a thinner, more waterproof cast that weighs less

---

•BOX 36.1   Contents of an Orthopedic Cart

- Suture removal supplies
- Webril and soft roll
- Assorted gauze dressings and bandages
- Sterile and nonsterile gloves
- Skin antiseptic agents
- Clippers

Nonsterile Items on Another Shelf

- Pulleys and trapeze attachments for bed traction
- Ropes, weights, and carriers
- Felt padding and foam rubber
- Arm and shoulder immobilizers
- Pelvic slings and rods
- Assorted sizes of gauze bandages and stockinette
- Stapler
- Safety pins
- Disposable or reusable plaster bucket with plastic liner bag
- Plastic bag for trash
- Assorted sizes of plaster and/or fiberglass rolls and splints
- Cast cutters, knives, scissors, spreaders, and benders

and is as strong as a plaster cast. Because of these advantages, casting tapes are preferred by many orthopedic surgeons for extremity casts.

Plaster Casts

Plaster **cast material** is composed of gypsum or anhydrous calcium sulfate. It is finely ground to break up the crystals and is then heated to drive out the water. When water is added again, recrystallization takes place and the plaster sets. It was first used as a method of splinting fractures in the 19th century.

Plaster bandages and splints are made of crinoline or some other fabric, with the plaster powder entrapped in the mesh. These are available in rolls or strips 2 to 8 inches (5–20 cm) wide. Plaster splints are either supplied precut or made from rolls as the need arises. Usually six or eight thicknesses of the desired length are used. To provide added strength, splints are applied over areas that may weaken from extra strain. Plaster bandages and splints are available with the following three types of plaster:

- Slow-setting plaster requires up to 18 minutes to set. It is used in large casts requiring more time to apply and mold. It permits blending of the layers.
- Medium-setting plaster requires up to 8 minutes to set. This type is used in average-size casts.
- Fast-setting plaster requires 4 to 5 minutes to set. It is advantageous for small casts on children who are difficult to keep in position. Many surgeons prefer using the fast-setting type in all kinds of casts; it is the most universally used type of plaster.

Application of Plaster

1. Spread a disposable plastic or nonwoven fabric sheet on the floor around the OR bed to catch drips.
2. Protect the OR bed. If the fracture table is used, spread a sheet over table parts after the patient is suspended.
3. Protect the patient's hair with a cap.
4. Use a disposable plaster pail or a plastic liner bag in a plaster bucket.
5. Fill the bucket with water at room temperature. Water warmer than 70° F to 75° F (21–24° C) will speed up the setting time and may cause excessive loss of plaster from the fabric. More important, plaster will get even hotter than its normal exothermic reaction if it is dipped in warm water. The patient could get burned.
6. Don nonsterile disposable gloves to protect the hands from irritation by lime content.
7. Remove the outer wrapping of the plaster roll. Start soaking the plaster only when the surgeon is ready to apply it. Keep just ahead in soaking it. Have the next roll ready when needed, but do not prepare several rolls ahead of time. They may harden and, if used, can produce an ineffective laminated cast. Avoid waste.
8. Hold the plaster roll under water in a vertical position to allow air bubbles to escape from the rolled ends. When air bubbles stop rising, the bandage is soaked through. Compress the ends between the fingers and palm of each hand to remove excess water. This procedure prevents telescoping during use.
9. Unroll the end approximately 1 inch (2.5 cm), and hand the roll to the surgeon.
10. Fanfold a strip once toward the center, before soaking, leaving the ends free to grasp. When soaking, grasp an end in

each hand, press the hands together, and submerge the strip in water for a few seconds; remove it, and pull the strip taut by the ends. It may seem drippy, but the layers blend together well when wet.

11. Ask the surgeon if another roll will be needed before soaking it when the cast appears near completion.
12. Handle the cast with flat, open hands—never fingers—and support the patient in such a way that they cannot attempt to bend an incorporated joint. Wet plaster has only one-third to one-half of its ultimate strength when dry. The person who supports an extremity while a cast is being applied takes care not to make finger-pressure areas in the plaster that will damage the tissue under it. Handle only with the palms of the hands.
13. Elevate an extremity on a longitudinal pillow until the cast hardens. If it is laid on a hard surface, flat pressure areas may be pressed onto it, causing pain and tissue damage. The surgeon may want to x-ray the casted extremity after CR to assure alignment of bones.
14. Clean up as much as possible while the cast is being applied. Wipe plaster off equipment, as well as off the patient, before it dries. Plaster is easy to remove when still damp; after it dries, it must be scraped off. A cast dryer, if used, hastens drying.
15. Avoid splashing plaster on the furniture, walls, and floor.
16. Clean the equipment and table thoroughly. If the sink has a plaster trap, all plaster drip can be washed down the sink and the contents of the bucket poured into the sink. If there is no plaster trap, leave the bucket until the plaster in the bottom hardens; then empty the water and throw the plaster pail or plastic liner bag into the trash. Clean a reusable bucket as soon as you are finished with it.

Padding Under Casts

Padding is usually placed under casts and serves the following several functions:

- It absorbs inevitable ooze from the wound after an open surgical procedure. Sterile padding is put on over the dressing before applying the cast.
- It protects the wound and the patient's skin.
- It protects bony prominences.
- Materials used for padding include:
  - *Stockinette:* A seamless tubing of knitted cotton 1 to 12 inches (2.5–30.4 cm) wide, stockinette stretches to fit any contour snugly.
  - *Sheet wadding:* A glazed cotton bandage 2 to 8 inches (5–20 cm) wide is available as sheeting. It is used over stockinette or in place of it.
  - *Soft roll:* A soft roll of thin cotton batting that has some stretch for smooth contour.
  - *Felt:* Available in sheeting made of wool or blends of wool, cotton, or rayon in thicknesses ranging from $1/8$ to $1/2$ inch (3–13 mm), felt is cut into desired sizes to fit bony prominences. Felt pads are applied over sheet wadding. The plaster adheres to pads and prevents them from slipping.
  - *Foam rubber:* Available in sheets $1/4$ to 1 inch (6.4–25 mm) in thickness, foam rubber may be used in place of felt.
  - *Webril:* Webril is a soft, lint-free cotton bandage. The surface is smooth but not glazed, so that each layer clings to the preceding one and the padding lies smoothly in place.

Common Cast Configurations

- *Cylinder:* A circular cast, made by wrapping the plaster bandages around an extremity, is used after closed or open reductions of fractures, after some surgical procedures for immobilization, or for the purpose of resting a part of an extremity (Fig. 36.32).
- *Walking cast:* A rubber walking heel or polyurethane sole is applied to the sole of a cylinder cast for ambulation. Use of a lower extremity helps maintain strength and muscle tone and helps prevent atrophy.
- *Hanging cast:* A cylinder is applied to the arm with the elbow flexed. It extends from the shoulder to over the hand, leaving the thumb and fingers free. A wire loop is incorporated at the wrist. A strap through this loop and around the neck suspends the arm. The weight of the cast provides needed traction on the humerus.
- *Shoulder spica:* Applied to the trunk, arm, and hand, leaving the fingers and thumb free, a spica cast is used after some surgical procedures on the shoulder or humerus or for a fracture of the humerus. The OR bed may be used for its application, or the patient may sit on a stool with the surgeon supporting the arm in the desired position.
- *Hip spica:* A hip spica cast is applied to the trunk and one or both legs after some hip procedures and fractures of the femur. The orthopedic table is used. The sacrum rests on a sacral rest. The perineal post provides countertraction. Attachments may be used to support the legs of an adult.
- *Minerva jacket:* A Minerva jacket is applied from the hips to the head. If the head is to be completely immobilized, it is included in the jacket. The plaster is molded to fit around the face and lower jaw. A part of the plaster at the back of the head is cut out. It is used for fractures of the cervical or upper thoracic vertebrae. The orthopedic table is necessary.
- *Body jacket:* A body jacket extends from the axillae to the hips to immobilize vertebrae. Application of this cast usually requires the orthopedic or Risser table with the necessary attachments, although sometimes the patient may stand on the floor. Traction may be applied by an overhead sling. If an open surgical procedure is to be performed with the patient in a body cast, a cast cutter must be at hand in case of respiratory difficulty. However, a body cast is usually bivalved before a patient is given an anesthetic.

- An opening is always made over the abdomen of a Minerva or body jacket to allow space for lung expansion and decompression of abdominal distention that normally occurs with ingestion of food. A folded towel may be placed over the abdomen before the stockinette is pulled over the body. This is removed when the opening is made in the cast to allow more space between the body and cast.
- *Plaster shell:* A body jacket is cut along each side, into anterior and posterior parts. The parts may be fastened together by heavy straps with buckles, or the patient may rest in one while the other is removed temporarily.
- *Wedge cast:* A wedge-shaped portion is cut from the cast. The edges are brought together and held with plaster reinforcement. This cast is used to overcome angulation in a fracture.
- *Plaster splint:* Six or more thicknesses of plaster of the desired width and length may be applied to the posterior part of an extremity and secured with gauze or a cotton elastic bandage. Excess water is pressed from the plaster splint after it is immersed in water. A splint may be used for immobilization of a fracture of the ulna or fibula. Inflatable air splints are commercially available. Splints are not circumferential; therefore tissue swelling does not create increased pressure around the limb.
- *Hairpin or sugar tong splint:* A splint twice as long as the lower arm and hand is used for a fracture of the ulna or radius. After the plaster is soaked, it may be covered with stockinette. Starting with one end on the back of the hand, the splint is placed around the flexed elbow. The palm of the hand and fingers rest on the other end of it. It is secured with a bandage. It is commonly used to support distal radial and ulnar fractures, including Colles fractures.
- *Abduction hip splint:* An abduction hip splint keeps hips in constant abduction. If desired for postoperative management, it is applied immediately after a hip procedure.
- *Plaster rope:* Plaster rope may support the arm in a shoulder spica or join legs in a bilateral hip spica. It is made by twisting a wet roll of plaster bandage into a rope as it is unwound, fanfolding to the desired length and drawing it through a cupped hand to blend the strands. A wooden splint may be incorporated into the rope for reinforcement.
- *Molds:* Molds are made as plaster patterns for removable metal or leather braces for the body, neck, or extremities.

• **Fig. 36.32** Application of a short arm cast. Webril is applied as padding followed by the rolled casting material.

- *Waterproof cast:* A breathable synthetic liner made with expanded polytetrafluoroethylene (ePTFE) is used under fiberglass casting material instead of padding. The liner allows the skin to get wet and water to drain from the cast. The casting liner stays dry and body heat causes the cast to dry.[10] It is often used in children because it can be soaked while bathing or swimming and dries quickly without damage to the skin or shape of the cast. More information can be found at www.aquacastliner.com.

Trimming, Removing, and Changing Casts

Rough edges of plaster are trimmed off, and the edges of a cast are covered with stockinette or adhesive tape to protect the patient's skin. Instruments specifically designed for cutting through plaster must be used for trimming or removing casts. These include the following:

- Plaster knives, which have short, slightly curved blades.
- Plaster scissors, which are heavy bandage scissors.
- Electric cast cutter, which is an oscillating saw. It cuts the cast but not the stockinette or other padding under it because the padding moves with the oscillations. The patient's skin also moves somewhat and is not injured if touched lightly, although care always should be taken not to touch the skin. One model has a vacuum attached to pick up the plaster dust created by the saw (Fig. 36.33). A carbide steel blade is recommended for cutting a fiberglass cast. (A regular blade dulls quickly and can result in an inadvertent burn to the patient.)
- Cast spreader, which is a long-handled instrument that has thin, serrated jaws that can be inserted in the cutting line to pry open the cast.
- Cast bender, which is a heavy forceps-type instrument used to bend a small portion of the edge of a cast away from an area, such as a portion of a jacket away from the mouth and chin, to give freer movement.

Sharp plaster knives or scissors generally are used to trim casts. For large casts the electric cast cutter may be used, for example, to cut an opening over the abdomen of a body jacket. In a hip spica, adequate space is provided for use of the bedpan without soiling. If it is necessary to cut a window (i.e., a small opening in a cast to remove sutures or inspect an area), it is put back in place and secured with a few turns of the plaster bandage. An opening in a cast encourages swelling of the tissues under it, known as *window edema.*

• **Fig. 36.33** Cast cutter and oscillating blades with vacuum attachment.

When the edema in a wound under a cast recedes, the cast does not furnish as much immobilization as may be desired. The cast is usually changed at this stage. A cast may be changed periodically during long-term immobilization because muscles atrophy with disuse. The cast becomes loose as muscle size decreases.

Skin sutures are removed at the time of a cast change if the cast was applied after a surgical procedure such as ORIF. A sterile suture removal tray should be ready for use when requested. Sterile sheet wadding may be needed to cover the wound after sutures are removed and before another cast is applied.

If the patient has been in a cast for some time, the skin is apt to be oily, somewhat soiled, and rough. If the surgeon wants the skin cleansed before applying another cast, only superficial dirt can be removed. Scrubbing off oily scales may cause irritation. Usually skin is not washed before applying sheet wadding and a new cast.

A large, plastic-lined trash container is used for disposal of the wrappings, trimmings, and removed cast during cast application and removal. The knives, scissors, cutter, spreader, and bender are washed and dried promptly after use. Before instruments are put away, lubrication is applied to all instrument joints to prevent rust and corrosion.

Complications After Orthopedic Surgery

Thromboembolism is the most common postoperative complication of orthopedic surgery, particularly if the patient must be immobilized for an extended period. Pneumonia can be fatal for older patients. Urinary tract infection and skin breakdown also are potential problems, particularly in geriatric patients. As previously emphasized, wound infection can be devastating.

Embolus

Fat embolism is possible after fracture of a long bone or crush injury. The yellow bone marrow at the point of the fracture of the long bone releases adipose cells into the circulation. The fat emboli enter the pulmonary circulation and cause the release of fatty acids. The alveoli are damaged, and the lung surfactant is rendered ineffective.

Thromboemboli can result from deep vein thrombosis, causing pulmonary emboli. Any vessel wall injury can cause this event. Air can enter the lung, but gas exchange cannot take place because of vascular obstruction at the level of the pulmonary artery. A vena cava filter may be indicated.

Rarely a bolus of bone cement can enter the venous system and travel to the patient's lungs. Always be alert to signals from the anesthesia personnel that the patient may be having changes in vital signs during the surgical procedure, especially if bone cement is used.

Compartment Syndrome

Edema, hematoma, and seroma may form between tissue layers of the fascial plane, causing compartment syndrome. The pressure from prolonged swelling results in further tissue destruction and necrosis that can lead to toxicity and death (Fig. 36.34). The lymphatic system tries to compensate, but as swelling increases the load is more than the lymphatic vessels can transfer. The interstitium becomes engorged, causing increased arterial pressure. The increasing arterial pressure leads to loss of distal pulses. Critical aspects in the diagnosis of compartment syndrome are based on neurovascular status (pulses, sensation, and motor function).[11]

• **Fig. 36.34** Compartment syndrome.

The pressure is relieved by a series of two to four longitudinal incisions in the fascia (**fasciotomy** incisions) that are left open to drain. Circulation can be tenuous, and the potential for nerve injury is great. Closure is not attempted for weeks or months. Meshed split-thickness or full-thickness skin grafts may be needed to cover the defect. Healing is slow, with significant scar formation over the incision sites.

EVOLVE WEBSITE

http://evolve.elsevier.com/Hornacky/BerryKohn/

- Historical Perspective
- Tips for the Scrub Person and Circulating Nurse
- Student Interactive Questions
- Glossary

References

1. Meyers A, Marquart M: *Pediatric physeal injuries overview*, Treasure Island, FL, 2023, StatPearls Publishing. www.ncbi.nlm.nih.gov. (Accessed 5 June 2023).
2. Venkatesan V, Rangasamy J: Diabetic pedal osteomyelitis and its treatment, *Chonnam Med J* 59(2):109−114, 2023.
3. Antia C, Greyling LA, Davis LS: Creating a sterile field for plantar procedures, *J Am Acad Dermatol* 72(1):27−28, 2015.
4. Elbuluk A, Novikov D, Gotlin M, et al.: Control strategies for infection prevention in total joint arthroplasty, *Orthop Clin North Am* 50(1):1−11, 2019.
5. The Bonati Institute: www.bonati.com. Accessed June 5, 2023.
6. Basques BA, Toy JO: General compared to spinal anesthesia for total hip replacement, *J Bone Joint Surg Am* 97(6):455−461, 2015.
7. Ferguson R, Palmer A, Taylor A, et al.: Hip replacement, *Lancet* 392(10158):1662−1671, 2018.
8. Antonios J, Korber S, Sivasundaram L, et al.: Trends in computer navigation and robotic assistance for total knee arthroplasty in the United States: an analysis of patient and hospital factors, *Arthroplast Today* 5(1):88−95, 2019.
9. Mihalko W, Mont M, Krackow K. In *The technique of total knee arthroplasty*, ed 2, Philadelphia, PA, 2023, Elsevier.
10. AquaCast: www.aquacastliner.com. Accessed June 8, 2023.
11. Torlincasi A, Lopez R, Waseem M: *Acute compartment syndrome*, Treasure Island, FL, 2023, StatPearls Publishing. www.ncbi.nlm.nih.gov. (Accessed 6 June 2023).

37

Neurosurgery of the Brain and Peripheral Nerves

CHAPTER OUTLINE

Anatomy and Physiology of the Brain, 790

Special Considerations in Neurosurgery, 792

Patient Care Considerations for Craniotomy, 795

Surgical Procedures of the Cranium, 799

Peripheral Nerve Surgery, 806

CHAPTER OBJECTIVES

After studying this chapter, the learner will be able to:

- Identify the pertinent anatomy of the brain and spinal cord.
- Describe the significance of neurologic monitoring.

- Discuss the risks associated with neurosurgery.

KEY TERMS AND DEFINITIONS

Arteriovenous malformation An abnormal collection of vessels that is not clearly defined as arterial or venous.

Benign tumor Neoplasm or abnormal growth that is not malignant and usually contained. The location in a vital area could potentially cause death or permanent injury.

Craniotomy Procedure in which the bones of the skull are opened by powered or manual instrumentation.

Glioma Tumor that arises between the neurons in the connective tissue.

Malignant tumor Primary tumor that begins in the brain and can spread to other central nervous system (CNS) tissue.

Secondary tumor Tumor that spreads to the brain from another area of the body. Metastatic cells from breast or lung form multiple brain tumors, for example.

Shunt Temporary or permanent bypass of a vascular or drainage system.

Stereotactic surgery Use of a computer imaging system to pinpoint the location of a tumor.

Subdural hematoma A collection of blood under the dural layer of meninges.

Trephine Creation of a circular hole into the skull (sometimes referred to as trepan) to relieve pressure on the brain. The procedure is referred to as trephination.

Tumor A collection of cells that exhibit uncontrolled growth. Brain tumors are named for the type of cell that mutates or for the location of origin.

Anatomy and Physiology of the Brain

An understanding of basic anatomy and physiology is essential for preparing for the approach used to reach intracranial and spinal cord structures.

Cranium

The brain is enclosed within the bony vault of the cranium (skull). Eight bones form the cranium: the single frontal, sphenoid, and ethmoid bones anteriorly; the paired temporal and parietal bones that form the middle fossa; and the occipital bone posteriorly. Although these bones are fused together by synarthroses (nonmobile joints) referred to as sutures, the cranium is described as being divided into three areas: the anterior, middle, and posterior fossae. Galea (tough, highly vascular fascia-like tissue over the cranium) connects muscles of the temples, forehead, and base of the skull. The scalp (skin) covers the muscles and extracranial vessels and nerves in subcutaneous tissue.

Meninges

The membranous covering of the central nervous system (CNS), referred to as meninges, lines the cranium and covers the brain and spinal cord. The three distinct layers are the dura mater (in direct contact with the cranium), arachnoid (a weblike space), and pia mater (in direct contact with the surface of the brain).

Cranial dura mater, firmly attached to the inner aspect of the cranium, has two layers that separate in planes to form venous sinuses. The arachnoid, which lies under the dura mater, has weblike connections with the pia mater, which closely adheres to the gray matter of the brain.

Cerebrospinal fluid (CSF) circulates through the arachnoid layer to bathe the brain very slowly and absorbs at the same rate. At any given time, the CSF concentration is 75 mL in volume. The normal intracranial pressure (ICP) in adults is 8 to 14 mm Hg. Coughing or sneezing can cause a temporary ICP elevation between 30 and 50 mm Hg. Measurement of CSF and ICP values can help diagnose disease, response to treatments, or measure cerebral perfusion. Cardiac and respiratory activity creates pulsatile fluid movement and variation in cerebral perfusion. The pia mater is a meshlike vascular membrane that follows the convolutions of the surface of the brain. The pia derives its blood supply from the internal carotid and vertebral arteries.

The dura is arranged in three large folds: the falx cerebri, which covers the hemispheres; the falx cerebelli, which separates the lobes of the cerebellum; and the tentorium cerebelli, which supports the temporal and occipital lobes. The tentorium is a surgical landmark that denotes supratentorial structures and infratentorial structures, such as the brainstem and cerebellum.

Brain

The brain is divided into five main subdivisions composed of gray matter (neurons, cell bodies) and white matter (axons, dendrites, nerve fibers). The brain has three distinct anatomic units that consist of several subdivisions, as shown in Fig. 37.1. The cranial nerves (Table 37.1) originate from several locations in the brain and its subdivisions (Fig. 37.2). Cranial nerve V (trigeminal) innervates most of the face in correlation with cervical dermatomes (Fig. 37.3).

The blood supply to the brain is derived from the carotid and vertebral arteries. The arterial component collectively joins at the circle of Willis (Fig. 37.4).[1] The venous drainage is a series of valveless, bidirectional venous sinuses that communicate directly with the vertebral venous sinuses.[1] The patterns of infectious spread and metastasis can be easily noted via the venous system that ranges from the pelvis to the cranium.

Cerebrum

The right and left hemispheres of the cerebrum are connected centrally by the corpus callosum, a broad band of nerve fibers. The cerebrum, also known as the telencephalon, occupies most of the area within the cranium and is arranged into superficial folds (called gyri) and furrows (called sulci), which are surgical anatomic landmarks. The outer cerebral cortex is the gray matter; the inner tissue is the white matter. Cranial nerve I originates here. Each hemisphere of the brain is divided into four anatomic lobes, as follows:

1. The frontal lobe lies within the anterior fossa.
2. The parietal lobe lies in the superior and anterior portion of the middle fossa.

TABLE 37.1 Cranial Nerves

Number	Name	Origin	Action
I	Olfactory	Telencephalon	Smell
II	Optic	Diencephalon	Vision
III	Oculomotor	Mesencephalon	Somatic motor for eyeballs, iris, and ciliary body
IV	Trochlear	Mesencephalon	Somatic motor for eyeballs
V	Trigeminal	Metencephalon	Motor and sensory
VI	Abducens	Myelencephalon	Somatic motor
VII	Facial	Myelencephalon	Motor and sensory
VIII	Vestibulocochlear	Myelencephalon	Hearing and balance
IX	Glossopharyngeal	Myelencephalon	Visceral motor and sensory, general sensory
X	Vagus	Myelencephalon	Visceral motor and sensory, general sensory
XI	Spinal accessory	Myelencephalon	Visceral motor
XII	Hypoglossal	Myelencephalon	Somatic motor

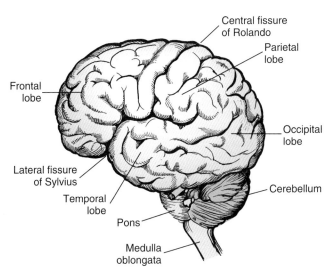

• **Fig. 37.1** Left lateral view of cerebral hemisphere.

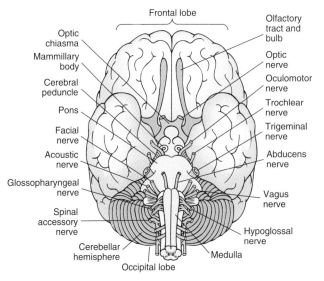

• **Fig. 37.2** Cranial nerves.

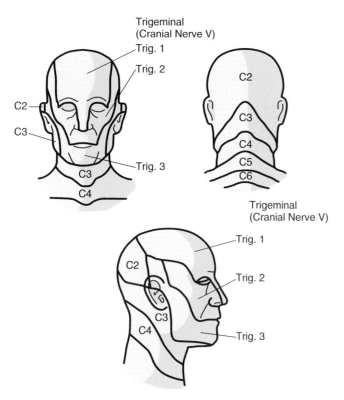

• **Fig. 37.3** Cranial nerve dermatomes.

3. The temporal lobe lies inferior to the frontal and parietal lobes within the middle fossa.
4. The occipital lobe lies posteriorly within the middle fossa.

The hypothalamus and thalamus, referred to as the diencephalon, also lie within the cerebrum to form the floor and lateral walls of the third ventricle. All afferent impulses, except smell, pass through here to the cerebrum. The optic chiasma forms the anterior border.

The diencephalon controls body temperature, emotion, hunger, thirst, sleep, and some hormones. Although it lies in the sella turcica outside the cerebrum, the pituitary body attaches to the inferior aspect of the hypothalamus.

The cerebral pedicles and the corpora quadrigemina form the midbrain, which is also referred to as the mesencephalon. The cerebral aqueduct runs through the full length of the structure. Cranial nerves III and IV originate here.

Brainstem

The brainstem lies anteriorly within the posterior fossa. It extends from the cerebral hemisphere to the base of the skull, where it merges with the spinal cord.

Pons and Cerebellum

The pons and cerebellum form the metencephalon. The pons is a bridge between the cerebrum and the medulla. It lies anterior to the bilobed cerebellum and is the origin of cranial nerves V, VI, VII, and VIII. The cerebellum lies below the occipital lobes of the cerebrum, posterior to the brainstem, within the posterior fossa. It is about one-fifth the size of the cerebrum. The cerebellum controls motion and equilibrium.

Medulla

The medulla oblongata forms the floor of the fourth ventricle and contains the origin of cranial nerves IX, X, XI, and XII. It contains the vital centers, such as cardiac, vasomotor, and respiratory function.

Ventricles

Four spaces within the brain are referred to as ventricles (Fig. 37.5). The lateral ventricles, one in each hemisphere of the cerebrum, drain into the foramen of Monro. The foramen of Monro opens into a central cavity, the third ventricle, which is connected by the aqueduct of Sylvius, with the fourth ventricle lying anterior to the cerebellum and posterior to the brainstem. CSF is a clear substance produced in the choroid plexuses, which are vascular extensions of the pia mater lining the ventricles. CSF is predominantly produced in the lateral ventricles and circulates through the subarachnoid space around the meninges covering the brain and spinal cord. The normal adult volume of circulating CSF is 125 to 150 mL. Obstruction of the CSF flow causes increased ICP.

Special Considerations in Neurosurgery

Neurosurgical procedures are classified according to the anatomic location in the nervous system: brain and cranial nerves, spinal cord and nerve roots, or autonomic and somatic peripheral nerves. Regardless of the location of the surgical site, neural tissue is handled gently to minimize functional disability from surgical trauma. Hemostasis is a critical factor to sustain the vital functions of circulation and respiration. The visibility of structures in the surgical site also should be ensured.

Diagnostics
Magnetic Resonance Imaging

Magnetic resonance imaging (MRI) provides a 3D image of the complex structures of the brain, revealing tumors and aneurysms. Intraoperative MRI (iMRI) is used during surgery. The unit can be mounted in the ceiling above the bed or in an adjacent room. The operating room (OR) bed can be moved sterilely into the MRI machine. Real-time MRI is used to see brain shift, bleeding, progress of tissue removal, or mapping for epilepsy. Magnetic resonance spectroscopy is a variant of MRI that can differentiate necrotic tissue from vital tissue after the application of radiation to reduce tumor size.

Computed Tomography

Computed tomography (CT) creates a detailed image of the brain with or without contrast media; however, CT is not as accurate as MRI for diagnosis of brain tumor types. CT is useful for diagnosis of trauma and bleeding into surrounding tissues. Three-dimensional CT-guided navigation systems are used for microsurgery for real-time images. Sometimes CT is used to observe for tumor recurrence.

Positron Emission Tomography

Positron emission tomography (PET) depicts brain activity more so than delineation of structure. It is used to distinguish living tissue from necrotic tissue and can be used to determine tumor grade after diagnosis. Interventional radiosurgery is facilitated by PET scan data.

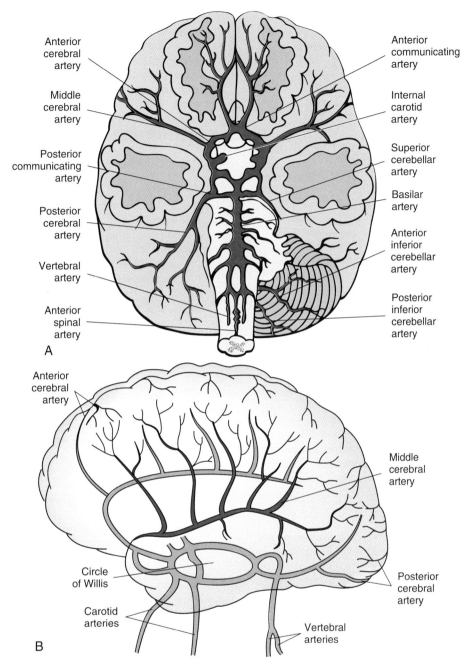

• **Fig. 37.4** Cerebral vasculature. **A,** Principal arteries of the brain. **B,** Circle of Willis and lateral view of cerebral circulation.

Digital Holography

Three-dimensional mapping is done with holograms. This technique is currently being used to produce 3D virtual reality (VR) images for brain mapping and tumor diagnosis.

Prognostics

The survivability of a brain tumor is determined by several factors:
- Malignant or benign
- Cell type and location
- Duration of cell growth
- Surgical or nonsurgical treatment
- Tumor grade (grades IV and V are the worst)

- Patient age; age extremes have worse prognosis
- Ability to function
- Symptomatic conditions

Methods of Hemostasis

The hemostatic methods commonly used by neurosurgeons for most procedures are detailed in the following sections.

Scalp Clips

The scalp is highly vascular. Bleeding is controlled with Leroy or Raney clips placed over the edges of the wound with a special clip applier as the primary incision is made. These disposable clips are

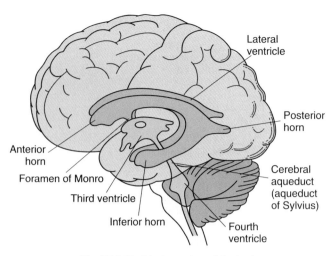

• **Fig. 37.5** Ventricular system of the brain.

[Labels in figure: Lateral ventricle; Posterior horn; Cerebral aqueduct (aqueduct of Sylvius); Fourth ventricle; Inferior horn; Third ventricle; Foramen of Monro; Anterior horn]

used as temporary wound pressure for hemostasis and are removed during closure of the wound.

Bone Wax

Bone wax is used on cranial and vertebral bones. The sterile wax is rolled into small 4 to 5-mm balls and placed on a smooth surface within reach of the neurosurgeon. Bone wax can act as a mechanical barrier to bone regrowth and healing.

Antibiotic Paste

Powdered antibiotic is mixed with saline solution or lactated Ringer's solution into a thick paste and smoothed over the cut ends of bones to seal off bleeders. Vancomycin powder is sometimes used in this way.

Compressed Absorbent Patties (Cottonoids)

Compressed absorbent patties, made of rayon, cotton, or polyester, rather than gauze sponges are used on fragile delicate neural tissues to absorb blood and fluids. They are also used for protection of wound edges and for hemostasis. Assorted sizes are moistened with normal saline solution, lactated Ringer's solution, or topical thrombin and pressed out flat on a smooth surface that is easily accessible to the neurosurgeon. Although the patties have no loose fibers, they could pick up lint if placed on a towel.

The standard for sponge counts includes counting these patties. They are retrieved before the surgical site is closed. Patties have a radiopaque thread securely attached to each one. This reminds the surgeon that they are in the wound and facilitates their removal. Care is taken not to suction patties into the suction tip. Some of the patties are as small as ¼-inch square. All patties are counted, although they are detectable by x-ray. The strings should not be cut off. Patties should not be cut and should be inspected to make sure they are intact upon return.

Chemical Agents

Chemical hemostatic agents may be used after resection to control bleeding from large vessels, sinuses, or the surface of a tumor bed. The scrub person moistens a gelatin sponge with normal saline solution or topical thrombin before handing it to the neurosurgeon. Microfibrillar collagen, supplied in fibers or knitted sheet form, is applied dry. The tips of tissue forceps should be dry to prevent this substance from adhering to them. Oxidized cellulose

also is applied dry but is removed after hemostasis has been attained because it can interfere with wound healing.

Ligating Clips

Clips are applied on larger vessels where electrocoagulation would be insufficient or its thermal effect would be hazardous. Some permanent clips, such as intracranial aneurysm clips, are specifically designed only for neurosurgical use. Titanium is preferred because it is nonmagnetic and causes less interference with diagnostic cranial studies, such as CT and MRI. Each type and size of clip requires a specific applier.

Electrosurgery

Monopolar electrosurgical unit (ESU) current is used to cut and coagulate tissue and small vessels of dermis and epidermis. Current is conducted through hemostatic forceps, fine smooth-tipped tissue forceps, or a metal suction tip to bleeding vessels. A combination suction-fulguration tip also may be used. The monopolar current passes through the patient's tissues and returns to the generator via the return electrode.

Bipolar current is frequently used for more precision in coagulation of tiny vessels without damage to surrounding tissue. The bipolar current does not travel through the patient's tissue to a return electrode.

Lasers

Argon, CO_2, potassium titanyl phosphate (KTP), neodymium:yttrium aluminum garnet (Nd:YAG), and tunable dye lasers are selectively used in neurosurgery in conjunction with the operating microscope, endoscopes, and stereotaxis. Each type has benefits, but all have definite limitations.

Depending on the type of laser and the location and type of tumor or vascular lesion, the laser may vaporize, shrink, or coagulate tissue. Precise hemostasis, minimal damage to contiguous structures, and visualization of effects are definite advantages of laser surgery for removal of brain and spinal cord tumors. Lasers are also used to assist in microvascular anastomoses.

Ultrasonic Aspiration

Although not technically a method of hemostasis, ultrasonic emulsification and aspiration devices fragment and remove tissue with minimal bleeding. The emulsification process assists in hemostasis of small vessels. The technique can be used to debulk or remove benign tumors in relatively inaccessible areas of the brain and intramedullary spinal cord. The high-frequency sound waves of the ultrasonic probe fragment the tumor while sparing adjacent structures, such as nerves and blood vessels. The tumor is emulsified and removed using suction. Various settings on the instrument allow the surgeon to adjust for removal of firm or calcified tumor or soft masses.

Interventional Neuroradiology

With fluoroscopy, a team consisting of a neurosurgeon and a neuroradiologist may insert a percutaneous transfemoral catheter into a strategic point in the intracranial circulation that feeds an arteriovenous malformation, an aneurysm, or a vascular occlusion. A substance such as silicone or isobutyl 2-cyanoacrylate or a detachable microballoon or coil is injected to effectively embolize the lesion or its major deep-feeding arteries. This facilitates surgical resection of the lesion by minimizing potential hemorrhage. The intravascular procedure may be done preoperatively or intraoperatively.

Adjuncts to Visibility

Neural tissues should be as clean, dry, and visible as possible without damaging them. Visibility is enhanced by the following procedures.

Irrigation

Most wounds are irrigated frequently with normal saline solution or lactated Ringer solution. The scrub person should keep a bulb syringe filled and ready for use. The solution should be maintained at close to body temperature or cooler to prevent vasodilation and excessive bleeding.

The tip of the bone drill burr should be irrigated during use to prevent overheating the tissues (Fig. 37.6).

Suction

Suction is necessary to evacuate blood, CSF, and irrigating fluid from the surgical site so the neurosurgeon can identify structures. Necrotic tissue, pus, or cystic matter also may be aspirated. A Frazier tip is usually used. Caution is taken to avoid applying vacuum directly on healthy neural tissue, especially brain tissue. This tissue is protected by compressed absorbent patties. Suction should be available for all neurosurgical procedures.

Retractors

A variety of self-retaining retractors, such as Leyla or Greenberg bed-mounted styles, are used to retract scalp or skin and muscles. Dura mater is usually retracted with traction sutures. Blunt, malleable, flat, and spoon-shaped spatulas are used to retract brain tissue. Because visibility of structures is critical, a retractor with a fiberoptic lighting system incorporated into it may be used, especially for intracranial procedures.

Headlight

A fiberoptic headlight is used by most neurosurgeons for supplemental lighting in the surgical site.

Endoscope

A side-viewing fiberoptic endoscope may be used to enhance visibility at obscure angles in otherwise visually inaccessible areas.

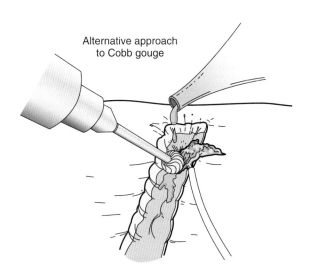

Alternative approach
to Cobb gouge

• **Fig. 37.6** Irrigation at the tip of the drill is important to prevent overheating the tissues. Eye protection is needed to prevent splash of bone chips and solution.

This endoscope is particularly useful for identification of lesions in the sella turcica, cerebral aneurysms, and intervertebral discs, for example. An endoscope may be used for placement of electrodes for stimulators or a catheter for radioisotopes.

The argon laser can be used through a ventriculoscope for intraventricular obliteration of the choroid plexuses and for intravascular treatment of lesions and neoplasms. The Nd:YAG laser can be used through a flexible or rigid neuroscope to vaporize a cyst. A straightforward, rigid, 0° scope may be used for electrocoagulation or laser obliteration of tissue and to obtain a CT-assisted stereotactic biopsy.

Neuro Intraoperative Viewing Systems

The NeuroGuide and NeuroNavigator intraoperative viewing systems provide capabilities for 3D viewing of structures through a tiny opening in the brain for diagnostic and therapeutic procedures with minimal trauma to tissues. Image-guided surgery provides preplanning maps, monitoring of brain activity, exact tumor location, smaller incisions, shorter recovery time, and less damage to surrounding tissue.[2]

Operating Microscope

The operating microscope provides an intense light and magnification for visualization of intracranial structures. Microsurgery permits removal of tumors and vascular lesions that are otherwise inaccessible or inoperable. The CO_2 laser may be used through a micromanipulator.

The microscope also is used for some spinal procedures and peripheral nerve repair. A fiberoptic camera attached to a microscope projects the surgical site onto a video monitor screen. This provides a clear view for the assistant and scrub person. In lieu of use of the microscope, the surgeon may wear binocular loupes to magnify the surgical site. Great care is taken not to bump or jar the instrument table or microscope during the procedure.

Patient Care Considerations for Craniotomy

The patient's fear of an inability to function independently as a result of intracranial surgery is paramount, either consciously or subconsciously. The brain is the core of one's being. Many neurosurgical patients do not undergo premedication, which allows neurologic assessment before induction of anesthesia or during a procedure performed with the patient under local anesthesia. The circulating nurse should be sensitive to the patient's fears and offer reassurance. Psychologic support is especially significant for a patient who is awake.

Patient Preparation

Preparation of the patient in the OR usually begins with clipping of hair with electric clippers. Hair on the head is considered the patient's personal property. When all of it is removed, it is saved. Hair removal and its disposition are documented on the patient's chart. Demarcation of the desired outline for the incision may be made on the scalp after the skin preparation and before draping. A sterile disposable skin marker is available (Fig. 37.7).

Prevention of peripheral nerve and circulatory damage requires that the circulating nurse check pressure points on the patient's body during prolonged procedures. Some microneurosurgical procedures take 10 hours or longer to complete. Gel pads or a foam mattress similar in configuration to an egg crate should be used if the patient is supine or prone on the OR bed.

• **Fig. 37.7** Craniotomy incision.

• **Fig. 37.8** Mayfield skull clamp stabilizes head for right frontotemporal craniotomy. Single pin on left and two spring-loaded pins on right penetrate outer table of skull.

Patient Positioning

The standard OR bed is used. A specialized head holder or frame is used. The incision and the type of procedure determine the head holder that is needed to position the patient. The basic support unit of a neurosurgical head-positioning device attaches in place of the headpiece on the standard OR bed. The Mayfield headrest or skull clamp fits into the basic frame to stabilize the head for cranial procedures.

The Mayfield headrest conforms to the contours of the patient's head like a horseshoe. The circular or horseshoe-shaped headrest equalizes weight distribution around the patient's face when in the prone position.

The Mayfield skull clamp provides stability that is necessary for microsurgical procedures and is desirable during lengthy procedures. This eliminates the risk for pressure-related complications around the face or eyes with the patient prone or in a lateral position. Three pins on the skull clamp partially penetrate the outer table of the skull. Pins on one side may be spring-loaded (Fig. 37.8) to join the skull and the clamp into one rigid mechanical unit. When pin fixation is used, antibiotic ointment is applied around each fixation pin to form an airtight seal. This reduces the risk for air embolism and infection. The circulating nurse should be familiar with the desired neurosurgical positions and the headrests, skull clamps, and attachments for each.

Supine Position

The supine position is used most commonly for approaches to the frontal, parietal, and temporal lobes within the anterior and middle fossae. A lateral position may be preferred for some of these surgical procedures, such as a unilateral approach to the right or left temporal lobe.

Prone Position

The patient is anesthetized in a supine position on the transport cart and turned prone onto the OR bed. A detailed description of prone positioning is found in Chapter 26 of this text. The eyes are lubricated, and the lids are taped closed for protection. The patient's transport cart should be immediately available in the event of the need for cardiac resuscitation. The patient needs to be placed supine in a rapid manner, and the nearby cart facilitates this maneuver.

• **Fig. 37.9** Neurosurgical sitting position for posterior approach. Frame of head holder is attached to side rails of back section of OR bed. Note that legs are flexed at thighs and are approximately at level of heart. Feet are padded at right angles to legs. Subgluteal padding protects sciatic nerves.

The prone position is used to access the occipital lobe. It also may be used for a suboccipital approach; however, many neurosurgeons prefer a sitting position to approach the posterior fossa.

Seated Position

The Mayfield basic frame is attached to the side rails of the OR bed to support the head for a posterior, unilateral, or nasal approach. In the seated position, the patient is at risk for pelvic venous pooling and air embolus.[3]

For a posterior approach, a head holder supports the forehead. The seated position allows greater torsion and flexion of the neck than either a lateral or the prone position and a more accessible approach to the cerebellopontine angle (Fig. 37.9).

Air embolus is a potential problem when a sitting position is used. The brain is higher than the heart in this position. Venous pressure is lower than atmospheric and can allow for entry of air into the heart via an open venous channel. Excess air in the right atrium can prevent blood from passing to the lungs for gas exchange.

The anesthesia provider may insert a central venous catheter in the subclavian or jugular vein before the procedure begins as a prophylactic measure in the event that air needs to be removed from the heart (Durant procedure).

A pneumatic counterpressure device may be used in some settings. An antishock garment (military antishock suit [MAST]) extends from the patient's rib margin to the ankles and is inflated if the patient's condition becomes hypotensive. The inflated garment raises the intracavitary pressures in the body. In lieu of a MAST garment, antiembolic stockings or sequential compression stockings are applied.

Controlled Hypothermia

Prevention of cerebral edema during craniotomy may be accomplished with hypothermia. Hypothermia also may be used to decrease cerebral blood flow and venous pressure, to decrease brain volume, and to control ICP. Patients are cooled to a core temperature between 57° F and 68° F (14° C and 20° C) with surface-induced hypothermia, intravenous (IV) cooling, or a combination of both. Core body temperature can be monitored via a thermal probe placed in the esophagus or rectum or contained within the indwelling Foley catheter.

Hypothermia with elective circulatory arrest and extracorporeal cardiopulmonary bypass is an alternative when conventional approaches to the control of blood loss are unsatisfactory. The desired core temperature before extracorporeal cardiopulmonary bypass begins is 64° F (18° C). The cooling process may take 1 hour. An 18 to 24-Fr arterial perfusion cannula is placed in the right femoral artery for oxygenated blood return, and a 28 or 32-Fr venous return cannula is placed in the left femoral vein for venous drainage.

Normally the brain cannot tolerate ischemia for more than a few minutes. This time is extended with lowering of body temperature. The average circulatory arrest time is between 12 and 45 minutes at 64° F (18° C). Hypothermia decreases cellular metabolism and therefore decreases oxygen consumption by the brain and heart during interruption of circulation. Intermittent administration of cold crystalloid cerebroplegia solution also may help protect the brain during cardiopulmonary bypass and profound hypothermia.

Blood viscosity increases as body temperature decreases. Two or three units of the patient's blood may be withdrawn and replaced with chilled normal saline solution. During rewarming, this blood is autotransfused. Crystalloid priming solution from the cardiopulmonary bypass machine also causes hemodilution.

Intracranial Pressure Control

Reduction of ICP and brain volume may be accomplished with withdrawal of spinal fluid. An intrathecal catheter or Touhy needle is inserted, before prepping and draping, for the anesthesia provider to remove CSF during the surgical procedure as desired by the neurosurgeon. ICP monitoring is discussed subsequently in this section.

Position of the Instrument Table

Instrumentation is usually arranged on a Mayfield or Phalen table or on a double Mayo stand set up over the patient positioned supine or prone. The scrub person stands on a tiered platform to easily set up and reach the instruments as they are needed. The instrument table surface can be raised or lowered.

The drapes over the patient's head are attached to the table drapes. Some surgeons use a skin stapler to attach drapes to the scalp. A one-piece sheet that provides a combined sterile table cover and the patient's cranial drape with a self-adhering circular incise area is available (Fig. 37.10).

If the patient will be in a Fowler or sitting position, the Mayfield instrument table is placed above and lateral to drape over the patient. The drapes form a tent on one side of the patient so the anesthesia provider can have access throughout the procedure.

Hemostasis

Infiltration of a local anesthetic agent with epinephrine beneath the scalp is desirable for many intracranial procedures. The epinephrine acts as a vasoconstrictor to control bleeding and the volume creates tumescence for a firmer incision line.

The scalp, extracranial arteries, and portions of the dura mater are the only structures covering the brain that are sensitive to pain; local anesthetic can provide some preemptive analgesia. Gelfoam or patties with topical thrombin may be used after the bone flap is opened. Some surgeons use rayon balls, but these are not usually radiopaque. Care is taken to account for all materials used in hemostasis.

Anticipation of difficulty in achieving hemostasis with the methods previously discussed is not unusual in some procedures for removal of vascular intracranial lesions. Controlled hypotension may be initiated by the anesthesia provider, with the concurrence of the neurosurgeon, to lower the blood pressure (BP).

The surgeon incises the scalp along the predetermined line. The scalp edges are highly vascular and require careful hemostasis. Excessive use of the ESU causes death of hair follicles, so temporary plastic Raney clips are placed along the skin edges for hemostasis (Fig. 37.11). These clips are applied individually with great care and with use of a special clip applier (Fig. 37.12). This same applier is used to remove the clips at the end of the procedure before skin closure. The Raney clips are disposable. Other styles are available preloaded in 10s and 20s in an applier that resembles a skin stapler.

• **Fig. 37.10** Neurosurgical team in place for craniotomy.

• **Fig. 37.11** Craniotomy scalp edge hemostasis with temporary plastic Raney clips.

• **Fig. 37.12 A,** Plastic Raney clips with applier. **B,** Application of temporary plastic Raney clips.

Physiologic Monitoring

Cerebral edema (brain swelling), cerebral arterial perfusion, and ICP can be safely controlled before, during, and after the surgical procedure. These parameters are continuously monitored. An intraarterial catheter is often inserted for continuous direct arterial BP monitoring and for drawing of samples for arterial blood gas analyses.

A central venous pressure line may be established also. A pulmonary artery catheter may be inserted to measure fluid volume and diagnose or aspirate an air embolus. Capnography is used routinely. Mass spectrometry is the most sensitive method of monitoring concentrations of inspired and expired gases. This sensitive device detects any type of gas, including nitrogen.

Doppler Ultrasound Scan

A precordial Doppler ultrasound transducer is secured over the precordium (i.e., over the right side of the heart to the right of the sternum between the third and sixth intercostal spaces). This is used primarily for continuous monitoring for air embolism in the patient in a sitting position. An altered ultrasound response results if air is present in the right atrium.

A sterile transcranial Doppler ultrasound transducer monitors changes in redistribution of cerebral blood flow, such as after obliteration of a large intracranial vascular malformation. This technique is also used to monitor cerebral vasospasm. Elevation of transcranial Doppler velocities precedes clinical signs of cerebral ischemia. The transducer also can be placed over the cerebral cortex to verify the location and depth of a tumor or cyst.

Evoked Potentials

Somatosensory evoked potentials guide the anesthesia provider in handling arterial BP, ventilation, inspired oxygen concentration, and patient positioning. Changes in cortical evoked potentials can indicate cerebral ischemia and systemic hypoxia. Both cortical and subcortical sensory evoked potentials can record surgical invasion of the spinal cord, peripheral nerve, nerve plexus, brainstem, or midbrain. To avert permanent injury to the patient, the surgeon may adjust retractors, alter the approach to a tumor, or perform a subtotal tumor resection on the basis of changes in evoked potentials. The anesthesia provider may adjust the depth of anesthesia.

Auditory brainstem evoked potentials, with a stimulus to the ear, may be used to monitor the eighth cranial nerve and brainstem during surgical procedures in the posterior fossa, if performed with the patient under local anesthesia.

Visual evoked potentials may be used during the surgical procedure for pituitary tumors, optic nerve decompression, aneurysms, and some other types of lesions. A strobe light flash is used to elicit responses. The light-emitting diodes are placed over closed eyelids and secured before the patient is prepped and draped.

Intracranial Pressure

ICP rises with an increase in volume of the brain, CSF, or cerebral blood supply or with decompensation (inability to compensate for pressure changes). When an abnormal elevation is sustained, ICP prevents adequate perfusion of the cerebral cortex. The brain is deprived of its blood supply. Pressure monitoring is the only exact method for determination of a rise in ICP and impending neurologic crisis during cranial procedures or after head injury. ICP monitoring is accomplished with implantation of a ventricular catheter, subarachnoid screw, or epidural sensor.

A ventricular catheter is invasive but is the most accurate method of ICP monitoring. The cannula and reservoir are inserted into the ventricle through a burr hole or twist drill hole in the skull. Proper positioning of stopcocks is important because incorrect placement may result in excessive CSF drainage with a sudden drop in ICP and possible brain herniation. This method evaluates volume and pressure responses and permits drainage of large amounts of CSF and instillation of contrast media and antibiotics. Catheter patency should be checked frequently. Postoperatively, the patient is observed for signs of infection, such as meningitis or ventriculitis.

A hollow steel subarachnoid screw is placed in the subdural space via a twist drill hole in the skull and a small incision in the dura mater. Although this method is used to measure ICP accurately and directly from CSF, it cannot be used to drain large amounts of fluid; it can provide access for CSF sampling. The screw may become occluded with blood or tissue. It should be checked frequently for patency.

A small epidural sensor is implanted in the epidural space of the brain through a small burr hole in the skull. The sensor is attached to a transducer, which converts CSF pressure to electrical impulses. The sensor cable is plugged into a monitor that produces a continuous readout. This is the least invasive method of ICP monitoring, but its accuracy is questionable.

Electroencephalogram

The function or organic activity of the brain may be monitored periodically throughout the surgical procedure with an electroencephalogram (EEG). Sterile subdermal needle electrodes may be inserted if surface scalp electrodes cannot be used.

Surgical Procedures of the Cranium

Craniectomy

Craniectomy is the removal (-ectomy) of a portion of the bones of the skull (cranium). After the scalp incision, the bone is perforated or removed to approach the brain. This may be accomplished through one or more (trephine) burr holes or twist drill holes. Each hole is drilled with an electrical or air-powered instrument or manually with a Hudson brace (Fig. 37.13). Burr holes are approximately ½ inch (13 mm) in diameter (Fig. 37.14). Some diagnostic and therapeutic procedures are performed through these holes. Additional bone may be removed with a rongeur to increase exposure of the brain for more extensive procedures, such as an approach to the cranial nerves or tumors in the posterior fossa or suboccipital region.

The bone may be cut between the burr holes with a flexible multifilament wire (Gigli saw) or air-powered craniotome. A dura guard attachment protects the dura mater. A large area of bone is raised for temporary or permanent removal. Attached to the muscle, which acts as a hinge, the bone may be turned back to expose the underlying dura, referred to as *raising a bone flap*. The bone flap may be removed and stored for later positioning.

• **Fig. 37.13** Hudson brace manual drill.

• **Fig. 37.14** Burr holes for craniectomy or craniotomy.

Storage can be done in a sterile container in a special refrigerator or placed in a tissue pocket created in the patient's abdominal wall.

Burr holes may be covered with a soft, pliable, silicone disc-shaped sheath, with or without a channel for introduction of a hypodermic needle for medication administration. The cover may be used to eliminate a cosmetically undesirable indentation of the scalp into the created bone defect.

Postoperative access to the cranial cavity through the hole or channel in the cover can be used for drainage of fluid or instillation of chemotherapeutic drugs. ICP monitoring devices can be attached. Other types of implantable infusion pumps also are inserted through a craniectomy.

Brain Pacemaker

Electrode plates of a brain pacemaker or cerebellar stimulator are implanted through small occipital and suboccipital craniectomies. Silicone-coated polyester fiber mesh plates, each with four pairs of platinum disc electrodes, are applied to the anterior and posterior surfaces of the cerebellum. One or two receivers, implanted just below the clavicle, are attached to the electrodes on the cerebellum by subcutaneously placed leads.

Stimulation of the pacemaker electrodes is controlled by an external transmitter through an antenna placed on the skin over the subdermal receiver. This device is used to control muscular hypertonia and seizures related to cerebral palsy, epilepsy, stroke, or brain injury.

Craniotomy

Scalp, bone, and dural flaps are raised to expose a large area of the cerebrum for exploration, definitive treatment, or excision of lesions within the brain. Raney clips are applied to the galea and over the edge of the scalp flap. The bone flap is turned as described for craniectomy by drilling four or five burr holes along the edge of the proposed bone incision and then cutting a line between the holes with a Gigli saw or a powered saw with a dural guard on the tip. Moistened sponges protect both the scalp flap and the bone flap. The dural flap is protected with large compressed patties.

For wound closure, the thin but tough fibrous dural flap is laid over the brain. Usually it is sutured with multiple interrupted stitches to provide a tight seal that prevents leakage of CSF. The bone flap may be repositioned and anchored with nonabsorbable sutures, silicone burr hole buttons, or titanium plates and screws. Absorbable screws can be used for aesthetic appearance. The galea is closed with interrupted sutures before the scalp is sutured or approximated with staples.

A silicone rubber suction drain may be placed in the subdural space to drain residual fluid from a subdural hematoma or the bed of a brain tumor or to remove red blood cells in CSF after a craniotomy.

Intracranial Tumors

Intracranial tumors can originate from the neural tissues of the brain, the meninges, glandular tissue, choroid plexuses, cranial nerves, blood vessels, embryonal defects, or metastatic lesions (Table 37.2). A craniotomy may be performed to remove a circumscribed, encapsulated, slow-growing, benign brain tumor. Some of these tumors, such as a meningioma, are highly vascular. Primary or secondary metastatic malignant tumors are broadly classified as gliomas. These have an unregulated cellular

<table>
<tr><td colspan="5">

TABLE 37.2 **Intracranial Neoplasms**
</td></tr>
</table>

Cell of Origin	Site	Age and Sex	Degree of Malignancy
Astrocytoma: Grades I and II			
Astrocyte	Cerebrum	Young adults Equal between sexes	Low malignancy; slow-growing tumor; becomes cystic; well-differentiated cell structure; average survival period is 6 years
			Most common brain tumor
Astrocytoma: Grades III and IV			
Astrocyte	Cerebrum, cerebellum, and white matter	Middle age Males > females	Highly malignant, slow-growing tumor; poorly differentiated cell structure; 20% of all brain tumors are this type; average survival period is 6 years
Ependymoma			
Cells lining ventricular system of brain and central canal of the spinal cord; most common in fourth ventricle	Fourth ventricle and distal spinal cord	Children and young adults Equal between sexes	Low malignancy; slow-growing tumor; variable differentiation of cell structure; may calcify; 10% of all brain tumors are this type; survival time is measured in months according to location of tumor
			30% of all spinal tumors
Glioblastoma Multiforme			
Glial cells	Cerebral hemispheres and corpus callosum	Middle age Equal between sexes	Highly malignant; infiltrative, rapidly growing; highly cellular with many necrotic foci; 50% of all brain tumors are this type; average survival period is 1 year
Medulloblastoma			
Uncertain, primitive bipotential cells	Cerebellum, fourth ventricle, and sub-arachnoid space	Children Males > females	Moderate malignancy; rapidly growing tumor; moderate differentiation of cell structure; 10% of all brain tumors are this type; average survival period is 15 months
Meningioma			
Arachnoid cell	Parasagittal and lateral convexities, sphenoidal ridge, and thoracic spinal cord	Middle age Females > males	Usually benign; encapsulated and easily separated from nervous tissue
Neurilemoma (Schwannoma)			
Schwann cells of cranial nerves and spinal nerve roots	Cranial nerve VIII in cerebellopontine angle and thoracic spinal cord	Middle age Equal between sexes	Usually benign; pain and paresthesia are common
Oligodendroglioma			
Oligodendrocyte	Cerebrum, white matter	Middle age Equal between sexes	Low malignancy; slow-growing tumor; moderate differentiation of cells; 5% of all brain tumors are this type; average survival period is 5 years

proliferation of rapidly growing cells, which invade surrounding brain tissue.

Glioblastoma multiforme, one of the most common brain tumors, is the most malignant type. Hemorrhagic and edematous effects of a rapidly growing tumor may be an indication for a lobectomy to give the brain an area for expansion and to impede mortality. The rigid characteristics of the skull prevent its expansion or contraction; however, the brain can expand or contract.

Subdural decompression by craniectomy for reduction of ICP and papilledema may be the palliative procedure of choice. As a result of anatomic location, some benign tumors are considered malignant because they cannot be safely removed without severe neurologic deficits or a threat to life-sustaining functions. Microneurosurgery and stereotaxis provide access to tumors in some anatomic locations that are otherwise impossible to reach, such as in third-ventricle and pineal regions.

Cranioplasty

Traumatic or surgically created skull defects are corrected with autogenous bone grafts or a synthetic or titanium prosthesis. Large defects in the anterior or middle fossae are covered for protection of the brain and cosmetic effect. The bone flap may be removed after an intracranial procedure to allow cerebral decompression postoperatively. It is stored under sterile conditions in the bone bank until it can be placed in the skull.

Bone removed because of an extensively comminuted fracture or bone disease may be replaced with sterile polymethylmethacrylate

(PMMA). This material contours better than preformed titanium plates. In sterile conditions, the sterile resin powder is mixed with the sterile liquid polymer to form a doughy mass. This is placed in a sterile plastic bag and rolled to the thickness of the skull with a roller.

While still pliable, PMMA is molded to the contour of the head and the size of the defect. When hardened, it can be trimmed with a rongeur, and the edges smoothed with a special small emery wheel mounted on the electric bone saw. The prosthesis is wired to the skull in several places. The brain expands to meet it and leaves no dead space between it and the dura.

Dural defects can be closed with autologous fascia graft, fibrin film, polyethylene film, synthetic absorbable mesh, or freeze-dried human cadaver dura mater grafts.

Intracranial Microneurosurgery

The magnification and lighting afforded by the operating microscope have refined intracranial microneurosurgical techniques and made possible approaches to many neurologic problems. A CO_2 laser may be adapted to the microscope for ablation of benign or malignant intracranial tumors. Discussions of some other microneurosurgical procedures follow.

Other Cranial Procedures
Excision of an Acoustic Neuroma

Retrosigmoid, middle fossa, or translabyrinthine approaches may be used by otologists for removal of acoustic neuromas. The surgical approach depends on the size and location of the tumor. A neurosurgeon resects an acoustic neuroma that more commonly extends into the posterior fossa of the cranial cavity. An acoustic neuroma can grow progressively into the trigeminal, facial, and abducens nerves and into the cerebellopontine angle (the area between the pons, medulla oblongata, and cerebellum). Potentially life-threatening, these involvements manifest symptoms of facial weakness, paresthesia, and dysphagia.

The patient is placed in a semi-Fowler or sitting position, with pin fixation in the Mayfield or Gardner-Wells frame. The operating microscope offers the potential for preservation of functional hearing. Particular caution is taken to obtain meticulous hemostasis, to spare the auditory artery if hearing is to be preserved, and to avoid trauma to or resection of the facial nerve. Facial nerve function is impossible to salvage in a percentage of patients. If the facial nerve is sacrificed, the patient may return for a facial–hypoglossal or facial–accessory nerve anastomosis 4 to 6 weeks postoperatively.

A retromastoid transtemporal approach with the patient in a lateral position or a subtemporal transtentorial approach with the patient supine may be preferred. The surgeon's decision to preserve or sacrifice the facial nerve or hearing influences the approach to an acoustic neuroma. The ultrasonic aspirator or CO_2 laser may be used to remove the tumor.

Decompression of Cranial Nerves

Microvascular decompression relieves the severe and disabling symptoms of some cranial nerve disorders, such as trigeminal neuralgia (tic douloureux), glossopharyngeal neuralgia, acoustic nerve dysfunction, and hemifacial spasm. Initial symptoms of hyperactivity in a cranial nerve can progress to loss of function. Some disorders are caused by mechanical cross-compression, usually vascular, of the nerve root at the brainstem. Symptoms depend on sensory and motor functions of the nerve.

With the patient in a sitting position, a retromastoid craniectomy is performed to explore the cerebellopontine angle. A supracerebellar exposure is used for the trigeminal nerve, and an infracerebellar exposure is used for the remainder of the cranial nerves. An artery or a vein that is compressing the nerve root may be mobilized away from the nerve. A tiny piece of silastic sponge may be placed between the vessel and nerve to relieve the pulsating pressure on the nerve. A tissue sling may be created to lift the vessel off the nerve. Tumors that were not diagnosed preoperatively are excised. If vascular decompression or another pathologic condition is not evident, the nerve may be sectioned to relieve pain.

Surgery of Cranial Blood Vessels
Cerebral Revascularization

For cerebral revascularization, an extracranial artery is anastomosed to an intracranial artery for bypass of stenotic or occlusive vascular disease distal to the bifurcation of the common carotid artery. This procedure provides an additional and significant source of blood to the cerebral circulation.

An artery in the scalp, such as the superficial temporal or occipital artery or another branch of the external carotid artery, is anastomosed to a branch of the middle cerebral artery or to a cortical branch of the cerebral artery. Vessels must be 1 mm in diameter or larger for the anastomosis to work. The procedure is primarily prophylactic to prevent development of a major brain attack (stroke) in patients who have had transient ischemic attacks or minor strokes with temporary disruption of brain function caused by blockage of the cerebrovascular system.

The patient is positioned supine with the head turned or is positioned laterally with the head stabilized flat on the OR bed for an approach through a temporal craniectomy. The anastomosis is made on the surface of the brain, end to end, side to side, or end to side of the arteries.

In some patients, plaque can be removed from the middle cerebral artery rather than the occlusion being bypassed. Cerebral embolectomy with a detachable balloon or other intravascular technique may be done to obliterate a carotid-cavernous fistula or arteriovenous malformation in conjunction with an extracranial-intracranial arterial bypass. Cranial bypass is the procedure of choice for cerebral revascularization in a patient who has a vascular lesion that cannot be treated with carotid endarterectomy.

Arteriovenous Malformation

An arteriovenous malformation (AVM) is an abnormal communication between the arterial and venous systems that involves many dilated blood vessels (Fig. 37.15). As the fistulous connections gradually enlarge under pressure, blood is diverted from surrounding brain tissue, causing scarring and compression as a result of poor perfusion. This process is accelerated by multiple small hemorrhages from the thin engorged vessels. Progressive neurologic deficits can cause seizures and life-threatening subarachnoid, intraventricular, or intraparenchymal hemorrhage.

A large diffuse AVM that involves multiple vessels and high-flow shunts can be difficult to excise. The strategy of the neurosurgeon may be to perform a staged resection with intraoperative embolization initially to reduce the number of fistulous arteries and size of shunts. For embolization, small silastic beads may be introduced into an AVM via a catheter placed into the internal carotid artery. This procedure usually is done a month before surgical resection.

Normal arteriovenous communication

Abnormal arteriovenous communication

• **Fig. 37.15** Arteriovenous malformation.

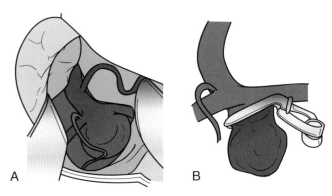

• **Fig. 37.16 A,** Middle cerebral artery aneurysm exposure. **B,** Middle cerebral artery aneurysm with clip to prevent rupture.

With the operating microscope, the surgeon carefully coagulates or clips the arteries as close to the AVM as possible. Healthy arteries that perfuse the brain beyond the AVM are preserved. At least one vein must remain patent to drain the AVM until other vessels are occluded. The preserved vein is then occluded, and the AVM is excised.

Occlusion of Aneurysms

Aneurysms of the cerebral and vertebral arteries vary from the size of a pea to the size of an orange. Most intracranial aneurysms are located near the basilar surface of the skull and arise from the internal carotid or middle cerebral arteries. Cerebral artery (berry) aneurysms are usually located on the circle of Willis at the base of the brain between the hemispheres of the cerebrum.

Most cerebral aneurysms are associated with a congenital defect of the tunica media of the intracranial vessel wall. Hemodynamic forces of pulsatile pressure cause enlargement, outpouching, and thinning of the arterial wall, which eventually ruptures. This is the most common source of subarachnoid hemorrhage. Most aneurysms seal spontaneously, but a surgical procedure may be indicated to prevent rebleeding. If diagnosed, an unruptured asymptomatic aneurysm may be occluded with Guglielmi platinum coils by a minimally invasive endovascular approach before rupture.

For open treatment, the patient is placed in a sitting position for suboccipital or subfrontal craniectomy and the aneurysm is exposed for occlusion. The neck (base) of the aneurysm is occluded with a low-pressure aneurysm clip or ligated if it can be isolated (Fig. 37.16). Microcoils can be placed in the aneurysm in the interventional radiation department to help prevent rupture (Fig. 37.17). If it cannot be isolated, the aneurysm and parent vessel may be wrapped in fine-mesh gauze and coated with PMMA, isobutyl 2-cyanoacrylate, or other epoxy resin to reinforce the wall.

More commonly, the aneurysm is coagulated with bipolar electrosurgery or a laser. Induced hypotension may be used to decrease blood flow in the artery feeding the aneurysm. This aids in dissection and occlusion. The operating microscope is used for delicate dissection of the arteries at the base of the brain.

Stereotaxis

Stereotaxis is the accurate location of a definite circumscribed area within the brain from external points or landmarks on the skull. It defines 3D coordinates (planes) with which one can approach

• **Fig. 37.17 A,** Cerebral aneurysm. **B,** Occlusive embolization coil placed in aneurysm to prevent rupture.

deep structures without damaging overlying structures. The technique is used to create or ablate a lesion in otherwise inaccessible parts of the brain. With determination of specific reference points on CT, PET, or MRI scans, the exact area for the target site of the lesion is calculated by a computer.[3] The computer, especially designed for stereotactic surgery, provides measurements for correct alignment of instrumentation and calculation of the depth of target tissue within the brain.

A stereoencephalotome, a specially designed mechanical apparatus, is attached to the skull with the patient in a sitting position. After this is in place, computerized data show localizers of the apparatus in relation to intracranial structures. The ventricular system provides the internal landmarks. Many models are available. The following basic types of stereoencephalotomes are used:

- *Semicircle arc system:* Steel screws are tapped through each of four burr holes for fixation of the head to a ring supported from a table attachment or a pedestal on the floor (Fig. 37.18). The ring is secured to arc plates. The head is moved rather than the apparatus.
- *Rectilinear system:* The apparatus can be moved back and forth and from side to side around the head to make adjustments.
- *Single arc system:* An arc over the head allows angular adjustments.
- *Custom face mask:* A premeasured face mask is made to hold the head in place.

• **Fig. 37.18** Stereotactic head frame.

The stereoencephalotome can obstruct the surgeon's access for an intracranial procedure. Frameless stereotactic systems or face masks enable the neurosurgeon to continually interact with CT scans and MRI displays via a computer linkage throughout an intracranial procedure. Known as an interactive image-guided stereotactic neurosurgery system, the system incorporates 3D images from cameras mounted over the OR bed, position-sensing probes and forceps, and a computer system. With a stereoencephalotome in place, stereotactic surgery can be performed through a burr hole, rigid or flexible endoscope, or open craniotomy.

A lesion may be made or removed by laser, high-frequency or radiofrequency electrocoagulation, cryosurgery, ultrasound, radiation, hyperthermia, or mechanical curettage. Procedures are performed with the patient under local anesthesia when patient cooperation to test motor or sensory function may be needed during the surgical procedure.[4] Various types of intracranial procedures are performed with computer-assisted stereotaxis.

Aspiration

A needle or cannula is placed into target tissue to aspirate a cyst, abscess, or hematoma. Tissue may be obtained for biopsy.

Functional Neurosurgery

For functional neurosurgery, lesions are created in the brain to reduce intractable pain or to control tremors or psychotic behavior.

Electrostimulation

Intermittent electrostimulation of the brain by stereotactically implanted electrodes can control a variety of benign intractable pain problems. One electrode is placed in the somatosensory system for evaluation of pain of central origin, and another is placed in the paraventricular gray matter for evaluation of pain of peripheral origin.

After postoperative evaluation of the effectiveness of electrical stimulation of each electrode, the patient returns to the OR to have a receiver placed under the skin on the anterior chest wall. A connecting wire is tunneled from the receiver to the electrode. An external transmitter and antenna placed over the receiver stimulate the electrode as desired by the patient.

Radiofrequency Retrogasserian Rhizotomy

Radiofrequency retrogasserian rhizotomy relieves the pain of trigeminal neuralgia, also known as tic douloureux. The fifth cranial (trigeminal) nerve carries sensory impulses for touch, pain, and external temperature from the face, scalp, and mucous membranes

in the head. Trigeminal neuralgia is an intense paroxysmal pain in one side of the face. It can be controlled by damaging the gasserian (trigeminal) ganglion.

An insulated cannula with an uninsulated tip is placed through the cheek and foramen ovale and is advanced to the gasserian ganglion. The ganglion is coagulated when a radiofrequency generator activates the tip of the cannula. Several lesions can be made to achieve the desired extent of paresthesia.

Thalamotomy

The forerunner of other stereotactic procedures, thalamotomy destroys a selected portion of the thalamus for relief of pain, epileptic seizures, and involuntary tremor or rigidity of muscles (e.g., in Parkinson disease) and occasionally for emotional disturbances. Functionally, the thalamus, located in the midbrain, is the principal relay point in the cerebrum for sensory impulses passing from lower parts of the nervous system to the cerebral cortex.

Cingulotomy

Bilateral symmetric radiofrequency electrolytic lesions are placed to disrupt pathways of the cingulum. The cingulum is a bundle of connecting fibers in the medial aspect of each cerebral hemisphere between the frontal and temporal lobes. Cingulotomies are performed for severe chronic pain, addiction, or some intractable psychoses that have not responded to other methods of treatment.

Pallidotomy

Stereotactic pallidotomy can be performed to decrease muscle rigidity associated with Parkinson disease.

Psychosurgery

Intractable depression, obsessive-compulsive disorders, and chronic anxiety may be treated with cingulotomy as described or with frontal lobotomy. With stereotactic control, a probe is inserted into the white matter of the frontal lobe of the brain to create a lesion via cryosurgery or electrocoagulation. The lesion disrupts neural cortical/subcortical connections in the frontal lobe anterior to the lateral ventricles that control emotions.

Some surgeons implant fine electrodes that remain indwelling for weeks to months. These can be used for chronic stimulation of surrounding tissue or to create additional electrocoagulative lesions. Complications include epilepsy, indecisiveness, and altered personality. Studies have shown that memory and intellect are not impaired. Psychosurgery is performed only if other treatments, such as medication or psychotherapy, have failed to provide relief.

Transcranial Magnetic Stimulation

Transcranial magnetic stimulation (TMS) is a noninvasive form of psychosurgery treatment for depression. An electromagnetic coil is placed against the scalp and delivers continuous or bursts of magnetic pulses.[5]

Theta burst stimulation (TBS) is intermittent or continuous delivery of lower magnetic energy designed to provide longer-lasting treatment for depression in patients not responding to TMS. Studies have shown safety for use in children and is under review by the U.S. Food and Drug Administration.

Intracranial Neoplasms

Computer-assisted stereotaxis helps locate and reach the margin of a deep-seated intracranial tumor either by open craniotomy or through an endoscope. Then a CO_2 or KTP laser beam or other agent can be directed to destroy the tumor while preserving healthy cerebral tissue.

Cryohypophysectomy

Creation of cryogenic lesions may be the procedure of choice for treatment of growth hormone—producing pituitary adenomas with no suprasellar extension. The cryosurgical probe is introduced into the sella turcica through a frontal burr hole. During creation of the lesion, ocular movements and visual acuity are carefully monitored.

Interstitial Radiation

Radioactive substances may be stereotactically implanted into malignant brain tumors. Multiple catheters can be placed throughout the target volume. The catheters are afterloaded with radioactive material such as iridium-192 or iodine-125 seeds. The catheters are inserted percutaneously through twist drill holes. Tiles made of collagen with radioactive seeds may be implanted.[6] For photoradiation therapy, a hematoporphyrin derivative may be injected preoperatively and activated by argon or a tunable dye laser to create a cytotoxic photochemical reaction in tumor cells.

Interstitial Hyperthermia

Catheters and remote sensors are implanted into the tumor volume. Sufficient heat is conducted through sensors to raise the temperature within the tumor to a degree that destroys its cells. This is effective against radioresistant hypoxic cells and poorly vascularized and metabolically inactive tumors.

Stereotactic Radiosurgery

Intense beams of high-energy gamma radiation or microwave-generated energy photons from a linear accelerator are directed to specific targets within the brain while sparing healthy brain tissue. Gamma knife stereotactic radiosurgery does not actually use a knife and is technically not surgery as the name implies.[7] This noninvasive procedure uses stereotaxis to identify the location of an intracranial tumor or AVM.

A specially designed helmet fits over the patient's head and the stereoencephalotome frame. A single high dose of cobalt-generated gamma radiation is directed through holes in the helmet. The beams are collimated and focused on the lesion. The gamma unit is a specific installation for this procedure. The treatment takes 5 to 30 minutes. It does not remove the lesion, but it can stop its growth and reduce its size.[7]

Control of Epilepsy

Epilepsy, caused by erratic electrical rhythms in the brain, manifests in a variety of intermittent disabling behaviors—most commonly, convulsive seizures. Epilepsy may result from a congenital anomaly within the brain or can develop after trauma, meningitis, or acute febrile illness. Patients with intractable seizures uncontrolled with medication may be candidates for surgery to remove the focal point of the seizures.

EEG monitoring and CT, PET, and MRI scans help with identification of the specific location of abnormal brain tissue that is causing seizures. One of two invasive procedures may be necessary if these tests are inconclusive:

- *Subdural grid implantation:* Via a frontotemporoparietal craniectomy, a silastic grid with metal discs attached to stainless steel or platinum electrodes is placed on the cortex of the brain. The grid size varies depending on the area to be monitored. The grid is anchored to the dura mater. The electrodes are tunneled under the skin to an area outside the incision before the dura, bone, and skin flaps are closed.

  Subsequently, seizure activity from the surface of the brain is monitored for several days with an EEG monitor connected to the electrodes. The grid also maps the brain to locate areas of motor, sensory, visual, speech, and memory control. The patient returns to the OR for removal of the grid. Cortical resection also may be performed at this time.

- *Stereotactic depth electrode implantation:* By correlating CT, PET, or MRI images with reference points on the stereotactic frame, electrodes are implanted directly into the brain. These are connected to an EEG to determine the focus of seizures within specific areas of the brain. After weeks of monitoring, the patient returns to the OR for removal of the electrodes. The epileptic focus may be destroyed by creating a stereotactic lesion at this time.

  After an epileptic focus is identified, a definitive surgical procedure can be performed to stop or reduce seizure activity. The objective is to maintain cerebral capabilities for language, speech, memory, vision, movement, and other sensory and motor neurologic functions.

Cortical Resection

Epileptogenic tissue is resected from the cerebral cortex where the epileptic focus is localized. An anterior temporal lobectomy is most commonly performed. Frontal and other extratemporal sites may be resected if the epileptic focus does not interfere with neurologic functions.

Corpus Callosotomy

The corpus callosum (a fibrous band of neurons) or the anterior commissure connecting the two hemispheres in the midline of the brain is severed. This prevents passage of neuronal discharges from a focal seizure between the hemispheres, thereby preventing secondary generalized seizures.

Hemispherectomy

A hemisphere severely damaged by widespread, persistent, multifocal seizures may be removed. This radical procedure is usually performed only on children with unilateral pathologic foci, including infantile hemiplegia (palsy), hemiparesis (paralysis), and hemianopia (loss of vision). The hemisphere (i.e., half of the brain) is resected with preservation of the basal ganglia. If an abnormal hemisphere is removed at an early age, the healthy half of the brain can take over much of the missing function.

Extracranial Procedures

The cranial procedures previously discussed include access to the surgical site through the skull. A few cranial neurosurgical procedures do not require craniectomy or intracranial incision.

External Occlusion of the Carotid Artery

When an internal carotid or middle cerebral artery aneurysm cannot be reached or controlled with other surgical techniques, a carotid clamp can be applied extracranially in the neck. Progressive turns on the clamp over several days cause occlusion of the carotid artery gradually until complete occlusion of the blood supply to the aneurysm is accomplished.

Endovascular Procedures

A thin catheter with a very fine guidewire can be advanced through a groin incision into a cerebral vessel to treat a problem within the brain. For example, using C-arm guidance, tiny platinum coils can be deployed or thrombotic material can be injected to seal off a cerebral aneurysm. Cerebral angioplasty uses a tiny balloon catheter to reopen the clogged or narrow lumen of a cerebral blood vessel. Stents can be placed to maintain patency.

Transsphenoidal Procedures

As a palliative surgical procedure, hypophysectomy (enucleation of the pituitary gland) may be performed for pain relief and endocrine ablation in patients with disseminated metastatic carcinoma of the breast or prostate gland or for relief of intractable pain from other types of disseminated carcinomas.

The microsurgical transsphenoidal approach also is used for removal of intrapituitary tumors or other lesions within the region of the sella turcica, a cavity of the sphenoid bone. Visual loss and endocrinopathy are the main symptoms of a pituitary tumor. Tumor tissue in the sella turcica is distinguished by both color and texture from the normal firm, yellowish anterior and red-gray posterior lobes of the pituitary.

The patient is placed in a semi-Fowler position with the head slightly flexed and tilted so that the patient's body is out of the way when the neurosurgeon sits in front of the face to work in the midsagittal plane. The image intensifier is positioned lateral to the patient's head with the horizontal beam centered on the sella turcica. A video monitor is placed behind and just above the patient's head so the surgeon can look at the screen in line with the binocular of the microscope.

Video radiofluoroscopy is used as an aid in placing instruments and resecting tissue. The image intensifier is switched on and off, as needed, to minimize exposure to radiation.

The floor of the sella turcica is exposed through the sphenoid sinus. The procedure can be performed transnasally (Fig. 37.19) or through a horizontal incision made under the upper lip at the junction of the gingiva and carried deep to the maxilla. Soft tissues are elevated; bone and nasal cartilage are resected. The resected nasal cartilage is preserved on the instrument table for possible replacement. A specially designed nasal speculum is inserted in the oral incision to visualize the sphenoid sinus. This is opened wide until the floor of the sella turcica can be identified. The floor is

• **Fig. 37.19** Transnasal hypophysectomy.

opened with an air-powered drill. The microscope is brought into position for visualization of the pituitary and other structures and lesions inside and around the sella turcica.

Treatment of Head Trauma

A patient with severe head injury first needs a patent airway. A relaxed jaw and tongue should be raised; if necessary, suction should be applied through the mouth. An endotracheal tube may be inserted. Ultimately, a tracheotomy may be necessary.

Vital signs, BP, dilation of pupils, and level of consciousness are checked frequently. An IV osmotic dehydrating solution, such as mannitol, may be ordered to reduce cerebral edema if no evidence of intracranial hemorrhage is found. After these supportive measures have been carried out, definitive treatment is initiated:

- Scalp lacerations are thoroughly cleansed, debrided, and sutured. Because the scalp is highly vascular, lacerations bleed profusely. Hypovolemic shock is rare but possible.
- Simple linear or comminuted fractures usually require no treatment. A depressed skull fracture must be elevated when bone is pressed 5 mm or more into any part of the brain.
- A compound fracture requires debridement. The extent of the surgical procedure depends on the specific extent of injury. Dura may need to be sutured. Some macerated brain tissue may have to be excised.
- An intracranial hematoma may be present. Depending on the location, intracranial hemorrhage may require an immediate emergency surgical procedure.
- Epidural hematoma. Bleeding caused by rupture or tear of the middle meningeal artery (or its branches) forms a hematoma between the skull and the dura. Usually associated with a skull fracture, signs and symptoms of increased ICP caused by rapid compression of the brain may occur immediately or within a few hours. An arterial hemorrhage presents an extreme surgical emergency to evacuate the clot and clip or electrocoagulate the bleeding vessel through a burr hole or small craniectomy.
- Subdural hematoma. Bleeding between the dura mater and arachnoid is usually caused by laceration of veins that cross the subdural space. A large encapsulated collection of blood over one or both cerebral hemispheres produces increased ICP and other neurologic changes. The onset and extent of these changes depend on the cause, size, and rapidity of growth of the hematoma. Treatment may necessitate a circular burr hole or trephination. A bone flap may be raised if more extensive exploration is indicated. Subdural hematoma may be:
  - *Acute:* Usually caused by arterial bleeding, symptoms occur rapidly. The vessel is ligated with clips or electrocoagulated.
  - *Subacute:* Usually caused by venous bleeding, symptoms appear within 24 to 48 hours to 5 days after the injury.
  - *Chronic:* Symptoms do not appear until 6 or more months after the injury.
- Intracerebral hematoma. Tears in the brain substance at the point of greatest impact most commonly occur in the anterior temporal and frontal lobes. Although it is usually absorbed, a hematoma may require evacuation and debridement of necrotic tissue.

Complications of Cranial Surgery

All cranial procedures present risks for postoperative seizures and neurologic deficits. Paralysis, muscle weakness, gait disturbances, and ataxia may be temporary or permanent. Neurologic damage can follow hemorrhage, occlusion of cerebral circulation, and increased ICP.[8]

Any sudden, sustained rise in ICP raises BP to maintain the cerebral blood flow and elevates pulmonary vascular pressure. This can lead to acute neurogenic pulmonary edema. This is also a complication of venous air embolism. Both venous and arterial air embolisms can result in ventricular dysrhythmias and fibrillation.[8] Infection is always a potential complication.

Peripheral Nerve Surgery

The peripheral nervous system (PNS) includes the cranial nerves, spinal nerves, and autonomic nervous system located outside the CNS. Ganglions, a group of nerve cell bodies also located outside the CNS, can transmit either autonomic (involuntary) or somatic (both reflex and voluntary) impulses. Somatic nerves supply voluntary muscles, skin, tendons, joints, and other structures that control the musculoskeletal system. Afferent nerve fibers carry sensory impulses from the organs and muscles to the CNS. Efferent fibers transmit motor impulses from the CNS back to them. Peripheral nerve procedures are performed on both the autonomic and somatic nervous systems. The neurosurgeon may identify nerves and test function with a nerve stimulator before or after dissection or repair.

Autonomic Nervous System

The autonomic nervous system is an aggregation of ganglions, nerves, and plexuses through which the viscera, heart, blood vessels, smooth muscles, and glands receive motor innervation to function involuntarily. This system is divided into the following:

- *Sympathetic nervous system:* This thoracolumbar division, which arises from the thoracic and first three lumbar segments of the spinal cord, includes the ganglionated trunk near the spinal cord, plexuses, and associated preganglionic and postganglionic nerve fibers. The efferent fibers transmit impulses that stimulate involuntary activity in the heart, blood vessels, smooth muscle of the viscera, and all the glands in the body.
- *Parasympathetic nervous system:* This craniosacral division includes the preganglionic fibers that leave the CNS with cranial nerves III (oculomotor), VII (facial), IX (glossopharyngeal), and X (vagus); the first three sacral nerves; outlying ganglions near the viscera; and postganglionic fibers. In general, this system innervates the same structures but has a regulatory function opposite that of the sympathetic nervous system. These efferent fibers act to restore stability for quieter activity.

Surgical procedures most frequently performed on the autonomic nervous system by neurosurgeons are discussed here, but surgeons in other disciplines do perform some of them.

Sympathectomy

Resection or division of the sympathetic ganglions and nerve fibers of the autonomic nervous system is performed in an attempt to increase peripheral circulation or to decrease the pain of peripheral vascular disease or intractable pain of other organic origin. It may be an emergency procedure to relieve severe vasospasm after arterial embolism or freezing of an extremity.

The paravertebral ganglionic chains or nerve fibers that innervate the affected area are resected or divided. The procedure may be termed *sympathetic ganglionectomy* or *splanchnicectomy*, but usually the surgical procedure is specified by the location of the ganglions and nerves. (General and vascular surgeons also perform some of the following surgical procedures.)

Upper Cervical Sympathectomy

Upper cervical sympathectomy is done to increase the blood supply in the internal carotid arteries. Through an anterior cervical approach in the neck, the superior cervical ganglion is resected. Ptosis of the eyelid may occur postoperatively because this ganglion innervates eyelid retraction.

Cervicothoracic Sympathectomy

Cervicothoracic sympathectomy may be performed to treat Raynaud phenomenon of the upper extremities by relieving the chronic vasoconstrictive process or to relieve angina pectoris or causalgia. Through a transaxillary-transpleural incision, the stellate ganglion of the middle cervical ganglionic chain is hemisected and the lower half resected along with the second through fifth thoracic nerve ganglions.

In select patients, video-assisted thoracoscopy is used to perform sympathectomy to treat Raynaud phenomenon, thoracic outlet syndrome, reflex sympathetic dystrophy, and hyperhidrosis of the upper limbs.

Thoracic Sympathectomy

Thoracic sympathectomy is usually done for relief of the chronic intractable pain of biliary and pancreatic disease. Through a posterior paravertebral incision over the transverse processes of the thoracic vertebrae, the ganglions of the 6th through 12th thoracic nerves are resected and the splanchnic nerves divided.

Thoracolumbar Sympathectomy

Thoracolumbar sympathectomy is performed for the treatment of essential hypertension. Usually done in two stages, bilateral resection is necessary to reduce BP by altering the vascular tone and denervating the viscera. With the patient prone or in a lateral position, a paravertebral incision parallel to the vertebral column extends from the ninth rib downward and then curves anteriorly toward the iliac crest. The lower half of the thoracic and the first through third lumbar chains with the ganglions and splanchnic nerves are resected.

Lumbar Sympathectomy

Lumbar sympathectomy may be of some value in the treatment of lower extremity vasospastic disease, such as Raynaud phenomenon and Buerger disease, ischemic ulcers as a result of vasospasm of the peripheral vessels, and some types of causalgia. Usually through a flank incision, the lumbar chain and ganglions located in the retroperitoneal space between the vertebral column and the psoas muscle are resected from above the second to below the third ganglions.

Presacral Neurectomy

The hypogastric nerve plexus may be resected for relief of idiopathic intractable dysmenorrhea and pelvic pain. Some gynecologists perform this procedure during pelvic surgery.

Vagotomy

Truncal vagotomy is total vagal denervation of all structures below the diaphragm. Selective vagotomy is performed more frequently to denervate a specific branch of the vagal nerve.

Somatic Nervous System

As cranial and spinal nerves extend out from the CNS into plexuses and peripheral nerve branches throughout the body, the somatic nervous system provides involuntary control over sensations and both voluntary and involuntary control over muscles. Loss of sensation and muscular control occurs distal to the site of severed or compressed nerve fibers. Sensation and function are restored only if regeneration of nerve axons takes place distally from an unobstructed axis cylinder proximal to the site of disruption.

Nerve injuries in the lower extremity tend to be a result of a major impact, such as an automobile accident; upper extremity injuries are more often associated with industrial accidents. Nerve injuries usually are associated with multisystem trauma such as fractures and lacerations. An injury may occur at any point along a peripheral nerve (e.g., from penetrating trauma that severs the nerve or blunt trauma that produces contusions or traction to the nerve). Lower extremity nerves do not recover as rapidly as do upper extremity nerves.

Most peripheral nerve surgery is performed to repair traumatic nerve injury in an extremity. Dissection is also done to remove tumors or relieve pain. Etiologic factors determine the location and length of the skin incision.

Neurorrhaphy

Neurorrhaphy (suturing of a divided nerve) must provide precise approximation of the nerve ends if function is to be restored. Primary repair may be accomplished by suturing the epineurium, or outer sheath. With magnification of the operating microscope, accurate fascicular alignment and epineural end-to-end suturing of larger nerve bundles constitute the desired technique to enhance regeneration of function. For a successful result, nerves are not repaired under tension. Primary repair soon after injury may be advantageous to align the fascicles.

A tumor, such as a neurofibroma or posttraumatic neuroma, is excised. If the nerve ends can be brought together without tension, they are anastomosed. Silastic membrane may be wrapped around the anastomosis to prevent adhesions with the surrounding tissue.

Neurolysis

Neurolysis (freeing of a nerve from adhesions) relieves pain and restores function. Release of the transverse carpal ligament overriding the median nerve in the wrist affords relief of carpal tunnel syndrome, for example.

Neurotomy, Neurectomy, and Neurexeresis

Neurotomy is division or dissection of nerve fibers. Neurectomy is excision of part of a nerve. Neurexeresis is extraction or avulsion of a nerve. These procedures may be performed to relieve localized peripheral pain.

ⓔ EVOLVE WEBSITE

http://evolve.elsevier.com/Hornacky/BerryKohn/

- Historical Perspective
- Tips for the Scrub Person and Circulating Nurse
- Student Interactive Questions
- Glossary

References

1. Bissacco D, Mandigers T, Romagnoli S, et al.: Acute venous problems: integrating medical, surgical, and interventional treatments, *Semin Vasc Surg* 36(2):307–318, 2023.
2. Roman A, Tufegdzic B, Lamperti M, et al.: Before the knife: a detailed step-by-step description of an optimized semi-sitting position in posterior surgery, *World Neurosurg* 172:e241–e249, 2023.
3. Barbagallo G, Morrone A, Certo F: Intraoperative computed tomography and awake craniotomy: a useful and safe combination in brain surgery, *World Neurosurg* 119:e159–e166, 2018.
4. Chua TH, See A, Ang B, et al.: Awake craniotomy for resection of brain metastases: a systematic review, *World Neurosurg* 120:e1128–e1135, 2018.
5. Croarkin P, MacMaster F: Transcranial magnetic stimulation for adolescent depression, *Child Adolesc Psychiatr Clin N Am* 28(1):33–43, 2018.
6. American Cancer Society: GammaTile. www.cancer.org. Accessed February 8, 2024.
7. Nicholls LW, Pinkham MB, Bernard A, et al.: Radiological kinetics of brain metastases and clinical implications for patients treated with stereotactic radiosurgery, *Oncology* 31(1):34–40, 2019.
8. D'Amico, Randy S, Jeffery B, et al: Management of injuries: complications of surgery for pineal regional tumors, *Complications in Neurosurgery* 24:125–131, St. Louis, MO, 2019, Elsevier.

Bibliography

Brennan P: Tumours of the central nervous system, *Surgery* 36(1):630–636, 2018.

Levy E, Ahmed A, Cappuzzo J: Recent advances in endovascular neurosurgery: pushing the envelope, *Neurosurg Clin N Am* 33(2):xi–xii, 2022.

Paulo D, Semonche A, Choudhry O, et al.: History of hemostasis in neurosurgery, *World Neurosurg* 124:237–250, 2019.

Whiting A, Catapano J, Walker C, et al.: Peri-lead edema after deep brain stimulation surgery, *World Neurosurg* 124:340–345, 2019.

38
Spinal Surgery

CHAPTER OUTLINE

Anatomy and Physiology of the Spinal Cord and Vertebral Column, 808

Special Considerations for Spinal Surgery, 811

Pathology of the Vertebrae and Spinal Cord, 816

Surgical Procedures of the Spine, 820

CHAPTER OBJECTIVES

After studying this chapter, the learner will be able to:

- Describe the anatomy of the vertebral column and spinal cord.
- Describe the implications of dermatome and myotome distributions.
- Discuss the implications of an individualized plan of care for each type of spinal surgery.

- Differentiate between the types of spinal positioning devices and operating room beds.
- Compare the salient points of spinal surgery that apply to orthopedic and neurologic procedures.

KEY TERMS AND DEFINITIONS

Anterior approach Entering the body through the front of the neck, chest, or abdomen.

Approach Method of incising and accessing the body. The approach is planned according to the type of procedure and location of the disease or injury. Knowledge of the approach helps the circulating nurse and scrub person plan the positioning and instrumentation for the surgical procedure.

Decompression Release of spinal pressure by cutting away of segments of the vertebral bone.

Dermatomes Levels of cutaneous sensory innervation from specific areas of the spinal cord to the peripheral nervous system.

Hemiplegia Injury to one side of the nervous system that results in decreased motion on the affected side of the body.

Idiopathic Unknown or uncertain origin.

Kyphosis Exaggerated thoracic curvature of the spine.

Lordosis Exaggerated lumbar curvature of the spine.

Myotomes Levels of muscle innervation from the spinal cord.

Osteoporosis Wasting and demineralization of bone.

Paralysis Decreased ability to move voluntarily.

Paraplegia Injury between the levels of T1 and T8; with injury between the levels T9 and T10, the individual may be able to sit up although lower limbs are affected.

Posterior approach Entering the body through the back of the neck, chest, or lower spine.

Quadriplegia Injury above the level of T1 that results in inability to move all four limbs.

Radiculopathy Pain that travels up or down a nerve pathway.

Reflex sympathetic dystrophy (RSD) Also known as complex regional pain syndrome (CRPS). Chronic intense pain from tissue damage, injury, or nervous system dysregulation.

Retroperitoneal Behind the peritoneal cavity without entering the sac.

Scoliosis Lateral curvature of the spine. Can be combined with kyphosis (kyphoscoliosis).

Spondylosis Bony degeneration of the vertebral column with mineral deposits.

Stagnara wake-up test The patient is awakened during the surgical procedure and asked to move their feet. The patient does not feel pain and is given an amnesic medication.

Stenosis Narrowing of a passage.

Thenar The web space between the index finger and the thumb.

Transoral approach Entering the body through the mouth to the back of the pharynx.

Transperitoneal Through the peritoneal cavity.

Anatomy and Physiology of the Spinal Cord and Vertebral Column

The vertebral column and spinal cord make up the posterior aspect of the trunk of the body. The relationship between the bones and nerves is evaluated first from a topographic perspective with assessment of the alignment of specific external landmarks (Fig. 38.1). The external dorsal musculature frames the margins of the surgical landmarks used in planning the posterior incision for spinal surgery (Fig. 38.2).

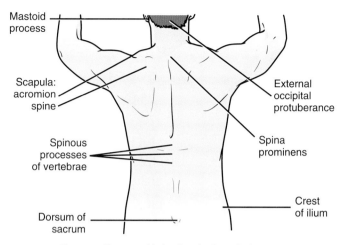

- **Fig. 38.1** Topographic landmarks for spinal surgery.

Mastoid process

Scapula: acromion spine

Spinous processes of vertebrae

Dorsum of sacrum

External occipital protuberance

Spina prominens

Crest of ilium

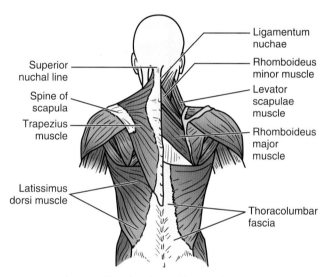

- **Fig. 38.2** Dorsal surface with muscular borders.

Superior nuchal line

Spine of scapula

Trapezius muscle

Latissimus dorsi muscle

Ligamentum nuchae

Rhomboideus minor muscle

Levator scapulae muscle

Rhomboideus major muscle

Thoracolumbar fascia

Curvatures of the Spine

The configuration of the spinal curvature depends on chronologic and **idiopathic** factors. Each age-group, as shown in Fig. 38.3, *A*, displays a different set of normal spinal curves based on physiologic development. Abnormal curvatures can be age related but sometimes are idiopathic without consideration for age. Examples include kyphosis and lordosis (Fig. 38.3, *B*).[1]

The Spinal Cord and Spinal Nerves

The spinal cord is between 17 and 20 inches (43—51 cm) long and passes through a central canal in the vertebral column to the level of the second or third lumbar vertebra (Fig. 38.4). Pairs of spinal nerve roots branch off to each side of the body from 31 segments of the spinal cord as it passes through the vertebrae.

The spinal nerves are as follows:

- Eight pairs cervical
- Twelve pairs thoracic
- Five pairs lumbar
- Five pairs sacral
- One pair coccygeal

The spinal nerves carry sensory and motor impulses between the central nervous system (CNS) and the peripheral nervous system (PNS). Reflex sympathetic dystrophy (RSD) or complex regional pain syndrome (CRPS) can cause chronic pain from dysfunction or interruption of the nervous system pathways. The cord is composed of gray matter (cell bodies) on the inside and white matter (nerve fibers) on the outside. This is the exact opposite of the substance of the brain. The ventral nerve roots are the motor axons to the muscles and glands, and the dorsal nerve roots are the sensory dendrites (Fig. 38.5). The dorsal root ganglion is easily entrapped by the bony vertebrae and causes pain and disability.

The cephalad portion of the cord begins at the base of the brain at the foramen magnum. The first thickened area of the spinal cord is at the C7-T1 junction, forming the brachial plexus. Compromise of the brachial plexus caused by bony impingement

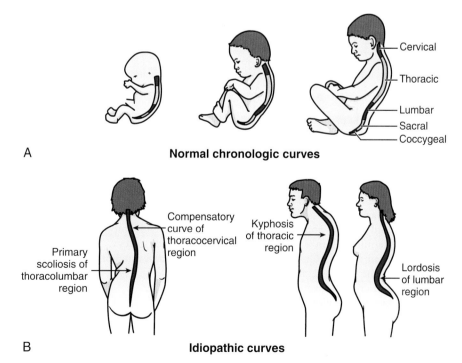

A   **Normal chronologic curves**

Cervical

Thoracic

Lumbar

Sacral

Coccygeal

Primary scoliosis of thoracolumbar region

Compensatory curve of thoracocervical region

Kyphosis of thoracic region

Lordosis of lumbar region

B   **Idiopathic curves**

- **Fig. 38.3** Natural and pathologic spinal curves. **A,** Normal chronologic curves. **B,** Idiopathic curves.

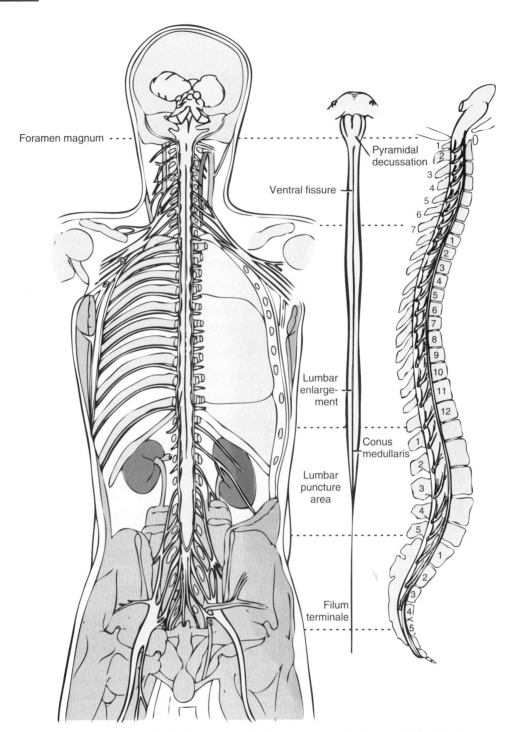

Foramen magnum

Pyramidal decussation

Ventral fissure

Lumbar enlargement

Conus medullaris

Lumbar puncture area

Filum terminale

• **Fig. 38.4** Spinal nerves. (Modified from Mettler FA: *Neuroanatomy,* ed 2, St. Louis, MO, 1948, Mosby.)

of the cervical or upper thoracic vertebrae results in arm and hand pain and muscular weakness with **thenar** wasting.

The caudal portion of the spinal cord thickens and ends at L1 to form the conus medullaris before terminating in a fibrous tail known as the cauda equina (horse's tail; Fig. 38.6). The nerve fibers that extend beyond L2-L3 form the lumbosacral plexus.

The blood supply to the spinal cord arises from the vertebral artery. The radicular artery of Adamkiewicz supplies blood to the lower third of the cord. Occlusion of this artery causes paraplegia. Venous drainage is through the intervertebral vein that drains into the azygous venous system.

The meninges cover the cord to the level of the second or third lumbar vertebra. They terminate in a fibrous band (filum terminale) that extends through the lumbar vertebrae and sacrum and attaches to the coccyx. The dura is not attached or continuous with the central canal of the vertebral column.

Vertebrae

All vertebrae have similar bony characteristics that form a circular canal to house the spinal cord.[1] The structure of a vertebra includes the following:

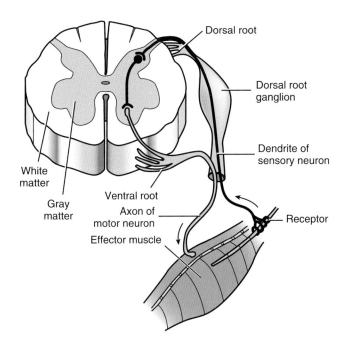

• **Fig. 38.5** Spinal innervation of the body.

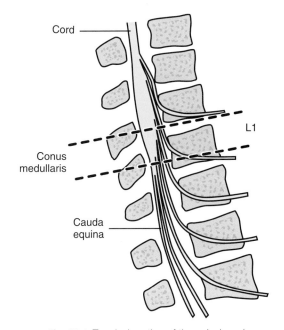

• **Fig. 38.6** Terminal portion of the spinal cord.

- A thick cylindric body that bears a portion of the weight of the torso.
- Two posterolateral extensions that form the proximal bony vertebral (neural) arch. These extensions form thick pedicles that connect to flatten laminae posteriorly. The laminae connect at the spinous process, forming a circle. Each pedicle has a notch superiorly and inferiorly to seat the vertebrae above and below.
- A transverse wing-shaped spinous process that is formed by the connection of the posterior laminae. The central foramen shapes the spinal canal.

The bony structure of the vertebral column extends from the foramen magnum at the base of the skull to the coccyx (Fig. 38.7, *A*).

The 33 vertebrae, which provide support for the body, vary in size and shape according to location and are separated by flexible discs over the anterior surface of the body (Fig. 38.7, *B*). Each disc is composed of two parts: an exterior annulus fibrosus and an interior gel referred to as the nucleus pulposus.

The seven cervical vertebrae are in the neck and form the secondary curvature. They are lighter weight with a smaller disc-bearing body. The top two cervical vertebrae, C1 atlas and C2 axis, have clearly distinct landmarks. The atlas laminae form a circle around the odontoid process of the axis so the head has a wide range of circular and linear motion (Fig. 38.8). The atlas-axis complex has no disc or spinous process and is considered to be the strongest vertebrae of the cervical portion of the vertebral column.

The 12 thoracic vertebrae articulate posteriorly with the ribs to form a cage around the thoracic organs, forming a primary curvature. The spinous processes are low profile and smaller than the lower vertebrae. The body and discs of the thoracic vertebrae are thinner and are designed to bear minimal weight.

The five lumbar vertebrae are posterior to the retroperitoneal cavity and are designed to carry the heaviest load of the entire vertebral column with the least amount of flexibility. The body and disc of each lumbar vertebra are thick and form a secondary curvature. Fig. 38.9 illustrates the combined lumbar vertebra-disc unit.

The five sacral vertebrae are fused in the adult to form the sacrum, and the four fused coccygeal vertebrae form the coccyx (Fig. 38.10). Collectively, these two sets of fused vertebrae form the posterior aspect of the pelvic girdle. Each vertebra is connected to the other by a series of ligamentous fibers (Fig. 38.11). The vertebral column measures about 28 inches (71 cm) in the average-size adult.

The physiologic relationship between the spinal cord, spinal nerves, and bony vertebral column affects multiple body systems if the curvature is misaligned or some pathology changes the size of a foramen or joint. Fig. 38.12 illustrates the major organ systems and the corresponding spinal nerves that can cause problems with physiologic functioning.

Special Considerations for Spinal Surgery

Because of the proximity of the vertebral column to the spinal cord, both neurosurgeons and orthopedic surgeons perform surgical procedures in this area. Many surgeons have attained subspecialty board certification in spinal surgery. Both disciplines use power drills, power saws, microscopes, and computer imaging to correct problems in the spinal column; however, many surgeons believe that spinal surgery is a specialty unto itself because of the multidisciplinary approaches applied in the correction of spinal problems.

Diagnostics

For diagnosis of spinal conditions, computed tomography (CT) is used to detect abnormal bone. CT and magnetic resonance imaging (MRI) are used to evaluate spinal injuries. MRI and myelography outline soft tissue abnormalities, such as disc degeneration, protrusion, or rupture.[2] Because it is noninvasive, MRI demonstrates improved diagnostic quality over myelography.

Positioning for Spinal Surgery

Positioning for spinal surgery can require the patient to be placed in either the supine or the prone position, depending on the type

• **Fig. 38.7** Vertebral column. **A,** Lateral view and posterior view. **B,** Differentiation of vertebrae.

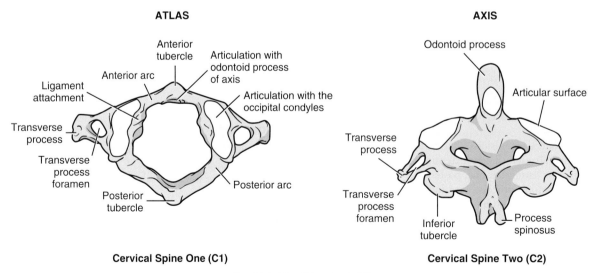

• **Fig. 38.8** Atlas C1 and axis C2.

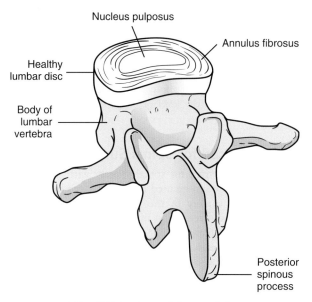

• **Fig. 38.9** Lumbar vertebrae and disc.

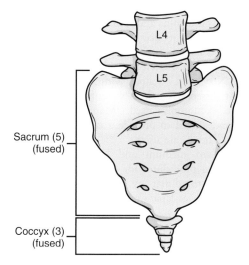

• **Fig. 38.10** Sacrum and coccyx.

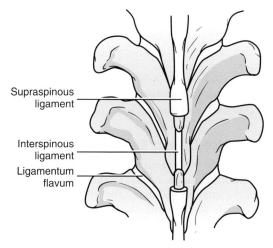

• **Fig. 38.11** Dorsal muscles and tendons.

• **Fig. 38.12** Physiologic relationship between the spinal cord, spinal nerves, and vertebral column.

of **approach** necessary for the planned procedure. Most facilities have specialized operating room (OR) beds that accommodate the modifications needed for adequate exposure of the surgical site. Some surgical body positions provide distraction of the vertebrae for more direct access to specific regions of the spine.

Considerations for patient positioning include prevention of untoward injury, such as pressure areas, pinch points on jointed tables, falls, wrong site surgery, and venous stasis. Ischemic pressure insult to the area around the eye can result in blindness.

Positioning a patient in the prone position is a multistep procedure. The patient is given general anesthesia on the transport cart, intubated, and catheterized. A minimum of four people is needed to turn the anesthetized patient into the prone position onto the specialized OR bed.

A few prone positions simulate kneeling or crouching, which means the patient may be in a full lift and body flexion before coming into contact with the surface of the OR bed. Fig. 38.13 shows the kneeling-crouching position used by some surgeons for lower spine procedures. This posture constricts the patient's circulation and increases the risk for embolization.

The Jackson table (Fig. 38.14) and the Jackson-Wilson table with the central arch (Fig. 38.15) are used for posterior spinal incisions. Each type of specialty spinal table allows the surgeon to position the patient for optimal vertebral position and exposure of the surgical site.

• **Fig. 38.13** Kneeling-crouching position for spinal surgery.

• **Fig. 38.14** Jackson spinal table.

• **Fig. 38.15** Jackson-Wilson spinal table.

Anesthesia Considerations

The anesthesia provider monitors and manipulates the patient's physiology. The patient's airway, breathing, and circulation are under constant surveillance by gross visual examination and by technologic devices. Airway and breathing are compromised by the prone positions used for the posterior spinal approach. The patient's chest excursion is decreased, and the intraabdominal pressure is released by allowing the abdominal cavity to rest in a dependent position. The loose abdomen permits the vena cava to remain at a low pressure, preventing excess venous oozing around the vertebral column and cord.

Airway

The patient under general anesthesia who is intubated and placed in a prone position is at high risk for loss of a patent airway. The shape of the trachea and the bifurcation of the bronchi create a complex scenario in which the tip of the endotracheal tube can slip into one bronchus, aerating only one lung. The opposite lung is not adequately ventilated, and the level of oxygen saturation decreases. The patient can become hypoxic. The anesthesia provider should remain vigilant about the endotracheal tube position within the trachea and the level of oxygen saturation in the patient's blood.

Instruments Used for Spinal Surgery

Surgical instruments used for spinal surgery with the **posterior approach** are designed to be used in narrow, deep incisions. The incisions used for surgery of the posterior spine involve paramedian dissection and retraction of several muscle layers. These incisions are very deep and do not always offer a visual advantage to the surgeon and team. The scrub person can prepare for this type of incision by providing medium to large self-retaining retractors in pairs because a matching pair is used in the cephalad and caudad margins. Some surgeons prefer an angled or jointed Weitlaner or Beckman style retractor.

An assortment of bone debulking rongeurs (Kerrison and Cloward) and curettes with a variety of jaw angles (forward biters, back biters, side biters, up biters, and down biters) are used to remove segments of lamina and spinous process. High-speed drills are sometimes used to reduce bony bulk.

Graspers used include bayonet-style forceps with and without bipolar energy. Sharp dissectors used for soft tissue such as the dura include No. 3 and 7 scalpels with several No. 10, 11, and 15 blades. Blunt dissectors such as a Penfield and other periosteal elevators are commonly used. Manual retractors are size-appropriate and angled to provide a clear field of vision for the surgeon. Nerve hooks are used.

Other standard medium and long instruments are used throughout spinal procedures for the posterior and anterior approaches. Keep in mind that any **anterior approach** requires basic soft tissue sets such as laparotomy instruments and retractors in addition to instruments specific to spinal procedures. Microinstruments are used for microscopic procedures.

Intraoperative Neural Monitoring of the Spinal Cord

Some spinal surgeons prefer to monitor sensory and motor activity of the brain and spinal cord during surgery (Fig. 38.16). Intraoperative neural monitoring during the procedure gives the surgeon an early indication of the condition of the cord and spinal nerves as each layer of soft or compact tissue is manipulated.[3]

Dermatomal mapping and **Stagnara wake-up tests** also are reliable techniques for monitoring of spinal cord function. In the latter test, the patient must be awake enough to respond to the surgeon's command to move the foot.

Radiologic Use During Spine Surgery

The surgeon usually has a scout x-ray performed. A spinal needle is inserted into the patient's back to the level of the vertebrae targeted for the surgical procedure. The needle serves as a marker and confirmation that the procedure is being performed at the correct level of the spine (Fig. 38.17). Some surgeons place an instrument in the intended spinal level and take a confirmation x-ray before proceeding with the surgical procedure.

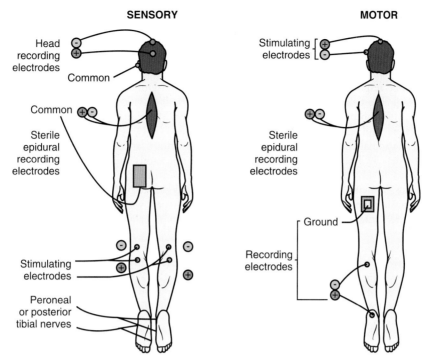

SENSORY

Head recording electrodes

Common

Common

Sterile epidural recording electrodes

Stimulating electrodes

Peroneal or posterior tibial nerves

MOTOR

Stimulating electrodes

Sterile epidural recording electrodes

Ground

Recording electrodes

• **Fig. 38.16** Intraoperative spinal cord monitoring.

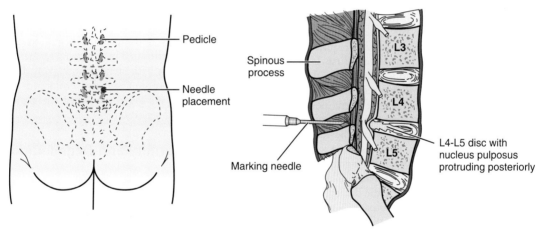

Pedicle

Needle placement

Spinous process

Marking needle

L3

L4

L5

L4-L5 disc with nucleus pulposus protruding posteriorly

• **Fig. 38.17** Needle localization of surgical level.

Additional x-rays may be taken during the procedure if hardware or appliances are implanted into the bone or surrounding tissue. Follow-up x-rays may be done before closure to provide documentation of the spinal procedure level and structural integrity of implants.

Modeling With Scans

Preoperative CT or MRI images can be used to create a three-dimensional computer model of the affected vertebrae and discs. The computer model allows the surgeon to see the target vertebrae and discs from all directions before incising the skin.

Microscope

The operating microscope was introduced in the late 1960s. Microdiscectomy is a discectomy performed with the operating microscope that is displayed on a video monitor. The video monitor enables the entire team to see the surgical site and anticipate the surgeon's next steps.

Robotic-Assisted Spinal Surgery

Precision tissue manipulation and dissection are made possible by robotic-assisted instrumentation.[4] Some of the systems in use offer the surgeon a greater freedom of hand and wrist motion in close quarters. Some maneuvers made with robotic instrumentation are not possible in the realm of human range of motion. The use of three-dimensional imaging can help surgeons place screws or disc implants into precise position. The surgeon's armamentarium is greatly expanded by using robotics for extremely delicate procedures.

Hemostasis

Meticulous hemostasis is necessary in the vertebral and spinal canals. Hematoma formation can create pressure and cause irreparable damage to the nervous system. Compressed cottonoids or patties are used for clearing blood and for applying topical agents such as thrombin. Cottonoids are counted and accounted for in the same manner as other sponges. Topical thrombin can be used for superficial oozing. Thrombin is never injected because it causes a fatal systemic thrombotic response.

Care is taken to avoid leaving absorbable hemostatic agents in any neural or bony space. Most absorbable agents swell in response to absorption of blood and cause compression in a constricted area. Pressure on the spinal cord or nerves can cause paralysis or other permanent deficit. The U.S. Food and Drug Administration (FDA) has issued an advisory concerning retained absorbable hemostatic materials in neural spaces. The material expands as it absorbs blood, causing pressure between the neural tissue and bone. Pressure on the neural tissue can result in permanent injury.

Bipolar electrosurgery is commonly used to minimize the amount of neural tissue involved with the effects of radio-frequency coagulation. Hemostasis for the cut edges of bone can be attained with bone wax or a paste made of powdered antibiotic and saline solution. Bone wax is not resorbed and can act as a mechanical barrier to osteogenesis in some individuals.

Graft Materials and Stabilization of the Vertebrae

Spinal fusion may be indicated to stabilize the vertebral column after spinal injury or excision of bone. Either a posterior or an anterior approach may be used to place the bone grafts. A combined anterior and posterior spinal fusion may be required for severe deformities. The anterior fusion is performed first. Unless the lesion or bone fragment to be removed is on the right side of the vertebral column, an anterior thoracolumbar approach is used through an incision with the patient in the right lateral position (left side up). A retroperitoneal incision is made for an anterior lumbar approach. These approaches are safer on the left side because the surgeon works near the aorta, which is more resistant to inadvertent injury than is the vena cava on the right.

Bone grafts are placed in the intervertebral spaces or along the spinous processes to bridge over or to stabilize the defect. The rib removed for an anterior thoracolumbar approach is used for grafting. Homogeneous cancellous bone from the bone bank may be needed to provide a larger quantity of bone than can be obtained from the rib or an autogenous graft from the crest of the patient's ilium.[5]

Cancellous bone rather than cortical bone is usually preferred for spinal fusion. Bone grafts may be used with or without internal fixation devices. The goals of spinal fusion are to achieve stability, rigidity, and correction of deformity. The combined use of internal fixation devices with bone grafts may facilitate postoperative care and early ambulation.

Complex procedures are performed for sublaminar wiring, pedicle screw fixation, and internal vertebral stabilization or fusion. Many spinal implant systems are available. All have the common goal of immobilizing spinal segments; each offers significant biomechanical advantages, but all have potential complications. The surgeon chooses the most appropriate device for the location, approach, and type of deformity and instability. For example, the posterior body and ligamentous structures in the cervical spine may be disrupted by a flexion-compression type of injury. Interspinous wiring and bone grafting provide posterior neck fusion for stability.

In the thoracolumbar spine, pedicular screw and plating systems can be used in conjunction with spinal fusion in treatment of fractures, spondylolisthesis, and idiopathic scoliosis. The following may be used to provide decompression of spinal nerve roots and vertebral alignment after posterior thoracolumbar spinal fusion:

- Cotrel-Dubousset rods, hooks, and screws
- The Texas Scottish Rite Hospital (TSRH) system of pedicle screw fixation with rods and cross-links
- TSRH 3D system of headless screws, smaller and stronger hardware, smaller incisions
- Luque rods and sublaminar wires
- Wisconsin spinous process wires
- PEEK interbody cage devices made from a high-performance polymer with carbon fiber (polyetheretherketone).[6] PEEK cages offer a hydrophobic surface; strong, flexible, and stable weight-bearing; and are radiolucent on x-ray, CT, and MRI. The cages are available in different sizes, heights, and shapes. PEEK is an alternative to titanium implants.

Kaneda, Zielke, Dwyer, or Dunn devices are used when an anterior approach is preferred. Each device has its own set of instrumentation for installation; these are not interchangeable.

Pathology of the Vertebrae and Spinal Cord

Disc Degeneration and Rupture
Compression on the Spinal Cord or Nerve Roots

The central canal of the vertebral column can become narrowed and cause compression on the cord (Fig. 38.18). Urgent decompression is necessary if the pressure begins to cause symptoms. Decompression is performed by removing segments of bone at the affected site. Patients with stenosis and spondylosis may be candidates for decompression surgery. Prolonged pressure on the spinal cord and nerves can cause permanent damage and loss of motor function and sensation.

Vertebral Deformity and Degeneration
Scoliosis

An idiopathic lateral curvature of the spine is scoliosis. It is more common in young females, although it can develop in later years with other bony deformities of the spine (Fig. 38.19). The diagnosis is made by having the individual bend forward and observing the linear direction of the spinal bones (Fig. 38.20). The curvature worsens with time. Any curvature of 40% or more requires correction. (Additional information can be found at www.scoliosis.org.)

Many body systems are affected by scoliosis. Digestion can be impaired. Chest excursion and respiratory effort are altered by the

Normal canal   Stenotic canal

• **Fig. 38.18** Stenosis of the vertebral canal.

• **Fig. 38.19** Scoliosis.

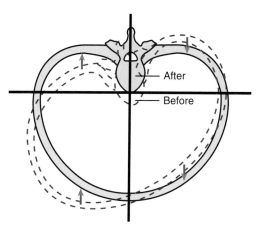

• **Fig. 38.21** Configuration of rib deformity in scoliosis.

• **Fig. 38.20** Abnormal vertebral alignment.

• **Fig. 38.22** Harrington rods.

deformity that occurs in the ribcage (Fig. 38.21). Extreme curves can cause disruption in lung growth, causing fibrosis of the lung tissue. The patient has an altered and unsteady gait.

Pediatric surgical patients are treated according to the curvature and age. Surgical considerations should not stunt the growth of the spine.[7] Surgical options include several types of rodding instrumentation, hardware systems, and biografting using allograft or autograft material. Each has a certain amount of failure risk and should not be used in the presence of osteoporosis. After a period of years, the graft material may be solid enough to remove the hardware.

Most surgeons prefer to leave the rods in place. The surgical approach can be anterior or posterior depending on the type of instrumentation used and the type of correction desired. The most commonly used surgical scoliosis correction systems are as follows:
1. Harrington rigid metallic rods used for the correction of spinal curvature greater than 60% were introduced in the 1960s. The rods are placed using a posterior approach. The patient is in a body cast for about 6 months postoperatively (Fig. 38.22). The rods can fracture over time because the main fixation is at the ends of the rods.
2. Luque rods are flexible L-shaped bilateral rods wired to the vertebral column to reverse the abnormal angle of the spine by 10%. A higher risk for injury exists because each custom curved segment is wired close to many levels of the spinal nerves. The patient does not need a brace postoperatively.

3. Cotrel-Dubousset features flexible rods with hooks and set screws that use biomechanical principles to reverse the abnormal spinal bends. This system preserves the natural curves of the spine. The system is complex and may require the patient to wear a brace after surgery. This system can be used for kyphoscoliosis.
4. Zielke instrumentation is similar to Cotrel-Dubousset but is used for double curvatures. An anterior approach is commonly used. A body brace is worn postoperatively.
5. The TSRH and TSRH 3D systems preserve the natural curves with a series of rods and hooks affixed with nuts and bolts to correct lateral rotation of the vertebrae. These rods can

be used for kyphoscoliosis. A brace is not always necessary postoperatively.

6. The Isola system is a series of rods and drop-in screws that provide a stable correction of spinal curvature using an anterior transthoracic approach with the patient in a lateral position. Each disc is removed and grafted. Each vertebral body is drilled and has a screw placed for fixation of the rods. These rods can be used for kyphoscoliosis of 40 degrees and may not require a body brace after surgery. This system can be used for adolescents and adults.

7. Drummond instrumentation uses a Harrington rod on the concave side of the spine and a Luque rod on the convex side. Each vertebra is individually wired. The patient wears a cast or brace postoperatively.

8. Vertical expandable prosthetic titanium rib (VEPTR) implants are used when the skeletal anatomy is immature and still growing. The distal aspect of the rods is affixed with screws, and the proximal ends are attached to pedicle hooks and distraction locks. The rod is cut longer than needed and bent into a corrective contour. Bone graft is used. These rods are also referred to as *growing rods* and can be used after 6 months of age.[8]

Postoperatively, the child wears a noncorrective body orthosis for 3 months. Every 6 months, the child is brought back to surgery and the proximal distraction locks are loosened and moved up the length of the rods to accommodate the increase in height. The VEPTR rods allow for spine lengthening and prevent thoracic instability.

9. Magnetic spinal growing rods for children with early-onset scoliosis have become popular because the lengthening process can be done without numerous invasive surgical procedures. After the initial rod placement, the rods can be adjusted as an office visit with an external magnet placed on the child's back. The rods can be lengthened in a few minutes and require lengthening every few months.[8]

Kyphosis

Osteoporosis is a degeneration and demineralization of bone that causes compression of the vertebral bodies at regions of spinal curvature (Fig. 38.23).[9] The flattening of the vertebral body causes a loss of height and decreases the accommodation of the movement of the spinal cord and major organ systems (Fig. 38.24). Respiratory effort can be compromised by a decrease in thoracic space.

Kyphoplasty is performed percutaneously with the introduction of a catheter and balloon assembly into the collapsed vertebral body (Fig. 38.25, *A*). The balloon is expanded with a radiopaque contrast media to reproduce and outline the vertebral height and then is removed and replaced with bone cement. The cement hardens to maintain the space created by the kyphoplasty balloon (Fig. 38.25, *B* and *C*).

Spinal Tumors

Spinal tumors may begin with slowly progressing problems such as bladder or bowel weakness and vague symptoms such as back pain and radiculopathy. Thoracic intraspinal tumors represent higher rates of morbidity in the presence of spinal cord atrophy and arachnoid scarring. The diagnostic process is prolonged because the symptoms are not consistent.

Most spinal tumors are readily diagnosed with MRI, and, if they metastasize, they travel to the bone first. Other cancers such

• **Fig. 38.23** Areas of compression treated with kyphoplasty.

• **Fig. 38.24** Compressed vertebral body.

as prostate, lung, and breast metastasize to the vertebrae through hematologic routes and can infiltrate the dura to the cord. About 55% of spinal tumors are metastatic in origin. Symptoms usually are related to spinal cord pressure.

The posterior segment of the vertebral arch is removed to expose the dura over the involved section of the spinal cord. The dura is incised and retracted with sutures. The tumor is excised, and the dura is closed tightly to prevent leakage of cerebrospinal fluid (CSF). Both intrinsic and extrinsic spinal cord tumors can be removed by laser with decreased tissue trauma. The laser is especially useful in areas difficult to reach by dissection, such as the foramen magnum or anterior spinal cord.

Tumors of the spinal area are classified as one of the following types:

1. *Extradural:* Outside the dural layer of the meninges. Many of these are benign, such as lipomas, chondromas, granulomas, and abscesses.

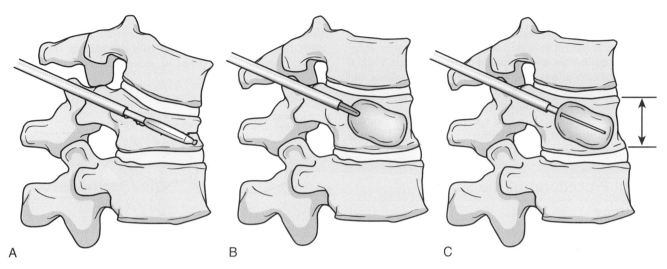

• **Fig. 38.25** **A,** Introduction of kyphoplasty catheter. **B,** The balloon on the kyphoplasty catheter is expanded. **C,** Bone cement is used to displace the kyphoplasty balloon and maintain vertebral height.

2. *Intradural:* Under the dural layer of the meninges, not invasive in the spinal cord. These tumors are frequently well circumscribed and slow growing. They arise from the cells of the proximal nerve roots. They can be noted with myelograms.
3. *Hemangioblastoma:* Vascular tumor in neural tissue. More common in 30 to 40-year-old men (2:1). These tumors can be associated with von Hippel-Lindau disease. Hemangioblastomas are more common in the cervical or thoracic areas.
4. *Astrocytoma (glial tumor):* This tumor of the spinal cord is rare and is more often found in 30 to 50-year-old men than in women. The appearance on MRI is very cystic and thickened. Large segments can be removed with irrigation-aspiration systems such as the cavitron ultrasonic surgical aspirator (CUSA).
   a. *Diffuse fibrous type:* More difficult to remove. Most spinal astrocytomas are this type.
   b. *Circumscribed:* More clearly defined and with a better prognosis for excision. Less invasive to surrounding tissue.
5. *Intraspinal intramedullary:* Slow-growing tumor inside the tissues of the spinal cord. More common in females. These grow more aggressively in children than in adults. Cervical and thoracic areas are the most common primary sites. Sacral tumors tend to metastasize readily to bone.
6. *Ependymoma tumors:* These tumors arise from the ependymal cells that line the central canal, from the ventriculus terminalis of the conus, and from the filum terminale with cells disseminated by the CSF. Some are encapsulated with many superficial vessels. Total removal of an encapsulated tumor may eliminate the need for postoperative radiation.
   a. Myxopapillary ependymal tumors arise exclusively in the filum terminale and the conus medullaris and are more common in young males.
   b. Metastasis from areas of the brain.

Spinal Trauma

During World War I, 80% of soldiers with spinal cord injuries died within the first 2 weeks of the wounding. Little was known about special spinal treatment and surgical decompression, so most of the wounded died of complications associated with the spinal cord injury, not the actual damage to the cord. Immobility and infection were leading causes of death. By World War II, specialized units were developed in response to scientific understanding of the cord and its function, greatly increasing the survival rate.

Vertebral fractures, with or without dislocation, can cause spinal cord compression that denervates nerve tracts below the injury. Spinal cord injury also may be caused by penetrating or stretching trauma or by damage to blood vessels that supply the cord. Spinal cord injuries are classified as follows:
• *Complete:* The patient lacks sensation, proprioception (position sense), and voluntary motor function below the level of the spinal cord damage. Lesions above the fifth cervical vertebra (C5) cause partial to complete diaphragmatic paralysis. Injury in the cervical region results in **quadriplegia** (i.e., functional impairment from the neck down). Lumbar cord injuries lead to **paraplegia** (i.e., excluding paralysis of the upper extremities). Spinal cord injuries and brain injuries such as a stroke can cause **hemiplegia** (i.e., paralysis on one side of the body).
• *Incomplete*: Some sensory, proprioceptive, and motor impulses are present. Loss of function depends on the extent and location of the injury. This is sometimes seen at the lower aspect of the cord below L1 in the region of the cauda equina. Bowel or bladder function can be affected without impairing mobility.

Spinal cord edema or hematoma can cause a cord lesion to ascend and worsen the neurologic deficit. Resultant paralysis may be relieved if the surgical procedure to remove bone fragments or to drain a hematoma compressing the spinal cord is done within a very short time after injury. Results are frequently discouraging.

Damage to the cord may be too extensive for return of function, or at best, return may be incomplete. Care is taken in moving and positioning the patient to avoid further paralysis. The patient should be log rolled (i.e., turned or lifted without flexing of the vertebral column).

A lumbar puncture with pressure readings may be done. If a block in the flow of spinal fluid is present, a laminotomy or laminectomy is done to decompress the spinal cord in a patient with complete paralysis or partial paralysis that is becoming progressively worse. A laminectomy also may be done to remove bone fragments. Internal fixation may be combined with decompression for thoracolumbar fractures.

Temperature control and monitoring of fluid and electrolyte balance are essential to the outcome for the patient with a spinal cord injury. The patient loses thermoregulatory ability after injury and tends to assume the temperature of the environment. Lack of vascular adaptation affects fluid balance. Pulmonary edema and left ventricular failure can occur. Pulmonary embolus also is a potential complication of immobility.

Technologic advances in surgical treatment, stabilization, and electrical stimulation have given patients with spinal cord injuries hope for regaining partial or full function.

Surgical Procedures of the Spine

Discectomy

Intervertebral disc injuries can happen anywhere along the vertebral column but usually occur between the lumbar vertebrae and are caused by lifting heavy objects or by twisting the spine. The nucleus pulposus can herniate or rupture through a tear in the annulus fibrosus and posterior ligament (Fig. 38.26). This protrusion, referred to as a herniated disc or ruptured or slipped disc, compresses the spinal nerve roots or spinal cord within the spinal canal against the vertebra. This causes pain along the dermatomes from the lumbar or sacral region to one or both lower legs (Fig. 38.27). Pain may radiate down the sciatic nerve pathway to the leg. Muscles can be affected causing multiple symptoms from weakness to paralysis when nerve impulses are disrupted from a myotome pathway. During the surgical procedure, the herniated nucleus pulposus or ruptured portion of the annulus fibrosus is excised (Fig. 38.28).

Microdiscectomy or percutaneous discectomy may be used to remove a herniated lumbar nucleus pulposus with minimal surgical manipulation. Microdiscectomy permits exposure of the herniated nucleus pulposus through a 1 or 2-inch (2.5- or 5-cm) incision without extensive manipulation of the paraspinal muscles or removal of a large section of lamina. The skin incision is shorter than required for a standard laminectomy; therefore recovery time is decreased.

Percutaneous Discectomy

Percutaneous lumbar discectomy (nucleoplasty) is an endoscopic procedure to remove a focal bulge—type herniated disc, usually at

the level of L4-L5. It is done with the patient under local anesthesia, usually with intravenous (IV) sedation because the patient must be alert enough to assess radicular pain in the leg. The patient may be either prone or in a lateral decubitus position.

• **Fig. 38.27** Ruptured disc.

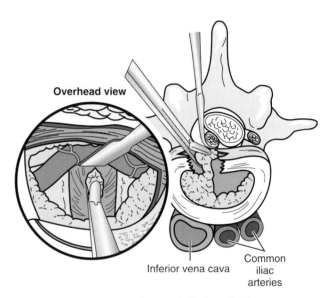

• **Fig. 38.28** Ruptured disc is excised.

• **Fig. 38.26** Herniated disc at L5-S1 causes pain along the associated dermatomes.

• **Fig. 38.29** Cervical dermatome.

A trocar is inserted through the skin and soft tissue into the disc capsule. Under fluoroscopic control, a cutting probe (Nucleotome) is inserted through the outer cannula. The herniated nucleus pulposus is excised and aspirated to relieve pressure on the spinal nerve root.

Total Disc Replacement

Total disc replacement (TDR) can be done for lumbar or cervical discs with an artificial material. Discs made from titanium, ceramic, and viscoelastic materials are available. Disc replacement has been approved for up to two levels. (More information can be found at www.spine.org.)

Cervical Spine

The cervical dermatome distribution is one of the prime indicators of the location of the injury or pathologic lesion (Fig. 38.29).

Transoral Approach

In the transoral approach the patient is positioned supine with the backrest of the OR bed elevated approximately 20 degrees. The head is stabilized in a headrest, and the airway is intubated with a nasotracheal tube (Fig. 38.30). The retractors are placed in the pharynx to retract the tongue and the soft palate. The uvula is retracted upward using a transnasal loop. The teeth are protected by tooth guards or moist sponges (Fig. 38.31). The transpharyngeal incision is made to access the retropharyngeal space. The high cervical spines C1-C2 can be repaired or stabilized.

Anterior Cervical Approach

The anterior cervical spine can be exposed through a transverse skin incision in the neck and dissection through the cleavage plane between the carotid artery and the esophagus (Fig. 38.32). The anterior cervical incision is created along the lateral muscular cleavage line or transversely across the anterior neck (Fig. 38.33). Medium self-retaining retractors are placed in the incision at right angles to provide exposure of the vertebral body while displacing the esophagus and trachea (Fig. 38.34). Care is taken to identify the nerves and vessels. Anterior cervical dissection can cause complications with speech and swallowing postoperatively.

The spinous processes and laminae remain intact when the anterior approach is used. A ruptured intervertebral disc or a

• **Fig. 38.30** Position for transoral cervical surgery.

• **Fig. 38.31** Transoral retractors.

fracture-dislocation with bone fragments compressing the cervical spinal cord or nerve roots can be completely explored at the level of the vertebral body (Fig. 38.35). Removal of the posterior margins of the vertebral bodies may be indicated to complete the decompression of the nerve root.

The operating microscope is a valuable adjunct to anterior cervical intervertebral discectomy and for an anterior approach to other cervical spinal lesions. A bone graft may be placed between the vertebral bodies for interbody fusion.

• **Fig. 38.32** Surgical landmarks for anterior cervical approach for cervical spine surgery.

• **Fig. 38.35** Cross-section of retracted tissue at the level of the cervical vertebrae.

• **Fig. 38.33** Anterior cervical incisions.

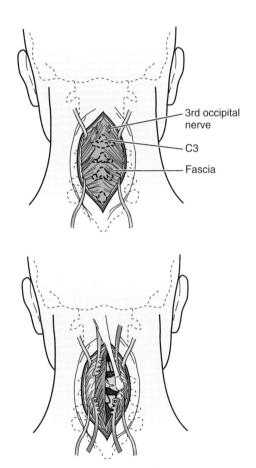

• **Fig. 38.36** Posterior cervical incision and laminectomy.

• **Fig. 38.34** Medium self-retaining retractors are placed at right angles.

Posterior Cervical Approach

The lower posterior cervical spine can be accessed with the patient in the prone position and the head stabilized in a head-positioning frame. The incision is made vertically over the cervical spinous processes (Fig. 38.36). The laminae are removed (Fig. 38.37), and the remaining cervical spinous processes are stabilized with plates and screws to minimize instability (Fig. 38.38).

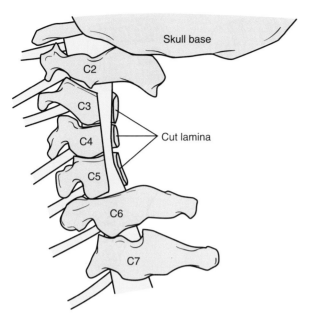

• **Fig. 38.37** Posterior cervical laminectomy at three levels.

• **Fig. 38.38** Posterior cervical stabilization after laminectomy.

• **Fig. 38.39** Supine anterior retroperitoneal approach.

Thoracic Spine
Anterior Thoracic Approach

An anterior approach is used for thoracic vertebral disc herniations, spinal cord tumors, or vertebral body fractures. A thoracic surgeon assists with a transthoracic approach. Fractured bone fragments can be stabilized with anterior spinal fusion or placement of posterior rods by costotransversectomy in the thoracic region. Thoracoscopic approaches can be used.

Posterior Thoracic Approach

Posterior thoracic spinal procedures do not involve a full thoracotomy. Positioning is similar to that used for lower posterior spinal procedures, and the incision is performed in the same manner as a lumbar incision.

Lumbar Spine
Anterior Transperitoneal Lumbar Approach

The anterior transperitoneal approach is performed on a supine patient through an abdominal incision, like a laparotomy, that enters the peritoneal cavity. Large table-mounted self-retaining retractors may be needed to provide exposure.

Anterior Retroperitoneal Lumbar Approach

The anterior retroperitoneal approach is performed on a patient in a supine or lateral position and involves an incision into the abdomen that is used to dissect the planes behind the peritoneal cavity from the abdominal wall (Fig. 38.39). The peritoneal cavity is displaced laterally and retracted away from the retroperitoneal space.

The retroperitoneal method is used for endoscopic spinal surgery and placement of interbody metallic cages for stabilization (Fig. 38.40). The cages are small titanium or carbon fiber frames packed with bone graft material and inserted between the bodies of the vertebrae. The graft-filled cages can be placed anteriorly (Fig. 38.41, *A*) or posteriorly (Fig. 38.41, *B*) through the disc space between the vertebral bodies or can be positioned vertically in the anterior interbody space (Fig. 38.41, *C*).

The endoscopic method of cage placement is commonly performed with the patient in a lateral position. The team is strategically positioned around the OR bed so the monitors are in a clear range of vision (Fig. 38.42).

Posterior Lumbar Approach

Removal of the spinous processes and lamina from one or more vertebrae is performed to expose an intervertebral or spinal cord lesion. A posterior laminectomy is usually carried out through a vertical midline skin incision with the patient positioned prone (Fig. 38.43). The patient may be positioned prone on a Jackson table or Wilson or Andrews frame to arch the spine forward for reduction of epidural blood loss by lowering the intraabdominal pressure on the vena cava. Overweight patients require additional consideration for redundant body tissues and the weight limits of special spinal frames.

The extent of the incision depends on the number of lumbar laminae to be removed. Fascia and muscles are retracted to expose

• **Fig. 38.40** Interbody cages.

A   B   C

• **Fig. 38.41** **A,** Anterior interbody cages. **B,** Posterior interbody cages. **C,** Open interbody cage in anterior placement.

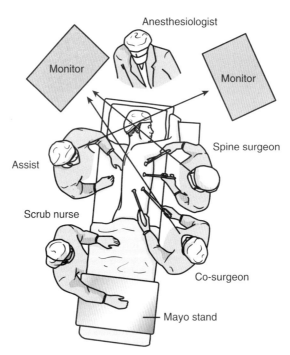

• **Fig. 38.42** Placement of the team for spinal endoscopy.

the spinous processes and laminae. These are sharply debulked and dissected with a rongeur, as necessary, for exposure of the spinal cord dura, spinal nerve roots, or an interlaminar lesion. An intervertebral disc, spinal cord tumor, bone fragments, and extradural or intradural foreign bodies are removed after the laminectomy is completed.

Cages can be placed during an open spinal procedure as part of the stabilization after a laminectomy. Fig. 38.44 shows an interbody cage packed with bone graft material and stabilization with plates and screws. Fig. 38.45 shows an L5-S1 fusion with bone graft for fusion with stabilization with short rods and screws.

• **Fig. 38.43** Lumbar incision for laminectomy.

• **Fig. 38.44** Interbody cage with plates and screws.

• **Fig. 38.45** L5-S1 fusion with bone graft and rods with screws.

EVOLVE WEBSITE

http://evolve.elsevier.com/Hornacky/BerryKohn/

- Historical Perspective
- Tips for the Scrub Person and Circulating Nurse
- Student Interactive Questions
- Glossary

References

1. Alkhalife Y, Padhye K, El-Hawary R: New technologies in pediatric spine surgery, *Orthop Clin North Am* 50(1):57–76, 2018.
2. Bhattacharyya S: Spinal cord myelopathy, *Am J Med* 131(11): 1293–1297, 2018.
3. Yoshida G, Ushirozako H, Kobayashi S, et al.: Intraoperative neuro-monitoring during adult spinal deformity surgery: alert positive cases for various surgical procedures, *Spine Deform* 7(1):132–140, 2018.
4. Le X, Tian W, Shi Z, et al.: Robot-assisted versus fluoroscopy-assisted cortical bone trajectory screw instrumentation in lumbar spinal surgery: a matched cohort from comparison, *World Neurosurg* 120:e745–e751, 2018.
5. Singh G, Hsu W: Biologics of lumbar interbody fusion, *Semin Spine Surg* 30(4):194–202, 2018.
6. Patel D, Yoo J, Karmakar S, et al.: Interbody options in lumbar fusion, *J Spine Surg* 5(1):S19–S24, 2019.
7. Mendenhall S, Mobasser D, Relyea K, et al.: Spinal instrumentation in infants, children, and adolescents, a review, *J Neurosurg Pediatr* 23:1–15, 2019.
8. Eltori A, Fuentes C: Magnetic growth modulation in orthopaedic and spine surgery, *J Orthop* 15(1):59–66, 2018.
9. Compston J, McClung M, Leslie W: Osteoporosis, *Lancet* 393(10169): 364–376, 2019.

Bibliography

Kaito T, Malsukawa K, Abe Y, et al.: Cortical pedicle screw placement in lumbar spinal surgery with a patient matched targeting guide: a cadaveric study, *J Orthop Sci* 23(6):865–869, 2018.

Ortiz AO, Moura A, Johnson B: Postsurgical spine: techniques, expected imaging findings, and complications, *Semin Ultrasound CT MR* 39(6):630–650, 2018.

Veeravagu A, Wang M: *Robotic and navigated spine surgery: surgical techniques and advancements*, Philadelphia, 2023, Elsevier.

39

Ophthalmic Surgery

CHAPTER OUTLINE

Anatomy and Physiology of the Eye, 826

Ophthalmic Surgical Patient Care, 827

Special Features of Ophthalmic Surgery, 829

Ocular Surgical Procedures, 832

Eye Injuries, 844

Ophthalmic Lasers, 845

CHAPTER OBJECTIVES

After studying this chapter, the learner will be able to:

- Identify the pertinent anatomy of the eye and surrounding structures.
- Describe the procedures performed on the eye for glaucoma.
- Discuss the advantages and disadvantages of intraocular lens implantation.
- Describe the actions of mydriatic and miotic drugs.

KEY TERMS AND DEFINITIONS

Aphakic Without a natural or prosthetic lens.
BSS Balanced salt solution used for eye irrigation.
Capsulorrhexis During cataract surgery a continuous circular opening is created in the anterior capsule to allow removal or phacoemulsification of the nucleus of the opacified lens.
Cataract Cloudy or yellowed lens of the eye.
Cyclodialysis Surgical opening between the anterior chamber and the suprachoroidal space to decrease elevated pressure within the eye of patients with glaucoma.
Discission Cut into soft tissue such as a cataract.

Gonioscopy Examination of the anterior chamber with a special lens.
Haptic Tiny flexible prong used to secure a prosthetic intraocular lens.
IOL Intraocular lens.
Phacoemulsification Irrigation and aspiration of a cataract using ultrasonic vibrations.
Pneumoretinopexy Repositioning of a detached retina by use of a gas or air bubble in the vitreous.

Anatomy and Physiology of the Eye

A thorough understanding of the anatomic structure and physiology of the eye is fundamental to a comprehension of the surgical procedures.

The eyeballs are framed bilaterally by the bony orbits. Each orbit comprises seven separate bones: the maxilla, palatine, frontal, sphenoid, zygoma, ethmoid, and lacrimal bones. Foramina, fissures, and grooves provide stability and access for vessels, nerves, and attachments. Adjacent anatomic structures include the lacrimal apparatus medially, the extraocular muscles and their attachments, and the sinuses.

The globe, or eyeball, is situated within the bony orbit and is surrounded by a padding of fatty tissue. Its position is maintained by extraocular muscles and fascial attachments. The sclera, the white outer tissue layer of the globe, is contiguous with the transparent avascular cornea anteriorly. The conjunctiva is the mucous membrane that lines the inner side of the upper and lower eyelids and the exposed portion of the sclera, except for the cornea (Fig. 39.1).

The eyeball is divided into two segments: anterior and posterior. The anterior segment of the eye includes the cornea, the anterior chamber filled with aqueous fluid (humor), the circular pigmented iris, and the lens. The lens consists of a clear, transparent, gelatinous protein encased in a capsule. It is supported by a series of suspensory ligaments called zonules. The posterior segment, the portion of the eye behind the lens, contains the vitreous fluid (which must be clear for vision), the retina, and the choroid linings, which are the vascular nourishing layers (Fig. 39.2).

Innervation of vision and sensory transmission is derived from the second cranial nerve (optic nerve) (Fig. 39.3). Motor innervation extends from the third cranial nerve (oculomotor nerve) to the rectus muscles. The superior oblique muscles are innervated by the fourth cranial nerve (trochlear nerve). The lateral rectus muscle is innervated by the sixth cranial nerve (abducens nerve).

The arterial supply of the eyeball, muscles, and eyelids comes from the ophthalmic artery, which is a branch of the internal carotid artery and drains into the superior and inferior ophthalmic

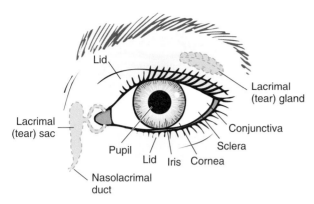

• **Fig. 39.1** Front view of eye.

• **Fig. 39.2** Anatomy of the eye. **A,** Anterior segment. *1,* Cornea; *2,* anterior chamber; *3,* pupil; *4,* iris; *5,* lens; *6,* ciliary body; *7,* zonule. **B,** Posterior segment. *8,* Vitreous body; *9,* retina; *10,* choroid; *11,* sclera; *12,* optic nerve; *13,* central retinal artery.

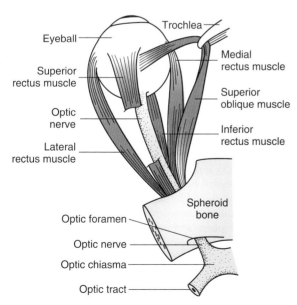

• **Fig. 39.3** Location of optic nerve in relation to eye muscles.

veins. The retina has a separate blood supply that is derived from the central retinal artery. Drainage is through the retinal vein.

The physiology of vision requires the following:
- Functioning visual apparatus
- Source of light
- Intact neurovascular communication with the brain
- Interpretation by the brain of what is seen

The eye resembles a camera with a compound lens system. Light rays emanating from an object in the field of vision are transmitted to the eye, where they traverse the optical system to reach the retina. The retina corresponds to the film of the camera. The area of highest sensitivity for details is called the *macula,* which is located approximately in the center of the retina at the posterior pole. The intensity of light is automatically determined by the size of the pupil, which is controlled by the iris muscles. The iris functions like the shutter of a camera.

The optical system comprises the transparent cornea, or window of the eye; the aqueous fluid behind the cornea; the pupil, or opening in the colored iris; and the lens. The naturally flexible lens focuses light rays by bending them to form an image on the retina—the innermost layer of the eye that contains the visual sensory nerve endings. These cells are connected to nerve fibers that converge toward the brain to become the optic nerve. The sensory cells translate patterns of light into nervous impulses, which are transmitted to the brain via the optic nerve. The occipital portion of the brain interprets the images of light rays registered on the retina.

Ophthalmic Surgical Patient Care

Impaired vision may produce prolonged severe stress and alter the patient's self-image. Most patients with impaired vision are older adults.[1] When caring for these patients, the health care provider should reassure them, exercise patience, give directions clearly, anticipate needs, and check their comfort level. Specific patient care considerations include, but are not limited to, the following:

1. Urinary urgency can be a problem in geriatric patients or in patients receiving diuretic medication. Although the patient should void before coming to the operating room (OR), offer the patient help to the bathroom if needed or the use of a bedpan or urinal before transfer to the OR. Severe urinary urgency can cause increased intraocular pressure (IOP) during the procedure. Strain and gross movement are dangerous and are to be avoided.
2. The surgeon and circulating nurse verify the intended surgical site with the patient and with the medical records. After confirmation and to avoid error, some surgeons place an indelible mark on the side of the patient's neck or a sticker above the affected eye. Care is taken to ensure that the sticker is not displaced by the patient.
3. The patient is placed in the supine position on the OR bed so the head and body are aligned. Most ORs use a dedicated ophthalmic OR bed that can be used during the procedure and to transport the patient to the postprocedural recovery area (Fig. 39.4). The top of the head is in line with the edge of the OR bed for accessibility. The head should not be turned greatly in either direction; the head is stabilized in a ring-shaped pillow (donut). The patient's gown is untied at the neck to prevent pressure. Any obstruction to venous circulation can cause undue increased IOP, which can produce a loss of vitreous humor when the eye is opened. To

• **Fig. 39.4** Dedicated ophthalmic bed.

• **Fig. 39.5** Creating a tent with the surgical drape and the Mayo stand for patient comfort.

assist venous return from the head, the OR bed is tilted so the patient's head is elevated by 5 to 10 degrees. For long procedures, an egg crate—type or gel pad mattress may be placed on the bed. Additional padding may be needed to position kyphotic or lordotic patients.

4. Skin preparation and draping procedures are performed according to routine. Sterile plastic drapes are often placed over woven textile drapes to contain lint, especially before lens implantation. A patient with a drape over the face is often apprehensive and afraid of suffocating. To help eliminate the feeling of claustrophobia, the drape can be placed over a Mayo stand or clipped to an intravenous (IV) pole to create a tentlike space above the patient's nose and mouth (Fig. 39.5). Oxygen is delivered if necessary via nasal prongs or insufflated to the facial area beneath the drape. An electrosurgical unit (ESU) is not to be used in an oxygen-rich environment because of the increased risk for ignition.

5. A quiet, stimulant-free environment is provided for the awake patient who is receiving a local anesthetic.

6. Because the patient has no defensive blink reflex to protect the retina from light exposure, some surgeons use a sterile, opaque pupillary shield to protect the patient's retina from phototoxic damage caused by prolonged exposure to illumination of the microscope. Some scopes have a sensor near the eyepiece that dims the light source when the

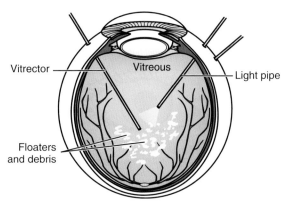

• **Fig. 39.6** Pars plana vitrectomy for emergency bleeding.

surgeon is not looking directly into the scope. The light reverts back to the desired intensity when the surgeon is positioned at the eyepiece.

7. The team should prepare for emergencies by anticipating problems. Fast action can make the difference between a seeing eye and a nonseeing eye postoperatively. The following are potential complications:
   a. A systemic reaction to medications or local anesthetic drugs and cardiac arrest.
   b. A loss of vitreous, which requires the removal of vitreous from the anterior chamber with a vitreotome to prevent prolapse of the wound, severe inflammation, or an updrawn pupil.
   c. An expulsive hemorrhage or an expulsion of ocular contents, which requires a sharp knife (e.g., Beaver blade, Wheeler knife) for fast cutdown into the pars plana area and an 18-gauge needle or cannula attached to a syringe to aspirate blood and reduce pressure in the vitreal compartment in an effort to save the eye and vision (Fig. 39.6).
   d. Instrument failure. Hand aspiration devices should be available for immediate use.

8. A wide variety of fine-size absorbable and nonabsorbable sutures may be used. The scrub person follows the manufacturer's recommendations for handling these delicate materials and needles with the appropriate needle holders. Many surgeons use sutureless techniques. Special techniques are used in microsurgery.

9. Hemostasis is attained with bipolar cautery and a bipolar eraser pencil. Sponges are spear shaped and consist of precut compressed cellulose on sticks (Fig. 39.7).

10. No foreign material should be introduced into the surgical site. Particulate matter from gloves, instruments, or sponges should be avoided. To remove any debris or impurity, intraocular lenses (**IOLs**) are soaked and rinsed in balanced salt solution (**BSS**) and sometimes lubricated with sodium hyaluronate (Healon) before insertion.

11. Inflammation should be kept as minimal as possible because even slight inflammation may result in total functional loss. Steroids are often administered locally, subconjunctivally, and sometimes systemically. The eye may respond violently to the slightest amount of trauma. All drugs and solutions should be clearly labeled.

12. Antibiotic drops are often instilled topically for 24 hours preoperatively and postoperatively.

McPherson bipolar ESU forceps   Bipolar ESU eraser pencil   Cellulose spears (absorbent)

• **Fig. 39.7** Instruments for hemostasis of the eye. *ESU,* Electrosurgical unit.

Solid Barraquer retractor   Open Barraquer retractor   Stevenson retractor

Wright orbit scissors   Castroviejo scissors   Heavy enucleation scissors   Fine enucleation scissors

Iridectomy scissors   Wescott scissors   Dewecker iridectomy scissors

• **Fig. 39.8** Eye instrumentation: self-retaining lid retractors and scissors.

13. A sterile eye pad is commonly applied at the conclusion of the surgical procedure. A protective plastic or metal shield may be secured over the eye pad to guard against mechanical injury. Absorbable corneal shields may be used.
14. The patient should not be permitted to participate in the move from the OR bed after intraocular procedures; this prevents a sudden rise in IOP and/or dislocation of the IOL implant.
15. Arm restraints are essential for infants and young children. Restraints are applied to adults only under extreme circumstances, such as disorientation. The use of side rails preoperatively and postoperatively is standard procedure for all patients undergoing ophthalmic surgery.

An important aspect of postoperative care is informing the patient not to get out of bed alone. A fall or injury to the eye can nullify an otherwise successful surgical procedure. The patient must not do anything to increase IOP (e.g., bend over at the waist, lift heavy objects). Deep breathing postoperatively is encouraged, but coughing is avoided because it could increase IOP and rupture the suture line. The patient should report any postoperative pain, swelling, redness, or discharge. The outcome of ophthalmic procedures includes a cosmetic as well as a functional aspect.

Special Features of Ophthalmic Surgery

The patient undergoing ophthalmic surgery faces impairment or loss of vision if the outcome of the surgical intervention is unfavorable. Special features of ophthalmic surgery aim to prevent such a loss. Surgical procedures on the eye are extremely delicate and require precision instrumentation, a steady hand, and quiet surroundings. The operating microscope, all accessory equipment, and microinstruments should be set up and checked before the surgical procedure. The outcome of the procedure depends on the condition of the instruments.

Ophthalmic Instrumentation

The tips of these expensive, fragile microinstruments should be protected and handled with extreme care before, during, and after use. Eye instrumentation is unique to the specialty. Only with rare exception are any of the following used in any other type of surgery:
- Self-retaining lid retractors and scissors (Fig. 39.8)
- Graspers and manual retractors (Fig. 39.9)
- Enucleation and measuring devices (Fig. 39.10)
- Punctum plug and forceps (Fig. 39.11)
- Corneal trephine (Fig. 39.12)

Desmarres chalazion forceps

Desmarres entropion forceps

Carter globe introducer

Elliott eye spatula

Treleats eye spatula

Macallens lid spatula

Rollet lachrymal hook

Jameson strabismus hook

Desmarres lid manual retractor

• **Fig. 39.9** Eye instrumentation: graspers and manual retractors.

Foster enucleation snare

Geissen eye ruler

Castroviejo calipers

Orbit sizers (sized 14 mm to 20 mm)

Shahl anterior chamber caliper

• **Fig. 39.10** Eye instrumentation: enucleation and measuring devices.

Operating Microscope

Ophthalmic surgeons use the operating microscope for intraocular procedures. When the operating microscope is used, the OR bed should be mechanically secure, and the patient's head should be stabilized. Inadvertent movement is not tolerated because of the minute surgical field. The headrest should be narrow so that it does not obstruct the surgeon's approach to the surgical site from the sides of the vertical column of the microscope. The patient is instructed about the importance of remaining still during the surgical procedure. Otherwise, the patient could easily move out of the field of vision under the microscope or precipitate a complication.

The assistant observes the surgical procedure through an assistant's ocular and irrigates the cornea with BSS to prevent drying (Fig. 39.13). The assistant should bring to the surgeon's attention any potentially unsatisfactory situation that the surgeon cannot

• **Fig. 39.11** Punctum plug and forceps.

observe from their position. Some scrub persons are trained to act as first assistants. The surgeon and the assistants should limit their caffeine intake before the procedure to promote steady hands when using microinstrumentation under the microscope.

• **Fig. 39.12** Corneal trephine for cadaver tissue procurement.

• **Fig. 39.13** Surgeon and first assistant using a ceiling-mounted microscope.

The surgeon will focus the microscope in a manner that permits a foot pedal–controlled zoom function without blurring the assistant's vision or the camera and video equipment. Many surgeons who use corrective eyewear will adjust the oculars for accommodation with the eyes against the eye cups to avoid having the discomfort of spectacles.

Ophthalmic Drugs

Many drugs are critical to the preparation of the eye for the surgical procedure. Orders for patient preparation often contain common abbreviations that identify the eye(s) to receive drops: OD (right eye), OS (left eye), and OU (both eyes); however, The Joint Commission (TJC) has advised that the use of abbreviations can lead to human error and recommends not using them in the interest of patient safety. Before skin preparation, the circulating nurse instills the medications and anesthetic drops as ordered. The following procedures should be observed when instilling eye drops:

1. Wash your hands.
2. Identify the correct medication, eye, and patient.
3. Check for allergy or sensitivity.
4. Explain the procedure to the patient.
5. Tilt back the patient's head and tell the patient to look up. While gently pulling down on the lower lid, instill the medication in the middle third of the inner aspect of the lower lid. Release the lid while the patient slowly closes the eye to retain the drop; let the patient close the eye between repeated drops. In a struggling child, have a parent tilt the child's head back

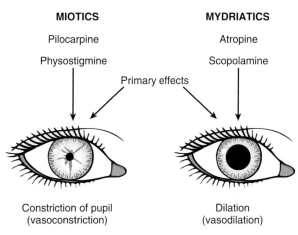

• **Fig. 39.14** Effects of miotic and mydriatic drugs.

and close both eyes. Instill the medication at the inner canthus. The drop will roll into the eye as the child opens it. Some medications, such as atropine, may have a systemic effect. To prevent drainage into the tear duct, nose, and stomach, gently blot excess fluid. In small infants or young children, systemic absorption is avoided by applying finger pressure over the lacrimal sac region (inner canthus) of both eyes simultaneously for 1 minute.

6. Administer only the specified number of drops.
7. Read the label on the vial before each instillation.
8. Each patient should receive a fresh, single-use, disposable vial of medication that is discarded after use.

Mydriatic and Miotic Drugs

Medications may be given to alter the size of the pupil (Fig. 39.14), including the following:

- *Mydriatic drops:* 2.5% or 10% phenylephrine (Neo-Synephrine) to dilate the pupil.
- *Mydriatic-cycloplegic drops:* 1% cyclopentolate hydrochloride (Cyclogyl), 1% atropine, 0.25% scopolamine, and 1% tropicamide (Mydriacyl) to dilate the pupil, paralyze the ciliary body, diminish the reaction to trauma, and prevent anterior synechiae (e.g., adherence of iris to the lens). These drugs are longer acting than phenylephrine.
- *Miotic drops:* 2% pilocarpine, carbachol (Miostat), and acetylcholine chloride (Miochol-E) to constrict the pupil.
- *Combination drugs:* Combination drugs may be used to limit the amount of drugs instilled into the eye. Examples of combination drugs include mydriatic/cycloplegic or hydroxyamphetamine/tropicamide (Paremyd).

Local and Topical Anesthesia

Except in children and select patients, local and topical anesthetics are commonly used for ophthalmic surgical procedures. Most surgical procedures are scheduled as monitored anesthesia care or attended local. Many short procedures are done without IV access. An anesthesia provider monitors the patient and administers oxygen and/or supplements the local anesthetic if necessary. IV midazolam (Versed) and/or fentanyl (Sublimaze) or propofol (Diprivan) is often given to relax the patient. The sedative effects of these agents increase the patient's tolerance to procedures. If a general anesthetic is used, the usual general anesthesia routines are followed.

Local anesthesia consists of the following:

1. Topical instillation of anesthetic drops. The drug used may be 0.5% proparacaine (Ophthaine), 0.5% tetracaine (Pontocaine), or 2% lidocaine (Xylocaine MPF [methylparaben-free]). Most surgeons prefer to use this method in combination with moderate sedation.
2. Local infiltration by injection of the lids and tissue around the eyes with anesthetic medication.
3. Retrobulbar block. An absolutely quiet eye is necessary, especially at high magnifications of the microscope. When general anesthesia is used, some surgeons administer a retrobulbar block for immobility and to lower IOP. A popular solution for this block consists of a mixture of equal parts of 2% or 4% lidocaine and 0.75% bupivacaine, 3.75 units/mL for penetration. A 25-gauge × 1½-inch (3.8-cm) needle with a sharp, rounded point (e.g., Atkinson needle) and a 5-mL syringe are used. The surgeon inserts the needle behind the eyeball to anesthetize the globe and paralyze the muscles. The patient is asked to look up and away from the injection site and is told that a slight burning sensation may accompany the injection. Up to 5 mL of solution may be slowly and carefully injected.

   Retrobulbar block may be followed by intermittent massage of the eye to soften it, lower IOP, and facilitate surgical manipulation during cataract extraction, especially when insertion of an IOL is being contemplated. Massage is continued until the IOP is lowered to a satisfactory level (e.g., 10–12 scale reading on sterile Schiøtz tonometer).
4. Peribulbar anesthesia. This is an alternative to retrobulbar injection. With this method, injections are made in the soft tissue superior and inferior to the globe rather than behind it. A greater amount of the same anesthetic solution used for retrobulbar injection is used for peribulbar anesthesia. With this procedure, adequate anesthesia is obtained without the risk for retrobulbar hemorrhage.

Ophthalmic Solutions

Extreme and constant care must be used with ophthalmic solutions. Nearly all these solutions are colorless and may be stored in similar receptacles. These solutions are immediately and individually labeled by the scrub person; the solution is discarded if the identification is missing. Solutions for intraocular use must be separated from all other solutions. Ideally, these solutions should be filtered with micropore filters before injection.

Epinephrine or other sympathomimetics may have side effects when used with some anesthetic agents. Therefore the surgeon should check with the anesthesia provider before using medications intraoperatively. Medications that may induce vomiting are also avoided. Any straining or gross movement may cause intraocular hemorrhage, a sudden rise in IOP that results in a loss of vitreous, or the expulsion of ocular contents through the wound; all these conditions can cause blindness.

Ocular Surgical Procedures

For convenience, surgical treatment of the eye can be divided into the following two main classifications:

1. *Extraocular:* Conditions affecting the exterior surface of the eye, eyelid, or orbit.
2. *Intraocular:* Conditions pertaining to the interior contents of the eye.

Extraocular Procedures

Eyelid

The anatomy of the upper and lower eyelids is described in Fig. 39.15.

Excision of Neoplasm of the Eyelid

Tissue may be excised with a knife, an ESU, diathermy, or cryosurgery. An extremely common but benign tumor of the lid is the chalazion—a cystic alteration of one of the oil-secreting meibomian glands in the lid (Fig. 39.16, *A*). The resulting accumulation of oil forms a hard tumor of the lid and requires excision. The excision is usually performed in an office or ambulatory surgical facility. Chalazion is differentiated from a stye (hordeolum) by the location on the lid. Styes are small, infected lash follicles along the lash line (see Fig. 39.16, *B*).

After removal of a malignant lesion of the lid, plastic procedures such as Z-plasty, sliding flaps from adjacent areas, or full- or partial-thickness flaps from the opposing lid are used to close the defect.

Correction of Ptosis

Ptosis, a drooping of the upper lid, may be acquired in adulthood but is more commonly congenital. For the levator aponeurosis procedure, an incision is made on the front surface of the lid to expose the tarsus and the aponeurosis. The tarsus is sutured to the aponeurosis, and the skin incision is closed.

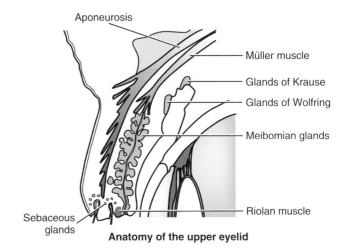

Anatomy of the upper eyelid

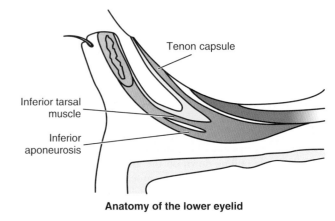

Anatomy of the lower eyelid

• **Fig. 39.15** Normal anatomy of the upper and lower eyelids.

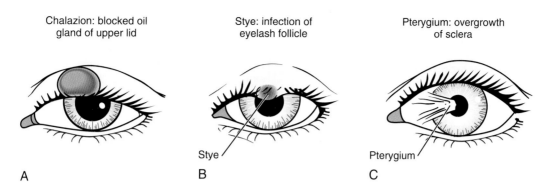

Chalazion: blocked oil
gland of upper lid

Stye: infection of
eyelash follicle

Pterygium: overgrowth
of sclera

Stye

Pterygium

A   B   C

• **Fig. 39.16** Common benign lesions of the eye commonly treated with surgery.

For the frontalis suspension procedure, the anterior surface of the upper lid is incised at the crease, and two smaller incisions are made above the eyebrow. A graft of fascia or synthetic material is attached to the tarsus and passed through the deep lid tissue and brought out through the eyebrow incisions. The graft material is secured, and the skin incisions are closed.

Repair of Acquired Malformation of the Eyelid

Conditions such as senile ectropion or entropion most commonly affect the lower lid (Fig. 39.17). Ectropion is a condition in which either the upper or lower lid is everted (turned out) to expose the conjunctival surface. Entropion is the opposite condition, in which the lid margin is inverted (turned in). As a result, the eyelashes often abrade the cornea. Various procedures may be used to correct both conditions.[2]

Blepharoplasty

A common result of aging is the stretching of the eyelid skin and the bulging of orbital fat from between the muscle fibers of the lids. Both conditions cause cosmetic disfigurement or baggy lids and, in extreme cases, may obstruct vision. In blepharoplasty, redundant folds of skin and herniated pockets of fat are removed, and defects in the muscle layer are repaired. Transconjunctival blepharoplasty is performed by making a small incision into the conjunctiva of the lower lid and removing fat pads. Small bleeders are cauterized with a disposable electrosurgical pencil. Blepharoplasty is commonly performed by plastic surgeons and is described in Chapter 40.

Lacrimal Apparatus

Lacrimal Duct Dilation

Lacrimal duct dilation is performed for excessive tearing. A series of probes, graduated in size, are introduced one by one into the duct system to permit freer drainage of tears. Dacryoadenitis is an inflamed lacrimal gland. Infection is usually caused by bacteria or viruses. Ophthalmologists recommend that patients with inflamed eyelids use diluted baby shampoo to cleanse lashes and lids.

Dacryocystectomy

Extirpation or removal of the lacrimal sac in the lower lid is performed for chronic dacryocystitis. This procedure does not reestablish the tear drainage system.

Dacryocystorhinostomy

Construction of a new opening into the nasal cavity from the lacrimal sac is performed to correct congenital malformation of or

Ectropion (turning out)
of lower lid

Entropion (turning in)
of lower lid

• **Fig. 39.17** Ectropion and entropion are surgically treated to realign the eyelash line for normal function.

trauma to the nasolacrimal duct. A new tear drainage system is constructed.

Extraocular Muscle

Procedures on the oculomotor muscles, which control eye movement, are performed to correct misalignment that interferes with the ability of the two eyes to remain in simultaneous focus on a viewed object. The surgical procedures correct muscle imbalance by strengthening a weak muscle or weakening an overactive one. Although commonly performed on children, these muscle procedures may be required in adult patients for the following:

- Untreated childhood strabismus (squint)
- Unsatisfactory result from a childhood surgical procedure
- Trauma to the brainstem or to the orbit with resultant muscle injury or paralysis
- Systemic disease (e.g., thyroid exophthalmos) and muscle paralysis
- Cerebrovascular accident with resultant muscle paralysis

Orbit

Decompression

Decompression is the treatment for severe exophthalmos, or a protrusion of the eyeball, that does not respond to medical treatment.

Orbital Tumors

Depending on the location of the orbital tumor, exploration may be approached through a lateral wall or the roof of the orbit. This procedure may involve a multidisciplinary team of surgeons.

Surgical Removal of the Eye

After removal of an eyeball, the patient is fitted with an artificial eye to restore cosmetic appearance. A spherical implant, such as silicone, plastic, tantalum, or hydroxyapatite, may be used to line the orbit and provide support for a prosthetic eye. The eye muscles are sutured to the implant, thereby providing natural movement, allowing the growth of surrounding tissue, and preventing the lower lid from sagging. The type of prosthesis that can be used depends on the procedure used to remove the eyeball.

Enucleation

Enucleation is the complete removal of the eyeball and the severing of its muscular attachments.[3] The muscle stumps are preserved, with the space between the stumps forming a pocket for the spherical plastic artificial eye. Overlying fasciae and conjunctivae are closed to hold the prosthesis in the socket. The contraction of eye muscles causes the prosthesis to move in the socket, simulating normal eye movements.

Eye prostheses are usually round or oval and can be textured or smooth. Some have pegs upon which the colored iris cap attaches. Others contain a magnet that adheres to the back of the visible colored iris portion. Sizes can be between 12 and 22 mm.

Evisceration

Evisceration removes the contents of the eyeball only; the outer sclera and muscles are left intact for attachment to a prosthesis. This procedure reduces the danger of transmitting an intraocular infection to the orbit and brain. Predisposing factors for evisceration include destruction of the eyeball by injury or disease and absolute glaucoma (hard blind eye).

Exenteration

Exenteration is the removal of the entire eye and orbital contents, including tendon, fatty, and fibrous tissues. This procedure is performed for a malignant tumor of the lids or eyeball that has extended into the orbit. Extensive plastic reconstruction is necessary before an artificial eye can be fitted.

Cornea

Although it consists of resilient tissue, the continually exposed cornea is especially susceptible to injury and infection.

Cauterization

Cauterization with chemicals or heat is sometimes used for a corneal ulceration that does not respond to antibiotics. This is sometimes performed for herpes simplex virus infections of the corneal epithelium. Cauterization may be used in conjunction with topical antiviral agents.

Pterygium

Pterygium is a benign growth of conjunctival tissue over the corneal surface. Although usually slow growing, pterygia can become fairly aggressive, especially in southern climates. A significant decrease in visual acuity secondary to induced astigmatism and corneal scarring can result from the abnormal growth. A popular surgical technique devised for the eradication of pterygia is the bare sclera method. This method involves excision of the entire pterygium, leaving an area of bare sclera. Beta radiation may be used as an adjunct to surgical treatment (see Fig. 39.16, *C*).

Corneal Transplantation (Keratoplasty)

With keratoplasty, a damaged cornea is removed and replaced with a healthy cornea from a human donor (Fig. 39.18). The cornea must be clear to permit light to enter and focus on the retina. Thus this procedure is indicated when scars or opacities on the cornea reduce or destroy vision by preventing the transmission of a clear image. Corneal opacity may result from degenerative changes, scars from chemical burns, perforated corneal ulcers, trauma, or edema after a cataract surgical procedure. In addition, ocular surgery, such as phacoemulsification, vitrectomy, and IOL implantation, has the potential to damage the corneal endothelium.

Because the cornea is avascular, keratoplasty is the most successful transplantation procedure and has considerably less rejection phenomena than all other tissues except bone. The greatest advance in technique to reduce the rate of rejection and the restriction of activity during convalescence has been the use of the operating microscope and microsutures. Continuous 10-0 or 11-0 nylon sutures are left in situ with minimal tissue reaction. The following two types of grafts are used:

1. *Full-thickness grafts:* The common type. The entire diameter of the corneal graft (6.5–8 mm) is replaced (penetrating keratoplasty).
2. *Partial-thickness or lamellar grafts:* Less popular. Only the top layer of the cornea, not its entire depth, is replaced (lamellar keratoplasty).

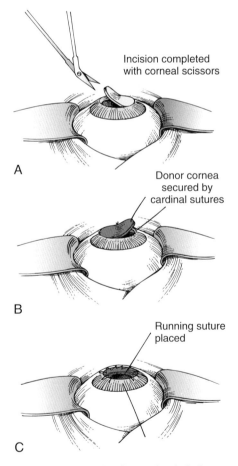

Incision completed with corneal scissors

A

Donor cornea secured by cardinal sutures

B

Running suture placed

C

• **Fig. 39.18** Corneal transplantation (keratoplasty). **A,** Damaged cornea is excised with corneal scissors. **B,** Donor cornea is secured by cardinal sutures. **C,** Continuous suture remains in situ.

An opaque cornea is an optically nonfunctioning one. The goal is to provide recipients with the highest-quality corneal tissue. A fresh, healthy cornea cut from the promptly enucleated eye of a relatively young donor within 4 to 6 hours of death is considered the best for transplantation. The cornea should be transplanted to the surface of the recipient eye, which has a healthy retina and optic nerve, as soon as possible to preserve viability and to prevent opacity. The acceptable times for collection of tissue after death and transplantation may vary among eye banks. The National Institutes of Health have established the National Eye Institute for further research.[4] (More information is available at www.nei.nih.gov.)

Donor tissue criteria include the following:

1. The consent for enucleation must conform to state laws. A certified eye bank technician may enucleate the eyes.

2. Medical information about the potential donor is evaluated. Some conditions that preclude the use of donor tissue are an unknown cause of death, previous intraocular surgery, Reye syndrome, lymphosarcoma, rabies, and transmissible diseases such as hepatitis, human immunodeficiency virus, and Creutzfeldt-Jakob disease. Donor information must be documented on the donor screening form that accompanies the tissue. A copy should be filed at the eye bank.

3. The endothelium, the very sensitive inner single layer of corneal cells, must be kept intact for eventual transparency of the graft. The entire donor globe is removed. Important factors to optimize the success of the transplant include sterile technique, the removal of as much conjunctiva as possible from the donor globe, avoidance of damage to or contamination of the removed eyes, and use of appropriate transport containers and preservation methods.

4. The donor's eyes are cooled as soon as possible to prevent deleterious effects. The placement of ice bags over the eyes promptly after death slows the metabolism of corneal cells. In general, the sooner the enucleated eyes are refrigerated, the better the quality of the donor tissue. Enucleated eyes are placed in a controlled environment at the eye bank.

5. The donor's cornea is carefully evaluated for epithelial defects, clarity, the presence of any foreign body, or any evidence of jaundice or infection. Endothelial cell count is a determining factor in estimating the prognosis of the transplant. The higher the count and the more regular the cellular pattern, the better the tissue. Age is not a deterrent if tissue is acceptable for transplantation, but donors younger than 65 years are preferred. The evaluation form must be completed and must accompany the tissue. The transplant surgeon also may receive specular microscopic photographs of the endothelium. Donor tissue preservation methods include:

   a. *Preservative medium.* Optisol-GS sterile buffered tissue culture contains the antibiotics gentamicin and streptomycin and allows refrigerated storage for 3 to 14 days. Tissue transplanted after 7 days has a higher risk for graft failure. Other solutions are available but Optisol-GS is the gold standard.[5] In the OR, the surgeon should inspect the container before using the cornea. If the cornea is cut to size for use with a trephine, the remaining corneoscleral rim should be placed in a culture medium and sent to the laboratory for culture. The incidence of positive cultures is low. The cornea should not be used, and the eye bank should be notified if the medium is turbid or contaminated, such as by a crack in the container.

   b. *Cryopreservation.* Both cryopreserved corneal and scleral tissue can be used for transplantation or for patching purposes. In general, their use is limited to emergency procedures when fresh tissue is not available. Usually this tissue is used less than 6 months after cryopreservation. Precise freezing and defrosting methods are of crucial importance in preventing injury to the endothelium. Corneal metabolism resumes with defrosting; therefore when the solution is thawed, the team should work rapidly because of the extreme time limitation. The tissue should be placed immediately within its natural anatomic environment to enhance the potential for successful grafting.

Regardless of the storage method, tissue preferably is used as soon as practical after donation. In the OR, adequate preparation, teamwork, and standardized transplantation procedures are imperative. The recipient eye is trephined to receive the donor cornea. A separate sterile donor table is set for the surgeon to use in preparing the donor tissue to the exact measurement needed for the recipient eye. During and after the procedure, topical antibiotics and steroids are administered under the conjunctiva to prevent infection and transplant rejection.

After the surgical procedure, a tissue recipient information form is completed to indicate how the tissue was used. This form is mailed to the eye bank, where it is kept on file. If the tissue is contaminated, the donor number and source can be easily traced. Information on the form includes recipient medical information; previous keratoplasties; the date, type, and details of the current surgical procedure; and the estimate of success.

The patient is instructed to report any symptoms, such as redness, light sensitivity, vision loss, or pain. A patch is worn for 1 to 4 days. Protective eyewear should be worn during the day, and a firm patch should be worn for sleeping for several months postoperatively. Sutures can be removed after a few months or may be left in permanently.

Suitable corneal tissue is in limited supply, which places restraints on transplantation. Numerous eye banks in the United States constitute the Eye Bank Association of America, which is tangentially associated with the International Eye Bank. These groups are central clearinghouses for the distribution of accessible tissue. They follow a stringent code of ethics in their functions to inform the public of the need for eye donations, to procure donated eyes, to assist in the optimal use of donor corneas locally, or to arrange for transportation to an area of greater need. More than 49,000 corneal transplants were recorded in the United States in 2022.[6] Tissue procurement is facilitated by the following:

- Distribution of donor forms from eye banks and organ donation organizations.
- Organ donation consent forms affixed to driver licenses. Family consent is still required before procurement.
- Education of medical and health care personnel to alert them to ask families of deceased patients for donations. Some state laws require a donation request.

Phototherapeutic Keratectomy

In phototherapeutic keratectomy (PTK), scar tissue is removed from the cornea with an excimer laser. This procedure restores vision that has been blocked by scars from an infection, injury, or inherited condition. PTK may obviate the need for a corneal transplant.

Refractive Keratoplasty

Refractive keratoplasty (corneal reshaping) includes a group of surgical procedures designed to alter the shape and refractive power (i.e., focusing power) of the cornea to minimize the optical problems of myopia, aphakia, keratoconus, hyperopia, and astigmatism:

1. Radial keratotomy reduces myopia (nearsightedness) by making multiple small radial incisions in the cornea to approximately 90% of its depth (Fig. 39.19). These incisions allow stretching and flattening of the anterior corneal surface, which corrects the refractive error by reducing corneal curvature and bringing light to a focus closer to or on the retina (Fig. 39.20).

   Radial keratotomy is performed on patients who have occupational requirements for a visual acuity level without the use of glasses or contact lenses, such as certain airline, police, and firefighter positions. The procedure also may be performed for cosmetic reasons. Potential complications include perforations of the cornea, permanent corneal scarring, glaring or variable vision, injury to the lens (causing cataract), and infection. Long-term results are somewhat unpredictable but are improved with microsurgical techniques. This procedure should be limited to patients with healthy eyes. Only low amounts of nearsightedness can be corrected with this procedure.

2. Keratomileusis and keratophakia procedures modify corneal refractivity by using a computerized technique to insert a lathed button of corneal tissue into the cornea. If the patient is the donor (keratomileusis), the anterior lamellae of the cornea are removed, reshaped by cryolathing, and then sutured in place. For keratophakia, the tissue is obtained from another donor and may be preserved.

   The lenticule is cryolathed during the surgical procedure, inserted intralamellarly into the recipient cornea, and sutured into place.

   Keratomileusis and keratophakia require a highly specialized, experienced team and costly equipment—the computer and the cryolathe for shaping the corneal button. With keratophakia, research is ongoing to develop other materials that may be used in place of human donor tissue. Plastic with a very high water content (similar to continuous-wear contact lens material) has been used.

3. Epikeratophakia is performed to correct extreme refractive errors such as aphakia (absence of lens, which induces extreme hyperopia), myopia, or keratoconus (cone-shaped cornea, which causes extreme astigmatism). The recipient corneal epithelium is removed, and a previously cryolathed and preserved donor button of corneal tissue is sutured onto the corneal surface of the recipient.

4. Corneal sculpting (photorefractive keratectomy [PRK]) is performed to reshape the corneal surface or to remove scars or other surface irregularities. The excimer laser is used to reshape the front corneal contour to correct nearsightedness, farsightedness, and astigmatism. The laser beam removes minute amounts of corneal tissue with each pulse wave without burning through or heating the tissue.

5. Laser-assisted in situ keratomileusis (LASIK) is performed to correct myopia (nearsightedness). A combination of excimer laser and keratome is used to remove layers of the cornea. A small flap is raised in the center of the corneal dome (Fig. 39.21). The laser is used to remove microlayers of tissue. The flap of corneal tissue is replaced without the need for suturing (Fig. 39.22).

6. Small incision lenticule extraction (SMILE) was approved by the U.S. Food and Drug Administration (FDA) in 2016 for correction of nearsightedness. The procedure can correct up to −10.00 diopters. The procedure is similar to LASIK but uses a femtosecond (FS) laser to make a tiny flapless incision into the corneal lenticule to reshape the cornea.[7] FS lasers are in the infrared light range and work similar to neodymium:yttrium-aluminum-garnet (Nd:YAG) lasers. The pulse duration is extremely short and precise. Healing requires no stitches and has few side effects.

7. Intrastromal corneal rings can be placed to elevate the border of the cornea, causing the central portion to recede (keratoconus). This implantable device was approved for use in 1998 and consists of two arc-shaped segments made of

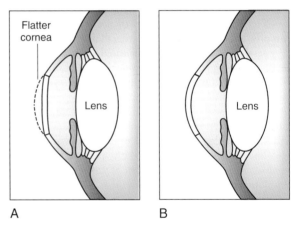

• **Fig. 39.20** Side view of incised corneas. **A,** Radial keratotomy (RK). **B,** Astigmatic keratotomy (AK).

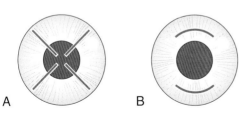

• **Fig. 39.19** Corneal incisions for visual improvement of myopia. **A,** Radial keratotomy (RK). **B,** Astigmatic keratotomy (AK).

• **Fig. 39.21** Keratotome used to raise the corneal flap for laser in situ keratomileusis (LASIK) surgery.

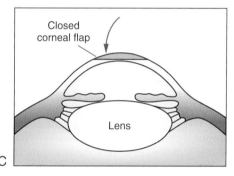

• **Fig. 39.22** Laser in situ keratomileusis (LASIK). **A,** Top layer of cornea is opened like a flap with keratome. **B,** Excimer laser removes thin layers of exposed corneal surface. **C,** Cornea is replaced.

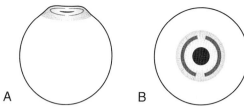

• **Fig. 39.23** Intrastromal corneal rings are used to form a depression in the center of the cornea for correction of myopia. **A,** Intrastromal corneal ring in place. The center of the cornea flattens. **B,** Two arcs form a circle under the edges of the cornea.

polymethylmethacrylate (PMMA) that are implanted in the circumferential stroma of the cornea. It can be removed surgically if vision correction is not satisfactory (Fig. 39.23).

Intraocular Procedures
Iris

Some ophthalmic surgeons subspecialize in anterior segment surgery on the iris and lens or in posterior segment surgery on the vitreous body, retina, and sclera. Both types of surgeries require specialized instrumentation. Most surgeons use the operating microscope for intraocular procedures.

Excision of Iris Prolapse
Prolapse may follow an eye laceration or a surgical procedure on the anterior segment. Fresh prolapses may be reduced mechanically during the surgical procedure or pharmacologically with drugs. Older prolapses should be excised to avoid an intraocular infection.

Glaucoma
Glaucoma is a disease characterized by abnormally increased intraocular fluid pressure; it often involves the iris. If uncontrolled,

glaucoma progresses to atrophy of the optic nerve, hardening of the eyeball, and blindness. The incidence of glaucoma in people older than 40 years increases with each decade. There is a familial predisposition to the disease.

IOP is estimated in one of the following three ways:
1. A Schiøtz tonometer records the depth of indentation of the cornea by a plunger of known weight. The degree of indentation is calibrated on the tonometer to correspond to the IOP. The normal numeric value is 10 to 22 mm Hg. The tonometer can be sterilized for use in the OR for preoperative pressure measurement.
2. An applanation tonometer attached to a biomicroscope (slit lamp) records the force required to flatten a specified area of cornea. This method is considered to be the most accurate. The normal value is 10 to 21 mm Hg.
3. An air-puff device measures the force of a reflected amount of air blown against the cornea.

Patients suspected of having glaucoma undergo additional testing. Tonography continuously measures the rate of aqueous outflow with an electric tonometer. Visual fields detect diminished peripheral vision. Gonioscopy determines the structure of the angle between the iris and the cornea. Two basic types of glaucoma are classified anatomically by the size of this angle: (1) narrow-angle or angle-closure glaucoma and (2) wide-angle or open-angle glaucoma.

If the angle is narrow, the iris may mechanically obstruct the outflow of aqueous humor. This will cause the pressure within the eye to rise and will precipitate an attack of acute glaucoma—an emergency situation that is very painful. Surgical intervention, usually a laser iridotomy, affords relief. It is always necessary to widen the angle for this condition and reduce pressure to avoid damage to the optic nerve. Surgical iridectomy occasionally is necessary.

Wide-angle or open-angle glaucoma is the most common type of glaucoma. It is a chronic type, is often of insidious onset, and may cause permanent visual loss before being detected. The obstruction is not mechanical but is a physiologic lack of ability to filter aqueous. Surgical procedures for this type of disease are performed only if medical and laser therapies are unsuccessful. Laser therapy to the trabecular meshwork (trabeculoplasty) offers an alternative to conventional surgical procedures for some glaucoma patients. One of the following surgical procedures may be preferred:
• Iridectomy (excising a sector of iris) or iridotomy (cutting a small opening in the iris) is performed to deflate the mechanical obstruction, thus increasing drainage by permitting the normal outflow of aqueous from the posterior to the anterior chamber. Another use of iridectomy is to create a new optical

pupillary opening to improve visual acuity for patients with corneal or lens opacity caused by injury or cataract not associated with glaucoma.

- Filtering-type procedures, of which there are many variations, such as trephining, trabeculectomy, or stent placement, create an artificial fistula between the angle of the anterior chamber and the subconjunctival space to bypass the usual blocked outflow channels. Iridectomy is usually performed as part of the procedure to eliminate blockage of the fistula by the underlying iris. The Nd:YAG laser may be used to reopen filtering sites that have scarred closed after previous surgery for glaucoma. The holmium:yttrium aluminum garnet (Ho:YAG) laser may be used to create an opening in the sclera (sclerostomy) to promote filtration.
- Cyclodialysis, cyclodiathermy, and cyclocryotherapy are performed to diminish aqueous secretion by the ciliary body. **Cyclodialysis** involves severing the blood supply of the ciliary body. Cyclodiathermy and cyclocryotherapy use the application of heat or cold, respectively, for the same purpose.

Secondary glaucoma is often a complication of an inflammation such as iritis, which usually responds best to medical treatment. On the other hand, neoplasm, vascular obstruction, trauma, or hemorrhage and other causes of obstruction to aqueous drainage may require surgical intervention. Treatment is directed to the primary cause.

Congenital glaucoma, from an inherent defect in the trabecular meshwork or a systemic disorder, manifests soon after birth.

Cataract

A cataract is an opacification of the crystalline lens, its capsule, or both. The more or less opaque lens does not transmit clear images to the retina. Symptoms are related to the location and configuration of the opacity. The cause may be a known metabolic or systemic disease, toxic material, radiation, trauma, or genetic factors, or the etiologic factors may be unknown. People are more prone to develop degenerative cataracts with advancing age. Although cataracts often develop in both eyes, each cataract tends to mature at a different rate, and only one is removed at a time. Most ophthalmologists perform cataract surgery as an ambulatory surgical procedure.

Cataracts may be classified as one of the following:
- Congenital
- Senile or primary
- Secondary, resulting from local or systemic disease or eye injury

Surgical removal, followed by appropriate optical rehabilitation, is the only treatment. The surgical procedure to be performed is determined by the patient's age and type of cataract. The procedure is selected according to visual requirements, general health, and the potential for rehabilitation. Cataract extraction with implantation of an intraocular lens is the most frequently performed surgical procedure in adults, and the advent of microsurgery has revolutionized this procedure (Fig. 39.24).

Extracapsular Extraction

With extracapsular extraction (ECCE), the lens is delivered through a small incision in the region of the limbus (the junction of the cornea and sclera). The anterior capsule is incised with a cystotome (a miniature hook-shaped knife) or with a **capsulorrhexis** forceps. The nucleus is delivered by manual expression, or it may be aspirated by phacoemulsification. The remaining cortex is extracted by irrigation-aspiration, sparing the posterior capsule, which is left in place. Automated mechanical irrigation-aspiration devices generally are used. Some surgeons prefer a manual technique using a two-way cannula and syringe. The wound is closed with a few sutures.

ECCE with preservation of the posterior capsule has revolutionized the practice of artificial lens implantation. The implant can be placed at the time of cataract extraction. It resides in the posterior chamber behind the iris and rests on the posterior capsule. The implant is therefore positioned in almost the identical location of the lens it replaces.

The physiologic advantage of ECCE, with or without phacoemulsification and/or lens implantation, is protection of the vitreous and retina by the clear posterior lens capsule, which then serves as an anatomic barrier between the posterior and anterior segments of the eye. Occasionally the posterior capsule remains opaque. Nd:YAG laser capsulotomy is performed at a later date to provide an optically clear opening.

The following innovations have enhanced the advantages of ECCE:

1. An operating microscope with coaxial illumination to clearly view the posterior capsule during aspiration.
2. A phacoemulsifier to remove the nucleus through a tiny (3.5 mm or smaller) incision. The smaller wound facilitates healing and causes less distortion of corneal curvatures.
3. An automated irrigation-aspiration system with an electronic sensor to remove all cortex remnants. This minimizes local foreign protein reaction.

Cornea
Cataract
Iris

Ultrasonic probe is used to break up the lens

The cloudy lens is removed

An intraocular lens is inserted

• **Fig. 39.24** Removing the cloudy lens and placing an intraocular lens in its place.

4. An Nd:YAG laser to atomize posterior capsule opacity. The laser achieves a better result than discission/needling, which requires a second surgical intervention. The laser can be used immediately postoperatively, or the procedure can be delayed. The laser can be used under a drop of local anesthetic without requiring an incision and without causing blood loss.

5. An intraocular foldable lens designed to achieve insertion into the posterior chamber through a small incision.

Intracapsular Extraction

Intracapsular extraction (ICCE) is not commonly used unless the natural lens is displaced. Advance planning is necessary on the rare occasions in which it is performed. The entire lens, intact within its capsule, is delivered through a moderate-sized incision made in the region of the limbus. Before delivery, an iridectomy or multiple iridotomies are performed, chiefly to prevent iris prolapse and preserve communication between the anterior and posterior chambers. Depending on the surgeon's preference, the lens is grasped by a forceps, suction device, or cryoextractor.

A miniaturized, sterile disposable cryoextractor facilitates removal of fragile or dislocated cataracts. The cryoprobe freezes onto the surface of the cataract, thus obtaining secure adherence. The freezing technique greatly reduces the inadvertent rupture of the capsule during extraction. The scrub person should have a BSS irrigator available for use in case it is necessary to unfreeze an unintentional attachment of the cryoextractor to the iris or cornea. The wound is closed watertight with multiple sutures, commonly 10-0 nylon.

With ICCE, the visual axis is free of remnants that might proliferate or opacify to obstruct vision. The success rate for regaining vision is high, but the popularity of this procedure has waned. Fluorescein angiography has identified a number of patients who developed cystoid macular edema postoperatively, resulting in marked loss of visual acuity. ICCE may also be followed by retinal detachment.

Linear Extraction

Linear extraction is performed in young adults. In this procedure, a small incision is made through the limbus. The anterior capsule is incised, and the major portion of it is excised with a cystotome. The soft cataract material is irrigated from the anterior chamber.

Phacoemulsification

Although the aspiration technique is commonly used in young people, it was not successful in older adults with senile cataracts until the late 1960s. At that time a sophisticated machine, the phacoemulsifier, was developed to break up (fragment) and remove firm, insoluble lens nuclei. This machine, with components for ultrasonic vibration and irrigation-aspiration, permits extracapsular extraction through a very small incision in the limbus. All functions are controlled by foot pedal.

The handpiece of the phacoemulsifier consists of a disposable, hollow, titanium alloy needle surrounded by a silicone sleeve. The needle is inserted into the anterior chamber after removal of the anterior capsule with a cystotome. The activated needle breaks up the lens with ultrasonic vibrations; the linear motion of the ultrasonic vibrations is created by electrical impulses. This process generates heat. A cooling pump circulates coolant, either fluid or air, through the power cord.

While the lens is thus emulsified, a constant flow of BSS irrigating solution through the sleeve prevents heat buildup. The irrigation-aspiration flow is automatically regulated to maintain anterior chamber depth. The aspirator removes the fragments. After the cortex (material surrounding the lens nucleus) is removed by irrigation-aspiration, the posterior capsule may be polished with an instrument to remove any residual cortex. The posterior capsule is left intact unless an opacity remains, in which case it may be incised during the initial surgical procedure or at a future time. The limbal incision can be closed with one stitch. Alternative methods do not require any suturing.

Appropriate checks should be made before use of the handpiece, and the integrity of the vacuum and irrigating systems must be confirmed. The handpiece should be disassembled for cleaning and sterilization and then reassembled on the sterile field before use. The handpiece can be steam-sterilized as a single unit. Care is taken to prevent biomaterials from being aspirated into the handpiece. Cleaning should be meticulous, and instrumentation must be sterilized after patient use.

In computerized machines, the phacoemulsification and aspiration settings are preset. To avoid error, the scrub person and circulating nurse work closely with the surgeon to monitor the various functions of the machine in use. They should also observe the transparent tubes for the flow of aspirate. Aspirated fluid is contaminated and is discarded postoperatively in the same manner as all blood or body fluid.

Phacoemulsification has the following advantages:
- It dramatically shortens convalescence time. The patient usually returns to full activity in 1 or 2 days.
- It uses a small incision and minimal sutures, which promotes healing.
- It retains the posterior capsule of the lens to preserve a more physiologically normal condition. The occurrence of post–lens extraction edema and retinal detachment is thereby diminished.
- The posterior capsule supports an implanted IOL. Postoperative astigmatism is minimized.[8]

Phacoemulsification also has the following disadvantages:
- It is not suitable for all patients. Contraindications are corneal disease, a dislocated lens, a shallow anterior chamber, difficult-to-dilate pupils, and completely hard, stonelike cataracts.
- It requires special techniques that, if not thoroughly mastered, may precipitate surgical complications such as temporary or permanent corneal damage (opacification), prolapse of the lens into the vitreous, and vitreous loss.
- It may injure the cells because of the necessary substantial amount of anterior chamber irrigation. Corneal cells are very sensitive to manipulation and can respond by loss of function.
- It requires meticulous technical monitoring of the machine. The usual precautions for the use of electrical equipment are also observed.

Clear Corneal Cataract Procedure

Foldable IOLs and topical anesthetic techniques have been integral with the use of "no stitch" corneal incisions. Patient selection includes the ability to fixate vision on a focal point and cooperate with commands from the surgeon. Tetracaine intraocular drops are used preoperatively and intraoperatively. Additional intraoperative anesthetics include injectable lidocaine without preservatives for infusion into the anterior chamber.

Rehabilitation After Cataract Extraction

Rehabilitation after cataract extraction consists of substitution for the missing part, the lens, so the optical system can function to focus incoming light on the retina. Patients with no optical substitute see only blurred objects of large size. Rehabilitation may be accomplished by spectacles (glasses), contact lenses, or IOL implantation.

Spectacle correction of aphakia, the absence of the lens, provides focusing of light. The spectacle lens is approximately 2 cm in front of the original lens and magnifies images so they are approximately 35% larger than those the patient saw before development and extraction of the cataract. This magnification requires considerable readjustment to judge distances. In addition, peripheral areas are distorted. The spectacle type of replacement is intolerable in patients who have good vision in the unaffected eye because an attempt to fuse the dissimilar images of the two eyes causes double vision.

A contact lens often is used to replace the optical deficiency caused by cataract extraction. This lens rests on the cornea only 2 to 3 mm from the original lens and thus causes only 7% magnification and provides a full, undistorted field of vision. It is difficult for some older adults to handle and care for contact lenses because of a lack of manual dexterity, arthritic hand and finger joints, or visual defects in the opposite eye. For these patients, an implanted IOL is a feasible and popular alternative.

Implantation of Intraocular Lens

IOL implantation is a microsurgical procedure in which an IOL is implanted in almost the identical position of the original lens and therefore does not change the size of the retinal image. Spatial displacement as seen by the aphakic eye and narrowing and distortion of the visual field are eliminated, thereby producing early visual rehabilitation. With spatial displacement, orientation in space is changed—objects are not where they appear to be.

An IOL is intended to remain in situ permanently. The implant is usually inserted through the same incision used to remove the defective, natural lens; this is called *primary insertion*. Some surgeons prefer to implant the lens at a later time; this is referred to as *secondary insertion*. The type of IOL used is contingent on the type of cataract extraction the surgeon chooses. Anterior chamber lenses are inserted in conjunction with ICCE or as secondary implants. Posterior chamber lenses are used after ECCE.

The prescription of the implanted lens (refractive power) involves complex preoperative calculations based on the patient's corneal curvature as determined by keratometer readings, anterior chamber depth, and eyeball axial length. Ultrasonography is helpful in making these determinations preoperatively. The information obtained is fed into a computer that automatically calculates the appropriate refractive power of the IOL.

Numerous IOLs of different shapes and sizes are available. Fig. 39.25 depicts a common type of implantable lens. The optical portion of a hard lens is made of an inert plastic (PMMA), with or without an ultraviolet blocker, that has been polished to a microscopic smoothness. Flexible and foldable lenses are made of silicone elastomer and acrylic resin.

The fixation portion has springlike supports or loops, called haptics, made of plastic (usually polypropylene). Some lenses are secured with polypropylene sutures. Lenses differ in design and method of fixation, and they can be classified according to placement or method of fixation.

Types of Intraocular Lenses

Fixed focus lens: A monofocal lens that corrects vision for near or far vision. Glasses may still be required.

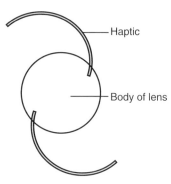

• **Fig. 39.25** Intraocular lens.

Accommodating lens: A multifocal lens that corrects near and far vision according to the patient's needs.
Toric lens: Corrects astigmatism and distance vision.
Light Adjustable Lens (LAL): Made of photosensitive material to allow UV light to enter the eye. After surgery, the patient undergoes two to four 90-second laser treatments. Unpolymerized macromers are photopolymerized to change the power and incoming light to enhance the patient's vision.

Anterior Chamber (Angle Fixation)

An anterior chamber lens consists of a band of plastic long enough to traverse the anterior chamber from one angle to the other. The optical portion is centrally located in the anterior chamber, in front of the pupil and iris. The pupil remains mobile because iris adhesions are not required for fixation. Although anterior chamber lenses are sometimes inserted primarily, they are popular lenses for secondary insertion.

Posterior Chamber (Capsular or Ciliary Body Fixation)

Posterior chamber lenses are placed behind the iris and pupil, where the patient's own lens used to be. Placement of the IOL in the most normal physiologic position results in stabilization of the iris; less irritation of the uveal tract; a reduced tendency for iritis, secondary glaucoma, and cystoid macular edema; and stabilization of the optics. Posterior lenses permit safe dilation of the pupil if necessary to examine or treat posterior structures of the eye, such as the retina.

With capsular fixation, the lower loop of the haptic is inserted into a pocket or capsule created during extraction of the cataract. The lens does not touch the iris, and the pupil is free to move. With ciliary fixation, the haptics are placed between the iris and the posterior capsule. They rest on the corona (inner rim) of the ciliary body.

Pros and Cons of Intraocular Lens Implantation

The final decision to implant an artificial lens rests with the surgeon, who should exercise good judgment to avoid serious complications.

Indications for implantation include the following:
- Older adult patients with disabling bilateral cataracts and others who cannot adapt to contact lenses
- Patients with occupations having specific visual requirements (e.g., airplane pilots) or a difficult working environment (e.g., ranchers in a dusty area)
- Children with a traumatic cataract, thus preventing amblyopia

Contraindications for implantation include the following:

- Impossibility for follow-up evaluation to observe patient for late complications
- Ocular conditions such as poorly controlled glaucoma or previous retinal detachment
- Diabetic proliferative retinopathy
- Poor result in previous implant
- Patient anxiety in regard to the procedure
- Young patients with congenital cataracts
- Endothelial corneal dystrophy
- Cataracts associated with recurrent iritis

Advantages to IOL implantation include the following:

- Superior spatial orientation and binocular vision
- Permanency of device unless complications develop
- Additional option for post–cataract extraction refractive correction
- Unrestricted pupillary dilation if necessary

Complications with IOL implantation include the following:

- Corneal damage or latent edema
- Prolonged inflammation such as iritis or vitritis
- Cystoid macular edema
- Secondary cataract (i.e., opacification of the anterior vitreous) from recurrent iritis
- Corneal opacity (rare with posterior implants)
- Dislocation or malposition of the lens, which can damage the cornea (fortunately rare)

The type of approach used to repair a dislocation depends on the amount of dislocation. With the anterior approach, an anterior vitrectomy is performed to remove the vitreous in front of the lens, followed by removal or repositioning of the lens. With the posterior approach, the vitrector is used to remove the lens and/or vitreous through the pars plana. The IOL can be repositioned or removed.

Retina

Defects in the continuity of the retina can occur after accidental or surgical trauma or as a result of certain degenerative diseases. The dense network of capillary vessels in the retina makes the eyes vulnerable to microvascular disease. Retinopathy is a noninflammatory degenerative disease of the retina.

Retinal changes can occur in patients with diabetes (i.e., diabetic retinopathy). Diabetes can affect every part of the eye, causing lens changes (cataract), palsied extraocular muscles, glaucoma, or corneal problems. A person who has had diabetes for more than 15 years has a significant likelihood of having some form of retinopathy, which generally occurs bilaterally. The severity of retinopathy may differ from one eye to the other. Retinopathy is classified as one of the following:

- *Background or nonproliferative:* With this type of retinopathy, disease is confined to the retinal surface. Bulges or microaneurysms form in retinal capillary walls, eventually permitting leakage and the deposition of exudates. Intraretinal hemorrhages occur and are reabsorbed. Progressive changes in capillary membranes lead to the blockage of capillaries, resulting in retinal ischemia. Deterioration then progresses to the proliferative stage.
- *Proliferative:* In the proliferative stage, new blood vessels emerge from the retina and form in the surrounding tissues in an effort to relieve retinal anoxia (i.e., neovascularization). These fragile vessels may rupture spontaneously, producing hemorrhage into the retina and/or vitreous humor. The eventual result may be partial or complete blindness. Panretinal photocoagulation (PRP) is one method of eliminating abnormal vascularization. PRP consists of the application of hundreds of laser burns to the peripheral retinal tissue to partially destroy it, thereby reducing the retinal metabolic need for oxygen. After neovascularization has occurred, laser therapy is less effective in delaying or stopping the destructive process. Therefore early diagnosis and treatment are crucial. In an effort to prevent the formation of new vessels, lasers are used to cauterize minute hypoxic areas of tissue before damage occurs.

A laser is used for cauterizing bleeding vessels, for diabetic retinopathy, and for other retinopathies such as central serous retinopathy with swelling of the macula, angiomas and hemangiomas, aneurysms, and small tumors. Laser is absorbed selectively by three pigments in the retina: macular xanthophyll, hemoglobin in the retinal and subretinal blood vessels, and melanin in the retinal pigment epithelium. Laser therapy is not effective in correcting severe retinal damage or detachment.

Repair of Detached Retina

The retina can become separated from its surrounding nourishing layer, the choroid (Fig. 39.26). This detachment may occur in any region of the retina. Primary retinal detachment is characterized by a hole in the retina.

Secondary detachment may result when blood, fluid, or a tumor gets behind and displaces the retina; this type of detachment is not necessarily accompanied by a hole. The seepage of vitreous fluid into the potential space between the retina and the choroid causes the retina to become detached, and a serious visual disturbance results such as full or partial blindness.

Enucleation is usually indicated for tumor-caused detachment.

Reattachment is effected only by surgical intervention. The retinal defect is sealed off, and often the subretinal fluid is drained. The specific procedure used to achieve retinal reattachment is determined by the type and location of the detachment. All or some of the following procedures may be used in combination:

- *Diathermy:* The traditional procedure involves diathermy coagulation to the area of the sclera overlying the region of the retinal defect. The resultant localized inflammation acts to seal off the break. Coagulation is delivered by a specialized short-wave diathermy unit.

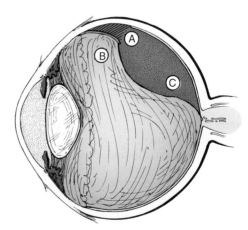

• **Fig. 39.26** Detached retina. **A,** Retinal break. **B,** Vitreous. **C,** Fluid or blood behind the retina. (From Ryan SJ, Wilkinson C, Schachat A, et al, editors: *Retina,* ed 4, vol 3, St. Louis, 2006, Mosby.)

- *Cryosurgery:* Some surgeons prefer cryosurgery because of the type of adhesion obtained. The therapeutic applications of cryosurgery are basically similar to those of diathermy, and the tissue reactions superficially resemble each other. Cryosurgery is often used for anterior tears.
- *Scleral buckling:* Internal elevation of the sclera may be increased by the scleral buckling procedure. This technique involves implantation of a wedge of silicone episclerally or intrasclerally. An encircling band of silicone may be used to keep constant external pressure on the buckle. Fig. 39.27 depicts the result of this procedure.
- *Intraocular gas tamponade:* Injection of room air or absorbable inert gas into the vitreous cavity can be used to create an intraocular tamponade. Room air absorbs after 5 days. Inert gases such as short-acting sulfahexafluoride (SF6), intermediate-acting perfluoroethane (C2F6), or long-acting perfluorooctane (C3F8) are sometimes used to approximate the retina to the choroid (i.e., flatten the retina against the choroid).

With **pneumoretinopexy**, the patient remains in a seated position for a superior tear or prone for a tear near the macula. This position is maintained for several weeks postoperatively so the gas bubble can successfully rise to close the retinal hole. The position and length of time in that position are determined by the ophthalmologist according to each patient's need. Pneumoretinopexy is less invasive than scleral buckling for securing a retinal detachment (Fig. 39.28).

- *Intraocular fluid tamponade:* Silicone oil has been approved by the FDA for use as a vitreous substitute in securing a retinal detachment that cannot be corrected through conventional surgical intervention.[9] Silicone oil is used for long-term intraocular tamponade. It is removed by the ophthalmologist several months postoperatively.

  Patients with proliferative vitreoretinopathy with inferior breaks benefit from a blended silicone solution that is heavier than the vitreous. A blend of perfluorohexyloctane and silicone (Densiron) has been shown to effect a repair to the detached lower retina in 90% of patients in clinical trials. The Densiron is removed between 12 and 14 weeks postoperatively.

- *Laser therapy:* Laser therapy can be used to secure the retina, except in severe detachment. A laser is often used to secure small posterior tears. (See the following discussion of laser therapy.)

Glaucoma and infection are potential postoperative complications of retinal reattachment. Glaucoma may be caused by congestion of the uvea by the buckle, increased IOP, or movement of injected gas from the desired site, causing blockage of outflow channels of aqueous humor. Infection is evident by swelling, purulent drainage, and a loss of optical clarity.

Laser Therapy

The laser delivery system uses the binocular microscope of the slit lamp, thus providing stereopsis and greater magnification. The nature of the laser beam permits extremely rapid delivery of radiant energy to produce a sharply defined burn. The small lesion it produces can be placed close to the macula.

Exposure can be as brief as 1/100 second and the treated area as small as 50 μm (less than 2/1000 inch) in diameter. Because of this short exposure time, immobilization of the eye is unnecessary unless the treated area is close to the macula, the central region of

Circumferential Silastic scleral buckle

• **Fig. 39.27** Compressive effects of scleral buckle. (From Ryan SJ, Wilkinson C, Schachat A, et al, editors: *Retina,* ed 4, vol 3, St. Louis, 2006, Mosby.)

the retina with the clearest visual acuity. Accidental injury of the macula may result in a loss of central vision. Pupillary dilation is essential to avoid macular burn.

The argon laser is effective in treating retinal holes or tears and diabetic retinopathy. The krypton laser can be used to treat lesions closer to the macula and to treat retinal bleeding because of its poor absorption of the yellow pigment of the retina. The krypton spectrum is poorly absorbed by the red pigment of hemoglobin. Therefore it may be used effectively to treat retinal bleeding in the presence of blood in the vitreous humor. Under these circumstances the argon blue laser is ineffective because of absorption by even a small amount of blood.

Photocoagulation

A retinal hole not surrounded by any detachment may be prophylactically sealed by xenon or laser photocoagulation. These therapeutic modalities, which are usually performed in an ophthalmic treatment area rather than the OR, were the outgrowth of traumatic retinal burns caused by watching an eclipse of the sun.

The xenon arc photocoagulator uses an intense source of multiwavelength light furnished by a xenon tube. The light is optically focused and concentrated into a delivering device that is basically an indirect ophthalmoscope. The latter can be used both to view the area to be treated and to aim the light beam. The light may be directed to any of the pigmented (light-absorbing) layers of the eye, such as the iris or retina. These darker layers readily absorb the white light of the xenon tube. The optical system of the eye is used in the process of focusing the light beam on the desired area.

The power setting and exposure time are completely controlled by the operating ophthalmologist. The pupil of the eye under therapy is dilated to give maximum visibility to the surgeon. The eye is immobilized by local anesthesia to prevent undesired movement, which could result in a burn to an area other than the one desired. Anesthesia also prevents pain from the intensity of the heat. Vitreous shrinkage that possibly leads to an inoperable detachment can be a complication.

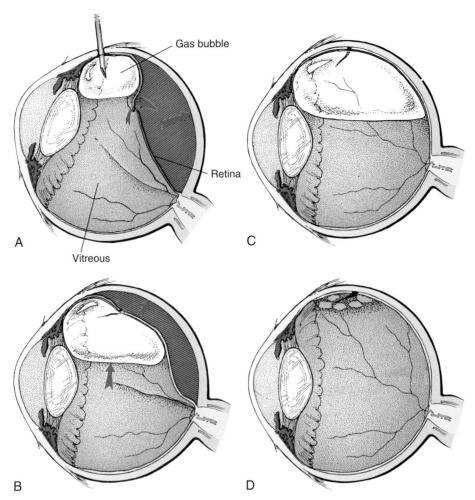

Gas bubble

Retina

Vitreous

A

B

C

D

• **Fig. 39.28** Pneumoretinopexy. **A,** Introduction of gas bubble. **B,** Gas bubble compresses retina. **C,** Tamponade formed by gas bubble. **D,** Gas bubble eventually absorbs. (From Ryan SJ, Wilkinson C, Schachat A, et al, editors: *Retina,* ed 4, vol 3, St. Louis, 2006, Mosby.)

Vitrectomy

Vitrectomy is the deliberate removal of a portion of the vitreous humor, also called vitreous body, that fills the space between the lens and the retina. Therapeutically it is performed for vitreal opacities, vitreal hemorrhage, and certain types of retinal damage or detachment. In addition to other causes, endophthalmitis (i.e., inflammation of the internal tissues of the eyeball) and the presence of an intraocular foreign body may result in vitreal opacity. In general, the candidates for vitrectomy have substantially impaired vision and complicated conditions preoperatively.

Whereas aqueous fluid is a clear liquid, vitreous is normally a transparent, gelatinous, viscid material containing fibrils. The vitreous helps give shape to the eyeball and serves a refractive function. It permits light rays to pass through it to the retina after the rays have traversed the lens. Diagnostically, the removal of a small amount of vitreous provides a sample for microbiologic study in suspected endophthalmitis. The procedure also provides tissue for biopsy to establish the diagnosis of intraocular tumors.

Alterations in the vitreous can have serious consequences. The loss of vitreous during surgical procedures is a dreaded complication, particularly of cataract extraction. Subsequent to retinal hemorrhage, which is common in patients with diabetes, bands of scar tissue may opacify the vitreous as well as adhere to the retina

near the original bleeding vessel. Traction on the retina by these bands or further cicatrization (scarring) can lead to retinal tears or detachment. A persistent hemorrhage, lasting more than 1 year, is permanent. It will not absorb spontaneously.

For years the vitreous was considered an inaccessible, inoperable area. Research and the advent of microsurgery have changed this belief. A loss of vitreous from the posterior segment during a cataract procedure is relatively innocuous if the anterior segment is cleared of vitreous. Thus no residual strands are present to cause traction effects or block visual function. In addition, the eye tolerates subtotal vitreal excision in the posterior segment if the vitreous body is proportionately replaced with BSS.

Vitrectomy is a microsurgical procedure that lasts 1 to 3 hours and requires a skilled retinal surgeon. It is performed using a vitreotome (vitrector). These devices, which incorporate a micromotor, terminate in a needlelike tube that contains a cutting mechanism for severing abnormal adhesions and cutting obstructive tissue into small pieces. In addition, the vitreotome has auxiliary connections for the aspiration of vitreous, debris, or blood from the posterior segment.

Vitreous is replaced with BSS via a separate infusion cannula to maintain adequate IOP. A fiberoptic light source or pic is inserted into the vitreous to illuminate the posterior portion of the globe.

Various vitrectomy systems are available, but all have cutting, suction, and illumination systems. The machine may have an automatic or hydraulic pole for rapidly regulating the height of the BSS bottle.

The scrub person and circulating nurse should assemble and check equipment before the surgical procedure begins. The vitreotome handpiece is attached to sterile tubing, which is connected to a power console. One person activates the various switches while the other tests the suction vacuum and cutting function. Suction is tested at maximum pressure. The tip is placed in sterile saline and activated until fluid reaches the collection bottle. The pressure is then lowered to the surgeon's preference.

To assess cutting, the switch is activated and the tip is checked visibly and audibly for movement. The infusion catheter is primed with a solution of the surgeon's choice to remove air bubbles that could disturb the view in the posterior segment. The manufacturer's manual should be consulted.

A local anesthetic is administered unless the patient's condition necessitates a general anesthetic. There are two approaches to the vitreous body, as follows:

1. Through the posterior segment via the pars plana (i.e., the anterior attachment of the retina). Because the pars plana has no visual function, entry here is relatively atraumatic and poses minimal risk for retinal detachment. The anterior segment remains intact, and IOP is maintained. This approach is used to incise opacified vitreous, old hemorrhage, or bands of scar tissue, thereby giving a clear view of the retina and restoring visual function.
2. Through the anterior segment via incision at the limbus (i.e., junction of the cornea and sclera). A small opening is made, and the tip of the vitrector is introduced. The vitreous is exposed through the pupillary opening. This approach is used to remove vitreous inadvertently displaced into the anterior chamber during cataract removal to avoid postoperative complications. The vitreous volume is replaced with BSS. Anterior vitrectomy also is used to correct retinal traction in retinopathy in premature infants (retrolental fibroplasia).

Vitrectomy is intricate and requires special equipment. The surgeon may request a bipolar cautery with a Charles clip attachment for actively bleeding intraocular vessels. A bipolar pencil or "eraser" may be used intraocularly. A handheld or "sew-on" contact lens placed onto the cornea enhances the view of the posterior chamber. A metal ring is sewn into place at two points around the limbus, encircling the cornea. Viscous material is placed on the cornea, and the lens of choice is placed down in the ring. Occasionally, a lensectomy is performed during vitrectomy to facilitate the view of the posterior segment.

After the removal of vitreous, before wound closure, and with the retina in clear view, the retina is inspected for defects such as holes or vascular abnormalities. If these are found, treatment is applied by means of endocryotherapy, a freezing application delivered by intraocular probe or a laser delivered by an intraocular device. These maneuvers may be accompanied by the injection of air or inert gas to push the retina into physiologic position.

Postoperatively, patients may experience considerable pain that requires medication, ice packs, and steroid eyedrops for treatment of inflammation. After vitrectomy, patients will experience aphakia if the lens was removed for visualization of the posterior segment, and they will eventually need optical correction such as that needed after cataract extraction. Vitrectomy can significantly improve vision.

Complications of vitrectomy include iatrogenic retinal damage, vitreous hemorrhage, or cataract formation from damage to the lens. A secondary surgical procedure may be required to repair the retina (e.g., a scleral buckling procedure or intraocular tamponade). No present treatment for retinopathy is free of danger. To save vision, some tissue is destroyed or sacrificed.

Eye Injuries

Various forms and degrees of trauma may occur as a result of injury. All types of injuries require immediate appraisal by an ophthalmologist.[10] A delay in treating even minor injuries may result in a temporary or permanent loss of vision. Complications include hemorrhage, infection, iritis or tears of the iris, retinal tears or detachment, macular edema, and secondary cataract.

Treatment may be immediate or secondary if a delay is necessary because of life-threatening injuries. Improved surgical management, such as vitrectomy and microsurgery, has reduced the loss of vision in severely injured eyes. An optimum result is especially crucial in patients with bilateral eye injuries. If possible, patients with eye injuries should be kept in the supine position until seen by an ophthalmologist.

Evaluation of the injury may necessitate sedating or anesthetizing the patient to prevent further damage at examination. Pressure to the eye must be avoided because bone fragments may be displaced or the globe contents emptied.

Injuries may be simple and involve only the external layers, or they may be compound and include the inner structures. They may be nonpenetrating (usually caused by a blunt object) or penetrating (caused by a sharp object). The more structures involved, the more difficult it is to salvage the eye.

Treatment is determined by the type or combination of injuries and aims to do the following:

- Promote healing and prevent anatomic distortion by reparative techniques
- Preserve and/or restore maximum vision
- Control pain by medication
- Prevent infection and inflammation through the administration of antibiotics and steroids

Nonpenetrating Injuries
Burns

Burns may be caused by ultraviolet radiation, such as sunlamps or sunlight, or by an electric flash. These types of burns are basically self-limited and are rarely surgical. A chemical burn constitutes an emergency. The initial treatment consists of flooding the cornea with water. Alkali burns may be further neutralized by prompt irrigation of the epithelium-denuded cornea with ethylenediaminetetraacetic acid (EDTA). This is especially important if discrete particles of alkali are superficially embedded within tissue. EDTA deactivates an enzyme (collagenase) and neutralizes soluble alkali such as sodium hydroxide (lye).

Severe burns may be treated with specific amino acids, EDTA, or acetylcysteine (Mucomyst) to inhibit the continued destruction of the cornea by collagenase; however, these burns often progress to corneal opacity and blindness.

Contusions of the Globe

Contusions of the globe may or may not require surgical treatment. If hemorrhage is present, treatment consists of bed rest and antiglaucoma therapy to control IOP. It is not unusual for a secondary hemorrhage to occur on the third or fourth day after injury.

If IOP remains high, blood staining of the cornea and damage to the optic nerve may result. It is then sometimes necessary to perform a paracentesis, in which an incision is made into the anterior chamber to drain the blood. If an organized clot is found, judicious irrigation may supplement the incision.

Penetrating Injuries

Lacerations of the globe may occur with or without a retained foreign body and with or without prolapse of the ocular contents. In injuries to the globe, an ophthalmic surgeon should repair both the eye wound and the tissues adjacent to the eye.

With a penetrating injury there is the possibility of an eventual sympathetic ophthalmia—an inflammation of the uninjured eye. Antitetanus therapy should be included in the treatment of these injuries.

Vitrectomy and lensectomy have rendered salvageable some massive injuries that formerly were inoperable. Such injuries include extensive lacerations with cataract formation, vitreous hemorrhage, and retinal damage.

Without a Foreign Body

Eyelid Laceration

Lacerations are repaired according to anatomic principles. Plastic repair involves approximation of the anatomic layers. Penetrating wounds, such as animal bites, are debrided. If the laceration includes the lacrimal canaliculus (duct for the passage of tears), special probes are used to identify the proximal portions for rejoining. Lacerations of the lacrimal canaliculus may be repaired by suturing over one of two types of stents.

The Quickert-Dryden tubing consists of a length of flexible silicone with a malleable metal lacrimal probe swaged onto each end. One end of the probe is inserted through the upper lid canaliculus, and the other end is inserted into the lower lid canaliculus. Both ends exit via the tear sac and nasolacrimal canal into the nose. The lacerated canaliculus is then sutured over the tubing, which is removed after healing takes place. Some surgeons prefer the rigid Veirs stainless steel rod, which is inserted into the lacerated canaliculus. A suture swaged to one end permits withdrawal of the rod after healing.

Conjunctival Laceration

Conjunctival laceration is usually debrided and, unless large, is permitted to heal without suturing. If the laceration is large and there is a loss of conjunctival tissue, sutures or rotating flaps of conjunctiva may be necessary for repair.

Corneal and Scleral Lacerations

A small corneal laceration may be covered with a protective soft contact lens to seal it and hold the edges together. A larger wound requires accurate appositional sutures that are best placed using the operating microscope. The microscope is especially useful for irregular, complicated, or multiple tears.

Some irregular corneal lacerations not easily closed by direct suturing may be closed and the leak stopped by the application of cyanoacrylate glue. A soft contact lens is usually placed as a bandage over the freshly glued cornea. A conjunctival flap can be placed to achieve a similar seal, but it is used less frequently.

A large laceration may require a penetrating keratoplasty as an emergency procedure to ensure the integrity of the eye.

Adequate exploration, particularly of a scleral wound, is necessary to both determine the extent of injury and ensure uncovering of the entire wound for repair. In instances of vitreous fluid presentation or loss, it is preferable to remove the fluid from the wound and the anterior chamber with the vitreotome before proceeding with repair. This is performed to prevent undesirable vitreous adhesions from developing postoperatively.

Posterior Rupture of the Globe

Rupture of the globe usually involves the herniation of retinal and uveal tissue into the orbit. Although such injuries are self-healing, the eye is irreparably damaged. This injury usually results in enucleation. Avulsion (tearing) of the optic nerve produces permanent blindness even though the rest of the globe may be intact.

With a Foreign Body

Extraocular injuries are usually not extensive. An intraocular foreign object is removed very gently under sterile conditions to avoid secondary infection and further trauma. A corneal foreign body is removed with a sharp probe (spud), and the surrounding rust ring is removed with a rotating burr. The type, size, and position of other intraocular foreign bodies should be determined accurately before removal. Localization is accomplished by the following:

- Direct vision with an ophthalmoscope
- Computed tomography scan
- Berman locator, a small but extremely sensitive version of a metal detector, which may indicate the exact location of a ferrous metallic foreign body
- X-ray study, using a contact lens containing radiopaque landmarks (Sweet localizer)

Fragments of ferrous metals often can be retrieved by using the attraction of a strong electromagnet. In some cases these foreign bodies can be withdrawn along the path of entry. Nonmagnetic foreign objects present a more serious problem. Often they are secured only by passing a delicate forceps into the globe. Such instrumentation is combined with a partial vitrectomy, thus obtaining satisfactory results.

In summary, traumatic injuries may introduce infection or produce a severe inflammatory reaction to a greater degree than do elective surgical procedures. Proper early treatment is indicated to save vision. Early intervention, before scar formation, may be necessary in some patients.

Ophthalmic Lasers

The use of an ophthalmic laser is often a safe alternative to conventional surgery for ablation of a pathologic condition. The color and wavelength of each laser determine which part of the eye it can best treat. Specific wavelengths destroy disease in tissues whose pigments are capable of discriminating absorption of that wavelength. Conversely, the selected wavelength should be only minimally absorbed by the vital adjacent tissues to be preserved. The ophthalmologist controls the power, intensity, and direction of the laser beam. The beam precisely cauterizes tissue and blood vessels, preventing bleeding. Each laser has selective uses:

- *Blue-green argon:* For a retinal detachment, tear, or hole; diabetic retinopathy; macular neovascular lesions; laser trabeculoplasty, to lower IOP and facilitate aqueous outflow in select patients with open-angle glaucoma; iridotomy, in place of iridectomy by incision; and to create a small opening in the iris that allows aqueous to enter the anterior chamber (angle-closure glaucoma). The use of this laser may reduce the threat of endophthalmitis, a serious postoperative complication.

Adherence of the iris to laser treatment sites (synechiae) is a complication of laser trabeculoplasty. A portable laser is available for intraoperative use. It permits surgeons to work inside rather than through the eye while the patient is under general anesthesia.

- *Red-yellow krypton:* For blood vessel aberrations of the choroid (common to senile macular disease) in which abnormal vessels damage adjacent nerve tissue; for lesions in the perimacular region (the laser beam passes through cloudy vitreous hemorrhage); and for retinal vascular diseases, such as proliferative diabetic retinopathy and retinal detachment.
- *Invisible pulsed Nd:YAG:* For preoperative anterior capsulotomy before extracapsular cataract extraction; posterior capsulotomy (**discission**) after extracapsular cataract extraction to make an opening in an opaque capsule and thus permit light to reach the retina; and lysis or severing of strands of vitreous and/or fibrous bands in the posterior segment that cause cystoid macular edema.

  Cloudy areas of tissue interfering with vision are painlessly pushed aside, resulting in immediate improvement in sight. Rather than producing the effect by absorption, energy is released almost entirely at the point of focus. Problems in both anterior and posterior parts of the eye are treatable (e.g., with optical iridectomy and photocoagulation of retinal disorders). Unlike with the visible light lasers, the Nd:YAG laser does not require the target tissue to be pigmented for effectiveness.
- *Visible excimer:* Argon-fluoride in the ultraviolet range. Used for shaping the cornea, as in lamellar keratectomy, to correct refractive disorders.
- *Invisible Ho:YAG:* For sclerostomy to create an opening in the sclera that promotes filtration for glaucoma. It also can be used for corneal sculpting.

  The following are advantages of laser therapy:
- Possibility of infection is minimal. Treatment is noninvasive and sterile, which is an advantage to diabetic and susceptible patients.
- Pain is minimal. Only a topical anesthetic is required unless many retinal areas are treated with a high-energy laser.
- It is performed as an ambulatory procedure.
- The appropriate amount of energy is concentrated in a very small area.
- The light is highly flexible, which seems to do little damage to the clear medium it traverses.
- The laser light is selectively absorbed. Ideally, only desired tissue is affected.
- It is useful in a poor-risk surgical patient or one who has had a previous unsuccessful surgical procedure.

ⓔ EVOLVE WEBSITE

http://evolve.elsevier.com/Hornacky/BerryKohn/

- Historical Perspective
- Tips for the Scrub Person and Circulating Nurse
- Student Interactive Questions
- Glossary

References

1. Shokri T, Lighthall J: periorbital rejuvenation, *Oper Tech Otolayngol Head Neck Surg* 29(4):243–251, 2018.
2. Beigi B, Degoumois A, Ogbuehi KC, et al.: Lower eyelid excursion: a functional and cosmetically relevant parameter in the treatment of lower eyelid retraction, *J Plast Reconstr Aesthet Surg* 72(2):310–316, 2018.
3. Reinheimer W: Techniques of enucleation and evisceration, *Oper Tech Otolayngol Head Neck Surg* 29(4):213–217, 2018.
4. National Eye Institute: www.nei.nih.gov. Accessed June 17, 2023.
5. Gimes I, Pintor A, DaSilva Sardinha M, et al.: Cold storage media versus Optisol-GS in the preservation of corneal quality for keratoplasty: a systemic review, *Appl Sci* 12:7079, 2022.
6. Eye Bank Association of America: www.restoresight.org. Accessed June 17, 2023.
7. Reinstein D, Cays G, Archer T, et al.: Inferior pseudo-hinge fulcrum technique and intraoperative complications of laser in situ keratomileusis retreatment after small-incision lenticule extraction, *J Cataract Refract Surg* 44(11):1355–1362, 2018.
8. Foster G, Ayers B, Fram N, et al.: Phacoemulsification of posterior polar cataracts, *J Cataract Refract Surg* 45(2):228–235, 2019.
9. Caporossi T, Franco F, Finocchio L, et al.: Densiron 68 heavy silicone oil in the management of inferior retinal detachment recurrence: analysis on functional and anatomical outcomes and complications, *Int J Ophthalmol* 12(4):615–620, 2019.
10. Heng LZ, Hamilton R: Ocular emergencies, *Medicine* 46(12):754–759, 2018.

Bibliography

Chansangpetch S, Larr K, Perez C, et al.: Efficacy of cataract surgery with trabecular micro bypass stent implantation in combined-mechanism angle closure glaucoma patients, *Am J Ophthalmol* 195:191–198, 2018.

40

Plastic and Reconstructive Surgery

CHAPTER OUTLINE

Special Features of Plastic and Reconstructive Surgery, 847

Skin and Tissue Grafting, 850

Head and Neck Plastic and Reconstructive Procedures, 858

Plastic and Reconstructive Procedures of Other Body Areas, 861

Burns, 867

CHAPTER OBJECTIVES

After studying this chapter, the learner will be able to:

- Identify pertinent anatomy of the integumentary system.
- List four primary reasons for plastic surgery.
- Differentiate autografts, allografts, and xenografts.

- Describe the techniques of skin and tissue grafting.
- Discuss the importance of fluid balance in the burn patient.

KEY TERMS AND DEFINITIONS

Aesthetic Pleasing visual form.
Composite graft Tissue graft composed of multiple tissue types. A composite graft can have skin, muscle, bone, and blood vessels in combination.
Debridement Removal of dead tissue from wound edges to reveal vital tissue.
Dermatome Instrument for graft procurement. Can be mechanized or freehand knife style.
Dorsal space The back of the hand.
Eschar Tissue layer that forms over a burn site.
Expander A silicone sac placed beneath the skin and gradually expanded to increase the surface area of the skin to cover a defect.
Flap A multilayer tissue segment used as a surface cover. Can remain attached to a vascularized pedicle or can be a separate segment anastomosed to a new vascular attachment.

Full-thickness skin graft (FTSG) Skin graft that consists of the epidermis and dermis.
Graft A portion of tissue used as a surface cover. Not vascularized.
Mesher A mechanical device used in the sterile field to cut slits into a split skin graft to expand the surface area.
Ptosis Drooping of a part such as an eyelid or breast.
Replantation Reattach a severed part. Involves the anastomosis of vessels, nerves, and compact tissue.
Split-thickness skin graft (STSG) Skin graft that consists of the epidermis and a thin layer of papillary dermis.
"Take" The process of physiologic acceptance and integration of a graft or flap.
Volar space Palm side of the hand.

Special Features of Plastic and Reconstructive Surgery

Plastic surgery has been called the "surgery of millimeters" because of the critical margin between good and poor cosmetic results. Each millimeter lack or excess of tissue can have a psychologic impact on the patient. If the patient thinks their appearance has improved, the patient's personality and self-image may improve and others may also respond positively. The term *plastic* means "to mold or give form."

Plastic surgeons practice their art on virtually any part of the body. They attempt to restore both form (**aesthetic** appearance) and function. Some plastic surgeons limit their practice to specific areas, such as the head and neck, hand, or breast. The surgeon specifically trained in the art of plastic surgery frequently is a member of a multidisciplinary team to assist with the repair of defects and/or restoration of function. The results depend not only on the skill of the plastic surgeon and the team but also on the age, health status, skin texture, bone structure, extent of the defect, and healing capacity of the patient. The use of technology such as lasers, computed tomography (CT), magnetic resonance imaging (MRI), robotics, and microsurgery can minimize incision sizes, offer faster healing, and provide better cosmetic appearances.

Many plastic and reconstructive surgical procedures are performed on an ambulatory basis; many are performed with the patient under local anesthesia with sedation. The surgeon performs the simplest and safest procedure that will provide a realistic outcome.

Scars are inevitable whenever skin is incised or excised. The incision is made along natural skin lines whenever possible. The plastic surgeon attempts to minimize scar formation by meticulous realignment and approximation of underlying tissues and wound edges. Many plastic procedures involve only the subcuticular tissues and skin. Reconstructive procedures may include manipulation of underlying cartilage, bones, muscles, tendons, nerves, and blood vessels.

Replacement tissues or other structural substances come from several sources as follows:

- *Autograft:* Use tissue from self
- *Isograft:* Use tissue from genetically identical person
- *Allograft:* Use tissue from same species
- *Xenograft:* Use tissue from different species
- *Bioengineered graft:* **Graft** source from combined biologic and synthetic materials
- *Synthetic graft:* Substance from nonbiologic source

Preoperative instructions to patients include avoiding aspirin and no smoking for at least 2 weeks before and during the healing process for an elective surgical procedure. Aspirin and other substances have an anticoagulant action that can affect bleeding, causing hematoma formation. Medications, herbs, dietary supplements, and other substances may promote postoperative bleeding. Smoking causes vasoconstrictive ischemia that can affect wound healing, causing tissue necrosis. Photographs are commonly taken preoperatively, intraoperatively, and postoperatively for planning, documentation, and teaching purposes.

General Considerations in Plastic Surgery

1. Pressure points are protected during prolonged procedures. Microvascular plastic and reconstructive surgical procedures may take several hours to complete. The patient should be positioned on a gel pad mattress. Bony prominences should be well padded to prevent tissue necrosis.
2. Sterile dye, such as methylene blue, indigo carmine, gentian violet, Bonney blue, or brilliant green, is often used to outline areas for incision. This can be done with a sterile marking pen or stylus before or after the skin is prepped. Some surgeons will use intravenous (IV) indocyanine green or fluorescent dye (fluorescein) and a black light (Wood lamp) to confirm vascularity of a **flap**.
3. Exposure of both sides for comparison is usually required for surgical procedures on the breast, face, ears, and neck. Photography is commonly used preoperatively, intraoperatively, and postoperatively. Equalization of tissue manipulation and excision is matched to preoperative measurements written on a full-size image of the body part undergoing the surgical procedure. Fig. 40.1 depicts the areas marked for facial procedures. The nose is measured in comparison to the distance between the zygomatic arches (Fig. 40.2). Contemporary surgeons are using terrain mapping for procedures such as facial allogenous transplantations (Fig. 40.3).
4. Draping often exposes much skin surface, which is unavoidable. A fenestrated sheet frequently cannot be used. The opening does not give adequate exposure, especially for skin grafting. Towels, self-adhering plastic sheeting, and minor and medium sheets under and around the areas according to need are used to drape as much of the patient as possible. Drapes can be secured with nonpiercing towel clips, skin staples, or sutures.
5. Local anesthesia is used for many surgical procedures on adults. Epinephrine may be added to help localize the agent,

• **Fig. 40.1** Facial measurement for plastic surgery.

• **Fig. 40.2** Nasal measurements are planned in relation to the zygoma for plastic surgery.

• **Fig. 40.3** Facial terrain measurements for full-face transplantation.

prolong the anesthetic action, and provide hemostasis by vasoconstriction. Care is taken not to use epinephrine in digits, ears, or other areas of terminal blood supply. Short 26 or 30-gauge needles are used for injection.

   a. The surgeon may administer a digital nerve block for procedures of the finger. The patient's hand is placed palm down, and a hypodermic needle is inserted through the webspace closest to the affected digit. The surgeon will aspirate to check clearance of all vessels. Then lidocaine 1% or 0.05% without epinephrine, 1 mL, is injected in the volar space (the region of the palmer surface). As the needle is withdrawn, 1 mL is injected at the level of the dorsal space (the region closest to the dorsum of the hand).

6. No. 15 and 11 scalpel blades are routinely used to cut small structures. Smaller blades, such as Beaver style, may be used.

7. An electrosurgical unit (ESU) pencil may be used to cut or coagulate during incision. Small, handheld battery-operated units are useful for tiny bleeders. Overuse of the ESU can cause devitalization of tissue and delay healing.

8. Instruments must be small for handling delicate tissues. Iris scissors, mosquito hemostats, fine-tipped tissue forceps, and other small-scale cutting, holding, clamping, and exposing instruments are part of the routine plastic surgery setup. Microinstruments are needed for microsurgical techniques.

9. Nerve stimulation may be used to help identify nerves, especially in craniofacial, neck, and hand reconstruction procedures.

10. Bone, cartilage, or skin grafts may be needed. Grafts and tissues can be used from several different sources for surface and subsurface modifications. Graft materials should not be allowed to dry out; these should be placed in a basin with a few drops of saline. Do not place in a folded moist sponge because the tissue could adhere to the sponge and be discarded from the field to the sponge bucket by accident.

11. Prosthetic implants may be used in plastic surgery to reconstruct subsurface soft tissue and cartilage defects. They cannot be used unless there is adequate soft tissue coverage. They cannot be used in an infected area.

12. Suture sizes range from 2-0 through 7-0, depending on the location and tissue, with size 8-0 through 11-0 sutures used for microsurgery. The material used varies according to the personal preference of the surgeon. Synthetic nonabsorbable and absorbable polymers are used more commonly than are natural materials because they cause less tissue reaction. Barbed suture has become popular because fewer knots are required and less suture material remains in the patient to resorb.

13. Atraumatic swaged-on needles of small diameter with sharp cutting edges minimize trauma to superficial tissues. A needle holder with an appropriately fine tip is used with these delicate, curved needles.

14. Skin staples may be used to close skin or secure skin grafts.

15. Wound closure strips may be used as skin dressings with sutures or to supplement closure with skin staples.

16. Closed-wound suction drainage is frequently used to drain flaps to prevent seroma and hematoma formation.

17. Fine mesh gauze may be used for the contact dressing. This may be impregnated with petrolatum or an oil emulsion, with or without medication, to cover denuded areas. Several types of sterile nonadherent dressings are commercially available. Dry gauze is not used on a denuded area because it adheres and acts as a foreign body, causing granulomas.

18. Pressure dressings may be used after extensive surgical procedures to splint soft tissues and prevent contractures. Even pressure keeps fluid formation in tissues or under a skin graft to a minimum. Commercial compression garments or dressings for various body areas are preferred by some plastic surgeons. Some dressings may be sutured into place. Donor graft sites require bulkier dressings because they have multiple pinpoint bleeders that ooze freely.

19. Stent fixation is a method of obtaining pressure when it is impossible to bandage an area snugly, such as the face or neck. A form-fitting mold may be taped over the nose like a splint. Long suture ends can be tied crisscrossed over a dressing to immobilize it and exert gentle, even pressure.

Tissue may be approximated, supplemented, excised, transferred, or transplanted. Many procedures are done in stages before complete reconstruction and restoration of function are achieved. Tissue flaps and grafts, prosthetic implants, and external prosthetic appliances may be required for functional and cosmetic restoration as a result of ablative surgery or trauma.

Psychologic Support for Patients Undergoing Plastic and Reconstructive Surgery

Physical appearance affects self-image and self-esteem. Patients can develop inferiority complexes and introverted personalities because of congenital or acquired alteration in body structure. The defect may not affect physiologic function but may predispose the person to psychologic crippling if it is not corrected to the individual's satisfaction.

Adults who are dissatisfied with their body image may believe a change in personal appearance will solve their social, marital, sexual, or business problems. The plastic surgeon assesses the patient's psychologic status, motivations, and expectations before scheduling a surgical procedure. Realistic, attainable outcomes are identified. The patient should be emotionally stable and aware of the potential outcomes. The surgeon should carefully obtain informed consent. Psychologic assessment and preparation are advisable preoperatively and are essential before surgical procedures that may result in disfigurement.

Extensive reconstruction for severe congenital deformities is done in stages, often over months or years. These patients require prolonged psychologic support and encouragement.

Plastic and reconstructive surgery, either therapeutic or cosmetic, evokes emotional responses from the patient, family or significant others, and the entire perioperative team. Anticipation of the final outcome, which can be seen by the patient and others, often creates temporary psychosocial reactions such as depression and isolation. Positive reassurance of progress in improvement of physical appearance and during emotional crises is essential throughout the perioperative period. Perhaps the surgeon-nurse-patient-family relationship is closer when a person undergoes alteration of physical appearance than with other types of surgeries.

The patient may be physically healthy but may suffer alterations in self-esteem related to a perception of a defect in appearance. Care must be given in a manner that protects the self-esteem of the patient and respects the dignity of family and significant others. This requires communication, understanding, and empathy. Preoperative teaching and discharge planning prepare the patient and the at-home caregivers for postoperative rehabilitation.

Categories of Plastic and Reconstructive Surgery

Four main categories of problems are treated by plastic surgeons:
1. *Congenital anomalies,* especially in the structure of the face and hands. Other disciplines may surgically treat genitourinary or orthopedic deformities.
2. *Aesthetic appearance,* especially of the body surface and subsurface, particularly the face and breasts.
3. *Benign and malignant neoplasms,* especially those leaving large soft tissue defects. Resection of extensive tumors other than those involving the skin or head and neck is not usually within the province of the plastic surgeon initially, but the patient may be referred for reconstructive surgery and rehabilitation. Frequently, reconstructive procedures are done in conjunction with another specialty surgeon at the time of tumor resection.
4. *Traumatically acquired disfigurements,* especially facial lacerations, hand injuries, and burns. The objective of the plastic surgeon is to restore function as well as body image.

Skin and Tissue Grafting

Denuded areas of the body are resurfaced by transplanting or transferring segments of skin and other tissues from an uninjured area (donor site) to the injured area (recipient site). The plastic surgeon prefers to transfer tissues of compatible color, texture, thickness, and hair-bearing characteristics. Soft tissue autografts are used whenever possible. They are classified as follows according to the source of their vascular supply (which is essential for viability):

- *Free graft:* Tissue is detached from the donor site and transplanted into the recipient site. It derives its vascular supply from the capillary ingrowth from the recipient site. Fig. 40.4 depicts regions of the body suitable for autologous graft procurement.
- *Pedicle flap:* Tissue remains attached at one or both ends of the donor site during transfer to the recipient site. The vascular supply is maintained from the vessels preserved in the pedicle of the donor site.[1] Advancement flaps, rotational flaps, rhomboid flaps, transverse rectus abdominis myocutaneous (TRAM)

flaps, and latissimus dorsi flaps (Fig. 40.5) are forms of pedicle flaps.
- *Free flap:* Tissue, including its vascular bundle, is detached from the donor site and transferred to the recipient site. Composite free flaps may include muscle, bone, and skin. Microvascular anastomoses between arteries and veins in the flap or autograft and recipient site establish the vascularity necessary for viability (Fig. 40.6).

Deformities caused by loss of soft tissue substance, such as trauma from accidental injury, tumor resection, or radiation therapy, may require a graft to fill in deficiencies and restore contours or to cover tendons and bones. Free grafts, pedicle flaps, and free flaps may be taken from various areas of the body to reconstruct soft tissue defects.

Grafting from one area of the body to another requires a process referred to as "take." The recipient site has to accept the donor tissue for the graft to take, or remain as a permanently viable tissue replacement. The skin graft take occurs in three steps. During the first 48 hours, plasma accumulates at the contact area of the graft. This keeps the tissue vitalized before circulation is established. The second phase is the start of capillary ingrowth. And the last step is the anastomosis of vascular channels. If the graft does not take, it sloughs off and necroses.

Skin Graft Knives and Dermatomes

A dermatome is a cutting instrument designed to excise split-thickness skin grafts (STSGs). The thickness of the graft can be

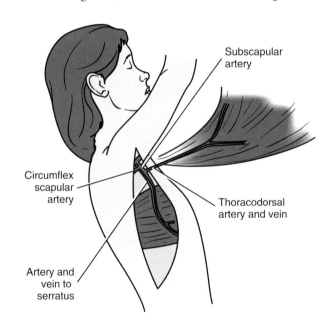

• **Fig. 40.5** Latissimus dorsi vascularized flap for breast reconstruction.

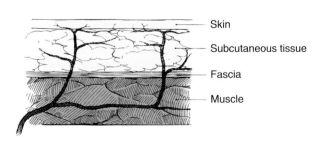

• **Fig. 40.6** Myocutaneous free flap.

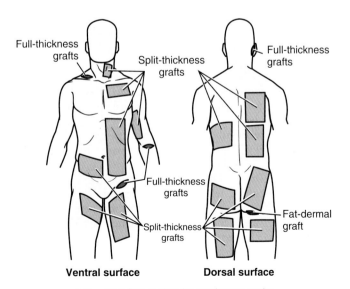

• **Fig. 40.4** Donor sites for autologous grafts.

calibrated by adjusting the depth gauge. The width of the graft is determined by the width of the cutting blade. Blades are detachable and disposable, which always ensures a sharp new blade for every patient. The cutting depth should always be reset at zero after changing blades. The length, width, and depth of the graft may be limited by the type of dermatome used and the surface from which the graft is procured (Fig. 40.7).

Freehand Skin Graft Knives and Dermatomes

Freehand knife dermatomes are used when the surface can be stabilized for precision cutting. The depth of the cut is determined by the setting on the blade gauge and adjusted by turning screws on the handle. Most styles have disposable blades. American surgeons Vilray Blair (1871–1955) and James Barrett Brown (1899–1971) developed a freehand knife that was modified by

• **Fig. 40.7** Dermatomes. **A,** Powered oscillating blade-type dermatome with depth gauges on each side of blade. **B,** Drum-type dermatome to manually cut skin graft. **C,** DeSilva freehand skin graft knife. **D,** Assistant provides countertraction for use of a manual Watson skin graft knife.

later plastic surgeons. The original style was designed like a straight razor but was later modified to include a roller for more accurate depth measurement (see Fig. 40.7, *C* and *D*).

Drum-Style Skin Graft Dermatomes

Padgett and Reese dermatomes consist of one-half of a metal drum, which forms half a circle (see Fig. 40.7, *B*). A metal handle through the center of the drum has an arm on each end. These arms hold the bar that carries the blade. The bar swings around the drum to cut the graft. The size of the graft is limited by the width and length of the drum. An adhesive is placed on both the skin surface and the drum to keep the skin in contact with the drum. The knife blade is moved from side to side as slight tension is exerted on the skin by rotating the drum. The drum-type dermatome is used on flat, open areas because it is bulky. Its use is limited by the body contour and the amount of suitable skin on the donor site.

Dermatome tape is used with the Reese dermatome. Packaged sterile, the tape has an adhesive coating on each side, covered with a paper backing. The backing is removed on one side and applied to the drum, taking care to line up the edges of the tape and the drum. After the backing paper is removed from the other side of the tape, the drum is placed on the skin, which adheres to it.

When a drum-type dermatome is being handled, the blade carrier is always grasped to prevent its swinging around the drum and seriously injuring the hands. The dermatome is left in the sterile rack when not in use or until the blade is removed.

Powered Skin Graft Dermatomes

Oscillating blade-type dermatomes may be electric or air powered with compressed nitrogen or air. The length of the graft is limited only by the donor site. The surgeon checks the adjustable-depth gauge before cutting the graft (see Fig. 40.7, *A*). The oscillating blade, free of vibrations, takes an accurate graft from donor sites that overlie firm structures, such as bone. The oscillating blade-type dermatome generally is not used on the abdominal wall, where underlying support is not firm.

Care is used in handling these precision dermatomes. If the dermatome is electric, the circulator should remove the foot pedal after the graft is taken. If the dermatome is air powered, the scrub person and surgeon should place a thumb under the lever on the handle while preparing the instrument for use. These dermatomes cannot be immersed in water or put in a washer-sterilizer or ultrasonic cleaner. The manufacturer's instructions should be followed for use, care, and sterilization.

Types of Skin and Tissue Grafts

Skin Grafts

The epidermis, including the basal layer of the dermis that generates new skin, is transplanted from a donor site to a recipient site, in which it becomes a part of living tissue in that area. Adherence to healthy underlying tissue and adequate vascularity are necessary for graft take (survival). A fibrin layer forms to bind the graft to the recipient site and to provide nourishment until vascularization is established in the graft. The depth of the graft (Fig. 40.8) varies according to its purpose, as follows:

- **Split-thickness skin graft (STSG):** The epidermis and half of the dermis to a depth of 0.010 to 0.035 inch (0.3–1 mm) are removed. The donor site heals uneventfully unless it becomes infected. STSGs are widely used to cover large denuded areas

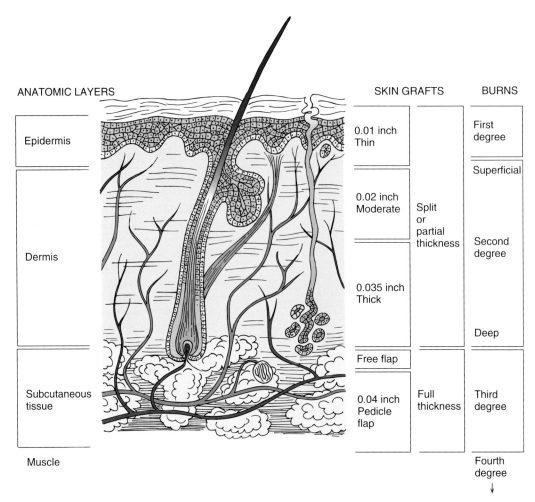

ANATOMIC LAYERS — SKIN GRAFTS — BURNS

Epidermis

Dermis

Subcutaneous tissue

Muscle

0.01 inch Thin — First degree

Superficial

0.02 inch Moderate — Split or partial thickness — Second degree

0.035 inch Thick

Deep

Free flap

0.04 inch Pedicle flap — Full thickness — Third degree

Fourth degree ↓

• **Fig. 40.8** Cross-section of skin and subcutaneous tissue, relative thickness of skin grafts, and categorization of burn injury.

on the back, trunk, and legs and can be meshed to cover larger areas. The donor site can be reused in 2 to 3 weeks after healing.

- Full-thickness skin graft (FTSG): The epidermis, dermis, and occasionally subcutaneous fat at a depth greater than 0.035 inch (1 mm) are removed or elevated. FTSGs inhibit wound contraction better than STSGs and generally are preferred on the face, neck, hands, elbows, axillae, knees, and feet. The donor site is either grafted or closed by primary intention. The donor site cannot be used again in the future.
- Composite graft: This graft includes epidermis, dermis, fat, and other structures such as bone, cartilage, nerve, or tendon.

The desired thickness of a skin graft is determined by the plastic surgeon before the skin is incised. The appropriate cutting instrument is selected to obtain the graft.

Split-Thickness Thiersch Graft

Removed with a freehand skin graft knife or dermatome, Thiersch grafts are used to cover superficial defects. The surgeon may use sutures or skin staples along the edges of the graft to hold it to underlying subcutaneous tissue. An even-pressure dressing is secured over the top of the graft. This prevents movement and helps obliterate dead space in the recipient site. The skin of the donor site regenerates rapidly, and the same area can be used again

in 2 or 3 weeks if necessary. If a thin graft is taken and the site remains free of infection, that donor site may be used again sooner.

Split-Thickness Mesh Graft

A mesh graft makes it possible to obtain a greater area of coverage from an STSG. After removal with a dermatome, the graft is placed on a plastic derma carrier, cut side down on the mesher platform. This is a rigid base to keep the graft spread out flat while it is put through a mesh dermatome. This instrument cuts small parallel slits in the graft. When expanded, the slits become diamond-shaped openings (Fig. 40.9). This permits expansion of the graft to cover an area three times as large as the original graft obtained from the donor site.

The mesh graft can be placed over the recipient site with slight tension. The increased edge exposures are conducive to rapid epithelialization. The mesh allows serum to escape through the openings. If a mesh dermatome is not available or is not feasible to use, slits can be made with a knife blade in the donor graft to accomplish the same purposes.

Although this method covers a larger area and contours well, much of the wound has to heal by secondary intention, causing scar contracture. The healed area maintains a "cobblestone" appearance.

• **Fig. 40.9** Split-thickness skin graft being passed through mesh derma-tome. Mesh graft expands to obtain greater coverage of recipient graft area.

Full-Thickness Wolfe Graft

The Wolfe graft is cut exactly to the size and shape of the recipient site with a skin graft knife. It is sutured into place under normal skin tension. FTSGs are used on the face, neck, or hands to fill in superficial denuded areas and over joints to prevent contractures. This graft does not become viable readily on granulated surfaces, and the amount that can be transferred is much more limited than with Thiersch grafts.

To ensure viability, the donor graft must be held in apposition to healthy tissue in the underlying recipient site. The surgeon tacks the edges of the graft with sutures or staples. The middle portion may be "quilted" (i.e., affixed) with sutures or staples. The graft is covered with an even-pressure dressing.

Free Composite Grafts

A composite graft usually includes skin, subcutaneous tissue and cartilage, bone, or other tissues. The viability of the graft depends on ingrowth of the vascular system from the recipient site.

Free Omental Grafts

A free graft of omentum can be used to provide contour in a soft tissue defect in the face or neck, to resurface an area such as the scalp, to provide vascular support for bone and skin grafts around prosthetic materials, and to control wound infection, such as in the chest wall. Omentum will localize inflammation and wall off infection.

It will not resorb when grafted. Omentum resected from the peritoneal cavity can be transplanted to an avascular area if sufficient blood vessels are available for microvascular anastomoses to the gastroepiploic artery and vein in the graft. STSGs cover the omental graft.

Pedicle Flaps

Creation of a pedicle flap may be the procedure of choice to reconstruct deformities of soft tissue loss that will create or that have created an obvious aesthetic or functional disability for the patient. The pedicle, which is the attachment of elevated tissue to the donor site, must contain a vascular bundle to maintain blood supply to the tissue. Pedicle flaps are constructed from several types of tissues and sources of vascular bundles. Nasal reconstruction is commonly done this way (Fig. 40.10).

• **Fig. 40.10** Pedicle flap nose reconstruction.

Flap survival seems to depend on a reduction in vascular resistance or an increase in arterial perfusion pressure, or both. Several techniques are used to monitor circulation in the flap intraoperatively and postoperatively.

Arterialized Tissue Flap

An FTSG contains a vascular bundle within subcutaneous tissue and skin. Arterialized flaps may contain the following:

- Axial vasculature from axial vessels that supply a fairly definite area of skin and subcutaneous tissue. A direct cutaneous artery flows through the length of the flap.
- Random or local vasculature from a subdermal plexus. Random flaps do not have a specific blood vessel within the flap. These are usually small flaps created around the head or neck.
- Both axial and random vasculature. A deltopectoral flap, for example, has axial vessels from the sternal region and random vessels in the deltoid area.

Depending on the proximity of the recipient site to the donor site, the pedicle flap will be one of the types discussed in the next three sections.

Rotational Flap. One end of the flap is rotated and sutured to the recipient site to cover a denuded area. The flap tissue is obtained from an area near the recipient site. Arterialized skin pedicle flaps with axial vasculature are rotated in a one-stage procedure. Random rotational pedicle flaps can be used in the face because vascularity is sufficient in the head and neck.

Cross-Finger Flap. Tissue at the donor site is undermined and rotated to cover a small defect in an adjacent digit.

Tissue Expansion Flap. The surface of the dermal-epidermal layer can be increased by implanting a tissue expansion device subcutaneously, close to the defect (Fig. 40.11). Available in many sizes and shapes, the device has a soft, pliable silicone pouch connected by tubing to a self-sealing inflation reservoir. After insertion under a designated area for creation of the skin flap, the pouch is filled with saline by injecting small amounts into the reservoir. Rapid expansion may be achieved immediately in the head or neck area or gradually over a period of weeks to months in other areas. Natural physiologic skin expansion occurs. The dermis stretches and thins while the epidermis duplicates itself without changing thickness. Tissue will increase to about 1.5 times the width of the device.

The vascular network that develops produces more viable tissue than that of other pedicle flaps. The tissue has similar color, texture, and thickness as the recipient site. The expanded tissue is advanced or transferred to cover the defect, helping minimize scarring and donor site deformity. Tissue expansion flaps are used for scalp and facial defects, breast reconstruction, and other soft tissue defects. They can be used for closure of large donor site defects.

Myocutaneous Flap

Pedicle myocutaneous flaps allow safe and rapid transfer of tissue over long distances to cover large defects and vital structures. They are used, for example, to close soft tissue defects in the lower extremities, to cover pressure sores, and to reconstruct contour after head and neck resection and mastectomy.

A myocutaneous flap incorporates the muscle with its overlying fascia, subcutaneous tissue, and skin. It receives a vigorous blood supply from the vascular pedicle that supplies the underlying muscle (see Fig. 40.6). It may include a neurovascular bundle with nerve fibers to innervate the muscle in the flap. Usually done as a one-stage procedure, myocutaneous flaps can be created from the following and other muscles:

- Trapezius
- Sternocleidomastoid
- Platysma
- Latissimus dorsi
- Pectoralis major
- Rectus abdominis
- Gracilis
- Gluteus maximus
- Tensor fascia lata
- Biceps or quadriceps femoris

Fasciocutaneous Flap

Mobilized fascia, subcutaneous tissue, and skin are transferred as pedicle flaps similarly to the way myocutaneous flaps are transferred. The donor site may need to be covered with an STSG.

Muscle Flap

A divided section of a muscle with its proximal blood supply intact can be rotated over a soft tissue defect, such as an ulcer on the leg or buttock. A vascularized muscle flap may be covered with an STSG.

Neurosensory Flap

Sensory nerves may remain intact in a flap with other tissues or be restored by microneural anastomosis or by nerve grafting. Preservation of nerves in a vascularized flap becomes important when sensation is critical to function, as in the hand or foot.

Omental Flap

Omentum is mobilized from the peritoneal cavity, without compromise of the vascular pedicle, to cover an infected mediastinal wound or a defect in the chest wall, such as after resection for irradiation necrosis or a neoplasm. The vascularity of donor omentum revascularizes the reconstructed chest wall recipient site. STSGs, which may be mesh grafts, cover the omental flap. If additional rigidity is needed to restore the chest wall, polypropylene mesh may be sutured inside the ribcage to supplement the strength of the omental flap.

Microsurgical Free-Flap Transfer

Composite free flaps or grafts of tissue are resected and transplanted from one area of the body to another to cover a denuded area or to restore function or body contour. Microsurgical

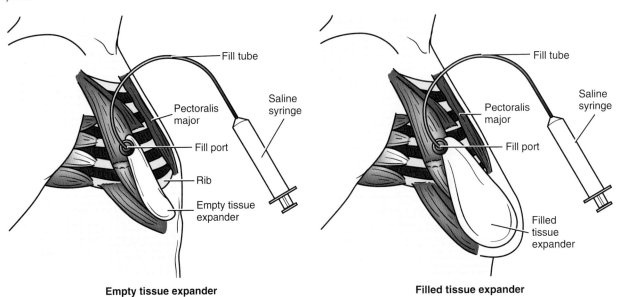

Empty tissue expander   **Filled tissue expander**

• **Fig. 40.11** Tissue expander under the pectoralis muscle.

techniques allow one-stage transfer of tissues.[2] The main artery and vein supplying donor tissues must be anastomosed to vessels in the recipient site under the operating microscope. Often two teams work simultaneously at donor and recipient sites. These are lengthy, tedious procedures, often taking many hours to complete.

Fasciocutaneous Graft

Free grafts of fascia with overlying skin, with or without underlying muscle, may be transferred. For example, temporalis fascia may be transplanted into another area in the face.

Free Muscle Graft

Free island grafts of functional muscle can be resected and transplanted to replace motor function in another area. Although only a small percentage of the graft survives, significant regeneration of muscle occurs. Free muscle, transferred by microvascular techniques and covered with an STSG, promotes healing of infected wounds.

Vascularized Muscle Pedicle Free Flap

In a multistaged procedure, a myocutaneous flap is raised at the donor site and allowed to develop a new, isolated vascular system before free transfer to a recipient site. The vascular system in the muscle underlying the skin flap branches out to supply the skin. At the final stage, the newly vascularized muscle pedicle is dissected free from the donor site. The donor site may need to be covered with an STSG.

Under the operating microscope, arteries and veins in the flap are anastomosed to vessels at the recipient site. Two teams may complete the final stage: one prepares and closes the recipient site and the other frees the flap and closes the donor site. The advantage of this type of flap is that the surgeon can select donor skin that will best provide color, texture, bulk, and contour at the recipient site, such as on the face.

Neurovascular Free Flap

Fascicles of nerves must be anastomosed to restore sensation; in addition, microvascular anastomoses of arteries and veins are needed to maintain viability of the donor tissue. A neurovascular free flap, also known as a sensate flap, may be taken from the scapular region. Many surgeons use the scapular flap because it is easy to dissect, has a long vascular pedicle, and creates a minimal donor site deformity. Other donor sites include the medial and lateral thigh and the lateral aspect of the upper arm.

Free Autologous Bone Graft

Vascularized autografts of bone are superior in strength and are less prone to deossification and structural weakness than are conventional bone grafts. Anastomosis of the vascular bundle with a free rib, for example, may increase the chance of survival of the donor bone graft in a poorly vascularized recipient site (Fig. 40.12).

Composite Myo-osteocutaneous Free Flap

A composite flap of skin, muscle, and bone provides soft tissue bulk, internal structural support, and external coverage in one-stage reconstruction of compound defects after head and neck resection. The skin and iliac crest on a vascular pedicle from the deep circumflex artery may be preferred. The scapula and tissue from the upper arm provide an alternative donor site. Or the skin, soft tissue, and latissimus dorsi muscle along with a portion of an underlying rib may be dissected free, preserving the thoracodorsal vessels for anastomosis at the recipient site. Other donor sites include the radial forearm and the fibula with the dorsalis pedis muscle.

Digital Transfer

Microneurovascular techniques are used for replantation of traumatically amputated digits. Less common is the toe-to-thumb

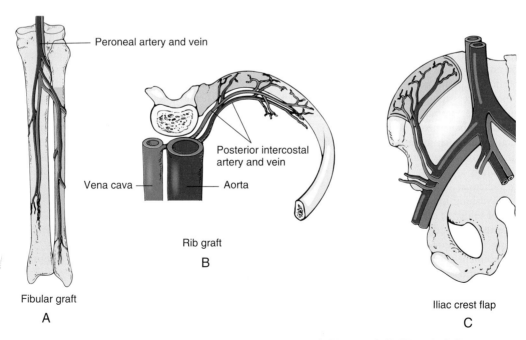

Peroneal artery and vein

Posterior intercostal artery and vein

Vena cava — Aorta

Rib graft

B

Fibular graft

A

Iliac crest flap

C

• **Fig. 40.12** Common donor sites for vascularized bone grafts. **A,** Fibular graft. **B,** Rib graft. **C,** Iliac crest graft.

transfer, called the free wraparound neurovascular flap, performed when an amputated thumb cannot be salvaged. Skin from the dorsum of the foot, the great toe (including tendons and bone), and the second toe web space are transferred as a sensate flap to the hand.

After bone fixation and tendon anastomoses, arterial circulation and venous drainage are established under the microscope. Digital nerves are anastomosed to reinnervate sensation and function. Other toes can be similarly transferred for finger reconstruction.

Replantation of Amputated Parts

Replantation may be attempted to salvage a traumatically amputated digit, hand, or entire upper extremity. A severed foot or lower extremity presents more formidable problems because of the functional necessity for weight-bearing. The victim of amputation of the scalp, nose, external ear, or penis also is a candidate for replantation. Using microsurgical techniques, replanted parts can survive with varying degrees of effectiveness.

Functional recovery, up to 80% of normal in some patients, may take up to a year or longer because it takes time for nerves to regenerate (approximately 2 inches [5 cm] per month). A team of specialists in hand surgery or of plastic surgeons with microvascular skill is vital to success in these arduous procedures.

Correct care and preservation of the severed part for transport with the patient is also vital to success. The amputated part should be placed dry into a plastic bag, which is then sealed and immersed in crushed ice inside an insulated container (e.g., Styrofoam) to retard melting of the ice during travel. The part should not be warmed, frozen, or packed in dry ice. Rapid transport and cooling with ice will buy time.

Initial treatment involves assessment of the total patient. The patient and family or significant others should be supported emotionally but not given definitive promises in regard to outcome. The surgeon considers numerous factors when planning for replantation: the need for the part, associated disease and injuries, economic and psychologic factors, and age. The following two criteria are of special significance:

1. The replanted part should have the potential for being useful.
2. There should be no undue risk to the general safety of the patient if the procedure is performed.

Replantation is more successful in young patients than in older patients. Also, incomplete amputations are more successful because they have intact subcutaneous venous circulation in the skin bridges. Restoration is much more difficult in crush injuries than in sharp, clean amputations. Contraindications to replantation include the following:

• Prolonged warm ischemia
• Severe bruising or crushing injury
• Multiple fractures or injury at different levels in the same digit
• Associated injuries that preclude the effort

Supportive therapy after injury includes tetanus toxoid, IV antibiotics, fluid replacement therapy, blood products, and judicious administration of anticoagulants.

Preoperative patient preparation is in anticipation of a long procedure. The surgical procedure may take from 4 to 16 hours. The patient is placed on a gel-filled mattress. The head, scapulae, sacrum, and heels are padded. A footboard may be used and antiembolic stockings or sequential compression devices applied. An indwelling Foley catheter is inserted if the procedure will take longer than 2 hours.

• **Fig. 40.13** Specialized hand table. The team is seated around the table.

Most replantations of the hand are done with the patient under moderate sedation and an axillary or supraclavicular block with a long-acting agent, such as bupivacaine (Marcaine, Sensorcaine) without epinephrine. General anesthesia is used for children and may be needed for adults for a long procedure.

These surgical procedures usually involve a two-team approach: one team prepares the recipient site with the patient's hand and arm positioned on a hand table (Fig. 40.13), and the other prepares the severed or distal part.

In the operating room (OR), the amputated part is cleansed with lactated Ringer solution or normal saline. Debridement of crushed tissue is carried out. Vessels are isolated for repair, and vessel patency is ensured. The basic steps of replantation of digits or extremities include the following (Fig. 40.14):

1. Identify proximal and distal tendons, nerves, and vessels.
2. Shorten bone within an acceptable limit necessary for tension-free repair of blood vessels, nerves, and soft tissues.
3. Stabilize the skeletal structure, such as with internal wire fixation techniques, to maintain joint continuity and fusion in functional position. Small plates and screws may be used.
4. Suture tendons and ligaments, both extensors and flexors, appropriately to lessen the junctional scar process that can inhibit motion.
5. Anastomose arteries and nerves. The vessels may be flushed with heparin solution, and systemic anticoagulants may be given. Antispasmodic agents may be needed.
6. Anastomose veins. A general rule is that more veins are anastomosed than are arteries to provide sufficient venous return and thereby minimize edema. Swelling creates pressure that impedes circulation, leading to necrosis. Leech therapy may be indicated to lessen the effects of diminished venous drainage and swelling.
7. Repair soft tissues and close the skin.
8. Perform a skin graft or tissue flap or transfer if necessary.

Microsurgical techniques are necessary for nerve, artery, and vein repairs of structures that have an external diameter of 1 mm or less.

To avoid constriction, a circumferential bandage is not applied. Instead, a foam bandage is used. The dressing is padded to prevent pressure sores and nerve damage. The original dressing is not changed for 10 days unless indicated.

Postoperative care is extremely important. Dressings must be checked carefully because even slight manipulation can cause great damage.

K-wire fixation

Bone alignment

Plate fixation

Plate and screw stabilization

Artery and nerve repair

Nerve repair   Flexor tendon repair

**Artery and nerve anastomosis,
flexor tendon repair**

Vein repair

Extensor tendon repair

**Extensor tendon repair,
vein anastomosis**

Skin repaired

Skin closure

• **Fig. 40.14** Steps in digit replantation.

Checking only the tip of the digit for circulation is not adequate. Circulation is verified by cautiously looking into the dressing to check the capillary refill, color, temperature, and drainage. Doppler imaging and a temperature probe may be used to evaluate arterial circulation. Patients are not permitted to smoke or chew tobacco because nicotine is a vasoconstrictor. Constriction of vessels may reduce circulation and cause devitalization of tissue.

The many hours expended by the OR team initially to achieve a successful repair of all structures can relieve the patient of subsequent procedures. The objective is to obtain maximal return of function by minimizing permanent disability. Physical and occupational therapies are important in rehabilitation.

General Considerations for All Tissue Autografts

1. Hypothermia is avoided. Room temperature should be increased to 75° F to 80° F (24–27° C).
2. For long procedures, the patient should be positioned on a gel pad mattress.
3. Skin may be prepped with a colorless antiseptic agent so that the plastic surgeon can see the true skin color and assess the vascularity of the donor graft.
4. Donor and recipient sites are prepped and draped separately but concurrently. Care is taken that cross-contamination does not occur from one site to the other.
5. The recipient site is covered with a sterile drape until the surgeon is ready to apply a free graft or pedicle flap if preparation of the donor site will be the first procedure. If the recipient site must be prepared or debrided to receive the donor graft or flap, the donor site is covered with a sterile towel.
6. A separate sterile instrument table is prepared for the donor site. This includes appropriate instruments for obtaining the graft or flap and dressings for the donor site. Two surgical teams may work simultaneously.

Place the dermatome on a separate, small sterile table, never on the recipient instrument table. Handle dermatomes carefully so the depth gauge is not disturbed. Care is taken to disconnect the power when loading the blades to prevent accidental activation of the device.

7. Grafts are kept moist by placing them in a basin and covering with normal saline. A free flap should be kept in cool saline until the recipient site is prepared. Ice may damage tissues and should be avoided.
8. The operating microscope and appropriate microinstruments must be in readiness for microvascular and neurologic anastomoses.
9. Tissue viability must be ensured. Some surgeons use CT angiogram or magnetic resonance angiogram (MRA) as a preplanning tool to assess blood flow. A sterile device may be needed during the surgical procedure to identify major blood vessels underlying a graft. Assessment of the patency of vessels and perfusion of the flap is possible through several types of monitoring.
   a. *Doppler probe:* A Doppler probe is placed on the recipient site preoperatively to obtain baseline measurements for comparison with postoperative measurements. The device has an audible pulsation sound and a digital readout. Ultrasonic Doppler probes also may be used for monitoring arterial vascularity of a part.
   b. *Photoplethysmographic disc:* A disc applied to the flap surface measures reflected light from pulsatile blood flow changes in tissue. A change in blood volume in tissue produces a corresponding change in the amount of light reflected. These changes are amplified and displayed on an oscilloscope.
   c. *Fluorometer:* A fluorescing dye is injected IV, and fluorescence is measured with a fluorometer to evaluate

perfusion of the flap. Fluorescein and an ultraviolet Wood lamp are used to check patency and perfusion. The room is darkened to see fluorescence. A photomultiplier may be used to amplify skin fluorescent emission.

d. *Thermocouple probe:* The patency of a microvascular anastomosis can be assessed by the temperature in surrounding tissues.

e. *Oxygen saturation:* Oxygen saturation of a flap can be monitored postoperatively with a probe similar to a pulse oximeter. ViOptix technology uses near-infrared spectroscopy to measure oxygen levels in real time or healing tissues.

10. Hemostasis is obtained during the surgical procedure with the use of warm saline packs, pressure, or thrombin.

11. An ESU is used very sparingly to prevent the devitalization of tissues.

12. Dressings over grafts vary by surgeon preference. Stent fixation to obtain pressure on the grafted area may be preferred. Some plastic surgeons omit pressure dressings and use an exposure technique on grafts so they can watch the graft and drain a hematoma or seroma if necessary.

The graft is kept covered with sterile, moist saline gauze dressings to keep the skin moist until revascularization occurs. Synthetic moisture- and vapor-permeable adhesive dressings are impermeable to liquid and bacteria. Healing under these occlusive dressings may be more rapid and less painful than at donor sites covered with fine mesh gauze. A cast may be applied to immobilize extremities for pedicle flaps.

Head and Neck Plastic and Reconstructive Procedures

Some plastic surgeons specialize in head and neck oncology or reconstruction, or both. Others limit their practice to aesthetic, or cosmetic, surgery.

Soft Tissue Reconstruction

Defects in soft tissues of the face or scalp, usually as a result of trauma, may be reconstructed by advancement of tissue expanded from an adjacent area. This technique ensures consistent skin color, texture, and hair-bearing characteristics. Other types of grafts or flaps may be necessary or preferred.

Craniofacial Surgical Procedures

The plastic surgeon usually heads the multidisciplinary team that performs the complex craniofacial procedures discussed in Chapter 41. Many of the concepts developed for these procedures are applied in less-complicated surgical procedures. A variety of extracranial osteotomies, with or without bone grafts, reshape the bony framework of the face and skull. The desired aesthetic and functional results can be obtained only by painstakingly careful planning, dissection, and repositioning.

Maxillofacial and Oral Surgical Procedures

Plastic surgeons reconstruct soft tissue defects around and in the mouth that are caused by trauma or surgical resection. Those maxillofacial procedures involving bony structures that may also be performed by plastic surgeons are discussed in Chapter 41. Congenital deformities are discussed in Chapter 8.

Facial Nerve Grafting

Restoration of the quality of facial expressions in a patient with severe facial nerve paralysis can be accomplished by transfacial nerve grafting. Segments of nerve grafts are brought through tunnels across the lips from the normal side of the face to the paralyzed side. These are anastomosed to the distal facial nerve on the normal side and then to the proximal branches of the injured nerve on the paralyzed side.

The overpull of the mouth and lower face toward the normal side is balanced when the nerve graft is anastomosed between fascicles of the intact facial nerve innervating the facial muscles to the same fascicles on the denervated side. If the facial muscle has been paralyzed for a prolonged period, the serratus muscle from the chest wall may be transplanted and innervated by the facial nerve.

Repair of Lacerations of the Lip or Mouth

Wound edges of the lips and/or mucosa in the mouth are carefully sutured to repair lacerations. The borders of the vermilion line are carefully realigned.

Excision of Leukoplakia

Chronic irritation can result in an abnormal whitening of the mucous membrane of the lip and tongue (leukoplakia), a lesion primarily seen in heavy smokers. Sharp dissection or a carbon dioxide (CO_2) laser is used to resect a precancerous lesion.

Excision of a Lip Tumor

Excision of a lip tumor may be minor, with V-wedge excision, or extensive, depending on the stage of malignancy. Extensive lesions require a flap procedure for reconstruction. Closure starts on the vermillion border of the lip.

Lip Reconstruction

Lips can be adequately reconstructed by a variety of techniques to restore sensation and motor function after trauma or surgical resection. Lip cancer is the most common type of cancer in the upper respiratory and digestive tracts. Surgical procedures to reconstruct lips may be classified as follows:

- Repair by primary closure of the remaining lip segments.
- Full-thickness cross-lip flaps from the opposite lip.
- Arterialized or myocutaneous flaps from adjacent cheek or nasolabial tissue.
- Distant flaps. Arterialized and innervated myocutaneous flaps from the forehead or deltopectoral region may be used. These require staged procedures. Free microvascular composite grafts are done in one stage.

The ideal repair yields a lip that is not tight and that has a good vermilion border, an adequate sulcus (philtrum), good sensation, and good muscle tone.

Aesthetic Procedures

Procedures are not always performed for aesthetic purposes alone. They may restore function as well as correct a facial deformity or defect.

Blepharoplasty

Redundant skin and/or protruding orbital fat is excised to correct deformities of the upper or lower eyelids of one or both eyes. Blepharochalasis (loss of elasticity of the skin of the eyelids) can occur at any age and usually is of unknown cause. Dermatochalasis primarily involves hypertrophy of the skin of the upper lids.

Resection of the excessive redundant skin removes the mechanical visual obstruction caused by these two conditions.

Protrusion of intraorbital fat into the lids is the most common eyelid deformity. It is often familial and is sometimes seen in patients as young as 20 years. This fat is removed from the compartments in the upper and/or lower lids to correct the deformity. This may be associated with dermatochalasis. A free graft of cartilage and mucosa from the nasal septum may be necessary to reconstruct lower eyelid defects after excision for tumor. Hypertrophy of the orbicularis muscle appears as a horizontal bulge below the lower lid margin. A skin-muscle flap resection may be performed. A surgical procedure for lifting the eyebrows will secondarily correct a hooding deformity of the upper lids caused by **ptosis** of the eyebrows.

These procedures are usually performed with the patient under local anesthesia. An upper lid incision is made in a natural skinfold; an incision in the lower lid is just under the eyelash line (Fig. 40.15). If the patient wears dentures, they should wear them to the OR because facial contour is distorted without them. The surgeon could remove too much or too little redundant skin.

Because of the proximity to the eyes, protrusion of periorbital fat may impair vision. Oculoplastic procedures may be performed by an ophthalmologist. Through a conjunctival incision, subconjunctival fat may be removed with a CO_2 laser. An eyelid procedure also may be necessary to protect the eye in a patient with facial nerve paralysis caused by trauma or tumor resection. A gold weight, between 0.05 and 1.2 g, or a spring can be inserted in the upper eyelid with the patient under local anesthesia. This protects the eye by allowing the eyelid to blink.

Otoplasty

Deformities of one or both external ears of an adult are usually the result of burns or traumatic avulsion. A segment of external ear that is partially or completely amputated often can be reattached to the remaining segment and buried beneath a flap of postauricular skin. The area over a completely severed auricular cartilage, which cannot be sutured back in place, is covered with an STSG initially.

• **Fig. 40.15** Incisions for blepharoplasty. **A,** Upper eyelid. **B,** Lower eyelid.

Later reconstruction may include insertion of cartilage autograft taken from the patient's ribcage, a cartilage allograft, or a porous polyethylene or silicone prosthetic implant. The porous implant allows vascular and soft tissue ingrowth that reduces the risk for infection and extrusion—potential complications with a silicone implant. The graft or implant is buried beneath a segment of turned-down temporoparietal fascia. Then the area is covered with an STSG from the scalp or an FTSG from the opposite postauricular area.

Rhinoplasty

Reshaping of the nose, although usually performed for cosmetic alteration desired by the patient, may be necessary to correct defects caused by trauma or surgical resection of neoplasms. Subtle changes with limited nasal reduction or augmentation of the nasal tip with the patient's own nasal cartilage can result in an aesthetically attractive and physiologically normal nose in most patients. Through an intranasal incision, the nose can be shortened or narrowed by rearranging, reshaping, and/or removing bone and cartilage. This may be done to relieve breathing problems. Nasal packing and a nasal splint support the structures postoperatively.

A free composite graft or pedicle flap may be necessary to close a large tissue defect. Bone or cartilage grafts may be needed for skeletal support. Prosthetic reconstruction for partial or total loss of the nose may be the procedure of choice.

Mentoplasty

The shape and size of the chin can be altered for aesthetics and/or functional bite disorders. The mandible can be repositioned forward or backward to change alignment in relation to the maxilla. Sections are removed to reduce size, or osteotomies are made to reshape the chin. An abnormally small jaw (micrognathia) is augmented with bone or cartilage grafts or a silicone implant or by advancing the mandible. Lip incompetence (inability to bring the lips together without tension) may be corrected during the same surgical procedure.

Rhytidoplasty

Commonly referred to as a face lift, rhytidoplasty involves extensive dissection from above the ear, both in front of and behind the pinna, downward along the jaw line and upper neck (Fig. 40.16, *A*). The skin is freed from underlying fascia. Wrinkles and folds caused by the normal aging process smooth out as the skin is lifted up and sutured in place. Dissection beneath the platysma muscle, referred to as the submuscular aponeurotic system (SMAS) procedure, minimizes the amount of skin undermined (see Fig. 40.16, *B*). The platysma is sutured back to the mastoid (see Fig. 40.16, *C*). Redundant skin is trimmed away.

A modified lift can be attained by using a clear barbed suture under the skin to lift the bilateral fascial planes. Using this suture is considered minimally invasive. Endoscopic methods can be used to elevate fascial planes. No excess tissue is trimmed away. Patients are advised to minimize the stress over the sutured areas for 3 months by wearing a chin strap at night and avoid traction on the tissues of the face. More discussion of barbed suture is found in Chapter 28 in the discussion of synthetic sutures (barbed polydioxanone: Quill suture, contour thread). This clear synthetic self-anchoring suture is approved for use by the U.S. Food and Drug Administration (FDA). It is used for dermal suturing without the need for knotted ends. The surface of the suture has

SMAS/platysma flap

• **Fig. 40.16** Rhytidoplasty (face lift). **A,** Incision from above ear and in front of and behind pinna. **B,** Dissection beneath and elevation of platysma flap (submuscular aponeurotic system [SMAS] procedure). **C,** Platysma muscle is sutured back to mastoid.

raised barbs that are angled from the center to the ends in both directions.

Frequently other procedures, such as blepharoplasty or rhinoplasty, accompany this surgical procedure. Meticulous hemostasis is essential to prevent hematoma formation, the foremost complication of rhytidoplasty. Hypotensive anesthesia may be used to help reduce this incidence. Closed-wound suction drainage is frequently used with or without a pressure dressing applied after the surgical procedure.

Face Transplantation

Surgeons in France and China performed successful partial face transplantations in 2006. Full-face transplantations were performed in 2010 in Spain and France. The first full-face transplantation in the United States was performed in 2011 in Boston. Traumatic injury to the face can cause massive facial tissue loss for which there is no cosmetic or functional replacement. Microvascular anastomosis has made free-flap allogeneic transfer possible, and antirejection drugs offer the promise of long-term take. A face transplant can cause emotional trauma.[3] The patient is counseled and may participate in surgical planning because they will no longer look the same as before the injury. Long-term success requires monitoring the graft for many years.[4]

Soft Tissue Augmentation

Fat transplantation may be done by mini-liposuction and injection of the patient's own tissue. Fat cells are withdrawn from the lower abdomen, hips, or thighs into a syringe through a hypodermic needle. The fat then is injected into areas around the lips or eyes to smooth wrinkles or into hollow spaces in the cheeks or other facial defects. This procedure may be done in conjunction with a rhytidoplasty. The correction is not permanent because the fat cells will die.

A purified form of bovine dermal collagen can be injected for the same purposes. A series of injections of small amounts of the collagen are deposited to fill small soft tissue defects or to smooth out wrinkles.

Hair Replacement

Hair follicles can be transplanted from the posterior aspect of the scalp to bald or balding areas. Hundreds of micrografts (4 μm) and minigrafts (4.5 μm) are implanted in staged rows over the entire bald area to change the hairline (Fig. 40.17). A new hairline

A. 1 hair follicular unit

B. 2-3 hair follicular units and linear grafts

C. Linear grafts

Map for hair graft transplants

Hair follicle grafts

Hair strip graft

• **Fig. 40.17** Hair transplantation.

can be initially established with rotational flaps from other parts of the scalp. This may necessitate tissue expansion. If hair loss is not complete, hair follicle grafts complement and thicken the existing hair. Several transplantation sessions may be necessary to achieve the final result the patient is seeking.

Plastic and Reconstructive Procedures of Other Body Areas

Adipose Tissue

Lipectomy is an excision of excessive fat and redundant skin from the upper arms, abdomen, buttocks, thighs, or other body areas.

Liposuction

Localized areas of fat deposits are removed by suction-assisted lipectomy, known as liposuction, to alter body contours. Males and females differ in areas of localized fat deposits (Fig. 40.18). Most surgeons prefer to inject target tissue with 1% lidocaine with 1:100,000 epinephrine in saline to create a tumescent effect to plump up the fat and firm the surface. This solution also reduces blood loss during the surgical procedure. The average adult dosage range for tumescent injection should not exceed 7 mg/kg of lidocaine and in general should not total more than 500 mg.

A blunt, hollow, curved or straight metal cannula (Mercedes cannula) measuring 1.5 to 6 mm with multiple openings in the distal shaft connected to a suction machine is inserted through small skin incisions (Fig. 40.19). The cannula is moved back and forth along the axial plane, parallel to the skin surface, to bluntly dissect and aspirate cores of fat in a honeycomb pattern. This pattern allows for uniform tissue contouring. A laser may be used through the cannula to vaporize fat rather than suction it out. The laser diminishes bleeding by coagulating vessels. The patient's hematocrit level decreases by 1% for each 150 mL of fat removed by conventional liposuction.

Suction-assisted lipectomy may be used in conjunction with conventional abdominoplasty. It is also used to remove fat from the neck and chin, upper arms, breasts, flanks, buttocks, thighs,

knees, and ankles. It can be used to defat transfer flaps and treat some forms of lymphedema and lipomas. The amount of fat removed should not exceed the ability of the overlying skin to contract and may be between 1500 and 2000 mL.

If tumescence is used, 2500 to 3000 mL may be removed without complications. Large fluid volume shifts follow lipectomy, so the inflow and suction contents should be monitored closely. The incisions are sutured and reinforced with wound closure strips, and compression garments are worn for 10 days to 2 weeks postoperatively to control edema and help skin remodeling.

Postoperative discharge planning should include advising the patient that each cannula port site will ooze serosanguineous fluid for a few days. Padding the bed at home is recommended. Removing and donning the compression garment can be difficult because of the tightness required for the synthetic elastic to be effective.

The patient can shower with the compression garment on using a liquid antibacterial soap and dry the garment area with a cool hair dryer. If the garment is removed, the reapplication is easier if the patient's body is completely dry.

Abdominoplasty

Abdominoplasty includes excising excess, lax abdominal wall skin and adipose tissue, and tightening abdominal wall musculature. This is usually a cosmetic procedure referred to as a "tummy tuck." Physical discomfort or the inability to perform personal hygiene because of a large pannus that hangs like an apron over the lower abdomen and genital region may be a functional indication for the procedure. Its purpose is not to make an obese person thin. The most suitable patient is of ideal weight and in good health. Causes of the abdominal wall laxity include pregnancy, marked weight loss, and the aging process.

Preoperatively, the primary incision line is marked along a natural skinfold using a marking pen with the patient in a standing position. After the administration of the anesthetic agent, the head and foot of the OR bed are elevated 15 to 20 degrees to anteflex the patient's torso and decrease abdominal tension

• **Fig. 40.18** Fat distributions differ between males and females.

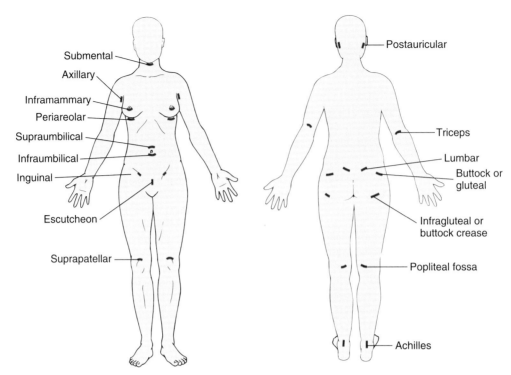

• **Fig. 40.19** Incision areas for suction-assisted lipectomy.

• **Fig. 40.20** Patient positioning for abdominoplasty.

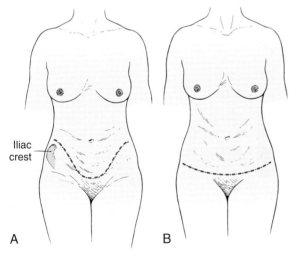

• **Fig. 40.21** Abdominoplasty incisions. **A,** Medial to iliac crest for patient who desires high "French cut" swimsuit. **B,** Natural abdominal skin crease fold below iliac crest.

(Fig. 40.20). The surgeon chooses either a low transverse incision from one anterosuperior iliac crest to the other or a combination transverse secondary vertical incision in a fleur-de-lis pattern (Fig. 40.21). The typical area of dissection extends subcutaneously to the costal margins and xyphoid process superiorly and to the midaxillary to lateral axillary lines laterally.

The umbilicus is preserved on a vascularized stalk and repositioned in the abdominal wall after the rectus muscle is tightened (plicated) and excess skin, subcutaneous tissue, and fat are resected. When wound closure is completed, the abdominal wall should be flat and smooth. Closed-suction drainage, a bulky pressure dressing, and an abdominal binder are used to prevent hematoma formation and eliminate dead space.

Postoperatively the patient is positioned with the head and foot of the bed flexed and then may ambulate progressively upon recommendation. Some surgeons will have a trapeze bar attached to the postoperative bed so the patient can shift positions easily. The patient will be instructed to maintain the flexed position while sleeping until the incision starts to heal.

Breast

Breasts can be enlarged, reduced, or reconstructed. Unilateral augmentation or reduction is sometimes performed to correct asymmetry of the breasts.

Augmentation Mammoplasty

A bilateral mammoplasty usually is performed for aesthetics on a woman who desires larger breasts. Inflatable implants are inserted under breast tissue or the underlying pectoralis muscles and then filled with sterile saline solution through self-sealing valves.

The breast implant can be inserted through a periareolar, transaxillary, inframammary, or supraumbilical endoscopic approach (Figs. 40.22 and 40.23). The periareolar incision, made around the outside border of the lower half of the areola, is the most difficult for insertion of the implant, but it leaves the most inconspicuous scar. The transaxillary incision in the axilla does not scar the breast. The inframammary incision, the most common, is

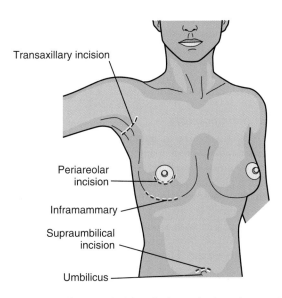

Transaxillary incision

Periareolar
incision

Inframammary

Supraumbilical
incision

Umbilicus

• **Fig. 40.22** Common incisions for breast implant placement.

• **Fig. 40.23** Transumbilical breast augmentation (TUBA).

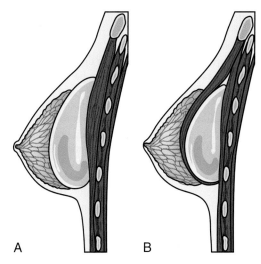

A   B

• **Fig. 40.24** Placement of breast implants. **A,** Placement of implant under the mammary gland and above the pectoralis muscle. **B,** Placement of implant under the pectoralis muscle.

made transversely along the submammary fold. The implant is inserted into a pocket formed between the mammary gland and pectoralis muscle or under the muscle (Fig. 40.24).

An implant also can be inserted through a supraumbilical endoscopic approach (transumbilical breast augmentation [TUBA]). This technique eliminates an incision into the breast. A single incision is made in the superior border of the inner aspect of the umbilicus. An endoscope is tunneled between the fascia and subcutaneous tissue up to the breast.

Subpectoral pockets are dissected to accommodate breast implants. The dissection can be performed bluntly or by saline balloon expansion. The endoscope permits visual placement of a deflated **expander** between the breast tissue and the pectoralis muscle. The expander is filled with sterile saline solution, through a fill tube, to create a pocket for the implant. After insertion through the endoscope into the pocket, the deflated implant is inflated with sterile IV saline solution, and the fill tube is removed.

Implants are supplied sterile by the manufacturer. The manufacturer's instructions for sterilization of nonsterile implants must be followed. Sterile packages should not be opened by the circulating nurse until the surgeon selects the appropriate-sized implants. Silastic sizers are frequently used to make this determination. The implant identification card should be put in the patient's chart and each implant's catalog and lot number recorded.

The woman with breast implants is not excluded from routine screening mammography programs. Additional radiologic images may be taken to visualize all of the breast tissue. Ultrasonography may be performed at the same time to confirm the integrity of the implant. Studies have shown that the risk for rupturing the implant is not increased by compression during mammography if performed according to the American College of Radiology standards.

Capsular contraction, hematoma, infection, and skin necrosis are potential complications after prosthetic implantation for breast augmentation performed either unilaterally or bilaterally. Because of reported incidences of rupture and leakage, with the possibility of the development of autoimmune disease, implants containing silicone gel are not used for breast augmentation or reconstruction unless women are enrolled in a controlled clinical study.

Explantation, or removing a ruptured or leaking silicone implant, frequently is complicated by intracapsular adhesions, also referred to as capsular contractures. Control of bleeding points is critical, to prevent silicone emboli in open blood vessels. This necessitates meticulous capsular dissection and hemostasis during removal of the implant shell, as well as irrigation with copious amounts of sterile saline solution to remove viscous silicone from the wound.

Reconstructive Mammoplasty

Breast reconstruction after mastectomy psychologically helps the patient cope with an altered body image. The type and timing of reconstruction are influenced by the patient's psychologic response to the mastectomy, the type of mastectomy, and the patient's diagnosis and prognosis.[5] Technical maneuvers of the general surgeon at the time of mastectomy will influence the possibility of an aesthetically acceptable result after breast reconstruction by the plastic surgeon. To reconstruct breast contour, an implant may be inserted beneath the muscle layers at the time of subcutaneous mastectomy in patients having prophylactic mastectomies.

After modified radical or radical mastectomy, the wound should be well healed, the scar mature, and the skin well vascularized before implantation. A prosthesis can be implanted only when reliable skin is available to cover it. Skin flaps should be cut as thickly as is consistent with a curative mastectomy. If sufficient skin flaps are not available, the plastic surgeon may use a tissue expander or transfer a pedicle skin flap from the abdomen or back to the chest wall.[6]

Immediate breast reconstruction, or a delay of only a few days, after a modified radical mastectomy can be psychologically advantageous in women who have small lesions and no metastases. A latissimus dorsi myocutaneous flap may be used with an inflatable implant. A vertical or TRAM island flap with the vascular bundle from the superior epigastric vessels, deep inferior epigastric perforator (DIEP) flap, or superficial inferior epigastric artery (SIEA) flap can be used without an implant (Fig. 40.25).[7] These flaps also can be used immediately or weeks to months after mastectomy for reconstruction. Aesthetically, the end result is a semblance of a breast in weight and consistency. The goal is fullness rather than projection from the chest. An areola and nipple complex may be constructed in a second-stage surgical procedure. Dermapigmentation (a form of tattooing) may be used to create natural color and shading resembling the nipple-areola complex. The initial tattoo may appear darker, but becomes lighter in color over time.

The techniques described may be contraindicated in markedly obese patients and in some patients who do not have a sufficient amount of autogenous tissue for breast reconstruction. Another option is to place a tissue expander under the pectoralis muscle (see Fig. 40.11). When the desired expansion is achieved, usually slightly larger than the other breast, the expander can be replaced with a permanent prosthesis.

One type of expander/mammary prosthesis has a detachable reservoir and tubing to convert the expander into a permanent prosthesis. If this technique is not an option and the patient does not have adequate tissue in the lower abdomen or back, transfer of a microvascular free flap may be the procedure of choice. The vascular pedicle from a transverse abdominis rectus, superior gluteal, or inferior gluteal myocutaneous free flap may be anastomosed to the axillary or thoracodorsal vessels.

Reduction Mammoplasty

Hyperplasia of the breasts is reduced by resection of skin and glandular tissue. Reduction mammoplasty is usually sought by women for comfort as well as aesthetic improvement of body image. The nipple-areola complexes are mobilized and transferred intact with the underlying breast tissue, maintaining the blood and nerve supply (Fig. 40.26). The excess skin and glandular tissue may be excised with a scalpel, dermatome blade, or laser (Fig. 40.27). Because breast tissue is very vascular, attention to hemostasis is important. The CO_2 laser offers the advantage of coagulating small blood vessels and sealing lymphatics as tissue is incised. A hemostatic scalpel can be used for the same purposes.

Reduction of the Male Breast

Reduction of the male breast is carried out for gynecomastia, a pathologic condition that consists of bilateral or unilateral enlargement of the male breast.[8] Gynecomastia occurs primarily after 40 years of age or during puberty and is usually related to alterations in the normal hormonal balance. All subareolar fibroglandular tissue is removed, followed by reconstruction of the resultant defect. Some surgeons perform liposuction-assisted procedures to debulk the male breast (Fig. 40.28). If liposuction is used, a compression vest is worn for 4 to 6 weeks postoperatively. Carcinoma can occur in the male breast.

Scars

Scar formation, the body's mechanism for healing wounds, is inevitable whenever skin is incised or injured. The plastic surgeon attempts to make a scar a fine line and as level and smooth as possible at the time of primary wound closure or as a secondary scar revision.

Scar Revision

The plastic surgeon can excise an aesthetically displeasing scar and then realign wound edges and close them with anticipation of a better cosmetic result. The direction of a scar can be changed to be less conspicuous in the natural skin lines. Scars are frequently revised after extensive reconstructive procedures or after a laceration with or without soft tissue trauma, particularly a facial scar. Z-plasty, W-plasty, M-plasty, lazy-S, Y-V-plasty, and other techniques are used to improve the appearance of a hypertrophied or prominent scar (Fig. 40.29).

Keloid formation, an abnormal deposition of collagen in healing skin wounds, presents a particularly difficult problem for the plastic surgeon and a psychologic problem for the patient. Keloids may require excision and grafting. The administration of a lathyrogenic agent and colchicine to inhibit cross-linking of newly synthesized collagen after grafting may prevent the development of recurrent keloid formation. Silicone sheeting sometimes helps reduce the bulkiness. The argon laser also is used in treating keloid scars to reduce the blood supply to the scar and to alter the balance of collagen synthesis and lysis.

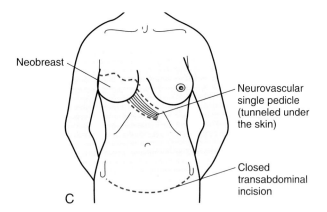

• **Fig. 40.25** Transverse rectus abdominis myocutaneous (TRAM) flap. **A,** Single TRAM flap with one rectus muscle used for neobreast. **B,** Both rectus muscles can be dissected for neobreasts if bilateral mastectomy is performed. **C,** Closed abdominal incision spans transversely from iliac crest to iliac crest. The neobreast remains attached to the vascular stalk to preserve viability of the breast mound created by the TRAM flap.

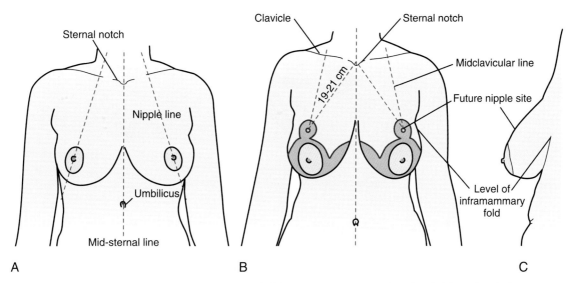

• **Fig. 40.26** Nipple symmetry measurement. **A,** Measurements are taken from the clavicle to the nipple. The midline is marked from the sternal notch to the umbilicus. **B,** The desired placement of the elevated nipple line is measured in a triangulated line based on the midline sternal notch. The average distance is 19 to 21 cm. **C,** The final measurement is taken laterally from the inframammary fold to the central breast anteriorly.

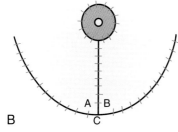

• **Fig. 40.27** Breast reduction. **A,** A keyhole incision is made in the breasts bilaterally. The tissue is deepithelialized, and the nipple is repositioned at the apex of the keyhole. **B,** The nipple is circumferentially sutured in place. The inframammary tissue is approximated vertically, followed by closure of the inframammary fold.

Dermabrasion

Dirt and cinders can become embedded in the dermis from a brush burn injury. The plastic surgeon may use a stiff nylon brush to scrub out dirt and irrigate it from the area with warm saline

• **Fig. 40.28** Contours for male breast reduction by liposuction.

solution. Medical sandpaper sometimes can be used. This procedure is not always satisfactory if many pitted scars are too deep to reach or there are changes in the pigment of scars. Some plastic surgeons prefer to use chemical preparations, such as phenol, trichloroacetic acid, or alpha hydroxy acid (glycolic acid), to produce dermal peeling for a skin-smoothing effect in select patients with facial scars or fine wrinkles.

The patient is advised to avoid direct sun exposure for at least 6 months. Patients with fair complexions and thin skin have more favorable results than do patients with dark, oily complexions because the chemicals used decrease melanin in the skin and cause discoloration.

A high-speed dermabrader with rotating tips covered with diamond dust can be used on moderately damaged or tattooed skin. The rotating speed is controlled by regulation of pressure from the compressed nitrogen gas power source. Older dermabraders have narrow bands of waterproof, steam-sterilizable sandpaper mounted on an electric, air-powered, or battery-operated drill. Care is taken by the team to wear appropriate eye protection

• **Fig. 40.29** Z-plasty technique of scar revision.

CO_2, Carbon dioxide; *KTP:YAG*, potassium titanyl phosphate:yttrium aluminum garnet.
From Fortunato NM, McCullough SM: *Plastic and reconstructive surgery*, St. Louis, 1998, Mosby.

TABLE 40.1	**Examples of Lasers Used for Skin Surface Modifications**	
Type of Laser	**Spectrum of Light**	**Notes**
Argon	Blue-green	Used for treatment of superficial vascular lesions, pigmented areas, and some inflammatory lesions; absorbed by hemoglobin
CO_2	Infrared	Has a red aiming beam to make the invisible infrared laser visible; absorbed by water
Tunable dye (Candela)	Yellow	Used to treat port-wine stains and vascular ectasia; very selective vascular destruction; absorbed by pigmented tissues
KTP:YAG	Green	Used to treat tattoos, vascular lesions, and pigmented lesions; good for removal of black, yellow, or blue; works well for dark-skinned patients; articulated arm
Alexandrite	Red	Used to treat tattoos, particularly blue, black, and green; not good for orange or yellow; fiberoptic: flexible arm

to shield against splashes and aerosolization of tissue, blood, and fluids.

Facial resurfacing also can be accomplished with the CO_2 laser. The depth of laser penetration is controlled by the focus of the beam. Full-face laser resurfacing promotes continuity of skin color and texture rather than spot removal of facial scars (Table 40.1).

Skin Cancer

Basal cell carcinoma, squamous cell carcinoma, and malignant melanoma are the three most common types of skin cancers.

Because overexposure to ultraviolet (UV) rays in sunlight is the primary cause of skin cancer, most skin cancers occur on exposed areas of the face, head, neck, and ears. Certain types of nevi are skin lesions that may be precancerous and therefore should be removed.

Non-UV skin cancers such as epidermolysis bullosa (EB) are inherited skin disorders that cause fatal metastatic cancers in young patients. The usual site of EB is chronic wounds that develop into long-term cutaneous scars. Poorly healing burns are frequently sites for EB that develop squamous cell cancers. One theory suggests that the constant process of healing triggers the cancer in susceptible patients. Surveillance of potential EB in these patients is recommended every 3 to 6 months from the age of 10 years and every 3 months from the age of 16 years. Squamous cell cancers discovered during the examinations are excised widely and full thickness. The extent of excision depends on whether lymphatic involvement can be identified. Treatment can involve chemotherapy, radiation, or amputation.

Suspicious UV and non-UV lesions may be removed by the following methods:
- Excision and closure with sutures, grafts, or flaps
- Punch biopsy with closure by second intention
- Cold-knife excision for frozen section
- Electrosurgical curettage and electrodesiccation
- Cryosurgery
- Laser surgery
- Radiation therapy

Mohs Micrographic Surgery

Mohs micrographic surgery is a technique used to excise advanced, recurrent, or poorly defined basal cell or squamous cell carcinomas of the skin with minimal excision of normal tissue. The bulk of the clinically evident tumor is excised initially. Then the lesion is resected by serial tangential excision (i.e., underlying tissue layers are removed with 1–3-mm borders). Each layer is numbered and charted for size and location. A map of the corresponding margins of each layer is drawn. The tissue is frozen, cut into sections, and examined microscopically (Fig. 40.30).

The patient may be allowed to leave the OR and wait in a waiting room for the results. The surgeon removes additional layers of tissue or extends dissection until microscopic examination determines that all cancer cells have been removed. A map of the excisional area is created and then the wound is closed.

Small wounds may be left open to heal by second intention. Others may be sutured or covered with a rotational myocutaneous flap from an adjacent area. Large denuded areas may require an STSG or FTSG. If a cartilage graft is needed, cartilage may be transferred from the auricle (pinna) of the ear to the transplantation site.

Mohs surgery is not used for excision of malignant melanomas. Primary melanomas are treated according to their anatomic site and level of cutaneous penetration. A wide margin of normal tissue is excised around the melanoma. Skin grafts often are

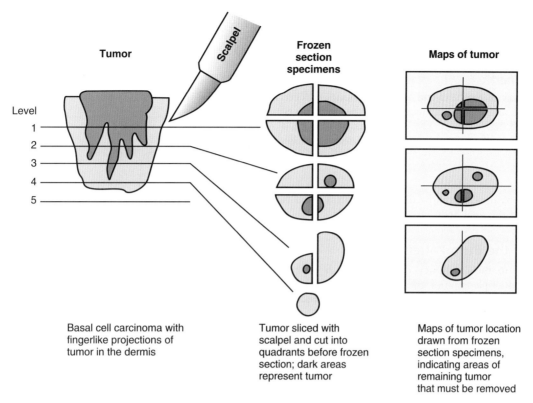

Tumor

Scalpel

Frozen section specimens

Maps of tumor

Level
1
2
3
4
5

Basal cell carcinoma with fingerlike projections of tumor in the dermis

Tumor sliced with scalpel and cut into quadrants before frozen section; dark areas represent tumor

Maps of tumor location drawn from frozen section specimens, indicating areas of remaining tumor that must be removed

• **Fig. 40.30** Mohs microscopic excisional tissue mapping.

required. Regional lymph node dissection may be indicated to control metastatic disease.

Burns

Skin and underlying tissues can be destroyed by thermal, chemical, or electrical injury. Burns are open wounds. As with other injuries, initial treatment is aimed at saving the patient's life. Then the treatment is directed toward preserving or restoring to normal, or as nearly normal as possible, the patient's bodily functions and appearance as rapidly as possible. The depth of the burn will determine how well cell regeneration presents and forms scar tissue. Researchers are working on various cell-regenerating processes to grow autografts from the patient's own cells.[9]

Depending on the depth, extent, and location of the burn, reconstruction may extend over long periods, from months to years. The patient must be helped to accept the disfigurement; thus rehabilitation from a psychologic standpoint is important. Psychotherapy, as well as surgery and physiotherapy, may be necessary to promote as early a return to normalcy and usefulness as possible.

Classification of Burns

The severity of the injury is determined by the location and the cause of the burn. The Abbreviated Burn Severity Index (ABSI) is a five-variable scale used to evaluate burn injury severity and the probability of survival.[10] The five variables are sex, age, presence of inhalation injury, presence of full-thickness burn, and percentage of total body surface burned. An ABSI score of 2 to 18 is calculated by the summation of coded values for each variable. Burns are classified by depth and extent as soon after injury as possible. Many burns are a combination of depths. The depth of a burn is classified by the degree of tissue involvement:

- *First-degree superficial burn:* Only the outer layer of the epidermis is involved in a first-degree burn. Superficial erythema, redness of the skin, and tissue destruction occur, but healing takes place rapidly.
- *Second-degree partial-thickness burn:* All of the epidermis and varying depths of the dermis are destroyed in a second-degree burn. This is usually characterized by blister formation, pain, and a moist, mottled red or pink appearance. Hair follicles and sebaceous glands may be destroyed. Reepithelialization can occur provided the deepest layer of the epithelium is viable. Superimposed infection can interfere with healing. Thickened scars form after healing of deep second-degree burns.
- *Third-degree full-thickness burn:* The skin, with all of its epithelial structures and subcutaneous tissue, is destroyed in a third-degree burn. This is characterized by a dry, pearly white or charred-appearing surface void of sensation. The destroyed skin forms a parchment-like eschar over the burned area. If removed or left to slough off, eschar leaves a denuded surface that can extend to the fascia. Third-degree burns require skin grafts for healing to occur unless the area is small enough for closure by reepithelialization.
- *Fourth-degree burn:* Sometimes referred to as char burns, fourth-degree burns may damage bones, tendons, muscles, blood vessels, and peripheral nerves. An electrical burn, for example, causes damage much deeper than is apparent on the skin surface. Often, necrotic muscle and bone must be excised.

Estimation of Burn Damage

Two methods are used to estimate the total percentage of body surface burned and the percentage of each degree of burn.

Lund-Browder Chart

The percentage sizes of the head and lower extremities differ in infancy, childhood, and adulthood. According to the guidelines of the Lund-Browder chart (Fig. 40.31), the percentage of burn is estimated on the basis of age in addition to the anatomic location of the burn.

Rule of Nines

The body surface of an adult can be divided into areas equal to multiples of 9% of the total body surface (Fig. 40.32).

Initial Care of the Burn Patient

Patients admitted to the emergency department with obvious burns may have multiple injuries and/or a pretrauma medical history that will complicate treatment. Initial care must include the following measures:

1. *Stop the burning process:* All clothing, jewelry, and metal and synthetic objects in contact with the patient's skin are removed.
2. *Ensure a patent airway:* The respiratory system may be damaged from inhalation of superheated air or toxic gases. Immediate nasotracheal intubation with assisted mechanical ventilation may be necessary. Soft endotracheal tubes are

preferred for prolonged intubation. Tracheotomy may be required several days later for prolonged respiratory assistance if the patient cannot be weaned from the ventilator. Bronchoscopy is performed routinely to evaluate the extent of tracheobronchial damage.

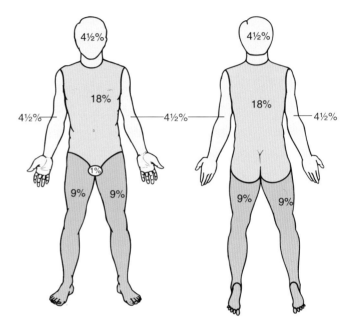

• **Fig. 40.32** Rule of nines chart to estimate burn injury to an adult.

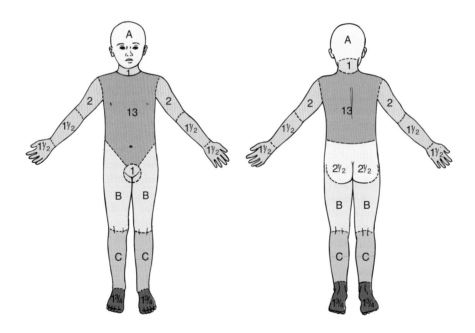

Relative percentage of areas affected by growth	Age in Years					
	0	1	5	10	15	Adult
A—½ of head	9½	8½	6½	5½	4½	3½
B—½ of one thigh	2¾	3¼	4	4¼	4½	4¾
C—½ of one leg	2½	2½	2¾	3	3¼	3½
Total percent burned		2°+		3°−		

• **Fig. 40.31** Lund-Browder chart to determine relative percentage of areas of burns on child's body.

3. *Establish IV fluid therapy:* Blood samples are drawn for laboratory analysis and type and crossmatching when a venipuncture, cutdown, or central line initiation is performed to establish an IV route for fluid and nutritional administration. Fluid and electrolyte balance must be restored as quickly as possible. Fluid, electrolytes, and protein are lost through changes in capillary permeability, causing intravascular volume shifts to interstitial tissues (third spacing). Fluid shifts are directly proportional to the depth and extent of the burn. Several formulas for determining fluid replacement have been developed to maintain plasma volume during the first 24 hours (Table 40.2). The calculated fluid replacement time begins at the time of injury, not when the patient arrives in the emergency department. A crystalloid solution of lactated Ringer's solution is infused initially because its hypertonic state decreases fluid loss from the intravascular space. Colloid-containing fluid, fresh frozen plasma, and other nutrients may be infused after the first 24 hours. The colloids will provide essential proteins to maintain balance in the intravascular compartment.

TABLE 40.2 — Fluid Replacement Formulas[a] for Burn Patients Developed at Major Burn Centers

First 24 Hours	Second 24 Hours
Parkland Hospital	
Crystalloid	
4 mL Ringer's lactate/% burn/kg	Dextrose 5% in water
Half during first 8 hours	Maintenance
Half during next 16 hours	
Colloid	
None	0.5 mL/% burn/kg
Brooke Army Hospital	
Crystalloid	
2 mL Ringer's lactate/% burn/kg	Dextrose 5% in water
Half during first 8 hours	Maintenance
Half during next 16 hours	
Colloid	
None	0.5 mL/% burn/kg
Massachusetts General Hospital	
Crystalloid	
1.5 mL Ringer's lactate/% burn/kg	None specified
Half during first 8 hours	
Half during next 16 hours	
Colloid	
0.5 mL/% burn/kg	None specified
None during first 4 hours	
Half during second 4 hours	
Half during next 16 hours	

[a]Formula is calculated as percent of total body surface area (% TBSA) × each kilogram (kg) of body weight × milliliters (mL) of fluid.

---

4. *Insert an indwelling Foley catheter:* Renal function is monitored closely. Urine specimens are sent for analysis. Urine is checked for pH and specific gravity at frequent intervals. The hourly output is recorded. Adequate fluid replacement should maintain an output of at least 30 mL/h.

5. *Cleanse the wound:* All burns are treated with sterile technique. A mild cleansing agent, such as povidone-iodine, and warm water or saline solution are used to gently remove debris and loose, devitalized tissue. Copious amounts of water, along with appropriate neutralizing agents, are used to cleanse and irrigate chemical burns. After cleansing, wet sheets under and around the patient must be removed and dry, sterile sheets applied. Nonwoven sheets specifically designed for burn care are commercially available.

6. *Estimate the percentage and depth of the burn:* Definitive treatment may be completed in the emergency department, or the patient may be transported to an immersion tank for further cleansing and debridement or to the OR for initiation of further therapy as indicated by assessment of the burn. The burned area is covered with sterile or clean linen for transfer of the patient from the emergency department.

7. *Assess the patient's preexisting medical history and other injuries:* The patient may have a chronic illness, such as diabetes or heart disease, that must be stabilized as part of the treatment regimen. Withdrawal from alcohol or drugs may cause physiologic disturbances. The patient may have suffered other injuries in the accident causing the burn. Abuse may be suspected, particularly in a child or older person. Appropriate interventions must be taken. The burn may not be the first priority if, for example, the patient has a head injury, ruptured internal organs, or fractures.

8. *Prepare the patient for transport:* The patient may go from the emergency department directly to a burn unit, the OR, or some other care area. The attending physician may initiate therapy before referral to a plastic surgeon. If available, hyperbaric oxygen (HBO) therapy may be used. HBO produces marked vasoconstriction, decreasing the loss of serum through the burn surface. This may reduce the need for fluid replacement.

Oxygen in cells around the burn may positively affect burn tissue to regenerate and begin healing. Partial-thickness burns may be prevented from progressing to full-thickness burns.

Methods of Surgical Treatment

Prevention of infection and promotion of healing are of utmost concern in the treatment of burn patients. The probability of infection developing increases in proportion to the percentage of body surface burned. Colonization of microorganisms may begin as early as 24 hours after the burn.

Excisional Debridement

Primary excision of necrotic tissue from deep second-degree and all full-thickness third-degree burned areas, followed immediately by skin grafting, is performed as soon as possible after the injury. Debridement can be accomplished with a scalpel, scissors, or other specialized instrument. The surgeon selects the most appropriate instrument for the particular burned area to be excised. Layers of burned tissue are removed sequentially until capillary bleeding indicates that tissue is viable. Hypotensive anesthesia may help control massive blood loss during extensive excisions.

Wound Bed Cover After Debridement

Areas of denuded tissue lose large amounts of fluid and provide a portal of entry for microorganisms. Skin replacement includes the use of natural and synthetic materials. First-line natural material is the patient's own skin and tissue (autograft). The availability of donor skin on the patient's body depends on the extent of injury and location of the recipient site. Meshed grafts are frequently used to expand coverage with small amounts of autografted skin. The patient's own skin (keratinocytes and fibroblasts) can be cultured and grown for placement over a wound (Epicel). Other techniques include growing autologous cells in a suspension and spraying them over the recipient site. Autologous fibroblasts can be incorporated into a hyaluronic matrix and placed over a wound.[8]

Allogeneic epidermal keratinocytes and dermal cells can serve as a biomaterial wound cover, but are not permanent. The recipient wound bed granulates and eventually rejects the allograft, requiring excision and regrafting with available autograft. Biologic materials used include neonatal skin cells from newborn circumcisions (Celaderm, OrCel), and cadavers. Allograft cells can be used alone (AlloDerm) or grown into porcine or bovine collagen or into synthetic materials such as silicone (TransCyte), polyglactin mesh (Dermagraft), and collagen (Apligraf and StrataGraft). Duration of allograft effectiveness can last for several weeks before rejection.

Xenograft of bovine or porcine collagen is derived from dermis and submucosa (Permacol, EZ Derm, Matriderm, and Oasis). A composite acellular silicone-nylon membrane with a chemically bonded polypeptide of porcine collagen, such as Biobrane, Suprathel, or Omiderm, will adhere to the wound surface to inhibit infection and control fluid loss for 7 to 10 days, stimulating granulation tissue and preparing the wound bed for autologous grafting.

Tangential Excision

Burned tissue is excised until normal dermal tissue is reached below the depth of the wound. Tangential excision is usually the procedure of choice for deep partial-thickness burns of the dorsum of the hands or on the arms or legs. It is advantageous to minimize contractures. The wound base, containing some viable dermal structures necessary for regeneration, is covered with a split-thickness autograft. Early tangential excision and grafting in one procedure for body surface burns can reduce mortality and septic complications and shorten hospitalization.

Escharectomy

Full-thickness eschar is excised down to the fascia when viable tissues in more superficial layers are not evident, except on the hands, neck, or face. All denuded areas created by excision are covered with a biologic dressing for 3 to 5 days. They are then grafted with full-thickness autografts. Frequently, split-thickness mesh grafts must be used to spread over large areas and allow seepage of serous fluids. These are not placed on the face and neck or over joints. If sufficient skin is not available for autografting, allografts or xenografts continue to be used as biologic dressings for short periods. They are changed every 3 to 5 days.

Other Surgical Procedures

During the course of hospitalization, a burn patient may come to the OR for one or many procedures. The patient is compromised and may be given a tetanus shot during treatment.

Escharotomy

Shrinkage of eschar may occur and cause a tourniquet effect in circumferential burns of the extremities or thorax. Bilateral incisions through the eschar, not including the fascia, are made to improve circulation to a lower extremity. Multiple incisions on the chest wall relieve respiratory distress. Sites of incisions avoid major peripheral nerves to prevent irreversible neurologic complications.

Fasciotomy

If adequate decompression does not occur after escharotomy, the incision may be extended into underlying fascia. Compartment syndrome can develop as blood or serum effuses between the fascial layers. The fascia may need to be incised in the body part if compromised circulation is evident. The incised layers will remain open for weeks or months and may need skin grafts to completely heal.

Amputation of Digits

Amputation may be necessary to control infection in the extremity and prevent septicemia if escharotomy is unsuccessful.

Debridement

Debridement of underlying tissues helps prevent extension of tissue loss. Nonviable tendons, cartilage, or bone may be excised, such as from the hand, ear, or skull.

Full-Thickness Skin Grafts

With or without tarsorrhaphy, FTSGs are used to prevent contracture of the eyelids. The cornea must be protected from exposure with corneal shields and lubrication.

Split-Thickness Skin Grafts

Autografts are applied to debrided areas as rapidly as possible. The hands and face are the first priority to restore function; joints and flexion creases are second to prevent contractures; and the extremities and trunk are the lowest priority. Skin from donor sites is cut thin if the site will be used again. Mesh grafts are frequently used to cover very large surfaces or irregular areas such as the perineum. Grafts are held in place with staples or sutures and dressings to achieve apposition and immobilization.

Tissue Expansion

If sufficient normal skin is available, a tissue expander may be placed beneath subcutaneous tissue to broaden the width for future use as a local flap to cover an adjacent burned area after excision of scar tissue or for better closure of the donor site.

Myocutaneous Flaps

Myocutaneous flaps, either on a pedicle or by free microvascular transfer, may be used in the reconstruction of burn wounds.

Biologic Dressing Changes

Instead of leaving a biologic dressing in place until rejection, with attendant inflammatory reaction, a biologic dressing is usually replaced as often as needed until the area is ready for an autograft or skin for an autograft is available. Biologic dressings may be allografts of human skin from a living or cadaver donor, placental or amniotic membranes, or a xenograft of porcine skin. Porcine dressings are applied initially on second-degree burns as a temporary dressing or used in conjunction with extensive excisional therapy. Synthetic skin substitutes may be preferred. A biologic dressing is used for the following several reasons:

- It helps control infection by covering denuded areas.
- It prevents loss of serum.
- It decreases pain.
- It seems to stimulate the formation of epithelium in dermis under it.
- It promotes growth of granulation tissue.

Dressing Changes

Occlusive dressings, if used, must be changed frequently to control infection harboring under them. An antimicrobial or chemotherapeutic agent may be applied as an integral part of the dressing. The following considerations apply:

1. *Silver sulfadiazine (Silvadene 1%) cream* applied directly to the burned area makes removal of a dressing less painful and does not disturb the healing process as it is removed. It is an effective topical antimicrobial and produces no metabolic side effects; some patients have developed neutropenia and delayed wound healing after its use. Some patients may develop a fungal infection.

Fresh cream is applied after cleansing and debridement. A layer of fine mesh gauze is laid over it (unless the open-exposure method will be used for further healing). Then soft, absorbent material, such as fluffed gauze, and a preformed splint may be used. These are held in place by a cotton elastic bandage. An occlusive dressing may be used to hold a hand, foot, or joint in functional position.

Silver sulfadiazine is a pregnancy class B drug and is not used if the patient has a sulfa allergy or is pregnant. The use of the cream is contraindicated on a pregnant woman near term because of the risk for kernicterus in the fetus. It should not be used on infants younger than 2 months of age.

2. *Mafenide acetate (Sulfamylon 5%) cream* penetrates intact eschar rapidly and is quite successful in reducing bacterial counts to optimal levels for skin grafting. Application directly on the burned area is painful for the patient after cleansing and debridement. It may cause maceration under the dressing. Absorption may result in metabolic acidosis; thus the acid-base balance must be closely monitored. Prolonged use may lead to renal or pulmonary complications.

Sulfamylon is available in a topical solution form. It is supplied in a 50-g package that can be added to a 1000-mL bottle of sterile saline or water for irrigation. Once prepared, the solution should be discarded after 48 hours. The solution is used to keep grafted skin dressings moist. Irrigation should not be done longer than 5 days because it can inhibit epithelial regeneration.

3. *Silver nitrate solution 0.5% in sterile distilled water* is used infrequently. After cleansing and debridement, multiple-thickness dressings are applied to the area. These are kept saturated with 0.5% silver nitrate solution and changed every 12 hours. For debridement, sterile distilled water is used for irrigation because saline may cause the precipitation of silver salts. It is ineffective in treating established wound infection because it does not penetrate intact eschar.

Care is taken to avoid splashing silver nitrate solution onto walls and floors because staining can occur. If disposable drapes and gowns are not used, stained linen must be laundered separately from other linen.

Serial Biopsy Cultures

Through two linear incisions, a biopsy of tissue, including subcutaneous fat, is excised for culturing. This is done every 2 or 3 days, until the eschar begins to separate, to monitor the colonization of microorganisms in the wound. The results of serial biopsy culture enable the surgeon to make decisions specific to the therapeutic needs of the patient. An antimicrobial or chemotherapeutic topical agent is selected or changed according to these results.

Treatment of Curling Ulcer

Gastrointestinal complications may occur any time from the early postinjury period through rehabilitation. Complaints must be carefully evaluated. The patient who develops massive bleeding from a stress ulcer in the stomach and duodenum (Curling ulcer) must be operated on. Vagotomy with antrectomy are most frequently performed by a general surgeon.

Treatment of Marjolin Ulcer

An ulceration caused by malignant changes (Marjolin ulcer) can develop in the surface area of a burn scar. As long as 20 years after the burn, a prolonged ulceration can lead to squamous cell carcinoma of the skin. The ulcer should be excised.

Environmental Considerations for Burn Patients

1. Environmental control is perhaps the essence of burn therapy. The environment must protect the wound from further injury and microbial invasion. A burn wound is always potentially contaminated until epithelialization occurs. Open exposure of the wound to room air may be the choice of the plastic surgeon for select patients. Regardless of the method of treatment, the following adjuncts are used, if the equipment is available, in the care of burn patients, in addition to strict adherence to all the principles of aseptic technique:
   a. Reverse isolation technique may be practiced to protect the patient, whose resistance is low, from infection from personnel. Caps, masks, shoe covers, sterile gowns, and sterile gloves are worn by all personnel attending the patient. This may be referred to as protective isolation.
   b. Laminar, or downward unidirectional, airflow away from the wound helps minimize airborne contamination.
   c. A plastic isolator protects the patient. Personnel do not directly enter this isolation unit. Patient care is given through clear plastic access walls. The environment around the patient inside the isolator is controlled at 90° F (32° C) and 94% relative humidity to conserve heat loss by evaporation.
2. Patients with extensive burns may be placed on a multifunction suspension bed specially designed to facilitate handling and turning. They are transported to the OR on these frames or beds. Patients must be turned slowly and gently because they are often hypovolemic after the injury.
3. Hypothermia must be prevented. The patient's thermoregulatory mechanism is altered by the destruction of skin that normally acts as an insulator. Heat loss is the greatest single problem the burn patient faces in the OR.
   a. The room temperature should be increased to between 80° F and 90° F (27−32° C) with low relative humidity of about 30% to 40%.
   b. The OR must be ready to receive the patient directly from the burn unit. The patient should not wait in a cool

holding area or corridor. Concern is for the patient's thermoregulation and potential for infection.

c. A warm hyperthermia blanket should cover the OR bed. The patient should be exposed as little as possible. Cover with warm blankets.

d. The patient's temperature should be monitored with a rectal or esophageal probe. Affixing skin probes may be contraindicated when large areas of tissue are damaged.

e. Solutions should be warmed before irrigation or infusion.

f. Operating during nighttime hours is advantageous for the patient because the normal schedule for oral intake is not interrupted.

4. Hypnosis and biofeedback techniques can reduce potential postanesthetic complications when many surgical procedures are necessary to achieve acceptable functional and aesthetic results after a burn. The OR environment must be quiet to be conducive to hypnotic suggestions given to the patient.

After the initial assessment of a severely burned patient, a prolonged period of treatment begins. A multidisciplinary team must coordinate the treatment plan to achieve the best possible clinical outcome for the patient. As with all plastic surgery patients, both physiologic support and psychosocial support are essential to successful rehabilitation.

EVOLVE WEBSITE

http://evolve.elsevier.com/Hornacky/BerryKohn/

- Historical Perspective
- Student Interactive Questions
- Glossary

References

1. Ogawa R: Surgery for scar revision and reduction: from primary closure to flap surgery, *Burns Trauma* 7(1):1–8, 2019.
2. Kollar B, Tasigiorgos S, Dorante MI, et al.: Innovations in reconstructive microsurgery: reconstructive transplantation, *J Surg Oncol* 118(5):800–806, 2018.
3. Lemogne C, Bellivier F, Fakra E, et al.: Psychological and psychiatric aspects of face transplantation: lessons learned from the long-term follow-up of six patients, *J Psychosom Res* 119(4):42–49, 2019.
4. Rifkin WJ, Manjunath A, Kimberly L, et al.: Long-distance care of face transplant recipients in the United States, *J Plast Reconstr Aesthet Surg* 71(10):1383–1391, 2018.
5. Chung AM, Stein MJ, Ghumman A, et al.: The effect of post mastectomy radiation therapy on breast reconstruction with and without acellular dermal matrix: a systematic review and meta-analysis protocol, *Syst Rev* 8(1):1–4, 2019.
6. Ding J, Lei L, Liu S, et al.: Macrophages are necessary for skin regeneration during tissue expansion, *J Transl Med* 17(1):1–10, 2019.
7. Speck N, Grufman V, Farhadi J: Trends and innovation in autologous breast reconstruction, *Arch Plast Surg* 50:240–247, 2023.
8. Salzillo R, Barone M, Cogliandro A, et al.: Evaluation of glandular liposculpture as a single treatment for grades I and II gynecomastia, *Aesthetic Plast Surg* 43(2):546–547, 2019.
9. Shpichka A, Butnaru D, Bezrukov EA, et al.: Skin tissue regeneration for burn injury, *Stem Cell Res Ther* 10(1):1–16, 2019.
10. Usmani A, Pipal D, Bagla H, et al.: Prediction of mortality in acute burn patients using the Abbreviated Burn Severity Index score: a single-center experience, *Cureus* 14(6):e26161, 2022.

41

Otorhinolaryngologic and Head and Neck Surgery

CHAPTER OUTLINE

General Considerations in Ear, Nose, and Throat Procedures, 873

Ear, 876

Nose, 881

Oral Cavity and Throat, 885

Neck, 889

Face and Skull, 897

CHAPTER OBJECTIVES

After studying this chapter, the learner will be able to:

- Identify the pertinent anatomy of the ear, nose, and throat.
- Describe the care of the patient having an otorhinolaryngologic procedure.
- List the main types of hearing loss and the treatments.
- Discuss the psychologic effects of head and neck surgery.
- List the precautions of caring for the patient with a tracheostomy.

KEY TERMS AND DEFINITIONS

Anomaly Abnormal development.

Cholesteatoma A mass of cholesterol and epithelial cells in the middle ear.

Cleft A separation of tissue.

Congenital Condition present at birth.

Deglutition Swallowing.

Glossoptosis Prolapsed tongue.

-Gnathia Jaw structure.

Suture Joint between skull bones that ossifies with age under normal circumstances.

General Considerations in Ear, Nose, and Throat Procedures

Surgical procedures of the structures of the head and neck region are not within the province of any one surgical specialty. Subspecialists from many disciplines, most notably general surgeons, plastic surgeons, otolaryngologists, and dentists, limit their surgical practice to specific types of problems involving areas of the head and/or neck. Training in these subspecialties is included in specialty postgraduate programs.

Otorhinolaryngology has traditionally been concerned with research and surgical treatment of diseases of the ear (oto), nose (rhino), and throat (laryngo). Advances in scientific knowledge, diagnostic capabilities, and technology have broadened the scope of this field, which has led to subspecialization. General otorhinolaryngologists, commonly called ear, nose, and throat (ENT) surgeons, practice within the total scope of this specialty. Other surgeons confine their practice to one of the subspecialties: otology, facial surgery, or head and neck oncology. The certifying body for this specialty is the American Board of Otolaryngology.

Dental and skeletal deformities of alignment and function coexist with aesthetic appearance. These deformities may be congenital, or they may be caused by trauma or disease. They may interfere with breathing, eating, swallowing, speaking, seeing, balance, or hearing. A multidisciplinary team of surgical specialists is often required to reconstruct complex deformities. This team may be all-inclusive with a plastic surgeon, neurosurgeon, oral surgeon, orthodontist or prosthodontist, otolaryngologist, ophthalmologist, radiologist, and general surgeon, or it may be limited to two or three specialists. The team may also include a psychiatrist or psychologist, speech pathologist, and social worker. A team includes all the specialties needed for complete preoperative assessment, intraoperative care, and postoperative rehabilitation of the individual patient.

Specific considerations include the following:

1. Preoperative explanations and postoperative instructions are vital to the outcome. For example, after ear or nasal procedures the patient must avoid blowing the nose, which would force air up the eustachian tube, potentially causing infection; force air through the incision; or dislodge a graft. To sneeze, both the nose and mouth should be open.

2. Communication is a major problem for patients with loss of hearing or voice. Touch is an effective means of conveying concern and letting the patient know they are not abandoned. A form of communication should be established such as pencil and paper, an erase board, or a tablet for the patient to communicate.

Anesthesia Considerations

Anesthesia can be local or general. Use of local anesthesia minimizes bleeding and postoperative discomfort in addition to affording the surgeon observation of patient response. It allows patient cooperation. A qualified perioperative nurse may deliver moderate sedation and monitor vital signs, including cardiac function with electrocardiogram (ECG) and oxygenation with a pulse oximeter in the absence of an anesthesia provider. The nurse records the amount of local anesthesia administered and documents the patient's intraoperative responses.

Monitored anesthesia care (MAC) may be used with an anesthesia provider in attendance for more complicated patients who need additional adjunctive medication and monitoring.

General anesthesia requires good control of the airway. The presence of an endotracheal tube in the mouth during general anesthesia can distort features during a surgical procedure in the oral cavity. Nasotracheal intubation may be necessary. Special endotracheal tubes are used if a laser is used. The use of methylene blue dye in sterile saline for filling the endotracheal tube cuff is recommended. If the cuff is perforated, the dye acts as an indicator.

In complex cases involving large areas of the head and neck, the patient may have a tracheostomy created and sutured in place for the duration of the procedure. The tracheostomy may be permanent or temporary depending on the procedure performed. Great care is exercised when using a surgically created airway. Tissue manipulation can dislodge the tracheostomy tube or serious bleeding can occur. Some anesthesia providers may hyperinflate the cuff on the tube to tamponade areas of bleeding. Hyperinflation of the cuff can cause tissue ischemia and is done with great care.[1] A fiberoptic laryngoscope or lighted bougie should be on hand to monitor the status of the airway when a tracheostomy tube is used during a surgical resection.

The anesthesia provider requires periodic access to the patient's head and neck, as do the surgeon and sterile team. Positioning of the operating room (OR) bed must provide space for the anesthesia machine and other equipment, such as the microscope. The anesthesia machine may be positioned near the patient's side or feet. The endotracheal tube is taped to prevent becoming dislodged during the procedure; all connections must be tight, and tubes must be unkinked. Breathing circuits may need an extension hose if the anesthesia machine is at the foot of the OR bed. The anesthesia provider usually sits alongside the OR bed near the lower half of the patient on the side opposite the surgeon (Fig. 41.1). Provisions are made for the anesthesia provider to have access to the intravenous (IV) line when the patient's arms are tucked in at the sides. Extension IV tubing is used.

Pharmacologic Considerations

Epinephrine in a local anesthetic, such as lidocaine, is frequently used as a vasoconstrictor in ENT procedures. The epinephrine in the local anesthetic can cause cardiac dysrhythmias, and the anesthesia provider should be alerted when it is injected.

Nitrous oxide diffuses into the middle ear, causing pressure. During ear procedures, such as tympanoplasty, the nitrous oxide is decreased or discontinued once the tympanic graft is placed, to minimize inner ear pressure that could displace the graft.

Neuromuscular blockade affects the nerves of the head and neck. The use of nerve conduction monitoring or nerve stimulators is adversely affected by strong skeletal relaxation drugs.

Positioning, Prepping, and Draping

Although the oral cavity is considered contaminated, sterile equipment and sterile technique are preferred to avoid introducing exogenous bloodborne microorganisms.

The patient is positioned supine. The arms are usually tucked in at the sides or secured over the abdomen. The patient's head is positioned in a donut or horseshoe headrest to prevent movement

• **Fig. 41.1** Room setup plan for ear, nose, and throat (ENT) cases. *ESU,* Electrosurgical unit.

during the procedure. Many procedures are done with the patient in a slight reverse Trendelenburg position or with a roll under the shoulders to hyperextend the head. Some surgeons prefer to have the patient in a modified beach-chair position. This helps anatomic positioning and controls bleeding.

The patient's eyes should be protected by corneal shields and sterile ophthalmic lubricant. Care is taken not to lean on the patient's draped face during the procedure. Pressure on the patient's eye can cause eye damage and cardiac dysrhythmias.

Care with antiseptic solutions during a facial prep is necessary because they are painful and irritating if they are allowed to touch a perforated eardrum or get into the eyes. A cotton or rayon ball can be used to occlude the ear during facial prepping. Cotton fibers can stick inside the ear, causing itching and discomfort postoperatively, and a small nonradiopaque gauze (2×2 inches) can be used instead. Some solutions, such as chlorhexidine or hexachlorophene, can cause permanent damage. Consult the manufacturer's recommendations before use.

The awake patient under local anesthesia may experience anxiety with drapes over the head. Oxygen ($6-8$ L/min) administered during the procedure affords relief. A patient with chronic lung disease should be given oxygen at 3 L/min.

Care is taken not to permit the use of cautery in an oxygen-rich environment. Oxygen builds up under the drapes and could create a fire hazard. Oxygen is combustible.

A patient having a procedure longer than 2 hours should have a Foley catheter inserted to monitor urine output. The drainage bag should be positioned in the view of the anesthesia provider.

Some surgeons prefer a turban-style head drape. Fig. 41.2, $A-E$ depicts the method used to create a turban from a drape. Patients undergoing local anesthesia may wear pajama-type bottoms or underpants to the OR in some facilities. Patients having general anesthesia should wear only a gown.

Equipment and Instrumentation

Illumination is provided by the overhead spotlight, the operating microscope, the endoscope, or the surgeon's fiberoptic headlight. Some surgeons want the room darkened during endoscopy. Various types of fiberoptic endoscopes with appropriate accessories are used. The diameter of aspirating tubes and forceps is small enough to pass through small lumens, and the length is long enough to extend beyond the end of the scope. The lighting mechanism and all accessories should be checked for working order before the patient is brought to the room.

Suction should be available at all times and should include several patent cannulas. The degree of suction should be variable and usually includes a thumbhole for intermittent release of the vacuum. Cannulas with very fine suction tips should be irrigated frequently to avoid blockage. Fine suction tips are equipped with stylets for clearing the lumens.

Suction irrigators are used with sinus endoscopes. Irrigation equipment and solution at body temperature should be available to remove bone dust, clean burrs, and rinse suction apparatus. Warm solutions would cause vasodilation, with the potential for obscured vision by venous bleeding.

Special care with electrical appliances is indicated. Bipolar and monopolar electrosurgery are used to control bleeding. Many ENT surgeons use coblation technology, which is a form of high-frequency bipolar energy in a conductive medium, usually saline. The target tissue is removed using a lower temperature than traditional electrosurgery devices.

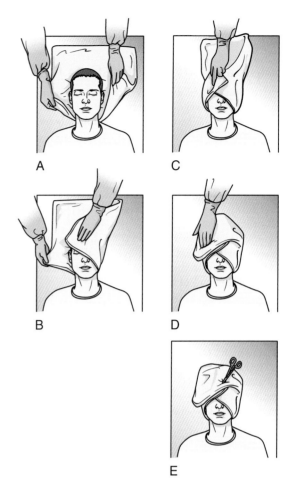

• **Fig. 41.2 A–E,** Making a head drape turban.

Compressed air or nitrogen drills with a foot-pedal control are used on bone, such as the mastoid area. Only the operator should activate the foot pedal. A number of drills for extremely delicate structures, such as stapes sculpturing, are powered by small electric motors fitted into a handpiece. The tip of the drill is cooled by small drips of irrigation solution during use.

Instrumentation is varied to suit the area. It includes very delicate, small endoscopic and microsurgical implements in addition to various-sized bone instruments because of the extensive involvement of cartilage and bone in the facial structures and skull. These areas have relatively little soft tissue. Many instruments are angled with small jaws to permit insertion without obscuring visualization.

Lasers may be used. Carbon dioxide (CO_2) lasers are used to vaporize tissue. Argon lasers coagulate tissue by heat generation. Potassium titanyl phosphate (KTP) lasers coagulate to shrink or debulk tissues. Neodymium:yttrium-aluminum-garnet (Nd:YAG) lasers cut and coagulate to minimize bleeding. Appropriate ebonized or dulled instrumentation and attachments must be available for each type of laser.

Laser surgery is usually done in conjunction with the operating microscope, endoscope, or computed tomography (CT)–guided systems. Microsurgical techniques are used because they facilitate distinction between normal and diseased tissue and allow more accurate dissection. All safety precautions are taken to avoid ignition and injury when a laser is used. Team members must wear protective eyewear of the correct optical density for the type of laser in use.

Cryosurgery may be used to destroy tissue in accessible areas, especially those that bleed profusely if incised.

Hemostasis and Drugs on the Sterile Field

One or two drops of blood can obscure a microsurgical field. Hemostatic aids and sponges should be ready at all times. Gelfoam pledgets soaked in 1:1000 epinephrine are commonly used. Soaked pledgets are kept in a labeled Petri dish or basin and passed only with forceps. Press the saturated pledget against the side of the dish to wring out some of the moisture before passing to the surgeon.

Various solutions and medications are on the sterile field, such as lidocaine, and epinephrine. Each container and delivery device should be clearly labeled for distinction between irrigation solutions and drugs.

Sponges and compressed patties are relatively small and are a distinct hazard when blood soaked because they can occlude an airway. All items used in the OR are counted or accounted for in their entirety at the end of the procedure.

Tissue Grafts and Implants

Handle tissue grafts only with forceps, taking care not to crush the tissue. Tissue grafts must be kept from drying out before use. A convenient method is to place the graft on a moist cellulose sponge in a sterile, covered Petri dish. Some surgeons intentionally dry a temporalis fascia graft to facilitate handling. This type of graft, as well as cartilage, may be flattened and thinned in a small sterile press.

Ear

Anatomy of the Ear

The structures of the outer and inner ear (Fig. 41.3, *A* and *B*) are concerned with two functions:
1. Hearing (i.e., receiving sound, amplifying it, and transmitting it to the brain for interpretation)
2. Maintaining body equilibrium

Anatomically, the ear is divided into three parts: external, middle, and inner.

External Ear

The external, or outer, ear consists of the auricle, or pinna, composed of cartilage except for the lobe; the skin; and the external auditory canal. The meatus of the auricle leads, via the ear canal, to the tympanic membrane or eardrum. This membrane separates the external and the middle ear. A color change of the translucent eardrum, visible through a speculum, may be indicative of middle ear disease. The outermost lining of the tympanic membrane is derived from tissue of the ear canal. The inner lining is continuous with the middle ear mucosa. The eardrum protects the middle ear but may be perforated by injury or pressure built up in the middle ear by infection.

Middle Ear

The middle ear consists of the tympanic cavity, a closed chamber that lies between the tympanic membrane and the inner ear. Within this cavity are the three smallest bones in the body—an ossicular chain comprising the malleus, incus, and stapes. They resemble a hammer, anvil, and stirrups, respectively. The malleus, which is attached to the eardrum, joins the incus, the extremity of which articulates with the stapes, the innermost bone. The footplate of the stapes fits in the oval (vestibular) window, an opening in the wall of the inner ear.

The bones of the ossicular chain must be able to move mechanically to conduct sound from the eardrum to the inner ear. The round (cochlear) window, also between the middle and the inner ear, equalizes pressure that enters through the oval window.

The middle ear opens into the nasopharynx by way of the eustachian tube. Normally closed during swallowing or yawning, the eustachian tube aerates the middle ear cavity. This mechanism is essential for adequate hearing.

Posteriorly the middle ear exits to the mastoid process. This inferior projection of the temporal bone is a honeycomb of air cells lined with mucous membrane. Because the antrum of the mastoid process connects with it, middle ear infection may

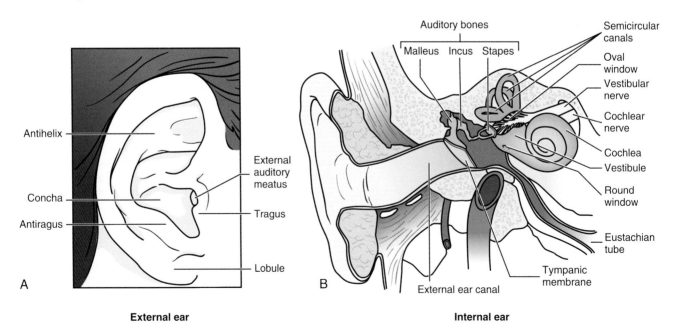

External ear

Internal ear

• **Fig. 41.3 A,** Anatomy of the outer ear. **B,** Anatomy of the inner ear.

produce mastoiditis. The middle ear is situated in the tympanic portion of the temporal bone; the inner ear is situated in the petrous portion, which integrates with the base of the skull. The tympanic portion also forms part of the ear canal.

Inner Ear

The end organs of hearing and equilibrium are situated in the inner ear. The two main sections—cochlear and vestibular—have distinct, although coordinated, functions. The cochlea, a bony spiral, relates to hearing. The vestibular labyrinth, which is composed of three semicircular canals, relates to equilibrium. These structures house two separate fluids—endolymph and perilymph—which nourish and protect the hearing receptors.

The neuroepithelium of the organ of Corti, the end organ of hearing, holds thousands of minute hair cells, which respond to sound waves that enter the cochlea via the oval window. The neuroepithelium of the vestibular portion also contains hair cells. Rapid head motion produces current in the endolymph that may result in nausea or vertigo. The eighth cranial (vestibulocochlear) nerve governs reflexes to muscles to maintain equilibrium and controls hearing.[2]

Proximal Structures

The middle and the inner ear are adjacent to many important structures. The seventh cranial (facial) nerve is enclosed in a bony canal running through the tympanic cavity and mastoid bone. The meninges of the temporal lobe of the brain are also near the middle ear and the mastoid. Facial paralysis, meningitis, and intracranial infection, such as brain abscess, are potential complications of ear infection.

The major blood vessels are the internal carotid artery and internal jugular vein, as well as the lateral sinus. Thrombosis and infection of the lateral sinus of the dura mater are potentially lethal complications of otitis media, with or without mastoiditis.

Physiology of Hearing

Sound or pressure waves enter the auricle. They pass along the ear canal to the tympanic membrane. The vibration of the waves is transmitted across the middle ear sequentially by the ossicles. Amplification of sound is enhanced to some extent by mechanical action of the ossicles but mainly by aerial ratio. A large volume of sound wave pressure from the tympanic membrane funnels to a small reactive area, the stapedial footplate, intensifying sound. At the stapedial footplate, sound pressure is transferred to the inner ear via the oval window. The hair cells of the organ of Corti are set in motion by disturbance of the inner ear fluids as sound wave pressure moves from the oval to the round window. Mechanical energy is converted to electrical potential, which is delivered to the brain along the eighth cranial nerve. The brain interprets the impulse (sound) as hearing.

Pathology of Hearing

Hearing affects the quality and quantity of interpersonal interactions. It is a major sense for communicating within one's environment. Loss of hearing therefore affects social relationships. The type of deafness or hearing loss in varying degrees may result from the following:

1. *Disease,* such as otosclerosis, in which changes in the bony capsule of the labyrinth occur. Otosclerotic bone invades the stapedial footplate, resulting in its fixation and ultimate inability to vibrate in the oval window. Hearing loss is gradual but progressive. This type of deficiency can be surgically corrected when auditory nerve endings are not destroyed.
2. *Trauma,* such as a perforated eardrum, requiring repair to restore function and aerial ratio.
3. *Infection,* usually controlled by antibiotics. Although it is more common in children, infection may also occur in adults. It may cause accumulation of fluid in the middle ear. Mastoiditis results from extension of otitis media.
   a. Serous otitis media may result from obstruction of the pharyngeal orifice of the eustachian tube. If blocked, for example, by hypertrophied adenoid tissue, infection, or allergic swelling, the eustachian tube is unable to equalize pressure because air cannot enter the middle ear from the pharynx. The vacuum or negative pressure thus created causes serum to be drawn into the tympanic cavity from blood vessels in the middle ear mucosa. Recurrent otitis media may require drainage of purulent exudate if conservative treatment fails.
   b. Acute otitis media may require drainage of purulent exudate if conservative treatment fails.
   c. Chronic otitis media with or without mastoiditis may follow recurrent otitis media with tympanic membrane perforation. It can produce a chronically draining ear.

Differential Diagnosis

Measurements that compare bone conduction with air conduction are important in differential diagnosis. Bone conduction refers to hearing as transmitted through the skull; air conduction refers to transmission of sound waves from the tympanic membrane to the inner ear via air. Hearing loss caused by a defect in the external or middle ear, referred to as conductive loss, is a mechanical obstruction of air conduction that usually can be helped by surgical intervention. When the decrement is in the inner ear, referred to as perceptive or sensorineural loss, damage to nerve tissue and/or sensory paths to the brain is not benefited by a surgical procedure. Cochlear nerve endings are the main component of sensorineural hearing (Fig. 41.4).[2]

Auditory acuity and function are measured by various tests. The audiogram is one measurement tool. Computer-averaged tomography is used to measure and analyze electrical impulses,

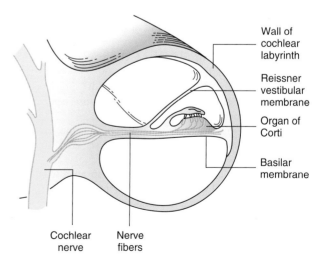

Labels: Wall of cochlear labyrinth · Reissner vestibular membrane · Organ of Corti · Basilar membrane · Cochlear nerve · Nerve fibers

• **Fig. 41.4** Cross-section of cochlear labyrinth with sensory neural mechanism.

known as auditory brainstem responses, from the brain and cortical auditory pathway. An acoustic reflex latency test of the stapedius reflex provides information about hearing sensitivity. Auditory brainstem evoked potentials assess the patient's hearing threshold.

Surgical Procedures of the Ear

Current techniques, instrumentation, lasers, and the operating microscope have enhanced the capability of otologists.

General Considerations

1. Local anesthesia may be used for a minor procedure on the external ear, but general anesthesia is used to avoid patient movement while the surgeon is manipulating delicate structures in the middle or inner ear.
   a. Inhalation anesthesia may be given by facemask for a short procedure, with the anesthesia provider seated at the head of the OR bed.
   b. The anesthesia provider sits alongside the OR bed with the patient facing them when the patient is intubated for a major procedure.
   c. Hypotensive anesthesia may be used to create a bloodless field, especially during microsurgery.
   d. Nitrous oxide is discontinued before placement of a graft in the middle ear to minimize the risk for increased pressure in the inner ear.
   e. General anesthesia may be supplemented with a local agent in some procedures, often with epinephrine to control bleeding.
2. The patient's head is turned with the affected side up and stabilized in a donut. The pinna on the unaffected side should be protected from pressure.
3. Lint-free drapes are preferred. It is mandatory that gloves be free of powder and lint. The formation of a powder granuloma in the oval window can cause irreversible sensorineural hearing loss.
4. The operating microscope is used for many otologic procedures. The light source must be carefully observed during the procedure. Strong lights from the microscope can cause tissue burns of the external auricle. Placing a moist sponge over the tissue can increase the effect of the heat and is not advised.
   a. The surgeon sits at the head or side of the OR bed to use the microscope.
   b. Microinstruments should be carefully handled before, during, and after use.
5. Compressed absorbent patties (cottonoids) moistened with normal saline solution, rather than gauze sponges, are frequently used. They must be counted.
6. Hemostasis may be achieved with epinephrine, absorbable hemostatic sponges or oxidized cellulose, laser, and bone wax.
7. Prosthetic devices should be available in an assortment of types and sizes. Tissue allografts may be used.
8. A nerve stimulator may be used to identify facial, acoustic, cochlear, and/or vestibular nerve branches. Evoked potential audiometry also may be used to monitor the seventh and eighth cranial nerves.
9. Bone instruments, including powered drills, are used for opening the temporal bone.
10. CO_2, Nd:YAG, argon, and KTP lasers are used during otologic procedures to control bleeding, divide nerves, and/or vaporize tissues.
11. Pressure dressings are usually applied. Some surgeons place 1 drop of phenylephrine (Neo-Synephrine) in the ear canal postoperatively.

External Ear Procedures

Removal of a Foreign Body

Removing a foreign body from the outer canal is performed most frequently in children. The object is washed out or removed to prevent purulent infection. A plant seed or vegetable foreign body, such as a pea, is not irrigated because it may swell in the ear and increase the difficulty of removal.

General anesthesia sometimes may be required. Trauma should be minimal during removal of a foreign body to prevent stenosis of the canal or perforation through the eardrum.

Drainage of a Hematoma

Usually a result of injury, a hematoma is drained to avoid infection with subsequent chondritis and deformity of the auricle.

Excision of a Tumor

The extent of the surgical procedure to excise a tumor, either benign or malignant, depends on the size and type of tumor. The skin of the pinna is vulnerable to actinic (chemical) changes caused by radiant energy during exposure to the sun. Basal cell lesions do not metastasize, but squamous cell carcinoma often does. Primary cancer may be excised by a wide or wedge excision with primary closure or a wide excision with a skin graft. If the lesion is extensive, partial or total pinnectomy may be necessary. The area can be skin-grafted and reconstructed cosmetically with a prosthesis. Radical temporal bone resection is indicated if the bone (canal) is involved. Neck dissection may be indicated if nodal metastases are present.

Middle Ear Procedures

Mastoidectomy

Mastoidectomy, the eradication of mastoid air cells, may be indicated to relieve complications of acute or chronic mastoiditis. Mastoidectomy is more commonly performed in conjunction with a reconstructive procedure (see "Tympanomastoid Reconstruction"). A cholesteatoma can form after repeated infections (Fig. 41.5).

Simple Mastoidectomy. The mastoid process is opened behind the ear. Air cells are removed by drilling through bone with small burrs, without involving the middle ear or external canal.

Modified Radical Mastoidectomy. Simple mastoidectomy and removal of the posterior wall of the ear canal provide drainage from the mastoid into the canal. The tympanic membrane and middle ear ossicles are preserved.

Radical Mastoidectomy. A radical mastoidectomy is performed for chronic mastoiditis. The middle ear cavity and mastoid antrum are combined into a single cavity for inspection and cleaning. Mastoid air cells are removed. The ossicles and tympanic membrane are partially removed. The stapes and facial nerve are preserved.

Tympanoplasty

Tympanoplasty, as a general term, refers to any procedure performed to repair defects in the eardrum and/or middle ear

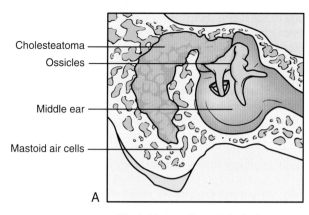

Mastoid air cells and cholesteatoma

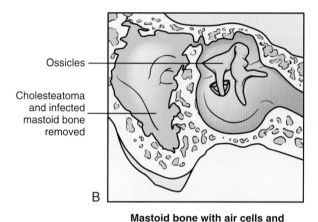

**Mastoid bone with air cells and
cholesteatoma removed**

• **Fig. 41.5 A,** Mastoid air cells and cholesteatoma. **B,** Mastoid bone with
air cells and cholesteatoma removed.

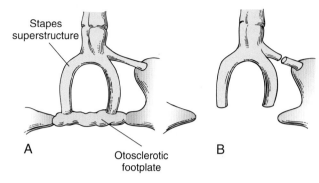

• **Fig. 41.6** Partial stapedectomy. **A,** Stapes superstructure attached to
fixed otosclerotic footplate. **B,** Footplate removed; superstructure remains.

structures for the purpose of reconstructing sound conduction
paths. The degree of hearing improvement after tympanoplasty is
related to the degree of damage. Preferably, the ear should be
uninfected at the time of the surgical procedure. If not, infected
tissue is debrided. As microsurgical procedures, tympanoplasties
are classified into the following five types:

1. *Type I* (myringoplasty) is closure of a perforation in the tympanic membrane caused by infection or trauma. The ossicular
chain is normal. Autologous fascia or a vein is used to repair
the perforation. A vein graft is taken from the patient's forearm or hand. Fascia, more commonly used as a patch over a
perforation, is obtained from the temporalis muscle.
2. *Type II* is closure of a perforated tympanic membrane with
erosion of the malleus. The graft is placed against the incus
or remains of the malleus.
3. *Type III* replaces the tympanic membrane to provide protection for the stapes and round window. The tympanic membrane, malleus, and incus have been destroyed by disease.
The stapes is intact and mobile. A homograft of tympanic
membrane with attached malleus and incus is placed in contact with the normal stapes, permitting transmission of
sound.[3]
4. *Type IV* is similar to type III except that the head, neck, and
crura of the stapes are missing. The mobile footplate may be
left exposed with the graft placed around it. The air pocket between the graft and the round window provides sound protection for the round window. To conserve the middle ear

hearing mechanism, homograft transplantation of tympanic
membrane and ossicles may be used to rebuild the chain.
5. *Type V* is similar to type IV except that the stapedial footplate
is fixed because of otosclerosis (otospongiosis). A fenestra
(small opening) is made in the horizontal semicircular canal.
The homograft seals off the middle ear to provide sound protection for the round window.

Reconstruction of the middle ear may be done with a prosthesis made from synthetic bioinert material such as high-density
polyethylene sponge (Plasti-Pore), hydroxyapatite, cement, glass
ionomer, stainless steel, titanium, tantalum, or fibrin glue.[3] Partial
and total ossicular replacement prostheses have been developed.

Tympanomastoid Reconstruction

Tympanoplasty may be combined with either simple or radical
mastoidectomy. The mastoid is drained and cleaned before
reconstruction of the eardrum or middle ear ossicles. After incision
behind the auricle, the tympanic membrane and tympanic cavity
are inspected. The mastoid antrum is entered by drilling through
mastoid bone.

Sometimes in chronic otitis media the mucous membrane of
the tympanic cavity is replaced by epithelium from the ear canal as
it grows through a perforation in the eardrum. Desquamated skin
cells that cannot escape form a ball or cyst, known as a cholesteatoma. If present in the middle ear or mastoid, a cholesteatoma
is removed during mastoidectomy and/or tympanoplasty. If left
intact, a cholesteatoma can cause permanent hearing loss, balance
disturbance, infection, and facial nerve paralysis.

Stapedectomy and Stapedotomy

Conductive hearing loss can result from fixation of the stapes,
most often caused by otosclerosis. The surgeon aims to restore
vibration from the incus to the mobile oval window membrane to
transmit sound. A stapedectomy involves partial or total removal
of the stapes.

A partial stapedectomy removes only the fixed footplate
(Fig. 41.6); a total stapedectomy removes the entire stapes,
including the footplate. A stapedotomy (small opening into the
footplate) may be the preferred procedure. The opening is made
with a handheld perforator, microsurgical power drill, or laser.
Argon, CO_2, or KTP lasers may be used for this purpose. A low-
wattage laser beam avoids thermal damage to the perilymph and
inner ear structures. After partial or total stapedectomy or stapedotomy, the remaining superstructure is used to reconstruct the
sound-conducting mechanism.

An incision is made deep in the canal near, but not in, the eardrum. The eardrum is folded over, giving access to the middle ear. The stapes is disconnected from the incus, fractured by fine microinstruments, and removed. The oval window is sealed by a graft of vein, perichondrium, fascia, fat, or an absorbable hemostatic sponge over the oval window. A prosthesis is inserted and connected to the incus and to the graft, thus restoring sound conduction. Prostheses are made of various inert materials such as polyethylene, stainless steel, or tantalum.

By performing the microsurgical procedure with the patient under local anesthesia, the surgeon can reposition the eardrum and speak to the patient to test whether their hearing is improved. Otosclerosis usually involves both ears, but stapedectomy is performed on only one ear at a time.

Stapes Mobilization

The stapes is manipulated at the footplate to restore normal function. A break through an otosclerotic lesion is achieved by means of transcrural pressure or direct application of chisels and picks to the footplate. A mobile, unaffected portion of a functioning stapes remains. Various techniques are used, with or without the use of prosthetic devices. The advantage of the procedure is that the preserved stapedial footplate provides natural protection for the inner ear. The disadvantage is that frequently a continuing otosclerotic process causes the footplate to become refixed. Therefore stapedectomy is more popular because it produces long-lasting results.

Stapes procedures are performed under direct vision with the operating microscope. The procedures do not disturb the integrity or position of the eardrum.

Removal of Middle Ear Vascular Tumors

The argon laser is absorbed by red pigment. Therefore it is suited for removal of small vascular tumors in the middle ear, such as glomus tympanicum tumors. The argon laser acts by photocoagulation.

Inner Ear Procedures

Endolymphatic Sac Shunt

The endolymphatic sac is an appendage of the membranous inner ear located in the posterior fossa, anterior to the lateral sinus and posterior to the semicircular canals. An excessive accumulation of endolymph in this sac causes the episodic vertigo (dizziness), tinnitus (ear ringing), and sensorineural hearing loss of Ménière disease. Through a simple mastoidectomy approach, the sac is opened and the inner ear is drained into either the subarachnoid space or the mastoid. A shunt tube is inserted to maintain drainage.

Labyrinthectomy

In labyrinthectomy the vestibular labyrinth is removed from the inner ear to correct incapacitating vertigo. This results in loss of vestibular function and hearing.

Vestibular Neurectomy

A middle fossa approach to the internal auditory canal for vestibular neurectomy combines otologic and neurosurgical procedures. Through a temporal bone craniotomy incision, dura of the floor of the middle fossa is elevated to expose structures in the superior portion of the internal auditory canal. The superior and inferior vestibular nerves, which control equilibrium, are sectioned to control intractable vertigo. The cochlear nerve, the hearing

portion of the eighth cranial (acoustic) nerve, is not damaged, thus preserving hearing. A graft of temporalis muscle is placed over the exposed internal auditory canal to prevent leakage of cerebrospinal fluid.

Removal of an Acoustic Neuroma

Acoustic neuroma resection may be performed by an otologist and/or a neurosurgeon, depending on its location and the extent of neurologic involvement. An acoustic neuroma is a slow-growing, encapsulated, benign tumor of the eighth cranial nerve. It originates in the neural sheath in the internal auditory canal but grows to involve nerve fibers in the posterior fossa. Initially the patient experiences unilateral hearing loss and disturbances, especially tinnitus, and equilibrium problems such as mild vertigo.

The syndrome may resemble Ménière disease or an expanding intracranial tumor. Early differential diagnosis is enhanced by brainstem evoked response audiometry, vertebral angiography, and small-volume air-contrast CT.

A small neuroma, confined to the internal auditory canal, may be resected by the otologist using a microsurgical technique through a middle fossa approach to preserve hearing. If a translabyrinthine approach is used to gain access to the internal auditory canal posterior to the inner ear structures, the patient will have total hearing loss after the surgical procedure. Acoustic neuromas extending into the cranial cavity are resected by the neurosurgeon. The CO_2 laser may be used to excise acoustic neuromas through a transmastoid or craniotomy approach. Cerebrospinal fluid leak and meningitis are complications of the craniotomy approach.

For select patients, stereotactic radiosurgery can be performed on an outpatient basis with local anesthesia. Hearing is preserved in 50% of these patients.

Implantation of a Cochlear Prosthesis

Cochlear implants have been used for adults since the 1980s, but it was not until the 1990s that they were used for children. Children as young as 9 months old can be candidates for implantation.[4] Placement in a young child can assist in speech development when a conventional hearing aid does not provide adequate sound perception. A cochlear implant can restore perception of sound to patients who have profound sensorineural deafness not responsive to external amplification of a hearing aid. They are indicated for use in patients who have intact eighth cranial nerve function.

The implant is an electronic device that converts sound waves into electrical signals to stimulate cochlear nerve fibers in the absence of functioning hair cells. Several devices are available. All have external and internal components (Fig. 41.7). The external part, which is attached behind the ear, has a microphone/transmitter and a speech processor/receiver. The internal part has a receiver/stimulator and electrode/channel that is threaded through the cochlea.

The internal electrode attaches to wires permanently implanted in the cochlea. Through a postauricular incision, a simple mastoidectomy is performed. Under the operating microscope, the facial recess between the posterior canal and the facial nerve is enlarged to expose the chorda tympani nerve and the middle ear. The electrode is securely seated in the mastoid cavity and placed through a recess into the middle ear. It is directed through an opening made in the round window into the scala tympani until it

Internal components
- Implanted receiver
- Electrode system

External components
- Transmitter system
- Sound processor
- Microphone

• **Fig. 41.7** Cochlear implant.

meets resistance. Placement is critical. A plug of fascia from the temporalis muscle is placed around the electrode at the round window to prevent perilymph leakage.

The internal electrode stimulates the auditory nerve to interpret sound. The single-channel model stimulates the nerve randomly so the patient can discern environmental sounds but not speech. A multichannel electrode enables the patient to distinguish environmental sounds and some speech by differentiating the frequency, volume, and pitch of sound waves. With a single-channel electrode, a ground wire is placed under the temporalis muscle in the mastoid or middle ear. A multichannel electrode does not have a ground wire. The internal receiver is sutured in position over the temporal bone behind the ear.

Electromagnetic components and/or a titanium enclosure for the receiver may act as an electrical ground device. Only bipolar electrosurgery is used if additional surgery is needed after placement of the receiver. Patients with stainless steel cochlear implants should avoid magnetic resonance imaging (MRI) because of metal components within the implanted device. MRI can be done with implants made of other materials, but should be performed only as recommended by the manufacturer of the implant.[5]

The external microphone/transmitter component of the implant activates the internal receiver/stimulator. Transmission may be percutaneous or transcutaneous. In the percutaneous model, a direct wire to a receiver implanted behind the ear connects the transmitter. In the transcutaneous model, the transmitter converts electrical energy into magnetic currents that pass through intact skin to the receiver. In both models, sound enters the microphone and is transmitted to a speech processor, worn outside the body, where it is encoded into electrical signals or energy and amplified. The coded signals return to the transmitter and are passed to the internal receiver. The patient can adjust amplification of environmental sounds.

Robotic-assisted placement of cochlear implants may be performed using tiny incisions. Precise implant placement and avoiding delicate structures such as the facial nerve is done with CT scans.[5] In 2022, the U.S. Food and Drug Administration (FDA) approved a trial for a totally implantable cochlear device that uses vibration sensors implanted into the cochlea. This technology does not have any visible external components.[5]

Nose

Anatomy of the Nose

The supporting structures of the nose consist of two nasal bones and the nasal processes of the maxillary bones superiorly, the lateral cartilages and connective tissue inferiorly, and the septum. The septum, composed of bone posteriorly and cartilage anteriorly, divides the nose into two chambers lined by mucous membrane. The anterior portion, or vestibule, holds the nasal hairs. The external anterior orifices are called nares.

The internal portion of the nose, the nasal cavity (Fig. 41.8), extends to the nasopharynx, the space behind the choanae (funnel-like posterior nasal orifices). The nose communicates with the ear via the eustachian tube. The hard and soft palates divide the nasal and oral cavities. The ethmoid bone separates the nasal and cranial cavities.

The paranasal sinuses are the frontal, maxillary, ethmoid, and sphenoid. Ostia (openings from the sinuses and nasolacrimal ducts) are located in the nasal lateral walls. The ostia provide a drainage system for the sinuses, as well as aerate them. Three turbinate bones (superior, middle, and inferior) are also situated in the lateral walls. These bones are covered with a vascular mucosa. Beneath each turbinate is a corresponding meatus. Tears drain into the nose through the nasolacrimal duct that enters the inferior meatus. Drainage from the paranasal sinuses is passed to the nose through the middle and superior meatus.

External and internal carotid arteries and their branches supply blood to the nasal region. Because of the extensive vascularity, lymphatic supply, and proximity to the brain, infections on or about the face are potentially very dangerous. Microorganisms may readily be carried to the cavernous sinus, or thrombi may form in the cavernous sinus. The sense of smell is derived from the first cranial (olfactory) nerve. The sensory nerve supply of the nasal area is associated with the trigeminal or fifth cranial nerve.

Physiology of the Nose

- It provides filtered air to the respiratory system. Fine cilia in the mucous membranes propel mucus toward the nasopharynx. Air is warmed and moistened as it passes to the trachea and lower respiratory tract.
- It contains the end organs for smell in the olfactory epithelium, which differs from other nasal epithelia. When nasal obstruction blocks off the olfactory epithelium, loss of smell (anosmia) results. The senses of smell and taste are closely related.

Surgical Procedures of the Nose

Nasal procedures are concerned with two factors: adequate ventilation to accessory spaces and adequate drainage from them. Abnormalities in structure, congenital or traumatic, and disease processes hinder function. Corrective procedures are done to relieve obstruction, to ensure drainage, to resect tumors, or to control bleeding (epistaxis).

General Considerations

1. CT and rhinoscopy are often performed preoperatively to diagnose the nature and extent of pathologic conditions, especially in the paranasal sinuses.
2. Many nasal procedures are performed with the patient under local anesthesia with or without IV sedation.

• **Fig. 41.8** Regions of the head and neck.

a. Topical anesthetic agents may be sprayed on the nasal mucosa or applied with soaked, compressed, absorbent patties (cottonoids) or sponges put in the nostrils. The used patties must be accounted for at the end of the procedure.

b. A local agent, often lidocaine hydrochloride, 1% or 2%, is injected into the middle meatus. Epinephrine usually is used for vasoconstriction to control bleeding.

c. When general anesthesia is indicated, a pack is placed in the pharynx to prevent aspiration of blood after the patient is intubated. Reconciliation of the count and removal of the pack at the end of surgery is critical for prevention of retained foreign objects.

3. Paranasal sinuses and tissues underlying the mucosa are considered sterile. Therefore instrumentation must be sterile, although the nasal cavity is considered a contaminated area because the instrumentation is entering a vascular bed. Venous drainage could easily carry microorganisms to the cavernous sinus, causing an intracranial infection.

4. CO_2, Nd:YAG, and KTP lasers may be used. Endoscopes also are used. All equipment and accessories should be checked for working order.

5. Nasal packing is inserted at the end of most procedures except endoscopic sinus and laser procedures. A mustache dressing may be placed under the nose to act as a drip pad. Postoperatively the patient should be positioned in a head-up position to minimize edema and bleeding. Ice is placed over the nasal bridge for the first 48 hours in 20-minute intervals.

Nasal Cavity Procedures

The supporting structures surrounding nasal air passages can be injured or displaced. Acute or chronic disease processes can cause dysfunction or obstruction.

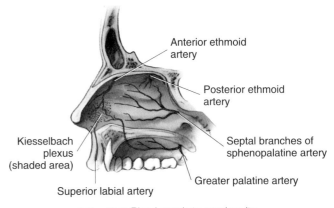

• **Fig. 41.9** Blood supply to nasal cavity.

Epistaxis

Most nosebleeds are caused by trauma, usually at the Kiesselbach plexus of arteries and veins (also known as the Little area) in the anterior part of the nasal septum (Fig. 41.9). Dehumidified air may cause changes in the mucosa and splitting of tiny vessels. Bleeding may be spontaneous, as in patients with arteriosclerosis, hypertension, or blood dyscrasia. Epistaxis is usually anterior and unilateral. In people with systemic disease, such as leukemia, or with severe fracture, the bleeding is frequently posterior and more severe. Management involves locating the precise bleeding site and promptly instituting appropriate therapy. Severe hemorrhage places the patient in a precarious condition. Hypovolemia should be corrected preoperatively.

Anterior Pack. Local vasoconstriction and pressure on the side of the nose will control most nosebleeds. Electrocoagulation or silver nitrate is used to provide hemostasis at the bleeding point as needed. When bleeding is from the anterior ethmoid artery, inaccessible to cautery, packing is applied to the area of depression between the septum and the middle turbinate.

Posterior Pack. A posterior pack may be necessary for constant pressure when bleeding is severe in the posterior part of the nose. The pack consists of rolled gauze securely tied to the middle of a length of narrow tape or strong string; commercial packs are available. To control infection and odor, gauze is lubricated with antibiotic ointment before insertion.

After a catheter is passed into the mouth via the nose, one end of the tape is tied to the oral end of the catheter. The catheter and attached tape are then drawn back through the mouth and out one nostril, thereby pulling the pack up into the nasopharynx. Thus one end of the tape comes out of the nose, the other end out of the mouth. These ends are secured to the patient's cheek with adhesive tape. The nasal end is taped to prevent the pack from slipping into the throat; the oral end facilitates removal of the pack. Some oozing may persist despite packing. The pack is left in place until bleeding is arrested, usually for at least 48 hours, but prolonged use can lead to otitis media or paranasal sinusitis.

Patients with postnasal packs are often apprehensive and uncomfortable. They must breathe through the mouth. Posterior packs tend to reduce arterial oxygen tension. All patients, especially geriatric patients and those with marginal pulmonary function, should be observed carefully for respiratory problems that may result from the pack dropping into the hypopharynx.

Artery Ligation. A microsurgical procedure is performed to control persistent nasal hemorrhage by reducing the blood supply to the posterior portion of the nose. Some surgeons prefer artery ligation to packing, or it may be performed with a pack in place. Through an incision in the oral mucosa, removal of the posterior wall exposes the maxillary sinus for transantral ligation. Terminal branches of the internal maxillary artery, a branch of the external carotid artery, are exposed, identified, and ligated with metallic clips. Electrocoagulation is used to control intraoperative bleeding, but if bleeding is excessive, creation of a nasoantral window establishes drainage. The replaced posterior mucosal flap is covered with an absorbable gelatin sponge, and the incision is closed.

Through an incision along the left side of the nose, ligation of the anterior and posterior ethmoidal arteries is helpful in controlling bleeding in the superior aspect of the nose.

The argon or KTP laser may be used to control severe epistaxis. If a laser is used to control bleeding, nasal packing usually is unnecessary.

Turbinectomy

Chronic engorgement of the middle and/or inferior turbinate causes nasal congestion and rhinorrhea. Rhinitis is frequently an allergic reaction. A KTP laser shrinks turbinates without removing normal mucosa. A CO_2 or Nd:YAG contact laser vaporizes the superficial layer of mucosa without injuring the turbinate or ablating the turbinate. The KTP or CO_2 laser fiber handpiece is directed through a nasal endoscope. Because bleeding is minimal, nasal packing is unnecessary. Electrocoagulation and cryosurgery also have been used to treat soft tissue obstruction and refractory allergic rhinitis.

Nasal Obstruction

Surgical intervention can provide relief for certain types of nasal obstructions. For example, after the mucosa is shrunk with a

vasoconstrictor and secretions are suctioned, a foreign body is removed with a forceps. An abscess or a hematoma may need to be drained to relieve pressure. Accumulation of pus or blood separates the perichondrium, the connective tissue, from underlying cartilage. This may cause necrosis of cartilage with resultant deformity. Infection must be eradicated to avoid extension to the brain.

Polypectomy. Polyps (soft, edematous masses) projecting from the nasal or sinus mucosa can obstruct the posterior choanae. Polyps usually are bilateral, but they may be unilateral, may be single or multiple, and frequently are infected. In addition to obstructing ventilation, they may obstruct the sense of smell if the olfactory epithelium is blocked.

Some polyps may be excised with a wire-loop snare through a nasal speculum or with forceps through an endoscope. Packing is inserted to control bleeding. The KTP laser coagulates the base to debulk multiple large polyps. The laser fiber can be directed through a straight or angled handpiece. A CO_2 laser can vaporize polyps. The laser is less invasive than other techniques.

Nasal Deformity

Surgical intervention can restore contour and/or improve function after an injury. A deformity in nasal structure also may be corrected to improve cosmetic appearance.

Reduction of a Nasal Fracture. Fracture of the septum or nasal bones often accompanies other trauma to the head. Intranasal manipulation is required to elevate depressed bone or cartilage that may be pushed into the paranasal sinuses. This should be performed as soon as possible to bring the parts into apposition. A delay of 7 to 10 days to permit edema to subside will not affect the outcome. Bleeding from a laceration must be immediately controlled and drained. Intranasal structure compatible with air passage must be preserved.

Septoplasty, Septal Reconstruction, and Submucous Resection. The terms *septoplasty, septal reconstruction,* and *submucous resection* are used interchangeably to describe correction of a deviated nasal septum. Often the result of injury, the condition interferes with breathing and drainage. With the patient under local anesthesia, one side of the septum is incised its entire length. Membranous coverings are detached from cartilage and bone. The deformed part of the septum is removed or straightened and replaced. Bilateral nasal packing is inserted to hold tissues in place and prevent bleeding. The procedure creates a patent airway and straight septal line, thereby reducing sinus disease and polyp formation.

Rhinoplasty. Rhinoplasty, a procedure to correct deformity of the nose, may be performed by a rhinologist or a plastic surgeon. It is a major procedure involving reconstruction and molding of the bones and cartilages. Septoplasty and rhinoplasty may be performed together; septorhinoplasty restores both function and cosmetic appearance. Local anesthesia and a vasoconstrictor are usually used.

Some surgeons prefer to use a nasal spray 30 minutes preoperatively. Both drugs decrease the risk for hypertension during the procedure, which could cause excessive bleeding. The skin is taped postoperatively to maintain the nasal structures in alignment. A rigid shield is applied for protection. This is not removed without a specific order from the surgeon. Temporary ecchymosis from surgical trauma surrounds the eyes postoperatively.

Repair of a Perforated Septum. Perforations occur most often in the anterior cartilage. If bleeding and crusting are severe, the perforation may be covered by rotated mucoperichondrial flaps or

• **Fig. 41.10** Paranasal sinuses.

the mucosa of adjacent intact septum may be denuded and a skin graft applied to cover the perforation. Nasal packing is inserted.

Paranasal Sinus Procedures

The paranasal sinuses are air-filled spaces in the skull (Fig. 41.10). Because the sinus mucous membrane lining is continuous with the mucous membrane lining of the nose, nasal infection may readily spread to the sinuses. Various procedures provide drainage for patients with chronic sinusitis that may result from allergies or repeated nasopharyngeal infection. Swelling of the nasal mucosa can trap microorganisms within a sinus cavity. Ostial occlusion and abnormalities in the walls of the nasal cavity interfere with breathing, drainage, and smell. Sinus procedures are executed through an external or an intranasal approach or through an endoscope.

Maxillary Sinus Procedure

The maxillary sinuses are located bilaterally between the upper teeth and the eyes.

Caldwell-Luc Procedure (Antrostomy). The maxillary sinus contents are approached through an incision of the oral mucous membrane above the canine teeth. The flap is retracted. A section of maxillary bone is cut out to create a large nasoantral window for aeration and permanent drainage by gravity into the nasal fossa under the inferior turbinate. Polyps and diseased tissue are removed, along with eradication of mucosa. At the completion of the surgical procedure, the sinus is packed with gauze impregnated with antibiotic ointment. One end of the gauze is brought through the window and into the nose. The incision under the upper lip is sutured. The packing is eventually removed through the nose. Antrostomy is usually limited to adults because of unerupted teeth in children. A Caldwell-Luc incision is also used for removal of a tumor in the maxillary sinus.

Ethmoid Sinus Procedures

The ethmoid sinus cells lie bilaterally between the nose and the orbits. The maxillary sinuses are below the ethmoid bones, and the frontal sinuses are above them.

Ethmoidectomy. Diseased tissue is removed from the ethmoid labyrinth, middle turbinate, and meatus. A large cavity is formed to facilitate aeration and drainage. Severe ethmoiditis can cause orbital abscess requiring drainage through an intranasal or external (Lynch) incision that extends from the inner half of the eyebrow down alongside the nose.

Turbinectomy. Removal of portions of the inferior and middle turbinates increases aeration and drainage. The cavity is packed at completion of the surgical procedure.

Frontal Sinus Procedures

The frontal sinuses are situated above the eyes. They are usually approached through the external incision described for ethmoidectomy, or a coronal incision may be made for exposure across the scalp from ear to ear.

Osteoplastic Flap Procedure. The bone covering the frontal sinus is exposed and incised. The contents of the sinus, such as a mucocele (a cyst lined with mucus-secreting glands), are extracted. The lining of the mucocele sac is removed and the cavity packed with fat (from the abdominal wall) to obliterate the sinus with fibrous tissue that fills in the cavity. The incised bone flap is then repositioned, and the incision is sutured.

Killian Procedure. A frontal sinus cavity is reached by removal of the floor or anterior wall of the sinus through an external incision above the eye. A large communication and drainage channel into the nose is formed.

Sphenoid Sinus Procedure

The sphenoid sinus is deep—almost in the center of the skull. It may be approached intranasally or via the external ethmoidectomy incision through the eyebrow.

Sphenoidotomy. Sphenoidotomy involves the creation of an opening into the sphenoid sinus for drainage.

Endoscopic Sinus Surgery

Sinuscopes permit direct visualization of the paranasal sinuses and the anatomy of lateral nasal walls. The site of diseased mucosa or obstructive tissue, such as polyps, can be localized for removal, with preservation of some mucosa and restoration of drainage (Fig. 41.11). The mucosa of each sinus has cilia that move air in waveforms. With an endoscopic approach, some ciliary motion may be retained for aeration. CT navigation systems are commonly used, especially for patients with a history of previous surgery or complicated anatomy.

The basic principle of endoscopic sinus surgery is that most sinus mucosal disease will resolve if aeration and drainage are reestablished. The extent of the procedure depends on the location of diseased mucosa and the resection necessary to establish drainage. Septal deformities or inferior turbinates causing nasal obstruction may be concurrently corrected (i.e., septoplasty and

• **Fig. 41.11** Sinusoscopy.

turbinoplasty). Minor procedures limited to removal of disease from maxillary or ethmoid sinuses usually can be done with topical and local anesthesia. IV sedation or general anesthesia is needed for more extensive procedures, such as ethmoidectomy or sphenoethmoidectomy.

The telescopes of sinuscopes are 2.7 and 4 mm in diameter with 0°, 25° or 30°, 70°, and 120° viewing angles. The quartz rod telescope has a solid quartz optical cone in the light post that attaches to a halogen light source. This system provides optimal light transmission through the fiberoptics of the miniaturized scope. An attached suction/irrigation device permits unobstructed viewing. The telescope is inserted intranasally and advanced into the frontal, ethmoid, or sphenoid sinus. It is inserted through a cannula in the canine fossa to reach the maxillary sinus.

Many accessory grasping and cutting instruments, including the KTP laser, are used to remove mucosa, lamina, osteum, and cells. Hemostasis is controlled with epinephrine and cautery or laser. Nasal packing usually is not required.

Functional Endoscopic Sinus Surgery. The functional endoscopic sinus surgery (FESS) procedure is also known as the Messerklinger technique. The surgeon begins at the ethmoid and works anteriorly to the frontal and maxillary sinuses to clear ethmoidal compartments of disease. If a minimal opening of the narrow osteomeatal tract at the anterior ethmoidal sinus will not achieve adequate drainage from other paranasal sinuses, a posterior ethmoidectomy and sphenoidotomy are included in the procedure.

Exenteration. Known as the Wigand procedure, total sphenoethmoidectomy and partial middle turbinate resection are performed, beginning with a sphenoidotomy and working anteriorly to the frontal sinus. This creates a broad opening of the sphenoidal, ethmoidal, frontal, and maxillary sinuses. To avoid the optic nerve, dissection does not extend beyond the lateral wall of the sphenoid. Visual evoked potentials monitor optic nerve function; the eyes are uncovered. The endoscopic procedure may be done bilaterally.

Resection of Tumors

Osteoma, a benign tumor, can arise from bones around the paranasal sinuses. Although rare, primary carcinoma and sarcoma do occur in the frontal, ethmoid, sphenoid, and maxillary sinuses. Most originate in the maxillary sinus. The incidence increases with age. The sinuses are proximal to the orbits, oral cavity, and base of the skull. A tumor in the maxillary sinus may be associated with oral or nasal symptoms, such as loosening of the upper teeth, bleeding from the nose, or asymmetry of the face. A malignant lesion in the ethmoid sinus may be accompanied by displacement of the eye, disturbance of smell, and nasal obstruction. Chronic sinusitis is thought to play an etiologic role because of an associated replacement of respiratory epithelium by stratified squamous cells.

Most sinus tumors are squamous cell carcinomas. Often the bony walls are invaded and destroyed by the time symptoms appear because the tumor tends to extend in all directions. Exploratory surgery by a Caldwell-Luc incision provides the best chance of early diagnosis. Radical craniofacial resection may be indicated.

Oral Cavity and Throat

Anatomy and Physiology of the Oral Cavity and Throat

The oral cavity is lined with thick mucous membrane. This squamous mucosa connects with the nasopharynx superiorly and the hypopharynx below. The hard palate, part of the maxillary bone, forms the floor of the nasal cavity and the anterior part of the roof of the mouth. The soft palate, a musculomembranous structure posterior to the hard palate, occludes the nasal cavity during speech and swallowing. These functions are aided by the uvula, a small conical appendage (tongue-like structure) that projects from the posterior free margin of the soft palate. It contains the uvular muscle covered by mucous membrane. The tongue, occupying much of the oral cavity, joins the soft palate and pharynx posteriorly by folds of mucous membrane.

The throat refers to space surrounded by the soft palate, the palatoglossal and palatopharyngeal arches, the base of the tongue, and the pharynx. The funnel-shaped pharynx is subdivided into the nasopharynx (above), oropharynx (middle), and hypopharynx (below). The nasopharynx communicates with the nasal cavity through the posterior choanae. The oropharynx includes the base of the tongue anteriorly, the tonsillar fossae laterally, and the oropharyngeal walls of the throat posteriorly. The hypopharynx leads from the oropharynx to the larynx, trachea, and esophagus. The pharynx, posterior to the larynx and the nasal and oral cavities, consists of constrictor muscles essential to swallowing. The proximity of food and air passages and the joint function of the pharynx in their passage contribute to the hazard of aspiration.

The nasopharynx and oropharynx contain masses of lymphoid tissue. The adenoids (pharyngeal tonsils) hang from the nasopharyngeal roof; the lingual tonsils are in mucosal crypts. The palatine tonsils lie on either side of the oropharynx. These, referred to as the tonsils, are supported in the tonsillar fossae by anterior and posterior pillars. A fibrous capsule adheres to each laterally.

The salivary glands are located in the soft tissue walls of the oral cavity. The six major paired glands are the submandibular, sublingual, and parotid glands. The parotid glands are the largest.

The ducts of these major glands, in addition to lesser glands, secrete saliva into the mouth. Saliva functions to moisten and lubricate food to aid in swallowing, to dissolve some substances and enzymatically digest starches, and to facilitate tasting.

Surgical Procedures of the Oral Cavity and Throat

Pathologic conditions may affect the lips, tongue, floor of the mouth, palates, salivary glands, or pharynx. The oral region is one of the most vascular areas of the body. Hemostasis may be achieved with an electrosurgical unit (ESU), hemostatic scalpel, argon beam coagulator, or laser. Lasers are used to vaporize both benign and malignant superficial and subepithelial lesions.

Abnormalities result from congenital malformation, improper occlusion or jaggedness of teeth, and infection, but most commonly they result from trauma and neoplasms. Adequate reconstruction restores the lining, internal structural support, soft tissue, and external coverage. Many of the craniofacial, maxillofacial, and dentofacial procedures previously described in this chapter are performed through intraoral incisions. Plastic surgeons, oral surgeons, laryngologists, or a multidisciplinary team may perform the following procedures through intraoral or extraoral incisions.

Excision of Salivary Gland Tumors

Benign mixed tumors of the salivary glands are more common than are malignant tumors and most frequently are located in a parotid gland. Most tumors can be removed by dissection, and some can be removed by cryosurgery. The incision is of adequate size to expose the entire gland and the facial nerve. A nerve stimulator is used to identify the nerve and its branches. Injury to the nerve results in postoperative facial paralysis.

Parotidectomy

Parotidectomy, excision of a parotid gland, is performed through an incision in the neck below the angle of the mandible and extending upward to one or both sides of the ear (Fig. 41.12). A swelling beneath the skin in the area in front of or below the ear is almost invariably within the substance of the parotid gland. This

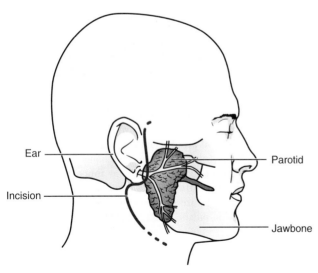

• **Fig. 41.12** Parotidectomy.

may be a benign, mixed, or malignant tumor. Benign lesions localized superficially may be excised by superficial subtotal parotidectomy. Lesions deep within the gland, extending under the mandible, frequently displace the soft palate in the oral cavity.

Radical neck dissection or hemimandibulectomy may be indicated to remove a highly invasive malignant tumor. For most parotid tumors the facial nerve can be isolated and preserved during total parotidectomy, unless the nerve is inextricably involved by the tumor. If the facial nerve is to be sacrificed, the nerve may be primarily grafted, with the great auricular nerve as a graft, to prevent total facial nerve paralysis.

Excision of Oral Carcinoma

Primary malignant lesions may occur in the lower lip, tongue, or floor of the mouth. Because of the proximity of cervical lymph nodes, metastasis occurs early. A painful bleeding ulcer is considered a suspicious symptom. Oral cancer in its earliest stages may be asymptomatic and painless. The human papillomavirus is a common cause. Small tumors may be treated with only irradiation, local excision with primary closure, or vaporization with a laser beam. Larger lesions compel more extensive procedures.

Subtotal Glossectomy or Hemiglossectomy

In subtotal glossectomy or hemiglossectomy, part (subtotal) or half (hemi-) of the tongue is removed (glossectomy). The extent of the resection will determine the type of reconstruction to resurface the oral cavity. Innervated free flaps may be used to maintain bulk and tone.

Total Glossectomy

All of the tongue and often the floor of the mouth are resected. A pectoralis major myocutaneous island flap is more advantageous than are the cervical, pectoral, or forehead flaps also used to restore the intraoral lining. Respiratory embarrassment and chronic aspiration are significant problems after glossectomy.

Cricopharyngeal myotomy may be performed to facilitate swallowing and reduce aspiration. The tip of the epiglottis is often sutured to the pharyngeal wall (epiglottopexy) to decrease aspiration. Unless it is involved directly with tumor, the larynx is preserved. Laryngeal suspension, achieved by placing a heavy suture around the mandibular ramus, holds the larynx laterally. Extension into the larynx and cervical metastases are indications for unilateral or bilateral neck dissection, usually with laryngectomy. A tracheotomy is always performed with a total glossectomy to maintain an airway.[6] For postoperative alimentation, a nasogastric tube is inserted before closing the pharynx.

Procedures of the Nasopharynx

Uvulopalatopharyngoplasty

Increasing the air space in the oropharynx corrects obstructive sleep apnea (OSA) caused by anatomic relationships in some patients. OSA can cause oxygen desaturation during apneic episodes that occur during sleep. This can lead to life-threatening pulmonary and systemic hypertension, cardiac dysrhythmias, and neurologic dysfunction if untreated. Upper airway obstruction may be caused by nasal obstruction, a deviated nasal septum, hypertrophied adenoids and/or tonsils, or mandibular retrognathism (overbite), which may be surgically corrected.

To diagnose OSA in patients who do not have obvious abnormalities, airway obstruction can be viewed during sleep with fiberoptic nasopharyngoscopy and fluoroscopy. Obstruction of the air passage for more than 10 seconds is diagnostic. Oxygen saturation of the blood is 85% in moderate cases and less than 60% in severe obstructive cases. Some of the oropharyngeal muscles may become atonic and collapse inward, and the soft palate may drop down. Patients who have a large, drooping soft palate and at least moderately redundant lateral pharyngeal walls or large tonsils are good candidates for uvulopalatopharyngoplasty. These patients have moderate apnea but do not have severe cardiac dysrhythmias.

The patient is continuously monitored during induction of anesthesia. The surgeon is present, and an emergency tracheotomy tray is available in case the patient's airway becomes obstructed.[6]

The full thickness of mucosa is resected from the posterior margin of the soft palate, including the uvula, and most of the anterior tonsillar pillar. The lesser palatine artery is ligated. The tonsils or mucosa of the tonsillar fossae is resected. The remaining posterior tonsillar pillar is sutured to the resected anterior pillar.[7] The palate is closed laterally. The extent of tissue removal varies according to the width and depth of the patient's oropharyngeal space.

Hypoglossal Nerve Stimulation

In 2019 the FDA approved a nerve stimulator for use in patients with OSA. A small generator, similar to a pacemaker, is implanted in the upper chest. An electrode is placed around the hypoglossal nerve and a sensor is implanted in the intercostal space. A lead from each is tunneled and connected to the generator. The generator can be programmed to stimulate the hypoglossal nerve during inspiration, preventing airway obstruction.[8]

Adenoidectomy

Adenoidectomy, the removal of hypertrophied adenoid tissue from the nasopharynx and behind the posterior choanae, may be performed in adults to relieve upper airway obstruction. This is more commonly performed in children, often to prevent recurrent otitis media. Adenoid tissue usually atrophies after adolescence.

The patient is supine. General anesthesia is administered, and the patient is intubated. Adenoids can be resected with an adenotome and curette or vaporized with a CO_2 laser. Bleeding is more easily controlled with the laser. Electrosurgery and/or gauze sponges soaked in epinephrine may be used after sharp dissection. Occasionally a posterior nasal pack is needed.

Procedures of the Oropharynx

Tonsillectomy

Chronically infected or hypertrophied tonsils are most frequently removed in childhood (Fig. 41.13). Even slightly enlarged tonsils can obstruct airflow to the lungs during sleep in an adult. Tonsillectomy may significantly improve symptoms of sleep apnea, with or without uvulopalatopharyngoplasty.

CO_2, Nd:YAG, argon, or KTP lasers may be used to excise tonsils from the tonsillar fossae.

The patient is supine. General anesthesia is administered. The endotracheal tube and cuff must be protected, and other laser precautions must be taken around the oral cavity. A smoke evacuator should be available with a CO_2 laser. A handheld laser may be used, or a beam may be directed through the microscope.

Local anesthesia is sometimes used for adult tonsillectomy. The patient is in the semi-Fowler or sitting position on the OR bed or sits in a specially designed chair. The throat is anesthetized with a

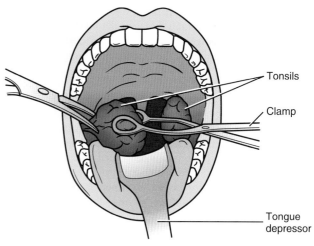

• **Fig. 41.13** Tonsillectomy.

topical agent and local infiltration. With sharp and blunt dissection, each tonsil is separated from the pillars and capsule and removed from the fossa with a tonsil snare.

Attention is given to hemostasis to prevent aspiration; suture ligatures, free ties, and/or absorbable ligating clips may be used. Bleeding can be difficult to control and can occur postoperatively with this technique. Less intraoperative bleeding occurs with laser tonsillectomy.

Incision and Drainage of a Peritonsillar Abscess

Less common since the advent of antibiotics, incision into the anterior tonsillar pillar may be necessary to drain purulent material posterior to the tonsillar capsule after acute tonsillitis.

Resection of a Tonsillar Tumor

A localized squamous cell carcinoma of the tonsil may be resected by dissection or with cryosurgery. An en bloc resection includes the primary tumor and nodes. Metastatic nodes are common. Superior progression of the tumor may reach the supratonsillar fossa, soft and hard palates, and uvula. Inferiorly the tumor may spread to the posterior and lateral walls of the larynx, base of the tongue, and pyriform sinus. Neck dissection may be indicated for regional disease. Surgery may be combined with preoperative or postoperative radiation therapy. The most common complications are fistula formation and delayed healing.

Pharyngeal Diverticulectomy (Zenker Diverticulum)

Pharyngeal diverticulectomy, or removal of sacs or outpouching of lower pharyngeal mucous membrane in which food collects, may be performed in extreme cases in which regurgitation presents a hazard of aspiration. The neck of the sac is dissected from the posterior pharyngeal wall and ligated. The stump of the excised sac is inverted into the pharyngeal wall. Diverticula may be removed endoscopically.

Dental Procedures

Just as the scope of many medical-surgical specialties, such as otolaryngology and head and neck surgery, has broadened, so has dentistry. Likewise, subspecialization within dentistry, through extensive specialized postgraduate education, has given OR practice privileges to dentists who perform surgical procedures in and around the oral cavity. Among these are the following:

- *Oral surgeon:* Oral surgery may be limited to exodontia (extraction of teeth) and minor surgery in the oral cavity. It may also include correction of dentofacial deformities (i.e., oral and maxillofacial surgery). A qualified oral surgeon is competent to complete a history and physical examination and thus determine the patient's ability to undergo the proposed surgical procedure.
- *Orthodontist:* Orthodontics focuses on irregularities of the teeth, malocclusion, and associated facial problems.
- *Prosthodontist:* Prosthodontics is concerned with artificial restoration of intraoral and external facial structures.
- *Periodontist:* Periodontics is the treatment and prevention of disease in the gingiva (gum), underlying soft tissues, and alveoli surrounding the teeth.

Patients with medical problems admitted to the hospital by oral surgeons and all patients admitted for dental care have an admission history, physical examination, and evaluation of their overall medical risk by a physician preoperatively. This physician is responsible for the care of a preexisting condition and any medical problem that arises during hospitalization.

Just as physicians from various specialties function as members of a multidisciplinary team, so do oral surgeons and dentists, each contributing to the dental health of the patient. Frequently they also function as collegial members of the teams involved in craniofacial or maxillofacial surgery. They assist with reconstruction of the face, correction of jaw deformities, and establishment of optimal dental occlusion. For example, the orthodontist may move teeth before a maxillofacial or oral surgeon repositions the jaws to correct malocclusion. Many patients undergo both preoperative and postoperative orthodontia. Prosthodontics may be necessary to replace missing teeth. Prosthodontists also may fit an artificial nose postoperatively after rhinectomy for a tumor or trauma.

Patients seeking dentofacial treatment usually have functional problems. These may include difficulty with mastication (chewing) and deglutition (swallowing), speech problems, abnormal tongue posture, or lip incompetence. A dental surgical procedure is defined as any manipulation, cutting, or removal of oral or perioral tissues and tooth structures where bleeding occurs. Oral surgeons and periodontists perform these procedures.

Periodontics

Diseases that affect the gingiva, bone, and supporting structures such as periodontal ligaments can occur at any age. Periodontal disease is the primary cause of tooth loss in adults older than 35 years. Treatment usually takes place in the periodontist's office. Patients who have medical problems, such as hemophilia or some other blood dyscrasia, severe diabetes, or heart disease, are admitted to the hospital. Periodontal plastic surgery encompasses resective, regenerative, and reconstructive techniques.

Gingivectomy

Portions of the gingiva, mucous membrane, and underlying soft tissue that covers the alveolar process and surrounds the teeth are excised to remove deep pockets of plaque, calculus, and inflamed soft tissue. The CO_2 laser may be used for this procedure.

Mucogingivoplasty

Plastic surgery around the teeth and gums is done primarily to reduce inflammation, prevent accumulation of bacteria, and stop sensitivity. Another indication is to rebuild bone and soft tissue destroyed by disease or trauma. Excessive gum tissue is excised to contour or reshape the gingiva for improved physiologic form or aesthetics. The alveoli may be reconstructed to change their shape and height. Gingival margins may be reshaped for the site of a false tooth or fixed bridge.

Gingival grafting or augmentation done before or during orthodontic treatment may reduce the risk for recession of gum tissue from around the roots of the teeth. Autologous mucogingival free grafts from the hard palate or pedicle flaps from adjacent tissues may be used to cover receded alveolar mucosa or an exposed tooth root. Flaps or grafts are used to augment inadequate zones of masticatory gingiva. Gingival onlay grafts are also used to enhance ridges where trauma or extraction has resulted in a reduced ridge, thus correcting an aesthetic defect.

Alveolar Ridge Reconstruction

The alveolar ridge is the bony remains of the alveolar process of the maxilla or mandible that formerly contained the teeth. Some edentulous patients have atrophic maxillae and/or mandibles or bony defects caused by trauma or tumor resection that will not support artificial dentures. The alveolar ridges can be augmented or reconstructed.

Inlay Bone Grafts

Bone grafts are used for augmentation of the maxillae and/or mandible. A prevascularized autologous rib graft may be transplanted into a maxillary defect; microvascular anastomoses revascularize the graft. Composite grafts of freeze-dried cadaver rib with autologous particulate cancellous bone and marrow may be preferred in the maxilla. Iliac bone used to augment the mandible calvaria may be harvested from the frontal, parietal, or occipital cranial bones for maxillofacial bone grafts. Calvarial bone undergoes less resorption than rib and iliac bone because of its dense blood supply; graft tissue revascularizes rapidly. Titanium osseointegration fixtures may be used to secure calvarial bone grafts in place.

Dental Implant

Fixtures are implanted into the gingiva and attached to bone to replace or augment lost dentition. Dental implants may replace a single tooth or missing teeth. They are made of biocompatible metals, most commonly titanium, and may be coated with ceramic, carbon, or sapphire. Several types are used:

- *Endosteal implant:* A threaded screw, cylinder, or flat blade is implanted in an alveolus in the maxilla or mandible. The number of implants placed depends on availability of bone and the number of teeth to be replaced. The fixture is covered with soft tissue. By the process of osseointegration, a perimucosal seal and bond develop between the gingiva and the surface of the implant. Some implants have small holes that allow bone to grow through them to secure the implant. After a minimum of 3 (for the mandible) to 6 (for the maxilla) months, a second-stage procedure is performed to connect a solid post to the implanted fixture. This extends slightly above the gingiva. The artificial tooth is attached to this post with tiny screws. Osseointegration provides firm, immobile support and distributes the stress of chewing evenly within the jaw.
- *Subperiosteal implant:* The implant is placed beneath the periosteum directly onto the alveolar bone. This type of implant is used when bone is insufficient to support an endosteal implant.

- *Transosteal implant:* A bone plate with retaining posts, similar to the mandibular staple (see following), is used when the patient has severe mandibular alveolar ridge atrophy.

Mandibular Staple

The staple fastener prosthesis is implanted as an alternative to bone grafting to restore the ability of the mandible to support a denture. The titanium alloy (Tivanium) device has two transosteal pins with a set of fasteners and lock nuts between them on the curved cross-arch connecting plate. The staple is inserted with a drill guide and twist drills specifically designed for it. The staple is evenly seated in the holes drilled in the mandible to the point of contact with the inferior border.

A scratch or bend may weaken the staple and may result in a fracture of the device. A deformed staple will not fit into the drill holes properly. The prosthesis is carefully protected and is handled very little before implantation.

Neck

Anatomy and Physiology of the Neck

The neck connects the head and trunk of the body. It is supported by the cervical vertebrae posteriorly and muscles anteriorly and laterally. The larynx, leading to the trachea, and the proximal end of the esophagus pass within the muscular structure. The vascular, nervous, and lymphatic systems leading to and from the head also pass through the neck. The thyroid and parathyroid glands lie along the trachea on the anterior aspect at the base of the neck.

Larynx

The larynx, situated anteriorly between the hypopharynx superiorly and the trachea inferiorly, consists of three major cartilages supported by ligaments and muscles: the thyroid cartilage, which protects the soft inner structures; the cricoid cartilage directly beneath it; and the paired arytenoid cartilages posterior to the thyroid and joined to the cricoid. The thyroid cartilage is incomplete posteriorly, but the cricoid is a complete ring. The cricothyroid space lies between the thyroid and cricoid cartilages.

The larynx functions as an organ for speech and for closure of the glottis during swallowing to protect the respiratory passage and prevent aspiration. The epiglottis, an elastic cartilage covered with mucous membrane at the root of the tongue in the hypopharynx, covers the superior opening of the larynx during swallowing.

Extrinsic muscles open and close the glottis, the space between the true vocal cords. Intrinsic muscles regulate vocal cord tension. Movement of the paired arytenoid cartilages opens and closes the glottis. Folds of mucous membrane covering muscle line the larynx. The two upper folds are the false cords; the two lower folds are the true vocal cords. The true vocal cords attach to the arytenoid cartilages posteriorly and to the thyroid cartilage anteriorly. The cords are an integral part of phonation. They vibrate to produce sounds by rhythmically moving air particles. Production of vocal sound involves coordination of the musculature of the lips, tongue, soft palate, pharynx, and larynx. The mouth and pharynx are the resonating cavities.

The tenth cranial (vagus) nerve innervates the larynx. Its major branch to the larynx is the recurrent laryngeal nerve (Fig. 41.14). Trauma to the nerve can result in laryngeal paralysis, which is devastating if both nerves are paralyzed.

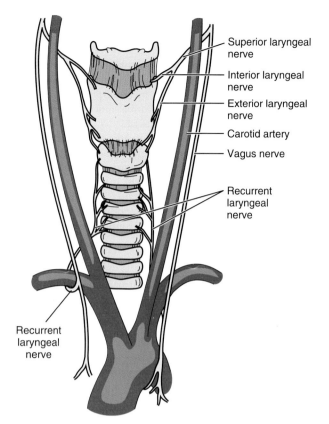

Superior laryngeal nerve

Interior laryngeal nerve

Exterior laryngeal nerve

Carotid artery

Vagus nerve

Recurrent laryngeal nerve

Recurrent laryngeal nerve

• **Fig. 41.14** Anatomy of the superior laryngeal and recurrent laryngeal nerves.

Trachea

The trachea is a 10 to 11-cm tube composed of rings of cartilage anteriorly and membrane posteriorly. This membrane also forms the anterior wall of the esophagus (the musculomembranous canal between the pharynx and the stomach). The trachea extends from the lower larynx to the carina in the chest, where it bifurcates to form the right and left main bronchi, leading to the lungs.

Surgical Procedures of the Larynx

Trauma or disease involving laryngeal cartilages, mucous membrane, or the vocal cords can obstruct respiration and/or speech. Surgical procedures are directed toward diagnosis of the cause and elimination of obstruction to maintain the larynx's dual functions in respiration and phonation.

Laryngoscopy

Laryngoscopy is a visual examination of the mucous membrane lining of the larynx and vocal cords with a lighted instrument, with or without the adjunct magnification of the operating microscope. Laryngoscopy is performed for diagnosis, biopsy, and/or treatment of laryngeal lesions, including the following:

- Foreign body, such as a coin, watch battery, or small toy.
- Papilloma of the vocal cords, which prevents accurate cord approximation and a normal voice.
- Laryngeal polyps, with stripping of polypoid mucosa to alleviate recurrence.
- Juvenile papilloma (multiple growths on the larynx, epiglottis, vocal cords, and trachea). These may be treated by cryosurgery or a laser in lieu of excision.

- Leukoplakia (a white thickening on the vocal cords, causing hoarseness). The lesion is examined histologically for differentiation from carcinoma.
- Laryngeal web (adherence of the anterior aspects of the vocal cords as a result of removal of mucous membrane or after inflammation). After excision, a metal or plastic plate may be placed between the cords until normal mucous membrane regenerates. The plate is then removed.

Preoperative preparation and endoscopic technique are similar for laryngoscopy, esophagoscopy, and bronchoscopy. General anesthesia usually is used, but local topical anesthesia may be preferred for some patients. The patient is supine with the neck hyperextended and head supported. As after any anesthetization of the throat, postoperative orders include nothing by mouth (NPO) status for a specific number of hours until throat reflexes have returned, to prevent aspiration.

Indirect Laryngoscopy

In indirect laryngoscopy, a laryngeal mirror is inserted through the mouth to the base of the tongue. With the patient in a sitting position, light is reflected to the area by the surgeon's headlamp. During this simple diagnostic procedure, a biopsy or polypectomy can be performed.

Direct Laryngoscopy

In direct laryngoscopy, a rigid, hollow, tubular laryngoscope is inserted into the larynx for direct visualization. Suction tubes and grasping forceps are maneuvered through the handheld laryngoscope. Fiberoptic light carriers are connected to a light source. Endoscopic principles as discussed in Chapter 32 are applicable.

Suspension Microlaryngoscopy

For microlaryngoscopy, the laryngoscope becomes self-retaining by suspension in a special appliance placed over the patient's chest. This gives the surgeon bimanual freedom in use of the operating microscope. The microscope provides binocular vision and magnification in critical inaccessible areas or areas difficult to visualize by direct laryngoscopy. A standard operating microscope with a 400-mm lens is used. Microlaryngeal instruments are added to the basic setup for direct laryngoscopy. Suspension microlaryngoscopy is used for most intralaryngeal procedures.

Laser Microlaryngoscopy

The CO_2 laser was introduced in laryngology by Jako and Strong in 1971. It was initially used for removal of recurrent laryngeal papillomas. Now CO_2 and other lasers are used to remove a variety of benign and malignant lesions in the respiratory tract, particularly in the larynx. For example, the argon laser may be used for treatment of hereditary hemorrhagic telangiectasia (dilated groups of capillaries) in the larynx.

A micromanipulator, used to direct the laser, is coupled to the operating microscope. The microscope lens focuses the beam. Reflecting mirrors defocus the beam to reach into otherwise inaccessible areas. Microlaryngeal instruments are used in addition to specific laser instruments. For example, anterior commissure vocal cord retractors with suction attachments are used to clear the smoke of tissue vaporization for visibility.

Laser Safety. The laser is a safe instrument when used around the oral cavity and neck only when the following safety precautions are taken:

1. The patient's eyelids should be taped shut and covered with moistened sponges to prevent injury from inadvertent reflection of the laser beam from a metal surface.
2. The patient's face should be covered with a moist towel so that only the oral cavity is exposed.
3. The patient's teeth should be protected from the pressure of the laryngoscope and from the laser beam.
4. Only noncombustible anesthetic gases are used. Anesthetic gases can be ignited by the laser. Nitrous oxide should not be used. Oxygen concentration may be decreased to between 21% and 30% during the lasing phase of the procedure.
5. A stainless steel or laminated aluminum and silicone endotracheal tube or a ventilating bronchoscope avoids the danger of ignition. Polyvinyl chloride and latex endotracheal tubes cannot be used because they are heat labile. Red rubber and silicone tubes may be wrapped with reflecting aluminum tape, but the tip is not always sufficiently protected if exposed to the laser beam. Ignition of endotracheal tubes has occurred. Moist gauze or compressed patties, attached to strings, are placed through the suspended laryngoscope to protect the balloon in the cuff of the tube from rupture by stray or reflected laser light. The balloon should be filled with sterile normal saline solution, which may be tinted with methylene blue dye, so the balloon will not ignite if ruptured. If a cuff does rupture, the blue dye will be immediately apparent. Rapid replacement of the endotracheal tube is necessary. A tracheotomy tray should be available for emergency use.
6. Combustible materials, such as sponges and drapes, are kept moist. Water effectively inhibits penetration of laser energy into surrounding tissue and materials.
7. Division of a blood vessel larger than 0.5 mm requires ligation or electrocoagulation.
8. All other precautions for laser surgery are taken.

Laryngeal Injuries

Patients with abnormal laryngeal conditions bear close watching for respiratory distress. The anterior, unprotected location of the larynx predisposes it to trauma, such as a crush injury. Treatment is concerned primarily with maintenance of the airway, which may be occluded by edema, hematoma, torn mucosa, or cartilaginous fragments.

Cricothyrotomy (emergency incision into the larynx) and/or tracheotomy (incision into the trachea) may be necessary to open the airway or to prevent asphyxia.[9] An intraluminal stent inserted into the larynx superior to the tracheostomy tube and fixed to it for stabilization may be worn for several months until the laryngeal laceration heals and an intralaryngeal airway reforms. The stent is used to mold the tissues.

Preservation of the voice is also a major concern. Severe laryngeal injury may result in permanent voice impairment. In unilateral vocal cord paralysis, because of muscle atrophy and muscle imbalance, a weak, hoarse ("air-spilling") voice is present. Inadequate glottic closure can be treated by injection of Teflon (Polytef) paste into the affected cord to augment its size and thus help bring the two cords into apposition. The injected material becomes firm and retains its shape. A functioning cord and marked improvement in voice quality result. This modality is used commonly when the recurrent laryngeal nerve is affected. It is not indicated for acute glottic incompetence. A suspension of Gelfoam powder in saline can be used for temporary augmentation until compensation or the need for permanent augmentation occurs.

Procedures for Carcinoma of the Larynx

Procedures vary depending on the size and location of the lesion, extent of invasion, and presence of regional or distant metastasis, as well as the patient's age, general condition, and rehabilitative capacity. Classification of malignant lesions by location includes glottic (true cords), supraglottic (above true cords), and infraglottic (below true cords) lesions.

In the early stages, cancer of the larynx is one of the most curable of all malignant tumors because of the sparse lymphatic supply in the region of the vocal cords. Radiologic study of the lesion by various methods, such as contrast laryngography, is a valuable adjunct in selecting an appropriate therapeutic modality. Laryngograms can identify mucosal irregularity, vocal cord thickening, or a tumor and can outline the lesion as well as portray functional alteration of laryngeal structures.

Symptoms vary as well. Hoarseness for more than 2 weeks' duration often is a result of cord fixation by a malignant glottic lesion. Dysphagia is suggestive of a tumor at the esophageal opening. Dyspnea from airway obstruction is a late manifestation.

Whenever possible, the surgeon will perform a conservative laryngectomy to retain some natural voice. These procedures yield the same rate of cure of selected cancers as a radical procedure—total laryngectomy—without sacrificing phonation, deglutition, or respiratory function. A neck stoma is usually necessary for breathing.

Laryngofissure With Partial Laryngectomy

Laryngofissure (division of or opening into the larynx) may be necessary to remove a foreign body or tumor. Laryngofissure with partial laryngectomy through an incision in the thyroid cartilage is performed to remove a large tumor confined to one vocal cord. A tracheotomy is performed to maintain the airway. Postoperative hoarseness may diminish as scar tissue forms to replace excised vocal cord.

Supraglottic Laryngectomy

The epiglottis, false cords, and hyoid bone are removed in a supraglottic laryngectomy when a tumor is located in the epiglottis (i.e., is supraglottic). A horizontal incision is made above the true vocal cords, thus preserving voice and a normal airway. Neck dissection may be done simultaneously. A temporary tracheotomy is always part of the procedure because of the danger of aspiration and postoperative edema. With the epiglottis removed, liquids in particular can easily spill into the trachea. A cuffed tracheostomy tube is a necessary precaution postoperatively.

Vertical Hemilaryngectomy

In hemilaryngectomy through a vertical incision, one true cord, false cord, arytenoid, and half of the thyroid cartilage are removed. The epiglottis, cricoid, and opposing cords are preserved. After healing, scar tissue fills in the surgical defect, almost approximating the remaining vocal cord. Thus the patient has a usable although hoarse voice and satisfactory airway and can eat normally. Sometimes a muscle flap is used for glottic reconstruction to improve voice quality. A prophylactic tracheotomy usually is done to protect the airway. Subcutaneous emphysema (i.e., infiltration of air under the skin) is a potential complication.

Total Laryngectomy

A radical procedure, total laryngectomy is performed for advanced lesions involving the larynx and/or hypopharyngeal area, with or without neck dissection. The entire larynx, hyoid bone, cricoid cartilage, two or three tracheal rings, and strap muscles are removed. This resection destroys the connection between the pharynx and the trachea. Pharyngeal walls and the lower trachea are preserved. The pharyngeal opening to the trachea is closed, leaving the pharynx open only to the esophagus.

The patient breathes and expels bronchial secretions through a permanent stoma at the base of the anterior neck postoperatively. This is created by suturing the tracheal stump to the skin (tracheostomy). The size of the stoma should be recorded on the patient's record in the event of emergency need for a tube at a later time. In patients with a permanent stoma, resuscitation is always via the stoma.

The nose no longer humidifies the air to the lungs. The sense of smell is also lost because the nasal olfactory epithelium is not stimulated by inhalation.[10] Acclimatization to air intake through the neck constitutes a major adjustment for the patient.

A nasogastric tube is inserted during the surgical procedure for temporary feeding. Although the patient no longer has a normal voice, normal eating is resumed after healing takes place.

The formation of a salivary fistula is one complication of laryngectomy. Swallowed saliva leaks out through a weakness in the pharyngeal suture line and through the skin. Rupture of the carotid artery, especially in preirradiated patients, is another complication. This may occur if radical neck dissection was also performed, which places the artery in the surgical area.

Rehabilitation should begin preoperatively at the time of diagnosis and include the family/significant others. It incorporates input from many professional disciplines because major disability results from the surgical procedure. In working with a speech pathologist, some patients develop esophageal speech. By intake of a bolus of air into the esophagus and vibration by cricopharyngeal muscles, sound is produced to articulate speech. Patients unable to perfect the technique may use an artificial larynx—an electronic device that includes pitch and volume.

Many patients are unable to acquire usable esophageal speech, with or without the artificial larynx. Some of these patients have undergone surgical procedures to rebuild a functioning glottis or create a permanent tracheoesophageal fistula to shunt pulmonary airflow to the pharynx for phonation. Aspiration pneumonia caused by leakage of saliva and food is a major problem after these procedures.

In addition, pharyngeal constrictor muscle spasms or stenosis may inhibit speech rehabilitation. Voice restoration for these aphonic patients may be enhanced by a valved prosthesis. This is inserted through a tracheoesophageal fistula to allow free flow of air into the esophagus for phonation, to prevent aspiration, and to maintain patency of the fistula. Examples of one-way valve voice prostheses used include:

- The Blom-Singer duckbill prosthesis, so named from the shape of the slit valve, is a silicone tube with retention flanges (collar-like projections). The fistula for the prosthesis is created through an esophagoscope inserted into the cervical esophagus. A needle is introduced to puncture the posterior tracheal wall and anterior esophagus at the superior aspect of the laryngectomy stoma. A rubber catheter stent is inserted through the puncture to maintain patency during healing. When the prosthesis is fitted, the flanges are taped to the peristomal skin. The patient occludes the stoma to produce a voice.

- The Blom-Singer tracheostoma valve and low-pressure prosthesis has a diaphragm that opens during normal respiration and closes in response to expiratory airflow for speech. The circular valve is recessed slightly into the tracheostoma, with the housing fixed to the peristomal skin with a hypoallergenic adhesive. The patient does not manually occlude the stoma during speech.
- The Panje voice prosthesis, commonly known as the voice button, is a biflanged silicone valve inserted into a simple tracheoesophageal stab wound. An insertion guide is used to place the prosthesis through the tracheostoma into the created fistula. The patient occludes the stoma to speak.

Practical help and moral support are offered to the newly laryngectomized patient by others who are members of support groups, such as the International Association of Laryngectomees and the Lost Chord Club. The American Cancer Society is also a resource for assistance.

Laryngeal Transplantation

In January 1998, Marshall Strome, formerly of the Cleveland Clinic Foundation, transplanted a larynx and a portion of a trachea into a 40-year-old man whose larynx was crushed in a motor vehicle accident 19 years previously. He was able to speak a few words within 12 hours of the procedure. The full extent of recovery will not be known for years; however, the patient, Timothy Heidler, has since become a motivational speaker and has joined the church choir.

The second successful larynx recipient was Brenda Charett Jensen in 2010 by Gregory Farwell at the University of California–Davis Medical Center. The surgical procedure took over 18 hours. She also received part of the donor's trachea and thyroid gland. After her surgery she was able to smell for the first time since her initial laryngeal injury. Jensen had a kidney-pancreas transplant in 2006.

Both patients have to take antirejection drugs for the rest of their lives. The earliest documented previous attempt to transplant a larynx was in 1969 in Belgium.

In 2023, the Mayo Clinic started the first program for laryngeal and trachea transplant using 3D models. The printed models are implanted to restore mouth breathing, swallowing, and speech. More information can be found at www.mayoclinic.org.

Surgical Procedures of the Esophagus

Esophageal disorders may be acquired or congenital. Abnormalities result from trauma, inflammation, neoplasm, or dysgenesis. A gastroenterologist and/or laryngologist may study them.

Esophagoscopy

Endoscopic direct visualization of the interior of the esophagus is performed to remove foreign bodies; to obtain biopsy, brush cytologic, or secretion specimens for diagnosis; and to examine the esophagus and esophageal orifice of the stomach for organic disease. Inspection is made for diverticula, varices, strictures, lesions, or a hiatal hernia, which may manifest as symptoms of obstruction, regurgitation, or bleeding.

Esophagoscopes are either rigid, hollow metal tubes or the flexible fiberoptic type of scope that reduces discomfort and trauma. Accessory instruments, such as aspiration tubes and biopsy forceps, are similar for all endoscopes. Removal of an obstructing mass, such as a steak bolus in the esophagus, is better accomplished with the rigid metal scope. Various sizes of scopes are available to suit the individual patient's situation.

The patient is positioned with the shoulders even with, or a little over, the edge of the body section of the OR bed. The head section is lowered. An assistant holds the patient's head. The patient is encouraged to relax by breathing deeply if the procedure is done with local topical anesthesia. The head is raised or lowered slowly, at the direction of the endoscopist as the esophagoscope is passed, until the neck is hyperextended. The esophagoscope is passed through the mouth and cricopharyngeal lumen to the cardiac sphincter at the esophagogastric junction. The entire area is carefully scrutinized. The esophagus may be distended by insufflation of air to assist in viewing in the presence of stenosis, or a lumen finder may be necessary. The scrub person introduces tips of aspirating tubes, grasping forceps, bougies, and other long accessories into a rigid esophagoscope for the endoscopist.

Removal of Foreign Bodies

Removal of foreign bodies from the pharynx and/or esophagus is relatively common. People who wear upper dentures are especially prone to swallowing sharp bones that cannot be felt against the covered palate. Pieces of meat or dental bridgework may lodge or become impacted in the food passage, occluding the airway by pressure. This is an emergency situation necessitating provision of a patent airway by endotracheal intubation or tracheotomy and endoscopic removal of the bolus or foreign object. Acute esophageal obstruction increases salivation, creating the danger of tracheopulmonary aspiration.

Children frequently swallow objects, such as watch or toy batteries, coins, buttons, parts of toys, or safety pins that may remain in the throat. Metallic objects are visible on radiographs, but many others are not.

It is dangerous to attempt to push an object toward the stomach because esophageal perforation can result. Esophagoscopy is the method of choice for removal, although the procedure is often difficult and painstaking. All effort is made to prevent trauma with resultant mediastinitis. Sometimes a small Foley catheter can be passed into the passage beyond the obstruction and the balloon inflated. This can aid in delivering oxygen to the patient and prevent the object from moving deeper into the passage.

Dilation of a Stricture

The esophageal lumen can narrow because of the formation of scar tissue resulting from inflammation or a burn at any level. Treatment consists of regular dilation with bougies of graduated sizes. Steroid administration is adjunctive therapy.

When an individual suffers a severe burn, such as from swallowing a caustic material, gastrostomy may be indicated to bypass the esophagus until it heals. Dilation of such strictures uses retrograde fusiform bougies with spindle-shaped shafts that are linked together. They are carried through the gastrostomy, up the esophagus, and out the mouth. The treatment is continued for an extended period.

Dilation of a stricture at the cardioesophageal junction may be necessary in patients with cardiospasm (achalasia). Gross dilation above the stricture, often a result of muscular atrophy, leads to regurgitation. Diagnosis is made by x-ray, esophagoscopy, or gastroscopy. If dilation is unsuccessful, a myotomy at the esophagogastric junction (Heller procedure) is performed to enlarge the opening into the stomach. Severe, unyielding strictures may necessitate stent placement, resection, or esophageal replacement.

Neoplasms of the Esophagus

Most often malignant, neoplasms of the esophagus are treated by resection, photodynamic therapy, or irradiation. Dysphagia or obstruction demands immediate investigation. Surgical procedures of the esophagus fall under the classification of gastrointestinal surgery and may involve a thoracoabdominal incision.

Cervical Esophageal Reconstruction

Restoration of continuity of the alimentary tract is a major challenge after ablative surgery of the neck, particularly after cervical esophagectomy or circumferential pharyngectomy. The location of the primary tumor and its extension and the extent of resection are contributing factors in determining the most satisfactory reconstruction. A pectoralis major myocutaneous flap or a free revascularized intestinal autograft will satisfactorily restore continuity in some situations.

Transposition of the mobilized stomach, jejunum, or colon into the neck may be performed when the entire esophagus is resected. Two teams working simultaneously perform this pull-up procedure. The team of general surgeons performs the abdominal dissection to mobilize the stomach or intestine while the other team resects the primary tumor in the neck. The tumor may arise from the hypopharynx, cervical esophagus, or thyroid gland. Radical neck dissection is carried out for extension into the cervical lymph nodes. Anastomosis of the stomach or intestine to an esophageal remnant may be accomplished with a circular intraluminal stapler if the primary esophageal tumor is above the level of the thoracic inlet. Primary pharyngogastric anastomosis may be required for high transection of the pharynx.

Surgical Procedures of the Trachea

Upper respiratory tract obstruction and ventilatory failure may require surgical intervention when the need for intubation or positive pressure ventilation would be long term or of indefinite duration or when severe laryngeal obstruction is present. The obstruction is bypassed or resected.

Historically, opening the trachea was recorded in Egypt in 36 BCE. Legends report that Alexander the Great (356–323 BCE) opened the neck of one of his choking soldiers with the tip of his sword. Contemporary tracheostomy involving an artificial airway tube was not common until the 20th century. One of the treatments for polio in 1930 used a tracheostomy for clearing the bronchial tree in paralyzed patients.

Tracheotomy and Tracheostomy

Tracheotomy is an incision into the trachea below the larynx. Tracheostomy is the formation of an opening into the trachea in which a tube is inserted to help the patient breathe. Performed in any age-group to improve or maintain patency of the airway or relieve obstruction, the opening in the trachea provides easy accessibility for suctioning secretions from the tracheobronchial tree or administering anesthetic to patients with facial trauma or burns.

A tracheotomy is commonly a controlled prophylactic procedure but can be an acute emergency. An endotracheal tube may provide temporary airway relief before and during the tracheotomy. Indications for tracheotomy include severe trauma to the hypopharynx or larynx, acute laryngotracheal bronchitis or epiglottitis in infants and children, laryngeal edema, prolonged intubation, or any other condition that obstructs respiration.

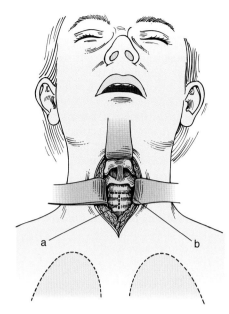

• **Fig. 41.15** Tracheotomy incisions. Midline vertical incision *(a)* is made between cricoid cartilage and suprasternal notch. Transverse incision *(b)* is used for emergency tracheotomy and cricothyrotomy.

Tracheotomy is often done with the patient under local anesthesia. The patient is supine with support under the shoulders to hyperextend the neck. A transverse incision is made, producing a better cosmetic result, or a midline vertical incision is made between the cricoid cartilage and the suprasternal notch. The overlying isthmus of the thyroid gland is retracted or divided, and the exposed third and fourth tracheal rings are incised through a midline vertical incision (Fig. 41.15). Use of cautery is avoided near the open trachea because the oxygen-rich environment supports combustion.

After tracheal suctioning to remove blood and secretions, a tracheostomy tube is inserted with the obturator in place. Immediately after insertion of the tube, the obturator is removed to open the airway. (This remains with the patient constantly in case of future need to reposition the tube.) The outer cannula is fixed in place, and the inner cannula can be suctioned or removed for cleaning. The wound is closed with a few sutures, or the superficial edges of the area above the tube may be sutured and the area below left with natural tissue approximation to facilitate drainage. A smooth-edged dressing split around the tube protects the skin. Commercial tracheostomy dressings are available.

Tapes tied to the ends of the outer cannula are secured around the neck. Proper tension allows insertion of one finger between the tape and skin. If the tapes are tied too tightly, they may compress the jugular vein; if the tapes are tied too loosely, the tube can obtrude with coughing. The tube should not be removed during the first 24 to 48 hours by any person unable to perform a tracheotomy because the tract to the trachea may occlude and not be immediately located.

A sterile tube identical to the one inserted and a tracheotomy set accompany the patient from the OR and constantly remain with them until otherwise indicated by the surgeon's order.

A tracheotomy is the creation of an open wound. Although rigid sterile technique is not possible, every effort is made to keep contamination to a minimum. Only sterile equipment with minimal handling is used to prevent infection. Suctioning through a tracheostomy tube is done as a sterile procedure with a sterile catheter and gloves. Careful suctioning prevents trauma. The catheter is inserted without application of suction, which could injure the tracheal walls and suction out oxygen in the patient with borderline oxygen saturation levels. Suction is applied as the catheter is withdrawn. Sterile solution is run through the catheter after use to clean it and maintain patency. Disposable catheters are recommended; they are used once and discarded.

Some patients who have undergone tracheotomy come to the OR for a change of the tube or other procedure. These patients may require suctioning while waiting in the holding area. Knowledge of and preparation for each patient is a prime responsibility of the circulator. These patients require humidified air, which can be delivered by various devices, to keep secretions liquefied and prevent drying of tissues. Other needs are constant observation and special communication (e.g., pencil and paper, dry erase board, and/or picture board).

Tracheostomy Tubes

Although an endotracheal tube may provide ventilation for short-term therapy, a tracheostomy tube is easier to suction and immobilize for extended use. It also reduces the possibility of laryngeal injury and tracheomalacia.

Most tubes have three parts—the outer cannula, inner cannula, and obturator (Fig. 41.16). The inner cannula is periodically removed and cleaned to prevent blockage by crusting of secretions. It is replaced immediately within the outer cannula so that the latter remains free of crusting. The obturator provides a smooth tip during tube insertion to prevent trauma to the tracheal wall. Some plastic tubes do not require an inner cannula because they remain relatively free of crust. If crusts do form, the tube is changed.

Some tubes have a built-in soft cuff that is inflated to eliminate any free space between the tube and the tracheal wall, thus preventing aspiration of drainage down the trachea. Cuffed tubes also facilitate function of any ventilatory apparatus.

A pilot balloon in the inflation line, attached to the outer cannula, indicates cuff inflation or deflation. Proper cuff inflation-deflation is very important. Irritation and pressure of the cuff against the tracheal wall can cause damage such as ulceration and necrosis of the mucosa, which can lead to infection, tracheobronchial fistula, erosion into the innominate artery, or stenosis from scarring.

Precautionary measures include deflation at regular intervals, by the physician's written order, to increase blood flow to the cuff

• **Fig. 41.16** Tracheostomy tube. **A,** Outer cuffed cannula. **B,** Inner cannula. **C,** Obturator. **D,** Pilot balloon in inflation line.

site; use of a low-pressure or controlled-pressure cuff; constant monitoring of intracuff pressure; and minimum inflation to ensure a leak-free system. Overinflation can reduce the tube diameter, as well as cause the cuff to extend over the tip of the tube, thus obstructing ventilation. Or the tracheal wall may herniate over the tube end. Underinflation may cause subcutaneous emphysema. Cuffs also should inflate symmetrically. The amount of air needed for inflation varies with the size of the trachea and the tube. Understandably, less air is needed for larger tubes. Usually 2 to 5 mL of air provides a closed system.

Specific tubes have special variations, such as an opening in the wall opposite the bevel to permit ventilation in case of bevel occlusion. Others have a radiopaque tip that allows x-ray visualization of the tube position. Many have connectors, some of which are a built-in swivel type, permitting lightweight, flexible, easy connection to a ventilating system. These connectors reduce the hazard of accidental disconnection. Still others have a fenestration in the outer cannula, permitting air to flow through the larynx. These tubes are used to allow assessment of spontaneous breathing and coughing in preparation for decannulation in patients no longer requiring mechanical ventilation.

With air passing through the larynx, the patient can speak with the proximal end of the cannula plugged. A so-called speaking tube permits introduction of humidified air and oxygen through a special line, and with upward flow of the gas through the larynx, the patient can speak.

Tracheal Resection

Tracheal obstruction can result from trauma or a tumor, thus occluding the patient's airway. Localized erosion and scarring, causing narrowing and breakdown of the trachea, can develop from prolonged endotracheal intubation or a tracheotomy. An obstructive or stenotic lesion can be resected and the trachea reconstructed by end-to-end anastomosis.

Through a cervical, low-collar skin incision, the upper trachea and subglottis are mobilized. A right posterolateral thoracotomy incision is used for lesions in the distal trachea near the carina, where the trachea bifurcates into the right and left bronchi. A longitudinal incision is made in the stenotic area, and an anode tube (a flexible wire-reinforced endotracheal tube) is inserted into the distal trachea to maintain respiration. The trachea is transected circumferentially above and below the obstructed segment. The laryngeal attachments to the trachea are released, and the suprahyoid muscle is transected. Up to 5 to 6 cm of trachea can be resected and closed by primary anastomosis. The neck is flexed so that the edges of the trachea can be approximated without tension.

The neck may be kept flexed during postoperative healing by a heavy suture from the chin to the chest. The patient remains intubated, with the end of the tube located beyond the anastomosis at the carina (as a stent), for 1 or 2 days. Care is taken to prevent the endotracheal tube from entering the bronchus and only using one lung. Epidural anesthesia is often used because using opioids can cause periods of apnea.

Surgical Procedures of the Anterior Neck

Many laryngologists and plastic surgeons, as well as some oral and general surgeons, perform neck dissection when cervical lymph nodes are involved in cancer of the head and neck. A multidisciplinary team, including a thoracic and/or general surgeon, may perform some complex resections and reconstructive procedures.

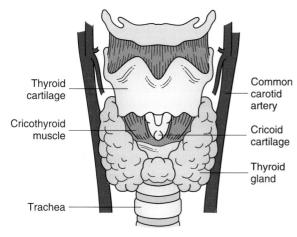

• **Fig. 41.17** Anterior view of thyroid gland.

Thyroid cartilage

Cricothyroid muscle

Trachea

Common carotid artery

Cricoid cartilage

Thyroid gland

The patient may be positioned with the neck extended, usually over a thyroid elevator. The arms are secured at the sides of the body and not on armboards, thus preventing distortion of the body contour in the neck region. The OR bed may be tilted into reverse Trendelenburg position.

Thyroid Procedures

The thyroid gland, located in the anterior aspect of the neck, is composed of two vascular lobes that lie on either side of the trachea and are united by a narrow band, the isthmus (Fig. 41.17). The thyroid hormone controls the rate of body metabolism and may influence physical and mental growth.

Hyperthyroidism (Graves disease), hypothyroidism, and an enlarged gland (goiter) are the main disorders of the thyroid gland. Drugs, radioactive iodine, and/or surgical resection are used to treat hyperthyroidism. This disease, which is rare in geriatric patients or the very young, affects women more frequently than men. Replacement of the thyroid hormone with drug therapy is the specific treatment for hypothyroidism. Oral administration of thyroid extract or iodine may reduce the size of the gland, but surgical excision is frequently necessary to remove benign or malignant tumors.

Emil Theodor Kocher (1841−1917), a Swiss surgeon, revolutionized thyroid surgical procedures for which he won the Nobel Peace Prize in 1909. Thanks to Jules Pean (1830−1898), who invented the hemostat in 1874 to control bleeding, Kocher demonstrated that if bleeding were controlled, patients would survive thyroidectomy. Before hemostasis, death from the procedure was around 70%. Kocher improved on the hemostat in 1882 with the development of the Kocher clamp and further increased the odds of many surgical procedures' success with advanced hemostasis. Preservation of the parathyroid glands in 1891 became an additional focus of thyroidectomy that enhanced the patient's metabolic physiology.

Thyroid Biopsy

A needle biopsy or an excisional biopsy may be performed to aid in establishing a diagnosis of thyroiditis or in differentiating between nodular goiter and carcinoma.

Thyroidectomy

During all thyroidectomy procedures, care is exercised not to damage the laryngeal nerves and parathyroid glands. The patient is

• **Fig. 41.18** Position and incision for thyroidectomy.

positioned supine with the neck hyperextended to provide good exposure of all structures (Fig. 41.18). A transverse collar incision is made in a natural skin crease about 1 inch (2.5 cm) above the clavicle. The cervical fascia is incised vertically in the midline.

Throughout the surgical procedure, meticulous hemostasis is maintained. Blood supply arises from the external carotid arteries to the upper poles of the thyroid gland and from the subclavian arteries to the lower poles. The superior laryngeal nerves, which innervate the cricothyroid muscles, and recurrent laryngeal nerves, which innervate the vocal cords, are identified. Trauma to these nerves can result in temporary or permanent laryngeal paralysis. Voice disturbances with hoarseness occur with paralysis of one vocal cord.

Postoperative complications of thyroidectomy include hematoma, edema of the glottis, injury to a recurrent laryngeal nerve, muscle rigidity and spasm (tetany), and acute thyrotoxicosis. A tracheotomy set should remain at the patient's bedside postoperatively for at least 24 hours in the event of respiratory obstruction.

A general surgeon usually performs thyroidectomy. Depending on the pathologic diagnosis, the surgeon chooses the most appropriate procedure for removal of a part of or the entire thyroid gland.

Thyroid Lobectomy. An entire lobe is removed, especially for toxic diffuse goiter, which is usually benign. In case of malignant growth, the lobe and lymph nodes in the neck that drain into the involved area may be dissected.

Subtotal Thyroidectomy. The usual procedure for hyperthyroidism is removal of approximately five-sixths of the thyroid gland. This procedure generally relieves symptoms permanently because the remaining thyroid tissue secretes sufficient hormone for normal function.

Total Thyroidectomy. Excision of both lobes plus the isthmus may be the procedure of choice for palpable disease in both lobes.

Substernal Intrathoracic Thyroidectomy. Invasion of the gland into substernal and intrathoracic regions can cause tracheal obstruction. The sternum may have to be split to remove a large, adherent intrathoracic goiter.

Parathyroid Gland Procedures

The parathyroid glands are small endocrine glands that regulate metabolism of calcium and phosphorus. Four or more glands are located within or are attached to the substance of the thyroid gland (two on each side), or they may migrate into the neck or mediastinum. Primary hyperparathyroidism is associated with hypercalcemia, which may be secondary to renal, skeletal, or gastrointestinal disease. A single gland or multiple glands may be diseased and surgically excised. The incision and exposure are the same as described for thyroidectomy.

Subtotal Parathyroidectomy

A single diseased gland, confirmed by frozen section, is excised. Up to three and a half glands may be removed if all glands appear to be involved, as in diffuse hyperplastic disease. Parathyroid glands are handled by their pedicles to avoid crushing, suturing, or violating the capsule. Inadvertently implanted parathyroid tissue may cause recurrence of disease or persistent or recurrent hypercalcemia. A remnant of normal tissue is left to prevent hypoparathyroidism, which may cause severe tetany. Removed normal tissue may be cryopreserved for autotransplantation in muscle, usually in the forearm, if hypoparathyroidism develops or reoperation is necessary for recurrent or persistent hyperparathyroidism.

Total Parathyroidectomy With Autotransplantation

All parathyroid tissue is removed when all glands are abnormal. First described by William Halsted in 1907, a portion of a gland is immediately transplanted into a vascularized muscle, usually the sternocleidomastoid, which is in the surgical field. Some surgeons prefer to put the transplant in a forearm muscle. This procedure may be done when embedded parathyroid glands are removed in conjunction with a total thyroidectomy. Postoperative supplemental calcium and vitamin D should be considered for treatment of hypoparathyroidism.

Thyroglossal Duct Cystectomy. During fetal development, the thyroid gland descends through the thyroglossal duct from the foramen cecum near the base of the tongue to the neck below the larynx. In adulthood, remnants of this embryonic duct may form a cyst in the anterior midline of the neck. Excision requires removal of the entire cystic sac and a portion of hyoid bone that surrounds the duct.

Cervical and Scalene Lymph Node Biopsy. Biopsy specimens are taken of the cervical and/or scalene nodes for diagnosis of metastatic extension of cancer or tuberculosis into these lymphatic nodes. A thoracic surgeon may perform the procedure.

Neck Dissections

Tumors, benign and malignant, occur in the head and neck regions. Although the origin of many of these neoplasms is technically in the head, the cervical lymph nodes frequently are involved secondarily by metastases from a primary head or neck malignant tumor. Treatment is directed toward definitive management for eradication of the tumor and metastases, with consideration for rehabilitation. In an attempt to eradicate all cancer foci, neck dissection may be performed at a time later than removal of a primary lesion of, for example, the parotid gland or tongue or simultaneously as a one-stage procedure. This composite resection removes the primary tumor and metastatic lesions at the same time en masse. Sometimes metastasis occurs before a primary lesion is discovered.

Various reconstructive techniques provide immediate restoration to improve speech, reestablish oral function, or prevent airway obstruction. Others involve delayed reconstruction. The method of repair depends on the type of defect resulting from excision of the lesion. Preoperatively, the patient's emotional stability is analyzed if the surgical procedure will result in a cosmetic deformity. Reconstruction is planned so that local tissue can be used whenever feasible and normal function is preserved whenever possible. The aim of reconstruction is to restore function and appearance.

Radical Neck Dissection

Malignant tumors of the oral or pharyngeal cavities, cutaneous malignant melanoma, and skin cancer in the head and neck region often require wide resection of the primary lesion and excision of all of the cervical lymph nodes on one or both sides of the neck. This procedure gives the patient with cancer of the cervical lymphatic chain a chance for cure and arrest of spread. When metastasis is known to be present or is highly suspected because of the location or stage of the malignancy, the surgical procedure is predicated on the assumption that metastases are regional and not distant.

A predominant cause of throat cancer is the human papillomavirus (HPV).[11] Current literature reflects that HPV-related cancer of the throat is found in a younger population of relatively otherwise healthy males. According to the Centers for Disease Control and Prevention (CDC), HPV cancers are decreasing since the introduction of the HPV vaccine. (More information can be found at www.cdc.gov.)[11] Many of these tumors present at the base of the tongue or near the tonsils. The scrub person should carefully keep all tonsillar specimens separate as left and right when sending them to pathology because lymphatic spread of cancer is specific to the side of the throat affected. Correct identification of which side is involved can spare the patient a more extensive radical procedure.

The head and neck surgeon plans the surgical procedure with reconstruction in mind, so that the incisions will allow good exposure but provide as much local flap tissue as possible for reconstruction. Incisions used for the tumor resection will necessarily vary according to the type of reconstruction planned. No single surgical procedure can be used to treat all lesions, but certain basic features remain common to all neck dissections (Fig. 41.19).

All lymph-bearing tissue from the midline anteriorly to the trapezius muscle posteriorly and from the mandible superiorly to the clavicle inferiorly is removed. All tissue between the deep cervical fascia and the platysma muscle externally is removed except the carotid artery system; the vagus, phrenic, and hypoglossal nerves; and the brachial plexus.

The massive tissue resection (removal en bloc) includes the jugular vein, 11th cranial (spinal accessory) nerve, sternocleidomastoid muscle, and submandibular salivary gland. Elimination of

C

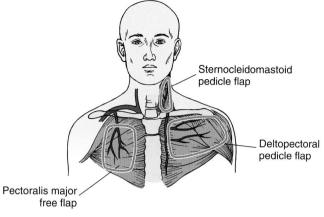

- **Fig. 41.19** Neck incisions for radical neck dissection. **A,** Block dissection. **B,** Modified Y-incision for block dissection to include radical parotidectomy. **C,** Submandibular surgical anatomy.

the motor nerve to the trapezius muscle contributes to muscular atrophy, subsequent shoulder drop on the affected side, and possibly decreased strength in raising the arm.

Various techniques are used to close the large defect in the anterior neck. When the occipital, posterior auricular, facial, and superior thyroid arteries can be preserved, arterialized skin flaps designed to incorporate branches from these vessels can be constructed with the length up to three or four times the width. Otherwise, the length of a flap should not exceed twice the width.

A deltopectoral pedicle flap or a pectoralis major myocutaneous free flap may be needed (Fig. 41.20). An exposed carotid artery is covered. Cervical flaps carrying their own blood supply may be used for this and to restore the oropharyngeal lining intraorally. A pedicle flap of sternocleidomastoid muscle from the clavicle may be an alternative.

The mandible is preserved unless it is involved by direct extension of the tumor into the bone. Access through a mandibular osteotomy or partial mandibulectomy is usually required for effective resection in the posterior oral cavity. Solid bony continuity and realignment of the dental arches are established for functional restoration of speech and chewing. A revascularized free fibular graft, a bone graft from the rib or iliac crest, cancellous bone chips, or a composite graft may be used to stabilize the mandible.

Effective drainage of the wound is important to healing. This is accomplished by use of closed-wound suction drains inserted through stab wounds below the clavicle. Prevention of hematoma protects the viability of the thin skin flaps and facilitates approximation of wound surfaces.

- **Fig. 41.20** Myocutaneous flap to close defect after radical neck dissection may be deltopectoral pedicle flap, pectoralis major free flap, or sternocleidomastoid pedicle flap.

A tracheotomy may be performed to protect the patient from respiratory distress in neck dissection alone. A tracheostomy is always done in a composite radical neck resection.

A feeding gastrostomy tube may be inserted for anticipated extended feeding. This permits suction to avoid aspiration and gastric distention in addition to providing a feeding route. The tube is usually inserted in the OR.

Potential complications of neck dissection are numerous, depending on the tumor itself, irradiation therapy, or necessary sacrifice of vital structures. Intraoperatively, hemorrhage may occur from injury to a major vessel or the thoracic duct. Postoperatively, invasion of overlying skin necrosis into a major vessel wall, such as the carotid artery, can cause an often-fatal blowout of the vessel. Slight previous bleeding may be a forewarning. Balloon occlusion of the carotid artery may be used to prevent hemorrhage.

Although reconstruction begins at the time of primary neck dissection, the patient usually requires considerable postoperative rehabilitation psychologically and staged procedures before cosmetic and functional reconstruction is complete.

The advent of robotic surgery has improved the process and outcome of throat cancer surgery. Transoral procedures are more refined using robotics and minimize the need for the disfigurement associated with radical neck surgery.

Face and Skull

Anatomy and Physiology of the Face

The face is the anterior part of the head, including the forehead, cheeks, nose, lips, and chin, but not the ears. The eyes, situated in the bony orbits, contribute to the features of the face, although they are not technically a part of the face.

The skeletal structure of the face and skull (Fig. 41.21) includes the frontal bone of the forehead. It forms the upper part of the orbits. Divided by sutures (i.e., lines of union between bones), the frontal bone joins the sphenoid and ethmoid and the paired nasal, lacrimal, maxilla, and zygomatic bones. The posterior orbits are formed by the sphenoid bone, which is shaped like a butterfly with extended wings, and the palatal bones. The medial walls are formed by the ethmoid, lacrimal, and nasal bones and maxilla. The lateral aspect is formed by the zygoma (malar bone),

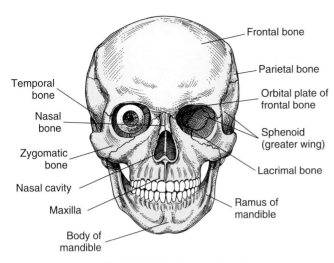

Temporal bone
Nasal bone
Zygomatic bone
Nasal cavity
Maxilla
Body of mandible
Frontal bone
Parietal bone
Orbital plate of frontal bone
Sphenoid (greater wing)
Lacrimal bone
Ramus of mandible

• **Fig. 41.21** Anterior view of skull.

or the cheekbone. The irregularly shaped ethmoid bone also forms the roof and posterior lateral wall of each nasal cavity. The nasal bones form the bridge of the nose between the orbits.

The maxilla (the upper jaw that holds the palate) extends laterally to the zygoma and temporal bone, under the orbit, and along the anterior nasal cavity. The maxillary bones are paired and join in the midline between the nose and the oral cavity. The alveoli that hold the teeth are along the alveolar processes of the maxillae.

The ramus of the mandible (the arch-shaped bone of the lower jaw) articulates with temporal bones at the temporomandibular joints in front of the ears. The alveoli, the tooth-bearing bodies, meet at the alveolar process to form the chin (mental region).

The bony structure of the face is covered with muscles, superficial blood vessels and nerves, epidermis, and dermis. Other structures (i.e., ducts and sinuses [air spaces]) are also in the soft tissues or bony structure of the face.

Considerations for Craniofacial Surgery

The term *craniofacial* refers to the cranium and face. Craniofacial surgery of increasing complexity has been performed since World War II. The approaches and techniques developed by French plastic surgeon Paul Tessier (1917–2008) have led to previously inaccessible anatomic areas. Tessier's accomplishments included the use of autologous bone and transcranial approach for correction of bony deformity of the eye orbits. He performed the first successful LeFort III osteotomy in 1958 that earned him the title of father of craniofacial surgery.

Exposure for dissection of soft tissues and bone to restore contour and symmetry in practically every type of facial deformity, whether congenital, neoplastic, or traumatic in origin, can be accomplished by a multidisciplinary team of surgeons. This team may include a plastic surgeon, neurosurgeon, anesthesia provider, ophthalmologist, oral surgeon, and otorhinolaryngologist. Some procedures require more than 100 separate maneuvers and may take as long as 14 to 16 hours to complete.

Many of the concepts developed for these very complex procedures are applied in the more common and less complicated procedures to reshape sections of the skull or reconstruct soft tissues. Craniofacial reconstruction should be performed as soon as indicated by the physiologic and psychologic effects of the

deformity on the patient, regardless of age. An early surgical procedure not only decreases psychologic trauma but also may prevent craniofacial distortion caused by brain and nerve damage of a disease process or traumatic injury.

Analysis of three-dimensional CT scans and cephalometric tracings accurately superimposed on transparent photographs of the patient preoperatively is essential to determine the extent of the facial deformity and the plan for skeletal rearrangement. The exact size of the defects that will need bone grafts can be determined.

Many procedures involve correction of malocclusion of the mandible at the same time that the orbitocranial skeleton is restructured. Dental models are cut and mounted on an articulator for reference.

Hypotensive anesthesia reduces blood loss during these extensive procedures. The patient is continuously monitored throughout the procedure to estimate blood loss. A preoperative tracheotomy may be necessary to maintain an adequate airway postoperatively.

Craniofacial Anomalies

Congenital craniofacial anomalies have a monumental effect on the life and activities of children their families and caregivers. These children spend much of their early lives in medical and surgical treatment followed by psychosocial therapy. Not only are these children physically deformed in appearance, but they also often have impaired vision, speech, and hearing and difficulty with nutritional intake. In some circumstances the child may be mentally disabled or have other brain injury that results in seizures. Correction of the anomaly can preserve normal intelligence in an estimated 77% of neonates affected when other genetic problems are not involved. Most craniofacial defects are not genetic in origin.

Some of the anomalies are extreme and visually gruesome, but defects that are incompatible with life are complex critical issues to correct in the first few hours or days after birth. The first objective of surgical intervention is to support the child's life functions such as breathing, eating, communicating, and vision. The second objective is to bring the child's form into a more natural appearance. Fig. 41.22 depicts the primary areas of the infant's skull that are involved with craniofacial deformity.

The entire therapeutic process is a multidisciplinary effort of many specialized team members. Another issue to consider is that the child may have additional congenital defects of the internal organs or limbs that need to be addressed simultaneously with the head and neck.

Most of the anomalies associated with the head and neck have been categorized by the type of defect and its effect on the development of the face and skull.[12] The main syndromes are as follows:

1. *Craniosynostosis:* Premature fusion of one or more sutures of the skull. Can be unilateral or bilateral, causing facial abnormalities and increased intracranial pressure. Diagnosis is made via x-ray, cranial ultrasound, and three-dimensional CT imaging. Congenital craniosynostosis occurs in 5:10,000 births.[11]
    a. *Scaphocephaly:* Most common type. Closure of the sagittal suture causes an increased anteroposterior length (Fig. 41.23, *A*).
    b. *Plagiocephaly:* Caused by unilateral or unequal coronal synostosis and may involve the lambdoid suture. The face and head are asymmetric (Fig. 41.23, *B*).

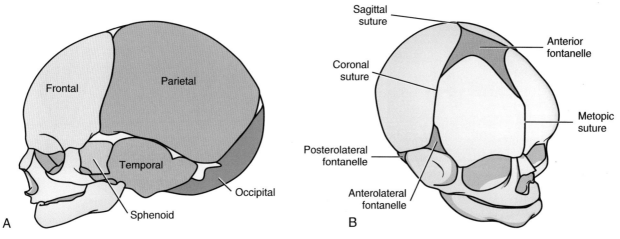

• **Fig. 41.22 A,** Bones of the infant skull. **B,** Suture synarthroses of the infant skull.

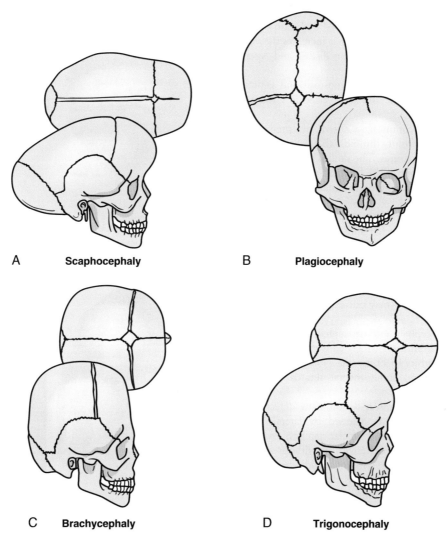

• **Fig. 41.23** Examples of craniosynostosis. **A,** Scaphocephaly. **B,** Plagiocephaly. **C,** Brachycephaly. **D,** Trigonocephaly.

• **Fig. 41.24** Hypertelorism. (From Martin R, Fanaroff A, Walsh M: *Fanaroff and Martin's neonatal-perinatal medicine,* ed 10, Philadelphia, 2015, Elsevier.)

• **Fig. 41.25** Pierre Robin syndrome. (From Martin R, Fanaroff A, Walsh M: *Fanaroff and Martin's neonatal-perinatal medicine,* ed 10, Philadelphia, 2015, Elsevier.)

c. *Acrocephaly/oxycephaly/turricephaly:* Caused by fusion of the coronal and frontoethmoidal sutures that increases the vertical axis of the skull. Seen in Crouzon disease and Apert syndrome.

d. *Brachycephaly:* Caused by bicoronal synostosis and sagittal shortening. The head is wide and short. Seen in Crouzon disease (see Fig. 41.23, *C*).

e. *Trigonocephaly:* Least common. Caused by premature closure of metopic and frontoethmoidal (between the frontal and ethmoid bones) sutures. The skull is triangle shaped with the apex on the front of the forehead with hypotelorism (abnormal decrease in the bony distance between the eyes) (see Fig. 41.23, *D*).

2. *Hypertelorism:* A genetic defect that may appear independently or as a result of a midline facial cleft and/or encephalocele and causes an abnormal increase in the bony distance between the eyes measured between the medial orbital walls. Problems with binocular vision and an absent sense of smell (Fig. 41.24).

3. *Pierre Robin syndrome:* Micrognathia, mandibular hypoplasia, wide cleft palate, glossoptosis (may cause apnea), and feeding difficulties (Fig. 41.25).

4. *Crouzon disease:* Brachycephaly and turricephaly caused by craniosynostosis, midfacial retrusion associated with maxillary hypoplasia, shallow eye orbits to house the globe, optic nerve damage, "bird beak" nose, some mental retardation, and airway difficulty (Fig. 41.26).

5. *Treacher Collins syndrome:* Autosomal dominant defect that causes mandibulofacial dysostosis. Caused by lateral facial clefts through the maxilla and malar arches; narrow oropharynx and a high-arched palate with or without a cleft; external ear deformities with or without middle and inner ear defects and conductive hearing loss; lower eyelid deformities, including coloboma (notching of the iris) and partial to total absence of lower lashes; and nasal deformity. May result in esophageal collapse requiring a feeding tube and apnea requiring a tracheostomy (Fig. 41.27).

6. *Craniofacial microsomia:* Caused by the intrauterine interruption of the development of the first and second branchial arches. Also known as oral-mandibular-auricular syndrome. Most common in males. Usually unilateral, but can be

• **Fig. 41.26** Crouzon disease. (From Posnick JC, editor: *Craniofacial and maxillofacial surgery in children and young adults,* vol 1, Philadelphia, 2000, Saunders.)

• **Fig. 41.27** Treacher Collins syndrome. (From Neligan PC: *Plastic surgery,* ed 3, Philadelphia, 2013, Elsevier.)

bilateral. Can accompany many other defects such as torticollis, craniosynostosis, microtia, facial clefts, absent lung or kidney, cranial nerve abnormality, vertebral malformations, eye malformation, oral feeding problems, and airway collapse.

• **Fig. 41.28** Apert syndrome. (From Posnick JC, editor: *Craniofacial and maxillofacial surgery in children and young adults,* vol 1, Philadelphia, 2000, Saunders.)

7. *Apert syndrome:* Also known as acrocephalosyndactyly (autosomal dominant syndrome of anomalies of the extremities, head, and hands). The syndrome is characterized by coronal craniosynostosis; exorbitism; hypertelorism; maxillary hypoplasia; wide, hooked nose; narrow palate with median groove, with or without cleft; bilateral symmetric syndactyly of the hands and/or feet; and ankylosis of the elbows, shoulders, and hips. Airway obstruction is secondary to midface hypoplasia, necessitating a tracheostomy, and anomalies of the heart, lungs, and kidneys can be life-threatening. Hearing can be a problem because of malformed eustachian tubes (Fig. 41.28).

8. *Microtia:* Small or absent ears.

Congenital craniofacial deformities are surgically treated by several types of cranial remodeling procedures. Some procedures require the child to wear midface external distraction devices that are tightened daily to cause the face to shift into a forward position. In some conditions the dome of the skull is reshaped by opening the fused sutures and wearing a helmet. Each congenital condition has varying degrees of intellectual disability associated with compression of the brain that must be released to minimize the damage.

Craniofacial Procedures

Midface Advancement

The base of the anterior cranial fossae can be exposed through a bifrontal incision to elevate a frontal bone flap. While the neurosurgeon is raising the flap, the plastic surgeon may take donor bone from a rib and/or the iliac crest if autologous bone grafts will be needed. Harvesting of bone from the calvaria (the upper, dome-like portion of the skull) may be preferred.

The facial skeleton is separated from the cranial base. The plastic surgeon raises the periorbita, orbital contents, and soft tissue over the dorsum of the nose. The subperiosteum of the anterior maxillae is elevated. Osteotomies are cut in the supraorbital region to mobilize the lateral walls. An anterior maxillary osteotomy, through an infraorbital approach, extends across and below the frontal processes of the maxillae. Osteotomies of the anterior cranial fossae and the medial and lateral orbital walls and floors are completed. The mobilized bones can be functionally advanced in three dimensions as desired. They are then stabilized with a plating system or wired into position.

To maintain stability, bone grafts also are wired into place in the resulting defects. Resorbable plates and fixation are available for use. Demineralized bone blocks, chips, or powder often is preferred to bone grafts to induce osteogenesis. The frontal bone flap is replaced, and the incision is closed.

Mandibular osteotomies may be done before closure to correct alignment of the jaws. Regardless of whether necessary, the mandible is stabilized after closure with intermaxillary wires and suspension wires to the zygomatic arch.

Depending on the deformity, variations of the intracranial and extracranial osteotomies are done to advance, align, or reposition the facial bones and reconstruct soft tissues. Many patients return to the OR for additional corrective procedures: eyelid ptosis and/or extraocular muscle surgery performed by the ophthalmologist; dacryocystorhinostomy and/or nasal reconstruction performed by the rhinologist; and bone augmentation or resection of the maxillae and/or mandible for repositioning by the plastic surgeon or oral surgeon. During all procedures the surgeons avoid injury to optic and facial nerves and to arteries and veins.

Procedures of the Orbit

An abnormally wide space between (hypertelorism) or malposition (dystopia) of the bony orbits is usually secondary to other craniofacial malformations. The medial orbital walls by themselves may be moved to correct minimal hypertelorism. Advancement of the superior and lateral walls, rather than total orbit advancement, may suffice to correct a dystopia. A combined intracranial and extracranial approach may be necessary to change the angle of the orbits and reposition the medial canthal ligaments of the eyes.

Resection of Nasal or Paranasal Sinus Tumors

Radical craniofacial resection may be indicated to remove gigantic benign nasal dermoid tumors and malignant tumors of the paranasal sinuses. In a one-stage procedure, all involved soft tissue is excised with simultaneous correction of the underlying skeletal structure.

Basal cell carcinoma is a common type of nasal tumor. The surgical procedure may be performed alone or as combined therapy. Immediate repair by skin graft or pedicle flap accompanies excision of well-defined lesions. Reconstruction is postponed in multicentric (many-centered) cancer or if there is doubt regarding extension of the tumor. More advanced lesions require replacement of the nose by a prosthesis or a tissue flap.

Erosion of a growth in one of the sinuses into an adjacent nasal wall can occlude the air passage. Resection may include partial or total maxillectomy and removal of surrounding tissues. The cavity usually is covered by a skin graft. Unilateral enucleation of the eye may be necessary. A radical surgical procedure for an ethmoid tumor also may involve removal of part of the base of the skull and excision of the maxillary antrum and the palate on the affected side.

In providing maxillofacial prostheses to replace facial structures after various procedures, the prosthodontist works closely with the surgeon and radiation therapist. Splints or stents hold tissue grafts in place, seal cavities from each other, or unite bony segments. A dental prosthesis to close the defect in the upper jaw and an eye prosthesis after enucleation contribute to the patient's rehabilitation after an extensive surgical procedure.

Resection of Craniofacial Tumors and Dysplasia

Malignant tumors can originate from soft tissues of the face and scalp, the oropharyngeal mucosa, the ear canal, or the lacrimal gland. They can invade the base of the skull. Fibrous dysplasia, a congenital metabolic disturbance that causes an abnormal proliferation of fibrous tissue, can result in asymmetric distortion and expansion of craniofacial bones.

These conditions can collapse the paranasal sinuses; compress the optic nerve or chiasm, causing loss of vision; and cause other functional disabilities. An acute epistaxis (nosebleed) can be life-threatening. A combined intracranial and extracranial approach may be used to completely remove the tumor or dysplastic bone. The remaining bony structures may be reshaped or repositioned. Bone grafts and/or prosthetic implants may be used for reconstruction of the forehead, orbits, nose, maxilla, and mandible.

Midfacial Fractures

The facial bones provide a shield for the brain. They also protect the senses of sight, smell, hearing, and taste. Although midfacial fractures and soft tissue injuries are seldom fatal, inadequate treatment can result in disfigurement and sensory impairment. For example, virtually all blindness secondary to trauma is permanent.

Facial fractures should be suspected when the patient complains of pain, malocclusion of the jaws, or diplopia (double vision). Swelling and asymmetry of the face may be obvious. Diagnosis is confirmed by x-ray or a CT scan to identify the bones involved. Rene Le Fort (1869–1951), a French plastic surgeon, pioneered fixation of midface fractures. The Le Fort classification of fractures, which is useful in determining the appropriate method of reduction and stabilization (Fig. 41.29), is as follows:

- *Le Fort I* fracture is a horizontal fracture of the maxilla, fragmenting the upper alveoli and palate.
- *Le Fort II* fracture is a pyramidal fracture of the frontal processes of the maxillae, the nasal bones, and the orbital floor. The maxillae are freely movable.
- *Le Fort III* fracture is a transverse fracture that includes zygomas, maxillae, and nasal bones and the ethmoid, sphenoid, and other orbital bones. This creates a craniofacial disjunction (separation).

Facial fractures are reduced, stabilized, and immobilized. Priorities of initial treatment after injury concern airway obstruction, possible cervical spine injury, and hemorrhage. Treatment of the fracture may be delayed. The surgeon follows the principles of approaching fractures from "inside out, downward up." This means that bony structures are repaired first, then the soft tissues;

the mandible or most distal fracture is reduced first before working upward toward the cranium.[13]

The method of bony repair is determined by the complexity of the fracture. Intermaxillary fixation combined with interdental wiring, external pin fixation, or rigid internal fixation effect stabilization. Minifacial and midfacial plates, microplates, and mandibular plates may be combined with arch bars or bone grafts.

Reduction of Orbital Fractures

If orbital contents are depressed into the maxillary sinus, surgical exploration through an orbital or a transspinal approach is indicated. The extent of the trauma should indicate the most appropriate surgical management. The injury may involve the rim or the floor of the orbit, or both, as follows:

- Fractures of the orbital rim, frequently associated with fractures of the zygoma, are usually detected by the resulting deformity. The fracture is reduced by appropriate means. Fragments are wired into place as necessary.
- A blowout fracture of the orbit may result from a direct blow to the eyeball, which is, in turn, transmitted to the very thin floor of the orbit. A typical fracture is in the medial third of the floor with dislocation of floor fragments into the maxillary sinus. The fracture occasionally may extend into the ethmoid plate. Consequently, orbital contents, which may include the inferior extraocular muscles, are usually herniated into the antrum. This produces limitation of upward gaze and some degree of enophthalmos (recession of the eyeball into the orbit).

The herniated orbital contents are reduced from the antrum back into the orbit with special attention to freeing the entrapped muscles. Plastic or silicone sheeting may be used to close the defect in the floor, or the fragments may be elevated by packing the antrum through a Caldwell-Luc (sinus) approach. The diagnosis may be overlooked unless a laminogram is taken.

Reduction of Nasal Fractures

Fracture of the nasal bones and septum often accompanies other trauma to the head, such as a blowout fracture of the orbit (see earlier). If the zygoma or maxilla is involved, reduction may be accomplished through a small incision anterior to the ear and superior to the zygomatic arch. Periosteal elevators are used to raise depressed bone and cartilage fragments. Nasal fractures are splinted with nasal packs and an external splint.

Reduction of Zygomatic Fractures

Dislocations of the zygoma are more common than fractures of the cheekbone (malar bone). Zygomatic fractures always involve the orbital bones. Those of the zygomatic arch are particularly unstable and require intraosseous or transosseous wire fixation after internal reduction with counterpressure from underneath the arch. Transantral Steinmann pinning may be necessary to maintain reduction of fragments in severely fragmented fractures. Absorbable plates composed of biodegradable polymers for zygomaticomaxillary fractures are commercially available. The plates are usually resorbed by the body after 1 year.[14]

Maxillofacial and Mandibular Procedures

The term *maxillofacial* pertains to the part of the face formed by the upper and lower jaws. Most maxillofacial procedures are designed to reconstruct defects in the lips, buccal sulcus, maxilla, alveolar ridge, floor of the mouth, mandible, or chin. These defects may be a result of trauma or resection of tumor. Whenever feasible, intraoral incisions are used to minimize facial scarring.

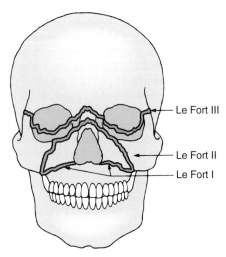

• **Fig. 41.29** Le Fort facial fractures.

Le Fort III
Le Fort II
Le Fort I

Intermaxillary Fixation of Fractures

After closed or open reduction, fractures of the maxilla and mandible are usually immobilized by interdental wiring if the patient has upper and lower teeth. If the patient is edentulous (without teeth), open reduction and skeletal fixation by circumferential wiring over an intraoral splint or screws and connecting bars may be necessary.

Erich arch bars are shaped along the dental arches. Wires are passed between the teeth to anchor the splints on the upper and lower jaws. Each splint contains a series of small lugs. Tiny rubber bands, placed around opposing lugs, hold the teeth in occlusion. Splints frequently are not used for fixation of these fractures. The teeth may be held in occlusion by wires passed around opposing teeth. After fixation of the mandible or maxilla, wire cutters accompany the patient from the OR and remain at the bedside as long as wires or rubber bands are in place. If the patient experiences respiratory difficulty or vomiting, the wires may have to be cut to prevent aspiration. Fluids may be difficult to swallow.

If microplates can be used for rigid fixation, the interdental wiring may be released after the fixation procedure is completed.

Mandibular Fractures

Some fractures of the mandible can be immobilized by transoral placement of noncompression miniplates. This technique obviates the necessity of interdental wiring. Vitallium, titanium, or stainless steel plates and screws are used for rigid fixation.

Mandibular Reconstruction

Skeletal defects creating loss of mandibular continuity are usually a result of trauma or benign disease. Bone replacement is the most common method of restoring function and contour. The patient's own ilium provides cancellous bone that can be shaped into the configuration of the jaw. A composite graft of a freeze-dried cadaver mandible packed with autologous cancellous bone chips also can be used. These grafts fill a bony defect but do not provide soft tissue coverage. A vascularized iliac graft is preferable to reconstruct the mandible and a large intraoral defect.

Temporomandibular Joint Syndrome

Persistent pain and dysfunction of the temporomandibular joint (TMJ) can be associated with stress-related bruxism (tensing muscles and grinding teeth), the position of teeth, malocclusion, trauma, arthritis, and other degenerative changes in one or both joints. If TMJ syndrome is unresponsive to conservative treatment, surgical intervention may be indicated.

Arthroscopy. Arthroscopy, usually performed bilaterally, is used to diagnose problems such as scarring or adhesions that do not show up on a CT or an MRI. Lysis of adhesions, mechanical debridement, and lavage of the TMJ may relieve symptoms. Repositioning or release of the fibrocartilaginous articular disc (meniscus) between the mandibular condyle and the glenoid fossa of the temporal bone may restore function.

A 1.7 or 1.9-mm arthroscope with a fiberoptic camera attached is locked into a cannula sheath inserted through an inferolateral puncture wound into the joint capsule. Continuous inflow and outflow of fluid, usually iced lactated Ringer's solution, is necessary to keep the joint distended for visibility and lavage. Therapeutic synovectomy and partial or complete meniscectomy may recontour the joint. A rotary shaver and/or the holmium:yttrium aluminum garnet (Ho:YAG) laser may be used. The laser rapidly resects and vaporizes cartilaginous tissue and coagulates bleeding vessels.

Arthroplasty. Open, direct visualization of the disc and condyle may be necessary to correct abnormal relationships. Either a preauricular or postauricular incision may be used to approach the TMJ. The condyle, fossa, and/or articular eminence may be reshaped or resurfaced. A damaged or displaced articular disc can be recontoured and repositioned. It is recontoured with a scalpel or by electrosurgical cutting and then repositioned and sutured in place. If the disc is torn or perforated, it is usually removed. A silicone elastomer implant or titanium alloy prosthesis may be used to reconstruct the joint. The jaw may be immobilized with interdental wiring to stabilize the TMJ during healing.

Orthognathic Surgery

The jaws can be reshaped or repositioned to correct functional bite disorders and/or for aesthetics. Occlusion (closure of teeth) depends on the anteroposterior relationship of the upper and lower jaws. The term *orthognathia,* derived from the Greek words *orthos,* meaning "straight," and *gnathos,* meaning "jaw," relates to treatment of conditions involving malposition of the maxilla or mandible, or both. Malocclusion occurs when teeth do not close together properly. It can cause difficulty in chewing and speaking, periodontal disease, and TMJ dysfunction. Psychologically debilitating facial deformity and bite disorders of genetic origin or as a result of growth disturbances or trauma include the following:

- *Prognathism:* One or both jaws project forward beyond the normal relationship with the cranial base. If the mandible (lower jaw) protrudes beyond the maxilla (upper jaw), it creates a prominence of chin, concave profile, and underbite. If the maxilla grows beyond the mandible, it creates an overbite.
- *Retrognathism:* One or both jaws are positioned posterior to the normal craniofacial relationship (i.e., behind the frontal plane of the forehead). In reference to the mandible, the condition is commonly known as a receding chin; this may create an overbite.
- *Apertognathia:* The front teeth do not close because the back teeth come together first, creating an open bite.
- *Micrognathia:* The dental arch, usually of the mandible, is too small to accommodate the teeth. Teeth are pushed out of alignment because they are crowded together.
- *Asymmetry:* A discrepancy in size, shape, or position of the jaws creates an imbalance between the right and left sides of the face.

Preoperative orthodontia may be required to align and level the teeth. The ultimate goal is to achieve functional stability of dentofacial structures with acceptable facial aesthetics. Surgical correction may include extraction of one or more teeth, maxillary and/or mandibular osteotomies with repositioning of bone segments, and/or repositioning of alveoli. Intraorally, bilateral maxillary osteotomies may be performed in conjunction with mandibular osteotomies, or either of these procedures can be done independently to change the shape of the facial contour.

Le Fort Osteotomy. For maxillary deformities, an incision is made in the mucosa of the upper lip. Osteotomies (i.e., bone cuts) are made in the medial and lateral maxillary sinus walls. The vomer is cut just above the floor of the nose. Pterygoid plates are sectioned from the maxilla. The maxilla is movable for reduction, augmentation, or repositioning. The maxilla can be detached from the base of the skull, maintaining vascular supply via the soft palate, and cut into segments to reconstruct the lower face as described for midface advancement. Usually miniplates anchored with screws bridge the osteotomy cuts.

Mandibular Osteotomy. Sagittal split osteotomies through the ramus and vertical osteotomies through the molar region on each side allow backward or forward repositioning of the mandible. If moved posteriorly, bone on the anterior aspect is trimmed for good medullary bone contact. Rigid fixation may be obtained with miniplates or with screws placed percutaneously through stab wounds. The latter are stabilized with an external fixator. If plates and screws are used, intermaxillary fixation as described for fractures may not be necessary.

Postoperative orthodontia may be required to complete closure of spaces around the osteotomies and thus stabilize occlusal function.

Mandibulectomy. Partial or total removal of the lower jaw is performed for extension of a tumor into the bone of the floor of the mouth. It may be performed with glossectomy and radical neck dissection for wide excision. The resultant chin recession is referred to as an Andy Gump deformity. Mandibular replacement combines bone graft and synthetic materials for restoration of speech and appearance.

A compound osseocutaneous flap from the iliac crest, with microvascular anastomosis of the deep circumflex iliac artery vascular pedicle, may be transferred for reconstruction. If the patient is dentulous, the relationship of opposing teeth is maintained; if edentulous, the patient wears a denture. Whenever possible, mandible-sparing procedures are done for carcinoma of the tongue.

ⓔ EVOLVE WEBSITE

http://evolve.elsevier.com/Hornacky/BerryKohn/

- Historical Perspective
- Tips for the Scrub Person and Circulating Nurse
- Student Interactive Questions
- Glossary

References

1. Estime S, Kuza C: Trauma airway management, *Anesthesiol Clin* 37(1):33–50, 2018.
2. Rhodes R, Tsai B: Future of implantable auditory devices, *Otolaryngol Clin North Am* 52(2):363–378, 2018.
3. Elaprolu S, Alexander A, Ganesan S, et al.: Effect of a boomerang-shaped conchal cartilage graft for type three tympanoplasty on hearing, *Int Arch Otorhinolaryngol* 25(2):e289–295, 2020.
4. Oehlerking R: *Cochlear receives FDA approval to lower the age of pediatric cochlear implantation to 9 months.* www.pronews.cochlear.com. Accessed July 5, 2023.
5. Food and Drug Administration: *Cochlear implants and MRI safety.* www.fda.gov. Accessed July 5, 2023.
6. Marvin K, Bowman P, Keller M, et al.: Effectiveness of an advanced airway training "boot camp" for family medicine physician trainees, *Otolaryngol Head Neck Surg* 16(2):204–208, 2020.
7. Hsueh YL: Palatal surgery for obstructive sleep apnea, *Sleep Med Clin* 14(1):51–58, 2018.
8. Gupta RJ, Kademani D, Liu SY: Upper airway (hypoglossal nerve) stimulation for treatment of obstructive sleep apnea, *Atlas Oral Maxillofac Surg Clin North Am* 27(1):53–58, 2019.
9. Louie M, Chang T, Grundmeier R: Recent advances in technology and its applications to pediatric emergency care, *Pediatr Clin North Am* 65(6):1229–1246, 2018.
10. Wong E, Smith M, Buchanan M, et al.: Smell-related quality of life changes after total laryngectomy: a multi-centre study, *Eur Arch Otorhinolaryngol* 280:3861–3866, 2023.
11. Centers for Disease Control and Prevention: *HPV.* www.cdc.gov. Accessed July 5, 2023.
12. Hamm JA, Robin NH: Newborn craniofacial malformations, *Clin Perinatol* 42(2):321–336, 2015.
13. Chukwulebe S, Hogrefe C: The diagnosis and management of facial bone fractures, *Emerg Med Clin North Am* 37(1):137–151, 2018.
14. Chu SG, Lee JS, Lee JW, et al.: Comparisons among four types of absorbable plates used for internal fixation of zygomaticomaxillary complex fractures, *J Craniomaxillofac Surg* 47(3):383–388, 2019.

42

Thoracic Surgery

CHAPTER OUTLINE

Anatomy and Physiology of the Thorax, 905

Physiology, 908

Special Features of Thoracic Surgery, 908

Thoracic Surgical Procedures, 916

Chest Trauma, 919

Intrathoracic Esophageal Procedures, 920

Complications of Thoracic Surgery, 920

CHAPTER OBJECTIVES

After studying this chapter the learner will be able to:

- Identify the pertinent anatomy of the thoracic cavity.
- Describe patient positioning for each type of thoracic incision.

- Discuss the setup of water-seal chest drainage.

KEY TERMS AND DEFINITIONS

Bougie Long, tapered, flexible dilator. Some bougies can be lighted for transillumination of a tubular anatomic structure, such as the esophagus.

Decortication Stripping adhesions from the surface of the pleura.

Fundus Dome-like top of stomach near where the esophagus inserts.

Lobectomy Removal of a lobe of the lung.

Mediastinum Cavity within the chest, between the pleura, that contains the esophagus, trachea, pericardium, and great vessels.

Pleurodesis Introduction of a chemical sclerosing agent into the chest. A powdered antibiotic, talc, or caustic chemical is instilled between the parietal and visceral layers of the pleura to fuse them by creating fibrous adhesions. The procedure can use dry chemicals or wet paste.

Plication Systematic rows of sutures that stabilize and secure a muscular region such as the diaphragm.

Pneumonectomy Removal of a lung.

Poudrage Full-strength dry powder is placed between pleural tissue layers to create adhesions.

Slurry Loose, moist paste made of fluid and powdered agent; used to intentionally create adhesions between two serous surfaces inside a cavity.

Thoracoscopy Rigid endoscopic procedure performed by percutaneous puncture of the thorax.

Anatomy and Physiology of the Thorax

An essential balance must be maintained between atmospheric pressure outside the chest and internal pressures within the thoracic cavity to sustain the vital function of respiration. Knowledge of the anatomy and physiology of the chest and thoracic cavity is necessary for an understanding of thoracic surgery.

Thoracic Cavity

The thorax, or chest, is the portion of the trunk between the neck and the abdomen. The thoracic cavity is divided into right and left pleural compartments separated by the mediastinum, which is a separate enclosed space located centrally. Alterations in pressure affecting one side of the thoracic cavity or the mediastinum cause a positional shift of the other compartments.

The bony framework of the thoracic cavity consists of the sternum and costal cartilage anteriorly, 12 pairs of ribs laterally, and 12 thoracic vertebrae posteriorly, all encased within soft tissue. The framework is bounded superiorly by structures of the lower part of the neck and inferiorly by the diaphragm. Eleven external and internal intercostal muscles, which lie between the ribs, have a corresponding artery, vein, and nerve, which require meticulous dissection to avoid inadvertent injury. The arterial blood supply is derived from the subclavian artery, internal thoracic artery, and the thoracic aorta. Venous drainage is through the mammary veins anteriorly and the azygos and hemiazygos veins posteriorly. Lymphatic drainage is through the parasternal nodes that follow the internal thoracic artery. Innervation is from the anterior roots of the thoracic spine (T1–T11) to the parietal pleura.

The first seven ribs articulate anteriorly in the midline with the sternum, which is composed of three parts: the manubrium

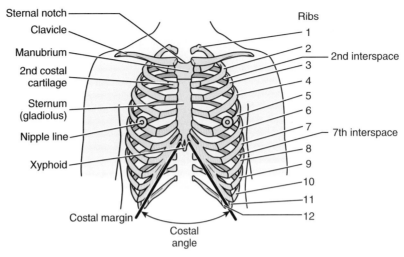

• **Fig. 42.1** Surgical landmarks of the bony ribcage.

Sternal notch
Clavicle
Manubrium
2nd costal cartilage
Sternum (gladiolus)
Nipple line
Xyphoid
Costal margin
Costal angle
Ribs
1
2
3
4
5
6
7
8
9
10
11
12
2nd interspace
7th interspace

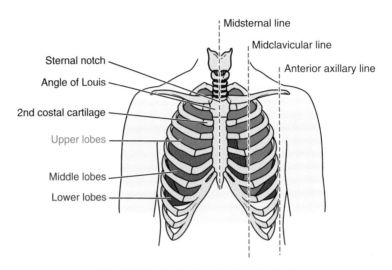

• **Fig. 42.2** Surgical landmarks: lines of direction.

Midsternal line
Midclavicular line
Anterior axillary line
Sternal notch
Angle of Louis
2nd costal cartilage
Upper lobes
Middle lobes
Lower lobes

(superiorly), the gladiolus (medially), and the xyphoid process (inferiorly). Ribs 1 and 2 articulate with the clavicle and the manubrium. The manubrium and gladiolus join in a projection referred to as the angle of Lewis, a surgical landmark (Fig. 42.1).

Ribs 3 through 7 articulate with the gladiolus (the main sternal body) via the costal cartilage. The 8th, 9th, and 10th ribs are joined anteriorly to the cartilage of the rib above each; the 11th and 12th ribs have no anterior fixation. The surgical incisional lines of direction in Fig. 42.2 bilaterally overlie the lobes of the lungs on a vertical axis, with the sternum (gladiolus) as the thoracic reference point.

The ribs articulate posteriorly with the thoracic vertebrae. The esophagus, trachea, and great vessels leading to and from the neck and arms pass through the small space between the manubrium and the vertebrae. Any structure pushing into this narrow opening (e.g., a mediastinal tumor) may obstruct breathing, venous return from the neck and arms, and swallowing.

Lungs

The lungs lie in the right sand left pleural cavities (Fig. 42.3). The main function of these porous, spongy, conical organs is oxygenation of the blood with inspired air and expiration of carbon dioxide. The apex of each extends to the neck; the base rests on the superior surface of the diaphragm.

The right lung, which has three lobes, an oblique fissure, and a straighter bronchus, is larger than the left lung, which has two lobes and a more angled bronchus. Blood supply is derived from the two pulmonary arteries and drains into the four pulmonary veins. Lymphatics drain into the bronchopulmonary nodes and into the thoracic duct. Innervation is through the pulmonary plexuses.

The lungs are enveloped by a serous membrane, referred to as the pleura. The pleura has two layers. The external parietal layer lines the inner surface of the thorax. The inner visceral layer covers the surface of the lung. Small amounts of serous fluid (transudate) are secreted between these layers to allow for smooth interface without friction. Excess inflammation or fluid accumulation causes pain and impaired respiratory effort. If infected, the transudate becomes exudate containing increased numbers of white blood cells. Severe inflammation causes fibrosis and adhesions of the pleural tissues.

The trachea divides at the carina into two main branches—the bronchi—leading to the right and left lungs. The right lung, with

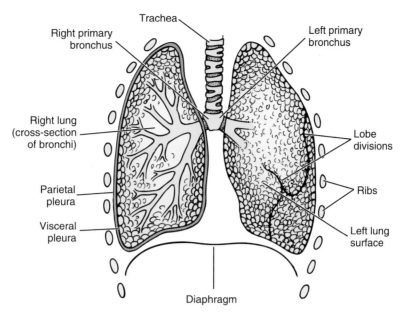

• **Fig. 42.3** Respiratory system within thoracic cavity.

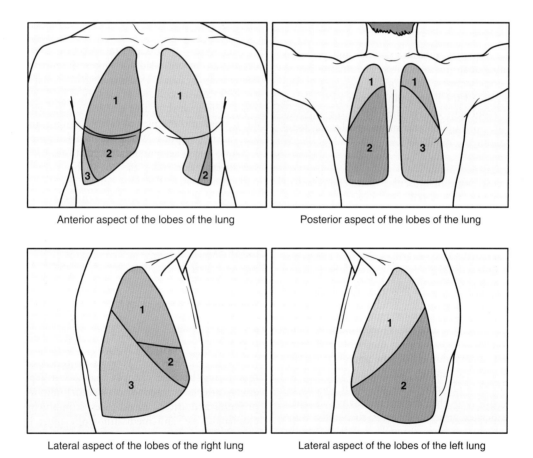

Anterior aspect of the lobes of the lung

Posterior aspect of the lobes of the lung

Lateral aspect of the lobes of the right lung

Lateral aspect of the lobes of the left lung

• **Fig. 42.4** Location of the lobes of the right and left lungs. Patient positioning will be determined for optimal access of the affected lobes or entire lung.

three lobes, is wider and broader than the left lung. This is because the liver is positioned beneath the diaphragm directly below the base. The left lung has only two lobes and is thinner, longer, and narrower. It shares space in the left side of the chest with the heart, which rests in an area of the left lung referred to as the cardiac notch (Fig. 42.4).

The bronchopulmonary segments within each lung are wedges of tissue separated by veins and thin connective membrane.

Although configuration of the segments differs, and variations in the bronchi and blood vessels exist between the right and left lungs, it is generally accepted that both lungs normally have 10 bronchopulmonary segments. Despite not being demarcated by surface fissures, these segments represent zones of distribution of the secondary bronchi and may be excised individually when the segment contains a small lesion, thus preserving the uninvolved portion.

Each segmental bronchus subdivides into numerous, increasingly smaller branches that eventually end in terminal bronchioles. These fine tubules invested by smooth muscles can constrict to close off the air passage, as in asthma. The terminal bronchioles give rise to respiratory bronchioles from which arise the alveoli. The approximately 300 million alveoli are the functional units wherein oxygenation takes place at the capillary level.

The hilus of the lung, on the mediastinal surface, is the point of entry for the primary bronchus, nerves, and blood vessels. The right primary bronchus is straighter and is a more direct continuation of the trachea. Arterial supply to the lung tissue is derived from the bronchial arteries. Venous drainage is through the bronchial veins, which empty into the azygos system. The pulmonary veins and arteries to and from the heart provide systemic pulmonary circulation. Innervation of the breathing mechanism is by the autonomic nervous system.

Mediastinum

The mediastinum has superior, anterior, middle, and posterior sections, each containing anatomic structures. The thymus lies in the anterior and superior sections, the thoracic aorta lies in the posterior section, the base of the heart and the great vessels lie in the middle, and the esophagus and trachea lie in the superior section. The organs are surrounded and suspended by the loose tissue diffused throughout the mediastinum.

Diaphragm

The diaphragm is a half dome of muscular tissue composed of four embryonic segments: (1) dorsal mesentery, (2) septum transversum, (3) two pleuroperitoneal folds, and (4) cervical myotomes that border the inferior aspect of the thoracic cavity. It originates from the six lower ribs on each side and attaches to the xyphoid and the external and internal arcuate ligaments. Abnormal separation of any of these layers changes the pressure gradient between the peritoneal cavity and the thorax, causing a shift of intraabdominal organs cephalad into the chest.

The arterial blood supply arises from the right and left phrenic, intercostal, and internal thoracic arteries. Venous drainage is via the inferior vena cava, the azygos vein on the right, and hemiazygos veins on the left. Innervation is from the phrenic nerve that arises from the fourth cervical ramus.

The esophagus, aorta, and vena cava pass from the thorax through the diaphragm into the abdominal cavity via three separate openings. Associated vessels and nerves, such as the vagus nerve, follow these three structures through the diaphragm to major organ systems (Fig. 42.5).

Physiology

The size of the thorax varies with the bellows action of the thoracic wall and diaphragm, increasing with inspiration and decreasing with expiration. A partial vacuum between the parietal and visceral pleurae expands the lungs. A negative (subatmospheric) pressure normally within the thorax is essential to life.

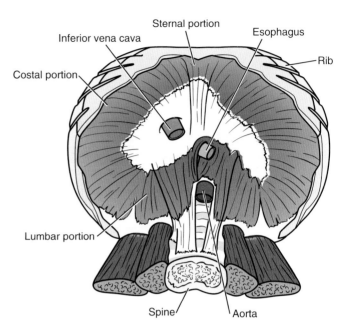

• **Fig. 42.5** Inferior view of diaphragm with orientation of vena cava, aorta, and esophagus.

Alterations of intrapleural pressure are of major concern because an uncontrolled opening in the thoracic wall and pressure change can be fatal. Uncontrolled increased positive pressure in one side causes a collapse of the lung on the other side. Referred to as a mediastinal shift, this reaction occurs with entrance of either air or fluid into the pleural cavity, compressing the opposite lung and causing dyspnea. When the mediastinum has moved its limit, it can no longer accommodate a great pressure change; the lung on the affected side collapses. Air in the pleural space between the parietal and visceral pleurae constitutes pneumothorax. Blood in the pleural space constitutes hemothorax.

A mediastinal shift disturbs heart action and circulation. Changes in pressure balance within the thorax reduce vital capacity—the greatest amount of air that can be exchanged in one breath. Many diseases and conditions (e.g., anesthesia, thoracic tumors, chest trauma) alter vital capacity.

Special Features of Thoracic Surgery

Entry into the thoracic cavity can be accompanied by pulmonary distress. Team members especially skilled in meeting emergency situations are essential. Patients require close observation and monitoring because changes may occur rapidly. A pulmonary artery catheter is inserted to monitor pulmonary capillary wedge pressures and arterial blood gases. Equipment for bronchoscopy, esophagoscopy, and mediastinoscopy must be readily available. Other preparations are routinely completed for entry into the chest for intrathoracic procedures, as follows:

1. Endotracheal anesthesia permits the lungs to expand and function even when subjected to atmospheric pressure. Administration of anesthesia under controlled positive pressure prevents physiologic imbalance and lung collapse in the presence of controlled pneumothorax. Use of a double-lumen endotracheal tube permits expansion of the unaffected lung and collapse of the lung on the surgical side (Fig. 42.6). At the conclusion of the surgical procedure the affected lung is

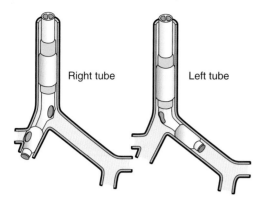

• **Fig. 42.6** Double-lumen endotracheal tube.

reexpanded by the anesthesia provider, and negative pressure in the chest is restored. Portable chest x-rays may be taken immediately to assess the status of the surgical area, pleural cavities, and lung reexpansion.

2. Instrumentation includes a basic laparotomy setup with the addition of thoracic instruments. These include bone instruments and a power saw (Fig. 42.7 shows rib strippers/rasps, shears, and an approximator/contractor); a large self-retaining chest retractor/rib spreader (Fig. 42.8); bronchus clamps and lung forceps (Fig. 42.9); and long instruments for work in a deep incision. Specialty retractors are used to hold lung tissue and displace the bones of the shoulder girdle (Fig. 42.10).

3. A variety of sutures may be used for soft tissues, vessels, and bone. The bronchus usually is closed with staples.

4. Sponges for hemostasis or blunt dissection are placed on long ring-handled forceps. Periosteal bleeding may be controlled by electrocoagulation. Bone wax may be needed to control bone marrow oozing.

5. Blood for transfusion should be available at all times. Hemorrhage is a major threat intraoperatively and postoperatively. Blood may be salvaged for autotransfusion by cell saver, and a postoperative drainage salvage reservoir and autotransfusion drain may be used.

6. The surgical field is potentially contaminated by secretions and contact with open air passages when a bronchus is opened and sutured. Used items and instruments are isolated in a discard basin. Maintenance of a dry field is important to prevent aspiration of blood and fluid, which predisposes the patient to postoperative pneumonia.

7. An airtight pleural cavity must be restored and negative pressure maintained for maximum pulmonary function postoperatively. Except after a few specific procedures, a sterile, closed water-seal drainage system is essential. Chest tubes are inserted through a stab wound and anchored to the chest wall with suture and tape. Two or three tubes are sometimes inserted into the pleural space and connected to separate drainage systems (Fig. 42.11, *A*). The tube at the base of the pleural space is usually inserted at the seventh costal interspace, near the anterior axillary line, to evacuate fluid. An upper tube, if indicated, is inserted at the apex through the anterior chest wall at the third costal interspace to evacuate air leaking from the lung. Positioning of the chest tubes can vary if the patient has a pneumothorax (Fig. 42.11, *B*). Key points to remember include:

• **Fig. 42.7** Rib instruments. **A,** Strippers/rasps. **B,** Shears. **C,** Approximator/contractor.

• **Fig. 42.8** Self-retaining chest retractor/rib spreader.

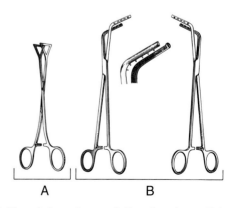

• **Fig. 42.9** Thoracic tissue forceps. **A,** Bronchus clamps. **B,** Lung forceps.

a. Connections must be physically tight and securely taped at the time of dressing application. The taped connections should not obscure the observation of drainage.

• **Fig. 42.10** Specialty lung and thoracic retractors.

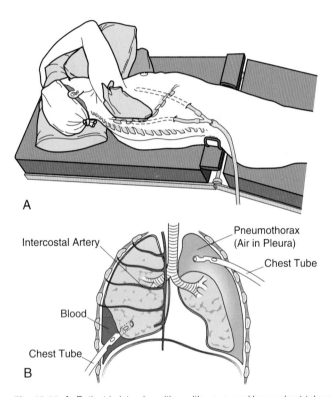

A

Pneumothorax
(Air in Pleura)

Intercostal Artery

Chest Tube

Blood

Chest Tube

B

• **Fig. 42.11** **A,** Patient in lateral position with upper and lower chest tubes in place. **B,** Placement of chest tubes for air evacuation and blood drainage in pneumothorax.

b. System components must be kept below the level of the patient's body to prevent reentry of air or fluid from the drainage collection system into the pleural cavity.

c. Tubes may be clamped before insertion and connection to the drainage system, depending on the surgeon's preference. Tubes are not routinely clamped at other times unless the surgeon specifically requests them. Specialized tube clamps are used for this purpose.

Access to the Thorax

Surgeon preference and the procedure determine the method of entrance into the thorax. Access may be gained by an anterior, lateral, or posterior approach, or a combination of these. Entrance through the ribcage may be intercostal between the ribs, through the periosteal bed of an unresected rib, or by rib resection. By

incising near the top of a rib the surgeon protects nerves and vessels that lie in the intercostal spaces. An intercostal approach may be used to drain an empyema pocket or mediastinal abscess or to obtain a biopsy specimen of lymph nodes or of a lung.

To enter the thorax via the periosteal bed, the periosteum of the rib is incised and removed from the unresected rib, and an incision is made through the bed. For entrance via a rib resection, the periosteum is incised and removed superiorly and inferiorly with a periosteal elevator and the rib is divided. Rib spreaders increase exposure, but if the exposure is still inadequate, the rib located above or below the incision also may be resected.

Endoscopy

Elective surgery depends on accurate diagnosis by radiologic and physiologic pulmonary function studies and by biochemical, cytologic, and histologic determinations and evaluations. Frequently, endoscopic procedures are performed to obtain secretions and tissue biopsy specimens.[1] Some lesions can be treated endoscopically.

Bronchoscopy

Disorders of the bronchus are most commonly infection, the presence of a foreign body, trauma, or neoplasms. Diagnosis is made by radiologic study and endoscopy. Bronchography (x-ray study of the tracheobronchial tree) is frequently done in conjunction with bronchoscopy. Bronchoscopy (direct visualization of the tracheobronchial tree through a bronchoscope) is done for the following purposes:

- *Diagnosis:* Securing an uncontaminated secretion for culture, obtaining a biopsy specimen, or finding the cause of a cough or hemoptysis
- *Intervention:* Removing a foreign body, excising a small tumor, applying medication, aspirating the bronchi, or providing an airway during performance of a tracheotomy

Foreign bodies in the trachea and bronchi are very serious, requiring a careful history and immediate bronchoscopy with preparation for a potential tracheotomy. Maintaining a safe airway during extraction is a major risk. If the airway is not seriously obstructed, the aspirated foreign body may remain in the bronchus for months without producing symptoms until suppuration develops. Coughing and hemoptysis bring the patient to the physician. Snares and graspers can be used to retrieve foreign bodies.

Bronchoscopes are of two types: a rigid hollow metal tube and a flexible fiberoptic type. The rigid bronchoscope commonly

Bronchoscope

Camera fits on this end

This end goes into video and the light source

Bronchoscope

Trachea

Left primary bronchus

• **Fig. 42.12** Flexible bronchoscopy.

uses a fiberoptic light carrier attached to a light source to allow visualization of the trachea and primary bronchi. It is the scope of choice for foreign body retrieval and determination of persistent bleeding. It has a side channel incorporated into the length of the instrument and perforations along the sides of the tube to allow oxygenation of bronchi and administration of anesthetic gases if general anesthesia is used.

Aspirating tubes, foreign body or biopsy forceps, and carbon dioxide (CO_2) lasers are manipulated through the rigid bronchoscope. Both rigid and flexible fiberoptic bronchoscopes are used for diagnostic and therapeutic procedures.

Flexible bronchoscopy is used frequently for the patient with decreased range of neck motion. Flexible bronchoscopy can be performed via the nasopharynx or orally to the trachea and into the bronchial tree (Fig. 42.12).

Tiny forceps and biopsy brushes can be inserted through the working channel of the flexible fiberoptic bronchoscope to obtain a tissue biopsy specimen. Because the diameter is smaller, the flexible fiberoptic scope reaches into the bronchi of the upper, middle, and lower lobes for examination and/or biopsy. Diagnostic needle aspiration, forceps biopsy, and bronchial brushings and washings are performed in accessible areas. Mediastinal lymph nodes can be aspirated through the flexible bronchoscope. Various types and lengths of aspirating tubes, forceps, and brushes are used to remove tissue and secretions. The neodymium:yttrium-aluminum-garnet (Nd:YAG) or argon laser can be used with either a rigid or a flexible bronchoscope.

Electromagnetic navigation bronchoscopy (ENB) uses preoperative CT scans to plan a real-time navigation path.[2] A steerable sensor can target the lesion even if it is in a difficult to reach location. The sensor can be locked in place, and the surgeon may identify it using blue or green dye or a microcoil can be deployed as a marker. Resection can take place using bronchoscopic instrumentation.

If the gag reflex can be controlled, oral rigid bronchoscopy can be performed with the patient under local anesthesia and intravenous sedation. General anesthesia may be necessary. The bronchoscope is inserted over the tongue and through the vocal cords to the trachea. The patient's head is turned to the right to visualize the left bronchus and to the left for the right bronchus (Fig. 42.13).

The bronchi may be examined to ascertain the patency of the tracheobronchial tree or to locate the source of an obstruction or bleeding. The person who assists the bronchoscopist introduces tips of instruments into the scope. Everyone involved with bronchoscopy should wear personal protective equipment (gown, gloves, mask, hair cover, and eye protection) to protect themselves from bronchial secretions and blood.

Some pulmonary lesions are treated by laser. The CO_2 laser is used for stenosis, granulation tissue, or other obstructive lesions that are not highly vascular. Video-assisted, flexible, fiberoptic laser bronchoscopy is more commonly performed using the Nd:YAG laser. This laser is preferred for vascular lesions, such as neoplasms, to produce hemostasis as it cuts. The argon laser is used for photodynamic therapy to shrink or destroy bronchial tumors. Everyone in the room, including the patient, is required to wear appropriate eye protection of the correct optical density for the type of laser in use.

Airway Stents

Airway obstruction can be relieved by insertion of metal mesh or silicone rubber stents.[3] These may be straight configuration, T-shaped, or T-Y bifurcation prostheses (Fig. 42.14). Metal stents are permanent and deployed via a rigid bronchoscope over a guidewire. The interstices of the mesh allow for tissue ingrowth, providing long-term palliation. Silicone stents are also deployed through a rigid bronchoscope but are removable.

Positioning is confirmed with x-rays or bronchoscopy. Daily moisture inhalation with a nebulizer is necessary to keep the area moist. Frequent suction may be necessary if the patient cannot clear secretions. Lasers cannot be used in the presence of the stent. They will cause overheating of the tissues as well as uneven pressure and distortion of the lumen of the stent.

The most common reasons for using airway stents are for palliation of obstructing neoplasm, postradiation therapy, after lung transplantation, and after fistula repair. Postoperative

Rigid bronchoscope and sheaths

A

Bronchoscopy under general anesthesia
using rigid bronchoscope

B

• **Fig. 42.13** Rigid bronchoscopy.

• **Fig. 42.14** Tracheal and bronchus straight stents.

complications can include stent migration, avulsion, fistula formation, bleeding, and infection.

A sterile bronchoscope should be used for each patient. Thorough cleaning of the bronchoscope and instrumentation is necessary immediately after the procedure. Terminal sterilization is recommended before storage.

Bronchoscopic Lung Volume Reduction (BLVR)

Patients between the ages of 45 and 75 years with chronic obstructive pulmonary disease (COPD) and emphysema may be candidates for the noninvasive placement of implanted lung valves. The lung implant is a one-way valve system made of silicone with a small expanding cage covered in silicone. Three to five valves can be inserted into the lung through a bronchoscope. The implanted valves close off the airways leading to diseased areas and remove the trapped air. This allows the healthy tissue to expand to improve breathing. The valves can be moved, replaced, or

removed. Complications such as dyspnea, pneumonia, pneumothorax, or hemoptysis can occur.[4]

Mediastinoscopy

Mediastinoscopy may immediately follow bronchoscopy. To prevent needless thoracotomy, mediastinoscopy is performed for assessment of resectability in patients with suspected bronchogenic carcinoma and for diagnosis of mediastinal lesions.

Mediastinoscopy uncovers mediastinal lymph nodes for direct visualization and biopsy.[5] Subaortic nodes draining the left lobe of the lung may be out of reach for biopsy with this technique. With the scope the mediastinoscopist can see down to the carina and about 4 cm distal to it along each bronchus. If more than one biopsy specimen is obtained, each specimen should be placed in a separate container and identified by location. The procedure gives a high percentage of accurate diagnoses and information in staging the extent of a lesion and determining its operability for curative resection. Sometimes a frozen section is done while the patient is in the OR, with resection performed immediately after a report from the pathologist.

General endotracheal anesthesia is used. The patient is supine with the neck hyperextended and the head turned slightly to the right. A small transverse incision is made in or about 2 cm above the suprasternal notch between the borders of the sternocleidomastoid muscle (Fig. 42.15).

Dissection is carried down to the pretracheal fascia. After blunt dissection the sterile mediastinoscope is passed behind the suprasternal notch and advanced behind the aortic arch into the superior mediastinum to the level of the carina. Care is exercised because of the proximity of the great vessels to the insertion point of the scope.

Bleeding is controlled by coagulation with an insulated electrosurgical suction tip. Although mediastinoscopy usually is performed without complication, major bleeding may require immediate thoracotomy. A chest x-ray frequently is obtained after mediastinoscopy.

Thoracostomy

Closed thoracostomy is performed to establish continuous drainage of fluid from the chest (usually purulent from sepsis or

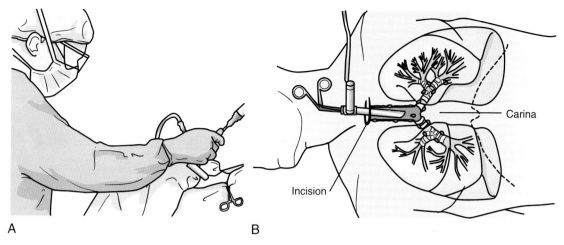

• **Fig. 42.15** Mediastinoscopy through incision at sternal notch. **A,** Insertion of mediastinoscope through suprasternal notch incision. **B,** Mediastinoscope in position.

drainage of blood) or to aid in restoring negative pressure in the thoracic cavity. It involves insertion of a tube through an intercostal space via a trocar and cannula.

Thoracoscopy

Thoracoscopy provides visualization of the pleural space, parietal and visceral pleurae, mediastinum, pericardium, and thoracic wall. The need for evaluation of pleural effusion (i.e., the accumulation of fluid, pus, or blood in the pleural space) and the need for obtaining biopsy specimens of pleural or lung tumors are the most common reasons for thoracoscopy.[6]

Definitive treatment of spontaneous pneumothorax (e.g., in patients with cystic fibrosis or in pleural effusion from cancer), using a sclerosing agent for chemical pleurodesis such as a slurry mixture or powder (poudrage), may be performed under thoracoscopic guidance. Materials used for pleurodesis include one or more of the following agents placed through a port or chest tube[7]:

- Erythromycin
- Bevacizumab
- Bleomycin
- *Corynebacterium parvum*
- Doxycycline
- Doxorubicin
- Fluorouracil
- Iodopovidone
- Cisplatin
- Minocycline
- Mitoxantrone
- Radioisotopes
- Silver nitrate
- Talc slurry or plain talc powder
- Cytarabine
- Etoposide

Fusion of the two pleural layers with a sclerosing agent prevents serous fluid production and accumulation in the chest.

Some of these agents can become systemic, causing side effects such as bone marrow depression. Several types of sclerosing agents, such as *C. parvum*, work only in the presence of malignancy and are not effective for pneumothorax and normal pleura. Talc can have a residual radiolucent quality that can interfere with chest x-rays.

• **Fig. 42.16** Thoracoscopy for lung biopsy.

In patients with empyema and adhesions a fibrous thickening on the visceral or parietal pleura may restrict pulmonary ventilation. Pulmonary decortication (membrane stripping) removes the restrictive layer or membrane over the lung to reexpand the entrapped lung and fill space remaining after drainage of an empyemic cavity (Fig. 42.16).

Thoracoscopic techniques include video-assisted thoracic surgery (VATS) and robotic single-port VATS for bullous emphysema, pneumonectomy, and debulking of thoracic tumors. Single-port robotics are used for selected cases in which instrumentation can be easily maneuvered.[8] Some procedures incorporate aspects of endoscopic and open techniques. An axillary approach to thoracoscopy provides good access to the apex of the lung and satisfactory aesthetic incisional closure. An intercostal incision for thoracoscopy is usually preferred, but resection of a rib may be necessary for some patients to facilitate access to the intrapleural space.

A laser can be used to vaporize thickened tissues between the visceral pleura and the lung or between the parietal pleura and the chest wall that impede breathing. Thoracoscopy is used effectively for separation of tissue layers.

General anesthesia is necessary. The patient is in a partial or full lateral thoracotomy position, depending on the preferred access portal sites that the surgeon selects. A small skin incision is made over and carried through the intercostal space of choice. The surgeon incises the parietal pleura to enter the pleural cavity.

After the anesthesia provider deflates the lung, the sterile thoracoscope is inserted into the pleural cavity. Pressures should not exceed 10 mm Hg. When the procedure is completed, the scope is removed and a chest tube is inserted and connected to a sterile, closed water-seal drainage system to remove residual air and fluid.

Complications of thoracoscopy include bleeding; injury to thoracic nerves, ducts, or vessels; atelectasis; and respiratory failure. Contraindications to the procedure are a fused lung, inability to tolerate a unilateral deflated lung, and cardiac instability.

Thoracic Incisional Approaches

Factors influencing the location of the thoracic incision include the following:
- Adequate exposure into the thoracic cavity
- Physiologic intrapleural pressure changes and constant movement of the chest
- Maintenance of integrity of the chest wall and diaphragm
- Condition of the underlying pleura and lung
- Objective of a minimally invasive procedure, if possible

Because of its continuity with the neck and abdominal structures, the thoracic cavity may be entered for neck and upper abdominal procedures as well as for thoracic procedures. Examples include a thoracic aortic aneurysm and pathologic conditions of the esophagus.

Posterolateral Thoracotomy

With the patient in a lateral chest position, a posterolateral incision permits maximum exposure to the lung, esophagus, diaphragm, and descending aorta for exploration of the thoracic cavity. Beginning anteriorly in the submammary fold, about at nipple level, a curved incision is made, extending below the scapular tip, following the course of the underlying ribs. Then curving upward and posteriorly, the incision may be carried as high as the spine of the scapula. Subcutaneous tissue is incised; the latissimus dorsi, lower margin of the trapezius, rhomboideus, and serratus muscles are divided; and bleeders are ligated. In dividing the serratus muscle, special precaution is taken to avoid the neurovascular bundle on the surface.

During closure the ribs are reapproximated with a rib approximator/contractor and sutures, the intercostal muscles are sutured, and the incision in the periosteal bed and pleura is closed (Fig. 42.17). Muscles are reapproximated anatomically and sutured; subcutaneous tissue and skin are closed.

Posterolateral thoracotomy is used for pulmonary resections, repair of a hiatal hernia, and procedures on the thoracic esophagus or posterior mediastinum.

Anterolateral Thoracotomy

For an anterolateral incision the patient is supine. Supports are placed under the affected side to tilt the shoulder 20 to 45 degrees for extension of the incision posteriorly. A pad behind the buttocks may rotate the hips slightly.

A submammary incision, directly below the breast but above the costal margin, extends from the anterior midline to the midaxillary or posterior axillary line. To avoid the axillary apex and a painful scar, the posterior end of the incision is curved downward. Superiorly, access is desired at about the fourth

• **Fig. 42.17** Rib approximation at closure of thoracotomy.

• **Fig. 42.18** Left thoracoabdominal incision with patient in lateral position.

interspace. Further anterior exposure can be gained, if desired, by transecting the sternum and continuing the incision to the contralateral interspace. The pectoralis muscles are divided, the serratus anterior fibers are separated, the intercostal muscles are divided, and the thorax is entered through an intercostal space. When an anterior incision extends to the sternal border, internal mammary arteries and veins are ligated and divided. If the incision is carried far laterally or posteriorly, injury to the long thoracic nerve must be avoided to prevent a winged scapula.

During closure the sternum is reapproximated with heavy suture, the ribs are approximated with pericostal sutures, and the muscles, subcutaneous tissue, and skin are closed.

Anterolateral thoracotomy is used for resection of a pulmonary cyst or a local lesion or for open lung biopsy.

Thoracoabdominal Incision

With the patient in a lateral position the thoracoabdominal incision extends from the posterior axillary line to the abdominal midline, paralleling the selected interspace (usually the seventh or eighth). After insertion of a rib spreader the incision in the intercostal muscles and pleura may be extended posteriorly from within for added exposure. The diaphragm may be divided peripherally. This incision exposes the upper abdomen, retroperitoneal area, and lower aspect of the chest (Fig. 42.18).

In closure the diaphragm is closed with interrupted sutures. The costal margin is secured by approximating the margins of the divided costal cartilages with suture. Tissue layers are closed in reverse order of incision.

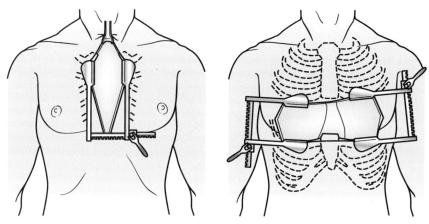

• **Fig. 42.19** Median sternotomy for lung procedures.

A thoracoabdominal incision is used for repair of a hiatal hernia, for esophagectomy, and in general surgery for resection of retroperitoneal tumors and cardioesophageal lesions.

Median Sternotomy

The patient is supine for a median sternotomy. A vertical incision extends through the midline from the suprasternal notch to the xyphoid process (Fig. 42.19). A power reciprocating saw is used to split the sternum in primary incisions. A median sternotomy incision is used for simultaneous bilateral pulmonary surgical procedures, treatment of mediastinal neoplasms or trauma, pulmonary embolectomy and cardiac and aortic procedures, and access to the lower cervical and upper thoracic vertebrae. This incision may be preferred for resection of peripheral neoplasms in patients with impaired pulmonary function, particularly in the upper and middle lobes of the lungs. Reoperative procedures require the use of an oscillating saw to open the sternum.

In closure, heavy-gauge stainless steel sutures are often used to close the sternum. Alternative techniques incorporate the use of implantable titanium locking clips (e.g., Sternal Talon) for rigid fixation of the sternum. The clips and instrumentation are supplied nonsterile and must be processed in the same manner as screw and plate sets.

For the use of locking clips the patient's sternum is measured for depth and width with calipers. The clips are two-part interlocking devices (male and female ends) that are seated in the split sternum with aligning forceps and snapped together using reduction clamps to join the bone segments together. As the clip components are united, ratcheted teeth hold the two parts together. Care is taken to ensure that underlying tissue is not entrapped in the clip assembly. The surface of the united clip is marked with margins along the ratchets indicating a "safe zone," which means that the clip is correctly placed and snapped together. A small screw on the female half is turned to physically lock the clip. Three locking clips are usually used.

For emergent reentry into the sternum the screw can be turned to release the ratchets and open the closed clip. The clips can be removed after the bone has healed. Sternal locking clips are implants and should be documented in the patient's record. The locking clip components should be restocked in the set according to size. The clips are for single use only and not reprocessed after individual patient use.

Partial Sternotomy

When partial sternotomy is used the distal sternum is cut vertically to the level of the manubrium. The patient has a smaller incision and becomes ambulatory sooner postoperatively.

Parasternotomy

Parasternotomy incisions are being used more frequently for minimally invasive cardiac procedures. An incision to the left or right of the sternum, without splitting the sternum, allows for visualization of the inner thorax.

Alternative Thoracotomy Incisions

The following alternative incisions may be used:

- A transaxillary approach for lung biopsy or wedge resection, particularly in the lower lobe, thoracic sympathectomy or exposure of the second to fifth thoracic ganglia, or exposure for thoracic outlet syndrome. This vertical incision causes minimal injury to muscles of the chest wall and preserves muscles of the shoulder.
- A supraclavicular (scalene) approach for phrenic nerve section, cervicothoracic sympathectomy, axillary vein thrombosis, or thoracic outlet syndrome. The incision is parallel to the clavicle. The first rib may be resected.
- Cervical mediastinotomy for drainage high in the mediastinum, such as after esophageal perforation.
- Anterior approach for upper dorsal sympathectomy, exposing upper thoracic ganglia.

Lung-Assist Devices

Extracorporeal Membrane Oxygenator

An extracorporeal membrane oxygenator (ECMO) is used as a resuscitative device for adults or children who have potentially reversible respiratory and/or cardiac failure.[9] It also is commonly used to prolong extracorporeal circulation when the patient is in distress after removal from cardiopulmonary bypass. The machine is designed like a cardiopulmonary bypass machine. ECMO was developed and first used to sustain neonates in 1975 by Robert H. Bartlett, MD (1939–), from the University of Michigan Health System. The use of ECMO has decreased the loss of cognitive function caused by anoxic brain damage. When used in combination with intentional controlled hypothermia, ECMO offers a better chance of little or no cognitive deficit.

The patient's hemoglobin is maintained at 12 to 15 g/dL during treatment by administration of packed red blood cells. Adequate platelet volume is augmented by administration of platelets and monitoring clotting times. Renal protection is critical because while on ECMO the body begins an inflammatory response followed by a diuretic phase within 48 hours. During this period the patient's body weight increases because of retained fluids. If urine output is low, the patient is given diuretics to stimulate the renal tubules and minimize fluid retention. Some patients require adjunct hemodialysis to give the kidneys a rest period. Periodic blood cultures are done. Hyperalimentation is done to ensure nutritional status.

ECMO also can be used for a short interim period (several days) to sustain the patient's life while waiting for an organ transplant or after major trauma. Potential complications include bleeding caused by the high-dose anticoagulants required to minimize clotting.[10] Survival rates increase to 44% for pediatric patients and 20% to 40% for adults when used as a resuscitation measure, as compared with the 10.7% cardiopulmonary resuscitation survival rate.[11] Activating ECMO immediately increases the chance for survival. Children in distress and arrest greater than 13 minutes before implementation of ECMO have not been successfully resuscitated.

The following are two methods of extracorporeal membrane oxygenation:

- *Venoarterial bypass:* Cannulation points include the common carotid artery and the internal jugular vein or the femoral artery and the femoral vein. Venoarterial bypass supports both the heart and lungs by removing deoxygenated venous blood via a vein, removing carbon dioxide, adding oxygen, and returning the oxygenated blood to the body via an artery. The device is used for patients of all ages. It is the method of choice for cardiopulmonary assistance in the preterm neonate because other appropriately sized assistive devices are unavailable.
- *Venovenous bypass:* The right atrium and the femoral vein are common sites for cannulation. Venovenous bypass supports pulmonary function by oxygenating venous blood and decreasing the circulating venous carbon dioxide level. The advantages are lower mechanical flow rates and decreased risk for arterial emboli. The patient receives ventilatory assistance, which supplements the oxygenation process.

Intravascular Oxygenator

A lung-assist device such as an intravascular oxygenator (IVOX) may be used temporarily to assist the adult patient with respiratory failure or acute respiratory distress syndrome (ARDS). The IVOX allows the patient's damaged lungs to heal. The device is inserted into the common femoral vein and advanced into the vena cava. A chest x-ray is performed to verify placement. It has hundreds of thin-walled hollow fibers made of polypropylene coated with gas-permeable membranes. The gas conduit that exits from the skin has two tubes: one delivers oxygen, and the other removes carbon dioxide via diffusion.

The oxygen inlet tube is connected to a pump to produce a flow of oxygen through the lumina of the fibers into venous blood. Carbon dioxide transfers through the outflow membrane, controlled by a vacuum pump. It can provide up to 50% of the patient's gas exchange requirements by bypassing the volume of oxygen to the lungs. By decreasing the airway pressure in the lungs, damaged tissue has a better chance to heal. The IVOX requires minimal anticoagulation and can remain in place for several weeks.

IVOX is less expensive and simpler to operate than ECMO. It is useful for patients who have had lung transplantation and cannot withstand the ventilating pressures associated with oxygenation.

Thoracic Surgical Procedures

Pulmonary resection often is the procedure of choice for malignant tumors and benign diseases such as bullous emphysema and tuberculosis. A bronchopleural fistula and pulmonary fibrosis are also among concerns of the thoracic surgeon.

Rib Resection

Rib resection for donor bone procurement requires much of the same instrumentation used for open thoracotomy. A segment of rib is removed (Fig. 42.20). Reconstructive procedures of the ear, mandible, or facial structures commonly use autologous rib grafts. Equipment and supplies should be immediately available for open thoracotomy or closed chest drainage if hemothorax or pneumothorax should occur.

Mediastinotomy

Anterior mediastinotomy may be indicated when radiographs show hilar or mediastinal nodal involvement inaccessible to mediastinoscopy. With the patient supine and under general anesthesia, an incision is made over the right or left third costal cartilage. The cartilage bed is incised. Extrapleural dissection is carried toward the hilus of the lung, and a biopsy specimen is obtained. If the desired nodes are deep, a mediastinoscope may be inserted through the incision to obtain the biopsy specimen. Alternatively, the pleural space may be entered for a lung biopsy. If this space is entered, closed water-seal chest drainage is required. If it is not entered, the incision is closed in layers without drainage. Mediastinotomy allows assessment of the extent of a lesion or a deformity.

Excision of Lesions

A median sternotomy (i.e., a vertical sternal splitting procedure) may be necessary to resect a cyst or a benign or malignant tumor in the upper anterior mediastinum. Through a posterolateral thoracotomy incision, a tumor may be resected or an abscess drained in the posterior mediastinum.

• **Fig. 42.20** Segmental rib resection.

Correction of a Pectus Deformity

Congenital deformities of the chest wall are usually corrected in childhood. Pectus carinatum (pigeon chest) is forward projection of the sternum, resembling the keel of a boat. Pectus excavatum (funnel chest), which is more common, is caused by elongation of costal cartilages, which pushes the sternum back toward the spine.

Surgical correction of pectus excavatum, sometimes delayed until adolescence or adulthood, is performed to relieve respiratory distress or pressure on the heart from mechanical compression or for cosmetic improvement. Various techniques may be used.

Usually with the patient supine and the upper chest slightly hyperextended, costal cartilages are exposed by muscle splitting and/or division through an anterior midline or horizontal inframammary incision. Involved costal cartilages and deformed rib ends are freed from sternal attachments and resected or straightened. The sternum is mobilized and restored to normal position, and its corrected position is maintained by fixation. An alternative method corrects the contour deformity with a prosthesis introduced through an inframammary incision. Dacron patches on the posterior surface stabilize the prosthesis. Additional discussion of corrections for pectus deformity can be found in Chapter 8.

Thoracotomy

An incision through the thoracic wall (i.e., thoracotomy) is indicated for drainage of pleural spaces, exploration of the thoracic cavity, or cardiac and pulmonary procedures. Thoracic surgical procedures, exclusive of cardiac procedures, include exploratory thoracotomy, open thoracotomy, and open chest drainage.

Exploratory Thoracotomy

Exploratory thoracotomy is performed as an open procedure to confirm the diagnosis and extent of involvement of bronchogenic carcinoma or other chest disease, such as a mediastinal lesion, when the pathologic process cannot be confirmed by endoscopy. A biopsy specimen is obtained, most often from the lower margin of the upper lobe, for disseminated lung disease. This may be done through an anterior thoracotomy with the patient under local anesthesia.

Biopsy specimens are also usually obtained from the mediastinal lymph nodes. Through a posterolateral incision, the lungs and hemithorax are exposed after the ribs are spread and the pleura is opened. Interstitial bleeding and chest trauma are other indications for exploration.

Open thoracotomy may be used for spontaneous pneumothorax, large air leaks that prevent reexpansion of the lung, or persistent leaks and incomplete lung reexpansion. This type of pneumothorax usually occurs from rupture of a bleb on the lung surface. By posterolateral incision through the fourth interspace, an apical bleb may be ligated or the involved segmental area of the lung resected. Abrasion or cauterization of the parietal pleura effects adhesion to the visceral pleura, thereby eliminating future rupture of blebs.

Open chest drainage also is used to eliminate an empyemic cavity, which accompanies chronic disease and lung adherence to the chest wall. With this procedure, portions of one or two ribs are removed to aid in the establishment of drainage.

Lung Resection

All or part of a diseased or traumatized lung may be resected (Fig. 42.21). Generally the indications are neoplasms; emphysematous blebs; and fungal infection, localized residual lung abscess, tuberculosis, and/or bronchiectasis resistant to nonsurgical treatment.[12] Neoplasms are the predominant indication. An anterior intercostal incision with division of costal cartilages above and below the incision may be used for excision of pulmonary nodules or lung biopsy.

A posterolateral incision is commonly used for lobectomy and pneumonectomy. Endotracheal anesthesia is used. Special precautions in pulmonary resection include meticulous hemostasis and closure of the bronchus, as well as continual attention to cardiopulmonary function preoperatively, intraoperatively, and postoperatively. Particular hazards are hemorrhage, which is difficult to control because of the size and friability of major pulmonary vessels and the proximity of the lungs to the heart; cardiopulmonary insufficiency; and the risk for injury to other intrathoracic structures, such as the vagus, phrenic, and left recurrent nerves and the esophagus. Specific resections include surgical resection, wedge resection, lobectomy, bronchoplastic reconstruction, and pneumonectomy.

Segmental Resection

Removal of individual bronchovascular segments of a lobe is preferred when wide excision is not necessary, such as for a pathologic process confined to a segment or acute hemorrhage. The arteries, veins, and bronchus of the involved segment are ligated and divided. The segment is separated from surrounding lung tissue and removed. The proximal bronchial stump is closed with sutures or staples.

Wedge Resection

Wedge resection is a conservative procedure performed when a lesion is thought to be benign. Along with an adequate margin of normal lung tissue, the diseased peripheral portion of a lobe is removed, and the lung tissue is sutured. A stapler may expedite removal and closure. A frozen section is done. If a benign

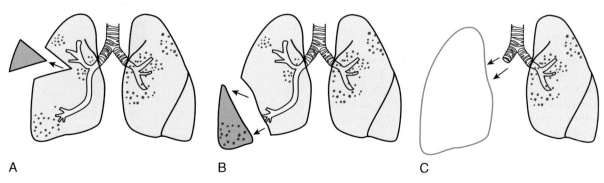

• **Fig. 42.21** Types of lung resections. **A,** Wedge resection. **B,** Lobectomy. **C,** Pneumonectomy.

A   B   C

diagnosis is confirmed, the wound is closed in layers, and a chest tube is inserted for closed water-seal drainage. If the lesion proves to be malignant, lobectomy or another appropriate procedure may be done. The advantage of wedge resection is its simplicity, with minimal blood loss and procedure time.

Lobectomy

One or more lobes of a lung are excised when disease or neoplasm is confined to the lobe. The remaining portion of the lung expands to fill the space formerly occupied by the removed lobe. Through a posterolateral incision, entrance to the chest may be intercostal or by rib resection. The pulmonary pleura is incised and freed from the hilus of the lobe. The arteries and veins to the pulmonary tissue being resected are ligated and divided. The bronchus of the lobe is identified by lung inflation while the bronchus to be resected is clamped.

Suction of blood and secretions from the open bronchus may precede closure of the bronchus by sutures or staples. A suture line in the bronchus is covered with a flap of parietal pleura to prevent leakage. Dissection is completed, the specimen is removed, and the chest is closed.

Bronchoplastic Reconstruction

Extensive partial pulmonary resection may be followed by bronchoplastic reconstruction to ensure maximum preservation of residual pulmonary tissue. These techniques require successful bronchial anastomoses to retain a patent airway to the bronchioles.

Pneumonectomy

Major indications for excision of an entire lung are malignant neoplasms and extensive unilateral pulmonary disease. The chest wall is opened by a posterolateral incision, the pleura is incised, the lung is exposed, and the pleural cavity is examined. After immobilization of the lung the hilus is dissected free on all sides. The pulmonary artery and veins are ligated and divided. The bronchus is clamped, divided, and closed with sutures or staples. The bronchus is checked for air leaks by instillation of normal saline solution, and the bronchial stump is covered with surrounding pleura. After wound closure, intrathoracic pressure is measured and residual air aspirated from the hemithorax until the desired pressure is reached. Use of chest drainage is governed by surgeon preference, but usually no chest tube is inserted.

Sacrifice of one lung places the entire responsibility for respiratory and circulatory function on the remaining lung. Potential complications are respiratory insufficiency, cardiac dysrhythmia, and a predisposition for infection because of dead space. The empty hemithorax gradually fills with fluid and eventually consolidates, thus preventing a mediastinal shift. Dehiscence of the bronchial closure may produce a bronchopleural fistula.

Lung Reduction

Lung reduction can be performed for patients who have emphysematous lung disease. In emphysema the lungs have become enlarged because the air sacs are destroyed. By reducing the size of the lungs, efficiency is improved. Minimally invasive techniques have been used with great success. Clinical trials are in process to validate the efficacy of the techniques.

Patient selection for the procedure is based on the patient's cardiac profile, pulmonary function, and exercise tolerance. Patients with severe disease of the heart or lungs and those who are older than 70 years are usually poor surgical risks for the procedure and are not surgical candidates.

Thoracoplasty

Thoracoplasty is usually done extrapleurally. The chest wall is mobilized to obliterate the pleural cavity or reduce thoracic space by resection of one or more ribs. Indications are inadequate expansion of the lung to fill the pleural space after resection, persistent shift of the mediastinum to the empty space after pneumonectomy, or chronic empyema. Tissue fibroses, contracts, and eventually obliterates the space. Thoracoplasty is reserved for patients in whom excessive space in the chest cannot be eliminated satisfactorily by other means to maintain the mediastinum in the midline.

Transplantation of Thoracic Organs

Transplantation of either a single lung or both lungs may be an option for the patient with end-stage pulmonary fibrosis, obstructive lung disease, or cystic fibrosis.

Thymectomy

The thymus gland lies on the pericardium in the anterior mediastinum from its origin in the cervical region around the trachea (Fig. 42.22). The two lobes are separated from the arch of the aorta and great vessels by a layer of fascia. In an adult the thymus has become smaller and, in some cases, negligible in size.

Thymectomy is usually performed through a median sternotomy, but the gland may be excised through a transcervical incision. The pericardium, the innominate vein, a portion of the superior vena cava, and a portion of the lung are removed en bloc to resect a thymoma. The phrenic nerve is spared to prevent diaphragmatic paralysis. Thymectomy without en bloc resection may be done to relieve symptoms of myasthenia gravis.

Thoracic Outlet Syndrome

The thoracic outlet is an area bordered by the manubrium anteriorly, the first rib anterolaterally, and the first thoracic vertebra posteriorly.[13] The subclavian artery and vein, the vertebral artery, and the brachial plexus pass through this space (Fig. 42.23). After

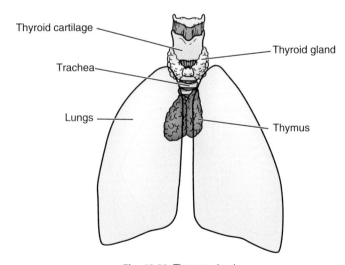

• **Fig. 42.22** Thymus gland.

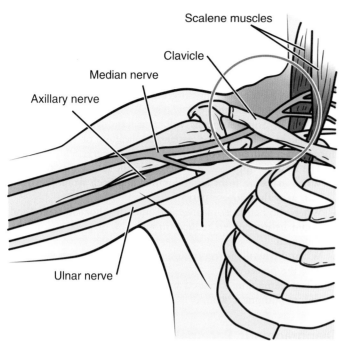

Scalene muscles
Clavicle
Median nerve
Axillary nerve
Ulnar nerve

• **Fig. 42.23** Thoracic outlet syndrome.

a neck injury or other postural deformity, changes can occur in the anterior and/or middle scalene muscles, causing intermittent pressure on these vessels and nerves. Symptoms include swelling, sweating, and pain and paresthesia of the upper extremities extending into the fingertips.

Diagnosis is made by having the patient raise the arms over the head and simultaneously observing for the Selmonosky triad, which is supraclavicular tenderness, pallor and paresthesia of the affected hand, and weakness of the fourth and fifth digits.[13]

When conservative treatment fails to relieve pain, scalenectomy or scalenotomy is performed. A supraclavicular incision with resection of the first rib or a transaxillary incision is used. In extreme circumstances, bilateral resection of the first rib may be necessary.[13]

Chest Trauma

Trauma to the chest varies in severity and may result in injury to the thoracic wall or intrathoracic organs such as the heart and lungs. If the trauma is severe, the patient is plunged into a critical condition. Rapid initial evaluation of the extent of injury is necessary to preserve life, with priority needs met first. These include resuscitation with relief of airway obstruction, treatment of shock and blood loss, and restoration of normal cardiorespiratory dynamics to the extent possible. Impairment of these dynamics may be caused by various factors such as disturbance of lung expansion or cardiac tamponade.

Trauma is categorized as blunt or penetrating. Blunt trauma usually results from a fall, blow, severe cough, blast, or deceleration injury. The patient may have little overt evidence of chest injury, even though they may be bleeding internally from pulmonary contusion. Penetrating wounds are usually caused by a low- or high-velocity missile, such as a knife stab or bullet. Surgical exploration may be required to control bleeding and/or air

leak. Open thoracotomy may be performed in the emergency department and the patient is brought to the operating room (OR) with the chest open for further exploration of the wound and closure.

Blunt Trauma

Fractured Ribs

Rib fracture is the most common injury to the chest wall, and the fourth to the eighth ribs are the ones mainly involved. Pain may be relieved by an intercostal nerve block. Surgical treatment is usually not required unless sharp edges or displaced bone fragments puncture the pleura or lung. Extensive pneumothorax requires immediate reexpansion of the lungs.

Multiple rib or sternal fractures often produce an unstable chest wall, resulting in flail chest. Normal respiration changes to paradoxic motion of the chest wall. The chest wall collapses on inspiration and expands on expiration. This results in ineffective respiration and coughing. As the chest wall expands, the free-floating sternum is sucked inward, thus impairing ventilation and producing hypoxia. The following measures are used to stabilize the chest wall:

1. Internal stabilization is achieved by controlled mechanical ventilation. An endotracheal tube or tracheostomy tube may be necessary to decrease pulmonary resistance and increase perfusion. Frequent suctioning maintains a clear airway; thus paradoxic motion and dead air space decrease.
2. Surgical stabilization is achieved by inserting pins or wiring fractures together. Fracture of the sternum, scapulae, and clavicles also may be involved in the injury.

Ruptured Organs

Blunt trauma can cause rupture of the diaphragm, aorta, or thoracic tracheobronchial tree, necessitating emergency thoracotomy. Contusions of the lung and pericardium may cause hemorrhage.

Penetrating Wounds

Anatomic visualization of the path of the projectile or instrument producing injury is important. A knife, for example, should not be removed except under the direction of a physician because it may be penetrating the heart or a major vessel.

Sucking Chest Wound

An open chest wound must be converted to a closed chest wound. Air rushes into an open wound, building up atmospheric positive pressure inside the pleural space. Pneumothorax followed by a mediastinal shift ensues.

Pneumothorax is relieved and further air prevented from entering the chest during respiration by suturing the wound and inserting one or more chest tubes.

Thoracentesis

Air or blood in the pleural cavity may be detected on x-ray and aspirated by a needle and syringe. A chest tube may be inserted into the pleural space percutaneously for closed thoracostomy drainage. If bleeding persists, the chest is opened and vessels are ligated or repaired.

Intrathoracic Esophageal Procedures

Esophageal disorders may be congenital, or they may be acquired by trauma or disease. Thoracic surgeons may perform esophageal resections for a benign tumor (e.g., leiomyoma) or relief of obstruction in the thoracic esophagus (e.g., stricture, stenosis, achalasia). Esophageal myotomy with or without fundoplication may relieve obstruction in the lower segment. Resections are performed for malignant tumors.

Early detection of esophageal carcinoma increases the rate of cure by surgical resection. Unfortunately, symptoms are not usually apparent in the early stages, so carcinoma of the esophagus generally presents a poor prognosis. Most surgical procedures provide palliation rather than cure. Radical en bloc mediastinectomy may become the procedure of choice, but esophagectomy is more commonly performed.

Esophagectomy

For esophagectomy the patient is in a lateral position. A posterolateral thoracotomy or thoracoabdominal incision is extended across the chest wall to expose the affected segment of the esophagus (i.e., upper, middle, or lower third). The thoracic cavity is opened, and the mediastinal pleura is incised. The esophagus is dissected away from the aorta and transected above and below the lesion.

For combined thoracoabdominal exposure of a lesion in the lower third of the esophagus, the diaphragm is opened and the stomach mobilized for transection and intrathoracic esophagogastrostomy. In some patients, resection and anastomosis may be performed without thoracotomy by means of a substernal resection to avoid morbidity associated with thoracoabdominal exposure.

High esophageal resection followed by hypopharyngeal reconstruction may be the procedure of choice for tumors in the upper third of the esophagus. Total esophagectomy for tumors in the middle third may be carried out through abdominal and cervical incisions, without thoracotomy. The stomach is mobilized for esophagogastric anastomosis in the neck. Examples of esophageal autologous tissue replacement are depicted in Fig. 42.24.

Repair of a Hiatal Hernia

Repair of herniation of the stomach through the diaphragm may be performed by a general surgeon or by a thoracic surgeon using thoracic routines, such as chest tube insertion with closed waterseal drainage. Plication (stitching) the fundus of the stomach is part of the procedure. The surgeon will use a full fundal wrap (Nissen fundoplication) or a partial fundal wrap (Toupet) (Fig. 42.25). Some surgeons will transilluminate the esophagus with a lighted bougie for easier visualization of the structure during open and endoscopic hiatal hernia surgery.

The thoracic approach is preferred in the following situations:
- When exposure from an abdominal approach would be difficult, as with an obese patient
- When the hernia is incarcerated into the thoracic cavity and would be difficult to reduce through the diaphragm into the abdomen
- When the hernia is recurrent and direct visualization will facilitate the procedure
- When herniation is caused by blunt trauma or a penetrating abdominothoracic wound

Diaphragmatic Pacemaker

Injury to the phrenic nerve can cause full or partial paralysis of the diaphragm. A battery-powered pacing device can be used to stimulate nerve impulses that cause the diaphragm to contract and relax. The device is partially external and partially internal with leads (Fig. 42.26).

Complications of Thoracic Surgery

Continuous movement of the chest causes postoperative pain. The patient is likely to breathe shallowly and not adequately raise secretions that accumulate as a result of inhaled anesthetics and sedation. Obstruction in the bronchi from retained secretions can lead to pneumonia and/or atelectasis. The plan of care should include preoperative teaching of breathing techniques to assist the patient in clearing airway secretions.

Development of one pulmonary complication frequently predisposes the patient to development of another. Other potential complications are pneumothorax from an air leak, hemothorax

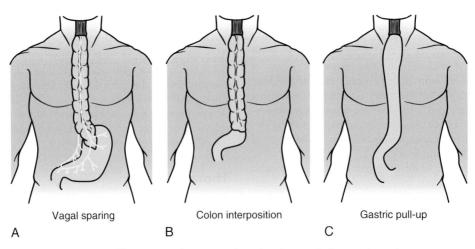

Vagal sparing Colon interposition Gastric pull-up

A   B   C

• **Fig. 42.24** Three approaches to esophageal replacement after esophagectomy.

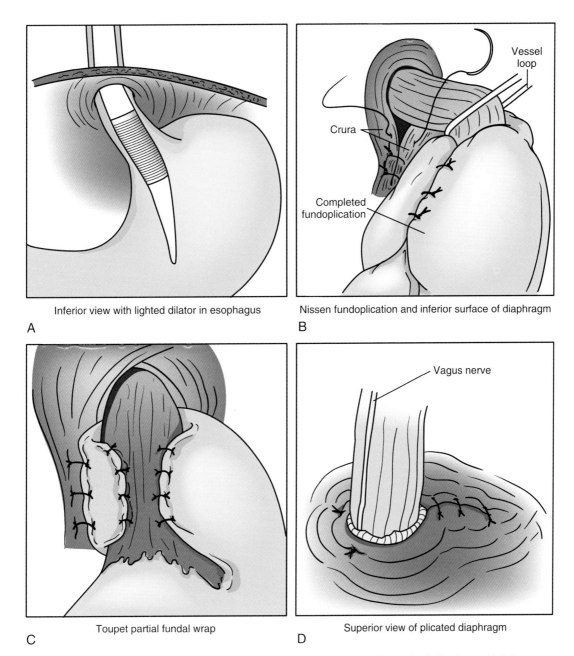

Inferior view with lighted dilator in esophagus

A

Nissen fundoplication and inferior surface of diaphragm

B

Vessel loop

Crura

Completed fundoplication

Toupet partial fundal wrap

C

Vagus nerve

Superior view of plicated diaphragm

D

• **Fig. 42.25** Hiatal hernia repair. **A,** Inferior view with lighted dilator. **B,** Nissen fundoplication and inferior surface of diaphragm. **C,** Toupet partial fundal wrap. **D,** Superior view of plicated diaphragm.

from hemorrhage, and pleural effusion. Empyema and persistent undrained fluid or air pockets can develop in intrathoracic spaces. A bronchopleural fistula may necessitate closure. Pulmonary shunting is also a major complication.

Chylothorax, the leakage of chyle from the thoracic duct of the lymphatic system into the pleural space, is a potential complication of thoracic surgery. This complication may occur in response to trauma or neoplasm, or after a surgical procedure in the chest cavity. Surgical repair of the thoracic duct is performed.

ARDS, also known as progressive pulmonary insufficiency or shock lung, may develop in the first 24 to 48 hours after a traumatic injury, such as pulmonary contusion or from diffuse or aspiration pneumonia. Beginning with dyspnea, grunting respirations, and tachycardia, signs progress to cyanosis, hypoxemia, and alveolar infiltration. Mortality is high. An IVOX/intravenacaval blood gas exchanger may be used as a temporary booster lung for a patient with ARDS or acute respiratory failure.

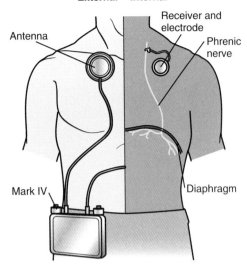

External Internal

Antenna

Receiver and electrode

Phrenic nerve

Mark IV

Diaphragm

• **Fig. 42.26** Diaphragmatic pacer for paralyzed diaphragm.

ⓔ EVOLVE WEBSITE

http://evolve.elsevier.com/Hornacky/BerryKohn/

- Historical Perspective
- Student Interactive Questions
- Glossary

References

1. Lin J, Fernandez F: Indications for invasive mediastinal staging for non-small cell lung cancer, *J Thorac Cardiovasc Surg* 156(6):2319–2324, 2018.

2. Hsu PK, Wu YC: The feasibility of electromagnetic navigation guided percutaneous microcoil localization for thoracoscopic resection of small pulmonary nodules, *J Thorac Cardiovasc Surg* 157(4):e211–e214, 2019.

3. Bozzo C, Profili S, Masala S: Successful use of self-expandable metal stents in a case of iatrogenic tracheal rupture, *Radiol Case Rep* 14(3):377–380, 2018.

4. American Lung Association: Endobronchial valve (EBV) therapy. www.lung.org. Accessed July 8, 2023.

5. Handy J, Bremner R, Crocenzi T, et al.: Expert consensus document on pulmonary metastasectomy, *Ann Thorac Surg* 107(2):631–649, 2019.

6. Allakhverdiev A, Davydov M, Akhmedov P: Thoracoscopic lobectomy with mediastinal lymph node dissection as a standard surgery for T1-2NoMo non-small cell lung cancer (>300 surgeries experience), *Ann Med Surg* 35:169–172, 2018.

7. Ali M, Surani S: Pleurodesis, *StatPearls*. www.ncbi.nlm.nih.gov. Accessed July 8, 2023.

8. Park SY, Kim HK, Jang DS, et al.: Initial experiences with robotic single-site thoracic surgery for mediastinal masses, *Ann Thorac Surg* 107(1):242–247, 2019.

9. Guglin M, Zucker M, Bazan V, et al.: Venoarterial ECMO for adults, *J Am Coll Cardiol* 73(6):698–716, 2019.

10. Raman J, Alimohamed M, Dobrilovic N, et al.: A comparison of low and standard anti-coagulation regimens in extracorporeal membrane oxygenation, *J Heart Lung Transplant* 38(4):433–439, 2019.

11. Charriere A, Assouline B, Scheen M, et al.: ECMO in cardiac arrest: a narrative review of the literature, *J Clin Med* 10(3):534, 2021.

12. Yablonskii P, Kudriashov G, Avetisyan A: Surgical resection in the treatment of pulmonary tuberculosis, *Thorac Surg Clin* 29(1):37–46, 2019.

13. Smith F, Winterborn R: Thoracic outlet syndrome, *Surgery* 37(2):112–118, 2019.

43

Cardiac Surgery

CHAPTER OUTLINE

Anatomy of the Heart and Great Vessels, 923

Physiology of the Heart, 925

Cardiac Cycle, 925

Special Features of Cardiac Surgery, 926

Cardiac Surgical Procedures, 933

Mechanical Assist Devices, 940

Complications of Cardiac Surgery, 945

CHAPTER OBJECTIVES

After studying this chapter, the learner will be able to:

- Identify the pertinent anatomy of the heart and great vessels.
- List the types of conduits used for coronary artery bypass grafting.

- Describe the function of a cardiac pacemaker.

KEY TERMS AND DEFINITIONS

Ablation Intentional destruction of tissue for therapeutic purposes.

Bicaval Two places on the vena cava.

Biventricular Both ventricles are affected.

Cardioplegia Solution infused into the heart for myocardial preservation during surgery.

Cardiopulmonary bypass Oxygenation of blood during heart surgery.

Conduit Tubular passage for blood.

De-airing Venting air from the chambers of the heart.

Echocardiography Means of observing the heart through sound waves displayed on a screen by using a probe.

Euvolemic Equilibrium of fluid balance in the body.

Ostia Natural opening into the coronary arteries.

Pedunculated Attached by a vascular stalk.

Pledget A Teflon felt attached to a suture to prevent tissue tearing during stitching.

Redo Return to the operating room for additional surgery during the postoperative phase. Usually denotes an emergency such as bleeding.

Tamponade The pericardium and surrounding tissue fills with blood and fluid causing restricted heart motion. Cardiac output is diminished.

Anatomy of the Heart and Great Vessels

Cardiac procedures involve the heart and associated great vessels. To understand diagnostic procedures, hemodynamic monitoring, myocardial preservation techniques, and cardiopulmonary bypass (CPB) used in conjunction with cardiac surgery requires knowledge of the normal anatomy and physiology of the heart.

The cardiovascular system supplies oxygen and nutrients to body cells and carries waste away from cells by the flow of blood through the system. The heart, blood, and lymph vessels constitute this circulatory system. The heart—the hollow muscular organ located in the thorax—maintains the circulation of blood throughout the body.

Heart

The heart is located in the middle mediastinum slightly left of midline. The heart is a four-chambered muscular "pump" enveloped by a closed, double-layered fibroserous sac—the pericardium. The outer parietal layer forms the sac that contains a small amount of clear serous fluid that lubricates the heart's moving surfaces. The base of the pericardium is attached to the diaphragm; the apex surrounds the great vessels arising from the base of the heart (Figs. 43.1 and 43.2).

The layers of the heart are the epicardium (outer visceral pericardium), myocardium (muscle fibers), and endocardium (inner membrane lining) (Fig. 43.3). Divided into right and left halves by an oblique longitudinal septum, each half of the heart has two chambers: a thin-walled upper atrium and a thick-walled lower ventricle. The right side of the heart pumps the pulmonary circulation, and the left side of the heart pumps blood into the systemic circulation. The right atrium receives desaturated blood from the inferior and superior venae cavae and the coronary veins.

The left atrium receives oxygenated blood from the pulmonary veins. The left ventricle pumps blood into the aorta and the coronary arteries. The heart's rounded apex, formed by the left

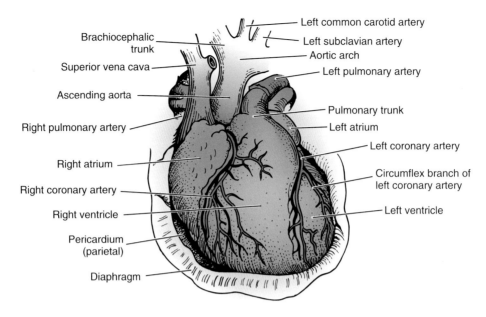

• **Fig. 43.1** Anterior view of the heart and great vessels.

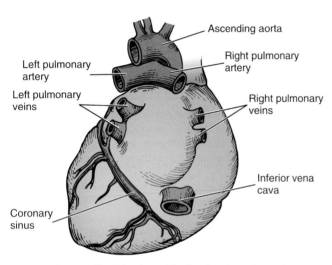

• **Fig. 43.2** Posterior view of the heart and great vessels.

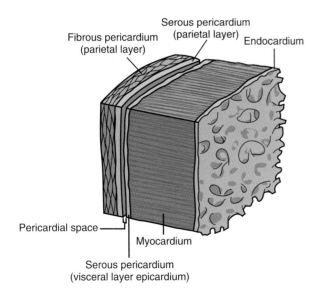

• **Fig. 43.3** Cross-section of the cardiac wall.

• **Fig. 43.4** Cardiac valves: superior view with atria removed.

ventricle, is behind the sixth rib slightly to the left of the sternum. The base is formed by the atria and great vessels.

Valves

Four heart valves promote unobstructed unidirectional blood flow through the chambers (Fig. 43.4). These valves are of the following two types:

1. *Atrioventricular (AV) valves:* The bases of the cusps (the endocardial leaflets) of these valves attach to the fibrous ring that surrounds their opening between the atrium and ventricle on each side of the heart.
   a. The right tricuspid valve has three cusps and lies between the right atrium and ventricle.
   b. The left mitral valve has two cusps and lies between the left atrium and ventricle.
2. *Semilunar valves:* These valves open to allow blood to flow from the heart chambers into the great vessels.
   a. The pulmonary valve between the right ventricle and the pulmonary trunk has three cusps.
   b. The aortic valve between the left ventricle and the aorta has three cusps.

When the ventricle begins to contract, the AV cusps float up to close the opening, preventing a backflow of blood, as the semilunar valves open. Sequential heart sounds (S1 and S2) are heard by stethoscope as the valves open and close.

Coronary Circulation

Coronary circulation supplies oxygen directly to the heart muscle and is predominantly anatomically right or left. The coronary arteries arise from the aorta just above the aortic valve and, with their branches, supply oxygen and nutrients to the heart muscle. The coronary arteries fill during the diastolic, or relaxation, phase. The left coronary artery divides shortly after its origin into two main trunks:

1. The anterior descending or interventricular branch courses toward the apex of the heart. Its branches distribute over the anterolateral wall of the left ventricle. Septal branches supply the anterior interventricular septum.
2. The circumflex branch passes posteriorly. Following the AV groove and passing under the left atrial appendage, it meets the right coronary artery at the base of the junction of both ventricles.

The right coronary artery is directed to the right, passing to the posterior aspect of the heart and eventually running between the two ventricles. Its branches supply the posterior interventricular septum. The desaturated coronary blood returns to the venous circulation through the coronary sinus.

The vagus nerve (parasympathetic nervous system) and cardiac branches of the cervical and upper thoracic ganglia (sympathetic nervous system) innervate the heart.

Physiology of the Heart

Electrical Conduction System

The conduction system of the heart (Fig. 43.5) permits synchronous contraction of the atria followed by contraction of the ventricles. The right and left sides of the heart function simultaneously but independently. Muscular contractions of the atria and ventricles are controlled by an electrical impulse that originates in the sinoatrial (SA) node. This "pacemaker" is a dense network of specialized Purkinje fibers that begin at the junction of the right atrium and superior vena cava. These fibers become continuous with muscle fibers of the atrium at the node's periphery. The stimulus is passed to the smaller AV node beneath the endocardium in the interatrial septum. A mass of interwoven conductive

tissue, this node's specialized fibers are continuous with atrial muscle fibers and the AV bundle of His.

The bundle of His provides conduction relay between the atria and ventricles. Arising from the AV node, the band of conducting tissue passes on both sides of the interventricular septum, its branches dividing and subdividing to penetrate every area of ventricular muscle and to transmit contraction impulses to the ventricles. Extensions of conductive tissue provide coordinated excitation of myocardium in both atria and ventricles. Each atrial contraction (depolarization) is followed by a period of recharging (repolarization) during which the ventricles contract. Ventricular contraction is followed by a period of recovery while the chambers fill with blood as the atria contract.

Cardiac Cycle

Myocardial contraction is referred to as *systole*; cardiac relaxation is referred to as *diastole*. Venous blood from the entire body enters the right atrium via the superior and inferior venae cavae and passes through the tricuspid valve to the right ventricle, from which it is ejected through the pulmonary valve into the pulmonary arterial trunk (Fig. 43.6). Right and left pulmonary arteries originating from the trunk carry the blood to the lungs, where it takes up oxygen and gives off carbon dioxide. Oxygenated blood is transported from the lungs to the left atrium by the pulmonary veins and enters the left ventricle through the mitral valve. Contraction of the left ventricle propels blood through the aortic valve into the aorta, from which it is carried to all parts of the body by arterial branches.

The highest pressure reached during left ventricular systole is the systolic blood pressure. After contraction the ventricle relaxes, during which time systemic intraarterial pressure falls to its lowest level—the diastolic blood pressure. Each contraction of the right ventricle forces blood through the pulmonary valve into the pulmonary arteries to the lungs. In summary, there are two circulations, as follows:

1. *Pulmonary:* From the right ventricle to the lungs and back to the left atrium.
2. *Systemic:* From the left ventricle to the aorta, to body tissues and organs, and back to the right atrium.

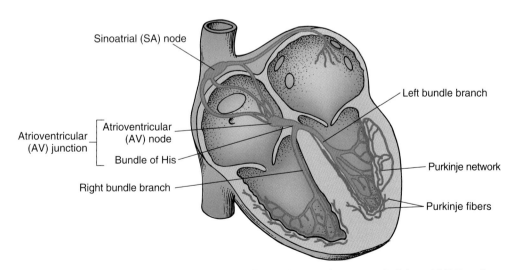

• **Fig. 43.5** Conducting system within the heart. Electrical system is composed of sinoatrial (SA) node; atrioventricular (AV) node and bundle of His at AV junction; left bundle branch; right bundle branch; and Purkinje network of Purkinje fibers.

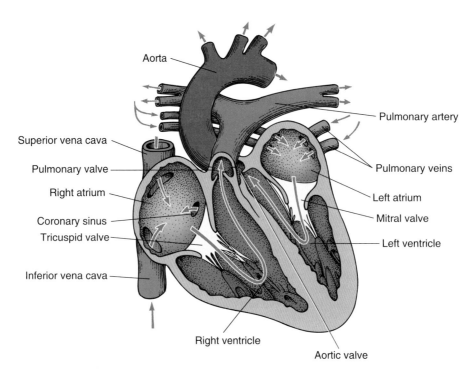

Aorta

Pulmonary artery

Superior vena cava

Pulmonary valve

Right atrium

Coronary sinus

Tricuspid valve

Inferior vena cava

Pulmonary veins

Left atrium

Mitral valve

Left ventricle

Right ventricle

Aortic valve

• **Fig. 43.6** Circulation of blood through heart. Arrows indicate direction of flow from superior vena cava and inferior vena cava into right atrium, through tricuspid valve into right ventricle, and through pulmonary valve into pulmonary artery. Blood flows from pulmonary veins into left atrium, through mitral valve into left ventricle, and through aortic valve into aorta.

Special Features of Cardiac Surgery

Cardiovascular surgery encompasses the spectrum of clinical pathologic processes associated with congenital anomalies and acquired diseases of the circulatory system. The often-complex surgical procedures involving the heart, great vessels, and peripheral blood vessels mandate the need for experienced operating room (OR) teams with special education and training.

The goal of cardiovascular surgeons is to restore or preserve adequate cardiac output and circulation of blood to the brain and tissues throughout the body. Technologic advancements in diagnosis, anesthesia, hemodynamic monitoring, extracorporeal circulation, myocardial preservation, prosthetic devices, and transplantation have made possible the correction of many defects and the treatment of cardiovascular diseases.

Cardiac surgery, more than any other surgical specialty, owes its success to teams of experts in chemistry, biology, immunology, biomedical engineering, and electronics, who work cooperatively with courageous surgeons and cardiologists.

Congenital malformations corrected in infancy or early childhood are discussed in Chapter 8. This chapter focuses on surgical procedures performed for acquired heart diseases in adults. The principles of general and thoracic surgery apply to cardiac surgery, but the following factors require emphasis:

- Extra minutes are not available, and seconds save lives.
- The team concept is of utmost importance. An experienced team working together can handle emergencies expeditiously.
- Comprehensive physical and psychologic preparation of the patient precedes a surgical procedure. Postoperatively the patient is taken to an intensive care unit (ICU). The patient is continuously monitored intraoperatively and postoperatively, including during transport to the ICU.

1. The OR for cardiovascular surgery should be equipped with the following:
   a. Cardiac defibrillator, pacemaker, and intraaortic counterpulsation devices.
   b. Cardioplegia (to induce cardiac arrest) and inotropic (to modify cardiac muscle contractility) drugs, including, but not limited to, the following[1]:
      (1) Calcium channel blockers
      (2) Dopamine (Intropin)
      (3) Dobutamine (Dobutrex)
      (4) Epinephrine (Adrenalin)
      (5) Intravenous (IV) nitroglycerin
      (6) Milrinone (Primacor)
      (7) Cardioplegic solution
   c. Laboratory facilities for blood gas, acid-base balance determinations, potassium, glucose, and hematocrit. Modern analyzers have microprocessors to determine values.
2. The basic thoracic setup is used with the addition of cardiovascular instruments (i.e., various noncrushing vascular and anastomosis clamps, cardiotomy suction tips and sump tubes, and cardiovascular sutures).
3. Prosthetic devices are sterilized by the manufacturer. Care is taken to maintain sterility during placement in the patient. Many types of valves, patches, grafts, and catheters are available. They should be biocompatible, nonthrombogenic, and nonbiodegradable.

   Valves are made of either a bioprosthetic (bovine, porcine, or cadaver) component or metal. Some bioprosthetic valves are preserved with glutaraldehyde. They are rinsed in fresh sterile saline three times to remove the preservative. Some surgeons culture the valve before implantation.

4. Local and/or systemic hypothermia may be used intraoperatively to reduce the body's need for oxygen and to preserve myocardial function. Commercial preparations of sterile slush for local hypothermia are convenient.

5. Intraoperative autotransfusion is often used for blood volume replacement. Blood substitutes such as hetastarch, an albumin substitute for plasma expansion, may be administered. Properly crossmatched blood should be available for transfusion in the event of excessive blood loss. Platelets, stored at room temperature, may be given after CPB to enhance clotting. Often little or no blood is needed for transfusion in many procedures when CPB is used. Also, medications may be infused to protect platelet function during CPB.

6. Closed water-seal drainage or suction drainage is used postoperatively to drain the mediastinum and/or pleural space(s) (Fig. 43.7).

7. Many devices are available for cardiac pacing, ventricular support, and treatment of cardiogenic shock. A portable cardiopulmonary support system, external pulsatile pump, and other devices are used. It is critical that these devices be properly sterilized and handled. Read package labels and inserts for the specific manufacturer's instructions.

The circulating nurse should affix labels and record serial numbers and identifying data in the patient's chart. In the event of a mechanical failure, this information becomes important. Lot numbers are logged according to facility policy and procedure.

8. The scrub person should set up a separate table for assembling devices. Check to be certain that all parts are available and functional. A missing component could be catastrophic.

Commonly Used Incisions for Cardiac Surgery

Several different approaches can be used for entering the chest cavity for cardiac surgery (Fig. 43.8).

Median Sternotomy

For median sternotomy the patient is supine. A median sternotomy incision is used for operations of the heart, ascending aorta, and anterior mediastinal structures, including the thymus and tumors that lie anterior to the heart.

A vertical incision extends through the midline from the suprasternal notch to approximately 2 inches below the xyphoid process (Fig. 43.9). Retrosternal tissue is dissected. The bony sternum is split (divided) with a powered sternal saw. Caution is used to avoid injury to underlying mediastinal structures, especially if the chest has been opened before. The blade has a safety guard to prevent penetration into the mediastinum.

At closure, heavy-gauge stainless steel wires are placed around or through the sternum, tightly pulled together, and twisted (Fig. 43.10). The ends are buried in the sternum. Other nonabsorbable sutures or closure devices may be used to provide firm fixation. The linea alba, subcutaneous tissue, and skin are sutured.

Complications are brachial plexus injury from bed-mounted retractors, costochondral separation caused by retraction, infection, nonunion, and keloid formation.

Paramedian Thoracotomy

An incision is made to either the immediate left or right of the sternum for minimally invasive cardiac procedures. A paramedian incision on the left side also may be used to perform a biopsy of lymph nodes that reside in the aortopulmonary window that cannot be reached with a mediastinoscope or computed

• **Fig. 43.7** Chest tube insertion.

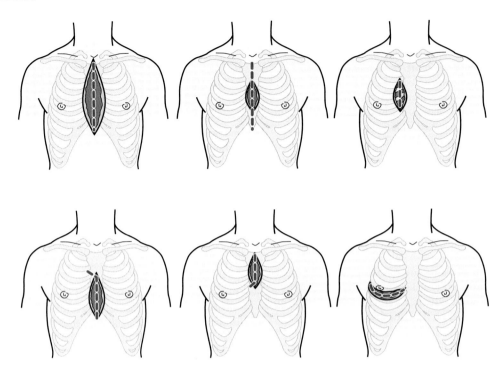

• **Fig. 43.8** Incisional approaches for cardiac surgery.

• **Fig. 43.9** Median sternotomy. (From Waldhausen JA, Pierce WS, Campbell DB, editors: *Surgery of the chest,* ed 6, St. Louis, 1996, Mosby.)

• **Fig. 43.10** Sternal closure with wire.

muscles. The internal mammary arteries and veins are ligated and divided. The sternum is divided horizontally.

At closure, the sternum is reapproximated securely, the ribs are approximated with pericostal sutures, and the remaining tissue layers are closed.

This incision is referred to as a clamshell and is mostly used for bilateral lung transplants. This incision is less commonly used and causes more discomfort for the patient.

Anterolateral or Posterolateral Thoracotomy

Anterolateral or posterolateral incisions may be preferred for some cardiac procedures such as valve procedures. For some procedures involving the posterior aspect of the heart, the thoracotomy incision is made on the right side (opposite side) of the chest.

Invasive Hemodynamic Monitoring

Although placement of invasive pressure monitoring lines is not their responsibility, perioperative nurses must document all access

tomography (CT)-guided percutaneous needle. This approach is the Chamberlain procedure.

Transsternal Bilateral Thoracotomy

A bilateral submammary incision is made with the patient supine for transsternal bilateral thoracotomy. In the midline the incision curves superiorly to cross the sternum at the fourth intercostal space level. Lateral extension is to the midaxillary line. The pleural cavity is entered via the interspace after division of the pectoralis lines and should be aware of the implications of data and the potential for complications, such as thrombus, dysrhythmias, embolus, cardiac arrest, and postoperative infection. For assessment of tissue perfusion, invasive hemodynamic monitoring is used to determine blood pressure in major arteries, veins, and the heart chambers. Indwelling catheter lines are inserted to measure the following:

- Radial and femoral artery pressures
- Central venous pressure (CVP)
- Pulmonary artery pressure. The Swan-Ganz catheter line determines right atrial, right ventricular, and pulmonary capillary wedge pressures of left ventricular function. It is also used to determine cardiac function as it measures cardiac output, index, oxygen saturation of the central venous system, and systemic vascular resistance that, along with pulmonary artery pressures, helps determine whether a patient is hypovolemic, hypervolemic, or euvolemic.

Indwelling intravascular catheters are inserted preoperatively. During a surgical procedure they provide information relative to the effects of anesthetic agents, surgical manipulation of the heart, hypothermia, extracorporeal circulation, induced ischemia, and cardiac arrest. A registered nurse may draw blood samples from the pressure lines at intervals during CPB perfusion for blood gas analysis. Catheter patency is maintained with heparinized flush solutions.

The catheter is flushed with heparinized saline or other recommended solution. Also, an air filter is attached to the end of the pressure tubing as a precaution against fatal air embolism. Every part of the line and filter must be flushed and free of air, or the pressure bag could force a bubble into the left atrium, causing an embolus. In the absence of mitral valve disease, left atrial pressure at the end of atrial diastole, just before the mitral valve opens, indicates left ventricular end-diastolic pressure and therefore left ventricular filling pressure and function.

Postoperatively, hemodynamic monitoring detects dysrhythmias caused by impaired myocardial perfusion, transient reduction in cardiac output with subsequent hypotension, hypovolemia secondary to hemorrhage, and tamponade. Circulating blood volume, pulmonary volume overload leading to pulmonary edema, and reactions to titrated vasopressor drugs also can be identified.

Intraoperative Monitoring

Noninvasive technologies are used intraoperatively to evaluate the effectiveness of some repairs and/or tissue perfusion. These technologies include the following:

- *Transesophageal echocardiography (TEE):* A transesophageal ultrasound probe is used for assessment of graft patency, myocardial perfusion, adequacy of valve replacement, or ventricular function. A Doppler color flow probe also may be useful to quantitatively assess other repairs.
- *Electrophysiologic measurements:* A computerized mapping system is used to identify the focus of dysrhythmias.
- *Near-infrared reflectance spectroscopy:* A device equipped with a sensor is attached to the patient's head. Light transmitted through the skin and skull to the brain is reflected to light detectors in the sensor. Changes in oxygen levels in the brain change light absorption. These changes may alert the anesthesia provider and surgeon to a developing oxygen deficit.

Cardiopulmonary Bypass

CPB is the technique of oxygenating and perfusing blood by means of a mechanical pump-oxygenator system. This apparatus temporarily substitutes for the function of the patient's heart and lungs during cardiac surgery. CPB is used for most intracardiac (open heart) and coronary artery procedures. Venous blood is diverted from the body to the machine for oxygenation (extracorporeal circulation) and is pumped back to the patient (Fig. 43.11).

In preparation for bypass, the patient is systemically heparinized to prevent clot formation within the CPB circuit. Two- or three-stage venous cannulas are inserted into the right atrial appendage and the inferior vena cava.

Venous and arterial cannulation for CPB can be achieved with cannulation of the femoral or subclavian artery and femoral vein. Special arterial cannulas are available for this, and a large-bore chest tube may be used for the femoral venous cannulation.

Bicaval cannulation is done by inserting venous cannulas into the inferior and superior venae cavae. A cannula for return of oxygenated blood to the systemic circulation is placed in the ascending aorta. The femoral or subclavian artery can be used as an alternative site in the presence of an ascending aneurysm, extensive adhesions, or severe calcification of the aorta. Cannulas are connected to the machine by sterile tubing before institution of bypass. During bypass, the lungs are kept deflated and immobilized.

Minimally invasive surgery has given rise to vacuum-assisted venous drainage (VAVD) for the attainment of a bloodless field. This method requires less priming medium for the machine and uses smaller cannulas. VAVD adds negative pressure of 225 to 240 mm Hg to the venous lines for faster decompression of the heart.

The perfusionist who operates the CPB machine must be familiar with its function, care, and operation. The perfusionist may be employed by the cardiac surgeon, a group practice, or the hospital.

Components of a Bypass System

Oxygenator

Oxygen is taken up and carbon dioxide is removed from the blood. The types of oxygenators include the following:

- *Bubble:* Bubbles of oxygen are supplied to the blood by direct blood/gas contact.
- *Membrane:* Oxygen and carbon dioxide diffuse through a permeable Teflon or polyethylene membrane that contains the blood. This method diminishes blood-gas interface. Several types of disposable membrane oxygenators are available.
- *Microporous membrane:* Blood film is separated from ventilating gas by a microporous polypropylene membrane folded like an accordion and operated like a bubble oxygenator. BP in this oxygenator exceeds gas pressure at all times, thus precluding gas bubbles passing through the microporous membrane.

Heat Exchanger

Incorporated in the circuit, a heat exchanger regulates blood temperature. Water at a thermostatically controlled temperature circulates through the exchanger, which can rapidly produce, control, or correct systemic hypothermia. Hypothermia is often used in conjunction with bypass to reduce oxygen demands of tissues and protect the myocardium during arrest.

• **Fig. 43.11** Cardiopulmonary bypass circuit. (From Waldhausen JA, Pierce WS, Campbell DB, editors: *Surgery of the chest,* ed 6, St. Louis, 1996, Mosby.)

Pump

Rollers turning over sterile plastic tubing propel reheated oxygenated blood in a relatively nonpulsatile flow through a blood filter and bubble trap to the arterial cannula for recirculation through the body. The rate of flow can be varied. It is calculated according to patient weight or body surface area. Reduced flow accompanies hypothermia.

Perfusion

Immediately before the surgical procedure, the machine is primed (filled) with a combination of crystalloid and colloid solutions, a balanced electrolyte component, and a cardiopreservative solution including sodium bicarbonate and heparinized plasma volume expander. Some circuits are heparin-coated by the manufacturer.

For a hemodilution technique of priming, the system is filled with fluid that will replace blood diverted to the pump-oxygenator system and is recirculated through the circuit to remove air bubbles. The priming solution should be of sufficient volume and of a suitable hematocrit level so that when mixed with the patient's blood, the resultant buffered plasma will be capable of achieving adequate perfusion and preventing myocardial acidosis. Blood is added as needed to maintain an adequate oxygen-carrying capacity and perfusion rate.

The bypass may be partial or total. In a partial bypass, only a portion of venous return is routed to the pump-oxygenator circuitry; the remaining portion follows the normal systemic circulation. In a total bypass, all venous return is diverted to the machine for total-body perfusion.

Umbilical tapes or silastic vessel loops are placed around the venae cavae and tightened like a tourniquet to ensure complete drainage and a bloodless field when bicaval drainage is used. The heart is arrested when perfusion tubing is secure.

During perfusion, the patient is monitored intensely (i.e., arterial and venous pressures, body and blood temperatures, blood gases and electrolytes, urinary output, and oxygen consumption). General anesthesia may be maintained by an anesthetic vaporizer that adds vapor to the oxygenating mixture or by IV anesthetic.

As the procedure nears completion, the patient is rewarmed to normal body temperature. The cross-clamp is removed from the aorta, and as blood fills the heart the heartbeat is restored. Mechanical ventilation is reestablished, and the patient is gradually weaned from CPB.

After discontinuance of bypass, the cannulas are removed and purse-string sutures around insertion sites are tied. A test dose of protamine sulfate is administered. If the patient is reaction-free, the full dose is continued until the heparin is completely reversed.

CPB may also be used in conjunction with deep hypothermia during neurosurgical procedures, in major organ transplantation, and for pulmonary embolectomy (Trendelenburg operation). It is also used to assist in the event of ventricular failure, to treat some types of pulmonary dysfunctions, and to perfuse an isolated segment of the body for cancer chemotherapy.

De-airing

If an open chamber procedure has been performed, de-airing (venting all the air from inside the heart) of the left ventricle is necessary before the aortic cross-clamp is removed. De-airing is done by placing a needle through the heart muscle into the left ventricle and removing the room air. Failure to remove room air from a heart chamber places the patient at risk for air embolus and possible stroke. Care is taken to include the needle in the final surgical count.

In redo heart procedures, the tip of the heart may be bound to the inner aspect of the chest, preventing adequate de-airing. Carbon dioxide (CO_2) is used to remedy this situation. CO_2 is heavier than room air and is prophylactically infused into the surgical site continuously during the procedure to minimize the need for de-airing by displacing room air in the chambers of the heart. Residual CO_2 is resorbed by the body without consequence to the patient. De-airing is still performed at the conclusion of the bypass procedure when CO_2 is used.

Myocardial Preservation

A bloodless, motionless field allows direct vision of the heart and its interior for repair of coronary circulation or intracardiac defects. CPB isolates the heart while the body is perfused with oxygenated blood. Cardiac arrest is purposely induced. During bypass, the perfusionist is in control of the patient's body temperature, oxygenation, and preservation of the body and brain. The surgeon assumes responsibility for preservation of the heart. Bypass time is kept to a minimum because injury from myocardial ischemia is time related.

Deliberate cardiac arrest may be effected by one or a combination of the following methods:

1. *Aortic cross-clamping:* The aorta is occluded with a vascular clamp proximal to the aortic cannula to block systemic circulation. Ischemic (anoxic) cardiac arrest occurs as the blocked systemic blood within the heart becomes deoxygenated and cardiac metabolic needs are depleted. This technique can be maintained for only a limited period because myocardial damage and necrosis will occur when the oxygen supply and energy required to maintain the subcellular system are depleted. Cerebrospinal fluid pressure may increase.

2. *Cardioplegia:* Most cardiac surgery is based on the use of cardioplegic solutions used alone or in combination with other techniques discussed. These are preparations of a small amount of potassium in crystalloid, blood, or other solution. Cardioplegia is delivered into the aortic root through the coronary ostia or into the coronary sinus through the right atrium.

   - *Antegrade infusion:* A catheter is placed into the coronary ostia via the ascending aorta above the aortic valve and below the aortic cross-clamp (Fig. 43.12). Cardioplegia is infused and flows into the coronary circulation. It is kept out of the left ventricle by a competent aortic valve and systemically by the aortic cross-clamp. Between 500 and 1000 mL of solution at 70 mm Hg pressure is initially used. Additional amounts are administered with each anastomosis. Severe coronary disease may cause uneven doses of cardioplegia and interfere with perfusion.

   - *Retrograde infusion:* A catheter is placed into the coronary sinus through the right atrium (Fig. 43.13). Cardioplegia is infused passively at 100 or 200 mL/min and is delivered to the myocardium by first traversing the venous system of the heart and then into the arterial system of the coronary circulation. This method is used during valve surgery and in bypass surgery when proximal lesions of the coronary arteries prohibit adequate antegrade delivery.

   - Retrograde cardioplegia does not perfuse the right ventricle or the capillary system of the left ventricle as well as antegrade methods. A better continuous flow is attained by placing a venous suction tip near the ostia.

   - When cardioplegic solution is injected into the coronary artery system, hyperkalemia immediately induces complete electromechanical cardiac arrest. The composition and temperature of the solution and infusion techniques can be

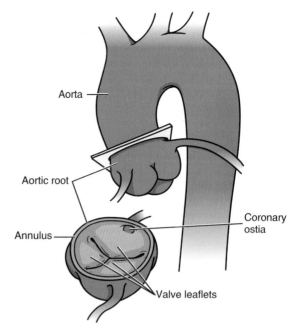

• **Fig. 43.12** Aortic root with coronary ostia of coronary arteries.

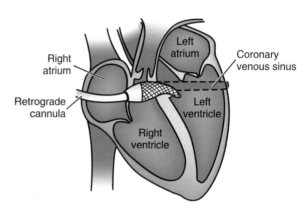

• **Fig. 43.13** Coronary sinus with retrograde cannula in place.

determined for each patient's disease process. Some solutions have a calcium antagonist, such as verapamil or nifedipine, to help prevent myocardial ischemia. Some are infused warm; others are infused cold for less myocardial ischemia. Infusion may be continuous or intermittent. In severe proximal coronary disease it may be necessary to give antegrade and retrograde for even distribution of the solution.

   - Coronary perfusion pressure during administration of the cardioplegic solution may influence regional delivery. When the solution is flushed out of the collateral circulation at the end of the surgical procedure, the heartbeat may resume spontaneously. If not, ventricular fibrillation is treated with countershock.

3. *Hypothermia:* Hypothermia reduces systemic metabolic needs and oxygen requirements. It exerts a protective effect during CPB through a temperature-related decrease of intracellular metabolism, thus allowing tissues to tolerate a prolonged period of decreased perfusion. Hypothermia is an essential component to ischemic myocardial preservation, but because of its calcium-loading effect, cardioplegic arrest precedes initiation of hypothermia.

Local hypothermia can be induced by topical application of iced saline slush around the heart or iced lactated Ringer solution to the heart externally and/or internally. Cardiac arrest also can be induced by deliberately lowering systemic body temperature moderately to 78.8° F to 89.6° F (26–32° C) or deeply to below 78.8° F (26° C). This is achieved by a cooling perfusate in the heart-lung machine.

Complications of Cardiopulmonary Bypass

Although excellent results are obtained with most procedures, significant derangements can occur after CPB. These are most obvious in infants or after prolonged surgical procedures in adults. Alterations in clotting may occur as a result of heparinization of blood, mechanical damage to platelets and clotting factors, and direct exposure of blood to oxygen. If trauma or transfusion reaction hemolyzes red blood cells, viscosity in renal tubules may cause tubular necrosis and renal failure.

Inadequate or extended perfusion and oxygenation may promote tissue anoxia and metabolic acidosis. Fluid and electrolyte balance merits close watching, particularly for hypervolemia. The patient must remain in a euvolemic state to prevent fluid overload. When nonblood fluids are used to prime the pump, they may diffuse into interstitial spaces. As this fluid returns to circulation postoperatively, hypervolemia may result. Furthermore, increased levels of aldosterone and antidiuretic hormone induced by the stress of surgery cause retention of sodium and water. Fluids are restricted for 24 hours postoperatively. Cerebral edema and encephalopathy at times ensue, for unknown reasons. These developments are generally temporary.

Postpump psychosis consists of visual and auditory hallucinations and paranoid delusions. This often terminates when the patient is transferred from the ICU.

The most severe pulmonary complication of extracorporeal circulation is postperfusion lung syndrome. Its cause is unknown. It is often fatal because of the development of atelectasis, pulmonary edema, and hemorrhage. Metabolic acidosis during bypass may lead to low cardiac output syndrome postoperatively. This occurs most frequently in patients with long histories of cardiac disease.

Diagnostic Procedures

Interference in any part of the circulatory system can jeopardize survival. A surgical procedure is preceded by extensive cardiovascular assessment on the basis of noninvasive and invasive studies that dictate subsequent treatment.

Noninvasive Procedures

Routine examination and electrocardiography are augmented by determination of venous pressure, cardiac output, circulation time, and blood chemistry studies. Chest x-ray reveals the heart's size, position, and outline. Screening or functional capacity testing, such as stress testing, is informative. Pulmonary function tests may detect left ventricular failure. Echocardiography with ultrasonic waves reveals the heart structure and gives information pertinent to congenital heart disease and valvular disease.

Invasive Procedures

X-ray visualization after injection of a nontoxic radiopaque substance permits study of the heart chambers, great vessels, and coronary circulation.

Radionuclide Imaging

Radionuclide imaging may be used to detect regional reductions in myocardial blood flow and thus help confirm or deny the diagnosis of myocardial infarction (necrosis of a portion of the myocardium caused by obstruction in a coronary artery). When a patient has "balanced disease," meaning equally blocked throughout all coronary distributions, the radionuclide uptake may be evenly distributed and be questionably interpreted as "normal." The cardiologist will compare all diagnostic findings and determine whether cardiac catheterization is the next step to definitive diagnosis despite a "normal" test.

Calcium scoring is also used to determine coronary lesions. This test measures the amount of calcium present in the coronary arteries and is graded to determine the severity of disease.

Angiography

Angiocardiography with intravascular injection of a radiopaque substance permits x-rays of the heart chambers, thoracic vessels, and coronary arteries. Rapid serial x-rays or motion pictures on an enlarged fluoroscopic screen show the heart's outline and the passage of contrast materials in the great vessels. Selective angiocardiography or coronary angiography is done in association with cardiac catheterization to evaluate coronary artery disease and determine the extent of obstructive disease in the coronary vessels. Aneurysms also may be diagnosed by angiography.

Cardiac Catheterization

Under image intensification fluoroscopy, a sterile catheter is introduced through a cutdown into a brachial vessel in the arm or percutaneously into a femoral vessel in the groin and is passed into the heart or a coronary artery (Fig. 43.14). The procedure permits the following:

- Evaluation of heart function
- Measurements of intracardiac and aortic pressure

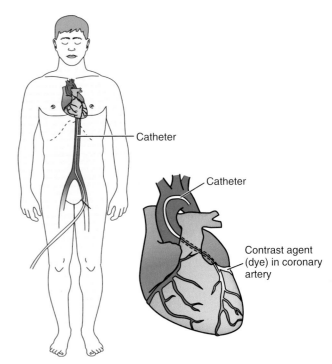

Catheter

Catheter

Contrast agent (dye) in coronary artery

• **Fig. 43.14** Cardiac catheterization through the femoral artery with the injection contrast agent.

- Visualization of the heart chambers
- Calculation of a valve area to determine stenosis

Catheterization is used to diagnose coronary artery disease, valvular heart disease, myocardial disease, or congenital anomalies. It is the ultimate tool for diagnosis of ischemic heart disease.

For study of the coronary arteries, a single catheter is passed and its tip is inserted into the ostia of the arteries for injection of contrast medium and tracing of solution flow. Cinefluorograms record findings. After removal of the catheter, the incision is closed and pressure dressings are applied.

For right-sided heart catheterization, a pulmonary artery catheter is inserted through the vein to obtain pressures in the right atrium and ventricle, pulmonary artery, and pulmonary artery wedge. Measurements of thermodilution, cardiac output, and oxygen saturation also may be obtained. The right internal jugular vein may be cannulated, and a bioptome (a specially designed biopsy forceps) may be advanced to obtain a right endomyocardial biopsy specimen. For left-sided heart catheterization, a catheter is inserted into an artery and advanced through the aortic valve into the left ventricle.

Physiologic monitoring with a multichannel recorder is continuous during the procedure. Potential complications include dysrhythmias, air embolus, thrombosis, and vascular and/or cardiac perforation.

Cardiac Surgical Procedures

The purposes of heart surgery are to correct acquired or congenital anatomic abnormalities, repair or replace defective heart valves, revascularize ischemic myocardium, and improve or assist ventricular function. The hours immediately before the surgical procedure can be a highly stressful period for the patient.

Mental stress can cause myocardial ischemia (inadequate blood supply to the heart) without symptoms of chest pain. Therefore the patient should be monitored from arrival in the OR suite, through induction of anesthesia, and throughout the surgical procedure. Administration of oxygen before induction of anesthesia may be indicated to help reduce stress. Procedures may be performed with or without CPB.

Valvular Heart Disease

Valvular heart disease may arise from a congenital abnormality or can be acquired. Abnormal vibrations or heart murmurs, referred to as S_3 or S_4, may be congenital or the end result of disease such as rheumatic fever or degenerative change.

Valves can become thickened and calcified, resulting in loss of valve substance, narrowing of the orifice, and immobility (Fig. 43.15). They then develop aortic insufficiency, fail to close completely, and permit blood leakage or regurgitation. Failure to open completely is caused by stenosis, which impedes blood flow. A defective valve is reconstructed if possible. If the valve is not repairable or if symptoms return after repair, a prosthetic valve is implanted.

Incisional approaches for valve surgery include median sternotomy, anterolateral thoracotomy, and other modifications of lateral thoracotomy. CPB is used for all valve procedures to create and maintain a bloodless field. Robotic-assisted approaches with the placement of multiple trocars can be performed for select valve replacements such as mitral valve replacement.[2] With the use of high-definition imaging, instrumentation can be maneuvered in tight spaces within a closed chest.

Normal aortic valve

Stenotic aortic valve

Aortic insufficiency

• **Fig. 43.15** Aortic valve disease.

Cardioplegia perfusion and administration can be affected by diseased valves. A continual flow of antegrade cardioplegia is given during aortic valve surgery unless the flow obstructs vision. Cannulation of the ostia can cause ostial stenosis. For mitral valve surgery the antegrade flow is interrupted by the mitral valve retractor and requires the aortic root to be de-aired before the procedure can resume.

Restorative Valve Procedures

Restorative and reparative valve surgery is the preferred procedure for most valve diseases. Reconstruction of the patient's own valve may restore normal valve function. Valvuloplasty and annuloplasty are valve-sparing procedures to maintain structural integrity and ventricular function. In valvuloplasty the leaflets are repaired and calcium deposits removed.

Some surgeons tuck a Raytec into the ventricle under the valve being repaired. Care is taken to account for this sponge and the particulate during the count performed at closure of the heart.

An annuloplasty ring, either flexible or nonflexible, may be used for support and to provide continuity and permanence of repair. Thromboembolism is less of a threat than it is after valve replacement; thus anticoagulant therapy is not indicated postoperatively.

Valve Replacement

A diseased mitral or aortic valve may be excised and replaced. The surgeon selects the most appropriate procedure and approach—repair versus replacement—and then the type and size of prosthesis to be used. Minimally invasive techniques are commonly performed.

Several factors are used to determine repair versus replacement of the valve with a mechanical or bioprosthetic valve. These include, but are not limited to, age, life expectancy, body surface area, contraindication to long-term anticoagulation, pathology of the valve, general health and lifestyle of the patient, and comorbidities.

The appropriate valve replacement prosthesis is nontoxic to the patient's system and has an effective valve area to accommodate the patient's body size. Several types of prosthetic heart valves are available.[3] They may be mechanical or biologic.

Mechanical Valves

One type of mechanical valve has discs resembling leaflets of human valves. The discs of some are tilted. The metal ring at the base of the cage may be covered with polyester fabric to facilitate suturing. It also encourages tissue ingrowth, an aid to long-term fixation.

All mechanical valves require long-term anticoagulation with warfarin (Coumadin) and monitoring of blood levels. Tissue valves may require short-term anticoagulation for 3 to 6 months while endothelialization of the annular ring is being undertaken by the body. Some may elect platelet inhibition with aspirin and a platelet inhibitor of choice. However, all tissue valve recipients will require long-term anticoagulation in the presence of atrial dysrhythmias such as atrial fibrillation and atrial flutter.

Biologic Valves

Biologic valves are made from allograft or xenograft (porcine bioprosthesis or bovine pericardial xenograft) donor material. Cryopreserved fresh aortic valve allografts are carefully thawed before use. Many bioprosthetic valves are preserved with α-oleic acid (AOA), which reduces calcification. If glutaraldehyde storage solution is used, it should be thoroughly rinsed from xenografts with sterile saline before implantation.

Mitral Valve Replacement

Open mitral valve surgery is accomplished through either a medial sternotomy or right thoracotomy. Whichever is used, the pericardium is entered and venous CPB cannulas are placed in the inferior and superior venae cavae. This keeps the surgical site free of blood from the CPB. However, during cardioplegia instillation, blood may inadvertently enter the field. Suction should remain handy.

The atrium is opened and the mitral valve is exposed, inspected, and removed by the circumferential excision and severance of muscular attachments to the ventricular wall. The surgeon usually leaves the annulus, chordae tendineae, and papillary muscles intact. Once the valve has been sized by the surgeon and an appropriate valve placed on the field, interrupted nonabsorbable sutures are placed all along the annulus in alternating colors, commonly blue and white. Teflon felt pledgets are commonly used as a buttress under the sutures to prevent the annulus from tearing when the prosthetic valve is seated and the sutures are tied.

Once all sutures have been placed, the valve is lowered into the space formerly occupied by the diseased valve and the sutures are tied (Fig. 43.16). After the newly implanted valve has been inspected and its proper functioning ensured, the atrium is closed while blood is allowed to fill the heart, displacing the room air. This begins the de-airing process.

Temporary pacing wires may be placed on the epicardium of the right ventricle and atrium. These are brought out through the

• **Fig. 43.16** Suturing the annulus of the valve.

skin and may be attached to an external pulse generator in the event bradycardia or other dysrhythmia requiring pacing is encountered during the immediate postoperative course. These are easily removed with gentle traction when deemed appropriate by the surgeon.

Aortic Valve Replacement

The surgical procedure for aortic valve replacement is basically the same as that described for mitral valve replacement except that the aortic valve is exposed through a transverse incision in the aorta. The surgical site can be kept free from blood by placing a plastic suction tube into a pulmonary vein and directed backward into the left atrium, across the mitral valve, and into the left ventricle.

Either a mechanical valve or bioprosthesis may be used. Biologic prostheses offer the advantage of a low embolic rate and obviate the need for prolonged anticoagulation therapy. Cryopreserved fresh aortic valve allograft, from either a donor bank or commercially available allograft, may be preferred. The aortic valve may be replaced with the patient's own pulmonary valve (i.e., an autograft known as the Ross procedure).

Transcatheter Aortic Valve Replacement

Many high-risk patients with severe aortic stenosis are not candidates for traditional open heart surgery.[4] A transcatheter aortic valve replacement (TAVR) may be their only option for improving valve function. TAVR is performed under fluoroscopy, using a compressed biologic valve that is introduced via catheter into the stenotic aortic valve. Once in position, a balloon is expanded to secure and deploy the valve.[4] There are three approaches, depending on what is best for the patient.

Transfemoral

The valve is introduced via the femoral artery.

Transapical

A small right thoracotomy is made, and the valve is introduced through the apex of the heart.

Transaortic

A mini-sternotomy is made, and the ascending aorta is exposed. The valve is introduced through an aortotomy in the ascending aorta.

Percutaneous Transluminal Balloon Valvuloplasty

An interventional cardiac catheterization procedure, balloon valvuloplasty may be an option to treat valvular stenosis in a high-risk patient who cannot tolerate valve replacement. A catheter with a deflated balloon is inserted under fluoroscopy across a stenosed aortic, pulmonary, tricuspid, or mitral valve. The balloon is repeatedly inflated until the valve is opened.

Coronary Artery Disease

Coronary arteries supplying the myocardium may become stenosed or obstructed, which is referred to as occlusive coronary artery disease or ischemic heart disease. Resultant myocardial ischemia may result in angina or myocardial infarction. Occlusive disease of the coronary arteries characteristically affects vessels in their proximal segments and at the origin of major branches. Significant obstructions can occur in one or all of the coronary arteries simultaneously.

The coronary circulation has four major arteries. The left main coronary artery is the shortest and gives rise to the left anterior descending (LAD) and circumflex (CX) coronary arteries. The right coronary artery (RCA) is the other major coronary artery. The RCA, LAD, and CX arteries also can have major branches arising from them. Revascularization to improve blood supply to the myocardium is possible by surgical intervention in selected patients.

Coronary Artery Bypass Graft

For coronary artery bypass grafting (CABG), single or multiple arterial bypasses are done, depending on the number of vessels affected and the degree of obstruction present. The internal mammary (thoracic) artery is the preferred vascular conduit in most patients. Segments of greater saphenous and lesser saphenous veins also are used to bypass coronary artery obstruction. The gastroepiploic, inferior epigastric, and radial arteries also may be used as free grafts. Because the patency rates of cryopreserved saphenous vein and umbilical vein allografts are poor, they are used when no other conduit of choice is available.

The chest is opened by median sternotomy or some other thoracotomy incision for minimal access, and the pericardium is incised. CPB may be used. Most cardiac surgeons wear loupes for magnification while constructing an anastomosis between the graft and the coronary artery. Techniques are influenced by the surgeon's preferred procedure and the extent of grafting.

After the conduit or graft is anastomosed, CPB is discontinued (if used); all incisions are closed and checked for leaks. The pericardium may be left open. The patient is hemodynamically stabilized. The wound is closed in the usual manner for sternotomy with closed water-seal chest drainage.

Off-pump CABG procedures are becoming increasingly popular. The use of a stabilizing retractor assists the surgeon by creating a still area at the site of the distal anastomosis (Fig. 43.17). The use of a CO_2 and saline mister-blower helps keep the anastomosis site clear of blood for enhanced vision. Temporary miniature penetrating "bulldog"-style clamps can be inserted into the myocardium and used to occlude the artery by gentle, even compression.

Once the anastomosis is completed, the stabilizer and bulldog clamps are removed and relocated to the next vessel. The heart is closely monitored for ischemia. CPB is instituted as an emergency measure via the femoral artery and vein if the heart tissue fails to

• **Fig. 43.17** Stabilizing retractor for "off-pump" cardiac procedures.

perfuse adequately during the procedure. This approach to coronary artery bypass is especially useful in patients with a calcified ascending aorta where cross-clamping would be contraindicated.

Internal Mammary Artery Conduit

The chest has right and left internal mammary arteries (IMAs). Because of the potential for a long-term patency rate, at least one IMA can be used as a conduit for myocardial revascularization when the proximal stenosis is greater than 70%. The right IMA will reach the RCA. The left IMA can be used for revascularization of the LAD but can also reach the diagonal vessel (branch of LAD) and the circumflex. Segments of either right, left, or both IMAs also are used as free grafts to bypass other diseased coronary arteries.

The IMA may become occluded and threadlike caused by what is termed *competitive flow*, when the intact artery senses an equalized flow in minimally occluded vessels. A significant proximal lesion must be present for the patient to reap the benefits of the IMA conduit. If the chest is reopened at a later date, care is taken not to transect the IMA.

The left IMA is dissected up to its origin (termed *taken down*) from the subclavian artery, freeing it from the retrosternal aspect of the chest wall (Fig. 43.18). A small amount of tissue is left around the circumference of the artery. After mobilization, the pericardium is notched or opened to minimize tension and distance to the diseased coronary artery. The goal is to prevent tension on the anastomosis, which can cause stenosis or possibly occlusion. Side-to-side or end-to-side anastomosis is performed primarily between IMA and the LAD coronary artery, distal to the obstruction (Fig. 43.19).

Saphenous Vein Conduit

The procedure for a saphenous vein bypass graft is expedited by two teams: one harvests the greater and lesser saphenous veins for use as conduit, and the other opens the chest and prepares for CPB. Methods for saphenous procurement include the open

• **Fig. 43.18** Internal mammary artery procurement using mounted self-retaining retractor. (Courtesy Rultract, Inc., Cleveland, OH.)

• **Fig. 43.19** End-to-side anastomosis of the internal mammary artery to a diseased coronary artery.

• **Fig. 43.20** Open saphenous vein procurement. (From Waldhausen JA, Pierce WS, Campbell DB, editors: *Surgery of the chest,* ed 6, St. Louis, 1996, Mosby.)

• **Fig. 43.21** Endoscopic saphenous vein procurement.

method (Fig. 43.20) and the endoscopic approach (Fig. 43.21). An adequate length of vein is removed to obtain sufficient graft material. The distal end of each vein segment is identified, and the graft is placed in heparinized normal saline solution after it has been harvested. It is handled gently to avoid trauma to the intima.

The vein is reversed to permit a normal direction of blood flow through the venous valves into the coronary artery.

The affected coronary artery is opened distal to the obstruction; the proximal end of the saphenous vein is anastomosed end to side to the artery, creating the distal anastomosis, thus bypassing the obstruction. Usually a fine 6-0 or 7-0 monofilament nonabsorbable suture is used. The proximal anastomosis is established by creating a small opening in the aorta with a punch and suturing the distal end of the vein to the aperture (Fig. 43.22).

Saphenous or other vein or artery bypass grafts are completed before the IMA is anastomosed to form a vascular conduit.

• **Fig. 43.22** Aortic punch.

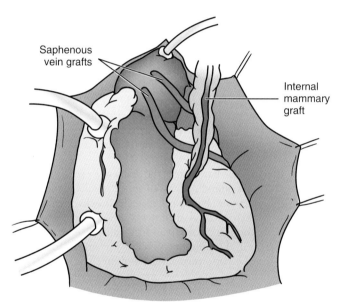

Saphenous
vein grafts

Internal
mammary
graft

• **Fig. 43.23** Triple conduit bypass. Two saphenous vein grafts with the left internal mammary arterial graft.

Manipulation of the heart could stress the arterial anastomosis of the IMA (Fig. 43.23).

Radial Artery Conduit

An arterial conduit is preferred for most patients because the patency rate remains higher for a longer period. The radial artery can be harvested either via a single incision or endoscopically. The radial artery arises 1 cm distal to the brachial artery and terminates at the distal aspect in the palmar artery. The harvested segment may measure between 4.7 and 9.9 inches (12–25 cm). The end diameters measure between 3 and 5 mm. The procured segment is usually taken from the patient's nondominant hand.

In patients undergoing bypass with radial artery conduit harvest, an Allen test or other test deemed appropriate by the surgeon

must be undertaken to ensure adequate perfusion of the hand via the ulnar artery.

Although surgical practices vary, a calcium channel blocker is administered preoperatively to avoid vasospasm of the radial artery during procurement. This is usually continued IV through post-operative day 1, when the patient can be switched to an oral form. Many types of calcium channel blockers are available for use (verapamil [Calan], diltiazem [Cardizem], amlodipine [Norvasc]) or combination calcium channel blocker and angiotensin-converting enzyme (ACE) inhibitor medications may be used (benazepril [Lotrel]).

Coronary Artery Angioplasty

Restoration of perfusion from the left coronary system is possible by direct enlargement of the left main coronary artery lumen in select patients in whom clinical circumstances preclude bypass grafting. A curved incision is made in the lateral aortic wall. Either the posterior or anterior aspect of the left main coronary artery is incised across the stenosis. An autologous onlay pericardial or onlay saphenous vein patch is sutured between the artery and the aortic wall.

Endarterectomy (removal of an organized thrombus and attached endothelium or atherosclerotic fatty plaques from the arterial wall) may be performed in conjunction with left coronary angioplasty or right CABG. Small spatulas, wire loops, miniature abrasive drills, or ultrasonic devices may be used to remove plaque.

Coronary artery angioplasty procedures usually are performed in the cardiac catheterization laboratory (cath lab) or special interventional procedures room in the radiology department. A standby OR team should be available for emergency coronary artery bypass in the event that acute coronary artery obstruction or perforation occurs.

Percutaneous Transluminal Coronary Angioplasty

Percutaneous transluminal coronary angioplasty (PTCA) is performed under fluoroscopy with image intensification. Balloon dilation of the coronary arteries may be the procedure of choice for select patients with significant atherosclerotic narrowing in a major coronary artery (Fig. 43.24). The coronary arteries are approached by either percutaneous femoral artery entry or brachial artery cutdown. A balloon-tipped catheter is passed through a guiding catheter into the area of the coronary artery with atherosclerotic material (plaque). The balloon is inflated with a saline-based contrast medium using a syringe or hydraulic pump. The expanded balloon compresses the plaque against the arterial lining and dilates the arterial wall, thus enlarging the lumen.

During the time the balloon is inflated, normal flow of oxygen supplied by the artery to the myocardium is interrupted. Oxygenation distal to the balloon may be maintained with oxygenated perfluorochemical emulsion (Fluosol) flowing through the catheter.

Catheters with ultrasonic devices or tiny drill heads may be used to pulverize atherosclerotic plaque before balloon dilation. Other procedures may be performed as an alternative to or in conjunction with balloon angioplasty.

Laser Angioplasty

An argon laser probe, a neodymium:yttrium-aluminum-garnet (Nd:YAG) optical fiber, or a pulsed excimer laser may be used for laser angioplasty. An integrated system combines direct laser energy and fiberoptics with a balloon angioplasty catheter. The

Diseased artery

Balloon catheter positioned in stenotic area

Inflated balloon presses plaque against arterial wall

Balloon is deflated and blood flow is reestablished

• **Fig. 43.24** Balloon angioplasty. (From Canobbio MM: *Cardiovascular disorders,* St. Louis, 1990, Mosby.)

catheter positions the laser fiber, which then vaporizes the plaque or thrombus obstructing the coronary vessels.

Intracoronary Stent

A stent may be inserted to act as a buttress to keep an artery open. The coronary artery to be stented should be at least 3 mm in diameter. The stent, which is permanently implanted at the site of the stenosis, widens the arterial lumen by compressing atherosclerotic plaque against the arterial wall. The stainless steel mesh or springlike coil stent is tightly wrapped around a balloon catheter. As the balloon is inflated, the stent expands. After the balloon is deflated and removed, the stent remains in place to provide structural support and keep the artery from collapsing.

Transmyocardial Revascularization

The myocardium can be revascularized with the creation of a series of channels in an ischemic area of the left ventricle. This procedure is performed through a left thoracotomy incision without the use of CPB. Using a CO_2 or holmium:yttrium-aluminum-garnet (Ho:YAG) laser, three to five channels are placed in the distal segment of the left ventricle. Hemostasis is

usually established within 45 to 60 seconds. This procedure is used when other conventional therapies cannot be used.

Cardiac Dysrhythmias

Some cardiac rhythm disorders are unresponsive to drug therapy. Normally the electrical cardiac impulse begins at the SA node, thus controlling the rhythm of the heart rate. Fibers from the SA node conduct the impulse through the atria into the AV node and then transmit it along the bundle of His into the ventricles, ending in Purkinje fibers.

Occasionally some other part of the heart develops a rhythmic discharge with a rate more rapid than the SA node. This causes tachycardia (a rapid heartbeat). The impulse also may repeatedly reenter the system, most often at the AV node—bundle of His junction (AV junction), causing overstimulation of the heart.

With epicardial and endocardial mapping techniques, the surgeon is able to pinpoint electrical activity causing dysrhythmia. Preoperatively the mapping procedure is done under fluoroscopy. Electrical impulses from electrode catheters, placed in the heart via a femoral vein, activate sites in the heart to reproduce the abnormal rhythm and obtain a direct electrocardiogram. Premature cycles, the origin of electrical signals, and accessory pathways can be pinpointed.

Intraoperative mapping may be needed to correlate preoperative studies or to identify other sites or pathways masked by antidysrhythmia drugs. The origin and site of a dysrhythmia determine the surgical procedure.[5]

Atrial fibrillation (AF) is one of the most common cardiac dysrhythmias, particularly in patients 50 to 60 years of age. Following cardiac surgery, about 30% of patients will convert to this rhythm. Patients with AF are at very high risk for stroke caused by an embolus, congestive heart failure, cardiomyopathy, and death.

Drug therapy is based on the patient's condition, but commonly includes quinidine, procainamide, sotalol, amiodarone, dofetilide, propafenone, beta-blockers, calcium channel blockers, and digoxin. When medical treatments are no longer effective, surgical intervention is necessary. Most patients have left-sided initiating foci near the pulmonary veins, but any of these procedures also can be performed for atrial flutter that is caused by right-sided initiating foci. Ablative treatment near the pulmonary veins causes the risk for pulmonary vein stenosis.

Maze Procedure

The maze procedure, named for the puzzle-like pattern appearance of the incisions introduced by James Cox in 1987, is a cure for AF by interrupting the impulses that cause the dysrhythmias and preserves the contractility of the atria. The procedure requires CPB because both atria are opened and a series of small incisions are made to interrupt the electrical pathways.

The scar tissue that forms as a result of the procedure causes the interruption in the pathways. A mitral valvuloplasty is done in conjunction with the maze procedure to improve cardiac performance.

This method has significant success rates for restoring regular sinus rhythm without the use of a pacemaker. Research is being done to develop a minimal access procedure that would not require CPB using saline and epicardially applied bipolar radiofrequency energy. Patients may experience difficulty in increasing their heart rate on exertion and the potential for prolonged conduction, leading to ineffective left atrial contraction.

Maze III Procedure

The maze III procedure incorporates similar techniques to the original maze procedure but requires the removal of both atrial appendages, isolation of the pulmonary veins, and application of cryoablation. Minimally invasive procedures are under development.

Mini Maze Procedure

The mini maze procedure uses high-radiofrequency ablation. It is similar to the maze III in that it requires isolation of the pulmonary veins altogether or in pairs in conjunction with ablation from the pulmonary veins to the annulus of the mitral valve. This is done without CPB and is highly successful in patients who experience intermittent atrial fibrillation and to a lesser extent in patients with chronic atrial fibrillation.

Radiofrequency Ablation

This treatment for AF involves the use of a surgical probe that creates a series of linear lesions. These lesions encircle the four pulmonary veins and left atrial appendage. The generator supplies temperature-controlled radiofrequency. The surgeon controls the power output.

Cryoablation

This procedure is used to treat the same dysrhythmias as radiofrequency ablation but uses a refrigerant to freeze the affected area to −112° F (−80° C). The maze III procedure can be modified to incorporate cryoablation that requires less aortic clamp time and decreased chest tube drainage postoperatively. A mitral valve procedure is performed in conjunction if necessary.

Ventricular Aneurysm

Atherosclerotic coronary disease predisposes an individual to myocardial infarction. Ventricular aneurysm (a segmental dilation of the ventricular wall) may develop any time from a few weeks to years after infarction. Predominantly occurring in the left ventricular wall, the aneurysm results from ventricular force on an area of nonfunctioning scar tissue.

The thin-walled fibrous aneurysm often contains clots within it. A left ventricular aneurysm usually produces hemodynamic instability manifested by congestive heart failure and ventricular dysrhythmia. The surgeon can excise the aneurysm and reconstruct the ventricle (Fig. 43.25).

The chest is opened by median sternotomy. CPB is established before the adhesion between the aneurysm and pericardium is detached. The ascending aorta is cross-clamped. The aneurysmal sac is opened with a vertical incision, and the area is cleared of thrombus. Fibrotic myocardium is excised circumferentially. Strips of Teflon felt are used as pledgets to prevent tearing of the suture through the ventricle (Fig. 43.26). Before completion of closure, air is removed from the ventricle by suction. The heartbeat is restored, decannulation is performed, and all incisions are closed.

Aneurysmectomy may be done as a single procedure or in conjunction with cardiomyoplasty, valve replacement, coronary artery bypass, or endocardial resection.

Modified Endoventricular Circular Patch Plasty (Dor Procedure)

Reconstructive surgery of the transmural anterior ventricular wall with a circular patch plasty was introduced by French surgeon Vincent Dor in 1984. This two-layer closure method uses a purse-string suture in the viable inner layer of the myocardium around a scarred aneurysm to minimize the dead area. The dead tissue is excised, and the purse-string is closed to restore the geometry of the ventricle.

Any remaining defect larger than 1.2 inches (3 cm) can be patched with Dacron. The remaining edges are closed with an interrupted mattress stitch over the outside of the patch with pledgeted nonabsorbable sutures to make it more stable. The result is a more normal left ventricular shape and size.

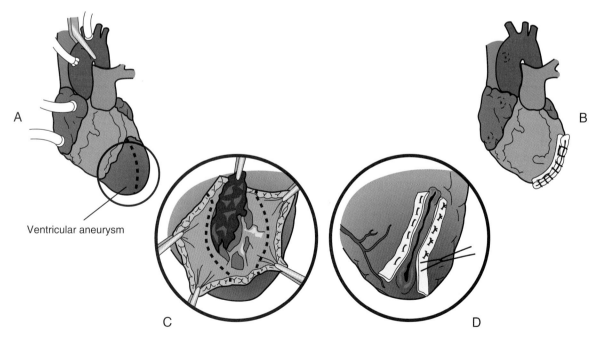

• **Fig. 43.25** Ventricular aneurysm repair. **A,** Aneurysmal sac is incised. **B,** Clot and excess tissue are removed. The circumscribed area is reinforced with suture. **C,** The edges of the trimmed myocardium are approximated and sutured with felt pledgeted suture bolsters. **D,** The closed myocardium is shown with felt pledgets left in place.

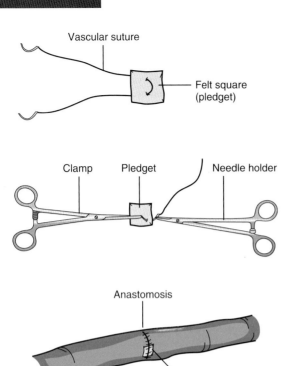

• **Fig. 43.26** Pledgeted suture preparation.

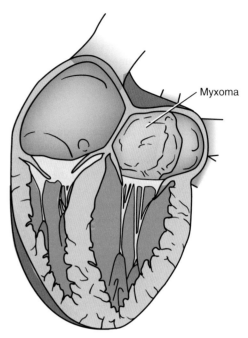

• **Fig. 43.27** Myxoma: primary cardiac tumor.

Septal Myectomy

Patients with hypertrophic cardiomyopathy have a thickened septal wall that impedes the outflow tract between the left ventricle and aortic valve. Surgical intervention is needed when medications are no longer effective. A median sternotomy is made, the pericardium is opened, and the heart is prepared for cannulation. After CPB is initiated and cardioplegia given, an incision is made in the ascending aorta. The septal wall can be accessed through the aortic valve. Portions of the septal wall are excised and carefully measured and weighed to confirm the amount of muscle removed. The aorta is then closed with nonabsorbable sutures. No sutures are needed within the ventricle because the endocardium will heal on its own. In many of these cases, the mitral valve needs repair or replacement, which will be done in conjunction with the myectomy.

Atrial Myxoma

Atrial myxoma is a primary cardiac tumor resembling a "cluster of grapes" that usually extends from the endocardium inside the atrium via a pedunculated stalk (Fig. 43.27). Myxomas are benign and most commonly found in the right atrium but can occur in the left atrium as well as simultaneously in both atria. These benign lesions are dangerous because of their embolic potential and possibility of decreasing the cardiac efficiency. Portions of the myxoma can become dislodged and embolize. If an embolus enters the left atrium, it can lead to a stroke or acute arterial ischemia of a limb or organ.

A myxoma can become enlarged and prolapse into the ventricle, causing incompetence of the tricuspid or mitral valve and leading to heart failure. Removal of a myxoma requires CPB. The entire pedicle stalk must be removed to prevent regrowth.

Cardiac Transplantation

Cardiac transplantation may be an acceptable option for the patient with limited life expectancy who is incapacitated by end-stage myocardial disease secondary to the following:

- Valvular disease with cardiomyopathy
- Coronary artery disease
- Ischemic cardiomyopathy
- Post—myocardial aneurysm
- Idiopathic cardiomyopathy
- Congenital heart disease
- Cardiac tumor

Cardiac transplantation is discussed further in Chapter 45.

Mechanical Assist Devices

Mechanical assist devices may be indicated for patients with cardiac dysfunction. These devices may be implanted in conjunction with other cardiac surgical procedures or to provide long-term assistance for life-sustaining cardiac function.

Cardiac Pacemaker

The conducting system of the heart may be altered or interrupted at any point by degenerative disease, drugs, or surgical trauma. This may cause syncope, diminished cardiac output, hypotension, dysrhythmias, partial or complete heart block, or sinus bradycardia (sick sinus syndrome). Patients with these conditions may be treated by artificial pacing (i.e., delivery of an electrical impulse by a pacemaker) to correct atrial and ventricular dysrhythmias and interrupt chronic atrial fibrillation.[6]

A pacemaker usually consists of a pulse generator, which produces electrical impulses, and leads to carry impulses to stimulating electrodes placed in contact with the heart (Fig. 43.28). A pacing system includes electromyocardial conduction.

Effective external pacing for ventricular standstill led to the development of partially implanted electrode leads connected to an external stimulator for long-term pacing for other conditions. Fully implantable pacemaker systems for long-term use have been available since 1960. An implantable microprocessor generator is hermetically sealed in a metallic container impermeable to body fluids.

Selection of a system depends on the specific pacing requirements of the individual patient. Pacemakers may be temporary or permanent. Endocardial (transvenous) or epicardial (myocardial) electrode leads may be used. Most of these units are programmable to alter pacing function.

Temporary pacing is often necessary before and during permanent-system implantation. Systemic complete heart block and sinus bradycardia are the most frequent indications for permanent-system implantation. A single-chamber ventricular pacemaker may be implanted. The dual-chamber pacemaker is commonly programmed in the DDD mode (Table 43.1). DDD mode senses and synchronously paces both chambers and triggers or inhibits the response to vary the ventricular rate with the atrial rate. Permanent pacing may be initiated by the following devices.

Endocardial Pacemaker

A transvenous electrode lead is placed in the endocardium and attached to a pulse generator. With the patient under local anesthesia, an incision is made just beneath the clavicle or in the deltopectoral groove, preferably on the side of the chest opposite the patient's dominant hand. The subcutaneous tissue is opened to underlying fascia to create a pocket for the pulse generator.

The lead may be inserted through the cephalic, subclavian, or internal or external jugular vein. Under fluoroscopy, the endocardial electrodes (leads) are advanced via the superior vena cava into the apex of the right ventricle. The leads are attached to the endocardium by one of two ways—passive or active fixation.

In passive fixation, the pacemaking electrode tip has small flexible plastic tines that become attached to the trabeculae of the right ventricle. The endocardium will overgrow these leads, causing a firm attachment.

The electrode used during active fixation has a small threaded tip that is deployed into the endocardium by the surgeon. Atrial leads are directed into the right atrial appendage. The lead is

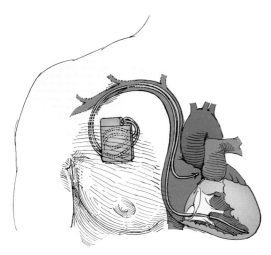

• **Fig. 43.28** Cardiac pacemaker. (From Waldhausen JA, Pierce WS, Campbell DB, editors: *Surgery of the chest,* ed 6, St. Louis, 1996, Mosby.)

Lithium batteries supply power for 5 to 10 years to the microprocessor of the pulse generator. Platinum alloy or stainless steel electrodes, with leads encased in plastic, may be unipolar or bipolar. Components with nickel alloy can cause reactions in allergic patients. With bipolar systems, electric current flows between two electrodes during pacing; it flows between the electrode tip and the pulse generator in unipolar systems. There are three varieties of pacemakers: (1) single chamber with leads to the right ventricle, (2) dual chamber with leads to the right atrium and right ventricle, and (3) biventricular with leads to the right atrium, right ventricle, and the coronary sinus.

A pacemaker may be either a standby ventricular demand type or a physiologic type. Both types are intermittent and noncompetitive with the patient's own pacing system. They monitor the heart's normal activity. The impulse to stimulate the heart is not emitted unless the rate of the heartbeat falls below a preset level. Also known as the R wave—inhibited or QRS-inhibited pacemaker, electrodes of the ventricular demand pacemaker are placed in the ventricle. Stimulating electrodes are placed in the atrium or ventricle, or both, depending on the type of physiologic pacemaker to be used.

TABLE 43.1 Identification Code for Cardiac Pacemakers[a]

First Letter (Chamber Paced)	Second Letter (Chamber Sensed)	Third Letter (Mode of Response to Sensing of Patient's Heart Rate)	Fourth Letter (Programmable Functions)	Fifth Letter (Tachyarrhythmia Function)
A = Atrium	A = Atrium	I = Inhibited response	P = Programmable rate and output only	N = Normal rate
V = Ventricle	V = Ventricle	T = Triggered response	M = Multiprogrammable	B = Bursts
D = Dual/both chambers	D = Dual/both chambers O = No sensing	D = Dual function/inhibited and triggered response R = Reverse response O = No response	C = Communicating noninvasive program O = Nonprogrammable	S = Scanning E = External

[a]Sequence of letters describes parameters and functions.

connected to the pulse generator, which in turn is placed into a previously prepared subcutaneous pocket. The incision is primarily closed with or without suction drainage.

Epicardial Electrodes

With the patient under general anesthesia, epicardial electrodes are placed via a transthoracic approach to the myocardium. For an extrapleural parasternal approach, the pericardium is entered by subperichondrial resection of the fifth costal cartilage. Two sew-on or screw-in type electrodes are implanted 1 cm apart in the myocardium of the right or left ventricle and/or atrium.

After the pacing thresholds are measured from an external source, electrode leads are tunneled under the costal margin to the pulse generator implanted in a subcutaneous pocket in the left upper quadrant of the abdominal wall. Water-seal chest drainage is necessary only if the pleura were entered.

Precautions With Pacemakers

A trauma or emergency patient may arrive in the OR with a pacemaker in place. A chest x-ray should be done to determine whether the leads are intact. If the manufacturer of the pacemaker is unknown, most have a marker that is visible on x-ray to provide the company name. If the function of the pacemaker is questionable, blood work should be done and a complete medication history taken. Some cardiac drugs and electrolyte imbalance can interfere with contractility. A special magnet can be positioned over the pacer pocket to cause the device to default at 60 to 80 beats/min in a fixed synchronous pattern. If the patient goes into cardiac arrest, the defibrillator pads should not be placed over the pacemaker pocket. The pads should be positioned on the anterior and posterior chest.

Use of a monopolar electrosurgical unit (ESU) is usually avoided during placement of a pacemaker or when a surgical procedure is performed on a patient with a pacemaker. Electromagnetic interference may affect the pulse generator, depending on the type of pacemaker. If it is necessary to use a monopolar ESU, the current should be kept as far away from the pulse generator as possible. The return electrode should be placed on the thigh area, not near the chest. Bipolar ESU may be a safer alternative because the current does not pass through the patient's body to a return electrode.

A pacing system analyzer measures the amount of energy in milliamperes (mA) needed to stimulate the heart. It is used to locate the area of the myocardium where the least amount of energy will be needed (generally 0.4–0.8 mA) and to test functioning of the electrode and pulse generator before placement. Telemetric communication capabilities of some pacemakers allow the surgeon to obtain direct evidence of battery output.

The patient with a pacemaker requires adequate follow-up care. An identification card containing the serial number, model, rate, manufacturer's name, and date of insertion should be carried with the patient. The circulating nurse records this information in the patient's medical record, along with the time of insertion. Patients with demand or radiofrequency units should be warned to avoid proximity to electromagnetic devices, such as magnetic resonance imaging (MRI) machines, because magnetic interference will interfere with the pacemaker function.

Battery depletion is the most common indication for replacement of the pulse generator. The old generator is removed from the subcutaneous pocket. A new one is connected to the electrode and inserted into the pocket. Occasionally, electrode problems

and/or erosion of or infection around the generator require surgical intervention.

Cardioverter-Defibrillator

The automatic implantable cardioverter-defibrillator (ICD) has the capability of recognizing potential life-threatening episodes of ventricular tachycardia or fibrillation. The system has a pair of sensing electrodes to monitor changes in the heart rate, cycle length, and waveform (Fig. 43.29). After the onset of ventricular tachycardia, two defibrillating electrodes deliver a synchronized shock to terminate it. The electrical conduction pattern of the heart is converted to a more normal pattern.

Newer models are capable of pacing, as well as defibrillating. Supplied sterile, the pulse generator of the device is powered by lithium batteries hermetically sealed in a titanium case. The device may be implanted in addition to endocardial resection or other ablation or instead of a surgical procedure for dysrhythmia. Placement of this device is similar to procedures described for implantation of cardiac pacemakers. If the ICD malfunctions and delivers more shocks than necessary, a magnet can be placed over the unit to stop the discharges without interrupting the pacing activity.

The wavelength of the ESU or magnetic field of MRI can deprogram the ICD and cause the device to discharge aberrant electric current into the myocardium. A specialized electromagnetic wand can be placed over the chest to deactivate the device for subsequent surgical procedures requiring the use of electrosurgery. The same electromagnetic wand can be used to reactivate and reprogram the ICD. ICDs are not affected by household appliances, such as microwave ovens, computer terminals, or television sets.

Intraaortic Balloon Pump

An intraaortic balloon pump (IABP) is a left ventricular supportive device used to assist a patient with prolonged myocardial ischemia, reversible left ventricular failure, or cardiogenic shock.

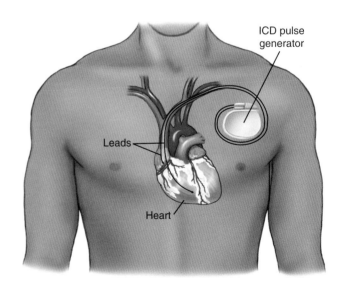

• **Fig. 43.29** Implantable defibrillator. (Modified from Goldberger A: *Clinical electrocardiography: a simplified approach,* ed 7, Mosby, St. Louis, 2006.)

The IABP can be inserted in the OR in conjunction with an open-heart procedure for circulatory support during weaning from CPB. Because the IABP can be inserted percutaneously via the femoral artery, it can be inserted in an interventional area such as the cardiac catheterization laboratory or the ICU when necessary. An IABP reduces left ventricular workload and increases delivery of oxygen to the myocardium, thereby increasing cardiac output and systemic perfusion. An IABP cannot be effective without partial ventricular function.

The cylindrical balloon is inserted into the descending thoracic aorta, just below the left subclavian artery, by way of a femoral artery (Fig. 43.30). The balloon catheter may be inserted percutaneously or by direct vision, or it can be inserted via a prosthetic arterial graft anastomosed end to side to the femoral artery. After insertion, the balloon catheter is connected to a pump console.

The IABP uses principles of counterpulsation. In contrast with systemic arteries, coronary arteries are constricted during systole and fill during diastole. Therefore inflating the balloon during diastole increases coronary perfusion, aiding contractility and oxygen transport. When the balloon is inflated, the blood volume displaced increases coronary artery pressure. When the balloon deflates during systole, the resistance against which the ventricle pumps is decreased. Balloons vary in size to provide 20, 30, or 40 mL of volume displacement, thus giving a maximum assist without total aortic occlusion. When the balloon is placed and the position is verified by chest x-ray, the complete system is vented of air and filled with either helium or carbon dioxide for balloon inflation, depending on the type of counterpulsator. The ratio of ventricular assist is determined by the individual patient's hemodynamic status.

The pump can be regulated automatically, triggered by an electrocardiogram signal, or operated manually. To prevent potential thrombi, pumping should be continuous. Intraaortic balloons are made of antithrombotic material. The manufacturer's

instructions for use should be followed. Pumps are equipped with sensors (e.g., alarm and automatic shutoff) to minimize danger.

Weaning from the IABP is usually gradual, as tolerated by the patient. Lower extremity pulses are checked during and periodically after balloon catheter removal to assess circulation in the foot on the side of the catheter insertion and to check for the presence of clots. Complications associated with an IABP include distal extremity ischemia, compartment syndrome, thrombus or emboli, gas embolism, arterial or aortic perforation, bleeding, and infection.

Ventricular Assist Device

A powered ventricular assist device (VAD) can be used to wean patients from CPB when the IABP, drugs, and/or cardiac pacing are ineffective, to support circulation after postinfarction cardiogenic shock or traumatic myocardial contusion, and to provide a temporary bridge for support before transplantation (Fig. 43.31). The VAD has been a significant bridge to transplantation and is useful for cardiac support until a suitable donor is available. The mechanical device maintains systemic and myocardial perfusion while promoting metabolic and hemodynamic recovery of a reversibly damaged myocardium.

The VAD does not depend on cardiac contractility or electrical conduction. It acts as an artificial ventricle. The VAD consists of a flexible polyurethane blood sac, a flexible diaphragm, and a pump assembly enclosed within a rigid polysulfone housing. Inlet and outlet valves maintain unidirectional blood flow. The VAD is attached to the patient via inflow and outflow cannulas. Support can be to the left, right, or both ventricles:

- *Left ventricular assistance (LVA):* Blood is withdrawn from the left atrium into a left ventricular assist device (LVAD) and returned to the ascending aorta. The polyurethane inflow cannula can be inserted into either the left atrium or the left

• **Fig. 43.30** Intraaortic balloon catheter positioned in descending thoracic aorta, above renal artery and below left subclavian artery, via femoral artery.

Left subclavian artery

Descending thoracic aorta

Renal artery

• **Fig. 43.31** HeartMate ventricular assist device. (Reprinted with the permission of Thoratec Corporation, Pleasanton, CA.)

ventricle. The outflow cannula has a segment of woven polyester that is anastomosed end to side to the thoracic aorta.

- *Right ventricular assistance (RVA):* Blood is withdrawn from the right atrium into the right ventricular assist device (RVAD) and is returned to the pulmonary artery. The inflow cannula is placed in the right atrium. The outflow cannula is anastomosed end to side to the main pulmonary artery.
- *Biventricular assistance (BVA):* Both an LVAD and RVAD can be used to support both ventricles simultaneously. The cannulas exit the pericardial sac below the costal margin. They are connected to parts of the VAD after removal of all air. Depending on the intended duration of support, the housing is exteriorized or implanted.
- *Extracorporeal VAD:* The extracorporeal VAD is used for short-term ventricular assistance and is externally powered pneumatically with compressed air or electrically with centrifugal force. The housing rests on the patient's chest, with the inflow and outflow cannulas passing through the chest wall. The power source is attached to the air-inlet port or pump head. The skin is approximated, or the chest is left open and covered with sterile material sutured to the wound edges. Then the chest is covered with a sterile occlusive dressing. The patient returns to the OR for removal of the device and chest closure or heart transplantation, usually within 10 days.
- *Implantable VAD:* The implantable VAD is for long-term use and is an electrically activated pump implanted in the left upper quadrant of the abdomen. The internal battery pack and control unit in the housing are connected to an external battery pack. The cannulas pass through the diaphragm.

The rate of pumping and movement of the diaphragm inside the VAD are programmed by the power console. Another type of LVAD is mounted on a catheter connected to a pump and external motor. The catheter, inserted via the femoral artery or by transthoracic or retroperitoneal approach, draws blood out of the left ventricle and returns it to the descending aorta.

Extracorporeal Membrane Oxygenator

An extracorporeal membrane oxygenator (ECMO) is used as a resuscitative device for patients who have potentially reversible respiratory and/or cardiac failure. It is also commonly used to prolong extracorporeal circulation when the patient is in distress after removal from CPB.

Artificial Heart

Clinical trials are in process to test an artificial heart that can be permanently implanted to maintain circulation in the patient with irreparable myocardial damage or end-stage cardiac disease who does not meet the criteria for cardiac transplantation. A total artificial heart also could be used as temporary support while the patient is awaiting a transplant.

Artificial Heart History

In 1982, William DeVries implanted the first total artificial heart into patient Barney Clark, who lived for 112 days with the device. In 1984, DeVries implanted an artificial heart into a second patient, William Schroeder, who lived 620 days. The Jarvik-7 was an air-driven, double-chambered device that replaced the ventricles. Connector cuffs were sutured to the atria, pulmonary artery, and aorta. These cuffs attached to rims of openings on the device. Power was supplied to the pumping chamber through

percutaneous tubes to an external source of compressed air. The patient was essentially tethered to a machine. Many complications, such as emboli, hemorrhage, and infection, were associated with the device.

Recent Advances in Artificial Heart Technology

The German Heart Institute Berlin developed a pediatric bridge to transplant approved by the U.S. Food and Drug Administration (FDA) in 2011. The Berlin Heart EXCOR works with the patient's failing heart by supporting the right and/or left side of the heart. The device is powered by an air pump that is not implanted in the child's body but is connected to cannulas in the heart. The sizes range from 10 to 60-mL capacity. The pulsatile chambers are maintained outside the body, where they can be continually assessed for blood quality and the presence of clots. EXCOR is contraindicated in babies who either cannot receive anticoagulants or must be examined by MRI. More information can be found at www.berlinheart.com.

Abiomed developed the AbioCor, a fully implantable artificial heart that has been granted permission by the FDA for use in clinical trials on humans since 2001. It is a softball-size self-contained unit with internal rechargeable batteries that can run independently for 30 minutes at a time. The implantable component of the device weighs around 2 lbs and is made of titanium and plastic. There are no external wires; however, an external power pack passes energy through the skin to an internal coil. The external power pack weighs 4 lb and is recharged every 4 hours.

The AbioCor is able to provide complete circulatory support with normal tissue perfusion and no hemolysis, according to current studies. Criteria for use of the AbioCor include biventricular failure without viable treatment alternatives and imminent death within 30 days. The patient's diseased heart is removed with the exception of small atrial attachments.

The first patient to receive the AbioCor implant was Robert Tools, age 59. The implantation was performed in July 2001 at Jewish Hospital in Louisville, Kentucky, by Laman Gray Jr. and Robert Dowling. Mr. Tools lived for 5 months with the device. The second recipient, Tom Christerson, age 71, had the device implanted in September 2001 at the same facility and lived for 512 days with the device. He lived at home and had the opportunity to celebrate his 55th wedding anniversary and the birth of his first great-grandchild. Additional patients have had the device implanted at several heart centers in the United States since, with little success. The company decided not to continue the project.

Patients in biventricular failure who need a heart transplant can have a SynCardia total artificial heart (TAH) as an immediate replacement bridge to transplant. The TAH replaces both ventricles and all four valves (Fig. 43.32). The atria remain intact. The SynCardia TAH 70 cc is the most commonly used bridge to transplant. SynCardia is the only FDA-approved artificial heart available. Some patients had replacement TAH implanted for adjustments to the system. The longest use by one patient was close to 4.5 years before his heart transplant was available.

Patient selection for TAH includes being a current transplant candidate, appropriate anticoagulation, and physiologic space in the chest (sternum to vertebrae) to accommodate the TAH device. The 160-g weight TAH device moves 9.5 L of blood through each ventricle and responds to resting needs or increases during exercise when muscular activity increases. The heart pump rate does not increase, but can increase ventricular blood capacity by 30% to

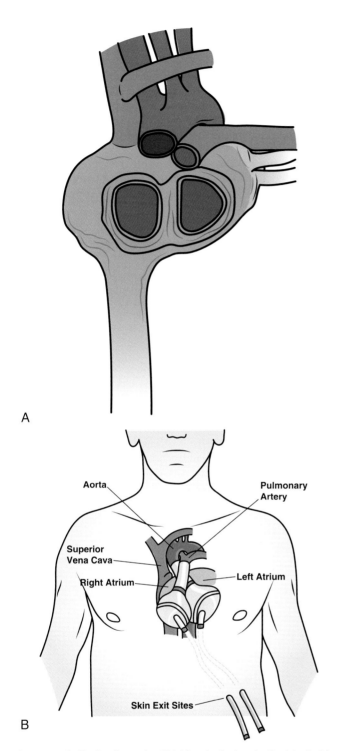

A

B

Aorta

Pulmonary Artery

Superior Vena Cava

Right Atrium

Left Atrium

Skin Exit Sites

• **Fig. 43.32 A,** SynCardia total artificial heart attaches to the intact atria with connection rings after removal of both ventricles and all four valves. The superior cardiac anatomy (arterial and venous) remains intact. **B,** SynCardia artificial heart biventricular device in place.

meet the body's needs. The improvement in blood flow to major organs improves the outcomes of health, leading to better outcomes as a transplant candidate.

The mechanism is powered by lithium ion batteries that are recharged easily with any available electrical outlet or the lighter system in a car. The two replacement ventricles each contain a diaphragm that responds to a pneumatic air power shift provided

by the power pack. The tubing to the power device exits the patient's body via the midabdomen. Patients are able to ambulate when stable after placement of the TAH. Any change in performance of the device sounds an alarm and flashes a light.

A clinical study started in 2015 with patients permits humanitarian or compassionate use for patients who are not transplant candidates. This study has permitted an improved quality of life for patients with a short life expectancy. These patients are able to go home with a portable power supply encased in a shoulder bag or backpack. The hope is to use the TAH as a permanent replacement in the future for the failed native heart.

A smaller 50-cc model is available for smaller patients. The criteria for the clinical investigation are age 10 to 79 years with functional atria. Body size and coagulation studies are some of the criteria for use of the 50-cc TAH and are similar to those used for the larger 70-cc TAH, already approved by the FDA. More information about the SynCardia TAH can be found at www. syncardia.com.

Surgeons at Duke University in Durham, North Carolina implanted an artificial heart by Carmat into a 39-year-old man. This was the first successful artificial heart to be implanted in the U.S. trial.[7] Several European countries and China are in the clinical trial phase of testing redesigned artificial hearts with hope of market approval by 2026.

Complications of Cardiac Surgery

Prevention of complications is a collaborative effort of the surgeon, anesthesiologist, scrub person, and circulating nurse. The care continuum continues through the patient's stay in the ICU and later in the stepdown area. Careful monitoring and management of BP are critical throughout the perioperative care period. Aggressive preoperative evaluation is necessary to screen for patients who are at high risk.

The most common complication of cardiac surgery with or without CBP is stroke. In a patient with atherosclerosis of the coronary arteries, the arterial supply of the brain is usually affected. Air embolus is a common complication during valve procedures. Meticulous de-airing of the heart is done by the surgeon before removal of the aortic cross-clamp in an attempt to prevent air embolus.

Low BP (50–60 mm Hg) during bypass can lead to ischemic cerebrovascular accidents of the brain. Hypertensive episodes can lead to hemorrhagic brain insults. Calcium deposits and atheroma that can line the intima of the aorta can embolize during the application and removal of the aortic cross-clamp. The surgeon inspects and palpates the aorta to find a section amenable to cross-clamping. There is no guarantee that plaque will not be dislodged by manipulation of the instrument.

Excessive bleeding can result in cardiogenic shock and alteration of the body's clotting mechanism. Factors that influence clotting include preoperative use of antiplatelet agents, occult liver disease, disruption of an anastomosis caused by hypertension or technical malfunction of a suture line, prolonged use of CPB, and ineffective use of protamine for reversal of heparin.

Mediastinal and/or pleural chest tubes are placed to monitor the amount of drainage and, if excessive, may warrant a return to the OR for exploration or redo.

Postoperative myocardial infarctions (MIs) are infrequent; however, an MI can lead to cardiogenic shock. Postoperative MI can be caused by a kink or acute thrombosis in the newly placed bypass conduit or an air embolus. Acute restrictive pericarditis can obstruct blood flow in a new graft, causing myocardial ischemia.

Organ failure is always a concern with cardiac surgery and CPB. Organ failure can affect any organ system but is most commonly seen in the kidneys. Low BP caused by an ineffective pump prevents the kidneys from functioning.

Acute tubular necrosis (ATN) can result from atherosclerosis of the renal arterial system, leading to kidney failure. Patients may need hemodialysis for a short time or for life, depending on the extent of renal damage. Some patients, who continue to have adequate urine output, may have only a transient rise in their blood urea nitrogen (BUN) and creatinine levels with quick return to normal without the assistance of hemodialysis.

Acute respiratory distress syndrome (ARDS) and other respiratory disorders complicate the postoperative outcomes of some patients undergoing cardiac surgery. Preoperative evaluation, especially in smokers, is essential to try to predict and prevent the incidence of postoperative pulmonary disorders.

The bowel and liver are occasionally affected by the surgical experience. Acute liver failure can be first noticed with postoperative blood work. A rise in liver function studies (aspartate aminotransferase [AST], alanine aminotransferase [ALT], bilirubin, alkaline phosphatase) can lead to coagulopathies. Bowel that becomes ischemic during bypass can become necrotic in the postoperative course and lead to profound sepsis and death.

Wound infections of the sternum can also lead to horrific sepsis and are managed surgically. The sepsis can result in a prolonged hospital stay or even death. Removing the sternum (sternectomy) is a procedure usually performed by a multidisciplinary team of both cardiac and plastic surgeons. Once the sternum is removed, the plastic surgeon creates a vascularized pedicle flap from the pectoralis muscles or omentum to create a tissue cover for the defect left by the missing sternum. The skin is closed over the flap. The ample blood supply of the muscles and omentum assist with the evacuation of any remaining pathogens and promote wound healing.

Cardiac tamponade occurs when blood and fluids build up around the heart. When blood collects in the pericardium and is not adequately evacuated by the drains, it can collect and begin to compress and compromise the function of the heart. This life-threatening event is first observed when there are increasing right atrial and right ventricular pressures. It is also reflected in a drop of more than 10 mm Hg in systolic blood pressure during the patient's inspiration (pulsus paradoxus). If left untreated, cardiac tamponade can lead to hypotension and fatal dysrhythmia.

Electrolyte imbalance in magnesium, potassium, and, to a lesser extent, calcium can lead to serious cardiac dysrhythmias such as sinus bradycardia, supraventricular tachycardia (SVT), ventricular tachycardia (VT), atrial fibrillation, atrial flutter, and ventricular fibrillation (VF). High levels of potassium will cause a fatal dysrhythmia if not medically corrected with medications such as glucose or insulin, furosemide (Lasix) or sodium polystyrene (Kayexalate), or hemodialysis.

Cardiogenic shock may be precipitated by coronary air embolism, pulmonary embolism, myocardial contusion, mechanical venous obstruction, or hypothermia. Precautions are taken intraoperatively to avoid postoperative cardiogenic and/or hemorrhagic shock. Excessive bleeding can result from stress to the clotting mechanism.

Cardiac surgery can be a lifesaving procedure if carefully managed by the entire perioperative team. Attention to sterile technique and patient monitoring are especially critical.

ⓔ EVOLVE WEBSITE

http://evolve.elsevier.com/Hornacky/BerryKohn/

- Historical Perspective
- Tips for the Scrub Person and Circulating Nurse
- Student Interactive Questions
- Glossary

References

1. Min J, Hong J: A cardioplegic solution with an understanding of a cardiochannelopathy, *Antioxidants (Basel)* 10(12):1878, 2021.
2. Sellke F, Ruel M: Robotic mitral valve surgery. In *Atlas of cardiac surgical techniques,* ed 2, St. Louis, MO, 2018, Elsevier, pp 347–382.
3. Sathananthan J, Sellers S, Barlow A, et al.: valve-in-valve transcatheter aortic valve replacement and bioprosthetic valve fracture comparing different transcatheter heart valve designs: an ex vivo bench study, *Cardiovasc Interv* 12(1):65–75, 2019.
4. Zoghbi W, Asch F, Bruce C, et al.: Guidelines for the evaluation of valvular regurgitation after percutaneous valve repair or replacement, *J Am Soc Echocardiogr* 32(4):431–475, 2019.
5. Chadda K, Ajijola O, Vaseghi M, et al.: Ageing, the autonomic nervous system and arrhythmia: from brain to heart, *Ageing Res Rev* 48:40–50, 2018.
6. Mehmood H, Goyal A: *Pacemaker types and selection,* Treasure Island, FL, 2023, StatPearls. www.ncbi.nlm,nih gov. Accessed July 12, 2023.
7. Duke U: *New generation artificial heart implanted in patient at Duke—first in U.S.* www.dukehealth.org. Accessed July 12, 2023.

Bibliography

Belott P: Cosmetic aspects of device implantation, *Heart Rhythm* 16(2):308–311, 2018.
Townsend C, Beauchamp D, Evers M, et al. In *Sabiston textbook of surgery,* ed 21, St. Louis, MO, 2022, Elsevier.

44
Vascular Surgery

CHAPTER OUTLINE

Anatomy and Physiology of the Vascular System, 947

Vascular Pathology, 949

Diagnostic Procedures, 951

Special Features of Vascular Surgery, 952

Composite Vein Grafts, 955

Conservative Interventional Techniques, 955

Laser Angioplasty, 956

Vascular Surgical Procedures, 958

CHAPTER OBJECTIVES

After studying this chapter the learner will be able to:

- Identify the pertinent anatomy of the peripheral vascular system.
- Describe the potential complications associated with peripheral vascular disease.

- Describe care of the patient with peripheral vascular disease.
- List the differences in aneurysms and their treatment.
- Discuss the vascular access options for hemodialysis.

KEY TERMS AND DEFINITIONS

Aneurysm Abnormal outpouching or bulging of an artery.

Anticoagulation Alteration in the cellular activity associated with clotting.

Dissecting aneurysm Occurs when the intima separates from the media. A false passage fills with blood, causing further separation of intima and media.

Embolize Material (e.g., fat, plaque, vegetation, or clot) in a blood vessel becomes bloodborne with the potential for lodging in smaller vascular tributaries.

Endarterectomy Removal of clot or other material from an artery.

Hemangioma Vascular lesions classified as tumors or malformations.

Hemodialysis Vascular system is accessed for the purpose of removing chemicals and other solutes from the blood.

Iatrogenic Condition inadvertently caused by the medical or surgical treatment performed by a physician.

Interstices Spaces in a woven surface or between the strands of a braided suture.

Mycotic aneurysm Bacterial vegetation embolizes from the valve of the heart to the arteries, where it implants and grows, causing the weakened artery to distend and rupture.

Pseudoaneurysm (false aneurysm) Injury to all three layers of the arterial wall that permits blood to accumulate in the connective tissue.

Thrombose Blood within a vascular structure clots and occludes the lumen.

True aneurysm Progressive dilation of an artery.

Anatomy and Physiology of the Vascular System

Vessels in the thorax, abdomen, extremities, and extracranial cerebrovascular area constitute the circulatory system (Fig. 44.1). The ascending aorta, which originates from the left ventricle, carries oxygenated blood from the heart to the arteries. The major arteries leading to the head and upper extremities—the brachiocephalic trunk, left common carotid, and subclavian arteries—branch off from the aortic arch in the middle mediastinum above the heart. The thoracic aorta then descends through the posterior mediastinum at the left side of the vertebral column.

Passing through the diaphragm, the abdominal aorta descends to the level of the fourth lumbar vertebra, where it bifurcates (i.e., divides) to form the common iliac arteries that lead to the lower extremities. Arteries from the abdominal aorta carry blood to the kidneys and the abdominal and pelvic organs. The femoral artery, which originates from the iliac artery, is the main artery in each leg.

Oxygenated blood flows from the arterial system through the capillary network and returns deoxygenated to the heart via the venous system (Fig. 44.2). The superior and inferior venae cavae enter the right atrium. The superior vena cava, formed by the union of the two brachiocephalic veins, returns deoxygenated venous blood from the head, neck, upper extremities, and chest.

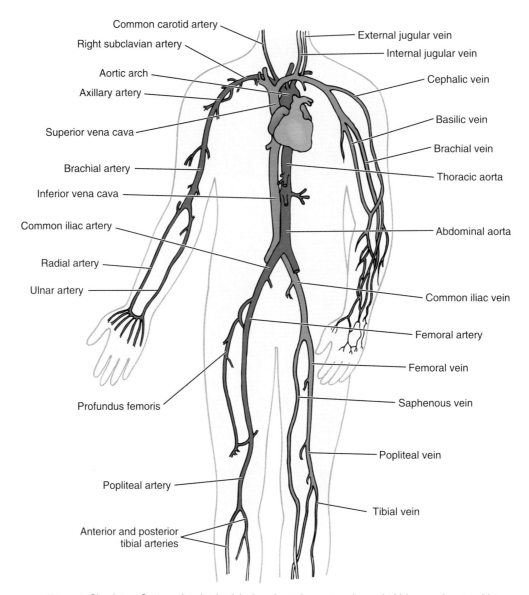

Common carotid artery
Right subclavian artery
Aortic arch
Axillary artery
Superior vena cava
Brachial artery
Inferior vena cava
Common iliac artery
Radial artery
Ulnar artery
Profundus femoris
Popliteal artery
Anterior and posterior tibial arteries

External jugular vein
Internal jugular vein
Cephalic vein
Basilic vein
Brachial vein
Thoracic aorta
Abdominal aorta
Common iliac vein
Femoral artery
Femoral vein
Saphenous vein
Popliteal vein
Tibial vein

• **Fig. 44.1** Circulatory System. Arteries (and the heart) are shown as red vessels. Veins are shown as blue vessels.

The inferior vena cava, which begins at the level of the fifth lumbar vertebra, returns blood from the lower extremities, pelvis, and abdominal organs. There are two exceptions to this oxygenation/deoxygenation pattern, as follows:

1. The pulmonary arteries carry deoxygenated blood to the lungs, and the pulmonary veins carry oxygenated blood to the heart.
2. In fetal umbilical circulation, one vein carries oxygenated blood and two arteries carry mixed blood. These three vessels, surrounded by Wharton jelly, traverse the umbilical cord to the placenta.

Innervation of the arteries and veins is controlled by the efferent vasomotor fibers of the autonomic nervous system. The nerve fibers enter the vessel adventitia (i.e., covering) along the same route as the blood supply. Stimulation of these nerves can cause vasoconstriction that shunts blood to larger organ groups, such as the skin or gastrointestinal tract. Some medications cause vasodilation, which relaxes the vessels and slows heart rate to decrease intraluminal pressure.

The vessels are lined with endothelial cells, which when intact do not support platelet aggregation. This property is interrupted when a vessel is injured, and a clot is allowed to form. The endothelial lining also secretes factors that resist clotting, stimulate tissue repair, and synthesize clotting factors.

Arterial Anatomy

Arteries are elastic and constrict in response to hemorrhage. The arterial walls are made up of three layers separated by internal and external elastic membranes (Fig. 44.3). The innermost layer is the intima (tunica intima), a single layer of endothelial cells on a thin matrix of hyaluronic acid, collagen, and elastic fibers. The middle layer is the media (tunica media, or yellow fibrous). It is the thickest of the layers and is composed of a combination of smooth muscle fibers, yellow collagen, and some elastic fibers. The medial layer gives the arterial wall the flexibility and strength to withstand higher internal pressure.

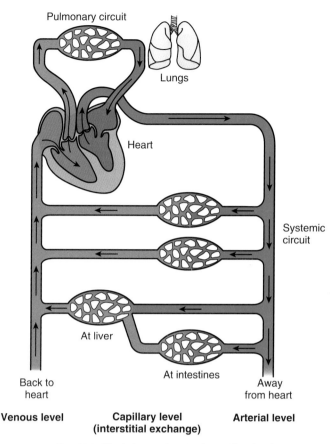

• **Fig. 44.2** Circulatory system to the capillary level.

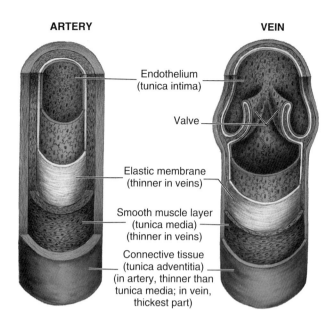

• **Fig. 44.3** Cross-section of an artery and a vein showing the three layers: tunica intima, tunica media, and tunica adventitia.

The outermost layer is the adventitia (tunica adventitia, or white fibrous connective tissue). It is the thinnest layer but provides most of the external support for the arterial wall and resistance to overexpansion.

The tissues of the adventitia and the outer third of the media are nourished by a series of capillaries called the vasa vasorum. The rest of the medial layer and the intimal layer are nourished by diffusion from the luminal flow. Terminal arteries, referred to as arterioles, end at the level of the capillary beds in the tissues.

Venous Anatomy

Venous walls are structured in three layers. The innermost layer, the intima, is composed of endothelial cells that produce coagulation factors. The middle layer, or media, is much thinner in the deep venous system and may even be hard to identify microscopically. The superficial veins have a thicker medial layer composed mainly of smooth muscle fibers. This provides some resistance and response to intraluminal pressure changes. The external layer, or the venous adventitia, is composed of loose connective tissue (see Fig. 44.2). Because of lower flow pressure, larger veins have internal semilunar valves to maintain the direction of the blood flow.

The muscular component of the lower extremities provides force during contraction of large muscle groups, which facilitates venous return from the larger peripheral sinusoids. The cerebral veins are an exception; they have no valves. Veins are less elastic than arteries and tend to ooze instead of contract in response to hemorrhage.

Venous anatomy has three structural components: superficial veins, deep veins, and perforators (also known as communicating veins) (Fig. 44.4). The venous structure and flow of the lower extremities are examples of this system. At the tissue level the origin of the venous system at the capillary bed is referred to as venules. The venous drainage of deoxygenated blood from the superficial veins returns through the perforators to the deep veins during muscular contraction. The deoxygenated blood then passes from the deep veins to the inferior vena cava.

Capillary Anatomy

Capillary beds are the vascular nutrition and waste exchange points of the arterial and venous systems. Capillaries are the diameter of a red blood cell and form a network throughout body tissues. Structurally they are a single epithelial cell layer thick, which facilitates the exchange of oxygen and carbon dioxide at the tissue level. They are semipermeable to water and crystalloids but are impermeable to larger molecules such as proteins. Oxygenated blood enters the capillary bed via the arterial system, and deoxygenated blood passively drains into the venous system.

There are no fibrous or muscular layers of the vessels at this level. Lymphatic vessels passively exchange lipids, debris, fluids, proteins, antibodies, and other nutrients at this level in response to skeletal muscle contraction. This fluid is filtered by the lymphatics and is transported through the thoracic duct to the vena cava. The lymphatic vessels are structurally very pliable and have valves to maintain a unidirectional flow.

Vascular Pathology

Vascular diseases that cause occlusion or stenosis are usually acquired diseases. Inadequate arterial blood supply causes ischemia in tissues and complete organ systems. If left untreated, this can lead to thrombus, embolus, ulceration, necrosis, or gangrene. Vessels are repaired, reconstructed, or replaced to improve peripheral (systemic) circulation.

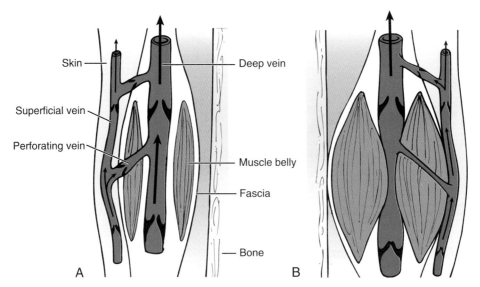

• **Fig. 44.4** Structural Components of Deep Venous Anatomy in Lower Extremity. **A,** Relaxed state. **B,** With muscle contraction, the perforating veins are squeezed closed.

Atherosclerosis is the most common arterial disease. It is a diffuse disease and begins as a disruption of the intima of a large artery. Cholesterol enters the media to stimulate muscle growth, and platelets accumulate around the disruption of the endothelial intima to form plaque or a thrombus. Often this process becomes localized around vessel orifices and branches (i.e., at bifurcations). The disease may produce stenosis (narrowing) and subsequent occlusion or ectasia (dilation) and aneurysm. The most common procedures are performed to revascularize a lower extremity for limb salvage, repair an aortoiliac aneurysm, and improve cerebral blood flow through the carotid arteries.

Atherosclerosis is the principal factor in transient ischemic attacks (TIAs; "mini strokes"), cerebrovascular accidents (strokes or "brain attacks"), myocardial infarctions (heart attacks), and aortic stenosis. Risk factors include familial history, a high level of serum cholesterol, smoking, and hypertension (Box 44.1).

Venous stasis disease or obstruction of venous return can cause hemodynamic imbalances that affect distal structures. Arterial blood enters the area, but cannot return through the venous system. Superior vena cava (SVC) syndrome is one example. Patients with compression on the SVC caused by benign or malignant tumors or mediastinal fibrosis have serious venous drainage obstruction of the head and upper extremities. SVC syndrome can be caused by venous thrombosis associated with pacer wires or central venous catheters. Patients experience visual disturbances and dyspnea.

Relief of the obstruction by conservative medical management is not always successful. SVC syndrome can be a surgical emergency. Endovascular treatment is usually the best choice. In select patients a surgical bypass may be necessary.

Hemangiomas are tangled masses of malformed blood vessels. They can be found anywhere in the body. These vascular dysmorphic structures are congenital and are classified as (1) low-flow venous/lymphatic or (2) high-flow arterial or combined venous-arterial. Low-flow hemangiomas are soft and compressible and appear bluish. They can cause disfigurement and an aching discomfort. The size ranges from small to large. Larger venous

• **BOX 44.1** **Risk Factors for the Development of Peripheral Vascular Disease**

- Advanced age
- Diabetes
- Familial predisposition
- Habitual long periods of standing
- High-fat diet causing high serum cholesterol
- Hypertension
- Obesity
- Repeated pregnancies
- Sedentary lifestyle
- Smoking
- Stress

hemangiomas can expel clots, bleed, and lead to multisystem organ failure based on the location. If located on an organ, the treatment must be surgical.

Low-flow lymphatic masses are referred to as lymphangiomas. Deeper lymphangiomas can lead to cystic hygromas of the neck. The treatment can be sclerotherapy or excisional surgery. Common postoperative complications include seroma formation and infection.

High-flow arterial or arteriovenous hemangiomas are very aggressive and are not cured despite surgical intervention. They appear as purple masses anywhere on the body or on internal organs. Fistulas form around arterial feeder vessels and establish new pathways continually. Growth of the hemangioma is stimulated by puberty, pregnancy, or physical trauma. The mass becomes pulsatile, and a bruit can be heard with a Doppler. Loss of a limb can be caused by a mixed hemangioma that impairs circulation and mobility. Treatment is aimed at the origin of the arterial feeders. This area may require repeated arterial embolization with ethyl esters, cyanoacrylate, or liquid vinyl alcohol polymer. High-flow hemangiomas may require life-long treatment.[1]

Diagnostic Procedures

Preoperative assessment of cardiac risk is critically important in planning the care of a patient who requires major vascular surgery. Peripheral arterial and venous diseases are assessed by auscultation, palpation, and observation.

Table 44.1 compares the assessment factors of peripheral arterial and venous obstructive diseases in an extremity. Peripheral vascular laboratories, which are similar to cardiac catheterization laboratories, have been established in many health care facilities to perform noninvasive and invasive studies before and after surgical intervention. Interventional radiologists perform many of the diagnostic tests. X-ray studies, scans, imaging, ultrasound, and Doppler assessment reveal most pathologic conditions.

Computed tomography (CT) and magnetic resonance imaging (MRI) are noninvasive techniques of choice to confirm a diagnosis of aortic aneurysm, thrombus, or atherosclerotic plaque in arterial walls, especially in the abdominal and carotid circulation. CT scans are a good way to assess the sizes and stages of vessel occlusions. They can be performed with or without a contrast medium and very quickly in emergency situations. CT scans are somewhat expensive and expose the patient to x-rays.

MRI is useful for evaluating a three-dimensional image of the vessel being studied. This method is contraindicated for patients with stainless steel pacemakers, vena cava filters, or vessel clips, but many patients can benefit from its use. Nonmagnetic materials are not contraindicated. MRI is more expensive than CT scans and takes longer to perform.

Carotid phonoangiography and oculoplethysmography (OPG) are techniques to obtain cerebral blood flow measurements to localize obstructions in the vessels of the head and neck. OPG is contraindicated in patients with intraocular lens implants.

Pulse volume recording (PVR) or photoplethysmography is used to measure systolic pressure in the extremities and digital arterial systems. This test is affected by artifacts and patient positioning. A diagnosis of deep vein thrombosis (DVT) may be made by phleborheography (PRG), a plethysmographic technique that records the rhythmic changes in venous volume in the legs; these changes are associated with respiration. PRG is not useful for small thrombi or deep iliac or femoral veins, and the process is time-consuming and expensive.

Ultrasonography is a major diagnostic tool for measuring segmental arterial pressures and venous patency in the extremities; it also may be used for abdominal circulation. Doppler color-coded flow imaging and transcranial Doppler imaging has mostly replaced carotid phonoangiography and OPG in the evaluation of carotid circulation. High-resolution, B-mode ultrasound provides real-time images of venous systems in the upper and lower extremities.

Saphenous and cephalic vein mapping accurately measures vein diameter, location, and quality to determine preoperatively if the vein is suitable for use as an arterial conduit in arterial reconstruction. Ultrasound also detects venous thrombosis. With a pulse Doppler blood flow detector, longitudinal and/or transverse cross-sectional scans are obtained and the images are recorded by oscilloscope. A computer-generated print of the image on the screen provides a permanent record of the arteriograph or venograph.

Intraoperative assessment of shunt performance or vessel patency or stenosis, as well as identification of an arteriovenous fistula (AVF), is easily performed with a sterile Doppler probe (Fig. 44.5). An audible signal is transduced and is similar to the sounds transmitted by a Geiger counter.

Invasive Procedures

Selective angiography permits the x-ray study of a particular segment of the vascular system. Aortography visualizes the aorta

---

TABLE 44.1   Comparison of Peripheral Arterial and Venous Obstructive Diseases in an Extremity

Assessment of Extremity	Arterial Obstructive Disease	Venous Obstructive Disease
Color	Dusky, blue, gray, mottled, pallor distal to obstruction	Red, purple, brown hemosiderin spots, brawny
Temperature	Cool, cold	Warm, hot
Visual and palpable characteristics	Dry, shiny, flaking skin; vessels not obvious Lack of hair on affected part Thick nails	Moist, peeling skin Vessels may be tortuous and inflamed Thickened tissue Hair present on affected part Normal nails
Sensation	Numbness, tingling, pain during exercise (intermittent claudication) Pain at rest in severe disease Increased pain when exposed to cold Pain can be acute and severe	Aching, throbbing, tightness, feeling of heaviness; muscles feel fatigued Pain decreased by motion or elevation of legs Feels worse at end of day
Mobility	Painful range of motion; limited flexion and extension caused by avascular necrosis at the tissue level	Painful range of motion; limited flexion and extension caused by congestive edema in joints
Size	Not enlarged, average for body build	Swollen, edematous
Integrity of surface layer	Peeling; infarcted; painful, deep, serous, oozing ulcers with defined edges on or between toes	Stasis ulceration; open, draining, shallow ulcers with irregular borders
Pulses	Weak or absent	Present
Condition of digits	Mottled, blackened, fragile, painful; can become gangrenous	Edematous, reddened, painful; can become gangrenous

• **Fig. 44.5** Doppler box and probe.

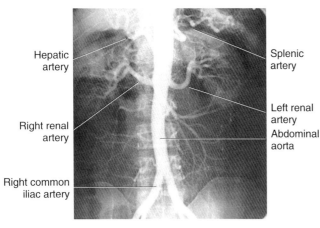

Hepatic artery

Right renal artery

Right common iliac artery

Splenic artery

Left renal artery

Abdominal aorta

• **Fig. 44.6** Normal abdominal aortogram.

(Fig. 44.6). Arteriography shows the patency of an artery or a branch of the aorta and its collateral circulation.

Phlebography detects DVT, and a venogram visualizes the veins. An angiogram requires the injection of a nontoxic contrast medium. The pain associated with injection of intravascular contrast material can be intense. The procedure may be performed under continuous epidural anesthesia or general anesthesia.

Angioscopy is an endoscopic technique used to visualize the interior of vessels. A small (1.5–3 mm), flexible fiberoptic angioscope is coupled to a camera, which allows the view from the angioscope to be seen on a monitor. The lining and structures within the blood vessels are visualized as the scope is advanced within each vessel. For many patients, angioscopy is an alternative preoperative diagnostic technique to angiography and may be used to evaluate the effectiveness of therapy intraoperatively. It can reveal retained atherosclerotic plaque or thrombi and suture lines.

Intravascular ultrasonic scanning of the coronary or peripheral vasculature uses a miniaturized ultrasonic probe at the end of a 3.5-Fr catheter. The probe is introduced over a guidewire. The probe is irrigated with heparinized saline as it is introduced into the vessel percutaneously. Images of the entire circumference are obtained and viewed on a monitor to determine the thickness of the vessel wall and the distribution of plaque within the wall. This technique may be performed percutaneously or during a surgical procedure. This device is single use and not reprocessed. This device is not recommended for use on cerebral vessels.

Special Features of Vascular Surgery

Circulation within the peripheral vascular system affects the brain, internal organs, and extremities. An expanding body of knowledge relating to vascular physiology and the development of the art of vascular surgery has improved the quality of life for many patients with peripheral vascular diseases. Circulatory problems may affect any part of the body, but this discussion focuses on the most common pathologic conditions amenable to vascular procedures performed by vascular surgeons and interventional radiologists. Current surgical trends include open procedures and endovascular techniques.

Vascular injury can occur during invasive diagnostic tests, intravascular monitoring, or therapeutic procedures. Iatrogenic arterial injuries, those resulting from an unexpected outcome of a procedure, can cause loss of function or even death from ischemia, hemorrhage, or embolus. The patient must be carefully observed and monitored for signs of complications during and after vascular procedures. Infection is a devastating postoperative complication that must be avoided through strict adherence to aseptic and sterile techniques. Other considerations include the following:

- A thorough understanding of the principles of general surgery should be combined with special training in vascular surgical techniques. Speed and accuracy are imperative.
- Local or monitored anesthesia care (MAC) is usually preferred for most conservative interventional procedures. General anesthesia or regional block is used for longer or more extensive procedures.
- Skin preparation is performed very gently. Vascular pathology (i.e., carotid stenosis, aneurysms, or venous thrombosis) should never be rubbed or pressed during the prep because plaque or clots could embolize, causing serious limb or brain damage. Aneurysms could rupture.
- Temperature regulation may be a problem during long procedures or when multiple blood transfusions are given. Warmed fluids can be administered via rapid infusing pumps. Forced-air warming blankets provide a normothermic temperature. Intentional hypothermia can be used to preserve the spinal cord during aortic surgery. The low temperatures decrease the metabolic needs of the cord by minimizing the effects of temporary ischemia during cross-clamping of the aorta.
- During anastomosis of vessels, meticulous care is exercised to avoid the danger of postoperative thrombosis and stenosis. To prevent undue trauma to vessels, an assortment of curved and angled scissors, noncrushing vascular clamps, and forceps specifically designed for vascular surgery is included in the instrument setup (Fig. 44.7). Umbilical tape (also called hernia tape) or synthetic vessel loops are used for retraction and vessel control (Fig. 44.8). An operating microscope may be used for anastomosis of vessels. Appropriate instrumentation for microsurgery is made available. Synthetic nonabsorbable monofilament suture materials are preferred because they are strong and pass through vessel walls and grafts easily with minimal trauma and tissue reaction. Uncoated braided suture has interstices (spaces) that cause trauma by abrasion and can harbor microorganisms.

A Cosgrove vascular clamp with cushioning jaw inserts

B Placing jaw inserts

C Jaw inserts in place

D Temporary vessel occlusion clamp and ring-handled applier

E Close-up of temporary occlusion clamp (disposable)

F Cooley bulldog

G Dietrich bulldog

• **Fig. 44.7** Specialty vascular instruments.

• **Fig. 44.8** Vessel loops in place for retraction of arteries and venous structures.

Swaged needles also minimize trauma. A larger swaged suture-to-needle ratio is advantageous to avoid leakage. Holes made in graft materials by the needle are occluded by the larger suture. Double-armed needle sutures are often used for vessel anastomosis.

Structurally the surgeon may use a triangulating technique in which three vessel edges are gently straightened to create a straight sutured angle with three separate sutures instead of suturing a circular stitch with one suture that could stricture.

• Heparinized solution is available for use as an anticoagulant irrigation. Preoperatively, heparin (5000 units) may be given subcutaneously (SQ) for DVT prophylaxis 1 hour before the surgical procedure. Intraoperatively the optimal dose is 70 to 100 units/kg of body weight if given intravenously (IV) for immediate systemic effect. Thromboelastography may be used intraoperatively to monitor the effects of heparin administration. Sensitivity to bovine sources of heparin can result in heparin-induced thrombocytopenia (HIT), also known as white clot syndrome. Clots composed of fibrin and platelets form after 4 to 15 days of heparin therapy. A severe decrease in the platelet count predisposes the patient to thrombosis and acute arterial occlusion.

• Patients with preoperative anticoagulation with warfarin for known blood coagulation pathology are at risk for extreme blood loss. Temporary reversal of the therapeutic anticoagulation for the duration of an emergent surgical procedure is accomplished by the administration of fresh frozen platelets (FFPs). Onset of FFP action is immediate and easily amenable to postoperative anticoagulation as necessary. The activity of FFP is short term.

Less urgent surgical procedures for the anticoagulated patient can be performed with minimal blood loss after the administration of vitamin K. Studies have shown that 1 mg of IV vitamin K reversed the effects of therapeutic anticoagulation within 27 hours of administration. SQ vitamin K injections are absorbed at an unpredictable rate and are rarely used. Low-dose vitamin K does not interfere with postoperative therapeutic anticoagulation regimens.

• Before closure at the end of the procedure, protamine sulfate, a heparin antagonist, is given to reverse the anticoagulant effect; 1 mg of protamine is given to counteract 100 units of heparin. Protamine is derived from fish semen and testicular tissue and may elicit a sensitivity reaction in patients who are allergic to fish. Patients with type 1 diabetes who take NPH (neutral

• **BOX 44.2** **Hemostatic Agents Used in Vascular Surgery**

- Absorbable gelatin sponge (Gelfoam) can be used dry or dipped in saline. According to the manufacturer, the patient may have an antigenic reaction when the sponge is soaked in thrombin. The sponge can be applied to the site and removed after 20 seconds or left in the wound; it is absorbed after 4 to 6 weeks. Gelfoam should never remain in a closed cavity because it greatly increases in size and can cause pressure on tissues. Because it may provide a favorable microbiologic growth medium, it is not used in the presence of infection. It is derived from porcine gelatin and has more of a mechanical than a chemical hemostatic property.
- Absorbable collagen (e.g., Avitene, Hemopad, Helistat)—either in powder, foam, woven, or nonwoven form—induces platelet adhesion and results in the formation of fibrin. It provides both a chemical and a mechanical hemostasis. Because it may provide a favorable microbiologic growth medium, it is not used in the presence of infection. The long-term effects of an in situ collagen hemostat are unknown, but animal studies indicate that it absorbs. It is of bovine origin and can be moistened, but it works better when dry.
- Oxidized cellulose (Surgicel, Oxycel) is applied dry over a bleeding site for hemostasis. Although a single layer can be left in the wound and absorbed, it is preferred that a large wad be removed because it may interfere with healing or cause pressure. It chemically destroys thrombin and is not used concurrently with it. Because it may provide a favorable microbiologic growth medium, it is not used in the presence of infection. It has some bactericidal properties against gram-positive and gram-negative microorganisms. The mode of action is mechanical hemostasis when applied to an area of bleeding.
- Fibrin glue is applied by simultaneously placing a combination of cryoprecipitate, bovine thrombin, and/or calcium chloride on the bleeding tissue surface to form a fibrin patch.
- Topical thrombin should be available. Preparations from bovine origin are contraindicated in patients who are sensitive or allergic to these products. Thrombin is never injected.

protamine Hagedorn) insulin also may be predisposed to a sensitivity reaction to protamine. Some men who have had a vasectomy may exhibit allergic or hypersensitivity reactions.

- Hemostatic agents can be used independently or in combination (Box 44.2). Care is taken not to permit hemostatic materials to be suctioned into the blood-salvage or cell-saving device. These products can be hazardous if permitted to enter the patient's vascular system. Containers and delivery devices for thrombin should be carefully labeled with concentration and dosage to prevent accidental injection.
- A vasodilator such as papaverine is used to relax the smooth muscle of the vessel. This prevents endothelial damage during intraluminal irrigation. Vasopressors should be available. Some surgeons use 1% lidocaine without epinephrine.
- Blood is lost by the flushing of clots and debris. Blood loss should be calculated, and blood should be available for replacement if the hematocrit level falls below 26%.

During procedures on the great vessels, blood may be salvaged from the thoracic or abdominal cavity for autotransfusion. An autologous blood salvage machine (cell saver) may be used to collect the patient's own blood for autotransfusion. Care is taken not to aspirate hemostatic materials or other debris into the blood suction-salvage device. A separate suction tip for blood salvage should be labeled and not used for suction of irrigation solutions.

Blood should be warmed before transfusion to help prevent inadvertent hypothermia. Consideration is given to the patient who does not want a blood transfusion. Patients undergoing nonemergent procedures should be given the option of donating autologous blood in advance of the procedure.

- For DVT prophylaxis, antiembolic stockings or sequential compression devices should be worn by the patient during and after the surgical procedure, in addition to therapeutic anticoagulant therapy.
- For vascular monitoring, Doppler ultrasound, pulse volume recorder, and/or intravascular imaging techniques are used intraoperatively to monitor hemodynamic changes and assess blood flow after peripheral vascular reconstruction. A pulmonary artery catheter (e.g., Swan-Ganz) is usually inserted to monitor pulmonary artery pressures during and after the procedure.

The most serious immediate postoperative complications are thrombus and hemorrhage. The patient may need to return to the OR for immediate correction of these problems. Long-term complications include infection and graft failure by occlusion.

Vascular Grafts

Biologic or synthetic prosthetic vascular grafts are required to bypass a vascular obstruction or reconstruct vessels. These substitute conduits for blood flow vary in length, diameter, and configuration to meet the requirements of each situation. A graft may be straight or bifurcated into a Y shape. Pieces of biologic or synthetic material may be cut to size for use as patch grafts.

The American National Standards Institute (ANSI) has established requirements for product characteristics and the labeling of textile and nontextile synthetic grafts, vascular allografts, and vascular xenografts. Grafts sterilized in see-through containers or packages permit the surgeon to select the appropriate size after exposure of the surgical site. Manufacturers' instructions for use and handling are strictly followed.

Biologic Vascular Grafts

Autografts, allografts, and xenografts have been used for arterial or venous conduits, but autologous grafts have a higher success rate. Allografts and xenografts have a higher failure rate.

Arterial Conduit

Autologous arteries are procured for coronary artery bypass grafting. The radial, gastroepiploic, or internal mammary arteries are commonly used. Arterial grafts do not **thrombose** and occlude as readily as do venous grafts.

Venous Conduit

An autologous vein is a suitable graft conduit because it is lined with endothelial cells that inhibit clotting. These cells produce fibrinolytic substances and the plasminogen factor essential to maintain patency. The saphenous vein is commonly used for an autologous arterial bypass or vein graft. If the saphenous vein is not suitable, the basilic or cephalic veins of the arm are sometimes used. A vein graft is used as a conduit in one of the following three ways:

1. *In situ conduit/bypass:* To revascularize a lower extremity, the saphenous vein is exposed at the proximal and distal aspects

but is left in place. The surgeon performs a venotomy at each end of the vein, inserts a valvulotome and/or a disposable valve cutter, and disrupts the internal valves. The occluded artery to be bypassed is ligated distally and proximally and then anastomosed proximally and distally to the saphenous vein. This technique reverses blood flow in the vein and reestablishes the flow of oxygenated blood beyond the level of arterial occlusion. Decreased manipulation and not excising the length of vein minimizes endothelial trauma and preserves antithrombogenic properties. The vasa vasorum and neurovascular components of the vessel remain intact.

2. *Nonreversed vein graft:* Renal and mesenteric revascularization also can be accomplished by grafting nonreversed segments of the saphenous vein.

3. *Reversed vein graft:* When a segment of saphenous vein is harvested for placement in the arterial system, the vein is reversed from its normal anatomic position so the valves will not obstruct arterial blood flow. Intact valves are used to keep the blood flow unidirectional after anastomosis. Endothelial integrity is maintained by gentle dissection and handling. The surgeon exposes the surgical site while the first assistant, resident, or another surgeon—working at a separate sterile table supplied with fine vascular instruments, ties, and vascular clips—prepares the vein for grafting.

Magnification loupes are worn to check for imperfections in the vein and tie off leaking perforators. The valves may be cut, especially in small-diameter segments. The vein is flushed with sterile, cold solution (commonly heparinized saline or Plasma-Lyte with papaverine hydrochloride) and immersed in this solution until the recipient site is prepared.

The saphenous vein decreases in diameter as it courses distally. A size discrepancy may cause difficulty at the anastomosis attachment sites.

Synthetic Vascular Prostheses

Various forms of synthetic materials are used to construct arterial vascular prostheses. Certain materials are more suitable than others for specific applications. The surgeon selects the most appropriate graft for each patient. Rejection and tissue reaction are minimized if Dacron or Teflon is used.

Knitted Polyester

Knitted polyester (Dacron) grafts are porous enough to allow the ingrowth of fibrous tissue into the interstices. They also are porous enough to allow blood to seep through the material and are therefore preclotted before insertion. Preclotting causes the wall of the graft to become impervious to blood by filling the interstices with fibrin. For the preclotting process the surgeon withdraws blood from the patient at the surgical site before anticoagulation therapy. The scrub person places the blood in a sterile basin containing the graft material. The blood saturates the lumen and all surfaces of the graft. The fabric-fibrin conduit later becomes firmly placed in tissue and provides a hypothrombogenic flow surface.

Filamentous Velour

Knitted velour construction of polyester grafts has uniform porosity for easy preclotting and ensures rapid tissue ingrowth. These types of grafts may be crimped or noncrimped, with velour inside and/or outside. One type, the exoskeleton (EXS) prosthesis, has a spiral polypropylene support fused to the outer surface of noncrimped velour. This graft was developed specifically for use across the knee joint. Another type, in which amikacin is bonded to knitted filamentous velour polyester with a bovine collagen matrix, provides an antibiotic in the prosthetic wall. This type of construction also renders the porous graft impervious to leaks, which eliminates the need for preclotting.

Bonded albumin also reduces porosity and potential thrombosis. Older style porous grafts required bonding. This was achieved by "baking on" autologous plasma. A porous graft was soaked in the patient's plasma or in allogeneic albumin and was then steam sterilized. This thermal process altered the fibrin and protein elements in plasma.

Woven Polyester

The weave of woven polyester (Dacron) grafts is tight enough to be leakproof; therefore these grafts do not require preclotting. Dacron is strong, flexible, and can be collagen coated. Dacron grafts are durable and usually do not need to be replaced.[2]

Polytetrafluoroethylene

The microporous wall of polytetrafluoroethylene (PTFE) serves as a lattice framework into which cells grow to become a microthin lining for contact with blood. These prostheses (Gore-Tex) do not require preclotting. Vascular grafts that are constructed of expanded and reinforced PTFE maintain dimensional stability. Configuration may be straight, tapered, or bifurcated. It may be supported by external rings to resist compression.

During the surgical procedure the inside lumen of the graft may be seeded with the patient's own endothelial cells to sustain patency. The graft may be bonded with an antibiotic before implantation to prevent infection.

Composite Vein Grafts

A composite graft of autogenous vein and synthetic, usually PTFE, may be the surgeon's choice as a substitute for an insufficient length of saphenous vein. The prosthetic graft is anastomosed to a segment of reversed or in situ autogenous vein. The prosthetic graft is cut to match the diameter of the vein.

Conservative Interventional Techniques

Peripheral vascular disease is often managed by a team of collaborating vascular surgeons, cardiologists, and radiologists. Multifaceted care encompasses invasive interventional procedures to treat occlusive disease conservatively. Endovascular procedures are considered minimally invasive conservative management. Vascular instruments and supplies for an open surgical procedure should be immediately available in the event a vessel is perforated or injured during any of the conservative interventional techniques. A perforation may be closed with sutures; a patch graft, in situ conduit, or synthetic prosthesis may be required.

Percutaneous Transluminal Angioplasty

Severe ischemia or incapacitating claudication (pain in a limb) resulting from localized or segmental stenosis or occlusive disease can be conservatively treated by recanalization to restore the lumen in the obstructed vessel.

Atherosclerosis in the iliac, femoral, and popliteal arteries is the most common indication for percutaneous transluminal angioplasty (PTA). Cardiac stents can be placed for coronary artery blockages. Stenosis in the renal arteries also can be treated. Stenotic renal arteries cause hypertension.

PTA is performed under local anesthesia and fluoroscopy, often in the interventional radiology department by a radiologist, in the angiography or cardiac catheterization laboratory by a cardiologist, or in the OR by a surgeon.

The area over the target vessel is anesthetized by local infiltration. In the Seldinger technique the artery is punctured percutaneously with a large-bore needle and a guidewire is introduced through the lumen of the needle. The needle is withdrawn and a plastic dilator sheath is advanced over the guidewire into the vessel. The guidewire is removed once the dilator sheath is seated in the vessel. Care is taken to secure the guidewire on the sterile instrument table in case it is needed again. The endovascular device is passed through the dilator sheath for the performance of several types of percutaneous intravascular procedures. The sheath can be peeled back and removed once the endovascular device is in place. Various techniques are used to dilate a stenotic lesion or displace or ablate a plaque by endovascular methods.

Balloon Angioplasty

A Gruentzig or other type of balloon dilation endovascular catheter is passed over the guidewire and positioned across the lesion. Catheters of several diameters with balloons of various widths and lengths are available. Determination of the appropriate balloon size and length is made on the basis of angiogram findings. When the balloon is inflated with a saline-based contrast medium, atheromatous material is compressed and displaced against the arterial wall. It remolds and cracks, splitting the plaque and intima (inner lining) and stretching the media (middle layer) and adventitia (outer layer), thus dilating the lumen of a stenosis or recanalizing an occlusion. The balloon is repeatedly inflated and deflated until the lumen is dilated. Balloon angioplasty is done before expanding a stent in the dilated lumen to maintain patency.

Intraluminal Stent

A prosthetic stent may be placed along the vessel wall to maintain patency after endovascular balloon dilation. The Palmaz stent, for example, is a stainless steel or cobalt chromium mesh tube mounted coaxially on a balloon angioplasty catheter. After the stent is positioned in the artery the balloon is inflated to expand the stent. The stent remains in place when the balloon is deflated and removed. Stents made of titanium, polypropylene, or other materials either operate in a similar manner or are self-expanding (Fig. 44.9).

A specialized method of performing carotid stenting uses a cerebroprotective guidewire and netlike sheath to prevent migration of particulate to the brain (Fig. 44.10). The protective net is positioned before the stent is inserted and deployed. Carotid stents are not always as effective as stents used in other vessels. The postoperative complications such as ischemic stroke are shown in studies to be higher in endovascular patients than in those who had conventional open endarterectomy.[3]

Laser Angioplasty

With laser angioplasty a laser fiber is introduced into an occluded artery to destroy plaque or thrombi. The laser usually is used to

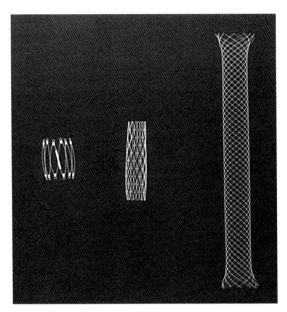

• **Fig. 44.9** Examples of intraluminal vascular stents.

supplement balloon angioplasty. The procedure may be done percutaneously or as an open surgical procedure via an angioscope. Several different types of laser probes are available. The physician selects the most appropriate probe on the basis of the location and size of the artery and the determination of the degree of calcification in plaque or other cause of obstruction. The delivery system determines the mechanism of action, as follows:

- *Thermal laser:* A thermal laser uses argon or neodymium:yttrium-aluminum-garnet (Nd:YAG) laser energy to heat the tip of a metal probe at the end of a fiberoptic catheter to a temperature between 392° F and 752° F (200−400° C). Plaque is vaporized as the tip is moved through the obstruction. This "hot tip" technique may cause some damage to vessel walls. The laser fiber may be positioned within a balloon to destroy the thrombus selectively or seal the arterial wall while the vessel is dilated. A temperature between 203° F and 230° F (95−110° C) in the surrounding tissues dries and disintegrates the thrombus. The combination of pressure from the inflated balloon and diffuse laser energy adheres the loose flaps of arterial tissue back onto the arterial wall; this process is known as *arterial welding.*

- *Photothermal laser:* A photothermal laser uses contact Nd:YAG laser energy. A sapphire-tipped probe or catheter heats plaque by a photopic effect at the point of contact for vaporization of plaque. This is followed by rapid cooling to prevent damage to the intima.

- *Photochemical laser:* A photochemical laser uses an excimer laser with pulsed energy or a tunable dye laser to destroy plaque with minimal generation of heat. With the athermal action of a "cold laser," the intima is not damaged. Heavily calcified plaque cannot be ablated by an excimer laser.

- *Photoablation:* An excimer laser with a special catheter can vaporize plaque by advancing the catheter into the plaque and ablating it with short bursts. The plaque is reduced to tiny particles and absorbed by the surrounding tissue. The use of the excimer laser prevents widespread thermal tissue damage and subsequent stenosis of the vessel.

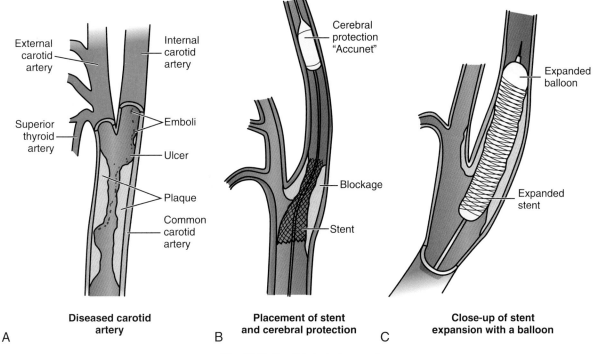

* **Fig. 44.10** Carotid stent placement.

Intravascular Ultrasonic Energy

An ultrasonic probe on the tip of a catheter can be used to recanalize occluded or stenosed peripheral vessels. Ultrasound can be used in combination with low-power lasers.

Atherectomy

In an atherectomy, catheter-mounted instruments are used for transluminal removal of atherosclerotic plaque. A high-speed rotating cam, burr, or side cutter is positioned under fluoroscopic guidance. The plaque is pulverized and retrieved to restore the patency of the vessel. These instruments may be used intraoperatively.

Thrombectomy and Embolectomy

For a thrombectomy and embolectomy a local anesthetic is infiltrated percutaneously. A 2 to 7-Fr Fogarty catheter is inserted proximally and advanced into a vessel distally beyond a soft thrombotic obstruction. The catheter stylet is removed. The balloon on the tip is then inflated with 0.05 to 2 mL of injectable heparinized saline solution according to the size of the balloon diameter. The amount of solution that can be safely used to inflate the balloon is listed on the inflation port. The balloon diameters range between 4 and 14 mm. As the catheter is withdrawn, thrombotic or embolic material is removed to restore blood flow to an extremity. Complications of catheter treatment include perforation of the vessel leading to a fistula formation that may need surgical repair.[4]

This procedure may be performed with fluoroscopy to selectively cannulate vessels. Different types and sizes of catheters and balloons may be used when the blockage is in a native vessel or an artificial graft (Fig. 44.11). Care is taken to use latex-free catheters when a patient is sensitive to latex products.

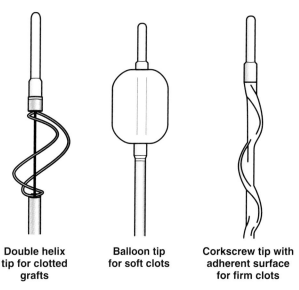

| Double helix tip for clotted grafts | Balloon tip for soft clots | Corkscrew tip with adherent surface for firm clots |

* **Fig. 44.11** Fogarty embolectomy catheter tips in close-up view.

Chronic venous insufficiency can develop with repeated venous thrombosis. This is more common in males than females. If the thrombus forms in the deep veins of the leg, valves can be destroyed, resulting in 30% recurrence within a year. The risk for forming venous stasis ulcers is high.

Closure Devices

Arterial closure devices are commonly used to close percutaneous puncture sites in place of manual compression.[5] Closure devices come in a variety of sizes and can be specific for an area, such as the femoral artery. Various size sheaths contain hemostatic agents or devices. A closure device may deploy suture, sealants, clips, a plug, or a disc. Complications include device failure, infection, and thrombosis.

Thrombolytic Therapy

In thrombolytic therapy, streptokinase, urokinase, or tissue-type plasminogen activator (t-PA) may be administered by local bolus infusion or x-ray—directed catheter into the occluded vessel or directly injected into the thrombus over 12 to 24 hours. Most clots break up within 24 hours. The patient is given IV sedation and local infiltration anesthesia. As the thrombolytic drug enters the vessel, the patient will feel a systemic warm feeling. An x-ray contrast medium will be used to monitor the position of the clot. Streptokinase is contraindicated in patients with a streptococcal infection.

The thrombolytic drugs activate plasminogen and cause liquefaction of fibrin, thus dissolving the clot or loosening it for removal by a balloon catheter. Thrombolytic therapy may be used in conjunction with angioplasty or infused intraoperatively, especially in tibial vessels, for lower limb salvage.

Streptokinase

Treatment for DVT, pulmonary embolus, or another clotted vessel is facilitated by the use of streptokinase. Streptokinase is derived from a form of β-hemolytic streptococci and has an indirect effect that breaks down fibrin. It may not be effective for patients who have antibodies against streptococcus infections. Clots more than 1 week old are not treated with this drug.

The maximum effectiveness of streptokinase is evident within 10 minutes. Reversal of the anticoagulant effect can be accomplished by administering cryoprecipitate or fresh frozen plasma. Some patients have a sensitivity reaction that can progress to anaphylaxis. Pretreatment with antihistamines and steroids may be indicated.

Urokinase

Urokinase is administered directly into the clot with a catheter in an interventional procedure room equipped with x-ray and fluoroscopy capabilities. Care is taken not to damage the endothelial lining of the vessel. Urokinase causes fewer sensitivity reactions than streptokinase, but it is expensive to produce. It is derived from fetal kidney cells and urine, and it is reconstituted with sterile water without a bacteriostatic agent.

Tissue-Type Plasminogen Activator

More recent advances in thrombolytic therapy include t-PA, a chemical that occurs naturally as a secretion of the endothelial cell lining of vessels. Several t-PA activators include tenecteplase, alteplase, and reteplase. These agents can be given as a bolus injection or an infusion.[6] However, there is a risk for bleeding when t-PA is used.

Vascular Surgical Procedures

If conservative therapy is unsuccessful or contraindicated, an open surgical procedure may be indicated.

Arterial Bypass

Occlusive disease or trauma may cause arterial blockage, or arterial injury may indirectly occur near the site of a fracture. The vessel lumen located above and below the lesion is usually normal. Vascular reconstruction is performed in an attempt to restore normal circulation. The surgeon selects an appropriate method to bypass the obstruction, as follows:

- The involved segment may be excised and the ends anastomosed if they can be approximated without tension.
- If direct anastomosis is impossible, the involved segment is excised, and an autograft or synthetic prosthetic graft is used as a replacement.
- The lesion can be bypassed using the long saphenous vein from one thigh as a vein graft, or a synthetic prosthetic graft may be used. The ends of the graft are anastomosed to the artery proximal and distal to the lesion. The obstructed segment of the artery is not resected.
- The lesion can be bypassed by interposing a prosthetic graft through the subcutaneous tissues between a patent artery and the artery distal to the lesion; this procedure is known as an extraanatomic bypass. For example, in a femoral-femoral bypass the graft is placed from the femoral artery of the unaffected leg to the femoral artery of the ischemic leg. In an axillofemoral bypass the graft is placed from the axillary artery to the femoral artery of the ischemic leg.

Femoropopliteal Bypass

The femoral artery is most prone to obstruction by occlusive vascular disease in a lower extremity. A femoropopliteal bypass, the most commonly performed bypass procedure in an extremity, may be the procedure of choice for severe ischemic disease and limb salvage (Fig. 44.12).

The patient is placed in the supine position on the OR bed with the thigh of the affected leg slightly abducted and the knee flexed and supported. The entire extremity is prepped and draped to allow adequate exposure. Incisions are made over the femoral

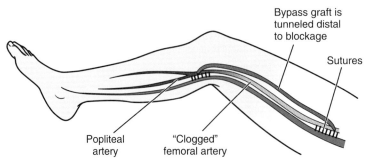

• **Fig. 44.12** Femoropopliteal bypass graft.

and popliteal arteries to expose them and explore the area before bypassing the obstruction in the femoral artery. An autogenous in situ saphenous vein graft, PTFE or noncrimped velour graft, or composite graft may be used.

Anastomoses may be visualized with an angioscope. During the surgical procedure, pulsations of the proximal and distal popliteal artery, as well as pulsations in the foot, are checked with a sterile Doppler pulse detector. A skin marker may be used to mark the location of the distal pulses for quick assessment.

Endarterectomy

Atherosclerotic plaque may cause localized stenosis in the major peripheral arteries. An endarterectomy involves the excision of the diseased endothelial lining of the artery and the occluding atheromatous deposits; this leaves a smooth lining (Fig. 44.13). Loosely attached plaque may be removed by dissection in the media with wire-loop strippers, spatulas, and/or catheters.

A long-segment endarterectomy may be facilitated in the iliac, femoral, and popliteal arteries with a powered oscillating endarterectomy valvulotome or other high-speed drill, to pulverize plaque as described for atherectomy. A saphenous vein or patch graft may be used to close the arteriotomy site. Plaque also can be vaporized from femoral and carotid arteries with a laser or laser/ultrasound. Subsequent inflammation and fibrosis are minimal, and healing is rapid.

Carotid Endarterectomy

One of the most common vascular procedures, a carotid endarterectomy, is performed to prevent a brain attack (stroke) in a patient with severe carotid artery insufficiency. Atherosclerotic plaque at the bifurcation of the common carotid and/or in the internal and external carotid arteries causes localized stenosis or ulceration that impedes cerebral blood flow. Endarterectomy is indicated when this stenosis causes TIAs.

This procedure can be performed with the patient under superficial and deep regional cervical block, or a general anesthesia may be preferred to preserve metabolic demands. The patient

should be continuously monitored by electroencephalogram (EEG) or computerized EEG topographic brain mapping (CETBM) to assess cerebral circulation and neurologic deficits.

The patient is placed in the supine position with the head turned away from the affected side. The head is placed in a donut, and a small roll is placed behind the shoulders to hyperextend the neck. Care must be taken not to place undue extension on the neck because such pressure may occlude vertebral arterial blood flow. The skin is prepped without causing excessive pressure or massage over the carotid artery, which could dislodge the plaque and cause an embolic event in the brain.

An oblique, 4-inch incision is made over the lateral neck on the affected side. The subcutaneous tissue, the platysma muscle, and the anterior border of the sternocleidomastoid muscle are incised. Retraction of the sternocleidomastoid muscle and jugular vein allows exposure of the common carotid artery and its internal and external branches.

After systemic heparinization administered by the anesthesia provider, angled vascular instruments are used to clamp above and below the occluded area. In certain instances an intraluminal shunt is inserted in the artery above and below the clamp to bypass blood flow to the brain while the artery is opened and the plaque is removed. Many surgeons routinely use a shunt, whereas other surgeons prefer an alternative means of cerebral protection, such as deliberate production of mild to moderate hypertension or hypercapnia. Cerebral protection during carotid cross-clamping is a primary concern to prevent serious postoperative neurologic complications.

An arteriotomy (incision in an artery) is made in the common carotid artery below the plaque and is extended upward; in the internal and external carotid arteries it begins above the plaque and extends downward. The plaque is dissected free with a swivel-knife or elevator and is removed in its entirety. In addition, most of the underlying media layer is removed. A headlight and magnifying loupes are worn by the surgeon to enhance visibility during dissection and closure of the arteriotomy. To check blood flow, a Doppler pulse detector is used after the artery is closed.

A PTFE or saphenous vein patch graft angioplasty or bypass grafting is occasionally necessary if an adequate lumen cannot be established. Bilateral endarterectomies may be indicated for severe bilateral occlusion, but the surgical procedures are performed at least a week apart. Complete occlusion is not amenable to surgical treatment because the pressure in the restored artery can be greater than the distal tissue can tolerate, causing severe damage.

Aneurysmectomy

An aneurysm is a localized abnormal dilation in an artery that results from the mechanical pressure of blood on a vessel wall that has been weakened by biochemical alterations. There are three types of aneurysms—pseudoaneurysms, true aneurysms, and dissecting aneurysms.

A pseudoaneurysm is usually caused by a break in the integrity of the vessel wall. The integrity can be breached by iatrogenic treatment during vascular procedures such as passing a stent or embolectomy. The pressure from inside the vessel causes all the layers of the vessel to separate and bulge. This can happen in any artery and requires an open surgical repair.

A true aneurysm does not separate all the layers of the arterial wall. The aneurysmal bulge forms in the media layer. These can take two forms—saccular or fusiform. A fusiform aneurysm is a uniform circumferential dilation. Less common is a saccular

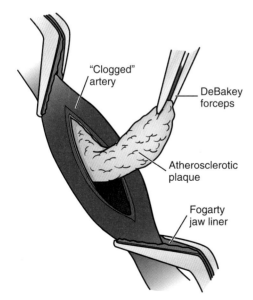

• **Fig. 44.13** Endarterectomy. Removing atherosclerotic plaque from an artery with Fogarty clamps in place.

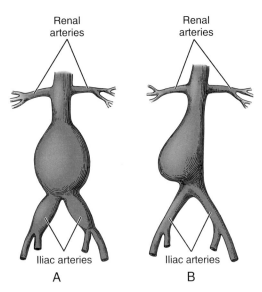

• **Fig. 44.14** Abdominal Aortic Aneurysm Between Renal and Iliac Arteries. **A,** Fusiform (circumferential) type. **B,** Saccular (saclike) type.

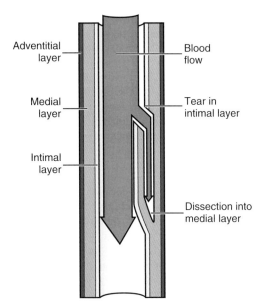

• **Fig. 44.15** Arterial Dissection. The intimal layer tears, and a false passage develops and fills with blood.

aneurysm, a saclike outpouching in the media of the vessel wall (Fig. 44.14).

An infection of the lining of the heart (bacterial endocarditis) can predispose the patient to the formation of a mycotic aneurysm. The microorganisms form vegetations on the leaflets of the heart valves that are ejected into the arterial circulation. The vegetations attach to a normal or diseased artery wall, causing an aneurysm to form and expand. Mycotic aneurysms can occur in true aneurysms or pseudoaneurysms, particularly at a point of bifurcation. Most mycotic aneurysms are found in the aorta, but they can occur in the femoral, carotid, cerebral, or brachial arteries. Multiple sites have been found in the same patient and can persist despite surgical treatment.

A dissecting aneurysm creates a false passage for blood between the intima and the media. The dissection can extend the full length of the aorta, causing damage to the vascular attachments of major organs such as the bowel and kidneys. Cystic medial necrosis causes a dissecting aneurysm, usually in the thoracic aorta, in which the media separates from the intima (Fig. 44.15).

Thoracic dissection requires a thoracotomy and replacement of the diseased portion of the aorta. Fig. 44.16 depicts the repaired ascending and descending aorta using synthetic graft material.

Atherosclerosis is the most common cause of a true aneurysm, but trauma also may be a factor. The abdominal aorta, thoracic aorta, aortic arch, and popliteal arteries are the vessels most often affected. Diagnostic evaluation combines a physical examination, laboratory findings, and the results of ultrasonography, CT scan, MRI, and aortography and/or angiography.

The location and extent of the lesion determine the operability of the aneurysm and the type of reconstruction.[7] For example, cross-clamping of the descending thoracic aorta to remove an aneurysm will impair blood supply to the spinal cord. Preservation methods must be used.

Repair in the arch or ascending aorta can impair cerebral and coronary perfusion. Descending and abdominal aortic aneurysms affect blood flow through the visceral, mesenteric, and renal arteries. Vital structures must be protected during aneurysmectomy.

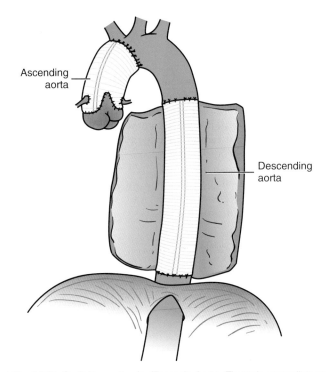

• **Fig. 44.16** Graft Examples for Thoracic Aorta. Thoracic ascending and thoracic descending repairs.

A ruptured aneurysm is a surgical emergency and precludes further evaluation. A transbrachial or transfemoral occluding balloon catheter may be placed in the aorta to prevent an exsanguinating hemorrhage. The surgical procedure is performed immediately. A ruptured abdominal aortic aneurysm (AAA) has a mortality rate over 80%.

Open Resection of an Abdominal Aortic Aneurysm

An AAA usually develops between the renal and iliac arteries (infrarenal), although it can occur anywhere along its course. An abdominal aneurysmectomy may be a lifesaving procedure. Serious hazards, including massive hemorrhage, ischemic organs, and injury to ureters and other nearby structures, are associated with the procedure. Renal failure is a potential complication. Modern techniques have greatly reduced elective AAA open resection 30-day mortality to between 4.4% and 8.6%.[8] Survivors of the procedure enjoy the same life expectancy as do other patients with comparable atherosclerotic disease. Early detection is key. Resection at 1.8 to 1.9 inch (4.5–5 cm) is usually successful.

Constant monitoring of cardiac function with a Swan-Ganz pulmonary artery catheter is used in these high-risk patients. Patients in an unstable condition may require frequent blood gas determinations. Central venous pressure monitoring is a guide for regulating fluid replacement. Blood must be available for transfusion. Autotransfusion may be used if massive hemorrhage is encountered, such as with a ruptured AAA. An indwelling Foley catheter is inserted preoperatively, and urinary output is monitored by the anesthesia provider. Mannitol can be infused before aortic cross-clamping to prevent ischemic renal failure. Prolonged cross-clamping can lead to spinal cord or bowel ischemia.

Somatosensory evoked potential (SSEP) monitoring measures primarily dorsal column (sensory) function and minimal anterior cord (motor) function. A time clock should be used to measure the amount of time the aorta is clamped.

Blood flow in the extremities should be checked immediately preoperatively and postoperatively to detect embolic or occlusive problems. Marking the location of the posterior tibial and dorsalis pedis pulses with a marking pen enables rapid location of the appropriate site when they need to be checked intraoperatively. An audible Doppler device generally is used.

In an open AAA resection, a long midline incision from the xyphoid process to the pubis is used. During surgery for an AAA, the abdomen is thoroughly explored, the small intestinal mesentery is mobilized, and the posterior peritoneum overlying the aorta is incised to expose the aneurysm. A bed-mounted, self-retaining abdominal retractor and blades helps provide needed exposure (Fig. 44.17).

The small intestine and ascending colon are delivered outside the abdomen to increase exposure and prevent injury. Warm moist tapes, moist radiopaque towels, silastic sheeting, or a Lahey (bowel) bag may be used to protect these structures. The incisions will extend into the anterior thighs for exploration of the femoral arteries.

Although the situation may be urgent or emergent, care is taken to account for any item placed in the abdomen. If counts are aborted because of the patient's condition, documentation in the patient's permanent record should include that the count was not performed, as well as the reason for not performing it. The count should not be listed as incorrect. An abdominal x-ray should be obtained as the patient's condition permits. If known items are packed into the patient for later removal, the numbers and types of items should be documented on the patient's record and reported in the handover report to the postanesthesia care unit (PACU).

An extended posterior retroperitoneal approach may be preferred, especially in a patient who is obese or has had previous abdominal surgery. The patient is placed in the right lateral position with the left side up. An oblique flank incision is extended along the superior margin of the 12th rib, which may be resected. The entire abdominal aorta and left renal artery are exposed by

• **Fig. 44.17** Abdominal aorta exposure for resection.

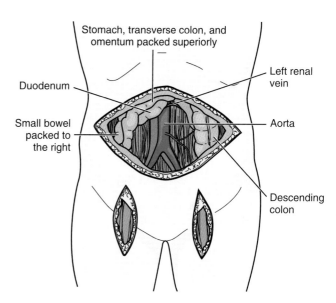

• **Fig. 44.18** Incisions used for aortic aneurysms that involve the femoral arteries.

opening the retroperitoneum without needing to enter the pleural or peritoneal cavities.

The kidney, ureter, and peritoneal sac are reflected anteromedially and packed with moist tapes. Exposure is maintained with self-retaining and handheld retractors. If access to the iliac or femoral arteries is required, the patient's hips are rotated to a semiprone position, and longitudinal incisions are made in the bilateral groins (Fig. 44.18).

Before occlusion of the aorta, blood is drawn if needed for preclotting the graft. Heparin is injected by the anesthesia provider for anticoagulation. Aortic clamps are placed proximal to the aneurysm, and the iliac arteries are clamped distally. The distal aortic stump or iliac arteries may be closed with staples. If the aneurysmal wall is opened, clots and loose intraluminal debris are

• **Fig. 44.19** Abdominal Aortic Graft Example. The abdominal aorta and bilateral femoral arteries have been repaired with synthetic graft material.

• **Fig. 44.20** Pseudoaneurysm. The endothelial (tunica intima) and the muscular (tunica media) layers separate, causing a bulge in the outer connective tissue layer of the artery.

removed. A tube graft is used if the aneurysm is confined to the aorta. More commonly, a bifurcated graft is sutured in place above the aneurysm and to the common iliac or femoral arteries distally (Fig. 44.19).

Branches of other arteries are anastomosed to the graft as necessary, depending on the segment of aorta being replaced. The graft is commonly placed inside the aneurysm (open inclusion method), and the sac is closed over the graft. With the less commonly used closed exclusion method, the graft is placed beside the unopened aneurysm sac.

Living tissue, either the aneurysm sac or the mesentery, must cover the prosthesis to prevent contact of the prosthesis with the intestines; otherwise a fistula can develop. After the aortic clamps are released, the anastomoses are checked for leakage. The incision is usually closed with nonabsorbable sutures; retention sutures are commonly used to support a long midline abdominal incision.

Pseudoaneurysm

Injury to the arterial layers causes blood to accumulate in the local connective tissue surrounding the vessel, forming an enlarging bulge that can rupture and hemorrhage. Pseudoaneurysm, sometimes referred to as a false aneurysm, commonly arises from an iatrogenic source. One example is an arterial intravascular procedure such as cardiac catheterization. The most common site is the femoral artery. Pseudoaneurysm differs from true aneurysm because it is caused by an outside source rather than vascular pathology (Fig. 44.20).

Repair of a pseudoaneurysm is performed in the OR and may require the use of a small patch of natural or synthetic graft. Some success has been achieved with localized thrombin injection under ultrasound guidance. Complications include embolization and compression of nerves and tissues in the area.

Endovascular Abdominal Aortic Aneurysm Repair

Endovascular aneurysm repair (EVAR) or AAA repair has the same indications as an open repair. The risk for rupture increases as the diameter of the aneurysm expands, especially if the diameter exceeds 0.5 cm per year. Not all AAAs can be repaired via the endovascular route. Anatomic criteria include having an adequate length of aorta between the renal arteries, the iliac arteries, and the aneurysmal bulge. If the anatomic diameter of the aorta exceeds 28 mm, the graft will not work.

Endovascular grafts can be modular or one piece with limbs that extend into the iliac arteries (Fig. 44.21).[9] The procedure is done by performing bilateral femoral cut-downs and placing guidewires cephalad into the aorta through the femoral artery on the ipsilateral (closest) side.

Aortograms are performed using full-strength contrast medium and a power injector. For a modular aortic stent, the first limb and body of the graft are placed up the guidewire using C-arm guidance and deployed into position. It is pulled caudad into position in the ipsilateral iliac artery and expanded with a balloon filled with half-strength contrast medium to seat the anchors. The second limb is introduced via the contralateral femoral artery and deployed. A unibody design with both limbs attached is positioned in the same manner; however, both distal limbs are seated into the iliac arteries at the same time and expanded.

Advantages of endovascular repair include smaller incisions, less blood loss, and shorter hospital stay. Disadvantages include the possibility of converting to an open method if a complication arises, endo leak, embolism, and renal artery occlusion.[9] Graft-related complications can lead to the need for additional procedures.

Standby instrumentation for an open procedure is a must. Blood salvage devices should be used. Doppler and warming/cooling

• **Fig. 44.21** Endovascular repair (ipsilateral and contralateral) of abdominal aortic aneurysm with a modular endograft.

devices should be used as needed throughout the procedure. The team should exercise all precautions for blood and radiation exposure. The guidewires and graft deployment devices are very long and require an extended sterile table setup.

Embolectomy

An embolus is a mass of undissolved matter carried by the bloodstream until it lodges in a blood vessel and occludes it. An embolus may be an air bubble, fat globule, blood clot, clump of bacteria, piece of tissue, or foreign body. The occlusion of a blood vessel by an embolus causes various symptoms depending on the size and location. The occlusion of a vessel in the brain, lungs, or heart can cause rapid and sudden death.

Surgical intervention is the primary treatment for an embolus unless contraindicated. Select patients may be treated with heparin, vasodilators, and perhaps sympathetic blocks. Renal or mesenteric emboli are usually treated by surgical embolectomy or bypass grafting. With an embolectomy the affected blood vessel is incised and the embolus is removed.

Pulmonary Embolus

The occlusion of a pulmonary artery or one of its branches usually occurs with emboli that originate from veins in the lower extremities or pelvis. Emboli pass up the inferior vena cava to the right side of the heart and are ejected from the right ventricle into the pulmonary artery. A pulmonary embolism may be diagnosed by lung scans, pulmonary angiograms, and phlebograms.

Pulmonary Embolectomy

A massive pulmonary embolism can cause irreversible cardiac arrest or profound refractory hypotension and hypoxemia. If portable cardiopulmonary bypass equipment is available, cannulas can be inserted at the patient's bedside or in the emergency department or intensive care unit. The patient is then transported to the OR. A median sternotomy is performed to establish total cardiopulmonary bypass and allow access to the pulmonary artery.

Large pulmonary emboli are removed by manual extraction (Trendelenburg operation), the passage of forceps into both the right and left pulmonary arteries, the passage of balloon catheters into pulmonary arterial segments, and squeezing both lungs to force peripheral thrombi through a pulmonary arteriotomy. The incision can be extended for vena cava ligation to prevent recurrent embolization.

Pulmonary Thromboendarterectomy

Chronic pulmonary thromboembolic disease may develop from failure to resolve a massive pulmonary embolus, repeated embolic episodes, or a combination of both. The removal of obstructions in the main pulmonary arteries by thromboendarterectomy improves right cardiac hemodynamics. The procedure is performed with the patient under induced hypothermia and cardiopulmonary bypass; thrombi are removed from the upper, middle, and lower branches of the right pulmonary artery and then from the left pulmonary artery.

Vena Cava Filter

Venous stasis in the deep veins of the lower extremities and pelvis can cause clotting and the potential for embolization via the vena cava through the right atrium to the lungs. Patient conditions that require prophylactic protection from venous embolization are described in Box 44.3. A specialized endovascular filter can be placed via the right jugular or femoral vein under fluoroscopic visualization into the vena cava to prevent emboli from traveling to the lungs (Fig. 44.22). The filter is seated above or below the renal arteries depending on the location of the venous thrombus. The ideal filter should have the following characteristics:

- Cost-effective
- Lifetime of device is not time limited
- High filtration without flow interruption
- Low access site thrombosis
- Small-caliber percutaneous insertion and deployment devices
- Repositioned or removed easily
- Secure fixation to vessel wall
- MRI friendly (nonmagnetic)

Vena cava filters are classified as permanent or temporary. Permanent titanium filters are designed to endothelialize to the vessel wall in as soon as 12 days. A clot that is ensnared in the filter eventually dissolves. The Greenfield filter is a permanent implant that traps and holds clots of 3 mm or larger. If preferred, it can be placed through the femoral vein over a guidewire to the level of L2-L3. Greenfield offers filters made of different materials and sizes to accommodate the patient's needs.

Permanent filters are manufactured by many companies. Filters are shaped differently, such as a cone-shaped stainless steel,

---

> **• BOX 44.3 Patient Conditions That Require Prophylactic Protection From Venous Embolization**
>
> - Anticoagulants are contraindicated
> - History of pulmonary embolus
> - Closed-head injury
> - Paralytic spinal cord injury and immobility
> - Pelvic fractures
> - Long-bone fractures
> - Poor cardiovascular reserve
> - Malignancies that cause hypercoagulation

titanium, Phynox (metal alloy), cobalt, or nitinol filter. Filters come in various sizes and lengths, measured from the apex to the base, and are ejected and fixed in position below the renal veins and above the point of juncture of the iliac veins. Hook-like prongs anchor the device in the correct orientation to collect clots.

Angiography is usually performed during the vena cava filter placement procedure, and the appropriate contrast medium should be readily available. For a high-risk patient a filter may be placed at the completion of a diagnostic angiogram. A patient with an enlarged, dilated caval lumen 0.3 mm in diameter caused by right heart failure may require placement of a filter in each iliac artery.

Temporary vena cava filters can be repositioned or removed. The Gunther Tulip vena cava filter manufactured by Cook allows percutaneous insertion and retrieval from 10 to 14 days after insertion and may be useful for either permanent or temporary prophylaxis against pulmonary embolism. Temporary filters can be placed through the brachial or femoral arteries. Prolonged placement may result in unsuccessful retrieval.

A titanium filter does not interfere with CT scans or MRI, but the radiologist should be informed of its presence before any imaging procedure is performed. Older stainless steel models cause distortion on imaging scans and are not safe during MRI because of the magnetic qualities and superheating of the metal. Patients with vena cava filters should be instructed to carry wallet cards with the make and model of filter implanted. After filter placement the patient usually begins anticoagulant therapy.

Complications include lower extremity edema, which may indicate an obstruction in the filter that requires prompt medical thrombolytic attention. Other potential complications include premature deployment of the device, migration toward the right atrium, or fracture of pieces.[10] If the device cannot be repositioned by endovascular methods, an open surgical procedure may be performed.

If a vena cava filter cannot be placed, the blood flow within the vena cava may be partially interrupted or plicated with specialized Moretz clips using an open abdominal retroperitoneal approach. This allows blood to return to the right ventricle of the heart without passage of the emboli to the lungs.

Venous Stasis Disease

When the valves of the veins fail to function normally, increased back pressure of blood causes the veins to become dilated, tortuous, or elongated. These are known as varicose veins. Pain and secondary complications, such as thrombophlebitis and venous stasis ulcers, may follow. It is believed there is a familial

• **Fig. 44.22** Vena Cava Filters. *Left to right:* Kimray-Greenfield, Titanium Greenfield, Simon-Nitinol, Gianturco Bird's Nest, Vena Tech. **A,** Actual filters. **B,** Radiographic images.

tendency toward varicosities caused by incompetent valves, which afflicts both males and females. Habitual long periods of standing, repeated pregnancies, and obesity are other predisposing factors.

A procedure may be performed to bypass a venous obstruction, such as iliac-venous occlusion or femoropopliteal occlusion. Venous valve repair (valvuloplasty) or venous valve transposition may be performed to correct femoral valvular incompetence and severe venous stasis and to salvage the saphenous vein. The perforator or superficial femoral veins may be ligated for severe venous stasis with marked fibrosis and ulcerations. Injection-compression sclerotherapy or laser use to treat varicose veins may be preferred to surgical treatment.

Ligation and Stripping of Varicose Veins

For ligation and stripping of varicose veins in a leg, the saphenous vein is excised in toto with the aid of a semiflexible stripping device; this procedure begins at the ankle. Additional incisions are made along the course of the vein to ligate perforator branches as the stripper is moved upward toward the groin. Perforators and branches are occluded with ligating clips and transected. At the groin an incision is made over the palpated stripper, and the vein is ligated at the saphenofemoral junction.

Preoperatively the surgeon may mark areas of varicosity for incision with the patient standing at the bedside. Some surgeons use indelible markers. During the skin prep, care is taken not to wash away the markings and not to massage areas of potential

thrombus accumulation. After closure of the incisions and the application of dressings, the full length of the leg is wrapped in cotton elastic bandages for compression.

Fasciotomy

Decompression by fasciotomy is the treatment of choice for the prevention of compartment syndrome after acute ischemia in the upper or lower extremity. Vascular compromise can occur after a penetrating or crush injury. Release of the overlying fascia may be indicated for clinical evidence of increased pressure, such as pain, edema, pallor, and diminished sensation.

Epidural Spinal Electrical Stimulation

Epidural spinal electrical stimulation (ESES) may be used to improve nutritional blood flow in patients with severe lower limb ischemia. This can lead to the healing of ischemic ulcers. ESES uses a microscope connected to a television camera, television monitor, and video recorder. Intravital capillary microscopy is performed before and after ESES to measure red blood cell velocity in skin capillaries. With the patient in a sitting position, the dorsum of the foot is placed over the microscope. Fluorescein dye is injected IV, and the time for perfusion of the capillaries is measured. With the patient under local anesthesia and x-ray control, an epidural electrode is placed parallel to the spinal column. After stimulation of the electrode, perfusion in the foot is tested again.

Vascular Shunts

Normal circulation can be altered to increase or decrease blood flow to a specific organ, either temporarily or permanently. A vascular anastomosis or prosthetic device may be used to establish a route for the diversion of blood flow. For example, vascular isolation of the liver can be achieved with an atrial caval shunt. This shunt permits continuous venous return to the ventricle to sustain cardiac output during the repair of traumatized suprahepatic or retrohepatic vena cava and/or hepatic veins. A straight tube or inflatable balloon catheter may be inserted to establish the shunt.

Portosystemic Shunts

A shunt between the portal and systemic venous systems is definitive treatment for esophageal varices complicated by portal hypertension. This surgical procedure may be only palliative. Many patients have progressive liver disease that eventually leads to liver and right-sided heart failure. Shunting does not repair an already damaged liver but can prevent further hemorrhage. Portal hypertension is an increase in portal venous pressure and is caused by the obstruction to intrahepatic blood flow as a result of cirrhosis, hepatitis, or thrombosis. The increased pressure results in venous dilation that causes esophageal varices. The patient also may have ascites. The purpose of the surgical procedure is to reduce portal hypertension and/or portal venous blood flow. The surgeon selects the most appropriate type of shunt to achieve the purpose.

Distal Splenorenal Shunt

Known as the Warren shunt, this procedure involves anastomosis between the splenic vein and the left renal vein. The hilum of the spleen and the tail of the pancreas are exposed through a left subcostal incision. The splenic vein is completely dissected from the pancreas to its bifurcation at the splenic hilum. This technical maneuver preserves portal profusion but eliminates collateral circulation to control bleeding from gastric and esophageal varices by decompression. The splenoportal system must be patent, and there must be adequate distance between the splenic and renal veins for the anastomosis.

An autogenous jugular or external iliac vein graft may be interposed to ensure a tension-free splenorenal anastomosis. A splenectomy may be performed. Other modifications may be made to meet specific patient circumstances.

Mesocaval Shunt

A mesocaval shunt is an option if a splenic vein is too small for a successful splenorenal shunt. A superior mesenteric inferior vena caval shunt is well tolerated by young patients. With a mesocaval shunt the side of the superior mesenteric vein may be anastomosed to the proximal end of the divided inferior vena cava. An interposition autologous vein or synthetic H-graft also may be used to create a shunt between the inferior vena cava and the superior mesenteric vein.

Portacaval Shunt

A portacaval shunt may be performed with end-to-side or side-to-side anastomosis between the portal vein and inferior vena cava, or with an interposition H-graft inserted between the portal vein and inferior vena cava. A ringed PTFE graft may be used, or an autologous graft may be obtained from an internal jugular or saphenous vein. The shunt relieves hypertension by bypassing the obstruction and diverting the return flow of blood to the liver from the portal vein, thus decompressing esophageal varices.

Depending on the type of portosystemic shunt planned by the surgeon, either a subcostal or transabdominal incision may be used. Two suction setups should be available to evacuate the copious amounts of ascitic fluid that can be anticipated when the peritoneum is opened. Both abdominal and vascular setups are prepared.

Pressure within the portal vein is measured with a manometer, via a cannulated branch of the superior mesenteric vein, at the beginning and at the conclusion of the surgical procedure. Because of venous distention and the vascularity of the surgical area, hemorrhage is a major intraoperative hazard. Care is taken to avoid injury to adjacent structures, including the hepatic artery and the common bile duct.

Arteriovenous Shunts and Fistulas

With arteriovenous shunts and fistulas, blood flow from an artery to a vein is established directly and without going through the capillary network. Access to the vascular system through an arteriovenous shunt or fistula is necessary for a patient who is suffering from end-stage renal disease and who is being maintained on long-term chronic hemodialysis.

With the patient under local anesthesia, the endogenous Cimino-Brescia arteriovenous fistula is established internally at the wrist by anastomosis between the radial artery and cephalic vein (Fig. 44.23). This method has the longest functional life of dialysis methods with fewer infections and thrombotic events. This method takes 3 to 4 months to mature before the fistula can be used for dialysis. Creation of a fistula is contraindicated in diabetic patients and patients with peripheral vascular disease.

If the vessels of the wrist and arm are inadequate, a synthetic PTFE graft may be interposed between the artery and vein (Fig. 44.24). A loop fistula may be created with a graft from the brachial artery to the cephalic or basilic vein in the antecubital fossa or from the brachial artery to the axillary vein in the upper arm. A graft access must mature for 3 to 6 weeks before use. The incidence of thrombosis is high.

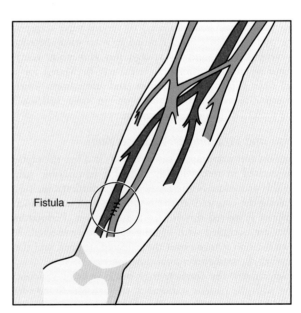

• **Fig. 44.23** Internal arteriovenous dialysis fistula.

• **Fig. 44.24** Internal dialysis graft.

• **Fig. 44.25** External dialysis catheter.

• **Fig. 44.26** Internal dialysis port system.

Enzymatically treated bovine carotid artery xenografts are used occasionally to create arteriovenous shunts or fistulas. Thrombosis and infection are the most common complications. Using a Fogarty balloon catheter, a thrombectomy may reestablish patency. Total explantation of the graft is necessary in the event of a generalized infection.

An external double-lumen dialysis catheter with inflow and outflow tubing that is inserted in the jugular vein to the right atrium can be used for hemodialysis (Fig. 44.25). This type of access is easily inserted and can be used immediately after placement. There is no pain associated with connecting as with percutaneous puncture to access a subcutaneous graft or fistula. Care is taken because these catheters are easily infected and thrombosed. The average usefulness of a catheter is 3 to 6 months. They can be replaced quickly when a problem occurs.

A hemodialysis double-port valve system can be implanted in the anterior chest with two catheters into the right jugular vein to the right atrium (Fig. 44.26). If the right jugular cannot be used, the catheters are passed through the right subclavian vein instead. Placement of the port valves should be planned for patient comfort and tissue stability at 10 or 15 mm beneath the surface of the skin. Pockets are created under the skin in an area that is not compressed by clothing or shoulder straps of handbags.

The exit valve is place laterally and the return valve is placed medially. Standardized placement helps prevent errors during cannulation of the valves during dialysis.

Vascular Anastomosis

The operating microscope is needed for microvascular anastomosis of small vessels to revascularize tissue. Patency of the anastomosis depends on factors related to blood flow, coagulation, and vessel spasm. The vessels must be approximated without trapping adventitia in the lumen. Collagen fibers, tissue thromboplastin, and other thrombogenic factors in the adventitia predispose the patient to rapid platelet aggregation that may cause thrombus formation. Interrupted sutures are placed through the full thickness of the vessel wall (i.e., adventitia, media, and intima).

Veins are technically more difficult to anastomose than are arteries because their walls are thinner and have less substantial muscularis. Anastomoses may be end to end or side to side. An interpositional vein graft may be needed to add length or to bridge a gap between the ends of either an artery or a vein. A patent artery should pulsate distal to the anastomosis. Although this procedure is used most commonly for tissue transplantation (e.g., vascularized free flaps or replants such as severed digits), the peripheral vascular surgeon may be needed to assist with vascular problems that require microvascular techniques.

Laser-assisted vascular anastomosis, also referred to as vascular tissue welding, fuses medium-size (6–8 mm) vessels together to form an anastomosis. The adventitial surface is less thrombogenic than it is after suturing and heals faster with less scar tissue. The argon laser is used for this technique. It may be used to create an arteriovenous shunt at the wrist for hemodialysis, to reattach severed limbs, and to repair damaged vessels.

Limb Salvage

Amputation of a lower extremity may be required for peripheral vascular disease or lymphedema with lymphangitis. All efforts are made to salvage the limb; amputation is the last resort. Ischemia can cause debilitating pain, skin ulcers, and gangrene, often secondary to smoking or diabetes. Revascularization by the techniques described in this chapter may save the patient from the emotional trauma of amputation. This is a prime objective of the peripheral vascular surgeon.

ⓔ EVOLVE WEBSITE

http://evolve.elsevier.com/Hornacky/BerryKohn/

- Historical Perspective
- Tips for the Scrub Person and Circulating Nurse
- Student Interactive Questions
- Glossary

References

1. Jiang Y, Zhang Y, Lu Z, et al.: Liquid embolic agents for interventional embolization, *ChemPhysMater* 1(1):39−50, 2022.
2. Russu E, Muresan A, Ivanescu A, et al.: Polytetrafluorethylene (PTFE) vs. polyester (DACRON) grafts in critical limb ischemia salvage, *Int J Environ Res Public Health* 20:1235, 2023.
3. Saleem T, Baril D: *Carotid stenting*, Treasure Island, FL, 2023, StatPearls. www.ncbi.nlm.nih.gov. (Accessed 1 July 2023).
4. Winters A, McDaniel M, Binongo J, et al.: A comparison of surgical pulmonary embolectomy and catheter-directed lysis for life-threatening pulmonary emboli, *Interact Cardiovasc Thorac Surg* 30(3):388−393, 2020.
5. Moore W, Lawrence P, Oderich G: Atherectomy and arterial closure devices: selection, technique, and results. In *Vascular and endovascular surgery*, ed 9, St. Louis, MO, 2019, Elsevier, pp 271−280.
6. Talha J, Siddiqui A: *Tissue plasminogen activator*, Treasure Island, FL, 2023, StatPearls. www.ncbi.nlm.nih.gov. (Accessed 1 July 2023).
7. Hsu M, Su TW, Su IH, et al.: Use of octopus technique for endovascular treatment of complex aortic lesions, *J Vasc Interv Radiol* 30(4):495−502, 2019.
8. Hammo S, Grannas D, Wahlgren C: Time distribution of mortality after ruptured abdominal aortic aneurysm repair, *Ann Vasc Surg* 86:313−319, 2022.
9. Yei K, Mathlouthi A, Naazie I, et al.: Long-term outcomes associated with open vs endovascular abdominal aortic aneurysm repair in a Medicare-matched database, *JAMA Netw Open* 5(5):e2212081, 2022.
10. Bajda J, Park A, Raj A, et al.: Inferior vena cava filters and complications: a systemic review, *Cureus* 15(6):e40038, 2023.

45

Organ Procurement and Transplantation

CHAPTER OUTLINE

Types of Transplants, 969

Tissue Transplantation, 969

Organ Transplantation, 972

CHAPTER OBJECTIVES

After studying this chapter, the learner will be able to:

- List the criteria for validating brain death.
- Describe the testing performed on tissue before it is suitable for transplantation.
- Discuss the role of the host procurement facility.
- Discuss the psychologic effect of a transplant on the donor and recipient families.

KEY TERMS AND DEFINITIONS

Apnea The absence of breathing.

Benching The sterile process of preparing an organ or tissue for transport to a receiving facility for transplant.

Benching table A sterile field established away from the primary sterile field for the preparation of an organ or tissue for transplant.

Brain death No brain function and no reflexes.

Donor Person, living or dead, who gives an organ or tissue to another person.

En bloc Multiple organs are procured from a donor with vascular and other communications intact.

Procurement The process of surgical removal of an organ or tissue from a donor.

Recipient The person who receives tissue or an organ from another person.

Transplant The process of taking tissue or an organ from one person and surgically placing it into another person.

Types of Transplants

Transplantation is the transfer of an organ or tissue from one person to another or from one body part to another. Concentrated efforts continue in search of compensation for or suitable replacements for deficient tissues and organs. The indication for organ transplantation is irreversible functional failure of the organ. The goals of transplantation include changing appearance, restoring function, or improving quality of life. (More information is available at www.unos.org and www.organdonor.gov.)

Certain tissues and whole organs can be transplanted and grafted to restore bodily function. The type of transplant selected depends on the purpose of the graft, anatomic function, and availability of the tissue or organ. The types of biologic transplants are listed in Box 45.1.

Tissue Transplantation

Some tissues can function normally even after being moved from one area of the patient's body to another (autologous) or after being obtained from another human donor (allogenous), as follows:

- Skin grafts provide a protective surface covering, initially acquiring and then eventually losing vascular connection with the host.
- Corneal grafts replace nonfunctioning corneal tissue.
- Bone grafts afford temporary structural supports and a pattern for regrowth of the host's bone; the grafts are then resorbed.
- Ossicles and the tympanic membrane in the ear can be transplanted to restore bone-conduction hearing loss.
- Cartilage restores contour in a defect of cartilaginous facial structures.

- Blood vessel grafts bypass or replace diseased or obstructed segments of vessels.
- Bone marrow restores hematologic and immunologic functions.
- Heart valves replace stenosed or diseased valves.

Tissue transplants can be either autografts or allografts. Xenograft (from another species) transplants are in the research phases. The American Association of Tissue Banks sets standards for retrieving, processing, storing, and labeling tissues and for donor criteria for allografts (Box 45.2). Tissue for transplantation is procured from suitable cadaver (nonliving or brain dead) donors, either heartbeating or non-heartbeating, or from a living donor. Table 45.1 details the procurement parameters for tissue allografts. (Additional information is available from the National Institute of Transplantation at the United Network for Organ Sharing at www.unos.org.)

Potential donors are screened to avoid the transmission of infection or disease. Multiple cultures are taken at the time of procurement for microbiologic and serologic testing. Tissue is not transplanted until negative test results are obtained; tissue is discarded if the test result is positive. Living bone donors are tested for human immunodeficiency virus (HIV) immediately after donation and again after 90 days because seroconversion can be delayed. Recipients also should be tested and should be negative for HIV, hepatitis B virus (HBV), and hepatitis C virus (HCV). A baseline is essential to establish that the patient was not infected by the act of grafting. Patients with HIV, HBV, or HCV are not barred from receiving an allograft, but baseline data can help rule out causes for rejection or infection. Incidences of graft failure and superinfection are high in patients who are immunocompromised with HIV.

Banked tissues are labeled with the donor's name and identification number, pertinent medical history, the pathology report of the donor, final culture and serology reports of donors, type and site of donation, date and time of procurement, and method of procurement and preservation.

Bone Marrow Transplantation

Bone marrow transplantation is essentially a tissue transplant. However, because this type of transplantation is fraught with the hazards of rejection, bone marrow is procured and transplanted with a protocol similar to that of solid organ procurement and transplantation. Bone marrow is transplanted only after conventional treatments have failed to replenish depleted bone marrow cells. The marrow given via infusion restores hematologic and immunologic functions. Indications for treatment are acute myelodysplastic syndrome, lymphoblastic leukemia, myelogenous leukemia, aplastic anemia, and certain other blood diseases.

Bone marrow transplantation is the only cure for severe combined immunodeficiency disease—a genetic disorder in which a child lacks adequate immune defenses to fight infections. Bone marrow transplants also are given to victims of severe radiation exposure. Contraindications to transplantation are renal or cardiac diseases.

With bone marrow transplantation, blood type and human leukocyte antigen (HLA) compatibility are essential. A bone marrow transplant may be one of the following three types:

1. *Autologous:* The donor is the recipient. Stem cells are collected from the patient with leukemia that is in remission, cryopreserved, and stored to be infused during a subsequent relapse.
2. *Allogeneic:* The donor is HLA-compatible with the recipient. Marrow is procured for immediate infusion into the recipient.
   a. A syngeneic donor, an identical twin, is preferred.
   b. A genotypically compatible sibling or parent has the identical tissue type.
   c. An unrelated allogeneic donor must be HLA-compatible. Graft-versus-host disease (GVHD) is unique to allogeneic bone marrow transplantation. With GVHD, donor T cells immunologically attach to recipient cells and cause tissue damage at the site of antigen localization.
3. *T cell–depleted marrow:* For prevention of GVHD, mature T lymphocytes are removed from donor marrow before infusion into the recipient.

Before transplantation, the recipient is given a high-dose regimen of immunosuppressive chemotherapy to eradicate leukemic, lymphoid, and bone marrow cells, thereby inducing marrow depression. The recipient also receives total body irradiation (TBI) to penetrate the areas resistant to the drugs. During this period of pretransplant preparation, the patient is placed in reverse isolation, preferably in a laminar airflow clean or sterile (germ-free) environment. The patient is closely monitored for the side effects of immunosuppressive chemotherapy and TBI.

After pretransplant protocols have been completed, the donor is hospitalized before the scheduled transplantation. In the OR, with the patient under general or spinal anesthesia, 500 to 700 mL of bone marrow is aspirated at multiple sites from the iliac crests; the sternum also may be used. The marrow is filtered,

TABLE 45.1 Tissue/Allograft Procurement Parameters[a]

Donor Tissue	Physiologic Status of Donor	Time Between Procurement and Grafting	Other Considerations
Cornea			
	Non-heartbeating cadaver donor	Procured 6—8 hours postmortem at room temperature	Corneas are not perfused tissue. Heartbeating status is unimportant. Tissue may be procured in morgue or setting other than OR, under sterile conditions.
		Procured 48 hours postmortem if donor has been refrigerated at 39.2° F (4° C)	Corneas are usually used fresh rather than in cryopreserved state.
		Transplanted fresh 7—10 days after procurement	Corneal tissue is not commonly cryopreserved.
		Cryopreserved cornea may be stored for 1 year	
Skin			
	Non-heartbeating cadaver donor	Procured 6—8 hours postmortem at room temperature	At least 75% of skin surface should be free of abrasions, scars, and deformities to qualify as donor.
		Procured within 24 hours postmortem if refrigerated at 39.2° F (4° C)	Skin is procured before bone and is taken only from below nipples to knees on ventral surface and from scapulae to popliteal area on dorsal surface. Tissue is taken to the depth of dermal layer (split thickness). A 70-kg donor can provide 7—8 ft² of skin.
		Cryopreserved skin can be stored for 5 years at −238° F (−150° C)	Newly procured skin is stored at 39.2° F (4° C) in preservation medium for a maximum of 24 hours. Cryopreserved skin is thawed at room temperature not to exceed 59° F (15° C) for use on recipient.
			Allograft skin is commonly used as a biologic dressing in combination with autograft skin. The recipient autograft is meshed 6:1 and then covered by allograft that has been meshed 2:1. Allograft skin is temporary and is replaced on the recipient every 48—72 hours until natural reepithelialization at the autograft site begins.
Iliac Crest			
	Non-heartbeating cadaver donor	Procured within 12 hours postmortem at room temperature	Bone is procured after the recovery of any other internal organs and skin. Preferably, bone is procured under sterile conditions; however, it may be procured under clean conditions in a setting such as the morgue and secondarily sterilized by ethylene oxide followed by aeration. Sterile bone can be freeze-dried and stored at room temperature.
		Procured within 24 hours postmortem if refrigerated at 39.2° F (4° C) Cryopreserved bone can be stored for 3 years at −112° F (−80° C)	
Joints and Long Bone			
	Non-heartbeating cadaver donor	Procured within 12 hours postmortem at room temperature	Bone is procured after the recovery of any other internal organs and skin. Preferably, bone is procured under sterile conditions; however, it may be procured under clean conditions in a setting such as the morgue and secondarily sterilized by ethylene oxide followed by aeration. Sterile bone can be freeze-dried and stored at room temperature.
		Procured within 24 hours postmortem if refrigerated at 39.2° F (4° C) Cryopreserved bone can be stored for 3 years at −112° F (−80° C)	Joints are not used as joints per se but are cut into pieces to fit a defect. Living nonrelated donor femoral head can be salvaged during total joint arthroplasty procedure and processed for use as bone plug or ground bone grafting tissue.
	Living nonrelated donor (femoral head or rib)		
Heart Valves			
	Non-heartbeating cadaver donor	Cryopreserved valves can be used within 1—2 years	Size match is important.

[a]Tissues are evaluated by condition. Age is not a barrier. For additional information, see www.organdonor.gov.

heparinized, and placed in sterile containers for infusion. The donor is watched for bleeding and may need blood and fluid replacement.

Marrow is infused into the recipient intravenously (IV) or via a Hickman or Broviac catheter over several hours. During this time, the patient is constantly attended and closely monitored for adverse reactions. By an unknown process, the marrow migrates into the marrow cavities of the bones. For 10 to 30 days after transplantation, the recipient may receive daily transfusions of lymphocytes, platelets, and granulocytes, preferably taken from the donor, to counteract the predictable side effects of pretransplant immunosuppressive therapy (mainly hemorrhage and infection).

If the marrow is not from an identical twin, blood is irradiated before transfusion to destroy the lymphocytes. Mature blood cells and platelets are unaffected by the irradiation process. Daily marrow aspirations and complete blood counts are performed on the host. The success or failure of transplantation is usually decided after 10 to 20 days, when the new marrow begins to function.

Organ Transplantation

Organ transplantation can be a lifesaving treatment for some end-stage diseases. More than 42,000 transplants were done in 2022, according to www.organdonor.gov. Although tissue grafts are commonplace, transplantation of functional, whole, vital organs presents physiologic, philosophic, and ethical dilemmas. A biologically related donor (referred to as a living related donor) makes a supreme sacrifice to become an organ donor; therefore cadavers are the primary source of organs for transplant. Organ donation is the ultimate gift of life and is given by the donor to the recipient. Transplantation can restore the recipient to near-normal physiologic status.

Ethical concerns cross religious and cultural boundaries.[1] Table 45.2 gives examples of religious and cultural groups and their positions about organ donation and transplantation. Some traditionalist beliefs do not support donation because the body of the dead should not be altered in any way. Modernist beliefs have transcended many old ways by pointing out that the body is not needed for passage into the afterlife. Information about religious and cultural views about donation can be found at www.organdonor.gov and www.lifebanc.org.

Kidney transplantation was initially the most successful and principal clinical application of organ transplantation. If a kidney graft fails, the patient may survive by returning to hemodialysis indefinitely before receiving another transplant. This option does not exist for transplants of the heart, liver, pancreas, lungs, or digestive system. No practical prolonged artificial support exists for these organs in the event of an allograft failure.

Transplantation of each organ involves unique technical and physiologic problems, but the major barriers and causes of

TABLE 45.2 Organ Donation and Transplantation Beliefs According to Religious or Cultural Groups

Religious or Cultural Group	Donate Organs	Accept Transplant	Notes
African Methodist Episcopal Zion (AME)	Yes, encouraged	Yes	See donation as a way of helping others
Amish	Yes, if assured of successful procedure for recipient	Yes	Use modern medical services
Anglican	Yes	Yes	Church of England stated that donation was a Christian duty
Assembly of God	Individual choice	Individual choice	No official policy
Baha'i	Yes	Yes	Very supportive
Baptist	Individual choice	Individual choice	Process must offer improvement and extension of life
Brethren	Yes	Yes	See donation as a way of helping others
Buddhism	Yes, donors are honored Individual choice	Yes	See donation as an act of compassion
Catholicism	Yes, encouraged as an act of charity and love	Yes	Pope Benedict XVI was an organ donor when serving as Cardinal; not permitted as Pope
Christian Church (Disciples of Christ)	Yes, encouraged to share God's love	Individual choice	Humans were created for the glory of God
Christian Science	Individual choice	Individual choice	Prefer to use spiritual means of healing over medical
Church of the Nazarene	Individual choice	Individual choice	No official policy
Confucianism	Traditional: No Modern: Individual choice	Individual choice	The body was a gift from parents and must not be violated
Episcopal	Yes, encouraged	Yes	Donation part of self-sacrifice for others
Evangelical	Individual choice	Individual choice	No official policy
Greek Orthodox	Yes	Yes	Donation is used to better human life
Gypsy (Romany)	No	Individual choice	Body should be intact at burial for the afterlife
Hinduism	Individual choice; one of the gods, Ganesha, was a young male with an elephant head transplant	Individual choice	No prohibitions; belief in reincarnation is not hindered by donation

TABLE 45.2   Organ Donation and Transplantation Beliefs According to Religious or Cultural Groups—cont'd

Religious or Cultural Group	Donate Organs	Accept Transplant	Notes
Islam	Individual choice	Individual choice	Priority to save human life is supported by Shariah law
Jehovah's Witnesses	Individual choice	Individual choice	Will accept an organ that has been drained of blood
Jesus Christians	Yes, encouraged	Yes	Very small sect; strongly encourage both living and after death donation
Judaism	Yes, encouraged to save a life	Yes	*Pikuach nefesh* is a Halakhic legal concept that permits organ donation to save a life
Lutheran	Yes	Yes	An expression of sacrificial love
Mennonite	Individual choice	Individual choice	No official policy
Moravian	Individual choice	Individual choice	No official policy
Mormon (Church of Jesus Christ of Latter Day Saints)	Individual choice	Individual choice	Encouraged to view the pros and cons before making decision
Pentecostal	Individual choice	Individual choice	No official policy
Presbyterian	Individual choice	Individual choice	No official policy
Protestantism	Yes, encouraged	Yes	Encouraged to donate
Quakers (Society of Friends)	Individual choice	Individual choice	No official policy
Rastafarianism	Not prohibited, but extremely rare	Not accepted because of fear of contamination of the body	Prefer all natural ways of life; the body is only a shell for the spirit
Seventh-Day Adventist	Yes, encouraged	Yes	Sect operates several specialized transplant hospitals
Shinto	No donation from dead bodies; permit living donation	Individual choice, but prefer living donor	The dead body is considered impure and must not be interfered with
Sikhism	Individual choice	Individual choice	The body is of no use when dead; the spirit is reborn into a new body at death; no prohibitions
Taoism	Traditionalist: No donation Modernist: Individual choice; the body is only a shelter for the spirit	Individual choice	Emphasis on natural ways; spirit is unchanged by changes in the body
United Church of Christ	Yes, encouraged	Yes	Very supportive
Unitarian Universalist	Yes, encouraged	Yes	Seen as an act of love
United Methodist	Yes, encouraged	Yes	Suggest all members carry donor cards
Wesleyan Church	Yes, encouraged	Yes	Seen as a Christian act of love

transplant failure are immunologic rejection and infection. Immunodeficiency depends on the amount of immunosuppression the patient receives to prevent rejection. Immunosuppressive agents leave the patient prone to opportunistic infection.[2] Reverse protective isolation may be advisable if the patient has development of leukopenia, a decrease in white blood cells. In other aspects of care, transplant recipients are similar to other critical surgical patients with severe chronic illnesses who need measures that minimize the risk for infection.

The American Society of Transplant Surgeons (www.asts.org) and the International Society of Transplantation meet regularly to exchange ideas and information among people of different scientific backgrounds. The aim is to achieve the best possible patient survival rather than merely transplant survival.

The Organ Transplant Registry of the American College of Surgeons, in conjunction with the National Institutes of Health, collects data on transplantation procedures and approves and funds various registries. The Federal Organ Transplantation and Procurement Act of 1983 provided financial grants for the initial development of regional organ procurement centers and a transplant registry.

A national task force has been established to analyze medical, legal, ethical, economic, and social issues of concern in organ procurement and transplantation.

Organ procurement organizations (OPOs) are regulated by government agencies; they collect organs and tissues from donors, exchange organs geographically, and register patients in need of a transplant. The registry includes information about the patient's blood group and tissue typing. Computer lists of patients waiting for donor organs are maintained by the Organ Procurement and Transplantation Network (OPTN), United Network for Organ Sharing (UNOS), and the North American Transplant Coordinator Organization 24-Hour Alert. Regional organ procurement organizations coordinate with these registries to match donated organs with compatible recipients nationwide. The position of the recipient on the waiting list is determined by the severity of the illness. Pediatric patients are given additional consideration.

Other countries have similar mechanisms. For example, the United Kingdom Transplant Register has membership in the Euro Transplant Register. Organs procured within the United Kingdom can be transported by air to another country in Europe, and vice versa, for a histocompatible recipient. The number of patients awaiting transplants exceeds the supply of available donor organs. As a result, many patients die while waiting for a suitable organ to become available.

Many people carry a signed Uniform Donor Card or other identification (e.g., the reverse side of a driver's license) that states that certain or all organs and tissues may be removed for transplantation in the event of death. Such cards, or a living will, constitute legal written consent under the Uniform Anatomical Gift Act enacted by all 50 states. Written or telephone consent is still obtained from the family of a potential donor before procurement may commence.

Time is paramount when critical organs are involved because their value depends on preservation of maximum functional viability. The time factor is less urgent with less critical tissue. When a potential donor has been identified, a transplantation coordinator contacts the regional registry and procurement team.

Organ Procurement

Immunologic rejection and the shortage of donor organs remain the principal deterrents to transplantation. The goal is selection of a donor-recipient match with adequate histocompatibility to permit an organ to function without complications. Organs and tissues come from two primary sources: cadaver (heartbeating and non-heartbeating) and living related donors (Table 45.3).

Tissue donors are between newborn and 80 years of age. All donors of vital organs must be free of sepsis or malignant processes, between newborn age and 65 years of age, and with good function of the donor organ. Technical aspects of the procurement procedure must ensure the viability of organs throughout the entire period between procurement and transplantation.

Cadaver Donor

Death is confirmed with irreversible cessation of all functions of the brain and brainstem. The criteria for brain death are listed in Table 45.4. For suitability for organ or tissue donation after death, cadaver donors are classified as either heartbeating or non-heartbeating.

Heartbeating donors are those with confirmed brain death in whom the vital organs can be preserved in vivo.[3] In these donors, brain death usually has resulted from severe neurologic trauma, such as head or spinal cord injury, hemorrhage, or anoxia. Death

TABLE 45.3	Organ Procurement Parameters[a]		
Donor Organ	Physiologic Status of Donor	Time Between Procurement and Transplantation	Other Considerations
Heart			
	Heartbeating cadaver donor	3–6 hours, fresh tissue	Heartbeating cadaver donor: total heart and segments of great vessels.
	Non-heartbeating cadaver donor	Cryopreserved valves can be used within 1–2 years	Non-heartbeating cadaver donor: heart valves only. Size match is important.
			Donor criteria include no cardiac disease and normal cardiac enzymes.
Lung			
	Heartbeating cadaver donor	1–4 hours	Heartbeating cadaver donor lung may be given en bloc to one recipient. The lungs may be separated or divided into segments (lobes) for several recipients.
	Living related donor		One lobe from living related donor is transplanted into recipient.
			Size match is important.
			Donor criteria include no evidence of trauma, negative sputum culture, normal chest x-ray.
Heart-Lung En Bloc			
	Heartbeating cadaver donor	1–4 hours	Heartbeating cadaver donor heart and lungs are transplanted en bloc into recipient.
			Size match is important. Donor criteria same as for individual heart or lung donation.
Liver			
	Heartbeating cadaver donor	8–24 hours	Heartbeating cadaver donor liver may be divided into two segments for two separate recipient patients.
	Living related donor		Small segment of living related donor's liver is transplanted into recipient.
			Size match is important.
			Donor criteria include normal liver function, normal liver enzymes and bilirubin, no evidence of trauma.

TABLE 45.3   Organ Procurement Parameters[a]—cont'd

Donor Organ	Physiologic Status of Donor	Time Between Procurement and Transplantation	Other Considerations
Kidney			
	Heartbeating cadaver donor	48–72 hours; ideally should be transplanted within 12 hours	Heartbeating and non-heartbeating cadaver donor kidneys are given to two separate recipients.
	Non-heartbeating cadaver donor in highly selected circumstances	Procured within 45 minutes of cardiac arrest, with immediate in situ cooling	
	Living related donor		One kidney from living related donor is transplanted into recipient.
			Donor criteria include normal renal function, normal serum creatinine, no evidence of trauma.
Pancreas			
	Heartbeating cadaver donor	12–24 hours	Heartbeating cadaver donor pancreas is transplanted as a whole or partial organ for one recipient.
	Living related donor		Tail segment of pancreas from living related donor may be transplanted into recipient.
			Donor criteria include normal pancreatic function, normal blood glucose regulation, normal serum amylase, no evidence of diabetes mellitus, no evidence of trauma.
Kidney-Pancreas			
	Heartbeating cadaver donor	12–24 hours	Heartbeating cadaver donor kidneys and pancreas are simultaneously transplanted into recipient. Usually performed for diabetic nephropathy. Donor criteria are the same as for individual kidney or pancreas donation.

[a]Organs are evaluated by condition. Age is not a barrier. For additional information, see www.organdonor.gov.

TABLE 45.4   Brain Death Criteria

Criteria	Clinical Assessment
Irreversible coma not caused by pharmacologic agent, hypothermia, or unknown cause	No response to external stimuli No cerebral brain activity on EEG over 10 minutes EEG activity has no prognostic value for estimation of cerebellar and brainstem activity
Absence of spontaneous movement, decerebrate posturing, and decorticate posturing Apnea with no spontaneous respiration not influenced by hypothermia or pharmacologic agent	Spinal nerve reflexes may be unaffected because these reflexes do not require cortical (brain) activity Elevated carbon dioxide in the blood is not a stimulus for breathing No spontaneous respiratory effort for 3 minutes when removed from ventilatory assist device $Pa_{CO_2} > 55$ mm Hg
No cranial nerve reflexes	Fixed and dilated pupils Pupils are unreactive to light No corneal reflex (no blinking when cornea is touched) No oculocephalic reflex (doll's eyes) No oculovestibular reflex (no response to ice water instilled in ear) No response to pain on face and head (pin prick, supraorbital pressure) No response to upper or lower airway stimulation (no gag or cough reflex when suctioned or stimulated by endotracheal tube)

EEG, Electroencephalogram.

must occur in a location in which a cardiopulmonary support system is immediately available (i.e., in the emergency department, operating room [OR], or other critical care unit).[3]

For organ donation, an individual who is brain dead is maintained on mechanical ventilation or cardiopulmonary bypass to prevent ischemic damage to the vital organs. Maintenance of a heartbeating donor before and during organ procurement includes the following:

- Systolic blood pressure above 90 mm Hg
- Central venous pressure of 5 to 10 mm Hg
- Hydration with crystalloids and colloids
- Urine output minimum of 100 mL/h (ideally, 200–300 mL/h)

- Ventilation with 100% oxygen
- Core body temperature of 98.6° F (37° C)

Non-heartbeating donors are not suitable for the procurement of parenchymal organs. With non-heartbeating donors, cardiopulmonary or ventilatory support was not provided after brain death. As a result, the major organs have suffered thrombosed vascular structures and ischemia. Skin, bone, heart valves, blood vessels, and corneas may be acceptable for procurement from select non-heartbeating donors (see Table 45.1).

Multiple Organ Procurement

The heartbeating donor is brought to the OR and treated with the same respect and care given to any other patient. A sample multiple organ procurement room setup is depicted in Fig. 45.1. Organs and tissues are removed under sterile conditions by a procurement team and preserved and transported to the recipient. The procurement team includes two surgeons, two assistants, and a scrub person. A circulating nurse and a scrub person from the host facility assist with the procedure. An anesthesia provider also

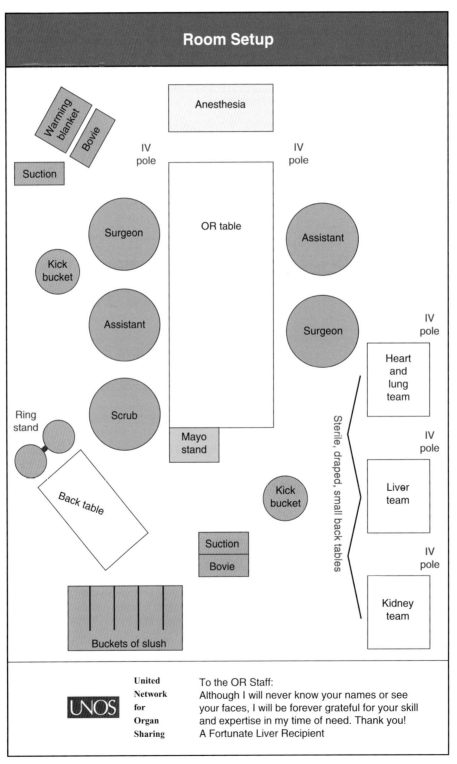

• **Fig. 45.1** Room setup for multiple organ procurement. (From Seifert PC: *Cardiac surgery: perioperative patient care,* St. Louis, 2002, Mosby. Courtesy UNOS, United Network for Organ Sharing.)

Procedure: Organ Recovery—Single or Multiorgan

Skin Prep:	Solution varies according to surgeon preference. Prep from clavicle to mid-thigh.	Position of Patient:	Supine with arms out or tucked, depending on organs to be recovered and surgeon preference. Place warming blanket under patient or use a lower-body Bear Hugger.
Drapes:	Laparotomy drapes are acceptable with a wider area of exposure. Free draping is also acceptable and may be preferred.		

Return electrode, ECG electrodes, and other devices should be placed on the posterior side of the body away from the sterile field.

Sutures and Needles
Depends upon surgeon preference—examples

Ties:	0, 2-0, 3-0, and 4-0 silk ties* #1 and #4 silk ties*
Suture:	2-0 silk on cutting or taper needle* 4-0 & 5-0 prolene on taper needle* 1 or 2 nylon on cutting needle for closure*
Other:	Ligaloops/endoloops, umbilical tapes* Vessel paws, bone wax*
Hold:	Large and small hemaclips Skin stapler with rotating head
Dressing:	Sterile 4x4s* Shroud kit*

* Some organ recovery agencies' customized packs will contain these items. Check with your recovery agency to prevent duplication.
** If no slush machine, contact your recovery agency for the formula for making slush. This procedure needs to be initiated at least one hour prior to the recovery case.

Instruments and Equipment
Specific tray names will vary according to institution

Basic:	Skin prep tray* Gowns × 5-10* Electrocautery units × 2 Lap tapes* Blades - #10 × 3, #15 × 2, #11 × 2* Suction sets × 2-3 (for large fluid volumes) Suction tips × 2 ea. Yankaur, Poole, or octopus Major laparotomy tray	Razors Towels × 5 Grounding pad × 2* Raytec sponges
Special:	Vascular tray Sternal saw Extra long balfour Vascular stapler (hold) Gallbladder dilators (hold)	Assorted vascular clamps Sternal retractor Mallet GIA, LDS (hold) Large basins × 2-3 (hold)
Extras:	Sterile ice Defibrillator with sterile internal paddles available Headlight available Ice machine available or several bags of unsterile ice IV poles (one for each organ to be recovered)	Slush (or capabilities)**

Visiting recovery teams may bring additional items, which you may need to autoclave.

• Fig. 45.1 cont'd

is necessary to maintain vital functions until the aorta is cross-clamped and cardiopulmonary support is no longer needed. A procurement coordinator from an affiliated organ procurement agency or organ bank usually accompanies the team and assists wherever needed throughout the procurement process. The procurement team brings the necessary supplies for packaging the organ and tissue for transport.

The procurement process includes the following functions:
1. The procurement coordinator facilitates the procurement process by:
   a. Obtaining blood samples and arranging tissue typing to assist the organ bank with the potential placement of procured organs.
   b. Documenting necessary information, making any needed phone calls, and coordinating the host facility personnel with the procurement team.
   c. Assisting the physician with communications with the donor family.
   d. Calling the procurement team.
   e. Assisting the circulating nurse and scrub person with the setup of the procurement room.
   f. Bringing the necessary cannulas for organ preservation.
2. The circulating nurse and scrub person assist in the procurement process by:
   a. Gathering sterile supplies, including:
      (1) Laparotomy drape pack and 10 extra medium drapes. Ten or more sets of gowns and gloves are needed.
      (2) Nonabsorbable sutures for ligating ties (usually 0, 2-0, 3-0, 4-0 silk) and for closure (usually a size 2

monofilament suture on a large cutting needle) as requested by the surgeon.
      (3) Ten umbilical tapes at least 30 inches long.
      (4) Four suction canisters and suction tubing with tips.
      (5) Two electrosurgical units, two dispersive electrodes, and handpieces with long and short blades.
      (6) Twelve scalpel blades, No. 10 and No. 15.
      (7) Two packs of bone wax.
      (8) Four Asepto syringes.
      (9) Twenty packs of laparotomy sponges.
      (10) Cold sterile normal saline solution, 6 L, for irrigation.
      (11) Autosuture cart (GIA and TA) for bowel or pancreas donors.
   b. Setting up sterile instrumentation, including:
      (1) Chest tray with sternal saw and self-retaining chest retractor.
      (2) Major abdominal laparotomy tray and large self-retaining abdominal retractor; some teams bring their own sterile instrument trays.
      (3) Vascular tray.
      (4) Minor tray for organ preparation table (benching table).
      (5) Basin set for main table and each benching table.
   c. Providing nonsterile equipment, including:
      (1) Two electrosurgical units and dispersive electrodes.
      (2) Suction containers to accommodate at least 24 L of fluid.
      (3) Power source for sternal saw.
      (4) One IV pole for each benching table.

(5) Warming blanket under the patient.

(6) Defibrillator.

(7) Skin preparation solution.

(8) Sterile saline to make slush, or slush machine if available.

(9) Crushed ice; dry ice is not used for organ preservation.

(10) Head lights for primary surgeons.

d. Medications and blood to have available:

(1) Heparin: 60,000 units.

(2) Furosemide (Lasix): 20 to 100 mg.

(3) Two units of packed red blood cells (typed and crossmatched).

3. The anesthesia provider assists in the procurement process by:

a. Ventilating the donor with 100% oxygen.

b. Monitoring electrocardiogram (ECG), blood pressure, urinary output, and fluid and electrolyte balance.

c. Administering drugs as necessary (e.g., dopamine or dobutamine for vasomotor regulation, muscle relaxants to neutralize spinal reflexes and relax the abdomen, osmotic diuretics for renal function, and heparin for anticoagulation).

d. Monitoring and replacing blood as appropriate.

e. Monitoring and maintaining core body temperature and initiating cooling: Cold fluids (usually saline, lactated Ringer's solution, or Collins solution with 30,000 units of heparin) are infused intravascularly 10 minutes before the aorta and vena cava are cross-clamped for heart removal. After the heart removal begins, the anesthesia provider turns off the anesthesia machine and leaves the room.

4. Incisions are made by the procurement surgeon to provide maximum access to organs and tissues:

a. A midline sternal-splitting incision is made from the suprasternal notch to the pubis to remove vital thoracic and abdominal organs (Fig. 45.2). It takes 2 to 3 hours to procure parenchymal (perfused) organs. Additional incisions are made as necessary.

b. Eyes are enucleated by an eye procurement specialist to preserve the corneas. Glass or plastic globes may be put in the sockets to maintain the shape. An ice pack is placed over the eyelids after procurement of the eyes, and the head is slightly elevated to minimize fluid accumulation. The patient is no longer on the ventilator, so the anesthesia provider is no longer at the head of the table.

c. Skin is taken with a dermatome from flat body surfaces, excluding the upper chest, neck, face, arms, lower legs, and feet (Fig. 45.3). Skin procurement may take 1 to 1.5 hours. Extra absorbent padding is advised because interstitial fluids seep from the tissues.

d. Skin is excised, and the muscles are separated. Long bones and iliac crests are removed in toto (Fig. 45.4) and are replaced with wooden, fiberglass, or metal dowels to maintain structural integrity. Bone procurement may take 5 to 6 hours to complete.

• **Fig. 45.3** For cadaveric allografts, skin is removed with dermatome from anterior and posterior flat surfaces between midchest and knees.

• **Fig. 45.2** Midline sternal-splitting incision from suprasternal notch to pubis is made for procurement of thoracic and abdominal organs from heartbeating cadaver donor.

• **Fig. 45.4** Long bones and iliac crests are procured for bone allografts. Humerus, tibia, and fibula are cut distally. Radius, ulna, and femur are disarticulated at both ends. Pelvis is cut at pubic and sacroiliac joints.

e. Multiple incisional closures may take 1 to 1.5 hours. Care is taken to close the incisions with regard to physical appearance. The family may want open viewing at a funeral home.

5. The sequence of organ removal is coordinated to maintain the viability of the organs. Several small sterile tables should be set up so organ and tissue packaging for transport can be completed away from the main sterile field. Minor dissection instrumentation may be needed for organ benching.

   a. Perfused tissues are taken first.

      (1) The kidneys and liver are mobilized and cannulated for in situ cooling.

      (2) The aorta is cross-clamped, and the heart is removed first, followed by the liver and then the kidneys, pancreas, and intestines. Mesenteric nodes and the spleen are sampled for tissue typing.

      (3) A combined heart-lung procurement (en bloc) may be performed after the other organs have been removed. The organs are removed with their vascular and structural attachments intact. A bronchoscopy may be necessary for assessment of the lungs. The lungs are ventilated during the procurement process, and a prostaglandin drip is infused.

   b. Nonperfused tissues are taken last.

      (1) Enucleation of the eyes for corneal procurement usually follows retrieval of the parenchymal organs.

      (2) Skin is taken, followed by vessels and bone.

6. Closure should be as aesthetic as possible for later viewing at funeral services. Most closures are done as single-layer closures. Prosthetic bone space-holders brought by the procurement team are placed. Ice packs are placed over eye sockets, and the head of the bed is elevated to minimize fluid accumulation around the eye sockets.

7. The procurement coordinator provides the necessary paperwork for the surgeons and team to use for documentation.

Additional Considerations in Cadaver Organ Procurement

The procurement coordinator remains at the host facility after the procurement team has departed. The coordinator's role extends into the aftercare given to the donor's body and the psychologic support and debriefing of the OR team. After the closure and dressing of all incisional wounds, the donor's body should be bathed and all drainage tubes and IV access lines removed. The patient's body should be treated respectfully at all times.

The body should be labeled with identification tags and placed on a clean transport cart. The head of the stretcher should be elevated 20 to 30 degrees. Ice packs should remain over the eye sockets to decrease serous pooling, for the benefit of the mortician who prepares the body for viewing. The donor's body is prepared as aesthetically as possible for the benefit of the family and loved ones.

Psychologic Support of the OR Team. The OR team may experience a sense of sadness and loss. These feelings are normal and to be expected. Death is not a common event in the OR. Although patients are technically brain dead before arrival in the OR, they give the outward appearance of being sustained on life support as in general anesthesia. After the aorta and vena cava are cross-clamped, ventilatory support is no longer needed and the anesthesia provider turns off the ventilator. The sudden silence can feel overwhelming.

The OR team may need the added support given by the procurement coordinator, who has experienced the same feelings and understands the psychologic impact of each stage of the procurement process. Personnel who specialize in procurement state that they feel the same sense of loss despite years of experience and exposure. An understanding of the outcome is important in the grieving process. Participation in the aftercare of the body helps provide the OR team with a sense of closure and completion of patient care.

Some of the same sadness may be shared by the critical care nursing staff members who helped monitor and maintain the donor's vital signs before transfer to the OR. Although the urge to be emotionally strong may exist, the shedding of tears of sorrow is therapeutic.

Psychologic Support for the Family of the Donor. The donor's family/significant others need support and communication from the procurement coordinator. The coordinator becomes known to the family/significant others and maintains communication with them for several months or longer as needed; the coordinator also provides referrals for follow-up counseling if the need arises. The coordinator informs the family/significant others of the progress of the recipients. In select situations, donor and recipient families may be brought together and may form lasting friendships.

The financial aspects of donor maintenance and subsequent organ procurement are paid by the procurement agency and are not the responsibility of the donor's family. Medical bills accumulated before the patient was identified as a potential donor are paid by the donor's family.

Living Related Donor

There are distinct advantages to procurement of a kidney, lobe of the liver or lung, tail segment of the pancreas, or marrow from a living related donor. The results are better than those with nonbiologically related cadaver organs because donor-recipient matches are usually good (identical twin sources are ideal for compatibility). Most live donors are healthy, which makes them good candidates for laparoscopic or robotic procedures.[4] Small incisions reduce postoperative pain, require use of fewer narcotics, and have a faster recovery. Waiting time is also reduced, and the procedure is planned and performed in controlled circumstances. The ethical concerns include the generalized risk of surgery to the donor.

The use of living donors involves the following special protocol:

1. Adult donors, who are preferred over adolescents or children, must be able to give informed consent voluntarily and without coercion. Children are used as donors only for a twin or for a patient with predictable results, which is sometimes the case between siblings for bone marrow donation. If the donor is a minor, court (legal) and parental or guardian consents are required to avoid bias. The donor must fully comprehend the sacrifice; if the physician deems it advisable, a psychiatric examination is included along with intelligence testing.

2. The donor must be in excellent health. The donor's physician confers with the donor and performs the preoperative physical examination to facilitate informed consent. Before a nephrectomy, renal arteriograms are performed to confirm the presence of bilateral kidneys and to identify the renal vasculature.

3. The donor should have no psychiatric complications. An extensive mental assessment is done.[5] Donor reactive depression may follow organ removal if adequate gratitude is not shown by all concerned.

Preservation of Organ Allografts

The successful use of donor tissue depends on rapid organ resection and cooling because the period of ischemia must be kept to a minimum. Long-term preservation of tissue remains a problem; current techniques use a variety of cryoprotective agents. Uncontrolled freezing may produce lethal cell injury; therefore this technique is used for skin, bone, semen, and blood suspensions but not for whole organs. Hypothermia above freezing at 39.2° F (4° C), with or without the perfusion with cold solutions, reduces general metabolic demands and thereby provides a safety margin. Methods of hypothermia include the following:

- Simple flush techniques with cold electrolyte solutions and storage via immersion in an electrolyte or flush-out solution in a plastic container that is kept at a hypothermic temperature.
- Hypothermic continuous pulsatile perfusion with an oxygenated electrolyte solution.

In 1987, potassium-based organ preservation solutions were developed at the University of Wisconsin by Dr. Folkert Belzer (1930–1995). These solutions are known as UW (Viaspan) and Belzer MPS solutions, and they extend the preservation time of the liver to 24 hours and of the kidney and pancreas to 72 hours. A total organ perfusion system (TOPS) consists of a machine that pumps an artificial blood substitute through the donor organ during transport. Minicomputers and microsensors regulate pH levels, blood pressure, and nutrient levels. The potential for altering the immunogenicity of an organ and improving its regenerative processes is the focus of research in perfusion techniques.

The organ is placed in a sterile container filled with perfusate. This container is placed in sterile double-plastic bags and packed in ice. Dry ice is not used. If the organ will be transported to another facility, a Styrofoam ice cooler generally is used as the outer container.

Immunologic Rejection

The body possesses an innate tendency to reject and destroy any foreign material except tissue from an identical twin; therefore transplanted cells from donors even slightly dissimilar to the recipient may be rejected.

Organ rejection involves the patient's immunologic system. Both the cellular and the humoral immune systems seem to be involved in the responses to transplanted cells. Activation of the immune system is a response to antigens introduced by the donor graft. An immunologic reaction usually is accompanied by a febrile systemic reaction, local inflammation, and deteriorating function of the graft.

A knowledge of antigens, individual-specific and species-specific, and their genetic transmission is important for the avoidance of violent reactions. Many factors influence the strength and rate of a rejection reaction: acquired immunologic tolerance, lymphatic depression, or previous sensitization by blood transfusions, pregnancies, or transplants. Rejection may be reversible with intensive therapy, or it may be progressive and lead to the cessation of transplant function.

Combating Rejection

Attempts must be made to find compatible donors and to minimize rejection. T cells can be spun from donor vertebral marrow and transfused into the recipient to prevent or minimize rejection. This action primes the recipient's system for organ acceptance.

The recipient's body can then recognize the transplanted organ as being familiar, which thus minimizes or prevents rejection.

Preoperative Matching of the Donor to the Recipient

Tissue typing and matching are used to determine the genetic disparity between the donor and the recipient. Histocompatibility implies acceptability by one individual of tissue from another. Histocompatibility tests, although not infallible, assist in donor-recipient selection and result in improved organ survival from both living and cadaver sources. The better the histocompatibility match and degree of genetic similarity between the donor and the recipient, the less serious the rejection.

Histocompatibility testing, or tissue typing, is based on the detection of cell-surface antigens known to affect rejection. Favorable results are expected when few histocompatibility antigens are detected. Preformed antibodies appear to have a harmful effect on graft survival. Histocompatibility testing uses serologic methods that include cell culture techniques and in vitro analysis for the study of cell-to-cell interaction and identification of the mediator of the interaction. Complex assay techniques measure the effects of antibodies and lymphocytes against donor tissue in a culture setup. Crossmatching between the recipient's serum and the donor's peripheral blood target cells is accomplished with multiple serologic reagents or flow cytometry with fluorescent-labeled monoclonal antibodies.

Immunosuppressive Therapy in the Recipient

Specific alterations in immune responses are produced by inactivating or destroying lymphoid cells that are capable of responding to the antigens. The goal is to selectively suppress antigenic reactions to the transplant without impairing the body's defense against pathogenic organisms. To allow the transplant to remain and function, an attempt is made to neutralize or modify the body's protective antigenic mechanisms through the use of various immunosuppressive agents. This barrier can be pierced at least temporarily by creating an increase in transplant tolerance or by paralyzing the recipient's immunologic system.

Because the lymphocytes and globulins seem to be mainly responsible for rejection, an attempt is made to vary their synthesis. Antibody formation and immune reaction can be suppressed by certain factors; the protocol for these methods is fairly standard in all transplantation centers.

1. Cyclosporine (Sandimmune), a soil fungus derivative, is a potent immunosuppressant that acts mainly on thymus-derived lymphocytes (T cells), the cells primarily responsible for rejection. This drug reduces rejection, especially in the early or inductive phase, without suppressing the entire immune system. It may be given orally or IV. It is always used with low doses of adrenal corticosteroids but usually not with other immunosuppressive agents. Its absorption rate is variable. The toxic effects on the kidneys must be monitored. Verapamil, a calcium channel blocker, may be given to reduce renal toxicity.
2. Immunosuppressive agents, such as FK-506 or 5R-506, may be preferred to cyclosporine to prevent rejection.
3. Monoclonal antilymphocyte globulin, muromonab-CD3 (Orthoclone OKT3), is derived from mouse antibodies and is used for the successful treatment of established allograft rejection without affecting the entire immune system. Monoclonal antibodies have the ability to reverse the initial episode of rejection by binding to specific targeted surface antigens on

mature T cells. They suppress only the activity of T cells that cause acute rejection.

4. Polyclonal antilymphocyte globulin, antibodies derived from horse serum, may be used for the induction of immunosuppression or for the reversal of rejection. It usually is given with other immunosuppressive agents.
5. Corticosteroids, such as prednisone, have an antiinflammatory effect that is useful in reversing early rejection reactions. There is an inverse relationship between steroids and lymphocytes. T cells migrate from the circulation to lymphoid tissue.
6. Agents cytostatic or cytotoxic to lymphatic tissue, such as azathioprine (Imuran), suppress the entire immune system and have serious side effects on other systems. They also interfere with DNA synthesis. Extracorporeal perfusion with these drugs and localized radiation to the transplant may be used either separately or concurrently.
7. Heterologous horse or rabbit antithymocyte globulin or antilymphocytic globulin or serum acts against circulating T cells and induces suppressor cells.

The use of immunosuppressive measures is not without complications. Leukopenia and susceptibility to infection are common sequelae. Therapy may not totally abolish rejection by the host but may delay the onset and decrease the incidence of rejection episodes during the crucial first month or two after transplantation.

Pretransplantation Transfusions

Blood transfusions from a living related donor expose the recipient to a limited number of leukocyte antigens and seem to reduce the risk for sensitization to the prospective donor transplant and thereby increase graft survival. Different blood products, including platelets, and pharmacologic conditioning may be part of a pretransplantation transfusion protocol to induce specific immune modification in the recipient. Random preoperative blood transfusions before cadaver organ transplantation may increase the risk for sensitization but may improve allograft survival.

Kidney Transplantation

Kidney transplantation has significantly improved the quality of life for many patients with chronic renal disease. Patients may choose to accept transplantation rather than remain on hemodialysis for the rest of their lives. Indication for transplantation is end-stage renal disease, most often glomerulonephritis, pyelonephritis, polycystic disease, or nephrosclerosis.

Recipients may be infants (at least 8–12 months with a body weight of 6–8 kg) to adults 70 years of age without severe extrarenal disease, malignant disease, or active sepsis. Nephrectomy is not performed before transplantation unless the patient has uncontrollable hypertension. Patients with detected presensitization states may need to wait longer for a suitably matched cadaver donor; statistically these patients have a lower 1-year graft survival rate than do unsensitized patients.

Recipients are carefully prepared preoperatively with kidney dialysis, regulation of fluid and electrolyte intake, pretransplantation blood transfusions, and control of hypertension. Proper donor-recipient matching is performed.

Donor preparation is equally important. The removal of a kidney is associated with low morbidity, but living related donors must guard against injuring the remaining kidney for the rest of their life. Donors are therefore advised to avoid body-contact sports.

Transplantation Procedure

Unless a cadaver donor organ is used, two adjoining ORs and teams are used for the transplantation procedure. One team procures and preserves the donor kidney, and the other team prepares the recipient site and transplants the kidney. The kidney is transplanted immediately after it is procured.

Donor Nephrectomy

In a living related donor, the kidney is removed through a flank incision (Fig. 45.5). Adequate renal perfusion and urinary output, maintenance of adequate blood pressure and ureteral blood supply, and gentleness in manipulation are extremely important intraoperatively. As soon as the kidney with its vascular attachments and ureter is excised, it is flushed with cold heparinized solution to remove red blood cells. Total ischemia time is usually less than 1 hour. The donor's incision is closed per routine technique.

Recipient Procedure

The iliac fossa is the standard site for transplantation in an adult patient (Fig. 45.6). The hypogastric artery is anastomosed to the

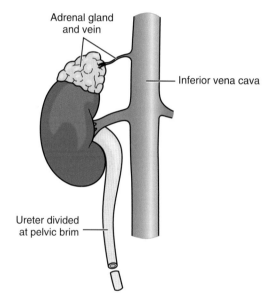

• **Fig. 45.5** Resection of right donor kidney.

• **Fig. 45.6** Kidney transplant is placed in the iliac fossa through a lower oblique abdominal incision.

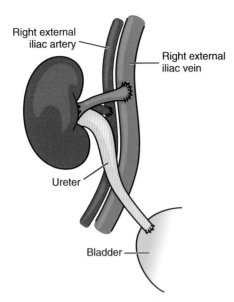

Right external iliac artery

Right external iliac vein

Ureter

Bladder

• **Fig. 45.7** Anastomosis of donor kidney to recipient site.

renal artery, and the common iliac vein is anastomosed to the renal vein (Fig. 45.7). Reconstruction of the urinary tract is the main technical problem. Ureteroneocystostomy, the implantation of a donor ureter into the bladder, is the preferred technique for urinary drainage. Alternative methods include ureteroureterostomy and ureteropyelostomy.

Complications of Renal Transplantation

The complications of renal transplantation may be renal-related or extrarenal. The most common renal-related complications include rejection (the dominant cause of graft failure), recurrent nephritis, acute tubular necrosis, and technical failure from genitourinary or vascular problems. Postoperative management is similar to that for other surgical patients, with emphasis on the initial adequacy of renal function, prevention of the hazardous effects of immunosuppressive therapy, and observation for allograft rejection. The following are the possible types of rejection:

- *Hyperacute, caused by presensitization:* Hyperacute rejection is an immediate acute rejection that occurs right after the anastomosis of blood vessels or within 24 hours. It includes thrombosis and extensive destruction of allograft vasculature.
- *Accelerated, caused by presensitization:* With accelerated rejection, the graft may function for up to 5 days, after which there is a rapid loss of renal function. Treatment for both hyperacute and accelerated rejection is immediate removal of the transplant.
- *Acute:* Acute rejection usually occurs 1 week to 4 months after transplantation and is often reversible unless the immune response is severe. Systemic and local symptoms, and reduced urinary output and abnormal laboratory findings, are present.
- *Chronic:* Antibodies that develop long after transplantation produce an insidious onset with mild hypertension and diminishing renal function. This type of rejection is not reversible. Acute and chronic rejection may be diagnosed by renal biopsy. Extrarenal complications are usually caused by immunosuppressive or corticosteroid therapy and include infection (the leading cause of death on a long-term basis), pneumonitis, hepatitis, gastrointestinal bleeding, and psychologic problems from a perpetual fear of rejection. Immunosuppressive therapy must be used with caution.

The results of kidney transplantation are gratifying; life can be significantly prolonged. Causes for concern are chronic liver failure and vascular disease (which is a major cause of death in patients on dialysis and may occur in a long-term transplant recipient). The incidence of malignant neoplasm in patients surviving renal transplantation more than 1 year exceeds that expected in the general population. More information about kidney procurement and transplantation is available from the National Kidney Foundation at www.kidney.org.

Heart Transplantation

Heart transplantation may be performed in select patients with end-stage cardiac disease such as irreversible extensive myocardial failure, widespread atherosclerotic deterioration, and ischemic disease with symptoms at rest.[6] Transplant recipients usually are younger than 55 years and have a life expectancy of less than 1 year. Patients may be following a regimen of dopamine infusion or supported by ventricular assist devices while waiting for a suitable donor.

A suitable heartbeating cadaver donor must have a blood type compatible with the recipient, be approximately the same weight and size as the recipient, and have no evidence of cardiac disease. Donors are usually younger than 40 years, but exceptions may be made.

Optimal preservation of the donor heart is crucial so it can resume full activity after transplantation.[7] Ischemia time must be less than 6 hours. After removal, the donor heart is rapidly cooled to 39.2° F (4° C) and is transported to the recipient.[7]

The transplantation team prepares the recipient while the donor heart is being procured in another OR or is being transported from another hospital. The recipient is brought to the OR. When the procurement team has inspected the donor heart and deemed it suitable, the transplantation team is notified by the procurement coordinator. After the induction of anesthesia, a pulmonary artery catheter and transesophageal echocardiography (TEE) probe are placed. A median sternotomy is performed.

Most recipients with long-standing cardiac disease have had previous sternotomies, and adhesions may be present. Careful dissection is necessary to avoid potential embolization from a dilated left ventricle. The myocardium is not manipulated until the aorta is cross-clamped, and the recipient's heart is not mobilized until the donor heart is ready for transplantation. The surgical procedure is similar to routine open heart procedures that use cardiopulmonary bypass. The following two surgical modalities are used for cardiac transplantation:

1. *Orthotopic heart transplantation:* The ventricles, atrial appendages, and most of the coronary sinus are excised from the donor heart. The opened atria, aorta, and pulmonary artery of the recipient heart are anastomosed to the donor heart. The sinoatrial nodes of both the donor and the recipient are left intact (Fig. 45.8). Spontaneous nerve regeneration is more likely to occur in younger patients who receive a younger donor organ. Studies have shown that 21% of heart recipients have some sympathetic nerve generation at the ventricular level. The amount of nerve regeneration improves exercise tolerance in the patient.

2. *Heterotopic transplantation:* The donor heart is inserted in an abnormal position in the right side of the chest as an assist device to enhance cardiac function. The recipient's heart is not removed. This less desirable alternative procedure may be indicated when increased pulmonary vascular resistance is a result

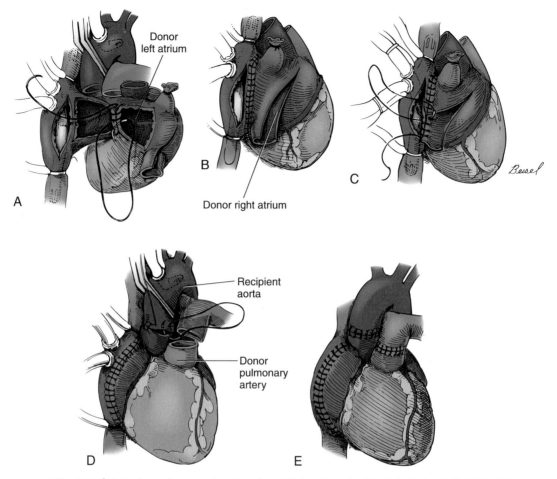

Donor
left atrium

A

B

Donor right atrium

C

Beisel

Recipient
aorta

Donor
pulmonary
artery

D

E

• **Fig. 45.8** Orthotopic cardiac transplantation. **A** and **B,** Anastomosis of the left atrial wall. **C,** Right atrial anastomosis. **D,** Aortic anastomosis. **E,** The pulmonary artery has been attached.

of left ventricular failure in the recipient's heart. The donor's right atrium is anastomosed to the recipient's right atrium. Anastomoses are completed between the aorta and pulmonary veins of the donor to the left atrium of the recipient (Fig. 45.9).

Most deaths occur in the first 2 postoperative months—the crucial period of immunologic rejection. Electrocardiographic changes, such as a drop in voltage, reduced cardiac output, arteritis, myocardial ischemia, and myocardial necrosis, occur during rejection. The diagnosis and monitoring of acute rejection may be facilitated with serial transvenous endomyocardial biopsies, which also may confirm the effectiveness of therapy. Using fluoroscopy, a forceps is passed through a catheter into the apex of the right ventricle via the right internal jugular vein and a small sample of myocardium is removed for histologic study.

A major obstacle to long-term survival is the development of obliterative coronary artery disease in the transplanted heart. The rejection process accelerates atherosclerosis. Improvement in survival rates is attributed to early and more accurate diagnosis of rejection and vigorous measures to prevent the atherosclerosis, which is thought to result from immunologic injury to the intima of the coronary vessels.

An increase in malignant neoplasms in heart transplant patients has been observed and attributed to immunosuppressive drugs.[7] Patients who have undergone a heart transplant need personalized

support to maintain a will to live and to adjust to psychologic problems that may arise at any time.

Combined Heart-Lung Transplantation

The organs of the cardiopulmonary system can be transplanted as an **en bloc** unit. Patients with primary pulmonary hypertension or pulmonary vascular disease secondary to congenital heart disease may be candidates for heart-lung transplantation. Patients with cystic or pulmonary fibrosis and chronic end-stage pulmonary disease also may receive combined transplants. If cardiac function in these patients has not been affected by the disease, their hearts may be used as heartbeating donor cardiac transplants for another patient.

In both the donor and the recipient, the trachea is transected above the carina and the heart and lungs are removed en bloc.[8] This surgical technique preserves the recipient's phrenic, vagus, and recurrent laryngeal nerves on pedicles, a portion of the right atrium and vena cava, and the aortic arch. A clamshell incision is the approach of choice (Fig. 45.10). The donor heart and lungs must fit without compression within the recipient's thoracic cavity. Size match is critical for the success of the procedure.[8] The donor trachea, right atrium, and aorta are anastomosed to corresponding structures in the recipient (Fig. 45.11).

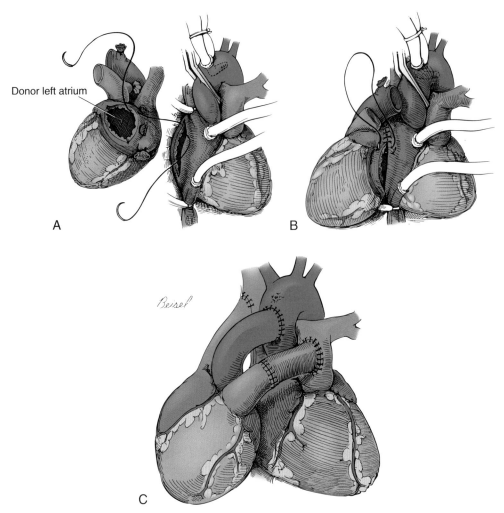

Donor left atrium

• **Fig. 45.9** Heterotopic cardiac transplantation. **A** and **B,** Left atrial anastomosis. **C,** A remnant of the donor superior vena cava (SVC) is anastomosed to the side of the recipient SVC. The donor ascending aorta and pulmonary artery are anastomosed end to side to their respective counterparts. A graft may be interposed between donor and recipient pulmonary arteries to provide additional length.

• **Fig. 45.10** Clamshell incision for double-lung transplant.

Cyclosporine given both preoperatively and postoperatively enhances healing of the tracheal anastomosis and combats cellular-mediated rejection. Bacterial pneumonia from subclinical bacterial contamination in the donor tracheobronchial tree is the most common cause of morbidity and mortality after heart-lung transplantation.

Lung Transplantation

Transplantation of a single lung, usually the left one, may be performed in a patient with end-stage pulmonary fibrosis who depends on oxygen therapy. Both lungs may be replaced sequentially as two single-lung transplants rather than as an en bloc combined heart-lung transplant. Children with broncho-pulmonary dysplasia, primary pulmonary hypertension, or congenital hiatal (diaphragmatic) hernia may benefit from a partial lung transplant. A lobe from a living relative may be transplanted instead of a whole lung from a cadaver source.

Optimal preservation of the donor organ is vitally important, and timing is critical. Ischemic time must be less than 4 hours; results improve as ischemic time decreases. Recipient preparation usually occurs simultaneously with donor procurement.

Single-lung transplantation involves bronchus-to-bronchus, pulmonary artery—to—pulmonary artery, and recipient pulmo-nary veins—to—donor atrial cuff anastomoses. The omentum is wrapped around the bronchus to provide additional blood supply and support the anastomosis.

Many special problems affect the success of clinical lung transplantation, as follows:

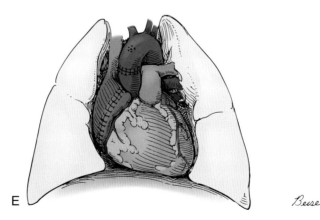

• **Fig. 45.11** Heart-lung transplantation. **A,** The recipient heart and lungs have been excised, exposing the posterior pericardium. Note the location of the phrenic, vagus, and recurrent laryngeal nerves and the right and left phrenic nerve pedicles. **B,** The recipient heart and lungs are brought onto the field; the right lung is passed beneath the recipient atriocaval remnant and right phrenic nerve to lie in the right pleura; the left lung will be placed beneath the left phrenic nerve and positioned in the left pleural space. **C,** The tracheal anastomosis is performed, followed by the right atrial anastomosis **(D)** and, finally, the aortic anastomosis **(E)**.

- Recipients usually have some degree of pulmonary infection at the time of the surgical procedure. The recipient's remaining lung, if diseased, may be a source of infection.
- Ventilation-perfusion imbalance between the transplanted lung and the remaining lung may result in reduced function of the transplant.
- Imminent rejection is not easily recognized.
- Vascular and fibrotic changes produced by rejection create ischemia and anoxia.
- Healing at the site of bronchial anastomosis is a problem, but less so with cyclosporine and an omental wrap.
- The procedure is technically difficult. The size of the donor lung, hilar structures, and bronchus must approximate those of the recipient.

Liver Transplantation

Hepatic transplantation may be performed in select patients with nonmalignant end-stage liver disease. The ideal recipients are patients with primary liver disease. Successful liver transplantation is performed on infants and children with biliary atresia who have development of chronic liver failure or on those with other liver or biliary problems. A preexisting infection in any part of the body is a distinct contraindication because the patient's preoperative status is poor and the patient lacks the protective proteins normally produced by the liver. Postoperative infection is always a marked danger.

The liver is susceptible to damage from ischemia. However, a donor liver can be preserved for up to 24 hours with the infusion of cold Belzer-MPS solution.

The liver may be separated into two sections and used for two recipients. The left lobe or a left lateral segmental graft may be transplanted into an infant or child; the right side, which is larger, can be transplanted into an adult.[8] For this reduced-size liver transplantation (RSLT) procedure, one team divides the donor organ while another team performs a hepatectomy on the recipient.

Successful living related liver transplantation is performed on infants and children with biliary atresia with development of chronic liver failure or on those with other liver or biliary problems. The adult donor gives the left lobe (the smaller lobe) if the recipient is an infant or a child. The liver grows as the child grows over time.

Anatomic complexity, friability of tissue, and vascularity of the liver contribute to the technical hazards of liver transplantation (Fig. 45.12). The surgical procedure may take more than 6 hours to complete and requires both extensive dissection and ligation of vessels to avoid postoperative hemorrhage. The vena cava must be mobilized. After it is divided, the diseased liver is removed and the donor organ anastomosed to the upper and then the lower vena cava as quickly as possible (Fig. 45.13).

During this critical period, venous return from the lower half of the body must be decompressed via a venovenous extracorporeal membrane oxygenation (ECMO) pump from the iliac to the axillary arteries. After anastomoses of the portal vein and hepatic artery, any bleeding must be controlled before reconstruction of the bile duct (Fig. 45.14).

Rejection may be noted by changes in laboratory findings, such as alterations in serum enzyme levels and elevated serum bilirubin values. Cellular infiltration of the graft causes impairment of clotting factors, liver cell necrosis, and impaired function. Complications from reconstruction of the biliary tract may lead to graft failure.

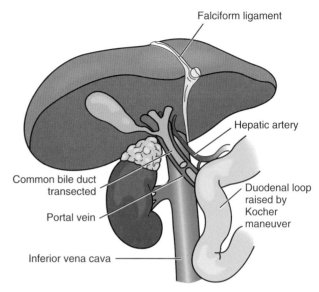

• **Fig. 45.12** Procurement of donor liver.

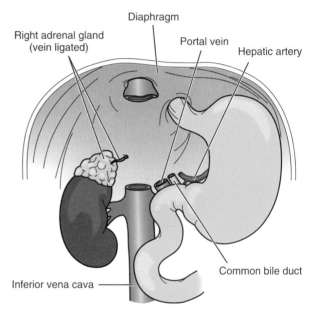

• **Fig. 45.13** Recipient liver resection.

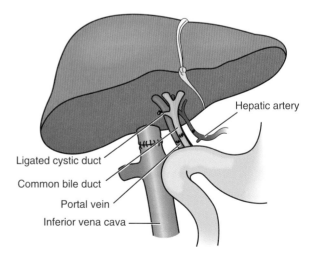

• **Fig. 45.14** Donor liver in situ after completion of anastomosis.

Pancreas Transplantation

Various techniques have been used in clinical pancreatic transplantation in the treatment of patients with severe diabetes and associated systemic complications. The goal is to provide physiologic islet function to achieve more satisfactory carbohydrate metabolism, to restore normal glucose homeostasis, and to prevent or halt secondary complications associated with diabetes mellitus. The whole pancreas, the distal segment, or isolated islets may be transplanted. The whole organ is obtained from a cadaver source. A kidney may be transplanted along with the pancreas en bloc with the associated segment of aorta and other structures.

A composite splanchnic organ graft may be obtained; this type of graft includes the entire pancreas, the spleen, and a segment of the duodenum. A segment of pancreas, usually the tail and body, can be obtained from a living related donor and placed into the extraperitoneal space in the iliac fossa. The splenic artery and vein of the donor segment are anastomosed to the external iliac artery and vein of the recipient. Islet cells or beta cells may be isolated for transplantation; beta cells are injected into the liver.

The transplantation procedure must allow exocrine secretions to drain from the pancreatic ducts. This is accomplished most commonly with pancreaticocystostomy for urinary drainage or pancreaticojejunostomy for enteric drainage. Insulin is secreted into the systemic circulation via arterial anastomoses between the donor organ and the recipient vessels.

Small Intestine Transplantation

The small bowel can be procured from a living related donor or cadaver donor. From a living related donor, a minimal segment of 39 to 59 inches (100−150 cm) of small intestine with a branch of the superior mesenteric artery and vein may be transplanted to correct short-bowel syndrome, genetic enzyme deficiencies, or malabsorption disorders in children. The whole small bowel alone or in combination with the liver and other digestive structures can be used from a cadaver donor. Because the body reacts to the lymphoid tissue transplanted with the intestine, the donor transplant organ may be irradiated to kill the lymph cells but not the mucosal cells.

Survival rates for intestinal transplant are around 50%. Most complications are related to reactions in the lymph tissue, heavy bacterial load of the gut, and technical graft failure.

Pediatric indications for intestinal transplant include the following:
- Volvulus
- Gastroschisis
- Necrotizing enterocolitis
- Intestinal atresia
- Trauma
- Hirschsprung disease
- Obstruction

Adult indications for intestinal transplant include the following:
- Crohn's disease
- Trauma
- Ischemia caused by thrombosis
- Familial polyposis
- Gardner syndrome
- Desmoid tumor
- Radiation enteritis
- Budd-Chiari syndrome

Multiorgan Transplantation

Modern medicine and techniques have enabled surgeons to transplant organs in patients who would otherwise die from organ failure. Organs and body parts such as the spleen, stomach, uterus, face, and hands have all been transplanted with some success. In 2022, the Cleveland Clinic completed the first multiorgan transplant on a 32-year-old male patient. The man received a stomach, liver, pancreas, small intestine, spleen, duodenum, and right colon. The surgery was successful, and the patient continues to improve.

With advances in technology, the Cleveland Clinic also performed the first single-port robotic kidney transplant. As these procedures are perfected, changes in instrumentation, sterile setup, and staff education will be needed for a successful minimally invasive transplant program. More information can be found at www.newsroom.clevelandclinic.org.

ⓔ EVOLVE WEBSITE

http://evolve.elsevier.com/Hornacky/BerryKohn/
- Historical Perspective
- Glossary
- Student Interactive Questions

References

1. Soylu D, Ozdemir A, Soylu A: Does religious attitude affect organ donation and transplantation? *Transplant Immunol* 71:10155, 2022.
2. Mella A, Mariano F, Dolla D, et al.: Bacterial and viral infection and sepsis in kidney transplanted patients, *Biomedicines* 10(3):701, 2022.
3. McLaughlin M, Miles B: Brain stem death, *Anaesth Intensive Care Med* 16(7):311−314, 2015.
4. Chow G, Shah P: Laparoscopic live donor nephrectomy. In *Atlas of laparoscopic and robotic surgery*, ed 4, St. Louis, MO, 2023, Elsevier, pp 139−154.
5. Sarkar S, Grover S, Chadda R: Psychiatric assessment of persons for solid-organ transplant, *Indian J Psychiatry* 64(2):S308−S318, 2022.
6. Chen Q, Emerson D, Megna D, et al.: Heart transplantation using donation after circulatory death in the United States, *J Thorac Cardiovasc Surg* 165(5):1849−1860, 2023.
7. Doyle MM, Collins K, Vachharajani N, et al.: Outcomes using grafts from donors after cardiac death, *J Am Coll Surg* 221(1):142−152, 2015.
8. Lesko M, Angel L: Organ donation, the non-perfect lung donor, and variability in conversion to transplant, *Clin Chest Med* 44(1):69−75, 2023.

Bibliography

Hasan A, Kittleson M: Heart transplantation in women, *Heart Fail Clin* 15(1):127−135, 2018.
Leland B, Wocial L: Exploring ethical dimensions of physician involvement in requests for organ donation in pediatric brain death, *Semin Pediatr Neurol* 45:101301, 2022.

Index

A

AAMI. *See* Association for the Advancement of Medical Instrumentation
Abandonment, 41–42
Abdominal aortic aneurysm, 960f
  endovascular repair of, 962–963, 963f
  open resection of, 960–962, 961f–962f
Abdominal approach, for gynecologic surgery, 701, 701f
Abdominal lift device, for endoscopy, 649–650
Abdominal positions, 501t–503t
Abdominal procedures, 670–674
  planning perioperative care for, 689
  systematic approach to evaluation, 689
Abdominal surgery, 557–559
  complications of, 691
  dissecting tissue layers of, 558f
  landmarks for, 557–559, 558f
  suturing, in tissue layers, 562f
  types of, 557–559, 558f
Abdominal trauma, 688–691
Abdominoperineal resection, 687–688
Abdominoplasty, 861–862, 862f
Abduct, 499
Abduction hip splint, 787
Ablation, 923, 939
Abortion, 52, 696, 716
  dilation and curettage, 709
  missed, 717
  spontaneous, 707
    due to occupational exposure, 235
  by suction curettage, 716–718
  threatened, 716
Above-knee amputation, 694
Abscess
  anal, 691
  mediastinal, 916
  peritonsillar, 887
Absorbable collagen, 590, 954b
Absorbable gelatin, 590, 954b
Absorbable suture(s), 562, 564–565, 564t
Absorption, 420, 422
Absorption rate, of local and regional anesthetics, 460–461
Abuse, of child, 122–123, 128, 703
Accessories, bed attachments and, 511, 512f
Accessory appendages, to integument, 556
Accountability, 16–18, 25b
  of accurate counts, 24–25
  counting and, 25b
Accreditation, 16, 91–92
Accreditation Council for Graduate Medical Education (ACGME), 664
Accreditation Manual for Hospitals, 90

Accreditation of schools and facilities
  for ambulatory surgery, 199–200
  for credentialing of qualified caregivers, 56
Accreditation Review Council on Education in Surgical Technology and Surgical Assisting (ARC-STSA), 34
Accrediting Bureau of Health Education Schools (ABHES), 56
Acetic acid, as sterilants, 332
Acetonuria, 106
Achilles tendon rupture, 785
Acholic stool, 125, 143
Acid-base balance, 632–633
Acidosis, 633
ACLS. *See* Advanced cardiac life support
Acoustic neuroma
  excision of, 801
  resection of, 880
Acquired disease processes, 126
Acquired immunodeficiency syndrome (AIDS), 118–119, 251
Active electrode, of electrosurgical unit, 360, 362
Active immunity, 240
Activities of daily living, of geriatric patient, 165
Acupuncture, 464–465, 464f–465f
Acute infection, of human immunodeficiency virus, 251
Acute respiratory distress syndrome (ARDS), 617, 619, 921
Adaptation to illness, 100–101
Additives, 429
  for local and regional anesthetics, 460–461
Adduct, 499
Adenoidectomy, 152, 887
Adenosine, 626
Adhesion barrier sheet, 605
Adhesions, 583, 605
  after abdominal surgery, 691
  pleural, 913
Adhesive tape
  anal procedures with, bed attachments and, 509
  pediatric, 141, 141f
Adhesive-backed strips, for skin closure, 581
Adhesives, tissue, 575–576, 575b
Adipose layer, subcutaneous, in skin, 555
Adjunct drug therapy, 623
Adjunct organ displacement, 654–655
Adjuvant therapy, 111, 117
  for cancer, 416
Administrative and management behaviors, 91–93
Administrative personnel, 81
  offices of, 181
Administrator, 79, 81
Admission
  and holding unit, preoperative, 180

Admission (*Continued*)
  to hospital, 379
  to operating room suite, 390–394
Adolescent gynecology, 703–704
Adrenal glands, 758
Adrenalectomy, 112, 413, 758
Adrenergic receptors, 625
Adrenocorticotropic hormone (ACTH), 106
Adson forceps, 342, 344f
Adult learner, 3, 4t
Advance directives, 37, 46
Advanced cardiac life support (ACLS), 630
  level, 71
  perianesthesia nurse in, 612
Advanced practice registered nurse (APRN), 71, 83
Adverse events, incident report for, 50
Advocacy, 16–17
Aeration, 312
  after ethylene oxide gas sterilization, 328t, 329–330
Aerobic bacteria, 238, 244
Aerosol, 260, 266
AESOP. *See* Automated Endoscopic System for Optimal Positioning
Aesthetic appearance, 847
AF. *See* Atrial fibrillation
Affector innervation, 555
Afterload, 547
Afterloading techniques, in radiation therapy, 115, 414
Aged, definition of, 161–162
Agency for Healthcare Research and Quality (AHRQ)
  clinical practice guidelines, 20
Agenda, setting of, 93
Aging. *See also* Geriatrics, perioperative
  cultural considerations in, 162
  myths about, 164
  perspectives on, 161–164
  process, adaptation to, 166
  theories of, 162–164
  wound healing and, 587
AIDS. *See* Acquired immunodeficiency syndrome
Air changes per hour (ACH), 184
Air conditioning system, 266
Air embolization
  in angiography, 403
  Doppler instrument in, 407
  Durant procedure for, 403, 407
Air embolus, 619
  in cardiac surgery, cardiopulmonary bypass and, 930
  central venous cannulation and, 545
  de-airing of heart and, 930–931, 945
  Doppler instruments and, 406
  pneumatic counterpressure device and, 593
  pulmonary artery cannulation and, 545
  in semi-Fowler's position, 514

Note: Pages followed by *b*, *t*, or *f* refer to boxes, tables, or figures, respectively.

988

Air embolus (*Continued*)
  sitting position, in neurosurgical patient, 796
  with valve procedures, 945
Air-conditioning grilles, cleaning of, 217
Air-powered instruments, 355
Air, contamination from, 263—264
Airborne contamination, 262b
  control of, 266
Airway
  of burn patient, 868
  cardiopulmonary resuscitation and, 628
  difficult, 435
  in head and neck surgery, 874
  in spinal surgery, 814
Airway obstruction, 618
Airway stents, 911—912, 912f
Alcohol
  as antimicrobial skin-cleansing agent, 286
  for disinfection, 306
  for skin preparation, 524
Alcohol-based preps, 66
Aldrete Postanesthesia Scoring System, 203, 204t
Alfentanil, 444
Alginate, 608t
Alimentary tract obstruction, in pediatric patients, 142
Alkalosis, 633
Allergic response
  to antibiotics, 255
  to local anesthetics, 462
  wound healing and, 588
Allergies
  identified by circulating nurses, 394
  to iodine, 524
  noted on chart and wristband, 390
  on patient's identification wristband, 421
  verifying, onto patient's chart, 485
Allergy band, 391—392
Allied health care personnel, 34—35
Allis forceps, 342, 344f
Allogeneic blood, 639—640
Allogeneic graft, 551, 576
Allogeneic transplant, 970
Allograft, 578
Allow-natural-death (AND) orders, 53
Alloy, 338
Alpha (α)-oleic acid (AOA), 934
Alpha particles, 113, 413
Alternating current, 356
Alternative surgical locations, 197—210.
    See also Ambulatory surgery
Aluminum chloride, 592
Aluminum foil, for dry heat sterilization, 326
Alveolar ridge reconstruction, 888—889
AM admission, 379
Ambulation, postoperative, 589
  teaching about, 386
Ambulatory care, 197
Ambulatory surgery
  alternative sites for, 197—210
  centers for, 197—210
  documentation of, 206
  facilities for
    accreditation of, 199—200
    licensure of, 199
    parking for, 198
    sample floor plan of, 198, 198f
    various terms for, 197
  future of, 198—199
  intraoperative patient care in, 202—203, 202f, 203b
  patient selection for, 200, 200b

Ambulatory surgery (*Continued*)
  postanesthesia care for, certification for, 612
  postoperative patient care in, 203—205, 204f
  preoperative patient care in, 200—202, 201f
  setting, 197—206
Amenorrhea, 696, 704
American National Standards Institute (ANSI)
    standards, 20
  laser hazards and, 368—369
American Nurses Association (ANA)
  code of conduct of, 51
  patient care standards of, documentation and, 47—49
American Nurses Credentialing Center, 80
American Society of Anesthesiologists (ASA), 433
  physical status classification of, 388—389,
    434, 610, 611t
American Society of PeriAnesthesia Nurses (ASPAN),
    610—611
American Society of Transplant Surgeons, 973
Amino amides, 461
Amino esters, 461—462
Amiodarone, 626
Amnesia, 432—433
  levels of, 434
  in moderate sedation, 452
  types of, 434—464
Amniocentesis, 722
Amniotic fluid, embolism of, 619
Amniotic membrane, 578
Ampule, drug, 420, 425, 426f
Amputated parts, replantation of, 856—857,
    856f—857f
Amputation
  of digits, in burn patient, 870
  of extremities, 694—695
    handling of, 398—399
    revascularization and, 968
ANA. *See* American Nurses Association
Anabolism, 105, 616, 643
Anaerobic bacteria, 238, 244
Anal procedures, positioning for, 509
Analgesia, 432—433
Anaphylaxis, 235, 624—625
  definition of, 218, 616
  vasogenic shock in, 642
Anaplasia, 395, 409
Anastomosis
  definition of, 64, 664, 673
  gastrointestinal, hand-sutured, 678
  in replantation, 856, 856f
  staplers, internal, 349
  vascular, 952—953, 967—968
ANCC's Nursing Administration: Scope and
    Standards of Practice, 80
Andragogy, 1, 3, 4t
Androgen deprivation therapy (ADT), 112
Anemia, 637—638
  definition of, 616, 637
  in geriatric patients, 171
Anesthesia, 432—433, 715—716
  alternatives to conventional, 464—465
  ambulatory surgery and, 199, 203, 203b
  art and science of, 433
  awareness, 220
  in children, induction of, 437
  choice of, 433
  considerations in pregnancy, 725—727
  equipment, 136
    for, pasteurization of, 308
  for geriatric patients

Anesthesia (*Continued*)
  general, 171
    intraoperative consideration of, 165, 175
  highly flammable, 229
  hypotensive, 637
  induction of, 434
    anesthesia providers duties prior to, 392—393
    by circulating nurse, 393—394, 487
  for ophthalmic surgery, 831—832
  for otorhinolaryngologic and head and neck
    of ear, 878
    surgery, 874, 874f
  of patient during, 109
  patient positioning and, timing of, 500
  pediatric, 135—140
    agents for, 139—140
    emergence from, 140
    equipment for, 136
    extubation and, 140
    induction in, 136—139
    intubation for, 136—139
    local, 139t
    maintenance of, 139—140
    premedication for, 136
    preoperative assessment by anesthesia provider,
      135—136
  for plastic and reconstructive surgery, 848—849
  preparations for, 391
  for spinal surgery, 814
  techniques and agents, 432—465
  for urologic examination, 733
Anesthesia department, offices of, 181
Anesthesia equipment, cleaning of, 215
Anesthesia machine, 438—440, 438f
  maintenance of, 438f
  monitoring, functions of, 536
Anesthesia provider, 55, 57—58
  handover report of, 612—613
  infections acquired by, 449—450
  for monitored anesthesia care, 453
  postanesthesia care unit and, 613
  preanesthesia duties of, 392—393
  preoperative visit by, 386
  for transfusion, of blood products, 639
Anesthesia screen, bed attachments and, 507, 508f
Anesthesia standby, 453
Anesthesia state, 433—434
Anesthesia technicians, 486
Anesthesia work and storage areas, 181—182
Anesthesiologist, 57
Anesthesiologist assistant (AA), 57
Anesthesiology, 433
Anesthetic administration, accessibility of, for
    positioning of patient, 506
Anesthetic agents
  and maintenance, 139f
  for malignant hyperthermia, 645—646
Anesthetic gases, 232
Anesthetics, knowledge of, 434
Aneurysm, 947, 959
  aortic, abdominal, 960—962, 960f—962f
  cause of, 959
  occlusion of, 802, 802f
  ruptured, 960
  thoracic, 960, 960f
  types of, 959
  ventricular, 939, 939f—940f
Aneurysm clip, 802
Aneurysm needle, 561
Angiography, 402—403, 932, 951—952, 952f
Angioplasty

Angioplasty (*Continued*)
  cerebral, 803, 805
  coronary artery, 937–938
  laser, 937–938, 956–958
  percutaneous transluminal, 955–956
Angioscopy, 952
Animal sources, of drugs, 427, 427b
Ankle
  arthrodesis of, 776
  procedure in, for draping of patient, 533
  skin preparation for, antiseptic, 527
  sports injuries to, 785
  total replacement, 780
Ankylosing spondylosis, 169
Anodized finish, 338–339
Anomalous venous return, 157
Anomaly, definition of, 873, 898
Anorectal procedures, 691–692
Anoscopes, 351f
Anoscopy, 691
Anoxia, 447, 620
  cerebral, 625
  definition of, 432, 616
Ansamycin, 257t
ANSI. *See* American National Standards Institute
Antagonist, 420, 430
Antegrade infusion, 931
Anterior, 499
Anterior approach, definition of, 808, 814
Anterior chest, surgical position, 518
Anterior colporrhaphy, 707
Anterior cruciate ligament injury, 784–785
Anterior resection, 684
Anterior spinal (nonfusion) tethering method, 150
Anterolateral thoracotomy, 914, 928
Antibiotic paste, in neurosurgery, 794
Antibiotic prophylaxis, 256
  preoperative administration of, 389
Antibiotics, 238, 243, 255–258
  inhibit cell wall synthesis, 255, 255t
  inhibit nucleic acid synthesis and replication, 255, 257t
  inhibit protein synthesis, 255, 256t
  potentiating neuromuscular blockers, 445
  resistance to, 258
  selection of, 258b
Anticholinergics, 432, 443, 627
Anticoagulants, for reduction of blood loss, 636–637
Anticoagulation, 947, 953
Antidysrhythmics, 626–627
Antiembolic measures, for geriatric patients, 175
Antiembolic stockings, 389, 592–593
  for neurosurgical patient, 797
Antiestrogen therapy, 112, 413
Antifolates, 257t
Antifungal drugs, 259
Antihistamines, for anesthesia reaction, 463
Antilymphocyte globulin, 981
Antimicrobial agent, 238, 256, 275
Antimicrobial skin-cleansing agents, 286–287
Antimicrobial therapy, 238, 255–259.
  See also Antibiotics
Antimuscarinics, 627
Antineoplastics, 429
Antisepsis, 260
Antiseptic rub, surgical hand hygiene with, 287
Antiseptic solution, 499
Antiseptics, 260, 262
  flammable, 230
  for skin cleansing, 286–287
  for skin preparation, 523–524

Antishock garment, 797
Antiviral drugs, 259
Antral stretch, 171
Antrostomy, 884
Anxiety, 379, 382
Anxiolysis, 434
AORN. *See* Association of Perioperative Registered Nurses
Aortic aneurysm, abdominal, 960–962, 960f–962f
  ruptured, 960
  thoracic, 960, 960f
Aortic cross-clamping, 931
  removal of, 945
Aortic valve
  disease of, 933f
  replacement of, 934
Aortography, 951–952, 952f
Apert syndrome, 901, 901f
Aperture drape, 527
Aphakic eye, 826, 840
Apligraf, 580
Apnea, 432, 435, 969, 975t
Appendectomy, 146, 685–686, 686f
  laparoscopic, 686
Appendix, anatomy of, 686f
Apprenticeships, 3
Approach, 808
Approximating, 338
Approximation instruments, 347–350
Approximation, definition of, 64, 342, 551, 553
Aprons, 267, 282
  of urologist, 733
Arched spinal frame, adjustable, bed attachments and, 509–510, 510f
Arcuate line, 555–556, 555f
ARDS. *See* Acute respiratory distress syndrome
Argon beam coagulator, 363, 598
Argon laser, 366
Arm scrub, with brush, 287
Arm strap, bed attachments and, 508
Armboards, 485
  bed attachments and, 508, 508f
  for safety measures, in positioning of patient, 504
Army military hospital, mobile, 206, 207f
Arrector pili, 556
Arterial blood pressure, monitoring, 541–542
Arterial bypass, 954–955, 958
  coronary artery, 935–937, 935f
  femoropopliteal, 958–959, 958f
Arterial conduit, 954
Arterial disease, Doppler studies of, 407
Arterial dissection, 960, 960f
Arterialized tissue flap, 853–854
Arteries, anatomy of, 948–949, 949f
Arteriography, 402–403
Arteriovenous malformation (AVM), 790, 801–802, 802f
Arteriovenous shunts
  fistulas and, 966–967, 966f–967f
  xenografts, 580, 967
Arthritis, 104
  osteoarthritis, 167, 169–170, 169f–170f
  rheumatoid, 169–170, 170f
Arthrodesis, 761, 776, 776f
Arthrography, 402
Arthroplasty, 776–782, 777f
  hip incisions, 777f
  humeral head replacement, 776–777, 777f
  patient care considerations in, 781–782
  of temporomandibular joint, 903
  total joint replacement, 777–781

Arthroplasty (*Continued*)
  elbow, 780–781
  hip, 778–780, 779f
  knee, 780, 780f
  metacarpophalangeal, 781
  metatarsophalangeal, 780
  shoulder, 780, 781f
  trapeziometacarpal, 781
  wrist, 781
Arthroscopy, 782–783, 782f
  of temporomandibular joint, 903
Arthrotomy, 783
Artificial heart, 944–945, 945f
Artificial insemination, 724
Artificial skin, 578
Artificial urinary sphincter, 748
ASA. *See* American Society of Anesthesiologists
Asepsis, 260
Aseptic technique, 24, 260–262
  surgical technologists, 35
  wound healing and, 588
Asepto syringe, 475, 479
ASPAN. *See* American Society of PeriAnesthesia Nurses
Aspiration, 803
  definition of, 616
  in geriatric patients, 175
  as respiratory complications, 617
  of stomach contents, cricoid pressure for prevention of, 436
  syringes for, 479
Aspiration biopsy, 397
Aspiration instruments, 351–352
Aspirin
  as anticoagulants, 637
  avoidance of, before plastic surgery, 848
Assault and battery, 41
Assertive behavior, 14
Assessment
  brief, by circulating nurse, 485, 486b
  of crime victim, 120–121
  pediatric, 127–128
  preoperative, for local or regional anesthesia, 451–452
  of wound, 607
Assisted reproduction, 722–725
Assisted respiration, 440
Association for the Advancement of Medical Instrumentation (AAMI)
  central service personnel credential from, 296
  device standards, 19
Association of Perioperative Registered Nurses (AORN), 509
  comprehensive surgical checklist, 23f
  on monitoring during local anesthesia, 452
  recommended practices, 21–26
  sales representatives and, 97
  skills checklist of, 6
  SYNTEGRITY standardized perioperative framework, 29f
Association of Surgical Assistants (ASA), 66
Association of Surgical Technologists (AST), 34, 62, 77–78
  Code of Ethics, 51
  skills checklist of, 6
  Standards of Practice, 18
Associations, in operating room team, 495–496
Asymptomatic infection, of human immunodeficiency virus, 251
Asynchronous cardioversion, 623
Atelectasis, 616, 620

Atherectomy, 957
Atherosclerosis, 950, 950b
Atracurium, 445
Atraumatic, term, 338, 342
Atresia, 125, 142
  in pediatric patients, 142
Atrial fibrillation (AF), 938
Atrial myxoma, 940, 940f
Atrial septal defect, 157, 157f
Atrioventricular (AV) valves, 924, 924f
Atrioventricular canal defect, 157–158
Atropine, 627
  in children, 133t–134t
    for premedication, 136
Attire, in operating room, 275–294
  components for
    body cover, 278
    gown, 283–284, 283f–284f
    head cover, 278–279, 279b
    mask, 280–281, 281b–282b
    personal protective equipment, 282–283, 282f
    restricted area, 179
    semirestricted area, 179
    shoe covers, 280
    surgical gown, 283–284
    unrestricted area and, 179
  consideration for, 277b
  criteria for, 285
  definition of, 275–276
  purpose of, 276
Audiovisual materials, 9
Auditory brainstem evoked potentials, 407–408, 798
Auditory evoked potentials, 549
Augmentation bladder, 747
Autistic spectral disorder, 104
Autoclaves, 321
Autograft, 578
Autologous blood, 640–641
Autologous graft, 551, 576
Autologous plasma, 575
Autologous transplant, 970
Automated cell salvage processor, 640
Automated Endoscopic System for Optimal Position-
  ing (AESOP), 660
Autonomic nervous system
  arteries and veins controlled by, 948
  nerve surgery and, 806–807
Autonomy, 37–38
Autotransfusion, 352, 927
Avascular necrosis, 761, 776
AVM. *See* Arteriovenous malformation
Awake intubation, 437
Axillary block, 459
Axillary lymph node dissection, for breast cancer,
  669f
Azathioprine, for transplant recipient, 981

B

Babcock forceps, 343
Bacillus, endospores of, 244
Back tables, 192
Backache, 220
Bacteria, 244–248, 244f
  aerobic, 244
  anaerobic, 244
  biofilm of, 239, 243, 243b
  characteristics of, 244–245
  endospore-forming, 213
  endospores of, 245–246, 245f–246f
  Gram stain of, 245
  growth of, 239, 240f

Bacteria (*Continued*)
  septic shock caused by, 246–247
  sexually transmitted diseases and, 248
  toxicity of, 246
  tuberculosis caused by, 247–248
  types of, 245–248
Bacterial pyrogens, 246
Bactericide, 295, 302
Bacteriostatic, 295
Balanced anesthesia, 434, 446
Balanced salt solution (BSS), 826, 828
Balloon ablation, intrauterine, 709, 709f
Balloon angioplasty, 956
  coronary, 937, 938f
Balloon pump, intraaortic, 942–943, 943f
Balloon septostomy, 159
Balloon valvuloplasty, percutaneous transluminal, 935
Barbed suture, 567, 567t
Bariatric surgery, 680–682, 681f
Barrett's esophagus, 676
Barriers, 6, 260, 262, 267, 275
  for geriatric patient, 166
Bartholin glands, 697, 706
Basic cardiac life support (BCLS), 203
Basin sets, steam sterilization of, 323
Bayonet forceps, 344f
BCLS. *See* Basic cardiac life support
Beam splitter, 360, 375
Behavioral objectives, 5–6, 9b
Behaviors, 1
  of patient, in response to illness, 100
  perioperative educator, 11–13
Below-knee amputation, 694, 694f
Benching, 969, 979
Benching table, 969, 977
Benchmarking, 16, 19, 35–36
Benign lesions, in children, 126
Benign neoplasms, 110
Benign tumor, 395, 408–409, 790, 800
Bentonite powder, 592
Beta particle sterilization, 333
Beta particles, 113
Between-case cleanup, definition of, 211
Bezoars, 146
Bicaval cannulation, 923, 929
Bier block, 459–461, 459f–460f
Bilateral adrenalectomy and oophorectomy, 112
Bilateral adrenalectomy and orchiectomy, 112
Biliary atresia, 143, 143f
Biliary tract procedures, 670–674
  cholecystectomy, 671, 671f
    laparoscopic, 671, 672f
  cholecystoduodenostomy/cholecystojejunostomy,
    673–674
  common bile duct exploration, 671–673
  endoscopic retrograde, 671
  hazards of, 670
Billroth I gastrectomy, 679f
Binocular, term, 360, 372
Bioabsorbable translucent spray, 605
Bioburden, 295, 298
  sterilization and, 313
Bioethical situations, 51–54
Biofeedback, for burn patients, 872
Biofilm, 239, 243
  definition of, 238, 295
  life cycle, 243f
Biohazards, 234–235
Biologic adhesives, 429, 575
Biologic hazards, 71, 219, 233–235
Biologic materials, 576

Biologic valves, 934
Biologic vascular grafts, 954–955
Biomedical engineering, clinical, 87
Bioprosthetic valves, 934
Biopsies, 395
  breast, 402, 666–667
  of burned tissue, 871
  endoscopic, 408
  excisional, 666
  frozen section and, 666
  incisional, 666
  liver needle, 674
  of thyroid, 895
Bioresistance, sterilization and, 313
Bioshielding, sterilization and, 313
Biostate, sterilization and, 313
Bioterrorism, 238, 259, 259b
Bipolar electrosurgery, 360, 364, 364f
Bispectral index monitoring, 549
Bivalved cast, 761, 770
Biventricular assistance (BVA), 944
Biventricular pacemakers, 923, 941
Bladder exstrophy, 146–147
Bladder flap urethroplasty, 748–749
Bladder neck suspension, transvaginal, 747–748
Bladder, urinary, 732
  anatomy of, 698f, 744–748
  voiding, preoperative, 389
Blades, 478, 478f. *See also* Sharps
  retractors and, 345–346, 346f
  scalpels and, 340, 340f
  ultrasonic, 377
Blalock-Hanlon procedure, 159
Blalock-Taussig procedure, 158, 158f
Bleeding. *See* Hemorrhage
Blended current, 360, 362
Blepharoplasty, 833, 858–859, 859f
Blindness, 103–104
Block charting, 47–48
Blocking quality, of local and regional anesthetics,
  460
Blood
  for autotransfusion, double-lumen suction tip for,
    352
  body fluids and, as sources of pathogens, 490
  drawing samples of, 538
Blood bank, 86
Blood chemistry, normal, values in, 633t
Blood gases, monitoring of, 542–543
  arterial, analysis, 543
Blood glucose levels, monitoring during surgery of,
  107
Blood loss
  categories of, 634
  considerations in, 634
  estimation of, 635, 636b
  fluid and electrolyte balance, 634
  measurement of, gastrointestinal decompression and,
    599
  monitoring of, 488
  pneumatic counterpressure device and, 593
  reduction of, 636–637
  in vascular surgery, 954
Blood loss replacement, 638–641
  allogeneic, 639–640
  autologous, 640–641
  complications of, 641
Blood patch, epidural, 458
Blood pressure
  arterial, monitoring of, 541–542
  of geriatric patient, 171

Blood pressure cuff, 593–595
Blood products, 639–640
  shelf life of, 639t
Blood substitutes, 641
Blood transfusion, 636
  autotransfusion, blood draw for, 380
  in children, 129
  by circulating nurse, 486
  pretransplantation of, 981
  in thoracic surgery, 909
  in vascular surgery, 954
Blood type and crossmatch, 380
Blood vessel grafts, 970
Blood volume
  in children, 129
  complications in, perioperative, 634–641
  total, 547
Blood volume expanders, 636
Blue babies, 158
Blue-green argon, 845–846
Blunt dissectors, 341, 342f
Blunt intracavitary applicator, 115
Blunt methods, 70, 70f
Blunt trocar, 649
Board certification, 56
Bodily kinesthetic learner, 4
Body habitus, 499
Body jacket, 787
Body mass index (BMI), 99, 108
Body mechanics, 220–221, 221f, 222b
Body restraint strap, bed attachments and, 509
Body rests, bed attachments and, 509
Body surface area, 626
Body, listening to, 14
Bogota bag, 581
Boiling water, for disinfection, 308
Bolsters
  for positioning, 511
  in sutures, 561
  for wound healing, 604, 604f
Bolus, 625–626
Bone bank, 579
Bone cement, 233, 576
Bone cement implantation syndrome (BCIS),
    761, 778
Bone cutters and saws, 341
Bone grafts, 578–579, 767, 969
  free autologous, 855, 855f
  for maxillae and/or mandible, 888
  procurement parameters for, 971t
  in total joint replacement, 778
Bone holders, 343, 345f
Bone hooks, 766, 766f
Bone implant, xenograft, 579
Bone marrow biopsy, 397
Bone marrow transplantation, 970–972
Bone procurement, rib resection for, 916, 916f
Bone wax, 596, 769
  alternatives, 596
  in neurosurgery, 794
  in spinal surgery, 816
  in thoracic surgery, 909
Bones, 762–764, 762f
  anatomy of, 763f
  healing of, 763–764, 764f
Boots, as personal protective equipment, 267
Borrowed servant rule, 39
Bougies, 676–677, 905, 920
Bowel gases (methane), flammable, 230
Bowel preparation, 382
Bowie-Dick test, 312, 321

Box, suture materials and, 571–572
Braces, orthopedic, 769
Brachial plexus, 809–810
Brachytherapy, 114–115, 395, 414
Brain, 790–792
  anatomy and physiology of, 790–792
  blood supply to, 791
  electrostimulation, 803
  oxygen reserves in, 542
Brain death, 54, 969–970
  criteria for, 975t
  organ procurement and, 974
Brain injury, in abused infant, 122
Brain pacemaker, 799
Brain tumors, 800
Brainstem, 792
Breast
  anatomy of, 667f
  of geriatric patients, 173
  procedure in, for draping of patient, 532
  skin preparation for, antiseptic, 525, 525f
Breast cancer, 173
  locations of, by quadrant, 667f
  stages of, 668t
  treatment options, 667
Breast procedures, 666–670
  biopsy, 666–667, 667f
  considerations for, in female, 670
  incision, and drainage, 666, 668f
  lumpectomy, 668, 669f
Breast self-examination, 402, 418
Breastfeeding, and medications, 421
Breathing circuit, 438, 451
  anesthesia, 439f
  contamination of, 450
  disposable, 450
Bretylium, 626
Broad ligaments, 698f, 699
Bronchoplastic reconstruction, 918
Bronchoscopic lung volume reduction (BLVR), 912
Bronchoscopy, 910–911, 911f–912f
Bronchospasm, as respiratory complications,
    617–618
Bronchus clamps, 909, 909f
Broviac catheter, 543
Brown-Buerger cystoscope, 735
Brush biopsy, 397
BSS. See Balanced salt solution
Budgeting, 95–97
Bugbee, 736
Bullets, X-rays of, 399
Bullying, 4
Bumpers, in sutures, 561
Bunionectomy, 783, 783f
Bupivacaine, 455t, 461
Burns, 867–872
  biologic dressings for, 870–871
  categorization of, 852f
  classification of, 867
  debridement of, 870
  dressing changes for, 871
  electrical, 229
  environmental considerations for patients with,
    871–872
  estimation of damage, 868
  estimation of percentage, 869
  fluid therapy for, 869, 869t
  initial care of, 868–869
  ocular, 844
  surgical treatment of, 869–871
  thermal, from equipment, 229

Burr holes, 799
Business manager, perioperative, 83
Buttonholes, 69
Buzzing, 362
Buzzing a forceps, 64, 66, 66f

C
C-arm image intensifier, 223, 223f, 400f
CABG. See Coronary artery bypass graft
Cabinets, in operating rooms, 192
Cadaver organ procurement, 979
Cages, interbody, 823, 825f
CAI. See Community-acquired infection
Calcium chloride, in malignant hyperthermia, 644
Calcium salts, 628
Calcium scoring, 932
Calcium, as electrolyte, 633
Caldwell-Luc procedure, 884
Calipers, 352, 353f
Call-light system, in operating room, 193
"Call out" feedback methods, 82
Camera operator, on laser team, 371
Cameras
  for endoscopy, 652, 653f
  ethylene oxide sterilization of, 329
  for operating microscope, 375
Camey pouch, 747
Cancer, 110–117, 395, 408–418
  causes of, 110, 408
  in children, warning signs of, 418
  clinical signs and symptoms of, 409
  extent of disease in, 110–111, 409
  familial syndromes of, 411t
  perioperative care for, 417
  risk avoidance behaviors for, 418
  risk avoidance for, 110
  risk factors for, 409
  risk-related factors for, 409, 411t
  screening for, 409, 410t
  staging of, 409
  tumor identification system for, 409
  tumor markers in, 412t
Cancer treatment, 111, 411–417
  adjuvant, 111, 117, 411–412
  by chemotherapy, 117, 411–412
  determining appropriate, 411–412
  by endocrine therapy, 112, 412–413
  intraoperative care for, considerations in, 111–112
  palliative, 111
  by photodynamic (laser) therapy, 112–113, 413
  preservation of reproductive system in, 412
  by radiation therapy, 113–117, 413–415
  by surgical resection, 111
    palliation and, 412
Candy cane stirrups, 510, 510f
Canister collection method, 640
Cannula, 352
  uterine, 344f
Cannulation, intravascular, monitoring of, 536–537
Capillary action, 312, 324
Capillary, anatomy of, 949
Capital budget, 79, 96–97
Capnometry, 542–543
Capsulorrhexis, 826, 838
Carbon dioxide laser, 366–367, 768
Carbon dioxide narcosis, 619
Carbon dioxide, monitoring of, 542
Carbon fiber, as synthetic material, for implants, 580
Carcinogenesis
  chemical, 411t
  viral-mediated, 411t

Carcinoma, 395
of larynx, 891–892
oral, 886
Carcinoma in situ, 110, 409
Cardiac arrest, 624–625
Cardiac catheterization, 932–933, 932f
electric shock hazard in, 228
Cardiac compression, 629, 629f
Cardiac dysrhythmias, 619, 622
during anesthesia, 436, 440, 487
procedure for, 938–939
Cardiac index (CI), 547
Cardiac output, monitoring of, 546–547
Cardiac pacemaker, 940–942, 941f, 941t
Cardiac surgery, 923–946
assist devices in, 940–945
artificial heart, 944–945
cardioverter-defibrillator, 942, 942f
intraaortic balloon pump, 942–943, 943f
pacemaker, 940–942, 941f, 941t
ventricular assist device, 943–944, 943f
cardiopulmonary bypass for, 929–932, 930f
complications of, 945–946
devices used in, 926
diagnostic procedures to, 932–933
extracorporeal membrane oxygenator and, 944
incisions for, 927–928, 928f
intraoperative monitoring in, 929
invasive hemodynamic monitoring in, 928–929
invasive procedures of, 932–933
noninvasive procedures of, 932
procedures in, 933–940
for atrial myxoma, 940, 940f
for coronary artery disease, 935–938
for dysrhythmias, 938–939
stress of, 933
valvular, 933–935, 933f
for ventricular aneurysm, 939, 939f–940f
special features of, 926–933
Cardiac tamponade, 923, 946
Cardiac transplantation, 940
Cardinal ligaments, 699
Cardiogenic shock, 642
Cardioplegia, 923, 926, 931, 931f
Cardiopulmonary bypass, 797, 923, 929–932, 930f
cardioplegia for, 931, 931f
complications of, 932
Cardiopulmonary resuscitation (CPR), 71, 628–632, 629f–630f
advanced cardiac life support in, 630
in ambulatory surgery, 203
basic cardiac life support in, 628–629
crash cart for, 630–631
duration of, 632
effectiveness of, 629
personnel responsibilities in, 631–632
postresuscitation care, 632
staff education, 632
Cardiopulmonary status, of pediatric patient, 131–132
Cardiopulmonary system, of geriatric patient, 168t, 170–171, 170f
Cardiotonics, 616, 627
Cardiovascular complications, perioperative, 620–632. See also Cardiopulmonary resuscitation
anxiety and, 620
cardiac arrest, 624–625
cardiac dysrhythmias, 622
coronary thrombosis, 621
deep vein thrombosis, 622

Cardiovascular complications, perioperative (Continued)
disseminated intravascular coagulation, 622
drugs for, intravenous, 625–626
hypertension, 621
hypotension, 620–621
venospasm, 621
venous stasis, 621
ventricular dysrhythmias, 622–624
Cardiovascular disease, 117
Cardiovascular surgery, 156–160
Cardioversion
asynchronous, 623
synchronized, 623
Cardioverter-defibrillator, implantable, 942, 942f
Caregiver, 161, 165
Carotid artery
blockage, of geriatric patient, 170, 170f
external occlusion of, 804
Carotid endarterectomy, 959
Carotid phonoangiography, 951
Carotid stenting, 956, 957f
Carpal tunnel syndrome, from holding retractors, 220
Carrier, 260
Carrier, as contamination source, 263
Cart system cleanup, 211, 216
Carts, in operating rooms, 192
Case cart system, 211, 216, 312, 316, 336, 336f
central processing department and, 336
checking, 466–474
decontamination of, 336
Case flow, maintaining of, 480–481, 482f–483f
Cassette, X-ray, 400
Cast material, 761
Cast room, 769
Casts, 769
application, 785–788
common configurations, 787–788, 787f
fiberglass, 785–786
material, 786
orthopedic cart and, 785b
padding under, 786
plaster, 786
trimming, removing, and changing, 788, 788f
Catabolism, 105, 616, 643
Cataract, 826, 838–840, 838f
extraction of, rehabilitation after, 839–840
in geriatric patients, 174
radiation protection and, 225
Cataract extraction, congenital, 150–151
Catecholamines, 627
Catheter insertion, 537–538
Catheterization, in geriatric patients, 175
Catheters, intravascular
in cardiac surgery, 929
monitoring of, 537–538
Cauda equina, 810, 811f
Caudad, 499
Caudal approach, 458
Causation, 37–38
Cauterization, 708
of cornea, 834
Cautery, ophthalmic, 828
Cavitation, 298
CBSPD. See Certification Board of Sterile Processing and Distribution
Cecostomy, 685
Cecum, anatomy of, 686f
Ceiling mount, 374
Ceiling-mounted endoscopic equipment, 653f
Ceiling, cleaning of, 217
of operating rooms, 187–188

Cellulitis, 241
Cellulose spears, 829f
Cellulose, oxidized, 954b
hemostasis and, 590–591
in neurosurgery, 794
Center for Devices and Radiological Health, laser hazards and, 368
Centers for Disease Control and Prevention (CDC), 90
wound classification of, 586
Centers for Medicare & Medicaid Services (CMS), 44, 89
Central command center, 91
Central processing area, 182
Central processing department, 87–88, 296
Central service personnel, 296–297
coordination of, with operating room staff, 296–297
Central storeroom, 87
Central venous cannulation, 543–544
for parenteral nutrition, 106
Central venous catheter, 416
Central venous pressure, monitoring of, 543–544
Cephalad, 499
Cephalic vein mapping, 951
Cephalocentesis, 154–155
Cerclage, 716, 716f
Cerebellar stimulator, 799
Cerebellum, 792
Cerebral blood flow measurements, 951
Cerebral function monitor, 548
Cerebral palsy, patient with, 104
Cerebral perfusion pressure (CPP), 549
Cerebral revascularization, 801
Cerebrospinal fluid (CSF), 791
Cerebrum, 791–792
Certification, 55–56
of central service personnel, 296
Certification Board of Sterile Processing and Distribution (CBSPD), 296
Certified nurse midwives (CNMs), 77, 85
Certified perioperative nurse (CNOR), 58–59, 71, 83
eligibility criteria, 60b
first assisting, 61
recertification, 60t
Certified postanesthesia care nurse (CPAN), 612
Certified registered central service technician (CRCST), 296
Certified registered nurse first assistant (CRNFA), 71, 76, 76b, 83
Certified sterile processing and distribution technician (CSPDT), 296
Certified surgical technologist (CST), 61–62, 77–78
calculating approved continuing education (CE) credits for, 62b
eligibility for certification by examination for, 62b
Cervical cancer, 702
Cervical dilators, 352, 353f
Cervical esophageal reconstruction, 893
Cervical spine
anterior approach of, 821, 822f
dermatome of, 820–821, 820f
nerves of, 812f
posterior approach of, 822, 822f–823f
transoral approach of, 821, 821f
vertebrae of, 810–811, 812f–813f
Cervicothoracic sympathectomy, 806
Cesarean birth, 696
Cesarean delivery, 177, 184

Cesarean delivery room, 194, 194f
  environmental controls in, 179t
Cesarean section, 177, 184, 719–721
  antibiotic prophylaxis and, 257–258
  father or support person at, 721
  perimortem, 718–719
  previous, 718
Chain of custody documentation, 399
Chain of evidence, skin preparation and, 520
Chain of specimen custody slip, 399
Chalazion, 832, 833f
Chaplain, hospital, 390
CHARGE association, 126
Charge nurse, 82–83
Charting modalities, 47–48
"Check back" feedback methods, 82
Check-in, 22
Check-off forms, 48
Check-off sheets for evaluation
  in circulating role, 5, 8f
  in scrub role, 6, 8f
Checklist
  Comprehensive Surgical, 23f
  preoperative, 390–391
Checkups
  annual, and cancer risk, 110
  regular, and cancer risk, 418
Chemical agents, in neurosurgery, 794
Chemical carcinogenesis, 411t
Chemical disinfectants, 302–308
  factors for selection of, 303
  influences on efficacy of, 302, 303b
  labeling of, 302, 302b
  liquid, 303, 304t–305t
  resistance to, 303, 306t
Chemical hazards, 71, 219, 231–233
Chemical hemostasis, 68–69
Chemical indicator tape, 317
Chemical sources, of drugs, 427
Chemical sterilants, in solution, 331–333
  advantages of, 331
  containers for, 332
  disadvantages of, 331–332
  preparing items for, 332–333
  rinsing after immersion in, 333
  timing of immersion cycle, 333
  types of, 332
Chemical sterilization, 326–333
Chemical wounds, intentional, 585
Chemotherapy, 117, 395
  indications for, 117
  intraoperative, 117
  postoperative, 117
  preoperative, 117
Chemotherapy, for cancer, 411–412, 416
  agents for, hazards associated, 233
  delivery devices for, 416–417
  indications for, 416
  infusion devices for, 417, 417f–418f
  intraoperative, 416
    for ovarian cancer, 714
  intraperitoneal, 233
  postoperative, 416
  preoperative, 416
Chest
  position, 518
  procedure in, for draping of patient, 532
  skin preparation for, antiseptic, 525, 525f
Chest drainage, 600–602, 601f
  thoracostomy for, 912–913, 919
Chest radiograph, monitoring of, 548

Chest rolls, for prone patient, 504
Chest trauma, 919
Chest tubes, 909–910, 910f
  in cardiac surgery, 927f, 945
  in chest trauma, 919
  in thoracic surgery, 909–910, 910f
Chest wound, sucking, 919
Chest x-ray, 401
  preoperative, 380
Chi points, 464, 465f
Chief executive officer (CEO), 84
Chief nursing officer (CNO), 80
Chief of surgery, 88
Child abuse, 122–123, 703
Chlamydia, 248
Chlorhexidine gluconate, 286
  for skin preparation, 524
Chlorhexidine, preoperative use by patient, 381
Chloride, as electrolyte, 633
Chlorine bleach, as presoak, 297
Chlorine compounds, for disinfection, 306–307
Chloroprocaine, 455t, 462
Choanal atresia, correction of, 151
Cholangiography, 403, 673
Cholecystectomy, 671, 671f
  laparoscopic, 671, 672f
Cholecystoduodenostomy, 673–674
Cholecystojejunostomy, 673–674
Choledochojejunostomy, 673–674
Choledocholithiasis, 670
Choledochoscopy, 673
Choledochostomy, 673
Cholelithiasis, 670
Cholelithotripsy, 673
Cholesteatoma, 873, 878, 879f
Cholinergic receptors, 625
Cholinergics, 446
Chorionic villus sampling, 721–722
Chromopertubation, 696, 703
Chronic obstructive pulmonary disease (COPD), 619, 912
Chronic wounds, 583, 586
Chylothorax, 921
Cicatrix, 583, 604–605
Cigarette drain, 599
CINAHL. See Cumulative Index to Nursing and Allied Health Literature
Cingulotomy, 803
Circular staplers
  end-to-end, 350
  intraluminal, 574
Circulating nurse, 6, 55, 58
  in anesthesia induction, 393–394
  assessment parameters, 28b
  in cardiopulmonary resuscitation, 631
  computer in operating room and, 193
  coordinated roles of, scrub person and, 466–498
  in counting
    sharps, 494
    sponges, 493–494
  in dispensing of medications, 425–426
  documentation by, 41
    of intraoperative patient care, 488, 489b
    of positioning, 519
  in dressings, application of, 604
  duties of, 466–495
    after the patient arrives, 485, 486b
    after the patient is anesthetized, 487, 487f
    after the scrub person scrubs, 484–485, 484f–485f
    after the surgeon and assistant(s) scrub, 487, 487f

Circulating nurse (Continued)
    after the surgical procedure is complete, 489–490
    during closure, 488–489
    entering the operating room with the patient, 485–486
    handover report to PACU nurse, 490
    in induction of general anesthesia, 487
    in intraoperative death, 124
    in patient transfer from the operating room, 490
    in starting the procedure, 487–488
    during the surgical procedure, 488–489
  handover report of, 612–613
  performance appraisal check-off sheet, 5
  roles of, as part of the nonsterile team, 468b
  in setting up the room, 466–474, 467f
    "eight P's" of, 476t–477t
    sterile supplies, opening of, 472–474
  specimen management by, 488
  sponge
    packaging increments of, 478b
    validating of, 472b–473b
  substerile room and, 184
  systematic activities for, 470t–472t
  transferring patient to operating room and, 391–394
Circulation, basic cardiac life support and, 629, 629f–630f
Circulatory considerations, for positioning of patient, 504–505
Circulatory status, wound healing and, 586–587
Circumcision, 147–148, 148f
  adult male, 756, 756f
Circumduct, 499
Circumferential, 499
  extremity prep, 526
Cisatracurium, 445
CJD. See Creutzfeldt-Jakob disease
Clamp and tie, 68
Clamping and occluding instruments, 343–345
Clamps, 69
  crushing, 343–345
  microsurgical, 353
  noncrushing, 345, 346f
  for orthopedic surgery, 766
Classroom, 181
Clean wounds, 586
Clean-contaminated wound, 587b
Cleaning
  of anesthesia equipment, 450–451
  of endoscopes, 658–659
  and sterilization, of powered instruments, 356
  of surgical environment. See also Surgical environment
    before first surgical procedure of day, 212
    guidelines for, 211
    preliminary preparations for, 212
    at room turnover, 212–216
Clear corneal cataract procedure, 839
Cleavage lines, 64
Cleft lip, 152–153, 153f
Cleft palate, 153, 153f
Clerk-receptionist, 180
Clinical competency, 13
  of perioperative nurse, 33–34
Clinical coordinator, 82
Clinical laboratory, 86
Clinical laser nurse, 371
Clinical nurse specialist (CNS), 83
Clinical pathology, 396
Clinical practice, realities of, 13–14

Clinical trials, of new drugs, 422
Clip appliers, 349–350, 595
  for endoscopy, 654
Clippers, for patient's skin, 521
Clips, 68, 575
  ligating, in neurosurgery, 794
Clitoris, 697
Cloaca, 125, 143
Clocks, for operating rooms, 192
Closed fracture, 771
Closed method, of incision, 648
Closed reduction, 761, 769
Closed water-seal drainage, in cardiac surgery,
    927, 927f
Closed wound suction systems, 600, 601f
Closed wounds, 585
Closed-assisted gloving, 275
Closed-circuit television, in operating room, 193
Closed-gloving, 275
Clostridium, endospores of, 245
Closure
  during
      circulating nurse duties, 488–489
      scrub person duties, 484
  after endoscopic procedures, 655
  in general surgery, 665
  instruments for, 347–350
Closure devices, arterial, 957–958
Clothing of patient, storing of, 389
Clubfoot deformity, 149, 149f
CMS. See Centers for Medicare & Medicaid Services
CNO. See Chief nursing officer
CNOR. See Certified perioperative nurse
CNS. See Clinical nurse specialist
Coagulating current, 360, 362
Coagulopathy, 616, 622
Coarctation of aorta, 157
Coaxial illumination, 360
Coaxial illuminators, 373
Cobalt-60, 333
Coblation, 364, 875
Cocaine, 455t, 461
Cochlear implants, 880–881, 881f
Cognition, 1, 3–4
Cognitive function, impairment of, patient with, 104
Colectomy, total, 684
Collagen
  for aesthetic procedures, 860
  hemostatic, materials for, 590
  microfibrillar, for hemostasis, 640
  in wound healing, 584, 587
  xenograft and, 580
Collagen sutures, 565
Colles fracture, 772
Colonoscopy, 687, 689f
Colorectal carcinoma, 686
  abdominoperineal resection for, 687–688
  low anterior colon resection for, 688, 689f
  rectal tumors, 692
Colorectal procedures, 686–688
Colostomy, 685, 686f
Colpocleisis, 708
  vaginal, 173
Colpoperineorrhaphy, posterior, 707
Colporrhaphy, anterior, 707
Colposcope, 122
Colposcopy, 702–703
Colpotomy, 703
  posterior, 703
Combat support hospital (CSH), 206–207
Combined internal-external disaster, 21

Commission on Accreditation of Allied Health Edu-
    cation Programs (CAAHEP), 34
Committees, 79, 88
Common bile duct exploration, 671–673
Common denominator, 423
Communicable infection, 264
Communication, 82, 91
  among ambulatory surgery caregivers, 199
  effective, 11
  with loss of hearing or voice, 874
  of nurse manager, 82
Communication systems, in operating room, 193
Communications, 81–82
Community-acquired infection (CAI), 238, 241, 264
Comorbidity, 99, 103, 161–162
Compartment syndrome, 606, 761, 788–789, 789f
Competency, 1, 13
Competency Statement, 16, 33–34
Competitive antagonists, 445
Competitive benchmarking, 35–36
Complicated wounds, 585–586
Complications, perioperative, 610–646
  after orthopedic surgery, 788–789
  of blood volume, 634–641
  cardiovascular, 620–632
  of cranial surgery, 805–806
  of fluid and electrolyte imbalances, 632–634
  as iatrogenic injury, 646
  as metabolic crises, 642–646
  potential for, during and after surgery, 616–617
  respiratory, 617–620
  scoring systems, to predict, 616–617
Composite graft, 847, 852–853, 955
Composite myo-osteocutaneous free flap, 855
Composite, wound care materials, 608t
Comprehensive Surgical Checklist, 23f
Compressed spectral array, 548–549
Compression devices, sequential, 593
Computed tomography (CT), 397, 402
  of brain, 792
  of spine, 811
  of vascular disease, 951
Computer information systems, 48
Computer-generated charting, 48
Computerized digital subtraction processor, 401
Computerized documentation, 48, 48b
Computers
  in control desk, 180
  in operating room, 193
    lines, 188–190
Conduction anesthesia, 432, 434
Conduction velocity, of local and regional anesthetics,
    460
Conduit, 923, 935
Condylomata, 250
Condylomata acuminata, ablation of, 749
Cone biopsy, cervical, 702, 702f
Conference room, 181
Confidentiality
  high-profile event, 123
  HIV infection and, 119
Conflict management, 94
Congenital anomalies, 125–126
  craniofacial, 898–901, 899f–901f
  definition of, 125, 873
  dislocated hip, 148, 148f
Congenital cataract extraction, 150–151
Congenital deformities, 873
  of chest wall, 917
Congenital obstruction, of nasolacrimal duct, 150
Conjunctival laceration, 845

Connell suture, 560
Consent, 37, 40, 44–46
  general, 44
  informed, 44–45
    for ambulatory surgery, 201–202
    for transfusion, of blood, 640
  for organ donation, 974
Constant gravity drainage, 599–600
Constipation, in geriatric patient, 171–172
Consultation room, 181
Contact contamination, 262b
Contact layer, dressing and, 602–603
Contact lenses, 104, 389, 392
Containers, rigid closed, 319–320
Contaminated, 260
Contaminated areas, preparing, 523
Contaminated items
  definition of, 262
  in general surgery, 665
Contaminated wounds, 586, 587b
Contamination
  of anesthesia equipment, 450
  definition of, 211
  human-borne sources of, 262–263
  nonhuman factors of, 263–264
  oral cavity and, 874
Continual performance evaluation and improvement,
    35–36
Continuing education (CE) credits, 62b
Continuous intravenous drip, 625
Continuous Performance Improvement Committee,
    90
Continuous running/locking, sutures, 560, 560f
Continuous, simple, sutures, 560, 560f
Contracted services, 39–40
Contracture, definition of, 583
Contralateral inguinal ring, 145
Contralateral, defined, 125, 145
Contrast media, 399–400, 399b
  in angiography, 403
  barium, 403
  in cholangiography, 403
  in CT, 402
  for endoscopy, 653
  in MRI, 404–405
  in myelography, 404
  in urography, 404
Contrast medium, 395, 420
Contraves stand, 360, 374
Control desk, 177, 179–181
Controlled homeostasis, 447–448
Controlled respiration, 440
Contusions, of globe, 844–845
Conus medullaris, 810, 810f
Convection oven, for sterilization, 325–326
Conversions
  definition of, 420
  pharmacologic, 424
Convulsions, 642
COPD. See Chronic obstructive pulmonary disease
Coping mechanisms, 100, 101t
Core biopsy, of breast, 666
Core temperature, 535, 547
Corium, in xenograft, 580
Cornea, procedures for, 834–837
  cauterization, 834
  laceration, 845
  phototherapeutic keratectomy, 835
  for pterygium, 834
  refractive keratoplasty, 836–837, 836f–837f
  transplantation, 834–835, 834f, 971t

Corneal grafts, 969
Corneal trephine, 829, 831f
Corneal ulceration, 834
Cornstarch powder, in surgical gloves, 284
Coronary artery angioplasty, 937—938
Coronary artery bypass graft (CABG), 935—937, 935f
Coronary artery disease, 935—938
Coronary circulation, 925
Coronary thrombosis, 621
Coroner's cases, 123—124
Corporate negligence doctrine, 40
Corpus callosotomy, 804
Cortical resection, for neurosurgery, 804
Corticosteroids, 112
    with cancer chemotherapy, 413
    for transplant recipient, 981
Cortisone, 112
Cotrel-Dubousset rods, 150f
Cottonoids, 492, 596, 794
Coumarin derivatives, 637
Count sheets, 357
    packed in instrument set, 320
    simplifying instrument counts in, 495
Counting and accountability, 25b
Counts, 490—495
    baseline, 491
    closing of, 491
    in establishing baselines, 477—478
    final, 491
    incorrect, 492
    initial, 491
    in instruments, 495
    in life-threatening emergency, 632
    of patties, 794
    procedures for, 490—492
    reasons for, 490b
    in sharps, 494
    in sponges, 492—494
Court-ordered procedures, 51—52
COVID-19, 252
    preventive measures, 252
    risk factors, 252
    symptoms, 252
    testing for, 252
CPAN. See Certified postanesthesia care nurse
CPP. See Cerebral perfusion pressure
CPR. See Cardiopulmonary resuscitation
Cranial blood vessels, surgery of, 801—802
Cranial nerves, 791, 791t
    decompression of, 801
Craniectomy, 799, 799f
Craniofacial anomalies, 898—901, 899f—901f
Craniofacial microsomia, 154, 900
Craniofacial surgery, 858, 898
    maxillofacial and mandibular, 902—904
    for midface advancement, 901
    for midfacial fractures, 902, 902f
    of orbit, 901
    for tumor resection, 901—902
Cranioplasty, 800—801
Craniosynostosis, 153—154, 154f, 898—900, 899f
Craniotomy, 790, 797
Cranium, surgical procedures of, 799—806
Crash cart, 630—631
CRCST. See Certified registered central service technician
Creams, 430
    dispensing to sterile surface, 426, 430
Credentialing, 56
Credentials, 55

Creutzfeldt-Jakob disease (CJD), 252—253, 320
    cottonoid and, contaminated, 490
    high-level disinfection and, 301, 302f
    new-variant, blood donation and, 639
Cricoid pressure, 436—437, 437f, 617
    for obstetric patient, 716
Crime victim, 120—121
Critical thinking, 1, 13
CRNFA. See Certified registered nurse first assistant
Cross clamping, of aorta, blood supply to spinal cord and, 959
Cross-contamination, 238, 248, 260, 264
Cross-finger flap, 854
Cross-infection, as contamination source, 263
Crosshatched jaws, needle holders with, 347
Crouzon disease, 900, 900f
Crushing clamps, 338, 343—345
Cryoablation
    for dysrhythmias, 939
    transperineal prostatic, 755
Cryoanesthesia, 459
Cryohypophysectomy, 804
Cryopreserved skin, 578
Cryosurgery, 597
    for otorhinolaryngologic and head and neck surgery, 876
Cryptorchidism, 125, 147
CSH. See Combat support hospital
CSPDT. See Certified sterile processing and distribution technician
CT. See Computed tomography
CT navigation systems, 884
Cul-de-sac hernia, 707
Culdocentesis, 703
Culdoscopy, 704
Cultures, 396
    of burned tissue, 871
Cumulative Index to Nursing and Allied Health Literature (CINAHL), 10
Curettes, 341, 343f
    for orthopedic surgery, 766
Curling's ulcer, 871
Current, 360
Current, electrical, 227
Cushing suture, 560
Custom packs, 211, 216, 312, 335—336
Cutaneous pressure photoplethysmography, 408
Cutaneous ureterostomy, 747
Cutting, 338
Cutting current, 360, 362
Cutting instruments, 339—341
    for orthopedic surgery, 766, 767f
Cutting sutures, 560—561
Cyanoacrylate, 575—576
Cyanosis
    central, 618, 621
    peripheral, 618
Cyclodialysis, 826, 838
Cyclosporine, 980
Cylinder cast, 787, 787f
Cystectomy, 745—747
    urinary diversion procedures for, 745—747
Cystocele, 707—708, 707f
Cystography, 404
Cystolithotomy, 744, 744f
Cystometrogram, 744
Cystoplasty, 745
Cystoscopy, 146, 744—745
    before abdominal procedure, 665
    patient preparation for, 733—734
    room for, 733

Cystoscopy room, 194
Cystotomy, 745
Cystourethrography, 404
Cytomegalovirus infection, 250
Cytoreductive debulking surgery. See Ultrasonosurgery
Cytoreductive surgery, 395, 412
Cytotoxic agents, 233

D

da Vinci robot, 662, 662f
Dacron cuff, 416f, 417
Dacron grafts, 955
Dacryocystectomy, 833
Dacryocystorhinostomy, 833
Daily terminal cleaning, 216—217
Damages, 37
Damp dusting, 213b
Dantrolene, for malignant hyperthermia, 644
De-airing, 923, 930—931
Dead space, 583
    in wound, 588
Deafness, 103
Death and dying, 54
Death of patient, in operating room, 123—124
Debridement, 64, 70, 583, 586, 607, 847, 856
    of burns, 870
    excisional, 869—870
    wet-to-dry dressing and, 604
    of wound, 523
    wound bed cover after, 870
Debulking cancer therapy, surgical, 111
Debulking instruments, 338, 341—342, 342f—343f
    for orthopedic surgery, 766, 767f
Debulking, surgical, 412
Decamethonium, 446
Decimals, 422—423
    addition of, 422
    division of, 423
    multiplication of, 422—423
    subtraction of, 422
Decision-making, moral principles in, 51, 51b
Decompression, 808, 816, 833
Decontamination,
    213, 260, 262, 295—311. See also Disinfection
    definition of, 211, 295
    of operating room contents, 213
    procedures for, 358
    standard precautions and, 268
Decortication, pulmonary, 905, 913
Decubitus ulcer, 583, 586
Deep, 499
Deep breathing, teaching about, 386
Deep sedation, 434
Deep vein thrombosis (DVT), 622
    in orthopedic surgery, 788
    phlebography of, 952
    phleborheography of, 951
    vascular surgery and, 953
Deep veins, 949, 950f
Deep wound infection, 606
Defendant, 37, 40
Defense, three lines of, 240
Defibrillation, 623—624, 626, 628
Defibrillator, implantable, 942, 942f
Deglutition, 873, 888
Degreasers, 430
Dehiscence, 583
    wound, 605
Dehydration, 634, 637
    in geriatric patient, 172

Deionized water, 295, 298
Delayed full-thickness injury, 586
Delayed primary closure, 584f, 585
Delegation, 55, 57−58
Delegation of duties, 94
Delicate forceps, 342
Denis Browne splint, clubfoot deformity, 149f
Density, sterilization and, 313
Dental implant, 888−889
Dental procedures, 887−889
Dentures, 389, 392
Departmental policies, 81
Departmental service divisions, 86−88
Deployable medical systems, 197, 206−209,
        207f−209f
Deployment, definition of, 197, 206
DEPMEDS, 197
Depolarization, 432, 446
Depolarizing neuromuscular blockers, 446
Deposition, 37, 39
Depression, local anesthetics and, 463
Depth of field, 360, 372
Dermabrasion, 865−866
Dermatographics, 553
Dermatome map, 610, 615
Dermatome tape, 851
Dermatomes, 454, 820, 850−851, 851f
    of cervical spine, 820, 820f
    definition of, 610, 808, 847
    perianesthesia for, personnel of, 612, 612f, 612b
Dermis, 554
Desflurane, 441t, 442
Desmopressin acetate, for reduction of blood loss,
        636
Detergent-disinfectants, 303
Deviated nasal septum, 883
Devitalized tissue, 583, 588
Dextran
    as blood volume expanders, 636
    in local anesthetic, 461
    low-molecular-weight, 637
Diabetes mellitus, 106−108, 107f, 107t
    common complications of, 107
    conditions caused by, 106−108
    in geriatric patient, 172
    management of surgical patient with, 106−108,
        107f, 107t
    preoperative assessment in, 107
    special considerations for, 108
    tissue perfusion deficiency in, 107
    types of, 106
Diagnostic chemical, 420, 430
Diagnostic procedures
    patient care considerations for, 396
    preoperative, 380
Diagnostics, 385
Dialysis, 739−741
    access modalities for, 740f, 966, 966f−967f
Diaphragm, 908, 908f
Diaphragmatic hernia, 145f
Diaphragmatic herniorrhaphy, 694
Diaphragmatic pacemaker, 920, 922f
Diathermy, 597
Diazepam, 441t
    for adverse effects of local anesthetic, 464
    in children, 133t−134t
        for premedication, 136
Dibucaine, 455t, 461
Dietary supplements
    pharmaceutical error and, 421
    potential complications with, 387, 388t

Digital chest drainage systems, 602
Digital compression, for hemostasis, 596
Digital holography, 793
Digital subtraction angiography (DSA), 401, 403
Digital subtraction processor, computerized, 401
Digital transfer, 855−856
Dilating instruments, 352, 353f
Dilating sleeve, 649
Dilation and curettage (D&C), 696, 709
        instruments for, 700t
Dilation and evacuation, 717−718
Dilation, definition of, 338, 352
Dilation, esophageal, 152
Dilation, of stricture, 892
Diluents, 420, 429
Diopter, 360, 372
Direct arterial pressure, monitoring of, 542
Direct laryngoscopy, 890
Director, of code, 631
Directories, 21
Directories hospital, 21
Dirty and infected wound, 587b
Disaster plan manual, 20
Disaster planning committee, 91
Disc regeneration and rupture, 816
Discectomy, 820−821, 820f
    micro, 820
Discharge instructions, for ambulatory surgery
        patient, 203, 205
Discharge, from hospital, 386
Discission, definition of, 826, 846
Disease, 1−2
Disinfectants, hazards associated with, 233
Disinfection, 260, 262, 295−311
    of anesthesia equipment, 450
    chemical disinfectants for, 302−308
        factors for selection of, 303
        influences on efficacy of, 302, 303b
        labeling of, 302, 302b
        liquid, 303, 304t−305t
        resistance to, 303, 306t
    of items used in patient care, 301−302
    levels of, 301−302
    methods of, 302−309
    physical disinfectants for, 308−309
    terminal, 266
Dislocated hip, congenital, 148, 148f
Dislocations, 776
Dispersing lint, 596b
Dispersive electrode, 363, 365
    placement of, 66, 487, 487f
Displacement, 148
Displacement ventilation, 177, 184
Disposable equipment, for anesthesia, 450
Disposable products, 309−311
Disruptive behavior (bullying), 1, 4
Dissecting aneurysm, 947, 960, 960f
Dissecting instruments, 339−341
    for orthopedic surgery, 766, 767f
Dissecting sponges, 492
Dissection, 69−70
    definition of, 64, 338−339
Disseminated cancer, 111, 409
Disseminated intravascular coagulation, 622
Dissociative anesthesia, 443
Distal, 499
Distance, from ionizing radiation, 224
Distilled water, 295, 298
Distress, 14
Distribution, 420, 422
Diuretics, 627

Diversion, 730, 739
Diverticulectomy, pharyngeal, 887
Diverticulosis, in geriatric patient, 171−172, 172f
Dividing stapler, 574
Do-not-resuscitate (DNR) orders, 53
Do-not-resuscitate (DNR) wristband, 391−392
Dobutamine, 627
Doctor of nursing practice (DNP) degree, 83
Documentation, 91, 95
    in ambulatory surgery, 206
    asset number of specialized equipment and, 361
    by circulating nurse, of positioning, 519
    computerized, 48, 48b
    to facility, benefits of, 47
    laser surgery and, 369
    of medications administered, 666
    of patient care, 47−49
        by circulating nurse, 488, 489b
    of perioperative patient care, 46−50
    PNDS, 32
    in postanesthesia care unit, 614
    standards and methods for, 47−49
Domain, 16
Domestic violence, 99, 121−122
    to pregnant women, 121
Donor, 969−970
Donut, 511, 511f
Doors, of operating room, 184
    control of airborne contamination in, 266
    kept closed, 266
Dopamine, 628
Doppler probe, 951, 952f
    color flow, in cardiac surgery, 929
    of vessels underlying graft, 857
Doppler studies, 406−407
Doppler ultrasound flowmeter, for arterial blood pres-
        sure, 541−542
Doppler ultrasound scan, physiologic monitoring and,
        798
Dor procedure, 939
Dorsal, 499
Dorsal position, 512−513, 512f
Dorsal recumbent position, modified, 512−513, 513f
Dorsal space, 847
Dorsal vein ligation, 757
    for erectile dysfunction, 757
Dosimeters, for radiation, 225, 225f
Double armboard, bed attachments and, 508, 509f
Double-gloving, 243, 267, 275, 283, 285
Doubling time, 239
Douglas, semicircular line of, 555−556, 555f
Downward violence, 94−95
Drains and drainage, 588−589, 597, 599−602
    active, 600−602, 601f
    in chest trauma, 919
    dressings for, 602−604
    intraoperative, 599
    passive, 599
    patient care considerations with, 602
    postoperative, 599−602
    in thoracic surgery, 909−910, 910f
Drape pack
    opening of, 473−474
    reusable woven fabric drapes in, arrangement of, 474
    steam sterilization of, 323
Drapes
    laser safety with, 369
    materials of, 527−529
        nonwoven disposable, 528
        self-adhering sheeting, 527−528
        woven textile fabrics, 528−529

Drapes (*Continued*)
  removing of, from patients, 484
  styles/types of, 529—530
    fenestrated sheets, 528f, 529
    separate sheets, 529—530
    towels, 529
Draping
  of equipment, 534
  of Mayo stand, 474—475, 475f
  of otorhinolaryngologic and head and neck surgery,
    874—875, 875f
  of patient, 479—480, 499—534
    materials in, 527—534
    planning the organization of, 501t—503t
    preliminary considerations in, 499—504
    principles of, 530
    procedures for, 530—534, 531f
    unusual circumstances in, 530
  for plastic surgery, 848
  of unsterile table, 271f
Drawsheet, bed attachments and, 508, 508f
Dressings, 602—604
  anatomy of, 603f
  application of, 484, 604
  for diabetic patient, 108
  functions of, 602
  for geriatric patients, 171
  material for, 608t
  in plastic and reconstructive surgery, 849
  types of, 602—604
Droperidol, 441t
Droplet contamination, 262b
Drops, eye, administering, 831
Drug administration, 26, 26f
Drug interactions, 625
  in geriatric patients, 175
Drugs and pharmaceuticals
  administration of
    abbreviations in, accepted, 424
    conversions of dosages in, 424
    dispensing to sterile field, 426
    mathematics of, 422
    routes of, 425, 429b
    seven rights of, 421
    weights and measures in, 425t
  in ambulatory surgery, safety with, 199
  breastfeeding and, 421
  in cardiac surgery, 926
  cardiovascular, intravenous, 625—626
  classification of, 626—628
  development of, 422
  effect on metabolism, 104, 104t
  in handling medications and solutions, on sterile
    field, 478—479
  legal aspects of, 50—51
  names of, 422
  ophthalmic, 831—832
  and other chemicals, 233
  in otorhinolaryngologic and head and neck surgery,
    876
  patient assessment and, 421
  pharmacodynamics, of local and regional anesthetics,
    460—461
  pregnancy, lactation and reproductive considerations
    with, 421—422
  sun exposure and, 110
  in surgery, 425—426
    administration routes for, 429b
    circulating nurse and, 425
    examples of, 428t—429t
    labeling of, 426

Drugs and pharmaceuticals (*Continued*)
    pharmacologic forms of, 428—430
    potential complications of, 430—431
    scrub person and, 426
    sources of, 426—428
    wound healing and, 588
Drum-style skin graft dermatomes, 851
Dry heat sterilization, 325—326
  biologic testing for, 326
Dry sterile dressing, 602
Ductoscopy, fiberoptic, 666—667
Duhamel procedure, 142
Dumping syndrome, 678
Dura mater, 579—580, 795
Durable power of attorney, 53—54
Durant position, 514
Durant procedure, 407, 619
Dust cover, 335
DVT. *See* Deep vein thrombosis
Dye, 420
Dyes, surgical, 398b, 421
Dynamic air removal, 321
Dynamic tension, 64
Dysplasia, 148
Dysrhythmias, 432, 436, 616, 618
  in geriatric patients, 170

E
Ear,
  876—881. *See also* Otorhinolaryngologic and
    head and neck surgery
  anatomy of, 876—877, 876f
  hearing loss and, 877
  infection of, 877
    cholesteatoma secondary to, 878, 879f
  physiology of hearing and, 877
  procedure in, for draping of patient, 532
  proximal structures of, 877
  skin preparation for, antiseptic, 525
  surgical procedures of, 878—881
    external ear, 878
    general considerations for, 878
    inner ear, 880—881
    middle ear, 878—880
Ear speculum, 351f
Ear, nose, and throat (ENT) surgeons, 873
Ebonized finish, 339
ECG. *See* Electrocardiogram
Echocardiogram, 540
Echocardiography, 406, 923, 932
ECMO. *See* Extracorporeal membrane oxygenator
Economy
  of motion, 496—497
  supplies and equipment in, 497—498
    avoid damage, 497—498
    for intended use, 497
    varieties and numbers of, 497
-ectomy, 664
Ectopic pregnancy, 718, 718f
Ectropion, 833, 833f
Edema, 583, 588, 634
Education coordinator, perioperative, 83—84
Education, perioperative, 1—15
  application of theory to practice in, 10—11
  behavioral objectives for, 5—6, 9b
  educator in, 5—10, 9b
  effective instruction, 6
  expected behaviors in, 11—13
  indications for surgical procedures in, 2t
  learner in, 3—5, 4t, 4b
  media and print learning resources for, 9—10

Education, perioperative (*Continued*)
  performance appraisal in
    in circulating role, 5
    in scrub role, 5
  personality traits in, 5
  practical experience in, 11
  realities of clinical practice in, 13—14
  reality shock in, 13
  structured curriculum in, 5
Educator, 5—10, 9b
EEG. *See* Electroencephalogram
Effective communication, barriers to, 82
Effector innervation, 555
Efficiency, of operating room team, 495—498
EHRs. *See* Electronic health records
Ejection fraction (EF), 546
Elastic bandage, for dressing, 603
Elbow
  procedure in, for draping of patient, 532—533
  skin preparation for, antiseptic, 526
  total joint replacement of, 780—781
Elective voluntary surgical ending of pregnancy, 696
Electric shock, 228
Electrical burns, 229
Electrical systems, for operating room, 188—190,
  189f—190f
Electrically powered instruments, 355—356
Electricity
  hazards in, 227—229
  parameters of, 227
Electrocardiogram (ECG),
  539—540, 540f, 540b, 541f
  continuous, 437
  preoperative, 380
Electrocautery, 362, 597
  of cervical abnormalities, 708
  hazard with, 364
Electroencephalogram (EEG), 548—549
  during neurosurgery, 799
Electrohydraulic lithotripsy, 742
Electrolytes, 633—634, 633t
Electronic health records (EHRs), 29, 41
Electronic medical records (EMRs), 379, 383
Electrophysiologic measurements, 929
Electrostimulation, of brain, 803
Electrosurgery, 361—365, 597
  argon beam coagulator in, 363
  bipolar, 364, 364f
  electrode tip for, 362
    debris from, discharged of, 362
  endoscopic, 654
  hazard of, 364
    burn, 364
  monopolar, 362—363
  in neurosurgery, 794
  with obese patient, 109
  for otorhinolaryngologic and head and neck surgery,
    875
  precautions with, 364—365
  in preparing sutures and ties, 478
  principles of, 361—362
  safety factors for, 364—365
  in spinal surgery, 816
Electrosurgical unit (ESU), 25, 69, 360, 362
  generator, 362
  providing, 480
Element, 16, 29
Elevators
  periosteal, 341, 342f, 766, 766f
  for transport to OR, 390
Ellik evacuator, 737, 737f

Embolectomy, 957, 957f, 963–964
    pulmonary, 963–964
Embolic phenomena, antiembolic stockings for, 389
Embolization, hemostasis and, 592
Embolize material, 947, 952
Embolus, 619
    after orthopedic surgery, 788
    aortic cross-clamp leading to, 945
    from atrial myxoma, 940
    definition of, 616
Embryo transfer, 724
Emergence, 432, 436, 446
Emergence and extubation, 140
Emergencies, gastrointestinal decompression and, 599
Emergency department (ED), 85
    on arrival to, 119–120
Emergency exploratory laparotomy, 690, 690f
Emergency situations, anesthesia procedures in, 389
Emergency surgical procedure, in newborns, 125
Emissions, 360, 365
Emotional preparation, of patient, 390
Emphysema, 912
Empirical quality results, 80
En bloc unit, 969, 983
Encephalocele, 154
End-of-life care, 123
End-to-end circular staplers, 350
Endarterectomy, 947, 959, 959f
    coronary, 937
Endobronchial intubation, accidental, 440
Endocardial pacemaker, 941–942
Endocrine ablation, 112, 413
Endocrine glands, 758
Endocrine system, of geriatric patient,
    168t, 172, 172f
Endocrine therapy, for cancer, 112, 412–413
Endolymphatic sac shunt, 880
Endometrial cancer, 701
Endometrium, 696, 698, 698f
Endorectal pull-through, 142
Endoscopes, 350–351, 351f
    camera and, 652, 653f
    care of, 658–659
    ethylene oxide sterilization of, 328
    fetoscope, 722
    flexible, 652, 652f
    high-level disinfection, 655–656
    instrumentation used in, 654f
    microscopic attachments, 653
    in neurosurgery, 795
    for otorhinolaryngologic and head and neck surgery,
        875
    radiographic assisted, 653
    rigid, 652, 652f
    rigid hollow, 652
    sterile, 656
    ultrasound transducer, 653
    wireless capsule, 652–653
Endoscopic procedures, 177, 194
    eight essential elements of, 647–655, 648b
        access portal into body, 647–649, 648f
        capture of specimens, within working space, 655
        closure or minimizing of access portal, 655
        evacuation of gases, fluids, and solids from body,
            655
        illumination, of working space, 651
        manipulation and maneuverability, within work-
            ing space, 653–655
        single port, 648, 648f
        vision, within working space, 651–652
        working space within body, 649–651, 650f

Endoscopic procedures (Continued)
    energy-driven devices, 654
    hazards of, 657–658
    for herniated disc, 820–821
    human intervention during robotic-assisted proce-
        dures and, 663
    instrument manipulating robot, and master console,
        661–662, 661f
    knowledge and skill for
        of surgeon, 655
        of team, 655
    pediatric, 657
    pelvic, 704–706
    robotic-assisted, 660–663
    spinal, 823, 824f
    of stomach, gastroscopy, 678
    suturing in, 654
    transanal microsurgery, 692
    transluminal, 647
    types of, 655–658
    virtual reality and, 662–663
Endoscopic retrograde cholangiopancreatography, 671
Endoscopic sinus surgery, of paranasal sinus,
    884–885, 885f
Endoscopic stapler, 574–575
Endoscopic suturing, 561
Endoscopic technique, angioscopy, 952
Endoscopy, 408
    considerations for patient safety, 659–660
    definition of, 647
    duties of assistant for flexible, 660
    hazards of, 657–658
    pediatric, 657
    and pregnant patient, 657
    robotic-assisted, 660–663
    thoracic, 910
    urologic, 733
Endoscopy room, 194
Endospores
    bacterial, 213, 245–246, 245f–246f
    definition of, 238, 242b, 244, 295
Endotoxins, bacterial, 246
Endotracheal administration, 432, 439–440
Endotracheal intubation, 138–139, 138t
Endotracheal tube, 435
    double-lumen, 908–909, 909f
    laser safety of, 369
Endotracheal tube, laser safety of, 890
Endovascular abdominal aortic aneurysm repair,
    962–963, 963f
Endovascular procedures, 955
    intracranial, 805
Enflurane, 442
Engineer, clinical, 87
Enhanced Nursing Licensure Compact (eNLC), 20
ENT. See Ear, nose, and throat (ENT) surgeons
Enteral feeding, 106
Enterocele, 707, 707f
Entropion, 833, 833f
Enucleation, 834
    instruments for, 829, 830f
Environment, in operating room, 394
Environmental controls
    for contamination prevention, 264–267
    by robotics, 660
    in surgical suite, 179t
Environmental factors, 1–2
Environmental services, 87
    infection control and, 265–266
Environmental theory, 17b, 163
Environmental tobacco smoke (ETS), 418

Enzymatic cleaner, 295, 297
Enzymatic detergent, for instruments, 359
EO/CO₂, 327
Ephedrine, for anesthesia reaction, 463
Epicardial electrodes, 942
Epidemiology, 238–239
Epidermis, 553–554
Epidermolysis bullosa (EB), 866
Epidural anesthesia, 139, 432, 434, 454–464,
    454f, 456f
    in obstetrics, 715
    thoracic and lumbar approaches, 458
Epidural block, pediatric anesthesia, 138
Epidural blood patch, 458
Epidural narcotic analgesia, 458
Epidural spinal electrical stimulation (ESES), 965
Epikeratophakia, 836
Epilepsy, control of, 804
Epinephrine
    with anesthetic, 460
        in ear, nose, and throat procedures, 874
    as cardiovascular drugs, 627
        in cardiopulmonary resuscitation, 630
    hemostasis and, 591
    to treat anesthesia reaction, 463
Epiphyseal cartilaginous growth lines, 148
Episiotomy, 718f
Epistaxis, 882–883, 882f
Epithelialization, 583
    of wound, 587, 607
Eponychium, 556
Equipment, 25
    adverse events related to, 49
    asset tag number of, 361
    capital budget for, 96–97
    economical use of, 497–498
    evaluation of, 97
    safe use of, 218–219
    specialized, surgical, 360–378
Equipment technician, biomedical, 87
Equipotential grounding system, 228
Erectile dysfunction, 173, 756
    after prostatectomy, 754
Ergonomics, definition of, 218, 222b
Ergonovine, oxytocin and, 591
Error, human, as contamination source, 263
Eschar, 583, 597–598, 847, 867
Escharectomy, for burns, 870
Escharotomy, of burns, 870
ESES. See Epidural spinal electrical stimulation
Esmarch bandage, 594
Esophageal atresia, 143, 143f
Esophageal dilation, 152
Esophageal hiatal herniorrhaphy, 677, 677f
Esophageal procedures, 676–677, 892–893, 920
Esophageal stethoscopes, 540–541
Esophageal varices, surgical procedures for, 677
Esophagectomy, 920, 920f
Esophagogastrectomy, 677
Esophagoscopy, 892
Estrogen, 699
    adrenal glands and, 758
Estrogen antagonist, 413
Estrogen replacement therapy, 173
Ethacrynate sodium, 627
Ethics
    bioethical situations in, 51–54
    issues in, 38
    professional codes of, 51
    surgical technologists, 35
    universal moral principles, 51

Ethics committee, 90—91
Ethmoid sinus procedures, 884
Ethmoidectomy, 884
Ethyl alcohol, for skin preparation, 524
Ethylene chlorohydrin, 329
Ethylene glycol, 329
Ethylene oxide, 233, 658
Ethylene oxide gas sterilization, 326—330, 359
    advantages of, 327
    aeration following, 328t, 329—330
    of anesthesia equipment, 451
    biologic testing of, 330
    disadvantages of, 327—328
    hazards of, 326—327
    loading the sterilizer for, 329
    packaging materials for, 329
    parameters of, 327
    preparing items for, 328—329
    timing of, 329
    types of sterilizers for, 328
Etidocaine, 455t, 461
ETS. *See* Environmental tobacco smoke
Eustress, 14
Euthanasia, 53
Euvolemic, term, 923
Evacuating, 338
Evacuation, definition of, 351
Evacuators, for urologic endoscopy, 737
Evaluation, 1, 6
Evert edges, definition of, 551, 560
Everting sutures, 560, 560f
Evidence-based practice, 27—28, 79—80
    vs. sacred cows, 92—93
Evisceration, 583, 605
    of eyeball, 834
Evoked potentials
    monitoring of, 549
    sensory, 407—408, 798
Ex vivo extracorporeal kidney surgery, 739
Excimer laser, 367
Excision, as intentional wounds, 585
Excisional biopsy, 397
    cervical, 702
Excretion, 420, 422
Exemplary professional practice, 80
Exenteration, 834
    of paranasal sinus, 885
    pelvic, 712
Exothermic reaction, 761, 778
Exotoxins, bacterial, 246
Expander, 847, 863
Expansion media, 429
Expiration, definition of, 535, 547
Exploratory laparotomy, emergency, 690, 690f
Exposing instruments, 345—347
    for orthopedic surgery, 766, 766f
Exposure, first assistant providing, 67, 68f
Exsanguination, 583, 594, 761, 770
Exstrophy of bladder, 146—147
Extend, 499
Extension doctrine, 40
External beam radiation therapy, 115—116
External defibrillation, 623—624
External disaster, 20
External ear, 876
External interactions, of geriatric patient, 166
External mechanical methods, hemostasis and,
    592—595
External respiration, definition of, 535, 542
Extracapsular extraction (ECCE), of cataract,
    838—839

Extracorporeal membrane oxygenator (ECMO),
    915, 944
Extracorporeal method, of sutures, 561
Extracorporeal shock wave lithotripsy, 742
Extracorporeal ventricular assist device (VAD), 944
Extracranial procedures, for neurosurgery, 804—805
Extraocular muscle procedures, 150
Extraperitoneal, defined, 730, 744
Extravasation, 583, 588
    in drug administration, 626
Extremity
    amputated, handling of, 399
    assessment of, for arterial and venous obstructive dis-
        eases, 951, 951t
    ischemia of
        epidural spinal electrical stimulation for, 965
        fasciotomy for, 965
    for neurovascular impairment, 771
    skin preparation for, antiseptic, 526—527
Extremity procedures, 770—771
    amputation, 694—695
    general considerations for, 770—771
    positioning for, 501t—503t
Extremity table, bed attachments and, 509
Extubation, 432, 436, 446
Exudate, 583, 599
    absorber, 608t
Eye, 826—846. *See also* Ophthalmic surgery
    anatomy and physiology of, 826—827, 827f
    injury in, iatrogenic, 646
    procedure in, for draping of patient, 532
    skin preparation for, antiseptic, 524—525
    surgical removal of, 834. *See also* Enucleation
Eye injuries, 844—845
Eye protection
    laser surgery and, for personnel safety, 370
    for patient, in head and neck surgery, 875
    as personal protective equipment, 282—283, 282f
Eyelid
    anatomy of, 832f
    malformation of, 833
    oculoplastic procedures, 150
    procedures, 832—833, 832f
Eyelid laceration, 845
Eyewear
    in laser use, 283
    for nonionizing radiation, 226b
    as personal protective equipment, 282—283, 282f
    protective, of scrub person, 474
    standard precautions in, 267

F

Face
    anatomy of, 897
    procedure in, for draping of patient, 531—532
    skin preparation for, antiseptic, 525
Face lift, 859, 860f
Face transplantation, 848, 848f, 860
Facemask, anesthesia administration via, 439
Facial cleft, 873, 900
Facial nerve grafting, 858
Facial resurfacing, 866, 866t
Facilities engineering department, 87
Facility-specific patient care standards, 20
Fallopian tubes, 698f, 699
    diagnostic procedures, 703
Falls
    of geriatric patients, 170, 174
    obese patient and, 108—109
    and physically challenged patients, 104
Falx cerebelli, 791

Falx cerebri, 791
Familial cancer syndromes, 411t
Family members
    nurse assistance of, 386
    postoperative care orders in, 614
    reassuring messages for, during surgery, 417
    staying with patient until surgery, 390
Family, of donor, 979
Family/significant others of patient, 102
    meeting room for surgeon and, 181
    viewing body of the deceased, 124
    waiting area for, 180
Fasanella-Servat operation, 150
Fascia lata, 576
Fascia, in skin, 555—556
Fasciculation, muscular, 432, 445
Fasciocutaneous flap, 854
Fasciocutaneous graft, 855
Fasciotomy, 761, 789
    in acute ischemia of extremity, 965
    of burn patient, 870
Fat deposits, of males and females, 861, 861f
Fat embolism, 619
    after orthopedic surgery, 788
Fat transplantation, aesthetic, 860
Fatigue, 496—497
FDA. *See* Food and Drug Administration
Federal Emergency Management Agency (FEMA), 91
Federal Medicare Act, 19—20
Federal Organ Transplantation and Procurement Act
    of 1983, 973
Feedback, 81—82
Felt casts, 786
Female genitalia, of geriatric patients, 174
Female reproductive system
    anatomy and physiology of, 697—700
    external genitalia, 697, 697f
    health implications, 235
    internal organs of, 697—699, 698f
    physiology of, 699—700
Female to male, of transsexual surgery, 759
Femoral head
    replacement, 777, 777f
    surface replacement, 777
Femoral hernias, 145
Femoral herniorrhaphy, 693
Femoropopliteal bypass, 958—959, 958f
Fenestrated sheets, as drapes, 528f, 529
Fentanyl, 441t, 444
    in children, 133t—134t
        for premedication, 136
    to induce hypotension, 448
    intercostal muscle spasm and, 620
Ferric subsulfate, 591
Fertilization, 723—725
    in vitro, 723
Fetal heart monitor, 728
Fetal surgery, intrauterine, 722
Fetal tissue, 52
Fetoscopy, 722
Fiber-optic light, 651
Fiber, dietary, and cancer risk, 418
Fiberoptic ductoscopy, 666—667
Fibrin glue, 575, 954b
Fibroids, uterine, 710
Fibroplasia, 584
    in drug therapy, 588
Fibrous dysplasia, craniofacial, 901—902
Field block, 460
Figure of 8, definition of, 551, 559
Filamentous velour, 955

Film badges, 225, 225f
Filter needle, 425
Filters, 964
Filters, inline, in changed between cases, 467
Financial responsibility, 95–97
Fine K-wire, 772
Fine needle aspiration, 397, 666
Fingernails, nail polish and acrylic nails, 381–382
Fire and explosion hazards, 229–231, 230f
    in ambulatory surgery, 199
    in laser surgery, 371
Fire extinguishers, 231
Fire safety, 231
Fire triangle, 218, 229–230, 230f
First assistant, 64–78
    disciplines associated with, 71–78
        certified nurse midwife, 77
        physician assistant, 77
        registered nurse, 71–76, 75f, 76b
        surgical technologist, 77–78
    functions of, 66–71
        in dissection, 69–70, 70f
        emergency situations, respond appropriately to,
            71
        in handle instrumentation, 66–67, 67f–68f
        in handling tissue with instrumentation, 69, 69f
        in hemostasis, 67–69
        patient assessment, 71
        in position, prep, and drape, 66
        providing exposure, 67, 68f
        surgical hazards, 71
        in suture, 70–71, 70f–72f, 74f
    knowledge and skill level of, 65–66
        in anatomy and physiology, 65
        in pharmacology, 65
        in procedure knowledge and techniques, 66, 66f
        in psychomotor dexterity, 65–66
        in surgical site management, 66, 66f
    surgical, 61
        certified nurse midwives, 85
        hazards to, 220
First intention/primary union, 584, 584f
Fissurectomy, 692
Fistula, 605
    procedures for repair of genital, 708
Fistulectomy, 691–692
Fistulotomy, 691–692
Fixation devices, orthopedic, 767
Fixatives, 429
FK-506, 980
Flammable agents, 230
Flap, 847–848
Flash sterilization, 272, 312, 321–322, 322t
Flat plate, 404, 742
Flexion, 499
Floor mount, 374, 374f
Floors
    cleaning of, 215, 217
    of operating rooms, 187
Florae, resident, 238–239
Flow sheets, 48
Fluid and electrolyte balance
    in geriatric patients, 172
    in pediatric patients, 128–130
    perioperative disorders of, 684
    wound healing and, 587
Fluid and electrolyte imbalances, 632–634
    acid-base balance and, 632–633
    electrolytes and, 633–634, 633t
    hypervolemia and, 634
    hypovolemia and, 634

Fluid overload, 634
Fluid replacement, in pediatric patients, 128–130
    by intraosseous infusion, 129, 130f
Fluid restriction, in children, 128
Fluid therapy, for burn patient, 869, 869t
Flumazenil, 444
Fluorometer, 857–858
Fluoroquinolones, 257t
Fluoroscope, 400–401
Fluoroscopy, radiation safety in, 225
    monitoring for, 225, 225f
Fluorovent, 641
Foam rubber casts, 786
Foam, wound care materials, 608t
Focal lengths, 360, 372
Focus charting, 47–48
Foley catheter, 519
    body temperature and, 547–548
    for burn patient, 869
    for cystostomy drainage, 747
    as urinary drainage, 599
Follow-up communications, in ambulatory surgery,
    205b
Fomites, 211, 213, 260, 263
Food and Drug Administration (FDA), 45
    drug safety during pregnancy and, 421
    laser regulations of, 369–370
    medical device regulations of, 368
Foot traffic, in operating rooms, 185b
Foot, skin preparation for, antiseptic, 527
Footboard, metal, bed attachments and, 510
Forceps, 69, 342
    bone-holding, 766, 766f
    microsurgical, 354, 354f
Forces of Magnetism, 80b
Forearm
    and forequarter amputation, 695
    skin preparation for, antiseptic, 526
Foreign body
    care for, 26
    in ear, 878
    in esophagus, 892
    removal, 151
    in traumatic wounds, 585
    unintentionally left, in patient, 490
Foreign substances, as areas considered contaminated,
    523
Forensic evidence, 120, 399
    skin preparation and, 520
    from traumatic wounds, 586
Formaldehyde, 233
    for disinfection, 307
Formalin, 398–399
Fractional curettage, 702
Fractions, 423, 423f
    to lowest terms, 423
Fracture table, 769–770
Fractures, 771–775, 771f
    in children, 148
    closed reduction of, 772
    external fixation of, 772
    in geriatric patient, 169f
    intermaxillary, 903
    mandibular, 903
    midfacial, 902, 902f
    nasal, 883, 902
    open reduction and internal fixation of, 772–775,
        773f–774f
        for Colles fracture, 772, 774f
        interlocking nail fixation for, 774–775
        intramedullary nailing for, 773–774, 775f–776f

Fractures (Continued)
        nails for, 773–775, 775f
        plates and screws for, 772–775, 775f
    ribs, 919
    skeletal traction on, 772
Frailty syndrome, 161–162
Frazier tip, 352
Fredet-Ramstedt procedure, 145
Free electron laser, 367
Free flap, 850, 850f, 854–856
    wraparound neurovascular, 855–856
Free graft, 850, 850f. See also Skin grafts
    free autologous, 855, 855f
    muscle, 855
Free tie
    definition of, 551, 559
    preparing, for use, 478
    standard length and, 572
Freehand skin graft knives and dermatomes, 851
Friable tissue, 583, 588–589
Frontal sinus procedures, 884
Frozen section, 397, 665
Fuel, 230
Fulguration, 597–598
Full anesthesia, 434
Full-thickness skin graft (FTSG), 847, 852, 852f,
    870
Functional activities, of geriatric patient, 165
Functional assessment, of geriatric patient, 165–166
Functional benchmarking, 35–36
Functional capacity, of geriatric patient, 165
Functional endoscopic sinus surgery (FESS), 885
Functional energy-driven devices, 654
Functional peripheral equipment, 660–661
Fundal pressure, 720f
Fundoplication, 920
    laparoscopic, 677
Fundus, 696, 698, 905, 920
Fungi, 253–254
Fungicide, 295, 302
Furniture
    cleaning of, 215
    in operating rooms, 192
Furosemide, 627
Fusiform (elliptical), 551
Fusiform aneurysm, 959–960, 960f
Fusiform incision, 553

G

Gallamine, 446
Gallbladder, 670, 670f–671f
Gallstones, 670
Gamete intrafallopian transfer (GIFT), 724
Gamma knife, 116, 415
Gamma rays, 113, 414
Gangrene, 146
Gas, 420
Gas cylinder, 430
Gas embolism, in endoscopy, 658
Gas plasma sterilizers, low-temperature, 330–331
Gas scavenger system, 438
Gas-sensitive tape, 317
Gases, 430
    piped-in, in operating room, 188–190, 189f
Gastrectomy, 679f
    subtotal, 679–680
    total, 679
Gastric banding, 681f
Gastric bypass, 681f, 682
Gastric procedures, 678–682
    bariatric surgery, 680–682, 681f

Gastric procedures (*Continued*)
  gastrointestinal, 679
  gastrojejunostomy, 680
  gastroscopy, 678
  gastrostomy, 678–679
  resections, 679–680, 680f
  vagotomy, 680
Gastrocystoplasty, 146–147
Gastrointestinal decompression, 599
Gastrointestinal procedures, 678
  intestinal, 682–686, 682f–683f
Gastrointestinal surgery, 677–682
  considerations for, 678
Gastrointestinal system, of geriatric patient, 168t, 171–172, 172f
Gastrointestinal X-ray studies, 403
Gastrojejunostomy, 680
Gastroplasty, 682
Gastroschisis, 145–146
Gastroscopy, 678
Gastrostomy, 678–679
Gastrostomy tube, 106
Gauss lines, 227
Gauze sponges, 492
Gauze, wound care materials, 608t
Gel pad, 509, 518
Gelatin, absorbable, 954b
  hemostasis and, 590
General anesthesia, 434
  adjunctive drugs used in, 444–446
  administration techniques for, 439–440
  agents for
    inhalation, 440–443, 441t
    intravenous, 443–444
  awareness during, 449
  care of patient during, 448–450, 452
  considerations with, 449, 454
  controlled homeostasis in, 447–448
    induced hypotension, 447–448
    induced hypothermia, 447, 447b
  depth of, 435t
    monitoring, 446
  emergence from, 446
  equipment for, 450–451
    care of, 450–451
    checking of, 451
    disposable, 450
    hazards of, 450
    reusable, care of, 450–451
  induced hypotension, 447–448
  induction of, 435–437, 435f
    by circulating nurse, 487
    key points during, 437
  inhalation systems for, 439
  intraoperative hypothermia and, 547
  large doses of, 620
  level of unconsciousness associated with, 435
  maintenance of, 437–440, 446–451
  objectives of, 437–438
  potentially lethal, 434
  rectal, 435
  safety factors in, 449–450
General surgery, 664–695
  for abdominal trauma, 688–691
  for amputation of extremities, 694–695
  anorectal, 691
  biliary tract, 670–674, 670f
  breast, 666, 666f
  colorectal, 686–688
  esophageal, 676–677
  gastrointestinal, 677–682

General surgery (*Continued*)
  hernia, 692–694
  liver, 674–675
  pancreatic, 675–676
  special considerations for, 664–666
  splenic, 675
General workroom, 182
Generation time, 239
Generator, 360, 362
Generic, definition of, 420, 422
Genetic mutation theory, 163
Genitourinary surgery, 146–148
Genitourinary system
  of geriatric patient, 163, 168t, 172–174, 173f
  surgical procedures of, 738–748
Geriatrics, perioperative, 161–176. *See also* Aging
  assessment of, 164–174
    functional, 165–166
    physical, 167–174, 168t
    psychosocial, 166
  intraoperative considerations in, 174–175
  postoperative considerations in, 175
Germicide, 302
Gerontology, 161
GIFT. *See* Gamete intrafallopian transfer
Gingival grafting or augmentation, 888
Gingivectomy, 888
Glaucoma, 837–838
Glenn procedure, 158, 158f
Glioma, 790, 799–800
Globe, posterior rupture of, 845
Glossectomy, 886
Glossoptosis, 873, 900
Gloves
  adhesions and, 605
  for cleaning, 212
  contaminated, removing or changing, 293–294, 293f–294f
  cornstarch powder on, 284
  double-gloving with, 243, 267
  latex, sensitivity/allergy to, 235, 236t
  lead-impregnated rubber, 225, 283
  opening, 286
  in operating room, 474
  as personal protective equipment, 283
  polymethylmethacrylate and, 233
  puncture to, 284–285
  removal of, by scrub person, 215
  surgical, 284–285
  types of, different uses of, 267
  for urinary catheterization, 519
  using the closed gloving method, 474
  utility, 283
Gloving, 269, 275–294
  closed technique, 289–291, 290f–291f
    of scrub person, 474
  drying hands and arms and, 287
  open technique, 288, 291–292, 291f–292f
  of team member, 292–293, 293f
GLP-1 and GIP, 106
GLP-1 receptors, 106
Glutaraldehyde, 233
  for disinfection, 307
  as sterilants, 332
  for sterilization, of anesthesia equipment, 451
Glycopyrrolate, in children, 133t–134t
  for premedication, 136
-Gnathia, 873
Golden period, 64, 70–71
Gonioscopy, definition of, 826, 837
Goniotomy, 151

Gonorrhea, 248
Goodsall's rule, of anal fistulas, 692, 692f
Gordon's functional health patterns, 31b
Gore-Tex soft tissue patch, 578
Gossypiboma, 490
Gown
  contaminated, removing or changing, 293–294, 293f–294f
  cuffs of, 283, 284f
  fire-resistant, 369
  fluid-resistant, 267
  opening, 286
  in operating room, 466, 474
  of patient, 389
    modesty and, 393–394
  steam sterilization of, 323
  of sterile personnel, 283f
  using the closed gloving method, 474
Gowning, 275–294
  assisted, 292–293
  closed-assisted, 288
  drying hands and arms and, 288, 288f
  open-assisted, 293
  self, 288–289, 288f–289f
  of team member, 292–293
  techniques in, 288–293
Graafian follicle, 696, 699
Grafts, 847
  as areas considered contaminated, 523
  in plastic and reconstructive surgery, 848
Gram stain, 245, 245t
  selection of antibiotics according to, 258b
Gram-negative bacilli, 258
  supported by water, 265
Granulation tissue, 583–585
Granulomas
  definition of, 583
  formation of, 585, 605
Grasping, 69, 338
Grasping instruments, 342–343, 344f
  for orthopedic surgery, 766, 766f
Gravid, 696, 727
Gravity convection oven, for sterilization, 326
Gravity displacement sterilizer, 312, 320, 325t, 359
  biologic testing of, 326
  loading of, 324
Great vessels, transposition of, 159, 159f
Grey-Turner suture, 560
Groshong catheters, 416
Grounding, electrical, 227–228, 360, 362
Guidance statements, 16, 18
Guidelines, 16, 18
Guidelines for Isolation Precautions in Hospitals, 266
Gunshot wounds, 121
Gynecologic diagnostic techniques, 701–706
  abdominal procedures in, 701–706
  cervical biopsy, 702, 702f
  colposcopy, 702–703
  colpotomy, 703
  culdocentesis, 703
  of fallopian tube, 703
  fractional curettage, 702
  general considerations, 700–701
  Papanicolaou (Pap) smear, 701
  pelvic examination, of anesthetized patient, 701
  Schiller test, 701
  vaginal procedures in, 707–710
    of cervix, 708
    of uterus, 709–710, 709f
    of vaginal wall, 707–708
  vulvar procedures in, 706

Gynecologic surgery, 696–729
  abdominal procedures
    of fallopian tubes, 712–713
    of ovaries, 713–714
    of pelvic floor, 714
  emotional preparation of patients for, 700
  pelvic exenteration, 712

H

Hair
  as contamination source, 263
  covered, for patient, 487
  of patient, 389
Hair follicles, 556
Hair patterns, of geriatric patient, 167
Hair removal, 391
  for craniotomy, 795
  for patient's skin, 521
Hair replacement, 860–861, 860f
Hairpin splint, 787
Halo traction, 149
Halogens, for disinfection, 304t–305t
Halothane, 442
Halsted suture technique, 559–560
Hammer toes, 783–784
Hand
  procedure in, for draping of patient, 533
  skin preparation for, antiseptic, 526
  surgical, 285–287
Hand hygiene, surgical, 275–294
  with antiseptic hand gel, 287
  preparations immediately before, 287
  purpose of, 285–286
  of scrub person, 474
Hand signals, of surgeons, 481, 482f
Hand surgery, 784
  amputations, 695
Hand table, 509
  for replantation of amputated part, 856, 856f
Hand-assisted access sleeves, 655
Handling powered instruments, 356
Handover report
  to PACU nurse, 490
  postoperative, 612–613
Handover, patient, 49b
Handwashing, 263
Hanging cast, 787
Haptics, 826, 840
Harmonic Scalpel, 377, 598, 654
Harrington rods, 150f, 817, 817f
Hasson blunt trocar, 656
Hazards
  biologic, 219, 233–235
  chemical, 219, 231–233
  classification of, 219
  environmental, 218–219
  physical, 219–231
    body mechanics and, 220–221, 221f, 222b
    environmental factors of, 219–220
    fire and explosion, 229–231, 230f
    ionizing radiation and, 222–225.
      See also Radiation safety
    magnetic resonance imaging, 227
    nonionizing radiation, 225–226, 226f
  regulation of, 219
  reproductive, 235
  risk management and, 236–237
Head cover, 278–279, 279b
Head nurse, 82–83
Head trauma, treatment of, 805
Head, procedure in, for draping of patient, 531

Headlight, 191
  in neurosurgery, 795
Headrests, bed attachments and, 510–511, 511f
Health care facility, sources of standardization data
    within, 20–21
Health care-acquired infection, 264
  endogenous, 264
  exogenous, 264
Health Information Technology for Economic and
    Clinical Health (HITECH) Act, 41
Health Insurance Portability and Accountability Act
    (HIPAA), 19–20, 41
  talking to patient's family and, 102
Healthcare ethics consultants (HEC-C), 90–91
Healthcare Infection Control Practices Advisory Com-
    mittee (HICPAC), 90, 243
Healthcare-acquired infection (HAI), 241
  definition of, 238
  mandatory reporting of, 243
Hearing
  differential diagnosis of, 877–878, 877f
  pathology of, 877–878
Hearing aids, 103, 389
  for geriatric patients, 174
Hearing impairment, 103
Hearing loss, 877
Heart
  anatomy of, 923–925, 924f
  artificial, 944–945
  diagnostic procedures to. *See* Cardiac catheterization
  physiology of, 925
    cardiac cycle, 925, 926f
    electrical conduction system, 925, 925f
Heart transplantation, 974t–975t, 982–983,
    983f–984f
  combine heart-lung, 983–984, 984f–985f
  heart-lung en bloc, 974t–975t, 979
  organ procurement for, 979
Heart valves. *See also* Valvuloplasty
  anatomy of, 924, 924f
  disease of, 933–935, 933f
  procurement parameters for, 971t
Heat exchanger, 929
Heat sterilization, moist, 320–325
Heating, ventilation, and air-conditioning (HVAC)
    system, 177, 183, 219
Hegar dilators, 352
Helminths, 254
Hemangioma, 153, 947, 950
Hematocrit
  hemodilution and, 636
  normal values of, 635t
Hematologic disorders, 637–638
Hematologic values, in pediatric patients, 129,
    129t
Hematology, wound healing and, 587
Hematoma, 583, 588, 604
  of external ear, 878
  subdural, head trauma with, 805
Hematoporphyrin derivative (HPD), 112
Hemicolectomy, 684
Hemilithotomy position, 516
Heminephrectomy, 738
Hemipelvectomy, 695
Hemiplegia, 808, 819
Hemispherectomy, 804
Hemodialysis, 740, 740f–741f, 947, 966
Hemodilution, 636
Hemodynamic monitoring
  invasive, 536–538
    cannulation for, 536–537

Hemodynamic monitoring (*Continued*)
  in cardiac surgery, 928–929
  catheters for, 537–538
  parameters, 539t
Hemodynamics
  definition of, 535–536
  Doppler instruments and, 407
Hemoglobin, normal values of, 635t
Hemoglobinopathies, 637
  definition of, 616
  sickle cell, 637–638
Hemolysis, definition of, 737
Hemolyze, 730
Hemophilia, 638
Hemopure, 641
Hemorrhage, 616, 619, 635
  in endoscopy, 658
Hemorrhagic disorders, 638
Hemorrhagic shock, 641–642
Hemorrhoid banding, 692f
Hemorrhoidectomy, 691, 691f–692f
Hemostasis, 64, 67–68, 583–609
  bleeding, types of, during surgery, 589
  in hepatic surgery, 694
  mechanism of, 590f
  methods of, 590–598, 793–794
    chemical, 590–592
    cold, 597
    hot, 597–598
    mechanical, 592–597
    thermal, 597–598
    wound healing and, 588
  in neurosurgery, 797
  in ophthalmic surgery, 828, 829f
  in otorhinolaryngologic and head and neck
    surgery, 876
  pharmacologic agents in, 636
  process in, 589
  in spinal surgery, 815–816
Hemostatic agents, in vascular surgery, 954, 954b
Hemostatic clamps, 343, 595
Hemostatic scalpel, 598
Hemostats, 343
  mosquito, 355
Hemothorax, 908
HEPA filter. *See* High-efficiency particulate air
    (HEPA) filter
Heparin, 636–637
  in vascular surgery, 953
Heparin-induced thrombocytopenia (HIT), 953
Hepatic artery catheter, 416–417
Hepatic resection, 674–675
Hepatitis A virus (HAV) infection, 249
Hepatitis B vaccine, for workers, 234
Hepatitis B virus (HBV) infection, 249
  anesthesia provider's exposure to, 450
  disinfectants and, 303
Hepatitis C virus (HCV) infection, 249
Hepatitis D virus (HDV) infection, 249
Hepatitis E virus (HEV) infection, 249
Hepatitis G virus (HGV) infection, 249
Hepatitis infection, 249
Herbal supplements, potential complications with,
    387, 388t, 430–431, 431b
Hernias
  direct, 693
  indirect, 693
  procedures for, 692–694, 693f
Herniated disc, 820f
  discectomy for, 820–821, 820f
Herniation, 605

Herniorrhaphy, 145
  esophageal hiatal, 677, 677f
Herpes infection, 249–250
Herpes simplex infection, 250
Herpetic whitlow, 250
Hetastarch, for blood volume expanders, 636
Heterotopic transplantation, 982–983, 984f
Hiatal hernia, 145, 171
  repair of, 694, 920, 921f
Hiatal herniorrhaphy, 694
Hickman catheters, 416, 416f, 543
HICPAC. *See* Healthcare Infection Control Practices
    Advisory Committee
Hierarchy of needs, 100–102, 100f
High-efficiency particulate air (HEPA) filter, 186
  in mask, 247, 266, 281, 450
High-fat diets, and cancer risk, 418
High-level disinfection, 295, 301, 302f
High-molecular-weight polyethylene orthopedic
    gloves, 285
Hip
  procedure in, for draping of patient, 533
  skin preparation for, antiseptic, 526, 526f
Hip abduction splint, 148f
Hip arthroplasty
  incisions for, 777f
  methods, 777f
  total joint replacement, 777–781
Hip disarticulation, 695
Hip restraint strap, bed attachments and, 509
Hip sheet, as drapes, 529
Hip spica, 787
Hip splint, abduction, 787
HIPAA. *See* Health Insurance Portability and
    Accountability Act
History and physical examination, preoperative, 380
Hit-and-run driving accident, 121
Hofmeister technique, 680
Holding area, presurgical, 390–391
Holding instruments, 342–343, 344f
Hollow endoscopes, 351
Holmium:yttrium aluminum garnet (Ho:YAG) laser,
    367, 768–769
Holocrine glands, 554–555
Holography, digital, 793
Home laundered scrubs, 278b
Homeostasis, 99–100
  controlled, 447–448
Homologous plasma, 575
Hooks, for retraction, 346, 347f
Horizontal airflow, 186, 186f
Horizontal mattress, sutures, 560, 560f
Hormonal receptor site studies, 112, 413
Hormonal therapy, for cancer, 112, 413
Hospital policy and procedure manual, 20
Hospital safety committee, 91
Hospital- (or health care) acquired infection (HAI),
    238
Housekeeping
  infection control and, 265–266
  services, 87
  storage areas, 182
Huber needle, 417, 418f
Hudson brace, 353
Hulka tenaculum, 343, 344f
Human dura mater, 579–580
Human experimentation, 52
Human immunodeficiency virus (HIV) infection,
    250–252
  bone donors and, 970
  disinfectants and, 303

Human immunodeficiency virus (HIV) infection
    (*Continued*)
  prevalence of, 53
  related clinical manifestations, 251–252
Human papillomavirus (HPV) infections, 250
  genital, wart secondary to, 749
  oral carcinoma associated with, 886
Human resources department, 88
Human skin equivalent, xenograft and, 580
Humeral head replacement, 776–777, 777f
Humidity
  ethylene oxide gas sterilization and, 327
  operating room, 183
HVAC. *See* Heating, ventilation, and air-conditioning
    (HVAC) system
Hybrid operating room, 177, 183
Hydrocele, 145
Hydrocelectomy, 750
Hydrocephalus, 154–155, 155f
Hydrocolloid, 608t
Hydrocortisone, 112
Hydrogel, 608t
Hydrogen peroxide
  for disinfection, 304t–305t, 308
  for plasma sterilization, 330–331
  for sterilization, 330–331
Hymen, 697, 697f
Hyperabduction, 499
Hyperadduction, 499
Hypercapnia, 432, 463, 618
Hyperextend, 499
Hyperglycemia, 106
Hypernatremia, 633
Hypersensitivity, predisposing factors for, 462
Hypertelorism, 900, 900f
Hypertension, 616, 621
Hyperthermia
  body temperature and, 547
  in children, 130–131
  interstitial, for brain tumors, 804
Hypertrophic scar, 583, 605
Hypervolemia, 634
Hypnoanesthesia, 464
Hypnosis, 464
  for burn patients, 872
Hypnotic, 432
Hypoallergenic milled gloves, 284
Hypochlorous acid, as sterilants, 332
Hypodermic needle, 420, 425, 426f
Hypoglossal nerve stimulation, 887
Hypoglycemia, 106
Hypoglycemic shock, 106
Hyponatremia, 633, 730, 737
  transurethral resection leading to, 737
Hypophysectomy, transnasal, 805f
Hypoplastic left heart syndrome, 159–160, 159f
Hypospadias, 147, 147f
Hypotension, 616, 620–621
  definition of, 616
  induced, 447–448, 637
  in infants, 129
Hypothermia, 432, 442
  for allograft preservation, 980
  for aortic surgery, 952
  body temperature and, 547
  controlled, for craniotomy, 797
  in endoscopic procedures, 658
  in geriatric patients, 174–175
  hemostasis and, 597
  inadvertent, 642–643
  induced, 447, 447b

Hypothermia (*Continued*)
  in pediatric patients, 130
  prevention of, in burn patients, 871–872
  reduced, for cardiac surgery, 927, 931
Hypoventilation, 616, 618–619
Hypovolemia, 634
Hypovolemic shock, 634, 641
Hypoxemia, 618
  from endotracheal administration, 440
Hypoxia, 449, 616–617
  from endotracheal administration, 440
  hypoxemia, 432
Hysterectomy
  abdominal, 711–712
  total abdominal, 710–711
  vaginal, 709–710
Hysteroplasty, 711f
Hysterosalpingography, 703, 703f
Hysteroscopy, 704–705

I

IABP. *See* Intraaortic balloon pump
Iatrogenic, 37, 583
Iatrogenic condition, 211, 213–214
Iatrogenic injury, 646
  arterial, 952–954
  definition of, 947
  in endoscopy, 658
Iatrogenic medical injury, 38
ICP. *See* Intracranial pressure
ICU. *See* Intensive care unit
Ideal body weight, 105
  obesity and, 108
Identifying the patient
  before administering medications, 421
  for ambulatory surgery, 199
Idiopathic, 808
Ignition sources, 230–231
Ileal conduit, 747, 747f
Ileorectal anastomosis, 685f
Ileostomy, 684–685, 685f
Iliac crest, procurement parameters for, 971t
Ilizarov external fixator, 772
Illegal drugs, use of, 421
Image intensifier, 401
  C-arm, 400–401, 400f
Immediate-use sterilization (IUSS), 25, 321
Immune response, wound healing and, 587–588
Immunologic sensitization, from local and regional
    anesthesia, 462
Immunosuppressed patient, protective isolation for,
    266
Immunosuppression, 118–119
  wound healing and, 588
Immunosuppressive therapy, for organ recipient,
    980–981
Immunotherapy, 112, 395, 411–412
Impairment of cognitive function, 104
Imperforate anus, 125, 143–144
Implant-related instruments, for orthopedic surgery,
    766–767
Implantable materials, 576–578, 577f
Implantable ventricular assist device (VAD), 944
Implantation, definition of, 551
Impotence, 730, 756–757
Improper fraction, 423
In situ vascular reconstructive techniques, 739
In vitro fertilization, 723
In-service education programs, 79, 84
Inactive dispersive return electrode, 360
Inamrinone, 627

Incandescent bulbs, 651
Incarcerated hernia, 693
Incident report, 50, 50b
Incidental wounds, 586
Incidental X-ray, 404
Incise cut, 64
Incise drape, 527
Incision, surgical, 551—556
  abdominal, 557—559
    types of, 557—559, 558f
  anterior surface, 557, 558f
  definition of, 583—584
  inguinal, 559
  in integument, 551—556
  as intentional wounds, 585
  landmarks for, 556—559, 556f
  Langer's lines and, 553
  lines in, 556, 557f
  McBurney's, 557—559
  midabdominal transverse, 559
  midline, 557
  paramedian, 557
  Pfannenstiel, 559
  placement of, 557
  subcostal upper quadrant oblique, 557
  thoracoabdominal, 559
Incisional biopsy, 397
  cervical, 702
Incisional herniorrhaphy, 693—694
Incisional infection, 606
Incomplete natural termination of pregnancy, 696
Incontinence, 147, 730, 738
Indiana pouch, 746
Indicator, 37, 39
Indicator gloves, 275, 283
Indicator tape, 312, 317
Indicators of sterilization
  biologic, 314—315
  chemical, 314, 315t
  mechanical, 314
Indirect laryngoscopy, 890
Individual positioning considerations, for positioning
    of patient, 506
Induction, 136—139, 432, 446
  types of, 137—139
Induction of ovulation, 723
Induction room, 180
Infants, gynecologic pathology in, 704
Infection
  after cardiac surgery, 946
  of breast, 666
  definition of, 238—239
  occupational exposure to, 53
  postoperative, of wound, 606
  processes of, 241
  risk of, in geriatric patients, 171, 175
  sources of, 264
  surgical site, 241
    criteria for defining, 264, 265t
Infection control
  in ambulatory surgery, 199
  environmental services/housekeeping, 265—266
  isolation precautions for, 266—267
Infection control committee, 89—90
Infection control coordinator, 89—90
Infection control manual, 21
Infection control nurse (ICN), 89—90
Infection control program, 90
Infectious waste, 214, 234
Inferior, 499
Infertility, male, 751

Infiltration, of local anesthetic, simple, 459
Inflammation, 583
  wound healing and, 585, 587—588
Information
  gathering, 384—385
  preoperative teaching and, 386
Informed consent, 44—45, 382
  in emergency situations, 46
  responsibility for, 45
  right to refuse surgical procedure, 46
  and second opinion, 46
  for surgical procedure, 45
  validation of, 45—46
  witnessing, 46
Infrared beams, for arterial blood pressure, 542
Infratentorial structures, 791
Infusion, 420, 426
Infusion catheters, 416
Infusion port, subcutaneous, 417, 417f—418f
Infusion pump, 626
  implantable, 417
Inguinal hernia, 145
Inguinal herniorrhaphy, 693
Inguinal incision, 558f, 559
Inhalant drug, 420, 430
Inhalation, 137
Inhalation anesthesia, 139
  administration techniques for, 440
  agents for, 440—443, 441t
  gas scavenger system, 184
Inhalation systems, for anesthesia, 451
Injection, 420, 425
Inner dispenser matrix, 572
Inner ear, 877
Inotropic drugs, 926
Inotropic effect, of drugs, 626—627
Inservice coordinator, 84
Inservice education, 84
Inspecting and testing, of instruments, 299—300
Inspiration, definition of, 543
Instillation, 338, 352
  instruments for, 351—352
Instrument book, 21
Instrument cleaning and decontamination, 297—301
  manual cleaning, 297—298
  prerinsing/presoaking, 297
  ultrasonic cleaning, 298—299
  washer-decontaminator, 298
  washer-sterilizer, 298
Instrument counts, 490—495. See also Counts
Instrument handling, 357—358
  dismantling the instrument table and, 359
  placing of used instruments and, 358
  setting up the instrument table and, 356—357
Instrument room, 182—183
Instrument set
  in case cart, 473—474
  standardization of, 475
Instrument sterilization
  assembly of sets for, 315—316
  packaging for, 316—320, 318f—319f
  preparation for, steam, 323
Instrument table
  arranging, 475, 476f, 476t—477t
  for craniotomy, 797, 797f
  dismantling of, 358—359
  moving of, into position, 487—488
  setting up, 356—357, 474
Instrumentation handling, by first assistant,
    66—67, 67f—68f
Instrumentation, for pediatric patients, 141—142

Instrumentation, surgical, 338—359
  classification of, 339—356
    accessory, 353
    aspiration, instillation and irrigation, 351—352
    clamping and occluding, 343—345
    closure and approximation, 347—350
    debulking, 341—342
    dilating and probing, 352, 353f
    dissecting and cutting, 339—341
    grasping and holding, 342—343
    measuring, 353
    microinstrumentation, 353—355
    powered, 355
    retracting and exposing, 345—347
    viewing, 350—351
  metal, fabrication of, 338—339
  for orthopedic surgery, 766—767
  types of finishes of, 339
Instruments
  for endoscopy, 654, 654f, 656
  for eye, cleaning of, 320
  inspecting and testing of, 299—300
  loaner, 335
  lubrication, 299
  marking for identification, 300
  for ophthalmic surgery, 829, 829f—830f
  for otorhinolaryngologic and head and neck surgery,
    875
  packaging of, 316—320, 318f—319f
  placing basket on sterile back table, 319
  prion-contaminated, 253
  repair of, 300
  replacement of, 301
  restoration and resurfacing of, 300—301
  for spinal surgery, 814
  for thoracic surgery, 909, 909f—910f
  for vascular surgery, 952—953, 953f
Insufflation pressures, 647—648, 656
Insufflator, 650
Insulin
  in geriatric patient, 172
  in malignant hyperthermia, 644
Insulin shock, 108
Insulin-dependent diabetes mellitus, 106
Integrator, 312, 314
Integument. See also Skin
  accessory appendages to, 556
  anatomy and physiology of, 551—556, 552t, 553f,
    553t
  glandular structures and ducts in, 554—555
  tissue layers under, 555—556
Integumentary system, of geriatric patient, 167, 168t,
    169f
Intensive care unit (ICU), 85
  overflow considerations of, 614
Intentional wounds, 585
Interbody cages, 823, 825f
Intercostal block, 460
Intercostal muscle spasm, 620
Interdepartmental relationships, 84—85
Interfacility transfer management, 205
Intermediate layer, dressing and, 603
Intermediate-level disinfection, 295, 302
Internal anastomosis staplers, 350
Internal beam radiation, 114—115
Internal benchmarking, 35—36
Internal cardiac compression, 629
Internal defibrillation, 624
Internal disasters, 20, 91
Internal indicator/integrator, 314
Internal mammary artery conduit, 935, 936f

Internal mechanical methods, hemostasis and, 595–597

Internal respiration, definition of, 535

Internal staplers, 574, 574f

International Association of Healthcare Central Service Material Management (IAHCSMM), instrument processing standards of, 296

International Code of Ethics for Nurses (INC), 51

International Standards Operations containers, 207–208, 208f

Interpersonal learner, 4

Interpreter, 103, 390

Interrupted sutures, 560, 560f

Interstices, 947, 952–953

Interstitial needles, 114, 414

Interstitial radiation therapy, 804

Interstitial seeds, 114, 414

Interventional neuroradiology, in neurosurgery, 794

Interventional radiographic procedure, 177, 183

Interventional radiography room, 193, 194f

Interventional radiology, 395, 404

Interventional techniques, 396, 955–956

Intestinal atresia, 146

Intestinal obstruction, 146
  in pediatric patients, 142

Intestinal procedures, 682–686, 682f–683f
  anorectal, 691–692
  appendectomy, 685–686, 686f
  colorectal, 686–688
  stomas, 684–685, 686f

Intraaortic balloon pump (IABP), 942–943, 943f

Intracapsular extraction (ICCE), of cataract, 839

Intracavitary capsules, 115, 414

Intracavitary colloidal suspensions, 115, 415

Intracorporeal method, of sutures, 561

Intracranial neoplasms, 803–804

Intracranial pressure (ICP)
  control of, 797
  monitoring, 549
  in neurosurgery, 798–799
  normal adult value of, 791

Intraepithelial cancer, 409

Intraluminal circular stapler, 574

Intraocular pressure (IOP), estimation of, 837

Intraoperative autotransfusion, 640

Intraoperative care, in perioperative pediatrics, 140–142

Intraoperative chemotherapy, 117

Intraoperative cholangiograms, 673, 673f

Intraoperative hepatic ultrasound, 674

Intraoperative phase, 30

Intraoperative radiation therapy, 116, 415

Intraoperative x-rays, 223, 223f

Intraosseous infusion, 129, 130f

Intraperitoneal catheter, 417

Intraperitoneal chemotherapy, 417

Intrapersonal learner, 4

Intrastromal corneal rings, 836–837, 837f

Intrathecal block, 456

Intrathecal injection, 432, 457

Intrauterine fetal surgery, 722f

Intravascular oxygenator (IVOX), 916, 921

Intravascular ultrasonic energy, 957

Intravascular ultrasonic scanning, 952

Intravenous anesthetic agents, 443–444

Intravenous cardiovascular drugs, 625–626

Intravenous drugs, 630

Intravenous infusion, 138

Intravenous infusion, in anesthesia induction, 435

Intravenous push, 626

Intravenous pyelography (IVP), 404

Intubation, 432, 435–436, 436f
  ambulatory surgery and, 203
  aspiration and, 617
  assessing difficulty with, 387
  awake, 437, 461
  in children, 138, 139f
  CPR and, 629
  cricoid pressure during, 436–437, 437f
  nasotracheal, 436

Intussusception, 125, 144, 144f

Invasive techniques, 396

Inverting sutures, 560

Iodine, for skin preparation, 524

Iodophors, 286
  for disinfection, 304t–305t, 307
  for skin preparation, 524

IOL, 826

Ionizing radiation, 113, 222–225, 333, 413–414
  definition of, 113, 218
  safety considerations in, 116, 223, 223b

IOP. See Intraocular pressure

Ipsilateral, 125

Ipsilateral periaortic lymph node dissection, 146

Ipsilateral, defined, 146

Iris
  intraocular procedures of, 837–838
  prolapse, 837

Irradiation sterilization, 333

Irreducible hernia, 693

Irreducible minimum, 260, 265, 273–274

Irrigating equipment, 736–737

Irrigation, 429, 596b
  before closure, in general surgery, 665–666
  for endoscopy, 654
  instruments for, 351–352
  in neurosurgery, 795
  solutions, 429, 475, 665–666
  suction with, 597
  sump drains with, 600
  of surgical site, 484
  syringes for, 479
  temperature of, in handling syringes, 479
  of traumatic wounds, 523

Ischemia, 583, 588

Isoflurane, 441t, 442

Isolated power system, 228

Isolation
  of burn patients, 871
  definition of, 260, 266

Isolation precautions, 266–267

Isopropyl alcohol, for skin preparation, 524

Isoproterenol, 626–627
  for anesthesia reaction, 463

Isosmotic, 730
  irrigating solutions, 737

-itis, 664

IVOX. See Intravascular oxygenator

IVP. See Intravenous pyelography

J

J-wire placement, in radiology, 666

Jackknife, surgical position, 517, 517f

Jatene procedure, atrial switch, 159

Jehovah's Witnesses, 640

Jewelry
  of patient
    instruction to leave at home, 382
    removed before leaving for OR, 389
    removed for electrosurgery, 364
  of personnel, removed for electrosurgery, 370
  of surgical personnel, 277, 277b

Joint procedures, 775–784
  arthrodesis, 776
  arthroscopy, 782–783, 782f–783f
  arthrotomy, 783
  bunionectomy, 783, 783f
  for dislocations, 776
  for hammer toes, 783–784
  neurolysis, 784
  in sports medicine, 784–785

Joints, procurement parameters for, 971t

K

Kahn uterine cannula and manipulator, 344f

Kaolin-based product, hemostasis and, 591

Kefauver-Harris Drug Amendments of 1962, 50

Keller arthroplasty, 783

Kelly procedure, 707

Keloids, 583, 605, 605f
  revision of, 864

Keratectomy
  photorefractive, 836
  phototherapeutic, 835

Keratomileusis, 836

Keratophakia, 836

Keratoplasty, 151
  corneal transplantation as, 834–835, 834f
  refractive, 836–837, 836f–837f

Kerr incision, 720

Ketamine, 441t, 443–444
  in children, 133t–134t
    for premedication, 136
  pediatric anesthesia, 138

Ketoacidosis, 106

Ketonuria, 106

Kevlar-woven glove liners, 283

Kick buckets, 488

Kidney rests, bed attachments and, 509, 509f

Kidney transplantation, 972, 974t–975t, 981–982
  complications of, 982
  donor nephrectomy for, 981, 981f
  organ procurement for, from cadaver for, 979
  recipient procedure in, 981–982, 981f–982f

Kidneys
  anatomy and physiology of, 730–731, 731f
  genitourinary system and, 738–748, 738f
  surgical position, 518, 518f
  surgical procedures of, 738–742

Killian procedure, 884

Killian's dehiscence, 677

Kirschner wire (K-wire), 772

Kittner dissectors, 492

Knee
  arthroscopy of, 782
  procedure in, for draping of patient, 533
  skin preparation for, antiseptic, 527, 527f
  in sports medicine, 784–785, 784f
  total replacement, 780, 780f

Knee-chest, surgical position, 517

Knitted polyester (Dacron) grafts, 955

Knives, 341
  microsurgical, 354
  skin graft, 850–851, 851f
  to surgeon, passing, 480, 480f

Knot placement, 560

Knot tying, 71

Knowledge, 1, 3

Kocher clamp, 343–345, 345f

Kock pouch, 746

Kraske (Jackknife), surgical position, 517, 517f

Kronig incision, 720

Kronner uterine manipulator for laparoscopy, 705f

Krypton laser, 367
KUB (kidneys, ureters, and bladder), 742
Kyphosis, 808, 818

L

Labeling, 317—318
Labia majora, 697, 697f
Labia minora, 697, 697f
Labor and delivery (L&D) unit, 85
Laboratory tests, preoperative, 380
Laboratory, in surgical suite, 181
Labyrinthectomy, 880
Lacrimal apparatus, procedures of, 833
Lacrimal duct dilation, 833
Lactated Ringer's solution
    as blood volume expanders, 636
Lactation, drug administration during, 421—422
Lahey forceps, 343
Laminae, vertebral, 811
Laminar air system, 266
    in orthopedic surgery, 769
Laminar airflow, 185
    for burn patients, 871
    definition of, 177, 761
    effectiveness of, obstacles to, 186—187, 188f
    for operating rooms, 185—186, 185f—187f
    for orthopedic surgery, 769
    special attire with, 284
Laminectomy
    cervical, 823f
    lumbar, 825f
Landmarks, surgical, 556—559, 556f
    abdominal, 557—559, 558f
        types of, 557—559, 558f
    for spinal surgery, 808, 809f
    for thoracic surgery, 905—906, 906f
Langer lines, 64, 553, 554f
Language barrier, 103
Lanz incision, 559
Lap pads, 492
Laparoscopes, 651
Laparoscopic procedures
    cholecystectomy, 671
    gynecology, 705—706
    repair, 693
Laparoscopic-assisted vaginal hysterectomy, 709—710, 710f
Laparoscopy, 656—657
    definition of, 647—648
    open, 656
    procedural considerations for, 657
Laparoscopy sheet, as drapes, 529
Laparotomy, 664, 675
    for draping of patient, 531, 531f
    emergency exploratory, 690, 690f
Laparotomy sheet, as drapes, 529
Laparotomy tapes, 492
Laryngeal mask airway (LMA), 439
Laryngeal papillomas, 152
Laryngeal transplantation, 892
Laryngoscope blades and handles, cleaning of, 215
Laryngoscopy, 889—890
Laryngospasm, 432, 436, 484, 487
    as respiratory complications, 617—618
Laryngotracheoplasty, 152
Larynx
    anatomy and physiology of, 889, 889f
    carcinoma of, 891—892
    injuries to, 890—891
    surgical procedures of, 889—892
Laser, 69, 360

Laser angioplasty, 937—938, 956—958
Laser beam, 360, 365
Laser lithotripsy, 743
Laser mask, 281
Laser microadapter, for operating microscope, 375
Laser nurse, 371
Laser plume, 267, 360, 370
    viral mutation in, 749
Laser resurfacing, 866, 866t
Laser safety committee, 89, 369
Laser safety officer (LSO), 89, 368
Laser surgery, 365—372
    advantages of, 371
    components of, 365
    disadvantages of, 371—372
    endoscopic, 377
        in urology, 736
    orthopedic, 768—769
    photodynamic therapy and, 368
    physical properties of, 365
    safety factors for, 368—371
        environmental, 370—371
        eye protection in, 370
        laser plume and, 370
        patient safety in, 369—370
        for personnel, 370
        policies and procedures in, 369
        regulatory agencies in, 368—369
        skin protection and, 370
    tissue effects of, 366
        factors associated with, 365b
    types of lasers for, 365—368, 365b
Laser team, 371
Laser therapy, 112—113
Laser-assisted in situ keratomileusis (LASIK), 836, 836f—837f
Laser-assisted vascular anastomosis, 967—968
Laser-resistant drape, 528
Lasers
    for cancer, 413
    definition of, 365
    hazards of, 226, 226f
    for hemostasis, 598
    in neurosurgery, 794
    ophthalmic, for retinal procedures, 842
    for otorhinolaryngologic and head and neck surgery, 878
    of larynx, 890
    of pulmonary lesions, 911, 913
    safety factors in, for head and neck procedures, 890
LASIK. See Laser-assisted in situ keratomileusis
Lateral chest (thoracotomy) position, 518
Lateral position, 499, 501t—503t
Lateral positioner (kidney rests), bed attachments and, 509, 509f
Lateral thoracoabdominal area, skin preparation for, antiseptic, 525, 525f
Lateral violence, 94, 94b
Latex sensitivity/allergy, 235, 236t, 284
    embolization and, 592
    syringes and, 479
    tourniquets and, 593
Latissimus dorsi flaps, 850, 850f
Laundry, 265
    cleaning of, 215
Laundry bag, for reusable woven fabric items, in operating room, 467
Laundry services, 88
Le Fort classification, 902, 902f
Le Fort osteotomy, 903—904
Lead aprons, 224—225, 224f

Lead shield, for patients, 223
Lead-impregnated gloves, 225
Leaded glasses, 225
Leaded gloves, 225
Leadership, 81
    qualifications and competency, 92
Learning organization, 79, 92
Learning styles, 1, 3—4
LeFort procedure, 173
Left atrial pressure (LAP), 545
Left ventricular assistance (LVA), 943—944
Left ventricular end-diastolic pressure (LVEDP), 545
Leg exercises, teaching about, 386
Leg length discrepancies, 148
Leg wraps, sequential compression, 593
Legal aspects, of drugs and pharmaceuticals, 50—51
Legal issues, 38
Leggings, as drapes, 530
Leiomyofibroma, 696, 710
Lens, intraocular, 828
    implantation of, 840—841, 840f
Lensed endoscopes, 351, 351f
Lensed instruments, ethylene oxide sterilization of, 328
Lesions, localization of, ultrasound imaging in, 407
Leukoplakia, excision of, 858
Liability, 37—42
    facility and team, prevention for, 38—39
    insurance, 39
    for retained surgical towels, 492—493
Licensed practical nurses/licensed vocational nurses (LPN/LVNs), 56
    circulating nurse duties of, 57
    Medicare regulation on role of, 57
    in postanesthesia care unit, 612
    as scrub person, 61
Licensure, 16, 55—56
Lidocaine, 455t, 461
    antidysrhythmics and, 626, 630
Life cycle, 161—162
Life expectancy, 161
Lift sheet (drawsheet), bed attachments and, 508, 508f
Lifting the patient, 489
    body mechanics in, 220—221, 221f
    obese, 109
Ligaments
    repair of, 784—785
    uterus, 699
Ligating clips, for hemostasis, 595
Ligating reels, 572
Ligating stapler, 574
Ligation, 64
Ligatures, 551, 559, 595
Light sedation, 434
Light source, 735
Lighting, in operating room, 190—191, 219
Limb salvage, 968
Linear array endoscope, 653
Linear extraction, of cataract, 839
Linear stapler, 574
Linen, 317
Linguistic learner, 4
Lint, 266
Lip
    reconstruction of, 858
    repair of lacerations of, 858
Lipectomy, 861
    suction-assisted, 861, 862f
Liposuction, 861, 861f—862f
Liquid drugs, 428—430

Liquid light, 373
Litho-, 730
Litholapaxy, 744, 744f
Lithotomy, surgical position, 514—516, 515f
Lithotripsy, transurethral ureteroscopic, 743—744, 743f
Lithotrity, 744
Liver function tests, 674
Liver procedures, 674—675
Liver transplantation, 974t—975t, 986, 986f
    from living, 984
    organ procurement for, from cadaver for, 979
Living will, 53
Load control number, 333
Loading dose, 420—421
Loaner instrumentation, 335
Lobectomy, 905, 917
Local anesthesia, 139, 432, 451—454
    actions of, 460—462
    administration of, 452
    advantages of, 454
    adverse reactions to, 463—464
    agents, 455t
    ambulatory surgery and, 203, 203b
    complications of, 460
    considerations in selection of, 454
    disadvantages of, 454
    in handling of, on sterile field, 479
    intraoperative patient care, 452
    local effects of, 462
    monitored care for, 453
    monitoring the patient during, 453—454, 463
    for nasal procedures, 881—882
    for ophthalmic surgery, 831—832
    patient preparation for, 451—452
    perioperative nurse's role during, 453
    precautions with, 462—463
    systemic effects of, 462—463
    toxicity and allergy caused by, 453t
    unrelated effects of, 464
Localized cancer, 111, 409
Localized drug effect, 420—421
Locker rooms, 181
Logical-mathematical learner, 4
Logs of bacterial growth, 238—239
Long bone, procurement parameters for, 971t
Longevity, 161, 163
Loose teeth, 392
Lordosis, 808
Loss of consciousness, induced, 435
Lotions, 430
Lounges, 181
Loupes, 372
Low-level disinfection, 295, 302
Low-temperature gas plasma sterilizers, 330—331
Lower extremity
    amputations of, 694—695
    procedure in, for draping of patient, 533
    skin preparation for, antiseptic, 527, 527f
Lower oblique incision, 559
Lubricants, 430
Lubricated instruments, ethylene oxide sterilization of, 328
Lubrication, of instruments, 299, 359
Luer slip tip syringe, 479
Luer-Lok tip syringe, 479
Lumbar approach, 458
Lumbar spine
    anterior retroperitoneal approach of, 823, 823f—824f
    anterior transperitoneal approach of, 823
    nerves of, 813f

Lumbar spine (*Continued*)
    posterior approach of, 823—824, 825f
    procedures of, 823—824
    vertebrae of, 811
Lumbar sympathectomy, 806
Lumens, ethylene oxide sterilization of, 328
Lumpectomy, 668, 669f
Lund-Browder chart, 868, 868f
Lung forceps, 909, 909f
Lung implant, 912
Lung reduction, 918
Lung resection, 917—918, 917f
Lung transplantation, 918, 974t—975t, 984—986
    combine heart-lung, 983—984, 984f—985f
    heart-lung en bloc, 974t—975t, 979
Lung-assist devices, 915—916
Lungs, 906—908, 907f
    collapse of, 908
Luque rods, 150
Lymph node biopsy, cervical and scalene, 896
Lymph node mapping, 405—406
Lymphadenectomy, 412
    pelvic, in prostatic carcinoma, 755
    retroperitoneal, in testicular cancer, 750
Lymphadenopathy, persistent generalized, 251
Lymphoscintigraphy, 405—406

M

MAC. *See* Monitored anesthesia care
Macroshock, 228
Mafenide acetate, 871
Maggot therapy, 584
Magill forceps, 436
Magnesium, as electrolyte, 633
Magnet recognition
    benefits of, 81
    eligibility for, 80
    maintaining, 80—81
    status, 80, 80b
Magnetic resonance imaging (MRI), 404—405, 405f
    of brain, 792
    hazards of, 227
    of spine, 811
    of vascular disease, 951
Magnifying power, 372
Mainz II pouch, 746
Male genitalia, of geriatric patients, 173
Male reproductive health implications, 235
Male reproductive organs, 749—757, 749f
    penis, 755—757
    prostate gland, 751—755
    testes, 749—750, 749f
    vas deferens, 750—751
Male to female, of transsexual surgery, 758—759
Malignant hyperthermia, 643—646
    etiology of, 643
    masseter muscle rigidity and, 436
    monitoring of, 644
    prevention for, 645—646
    supplies for, 645
    susceptible patients in, 643
    symptoms of, 643—644
    treatment of, 644—645
    triggers, 643
Malignant tumor, 395, 408, 790, 799—800
Mallampati classification, 435, 436f
Malleable retractors, 346
Mallet, 353, 353f
Malnutrition, 105
    in geriatric patients, 171
    wound healing and, 587

Malpractice, 37
Mammography, 401—402
Mammoplasty
    for augmentation, 862—863, 863f
    for male reduction, 864, 865f
    for reconstruction, 863—864, 864f
    for reduction, 864, 865f
Management, of surgical services, 81—82
    administrative personnel in, 81
        business manager, 83
        clinical coordinator, 82
        clinical nurse specialist (CNS), 83
        education coordinator, 83—84
        head nurse or charge nurse, 82—83
        nurse manager, 81—82
    budgeting and financial responsibility, 95—97
    of new products and equipment, 97
    patient services departments and, 85—86
    personnel management, 93—95
Manager, 79
    responsibilities, 82—84
Mandible
    anatomy of, 898, 898f
    bone grafts for, 888
Mandibular fractures, 903
Mandibular osteotomy, 904
Mandibular procedures, 902—904
Mandibular reconstruction, 903
Mandibular staple, 889
Mandibulectomy, 904
Mannitol, 632
    in malignant hyperthermia, 644
Manual cleaning, 297—298
Manual hemostasis, 68
Manual retractors, 345—346, 346f
MAP. *See* Mean arterial pressure
Marjolin ulcer, 871
Marking pens, sterile, 426, 478
Marlex mesh, 577—578
Marshall-Marchetti-Krantz vesicourethral suspension, 714
Marsupialization
    of Bartholin gland cyst, 706
    of cyst and sinus tract, 692
Mask image, 401
Mask inhalation, 439
Masks
    droplet transmission, 263
    high-efficiency particulate air (HEPA) filtration, 247, 266, 281
    laser and, 281, 370
    for operating room personnel, 281f, 281b—282b
    for patients and staff, 213
    plume particulate and, 234—235
    in restricted area, 179
Maslow's hierarchy of needs, 100—102, 100f
Mass casualties, microorganisms in, 259
Masseter muscle rigidity (MMR), 436, 643
MAST pneumatic counterpressure device, 593
Mastectomy
    extended radical, 670
    incisions, 669f
    modified radical, 669
    radical, 669—670
    segmental, 668
    simple, 668—669
    stage of cancer and, 668t
Mastoidectomy, 878, 879f
Mastoiditis, 878
Material safety data sheets (MSDS), 20, 231—232
Materials, 79, 82

Materials management, 87–88
Maxillae
anatomy of, 898, 898f
bone grafts for, 888
fractures of, 903
Maxillary sinus procedure, 884
Maxillofacial procedures, 858, 902–904
Mayfield headrest, 796
Mayo stand, 192
in application of dressing, 484
arranging, 475–477, 477f
draping, 474–475, 475f
Maze III procedure, 939
Maze procedure, 938–939
McBride operation, 783
McBurney incision, 557–559, 558f
McCarthy panendoscope, 735
McDonald procedure, 716
Mean arterial pressure (MAP), 542
Measuring devices
for ophthalmic surgery, 829, 830f
for orthopedic surgery, 766, 768f
Measuring instruments, 353
Meatotomy, 730, 742
Mechanical convection oven, for sterilization, 325–326
Mechanical valves, 934
Medial, 499
Median sternotomy, 915, 915f, 927, 928f
Mediastinal shift, 908
Mediastinoscopy, 912, 913f
Mediastinotomy, 916–917
Mediastinum, 905, 908
Medical Device Amendments of 1976, 50
Medical devices, legal aspects of, 50–51
Medical gas, terminology for, 430
Medical Literature Analysis and Retrieval System Online (MEDLINE), 10
Medical records department, 86
Medical students, 3
Medicare
ambulatory surgery and, 199
regulation on operating room team, 57
Medicare's "No Pay List," 19
Medication error, circulating nurse and, 394
Medications, 429
on sterile field, 478–479
Medicine cup, delivering drug to, 425
Medium, 360–362
Medium sheet, as drapes, 530
Medscape, 10
Medulla oblongata, 791f, 792
MedWatch program, 51
Meeting room, 181
Meetings, 93
MEGADYNE, 363
Melanoma, malignant, 866–867
Menarche, 696, 699–700
Meninges, 790–791
of spinal cord, 810
Meniscus injury, 785
Menometrorrhagia, 696
Menorrhagia, 696
thermal balloon ablation, 704, 709, 709f
Menstruating surgical patient, 389
Menstruation, 696, 699, 724
Mental models, 92
Mental relaxation, 14
Mentoplasty, 859
Mentoring, 1
Meperidine, 447

Mephentermine, 628
Mepivacaine, 455t, 461
Mersilene mesh, 577
Mesentery, 682
Mesh graft, 852, 853f
Mesh undergarments, 603
Mesher, 847
Mesher platform, 852
Mesocaval shunt, 966
Metabolic crises
definition of, 616, 643
perioperative, 642–646
Metabolic syndrome, in geriatric patients, 172
Metabolism, 420, 422
nutritional status and, 105–106
in pediatric patient, 128
stress and, 105–106
Metacarpophalangeal joint, total replacement, 781
Metal footboard, bed attachments and, 510
Metal, as synthetic material, for implants, 580–581
Metallic radium, 114
Metallurgy, 338
Metaraminol, 628
Metastatic cancer, 111, 409
Metatarsal osteotomy, 783
Methicillin-resistant *Staphylococcus* aureus, 258
Methohexital, 441t
Methoxamine, 628
Methyl methacrylate, 233, 576
as implant, 581
Metocurine, 446
Microdiscectomy, 820
Microfibrillar collagen
for hemostasis, 640
hemostasis and, 590
hemostatic, in neurosurgery, 794
Microinstrumentation, 353–355, 354f
Microlaryngoscopy, for otorhinolaryngologic and head and neck surgery, of larynx, 890
Microorganisms, 238
in biofilm, 239
body fluids and substances carrying, 241b
definition of, 238
epidemiology of, 239
identification of, 239
infectious, operating room cleanup and, 213–214
living conditions for, 240b
in mass casualties and bioterrorism, 259
nonpathogens *versus* pathogens, 239–243
pathogenic, 261
types of, 244–254, 244t.
See also Bacteria; Fungi; Helminths; Prions; Protozoa; Viruses
resistance levels of, 306t
risk for exposure and, 241–243, 242b
transmission of, 262
viability of, 239–240
Microscope, 361. See also Microsurgery
for ophthalmic surgery, 830–831, 831f
for spinal surgery, 815
Microshock, 228
Microsomia, craniofacial, 900
Microsurgery, 372–377
advantages of, 372
anesthesia for, 376
armrests and chair for, 376–377
considerations in, 376–377
for free-flap transfer, 854–856
microscope for, operating, 372–376
accessories for, 375–376
assistant's binoculars for, 375

Microsurgery (*Continued*)
broadfield viewing lens for, 375, 375f
cameras for, 375
care of, 376
components of, 372–373
couplings for, 375
drape for, 376
electrical system of, 375
focus of, 373
illumination system of, 373
laser beams and, 378
laser microadapter for, 375
lens system of, 372
magnification of, 373
mounting systems for, 373–375
remote foot controls for, 375–376
zoom lens of, 373
for otorhinolaryngologic and head and neck surgery, 878
for nasal hemorrhage, 883
patient preparation for, 376
scrub person's duties in, 376
stability of field for, 376
technique of, 372
transanal endoscopic, 692
Microtia, 901
Microwave sterilization, 333
Microwave thermotherapy, transurethral, 752, 752f
Midabdominal transverse incision, 558f, 559
Midazolam, 441t
in children, 133t–134t
for premedication, 136
for moderate sedation, 452
Middle ear, 876–877
Middle ear tympanoplasty, 151
Midline incision, 557
Military hospital, mobile, 206, 207f
Milwaukee brace, scoliosis, 149f
Mind relaxation, 14
Mineral sources, of drugs, 427, 428b
Minerva jacket, 149, 787
Mini maze procedure, 939
Minilaparotomy, 712
Minimal access procedure, 2–3
Minimally invasive surgery, 2, 177, 194
Minimally invasive surgery room, 194
Minimally invasive surgical (MIS) procedure, 177
Minimally invasive techniques, 933
Minor sheet, as drapes, 530
Minutes of meetings, 93
Miotic drugs, 831, 831f
Mirror finish, 339
Miscarriage, 716
Missed abortion, 696
Mitral valve replacement, 934, 934f
Mitrofanoff technique, 746
Mivacurium, 445
Mobile army military hospital, 206, 207f
Mobile hospital setting, surgery in, 209–210, 209t
Moderate sedation, 432, 434, 451
attended by anesthesia provider, 452
Modified endoventricular circular patch plasty, 939
Modified radical mastoidectomy, 878
Modified sitting position, 514
Mohs micrographic surgery, 866–867, 867f
Moist heat sterilization, 320–325
Molds, plaster, 787
Monitored anesthesia care (MAC), 453
Monitoring, 197, 203, 535
definition of, 197, 536
intraoperative

Monitoring (*Continued*)
  in ambulatory surgery, 203, 203b
  with geriatric patients, 175
  physiologic, 535—550
    arterial blood pressure, 541—542
    blood gases, 542—543
    body temperature, 547—548
    capnometry, 542—543
    cardiac output, 546—547
    central venous pressure, 543—544
    chest radiograph, 548
    echocardiogram, 540
    electrocardiogram, 539—540, 540f, 540b, 541f
    electroencephalogram, 548—549
    evoked potentials, 549
    functions, 535—549
    hemodynamic, parameters, 539t
    intracranial pressure, 549
    invasive hemodynamic, 536—538
    in neurosurgery, 798—799
    noninvasive methods of, 538b
    optode, 543
    oxygenation, 542—543
    parameters, 538—549, 538b
    pH, 542—543
    pulmonary artery pressure, 544—546
    pulse oximetry, 542
    respiratory tidal volume, 547
    stethoscopy, 540—541
    total blood volume, 547
    urinary output, 548
  postoperative, 613—614
Monitoring screens, in operating rooms, 191—192
Monoclonal antilymphocyte globulin, 980—981
Monocular, term, 361, 372
Monofilament suture, 563
Monopolar electrosurgery, 361—363
Monsel solution, 591
Montgomery straps, 603
Mops, cleaning of, 215—216
Moral principles
  in decision-making, 51b
  universal, 51
Morbid obesity, 108
Morning admission, 379
Morning-after pills, 121
Morphine, 444
Motion economy, 496—497
Movement, 266
Moving the patient, timing of, 500
MRI. *See* Magnetic resonance imaging
Mucogingivoplasty, 888
Multifilament suture, 563
Multiorgan transplantation, 987
Muromonab-CD3, 980—981
Muscle flap, 854
Muscle relaxants, 444—446
  reversal agents, 446
Muscle relaxation, 438
Muscles, 765
  uterus, 699
Muscular fasciculation, 445
Musculoskeletal considerations, for positioning of
    patient, 505
Musculoskeletal system
  anatomy and physiology of, 762—765, 762f
  of geriatric patient, 167—170, 168t, 169f—170f
Music
  for ambulatory surgery patient, 203
  in operating room, 220
  in surgical holding area, 391

Musical learner, 4
Mustard procedure, atrial switch, 159
Mutual support, 81—82
Mycotic aneurysm, 947, 960
Mydriatic drugs, 831, 831f
Myectomy, 150
Myelography, 404
Myelomeningocele, 155
Myocardial preservation, 931—932
Myocutaneous free flap, 850f, 854
  for burn patient, 870
Myomectomy, 710—711
Myometrium, 698
Myotomes, 610, 612, 808, 820
Myotomy, 150
Myringoplasty, 879
Myringotomy, 151, 151f

N

Nail polish and acrylic nails, 381—382
Nails, 556
  of geriatric patient, 167
Naloxone, 444
Naloxone hydrochloride, 619
NANDA International, human response patterns, 28b
Narcosis, 432
Narcotic analgesia, epidural, 458
Narcotic antagonist, 444
Narcotics, 139
  for general anesthesia, 444
  opioid, 433, 441
Narrative charting, 47—48
Nasal cavity
  blood supply to, 882f
  surgical procedures of, 881—885
Nasal deformity, 883—884
Nasal fracture, 883, 902
Nasal obstruction, procedures for, 883
Nasal reconstruction, 853, 853f
Nasal septum
  deviated, 883
  perforated, 883—884
Nasal speculum, 350, 351f
Nasal tumors, 901
Nasogastric tube, 106, 435
  for gastrointestinal decompression, 599
Nasolacrimal duct, congenital obstruction, 150
Nasopharynx, surgical procedures of, 886—887
Nasotracheal intubation, 436f
Nasotracheal tube, 138
National Assistant at Surgery Certification (NASC)
    organization, 71
National Board of Surgical Technology and Surgical
    Assisting (NBSTSA), 34, 56, 77—78
National Fire Protection Association (NFPA)
    standards, 19
National Patient Safety Goals (NPSGs),
    42—44, 43f
National Quality Forum (NQF), 20
Natural Orifice Transluminal Endoscopic Surgery
    (NOTES), 647—648
Naturalist learner, 4
NBSTSA. *See* National Board of Surgical Technology
    and Surgical Assisting
Near miss, 37, 42b
Near-infrared reflectance spectroscopy, 929
Neck
  anatomy and physiology of, 889
  anterior, surgical procedures of, 894—896
    dissections, 896—897
    parathyroid, 896

Neck (*Continued*)
    thyroid, 895—896, 895f
  skin preparation for, antiseptic, 524—525
Necrosis, 583, 586
Necrotizing fasciitis, 606
Needle holders, 347
  microsurgical, 354
  in suture and tie management, 483
  with tungsten carbide jaws, 347
Needles, surgical, 568—571
  body of, 568—569, 569f, 569t
  considerations in the choice of, 571
  eye of, 569—570, 569f
    free, 569—570
    French, 569f—570f, 570
    swaged-on, 570, 570f
  hypodermic
    anatomy of, 425, 426f
    for dispensing drug in vial, 425
    filter, 425
    size of, 479
  in managing sharps, 478
  packaging and preparation of, 571—573
  placement of, in needle holder, 570—571, 571f
  point of, 568, 568f
    blunt, 568
    conventional cutting, 568
    cutting, 568
    reverse-cutting, 568
    side-cutting, 568
    taper, 568
    trocar, 568
  reusable, preparation of, 571
Needlesticks, 234
  risk for patients of, 243
Needs
  Maslow's hierarchy of, 100—102, 100f
  of patient, addressing, 384
  patient's basic, 100—102
Negative pressure dressing, 604
Negligence, 37
  doctrine of corporate negligence, 40
  doctrine of *Res Ipsa Loquitur*, 40
  doctrine of *respondeat superior*, 40
Neobladder, 730, 746
Neodymium:yttrium aluminum garnet (Nd:YAG)
    laser, 367, 768—769
Neonate, 125—126, 721
Neoplasia, 696
Neoplasms, 395, 408, 702
  of esophagus, 893
  of eyelid, 832
  intracranial, 803—804
Neostigmine, 446
Nephrectomy, 146, 738—739
  donor, 981, 981f
Nephrolithotomy, 742
Nephrolithotripsy, percutaneous, 741—742
Nephron, 732f
Nephrostolithotomy, percutaneous, 741—742
Nephrostomy, 146, 739, 739f
Nerve blocks, 433, 451, 459
Nerve deficit, postoperative, 464
Nerve stimulator, in orthopedic surgery, 769
Nervous system, of geriatric patient, 168t, 174
Neurectomy, 807
Neurexeresis, 807
Neuroborreliosis, 244
Neurogenic, 730
Neurogenic bladder, 146
Neurogenic disorders, 730

Neurogenic shock, 642
NeuroGuide intraoperative viewing system, 795
Neurologic surgery, pediatric, 153—155
Neurolysis, 784, 807
Neurometrics monitor, 549
Neuromuscular blockers, 140, 445
    antibiotics that potentiate, 445, 445b
    in head and neck procedures, 874
    malignant hyperthermia and, 646
Neuroradiology, interventional, 794
Neurorrhaphy, 807
Neurosensory flap, 854
Neurostimulation, for bladder control, 748
Neurosurgeons, spinal surgery and, 811
Neurosurgery, 790—807
    adjuncts to visibility in, 795, 795f
    complications of cranial surgery in, 805—806
    cranial nerve, decompression in, 801
    craniectomy in, 799, 799f
    cranioplasty in, 800—801
    craniotomy in, 799—800
        controlled hypothermia in, 797
        hemostasis in, 797, 798f
        ICP control in, 798—799
        instrument table in, 797
        patient positioning for, 796—797
        patient preparation for, 795, 796f
        physiologic monitoring, 798—799
    diagnostics for, 792—793
    functional, 803
    for head trauma, 805
    hemostasis and, 793—794
    microneurosurgery in, intracranial, 801
    psychosurgery and, 803
    special considerations in, 792—795
    stereotaxis for, 802—804, 803f
    of tumors, intracranial, 799—800, 800t
    prognostic factors, 793
Neurosyphilis, 244
Neurotomy, 807
Neurovascular free flap, 855
New knowledge, innovation, and improvements, 80
New product evaluation, 97
Nightingale, Florence, 17, 17b
NIRS. See Near-infrared reflectance scope
Nitrofurantoin, 257t
Nitroglycerin, 627
    to induce hypotension, 448
Nitroimidazoles, 257t
Nitroprusside, 627
Nitrous oxide (N_2O), 137, 441—442, 441t
    during ear procedures, 874
    lines for, 188
    as occupational hazard, 232, 441—442
Noise, in operating room, 220
Nomenclature, 16, 31
Non-insulin-dependent diabetes mellitus, 106
Nonabsorbable sutures, 562, 565—567, 566t
Nonallergenic tape, 603
Noncritical items, cleaning of, 215
Noncrushing clamps, 345, 346f
Nondepolarizing neuromuscular blockers, 445—446
Noninvasive techniques, 396
Nonionizing radiation, 218, 225—226, 226f
Nonnursing administrative duties, 83
Nonpenetrating injuries, of eye, 844—845
Nonsterile latex gloves, 283
Nonsterile team members, 55, 57—62
    role of, circulating nurse as part of, 468b
Nonwoven fabrics, 317
    for ethylene oxide gas sterilization, 329

"No Pay List", 19—20
Norepinephrine, 627
Normovolemic hemodilution technique, 448
Nose,
    881—885. See also Otorhinolaryngologic and
        head and neck surgery
    anatomy of, 881, 882f
    physiology of, 881
    skin preparation for, antiseptic, 525
    surgical procedures of, 881—885
        general considerations for, 881—882
        nasal cavity, 882—884
        paranasal sinus, 884—885, 884f
NOTES. See Natural Orifice Transluminal Endo-
    scopic Surgery
"No touch" techniques, 417
    in handling syringes, 479
NPO (nothing by mouth), 128, 201
    after abdominal surgery, 691
    in geriatric patients, 171
    local or regional anesthesia and, 452
    in pediatric patients, 128
    written instructions to patient about, 380
NPSG. See National Patient Safety Goals
NQF. See National Quality Forum
Nuclear medicine departments, 85—86
Nuclear medicine studies, 395, 405—406
Nurse
    clinical laser, 371
    in holding area, 390—391
Nurse clinician, perioperative, 83
Nurse executive, 84—85
Nurse manager, perioperative, 81—82
Nursing diagnosis, 16, 28
Nursing Intervention Classification (NIC), 32
Nursing Outcomes Classification (NOC), 32
Nursing process, 16, 28—30, 28b, 615
Nursing student, perioperative, 3—5
Nutrition
    cancer risk and, 110
    patient with alteration of, 104—106
        drugs interfering with, 104, 104t
        head and neck procedures and, 104—105
        malnutrition, 105, 105b
        metabolism and, 105—106
        supplements and, 106
Nutritional alteration, 104—106, 104t, 105b
Nutritional status
    of patient, geriatric, 171
    wound healing and, 587

O
Obese patient, 108—110
    aspiration hazard in, 436
    common complications in, 108
    nutritional status of, 587
    physiologic dysfunctions impairments with,
        107, 107t
    positioning of, 500
    special considerations for, 108—110
        in positioning, 109f
Obesity, 107t, 108—110
Objective lenses, 372
Objectives, 1, 81, 361
    perioperative education and, 5
Obligation, 16—18
Obstetric services, 85
Obstetric surgery, 696—729
Obstetrics, perioperative, 714—718
    aborted pregnancy in, 716—718

Obstetrics, perioperative (Continued)
    complicated birth in, 718—722
        cesarean birth, 719—721, 720f—721f
        ectopic pregnancy in, 718, 718f
        vaginal, 718—719, 719f
    considerations for, 714—716
        in positioning, 714—715, 715f
    threatened abortion, 716
Obturator, 647
Occluding instruments, 343—345
Occlusion, 338, 349—350
Occlusion banding, 585
Occlusive dressing, 583, 602
Occupational hazard, 1—2
Occupational Safety and Health Administration
    (OSHA), 219, 231—232
    laser safety and, 369
    standards, 20
Ochsner clamp, 343—345
Oculars, 361, 372—373
Oculomotor muscles, procedures of, 833
Oculoplastic procedures on eyelids, 150
Oculoplethysmography (OPG), 408, 951
Offices, in surgical suites, 181
Oil glands, in skin, 554—555
Oils, dry heat sterilization of, 326
Ointments, dispensing to sterile surface, 426
-oma, 395
Omental flap, 854
Omental grafts, 853
Omphalocele, 145—146
Oncologic considerations, 395—419
Oncology, 408
One-hand placement, of tubing, 649
One-layer dressing, 602
Oophorectomy, 413, 713—714
Open abdominal cholecystectomy, 671
Open fracture, 771
Open laparoscopy, 656
Open method, of incision, 648
Open reduction and internal fixation (ORIF) of a
    fracture, 761
Open wounds, 585
Open-assisted gloving, 275
Open-gloving, 275
Opening sterile supplies, 472—474, 474f
Operating bed, 506—512, 506f—507f
    attachments of, special equipment and, 507—512
        accessories, 511, 512f
        adhesive tape, anal procedures with, 509
        anesthesia screen, 507, 508f
        arched spinal frame, adjustable, 509—510, 510f
        armboard, 508, 508f
        body (hip) restraint strap, 509
        body rests and braces, 509
        double armboard, 508, 509f
        extremity table, upper, 509
        headrests, 510—511, 511f
        lateral positioner (kidney rests), 509, 509f
        lift sheet (drawsheet), 508, 508f
        metal footboard, 510
        pressure-minimizing mattress, 512
        safety belt, 507
        shoulder braces, 509
        shoulder bridge (thyroid elevator), 509
        stirrups, 510, 510f—511f
        surgical vacuum positioning system, 512
        wrist or arm strap, 508
    for obese patient, 104
    ophthalmic, 827—828, 828f
    positioning at, 220, 221f

Operating bed mount, 375
Operating microscope, in neurosurgery, 795
Operating room, 179, 183—193, 183f
  basic layout of, 212, 212f
  cabinets or carts in, 192
  categories of, 183
  cleaning of
    daily terminal, 216—217
    for next patient, 216
    preliminary preparations for, 212
    weekly or monthly, 217
  clocks in, 192
  communication systems in, 193
  computer lines for, 188—190
  definition of, 177
  of deployable medical systems,
    206—209, 207f—209f
  doors of, 184
  electrical systems for, 188—190, 189f—190f
  entering, with patient, 485—486
  environmental controls in, 179t
  floors of, 187
  forensic evidence, 120
  furniture in, 192
  greening of, 217
  humidity in, 183
  individual patient setups of, 216
  laminar airflow for, 185—186, 185f—187f
  lighting in, 190—191, 219
  monitoring screens in, 191—192
  music in, 220
  noise in, 220
  other equipment, 192
  patient transfer from, 490
  piped-in gases for, 188—190, 189f
  radiograph screens for, 192
  safety committees, 89—90
  setting up, 466—474
    "eight P's" of, 476t—477t
    for organ procurement, 976—977, 976f
    sterile supplies, opening of, 474f, 487
  size determinations of, 183
  spotlights in, 467
  substerile room and, 184
  temperature of, 184
  transfer of patient to, 391—394, 392f
  ventilation in, 184—187, 185b, 219
  view boxes for, 192
  walls and ceiling of, 187—188
Operating Room Nurses Association of Canada
  (ORNAC), 18
Operating room team
  efficiency of, 495—498
    motion economy and, 496—497
    productivity and, 495
    supplies and equipment, economical use of,
      497—498
    time and, 495—497
  psychological support of, 979
Operational budget, 79, 96
Ophthalmic lasers, 845—846
Ophthalmic surgery, 826—846
  anesthesia for, 831—832
  complications of, 828, 828f
  draping for, 828
  drugs used for, 831—832
  extraocular, procedures in, 832—837
    of cornea, 834—837
    for eye removal, 834
    of eyelid, 832—833, 832f
    of lacrimal apparatus, 833

Ophthalmic surgery (*Continued*)
    of oculomotor muscles, 833
    orbit, 833
  hemostasis in, 828, 829f
  instrumentation for, 829, 829f—830f
  intraocular, procedures in, 832, 837—844
    for cataract, 838—840, 838f
    of iris, 837—838
    for lens implantation, 840—841, 840f
    of retina, 841—842
    vitrectomy, 843—844
  laser, for retinal procedures, 842
  microscope for, 830—831, 831f
  operating room for, 827—828
  patient care in, 827—829, 828f
  special features of, 829—832
Ophthalmologic surgery, pediatric, 150
Opiate receptors, 625
Opportunists, 238, 251
Optode, 543
Oral cavity and throat,
    885—889. *See also* Otorhinolaryngologic and
    head and neck surgery
  anatomy and physiology of, 885—886
  surgical procedures of, 886—887
    dental, 887—889
    of nasopharynx, 886—887
    for oral carcinoma, 886
    for oropharynx, 887
    for salivary gland tumors, 886
Oral surgeon, 888
Oral surgical procedures, 858
Orbit
  exenteration of, 834
  fractures of, 902
  procedures of, 833
    for craniofacial anomalies, 901
Orchiectomy, 413, 750
Orchiopexy, 147
Organ banks, 976—977
Organ donation, 54, 972
  donor cards and, 974
  in religious and cultural groups, 972,
    972t—973t
  tissue typing for, 980
Organ procurement, 974—979, 974t—975t
  with cadaver donor, 974—979, 975t
    brain death and, 974, 975t
  counting procedures in, 491
  with living related donor, 979
  multiple, 976—979, 976f, 978f
  preservation of organ allografts in, 980
  psychological support of OR team, 979
Organ Procurement and Transplantation Network
  (OPTN), 973—974
Organ Transplant Registry of the American College
  of Surgeons, 973
Organ transplantation, 54, 969—987
  immunologic rejection in, 972—973, 980—981
  types of, 982
Organ transplants, 579
Orientation, 1, 3
Orientation manual, 21
Orientation program of institution, 3, 83
  basic competency achieved in, 13
  policies and procedures in, 6, 21
  preceptors, mentors, and role models in, 13—14
ORNAC. *See* Operating Room Nurses Association of
  Canada
Oropharynx, surgical procedures of, 887
-orrhaphy, 664

Orthodontist, 888
Orthognathic surgery, 903—904
Orthopedic cart, 785, 785b
Orthopedic surgeons, spinal surgery and, 811
Orthopedic surgery, 761—789
  art and science of, 761—762
  attire used for, 284f
  in children, 148—150
  indications for, 771
  instrumentation for, 766—767
  materials and equipment and, 767—770
  special considerations in, 770
  special features of, 765—770
  in sports medicine, 784—785
Orthotopic heart transplantation, 982, 983f
Orthotopic neobladder, 730, 746—747
OSHA. *See* Occupational Safety and Health
  Administration
Osteoarthritis, 167, 169—170, 169f—170f
Osteoblasts, 761, 764
Osteoclasts, 761, 763
Osteomyelitis, 761, 765
Osteoplastic flap procedure, of frontal sinus, 884
Osteoporosis, 167, 169, 169f, 808, 818
Osteotomes, 341—342, 342f, 766
Osteotomy
  mandibular, 904
  maxillary, 903
Ostia, 923, 931
-ostomy, 664
Ostomy, intestinal, 684
Otitis media, 877
  cholesteatoma secondary to, 879
-otomy, 664
Otoplasty, 153, 859
Otorhinolaryngologic and head and neck surgery,
  873—904. *See also* Ear; Neck; Nose; Oral cavity
  and throat
  anesthesia for, 874, 874f
  communication with patients and, 874
  draping for, 874—875, 875f
  equipment and instrumentation for, 875—876
  eye protection in, 875
  general considerations in ear, nose, and throat
    procedures in, 873—876
  hemostasis in, 876
  pharmacologic considerations in, 874
  positioning for, 874—875
  prepping for, 874—875
  surgical specialty involved in, 873
  tissue grafts and implants in, 876
Otorhinolaryngologic surgery, 151—152
Outcome, 16, 18
Outer layer, dressing and, 603
Outpatient, surgery procedure for, 3
Outside air (OA), 179t, 184
Ovarian cancer, 713
Ovarian cystectomy, 713
Ovaries, anatomy of, 698f, 699
Overbed table attachment, 508f
Overdosage, from local and regional anesthesia, 462
Overhead operating light, cleaning of, 215
Overwrap, suture materials and, 572
Ovulation, 699
  induction of, 723
Ovum retrieval, 724
  in vitro fertilization, 723
Oxidized cellulose, 954b
  hemostasis and, 590—591
Oxidizer, 230
Oxycyte, 641

Oxygen
   administration of, during head and neck surgery, 875
   fire hazards and, 230
      in laser surgery, 371
   to ophthalmic surgical patient, 828
   supply line for, 188
Oxygenation, 619
   monitoring of, 542—543
Oxygenator, 929
Oxyglobin, 641
Oxytocin
   after cesarean delivery, 720
   hemostasis and, 591
Ozone gas sterilization, 331

P
Pacemaker, cardiac, 940—942, 941f, 941t
   precautions with, 942
Packaging materials
   for dry heat sterilization, 326
   integrity and handling of, 334—335
Packing, 595
   vaginal, 700—701
Packs, 492, 595
PaCO₂, 433
Padding of operating bed, 504b
   for diabetic patient, 108
Pain management, in pediatrics, perioperative, 132—134, 132t—134t
Pain, assessment for, in postanesthesia care unit, 613
Palatoplasty, 152—153
Palliation, 395
Palliative care, 123
Palliative measures, 412
Pallidotomy, 803
Palmed, 64
Pancreas transplantation, 974t—975t, 979, 987
Pancreatectomy, 676
Pancreatic procedures, 675—676
Pancreaticoduodenal trauma, 676
Pancreaticoduodenectomy, 676, 676f
Pancreaticojejunostomy, 676
Pancuronium, 445
PaO₂, 433
Papanicolaou (Pap) smear, 701
Papillomas, laryngeal, 152
Parachlorometaxylenol, 286
   for skin preparation, 524
Paradigm, 99—101
Paralysis, 104, 808, 816
Paramedian incision, 556f, 557
Paramedian thoracotomy, 927—928
Paranasal sinuses
   anatomy of, 881, 882f
   as sterile, 882
   surgical procedures of, 884—885, 884f—885f, 901
Paraplegia, 808, 819
Parasternotomy, 915
Parathyroid gland, procedures of, 896
Paravertebral block, 459
Paraxial illuminators, 373
Parenteral nutrition, 106
Park procedure, 159
Parotidectomy, 886, 886f
Pars plana vitrectomy, 828f
Partial laryngectomy, laryngofissure with, 891
Partial thromboplastin time (PTT), normal values of, 635t
PASS mnemonic, 231
Passive drains, 599

Passive immunity, 240
Pasteurization, 295, 308
PAT center, 197
Patent ductus arteriosus, 157, 157f
Pathogenic condition, 238—239, 260, 262—263
Pathogenic microorganisms, 260—261
Pathogens
   body fluids and substances carrying, 241b
   defense against, three lines of, 240
   pathogenic invasion by, 240—241
   viability of, 240b
Pathologic examination, definition of, 395, 397
Pathologic fracture, 771
Pathology department, 86
Patient, 99—124
   end-of-life care for, 123
   hospitalized, 379
   as individual, 99—102, 100f
      basic needs of, 100—102, 100f
      family/significant others, 102
      perception of care, 102
      reactions to illness, 101t, 102
   with individualized needs, 102—110
      cardiovascular disease, 117
      diabetes mellitus, 106—108, 107f, 107t
      immunosuppression, 118—119
      impairment of cognitive function, 104
      nutritional alteration, 104—106, 104t, 105b
      obesity, 107t, 108—110
      with patient having sensory impairment, 103—104
      physical challenge, 103—104
      pulmonary disease, 117—118
      sensory impairment, 103—104
   preoperative preparation of, 379—394
Patient advocacy, 17
Patient assessment, 71
Patient care departments, 85
Patient care division, 85
Patient handover, 49b
Patient identification, 22
   in minimizing potential hazard, 394
   preoperative, 390
   validating with parent in, 392
Patient monitoring, 26
Patient observation, 23—24
Patient positioning, 24
Patient return electrode, 363
Patient rights, 17
Patient roller, 489
Patient safety, 44
   considerations for, 659—660
   radiation exposure and, 223—224
Patient Safety and Quality Improvement Act of 2005, 42
Patient selection, in vitro fertilization, 723
Patient Self-Determination Act (PSDA), 46
Patient services departments, 85—86
Patient teaching, 26
   for adults, 3—4
Patient-nurse relationship, 27
Patties, 492, 794
   compressed absorbent, 596
PCWP. See Pulmonary capillary wedge pressures
PE. See Pulmonary embolus
Peanut sponges, 492
Pectus carinatum, 156, 917
Pectus excavatum, 155—156, 156f, 917
Pedagogy, 1, 3
Pediatric anesthesia, 135—140
   agents for, 139—140

Pediatric anesthesia (Continued)
   emergence from, 140
   equipment for, 136
   extubation and, 140
   induction in, 136—139
   intubation for, 136—139
   local, 139t
   maintenance of, 139—140
   premedication for, 136
   preoperative assessment by anesthesia provider, 135—136
Pediatric endoscopy, 657
Pediatrics, perioperative, 125—160
   advances in knowledge of, 126
   chronologic age in, 126—127, 127t
   common surgical procedures, 142—160
      cardiovascular, 156—160
      emergent, 142—146
      endoscopic, 142
      genitourinary, 146—148
      neurologic, 153—155
      ophthalmologic, 150—151
      orthopedic and spinal, 148—150
      otorhinolaryngologic, 151—152
      plastic and reconstructive, 152—153
      thoracic, 155—156
   considerations in, 126—127
   fluid and electrolyte balance considerations in, 128—130
   hematologic values, in pediatric patients, 129t
   indications for surgery and, 125—126, 129t
   infection risk in, 132
   intraoperative care in, 140—142
   metabolism and nutritional considerations, 128
   pain management in, 132—134, 132t—134t
   postoperative care in, 160
   preoperative psychologic preparation, 134—135
   psychological development and, 127t
Pedicle flaps, 850, 850f, 853—854, 853f
Pedunculated stalk, 923, 940
Peel packs or pouches, 317
   dispensing contents to sterile field, 425
   for dry heat sterilization, 329
   for ethylene oxide gas sterilization, 329
   in sterile supplies, 473
   storage of, 317
Peer review, 36
Pelvic examination, 701
Pelvic exenteration, 712
Pelvic lymph node dissection, radical hysterectomy with, 712
Pelvic outlet, procedures for repair of, 707—708
Penectomy, 757
Penetrating injuries, of eye, 845
Penetrating wounds, 919
Penile cancer, 757
Penile prosthesis, 757, 757f
Penis, anatomy and physiology of, 755—757
Penrose drains, 599
Peracetic acid, as sterilants, 333
Percent, 423
Perception, 99—100
Percutaneous, 338, 396, 647
Percutaneous discectomy, 820—821
Percutaneous endoscopic gastrostomy (PEG), 679
   tube placement, 144f
Percutaneous needle biopsy, 397
   of liver, 674
Percutaneous puncture, 397, 647—649
   ultrasonography and, 407

Percutaneous transluminal angioplasty, 955–956
 coronary, 937, 938f
Percutaneous transluminal balloon valvuloplasty, 935
Percutaneous, definition of, 350–351
Pereyra procedure, 747
Perfluorocarbon, oxygen-carrying, 641
Perforation, in endoscopy, 657
Performance appraisal check-off sheets
 in circulating role, 5, 8f
 in scrub role, 5, 8f
Performance improvement committee, 90
Performance improvement studies, 35
Perfusion, 429, 930
Perianesthesia nurse, 55, 57
 definition of, 610, 612
 postoperative patient care and, 612
 preoperative visit by, 382
Perianesthesia team, 57
Peribulbar anesthesia, 832
Perineal sheet, as drapes, 529
Perineal urethrostomy, 748
Perineum
 female, 697, 697f
 procedure in, for draping of patient, 533
Periodontics, 888
Periodontist, 888
Perioperative, 1
Perioperative administrative personnel, 81
Perioperative business manager, 83
Perioperative documentation, 48–49
Perioperative education coordinator, 83–84
Perioperative environment, care of, 535–550.
 See also Surgical environment
Perioperative nurse
 clinical competency of, 33–34
 patient's expectations from, 102
 role of, during local anesthesia, 453
Perioperative Nursing Data Set (PNDS),
 16, 18, 29–30, 47–49
Perioperative nursing practice
 documentation, 31
 evaluation, 32–33
 implementation, 32
 physiologic assessment, 31
 planning, 32
 psychosocial assessment, 31
 scope of, 34
 standards of, 30–33
Perioperative patient care, 3
 documentation of, 46–50
 nursing process into, 28–29
Perioperative patient care services, administration of,
 79–98
 and magnet recognition, 80b, 81
Perioperative patient care team, 56–62
Perioperative Patient Outcomes: Standards of Perioperative Care, 18
Perioperative patient, physiologic maintenance and
 monitoring of, 535–550
Perioperative policy and procedure manual, 21
Periosteal elevators, 342f, 766, 766f
Peripheral nerve considerations, for positioning of
 patient, 505
Peripheral nerve surgery, 806–807
Peripheral support areas, 180–183
Peritoneal cavity, 674f
Peritoneal dialysis, 740–741, 741f
Peritoneal lavage, 689–690
Peritoneum, in skin, 556
Peritonitis, 691
Peritonsillar abscess, 887

Periurethral injection of bulking agent, 748
Permanent filters, 964
Permanent section, 397
 dyes and stains for, 413
Perpendicular, 64
Perpetrator, 99, 119
Personal attributes, 11, 12t
Personal mastery, 92
Personal property of patient
 documenting, 49, 389
 protection of, 22–23
Personal protective equipment (PPE), 267, 275
Personal skills and communications, 81–82
Personnel management, 93–95
Personnel safety, 223b, 224–225, 224f
Pessary, 173, 173f
PET. *See* Positron emission tomography
Petrolatum-based lotions, 285
Pfannenstiel incision, 558f, 559
pH, 433, 460, 633
Phacoemulsification, 826, 838–839
Phantom limb pain, 694
Pharmaceutical error, avoiding, 421
Pharmacists, 86
Pharmacodynamics, 625–626
Pharmacokinetics, 420, 430
Pharmacologic agents, for reduction of blood loss,
 636
Pharmacology, 65
 surgical, 420–431
 baselines of, 421–424
Pharmacy, 86
Pharyngeal diverticulectomy, 887
Phenolic compounds, for disinfection, 304t–305t,
 308
Phenylephrine, 628
Philosophy, 81
Phimosis, 756
Phlebography, 952
Phone call
 for evaluation of expected outcomes, 615
 follow-up, 205
 by perianesthesia nurses, 611
 preoperative
 before ambulatory surgery, 202
 to review arrangements, 382
Phosphate, as electrolyte, 633
Photocoagulation, 598
 retinal, 842
Photodynamic (laser) therapy, 112–113, 368
 for cancer, 413
Photoplethysmographic disc, 857
Photoplethysmography, 951
Photoradiation, for cancer, 413
Photorefractive keratectomy (PRK), 836
Photosensitive drug, 113
Phototherapeutic keratectomy (PTK), 835
Physical assessment
 of geriatric patient, 167–174, 168t
 pediatric, 128–134
Physical challenge, 103–104
Physical disinfectants, 308–309
Physical facilities, 177–196. *See also* Surgical suites
Physical factor theory, 163–164
Physical hazards, 71
Physically challenged patient, 103
Physician Assistant National Certifying (PANC)
 exam, 77
Physician assistant, as first assistant, 77
Physician-assisted suicide, 53

Pia mater, 790
Pick-ups, 342
Pierre Robin syndrome, 900, 900f
Pilonidal cysts, excision of, 692
Pipecuronium, 446
Piped-in gases, in operating room, 188–190, 189f
Placebo effect, 420, 430
"Place it once" principle, 480
Placental problems, 718–719, 719f
Plain cysto, 744–745
Plaintiff, 37–38
Plan of care
 accompanying patient to operating room and, 390
 evaluation of expected outcomes, 614
 by holding area nurse, 391
 preoperative nurse interview and, 382
 reviewed by circulating nurse, 392
Plant sources, of drugs, 427
Plasma scalpel, 598
Plasma, as biologic adhesives, 575
Plaster casts, 786
Plaster room, 769
Plaster rope, 787
Plaster shell, 787
Plaster splint, 787
Plastic and reconstructive surgery, 847–872.
 See also Burns
 of adipose tissue, 861–862
 abdominoplasty, 861–862, 862f
 liposuction, 861, 861f–862f
 of breast, 862–864
 of augmentation, 862–863, 863f
 for male reduction, 864, 865f
 for reconstruction, 863–864, 864f
 for reduction, 864, 865f
 categories of, 850
 for facial resurfacing, 866, 866t
 general considerations for autografts, 857–858
 general considerations in, 848–849, 848f
 head and neck procedures in, 858–861
 pediatric, 152–153
 preoperative instruction to patients for, 848
 preoperative measurements for, 848, 848f
 psychological support for, 849
 replantation of amputated parts, 856–857,
 856f–857f
 for scar revision, 864, 866f
 skin and tissue grafting in, 850–858
 "take" of graft in, 850
 classification of, 850
 free flap, 850, 850f, 854–856
 pedicle flap, 850, 850f, 853–854, 853f
 skin graft, 850–851, 851f
 for skin cancer, 866–867
 special features of, 847–850
Plastic isolator
 for burn patients, 871
 draping of, 534
Plastics, steam sterilization of, 323
Plated instruments, 339
Platelets, normal values of, 635t
Pledgets, 595
 of Teflon felt, 923, 934, 939, 940f
Plethysmography, 396, 408, 951
Pleura, 906, 907f
Pleural effusion, 913
Pleurodesis, 905, 913
Plication, 905, 920
Plume
 electrosurgical, 365
 laser, 267, 370

Plume (Continued)
  surgical, 234–235
  thermal, 177, 185, 185f
PMMA. See Polymethylmethacrylate
PNDS. See Perioperative Nursing Data Set
Pneumatic counterpressure device, 593, 797
Pneumatic tourniquet, 593–595
Pneumatic tube system, 180
Pneumonectomy, 905, 913, 917f, 918
Pneumoperitoneum, for endoscopy, 142, 647, 649, 650f
Pneumoretinopexy, 826, 842, 843f
Pneumothorax, 619–620, 908
  chest wound with, 919
  controlled, 908–909
  fractured ribs with, 919
  open thoracotomy for, 917
  pleurodesis for, 913
Point of use cleaning, 297
Policies and procedures, 22
  administrative responsibility for, 81
Polyclonal antilymphocyte globulin, 981
Polydactyly, 153, 154f
Polyester fiber
  as implant, 581
  as mesh, 577
  as suture, 566–567
Polyethylene, as implant, 581
Polyglactin 910 mesh, 577
PolyHeme, 641
Polymethylmethacrylate (PMMA), 233
Polypectomy
  colorectal, 687
  nasal, 883
Polypharmacy, 99, 103, 420, 430
Polypropylene
  as mesh, 577–578
  as suture, 567
Polytetrafluoroethylene, 578
  in prosthetic devices, 581
  vascular grafts constructed of, 955
Pons, 791f, 792
Poole abdominal suction tip, 352
Pooled-donor plasma, 575
Pop-off needle, 570
Porcine dermis, 578
Portable X-ray machine, 400
Portacaval shunt, 966
Portosystemic shunts, 675, 966
Position statements, 16, 27
Positioning of patient, 499–534
  accessibility for anesthetic administration for, 506
  accessibility of the surgical site for, 506
  anatomic and physiologic considerations for, 504–506
  circulatory considerations for, 504–505
  complications caused by, 505b
  for craniotomy, 796–797, 796f
  equipment for, 506–512
  geriatric, 175
    hiatal hernia, 171
    musculoskeletal changes and, 169
  individual positioning considerations for, 506
  musculoskeletal considerations for, 505
  obese, 109, 109f, 500
  for otorhinolaryngologic and head and neck surgery, 874–875
  padding for, 504b
  pediatric, 140, 141f
  peripheral nerve considerations for, 505
  physically challenged patient, 103

Positioning of patient (Continued)
  planning the organization of, 501t–503t
  preliminary considerations in, 499–504
  preparations for, 500
  respiratory considerations for, 504
  responsibility for, 500
  safety measures in, 500–504, 505f
  soft tissue considerations for, 505–506
  for spinal surgery, 811–813, 814f
  timing of, anesthetic administration and, 500
Positions, surgical, 512–519
  anterior chest, 518
  beach chair, 514, 515f
  documentation of, 519
  kidney, 518, 518f
  knee-chest, 517
  Kraske (Jackknife), 517, 517f
  lateral, 518
  lateral chest (thoracotomy), 518
  lithotomy, 514–516, 515f
  modifications for individual patient, 518–519
  prone, 516, 516f
    modified, 516
  semi-Fowler, 514, 514f
  Sims recumbent, 517–518
  sitting, 514
    modified, 514
  supine (dorsal), 512–513, 512f
  Trendelenburg, 513, 513f
    reverse, 513–514, 514f
Positive reinforcement, 6
Positron emission tomography (PET), 406
  of brain, 792
Postanesthesia care, 610–612
  perianesthesia and, personnel of, 612, 612f, 612b
  phases of, 610–611
Postanesthesia care unit (PACU), 57, 160, 180, 610
  admission to, 612–614
  for ambulatory surgery, 203, 204f
  discharge from, 614–615
  documentation in, 614
  environmental controls in, 179t
  handover to, 612–613
  overflow considerations for, 614
Posterior, definition of, 499
Posterior approach, definition of, 808, 814
Posterior colpoperineorrhaphy, 707
Posterior spinal fusion, 149–150
Posterolateral thoracotomy, 914, 914f, 928
Postmortem patient care, 124
Postoperative autotransfusion, 640–641
Postoperative chemotherapy, 117
Postoperative evaluation program, 615
Postoperative patient care, 610–615
  activities for, 613–614
  in ambulatory surgery, 203–205, 204f
  documentation in, 614
  evaluation of expected outcomes in, 614–615
  handover report for, 613
  observation of, 611
  orders for, 613–614
  overflow considerations for, 614
  perianesthesia patient care personnel and, 611–612, 612f, 612b
  postanesthesia care unit, 611
    admission to, 612–614
    discharge from, 614–615
  professional activities and, 612
Postoperative pediatric patient care, 160
Postoperative phase, 30
Postoperative wound infection, 24

Postperfusion lung syndrome, 932
Postresuscitation care, 632
Posttraumatic stress disorder (PTSD), 210
Potassium titanyl phosphate (KTP) laser, 367
Potassium, as electrolyte, 633
Potential sources of injury, to caregiver and patient, 218–237. See also Hazards
Potentiation, 420, 430
Pott's fractures, 785
Potts-Smith-Gibson procedure, 158, 158f
Pouch of Douglas (retrouterine cul-de-sac), 698
Poudrage, 905, 913
Povidone-iodine, 286, 524
Powders, 430
Power, 361–362
Power sources, 355–356, 361, 365
Power-driven cutting instruments, for orthopedic surgery, 766
Powered equipment, steam sterilization of, 323
Powered instruments, 355
  microsurgical, 355
  sterilization of, 355
Powered skin graft dermatomes, 851
PowerPoint presentations, 4
PPE. See Personal protective equipment
Preadmission procedures, 380–389
Preadmission testing (PAT) area, 379–380
Preanesthesia medications, 389–390
Preanesthesia preparations, 391
Preceptor, 1, 4, 84
  collaboration with educator and manager, 12
  role of, 13–14
Precordial thump, 623
  in infant, 628
Precut lengths, of suture material, 572
Prednisone, 112
Pregnancy
  adolescent, 704
  altered laboratory values of, 715t
  anatomic and physiologic changes of, 726t–727t
  anesthesia considerations in, 725–727
  domestic violence during, 121
  drug administration during, 421
  ectopic, 718, 718f
  general anesthesia during, 449
  intraoperative care in, 727–728
  intrauterine fetal surgery in, 722
  nonobstetric surgical procedures in, 725–729
    intraoperative risks, 728
    plan of care, 725
    psychologic considerations, 728–729
  positioning of patient during, 437
  prenatal testing in, 721–722
  rape victims and, 121
  stages of fetal development, 725b
Pregnant employees, 235
Pregnant nonobstetric patients, hypotension and, 517–518
Preinvasive cancer, 409
Preload, 546–547
Preloading techniques, in radiation therapy, 115, 414–415
Premature ventricular contraction (PVC), 622, 622f
Premedication, for pediatric anesthesia, 136
Prenatal testing, 721–722
Preoperative admission and holding unit, 180
Preoperative blood donation, 640
Preoperative chemotherapy, 117
Preoperative matching, of donor, 980
Preoperative medication, in anesthetized patient, 487

Preoperative patient care, in ambulatory surgery, 200–202, 201f
Preoperative phase, 30
Preoperative preparation of patient, 379–394
  anesthesia assessment in, 382, 387
  bedtime sedation in, 382
  bowel preparation in, 382
  checklist for, 390–391
  emotional, 390
  history and physical examination as, 380, 380f
  informed consent in, 382
  nurse interview in, 382
  nurse phone call in, 382, 384
  for obese patient, 108
  to operating room, 389–390
  surgeon's specific orders in, 382
  teaching in, 386
  visit by perioperative/perianesthesia nurse in, 382–383
  written instructions as, 380–382
Preoperative visit, by perianesthesia nurse, 382–383
  cons of, 383
  interviewing skills in, 383
  pros of, 382–383
  structured, 383–384
Preoxygenation, 435
Preperitoneal insufflation, in endoscopy, 658
Prepping of patient, 499–534
  planning the organization of, 501t–503t
  preliminary considerations in, 499–504
Preprocedural testing and assessment area (PAT center), 197
Prerinsing, 297
Presacral neurectomy, 806
Prescriptive privileges, of advanced practice nurses, 83
Preservatives, 429
Presoaking, 297
Press cut, 64, 69
Pressure dressing, 595, 603
  keloid formation and, 605
Pressure injuries, 506
Pressure sores, 586
Pressure-minimizing mattress, bed attachments and, 512
Pressure-redistributing padding, 506
Pressure, interpretation of, 545–546
Presurgical holding area, 379, 390–391
Preterm infant, 126
  fluid replacement for, 128
Prevacuum sterilizer, 312, 320–321, 324–325, 325t, 359
  biologic testing of, 324–325
Preventive drug, 420
Prilocaine, 455t, 461
Primary sterile packet, suture materials and, 572
Printer toner, 316
Prions, 213–214, 238, 252–253
  disease, transmission of, 253
  sterilization and, 320
Privacy, invasion of, 41
PRK. See Photorefractive keratectomy
Probe, 352
Probing instruments, 352
Problem-oriented charting, 48
Problem-oriented medical record (POMR), 48
PROBOT, 662
Procainamide, 626
  for malignant hyperthermia, 644
Procaine, 455t, 462
Procedure knowledge and techniques, 66, 66f
Procedure rooms, 177, 179, 193–194

Process challenge pack/process challenge device (PCD), 312, 314
Processing equipment, X-ray, 400
Procidentia, 707, 708f
Proctoscopy, 691
Procurement, 969–970
Product evaluation, 97
Productivity, 495
Profession, 16
Professional credentialing, 55–63
Professional involvement, 93
Professional perioperative nursing, 27
Professionalism, 26–27
Progesterone, 699
Prolene, as mesh, 577–578
Prone position, 499, 501t–503t, 516, 516f
  for cranial procedures, 796
Prophylaxis
  for malignant hyperthermia, 645–646
  for personnel, 268
Propofol, 441t, 443
  hypothermia and, 642
Proportion, 423–424
Propranolol, 626
Prostate examination, 173
  biopsy of, 173–174
Prostate gland, 749f, 751–755
  benign enlargement of, 752
  biopsy of, 752f
Prostatectomy, 752, 753f
  nerve-sparing, 754
  perineal, 754–755, 754f
  radical retropubic, 754, 755f
  retropubic, 754
  robotic-assisted, 755
  suprapubic, 754, 754f
Prostatic carcinoma, 752
  cryoablation for, 755
  lymphadenectomy for, 755
Prostatic urethra, balloon dilation and stenting of, 752, 752f
Prosthesis, 551, 580
  eye, 834
  orthopedic, 768
  preoperative management of, asking patient about, 382–383
  removal for safekeeping, 389
Prosthetic vascular grafts, 954
Prosthodontist, 888
Protamine sulfate, 953–954
Protected health information (PHI), 41
Protein deficiency, 105, 105b
Protein, engineered, 427–428
Proteolytic enzymatic detergent, as presoak, 297
Prothrombin time (PT), normal values of, 635t
Protocol, universal, 22
Protozoa, 254
Proximal, 499
Proximate cause, 37, 42
Pseudoaneurysm, 947, 959, 962, 962f
  repair of, 962
Pseudomonas aeruginosa, in breathing circuit, 450
Psychological development, theories of, 127t
Psychological support, for plastic and reconstructive surgery, 849
Psychomotor dexterity, 65–66
Psychomotor learning, 1, 10
Psychosocial assessment
  of geriatric patient, 166
  pediatric, 127–128
Psychosocial support, preoperative teaching and, 386

Psychosurgery, 803
Pterygium, 833f, 834
PTK. See Phototherapeutic keratectomy
Ptosis, 832–833, 847, 859
PTSD. See Posttraumatic stress disorder
Puberty, 125–126
Pudendum, 697
Pulmonary artery banding, 159
Pulmonary artery cannulation, 544–545
Pulmonary artery catheters, 544
  complications of, monitoring, 546
Pulmonary artery pressure
  in cardiac surgery, 929
  monitoring, 544–546
Pulmonary capillary wedge pressures (PCWP), 544, 546
Pulmonary collapse, 620
Pulmonary disease, 117–118
Pulmonary edema, 620
Pulmonary embolus (PE), 619
  surgical procedures for, 963–964
Pulmonary thromboendarterectomy, 964
Pulse
  definition of, 535, 537
  in witnessed arrest, 628
Pulse oximetry, 542
Pulse volume recording (PVR), 951
Pump, 930
Punch biopsy, 397
Punches, 341
Punctum plug and forceps, 829, 830f
Puncture injuries, 234
  management of, 267–268
  prevention of, 267–268
Pupillary dilation, in cardiac arrest, 625
Pupillary distance, 361, 373
Purchasing department, 87
Purse string, 551
Purse string suture, 560, 569
Pus formation, 241
PVC. See Premature ventricular contraction
PVR. See Pulse volume recording
Pyelolithotomy, 742
Pyeloplasty, 739
Pyelostomy, 739
Pyeloureteroplasty, 146
Pyloric stenosis, 145
Pyloromyotomy, 145
Pyloroplasty, 680

Q

Quadriplegia, 808, 819
Qualified care givers, credentialing of, 56
Qualified team, patient dependence on, 56
Quality and Performance Improvement Standards for Perioperative Nursing, 18
Quality improvement coordinator, 90
Quality of life, ethical issues involving, 53
Quaternary ammonium compounds, for disinfection, 308
Quench button, 227
Quinolones, 257t
Quorum sensing, 244–245

R

RACE mnemonic, 231
Radial artery conduit, 937
Radial echoendoscope, 653
Radial keratotomy, 836
Radiation safety
  for patients, 223–224

Radiation safety (*Continued*)
  for personnel, 223b, 224—225, 224f
    monitoring exposure in, 225
  warning sign, 222f
Radiation safety committee, 89
Radiation sources, implantation of, 414—415
Radiation sterilization, 333
Radiation therapy, 113—117
  effects on perioperative patient, 117, 415
  external beam, 115—116
  implantation of sources of, 114
  intraoperative, 116, 415
  preservation of reproductive system in, 412
    safety rules for, 116
  sources of, 113—114
  stereotactic radiosurgery, 116
  wound healing and, 588
Radical mastoidectomy, 878
Radical neck dissection, 896—897, 897f
Radical nephrectomy, 738
Radiculopathy, 808, 818
Radiofrequency ablation, for atrial fibrillation, 939
Radiofrequency identification (RFID) technology, 492
Radiograph screens, in operating rooms, 192
Radioisotopes, 653
Radiologic examination, 399—404
  diagnostic
    angiography, 402—403
    arteriography, 402—403
    arthrography, 402
    chest X-ray, 401
    computed tomography, 402
    gastrointestinal X-ray studies, 403
    incidental X-ray, 404
    mammography, 401—402
    for trauma, 401
    urography, 404
    ventriculography, 402
  equipment and accessories for, 399—401
    C-arm image intensifier, 401
    cassette, 400
    computerized digital subtraction processor, 401
    contrast media, 399—400
    fixed X-ray equipment, 400
    fluoroscope, 400—401
    image intensifier, 401
    portable X-ray machine, 400
    processing equipment, 400
    radiolucent gases, 400
    table, 400
Radiologic table, 400, 400f
Radiology, 85—86
Radiology services, in surgical suites, 181
Radiolucent gases, 400
Radionuclide imaging, myocardial, 932
Radionuclides, 114, 405
  half-life of, 114
  irradiation with, 114
Radiosurgery, stereotactic, 415, 804
Radium, 113—114
Radon, 114
Raising a flap, 64
Rape, victim of, 121
Rapid-sequence induction, for obstetric patient, 716
Rashkind procedure, 159
Rasps, 341—342
Rat-toothed forceps, 342
Ratio, 423—424
Raytex (Raytec) sponges, 492

Razor, for patient's skin, 521
Reaction, definition of, 420—421
Reality shock, 13
Really Simple Syndication (RSS), 10
Reasonable man doctrine, 40
Receptor mechanisms, of drugs, 625
Receptor sites, 420—421
Recipient, 969—970
Recommended practices, 16, 18, 21—26
Recovery centers, freestanding, 205
Recovery period, in ambulatory surgery, 200
Recreational drugs, 421
Rectal induction, 137—138
Rectocele, 707, 707f
Rectoperineal area, skin preparation for, antiseptic, 525—526, 526f
Rectovaginal fistula, repair of, 708
Rectum, 698f
Recycling, 217
Red blood cells, normal values of, 635t
Red rubber catheter, hazardous as insulation, 230
Red rubber endotracheal tube, and laser safety, 369
Red-yellow krypton, 846
Redo heart procedures, 923, 930—931
Reducible hernia, 693
Reflex sympathetic dystrophy, 808—809
Refractive keratoplasty, 836—837, 836f—837f
Regional anesthesia, 433, 451—454
  actions of, 460—462
  administration techniques for, 458—460
  adverse reactions to, 463—464
    treatment of, 463—464
  agents, 455t
  complications of, 462—464
  local effects of, 462
  monitoring the patient during, 464
  patient preparation for, 451—452
  performed in holding area, 391
  precautions with, 462—463
  systemic effects of, 462—463
    signs and symptoms of, 463
  toxicity of, 461
  unrelated effects of, 464
Regional cancer, 111, 409
Regional drugs, choices in, 454—456
Regional injection, of anesthesia, 459—460
Registered nurse (RN), 81
Registered nurse first assistant (RNFA), 71, 83
Registered nurse, Medicare regulation on role of, 56
Registration, 55—56
Regulatory bodies, standards from, 19—20
Rehabilitation, 695
Rehabilitation Act of 1973, 103
Reimbursement sources, in ambulatory surgery, 200
Removable bridges, 389
Renal revascularization, 739
Repair, of instruments, 300
Replacement, of instruments, 301
Replantation, of amputated parts, 847, 856—857, 856f—857f
Reprocessing, of disposable products, 310
Reproductive hazards, 235
Reproductive sterilization, 52
Res Ipsa Loquitur doctrine, 40
Resection, 664—665
Resectoscope, 735—736, 736f
Resistance, electrical, 227
Resolving power, 372
  of microscope, 373
Resources, of geriatric patient, 166
Respiration, definition of, 535, 542

Respiratory complications, perioperative, 617—620
  airway and respiratory obstruction, 618
  aspiration, 617
  atelectasis, 620
  emboli, 619
  hypoventilation, 618—619
  intercostal muscle spasm, 620
  laryngospasm and bronchospasm, 617—618
  pneumothorax, 619—620
  pulmonary edema, 620
Respiratory considerations, for positioning of patient, 504
Respiratory obstruction, 618
Respiratory system, of geriatric patient, 168t
Respiratory tidal volume (VT), 547
Respondeat superior doctrine, 40
Responsibility, 16, 18
Resterilization, of disposable products, 310
Restoration and resurfacing, of instruments, 300—301
Restorative valve, procedures of, 933
Restricted area, 179
Restricted surgical suite, definition of, 177
Retained products of conception (RPOC)/retained secundus, 696
Retained secundus, 717
Retention bridges, in sutures, 561
Retention sutures, 561, 665
Retina
  detachment, repair of, 841—842, 841f
  procedures for, 841—842
Retinopathy, 841
Retracting instruments, 345—347
Retraction, 64—65, 338, 345—346
  in vascular surgery, 952—953, 953f
Retractors
  bed-mounted, 347
  in endoscopic field, 654—655
  malleable, 345—346, 346f
  microsurgical, 355
  in neurosurgery, 795
  for ophthalmic surgery, 829, 829f
  for orthopedic surgery, 766
  self-retaining, 346—347, 348f
  for thoracic surgery, 909, 909f
Retrobulbar block, 832
Retrograde infusion, 931
Retrograde pyelography, 404
Retroperitoneal incision, 808, 816
Retroperitoneal space, 730
Return electrode, 363, 363f, 365
Reusable woven textile gowns, 284
Reuse of disposable products, 310
Reverse Trendelenburg position, 499, 513—514, 514f
Rheumatoid arthritis, 169—170, 170f
  malignant hyperthermia and, 643
Rhinoplasty, 859, 883
Rhinoscopy, 881
Rhizotomy, radiofrequency retrogasserian, 803
Rhytidoplasty, 859—860, 860f
Rib fracture, 919
Rib instruments, 909, 909f
Rib resection, 916, 916f
Ribbon retractors, 346
Ribcage, 905—906, 906f
Right atrial pressure (RAP), 545
Right to die, 53—54
Right ventricular assistance (RVA), 944
Right ventricular pressure, 545—546
Rights, 16—17
Rigid closed containers, 319—320
Rigid container, 312

Ring control syringe, 479
Ring stand, 475
Ring-handled clamp, 343
Ringer's lactate solution, 632
    for blood volume expanders, 636
Risk management, 236–237
Risk management department, 50
Risk manager, 90
Risser jacket, 149
RNFA. *See* Registered nurse first assistant
Robert Jones dressing, 770
Robotic components, 662f
Robotic-assisted surgery
    advantages and disadvantages of, 663
    endoscopy and, 647–663
    human intervention during, 663
    spinal, 815
Robotics, 142, 655
    environmental control by, 660
Rockey-Davis incision, 559
Rocuronium, 445
Role model, 1, 13
Room turnover
    activities
        by scrub person, 214–215
        by team, 215–216
    assist in, 489
    definition of, 211, 216, 335
    between patients, 212–216
Root cause analysis, 37, 42
Ropivacaine, 455t, 461
Rotation of supplies, 335
Rotational flap, 853
Round ligaments, 699
Roux-en-Y gastroenterostomy, 680
Rubber band, tourniquets and, 594
Rubber bandage, tourniquets and, 595
Rubber goods, steam sterilization of, 323
Rubber tubing, tourniquets and, 595
Ruby laser, 367
Rule of nines, 868, 868f
Rule of tens, 125, 152
"Running the bowel", 690, 690f
Ruptured organs, 919

S

Saccular aneurysm, 959–960, 960f
Sacred cows, 79, 92–93
Safe environment, business manager's coordination
        of, 83
Safeguards
    biologic hazards, 233–235
    electrical, 228
    in fire and explosion, 230
    physical hazards, 219–231
Safety, 218–219
    with specialized equipment, 361
Safety belt, 485
    bed attachments and, 507
Safety data sheets (SDS), 20
    for chemical disinfectants, 302
Safety plan manual, 20
Sales representatives, 97
    loaner instrumentation from, 335
Salivary gland tumors, 886
Salpingectomy, 713
Salpingo-oophorectomy, 712
Salpingolysis, 713
Salpingostomy, 713
Salvage collection bag, 640
Saphenous vein conduit, 935–937, 936f–937f

Saphenous vein harvest, by balloon dissection,
        650–651, 651f
Saphenous vein mapping, 951
Sarcoma, 396
Sarcopenia, 161–162
Satin finish, 339
Sayre sling, 149
Scalp clips, 793–794
Scalpels, 69–70, 340
    loading, 478, 478f
    for skin incision, 480
Scar, 583, 604–605, 605f, 864
    formation of, 584
    silicone dressing and, 604
Scar revision, 864, 866f
Schauta procedure, 709
Schiller test, 701
Schoemaker procedure, 679–680
Scintigraphy, 396, 405–406
Scissors, 341, 341f
    hand signal for, 481
    microsurgical, 354–355
    for ophthalmic surgery, 829f
    ultrasonic, 377–378
Scleral buckling, 842, 842f
Scleral lacerations, 845
Sclerotherapy, 592
    for esophageal varices, 677
Scoliosis, 149–150, 808, 816–818, 817f
Scrape cut, 64
Screwdrivers, 353
Scrub person, 26, 55, 61, 62b
    in cardiopulmonary resuscitation, 631–632
    coordinated roles of, circulating nurse and, 466–498
    counting of
        sharps, 494
        sponges, 493
    drugs and pharmaceuticals and, 425
    duties of, 466–495
        after the surgeon and assistant(s) scrub, 479
        in arranging instrument table, 475, 476f
        in arranging Mayo stand, 475–477, 477f
        in basin setup, 475
        during closure, 484
        in draping Mayo stand, 474–475, 475f
        draping the patient, 479–480
        in establishing baselines, 477–478
        handling medications and solutions on the sterile
            field, 478–479
        in handling syringes, 479
        in loading scalpels, 478, 478f
        in managing sharps, 478
        in preparation of sterile field, 474–484
        in preparing sutures and ties for use, 478
        during surgical procedure, 480, 480f
    in microsurgery, 376
    nurse in hospital orientation program, 3
    performance appraisal check-off sheet, 5, 8f
    privately employed, 61
    role of, as part of sterile team, 467
    room turnover activities by, 214–215
    in setting up the room, 466–474, 467f
        "eight P's" of, 476t–477t
        sterile supplies, opening of, 472–474
    sponge
        packaging increments of, 478b
        validating of, 472b–473b
    sterile field and, surgical towels on, 481b
    surgical technology training as, 3
    systematic activities for, 469t–470t
Scrub room, 183

Scrub sinks, 285
    cleaning in area of, 217
Scrub suit, 275
Sealants, 317–318
Sebaceous glands, in skin, 554–555
Second intention, 584–585, 584f
Secondary tumor, 790, 799–800
Secondhand smoke, 418
Security systems, 181
Sedation
    bedtime, preoperative, 382
    in children, 133t–134t
Sedative, 433
Segmental resection, 917
Self-examination, for cancer signs, 110, 418
Self-perception of health, of geriatric patient, 166
Self-retaining retractors, 346–347, 348f
Sellick's maneuver, 436, 617
Semi-Fowler position, 514, 514f
    intracranial pressure monitoring and, 549
Semicircular line of Douglas, 555–556, 555f
Semilunar valves, 924
Semirestricted area, 177, 179
Semirestricted surgical suite, 177
Semisolids, 430
Semisynthetic sources, of drugs, 427–428
Senescence, 161
Senile, 161
Senile adults, 161, 164
Senning procedure, atrial switch, 159
Sensory evoked potentials, 407–408, 798
Sensory impairment, 103–104
    patient with, 103
Sentinel events, 37, 42–44
    institutional reporting of, 42
    reportable and nonreportable, 42b
    and TJC, 42–44
Sentinel node biopsy, of breast, 666
Sentinel node sampling, 405–406
Separate sheets, as drapes, 529–530
Sepsis, 239, 241, 260, 264
Septal defects, 157
Septal myectomy, 940
Septal reconstruction, 883
Septic shock, 241, 246–247, 642
Septoplasty, 883
Sequential compression device, 593
Sequential wrapping, 317
Seroma, 583, 595, 604
Serosa, 698f
Service elevators, 266
Sevoflurane, 441t, 442–443
Sex reassignment, 758–759
Sexual assault, victim of, 121–122
Sexuality, in geriatric patients, 174
Sexually transmitted diseases, bacterial, 248
SGLT2 inhibitors, 106
Shared vision, 92
Sharp instrument, 338–339
Sharp trocar, 649
Sharps, 494. *See also* Counts
    count of, 494
    disposal of, 214, 494
    managing, 478
    methods of accounting for, 494
Shedders, of skin, 262–263
Sheet wadding, 788
Shelf life, after sterilization, 334–335
Sherman plate and screws, 773, 775f
Shielding, from radiation, 224–225, 224f
Shirodkar procedure, 716, 717f

Shivering, postanesthesia, 642
Shock, 641–642
    cardiogenic, 642, 946
    hemorrhagic, 642
    hypovolemic, 634, 641
    neurogenic, 642
    vasogenic, 642
Shockwave therapy, 146
Shoe covers, 280, 280b
    as personal protective equipment, 267
Shoes, in operating room, 220
Shoulder
    procedure in, for draping of patient, 532
    skin preparation for, antiseptic, 525
    in sports medicine, 785
    total joint replacement, 780, 781f
Shoulder braces or support, bed attachments and,
        509
Shoulder bridge (thyroid elevator), bed attachments
        and, 509
Shoulder spica, 787
Shunts, 790, 801
    vascular, 966–967
Sickle cell hemoglobinopathies, 637–638
Side effect, definition of, 420–421
Sigmoidoscopy, 686–687, 691
Sign in, 22
Sign language, 103
Sign out, 22
Silicone dressing, 604
Silicone, as implant, 581
Silo, wound, 581
Silver bunionectomy, 783
Silver nitrate, 591–592, 871
Silver sulfadiazine, 871
Simple gastrostomy, 679
Simple local infiltration, 459
Simple mastoidectomy, 878
Simple wounds, 585
Sims recumbent position, 517–518
Single photon emission computed tomography
        (SPECT), 406
Single sheet, as drapes, 530
Single ultrasound probes, 653
Single wrap, 317
Sinus rhythm, 535, 540, 540b, 541f
Sinus tract, 605
Sitting position, 501t–503t, 514
    correct posture in, 220
    modified, 514
    for neurosurgical procedures, 796, 796f
    pneumatic counterpressure device and, 593
Situation monitoring, 81
Skeleton, human, 762, 762f
Skill, 1, 3
Skill training, preoperative teaching and, 386
Skin. See also Integument
    accessory appendages to, 556
    anatomy and physiology of, 551–556, 552t, 553f,
        553t
    blood supply of, 555
    as contamination source, 262–263
    dermis in, 554
    of diabetic patient, 108
    epidermis in, 553–554
    of geriatric patients, 167
    glandular structures and ducts in, 554–555
    Langer's lines in, 553, 554f
    laser safety and, 371
    microbiology of, 285
    oil glands in, 554–555

Skin (Continued)
    sweat glands in, 555
    tissue layers under, 555–556
Skin cancer, 866–867
    sun exposure and, 418
Skin cleansers, 430
Skin closure, 581–582
    dressing for, 602
    strips, 581–582
Skin degreasing, for patient's skin, 521
Skin grafts, 850–851, 851f, 969. See also Plastic
        and reconstructive surgery
    and dermatomes, 850–851, 851f
    procurement from cadaver, 978, 978f
    procurement parameters for, 971t
Skin injury prevention, 25–26
Skin preparation, 520–527
    antiseptic solutions for, 523–524
    of areas considered contaminated, 523
    cleansing fundamentals, 521–523
        one-step, 522–523, 522f
        two-step, 521–522, 521f–522f
    documentation of, 527
    preliminary, 521
    preoperative, 381
    for specific anatomic areas, 524–527, 525f–527f
    for vascular surgery, 952
Skin sealant, 608t
Skin stapler, 573
Skin tension, 64
Skin-cleansing agents, antimicrobial, 286–287
Skull, anatomy of, 897–898, 898f
    infant, 899f
Sled, 508, 508f
Sleep apnea, obstructive, 886
Sling stirrups, 510, 510f
Slippers, 390
Slurry, definition of, 905, 913
Small intestine, 682
    resection of, 682
    transplantation of, 987
Smears, 396
Smile, 393
Smoke evacuator, 235
Smoking
    cancer and, 110, 418
    wound healing and, 587, 848
Smooth jaws, needle holders with, 349
Smooth tissue forceps, 342
Snares, 342
Sneeze, in operating room, 281
Soap, antimicrobial, 287
    preoperative use by patient, 381
Sodium bicarbonate, 628
    in local anesthetic, 460
    for malignant hyperthermia, 644
Sodium carbonate, in boiling water, 308
Sodium hypochlorite, as presoak, 297
Sodium nitroprusside, 627
    to induce hypotension, 448
Sodium, as electrolyte, 633
Soft roll casts, 786
Soft tissue allografts, orthopedic, 767
Soft tissue considerations, for positioning of patient,
        505–506
Soft tissue reconstruction, 858
Solids, 430
Solution basin, 596b
Solutions, 425
    handling, on sterile field, 478–479
    IV crystalloid, 486

Solutions (Continued)
    IV, dispensing to sterile field, 425
    ophthalmic, 832
    preparations of, by circulating nurse, 485
    on sterile field, 478–479
Somatic nervous system, 807
Somatosensory evoked potentials, 407, 549, 798
Sonic energy, 356
Source, 361
Space allocation, in surgical suite, 178–179
Spark-gap generator, 736
Spastic cerebral palsy, 155
Spatial relationships, 260, 270
Spatulas, microsurgical, 355
Spaulding's classification of patient care items,
        261, 301
Special procedure rooms, 193–194
Specialized equipment, surgical, 360–378
    use of, 361
Specialized tray sets, 320
Specialty technicians, 57
Specimen preparation, 26
Specimens, 395–419, 398t
    endoscopic capture of, 655
    management of
        by circulating nurse, 488
        on sterile field, 483–484
    pathologic examination and, 396–399
    surgical, collecting, 398–399
SPECT. See Single photon emission computed
        tomography
Speculums, 350
Spermatocelectomy, 750
Sphenoid sinus procedure, 884
Sphenoidotomy, 884
Sphygmomanometer, 541
    for arterial blood pressure, 541
Spina bifida, 155, 155f–156f
    latex allergy associated with, 235
Spinal anesthesia, 433, 454–464
    advantages of, 457
    choice of agent for, 456
    disadvantages of, 457–458
    duration of agent for, 456–457
    landmarks for injection in, 455–456, 456f
    in lateral position, 457, 457f
    levels of, 456
    needles for, 455–456, 456f
    procedure for, 457–458, 457f
    in sitting position, 457, 457f
    subarachnoid space and, 456, 456f
Spinal cord, 808–825
    anatomy of, 808–811
    compression of, 816, 816f, 819
    monitoring of, during spinal surgery, 814, 815f
    pathology of, 816–820. See also Scoliosis
        kyphosis, 818, 818f–819f
        trauma, 819–820
        tumors, 818–819
        vertebral stenosis, 816f
Spinal frame, adjustable, bed attachments and,
        509–510, 510f
Spinal fusion, 149
    lumbar, 824
    materials for, 816
Spinal headache, 457
Spinal nerve roots, compression on, 816, 816f
Spinal nerves, 809–810, 810f–811f
Spinal surgery, 808–825
    anesthesia for, 814
    in children, 148–150

Spinal surgery (*Continued*)
diagnostics of, 811
graft materials in, 816
hemostasis in, 815–816
instruments for, 814
landmarks for, 808, 809f
monitoring of spinal cord during, 814, 815f
needle localization of level for, 815f
positioning for, 811–813, 814f
procedures in, 820–824. *See also* Spinal fusion
cervical, 821–822, 821f
discectomy, 820–821, 820f
lumbar, 823–824
thoracic, 823
radiologic use during, 814–815, 815f
robotic-assisted, 815
special considerations for, 811–816
stabilization in, 816
x-ray for, 814
Spinal tray, 457
Spine, curvatures of, 809, 809f
Splash basins, 475
Spleen, 675
Splenectomy, 146, 675
Splenorenal shunt, 966
Splenorrhaphy, 675
Splints, 786
Split sheet, as drapes, 529–530
Split-thickness mesh graft, 852, 853f
Split-thickness skin graft (STSG), 847, 851–852, 870
Split-thickness Thiersch graft, 852
Splitting, 64
Spondylosis, 808
Sponge buckets, 192, 488
Sponge sticks, 700
Sponges, 492–494. *See also* Counts
counting of, 493
management of, by circulating nurse, 488
methods of accounting for, 493
moistening, 475
packaging increments of, 478b
from prep tray, 487
providing, during surgical procedure, 480
types of, 492–493
validating of, 472b–473b
weighing, in estimation of blood loss, 636b
Sponging, 64, 66
Spontaneous abortion, 696
Spontaneous infection, 264
Sporicide, 295, 302
Sports medicine, 784–785
Spotlights, test of, in operating room, 467
Stab wounds, 121
Stabilization bar, for fracture, 772
Staff development programs, 84
Staff education, 632
Staffing, 93–94
Stagnara wake-up tests, 808, 814
Stainless steel boats, for dry heat sterilization, 326
Stainless steel instruments, 338–339
Stains, 420, 430
tissue, 398b
Stamey procedure, 747–748
Standard length, of suture material, 572, 572f–573f
Standard precautions, 260, 267–268
by anesthesia staff, 450
for bloodborne source, 253
definition of, 239, 263
Standardization of patient care, 18–21
for documentation, 47–49

Standardization of patient care (*Continued*)
within health care facility, sources of, 20–21
importance of, 18
professional sources of standards, 18–19
from regulatory bodies, 19–20
Standards, 16, 18
Standards of Perioperative Administrative Nursing Practice, 18
Standards of Perioperative Clinical Practice, 18
Standing, body mechanics of, 220
Stapedectomy, 879–880, 879f
Stapedotomy, 879–880
Stapes mobilization, 880
Staphylococcus aureus infection
methicillin-resistant, 258
toxic shock syndrome in, 246, 247f
Staplers, 349
for anastomosis, 350
linear, for endoscopy, 654
Staples, surgical, 573–575
Static electricity, 229
Static tension, 64
Steam sterilization, 269
advantages of, 320
basin sets in, 323
biologic testing of, 324
disadvantages of, 320–321
drape packs in, 323
drying the load after, 324
eye instrumentation and, 320
with gravity displacement sterilizer, 320–321, 324, 325t
for immediate use, 321, 322t, 356–357
loading of sterilizer for, 324
for powered equipment, 323
precautions with, 322–323
preparing surgical instruments for, 323
with prevacuum sterilizer, 320–321, 324–325
prions and, 320
rubber goods in, 323
thermoplastics in, 323
timing of, 324, 325t
types of sterilizers for, 321–322
wood products in, 323
Steam under pressure, 320–325, 321f, 322t
Steam-sensitive tape, 317
Stem cell research, 52
Stenosis, 808, 816f
Stent
airway, 911–912, 912f
intracoronary, 938
intraluminal vascular, 956, 956f
carotid, 956, 956f
Stent dressing, 603
Stent fixation, 849
Stereopsis, 361, 372–373
Stereotactic breast biopsy, 666
Stereotactic core breast tissue biopsy, 402
Stereotactic radiosurgery, 116, 415, 804
Stereotactic surgery, 790
Stereotaxis, 396, 415
Sterile, 260, 312
Sterile attire, 275, 283
Sterile core, 177, 192
Sterile field, 260, 272
aseptic transfer to, by circulating nurse, 484–488
definition of, 261
dispensing drug or material to, 425–426
"eight P's" of, 476t–477t
flipping items to, 484, 485f

Sterile field (*Continued*)
medications and solutions on, handling of, 478–479
preparation of, by scrub person, 474–484
during surgical procedure
specimen management on, 483–484
towels and, 480–484, 481b
Sterile supplies, opening of, 472–474, 474f
Sterile supply room, 182
Sterile table, setup for, 216
Sterile team, 55, 57–62
role of, scrub person as part of, 467b
Sterile technique, 24, 262
areas for personnel in, 270–271
in circulating nurse duties, 487
continuous viewing in, 272
definition of, 261
edges of sterile contents and, 271–272
gowns and gloves in, 269–270
integrity of sterile items in, 273
principles of, 269–274
questionable items in, 269
reaching or leaning and, 270–271, 271f
with seated surgical team, 270f
sterile areas to minimum, 273
sterile field and, 269–271
sterile items in, 269
tables in, 270
touching by personnel in, 270
unsterile personnel avoid sterile areas, 273
Sterility, of disposable products, 310–311
Sterilization, 312–337
administrative monitoring of, 314
of anesthesia equipment, 451
assembly of instrument sets for, 315–316
control measures for, 333–335
load number in, 333
shelf life in, 334–335
wet packs and, 334
of custom packs, 335–336
cycle of, 313
date of, 333
vs. disinfection, 313
of endoscopes, 659
of loaner instrumentation, 335
methods of, 313
chemical, 326–333
chemicals in solution, 331–333
dry heat, 325–326
ethylene oxide, 326–330
hydrogen peroxide plasma, 330–331
ozone gas, 331
radiation, 333
monitoring of, 313–315
packaging items for, 316–320, 318f–319f
of powered instruments, 356, 358
reliability parameters for, 313
reproductive, 52
of specialized tray sets, 320
terminal, 261
procedures for, 359
Sterilizers, cleaning of, 217
Sterilizing agents, 232–233
Sternotomy
median, 915, 915f, 927, 928f
partial, 915
Steroids, for anesthesia reaction, 463
STERRAD sterilizer, 330
Stethoscopy, 540–541
Stick tie, 551, 559, 595
Stimulation, local anesthetics and, 463
Stirrups, bed attachments and, 510, 510f–511f

Stockinette
 under cast, 786
 as drapes, 530
 in dressing, 603
Stoma, 664, 684–685
 as areas considered contaminated, 523
 intestinal, 686f
Stone forceps, 343
Storage, 182–183
 of endoscopes, 659
 of sterile packages, 335
Storage room, environmental controls in, 179t
Storage shelves, cleaning of, 217
Storeroom, central, 87
Strain-gauge plethysmography, 408
Strangulated hernia, 693
Stratum basale, 554
Stratum corneum, 554
Stratum granulosum, 554
Stratum lucidum, 554
Stratum spinosum, 554
Streptococcus infection, 244, 244f
Streptokinase, 958
Stress, 99, 101–102
 diabetes mellitus and, 105
 factors affecting, 101
 metabolism and, 105–106
 physiologic and psychologic response to, 101–102
 reduction, 14
Strike-through, 312, 324
Stroke volume (SV), 546
Structural empowerment, 80
Student, perioperative, working, policy for, 3–5,
  4t, 4b
Studer pouch, 746, 746f
Styes, 832, 833f
Styptics, 591
Subclavian catheters, 416
Subcostal upper quadrant oblique incision, 557
Subcutaneous adipose layer, in skin, 555
Subdural hematoma, 790, 805
Subhepatic abscess, 674
Subjective-objective assessment plan (SOAP), 47–48
Subjective-objective charting, 47–48
Submucous resection, 883
Subphrenic abscess, 674
Substerile room, 177, 179, 184
 basic layout of, 212f
Substernal intrathoracic thyroidectomy, 896
Subtotal gastrectomy, 679–680, 679f
Subtotal parathyroidectomy, 895–896
Subtotal thyroidectomy, 895–896
Subungual, 275
Succinylcholine, 446
 malignant hyperthermia and, 643
Suction, 64, 66, 597
 available when peritoneum is opened, 665
 closed wound, systems, 600, 601f
 connecting and checking of, 467
 flushing tip after surgery, 358
 flushing tip during surgery, 358
 instruments for, 351
 in neurosurgery, 795
 for otorhinolaryngologic and head and neck surgery,
   875
 through endoscope, 654
Suction drainage, in cardiac surgery, 927, 927f
Sudoriferous glands, in skin, 555
Sufentanil, 441t, 458
 in children, 133t–134t
  for premedication, 136

Sugar tong splint, 787
Suicide, 53
Suite, 177
Sulfonamides, 257t
Sump drains, 600
Sun exposure, and cancer risk, 418
Sunscreen, 110, 418
Superficial, 499
Superinfection, 239
Superior, 499
Superior vena cava (SVC) syndrome, 950
Supine position, 499, 501t–503t, 512–513, 512f
 for cranial procedures, 796
Supplements, nutritional, 106
Supplies
 economical use of, 497–498
 rotation of, 335
Support services, 181
Supraglottic laryngectomy, 891
Suprapubic cystostomy, 745
Suprapubic prostatectomy, 754, 754f
Supratentorial structures, 791
Surgeon, 55, 59–61
 hand signals of, 481, 482f
 handover report from, 613
 verbal abuse by, 95
Surgeon's preference cards/case cart sheet, 21
Surgery, 1–3
 art and science of, 2–3
 common indications for, in children, 125–126
 facilities for, 3
 improvements in, 2–3
 indications for, 2t, 125–126
 invasiveness of, 2–3
Surgical anatomy and physiology, 65
Surgical assistant (SA), 55, 57, 65, 77
Surgical conscience, 2, 13, 17, 17b
 elements of, 17b
Surgical cotton, 565
Surgical debulking (cytoreduction), 111
Surgical environment
 cleaning of. See Cleaning, of surgical environment
 establishing, 211–212
Surgical gut, 564
Surgical hand hygiene (surgical scrub), 275,
  285–287
Surgical hazards, 71
Surgical intensive care unit (SICU), 85
Surgical microbiology, 238–259.
  See also Microorganisms
Surgical nylon, 566
Surgical pathology, 396
 specimens for, 396, 398t
Surgical plume, 234–235
Surgical procedure, 2–3
 perioperative pediatrics, 142–160
  cardiovascular, 156–160
  emergent, 142–146
  endoscopic, 142
  genitourinary, 146–148
  neurologic, 153–155
  ophthalmologic, 150–151
  orthopedic and spinal, 148–150
  otorhinolaryngologic, 151–152
  plastic and reconstructive, 152–153
  thoracic, 155–156
Surgical resection, tumor, 111
Surgical scrub, 285. See also Hand hygiene, surgical
Surgical services committee, 88
Surgical services, management of, 91–95
Surgical silk, 565

Surgical site
 accessibility of, for positioning of patient, 506
 identifying, 22, 394
 irrigation of, 484
 marking, 392
 for ophthalmic surgery, 827
 preparation and draping of, 519–534
 "time out" for prevention of wrong, 23b
Surgical site infection (SSI), 89, 89b, 239, 241
Surgical site management, 66, 66f
Surgical smoke, 234–235. See also Plume
Surgical stainless steel, 565
Surgical suites
 construction or renovation of, 194–196
  considerations for, 194–195, 195b
  principles in, 195–196
 definition of, 177–178
 environmental controls in, 179t
 operating rooms in. See Operating room
 peripheral support areas of, 180–183
 physical layout of, 178–179
  location, 178
  space allocation in, 178–179
  traffic patterns in, 178–179
  type of, 178, 178f–179f
 special procedure rooms in, 193–194
 transition zones in, 179–180
Surgical technologist (ST), 57, 62b, 65, 77–78
 clinical competency of, 35
 guidelines for, 34–35
 in sterile processing, 336
Surgical technology, 34–35
Surgical technology student, 3
Surgical vacuum positioning system, bed attachments
  and, 512
Surveillance, 90
Suspension microlaryngoscopy, 890
Suture (verb), 65, 68, 70–71, 70f
Suture book, 494
Suture ligature, 559
Suture material
 absorbable, 564–565, 564t
  collagen, 565
  surgical gut, 564
  synthetic, polymers, 565
 barbed, 567, 567t
 choice of, 562–567, 563f
 definition of, 559
 gauge of, 562, 563b
 in hypertrophic scars, 605
 nonabsorbable, 565–567, 566t
  surgical cotton, 565
  surgical silk, 565
  surgical stainless steel, 565
  synthetic, polymers, 565–567
 packaging of, 571–572
 preparation of, 572–573, 572f–573f
 specifications for, 561–562
 for vascular surgery, 952–953
Suture passer, for cerclage, 716f
Sutures, 551, 873, 897–898
 basics, 559–567
 checking list of, in circulating nurse duties, 484
 considerations in the choice of, 571
 management of, 481–483, 483f
 in operating room, 473
 in orthopedic surgery, 769
 packaging and preparation of, 571–573
 preparing, 478
Suturing
 cutting sutures in, 560–561

Suturing (*Continued*)
    endoscopic, 561
    Halsted, technique of, 559–560
    knot placement in, 560
    methods of, 560, 560f
    principles of, 560–561
    retention bridges, bolsters, and bumpers in,
        561, 562f
    retention sutures in, 561
    techniques of, 559–560
    traction suture in, 561
    in vascular surgery, 953
SVR. *See* Systemic vascular resistance
Swaged needles, 570, 570f
    as suture, 572–573
    for vascular surgery, 952–953
Swan-Ganz catheter, 545
    in cardiac surgery, 929
Sweat glands, in skin, 555
Syme amputation, 695, 695f
Sympathectomy, 806
Sympathomimetics, 626
Symphysis pubis, 698f
SynCardia, 944
Syndactyly, 153
Synthetic adhesives, 575–576
Synthetic materials, 576–578
Synthetic meshes, 576–578
Synthetic polymers
    absorbable, 565
    nonabsorbable, 565–567
Synthetic sources, of drugs, 427–428
Synthetic vascular prostheses, 955
Syphilis, 248
Syringe, 425, 426f
    handling of, 479
    labeling of, 425
    types of, 426f
Systemic effect, 420
    of local and regional anesthesia, 462–463
Systemic vascular resistance (SVR), 547
Systems approach, 37
Systems thinking, 79, 92

T

T cell-depleted marrow, 970
t-PA. *See* Tissue-type plasminogen activator
Tachycardia, 433, 446, 460, 463
Tachypnea, 433
"Take", 847
Talc, 430
    dry heat sterilization of, 326
    for pleurodesis, 913
Talipes deformities, 148–149
Talipes equinovarus, 149
Talipes varus, 149, 149f
Tampons, 492
Tangential excision, of burns, 870
Tanner's stages, 696, 704
Tannic acid, 592
Tape, 492
    dressing and, 603
TASS. *See* Toxic anterior segment syndrome
Taxonomy, 16, 31
TBA (to be admitted), 379
TBV. *See* Total blood volume
TCI (to come in), 379
Teaching
    effective, 386–387
    preoperative, 386

Team
    operating room, efficiency of, 495–498
    perioperative
        assisting anesthesia provider, 433
        credentialing of, 56
        members of, 57–62
Team learning, 92
TeamSTEPPS, 81
Teamwork, 11–13
Technology, 361
TEE. *See* Transesophageal echocardiography
Teeth, loose, 392
Teflon, in prosthetic devices, 581
Telehealth, 197, 205
Telescope, 735f
    urologic, 735
TEM. *See* Transanal endoscopic microsurgery
TEMPER tents, 206–207, 208f–209f
Temperature
    body
        in children, 130
        monitoring, 547–548
        operating room, 184
    ethylene oxide gas sterilization and, 327
Temporomandibular joint syndrome, 903
Tenaculums, 343, 344f
Tenckhoff catheter, 117, 417
Tendon repair, 784–785
    in children, 148
Tendons, 765
Tenorrhaphy, 784
Tenotomy, 150
TENS. *See* Transcutaneous electrical nerve
        stimulation
Tensile strength, of wound, 583–584, 589
Tentorium cerebelli, 791
Terminal cleaning, 211–212, 312, 316
    daily, 216–217
    definition of, 211
Terminal end staplers, 350, 350f
Terminal sterilization, 261, 313, 316
    and terminal disinfection, 261
Testes, 749–750, 749f
Testicular self-examination (TSE), 410t, 750
Testicular torsion, 750
Tetanus bacillus immunization, 586
Tetracaine, 455t, 462
Tetralogy of Fallot, 158–159
Textiloma, 490
Thalamotomy, 803
The Joint Commission (TJC)
    accreditation by, 56, 80
    contracted services, 39–40
    factors contributing to wrong surgery and, 23b
    and sentinel events, 42–44
    standards of, 18
Thelarche, 696, 703–704
Thenar, 808–810
Thenar grip, 65
Thermal balloon ablation, intrauterine, 709
Thermal burns, 229
Thermal drape, 528
Thermal hemostasis, 69
Thermal plume, 177, 185, 185f
    airborne contamination and, 263–264
Thermal sterilization, 320–326
Thermocouple probe, 858
Thermodilution catheter, Swan-Ganz, 545
Thermodilution technique, 545
Thermoplastics, steam sterilization of, 323

Thiersch graft, 852
Thigh, skin preparation for, antiseptic, 526–527
Thiopental, 443
Thiopental sodium, 441t
Third intention/delayed primary closure, 585
Thopaz⁺, 602
Thoracentesis, 919
Thoracic approach, 458
Thoracic outlet syndrome, 918–919, 919f
Thoracic spine
    anterior approach of, 823
    posterior approach of, 823
    procedures of, 823
    vertebrae, 811
Thoracic surgery, 905–922
    access to thorax in, 910–914
    anesthesia for, 908–909
    approaches, incisional, 914–915
    blood transfusion in, 909
    bronchoscopic lung volume reduction, 912
    bronchoscopy in, 910–911, 912f
    complications of, 920–921
    contaminated secretions in, 909
    controlled pneumothorax for, 908–909
    drainage system for, 909–910, 910f
    endoscopy in, 910
    esophageal, 920
    instrumentation for, 909, 909f–910f
    landmark for, 905–906, 906f
    lung-assist devices in, 915–916
    mediastinoscopy in, 912, 913f
    monitoring in, 908–910
    pediatric, 155–156
    procedures in, 916–919
        by mediastinotomy, 916–917
        rib resection, 916, 916f
        for thoracic outlet syndrome, 918–919, 919f
        by thoracotomy, 917–918
        thymectomy as, 918, 918f
        for trauma, 919
    special features of, 908–916
    thoracoscopy in, 913–914, 913f
    thoracostomy in, 912–913
Thoracic sympathectomy, 806
Thoracoabdominal area, skin preparation for,
    antiseptic, 525, 525f
Thoracoabdominal incision, 559, 914–915, 914f
Thoracolumbar sympathectomy, 806
Thoracoplasty, 918
Thoracoscopy, 905, 913–914, 913f
Thoracostomy, 912–913. *See also* Chest drainage
Thoracotomy, 917–918
    alternative incisions, 915
    for cardiac surgery, 927–928
    for chest trauma, 919
    exploratory, 917
    for lung reduction, 918
    for lung resection, 917–918, 917f
    for pneumonectomy, 917f, 918
    surgical position, 518
    for thoracoplasty, 918
    for transplantation, 918
Thorax
    anatomy of, 905–908
        diaphragm, 908, 908f
        lungs, 906–908, 907f
        mediastinum, 908
        thoracic cavity, 905–906, 906f
    physiology of, 908
Threatened abortion, 696

Three-layer dressing, 602–603
Thrombectomy, 957
Thrombin, 592
    topical, 954b
Thrombocytopenia, heparin-induced, 953
Thromboembolism prophylaxis
    in diabetic patient, 108
    in obese patient, 108
Thromboembolism, after orthopedic surgery, 788
Thromboendarterectomy, pulmonary, 964
Thrombolytic therapy, 958
Thrombophlebitis, 619
Thrombose, 947, 954
Thrombus, 616, 619
Thumb forceps, 342
Thymectomy, 918, 918f
Thyroglossal duct cystectomy, 896
Thyroid elevator, bed attachments and, 509
Thyroid hormone, in geriatric patient, 172
Thyroid lobectomy, 895
Thyroid sheet, as drapes, 529
Thyroid, surgical procedures of, 895–896, 895f
Thyroid/sternal lead shields, 225, 225f
Thyroidectomy, 895–896, 895f
Tidal volume, respiratory, 547
Tie on a passer, 481, 483f
Ties
    definition of, 559
    managing of, 481–483, 483f
    preparing, 478
Time
    ethylene oxide gas sterilization and, 327
    ionizing radiation and, 224
    managing of, in operating room, 495–497
Time out, 22, 23b
Tissue allograft, procurement parameters for, 971t
Tissue approximation, wound healing and, 588
Tissue donors, 974
Tissue expander, for burn patients, 870
Tissue expansion flap, 854, 854f
Tissue grafts
    in otorhinolaryngologic and head and neck surgery, 876
    types of, 851–856
Tissue handling, wound healing and, 588
Tissue reaction, 583, 589
Tissue replacement materials, 578–581
    biologic, 578–580
    biologic wound cover and, 578
    synthetic, 580–581
Tissue transplantation, 969–972
    donor criteria for, 969–970, 970b
Tissue transplants, 579–580
Tissue-type plasminogen activator (t-PA), 958
Titanium, 339
Titration, 626
TJC. See The Joint Commission
TMR. See Transmyocardial revascularization
TNM categories, of cancer, 409
Toe, and transmetatarsal amputations, 694
Tolerance, 420, 430
Tomography, 396
Toner, 357
    printer, 316
Tongue, resection of, 886
Tonsil sponges, 492
Tonsillar tumor, 887
Tonsillectomy, 152, 152f, 887, 887f
Toomey evacuator, 737
Toomey irrigator, 737f
Toothed tissue forceps, 342, 344f

Topical anesthesia, 433, 459
Tort, 37–38
Total blood volume (TBV), 547, 634
Total disc replacement, 821
Total laryngectomy, 891–892
Total parathyroidectomy, with autotransplantation, 896
Total thyroidectomy, 896
Total-body scanning, 405
Touch, 385, 393
Tourniquets, 68, 593
    contraindications for, 595
    pneumatic, 770
Towels
    as drapes, 527
    in draping the patient, 479
    sterile field and, in surgical procedure, 480–484, 481b
Toxic anterior segment syndrome (TASS), 320
Toxic levels, 420–421
Toxic shock syndrome, 246
Trachea
    anatomy of, 889
    surgical procedures of, 893–894
Tracheal resection, 894
Tracheal/laryngeal stenosis, 152
Trachelectomy, 708
Trachelorrhaphy, 708
Tracheoesophageal fistula (TEF), 143
Tracheostomy, 893–894
Tracheostomy tubes, 894, 894f
Tracheotomy, 152, 893–894, 893f–894f
Traction countertraction, 69–70
Traction suture, 561
Traction-countertraction, 65
Traction, skeletal, 772
Traffic pattern, in surgical suite, 178–179
Traffic, contamination and, 266
Trailing the suture, 571
Transanal endoscopic microsurgery (TEM), 692
Transcatheter aortic valve replacement (TAVR), 934
Transcranial magnetic stimulation, 803
Transcutaneous electrical nerve stimulation (TENS), 770
Transection, 65
Transesophageal echocardiography (TEE), 929
Transfer zones, cleaning of, 217
Transfer, of patient, from the operating room, 490
Transfixion screws, 774–775
Transfixion suture, 595
Transformational leadership, 80
Transfusion, in cardiac surgery, 927
Transition zones, 179–180
Transitions of care, 82
Transmissible spongiform encephalopathy (TSE), 252
    postexposure prophylaxis for, 253
Transmyocardial revascularization, 938
Transoral approach, 808
Transparent film, 608t
Transperineal prostatic cryoablation, 755
Transperitoneal, 808
Transplant, 969
Transplantation. See also Organ transplantation
    types of, 969, 970b
Transportation, of patient
    obese, 109
    to operating room suite, 390
    using transfer device, 390
Transsexual surgery, 758–759
Transsphenoidal procedures, 805
Transsternal bilateral thoracotomy, 928

Transurethral microwave thermotherapy, of prostatic
    tissue, 752, 752f
Transurethral needle ablation (TUNA), 752–753, 753f
Transurethral resection of the prostate (TURP), 753, 753f
Transurethral resection syndrome, 737
Transurethral, defined, 730, 735
Transverse colectomy, 684
Transverse incision, midabdominal, 558f, 559
Trapeziometacarpal joint, total replacement of, 781
Trash
    collecting for removal of, 215
    disposal of, in operating room, 467
Trauma
    abdominal, 688–691
    chest, 919
    in children, 126
    head, 805
    intraoperative autotransfusion in, 640
    laryngeal, 890
    pancreaticoduodenal, 676
    renal, 739
    scrotal-testicular, 750
    spinal, 819–820
    X-ray studies for, 401
Trauma center, 85
Traumatic, 338
Traumatic clamps, 343
Traumatic fracture, 771
Traumatic injury, 739
Traumatic shock, 641
Traumatic wounds, 585–586
    as areas considered contaminated, 523
Tray sets, specialized, 320
Treacher Collins syndrome, 900, 900f
Trendelenburg position, 499, 513, 513f
Trephine, 790, 799
Triage center, 91
Triangulation, 65
Triclosan, 286
Tricuspid atresia, 159
Trimethaphan, to induce hypotension, 449
Trimethaphan, to induce hypotension, 449
Tripod grip, 65, 68f
Trismus, 436
Trocar, 338, 352
    definition of, 647
    and sheath, 649
True aneurysm, 947, 959–960
Truncus arteriosus, 159
Tubal anastomosis, 713
Tubal insufflation, 703
Tubal ligation, for reproductive sterilization, 712–713
Tubal perfusion, 703
Tuberculosis, 247–248
    anesthesia precautions with, 450
    disinfection and, 302
Tubing
    ethylene oxide gas sterilization of, 328
    steam sterilization of, 323
Tubocurarine, 445
Tuboplasty, 713
Tucking, 150
Tumescents, 429
"Tummy tuck", 861
Tumor, 396, 790, 792
    breast, 401
    craniofacial, 901–902
    of esophagus, 920
    of external ear, 878

Tumor (*Continued*)
intracranial, 799—800, 800t
of lip, 858
mandibular extension of, 904
mediastinal, 916—917
of middle ear, vascular, 880
nasal, 901
neck dissections for, 896—897
orbital, 833
of paranasal sinus, 885, 901
reconstruction after resection of, 850
of salivary glands, 886
size and location of, 117
of spine, 818—819
tonsillar, 887
type of, 117
Tumor identification system (TNM), 409, 412b
Tumor markers, monitoring, 409, 412t
TUNA. *See* Transurethral needle ablation
Tunable dye laser, 367—368
Tungsten carbide, 339
needle holders with jaws of, 347
Tunnel syndrome, 784
Turbinectomy, 883—884
Turbinoplasty, 884—885
Turnover, 211, 216, 313
TURP. *See* Transurethral resection of the prostate
Two-hand placement, of tubing, 649
Tympanomastoid reconstruction, 879
Tympanoplasty, 878—879
Tympanostomy, 151

U

U.S. Food and Drug Administration (FDA), 20
implantable cochlear device, 881
Ulcers
as chronic wounds, 586
definition of, 583, 586
stress of burns and, 871
venous stasis, 964—965
Ulnar nerve block, 459
Ultrasonic aspiration, 794
Ultrasonic aspirator, 674
Ultrasonic blade, and scissors, 377
Ultrasonic cleaning, 298—299
Ultrasonic dissectors, endoscopic, 654
Ultrasonic imaging, 653
Ultrasonic lithotripsy, percutaneous, 742
Ultrasonic scalpel, 598
Ultrasonic scanning, intravascular, 952
Ultrasonography, 406
in cesarean section, 721
intraoperative, 407
common bile duct exploration, 673
hepatic, 674—675
of peripheral vascular disease, 951
Ultrasonosurgery, 377
Ultraviolet irradiation, for disinfection, 308—309
Umbilical cord vein graft, 580
Umbilical herniorrhaphy, 693
Umbilical tape, 561
in vascular surgery, 952—953
Umbilicus, as areas considered contaminated, 523
Unconsciousness, induced, 435
Undermining, 551, 553
skin with scissors, 65, 70f
Ungues, 556
Unified team, motivation and building, 93—94
Union, 761, 763—764
Unit manager, 83
United Kingdom Transplant Register, 974

Universal Protocol, 22, 44
Unrestricted area, 179
Unrestricted surgical suite, definition of, 177
Unsterile, 261
Unsterile table, draping, 474
Upper arm, skin preparation for, antiseptic, 526
Upper cervical sympathectomy, 806
Upper extremity table, bed attachments and, 509
Upper extremity, amputations of, 695
Upper femoral epiphysis, slipping of, 148
Urachus, 125, 144
Ureter, 698f
Ureteral calculi, 742
Ureteral catheters, 665, 742—743, 743f
Ureteral reimplantation, 147
Ureteral stent, 743
Ureterolithotomy, 743
Ureteroneocystostomy, 744
Ureteroscopy, 742—743
Ureterosigmoidostomy, 746
Ureterostomy, cutaneous, 747
Ureteroureterostomy, 744
Ureters, 731
anatomy of, 742—744
procedures of, 742—744
Urethra, 748—749
anatomy of, 732—733
dysfunction of, 748
prostatic, balloon dilation and stenting of, 752, 752f
Urethral dilation, 748, 748f
Urethral repair, 147
Urethral stent, 748
Urethral suspension procedures, 714
Urethroplasty, 748—749
bladder flap, 748—749
Urethrostomy, perineal, 748
Urethrotomy, 748—749
Urinary bladder, 736—737
anatomy of, 698f, 744—748
surgical procedures of, 744—748
voiding, preoperative, 389
Urinary calculus, 741—742
Urinary catheterization, 519—520, 519f—520f
by suprapubic cystostomy, 745
Urinary diversion procedure, continent, 745—747, 746f
Urinary drainage, for intraoperative drainage, 599
Urinary incontinence, 747—748
in geriatric patient, 172—173
Urinary output, 548
of geriatric patients, 173
in young children, 129
Urinary sphincter, artificial, 748
Urinary stress incontinence procedures, 714
Urinary system, anatomy and physiology of, 730—733, 731f
Urine, color of, 548
Urography, 404
Urokinase, 958
Urolithiasis, 741—742, 741f
lithotripsy for
electrohydraulic, 742
ultrasonic, 742
percutaneous nephrostolithotomy for, 741—742
Urologic bed, 733, 733f
Urologic endoscopes
accessories for, 736—737
care and preventive maintenance, 737—738
types of, 735—736
Urologic endoscopy, 733

Urologic surgery, 730—760
of kidneys, 730—731, 731f
postoperative complications of, 759
of ureters, 742—744
Urticaria, 218, 235
Uterine anomalies, 711f
Uterine artery, fibroid embolization through, 710—711
Uterine cancer, 701
Uterine cannula, 343
Uterine cervix, 698f
Uterine clamps, 345, 345f
Uterine dilators, 353f
Uterine fibroids, 711f
Uterine fundus, 698f
Uterine procedures
dilation and curettage (D&C)
hysterectomy, vaginal, 709
instruments for, 700t
thermal balloon ablation, 709
Uterine prolapse, 173f
Uterine tenaculums, 343, 344f
Uterosacral ligaments, 699
Uterus, 698—699, 698f
laparoscopic view of, 710f
prolapsed, repair of, 707—708, 708f
Uterus transplants, 724—725
Utility gloves, 283
Utility room, 182
Uvulopalatopharyngoplasty, 886—887

V

VACTERL association, 125—126
Vacuum dressings, 604
Vacuum positioning system, bed attachments and, 512
Vacuum-assisted venous drainage (VAVD), 929
VAD. *See* Ventricular assist device
Vagina, 698, 698f
skin preparation for, antiseptic, 526, 526f
Vaginal approach, 700—701, 700t
Vaginal eversion, repair of, 708
Vaginal lesion, excision of, 707
Vaginal packing, 700—701
Vaginal plastic procedures, 707
Vaginal speculum, 351f
Vaginal-abdominal approach, combined, 701
Vaginectomy, 707
Vaginoplasty, 707
Vagotomy, 680, 680f, 807
Valve replacement, 933—934
Valvular heart disease, 933—935, 933f
Valvular stenosis, 159
Valvuloplasty
percutaneous transluminal balloon, 935
venous, 965
Van Buren sounds, 748, 748f
Vancomycin-resistant enterococci, 258
Vapor phase sterilizer, 331
Varicocele ligation, 750
Varicose veins, 964—965
Vas deferens, 749f, 750—751
Vascular diseases, 949, 950b
assessment of, in an extremity, 951, 951t
diagnostic procedures of, 951—952
invasive, 951—952, 952f
noninvasive, 951, 952f
Vascular grafts, 954—955
Vascular surgery, 947—968
complications of, 952—955
considerations for, 952—955

Vascular surgery (*Continued*)
  grafts used in, 954–955
  instrument for, 952–953, 953f
  procedures in, 958–968
    aneurysmectomy, 959–963, 960f–962f
    arterial bypass, 958
    embolectomy, 963–964
    endarterectomy, 959, 959f
    for limb salvage, 968
    for pseudoaneurysm repair, 962
    shunts, 966–967
    for vascular anastomosis, 967–968
    for venous stasis disease, 964–965
  retraction in, 952–953, 952f
  special features of, 952–955
Vascular system, anatomy and physiology of,
    947–949, 948f–949f
Vascular tissue welding, 967–968
Vascularized muscle pedicle free flap, 855
Vasectomy, 750–751
Vasoconstrictor, 616, 625
Vasodilators, 623, 627
  definition of, 616
  for reduction of blood loss, 636
  in vascular surgery, 954
Vasogenic shock, 642
Vasopressors, 627–628
Vasovasostomy, 751, 751f
VAVD. *See* Vacuum-assisted venous drainage
Vecuronium, 445
Vein graft, 954–955
Veins
  anastomosis of, 967
  anatomy of, 949, 949f–950f
Vena cava filter, 964, 964b, 965f
Vendors, 97
Venipuncture, percutaneous, 486
Venospasm, 621
Venous access device, 417
Venous conduit, 954–955
Venous cutdown, 486
Venous disease, Doppler studies of, 407
Venous impedance plethysmography, 408
Venous stasis, 621, 950
  causing ulcers, 586
Ventilation
  basic cardiac life support and, 628–629
  definition of, 543
  in operating rooms, 184–187, 185b, 219
    anesthetic gases and, 232
Ventilation/inspiration, 535
Ventral, 499
Ventral herniorrhaphy, 693–694
Ventricles, 792, 794f
Ventricular aneurysm, 939, 939f–940f
Ventricular assist device (VAD), 943–944, 943f
Ventricular dysrhythmias, 622–624
Ventricular fibrillation, 623–624, 623f
Ventricular flutter, 623
Ventricular septal defect, 157, 157f
Ventricular tachycardia, 622–623, 623f, 626
  inadvertent hypothermia and, 642
Ventriculoatrial shunts, 154–155
Ventriculography, 402
Ventriculostomy, for hydrocephalus, in pediatric
    patient, 154–155
Verapamil, 626
Verbal abuse, surgeons, 95
Veress needle, 647–649
Vertebral deformity and degeneration, 816–818
Vertical airflow, 186, 186f

Vertical banded gastroplasty, 682
Vertical hemilaryngectomy, 891
Vertical mattress, sutures, 560
Vesico-psoas hitch procedure, 744
Vesicostomy, cutaneous, 745
Vesicoureteral reflux, 147
Vesicovaginal fistula, repair of, 708
Vessel loops, 561, 952–953, 953f
Vest, sterile, 293
Vestibular neurectomy, 880
Vestibules, 207, 209f, 697, 697f
Veterinary surgical facilities, 210
Vials, drugs in, 420, 425, 425f
Vicryl mesh, 577
Victim, 99
Victimization, 123
Victims, 119
Video camera, for endoscopy, 652
Video monitor, for endoscopy, 652
Video-assisted laser endoscopy, 377
View boxes, radiographic, 192
Viewing instruments, 350–351
Vinyl gloves, 283
Violence, lateral, 94
Violent shaking, 122
Viral theory, 163
Viral-mediated carcinogenesis, 411t
Virtual reality, 662–663
Virucide, 295, 302
Viruses, 248–252. *See also* Human
    immunodeficiency virus (HIV) infection;
    Human papillomavirus (HPV) infections
  characteristics of, 248–249
  cytomegalovirus, 250
  hepatitis infection, 249
  herpes infection, 249–250
VISTASEAL, 575
Visual evoked potential, 408, 798
Visual impairment, 103–104
Visual-spatial learner, 3
Visualization agents, 430
Vital signs, pediatric ranges of, 131, 131t
Vitallium, 339
Vitamin K, 637, 953
Vitrectomy, 843–844
  for injury, 843–844
  pars plana, 828f
Voice intercommunication system, in operating room,
    193
Voice prostheses, 891–892
Voiding cystourethrography, 404
Voiding, preoperative, 389
Volar space, 847
Voltage, 227
Voluntary certification, 76
Voluntary reproductive sterilization, 52
Volvulus, 125, 144
Vulva, 697, 697f
  diseases of, 706
Vulvar procedures, 706, 706f

W

Wake-up tests, Stagnara, 814
Walking cast, 787
Wall mount, 375
Walls
  cleaning of, 216–217
  of operating rooms, 187–188
Wappler cystourethroscope, 735
Warfarin, 637
  vascular surgery in patient using, 953

Warts, venereal, 250
Washer-decontaminator, 298
Washer-sterilizer, 298
Waste gases, 438–439
Waste, standard precautions with, 268
Water bag lithotripsy, 742
Water, contamination associated with, 265
Waterston procedure, 158, 158f
Wavelengths, 361, 365
Wear-and-tear theory, of aging, 162–163
Webril, 786, 787f
Wedge body jacket, 149
Wedge cast, 787
Wedge resection, 917–918
Weight, of geriatric patient, 171
Wertheim procedure, radical, 712
Wet packs, 334
  definition of, 313
Wet steam, 334
Wet vacs, 216
Wet-to-dry dressing, 604
Wet-to-wet dressing, 604
Wheelchair, transportation by, 390
Whipple procedure, 676, 676f
Whitlow, herpetic, 250
Wicking, definition of, 313, 323
Wilms tumor, 146
Wolfe graft, 853
Wong-Baker FACES pain rating scale, 133f
Work and storage areas, 181–182
Workbench surgery, 739
Working distances, 361, 372
Workroom, general, 182
Worms, 254
Wound assessment, 607
Wound care, materials for, 608t
Wound classification, surgical, 586, 587b
Wound closure, 559–582
Wound contraction, 584–585
Wound disruption
  definition of, 583
  postoperative, 605–606
Wound healing, 583–609
  complications of, 604–606
  factors influencing, 586–589
    health condition, of patient, 586–588
    physical activity, 589
    postoperative complications, 589
    surgical technique, 588–589
    wound classification, 586, 587b
  mechanism of, 584–585, 584f
  wound care and, 607
Wound infections
  postoperative, 24, 606–607
  prevention of, 606–607
Wound management, 598–604
Wound security, wound healing and, 588–589
Wound silo, 581
Wounds, types of, 585–586
Woven fabrics, 317
  for dry heat sterilization, 329
  for ethylene oxide gas sterilization, 329
Woven polyester, 955
Wrapped trays, 318–319
Wrist
  arthroscopy of, 782
  total joint replacement of, 781
Wrist strap, bed attachments and, 508
Wristband
  allergies on, 421, 485
  checking of, 391–392

Written departmental instructions for personnel, 91
Written instructions, preoperative, 380–382, 381f
Wrong site surgery, 23b

X

X-ray equipment, in orthopedic surgery, 770
X-rays, 113, 399, 414

Xenograft, 551, 578
  biomaterials, 580
  bone implant, 579

Y

Y-tubing for cystoscopy, 736f
Yankauer tip, 352

Z

Zenker's diverticulum, 677, 887
Zeolite beads, hemostasis and, 591
Zinc chloride paste, 592
Zoom, 361, 373
Zygomatic fractures, 902